Handbuch der experimentellen Pharmakologie

Vol. 48 Heffter-Heubner New Series

Handbook of Experimental Pharmacology

Arthropod Venoms

Contributors

D.W. Alsop · R.L. Beard · S. Bettini · M.S. Blum
P.M. Brignoli · W. Bücherl · A. Delgado Quiroz · C.R. Diniz
H. Edery · P. Efrati · T. Eisner · S. Gitter · M. Goyffon
M.R. Gray · Y. Hashimoto · H.R. Hermann · K. Hicks
J. Ishay · H. Joshua · S. Konosu · J. Kovoor · G. Levy
Z. Maretić · M. Maroli · J. Meinwald · A. Minelli
F. Miranda · M.F. Murnaghan · R. O'Connor · F.J. O'Rourke
M.L. Peck · J.E. Percy · F.A. Pereira-Lima · W. Rathmayer
H. Rochat · L.M. Roth · S. Schenberg · H. Schenone
A. Shulov · H.L. Stahnke · G. Suarez · S.K. Sutherland
J. Weatherston · E. Zlotkin

Editor

Sergio Bettini

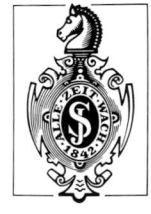

Springer-Verlag Berlin Heidelberg New York 1978

Prof. Dr. S. Bettini, Istituto Superiore di Sanità, Viale Regina Elena 299, Rome/
Italy

With 293 Figures

ISBN 3-540-08228-X Springer-Verlag Berlin Heidelberg New York
ISBN 0-387-08228-X Springer-Verlag New York Heidelberg Berlin

Library of Congress Cataloging in Publication Data. Main entry under title: Arthropod venoms. (Handbook of experimental
pharmacology: New series; v. 48) Bibliography: p. Includes index. 1. Arthropoda, Poisonous—Venom. I. Alsop, David W.,
1939— II. Bettini, Sergio, 1916— III. Series: Handbuch der experimentellen Pharmakologie: New series; v. 48.
QP905.H3 vol. 48 [QP941.A73]615′.1′08s [595′.2′0457] 77-24628

Typesetting printing, and bookbinding: Universitätsdruckerei H. Stürtz AG, Würzburg
2122/3130-543210

Preface

ה

Arthropod venoms have received much attention and have played an important role in folklore and medicine since ancient times. Scorpion envenomation, "tarantism," bee and wasp stings are among those subjects about which most has been speculated and written in the past. In the last 50 years or so, a great number of scientific papers have been devoted to arthropod venoms, but only a few volumes have been designed to collect this rapidly increasing material, and these are not recent. Of late, the chemistry and mode of action of several arthropod venoms have been thoroughly studied, and some of these substances will probably be used as pharmacological tools and also as therapeutic agents.

The aim of the present volume is to collect in manual form new information as well as the old notions on arthropod venoms.

Even though it was our intention to present a volume on arthropod venoms, and not on venomous arthropods, inevitably we were forced to include information on venom-producing organisms as well. We assumed, in fact, that those scientists for whom the present manual is primarily intended (biochemists, particularly comparative biochemists, and pharmacologists) should be familiar with the biologic elements concerning the venom-producing species; which should show them how important it is to operate in close collaboration with biologists specialized in venomous arthropod systematics and biology. Furthermore, the distribution, ethology, and ecology of venomous species should be thoroughly known if the specific therapy and prevention of envenomation are to be correctly undertaken by clinicians and public health specialists respectively. For these reasons the reader, besides an introductory chapter on arthropod systematics, will find in the first part of each chapter much space devoted to the distribution and biology of the venomous species.

The origin and nature of animal substances called venoms and the concept of toxicity have been much debated throughout the years and several definitions of the term "venom" have been given by different authors. In our volume the proposed definition is the old one of E.N. PAWLOWSKY (Gifttiere und ihre Giftigkeit. Jena: G. Fischer, 1927), later adopted by E. KAISER and E. MICHL (Die Biochemie der tierischen Gifte. Wien: F. Deuticke, 1958) which reads as follows: "Those substances are considered venoms which, due to their chemical characteristics, after their penetration into the human or animal body can cause, even in small doses, alterations in their health, or death." By following such a definition, the authors were allowed to include in this volume topics regarding all toxic substances derived from arthropods, even those not originating from venomous apparatuses.

The concept of toxic properties of tissues has been well treated already by M. PHISALIX (Animaux Venimeux et Venins. Paris: Masson, 1922) and recently by E. HABERMAN (Chemistry, Pharmacology, and Toxicology of Bee, Wasp, and Hornet Venoms. In: Animals and their Venoms, Vol. III, Eds. W. Bücherl and E. Buckley. New York: Academic Press, 1971). Obviously the limits of this concept are vague: many substances present in arthropods, for instance, may cause toxic phenomena if administered in high doses. As HABERMAN states, the frontier between "simple" body constituents and "venom" is not sharply marked: an example is given by biogenic amines which are present both in tissues and in venoms. On the other hand, in some cases (e.g., bee venom) when the venom is administered at very low doses, the original sense of the term gives way to its conceptual opposite, that of medicament.

We have deemed it useful to broaden the subject by also including in the volume the arthropod defensive substances, some of which are not to be considered as toxic *sensu stricto,* even though they do induce profound behavioral modifications in other species. This type of compound appears more puzzling if, for instance, we consider that some ketones are utilized by ants both for defensive and communicative functions (M.S. BLUM and H.R. HERMAN, Chapter 25).

The limits to be attributed to the term venom could not, therefore, be fixed *a priori,* but were left in each case to the judgment of the individual authors.

As initially planned, the volume should have also included chapters dealing with species belonging to orders less known for their poisonous characteristics. It is well known that the saliva of Diptera, for instance, often causes local and general toxic phenomena not to be attributed to allergic responses only (e.g., toxic reactions due to bites of tabanid larvae, asilids, simulids, ceratopogonids, etc.). Information in such a field, however, is so scanty that we had to abandon the idea. On the other hand, a great deal has already been published on insect allergy, a topic more pertinent to the field of immunology. On this subject, excellent reviews have been presented by S. SHULMAN (Allergic responses to insect bites. Annual Rev. Entomol. **12**, 323–346, 1967), B.F. FEINGOLD, E. BENJAMINI and D. MICHAELI (The allergic responses to insect bites. Annual Rev. Entomol. **13**, 137–158, 1968) and C.A. FRAZIER (Insect Allergy, St. Louis: W.H. Green, 1969), to which the reader is referred.

The volume has been divided into 26 chapters, each one related to a specific zoologic group, this being the only possible way of arranging the abundant material on the various subjects without risking many omissions or repetitions. Unfortunately, as will be noted by the careful reader, a few were unavoidable. The existence of a very large number of arthropod-borne toxic substances, and of even larger number of specialists, 43 of whom were invited to participate in the preparation of the present volume, made this drawback inevitable.

In order to cover the naturalistic as well as the biochemical and pharmacologic aspects of each chapter, more than one author was often needed. Though this represented an advantage as far as the thorough treatment of the subject was concerned, it negatively influenced the uniformity of the volume because of the diverse nature and amount of information available for each topic.

The authors of the volume are among the most qualified specialists in their fields. They were asked to include in their chapters all that is known on the subject, so as to match the purpose and tradition of the monographs published by the Handbook of Experimental Pharmacology.

Editing of the present volume started in January 1974. The mailing of the first group of invitations coincided with one of the most serious postal strikes in Italy, so that a great deal of mail went astray. This, plus the courteous declining by some scientists and the delay of others in providing the manuscripts caused the volume to be published at the end of 1977 and consequently a few of the chapters may be somewhat outdated.

I wish to express my gratitude to all authors who have taken on the burden of this task with enthusiasm and skill: they should be praised for the high standard of their reviews. Thanks are due to Professor P. BRIGNOLI for the time he has devoted to discussing some of the naturalistic problems of the volume. I am particularly indebted to Miss A.M. LOPOMO for her excellent secretarial work. I also wish to thank member of the staff of Springer-Verlag, who were extremely cooperative in the preparation of the volume.

In January of this year we received the very sad news that our Japanese colleague Professor Y. HASHIMOTO, who had prepared jointly with Professor S. KONOSU the chapter "Venoms of Crustacea and Merostomata", had died on 23 September 1976. I am sure that I share the feelings of all the other authors in expressing our deep sorrow and sympathy to Professor HASHIMOTO's family and to all those who have had the pleasure of working with him.

August 1977 SERGIO BETTINI

Table of Contents

CHAPTER 3

Defensive Secretions of Millipeds. T. EISNER, D. ALSOP, K. HICKS, and J. MEINWALD.
With 13 Figures

CHAPTER 4

Secretions of Centipedes. A. MINELLI. With 2 Figures

CHAPTER 5

Secretions of Opilionids, Whip Scorpions and Pseudoscorpions. T. EISNER, D. ALSOP,
and J. MEINWALD. With 7 Figures

CHAPTER 6

Review of the Spider Families, with Notes on the Lesser-Known Poisonous Forms.
S. BETTINI and P.M. BRIGNOLI

CHAPTER 7

Venoms of Dipluridae. M.R. GRAY and S.K. SUTHERLAND

CHAPTER 8

Venoms of Theridiidae, Genus Latrodectus

A. Systematics, Distribution and Biology of Species; Chemistry, Pharmacology and Mode of Action of Venom. S. BETTINI and M. MAROLI. With 8 Figures

CHAPTER 10

Venoms of Ctenidae. S. SCHENBERG and F.A. PEREIRA LIMA. With 15 Figures

CHAPTER 11

Venoms of Scytodidae. Genus Loxosceles. H. Schenone and G. Suarez. With 6 Figures

CHAPTER 12

The Genus Centruroides (Buthidae) and Its Venom. H.L. STAHNKE. With 2 Figures

CHAPTER 13

Venoms of Buthinae

A. Systematics and Biology of Buthinae. A. SHULOV and G. LEVY

B. Symptomatology and Treatment of Buthinae Stings. P. EFRATI

B. Chemical and Pharmacologic Aspects of Tityinae Venoms. C.R. DINIZ.
With 8 Figures

CHAPTER 15

Chactoid Venoms M. GOYFFON and J. KOVOOR. With 6 Figures

CHAPTER 16

Tick Paralysis. M.F. MURNAGHAN and F.J. O'ROURKE. With 3 Figures

CHAPTER 17

Toxins of Blattaria. L.M. ROTH and D.W. ALSOP. With 24 Figures

CHAPTER 18

Venoms of Rhyncota (Hemiptera). J. WEATHERSTON and J.E. PERCY

CHAPTER 19

Venoms of Coleoptera. J. WEATHERSTON and J.E. PERCY

CHAPTER 20

Venoms of Lepidoptera. A. DELGADO QUIROZ. With 19 Figures

CHAPTER 21

Venoms of Apidae. R. O'CONNOR and M.L. PECK. With 8 Figures

CHAPTER 22

Venoms of Sphecidae, Pompilidae, Mutillidae, and Bethylidae. W. RATHMAYER. With 8 Figures

CHAPTER 23

Venoms of Vespidae. H. EDERY, J. ISHAY, S. GITTER and H. JOSHUA. With 30 Figures

CHAPTER 24

Venoms of Braconidae. R.L. BEARD. With 13 Figures

CHAPTER 25

Venoms and Venom Apparatuses of the Formicidae: Myrmeciinae, Ponerinae, Dorylinae, Pseudomyrmecinae, Myrmicinae and Formicinae. M.S. BLUM and H.R. HERMANN. With 65 Figures

CHAPTER 26

Venom and Venom Apparatuses of the Formicidae: Dolichoderinae and Aneuretinae.
M.S. BLUM and H.R. HERMANN, JR. With 11 Figures

List of Contributors

D.W. Alsop, Dr., Department of Biology, Queen's College, City University of New York, Flushing, NY 11367, USA

R.L. Beard, Dr., 864 Mountain Road, Cheshire, CT 06410, USA

S. Bettini, Professor Dr., Istituto Superiore di Sanità, Viale Regina Elena 299, I-00161 Rome, Italy

M.S. Blum, Professor, Department of Entomology, University of Georgia, Athens, GA 30602, USA

P.M. Brignoli, Professor Dr., Università degli Studi di L'Aquila, Istituto di Zoologia, Piazza Regina Margherita 7, I-67100 L'Aquila, Italy

W. Bücherl, Professor Dr., Rua Sagarana 152, Vila Madalena, 0544 São Paulo, Brazil

A. Delgado Quiroz, Dr., Instituto de Medicina Tropical, "Daniel A. Carrion", Universidad Nacional Mayor de San Marcos, Casilla 10138, Lima 1, Perú

C.R. Diniz, Dr., Ministerio da Educação E Cultura, Universidade Federal De Minas Gerais, CP. 2486, Instituto De Ciencias Biológicas, Dept. Bioquîmica, 30.000 Belo Horizonte, M.G., Brazil

H. Edery, Professor, Department of Physiology and Pharmacology, Sackler School of Medicine, Tel-Aviv University, Ramat Aviv, Israel

P. Efrati, Professor, Kaplan Hospital, Rehovot, Israel

T. Eisner, Professor, Section of Neurobiology and Behavior, Cornell University, 139 Langmuir Laboratory, Ithaca, NY 14853, USA

S. Gitter, Professor, Department of Physiology and Pharmacology, Sackler Scholl of Medicine, Tel-Aviv University, Ramat-Aviv, Israel

M. Goyffon, Dr., Muséum National d'Histoire Naturelle, Laboratoire d'Etudes et de Recherches sur les Animaux Irradiés C.R.S.S.A. − C.N.R.S., 57 Rue Cuvier, F-75 Paris 5e, France

M.R. Gray, Dr., The Australian Museum, P.O. Box A 285, Sydney, N.S.W. 2000, Australia

Y. Hashimoto, Professor†, The University of Tokyo, Faculty of Agriculture, Laboratory of Marine Biochemistry, Bunkyo-ku, Tokyo, Japan

H.R. HERMANN, Professor, Department of Entomology, University of Georgia, Athens, GA 30602, USA

KAREN HICKS, Dr., Section of Neurobiology and Behavior, 139 Langmuir Laboratory, Cornell University, Ithaca, NY 14853, USA

J. ISHAY, Dr., Department of Physiology and Pharmacology, Sackler School of Medicine, Tel-Aviv University, Ramat-Aviv, Israel

H. JOSHUA, Dr., Clinical Laboratory, Beilinson Medical Center, Petah Tikva, Israel

S. KONOSU, Dr., The University of Tokyo, Faculty of Agriculture, Laboratory of Marine Biochemistry, Bunkyo-ku, Tokyo 113, Japan

JACQUELINE KOVOOR, Universite Pierre-et-Marie Curie, Laboratoire d'Evolution, 105, Bd. Raspail, F-75006 Paris, France

G. LEVY, Dr., Department of Entomology and Venomous Animals, The Hebrew University, Jerusalem, Israel

Z. MARETIĆ, Dr., Medicinski centar, Pula, Jugoslavia

M. MAROLI, Dr., Laboratorio di Parassitologia, Istituto Superiore di Sanità, Viale Regina Elena 299, I-00161 Rome, Italy

J. MEINWALD, Professor Dr., Department of Chemistry, Cornell University, Spencer T. Olin Laboratory, Ithaca, NY 14853, USA

A. MINELLI, Professor Dr., Istituto di Biologia Animale, Università degli Studi, Via Poredan 10, I-35100 Padova, Italy

F. MIRANDA, Dr., Laboratoire de Biochimie, Faculté de Medecine-Secteur Nord, F-13326 Marseille Cedex 3, France

M.F. MURNAGHAN, Professor, Department of Physiology, Earlsfort Terrace, University College, Dublin, Ireland

R. O'CONNOR, Dr., Chemistry Department, Texas University, College Station, TX 77843, USA

F.J. O'ROURKE, Dr., Department of Zoology, University College, Lee Maltings Prospect Row, Cork, Ireland

M.L. PECK, Ass. Professor, Department of Chemistry, Texas A+M University, College of Science, College Station, TX 77843, USA

J.E. PERCY, Dr., Canadian Forestry Service, Insect Pathology Research Institute, P.O. Box 490, Sault Ste. Marie, Ontario P6A 5M7, Canada

F.A. PEREIRA-LIMA, Dr., Servico de Fisiologia do Instituto Butantan, Caixa Postal 65, Sào Paulo, Brazil

W. RATHMAYER, Professor, Fachbereich Biologie, Universität Konstanz, Postfach 733, 7750 Konstanz, Germany

H. ROCHAT, Dr., Laboratoire de Biochimie, Faculté de Medecine — Secteur Nord, F-13326 Marseille, Cedex 3, France

L.M. ROTH, Dr., 81 Brush Hill Road, Sherborn, Massachusettes, USA 01770

S. SCHENBERG, Professor, Servico de Fisiologia, Instituto Butantan, Caixa Postal 65, São Paulo, Brazil

H. SCHENONE, Dr., Instituto de Parassitologia, Universidad de Chile, Cassila 9183, Santiago de Chile, Chile

A. SHULOV, Professor Dr., Department of Entomology and Venomous Animals, The Hebrew University, Jerusalem, Israel

H.L. STAHNKE, Professor, Poisonus Animals Research Laboratory, Department of Zoology, Arizona State University, Tempe, Arizona 85281, USA

G. SUAREZ, Dr., Department of Medicine, Albert Einstein College of Medicine, 1300 Morris Park Avenue, Bronx, NY 10461, USA

S.K. SUTHERLAND, Dr., Department of Immunological Research, Commonwealth Serum Laboratories, 45 Poplar Rd., Parkville, Melbourne 3052, Australia

J. WEATHERSTON, Dr., Forest Pest Management Institute, 1219 Queen Street East, Sault Ste. Marie, Ontario, Canada

E. ZLOTKIN, Dr., The Hebrew University of Jerusalem, Department of Entomology and Venomous Animals, Jerusalem, Israel

CHAPTER 1

Introduction to Venomous Arthropod Systematics

P.M. Brignoli

A. Introduction

The main purpose of this introductory chapter is to offer the reader some essential, general information on the systematics of the groups considered in the present volume, particularly to the reader with only a superficial zoological background. It must be understood that identification of arthropods presents difficulties when the level of species, or even genus, is reached. This can normally be done only by specialists. (Advice on identification is given under Sect. VII.)

I. What are Arthropoda?

By far the largest animal group, about one million species have already been identified, and hundreds of new ones are discovered every year. Arthropoda are ubiquitous, for they have become adapted to all kinds of environment.

Since the beginning of last century, they have been considered as phylogenetically related to the segmented worms (Annelida); recent findings indicate that a relationship also exists with the Mollusca. Arthropoda constitute an extremely old zoological group; fossils from the Palaeozoic era are known from most of its orders, but the origins of the whole group and the relationship between the different classes are uncertain and criticizable; a few authors consider them polyphyletic.

The main characteristics of Arthropoda are segmentation (internal and external) of the body, the usual presence of articulated appendages, and of a hard exoskeleton formed mostly by chitin. The combination of these characteristics is not to be found in any other animal; on this basis, all venomous Arthropoda can be easily identified.

II. The Main Divisions of the "Type"

Three large groups can easily be separated: Chelicerata, Crustacea, and Hexapoda or Insecta. The first, which includes a handful of recent Merostomata (the horseshoe "crab"), many Arachnida, and possibly the Pantopoda or Pycnogonida (the sea-spider), has in common a low number of appendages in the anterior part of the body and generally the absence of walking limbs in the posterior part of the body; Crustacea usually have a high number of appendages on each part of their body; most of the Hexapoda have three pairs of legs, differently modified mouthparts, and two pairs of wings.

There remain a few groups of terrestrial, elongated, wingless, and multilegged forms of discussed affinities, which have often been classed under the name of Myriapoda.

The general organization of these groups could be outlined as follows:

1) Chelicerata: body formed by two principal parts, *prosoma* (head + thorax) and *opisthosoma* (abdomen); 6 pairs of articulated appendages, inserted only on the prosoma; *chelicerae* (preoral in the adult), used especially for feeding; *pedipalpi,* modified in various ways; four pairs of *legs.*

2. Crustacea: body typically divided into three parts, *cephalon* (head), *pereion* (thorax), and *pleon* (abdomen); the head can be partially fused with the thorax but never so fully as in the Chelicerata; all parts of the body can bear appendages; noteworthy is the presence of two pairs of *antennae* on the head.

3. Hexapoda: body of the adult always clearly divided in three parts, *head, thorax,* and *abdomen;* articulated appendages are borne only by the first two; noteworthy is the presence of only one pair of *antennae* on the head; in most groups there are two pairs of *wings,* inserted on the thorax only.

4. Myriapoda: body divided into two parts, *head* and *trunk,* the latter formed by segments very similar to each other, most of which bear legs; one pair of *antennae* on the head.

III. The Chelicerata

Venomous forms of this group exist only in the class Arachnida (about 40,000 species described), which includes mostly terrestrial arthropods divided into many orders. The general form of the body ("compact" or clearly divided into two segments) and especially the modifications of the pedipalpi enable them to be readily identified and classified.

1. Scorpionida

There are about 600 known species of this well-known group divided mainly into six or seven families, which can be distinguished by the form of the sternum, the presence or absence of modified spines ("spurs") at the basis of tarsi or basitarsi (the last two articles of the legs) and peculiarities of the combs (a paired ventral structure of discussed function). Taxonomy at lower levels pays particular attention to the sensory setae (trichobotriae) of the "hand", the "pince" of the pedipalp. Theoretically, all species are venomous.

2. Uropygi or Thelyphonida

Only 85 species of whip scorpions are actually known; until recently, this order was united with the Amblypygi and the Schizomida in the heterogeneous order Pedipalpi. They are rather rare animals, somewhat similar to scorpions, but caudally have only a simple, harmless flagellum. They possess glands which excrete defensive, repellent secretions.

3. Pseudoscorpionida

The false-scorpions known so far number about 1100; most are very small (less than 5 mm). They can be easily identified by their similarity to a "tailless" scorpion. Their poison glands are located in the pedipalpi; their dimensions and way of life (in litter, under bark, in caves) prevent damage to man. They are divided into three suborders, and many of the families are not easy for the nonspecialist to distinguish. The classification at species level is based on the tricobothriae of the hand and the internal genitalia.

4. Opiliones

The more common forms of this relatively large order (about 2500 species) have a "compact", well-segmented body and relatively long legs. They are divided into three suborders: Cyphophthalmi (small, mite-like, edaphic forms), Laniatores (mostly tropical, often with curiously shaped body and legs), and Palpatores (most of which are the "typical" harvestmen with ovoidal body and long, thin legs). This group is essentially harmless, possessing only defensive repugnatory glands. Classification is based on external morphology and genitalia.

5. Acarina

It is impossible to give a simple definition of this large (more than 10,000 species) and heterogeneous order. As harvestmen they have a "compact" body, usually with no traces at all of segmentation; their legs are often reduced in size, and the mouthparts are transformed for piercing. Some parasitic species have only two pairs of legs; most of the larvae are three legged. The number of suborders is still under discussion, and the classification of the whole group (probably poly-phyletic) is in rapid evolution. The well-known ticks (Ixodides), the only group considered in this handbook, would belong, according to some recent authors, to the suborder Parasitiformes (Metastigmata).

6. Araneae

Currently, about 25,000 species of spiders have been identified; they are very uniform by general morphology, which makes it practically impossible for nonspe-cialists to distinguish between the many (about 70) usually accepted families.

All spiders produce silk with more or less developed spinnerets at the end of the opisthosoma; nearly all have poison glands in the chelicerae. Not considering the archaic Liphistiomorpha (of Southeast Asia) with a segmented abdomen, all spiders fall in two main groups: Orthognatha (Mygalomorphae), in which the claws of the chelicerae can move only in a plane vertical to the ground, and Labidognatha (Araneomorphae), in which the claws can move in a plane parallel to the ground. Classification at the lower levels is still an uncertainty; the problems (in the Labidognatha) are represented by the presence in many genera of a supple-mentary silk-producing plate (*cribellum*) anterior to the first pair of spinnerets and by the presence of forms with simple or complex genitalia in many phyletic lines.

At species level, the most-used characteristics for classification are the accessory copulatory organs of the male (*bulbi*), which are derived from a transformation of the extremity of the pedipalpi, and the external or internal genitalia of the females (*epigyne, vulva*).

IV. The Crustacea

The some 40,000 known species of this mostly aquatic group are actually divided into no less than ten subclasses (Cephalocarida, Anostraca, Phyllopoda, Ostracoda, Mystacocarida, Copepoda, Branchiura, Ascothoracica, Cirripedia, and Malacostraca) of which the first nine correspond to the "Entomostraca" of the old systems. The characteristics most useful for classification are the number of recognizable segments and the number, form, and function of the limbs.

The Malacostraca are by far the largest and highest developed group; to them belong most Crustacea of any importance to man. They can usually be distinguished from the other subclasses by the presence of appendages on the pleon. In modern systems, they are divided into six superorders (Phyllocarida, Hoplocarida, Syncarida, Eucarida, Pancarida, and Peracarida) with 13 orders, the more familiar of these being Stomatopoda (Hoplocarida), Euphausiacea ("krill") and Decapoda (both Eucarida), Mysidacea, Amphipoda, and Isopoda (all Peracarida).

Identification characteristics at the species level depend upon the group; the shape of the body and of some appendages are the most common.

V. The "Myriapoda"

Most recent authors consider this group to be heterogeneous. It unites superficially similar forms which share many generalized (primitive?) characteristics, a terrestrial way of life and a relatively elongated body. Of the four usually accepted groups, Symphyla and Pauropoda include small soil-living forms of no toxicological importance.

1. Chilopoda

A somewhat primitive group, about 3000 species, chilopoda have at most only one pair of legs for each segment. In common with insects, they have the position of the genital openings near the posterior end of the body. Most are active, predatory forms which inject poison with anterior modified limbs.

They are divided into two orders: Notostigmophora (few specialized species, with very long antennae and legs) and Pleurostigmophora (the "typical" centipedes). Classification at species level is based on sensory hairs, chaetotaxy, form of the *furcipolae* (the "fangs"), etc.

2. Diplopoda

More than 7000 species of millipedes are known; all are highly specialized from many points of view. Identification is easy through the presence of two pairs of legs on most segments. Nearly all are harmless soil-living forms with only defensive repugnatory glands. Only a few species belong to the order Pselaphognatha (small secretive forms with a soft exoskeleton covered by tufts of bristles), whereas most belong to the Chilognatha.

Their *gonopodia* (genital appendages) are widely used in taxonomy at species level.

VI. The Hexapoda or Insecta

It is very difficult to give in a limited space detailed information on this enormous group, the largest of the Arthropoda and of all living beings. It must also be recalled that most Insecta larvae are often not recognizable as arthropods by untrained persons. For a correct definition of most orders, therefore, the preimaginal instars (nonadults), should also be taken into consideration. This would be impossible in the present chapter.

The most primitive Insecta are the so-called Apterygota, e.g., the primary wingless forms; some of these (the orders Diplura, Protura, and Collembola) are sometimes even detached from the group Insecta. Only the old "Thysanura", now divided in Archaeognatha and Zygentoma, seem very near to the true Insecta.

All these groups include small, soil-living species of no toxicological importance, as are also the most primitive winged insects, the Ephemeroptera (mayflies), Odonata (dragonflies), and Plecoptera (stoneflies).

The Paurometabola are still primitive forms, with larvae very similar to the adults and mostly hardened anterior wings. To the Paurometabola belong the Blattodea (cockroaches) and Dermaptera (earwigs) as well as many other orders (Embioptera, Notoptera, Mantodea, Isoptera, Phasmida, Ensifera, Caelifera, e.g., praying mantis, termites, stickinsects, grasshoppers, crickets, etc.). All have simple mouthparts and most are harmless vegetarians.

Incomplete or no metamorphosis is one of the characteristics shared by all groups included in the Paraneoptera, which include the Rhynchota or Hemiptera (bugs, aphids, etc.), the Anoplura or Siphunculata (lice), as well as the Zoraptera, Psocoptera, Mallophaga, and Thysanoptera. Most of these orders have more specialized mouthparts and many are of considerable practical importance.

The taxonomical position of the fleas (Aphaniptera or Siphonaptera) and of the parasitic Strepsiptera is still discussed; both groups are highly specialized.

All other insects have complete metamorphosis and belong, therefore, to the Holometabola, Coleoptera (beetles), Hymenoptera (bees, wasps, ants, etc.), Lepidoptera (butterflies and moths), Diptera (flies, mosquitoes, etc.), and the minor orders Megaloptera, Raphidioptera, Planipennia, Mecoptera and Trichoptera.

1. Blattodea and Dermaptera

Both are small groups (for Insects), with only 3500 known species of the first order and 1300 of the second.

Many cockroaches are well known house pests, but most of the species live secludedly in the woods throughout the whole world; they have repugnatory glands such as some earwigs, which are relatively harmless edaphic forms easily identified by the well-developed, pince-like abdominal *cerci* (some Diplura are similar to them but are mostly whitish and much smaller).

2. Rhynchota and Anoplura

No less than 70,000 Rhynchota are known and are divided in many families. All have mouthparts modified for piercing animal and vegetal tissues. The related lice are only 400 species; in modern systems they are united to the Mallophaga in the order Phthiraptera. Through an adaptation to a parasitic life, they have completely lost their wings and undergo no apparent metamorphosis.

3. Aphaniptera

The some 1600 species of fleas are all very similar, with modified mouthparts and legs. They have wormlike larvae similar to those of the Diptera.

4. Coleoptera

It is impossible to give the exact number of known beetles; some sources report a total of 350,000. Most can be easily identified by the hardened anterior wings (*elytrae*). Some Rhynchota are superficially similar but have long, very visible mouthparts.

Many of the dozens of families into which this order is divided are enormous: 29,000 Carabidae, 30,000 Staphylinidae, 20,000 Scarabeidae, etc.

5. Hymenoptera

About 100,000 species of this order are known, most of which can be easily identified by the typical "wasp-waist." It should be noted that many other Arthropoda mimic them, even in behaviour.

Most forms have two pairs of well-developed transparent wings, but many are wingless.

6. Diptera

Most of the 85,000 Diptera have only two wings; a few are wingless. To this group belong many of the most specialized Insecta. Many larvae can be a riddle even for experienced zoologists. Most adults are shaped like typical flies or mosquitoes.

7. Lepidoptera

The small, often coloured, scales which cover the wings are the most apparent characteristic of the more than 100,000 butterflies and moths. The adults of many of these have strongly modified mouthparts and often do not feed at all; their larvae are the well-known caterpillars.

VII. Some General Advices

1. How to Identify an Arthropod

The few characteristics above listed for each group should enable anyone to determine an Arthropod at class level and, perhaps with the help of a general textbook, to order level.

It is obviously impossible to give in the present chapter keys to family level. For many groups keys can be found only in very advanced treatises, often old and difficult to find. Their use is often not easy, even for trained zoologists.

A list of all described animals nowhere exists; for a few groups there are catalogues of all species, but most of these are not up to date.

At regional level, there are many local faunae and catalogues; unfortunately, they are practically limited to some parts of the Northern Hemisphere (this applies naturally only to the groups of interest here).

A nonzoologist who needs to know what name to give to a certain Arthropod should normally ask the advice of a specialist. It is also to be noted that unfortunately there are no specialists for practically any group; most concentrate their interest on a single genus, a family, or an order (depending on the size) often limited to a geographical region or subregion. Furthermore, a specialist cannot always be found (and often, if found, it is not certain that he will accept material in study, as all active specialists are overburdened with work).

2. How to Conserve an Arthropod

It is significant here to remember that nearly all Arthopods can be killed and preserved for future taxonomical study in simple alcohol (70°–80°). This is the best method for all Arachnida, Crustacea, Myriapoda, and most Insecta. Of the latter, only the Lepidoptera cannot be preserved in this way; they are best killed by gentle pression on the thorax or by exposure to KCN or chlorophormium vapors and put with folded wings in small envelopes. Many Insecta should be preserved dry, but this requires some experience to obtain good results.

3. What to Expect From the Bibliography

It is impossible to list here all the many thousands of taxonomical papers written on the Arthropoda; most nonzoologists are unaware of the fact that by internationally long-accepted rules, every taxonomist must consider all the literature published on a given species since 1758 (no exclusions are allowed for uncommon languages and obscure periodicals).

It makes little sense to list many specialized taxonomical monographs, well known to the specialists and useless for the layman.

The works listed here are, therefore, general treatises, bibliographies, large catalogues from which most potentially useful information on morphology, biology, and taxonomy at the higher levels can be obtained.

References

A. General Works

I. The Zoological Record

This periodical, published since 1864 by the Zoological Society of London, is of paramount importance for any taxonomical study. All publications on taxonomy, morphology ecology, etc., are listed and analyzed in it, but unfortunately after an usual delay of three to four years. (The volume on publications of 1970 appeared in 1974.)

II. Treatises

Handbuch der Zoologie: original editors, Kükenthal, W. and Krumbach, Th.; Berlin & Leipzig: de Gruyter. A general zoological treatise covering all aspects of all groups. (Some parts are still to be published.)

Klassen und Ordnungen des Tierreichs: Original editor, Bronn, H.G.; Leipzig: Akademische Verlagsgesellschaft. (Much more ambitious than the preceding; all groups are treated monographically. Some parts are still to be published.)

Traité de Zoologie: Grasse, P.P., editor. Paris: Masson. (Intermediate in its dimensions between the first two. Soon to be beended.)

Das Tierreich: Eine Zusammenstellung und Kennzeichnung der rezenten Tierformen: Berlin: Friedländer & Sohn, and Berlin & Leipzig: de Gruyter. (Each part of this work is a strictly taxonomic monograph about a single group; most parts are now unfortunately very old. Still appears, but very rarely.)

III. Works on All Groups of Arthropoda

Kaestner, A.: *Lehrbuch der speziellen Zoologie, Teil I* (2—3). Stuttgart-Jena: Gustav Fischer 1957—73. (A modern, detailed, and practical work at university level; good bibliography.)

Sharov, A.G.: *Basic Arthropodan Stock.* Oxford: Pergamon Press, 1966. (Important discussion of the affinities between the groups.)

Snodgrass, R.E.: *A Textbook of Arthropod Anatomy.* Ithaca, N.Y.: Cornell Univ. Press, 1952.

B. Chelicerata

I. Works on All (or most) Orders

Berland, L.: Les arachnides. Paris: Lechevalier, 1932. (Somewhat old, but still useful.)

Kaestner, A.: Arachnida. In: Handbuch der Zoologie, 3(2). Berlin-Leipzig: de Gruyter, 1940.

Millot, J.: Classe des Arachnides. In: Traité de Zoologie, Tome VI. Paris: Masson, 1949.

Savory, Th.: Arachnida. London-New York: Academic Press, 1964. (Recent, but not rich in details.)

II. Scorpionida

Kaestner, A.: Scorpiones. In: Handbuch der Zoologie, 3(2). Berlin-Leipzig: de Gruyter, 1940.

Kraepelin, K.: Scorpiones und Pedipalpi. In: Das Tierreich, 8. Berlin: Friedländer & Sohn, 1899. (Old, but still important in taxonomy.)

Vachon, M.: Études sur les scorpions. Algiers: Institut Pasteur, 1952. (Very important as an introduction to the taxonomy of this group.)

Vachon, M., Millot, J.: Ordre des Scorpions. In: Traité de Zoologie, Tome VI. Paris: Masson, 1949.

Werner, F.: Scorpiones, Pedipalpi. In: Klassen und Ordnungen des Tierreichs, 5(IV)8. Leipzig: Akademische Verlagsgesellschaft, 1935.

III. Uropygi or Thelyphonida

Kaestner, A.: Pedipalpi. In: Handbuch der Zoologie, 3(2). Berlin & Leipzig: de Gruyter, 1932.
Kraepelin, K. (See above.)
Millot, J.: Ordre des Uropyges. In: Traité de Zoologie, Tome VI. Paris: Masson, 1949.
Werner, F. (See above.)

IV. Pseudoscorpionida

Beier, M.: Pseudoscorpionidea. In: Handbuch der Zoologie, 3(2). Berlin & Leipzig: de Gruyter, 1932.
Beier, M.: Pseudoscorpionidea. In: Das Tierreich, 57—58. Berlin-Leipzig: de Gruyter, 1932. (Somewhat old.)
Beier, M.: Ordnung Pseudoscorpionidea. In: Bestimmungsbücher zur Bodenfauna Europas, 7. Berlin: Akademie Verlag, 1963. (European fauna only.)
Roewer, C.F.: Chelonethi.: In Klassen und Ordnungen des Tierreichs, 5(IV)6. Leipzig: Akademische Verlagsgesellschaft, 1936—40.
Vachon, M.: Ordre des Pseudoscorpions. In: Traité de Zoologie, Tome VI. Paris: Masson, 1949.

V. Opiliones

Berland, L.: Ordre des Opilions. In: Traité de Zoologie, Tome VI. Paris: Masson, 1949.
Kaestner, A.: Opiliones. In: Handbuch der Zoologie, 3(2). Berlin-Leipzig: de Gruyter, 1935.
Roewer, C.F.: Die Weberknechte der Erde. Jena: Gustav Fischer, 1923. (Very old, but still fundamental for taxonomy.)
Silhavy, V.: Sekaci-Opilionidea. In: Fauna CSR, 7. Prague: Akademia Ved, 1956. (Abundant data; in Czech.)

VI. Acarina

André, M.: Ordre des Acariens. In: Traité de Zoologie, Tome VI. Paris: Masson, 1949.
Arthur, D.R.: Ticks and Diseases. Oxford: Pergamon Press, 1962.
Nuttall, G.H., Warburton, C., Cooper, W.F., Robinson, V.E.: Ticks, a monograph of the Ixodoidea. Cambridge University Press, 1908—1926.
Serdjukova, G.V.: Ixodidae. In: Fauna of the USSR, 64. Leningrad-Moscow: Izdatelstvo Academit Nauk SSSR, 1956. (In Russian.)
Senevet, G.: Ixodoidés. In: Faune de France, 32. Paris: Lechevalier, 1937.
Vitzthum, H.: Acarina. In: Klassen und Ordnungen des Tierreichs, 5(IV)5. Leipzig: Akademische Verlagsgesellschaft, 1943.

VII. Araneae

Bonnet, P.: Bibliographia araneorum. Toulouse: Douladoue 1945—61. (List and analysis of all papers published on spiders up to 1939.)
Bristowe, W.S.: The comity of spiders. London: Ray Society, 1939—41.
Gerhardt, U., Kaestner, A.: Araneae. In: Handbuch der Zoologie, 3(2). Berlin-Leipzig: de Gruyter, 1937—38.
Gertsch, W.J.: American spiders. New York: Van Nostrand Co., 1949.
Roewer, C.F.: Katalog der Araneae von 1758 bis 1940 bzw. 1954. Bremen-Bruxelles: Natura and Institut R. des Sciences Naturelles, 1942—54. (Very practical for taxonomy.)
Millot, J.: Ordre des Aranéides. In: Traité de Zoologie, Tome VI. Paris: Masson, 1949.
Simon, E.: Histoire naturelle des araignées. Paris: Roret 1892—1903. (Old, but still fundamental in taxonomy.)
Yaginuma, T.: Spiders of Japan in color. Osaka: Hoikusha, 1971. (Colored illustrations of many species.)

C. Crustacea

I. General Works

Gruner, H.E., Holthuis, L.B. (eds.): Crustaceorum catalogus. Den Haag: Dr. W. Junk. (Only
three parts of this work, begun in 1967, have so far been published.)
Zimmer, C.: Crustacea. In: Handbuch der Zoologie, 3(1). Berlin-Leipzig: de Gruyter, 1927.

II. Special Works

In: Handbuch der Zoologie: In this treatise all groups have been covered from 1926 to
27. (Out of date.)
In:KlassenundOrdnungendesTierreichs:
Balss, H.: Stomatopoda, 5(I)6(2), 1938.
Balss, H., Buddenbrock, W. von, Grunder, H.E., Korschelt, E.: Decapoda, 5(I)7. 1940—61.
(Very extensive.)
Graham Cannon, H.: Leptostraca, 5(I)4(1), 1960.
Gruner, H.E., Zimmer, C.: Euphausiacea, 5(I)6(3), 1956.
Hartmann, G.: Ostracoda, 5(I)2, 1966—67.
Krüger, P.: Ascothoracida, Cirripedia, 5(I)3, 1940.
Monod, Th.: Thermosbenacea, 5(I)4, 1940.
Siewing, R.: Syncarida, 5(I)4(2), 1959.
Zimmer, C.: Cumacea, 5(I)4, 1941.

D. Myriapoda

I. Chilopoda

Attems, C.: Chilopoda. In: Handbuch der Zoologie, 4(l). Berlin-Leipzig: de Gruyter, 1926.
Attems, C.: Chilopoda. In: Das Tierreich, 52—53. Berlin-Leipzig: de Gruyter, 1929—30.
Verhoeff, K.W.: Chilopoda. In: Klassen und Ordnungen des Tierreichs, 5(II). Leipzig: Akade-
mische Verlagsgesellschaft, 1902—25.

II. Diplopoda

Attems, C.: Diplopoda. In: Handbuch der Zoologie 4(1). Berlin-Leipzig: de Gruyter 1926.
Verhoeff, K.W.: Diplopoda. In: Klassen und Ordnungen des Tierreichs, 5(II). Leipzig: Akademische Verlagsgesellschaft, 1928—32.

E. Hexapoda

I. General Entomological Textbooks

Eidmann, H.: Lehrbuch der Entomologie, II Aufl. Hamburg: Parey, 1970.
Fox, R.M., Fox, J.W.: Introduction to comparative entomology. New York: Reinhold Publ.
Co., 1964. (Covers other groups also.)
Grandi, G.: Introduzione allo studio dell'entomologia. Bologna: Edizioni agricole, 1951. (Often
overlooked, but very extensive.)
Hennig, W.: Die Stammesgeschichte der Insekten. Frankfurt/Main: Kramer, 1969.
Imms, A.D.: *A General Textbook of Entomology,* 9th ed. London: Methuen & Co., 1969.
Ross, H.H.: *A Textbook of Entomology,* 2nd ed. New York: J. Wiley & Sons Inc., 1956.
Schroeder, C.: Handbuch der Entomologie. Jena: Gustav Fischer, 1912—29. (Old, but still
important.)
Snodgrass, R.E.: *Principles of Insect Morphology.* New York-London: McGraw Hill, 1935.
Weber, H.: Grundriß der Insektenkunde, III Aufl. Stuttgart: Gustav Fischer, 1954.
Wigglesworth, W.B.: The life of insects. London: Weidenfeld & Nicolson, 1964. (Principally
on biology.)

II. The Great Treatises

In: Handbuch der Zoologie:
Beier, M., Rohdendorff, B.B.: Allgemeines (Diagnose, Geschichte etc.). 4(2) II Aufl., 1969.
Handlirsch, A.: Allgemeine Einleitung in die Naturgeschichte der Insecta. 4(2) I Aufl., 1926—29.
In: Traité de Zoologie:
Bitsch, J., Denis, J.R., Seguy, E., Termier, M.: Insectes, tête, aile, vol. Tome VIII, 1973.
Jeannel, R.: Paléontologie, Géonémie. Tome IX, 1949.

III. Works About Single Groups

1. Blattodea and Dermaptera

Beier, M.: Embioidea, Orthopteroidea, Blattopteroidea, Mantodea. In: Klassen und Ordnungen des Tierreichs, 5(III)6. Leipzig: Akademische Verlagsgesellschaft, 1955—64.
Beier, M.: Blattariae. In: Handbuch der Zoologie, 4(2) II Aufl. Berlin: de Gruyter, 1974.
Chopard, L.: La biologie des Orthoptères. Paris: Lechevalier, 1938. (Abundant data)
Chopard, L.: Superordre des Dermapteroides. In: Traité de Zoologie. Tome IX. Paris: Masson, 1949.
Chopard, L.: Ordre des Dictyoptères. In: Traité de Zoologie, Tome IX. Paris: Masson, 1949.
Günther, K., Herter, K.: Dermaptera. In: Handbuch der Zoologie, 4(2) II Aufl. Berlin: de Gruyter, 1974.
Handlirsch, A.: Ordnungen der Dermaptera, Blattariae, etc. In: Handbuch der Zoologie, 4(2) I Aufl. Leipzig-Berlin: de Gruyter, 1929—30.
Harz, K.: Die Geradflügler Mitteleuropas. Jena: Gustav Fischer, 1957. (General.)

2. Rhynchota and Anoplura

Beier, M.: Ordnungen der Heteroptera und Homoptera. In: Handbuch der Zoologie, 4(2) I Aufl. Leipzig-Berlin: de Gruyter, 1937—38.
Ferris, G.F.: The sucking lice. Mem. Pacif. Coast ent. Soc. 1, 1—320 (1951).
Handlirsch, A.: Ordnung der Siphunculata. In: Handbuch der Zoologie, 4 (2) I Aufl. Leipzig-Berlin: de Gruyter, 1930.
Jordan, K.H.C.: Heteroptera. In: Handbuch der Zoologie, 4(2) II Aufl. Berlin: de Gruyter, 1972.
Miller, N.C.E.: The biology of the Heteroptera. London: Leonard Hill Ltd., 1956. (Not extensive.)
Pesson, P., Poisson, R.: Superordre des Hémiptéroïdes. In: Traité de Zoologie, Tome X(2). Paris: Masson, 1951.
Seguy, E.: Ordre Anoploures. In: Traité de Zoologie Tome X(2). Paris: Masson, 1951.
Weber, H.: Biologie der Hemipteren. Berlin: J. Springer, 1930. (Old, but still interesting.)

3. Aphaniptera

Beier, M.: Ordnung der Suctoria oder Siphonaptera oder Aphaniptera. In: Handbuch der Zoologie, 4(2) I Aufl. Leipzig-Berlin: de Gruyter, 1937.
Seguy, E.: Ordre des Siphonaptères. In: Traité de Zoologie, Tome X(1). Paris: Masson, 1951.
Wagner, J.: Aphaniptera. In Klassen und Ordnungen des Tierreichs, 5(III)13. Leipzig: Akademische Verlagsgesellschaft, 1939.

4. Coleoptera

Arnett, R.H.: The beetles of the United States. Ann Arbor: The Amer. Entomological Instit., 1971. (Useful for identification of most families.)

Jeannel, R., Paulian, R.: Superordre des Coléoptères. In: Traité de Zoologie, Tome IX. Paris: Masson, 1949.
Meixner, J.: Ordnung der Coleoptera. In: Handbuch der Zoologie, 4(2) I Aufl. Leipzig-Berlin: de Gruyter, 1934—36.

5. Hymenoptera

Berland, L., Bernard, F.: Superordre des Hyménoptéroïdes. In: Traité de Zoologie, Tome X(2). Paris: Masson, 1951.
Handlirsch, A.: Ordnung der Hymenoptera. In: Handbuch der Zoologie, 4(2) I Aufl. Leipzig-Berlin: de Gruyter, 1933.

6. Diptera

Goma, L.K.H.: The Mosquito. London: Hutchinson & Co., 1966. (Limited.)
Hendel, F., Beier, M.: Ordnung der Diptera. In: Handbuch der Zoologie, 4(2) I Aufl. Leipzig-Berlin: de Gruyter, 1936—37.
Hennig, W.: Diptera. In: Handbuch der Zoologie, 4(2) II Aufl. Berlin: de Gruyter, 1973.
Seguy, E.: La biologie des Diptères. Paris: Lechevalier, 1950.
Seguy, E.: Ordre des Diptères. In: Traité de Zoologie, Tome 10 (1). Paris: Masson, 1951.
Senevet, G.: Les Anophèles de la France et de ses colonies. Paris: Lechevalier, 1935. (Somewhat old.)

7. Lepidoptera

Bourgogne, J.: Ordre des Lepidoptères. In: Traité de Zoologie, Tome 10 (1). Paris: Masson, 1951.
Ford, E.B.: *Butterflies,* 3rd ed. London: Collins, 1957.
Hering, M.: Biologie der Schmetterlinge. Berlin: J. Springer, 1926.
Portier, P.: La biologie des Lepidoptères. Paris: Lechevalier, 1949.
Zerny, H., Beier, M.: Ordnung der Lepidoptera. In: Handbuch der Zoologie, 4(2) I Aufl. Leipzig-Berlin, 1936.

F. Local Faunae, Catalogues, Field Guides, etc.

It was impossible to list here all the works which would fall in this category; it shall be sufficient to list the most important faunae: Faune de France (Paris: Lechevalier), Die Tierwelt Deutschlands (Jena: Gustav Fischer), Fauna of the USSR (Leningrad), Fauna Japonica (edited by the Biogeographical Society of Japan), etc. Some of the volumes of these series are true monographs of whole families or orders. World catalogues (usually incomplete) of many groups of insects, have been published. Many field guides, especially on butterflies, exist; these works should normally be used only by taxonomists, as they require knowledge of the methods and principles of taxonomy.

CHAPTER 2

Venoms of Crustacea and Merostomata

Y. Hashimoto and S. Konosu

A. Introduction

Many intoxications have long been supposed to be related to the ingestion of toxic crustaceans, and a number of papers on this subject have been published and reviewed by Halstead (1965), Guinot (1967), and Holthuis (1968). These authors list more than 20 species that are suspected to be toxic. Among these crustaceans, however, the sand crab, *Emerita analoga,* is the only species whose toxin has been to some extent experimentally examined (Sommer, 1932; Sommer and Meyer, 1937). In this chapter only the reports based on experimental data will be reviewed; the older literature above will not be discussed, in order to avoid overlapping.

In recent years, several species of crab have clearly been shown to be toxic, while some of the previously suspected species have proven to be nontoxic. As was pointed out by Holthuis (1968), this may imply that the reputation of these crustaceans may have originated from unfounded tradition, bacterial infection, or allergic reactions of people who are sensitive to crustacean meat.

In a field investigation of ciguatera in the Ryukyu and Amami Islands, Hashimoto et al. (1969b) encountered the widespread belief that toxic crabs were the primary source of the toxin that caused fishes to become ciguateric. Residents also informed the field workers of sporadic outbreaks of intoxication in humans and domestic animals, following the ingestion of toxic crabs. A total of about 1000 specimens, covering 8 families and 72 species from the Ryukyu and Amami Islands were tested, and three xanthid crabs, *Zosimus aeneus, Platypodia granulosa,* and *Atergatis floridus,* were found to contain saxitoxin (Hashimoto et al., 1967; Inoue et al., 1968; Konosu et al., 1968; Noguchi et al., 1969; Hashimoto et al., 1969a). This study was followed by that of another group of the Japanese workers (Mori et al., 1968; Uwatoko-Setoguchi et al., 1969), who obtained the partially purified preparation of *Z. aeneus* toxin and detected some toxic substances in several species of crab collected from the same islands. The presence of a toxin different from saxitoxin has been noted by Teh and Gardiner (1970, 1974) in *Lophozozymus pictor.*

A few papers also suggest that the coconut and horseshoe crabs may be important from the standpoint of public health. These crabs are included in this chapter although their toxins have not yet been studied.

B. Crustaceans Suspected of Being Poisonous

The crustaceans reputed to be poisonous are:

Subclass Cirripedia
 Order Rhizocephala
  Family Sacculinidae   *Sacculina carcini* Thompson
Subclass Malacostraca
 Order Decapoda
  Family Coenobitidae   *Birgus latro* (Linnaeus)
  Family Hippidae   *Emerita analoga* (Stimpson)
  Family Raninidae   *Ranina ranina* (Linnaeus)
  Family Dromiidae   *Dromidiopsis dormia* (Linnaeus)
  Family Majidae   *Micippa philyra* (Herbst)
  Family Parthenopidae   *Parthenope longimanus* (Linnaeus)
                           Daldorfia horrida (Linnaeus)
                           Daira perlata (Herbst)
  Family Portunidae   *Thalamita prymna* (Herbst)
                           Thalamita danae Stimpson
  Family Xanthidae   *Carpilius convexus* (Forskål)
                           Carpilius maculatus (Linnaeus)
                           Liomera cinctimana (White)
                           Zosimus aeneus (Linnaeus)
                           Lophozozymus pictor (Fabricius)
                           Platypodia granulosa (Rüppell)
                           Atergatis floridus (Linnaeus)
                           Euxanthus exsculptus (Herbst)
                           Demania reynaudii (H. Milne Edwards)
                           (= *Xantho reynaudii* H.M. Edw.)
                           Demania toxica Garth
                           Etisus splendidus Rathbun
                           Eriphia sebana (Shaw and Nodder)
                           Eriphia scabricula Dana
                           Eriphia norfolcensis Grant and McCulloch
                           Pilumnus vespertilio (Fabricius)
  Family Gecarcinidae   *Ucides cordatus* (Linnaeus)
                           Cardisoma carnifex (Herbst)
  Family Ocypodidae   *Ocypode ceratophthalma* (Pallas)
  Family Mictyridae   *Mictyris longicarpus* Latreille

In addition, Halstead (1965) referred to the toxicity of some unidentified species of crab, crayfish, lobster, and shrimp.

Several species among the crabs listed above have received conflicting toxicity evaluations. The first one is *C. convexus*; its edibility is suspect in some districts (Cooper, 1964; Guinot, 1967). Mori et al. (1968) noted that the hot-water extract from a specimen of this species was fatal to mice and exerted some effects on the nerve membrane as described below. On the other hand, it was reported by Ehrhart and Niaussat (1970) that 2 specimens of this species from Clipperton

Island in the tropical Pacific did not show any toxic effect on mice. We also failed to detect the toxicity in 38 specimens from the Ryukyus, one from American Samoa, and 5 from Rangiroa, French Polynesia (HASHIMOTO et al., 1969 a; KONOSU et al., 1970). The next crab, *E. sebana,* is listed as poisonous by HOLTHUIS (1968) and reported by a native physician to have caused fatalities in Koror, Palau (MOTE and HALSTEAD: Private communication, 1969). MORI et al. (1968) stated that 2 specimens from the Ryukyus were fatal to mice. We found, however, 26 specimens from the Ryukyus and 2 from Rangiroa to be all nontoxic (HASHIMOTO et al., 1969 a; KONOSU et al., 1970). Six species of crab, *D. perlata, T. prymna, L. cincti-mana, E. scabricula, T. danae,* and *E. exsculptus,* were reported to be toxic by MORI et al. (1968), but the first 4 species collected from the same area were found to be entirely nontoxic in our test (HASHIMOTO et al., 1969 a). As described above, MORI et al. reported that the water extracts from 8 species of crab were toxic to mice. It is, however, most probable that the toxicity of some specimens is attributable to a high concentration of minerals present in the extracts, because they recognized the toxicity only at a very high dose.

A crab, *D. toxica,* was reported by ALCALA and HALSTEAD (1970) to have caused a human death in the Philippines; it was first described by Garth (1971) as a new species. Its toxicity, however, has not yet been studied. HOLTHUIS (1968) cited *D. dormia* and *P. vespertilio* as poisonous. Three specimens of the former and 61 of the latter from the Ryukyus were all nontoxic in our screening test (HASHIMOTO et al., 1969 a). At the same time, we recognized no toxicity in 4 species, *C. maculatus, E. splendidus, O. ceratophthalma,* and *M. longicarpus,* which are suspected to be dangerous to eat in some areas (HOLTHUIS, 1968; HASHIMOTO et al., 1969 a; KONOSU et al., 1970) and in 57 species, which have had no prior toxic history (HASHIMOTO et al., 1969 a).

C. Toxicity of Crabs

As mentioned above, the toxicity of most of the crustaceans suspected to be poisonous has not been studied adequately except for 5 species of crab, *Zosimus aeneus, Platypodia granulosa, Atergatis floridus, Emerita analoga,* and *Lophozozymus pictor.* This section is concerned with these 5 species. The first 4 species contain saxitoxin, while *L. pictor* possesses another toxin.

I. Crabs Containing Saxitoxin

In our toxicity study of *Z. aeneus, P. granulosa,* and *A. floridus,* we used the following method (INOUE et al., 1968), which is essentially identical with that for determining shellfish toxicity (PRAKASH et al., 1971). The specimen is minced thoroughly in a mortar and 1 g of minced material is heated with 9 ml of water in a boiling water bath for 5 min and occasionally stirred. After being cooled under running tap water, the mixture is centrifuged or filtered. By intraperitoneal injection of a 0.5-ml portion into mice weighing approximately 20 g, the dilution necessary to kill mice in 15 to 30 min is obtained. From the average death time observed in 2 or 3 mice at this dilution and the dose-death time curve (Fig. 1),

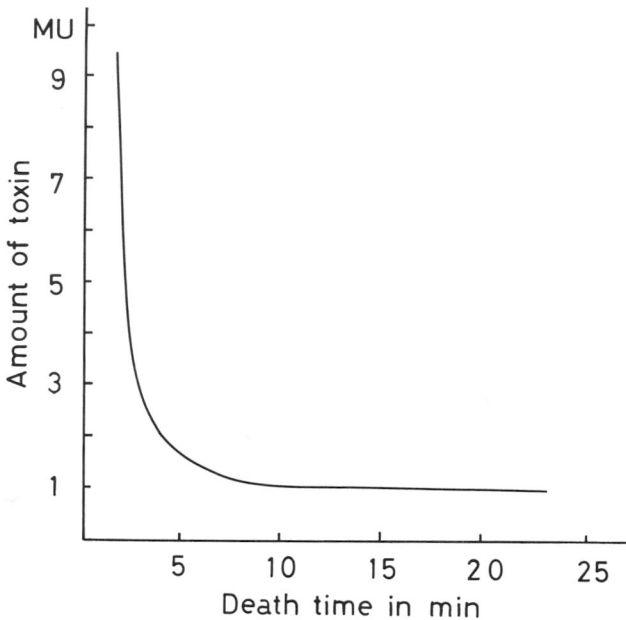

Fig. 1. Dose-death time curve for crab toxin

the minimum lethal dose is determined. To indicate the amount of toxin, the number of 20-g mice which will be killed is expressed as "mouse unit" (MU), following the method adopted for saxitoxin. When a 0.5-ml portion of the original extract did not kill the mice, the specimen was regarded as nontoxic (less than 20 MU/g).

It is noteworthy that the toxicity is kept unchanged when the crab samples are preserved frozen, but decreases remarkably or disappears completely when they are preserved in ethanol or by desiccation.

From the standpoint of public health, Z. aeneus may be far more important than the others, since it is larger in size, greater in toxicity (Konosu et al., 1969), and notorious in various islands of the Pacific (Holthuis, 1968; Hashimoto et al., 1967; Konosu et al., 1970). This species, however, is considered to be nontoxic in some areas and is consumed by inhabitants without harmful effects (Holthuis, 1968). Konosu et al. (1969, 1970) examined lethality to mice of the specimens collected from various parts of the Pacific. As shown in Table 1, all or at least part of the specimens are toxic in the Amami Islands, Ishigaki Island, Marcus Island, and Rangiroa in the Tuamotu Islands. The Gilbert Islands and Serua Island in the Fiji Archipelago may also be regarded as toxic areas because the evaporated ethanol residues, in which the specimens from the Gilbert Islands were preserved, showed weak toxicity (Konosu et al., 1969) and a poisoning due to Z. aeneus in Serua Island was confirmed by Schuierer (Private communication, 1968). Although it has been reported that this species is caught and used for food at Rangiroa (Holthuis, 1968), all 9 specimens from there show rather high toxicity. It is interesting that none of 38 specimens from Espiritu Santo exhibited

Table 1. Occurrence of toxic *Z. aeneus* in various islands in the Pacific

Location of catch	No. of crabs tested (No. of toxic crabs)[a]
Amami Islands	109 (79)
Ishigaki Island	27 (26)
Marcus Island	28 (5)
Espiritu Santo, New Hebrides	38 (0)
American Samoa	2 (0)
Rangiroa, Tuamotu Islands	9 (9)

[a] Specimens showing a toxicity of less than 20 MU/g are regarded as nontoxic.

any toxicity. This coincides well with the information from IIZUKA (Private communication, 1968) that inhabitants eat this species but intoxication has never occurred in the New Hebrides. Two specimens from American Samoa are also nontoxic, but the number of specimens is too small to regard it as a nontoxic area. The intestine of this species has been reputed to be poisonous in Samoa (HOLTHUIS, 1968). Thus, the diversity of opinion among the previous authors on the toxicity of this species may be attributable to individual and regional variations.

A. floridus was reported some time ago to be responsible for the death of a Filipino (BANNER: Private communication, 1968) and not to be used as food by the natives of Amboina (HOLTHUIS, 1968). Intoxication by this crab is unknown in Japan, probably due to the fact that this crab has never been a human food, although it is common in the southern parts of Japan and is often caught in tangle-nets that are used for spiny lobsters. Of the 144 specimens collected from 15 stations covering the whole range of its distribution in Japan, 102 specimens from 13 stations were found to be toxic, suggesting that toxic *A. floridus* is distributed throughout almost its entire range (INOUE et al., 1968; KONOSU et al., 1969).

No previous report on the suspected toxicity of *P. granulosa* had been available, but our screening test revealed that the crab from the Ryukyus contain a paralytic toxin similar to that of *Z. aeneus* (HASHIMOTO et al., 1967). The frequency of toxic individuals was much higher among the specimens from Ishigaki Island than those from Miyako Island (KONOSU et al., 1969).

Some examples indicating the pattern of toxicity in *Z. aeneus* are presented in Table 2. Great individual variation of toxicity is seen even among specimens collected at the same place at the same time. No obvious difference in lethality is observed between male and female. Although these results are somewhat inconclusive, there seems to be no significant seasonal variation of toxicity, so far as examined in Amami-Oshima Island (KONOSU et al., 1969). Two other xanthid crabs, *P. granulosa* and *A. floridus,* showed a quite similar pattern in individual and regional variations of toxicity, although their toxicity is generally lower than that of *Z. aeneus* (INOUE et al., 1968; KONOSU et al., 1969, 1970).

The distribution of toxin in various tissues is shown in Table 3, in which one specimen each of three xanthids is listed as an example. The most characteristic feature is that the appendages are usually more poisonous than the cephalothorax

Table 2. Toxicity of *Z. aeneus* (MU/g)

Location of catch	Sex	Date of catch (1969)	Body wt. (g)	Append- ages	Cephalo- thorax	Whole[a] body
Ishigaki Island	M	April 4	74	2000	400	1050
	M		44	1500	300	820
	M		28	2000	600	1100
	M		28	20	40	30
	F		31	2000	800	1260
	F		24	1500	100	740
	F		27	600	160	320
	F		34	600	300	420
	M	April 30	52	20	200	120
	M		54	400	40	190
	F		49	800	200	410
	F		78	150	40	80
Marcus Island	F	July 8	29	20	20	20
	F		29	20	(−)[b]	(−)
	M	July	16	20	(−)	(−)
	F		33	20	(−)	(−)
	F		52	20	30	30
	F		33	20	20	20
	M	Nov.	28	20	(−)	(−)
	F		29	20	(−)	(−)
	F		41	20	(−)	(−)
Rangiroa	M	March 19	32	150	100	120
	M		30	120	40	70
	F		101	200	30	120
	M	July 17	39	310	190	260
	M		22	120	60	90
	M		6	40	20	30
	F		95	240	40	140
	F		26	250	130	190

[a] Calculated value.
[b] Nontoxic(lessthan20 MU/g).)

in all three species and that an appreciable amount of toxin is detected in the exoskeleton of both appendages and cephalothorax, while the muscle of cephalo-thorax, gills, and endophragm are weakly toxic or nontoxic. The lethal dose of saxitoxin when used orally by humans is not accurately known, but SCHANTZ (1970) suggested that it may be close to 500 µg (equivalent to about 3000 MU). If this value is applied to *Z. aeneus* toxin, a 0.5-g portion of the muscle of the chela, as shown in Table 3, may contain enough toxin to kill a person.

Finally, the toxin of a sand crab, *E. analoga,* is concentrated in the digestive gland (SOMMER, 1932). The periodic toxicity of this decapod has been explained by the fact that it feeds on dinoflagellates (*Gonyaulax* spp.) which produce saxitoxin. The origin of the toxin in the three species of xanthid crab is still unknown.

Table 3. Distribution of toxin in the body of toxic crabs

Part of the body	Toxicity	Part of the body	Toxicity
Z. aeneus	(MU/g)	*A. floridus*	(MU/g)
Appendages		Appendages	
Exoskeleton of chela	2000	Exoskeleton	150
Muscle of chela	6000	Muscle	400
Exoskeleton of walking legs	2000	Cephalothorax	
Muscle of walking legs	3500	Exoskeleton	65
Cephalothorax		Muscle	45
Exoskeleton	2000	Viscera	25
Muscle	40	Gills	< 20
Viscera	1300	*P. granulosa*	
Endophragm	80	Appendages	
Gills	25	Chelae	400
		Walking legs	500
		Cephalothorax	110

The marked individual and regional variations may suggest that the toxin is of exogenous origin rather than endogenous. However, at least at the time of collection of toxic specimens there was no sign of a red tide of dinoflagellates. It is strange that the distribution of toxin is limited only to three species of the many members of the Xanthidae family.

II. Toxicity of L. pictor

HOLTHUIS (1968) cited earlier records that *L. pictor* is considered to be consistently harmful in Amboina, while it is one of the edible crabs in Indo-China. TEH and GARDINER (1970) found that the appendages, carapace, and flesh plus internal organs were all toxic and differed little in potency, in contrast to the three other xanthid crabs mentioned above.

One specimen of this species from Ishigaki Island was nontoxic in our test, but further study is necessary in view of the great individual variation of toxicity observed among the other xanthids.

D. Biology of Poisonous Xanthid Crabs

As described above, 4 species of crab, *Zosimus aeneus, Platypodia granulosa, Atergatis floridus,* and *Lophozozymus pictor,* all belonging to the Family Xanthidae, have recently been confirmed to be poisonous. In this section, a brief account of their biological characteristics is given.

I. Zosimus aeneus (LINNAEUS, 1758)
(Fig. 2)

Cancer aeneus LINNAEUS, 1758
Zozymus aeneus, ALCOCK, 1898
Zosimus aeneus, BUITENDIJK, 1960

1. Description

Carapace slightly convex in both directions; regions well indicated, especially protogastric, cardiac, intestinal, and branchial regions well defined by deep grooves; the posterior half strongly subdivided; lobules scale-shaped. Front not directed downward, divided into two lobes. Anterolateral margin four-lobed; the anterior three lobes broad, plate-like; the fourth smallest, projecting laterally.

Chelipeds subequal, stout; outer surfaces of wrist and palm with crests set off by rather deep furrows; inner angle of wrist armed with two blunt teeth; upper margin of palm crested. In walking legs, meri, carpi, and propodi very broad; upper margins of each segment crested; outer surfaces of these segments more or less rugose; inner surfaces of these crests with a thick fringe of hairs.

In the collection from the Ryukyu Islands, maximum carapace length 54.8 mm, its carapace breadth 82.5 mm (Miyake: Private communication, 1974).

2. Color in Life

Greenish blue with white, brown, and yellow patches irregularly. Movable and immovable fingers of chelipeds with dark brown.

3. Habitat and Distribution

The species is found on coral reefs near low tide mark, especially in crevices of flat reefs or under large coral masses. It apparently avoids living corals.

In the Ryukyu Islands people catch the crabs that live on the reef flats with the aid of an acetylene lamp at night, or collect them with tangle-nets set for spiny lobsters up to 10 meters deep.

It has been reported from the Red Sea to Hawaii, from the Ryukyus to New Zealand.

4. Feeding Habits and Spawning Season

The stomach contents of 6 individuals from Amami-Oshima Island were examined by Saisho and Ushio (1969) and found to contain the following algae: *Codium* sp., *Chlorodesnis comosa*, *Ectocarpus* sp., *Sphacelaria* sp., *Jania* sp., *Hypnea* sp., and *Polysiphonia* sp. In addition, spicules of two species of sponge and fragments of coral were found. In a rearing experiment in aquaria for about 3 months, the crabs took actively meat of fish, shrimp, and clam. These observations suggest that this species is omnivorous.

The spawning season in the Amami Islands is assumed to range from summer to autumn with a peak in August and September (Saisho and Ushio, 1969).

II. Platypodia granulosa (Rüppell, 1830)
(Fig. 3)

Xantho granulosus Rüppell, 1830
Cancer (Aegle) granulosus, De Haan, 1833
Lophoactaea granulosa, A. Milne Edwards, 1865

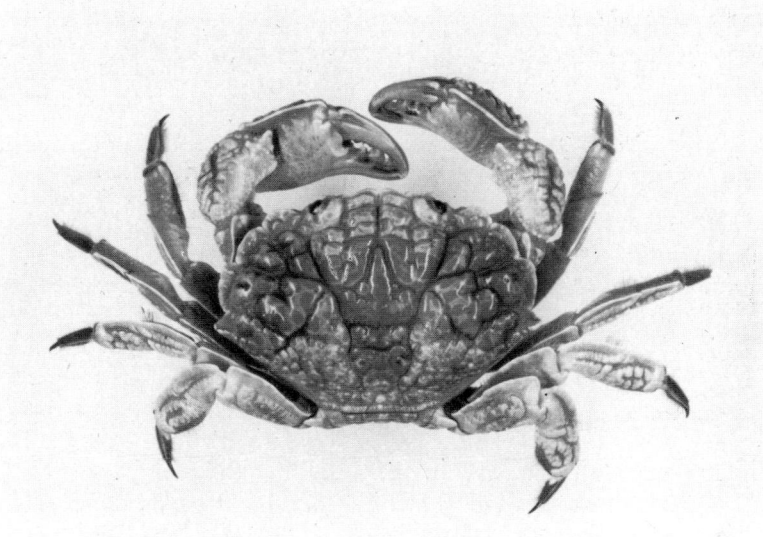

Fig. 2. *Zosimus aeneus* (LINNAEUS). (By the courtesy of Dr. S. MIYAKE)

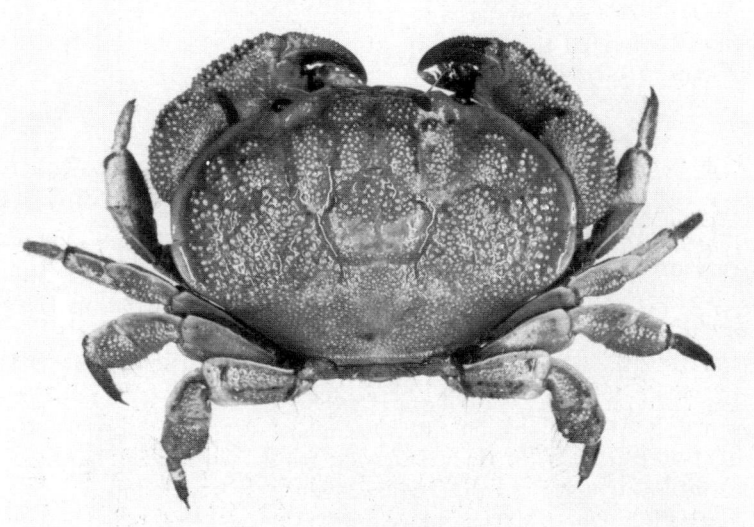

Fig. 3. *Platypodia granulosa* (RÜPPELL). (By the courtesy of Dr. S. MIYAKE)

Platypodia granulosa, RATHBUN, 1906
Platypodia granulosa, FOREST and GUINOT, 1961

1. Description

Carapace subovate, slightly convex longitudinally, and with distinct regions; lobulated, covered with equal-sized granules and a few short hairs; furnished with crested margins throughout the front, orbit, and anterolateral margin.

Chelipeds subequal, wrist and palm with granules on outer surface; palm moreover crested on upper margin. Meri, carpi, and propodi of walking legs flattened, each segment crested on upper margin; meri furnished with a deep furrow on the lower surface.

In the collection from the Caroline Islands, maximum carapace length 28 mm, its carapace breadth 42 mm (MIYAKE: Private communication, 1974).

2. Color in Life

Crabs commonly found to be dark yellowish green, rarely yellow or purplish brown.

3. Habitat and Distribution

Found on coral reefs with larger crabs near the low tide mark.

Common throughout the Indo-Pacific, from the Red Sea and East African coast to the Ryukyu Islands and Hawaii.

III. Atergatis floridus (LINNAEUS, 1767)
(Fig. 4)

Atergatis floridus, ALCOCK, 1898
Atergatis ocyroe, RATHBUN, 1902
Atergatis floridus, BUITENDIJK, 1960

1. Description

Carapace smooth, convex longitudinally; regions separated by shallow grooves. Front slightly shorter than one-third of the carapace breadth; frontal margin faintly bilobed. Anterolateral margin crested, divided into three successively broader lobes by three sutures; the posterior suture separates the blunt tubercle at epibranchial angle from third anterolateral lobe.

Chelipeds subequal; upper margin of palm strongly crested; movable and immovable fingers with three to four blunt teeth on each cutting margin. Meri, carpi, and propodi of walking legs broad, and crested on upper margins; meri also provided with a deep furrow on the lower surface; lower margin of propodi and upper and lower margins of dactyli furnished with tufts of hairs.

In the collection from the Ryukyu Islands, maximum carapace length 35.3 mm, its carapace breadth 52.3 mm (MIYAKE: Private communication, 1974).

2. Color in Life

Upper surface of carapace dark brownish purple or greenish purple or greenish purple with light-colored blotches somewhat irregularly distributed; fingers of chelipeds dark brown.

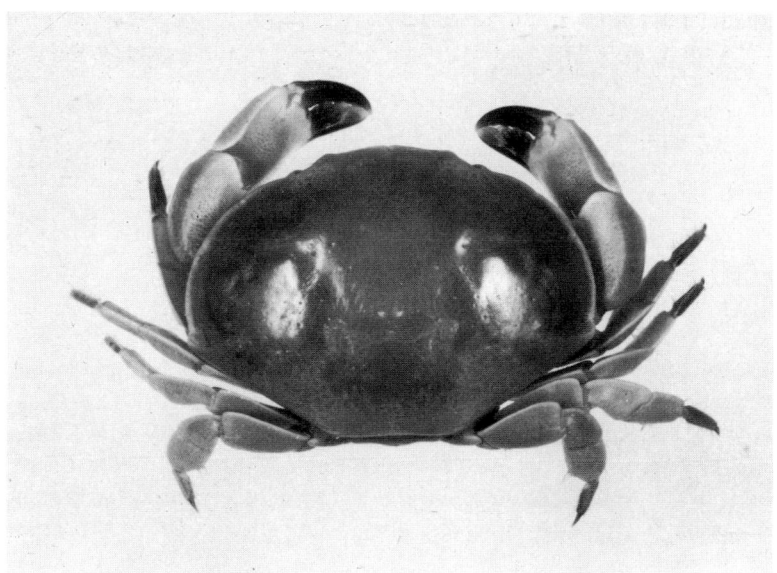

Fig. 4. *Atergatis floridus* (LINNAEUS). (By the courtesy of Dr. S. MIYAKE)

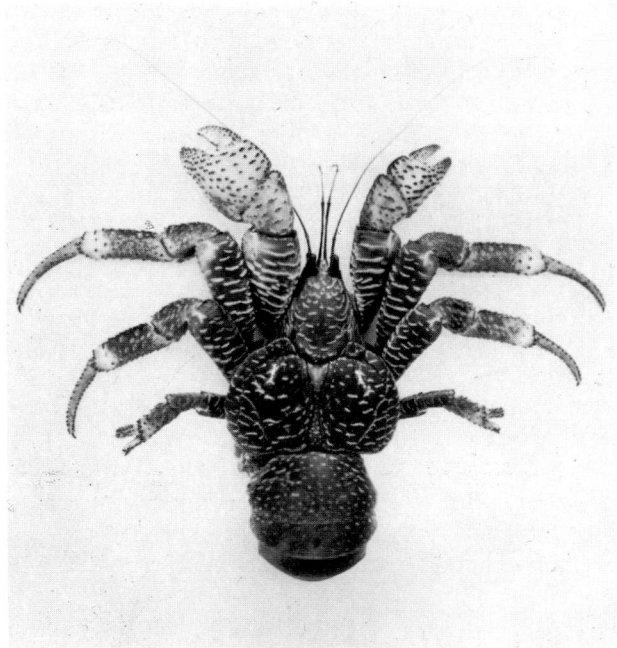

Fig. 5. *Birgus latro* (LINNAEUS). (By the courtesy of Dr. S. MIYAKE)

3. Habitat and Distribution

Commonly found on rocky shores and coral reefs. In Japan the crabs are collected by dredges or by tangle-nets set for spiny lobsters on the ocean floor at a depth of from 50 to 150 m.

From the east coast of Africa and the Red Sea throughout the whole Indo-Pacific to Hawaii and the South coast of Japan.

IV. Lophozozymus pictor (Fabricius, 1798)

1. Description

"Carapace rather broad, smooth, with only a few short hairs on the ridge of the fourth antero-lateral lobe and anterior to this ridge. Gastric region surrounded by grooves; lobe 3 and 4L separated from each other and from the antero-lateral margin. Front narrowly cleft in the middle, slightly convex to the orbits. Orbital margin with the three usual sutures and separated from the antero-lateral margin by a wide gap. Of the four antero-lateral lobes the third is the sharpest; the third and fourth are keeled."

"Cheliped equal; outer surface of the joints smooth; upper border of meri with a strong bilobed crest, the outer surface of the meri somewhat hairy near this crest and near the anterior margin. Wrist with two rather strong tubercles at the inner angle and a furrow in the anterior part of the outer surface; upper border of palm coarsely crested; fingers pointed, with some blunt teeth on their cutting edges. Upper borders of meri, carpi, and propodi of the walking legs strongly crested; on the inner surface some tufts of long hairs just behind the crest; outer surface of all these joints smooth. Lower and inner borders of meri crested and with some tufts of hairs; lower border of propodi hairy; dactyli hairy on upper and lower borders up to the claw." (Buitendijk, 1960)

2. Coloration

"On a yellow ground a network of red; gastric and branchial regions almost entirely red; on the chelipeds red spots arranged in blotches and separated by white." (loc. cit.)

3. Distribution

"Common in the eastern Indo-Pacific, from Singapore, the Philippines, and the Malay Archipelago through Australia (and there chiefly along the east coast) to Samoa and Marutea, Gambier Archipelago." (loc. cit.)

E. Chemistry of Toxins in Crabs

The presence of several toxins in crabs is indicated, but these toxins have been only poorly characterized, except for saxitoxin in a xanthid crab *Zosimus aeneus*.

Identity of *Z. aeneus* toxin with saxitoxin was demonstrated by our group (Konosu et al., 1968; Noguchi et al., 1969). During the purification process the

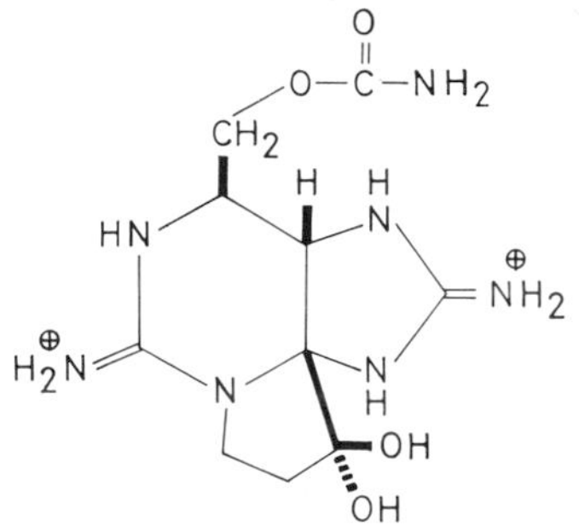

Fig. 6. Structure of saxitoxin

toxin behaved very similarly to saxitoxin but not to tetrodotoxin. The final preparation was indistinguishable from saxitoxin in all chemical properties examined so far. Saxitoxin is a powerful neurotoxin produced by the dinoflagellates *Gonyaulax* spp. (PRAKASH et al., 1971) and the most purified specimen of its dihydrochloride has a fromula $C_{10}H_{17}N_7O_4 \cdot 2HCl$ (SCHANTZ et al., 1966). It has recently been crystallized as *p*-bromobenzenesulfonate and its structure (Fig. 6) has been determined by x-ray diffraction (SCHANTZ et al., 1975).

I. Purification of Z. aeneus Toxin

KONOSU et al. (1968) found that the purification methods employed for tetrodotoxin (TSUDA and KAWAMURA, 1952) were inadequate for purifying the crab toxin, while the column chromatographic method devised by SCHANTZ et al. (1957) for saxitoxin was very effective. A typical purification run is as follows (NOGUCHI et al., 1969).

Strongly toxic specimens of *Z. aeneus* were crushed and extracted in the cold 3 times each with 2 volumes of water. The combined extracts were acidified with conc. HCl to pH 2 and heated rapidly. Immediately after the temperature reached 90° C the extracts were cooled in running tap water and the precipitates were removed by centrifugation. The resulting supernatant was concentrated under reduced pressure, adjusted to pH 5.5 with 1 N NaOH, and subjected to column chromatography using Amberlite IRC-50, Amberlite IRP-64, and activated alumina after SCHANTZ et al. (1957). The behavior of the toxin on the columns was similar to that of saxitoxin and a purified sample having a toxicity of 5100 MU/mg solid was finally obtained (Table 4).

Table 4. Toxicity of *Z. aeneus* toxin at each step in the purification process

Step	Total MU ($\times 10^3$)	Solid (mg)	MU/mg solid
Aqueous extract	280	43,000	6.5
Chromatography:			
1. Amberlite IRC-50	183	332	550
2. Amberlite IRP-64	101	117	860
3. Amberlite IRP-64	100	48.6	2060
4. Activated alumina	38.8	7.6	5100

Uwatoko-Setoguchi et al. (1969) also purified the toxin from *Z. aeneus* by employing columns of Amberlite CG-120 (Na$^+$ form) and Amberlite CG-50 (Na$^+$ and H$^+$ forms), and obtained a preparation showing a potency of 3000 MU/mg solid.

II. Chemical Properties of Z. aeneus Toxin

The toxin is soluble in methanol, slightly soluble in ethanol, and insoluble in diethyl ether, petroleum ether, hexane, chloroform, and 1-butanol. It is not partitioned into diethyl ether, petroleum ether, and chloroform from the aqueous solution adjusted to pH 2.0 or pH 10.0. The toxicity remains unchanged after heating on a boiling water bath for 15 min in neutral and acidic media, but is reduced to half at pH 10.0. It is easily dialyzable through a cellophane membrane (Hashimoto et al., 1967). The toxin is basic in nature as shown by an electrofocusing technique (Uwatoko-Setoguchi et al., 1969) and positive to Weber and Jaffé reagents (Konosu et al., 1968).

The most purified preparation of toxin showed a lethality of 5100 MU/mg solid and $[\alpha]_D^{27} + 117°$ C (in 0.001 N HCl). These values are close to those reported for the purified saxitoxin (5500 ± 500 MU/mg solid and $[\alpha]_D^{25} + 130 ± 5°$) (Schantz et al., 1957). The IR spectra in a KBr pellet are almost identical, as shown in Fig. 7 (Noguchi et al., 1969). These two toxins were indistinguishable in paper and thin layer chromatography (Konosu et al., 1968).

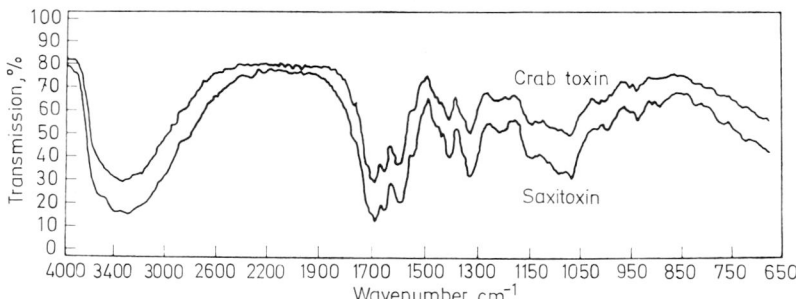

Fig. 7. Infrared absorption spectra of *Z. aeneus* toxin and saxitoxin in KBr pellets

III. Chemical Properties of Toxins from Other Crabs

The toxins of *Z. aeneus* and *Atergatis floridus* are identical in pharmacological and chemical properties so far examined (Inoue et al., 1968). Teh and Gardiner (1974) have recently reported that the *Lophozozymus pictor* toxin was partially purified by gel filtration on Sephadex G-50. The semi-purified toxin was soluble in water, slightly soluble in ethanol, and insoluble in n-pentane, benzene, and diethyl ether. The LD$_{50}$ for mice was 377 µg/kg. It had a molecular weight of between 1000 and 5000 and gave reactions that suggested the presence of free amino and phenolic groups. Mori et al. (1968) postulated the presence of several different toxic components in crabs based on solubility in organic solvents and effect on frog nerve membrane. The chemical properties of these toxic components other than solubility and heat stability are still obscure.

F. Pharmacology of Toxins in Crabs

As mentioned in the preceding sections, several toxins were postulated to be present in crabs, but only the pharmacological properties of *Zosimus aeneus* and of *Lophozo-zymus pictor* toxins have been studied to some extent.

I. Z. aeneus Toxin

Symptoms and signs in humans and test animals clearly showed that the toxin is paralytic in nature and close to saxitoxin (HASHIMOTO et al., 1967). Recently, its blocking activity to nerve excitation has been studied by DEGUCHI et al. (Unpublished data) in comparison with tetrodotoxin.

1. Poisoning Cases and Symptoms

We located 19 human intoxications following the ingestion of toxic crabs in the Ryukyu and Amami Islands. Fatal cases in domestic animals, chiefly pigs, were also reported. Symptoms include paralysis, resembling that in shellfish poisoning, as the following typical case report indicates (HASHIMOTO et al., 1967).

At around 6:30 a.m. a crab (*Z. aeneus*), 3 lobsters, and an unspecified edible crab were boiled in miso soup and served for breakfast. Soon after the meal, a man (Case A, aged 52), who had eaten 3 bowls of soup, gradually began to feel ill and was aware that he had been poisoned when he saw that a pig vomited and died after being fed the remnants of the soup. He was soon informed that his wife (Case B, aged 49), who had also eaten 3 bowls of the soup and left home after breakfast, had collapsed in the road. He went out to take care of her, but he too collapsed and was carried back to his house, where he died at about 11 a.m. before a doctor arrived. When the wife was found lying in the road, she could neither speak nor move and died at about 10 a.m. A son (Case C, aged 9), who ate the meat of the chelae and a small quantity of soup, experienced paralysis of the feet and felt ill. He was hospitalized with his relatives (Case D and E), who had eaten only the meat of the lobster. When he arrived at the hospital, he complained of numbness of the limbs. After several days he recovered completely. Cases D and E had slight numbness and aphasia, but treatment in the hospital contributed to their rapid recovery. Six domestic fowls which had ingested the vomitus of Case A were later found dead.

2. Signs in Test Animals

The intraperitoneal injection into mice of a lethal dose induced restlessness, paralysis in the hind limbs, and a wobbling gait followed by gasping, jumping, and death. On autopsy immediately after the respiratory arrest, no marked changes in the internal organs were found, and the heart continued to beat for more

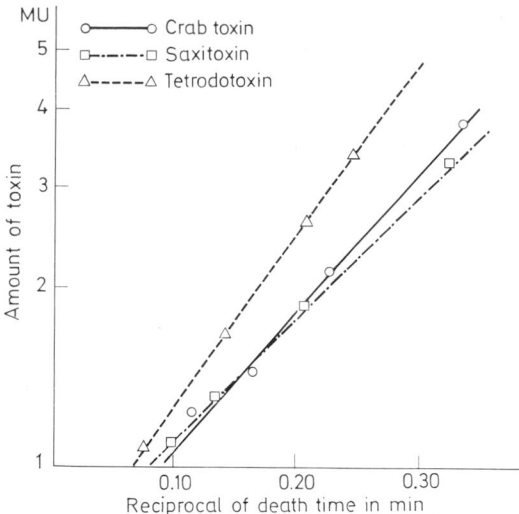

Fig. 8. Dose-death time relationship in mice for various marine toxins

than 30 min. The mice were usually dead within 30 min and those surviving the first 30 min continued to survive during subsequent observation for a week. The dose-death time relationship is shown in Fig. 8. The line for the crab toxin almost coincides with that for saxitoxin, but varies from that for tetrodotoxin.

A cat (480 g) showed mild paralysis of the hind limbs about 20 min after ingestion of 5 g of steamed crab meat (350 MU/g meat) and vomited repeatedly thereafter. This was followed by complete paralysis of the limbs, gasping, jumping, and death 54 min after ingestion. On subcutaneous injection of the hot-water extract containing 250 MU, a cat (960 g) vomited vigorously at 5 and 7 min, and died 12 min after injection. The signs were similar to those mentioned above.

3. Effects on Nerve Excitation

Effects of a partially purified toxin (4100 MU/mg solid) from *Z. aeneus* and crystalline tetrodotoxin were examined by DEGUCHI et al. on nerve excitation in the sciatic nerve of a frog *Rana brevipoda* and the giant axon of a crayfish *Procambarus clarkii* (Unpublished data).

When *Z. aeneus* toxin (0.05 MU/ml) was applied to the frog sciatic nerve in the sucrose-gap chamber, maximum block (87%) was attained in 5 min (Fig. 9). A 95% block occurred in 3 min at 0.1 MU/ml and complete block in 2.5 min at 0.2 MU/ml, as rapidly as in the case of tetrodotoxin (Fig. 10). The blocking activity of *Z. aeneus* toxin at 0.1 MU/ml is thus almost the same as that of 2×10^{-8} w/v crystalline tetrodotoxin. The block induced by the low concentrations of *Z. aeneus* toxin was extinguished fairly rapidly and almost completely by washing (Fig. 9), whereas the block induced at 0.2 MU/ml was only incompletely extinguished (Fig. 10). The block produced by tetrodotoxin was more completely extinguished in the nerve which had previously been treated with *Z. aeneus* toxin

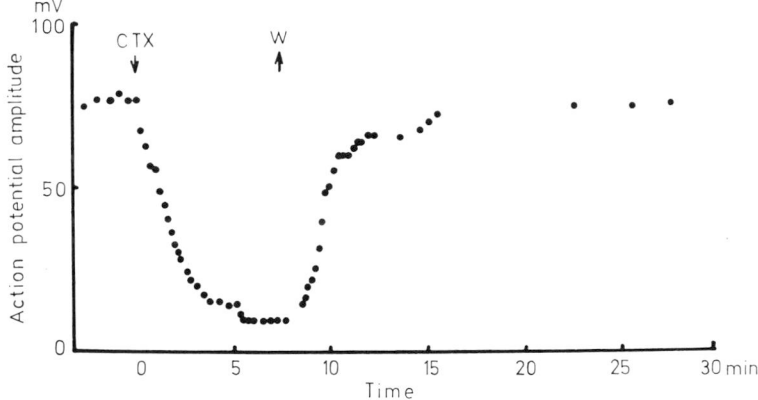

Fig. 9. Block of action potential in the frog sciatic nerve by *Z. aeneus* toxin. At CTX (time 0) the crab toxin solution (0.05 MU/ml) was introduced into the sucrose-gap chamber at a flow rate of 1.53 ml/min. The toxin solution was washed at W

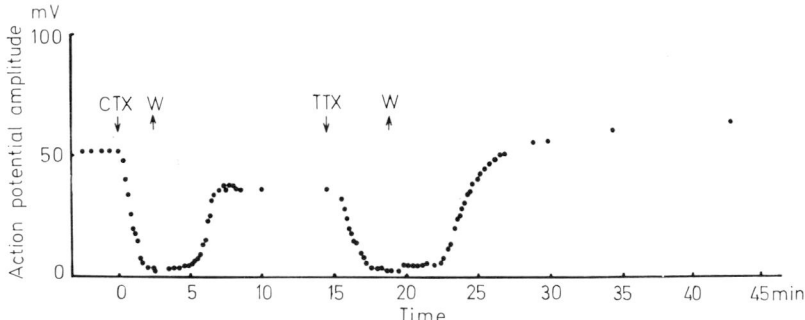

Fig. 10. Block of action potential in the frog sciatic nerve by *Z. aeneus* toxin and tetrodotoxin. At CTX (time 0) the crab toxin solution (0.2 MU/ml) and at TTX the tetrodotoxin solution $(2 \times 10^{-8} \text{w/v})$ were introduced into the sucrose-gap chamber, respectively. The toxin solutions were washed at W

(Fig. 10). A similar result has been noted for the combination of tetrodotoxin and saxitoxin by NARAHASHI et al. (1967). The EC_{50} value was estimated to be 0.0252 MU/ml for *Z. aeneus* toxin, corresponding approximately to 6×10^{-9} w/v. It may thus be reasonably stated that the nerve blocking activity of *Z. aeneus* toxin is comparable to that of tetrodotoxin.

Effects on the isolated giant axons of crayfish are shown in Figs. 11 and 12. In its blocking action, *Z. aeneus* toxin closely resembles tetrodotoxin; in both cases, the threshold potential for spike generation is elevated and the rate of rise in action potential is greatly diminished, while the delayed rectification is little affected even after the action potential is almost completely blocked (Fig. 11). These results suggest that the crab toxin might similarly block the initial conductance increase in excitation, leaving the delayed component unaffected, as was

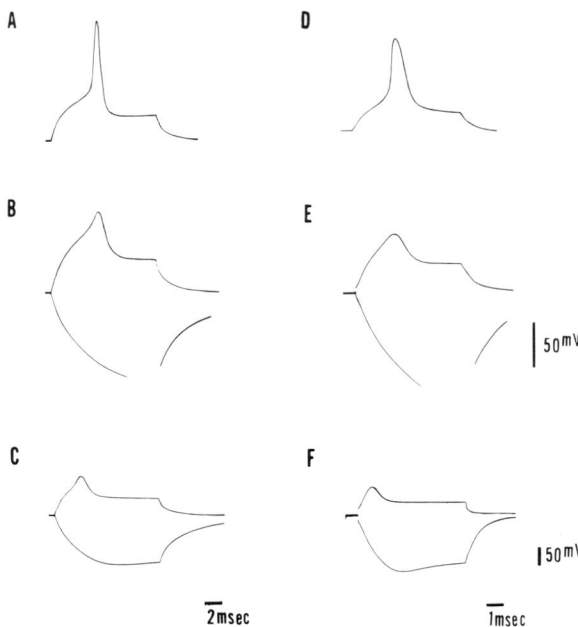

Fig. 11. Changes in potential in the crayfish giant-axon membrane by applied current. A~C and D~F are recorded from the same preparations, respectively. B and C, in the presence of Z. aenus toxin (0.1 MU/ml); E and F, in the presence of tetrodotoxin (1×10^{-8}w/v). A is obtained after washing the crab toxin, and D before treatment with the drug. The time scale for A~C is given in C, and that for D~F in F. The voltage scale for A, B, D, and E is given in E, and that for C and F in F

observed with tetrodotoxin (NARAHASHI et al., 1964; NAKAMURA et al., 1965). To confirm this assumption, the membrane current associated with depolarization of the membrane was measured under the voltage clamp arrangement in the presence and absence of toxin (Fig. 12). In physiological solution, the membrane current which results from a square, above threshold, depolarizing pulse comprises two components, an initial transient inward current and subsequent enduring outward current (Fig. 12-F). The initial component was extinguished either in Na-free solution or in the presence of tetrodotoxin, implying that this current is carried by Na ions. On the other hand, the delayed outwart current was diminished by 60 mM tetraethylammonium, indicating that this component might be carried by K ions. When Z. aeneus toxin above 0.05 MU/ml was applied to the axon, the initial transient inward current was progressively decreased and finally extinguished. By contrast the delayed outward current showed little if any change in the presence of the toxin (Fig. 12-E). Such a selective effect of Z. aeneus toxin is clearly seen in Fig. 13. These characteristics are also seen in the block induced by tetrodotoxin (Fig. 14) (NARAHASHI et al., 1964; NAKAMURA et al., 1965; TAKATA et al., 1966) and by saxitoxin (NARAHASHI et al., 1967). The recovery from the block on washing was faster in Z. aeneus toxin. NARAHASHI et al. (1967) have observed that saxitoxin is washed out much more easily than tetrodotoxin.

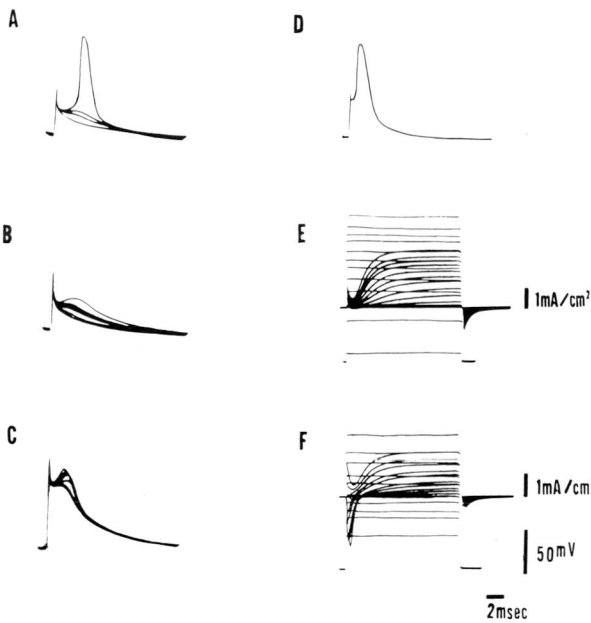

Fig. 12. Effects of *Z. aeneus* toxin on the action potential and membrane current in the crayfish giant axon. All records are obtained on the same preparation. A ~ D represent the action potentials, and E and F membrane currents. A, control record before treatment; B and C, in the presence of crab toxin (0.05 MU/ml); D and F, after washing; E, soon after C

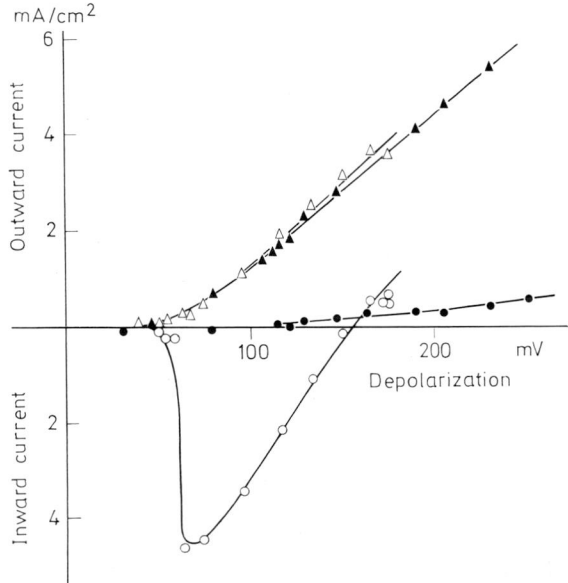

Fig. 13. V-I relations for the peak transient current and steady outward current, following step depolarization in voltage-clamped crayfish giant-axon membrane. ○ and ● represent the peak transient currents, and △ and ▲ the steady outward currents before and after treatment with *Z. aeneus* toxin (0.1 MU/ml), respectively

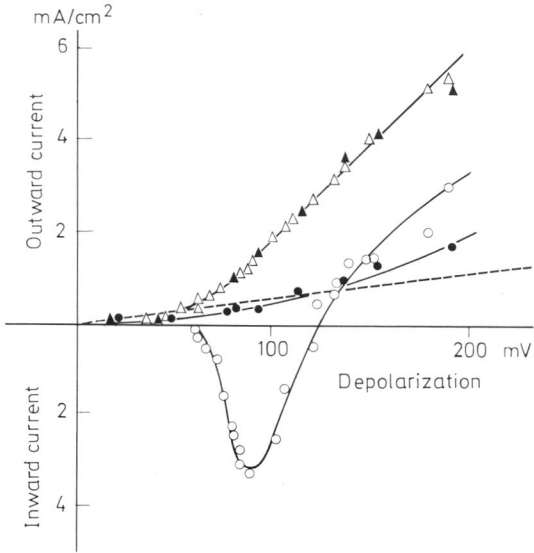

Fig. 14. V-I relations for the peak transient current and steady outward current, for step depolarization in voltage-clamped crayfish giant-axon membrane. The signs are the same as in Fig. 13, except that crab toxin is replaced by tetrodotoxin (1×10^{-8} w/v). The broken line shows the level of nonspecific leakage current

II. The Toxin of L. pictor

Using aqueous extracts from *L. pictor*, Teh and Gardiner (1970) investigated the lethality to mice and effects on respiration, blood pressure, and neuromuscular transmission in rats. Toxicity is defined by LD_{50} and expressed by mouse unit (MU) in these studies.

Oral administration to mice (18—20 g) of the aqueous extract from 1 g of whole crab produced sedation and partial paralysis of the hind limbs after about 1 h, followed by restlessness, labored respiration, convulsion, and death. Intraperitoneal injection of the same dose killed mice within a few min. Small doses corresponding to 2.5 to 3.3 mg of the crab killed mice in 20 to 30 h when administered intraperitoneally. The sequence of signs was the same regardless of the routes of administration. The dose-death time relationship for *L. pictor* toxin apparently differed from those for tetrodotoxin, saxitoxin, and the ciguatera-like poison obtained by McFarren (1967).

Using rats (300—400 g) anesthetized with pentobarbitone (35 mg/kg), effects of the toxin on respiration, blood pressure, and neuromuscular transmission were examined. Intravenous administration of a small amount of *L. pictor* toxin (0.6 MU) produced gradual increase in respiratory excursions for about 30 min. The respiration remained stimulated for 2.5 h and became irregular with severe gasping. At a dose of 3 MU, respiration was initially strongly stimulated in depth for 60 to 90 sec and then declined rapidly after a brief period of recovery.

Small doses had a very transient pressor effect or no effect on the blood pressure. A dose of 3 MU produced a transient rise in blood pressure for 10 to 15 sec, followed by a progressive fall to zero in 5 to 7 min. At a dose as large as 30 MU, a sharp but transient increase in blood pressure rapidly occurred, coinciding with a short period of apnoea followed by a few gasping movements. These events were almost immediately followed by cessation of respiration and the blood pressure dropping to zero. The contraction of the gastrocnemius muscle in response to stimulation of the sciatic nerve continued for 10 min after complete failure of respiratory and circulatory systems.

These effects of *L. pictor* toxin were quite different from those of tetrodotoxin; 1.08 µg of the latter toxin (*ca.* 7 MU) given intravenously produced an immediate fall in blood pressure, inhibition of respiration, and a decrease in the response of the gastrocnemius muscle to approximately half of the control. The effect on respiration lasted only for 2 to 3 min, but that on the blood pressure for 20 to 30 min.

III. Toxin in Other Crabs

Using the single node of Ranvier of a frog, Mori et al. (1968) examined the effects of hot-water extracts from 8 species of crab on the nerve membrane and observed that those of three species, *Carpilius convexus, Thalamita danae,* and *Eriphia sebana,* induced: depolarization of the membrane, a decrease in action potential amplitude, and elevation of the firing level. These effects disappeared almost completely immediately after washing out the extracts.

G. Coconut Crab Poisoning

Holthuis (1968) in his review briefly referred to Balss' report that on Yap Island in the Carolines the natives starve the coconut crab, *Birgus* sp., for a few days before eating it, so that no toxic substances remain in its intestinal tract. According to Bagnis (Private communication, 1968), a poisoning from eating the coconut crab occurred in the Tuamotu Islands, French Polynesia. It was also reported by Mote (Private communication, 1968) that in Palau the coconut crab is believed to be toxic. In the Ryukyu Islands, Hashimoto et al. (1969b) and Yonabaru (1974) found sporadic outbreaks of coconut-crab poisoning and some legends on the origin of the toxin. According to their reports, symptoms appear within several hours after ingestion and consist of languor of the whole body, vomiting, and diarrhea. Victims are usually forced because of exhaustion to lie in bed for several days. In 12 outbreaks of poisoning, 4 out of 51 patients died, according to the above investigators. Pigs were also intoxicated from eating leftovers of the crab and appeared to be very sensitive to the toxin.

The coconut crab that caused the poisoning was identified by Miyake as *Birgus latro* (Linnaeus, 1767) (Fig. 5).

I. Biology of Coconut Crab

Cancer latro Linnaeus, 1767
Birgus latro, De Haan, 1849
Birgus latro, Alcock, 1905
Birgus latro, Ward, 1942

1. Description

Carapace heart-shaped, well calcified; branchial regions strongly expanded. Antennular peduncle nearly as long as the carapace length. Antennal peduncle compressed, with short acicle which fused with second joint.

Chelipeds massive; left one larger than right; fingers move obliquely. Fourth and fifth legs cheliform; fourth much larger than fifth which lies concealed in the branchial chamber.

Abdomen broad, symmetrical, well calcified; second to fifth terga broad, overlapping plates with small pleura; sixth terga and telson reduced, very small, widely separated from fifth, and located ventrally; sixth terga with reduced uropods but symmetrical; pleopods missing in the male, but female carrying three hairy biramous ones on left side of second and to fourth segments.

In the collection from Yaéyama Group of the Ryukyu Islands, maximum carapace length 120 mm, its body weight 1.29 kg (Miyake: Private communication, 1974).

2. Color when Alive, Habitat, and Distribution

Red-brown and bluish, variegated.

This crab is best known for its feeding habits that have given it both of its common names, coconut crab and robber crab. The crabs live in burrows under coconut palms in tropical islands.

In southern Taiwan and in Yaéyama Group of the Ryukyu Islands, they inhabit *Pandanus* and *Diospyros* forests and feed on their fruits or occasionally on sweet potatoes and peanuts.

Madagascar, Réunion, Mauritius, Seychelles and Chagos Islands, to the Andamans and Nicobars, then through the East Indian Archipelago, to the Ryukyu Islands, and through Polynesia to Tuamotu Archipelago, Fanning and Sandwich Islands (Alcock, 1905).

II. Toxicity of the Coconut Crab

The toxicity of the coconut crab is reputed to show individual and regional variations and to be derived from some plants in the Ryukyus. One was identified as *Diospyros maritima* Blume in the Family Ebenaceae and the other as *Hernandia sonora* Linnaeus in the Family Hernandiaceae (Fig. 15). The crabs are believed by inhabitants to become toxic when they feed on fruits of the former plant or dwell under the latter. It is most likely that the toxic effect might be attributable to the gut contents rather than to the coconut crab itself.

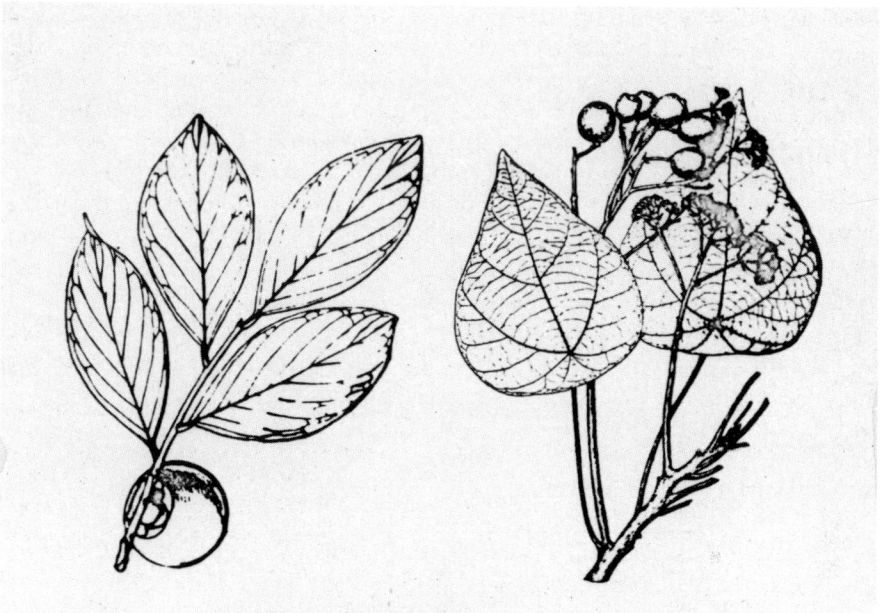

Fig. 15   *Diospyros maritima* Blume (left, taken from Kanehira, 1936)
            Hernandia sonora Linnaeus (right, taken from Kanehira, 1933)

Mori et al. (1968) reported that the methanol-soluble fraction of a hot-water extract of the crab from the Ryukyus killed mice in 7 to 12 min after intraperitoneal injection. The toxin was dialyzable. No other report of experimental work on the toxicity of coconut crab and its toxin is available.

H. Horseshoe-Crab Poisoning

Intoxication following the ingestion of horseshoe crab has been one of the long-standing problems of public health in Southeast Asia. The clinical characteristics of the poisoning have been well documented (Halstead, 1965), but little is known of the nature of the toxic principle.

I. Biology of Horseshoe Crabs

The horseshoe or king crabs belong to the Family Xiphosuridae in the Class Merostomata and are not true crabs. Only 5 species of 3 genera, *Limulus, Carcinoscorpius,* and *Tachypleus,* are known to live today. They have a characteristic arched cephalothorax and a horseshoe-shaped carapace. The abdomen is wide and unsegmented. They inhabit sandy or muddy bottoms in coastal waters and feed on polychaete worms, molluscs, miscellaneous small animals, and algae. Reproduction occurs in late spring and early summer.

In Thailand, where many cases of poisoning have been reported, two species are known, *C. rotundicauda* and *T. gigas*. Smith (1933) described that the former is called *mangda fai, mangda tuey,* and *hera,* and the latter *mangda tale.* Banner and Stephens (1966), however, cite Piyakarnchana who states that the species in Thai waters are distinguished by the names *mangda* for *C. rotundicauda* and *hela* or *hera* for *T. gigas*. They also quote the description of Chuang that *C. rotundicauda* is 35 cm in total length in the adult stage, has a smooth cylindrical caudal spine which exceeds half of the body length, and dwells in the littoral zone of sandy shores and estuarine mud flats. On the other hand, *T. gigas* dwells in depths up to 40 m, exceeds 50 cm in total length, and has a caudal spine, which is serrated dorsally and equals half the total length of the body. The eggs of this species are a delicacy. According to Smith (1933), *C. rotundicauda* is readily identified by the presence of conspicuous hairs on the back and tail.

II. Toxicity of Horseshoe Crabs

Three species, *C. rotundicauda* (Latreille), *T. gigas* (Müller), and *T. tridentatus* Leach, are listed by Halstead (1965) as toxic. There is some confusion about the toxicity of the two above species in Thailand. Smith (1933) stated that the flesh and eggs of *Carcinoscorpius* are highly poisonous and have been responsible for numerous deaths, while those of *Tachypleus* are not. Trishnananda et al. (1966) also noted that there is no report of poisoning following the ingestion of the latter, while the ingestion of the former is reputed to cause sporadic poisonings in some localities between February and June. On the other hand, Banner and Stephens (1966) state that *C. rotundicauda* is used for food, but *T. gigas,* which was reported by Chuang as a delicacy, is considered toxic and never eaten.

The toxic principle of these horseshoe crabs is still unknown. It was assumed by Smith (1933) to be a powerful alkaloid which acts very quickly on humans and domestic animals. According to Trishnananda et al. (1966), the toxin is heat-stable and does not appear to be a cholinesterase inhibitor, since serum cholinesterase activity was within normal limits in two patients who were severely affected. Based on the apparently seasonal appearance of poisoning in the same localities and the clinical findings, which are similar to those of paralytic shellfish poisoning, these investigators assumed that the toxin may originate in the food of the crab which may include poisonous dinoflagellates, as is the case with paralytic shellfish poison. They further observed that laboratory mice that were fed eggs of *C. rotundicauda,* died within 4 h. No further study on the nature of the toxic factor has been carried out.

Banner and Stephens (1966) examined the toxicity of *C. rotundicauda* on specimens obtained at a market in Bangkok, which were transported to Hawaii under preservation in 70% aqueous ethanol. The ethanolic preservative was concentrated under reduced pressure and the residue was fractionated into ether- and water-soluble fractions, which were injected intraperitoneally into mice after being homogenized in 0.9% saline solution with Tween 60. The results were baffling, but they concluded that at least some individuals of this species seemed to contain one or more substances toxic to mice.

III. Clinical Characteristics

HALSTEAD (1965) summarized the symptoms of the affected patients as follows. The onset of symptoms in Asian horseshoe-crab poisoning usually occurs within a period of 30 min. Initial symptoms consist of dizziness, headache, nausea, slow pulse rate, decreased body temperature, vomiting, abdominal cramps, diarrhea, cardiac palpitation, numbness of lips, paresthesias of lower extremities, and generalized weakness. In the more severe cases, symptoms occur in rapid succession, such as aphonia, sensation of heat in mouth, throat, and stomach, inability to lift arms and legs, generalized muscular paralysis, trisms, hypersalivation, drowsiness, and loss of consciousness. Mortality rate is unknown, but is reported very high. Death, if it occurs, takes place within a period of 16 h.

A detailed case report on poisoning by TRISHNANANDA et al. (1966) represents precisely the same clinical manifestations mentioned above and suggests a close resemblance between horseshoe-crab poisoning and paralytic shellfish poisoning.

I. Prevention and Treatment of Crab Poisoning

It is advisable not to eat tropical and subtropical shore crabs unless reliable information on their edibility is obtained. The usual method of cooking, such as boiling, steaming, and baking, do not completely destroy the toxin. The soup in which toxic crabs have been cooked may be also dangerous.

No report is available on the treatment for crab poisoning itself, but the treatment recommended for paralytic shellfish poisoning may also be useful here, since the crab toxin studied by us is identical to saxitoxin.

The treatment for paralytic shellfish poisoning is summarized by HALSTEAD (1965) as follows: For the most part, only symptoms can be treated and the poison has no specific antidote. Apomorphine is more effective than lavage in removing pieces of shellfish from the stomach. Lloyd's reagent and similar adsorbents may be tried. Alkaline fluids are of value since the toxin is unstable in alkaline media. Diuresis may be instituted with 5% ammonium chloride. Artificial respiration is an important adjunct and should be performed promptly if there is any sign of respiratory difficulty. The anticurare drugs, such as neostigmine, are useful in aiding artificial respiration. DL-Amphetamine, epinephrine, ephedrine, and DMPP (1,1-dimethyl-4-phenylpiperazinium iodide) are also recommended. Digitalis and alcohol are not recommended.

Acknowledgement: The authors are grateful to Drs. A.H. BANNER and P.J. SCHEUER, University of Hawaii, Dr. S. MIYAKE, Kyushu Sangyo University, and Dr. N. URAKAWA, The University of Tokyo, for assistance with this manuscript.

References

Alcala, A.C., Halstead, B.W.: Fatality to ingestion of the crab *Demania* sp. in the Philippines. Clin. Toxicol. **3**, 609—611 (1970).
Alcock, A.: Materials for a carcinological fauna of India. No. 3. The Brachyura Cyclometopa.

Part I. The Family Xanthidae. J. Asiat. Soc. Bengal, Calcutta **67**, Part 2, No. 1, 67—233 (1898).

Alcock, A.: Catalogue of the Indian decapod Crustacea in the collection of the Indian Museum. Part 2, Anomura, I. Pagurides. Calcutta: The Trustees of the Indian Museum 1905.

Banner, A.H., Stephens, B.J.: A note on the toxicity of the horseshoe crab in the Gulf of Thailand. Natural History Bull. Siam Soc. **21**, 197—203 (1966).

Buitendijk, A.M.: Biological results of the Snellius Expedition. XXI. Brachyura of the Families Atelecyclidae and Xanthidae (Part I). Temminckia **10**, 252—338 (1960).

Cooper, M.J.: Ciguatera and other marine poisoning in the Gilbert Islands. Pacific Sci. **18**, 411—440 (1964).

Deguchi, T., Kohri, S., Urakawa, N., Sakai, Y., Ikeda, M.: Unpublished data.

Ehrhardt, J.P., Niaussat, P.: De l'éventuelle toxicité du décapode brachyoure *Carpilius convexus* Forskal. Étude d'exemplaires provenant de l'atoll de Clipperton. Cah. Pacifique **14**, 105—116 (1970).

Forest, J., Guinot, D.: Crustacés décapodes brachyoures de Tahiti et des Tuamotu. In: Expédition française sur le récifs coralliens de la Nouvelle-Calédonie. Volume préliminaire. Paris: A. Lahure 1961.

Garth, J.S.: *Demania toxica,* a new species of poisonous crab from the Philippines. Micronesica **7**, 179—183 (1971).

Guinot, D.: Les crabs comestibles de l'Indo-Pacifique. Paris: Éditions de la Fondation Singer-Polignac 1967.

Haan, W. de: Crustacea. In: Fauna Japonica sive descriptio animalium, quae in itinere per Japoniam, jussu et auspiciis superiorum, qui summum in India Batava Imperium tenent, suscepto, annis 1823—1830 collegit, notis, observationibus et adumbrationibus illustravit, 1833—1850.

Halstead, B.W.: Poisonous and venomous marine animals of the world, Vol. 1. Washington, D.C.: U.S. Government Printing Office 1965.

Hashimoto, Y., Konosu, S., Inoue, A., Saisho, T., Miyake, S.: Screening of toxic crabs in the Ryukyu and Amami Islands. Bull. Japan. Soc. Sci. Fish. **35**, 83—87 (1969a).

Hashimoto, Y., Konosu, S., Yasumoto, T., Inoue, A., Noguchi, T.: Occurrence of toxic crabs in Ryukyu and Amami Islands. Toxicon **5**, 85—90 (1967).

Hashimoto, Y., Konosu, S., Yasumoto, T., Kamiya, H.: Ciguatera in the Ryukyu and Amami Islands. Bull. Japan. Soc. Sci. Fish. **35**, 316—326 (1969b).

Holthuis, L.B.: Are there poisonous crabs? Crustaceana **15**, 215—222 (1968).

Inoue, A., Noguchi, T., Konosu, S., Hashimoto, Y.: A new toxic crab, *Atergatis floridus.* Toxicon **6**, 119—123 (1968).

Kanehira, R.: Flora Micronesica. Tokyo: South Sea Bureau under the Japanese Mandate 1933.

Kanehira, R.: Formosan trees indigenous to the island. Tokyo: Dept. of Forestry, Govern. Res. Inst., Formosa 1936.

Konosu, S., Inoue, A., Noguchi, T., Hashimoto, Y.: Comparison of crab toxin with saxitoxin and tetrodotoxin. Toxicon **6**, 113—117 (1968).

Konosu, S., Inoue, A., Noguchi, T., Hashimoto, Y.: A further examination on the toxicity of three species of xanthid crab. Bull. Japan. Soc. Sci. Fish. **35**, 88—92 (1969).

Konosu, S., Noguchi, T., Hashimoto, Y.: Toxicity of a xanthid crab, *Zosimus aeneus,* and several other species in the Pacific. Bull. Japan. Soc. Sci. Fish. **36**, 715—719 (1970).

Linnaeus, C.: Systema Naturae per Regna tria Naturae, secundum Classes, Ordines, Genera, Species, cum Characteribus, Differentiis, Synonymis, Locis. ed. 10, 1758.

Linnaeus, C.: *ibid.* ed. 12, 1767.

McFarren, E.F.: Differentiation of the poisons of fish, shellfish and plankton. In: Animal toxins. Oxford: Pergamon Press 1967.

Milne Edwards, A.: Etudes zoologiques sur les crustacés récents de la famille des carcériens. Nouv. Arch. Mus. Hist. nat., Paris **1**, 177—308 (1865).

Mori, Y., Anraku, M., Yagi, K., Maeno, T., Hashimura, S., Obo, F., Tada, I.: On the venomous crustacea and fish from Amami-Oshima and Okinawa Islands–I. Med. J. Kagoshima Univ. **19**, 729—736 (1968).

Nakamura, Y., Nakajima, S., Grundfest, H.: The action of tetrodotoxin on electrogenic components of squid giant axons. J. gen. Physiol. **48**, 985—996 (1965).

Narahashi, T., Haas, H.G., Therrien, E.F.: Saxitoxin and tetrodotoxin: Comparison of nerve blocking mechanism. Science **157**, 1441—1442 (1967).

Narahashi, T., Moore, J.W., Scott, W.R.: Tetrodotoxin blockage of sodium conductance increase in lobster giant axons. J. gen. Physiol. **47**, 965—974 (1964).

Noguchi, T., Konosu, S., Hashimoto, Y.: Identity of the crab toxin with saxitoxin. Toxicon **7**, 325—326 (1969).

Prakash, A., Medcof, J.C., Tennant, A.D.: Paralytic shellfish poisoning in eastern Canada. Fish. Res. Board Can. Bull. **177** (1971).

Rathbun, M.J.: The Brachyura and Macrura of the Hawaiian Islands. U.S. Fish. Comm. Bull. Washington for 1903, Part 3, 827—930 (1906).

Rathbun, M.J.: Japanese stalk-eyed crustaceans. Proc. U.S. nat. Mus. Washington **26**, 23—55 (1902).

Rüppell, E.: Beschreibung und Abbildung von 24 Arten kurzschwänzigen Krabben, als Beitrag zur Naturgeschichte des roten Meers. Heinrich Ludwig Brönner: Frankfurt a.M. 1830.

Saisho, T., Ushio, Y.: A study on the distribution and ecology of toxic crabs in the Ryukyu and Amami Islands. Mem. Fac. Fish., Kagoshima Univ. **18**, 47—63 (1969).

Schantz, E.J.: Algal toxins. In: Properties and products of algae. New York, N.Y.: Plenum Press 1970.

Schantz, E.J., Ghazarossian, V.E., Schnoes, H.K., Strong, F.M., Springer, J.P., Pezzanite, J.O., Clardy, J.: The structure of saxitoxin. J. Amer. Chem. Soc. **97**, 1238—1239 (1975).

Schantz, E.J.: Lynch, J.M., Vayvada, G., Matsumoto, K., Rapoport, H.: The purification and characterization of the poison produced by *Gonyaulax catenella* in axenic culture. Biochemistry **5**, 1191—1195 (1966).

Schantz, E.J., Mold, J.D., Stanger, D.W., Shavel, J., Riel, F.J., Bowden, J.P., Lynch, J.M., Wyler, R.S., Riegel, B., Sommer, H.: Paralytic shellfish poison—VI. A procedure for the isolation and purification of the poison from toxic clam and mussel tissues. J. Amer. Chem. Soc. **79**, 5230—5235 (1957).

Smith, H.M.: A poisonous horseshoe crab. J. Siam Soc., Natural History Suppl. **9**, 143—145 (1933).

Sommer, H.: The occurrence of the paralytic shell-fish poison in the common sand crab. Science **76**, 574—575 (1932).

Sommer, H., Meyer, K.F.: Paralytic shell-fish poisoning. Arch. Pathol. **24**, 560—598 (1937).

Takata, M., Moore, J.W., Kao, C.Y., Fuhrman, F.A.: Blockage of sodium conductance increase in lobster giant axon by tarichatoxin (tetrodotoxin). J. gen. Physiol. **49**, 977—988 (1966).

Teh, Y.F., Gardiner, J.E.: Toxin from the coral reef crab, *Lophozozymus pictor*. Pharmacol. Res. Commun. **2**, 251—256 (1970).

Teh, Y.F., Gardiner, J.E.: Partial purification of *Lophozozymus pictor* toxin. Toxicon **12**, 603—610 (1974).

Trishnananda, M., Tuchinda, C., Yipinsoi, T., Oonsombat, P.: Poisoning following the ingestion of the horseshoe crab (*Carcinoscorpius rotundicauda*): Report of four cases in Thailand. J. Trop. Med. Hyg. **69**, 194—196 (1966).

Tsuda, K., Kawamura, M.: The constituents of the ovaries of globefish—VI. Purification of globefish poison by chromatography. J. Pharmacol. Soc. Japan **72**, 187—190 (1952).

Uwatoko-Setoguchi, Y., Obo, F., Hashimura, S.: Purification and chemical properties of the toxin of crab. Acta Med. Univ. Kagoshima. **11**, 35—42 (1969).

Ward, M.: Notes on the Crustacea of the Desjardins Museum, Mauritius Institute, with description of new genera and species. Mauritius Inst. Bull. **2**, 49—113 (1942).

Yonabaru, S.: Investigation on the coconut crab poisonings. Tech. Rep. XVI. Lab. of Marine Biochem., Fac. of Agr., Univ. of Tokyo (1974).

CHAPTER 3

Defensive Secretions of Millipeds

T. Eisner, D. Alsop, K. Hicks, and J. Meinwald

Introduction

The millipeds, comprising the arthropodan class Diplopoda, are a relatively uniform and unspectacular lot. Generally slow and sluggish despite their many legs, they are for the most part furtive vegetarian scavengers, active primarily at night. Only about 7500 species have been described (Kaestner, 1968). In a numerical sense, therefore, and certainly relative to the insects, they represent one of the less successful experiments in terrestrial arthropodan evolution. But in another sense they are all but unsuccessful. They are an ancient group dating back to Devonian times, and they have held their own to this day, despite the evolutionary diversification of those very animals, the vertebrates, insects, and arachnids, that have come to include the primary predacious enemies of millipeds. Survival under hazardous conditions presupposes the possession of effective means of defense, and millipeds do indeed possess such means. Anyone who has collected these animals in the field is familiar with the odorous and often noxiously irritating fluids that so many of them emit when handled. These fluids are the products of special exocrine defensive glands that have evolved, quite clearly, for protection against predation. Much has been learned about the chemistry and biology of these glands. It is our purpose here to summarize this work.

   Arthropods as a group are richly endowed with chemical defenses. Sometimes, as in the case of the venom glands of centipedes, or the stinging apparatus of Hymenoptera, this weaponry serves both offensively for incapacitation of prey, and defensively against predators. But purely protective weapons are also widespread, and they differ considerably in structure and operation. The urticating hairs of saturniid and other caterpillars are strictly defensive in function, as are the enteric discharges so commonly produced by herbivorous insects (Eisner, 1970; Eisner et al., 1974), and the sticky exudates found in certain cockroaches (Plattner et al., 1972). Glandular devices directly comparable to those of millipeds are also commonplace, particularly in insects (Eisner, 1970), but they occur also in such arthropods as whipscorpions and opilionids. Structurally, these glands are essentially sac-like invaginations of the body wall, filled with liquid secretion, and discharged by compression. The sacs are lined with a thin and flexible cuticular membrane that is continuous with the body wall, and the glandular cells that produce the secretions are diverse, and often highly specialized in cytological detail. In millipeds the glands are serially arranged as segmental pairs, with openings visible as tiny pores along the length of the body (Fig. 1). The pores were originally considered to be respiratory, until Savi (1823) called attention to their true nature.

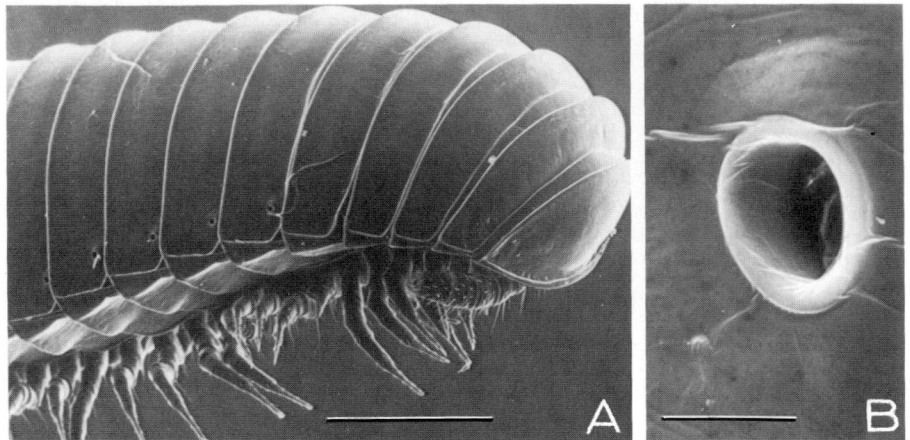

Fig. 1A and B. (A) Scanning electronmicrograph of front end of *Polyzonium rosalbum.* The gland openings are visible as small pores near the outer margins of the tergites. (B) Single gland opening, enlarged. (Reference bars: A, 0.25 mm; B, 0.02 mm)

Earlier studies made frequent reference to the presence of these glands in millipeds, but knowledge about the chemistry of the secretions stems mostly from work of the past two decades.

A. Distribution, Structure, and Mode of Operation of the Glands

As seen in Table 1, defensive glands are commonly but not invariably present in millipeds. In the large subclass Helminthomorpha, all orders except the Chordeumida have glands. In the Pentazonia, the Glomerida have glands, but the Sphaerotheriida appear to lack them (Eisner, T., unpublished observations on the South African *Sphaerotherium giganteum* and *S. punctulatum*), and there is uncertainty as to their presence in the Glomeridesmida. The single order of the Penicillata, the aberrant Polyxenida, have no glands. Secondary loss of glands has occurred in certain Polydesmida (Hoffman, R.L., personal communication).

The defensive glands of millipeds are of three primary types, which for the sake of simplicity we shall designate 1, 2, and 3.

Gland Type 1

This type is found in the order Glomerida, where it has been studied by Brandt (1839), Dohle (1964), Silvestri (1903), and Verhoeff (1928). It may be exemplified by the glands of the European *Glomeris marginata,* which we ourselves have examined (Figs. 2 and 3).

There are eight pairs of glands in *Glomeris,* located in segments 4—11. The slender elongated sacs merge middorsally, where each pair opens through a narrow slitlike orifice. *Glomeris,* like other members of its order, is a "pill" milliped, which coils tightly into a sphere when disturbed. The possession of middorsal

Table 1. Class Diplopoda: Distribution of Defensive Glands and State of Chemical Knowledge of the Secretions

Subclass[a]	Order[a]	Glands[b]	Secretion[c]
Penicillata	Polyxenida	—	
Pentazonia	Glomeridesmida	?	
	Glomerida	+	+
	Sphaerotheriida	—	
Helminthomorpha	Spirobolida	+	+
	Spirostreptida	+	+
	Julida	+	+
	Callipodida	+	+
	Chordeumida	—	
	Polydesmida	+	+
	Stemmiulida	+	—
	Platydesmida	+	—
	Siphonophorida	+	—
	Polyzoniida	+	+

[a] Classification according to Hoffman, R.L. (1969, and personal communication)
[b] present (+); absent (−); uncertain (?)
[c] chemical components characterized in some species (+); no species studied chemically (−)

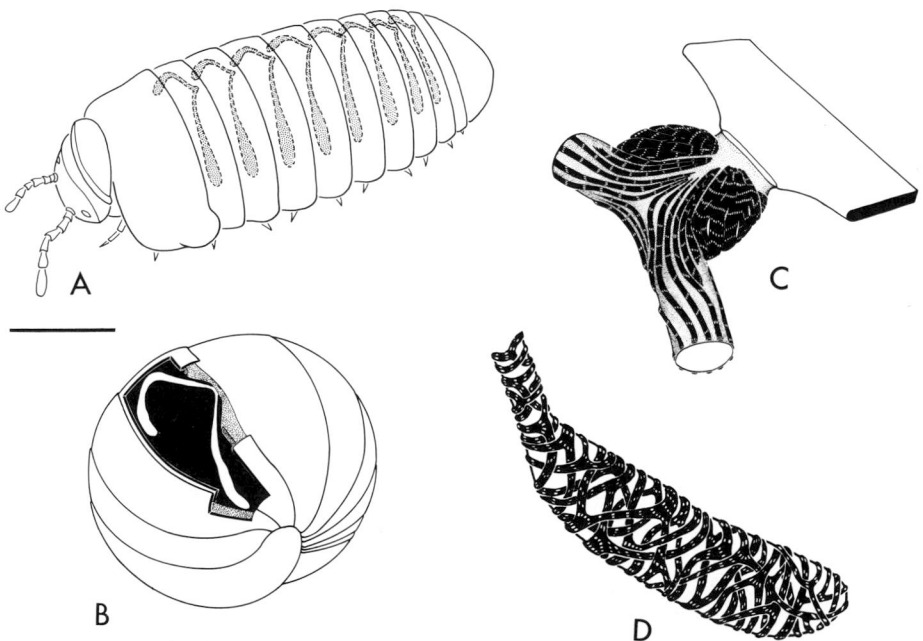

Fig. 2A–D. *Gland type 1.* (A) *Glomeris marginata*, showing location of the eight pairs of segmental glands. (B) Coiled *Glomeris*, showing cutaway with one gland pair in place. (C) Enlarged view of muscled junction of a gland pair at level of slit-like gland opening. (D) Portion of a glandular sac, showing arrangement of investing musculature. (Reference bar in A: 2 mm)

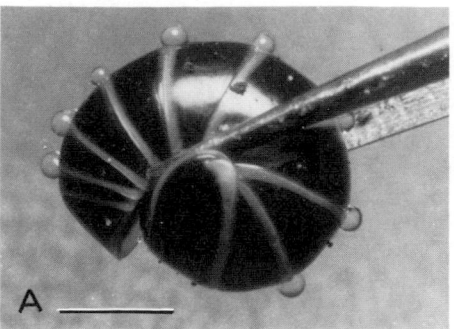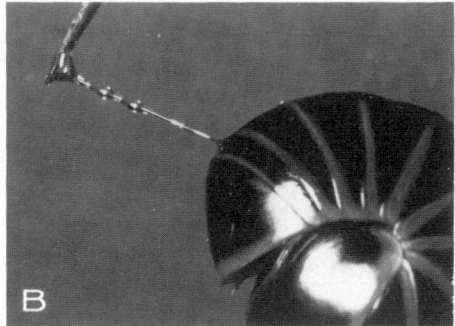

Fig. 3 A and B. (A) A specimen of *Glomeris marginata*, coiled while held in forceps, discharging droplets from its eight gland openings. (B) Sticky droplet of *Glomeris* secretion being drawn into a thread by a pin. (Reference bar in A: 2 mm)

gland openings insures maximal spacing of the sites of secretory emission when the coiled animal discharges. Gland compression is effected by an elaborate muscular network that envelopes each gland (Fig. 2D). Just inside the valvular orifice, the muscles are highly specialized (Fig. 2C). The secretion of *Glomeris* is a viscous, translucent, odorless fluid, emitted in the form of discrete small droplets (Fig. 3 A). The active principles in the fluid are quinazolinones (Tables 2 and 3).

Gland Type 2

This is the most widespread type, basic to the subclass Helminthomorpha. It occurs with more or less modification of detail in the orders Spirobolida, Spirostreptida, Julida, Callipodida, Platydesmida, and Polyzoniida. It may also occur in the Stemmiulida and Siphonophorida, but in these orders the glands appear not to have been studied. The Polydesmida stand alone in the subclass in having glands notably different in form (see gland type 3, below). Anatomical descriptions of gland type 2 abound (BARTH, 1967; EISNER et al., 1963b; LEIDY, 1849; ROSSI, 1903; SILVESTRI, 1903; VERHOEFF, 1928; VOGES, 1878; WEATHERSTON and PERCY, 1969; WOOD, 1975; WOODRING and BLUM, 1965).

The glands of *Narceus gordanus* (order Spirobolida) are representative of this type (Figs. 4 A − B, 5 A − C). They are present in all segments except the first five and the last. Each gland is a spherical sac (Fig. 5C), ordinarily lying embedded amid the muscles of the body wall. The sac has no compressor muscles of its own. A slender efferent duct leads from the sac to the outer orifice, which is porelike and situated at about the level of the lateral midline. The terminal portion of the efferent duct is ordinarily collapsed and occluded, and passively maintained in this condition by tight spring-like inflection of the duct wall. A special muscle that attaches to the body wall and inserts on the inflection serves to open this valve. Secretory discharge involves, presumably, a contraction of this muscle, plus simultaneous compression of the sac. Sac compression must be effected indirectly, possibly by increased hemocoel pressure, or by pressure from the integumental muscles that surround the gland, or by a combination of both these actions.

Table 2. Chemical Components in Defensive Secretions of Millipeds

	Chemical Components	Millipeds in Which Components are Found[a]
I	Hydrogen cyanide	37—41, 43—55
II	Formic acid	52
III	Acetic acid	52
IV	Isovaleric acid	52, 54
V	Myristic acid	54
VI	Stearic acid	54
VII	Hexadecyl acetate	30
VIII	Δ^9-Hexadecenyl acetate	30
IX	Δ^9-Octadecenyl acetate	30
X	*trans*-2-Dodecenal	8
XI	Benzaldehyde	37, 39, 40, 42—44, 48—50, 52, 54
XII	Benzoic acid	44, 48, 52, 54
XIII	Mandelonitrile	37, 39, 44, 54
XIV	Mandelonitrile benzoate	44, 52, 54
XV	Benzoyl cyanide	37, 39, 54
XVI	Phenol	48, 49
XVII	*o*-Cresol	34
XVIII	*p*-Cresol	36
XIX	Guaiacol (=2-methoxyphenol)	42, 43, 48
XX	1,4-Benzoquinone	28, 35
XXI	2-Methyl-1,4-benzoquinone	2—17, 19—21, 24—27, 29—33
XXII	2-Methyl-3-methoxy-1,4-benzoquinone	2—6, 10, 11, 13—20, 22, 23, 25, 26, 30—34
XXIII	2,3-Dimethoxy-1,4-benzoquinone	3, 35
XXIV	5-Methyl-2,3-dimethoxy-1,4-benzoquinone	3
XXV	2-Methyl-1,4-hydroquinone	33
XXVI	2-Methyl-3-methoxy-1,4-hydroquinone	33
XXVII	*Glomerin* (=1,2-dimethyl-4(3H)-quinazolinone)	1
XXVIII	*Homoglomerin* (=1-methyl-2-ethyl-4(3H)-quinazolinone)	1
XXIX	*Polyzonimine*	56
XXX	*Nitropolyzonamine*	56

[a] Numbers refer to millipeds listed in Table 3, which also gives pertinent references.

Table 3. Millipeds in Which Chemical Component of Defensive Secretions have been Identified

Millipeds[a]	Chemical Components Present in the Defensive Secretions[b]	Authority
Subclass Pentazonia		
Order Glomerida		
1. *Glomeris marginata*	XXVII, XXVIII	MEINWALD, Y.C. et al., 1966; SCHILDKNECHT and WENNEIS, 1966; SCHILD-KNECHT et al., 1966; SCHILDKNECHT et al., 1967

Millipeds[a]	Chemical Components Present in the Defensive Secretions[b]	Authority
Subclass Helminthomorpha		
Order Spirobolida		
2. *Chicobolus spinigerus*	XXI, XXII	Monro et al., 1962
3. *Epibolus pulchripes* (= *Metiche tanganyicense*)	XXI, XXII, XXIII, XXIV	Wood et al., 1975
4. *Floridobolus penneri*	XXI, XXII	Monro et al., 1962
5. *Narceus annularis*	XXI, XXII	Monro et al., 1962; Percy and Weatherston, 1971
6. *N. gordanus*	XXI, XXII	Monro et al., 1962
7. *Pachybolus laminatus*	XXI	Barbier and Lederer, 1957
8. *Rhinocricus insulatus*	X, XXI	Wheeler et al., 1964
9. *R. varians*	XXI	Moussatché et al., 1969
10. *Rhinocricus* sp.	XXI, XXII	Schildknecht and Weis, 1961
11. *Trigoniulus lumbricinus*	XXI, XXII	Monro et al., 1962
Order Spirostreptida		
12. *Aulonopygus aculeatus*	XXI	Barbier, 1959
13. *Archispirostreptus gigas*	XXI, XXII	Wood, 1974
14. *A. tumuliporus*	XXI, XXII	Smolanoff et al., 1975b
15. *Cambala hubrichti*	XXI, XXII	Eisner et al., 1965
16. *Collostreptus fulvus*	XXI, XXII	Perissé and Salles, 1970
17. *Doratogonus annulipes*	XXI, XXII	Eisner et al., 1965
18. *Orthoporus conifer*	XXII	Eisner et al., 1965
19. *O. flavior*	XXI, XXII	Eisner et al., 1965
20. *O. ornatus* (= *O. punctilliger*)	XXI, XXII	Eisner et al., 1965
21. *Peridontopyge aberrans*	XXI	Barbier, 1959
22. *P. conani*	XXII	Smolanoff et al., 1975b
23. *P. rubescens*	XXII	Smolanoff et al., 1975b
24. *P. vachoni*	XXI	Barbier, 1959
25. *Prionopetalum frundsbergi*	XXI, XXII	Wood, 1974
26. *P. tricuspis*	XXI, XXII	Wood, 1974
27. *Rhapidostreptus virgator* (= *Spirostreptus v.*)	XXI	Barbier and Lederer, 1957
28. *Spirostreptus castaneus*	XX	Barbier and Lederer, 1957
29. *S. multisulcatus*	XXI	Barbier, 1959
Order Julida		
30. *Blaniulus guttulatus*	VII, VIII, IX, XXI, XXII	Weatherston et al., 1971
31. *Chromatoiulus unilineatus* (= *Brachyiulus u.*)	XXI, XXII	Schildknecht and Weis, 1961
32. *Cylindroiulus londinensis* (= *C. teutonicus*)	XXI, XXII	Schildknecht and Weis, 1961
33. *Ommatoiulus sabulosus* (= *Archiulus s.*)	XXI, XXII, XXV, XXVI	Schildknecht and Krämer, 1962; Trave et al., 1959

Millipeds[a]	Chemical Components Present in the Defensive Secretions[b]	Authority
34. *Oriulus delus*	XVII, XXII	KLUGE and EISNER, 1971
35. *Uroblaniulus canadensis*	XX, XXIII	WEATHERSTON and PERCY, 1969
Order Callipodida		
36. *Abacion magnum*	XVIII	EISNER et al., 1963b
Order Polydesmida		
37. *Apheloria corrugata* (= *A. coriacea*)	I, XI, XIII, XV	CONNER et al., 1977; EISNER and EISNER, 1965; EISNER et al., 1963a; EISNER, et al., 1963; WEATHERSTON and GARDINER, 1973
38. *A. kleinpetri*	I	EISNER et al., 1975
39. *A. trimaculata*	I, XI XIII, XV	CONNER et al., 1977; EISNER, et al., 1975
40. *Astrodesmus laxus*	I, XI	EISNER, et al., 1975
41. *Cherokia geordiana*	I	EISNER, et al., 1963
42. *Euryurus australis*	XI, XIX	DUFFIELD et al., 1974
43. *E. leachii*	I, XI, XIX	DUFFIELD et al., 1974; HALL et al., 1969
44. *Gomphodesmus pavani*	I, XI, XII, XIII, XIV	BARBETTA et al., 1966
45. *Harpaphe haydeniana* (= *Leptodesmus h.*)	I	COOLIDGE, 1909
46. *Motyxia sequoiae* (= *Luminodesmus s.*)	I	DAVENPORT et al., 1952
47. *Nannaria* sp.	I	EISNER, et al., 1963
48. *Orthomorpha coarctata*	I, XI, XII, XVI, XIX	MONTEIRO, 1961
49. *Oxidus gracilis* (= *Fontaria g.*)	I, XI, XVI	BLUM et al., 1973; EISNER, et al., 1963; GULDENSTEEDEN-EGELING, 1882
50. *Pachydesmus crassicutis*	I, XI	BLUM and WOODRING, 1962
51. *Pleuroloma flavipes*	I	HALL et al., 1969
52. *Polydesmus collaris*	I, II, III, IV, XI, XII, XIV	CASNATI et al., 1963
53. *Pseudopolydesmus branneri*	I	EISNER, et al., 1975
54. *P. serratus*	I, IV, V, VI, XI, XII, XIII, XIV, XV	CONNER, et al., 1977; EISNER, et al., 1963 WHEELER, 1890
55. [= *Polydesmus (Fontaria) virginienses*][c]	I	
Order Polyzoniida		
56. *Polyzonium rosalbum*	XXIX, XXX	MEINWALD et al., 1975; SMOLANOFF et al., 1975a

[a] Terminology and classification according to HOFFMAN, R.L. (1969, and personal communication). When generic or specific names differ from those used by authorities cited, the terminology of the latter is given in parenthesis.
[b] Numerals refer to compounds listed in Table 2.
[c] It is impossible to know which species this might have been.

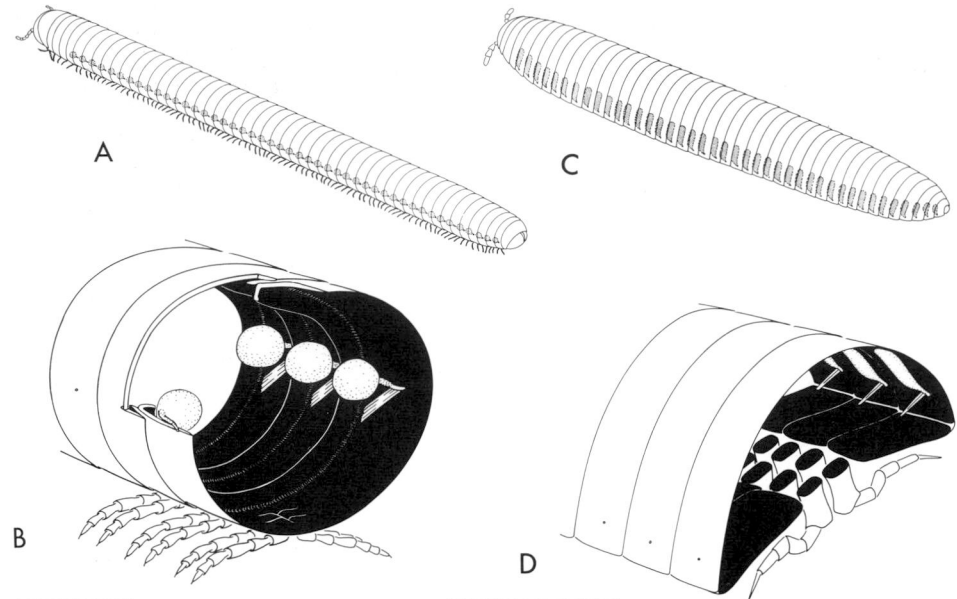

Fig. 4A–D. *Gland type 2.* (A) *Narceus gordanus,* showing segmental glands in place. (B) Portion of body of *Narceus,* cut away to show glands. (C) *Polyzonium rosalbum,* with glands drawn in. (D) Portion of body of *Polyzonium,* showing glands on right side. (Reference bars: B, 3 mm; D, 1 mm)

Narceus gordanus discharges its quinone-containing secretion (Tables 2 and 3) as a liquid ooze (Fig. 5A and B), as millipeds generally do. Some species, however, may on occasion discharge their fluid as a spray, sometimes with considerable force (Burtt, 1947; Haneveld, 1958; Loomis, 1936, 1941; Woodring and Blum, 1965). We ourselves have observed discharges of up to nearly 50 cm in *Narceus annularis,* but spraying is exceptional in this animal. The suggestion (Woodring and Blum, 1965) that the force for such ejections is somehow engendered within the terminal valves of the glands can probably be dismissed, if for no other reason than that not enough fluid could possibly be stored within the valvular portion of the glands to account for the volumes of fluid ejected.

In the Spirostreptida, Julida, and Callipodida, the glands are closely similar to those of *Narceus,* as we confirmed by dissection of *Orthoporus flavior* (Spirostreptida), *Oriulus delus* (Julida), and *Abacion magnum* (Callipodida) (Eisner, T. and Alsop, D., unpublished; Eisner et al., 1963b). In the Polyzoniida the glands are more elongate in shape, but otherwise also essentially similar (Fig. 4C and D), and the same seems to hold for the Platydesmida, in which the glands are slender lengthy tubes (Wood, 1864; Alsop, D., unpublished observations on *Brachycybe lecontei*).

Gland Type 3

This type (Effenberger, 1909; Eisner et al., 1963a; Silvestri, 1903; Weber, 1882; Woodring and Blum, 1963) is restricted to the helminthomorph order Polydes-

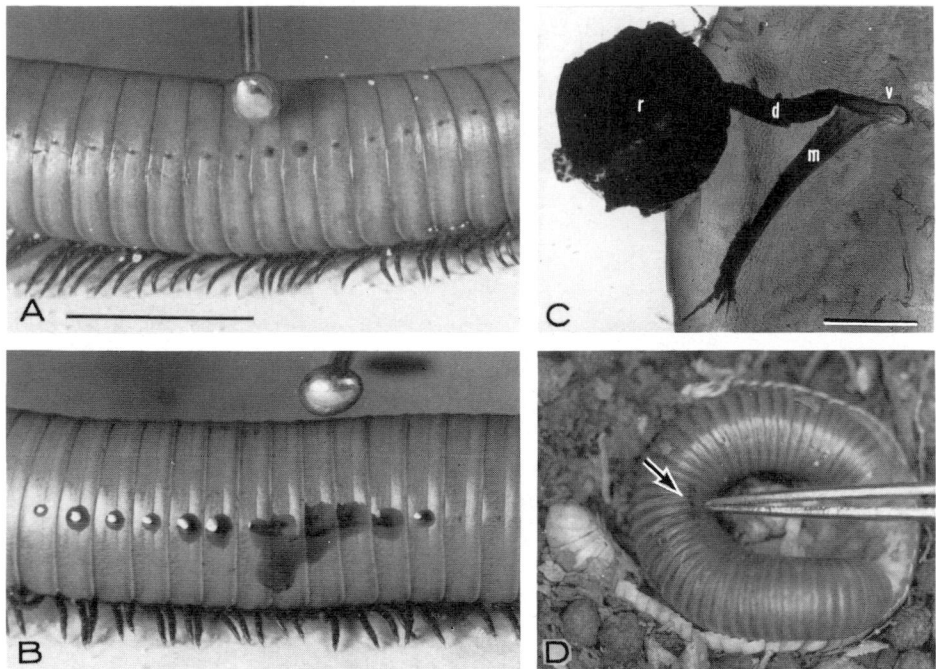

Fig. 5A — D. *Narceus gordanus* discharging quinonoid secretion in response to tapping with a metal mallet. The response is initially localized (A), and spreads to adjacent segments after persistent stimulation (B). (C) Gland of *Narceus gordanus,* showing spherical reservoir (*r*) in which secretion is stored, and slender efferent duct (*d*), with terminal valve (*v*), and valve-opener muscle (*m*). (D) Newly molted *Narceus annularis,* responding to prodding by discharging secretion (*arrow*) from the glands of the region prodded. The cast exoskeleton of the previous instar still surrounds the milliped. (Reference bars: A, 1 cm; C 0.5 mm)

mida, which includes the cyanogenetic species. Basically, a gland of this type (cf. *Apheloria corrugata,* Figs. 6 and 7) consists of the conventional membranous sac that also characterizes gland type 2, but interposed between this sac and the outer opening of the gland is a small, rigidly constructed, second compartment. The inner and outer compartments have been called reservoir and vestibule respectively (EISNER et al., 1963a). The functional significance of this bicompartmentalization is discussed in Section C, below. The reservoir, like its counterpart in the glands of type 2, lacks intrinsic compressor muscles. Moreover, the junction between reservoir and vestibule is valvular in nature, and similar in construction to the terminal valve in the efferent duct of gland type 2. Gland type 3 may, in fact, be no more than a gland type 2 with an added vestibule, an elaboration that may have evolved simply by secondary invagination of the body wall. Glands of type 3 are usually arranged in discontinuous rather than continuous sequence along the length of the millipeds (HANNUM, 1926). In *Apheloria corrugata,* as in most polydesmoids, the glands are in segments 5, 7, 9, 10, 12, 13, and 15 — 19. (Fig. 6A). The cyanogenetic secretion (Tables 2 and 3) oozes as droplets from the individual glands (Fig. 7A).

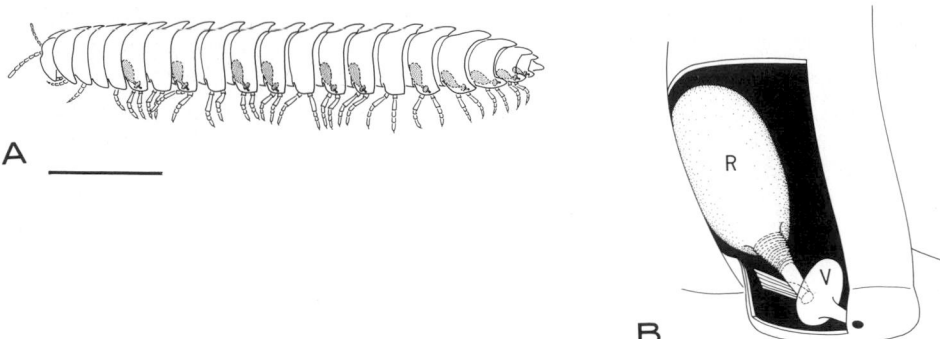

Fig. 6A and B. *Gland type 3.* (A) *Apheloria corrugata,* showing segmental arrangement of the glands. (B) Enlarged view of gland of *Apheloria* (*R*, reservoir; *V*, vestibule). (Reference bar in A, 1 cm)

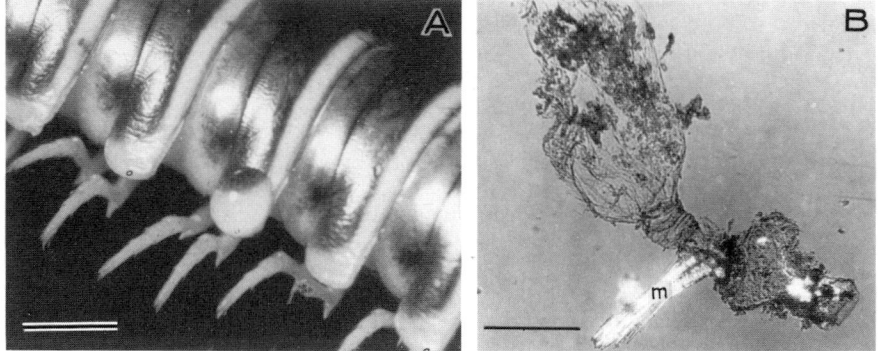

Fig. 7A and B. (A) Enlarged view of portion of left side of *Apheloria corrugata,* showing droplet of secretion discharged from one gland. Gland openings have been outlined in ink. (B) Isolated gland of *Apheloria corrugata,* showing revervoir and vestibule (compare with Fig. 6B). The muscle (*m*) that opens the valve between the two compartments is seen as bright band in partially polarized light. (Reference bars: A, 2 mm; B, 0.5 mm)

Cytology of the Glands

Relatively little is known about the cytology of the glandular tissue that produces the secretions. It is clear from conventional histological work that the gland cells are a part of the wall of the glandular sacs themselves, and that they may be more or less restricted to specialized portions of the wall (Barth, 1967; Rimsky-Korsakow, 1895; Silvestri, 1903). Weatherston and Percy (1969) have described the gland cells of *Uroblaniulus canadensis* (order Julida), which they found to contain specialized vesicles and cuticular ducts as are commonly present in exocrine cells of arthropods. In insects it has been postulated that such vesicles and ducts are the seat of the synthetic processes that lead to the production of the secretory constituents (Eisner, 1970). Intracellular cuticular ducts are also present in glands of Spirobolida (*Narceus* spp.), Callipodida (*Abacion magnum*), and Polydesmida (*Apheloria corrugata*), and can be readily demonstrated in KOH-treated glands from which all noncuticular components have been digested away (ALSOP, D., and EISNER, T., unpublished). WOODRING and BLUM (1965) who apparently missed the cuticular cellular elaborations in *Orthocricus arboreus*, speculate that secretion in this species occurs by holocrine action, but they present no convincing evidence. It is surprising that no electron-microscopic studies have been made of milliped glands, considering how often such studies have been made in insects.

B. Chemistry of the Secretions

Earlier claims about the chemistry of the secretions were usually little more than guesses, inspired by the frequently powerful and supposedly evocative odors of the fluids. The odors have been said in various species to be reminiscent of iodine, chlorine, camphor, acids, walnut, garlic, urine, and even feces! (BURTT, 1938; COOK, 1900; LISTER, 1670; SAVI, 1823; VERHOEFF, 1928, and references therein). But there were also two pioneering chemical studies, one reporting hydrogen cyanide emission by a polydesmoid milliped (GULDENSTEEDEN-EGELING, 1882) and the other claiming the presence of quinone (very likely 1,4-benzoquinone) in the secretion of a species of Julida (BÉHAL and PHISALIX, 1900). Some dozens of millipeds have been investigated since then, comprising representatives of most of the orders known to have glands (Table 1). The species, their compounds, and the pertinent literature references are listed in Tables 2 and 3. Some of the compounds are also shown by formula in Figure 8.

Defensive secretions have generally been obtained by disturbing the millipeds and gathering the resultant discharge on filter paper or other absorbent material. Extraction of these wipings with a solvent such as methylene chloride or carbon disulfide provides a solution suitable for standard chromatographic and spectral analyses. Thin layer chromatography and gas-liquid chromatography have proven especially useful in separating and purifying individual components from these secretions. In recent investigations gas chromatography coupled with mass spectrometry (MCFADDEN, 1973) has played an important role. In fact, those studies which were carried out before this technique was available may well have missed minor components which would now be readily detected. It should also be noted that polar and/or high molecular weight compounds are not well handled by these methods and require special techniques.

In most cases the structures of defensive compounds can be deduced from infrared, nuclear magnetic resonance, and mass spectral data; comparison with an authentic sample in the case of known compounds then provides a final confirmation of identity. When anomalous or previously unknown compounds were encountered (such as XXVII — XXX) structural confirmation was obtained by comparison with unambiguously synthesized material (MEINWALD, et al., 1966; MEINWALD et al., 1975; SMOLANOFF et al., 1975a). In the case of *nitropolyzonamine* (XXX), the unusual tricyclic component of the *Polyzonium rosalbum* secretion, both the structure and absolute configuration were based on x-ray crystallographic examination (MEINWALD et al., 1975).

The milliped compounds are, for the most part, of low molecular weight, in the range below 300. They include, in addition to hydrogen cyanide (I), several

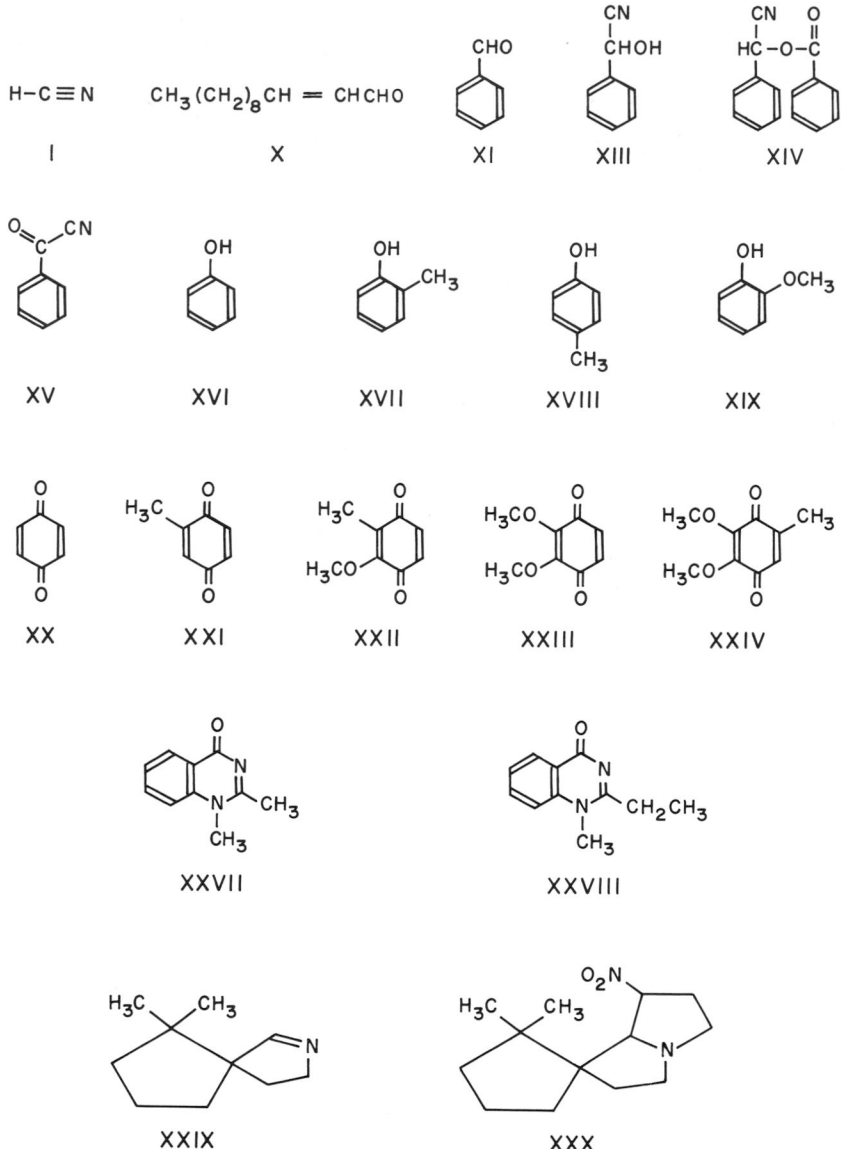

Fig. 8. Chemical components of defensive secretions of millipeds. Roman numerals correspond to compounds named in Table 2.

aliphatic acids (II — VI), three acetate esters (VII — IX), one aliphatic aldehyde (X), one aromatic aldehyde (XI), one aromatic acid (XII), two cyanogenetic compounds (XIII, XV) and the ester of one of them (XIV), four phenols (XVI — XIX), five benzoquinones (XX — XXIV), two hydroquinones (XXV, XXVI), two quinazolinones (*glomerin* and *homoglomerin*, XXVII and XXVIII), a nitrogen-containing monoterpene (*polyzonimine*, XXIX), and a related tricyclic nitro compound (*nitro-*

polyzonamine, XXX). Some components, such as the benzoquinones, hydrogen cyanide, and benzaldehyde, are known from an array of species, but the remaining compounds are known from few or single species only.

There is some phylogenetic pattern in the distribution of the compounds (Table 3). The benzoquinones all occur in species of three orders of the Helminthomorpha: the Spirobolida, Spirostreptida, and Julida. These orders might well be called the quinone millipeds, for although in some the secretion contains non-quinonoidal components (*trans*-2-dodecenal in *Rhinocricus insulatus;* o-cresol in *Oriulus delus;* acetate esters in *Blaniulus guttulatus*), all produce at least some quinones. Collectors who handle these animals are often left with their fingers stained intense purple for days. This discoloration is caused by the tanning action of the quinones, a reaction mistakenly assumed to indicate iodine in some early literature (VERHOEFF, 1928). The presence of minor quantities of hydroquinones reported for one of these millipeds (SCHILDKNECHT and KRÄMER, 1962), is not surprising, since hydroquinones may be expected to be the chemical precursors of the quinones in these secretions.

Hydrogen cyanide production is restricted to the helminthomorph order Polydesmida, which might be called the cyanogenetic order. Cyanogenesis in these animals appears to occur by dissociation of a cyanohydrin (see Section C, below), and it is therefore not surprising that an aldehyde, benzaldehyde, has been consistently found, together with hydrogen cyanide, where an appropriate chemical search for aldehyde was made. The undissociated cyanohydrin of benzaldehyde, mandelonitrile, has also been identified in several species. We have recently isolated a second cyanogenetic compound, benzoyl cyanide, from the secretion of three polydesmoids (CONNER et al., 1977). The compound was invariably present together with mandelonitrile, although always in lesser quantities, and must therefore serve as a supplementary source of the hydrogen cyanide released by the secretions. Whether benzoyl cyanide is a general constituent of polydesmoid secretion remains to be seen. Several non-cyanogenetic compounds have also been identified in polydesmoid secretions, including phenol, guaiacol, and a series of organic acids (formic, acetic, isovaleric, myristic, stearic, benzoic). One compound, mandelonitrile benzoate, previously known from two species, was thought to represent an artifact formed during isolation of the substance (BARBETTA et al., 1966), but it has now been shown in a third species to be a component of fresh secretion (CONNER et al., 1977).

In the remaining orders only single species have been studied. *Abacion magnum,* a member of the helminthomorph order Callipodida, produces a phenol, *p*-cresol, not yet found in any other millipeds. *Polyzonium rosalbum,* a helminthomorph of the order Polyzoniida, secretes the monoterpene *polyzonimine* along with the closely related *nitropolyzonamine. Glomeris marginata,* of the subclass Penicillata, order Glomerida, produces the quinazolinones *glomerin* and *homoglomerin.* The secretion of *Glomeris* is viscous and sticky, due to the presence of an ancillary proteinaceous material of known amino acid composition (SCHILDKNECHT et al., 1967). Proteinaceous components may also occur in the secretion of *Polyzonium rosalbum,* which is comparably sticky, but other millipeds generally produce mobile fluids, probably devoid of macromolecules.

Of the compounds found so far in milliped secretions, the most unusual are *polyzonimine* and *nitropolyzonamine*. No monoterpenes of natural origin are known to possess the carbon skeleton characteristic of these materials, nor have other natural products been previously characterized based on the 2-azaspiro[4.4]nonane ring system. While *nitropolyzonamine* resembles the pyrrolizidine alkaloids, none of these alkaloids have been found to contain either the additional spirocyclic ring or a nitro substituent (Bull et al., 1968). The quinazolinones of *Glomeris* are also unusual, inasmuch as no other animal quinazolinones are known. The other milliped components are all known to occur as such, or as closely related compounds, in the secretions of other arthropods. Benzoquinones are particularly widespread, having been isolated from the defensive fluids of opilionids, cockroaches, termites, earwigs, and grasshoppers, as well as from carabid, staphylinid, alleculid, and tenebrionid beetles (Eisner et al., 1971; Altman and Dittmer, 1973). Of the five benzoquinones in millipeds, only 2,3-dimethoxy-1,4-benzoquinone and 5-methyl-2,3-dimethoxy-1,4-benzoquinone (ubiquinone-0) appear so far to be restricted to these animals. Cyanogenesis as such is also not unusual, since it is known to occur in centipedes, moths, and chrysomelid beetle larvae (Jones et al., 1962; Jones et al., 1976; Moore, 1967; Schildknecht et al., 1968). Even benzoyl cyanide, the novel second cyanogenetic compound of millipeds (Conner et al., 1977) is now known also from the cyanogenetic secretion of geophilomorph centipedes (Jones et al., 1976). Phenols have also been reported from other arthropod sources, as have aliphatic and aromatic aldehydes and acids, and acetate esters (Altman and Dittmer, 1973). Hydroquinones may be generally present as minor components in quinonoidal secretions (Schildknecht and Krämer, 1962).

Plants also produce compounds of the categories secreted by millipeds. In plants, these compounds are part of the complement of so-called secondary metabolites, now widely believed to serve for the chemical defense of the plants (Eisner, 1970; Whittaker and Feeny, 1971). Thus, there are several quinazoline alkaloids, such as *arborine,* from an Indian medicinal plant, which are closely related to quinazolinones of *Glomeris* (Armarego, 1963; Chakravarti et al., 1961). The quinones, phenols, aldehydes, and aliphatic esters of millipeds all occur as such or have close counterparts in plants (Karrer, 1958).

We have omitted from our tabulations some of the compounds reported in the literature as occurring in millipeds. Thus, we have excluded the glucoside of *p*-isopropylmandelonitrile (Pallares, 1946), since this compound was isolated from whole milliped extracts rather than from the defensive secretion itself. Since the milliped is a polydesmoid, it is entirely likely that it does produce hydrogen cyanide, together perhaps with cuminaldehyde as the ancillary aldehyde, but we omitted the reference in order to preclude the inference that an undissociated cyanohydrin glucoside occurs in the secretion. In line with this omission, we also excluded another report, claiming, on the basis of inconclusive chromatographic evidence, that the secretion of the polydesmoid *Pachydesmus crassicutis* contains free sugar (Blum and Woodring, 1962). Absence of sugar in detectable concentrations has been proven for the secretion of the related species, *Apheloria corrugata* (Eisner, et al., 1963). Although it seems likely, therefore, that polydesmoid glands store cyanohydrins as such rather than as cyanohydrin glycosides, the ultimate systemic precursors of the compounds may yet turn out to be glycosides.

We have also excluded two quinones, 2-ethyl-1,4-benzoquinone and 2,3-dimethyl-1,4-benzoquinone, reported respectively from two and one species of Spirobolida (MOUSSATCHÉ et al., 1969; PÉRISSÉ et al., 1968). Since these are the only reports of the presence of these quinones in millipeds, and they are based on chromatographic evidence alone, the identifications seemed tentative. The classical first identification of a milliped quinone (BÉHAL and PHISALIX, 1900) is also omitted, since the precise nature of the quinone remains uncertain.

As indicated by many authors, unknown constituents remain to be identified in some of the secretions that have been studied. Future work is thus certain to amplify some of the listings given in Table 3.

We know little about the amounts of secretory material produced by the millipeds. In *Glomeris marginata,* individual specimens were estimated to contain an average of $30-40$ µg quinazolinones (MEINWALD et al., 1966; SCHILDKNECHT et al., 1967). Large tropical millipeds may contain as much as 200–300 mg benzoquinones, while smaller juloids may have only in the order of 1 mg or less (SCHILDKNECHT and WEISS, 1961). A medium-sized spirostreptoid (*Peridontopyge rubescens*) may contain upwards of 50 mg quinones, or somewhat more than 1% of body weight (EISNER, T., and HICKS, K., unpublished).

Precise measurements have been made of the cyanogenetic output of polydesmoid millipeds. In *Apheloria corrugata,* the cyanogenetic yield of individuals, assayed freshly after capture (without prior disturbance) was found to be highly variable, ranging from virtually 0 to over 600 µg per animal. Mean yield was 114 µg/animal (135 µg/gram body weight), while in the smaller *Pseudopolydesmus serratus* it was 41 µg/animal (280 µg/gram body weight) (EISNER, et al., 1967).

C. Biochemistry of the Secretions

The active principles of the defensive secretions of arthropods may originate in one of two ways. Either they are synthesized endogenously by the animals themselves, according to more or less conventional biosynthetic schemes, and at the expense of normally available metabolic precursors (i.e., amino acids, sugars, etc.), or they are appropriated from an exogenous source, usually their food, which provides the materials in essentially prefabricated form. Examples of both of these strategies have been documented for insects. Thus, the quinones and terpenes produced in the defensive glands of certain beetles, ants, and walking sticks are synthesized by the insects themselves, while the cardiac glycosides, aristolochic acid, terpenes, and resin acids, employed for defense by some butterflies and sawfly larvae are sequestered by these animals from plants (references in EISNER, 1970; EISNER et al., 1974).

Little is known about the biochemical origin of milliped secretions. However, two studies have given important results. In the earlier of these (SCHILDKNECHT and WENNEIS, 1967) it was shown that *Glomeris marginata,* when fed or injected with anthranilic acid ($^{14}CO_2H$), produces radioactive *glomerin* (XXVII) and *homoglomerin* (XXVIII). The specific activity of these products was about 1% of that present in the precursor. In the case of *homoglomerin,* a base hydrolysis was carried out to yield labeled N-methylanthranilic acid whose specific activity was the same

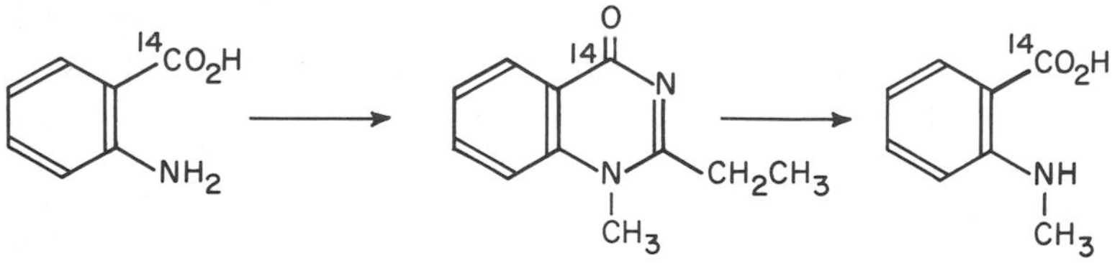

Fig. 9. Incorporation of anthranilic acid into *homoglomerin*. Details in text. After Schildknecht and Wenneis (1967)

as that of the *homoglomerin* itself, suggesting that the ^{14}C label remained in the expected position throughout this process (Fig. 9).

While this study, judged by modern biosynthetic standards, is far from detailed, it does provide answers to two basic questions. First, it establishes the fact that these millipeds are able to produce their quinazolinones from a simple precursor and, therefore, that the animals are not dependent on obtaining preformed alkaloids from their food. And second, it shows that anthranilic acid, a known precursor of quinazoline alkaloids in plants, can serve a similar role in an arthropod.

Another study has given some insight into the biosynthesis of hydrogen cyanide (I) and benzaldehyde (XI) in the polydesmoid *Oxidus gracilis* (Towers et al., 1972). It is well known that many plants contain cyanogenic glycosides. In the case of prunasin (mandelonitrile glucoside), it has been shown by isotopic tracer experiments that phenylalanine is the mandelonitrile precursor, via the corresponding N-hydroxyamino acid, the aldoxime, and phenylacetonitrile (Conn and Butler, 1969; Ben-Yehoshua and Conn, 1964; Tapper et al., 1972). Once again, either polydesmoids are able to perform an analogous synthesis, or they may acquire their cyanogenetic ability by sequestering plant-produced cyanogens. By means of feeding experiments in which D,L-phenylalanine, specifically labeled with ^{14}C, was administered to *O. gracilis,* it was possible to show that both hydrogen cyanide and benzaldehyde can be produced from this precursor. (Interestingly, tyrosine-2-^{14}C did not serve as a precursor for hydrogen cyanide, or, of course, benzaldehyde.) The incorporation results are compatible with the overall scheme shown in Figure 10, which at this level of detail is indistinguishable from the previously elucidated plant pathway. It would appear, therefore, that the polydesmoids have independently evolved the enzyme systems necessary for the production of their defensive secretions.

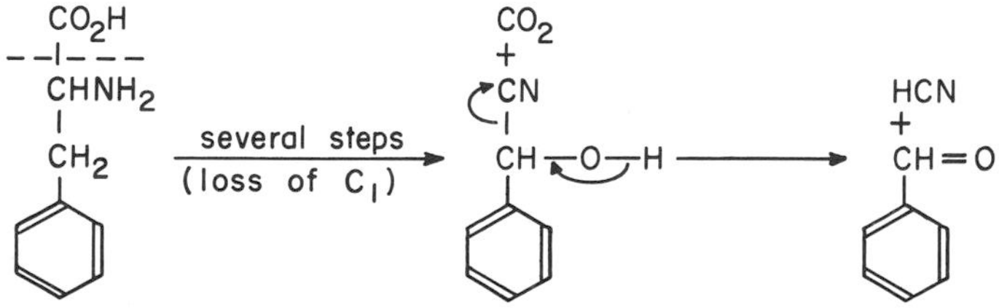

Fig. 10. Biosynthesis of hydrogen cyanide and benzaldehyde from phenylalanine *via* mandelonitrile. Details in text. After Towers et al. (1972)

The mechanism whereby polydesmoid millipeds exercise control over the activation of cyanogenesis has been elucidated, at least in its essentials. Polydesmoid millipeds have bicompartmentalized glands of the aforementioned type 3 (see part A, above, and Fig. 6). By means of microcolorimetric tests carried out on the contents of excised glands of *Apheloria corrugata*, it has been shown (EISNER et al., 1963a; EISNER, et al., 1963) that the inner compartment (reservoir) of the gland contains an aqueous emulsion of mandelonitrile, the adduct of benzaldehyde and hydrogen cyanide (Fig. 11). The smaller outer compartment (vestibule) contains a heat-labile factor, presumably enzymatic in nature, capable of promoting the dissociation of mandelonitrile. The two compartments are ordinarily sealed from one another by the intervening valve. When attacked, the milliped contracts the muscle that opens the valve, and by squeezing the reservoir (blood pressure?) forces its contents through the vestibule to the outside. The emergent droplet, consisting of aqueous emulsion of mandelonitrile plus enzyme, oozes from the pore. Hydrogen cyanide and benzaldehyde, the products of the dissociation, are released as vapors that protectively surround the milliped. Measurements made of the time course of cyanogenesis following discharge have shown the process to last for 30 min. or longer (EISNER et al., 1963a). In *Apheloria corrugata,* mandeloni-

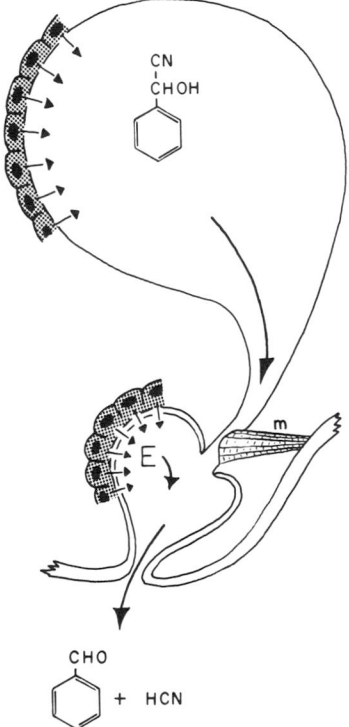

Fig. 11. Diagram of the two-chambered cyanogenetic glandular apparatus of the polydesmoid milliped, *Apheloria corrugata* (cf. gland type 3, Figs. 6, 7). The inner compartment (reservoir) stores mandelonitrile, while the smaller compartment (vestibule) contains an enzyme (*E*) that catalyzes the breakdown of mandelonitrile into hydrogen cyanide and benzaldehyde. A muscle (*m*) operates the valve between the two compartments

trile is the principal cyanogenetic compound, and the mechanism is uncomplicated by the additional presence, at the minimal concentration of 1%, of benzoyl cyanide (Conner et al., 1977). But in other polydesmoids there may be fully a third as much benzoyl cyanide as mandelonitrile (Conner et al., 1977), and any explanation of the cyanogenetic mechanism must take into account the presence of both compounds.

In summary, while no detailed study of defensive compound biosynthesis has been reported, it is clear that some millipeds have biosynthetic capabilities which seem closely analogous to those found in plants. Whether some of these syntheses are dependent upon symbiotic microorganisms remains unknown. From the viewpoint of an organic chemist, the two related spiro compounds secreted by *Polyzonium rosalbum* are especially interesting since they are the only milliped compounds which do not have close relatives among the secondary metabolites from plant sources. There are, of course, other biochemical questions that might be raised in connection with chemical defense mechanisms. For example, nothing is known about how the synthesis of defensive compounds is controlled, or what priority these syntheses are given when they might have to compete with other essential biochemical processes. For the biochemist, this entire field represents essentially virgin territory.

D. Defensive Effectiveness of the Glands

Encounters between millipeds and predators have generally not been witnessed under natural conditions, but they have been staged in the laboratory, with persuasive results. Many invertebrate and vertebrate predators have been tested against such millipeds as juloids, spiroboloids, callipodoids, polydesmoids, glomeroids, and polyzonioids, and rejections have been seen in tests with ants, cicindellid beetles, spiders, toads, lizards, birds, mice, grasshopper mice, a mouse opossum, an armadillo, and even a dog (Blum and Woodring, 1962; Cloudsley-Thompson, 1949 and references therein; Donisthorpe, 1927; Duffield et al., 1974; Eisner, 1970; Eisner and Eisner, 1965; Eisner and Meinwald, 1966; Eisner et al., 1963 b; Kafatos, 1961; Kinkel, 1955; Schildknecht et al., 1967; Smolanoff et al., 1975 a; Wheeler et al., 1964). Even such unnatural predators as fish have been said to reject millipeds (Cloudsley-Thompson, 1949). Some vertebrate predators accepted millipeds at first, as was the case with a mouse opossum and an armadillo (Kafatos, 1961), and with toads, birds, and mice (Schildknecht et al., 1967), but they tended to reject such prey on subsequent presentation. The millipeds used in all these tests included producers of virtually every major category of defensive compound known from these animals. There can be no doubt that the defenses are effective.

Milliped glands are specially refined for efficient operation. Rarely does a milliped discharge from all glands at once. As a rule it emits fluid only from the glands closest to the region of the body subjected to disturbance (Fig. 5A and B), and shows generalized emission only as a counter to generalized assault. Such control over the localization of the discharge has been demonstrated in a variety of millipeds, including spiroboloid, juloid, polydesmoid, and callipodoid species (EISNER and EISNER, 1965; EISNER et al, 1963b; KAFATOS, 1961; KINKEL, 1955; VERHOEFF, 1928; WOODRING and BLUM, 1965). The control mechanism is unaffected by decapitation (KINKEL, 1955).

Following a discharge, a milliped may be more or less persistently protected by the residual secretion that coats its body. Invulnerability against renewed assault has been demonstrated vis à vis ants in quinone-producing (juloid), cyanogenetic (polydesmoid), and phenol-producing (callipodoid) millipeds (BLUM and WOOD-RING, 1962; EISNER et al., 1963b; KAFATOS, 1961). The effect may be attributable, in polydesmoid species, to the ongoing cyanogenesis that takes place in the secretion after emission (EISNER et al., 1963a), but in other species may simply reflect the relatively moderate evaporative rates of the fluids.

The ability of some millipeds to spray their secretion, and to do so forcibly, must improve their defensive capabilities against vertebrates, whose most sensitive facial surfaces, the corneas of the eyes, may be hit as a result. Spraying millipeds all apparently eject quinones, substances which, to human eyes at least, are powerfully and painfully irritating (HANEVELD, 1958; LOOMIS, 1936; WOOD et al., 1975).

Millipeds need not even be chemically defenseless at the time of molting. A specimen of *Narceus annularis,* still soft-bodied and lying within its discarded integumental shell, responded to poking (Fig. 5D) by discharging quinonoidal secretion from its glands (EISNER, T., unpublished). Unlike other arthropods, which shed their glandular linings together with the secretory contents as part of the molt (e.g. the cockroach *Diploptera punctata;* ROTH and STAY, 1958), and need to replenish their secretion every time they cast their skin, *Narceus* manages somehow to conserve the fluid during the molt.

Few systematic studies have been carried out designed to clarify precisely how the defensive substances affect predators. Existing evidence suggests that a diversity of modes of action may be involved. Substances such as benzoquinones, cresols, and *polyzonimine,* appear to act as conventional repellents. This was demonstrated in tests with such major milliped enemies as ants. Presentation of a small capillary tube laden with *polyzonimine* to a group of ants feeding at a sugar source caused dispersal of the ants in a matter of seconds (SMOLANOFF et al., 1975a) (Fig. 12A–D). Comparable results were achieved with 1,4-benzoquinone, 2-methyl-1,4-benzoquinone, 2-methyl-3-methoxy-1,4-benzoquinone, o-cresol, and p-cresol (EISNER, T., unpublished). It has been postulated (EISNER, 1970) that such repellents may exert their deterrency by acting, via the so-called common chemical sense, as irritants (WEDDELL and MILLER, 1962). Ants, spiders, and even vertebrates commonly perform cleansing reactions when contacted by these substances or their vapors, (EISNER, 1970). Quinone vapors delivered to the eye of a mouse or bird induce blinking or wiping with the nyctitans, and application of benzoquinones to the integument of a frog elicits scratching (EISNER, T., unpublished). The pain caused by a quinonoid secretion to the human eye has been vividly described (LOOMIS, 1936). Preening reflexes have provided the basis for bioassays of the irritant effectiveness of *polyzonimine*. Application of the substance to the abdominal cuticle of cockroaches (*Periplaneta americana*) causes scratching at concentrations as low as 10^{-4}M (the concentration of the substance in the *Polyzonium* secretion is $> 10^{-1}$M) (SMOLANOFF et al., 1975a). Flies (*Phormia regina*) perform labellar cleaning in response to near-contact presentation of 10^{-1}M *polyzonimine* in a capillary tube (SMOLANOFF et al.,

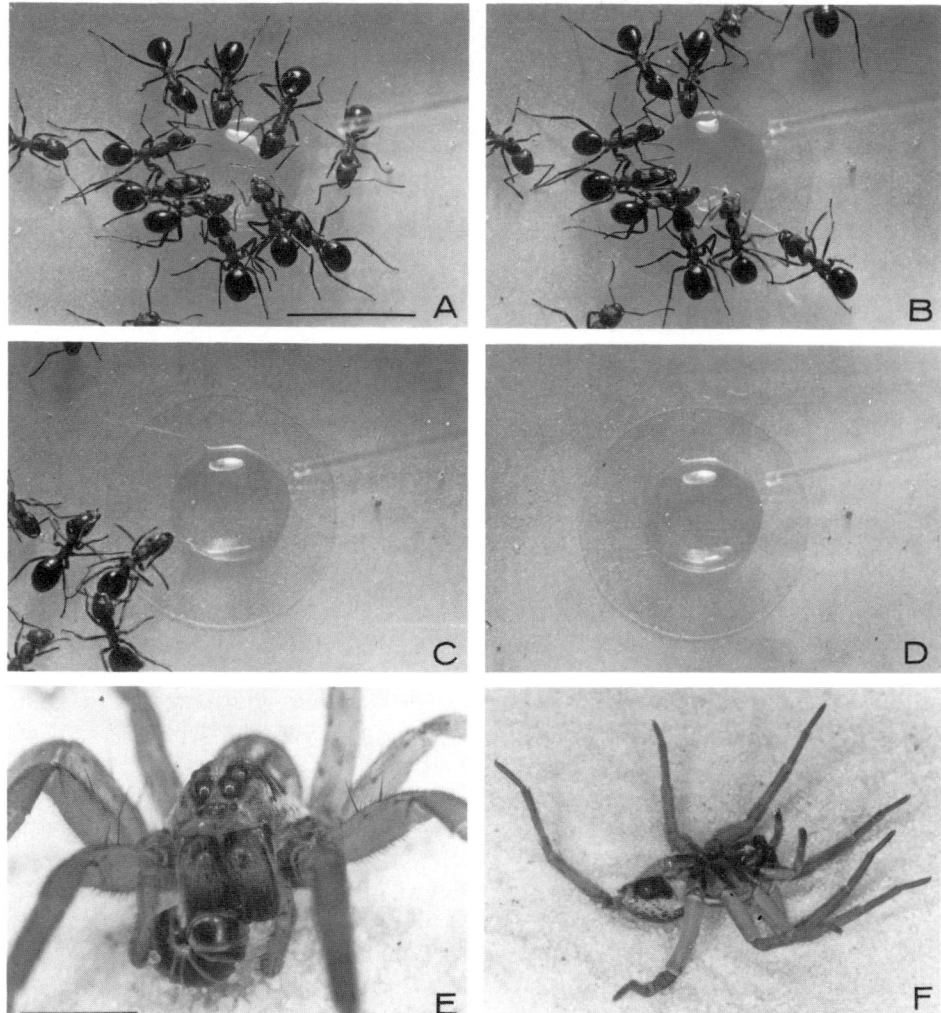

Fig. 12A—D. Dispersal of ants (*Formica exsectoides*) in response to *polyzonimine*. The ants are initially seen feeding on a drop of sugar solution, and the *polyzonimine* is presented to them in the capillary tube introduced from the right. The time course of the photographs (motorized 35 mm camera), beginning with time=0 in Fig. (A) is: (B) (0.5 sec); (C) (1.5 sec); (D)(2.5 sec). E—F. Fate of a lycosid spider that fed (E) on *Glomeris marginata*. The quinazolinones (*glomerin* and *homoglomerin*) in the secretion of the milliped induce a protracted immobilization of the spider. Laid on its back (F), the spider remains motionless, and non-responsive to prodding. (Reference bars: A, 1 cm; E, 5 mm)

1975a). Benzoquinones and cresols induce similar responses in cockroaches and flies (Eisner et al., 1963b; Eisner, T., unpublished).

Other secretory components of millipeds may act primarily as toxins. This is most probably true for hydrogen cyanide. The amounts of this substance produced by a polydesmoid milliped may be considerable. A single *Apheloria corrugata,* weighing 1 g and having a production capacity of 600 μg hydrogen cyanide (the near maximum capacity for the species), has an output equivalence of 18 times the lethal dose of a 300 g pigeon, 6 times the LD of a 25 g mouse, 0.4 times the LD of a 25 g frog, and 0.01 times the LD of man (EISNER et al., 1967). Confinement with a disturbed polydesmoid milliped can indeed be fatal to other animals, as has been noted with bees, flies, and cockroaches (DAVENPORT et al., 1952; EISNER, et al., 1967; HALL et al., 1969). Of course, predators do not normally attack under confined conditions, nor do they necessarily ingest a milliped, so deterrency may involve only relatively brief topical exposure to the secretion or its vapors. Hydrogen cyanide may still act as a poison under such conditions, perhaps to peripheral receptors only, whose total or partial "silencing" may temporarily disorient a predator. One might envision this sort of mechanism operating with insectan predators such as ants. A contributive repellent effect may be provided by the ancillary components (benzaldehyde, and in some cases phenols) which accompany the hydrogen cyanide in cyanogenetic secretions. Benzaldehyde does disperse ants (in the manner shown for *polyzonimine* in Fig. 12A – D), and it also induces scratch reflexes in cockroaches (EISNER, T., unpublished).

Of particular interest as regards mode of action are the two quinazolinones *glomerin* and *homoglomerin* (XXVII and XXVIII) produced by the pill milliped *Glomeris marginata.* These substances have been shown to be toxic to both vertebrates and arthropods. Within hours after consuming *Glomeris,* mice become lethargic, partly paralyzed, and tremorous. Two mice, having taken 6 and 11 *Glomeris,* respectively, died. Birds showed retarded alarm reactions, and toads vomited the millipeds (SCHILDKNECHT et al., 1967). Lycosid spiders are also affected by *Glomeris.* For minutes or even hours after an attack upon a milliped, a spider may appear normal, but it may then develop symptoms of motor impairment, and even eventual total paralysis (Fig. 12E and F). Although slow recovery occurred in the laboratory, it is doubtful that a paralyzed spider could long survive in nature. The effects could be duplicated with synthetic quinazolinones (CARREL, J.C., and EISNER, T., in EISNER, T., 1970). The biochemical basis of this toxicity is unknown, and clearly worthy of investigation. Mice are highly sensitive to quinazolinones: for *glomerin,* LD-50's are given as 17 – 34 mg/kg (oral dosage) and 9 – 17 mg/kg (intraperitoneal dosage) (SCHILDKNECHT et al., 1967). Quinazolinones need not only affect predators by delayed toxic action. In fact, in evolutionary terms, and without invoking kin selection, it is difficult to see how organisms may come upon the possession of poisons which, if they are to exert their defensive action, require the loss to predation of the individuals that carry them (discussion in EISNER, 1970). But quinazolinones are also notably bitter in taste, and this quality, which could cause *Glomeris* to be rejected merely on the basis of noninjurious oral inspection, could in itself account for the evolution of the toxins. Bitterness of *glomerin* to humans is said to be detectable at a concentration of 6×10^{-4}M in aqueous solution. *Brucine,* one of the bitterest substances known, has a detection threshold of 10^{-6}M (SCHILDKNECHT et al., 1966).

The *Glomeris* secretion has yet a third, strictly mechanical, mode of action. By virtue of the proteinaceous material that it contains (SCHILDKNECHT et al., 1967), the fluid is viscous and sticky, and readily pulled into threads (Fig. 3B), which harden quickly on exposure to air. Small predators are entangled and visibly

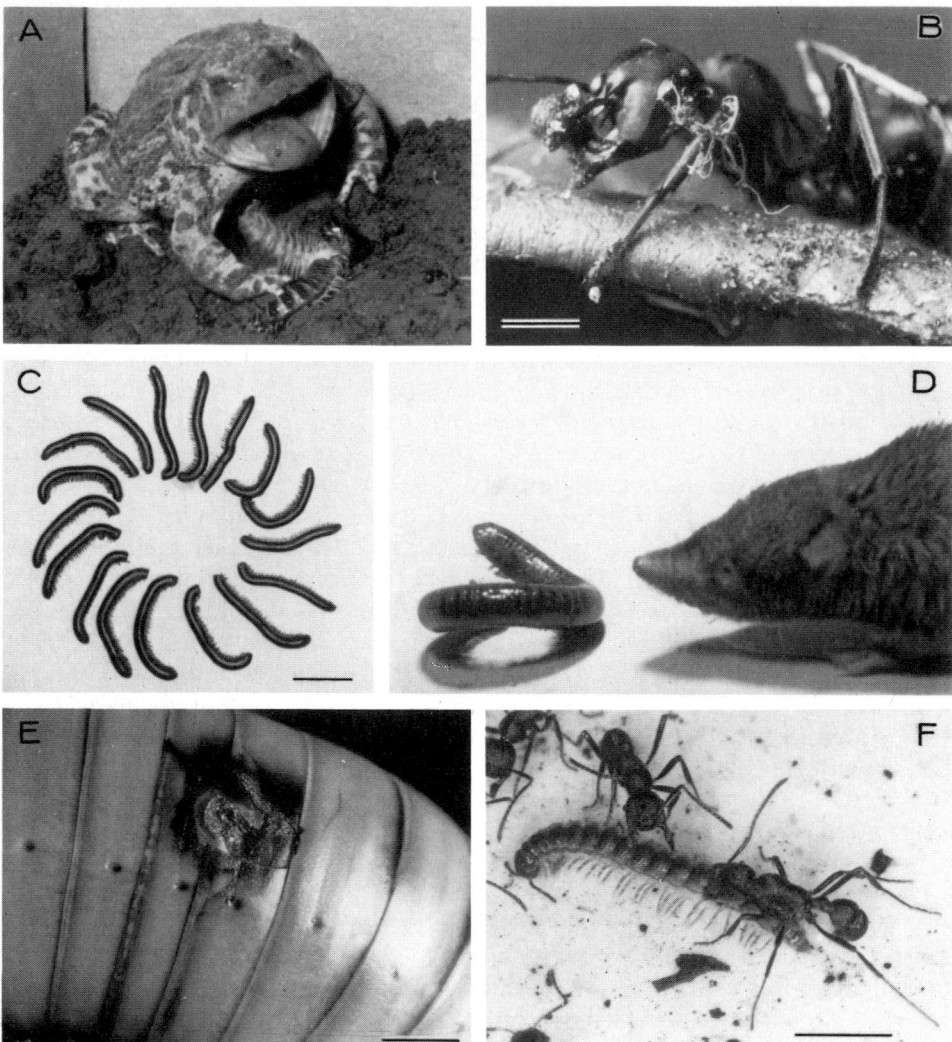

Fig. 13A — F. (A) A toad (*Bufo cognatus*) rejecting a polydesmoid milliped (*Apheloria corrugata*). (B) An ant (*Formica polyctena*), after having been contaminated with the sticky secretion of *Glomeris marginata* (see Fig. 3B); the left antenna is stuck to the cranium, together with a dislodged infrabuccal pellet; the left leg is fastened to the head by dried coiled threads of secretion. (C) Dead millipeds (*Narceus annularis*) found in the field near Ithaca, N.Y., decapitated by an unknown predator (see text for details). (D) A shrew (*Blarina brevicauda*) backing away from a milliped (*Narceus annularis*) that it just attacked. The milliped glistens with discharged quinonoid secretion. (E) Natural healed injury, presumably predator-inflicted, found in an otherwise fully normal *Narceus gordanus*. (F) Ponerine ants (*Gnamtogenys perspicax*) attacking a polydesmoid milliped (*Oxidus gracilis*). The ants are undeterred by the cyanogenetic secretion of the milliped (see text for details). (Reference bars: B, 1 mm; C, 5 cm; E, 2 mm; F, 5 mm)

handicapped by the material (Fig. 13 B), and may have difficulty ridding themselves of it (EISNER and MEINWALD, 1966; SCHILDKNECHT et al., 1967). This may well be the principal effect of the *Glomeris* secretion against ants. *Polyzonium rosalbum* has a comparably sticky secretion which may also act mechanically to incapacitate small predators. CHAMBERLIN (1923a), referring to a siphonophoroid (*Siphonophora pearsei*), calls attention to the animal's ability to "shoot out threads of slime when handled".

Other milliped secretions may also have more or less complex modes of action. Repellents such as quinones and phenols, for example, may be orally distasteful to some predators, in addition to being irritating. And they may also be toxic. Benzoquinones in particular are of high toxicity. Early investigators already noted that rats and guinea pigs cannot withstand subcutaneous or intraperitoneal injections of juloid secretions (PHISALIX, 1900, 1922; ROSSI, 1903). MOUSSATCHÉ et al., (1967, 1969) showed the LD-50 dosage of 1,4-benzoquinone in rats (intravenous injection) to be 15.8 ± 5.7 mg/kg, and 17.4 ± 4.7 mg/kg for 2-methyl-1,4-benzoquinone. In vitro effects of benzoquinones on guinea pig ileum could be prevented by addition of thiol-group protecting substances (glutathione, cysteine), a finding that supports the view (HOFFMAN-OSTENHOF, 1947; POTTER, 1942) that benzoquinones, as powerful oxidizing agents, act, in part at least, by inhibiting SH groups. But one wonders how much systemic exposure to quinones a vertebrate really gets when it ingests quinone-producing millipeds. Benzoquinones are highly reactive, and they may not readily withstand enteric exposure without alteration. It is interesting in this connection that enteric administration of benzoquinones to rats and mice caused no noticeable symptoms (KINKEL, 1955; ROSSI, 1903). Dogs, however, were said to vomit after being fed *Rhinocricus padbergi,* a spiroboloid (PENTEADO and MAUGÉ, 1974). Inhalation of quinones may be hazardous. We ourselves have found "milking" of large spiroboloid or spirostreptoid millipeds an annoying experience, and there is one report of a lizard having died as a result of confinement with a secreting spiroboloid milliped (STEBBINS, 1944).

Given the proven deterrency of the various milliped secretions, it is surprising that there should be predators that feed on millipeds, sometimes even as a matter of routine. There are several reports of ponerine ants that feed on millipeds, mostly, but not exclusively on polydesmoids (KEMPF and BROWN, 1970; SCHUBART, 1945, 1950; WHEELER and MANN, 1914). One of us (T.E.), in conjunction with Dr. W.L. BROWN, JR. at Cornell University, witnessed attacks of a Brazilian ponerine, *Gnamtogenys perspicax,* upon small polydesmoids offered to them in the laboratory. The ants seemed undeterred by the secretion, (Fig. 13 F) despite the release of hydrogen cyanide, which was demonstrated by the blue color that developed on pieces of filter paper impregnated with benzidine acetate-copper acetate reagent (FEIGL, 1966) held beside the millipeds while under attack. Some polydesmoid millipeds (family Stylodesmidae) are myrmecophiles of ecitonine army ants in the neotropics. The millipeds run with the emigration columns of the ants and are apparently capable of following the ants' chemical trails. They are occasionally even carried by the ants. It is suggested that the millipeds might be true symbionts that keep the area around the ant nest clean by feeding on organic debris. At no time did the ants appear to prompt a secretory release from the millipeds (RETTENMEYER, 1962). Some polydesmoid millipeds are also said to be termitophilous (CHAMBERLIN, 1923b).

Another group of insects that feed on millipeds are the larvae of beetles of the family Phengodidae, as was first reported by RIVERS (1886). These animals kill the millipeds in a remarkable way. As described by TIEMANN (1967), when a larva comes upon a milliped, it runs alongside it, until it can mount its back. Once it does so, it throws a coil around the milliped with its last abdominal segments, and by reaching forward with its head, uses its sickle-shaped mandibles to sever the milliped's nerve cord just behind the head. The milliped is paralyzed, whereupon the larva eats it, commencing with the head, and proceeding backward, cleaning out each segment from the inside, one at a time. Both quinone-producing and cyanogenetic millipeds are taken by these larvae. One of us (T.E.) has observed a phengodid larva feeding on a polydesmoid milliped in a field near Denton, Texas. LAWRENCE (1966) describes the behavior of certain African reduviid bugs of the genera *Glymmatophora* and *Cleptria,* the nymphs of which attack millipeds in groups, piercing them one at a time with their beaks until they are immobilized, and then proceeding to suck them dry.

Additional evidence of predation upon millipeds comes from literature on stomach or fecal contents, laboratory tests, and more or less incidental field observations. It is clear that some spiders can take millipeds, but apparently not as a rule (CLOUDSLEY-THOMPSON, 1949, and references therein). Certain African scorpions feed on millipeds, whose skeletal remains are found heaped beside the scorpions' burrows (COOKE, J.A.L., personal communication; LAWRENCE, 1966). One of these scorpions, *Opisthacanthus laevipes,* was observed feeding on a spirostreptoid milliped, seemingly unaffected by the "copious secretions" oozing from its glands (LAWRENCE, 1966). The South African dormouse *Graphiurus murinus* appears to live largely on spirostreptoids (LAWRENCE, 1966). Millipeds have also been found in the stomach or feces of salamanders, alligators, a turtle, birds, moles, an armadillo, and a skunk (CLOUDSLEY-THOMPSON, 1949, and references therein; LAWRENCE, 1966; MCATEE, 1932; SACHTLEBEN, 1926, cited in KINKEL, 1955; SCHUBART, 1947; STEBBINS, 1944). Some birds, such as starlings, may be major predators of millipeds, which are said to make up almost 12% of their annual diet, and as much as 55% of their early spring diet. The stomachs of some individuals were found to contain nothing but millipeds (KALMBACH and GABRIELSON, 1921). CLOUDSLEY-THOMPSON (1949), KINKEL (1955), and VERHOEFF (1928) found *Bufo* to take polydesmoid and juloid millipeds in the laboratory, a finding in line with the reported presence of diplopods in stomach contents of toads (KIRKLAND, 1904). Tests in our own laboratories (EISNER, T., unpublished; KAFATOS, 1961) have shown *Bufo cognatus* to take polydesmoid, juloid, and small spiroboloid millipeds readily, provided they flip them into the mouth and swallow them in one quick action. If the milliped was taken into the mouth crosswise so that considerable mouthing was required to reorient it in anticipation of swallowing, it was often rejected (Fig. 13 A). The reorientation, it seems, gives the milliped time to repel the toad by discharging its glands, something that it is not quick enough to do when it is simply gulped down. That anurans are indeed topically sensitive to milliped secretions, or at least their components, was readily evidenced by the scratch reflexes that they performed in response to topical application of benzaldehyde, o-cresol, and especially benzoquinones. Amphibia may not only be enterically tolerant of milliped secretions, but perhaps even somewhat systemically tolerant.

Injection of quinonoid secretion from juloid millipeds into frogs is said to have had no effect (KINKEL, 1955; PHISALIX, 1900).

Some predators appear to feed selectively on the glandless portions of millipeds, wasteful as this procedure may seem. In a wooded region near Ithaca, N.Y. (Taughannock State Park), where the spiroboloid *Narceus annularis* was occasionally very abundant and active in large numbers on the soil surface at night, we found on several consecutive dawns when we visited the site, the decapitated and still writhing bodies of dozens of these millipeds. Only the head and the few glandless postcephalic segments had been eaten (Fig. 13C). The suspected rodent responsible was never caught. Shrews (*Blarina brevicauda*) and field mice (*Peromyscus leucopus*) that were trapped in the area and tested in the laboratory, either ignored the millipeds, or if they attacked and killed them, found themselves repelled by the secretion as they bit into their bodies (Fig. 13D). "Robespierre", as we named the "culprit" (if indeed there was only one), remained a mysterious stranger (EISNER, T. and DEAN, J., unpublished).

A question of some interest concerns the millipeds' apparent insensitivity to their own secretions. HALL et al. (1971) have investigated this problem in *Euryurus leachii* and *Pleuroloma flavipes*, two cyanogenetic polydesmoid millipeds. These animals are highly resistant to hydrogen cyanide vapors. The insensitivity is not attributable to failure of hydrogen cyanide to penetrate the millipeds, or to an ability of these animals to tolerate anaerobiosis. The millipeds have a high systemic tolerance of injected cyanide, about 5−10 times the tolerance of cockroaches, and 30−6000 times the tolerance of mammals. The mitochondrial respiration is itself cyanide resistant in these animals. Whether this resistance is attributable to presence of excess cytochrome oxidase or an abnormally resistant terminal oxidase could not be distinguished with certainty, although the evidence favors the presence of a resistant oxidase.

E. Implications to Humans

Milliped secretions are not much of a hazard to humans. The substances are not injected, and contact with them, as a rule, is likely to cause more annoyance than harm, if indeed it is troublesome at all. Encounters with millipeds are likely to be fortuitous rather than commonplace, since most species are rather secretive in their habits. The more powerful irritating secretions, such as the quinonoid fluids, which some species are capable of spraying, can be the source of considerable pain if they impinge upon the eyes, but even these relatively severe effects are reportedly transient in humans (HANEVELD, 1958; LOOMIS, 1936). Indigenous populations are sometimes said to fear such species (BURTT, 1947; HANEVELD, 1958; KEEGAN, 1963; KOPSTEIN, 1932). On body skin, quinonoid secretions usually induce no more than local discoloration due to tanning, although "smarting", irritation, and a skin eruption have been reported (BURTT, 1938; HALSTEAD and RYCKMAN, 1949; WOOD et al., 1975). Wound contamination with milliped secretion reportedly induced a rash (VERHOEFF, 1928). More massive exposure to quinonoid secretion, resulting from the placement of a large African milliped in a hip pocket, caused inflammation and ulceration (BURTT, 1947). Spraying millipeds have been blamed for blindness of a dog (reference in Haneveld, 1958), and of chickens in Haiti (Loomis, 1936). The presumption that millipeds can parasitize the mammalian digestive tract is contraindicated by the findings of Penteado and Maugé (1974). Verhoeff (1928) and Kopstein (1932) called attention to the use of exotic millipeds for preparation of arrow poisons. Pallares (1946) isolated a cyanohydrin glucoside from body extracts of a polydesmoid milliped used for this purpose in Mexico.

F. Other Defenses of Millipeds

Defensive glands are not the only protective means of millipeds. Many are endowed with an extraordinarily tough integument, which may render them impregnable to some predators. Their resistance to compression may be considerable (Schild-knecht and Wenneis, 1966; Verhoeff, 1928). A 4 mg juloid (*Blaniulus*) can withstand 25,000 times its own weight (100 g) without being crushed (Kinkel, 1955). Special behavioral adaptations also contribute to defense. Many species become immobile when disturbed. Some respond to contact by simply halting in their tracks, a maneuver that can cause ants to ignore them (Eisner et al., 1963b). Coiling, either partial, with just the front end bent backward beneath the body, or total, with the entire body coiled into a flat spiral, is also a common stratagem (Eisner and Eisner, 1965; Eisner et al., 1963b; Kinkel, 1955; Verhoeff, 1928). Members of the Glomerida and Sphaerotheriida coil into a smooth tight sphere which predators may have difficulty grasping and crushing (Eisner and Davis, 1967; Schildknecht et al., 1967). The large African Sphaerotheriida lack glands and are particularly tough. Despite this armor, banded mongoose feed on the millipeds by hurling them backward between their hind legs and smashing them against an appropriately hard surface (Eisner and Davis, 1967; Eisner, 1968). Some millipeds wiggle when disturbed (Verhoeff, 1928), and there are even certain African Stemmiulida that jump. These remarkable animals effect their escape by combining a relatively quick gait with intermittent hops (Evans and Blower, 1973). A diversity of species defecate when handled (Lawrence, 1966; Verhoeff, 1928; Eisner, T. personal observation), a relatively common arthropodan (and particularly insectan) response, presumed to be defensive (Eisner, 1970). Some millipeds, particularly polydesmoids, are gaudily colored and clearly aposematic, at least when exposed in daylight. Other species, which are luminescent (Cook, 1900; Davenport et al., 1952), may essentially be nocturnally aposematic. In *Motyxia sequoiae,* a polydesmoid (cyanogenetic) species, the lumiscence is green (maximum emission 495 nm) and continuous (Hastings and Davenport, 1957), and the animals are clearly conspicuous on the open ground where they are active at night.

Some milliped secretions, particularly the benzoquinones, are relatively powerful antibiotics (Geiger, 1946). The possibility that vapors leaking from the defensive glands may act in some adaptive capacity to provide asepsis in the immediate environment of a milliped, perhaps at times when it is relatively sedentary, has been entertained, but not fully substantiated (Kafatos, 1961). The possibility has also been investigated that millipeds might impregnate their egg capsules with antimicrobial agents. These capsules, in which the emerged young spend the early part of their existence, are moulded primarily of soil and vegetable debris, and built with apparent addition of maternal enteric constituents, both oral and aboral in origin (Loomis, 1933; Shaw, 1966). No antibacterial or antifungal activity could be detected in extracts of egg capsules of *Glomeris marginata* or *Narceus annularis* (Eisner et al., 1970). However, antifungal activity is reported from the liquid excrement of an Indian milliped, *Cingalobolus bugnioni* (Rajulu, 1968).

Finally, attention should be called to the elaborate bristles on the bodies of the aberrant millipeds of the order Polyxenida, a group that may well deserve class status separate from the Diplopoda. It has been suggested, without evidence, that the bristles are protective against predation (Donisthorpe, 1927; Verhoeff, 1928). Whether they function as detachable entangling devices, as do the somewhat similar bristles of dermestid beetle larvae (Nutting and Spangler, 1969), remains to be determined.

Acknowledgements: This paper is dedicated to Dr. Hans E. Eisner, who collaborated in many of our joint studies of millipeds. Our work on the general subject of arthropod secretions has been supported by grants AI-02908 and AI-12020 from the National Institutes of Health, and grant BMS-74-15084 from the National Science Foundation. We thank Dr. Richard L. Hoffman, Radford College, Radford, Virginia for expert advice on millipeds and for comments on and criticism of the manuscript. Our colleague, W.T. Keeton, Jr., has offered helpful suggestions. Some of our studies of millipeds were done at the Archbold Biological Station, Lake Placid, Florida, and the Huyck Preserve, Rensselaerville, N.Y. We thank the late Mr. Richard Archbold, and Dr. Robert Dalgleish, the directors of these facilities, for their hospitality and kindness.

Note added in proof: Since the completion of this review, the defensive secretions of seventeen species of polydesmoid millipeds have been described (Duffey et al., 1977). Eleven of these species were found to produce benzoyl cyanide (XV).

References

Altman, P.L., Dittmer, D.S.: Biology Data Book. 2nd Ed. Bethesda, Md: Fed. of Amer. Socs. for Exp. Biol., 1973, Vol. II, Sect. 80, Part I.

Armarego, W.L.F.: Quinazolines. In: Advances in Heterocyclic Chemistry (Katritzky, A.R. ed.), New York, Academic Press, 1963, Vol. I, pp. 253—309.

Barbetta, M., Casnati, G., Pavan, M.: Sulla presenza di D-(+)-mandelonitrile nella secrezione difensiva del miriapode *Gomphodesmus pavani* Dem. Mem. Soc. Entomol. Ital. **45**, 169—176 (1966).

Barbier, M.: Séparations de p-benzoquinones naturelles par chromatoplaques. J. Chromat. **2**, 649—651 (1959).

Barbier, M., Lederer, E.: On the benzoquinones of the venom of three species of myriapods. Biokhimiya **22**, 221—225 (1957).

Barth, R.: Microanatomia e citologia das glandulas penconhentas de *Rhinocricus padbergii* (Diplopoda). Mem. Inst. Osw. Cruz **65**, 175—195 (1967).

Béhal, A., Phisalix, M.C.: La quinone, principe actif du vénin du *Julus terrestris*. C. R. Soc. Biol. (Paris) **52**, 1036—1038 (1900).

Ben-Yehoshua, S., Conn, E.E.: Biosynthesis of prunasin, the cyanogenic glycoside of peach. Plant Physiol. **39**, 331—333 (1964).

Blum, M.S., MacConnell, J.G., Brand, J.M., Duffield, R.M., Fales, H.M.: Phenol and benzaldehyde in the defensive secretion of a strongylosomid milliped. Ann. entomol. Soc. Amer. **66**, 235 (1973).

Blum, M.S., Woodring, J.P.: Secretion of benzaldehyde and hydrogen cyanide by the millipede *Pachydesmus crassicutis* (Wood). Science **138**, 512—513 (1962).

Brandt, J.F.: Rapport préalable relatif aux recherches ultérieures sur l'histoire, l'anatomie et la physiologie des Glomerides. Bull. Acad. Imp. Sci. St. Petersbourg **6**, 152—155 (1839).

Bull, L.B., Culvenor, C.C.J., Dick, A.T.: The Pyrrolizidine Alkaloids. Amsterdam: North-Holland Publishing Company, 1968.

Burtt, E.: Irritant exudation from a millipede. Nature (Lond.) **142**, 796 (1938).

Burtt, E.: Exudate from millipedes with particular reference to its injurious effects. Trop. Dis. Bull. **44**, 7—12 (1947).

Casnati, G., Nencini, G., Quilico, A., Pavan, M., Ricca, A., Salvatori, T.: The secretion of the myriapod *Polydesmus collaris collaris* (Koch). Experentia (Basel) **19**, 409—415 (1963).

Chakravarti, D., Chakravarti, R.N., Cohen, L.A., Dasgupta, B., Datta, S., Miller, H.K.: Alkaloids of *Glycosmis arborea* II. Structure of arborine. Tetrahedron **16**, 224 (1961).

Chamberlin, R.V.: Results of the Bryant Walker Expeditions of the University of Michigan to Colombia, 1913, and British Guiana, 1914. The Diplopoda. Occ. Papers Mus. Zool. Univ. Michigan **133**, 1—142 (1923a).

Chamberlin, R.V.: On four termitophilous millipedes from British Guiana. Zoologica **3**, 411—421 (1923b).

Cloudsley-Thompson, J.L.: The enemies of myriapods. Naturalist **831**, 137—141 (1949).

Conn, E.E., Butler, G.W.: The biosynthesis of cyanogenic glycosides and other simple nitrogen compounds. In: Perspectives in Phytochemistry (Harborne, J.B., Swain, T., eds.), pp. 47—74. New York: Academic Press, 1969.

Conner, W.E., Jones, T.H., Eisner, T., Meinwald, J.: Benzoyl cyanide in the defensive secretion of polydesmoid millipeds. Experientia (Basel) **33**, 206 (1977).

Cook, O.F.: Camphor secreted by an animal (*Polyzonium*). Science N.S. **12**, 516—521 (1900).

Coolidge, K.R.: Secretion of hydrocyanic acid by *Leptodesmus haydenianus*, Wood. Canad. Entomol. **41**, 104 (1909).

Davenport, D., Wootton, D.M., Cushing, J.E.: The biology of the Sierra luminous millipede, *Luminodesmus sequoiae*, Loomis and Davenport. Biol. Bull. **102**, 100—110 (1952).

Dohle, W.: Die Embryonalentwicklung von *Glomeris marginata* (Villers) im Vergleich zur Entwicklung anderer Diplopoden. Zool. Jb. Anat. **81**, 241—310 (1964).

Donisthorpe, H. St. J. K.: The Guests of British Ants, their Habits and Life Histories. London: Routledge, 1927.

Duffey, S.S., Blum, M.S., Fales, H.M., Evans, S.L., Roncadori, R.W., Tiemann, D.L., Nakagawa, Y.: Benzoyl cyanide and mandelonitrile benzoate in the defensive secretions of millipedes. J. Chem. Ecol. **3**, 101—113 (1977).

Duffield, R.M., Blum, M.S., Brand, J.M.: Guaicol in the defensive secretions of polydesmid millipedes. Ann. entomol. Soc. Amer. **67**, 821—822 (1974).

Effenberger, W.: Beiträge zur Kenntnis der Gattung *Polydesmus*. Z. Naturwiss. Jena **44**, 527—586 (1909).

Eisner, H.E., Alsop, D.W., Eisner, T.: Defense mechanisms of arthropods. XX. Quantitative assessment of hydrogen cyanide production in two species of millipedes. Psyche **74**, 107—117 (1967).

Eisner, H.E., Eisner, T., Hurst, J.J.: Hydrogen cyanide and benzaldehyde produced by millipedes. Chem. and Ind. 124—125 (1963).

Eisner, H.E., Wood, W.F., Eisner, T.: Hydrogen cyanide production in North American and African polydesmoid millipedes. Psyche **82**, 20—23 (1975).

Eisner, T.: Mongoose and millipedes. Science **160**, 1367 (1968).

Eisner, T.: Chemical defense against predation in arthropods. In: Chemical Ecology (Sondheimer, E., and Simeone, J.B. eds.), pp. 157—217. New York: Academic Press, 1970.

Eisner, T., Davis, J.A.: Mongoose throwing and smashing millipedes. Science **155**, 577—579 (1967).

Eisner, T., Eisner, H.E.: Mystery of a millipede. Nat. Hist. **74**, 30—37 (1965).

Eisner, T., Eisner, H.E., Hurst, J.J., Kafatos, F.C., Meinwald, J.: Cyanogenic glandular apparatus of a millipede. Science **139**, 1218—1220 (1963a).

Eisner, T., Hendry, L.B., Meinwald, J.: 2,5-Dichlorophenol (from ingested herbicide?) in defensive secretion of grasshopper. Science **172**, 277—278 (1971).

Eisner, T., Hurst, J.J., Keeton, W.T., Meinwald, Y.: Defense mechanisms of arthropods. XVI. Para-benzoquinones in the secretion of spirostreptoid millipedes. Ann. entomol. Soc. Amer. **58**, 247−248 (1965).

Eisner, T., Hurst, J.J., Meinwald, J.: Defense mechanisms of arthropods. XI. The structure, function, and phenolic secretions of the glands of a chordeumoid millipede and a carabid beetle. Psyche **70**, 94−116 (1963b).

Eisner, T., Johnessee, J.S., Carrel, J., Hendry, L.B., Meinwald, J.: Defensive use by an insect of a plant resin. Science **184**, 996−999 (1974).

Eisner, T., Meinwald, J.: Defensive secretions of arthropods. Science **153**, 1341−1350 (1966).

Eisner, T., Zahler, S.A., Carrel, J.E., Brown, D.J., Lones, G.W.: Absence of antimicrobial substances in the egg capsules of millipedes. Nature (Lond.) **225**, 661 (1970).

Evans, M.E.G., Blower, J.G.: A jumping millipede. Nature (Lond.) **246**, 427−428 (1973).

Feigel, F.: Spot Tests in Organic Analysis. New York: Elsevier, 1966.

Geiger, W.B.: The mechanism of the antibacterial action of quinones and hydroquinones. Arch. Biochem. **11**, 23−32 (1946).

Guldensteeden-Egeling, C.: Ueber Bildung von Cyanwasserstoffsäure bei einem Myriapoden. Pflügers Arch. ges. Physiol. **28**, 576−579 (1882).

Hall, F.R., Hollingworth, R.M., Shankland, D.L.: Cyanide tolerance in millipedes: comparison of respiration in millipedes and insects. Entomol. News **80**, 277−282 (1969).

Hall, F.R., Hollingworth, R.M., Shankland, D.L.: Cyanide tolerance in millipedes: the biochemical basis. Comp. Biochem. Physiol. **38B**, 723−737 (1971).

Halstead, B.W., Ryckman, R.: Injurious effects from contacts with millipedes. Med. Arts Sci. **3**, 16−18 (1949).

Haneveld, G.T.: Eye lesions caused by the exudate of tropical millipedes. I. Report on a case. Trop. geogr. Med. **10**, 165−167 (1958).

Hannum, C.A.: Anatomy of the millipede *Chonaphe armatus*. Publ. Puget Sound Biol. Sta. **5**, 109−123 (1926).

Hastings, J.W., Davenport, D.: The luminescence of the millipede, *Luminodesmus sequoiae*. Biol. Bull. **113**, 120−128 (1957).

Hoffman, R.L.: Myriapoda, exclusive of insecta. In: Treatise on Invertebrate Paleontology, Part R, Arthropoda 4 (Moore, R.C., ed.), pp. R572−R606. Boulder, Colo: Univ. of Kans. and Geol. Soc. Amer., 1969.

Hoffman-Ostenhof, O.: Mechanism of the antibiotic action of certain quinones. Science **105**, 549−550 (1947).

Jones, D.A., Parsons, J., Rothschild, M.: Release of hydrocyanic acid from crushed tissues of all stages in the life-cycle of species of the Zygaeninae (Lepidoptera). Nature (Lond.) **193**, 52−53 (1962).

Jones, T.H., Conner, W.E., Meinwald, J., Eisner, H.E., Eisner, T.: Benzoyl cyanide and mandelonitrile in the cyanogenetic secretion of a centipede. J. Chem. Ecol. **2**, 421−429 (1976).

Kaestner, A.: Invertebrate Zoology. New York: Interscience Publ., 1968, Vol. II.

Kafatos, F.C.: The chemical defense mechanisms of millipedes. Honors Thesis. Cornell Univ., Ithaca, N.Y. (1961).

Kalmbach, E.R., Gabrielson, I.N.: Economic value of the starling in the United States. Bull. U.S. Dep. Agric. **868**, 1−66 (1921).

Karrer, W.: Konstitution und Vorkommen der organischen Pflanzenstoffe, exkl. Alkaloide. Basel: Birkhäuser 1958.

Keegan, H.L.: Centipedes and millipedes as pests in tropical areas. In: Venomous and Poisonous Animals and Noxious Plants of the Pacific Region (Keegan, H.L. and MacFarlane, W.V., eds.), New York: Macmillan Co., 1963, pp. 161−163.

Kempf, W.W., Brown, W.L., Jr.: Two new ants of Tribe Ectatommini from Colombia (Hymenoptera: Formicidae). Stud. entomol. **13**, 311−320 (1970).

Kinkel, H.: Zur Biologie und Ökologie des getüpfelten Tausendfusses *Blaniulus guttulatus* Gerv. Z. angew. Entomol. **37**, 401−436 (1955).

Kirkland, A.H.: Usefulness of the American toad. U.S. Dept. Agr. Farmer's Bull., 196 (1904).

Kluge, A.F., Eisner, T.: Defense mechanisms of arthropods. XXVIII. A quinone and a phenol in the defensive secretion of a parajulid milliped. Ann. entomol. Soc. Amer. **64**, 314−315 (1971).

Kopstein, F.: Die Gifttiere Java's und ihre Bedeutung für den Menschen. Med. v. d. Dienst. d. Volksgezondheid in Ned. Indie. **21**, 222—256 (1932).

Lawrence, R.F.: The Myriapoda of the Kruger National Park. Zool. afr. **2**, 225—262 (1966).

Leidy, J.: On the characters and intimate structure of the odoriferous glands of the Invertebrata. Proc. Philad. Acad. nat. Sci. **4**, 234—236 (1849).

Lister, M.: Extract of a letter from Dr. Martin Lister, Jan. 25, 1670—71, relating partly to the same argument with that of the former letter, and alluding to another insect likely to yield an acid liquor; and partly to the bleeding of the sycamore. Phil. Trans. **5**, 556—558 (1670).

Loomis, H.F.: Egg-laying habits and larval stages of a milliped *Arctobolus marginatus* (Say) Cook, native at Washington. J. Wash. Acad. Sci. **23**, 100—101 (1933).

Loomis, H.F.: The millipeds of Hispaniola, with descriptions of a new family, new genera, and new species. Bull. Mus. Comp. Zool. Harvard **80**, 1—191 (1936).

Loomis, H.F.: New genera and species of millipeds from the southern peninsula of Haiti. J. Wash. Acad. Sci. **31**, 188—195 (1941).

McAtee, W.L.: Effectiveness in nature of the so-called protective adaptations in the animal kingdom, chiefly as illustrated by the food habits of nearctic birds. Smithsonian Inst. Misc. Coll. **85**, 22 (1932).

McFadden, W.H.: Techniques of Combined Gas Chromatography/Mass Spectrometry. New York: Wiley-Interscience, 1973.

Meinwald, J., Smolanoff, J., McPhail, A., Miller, R., Eisner, T. and Hicks, K.: Nitropolyzonamine: a spirocyclic nitro compound from the defensive glands of a milliped (*Polyzonium rosalbum*). Tetrahedron Lett. no. 28, 2367—2370 (1975).

Meinwald, Y.C., Meinwald, J., Eisner, T.: 1,2-Dialkyl-4(3H)-quinazolinones in the defensive secretion of a millipede (*Glomeris marginata*). Science **154**, 390—391 (1966).

Monro, A., Chadha, M., Meinwald, J., Eisner, T.: Defense mechanisms of arthropods. VI. Para-benzoquinones in the secretion of five species of millipedes. Ann. entomol. Soc. Amer. **55**, 261—262 (1962).

Monteiro, H.: Constituents of the secretion of *Orthomorpha coarctata* Schubart. An. Ass. bras. Quim. **20**, 29—31 (1961).

Moore, B.P.: Hydrogen cyanide in the defensive secretions of larval Paropsini (Coleoptera: Chrysomelidae). J. Aust. entomol. Soc. **6**, 36—38 (1967).

Moussatché, H., Lopez Cuadra, J., Ramos, P.R., Perissé, A.C.M.: Pharmacological experiments with benzoquinones. Rev. bras. Biol. **27**, 369—379 (1967).

Moussatché, H., Lopez Cuadra, J., Ramos, P.R., Perissé, A.C.M., Salles, C.A., Loureiros, E.G.: Chemistry and pharmacology of the venomous secretion of Rhinocricus varians. Rev. bras. Biol. **29**, 25—34 (1969).

Nutting, W.L., Spangler, H.G.: The hastate setae of certain dermestid larvae: an entangling defense mechanism. Ann. entomol. Soc. Amer. **62**, 763—769 (1969).

Pallares, E.S.: Note on the poison produced by the *Polydesmus (Fontaria) vicinus,* Lin. Arch. Biochem. **9**, 105—108 (1946).

Penteado, C.H.S., Maugé, G.D.: Tentativa de infestação do trato alimentar de cães pelo diplópode *Rhinocricus padbergi,* Verhoeff. Rev. bras. Pesquisas Med. Biol. **7**, 29—35 (1974).

Percy, J.E., Weatherston, J.: Studies of physiologically active arthropod secretions. V. Histological studies of the defence mechanism of *Narceus annularis* (Raf.) (Diplopoda: Spirobolida). Canad. J. Zool. **49**, 278—279 (1971).

Perissé, A.C.M., Salles, C.A.: Estudo químico de Diplopoda Brasileiros. III. *Collostreptus fulvus* (Schubart, 1960). Atas Soc. Biol. Rio de Janeiro **13**, 95—99 (1970).

Perissé, A.C.M., Salles, C.A., Moussatché, H.: Estudo químico de Diplopoda Braileiros II. *Spirostrophus naresi* (Pocock). Atas Soc. Biol. Rio de Janeiro **12**, 155—156 (1968).

Phisalix, M.C.: Un venin volatil. Secretion cutanée du *Julus terrestris.* C. R. Soc. Biol. (Paris) **70**, 1033—1036 (1900).

Phisalix, M.C.: Animaux Venimeux et Venins Vol. I. Paris: Masson, 1922.

Plattner, H., Salpeter, M., Carrel, J.E., Eisner, T.: Struktur and Funktion des Drüsenepithels der postabdominalen Tergite von *Blatta orientalis.* Z. Zellforsch. **125**, 45—87 (1972).

Potter, V.R.: The inhibition of sulphydryl-containing enzymes by split products of p-dimethyl-aminobenzene. Cancer Res. **2**, 688—693 (1942).

Rajulu, G.S.: Occurrence of an antimicrobial substance in the excrement of egg-laying millipedes *Cingalobolus bugnioni*. Sci. and Cult. **35**, 116 (1968).

Rettenmeyer, C.W.: The behavior of millipedes found with neotropical army ants. J. Kans. Entomol. Soc. **35**, 377—384 (1962).

Rimsky-Korsakow, M.: Über *Polyzonium germanicum* Brandt. Trav. Soc. imp. Nat. St. Petersbourg **25**, 21—28 (1895).

Rivers, J.J.: Description of the form of the female in a lampyrid (*Zarhipis riversi* Horn). Amer. Naturalist **20**, 648—650 (1886).

Rossi, G.: Le glandole odorifere dell' *Julus communis*. Z. wiss. Zool. **74**, 64—80 (1903).

Roth, L.M., Stay, B.: The occurrence of para-quinones in some arthropods, with emphasis on the quinone-secreting tracheal glands of *Diploptera punctata* (Blattaria). J. Insect Physiol. **1**, 305—318 (1958).

Sachtleben, H.: Untersuchungen über die Nahrung des Maulwurfs. Arb. biol. Reichsanstalt Land- u. Forstwirtschaft Berlin **14**, 77—96 (1926).

Savi, P.: Bemerkungen über *Julus communis*. Isis **12** and **13**, 214—222 (1823).

Schildknecht, H., Krämer, H.: Zum Nachweis von Hydrochinonen neben Chinonen in den Abwehrblasen von Arthropoden. XV. Mitteilung über Insekten-Abwehrstoffe. Z. Naturforsch. **17b**, 701—702 (1962).

Schildknecht, H., Maschwitz, U., Krauss, D.: Blausäure im Wehrsekret des Erdläufers *Pachymerium ferrugineum*. Naturwissenschaften **55**, 230 (1968).

Schildknecht, H., Maschwitz, U., Wenneis, W.F.: Neue Stoffe aus dem Wehrsekret der Diplopodengattung *Glomeris*. Über Arthropoden-Abwehrstoffe. XXIV. Naturwissenschaften **54**, 196—197 (1967).

Schildknecht, H., Weis, K.H.: Chinone als aktives Prinzip der Abwehrstoffe von Diplopoden. Z. Naturforsch. **16b**, 810—816 (1961).

Schildknecht, H., Wenneis, W.F.: Über Arthropoden-(Insekten) Abwehrstoffe. XX. Structuraufklärung des Glomerins. Z. Naturforsch. **21b**, 552—556 (1966).

Schildknecht, H., Wenneis, W.F.: Über Arthropoden-Abwehrstoffe. XXV. Anthranilsäure als Precursor der Arthropoden-Alkaloide Glomerin und Homoglomerin. Tetrahedron Lett. **1967**, 1815—1818 (1967).

Schildknecht, H., Wenneis, W.F., Weis, K.H., Maschwitz, U.: Glomerin, ein neues Arthropoden-Alkaloid. Z. Naturforsch. **21b**, 121—127 (1966).

Schubart, O.: Diplopodos de Monte Alegre. Papéis Avulsos Departm. Zool. São Paulo **6**, . 283—320 (1945).

Schubart, O.: Os Diplopoda da viagen do naturalista Antenor Leitão de Carvalho aos rios Araguaia e Amazonas em 1939 e 1940. Boll. Mus. Nac. Zool. Rio de Janeiro **82**, 1—74 (1947).

Schubart, O.: Ameisen und Diplopoden in ihren gegenseitigen Beziehungen Rev. Entomol. **21**, 615—622 (1950).

Shaw, G.G.: New observations on reproductive behavior in the milliped *Narceus annularis* (Raf.). Ecology **47**, 322—323 (1966).

Silvestri, P.: Acari Myriapoda et Scorpiones: Classis Diplopoda. Vol. I. Portìcì., 1903.

Smolanoff, J., Demange, J.M., Eisner, T., Meinwald, J.: 1,4-Benzoquinones in African millipedes. Psyche **82**, 78—80 (1975b).

Smolanoff, J., Kluge, A.F., Meinwald, J., McPhail, A., Miller, R.W., Hicks, K., Eisner, T.: Polyzonimine: a novel terpenoid insect repellent produced by a milliped. Science **188**, 734—736 (1975a).

Stebbins, R.C.: Lizards killed by a millipede. Amer. Midl. Natur. **32**, 777—778 (1944).

Tapper, B.A., Zilg, H., Conn, E.E.: 2-Hydroxyaldoximes as possible precursors in the biosynthesis of cyanogenic glucosides. Phytochemistry **11**, 1047—1053 (1972).

Tiemann, D.L.: Observations on the natural history of the western banded glowworm *Zarhipis integripennis* (LeConte) (Coleoptera: Phengodidae). Proc. Calif. Acad. Sci. **35**, 235—264 (1967).

Towers, G.H.N., Duffey, S.S., Siegel, S.M.: Defensive secretion: biosynthesis of hydrogen cyanide and benzaldehyde from phenylalanine by a millipede. Canad. J. Zool. **50**, 1047—1050 (1972).

Trave, R., Garanti, L., Pavan, M.: Ricerche sulla natura chimica del veleno del miriapode *Archiulus (Schizophyllum) sabulosus* L. Chim. et Ind. **41**, 19—29 (1959).

Verhoeff, K.W.: Klasse Diplopoda. In: Klassen und Ordnungen des Tier-Reichs (Bronn, H.G. ed.), Vol. 5 Part II Section 1 (1—6). Leipzig: Akademische Verlagsgesellschaft, 1928.

Voges, E.: Beiträge zur Kenntnis der Juliden. Z. wiss. Zool. **31**, 127—194 (1878).

Weatherston, J., Gardiner, E.J.: The defensive secretion of a polydesmoid millipede (Diplopoda). Canad. Entomol. **105**, 1375—1376 (1973).

Weatherston, J., Percy, J.E.: Studies of physiologically active arthropod secretions. III. Chemical, morphological, and histological studies of the defence mechanism of *Uroblaniulus canadensis* (Say) (Diplopoda: Julida). Canad. J. Zool. **47**, 1389—1394 (1969).

Weatherston, J., Tyrrell, D., Percy, J.E.: Long-chain alcohol acetates in the defensive secretion of the millipede *Blaniulus guttulatus*. Chem. Phys. Lipids **7**, 98—100 (1971).

Weber, M.: Ueber eine Cyanwasserstoffsäure bereitende Drüse. Arch. mikr. Anat. **21**, 468—475 (1882).

Weddell, G., Miller, S.: Cutaneous sensibility. Ann. Rev. Physiol. **24**, 199—222 (1962).

Wheeler, J.W., Meinwald, J., Hurst, J.J., Eisner, T.: Trans-2-dodecenal and 2-methyl-1,4-quinone produced by a millipede. Science **144**, 540—541 (1964).

Wheeler, W.M.: Hydrocyanic acid secreted by *Polydesmus virginiensis*, Drury. Psyche **5**, 442 (1890).

Wheeler, W.M., Mann, W.M.: The ants of Haiti. Bull. Amer. Mus. Natur. His. **33**, 1—61 (1914).

Whittaker, R.H., Feeny, P.P.: Allelochemics: chemical interactions between species. Science **171**, 757—770 (1971).

Wood, H.C.: Description of new genera and species of North American Myriapoda. Proc. Philad. Acad. Nat. Sci. **16**, 186—187 (1864).

Wood, W.F.: Toluquinone and 2-methoxy-3-methylbenzoquinone from the defensive secretions of three African millipedes. Ann. entomol. Soc. Amer. **67**, 988—989 (1974).

Wood, W.F., Shepherd, J., Chong, B., Meinwald, J.: Ubiquinone-O in the defensive secretion of an African millipede. Nature (Lond.) **253**, 625—626 (1975).

Woodring, J.P., Blum, M.S.: The anatomy and physiology of the repugnatorial glands of *Pachydesmus crassicutus*. Ann. entomol. Soc. Amer. **56**, 448—453 (1963).

Woodring, J.P., Blum, M.S.: The anatomy, physiology and comparative aspects of the repugnatorial glands of *Orthocricus arboreus* (Diplopoda: Spirobolida). J. Morph. **116**, 99—108 (1965).

CHAPTER 4

Secretions of Centipedes

A. Minelli*

A. The Centipedes

Centipedes are a well-characterized group within the "myriapods." Since Pocock's
(1887, 1893a, 1893b) and Kingsley's (1888) papers, they are recognized as a
separate class, Chilopoda.

Centipedes have a more or less elongated, usually flattened body, from 3 to
250 mm in length. The body includes a head and a trunk. The head bears a
pair of sensory appendages, the antennae, the eyes (often lacking), and the mouthparts, i.e., the mandibles (jaws) and two pairs of maxillae. The first trunk-segment
(forcipular segment) bears a pair of biting appendages, the forcipules (or toxicog-
nathes) used both as offensive and defensive weapons; and each of the following
segments bear a pair of legs.

The class includes some 3000 known species (Schubart, 1960), classified into
four orders: Scutigeromorpha (the house centipede and its allies) with shorter
body, compound eyes, very elongated antennae and legs, and dorsally placed spiracles; Lithobiomorpha (the lithobiids and their allies, very common under stones
in the Northern hemisphere) with a medium long, more or less flattened body,
medium-sized legs and antennae; Scolopendromorpha (the scolopenders and the
eyeless cryptopids) with more elongated but stout body, shorter antennae and
legs; and Geophilomorpha (the geophilids), always eyeless, with very elongated,
often wormlike body, very short antennae and legs (Fig. 1). A single genus *Crateros-
tigmus* from Tasmania may need to be placed in a separate order. The number
of walking legs varies from 15 pairs (Scutigeromorpha, Lithobiomorpha) to 21−23
(Scolopendromorpha) to 33−177 pairs (Geophilomorpha). A modern, though pro-
visory, scheme of centipede classification is given by Anonymous (1974).

Centipedes live mostly under stones and bark or in the litter between fallen
leaves, where they prey upon smaller animals; some species are ruin- or cave-
dwellers. As predators, they possess a pair of venomous glands connected with
an effective injecting device, the forcipules. Their bite may be also of medical
importance, if we look at the consequences of biting by the bigger species, mostly
scolopendrids. In addition to this well-known weapon, centipedes do possess a
wide repertory of defensive chemicals in the form of sticking substances (Geophilomorpha, Lithobiomorpha), of venomous (Geophilomorpha), or repugnant (Scolopendromorpha, one species) secretions.

We shall review the topography and histology of the exocrine glands of

*Istituto di Biologia Animale, Università di Padova (Italia)

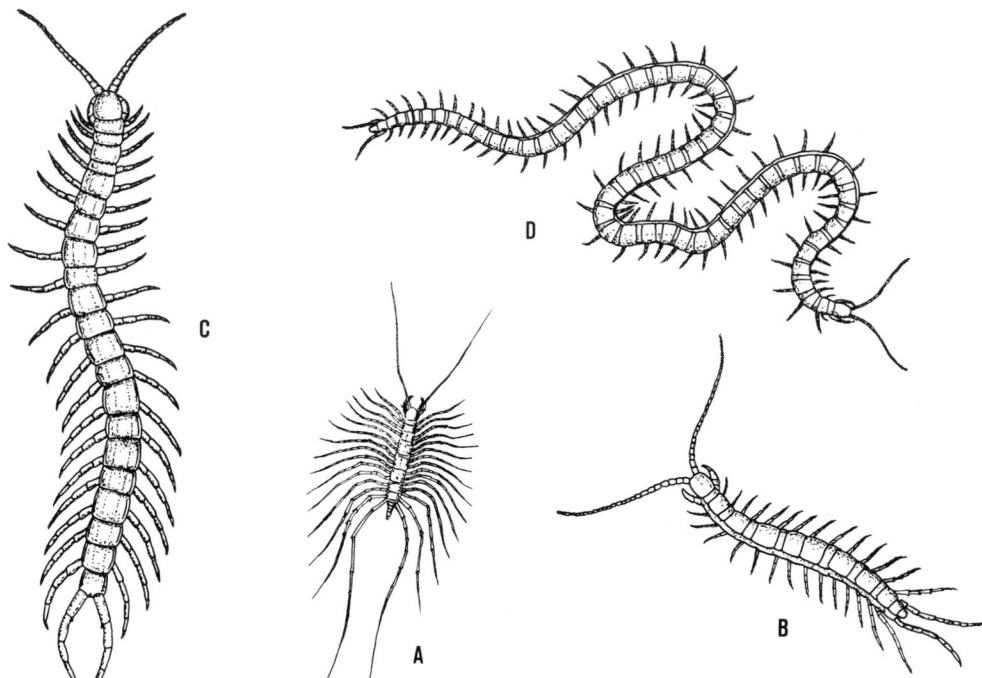

Fig. 1A–D. Habitus of scutigeromorph (A), lithobiomorph (B), scolopendromorph (C), and geophilomorph (D) (from various authors)

centipedes, the chemistry of the substances they produce, and the effects of these upon other animals, including man.

It is worth saying that we know very little about the nature of these substances, very few papers have appeared dealing with their chemistry or pharmacology. Our meager knowledge about these topics is only one aspect of our poor understanding of centipede biology. This may simply reflect the fact that centipedes are not arthropods of outstanding economic or medical importance.

In the modern literature we find very few papers dealing with the role of centipedes as predators in terrestrial ecosystems; on the other hand, most handbooks of medical entomology say very little about centipede secretions, whereas they give full account of the infrequent and little interesting cases of pseudoparasitism, centipedes having been occasionally found in the nose, in the frontal sinuses, in the external ear, or in the alimentary tract of humans (about 30 instances; for more comprehensive accounts see BLANCHARD, 1898, 1902; NEVEU-LEMAIRE 1907, 1938; GARZIA, 1938).

Large general works on centipede biology are very old (VERHOEFF, 1902–1925; ATTEMS, 1926); a short introduction to habits and behavior is given by CLOUDSLEY-THOMPSON (1958); a taxonomic account of the scolopendromorphs of medical importance is reported by BÜCHERL (1971).

B. Glands and Secretions

I. Defensive and Offensive Weapons of Centipedes

As opposed to millipedes, which as a rule are pacific devourers of decaying plant matter, centipedes are predators, often quite active and lively ones. We can also expect them to produce toxic, perhaps paralyzing substances to be injected into victims, but we do not expect they should discharge also smelling noxious secretions as those largely produced by millipedes (see EISNER et al., this volume). To a predator's survival a cryptic habit is of value; the hidden life is itself a mean for escaping predators and the offensive weapons may well be turned into defensive ones; occasionally, sticky or otherwise noxious secretions may occur, also provided they are not too diffusible or strong-smelling.

Such an expectation is well-fulfilled by centipedes, whose forcipules are always (with some reserve for the geophilids) the most valuable offensive and defensive weapon. Their nocturnal or subterranean life reduces the chance of meeting potential enemies and their numerous glands, distributed over the whole body, supply noxious or sticky (occasionally luminescent) secretions. However, an example of a centipede giving off a fetid odor when irritated is reported by LAWRENCE (1968) (see under V.IV.2).

II. Topography of the Exocrine Glands

It has been said (BLOWER, 1952) that "the epidermis of a centipede is virtually an epithelium of unicellular glands" in addition to which many groups of larger

Table 1. Occurrence of different exocrinous glands in the four orders of centipedes. (According to FAHLANDER, 1938; BLOWER, 1952; and others).

			Scutigeromorpha	Lithobiomorpha	Scolopendromorpha	Geophilomorpha
Unicellular glands		Head glands	+	+	+	+
		Ventral glands	−	−	−	+
		Telopodal glands	−	+	−	−
		Venom's glands	+	+	+	+
Multicellular glands	Anterior glands	Lateral buccal glands	+	+	+	−
		Medial buccal glands	+	+	+	±
		Mandibular glands	+	+	+	+
		I. Maxillar glands	+	−	−	−
		II. Maxillar glands	+	+	+	+
		Gl. of the Ist trunk segment	+	−	−	−
		Gl. of the IInd trunk segment	+	−	+	−
	Glands connected with genital apparatus		+	+	+	+
	Posterior glands	Coxal glands	−	+	+	+
		Anal glands	−	±	+	±

glands are distributed in different body districts. The histologic structure of the different glands and gland clusters seems to be quite uniform through the class.

According to their complexity, we can classify the exocrine glands of centipedes in two major classes: (1) unicellular glands and (2) multicellular glands. Each class includes, in turn, many groups of glands which can be arranged according to the body site. Their distribution and occurrence throughout the four orders of centipedes are summarized in Table 1.

In the following section we shall describe in some detail the venomous glands of the forcipular segment of all centipedes as well as the ventral and coxal glands of the geophilomorphs. For the other glands see Duboscq (1898) and Fahlander (1938).

III. Histology of the Glands

1. The Forcipular Gland (Fig. 2)

The venom's apparatus of a centipede consists of a pair of glands whose ducts open at the inner side of the apical segment of each forcipule, near its distal end, as first described by Newport (1844 – 1845). In most cases the gland occupies the proximal section of the appendage; in some genera, however, it is displaced backward: in the geophilid *Chaetechelyne vesuviana* Newp. the venom gland lies between the 12th and 18th trunk segment (Dubosq, 1896).

Histologic descriptions of the venom gland are given by Duboscq (1894, 1898), Pawlowsky (1913), Phisalix (1922), Bücherl (1946, 1971), and Barth (1967) for *Scolopendra* and allied genera; by Duboscq (1894, 1898) for *Cryptops, Lithobius, Scutigera, Chaetechelyne;* by Applegarth (1952) for *Pseudolithobius megaloporus* (Stuxberg). For details concerning the development of the forcipules and the forcipular glands see Heymons (1901).

The longitudinal axis of the gland is built up by the chitinous secretory duct which ends proximally in the shape of a porous bulb. As a rule, this bulb is little enlarged; however, size and shape may vary considerably within one genus (e.g., *Cryptops*) or even within one species (e.g., *C. parisi* Bröl.). Each porus receives the secretion of a glandular cell. As shown by Duboscq (1894) in *Scolopendra,* the bulb's surface is not uniformly porous: a stripe without pores runs on its external side: no glandular cells are lying along this stripe.

The glandular cells are radially arranged in a single layer around the chitinous duct. Their shape is pyramidal with the base lying on the basal membrane and the apex in contact with a porus. The nuclei are localized near the cell's base. The synthesis of the venom has been investigated by Duboscq (1894) and Launoy (1903). Launoy distinguished between (1) a nuclear secretive process, suggested *inter alia* by the increase in size of the nucleus; and (2) a subsequent cytoplasmic elaboration of the venom on the ergastoplasm. On the whole it is difficult to understand the secretory process along these old descriptions; we need observations involving histochemistry, electron microscopy, and autoradiography.

As shown by Pawlowsky (1913), the venom gland can be easily interpreted as an epithelial infolding whose specialized cells have all become secreting, whereas the invaginated cuticle has become the porous glandular duct.

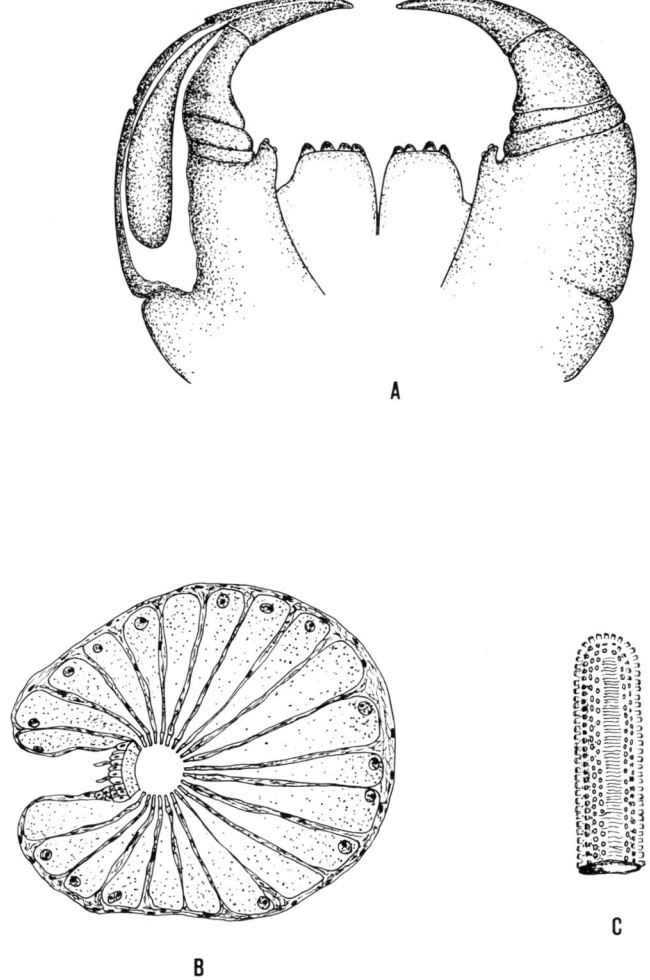

A

B

C

Fig. 2A–C. Forcipules and venom's gland of scolopender. A. Forcipules of *S. viridicornis* Leach, sectioned (*left*) to show venom's gland; B. Cross section of venom's gland of *S. cingulata* Latr.; C. Porous duct of venom's gland of same species (A after BÜCHERL, B and C after DUBOSCQ, all redrawn)

A sheath of striated muscular fibers envelops the gland; DUBOSCQ (1894) was able to distinguish there a superficial layer from a profound one.

2. Ventral and Coxal Glands of the Geophilomorphs

On the sternites of the geophilids there are large clusters of unicellular glands which open through characteristic porous plates whose form and arrangement along the ventral side vary greatly according to the genera and species. These glands were first illustrated by PASSERINI (1882) in *Geophilus Gabrielis* (now *Himantarium gabrielis* (L.), thereafter by DUBOSCQ (1896) in *C. vesuviana* Newp.

In the latter species the sternal plates are 0.2 mm in diameter; each plate is pierced by 100 — 300 pores 4 — 5 μm in diameter; in each pore a unicellular gland, up to 0.5 mm long opens. The secretion may occupy nine-tenths of the cell; the cytoplasm is reduced to a thin external layer. The glandular cells are surrounded by a connectival and muscular sheath to form a four-lobed gland mass.

The structure of the coxal glands of the geophilomorphs has been illustrated in some detail by TÖMÖSVÁRY (1885) for *G. flavidus* (now *Clinopodes flavidus* (C. Koch)).

These glands occupy the coxopleural region of the last legbearing segment and open through big cuticular pores at or near the coxae of the last pair of legs. Each gland is spherical or pear-shaped and consists of numerous elongated cells with a common secretory duct. The cell cluster is surrounded by a *tunica propria* perhaps identical with the basal membrane of the epithelium.

IV. Secretions

1. Sticky Secretions

Sticky secretions are produced by geophilomorphs and lithobiomorphs and are very useful to the centipedes as a defensive weapon against ants, carabid beetles, and other enemies (RIDLEY, 1936).

Geophilomorphs produce sticky secretions by means of the ventral glands as well as of the coxal glands of the last leg-bearing segment. The ventral secretion may be luminescent (see following section). In some species there are two "anal glands" near the anal opening. A first suggestion on the chemical nature and the possible meaning of the secretion was given by FANZAGO (1881), PASSERINI (1882), and TÖMÖSVÁRY (1885); subsequent accounts deal more with the luminescent properties of the secretion than with its sticking nature.

Sticky secretions are produced also by lithobiomorphs; very little is known about them. Ancient authors (WILLEM, 1897; VERHOEFF, 1902 — 1925; ATTEMS, 1926) said that the secretion is produced by the coxal glands (*glandes filières* of WILLEM, 1897, cfr. TÖMÖSVÁRY's *Spinndrüsen* = coxal glands of the geophilids). According to BLOWER (1952), this is incorrect, the secretion being produced by small glands placed on the femur, tibia, tarsus, and metatarsus of the last two pairs of legs; he calls them "telopodal glands." The secretion (BLOWER, 1952) appears to be a lipoid-protein complex.

Other arthropods and arthropodlike animals rely upon sticky secretions for defense. Two well-known examples are the pill millipedes (*Glomeris* spp.) (e.g., see EISNER and MEINWALD, 1966) and the onychophorans (e.g., see HOLLIDAY, 1942; EDWARDS, 1963): the latter use the secretion of the coxal glands also for prey immobilization.

A volatile compound found in the secretion of a geophilomorph, *Pachymerium ferrugineum* (Koch) is hydrocyanic acid (SCHILDKNECHT et al., 1968); this compound is a common defensive secretion of millipedes (EISNER et al., this volume). JONES et al. (1976) characterize the sticky and odorous secretion of *Geophilus vittatus* as proteinaceous and cyanogenetic. The secretion is shown to contain two cyanogenetic compounds, mandelonitrile and benzoyl cyanide, as well as two products derived from these compounds as a result of hydrogen cyanide production, i.e. benzaldehyde and benzoic acid.

2. Luminescent Secretions

HARVEY (1952) credits Oviedo as having first recorded a luminous centipede on the island of St. Domingo in 1520. The first modern accounts are those by DUBOIS (1886, 1887, 1893) on the geophilomorphs *Scolioplanes crassipes* (now *Strigamia crassipes* (Koch)) and *Orya barbarica* (F.)[1].

The subsequent bibliography on luminous centipedes and their luminescent secretions includes HUET (1886), MACE' (1886, 1887), BLANCHARD (1888), GAZAGNAIRE (1888, 1890), HAASE (1889), SINCLAIR (1895), THOMAS (1895, 1902), POCOCK (1896), BOZWARD (1896), PLOWMAN (1896), LUDWIG (1901), VERHOEFF (1902—25), BROCKHAUSEN (1903), HAUPT (1903), ROBERTS (1916), BRADE-BIRKS and BRADE-BIRKS (1920), HARVEY (1920, 1940, 1952), BUCHNER (1921), DAMMERMANN (1923), ARNDT (1924), ATTEMS (1926), KOCH (1927), PATTON (1931), STAMMER (1935), RIDLEY (1936), HANEDA (1939), AGUAYO (1951), GRUNER (1954), and ALLAN (1966).

The more interesting papers including histologic studies are those by BRADE-BIRKS and BRADE-BIRKS (1920) and KOCH (1927). A more recent and valuable complication is given by HARVEY (1952) who underlines the great incompleteness of our knowledge on the subject.

Luminescence occurs in many geophilomorphs; in addition, *Otostigmus aculeatus* Haase, a scolopendromorph occurring in Vietnam and other countries of Southeast Asia, is said by HOUDEMER (1926) and PATTON (1931) to emit "a phosphorescent vesicant fluid" causing painful blisters.

The light of the geophilids is undoubtedly due to chemiluminescence, but its chemistry is almost unknown.

A luminescent secretion is in fact produced by the ventral glands, opening in the sternites in genus- and species-specific arrangement. Histologic investigations have demonstrated the existence of two kinds of gland cells, opening on the ventral surface by separate pores; however, it is not clear whether the two kinds of cells are actually both involved in luminescence.

Geophilid luminescence may be used for protection against predators. Carabid beetles attacking geophilids have been recorded to be very intrigued by the ventral luminous secretion which is presumably noxious to them (RIDLEY, 1936).

3. Smelling Secretions

As reported by LAWRENCE (1968), the South African scolopendromorph *Cormocephalus nitidus* Porath gives off a fetid odor when irritated. The identity of the gland producing the secretion and its chemical nature are currently under investigation at the Rhodes University (LAWRENCE, personal communication).

---

[1] HARVEY credites PASSERINI (1882) as having studied the luminescence of *G. gabrielis*. This species, today placed in the genus *Himantarium*, does not seem to produce any luminescent secretion; the Italian entomologist described the ventral gland in that species as secreting a brightly colored and intensely smelling substance.

A more or less pleasant odor is perceived by humans when smelling the secretion of the ventral glands of some geophilomorphs but this smell is perhaps of little value to the centipede.

CLOUDSLEY-THOMPSON (1958) expresses the view that centipedes do not appear to be eaten by spiders and other predatory animals unless other food is lacking, because they are "probably distasteful." Centipedes are occasionally eaten by salamanders (AUERBACH, 1952), vipers (*Vipera ammodytes*) (CLARK, 1967), and flycatchers (*Muscicapa hypoleuca muscipeta*) (BERNDT and RAPSCH, 1958).

4. Venom of the Forcipular Glands

a) Effects of Bite on Humans

Scolopenders (*Scolopendra* spp.) biting humans are often recorded from tropical areas, more rarely from temperate ones. Many instances of death after scolopender bite have been reported in the older literature (e.g., FAUST, 1928); however, more recent authors (REMINGTON, 1950; BÜCHERL, 1946, 1971) are inclined to deny reliability to most reports, accepting as the unique authenticated example the death of a 7-years-old girl who was bitten on the head by a scolopender (perhaps *S. subspinipes* Leach) in the Philippines (see PINEDA, 1923; VENZMER, 1932; REMINGTON, 1950).

JOLIVET (1971) is correct in observing that the effect of scolopenders bites in tropical areas may vary very much, according to the animal species, the bitten person, and the body region affected.

Most authors agree in attributing to scolopenders' bite only a local effect, with erythema, edema, and a superficial necrosis which disappears in 1—3 weeks without cicatrizing (BÜCHERL, 1946; see also DUBOSCQ, 1894, 1898; PHISALIX, 1922; SCHNEE, 1911; BARTHMEYER and SCHMALFUSS, 1933; MACHADO, 1944; KEEGAN, 1963). A few more details are given be DE CASTRO (1921) who describes intense lymphangitis with edema as well as inflammation of the skin and subcutaneous tissues, which in some instances may progress to a condition resembling a phagedenic ulceration.

According to DUBOSCQ (1894, 1898), who studied *S. cingulata* Latr., the effect of the bite differs according to the season: winter (February) bites will cause a local burning distention which disappears within 1 h, whereas spring (March-April) bites will cause the characteristic painful inflammation and the distention described by many authors.

In some cases of repeated bites received by the same person (DUBOSCQ, 1894; SCHNEE, 1911) no immunity has been generally observed; however, some form of immunity seems to occur for the venom of an unidentified scolopendromorph common in the Barbados Islands (GARDNER, personal communication).

No serum has been envisaged against scolopender's venom (BÜCHERL, 1971).

As far as other centipede genera are concerned, our knowledge of the effects of their bites is far less than that for *Scolopendra*. However, it is certain that no other centipede is able to inflict very serious bites to humans, as confirmed by the observations concerning the following species:

Scolopendromorpha: *Theatops spinicauda* (Wood), body length 48 mm (BAERG, 1924); *Cryptops anomalans* Newp., body length 35 mm (MINELLI, unpublished observation).

Lithobiomorpha: *Polybothrus fasciatus* (now *Eupolybothrus fasciatus* (Newport)), body length 40 mm (ATTEMS, 1926); *Lithobius* sp. (WEBER, 1907).

Scutigeromorpha: *Scutigera coleoptrata* (L.) (often referred to as *Cermatia forceps* Raf. or *S. forceps* (Raf.)), body length 25 mm (KUNKEL D'HERCULAIS, 1911; EWING, 1928; HERMS, 1939; METCALFE and FLINT, 1951; JUDD, 1952).

For a full bibliography of envenomations by centipedes, see ROSENFELD and KELEN (1969).

b) Effects of Bite on Laboratory Animals

A scolopender's bite may be lethal to small mammals and birds. Among the published instances we may quote BRIOT (1904), according to whom the scolopender's bite may be lethal to the rabbit, and NORMAN (1897) who reports a scolopender from Texas killing mice but not small snakes and refusing to bite toads (whereas OKEDEN (1905) reports a scolopender eating a snake).

LD_{50} of scolopender venom injected in mice has been determined experimentally by BÜCHERL (1946) by employing five scolopendromorph species inhabiting Southern America. A crude venom preparation was obtained by crushing the venom gland in physiologic solution and then filtering the suspension. The more interesting results of the experiment are summarized in Table 2.

Other experimental researches have been carried out by LÉVY (1923a, 1923b, 1927a, 1927b) of different centipede species occurring in France (*S. coleptrata* (L.), *L. forficatus* (L.), *C. anomalans* Newp., *S. cingulata* Latr. and *H. gabrielis* (L.)). LÉVY did find hemolytic properties in the venom of the two scolopendromorphs, i.e., *C. anomalans* and *S. cingulata,* but was unable to demonstrate such properties in the venom of the other species. According to this author, the hemolytic properties, enhanced by addition of lecithin, are similar to those of the venom of cobra snakes. The hemolytic substance seems to be thermolabile.

Moreover, LÉVY demonstrated (1927b) that some centipedes are insensitive to their own venom: the blood (hemolymph) of *L. forficatus* seems to have antitoxic properties against the venom of the same species and that of *C. anomalans.*

Table 2. LD_{50} of venom of some scolopendromorphs for adult mice (body weight 20 g) expressed as number of individual glands killing half of tested animals (From BÜCHERL, 1946)

Species	Body length of centipede (cm)	Median lethal dose	
		Intra-venously	Intra-muscularly
Scolopendra viridicornis Newp.	16 — 19	0.030	0.250
S. subspinipes Leach	11 — 18	0.047	1.2
Otostigmus scabricauda Humb. & Sass.	6 — 7	0.012	0.070
Cryptops iheringi Bröl.	6 — 9	0.150	0.340
Scolopocryptops ferrugineus ferrugineus (L.)	5 — 7	0.160	0.390

Observations carried out by Bücherl (1946) on mice, where the bite of scolopenders causes death from respiratory paralysis and tetanus, suggest a neurotoxic effect of the venom.

c) Chemistry of the Venom

The chemistry of centipede venom is virtually unknown. A very old paper by Cornwall (1916) records the production of an "anticoagulin" and of various substances with enzymatic properties by the Indian scolopendromorph *Ethmostigmus spinosus* (Newp.).

In a recent paper the presence of 5-hydroxytryptamine in the venom of *S. viridicornis* Newp. is reported (Welsh and Batty, 1963; see also Pavan and Valcurone Dazzini, 1971). This widely distributed substance has been also found in other glands related to biting and feeding, namely in the salivary glands of cephalopods (e.g., *Octopus vulgaris,* see Erspamer and Asero, 1953). This may indirectly confirm the hypothesis that the venom of centipedes is primarily connected with prey immobilization and feeding (see also Freyvogel, 1972).

Acknowledgements: The author is indebted to prof. R.F. Lawrence (Grahamstown, S. Africa) and Dr. K.H. Gardner (Cape Town, S. Africa) for supply of unpublished observations, to Prof. S. Bettini (Rome, Italy) for bibliographicall aid and to Prof. F. Ghiretti and P. Omodeo (Padova, Italy) for a critical reading of the manuscript.

References

Aguayo, C.G.: Lamparas aimmadas. Boll Hist. nat. Soc., la Habana, **2**, 61−80 (1951).

Allan, P.B.M.: The Ignis fatuus. Entomologist's Rec. J. Var., **78**, 104 (1966).

Anonymous: Classification of the myriapoda. In: Myriapoda. Blower, J.G. (Ed.) Symp. zool. Soc. London, **32**, 709−712 1974.

Applegarth, A.G.: The anatomy of the cephalic region of a centipede, *Pseudolithobius megaloporus* (Stuxberg) (Chilopoda). Microentomology, **17**, 127−171 (1952).

Arndt, W.: Leuchtende Tausendfüsse in Schlesien. Jhr. Ver. Schles. Insektenk., **14**, 31−33 (1924).

Attems, C.: Chilopoda. In: Handbuch der Zoologie. Kükenthal, W. and Krumbach, Th. (Eds.) Bd. 4 (1). Berlin-Leipzig: De Gruyter 1926.

Auerbach, S.I.: Centipedes in the diet of salamanders. Nat. Hist. Misc., **103**, 1−2 (1952).

Baerg, W.J.: The effect of the venom of some supposedly poisonous Arthropods (Centipedes and Scorpions). J. Entomol. Soc. Amer. **17**, 343−352 (1924).

Barth, R.: Histologische Studien an den Giftdrüsen von *Scolopendra viridicornis* Newp. An. Acad. bras. Cienc. **39**, 179−193 (1967).

Barthmeyer, A., Schmalfuss, H.: Tausendfussbiss-Vergiftung. In: Samml. Vergiftungsf. **4**, 209−210 (1933).

Berndt, R., Rapsch, I.: Materialien zur Kenntnis der Ernährungsweise des Trauerschnäppers (*Muscicapa hypoleuca muscipeta* Bechstein) im Kiefernforst. Anz. Schädlingsk., **31**, 24−27 (1958).

Blanchard, M.R.: Sur la phosphorescence de *Geophilus*. Bull. Soc. Zool. Fr., **13**, 186 (1888).

Blanchard, R.: Sur le pseudo-parasitisme des Myriapodes chez l'homme. Arch. parasit., **1**, 452−490 (1898).

Blanchard, R.: Nouvelles observations sur le pseudo-parasitisme des Myriapodes chez l'homme. Arch. parasit., **6**, 245−256 (1902).

Blower, G.: Epidermal glands in centipedes. Nature (Lond.) **170**, 166—167 (1952).

Bozward, J.L.: A luminous centipede. Nature (Lond.) **53**, 223 (1896).

Brade-Birks, H.K., Brade-Birks, S.G.: Notes on Myriapoda. XX. Luminous Chilopoda, with special reference to *Geophilus carpophagus,* Leach. Ann. Mag. nat. Hist., (9) **5**, 1—30 (1920).

Briot, A.: Sur le venin des Scolopendres. C.R. Soc. Biol. (Paris) **57**, 476—477 (1904).

Brockhausen, H.: Über leuchtende Skolopender. Jh. Westfal. Ver., **31**, 163—164 (1903).

Buchner, P.: Tier und Pflanze in intrazellularer Symbiose. Berlin: Bornträger 1921.

Bücherl, W.: Açâo do veneno dos Escolopendromorfos do Brasil sobre alguns animais de laboratorio. Mem. Inst. Butantan, **19**, 181—197 (1946).

Bücherl, W.: Venomous Chilopods or Centipedes. In: Venomous animals and their venoms. Bücherl, W. and Buckley, E.E. (eds.). New York-London: Acad. Press, **3**, 169—196 (1971).

Clark, R.J.: Centipede in stomach of young *Vipera ammodytes meridionalis.* Copeia, **1967**, 224 (1967).

Cloudsley-Thompson, S.L.: Spiders, Scorpions, Centipedes and Mites. The Ecology and Natural History of Woodlice, "Myriapods" and Arachnids. London: Pergamon Press 1958.

Cornwall, J.W.: Some centipedes and their venom. Indian J. med. Res., **3**, 541—557 (1916).

Dammermann, K.W.: The fauna of Krakatau, Verlaten Island and Sebesy. Treubia, **3**, 61—112 (1923).

De Castro, A.B.: The poison of the Scolopendridae. Being a special reference to the andaman species. Indian. med. Gaz., **56**, 207 (1921).

Dubois, M.R.: De la fonction photogénique chez les Myriapodes. C.R. Soc. Biol. (Paris) **3**, 518—522, 523—525 (1886).

Dubois, M.R.: Note sur les Myriapodes lumineux (Réponse a M. Macé). C.R. Soc. Biol. (Paris) **4**, 6—7 (1887).

Dubois, R.: Sur le mécanisme de la production de la lumière chez l'*Orya barbarica* d'Algérie. C.R. Acad. Sci. (Paris) **117**, 184—186 (1893).

Duboscq, O.: La glande venimeuse de la Scolopendre. Arch. Zool. exp. gén., (3) **2**, 575—582 (1894).

Duboscq, O.: Les glandes ventrales et la glande venimeuse de *Chaetechelyne vesuviana,* Newp. Bull. Soc. Normand., **9**, 151—173 (1896).

Duboscq, O.: Recherches sur les Chilopodes. Arch. Zool. exp. gén., (3) **6**, 481—650 (1898).

Edwards, J.S.: Arthropods as predators. Viewpoints Biol., **2**, 85—114 (1963).

Eisner, T., Meinwald, J.: Defensive secretions of arthropods. Insects, millipedes and some of their relatives discharge noxious secretions that repel predators. Science, **153**, 1341—1350 (1966).

Erspamer, V., Asero, B.: Isolation of enteramine from extracts of posterior salivary glands of *Octopus vulgaris* and of *Discoglossus pictus* skin. J. biol. Chem., **200**, 311—318 (1953).

Ewing, H.E.: Observations on the habits and the injury caused by the bites or stings of some common North American Arthropods. Amer. J. trop. Med., **8**, 39—62 (1928).

Fahlander, K.: Beiträge zur Anatomie und systematischen Einteilung der Chilopoden. Zool. Bidr. Uppsala, **17**, 1—148 (1938).

Fanzago, F.: Sulla secrezione ventrale del *Geophilus Gabrielis.* Atti Soc. Ven.-trent. Sci. nat., (5) **7**, 641—646 (1881).

Faust, E.S.: Vergiftungen durch tierische Gifte. In: Lexicon der Toxicologie. Flury, F., and Zanger, G. (Eds.) Berlin: Springer 1928.

Freyvogel, Th.A.: Poisonous and Venomous Animals in East Africa. Acta trop. (Basel) **29**, 401—451 (1972).

Garzia, G.: Un caso di parassitismo accidentale da *Himantarium gabrielis* (L.) nell'intestino di un bambino. Riv. Parassit., **2**, 305—313 (1938).

Gazagnaire, J.: La phosphorescence chez les Myriapodes. Bull. Soc. Zool. Fr., **13**, 182—186 (1888); Bull. Soc. ent. Fr., **8**, XCIII—XCV (1888).

Gazagnaire, J.: La phosphorescence chez les Myriapodes de la famille des *Geophilidae.* Epoque et conditions physiologiques de l'apparition de la phosphorescence. Mém. Soc. Zool. Fr., **3**, 136—146 (1890).

Gruner, H.-E.: Leuchtende Tiere. Wittenberg 1954.

Haase, E.: Über das Leuchten der Myriapoden. Tag. dtsch. nat. Ver., **61**, 48—49 (1889).

Haneda, Y.: The terrestrial luminescent animals and plants in Palau and Yap Islands. Kagaku
   Nanyo (Sci. South Sea), **2**, 30—35 (1939).
Harvey, E.N.: The nature of animal light. Philadelphia-London: Lippincott 1920.
Harvey, E.N.: Living light. Princeton: Princeton University Press 1940.
Harvey, E.N.: Bioluminescence. New York: Academic Press 1952.
Haupt, H.: Leuchtende Organismen. Naturw. Wschr., **19**, 65—71 (1903).
Herms, W.B.: Medical entomology. New York: Macmillan 1939.
Heymons, R.: Die Entwicklungsgeschichte der Scolopender. Zoologica, **13**, 244 pp. (1901).
Holliday, R.A.: Some observations on Natal Onychophora. Ann. Natal Museum, **10**, 237—244
   (1942).
Houdemer, E.: Note sur un Myriapode vésicant du Tonkin, *Otostigmus aculeatus* Haase.
   Bull. Mus. Hist. nat., Paris, **1926**, 213—214 (1926).
Huet, M.: Note sur un Myriapode lumineux trouvé à la Fere (Aisne). C.R. Soc. Biol. (Paris)
   (8) **3**, 523—524 (1886).
Jolivet, P.: La toxicité des Myriapodes du Sud-Est asiatique. Entomologiste, Paris, **27**, 156—158
   (1972).
Jones, T.H., Conner, W.E., Meinwald, J., Eisner, H.E., Eisner, T.: Benzoyl cyanide and
   mandelonitrile in the cyanogenetic secretion of a centipede. J. Chem. Ecol. **2**, 421—429 (1976)
Judd, W.W.: House Centipede (*Scutigera forceps* (Raf.)) biting human. Entomol. New, **63**,
   238 (1952).
Keegan, H.L.: Centipedes and millipedes as pests in tropical areas, In: Venomous and poi-
   sonous animals and noxious plants of the pacific region. Keegan, H.L. and Macfarlane,
   W.V. (Eds.) Oxford: Pergamon Press 1963.
Kingsley, J.S.: The classification of the myriapoda. Amer. Nat., **22**, 1118—1121 (1888).
Koch, A.: Studien an leuchtenden Tieren. 1. Das Leuchten der Myriapoden. Z. Morph.
   Okol. Tiere, **8**, 241—270 (1927).
Kunckel D'Herculais, J.: Observations sur les moeurs d'un myriopode, la scutigère coléoptrée.
   Son utilité comme destructrice des mouches, action de son venin, légende de sa présence
   accidentelle dans l'appareil digestif de l'homme. C.R. Acad. Sci. (Paris) **153**, 399—401
   (1911); Bul. Soc. ent. Fr., **1912**, 193—198 (1912).
Launoy, L.: Contribution à l'étude des phénomènes nucléaires de la sécrétion (cellules à
   venin-cellules à enzyme). Ann. Sci. nat., (8) **18**, 1—224 (1903).
Lawrence, R.F.: Two new centipedes from southern Africa. Ann. Cape Prov. Mus., **6**, 77—79
   (1968).
Lever, R.A.: Irritant exudation from a centipede. Nature (Lond.) **143**, 78—79 (1939).
Lévy, R.: Sur le mécanisme de l'hemolyse par le venin de Scolopendre. C.R. Acad. Sci.
   (Paris) **177**, 1326—1328 (1923a).
Lévy, R.: Sur les propriétés hémolytiques du venin de certaines Myriapodes Chilopodes.
   Bull. Soc. Zool. Fr., **48**, 294—297 (1923b).
Lévy, R.: Intoxication de l'ecrevisse par le venins de deux myriapodes chilopodes. C.R. Soc.
   Biol. (Paris) **96**, 256—257 (1927a).
Lévy, R.: Action antitoxique du sang de *Lithobius forficatus* L. vis-à-vis du venin de la
   même espèce et vis-à-vis du venin de *Cryptops anomalans* Newp., C.R. Soc. Biol. (Paris)
   96, 258 (1927b).
Ludwig, F.: Phosphoreszierende Tausendfüssler und die Lichtfäule des Holzes. Zbl. Bakt.,
   Abt. 2, **7**, 270—274 (1901).
Macé: Sur la phosphorescence des geophiles. C.R. Acad. Sci. (Paris) **103**, 1273—1274 (1886).
Macé: Les glandes préanales et la phosphorescence des geophiles. C.R. Soc. Biol. (Paris)
   4, 37 (1887).
Machado, O.: Observaçoes sôbre as mordeduras das escolopendras. Bol. Inst. Vital Bresil,
   27, 5—7 (1944).
Metcalfe, C.L., Flint, W.P.: Destructive and useful insects: their habits and control. New
   York-London: McGraw Hill 1928.
Neveu-Lemaire, M.: Un nouveau cas de parasitisme accidental d'un myriapode dans le tube
   digestif de l'homme. C.R. Soc. Biol. (Paris) **63**, 307—308 (1907).
Neveu-Lemaire, M.: Traité d'entomologie médicale et vétérinaire. Paris: Masson 1938.
Newport, G.: Monograph of the class myriapoda, order chilopoda; with observations on

the general arrangement of the articulata. Trans. Linn. Soc. Lond., **19**, 265 – 302, 349 – 439 (1844 – 1845).

Norman, W.W.: The poison of centipedes (*Scolopendra morsitans*). Proc. Texas Acad. Sci., **1**, 118 – 119 (1897).

Okeden, W.P.: A centipede eating a snake. J. Bombay Soc., **15**, 135; **16**, 364 – 365 (1905).

Passerini, N.: Sull'organo ventrale del *Geophilus gabrielis,* Fabr. Boll. Soc. entomol. Ital., **14**, 323 – 328 (1882).

Patton, W.S.: Insects, ticks, mites and venomous animals of medical and veterinary importance. Part II. Public Health. Liverpool: Croydon 1931.

Pavan, M., Valcurone Dazzini, M.: Toxicology and Pharmacology (of Arthropoda). In: Chemical Zoology. Florkin, M. and Scheer, B.T. (eds.) New York-London: Academic Press. Vol. 6 1971.

Pawlowsky, E.: Ein Beitrag zur Kenntnis des Baues der Giftdrüsen von *Scolopendra morsitans.* Zool. Jb., Anat., **36**, 91 – 112 (1913).

Phisalix, M.: Animaux venimeux et venins. Paris, Masson. 2 vols. (1922). Pineda, in J. Philipp. med. Ass. **3**, 59, 93 (1923) (not seen; quoted from Remington, 1950).

Plowman, T.: A luminous centipede. Nature, **53**, 249 (1896).

Pocock, R.I.: On the classification of the diplopoda. Ann. nat. Hist., **20**, 283 (1887).

Pocock, R.I.: On the classification of the tracheate *Arthropoda.* Zool. Anz., **16**, 271 – 275 (1893a).

Pocock, R.I.: On the classification of the tracheate *Arthropoda:* a correction. Nature (Lond.) **49**, 124 (1893b).

Pocock, R.I.: A luminous centipede. Nature (Lond.) **53**, 223 (1896).

Remington, C.L.: The bite and habit of a giant centipede (*Scolopendra subspinipes*) in the Philippine Islands. Amer. J. trop. Med., **30**, 453 – 455 (1950).

Ridley, H.N.: The luminous secretion of the centipede Geophilus as a defense against the attack of beetles. Proc. roy. entomol. Soc. **A 11**, 48 (1936).

Roberts, F.M.: Luminous centipedes. Nature (Lond.) **98**, 269 (1916).

Rosenfeld, G., Kelen, E.M.A.: Bibliography of animal venoms, envenemations and treatments. Period 1500 – 1968. Sao Paulo (1969).

Schildknecht, H., Maschwitz, V., Krauss, D.: Blausäure im Wehrsekret des Erdläufers *Pachymerium ferrugineum.* XXXV. Mitteilung über Arthropoden-Abwehrstoffe. Naturwissenschaften **55**, 230 (1968).

Schnee: Sechs an mir selbst beobachtete Skolopenderbisse und einiges über Skorpionenstiche. Arch. Schiffs- u. Tropenhyg., **15**, 156 – 160 (1911).

Schubart, O.: Die Zahl der in 200 Jahren zoologischer Forschung (1758 – 1957) beschriebenen Myriapoden-Arten. Zool. Anz., **165**, 84 – 89 (1960).

Sinclair, F.G.: Myriopoda. In: The cambridge natural history. Vol. 5. London: Macmillan (1895).

Stammer, H.-J.: Leuchtende Tiere in Schlesien. Jber. schles. Ges. vaterl. Kult., **107**, 51 – 52 (1935).

Thomas, R.H.: A luminous centipede. Nature (Lond.) **53**, 130 (1895).

Thomas, R.H.: A luminous centipede. Nature (Lond.) **65**, 223 (1902).

Tömösváry, E.: Über den Bau der Spinndrüsen bei den Geophiliden. Math. Nat. Ber. Ung., **2**, 441 – 445 (1885).

Verhoeff, K.W.: Chilopoda, In: Bronn's Klassen und Ordnungen des Tierreiches. Bd. 5(2). Leipzig: Akademische Verlagsgesellschaft 1902 – 1925.

Weber, L.: Hautausschlag durch den Biss von *Lithobius.* Abh. Ver. Naturk., Cassel, **51**, 174 – 175 (1970).

Welsh, J.H., Batty, C.S.: 5-Hydroxytryptamine content of some arthropod venoms and venom-containing parts. Toxicon, **1**, 165 – 173 (1963).

Willem, V.: Les glandes filières (coxales) des Lithobies. Ann. Soc. entomol. Belg., **41**, 87 – 89 (1897).

CHAPTER 5

Secretions of Opilionids, Whip Scorpions and Pseudoscorpions[1]

T. Eisner[2], D. Alsop[3], J. Meinwald[4]

The opilionids (order Opiliones), whip scorpions (order Uropygi), and pseudoscorpions (order Pseudoscorpiones), all belong to the class Arachnida. Within the class, the three orders are not particularly closely related to one another, and they are treated together here merely as a matter of convenience. The opilionids, with some 3000 known species (Levi et al., 1968), comprise the largest of these orders. The pseudoscorpions include about 1500 described species (Weygoldt, 1969), and the whip scorpions only about 70 (Levi et al., 1968). The glands of opilionids and whip scorpions are purely defensive devices, whose dischargeable contents serve to repel enemies. Pseudoscorpions produce injectable poisons, employed supposedly only for immobilization of prey. Chemical studies have been done on the secretion of only one whip scorpion and relatively few opilionids. Nothing is known about the chemistry of pseudoscorpion venom. The summary that follows stresses the more recent work.

A. Order Opiliones

The opilionids or harvestmen live primarily in moist and shaded habitats and are active mainly at night. In the daytime they are usually found in hiding, mostly under logs and rocks, in leaf litter, or in dense vegetation. They feed primarily on live insects and occasionally on dead animals and plant juices. The members of the largest family, the Phalangiidae, are commonly known as daddy longlegs in the U.S.A. The biology of opilionids has been reviewed by Berland (1949), Cloudsley-Thompson (1968), and Kaestner (1968).

All three suborders of the Opiliones—the Cyphophthalmi, the Laniatores and the Palpatores—have defensive glands. These organs consist of a pair of compressible sacs, situated dorsally in the body and opening near the anterolateral margins of the carapace (Figs. 1, 2, and 4B). The openings were once thought to be spiracles or eyes (see historical review in Hansen and Sørensen (1904)). Despite some variation in structure, the glands are probably homologous throughout the order. Like many other exocrine glands of arthropods, they are essentially infoldings of the body wall, consisting of a glandular epithelium and an inner membranous

[1] Paper no. XLV of the series *Defense Mechanisms of Arthropods*
[2] Section of Neurobiology and Behavior, Division of Biological Sciences, Cornell University, Ithaca, N.Y. 14853
[3] Department of Biology, Queens College, Flushing, N.Y. 11367
[4] Department of Chemistry, Cornell University, Ithaca, N.Y. 14853

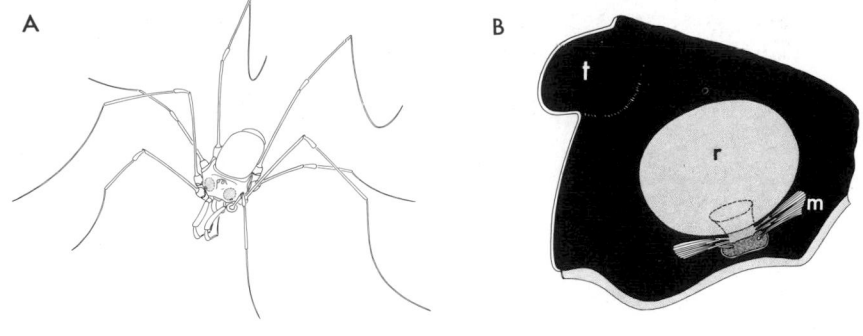

Fig. 1. (A) Diagram of an opilionid (Palpatores, Phalangiidae, *Leiobunum* sp.). The location of glands is indicated by two stippled circles. (B) Gland of *Leiobunum,* as it appears from beneath, attached to the inner surface of portion of carapace (*t*, eye turret). Special muscles (*m*) are associated with valvular opening of gland. There are no compressor muscles on the reservoir (*r*) of the gland. (Reference bars: A, 1 cm; B, 0.5 mm)

cuticular lining (Faussek, 1892; Juberthie, 1961 a; Krohn, 1879). The gland cells are endowed with tubular cuticular ducts (Krohn, 1879), such as are commonly found in secretory cells of arthropods (Eisner, 1970). The muscles associated with the glands are of more or less complex arrangement. According to Juberthie (1961 a, 1961 b), the most elaborate musculature is found in the primitive Cyphophthalmi, in which there are, in addition to special muscles associated with the valvular openings of the glands, compressor muscles of the sacs themselves. In the Laniatores, the musculature is somewhat reduced, and in the Palpatores the muscles of the sacs are missing altogether (Fig. 1 B). Such unmuscled sacs are presumably compressed indirectly, either by hemolymph pressure, or by pressure from adjacent organs. Some variation also prevails in the location of the gland openings, which in the Cyphophthalmi are placed atop small tubercles (Juberthie, 1961 a).

Chemical studies of opilionid secretions have not been extensive (Table 1, Fig. 3). No Cyphophthalmi have been investigated. The six Laniatores studied produce a variety of alkylated 1,4-benzoquinones and phenols. Quinones are widely distributed in the defensive secretions of other arthropods, including insects and millipeds (references in Altman and Dittmer, 1973; Eisner, 1970; Eisner et al., 1974). However, the particular alkylated quinones produced by opilionids appear to be of more restricted occurrence. 2,3-Dimethyl-1,4-benzoquinone is known only from the defensive secretion of certain Australian tenebrionid beetles (Eisner et al., 1974) and from some carabid beetles (Eisner, T. and Meinwald, J., unpublished observations on *Brachinus* and ozaenines) while 2,5-dimethyl-1,4-benzoquinone and 2,3,5-trimethyl-1,4-benzoquinone are known from no other arthropods. Of the two Laniatores phenols, 2,3-dimethylphenol has been found only in a single plant (Irvine and Saxby, 1968), while 2-methyl-5-ethylphenol has not previously been found in nature.

Eight congeneric species of Palpatores (and one additional species) produce an array of related volatile branched chain alcohols, ketones, and an aldehyde. Two ketones, 4-methylheptan-3-one and 4-methylhexan-3-one, present in six of these species, are known also from the mandibular glands of certain myrmicine

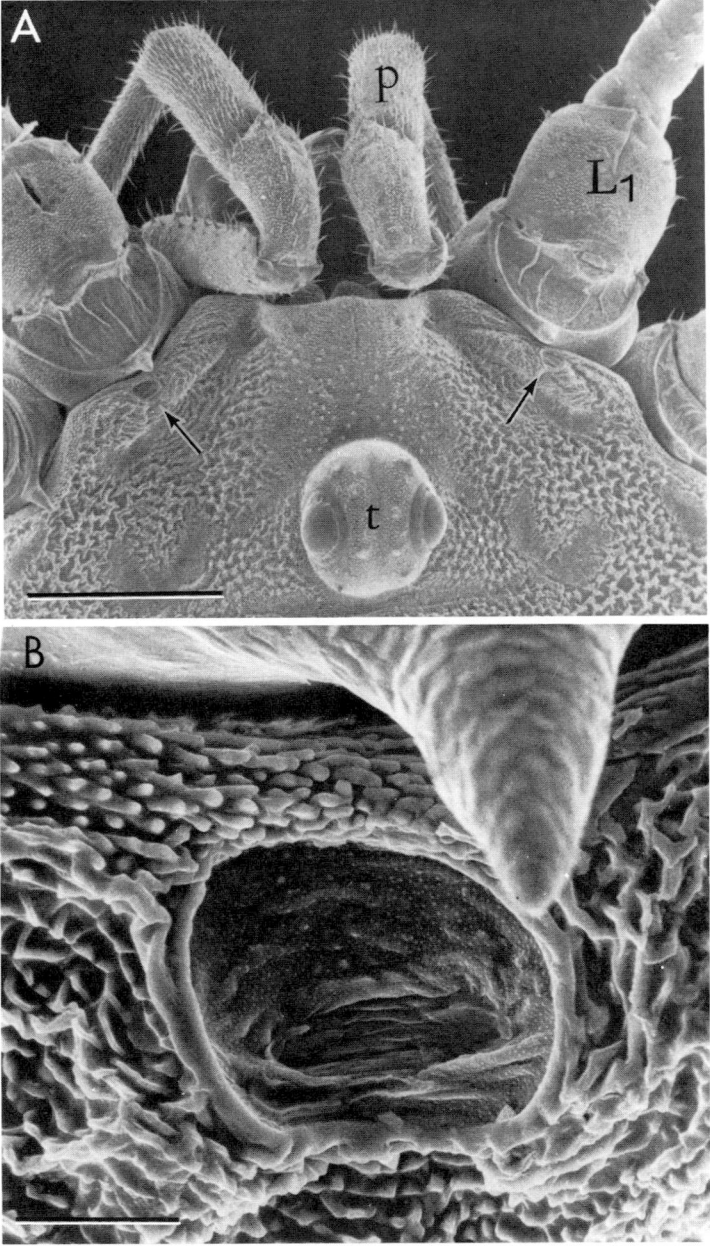

Fig. 2. (A). Dorsal view of front of body of an unidentified opilionid (Palpatores, Phalangiidae). Arrows point to gland openings; *t*, eye turret; *p*, pedipalp; L_1, leg 1. (B) Enlarged view of left gland opening. (Reference bars: A, 0.5 mm; B, 0.05 mm)

Table 1. List of Opiliones studied chemically, and compounds isolated from their secretions. The structure of the compounds is shown in Fig. 3.

Group and Species	Compound(s) in Secretion[a]	Authority
Order Opiliones		
Suborder Cyphophthalmi	none identified	
Suborder Laniatores		
Family Cosmetidae		
Vonones sayi	I, III	Eisner et al., 1971
Paecilaemella quadripunctata[b]	I, III	Eisner et al., 1977
P. eutypa[b]	I, II, III	Eisner et al., 1977
Cynorta astora[b]	IV, V	Eisner et al., 1977
Family Gonyleptidae		
Heteropachyloidellus robustus	I, II, III	Estable et al., 1955; Fieser and Ardao, 1956
Zygopachylus albimarginis[b]	I, V(?)[c]	Eisner et al., 1977
Suborder Palpatores		
Family Phalangiidae		
Leiobunum vittatum	X, XI	Meinwald et al., 1971
L. formosum	X	Blum and Edgar, 1971
L. speciosum	X	Blum and Edgar, 1971
L. ventricosum	X	Jones et al., 1976
L. calcar	XI, XIII	Jones et al., 1977
L. longipes	XII	Jones et al., 1976
L. nigripalpi	VI, VII, VIII, IX, XV	Jones et al., 1977
L. leiopenis	IX, X, XIII, XIV	Jones et al., 1977
Hadrobunus maculosus	X	Jones et al., 1976

[a] Numerals refer to compounds shown in Fig. 3.
[b] These identifications are tentative. Specimens are deposited under R.E. Silberglied label in National Museum of Natural History, Washington, D.C.
[c] Tentatively identified on basis of a mass spectrum indicative of a methyl-ethylphenol.

and ponerine ants (Blum et al., 1968; Duffield and Blum, 1973; Fales et al., 1972; McGurk et al., 1966). Of the two Laniatores phenols, 2,3-dimethylphenol 1972; McGurk et al., 1966). The remaining eight alicyclic components are apparently not known from other natural sources. From a consideration of the structures of these compounds, it is impossible to guess whether they are terpenoids from a biosynthetic viewpoint, or whether they represent methylated polyketides. In any case, they demonstrate an interesting range of biosynthetic abilities within this suborder.

Relatively little is known about the defensive effectiveness of the secretions, although such evidence as exists suggests that the fluids are indeed deterrent to some predators. Ants that attacked Vonones sayi or Leiobunum in laboratory tests were repelled by the secretory discharges that they elicited from the opilionids, and the repellent effect could be duplicated by subjecting the ants to vapors from authentic samples of the quinones or ketone present in the secretions (Blum and Edgar, 1971; Eisner et al., 1971). Some spiders are also deterred by opilionids (Cloudsley-Thompson, 1968), but others are not (Immel, 1954). Predators such

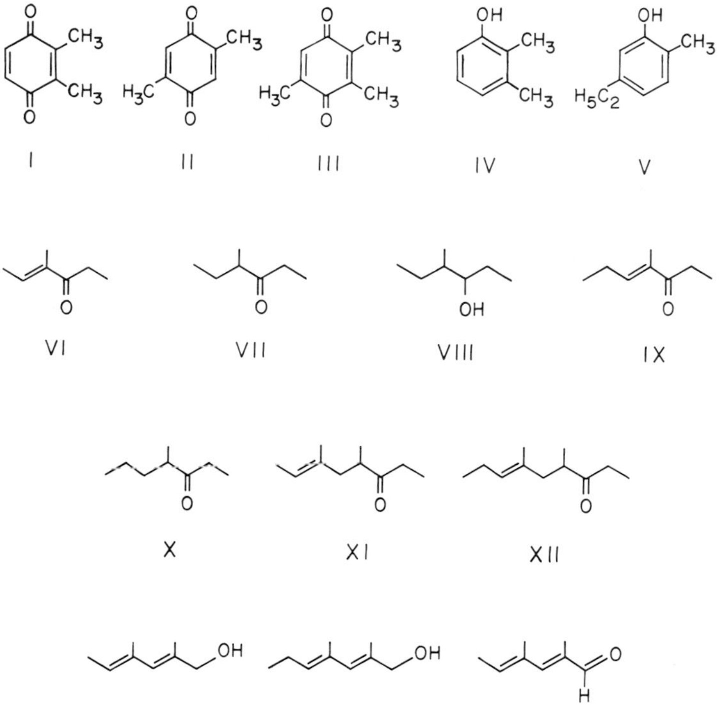

Fig. 3. Constituents identified in secretions of Opiliones. (I) 2,3-dimethyl-1,4-benzoquinone; (II) 2,5-dimethyl-1,4-benzoquinone; (III) 2,3,5-trimethyl-1,4-benzoquinone; (IV) 2,3-dimethylphenol; (V) 2-methyl-5-ethylphenol; (VI) E-4-methylhex-4-ene-3-one; (VII) 4-methylhexan-3-one; (VIII) 4-methylhexan-3-ol; (IX) E-4-methylhept-4-ene-3-one; (X) 4-methylheptan-3-one; (XI) E-4,6-dimethyloct-6-ene-3-one; (XII) E-4,6-dimethylnon-6-ene-3-one; (XIII) E,E-2,4-dimethylhexa-2,4-dien-1-ol; (XIV) E,E-2,4-dimethylhepta-2,4-dien-1-ol; (XV) E,E-2,4-dimethylhexadienal

as vertebrates might also be repelled, but this remains to be shown. Judging from the effectiveness of the quinone and phenol-containing secretions of other arthropods (EISNER et al., 1963; references in EISNER and MEINWALD, 1966), it seems likely that the quinone-producing Laniatores might be particularly well protected. The Palpatores appear to be more vulnerable, and a diversity of predators are said to take them (BISHOP, 1950; BRISTOWE, 1949; CLOUDSLEY-THOMPSON, 1968; EDGAR, 1960, quoted in BLUM and EDGAR, 1971).

Secretory emission in opilionids can occur in a diversity of ways (BISHOP, 1950; BLUM and EDGAR, 1971; JUBERTHIE, 1961a; LAWRENCE, 1938). Sometimes the fluids are ejected as a spray, but more commonly they merely ooze from the glands, and either accumulate as globular droplets over the gland openings, or spread from their sites of emission to other parts of the body. Special grooves along the margins of the carapace may serve to convey the fluids backward to the rear of the body, or the fluid may seep between the bases of the legs to the ventral surface. In Palpatores, where the discharged fluids may be more mobile,

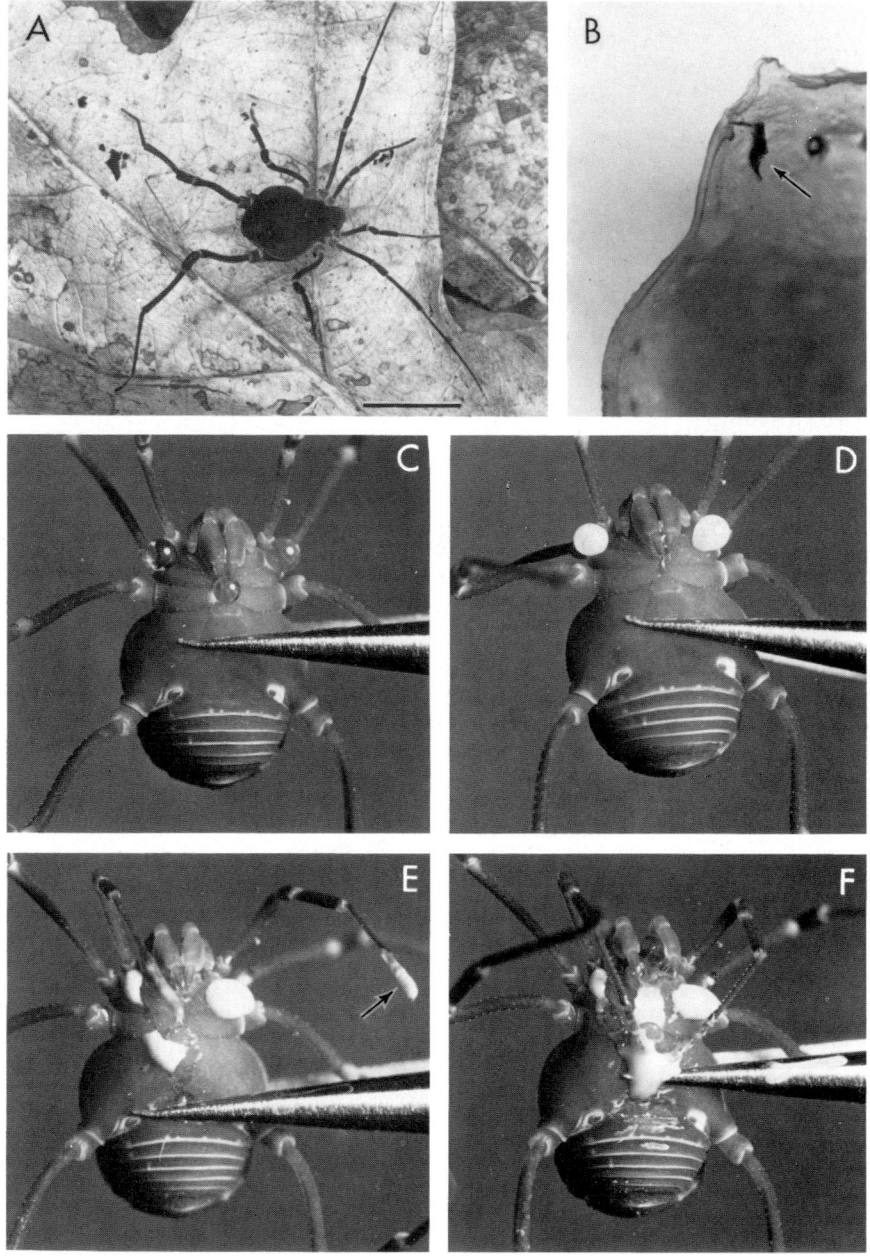

Fig. 4. (A) *Vonones sayi* (Laniatores, Cosmetidae) (reference bar: 0.5 cm). (B) Portion of carapace of *Vonones,* showing gland attached (*arrow*). (C–F) Ventral view of *Vonones,* held
in forceps, showing successive stages in the discharge and delivery of its defensive effluent.
The clear regurgitated fluid initially discharged (C) stems from the mouth (where excess fluid
has accumulated as a median droplet) and is conveyed to the margins of the body, where
it accumulates as two droplets. Quinonoid secretion is then injected into the droplets, which
tarnish as a result (D), and the fluid is administered to the offending forceps by brushing
of the forelegs (E, F). Note tip of foreleg coated with effluent in (E) (*arrow*)

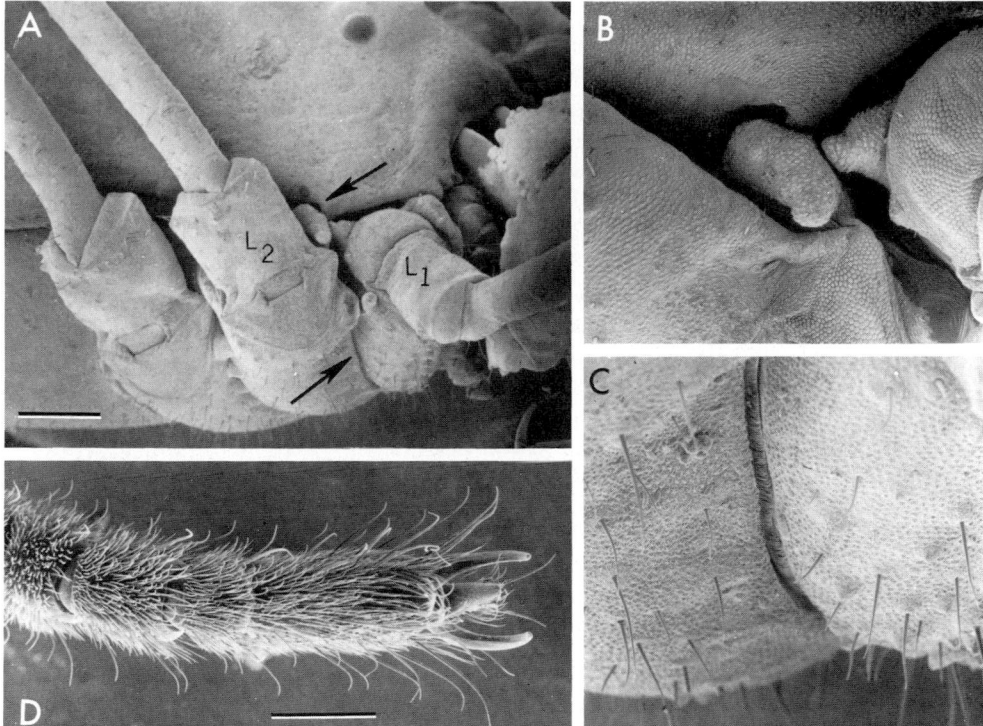

Fig. 5.(A). *Cynorta astora* (Laniatores, Cosmetidae): right lateral view of anterior portion of body. Upper arrow points to gland opening, lower arrow to groove along which oral fluid is conveyed (L_1, leg 1; L_2, leg 2). (B) Same, enlarged view of gland opening and surrounding area. (C) Same, enlarged view of groove. (D) *Paecilaemella eutypa* (Laniatores, Cosmetidae): Hairy tip of foreleg. The leg is used as a brush (as in Fig. 4E—F) for administration of defensive fluid to an enemy. (Reference bars: A, 0.5 mm; D, 0.25 mm)

spreading can occur sporadically over much of the microsculptured surface (see Fig. 2A) of the carapace.

Cyphophthalmi have a remarkable way of administering secretion with their legs (JUBERTHIE, 1961 b). When *Parasiro coiffaiti* is disturbed, as when one of its legs is seized in forceps, it discharges a droplet from the gland of the side of the leg seized, dips one of the free legs of that side into the droplet, and then transfers the secretion with this leg to the leg seized. *Siro rubens* behaves in a comparable way, although the defensive maneuvers differ in detail.

Vonones sayi (Fig. 4A), a member of the Laniatores, also administers secretion by leg dabbing (EISNER et al., 1971). This animal produces quinones (Table 1), which it stores in its glands in undiluted form. When disturbed, the animal first emits aqueous enteric fluid from the mouth, conveys this by way of two clefts between the bases of the 1st and 2nd legs to the sites of the gland openings, and then discharges quinones into the enteric fluid as this accumulates over the openings. The animal then dips the tips of its forelegs into the freshly formulated quinone solution and effects dosaged delivery of the fluid by brushing it against the offending agent with the wetted legs (Fig. 4C—F). Predators such as ants are effectively repelled in this fashion. In its tiny glands (Fig. 4B), *Vonones* stores only a few micrograms of quinones (the recorded maximum is 48 μg/animal), but since this material is used sparingly, it is actually enough to provision over 30 enteric loads of fluid, which has been estimated to suffice for defense against over 1500 individual ant attacks. *Vonones'* remarkable habit of mixing solute and solvent just prior to use may reflect the animal's functional need to do so. Benzoquinones are unstable in water, and hence unsuitable for long-term storage in aqueous solution. Other Laniatores of the family Cosmetidae, including the phenol-producing *Cynorta astora,* show comparable leg-dabbing behavior (EISNER et al., 1977). The scanning electronmicrographs in Fig. 5 show the brush-like tip of the foreleg, as well as the gland opening and its relationship to the groove that conveys the oral fluid.

Opilionids may also be protected by nonchemical means. They are generally cryptically colored and hence well camouflaged in a diversity of situations, and many of them "death-feign" when disturbed, assuming more or less rigid stances, with their legs pulled in or stretched out in characteristic fashion (EISNER et al., 1971; IMMEL, 1954; ŠILHAVÝ, 1956). It is also common for opilionids to autotomize a leg when seized by it. This mechanism, which is said to occur in all Palpatores except the Trogulidae, has recently been studied in some detail by WASGESTIAN-SCHALLER (1968). Following autotomy, the discarded leg may twitch rhythmically, thereby diverting the predator from pursuit of the opilionid itself. The diversion is effective, as was shown in tests with ants and spiders. Interestingly, the legs of Palpatores have special spiracular openings that provide the legs with a subsidiary respiratory supply of their own. Following autotomy, this supply contributes to maintenance of the twitch mechanism. Leg autotomy in opilionids is, of course, functionally comparable to the well known tail autotomy of lizards. Unlike lizards, however, which can regrow their tail, opilionids do not regenerate their discarded legs. Tropical Gonyleptidae have yet another defense: by drawing their short hind femora together behind them, they can administer a sharp pinch (CLOUDSLEY-THOMPSON, 1968).

Much remains to be learned about opilionids generally, and about their glands. Chemical studies alone are likely to prove fruitful, as would studies of the biosynthesis of the secretory components, of the ultrastructure of the glands, and of the mode of action of the secretions.

B. Order Uropygi

As is generally the case with lesser groups of arachnids, our knowledge of the natural history of whip scorpions is meager. We know that they date back to the Carboniferous, and that they have changed little since then. They are primarily tropical in distribution but extend also into parts of the northern subtropics. They live in cryptic habitats, under logs, rocks, bark, or leaf litter, and are active primarily at night. They appear to be exclusively carnivorous, feeding chiefly on live insects and other arthropods. Existing reviews of whip scorpion biology (CLOUDSLEY-THOMPSON, 1968; KAESTNER, 1968; MILLOT, 1949; WERNER, 1935), have been amplified by recent life history and reproductive studies (WEYGOLDT, 1971, 1972a, 1972b).

To naturalists, whip scorpions have long been of interest because of their ability to secrete a pungent and irritating fluid, which they discharge as a jetlike spray when disturbed (GRAVELY, 1915; STRUBELL, 1926; WERNER, 1935; WOOD-MA-SON, 1882). The spray can be the source of some annoyance and pain to humans if it impinges on sensitive areas (SANDERSON, 1939; STRUBELL, 1926) and in at least one instance is said to have elicited serious blistering of the skin (HOWARD, 1919).

Only one species, the North American *Mastigoproctus giganteus* (Fig. 6), appears to have been studied in some detail (EISNER, 1962; EISNER et al., 1961). This animal, which in parts of the U.S.A. is called vinegaroon or vinegarone, does indeed produce the·substance that gives rise to its name: the secretion contains acetic acid at an astonishingly high concentration of 84%! In addition, the mixture contains caprylic acid (5%) and water (11%). The glands, which have been described in this and in related species by EISNER et al. (1961), LAURIE (1894), SCHIMKEWITSCH (1906), WOOD-MASON (1882) and BÖRNER (1904), consist of a pair of voluminous sacs (Fig. 6), situated posteriorly in the opisthosoma, and opening at the end of the short segmented knob that forms the base of the flagellum (Fig. 7A). By rotating the knob, the animal can aim its spray, and it does in fact discharge with accuracy toward quarters of its body subjected to assault (Fig. 7C–D). Forward discharges are not directed by aiming of the knob alone, but require additional postural adjustments of the opisthosoma as a whole (Fig. 7B). *Mastigoproctus* sprays only in response to direct contact stimulation. Mere proximity of a potential threat evokes no discharges. As many as 19 ejections have been elicited from a single animal. The spray was shown to be effectively deterrent to a diversity

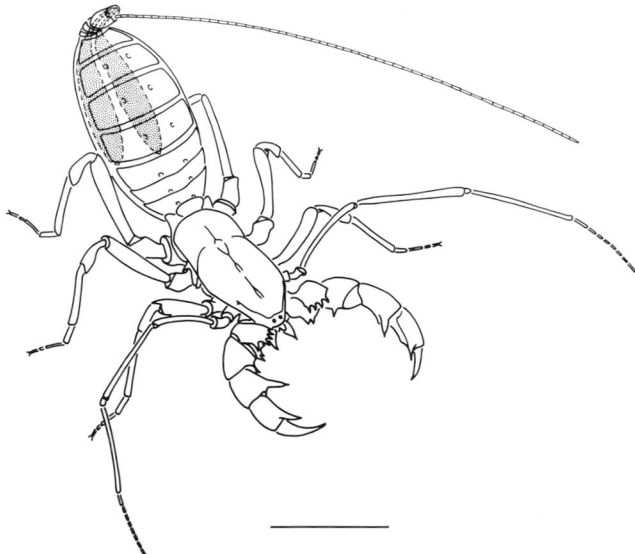

Fig. 6. Diagram of whip scorpion (*Mastigoproctus giganteus*). The glands are indicated by the two large stippled sacs. (Reference bar: 2 cm)

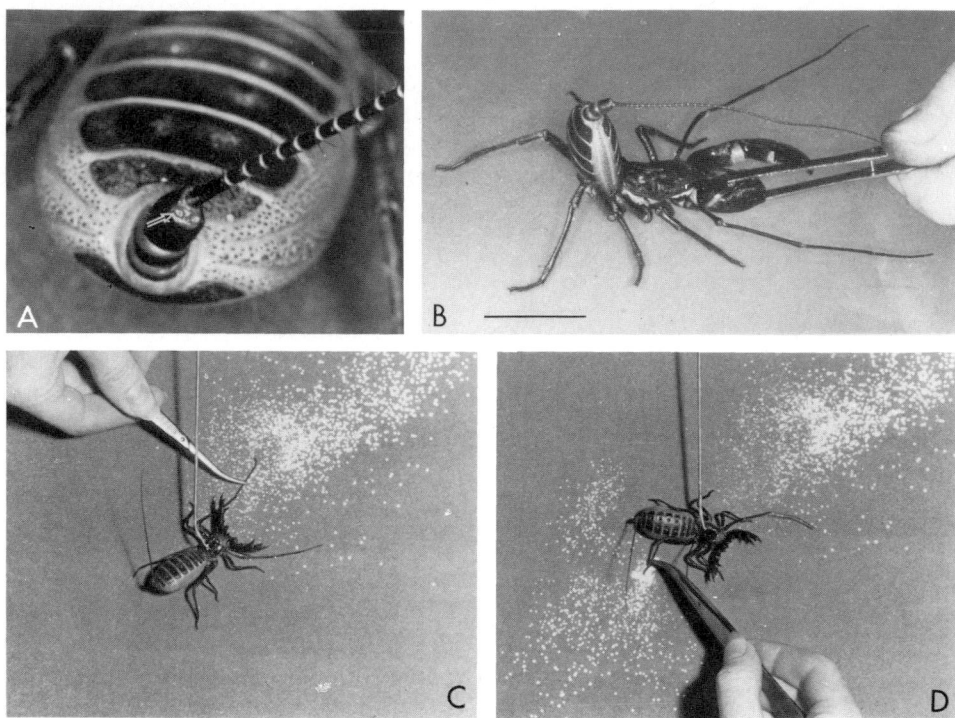

Fig. 7.(A). Rear view of *Mastigoproctus giganteus,* showing the revolvable three-segmented "spray nozzle" that bears the two slit-like gland openings (arrow points to left opening). (B) *Mastigoproctus* maneuvering in response to a frontal "assault" by raising its opisthosoma and deflecting its "nozzle" forward, preparatory to delivery of an anteriorly directed discharge. (Reference bar: 3 cm). (C – D) Two consecutive aimed discharges elicited from *Mastigoproctus* by pinching individual appendages as shown. The pattern of the spray is registered on filter paper impregnated with an alkaline solution of phenolphthalein

of predators, including ants (*Formica, Pogonomyrmex*), solpugids (*Eremobates*), and lizards (*Anolis*). Grasshopper mice (*Onychomys*) were persistent despite the spray, but were also noticeably affected by it.

Although the principal deterrent component of the secretion is undoubtedly the acetic acid, caprylic acid adds considerably to the effectiveness of the spray as it is used against arthropods. By acting as a wetting agent, caprylic acid promotes the spread of the spray droplets over the cuticle of the predator, thereby increasing the effective area of contact of the poison. In addition, the acid promotes the penetration of the secretion through the arthropod integument, presumably by increasing the permeability of the epicuticular lipid barrier.

When whip scorpions first emerge from the egg, their glands are incompletely developed (SCHIMKEWITSCH, 1906) and probably nonfunctional. The young at this stage do not lead a free life, but remain clinging to the mother's back (STRUBELL, 1926; WEYGOLDT, 1972a), and are presumably dependent on her defenses. It is not until after the second molt, when the young metamorphose into miniature adults, that they leave the parent (STRUBELL, 1926). By that time their glands are fully developed (SCHIMKEWITSCH, 1906).

Anecdotal evidence suggests that other whip scorpions may also produce acetic acid-containing secretions. In Martinique, whip scorpions are known as "vinai-griers" (POCOCK, 1895; WOOD-MASON, 1882), and Brazil they are called "escor-piões vinagre" (VANZOLINI, P.E., personal communication). But in some species the secretions supposedly have aberrant odors (GRAVELY, 1915; STRUBELL, 1926), and their chemistry may yet turn out to be different.

C. Order Pseudoscorpiones

These fascinating but secretive animals are scarcely known to most biologists. An informative booklet has recently been written about them (WEYGOLDT, 1969). Two suborders of pseudoscorpions, the Diposphyronida and the Monosphyronida, have poison glands in their pincers (=the chelae of the pedipalps). The glands are located in either the fixed or the moveable finger of the pincers, or occasionally in both fingers (VACHON, 1949). The chemistry and pharmacology of the venom of these glands, which is employed for immobilization of prey, is unknown. In at least one species, *Dactylochelifer latreillei,* the venom is quick in its action: a captured fruit fly ceased moving within seconds, and died after some minutes (WEYGOLDT, 1969). The venom of pseudoscorpions is innocuous to humans, at least in the amounts that these small animals are capable of injecting it (VACHON, 1949).

Acknowledgments: Our own research on arthropod secretions has been supported by grants AI-02908 from the National Institutes of Health and BMS-74-15084 from the National Science Foundation. The scanning electronmicrographs in Fig. 2 were taken by T.E. while a Fellow of the John Simon Guggenheim Foundation at the laboratories of Barry Filshie and Colin Beaton, Division of Entomology, C.S.I.R.O., Canberra, whose help is also gratefully acknowledged. Some of our chemical work on Palpatores was done with specimens taken at the Huyck Preserve, Rensellaerville, N.Y., where some of our field work is conducted.

References

Altman, P.L., Dittmer, D.S.: Biology Data Book. 2nd Ed. Bethesda, Md: Federation of American Societies for Exp. Bio., 1973, Vol. II, Sect. 80, Part I.
Berland, L.: Ordre des Opilions. In: Traité de Zoologie (Grassé, P.P. ed.) Paris: Masson et Cie, 1949, Vol. VI, pp. 761–793.
Bishop, S.C.: The life of a harvestman. Nature Mag. **276**, 264–267 (1950).
Blum, M.S., Edgar, A.L.: 4-Methyl-3-heptanone: identification and role in opilionid exocrine secretions. Insect Biochem. **1**, 181–188 (1971).
Blum, M.S., Padovani, F., Amante, E.: Alkanones and terpenes in the mandibular glands of *Atta* species. Comp. Biochem. Physiol. **26**, 291–299 (1968).
Bristowe, W.S.: Distribution of harvestmen in England and Ireland with notes on their environment, names, and food. J. Anim. Ecol. **18**, 100–114 (1949).
Börner, C.: Beiträge zur Morphologie der Arthropoden — I. Ein Beitrag zur Kenntnis de Pedipalpen. Zoologica, Stuttgart **42**, 1–174 (1904).

Cloudsley-Thompson, J.S.: Spiders, Scorpions, Centipedes, and Mites. London: Pergamon Press, 1968.

Duffield, R.M., Blum, M.S.: 4-Methyl-3-heptanone: identification and function in *Neoponera villosa* (Hymenoptera: Formicidae). Ann. Entomol. Soc. Amer. **66**, 1357 (1973).

Edgar, A.L.: The biology of the order Phalangida in Michigan. Thesis, Ann Arbor, Mich: Edwards Bros, 1960.

Eisner, T.: Survival by acid defense. Natural History **71**, 10–19 (1962).

Eisner, T.: Chemical defense against predation in arthropods. In: Chemical Ecology (Sondheimer, E. and Simeone, J.B. eds.). New York: Academic Press 1970, 157–217.

Eisner, T., Aneshansley, D., Eisner, M., Rutowski, R., Chong, B., Meinwald, J.: Chemical defense and sound production in Australian tenebrionid beetles (*Adelium* spp.). Psyche **81**, 189–208 (1974).

Eisner, T., Hurst, J.J., and Meinwald, J.: Defense mechanisms of arthropods. XI. The structure, function, and phenolic secretions of the glands of a chordeumoid millipede and a carabid beetle. Psyche **70**, 94–116 (1963).

Eisner, T., Jones, T.H., Hicks, K., Silberglied, R.H., and Meinwald, J.: Quinones and phenols from neotropical opilionids. J. Chem. Ecol., in press (1977).

Eisner, T., Kluge, A.F., Carrel, J.C., Meinwald, J.: Defense of phalangid: liquid repellent administered by leg dabbing. Science **173**, 650–652 (1971).

Eisner, T., Meinwald, J.: Defensive secretions of arthropods. Science **153**, 1341–1350 (1966).

Eisner, T., Meinwald, J., Monro, A., Ghent, R.: Defence mechanisms of arthropods. I. The composition and function of the spray of the whipscorpion, *Mastigoproctus giganteus* (Lucas) (Arachnida, Pedipalpida). J. Ins. Physiol. **6**, 272–298 (1961).

Estable, C., Ardao, M.I., Brasil, N.P., Fieser, L.F.: Gonyleptidine. J. Amer. Chem. Soc. **77**, 4942 (1955).

Fales, H.M., Blum, M.S., Crewe, R.M., and Brand, J.M. Alarm pheromones in the mandibular glands of *Manica*. J. Ins. Physiol. **18**, 1077–1088 (1972).

Faussek, V.: Zur Anatomie und Embryologie der Phalangiden. Biol. Zentralbl. **12**, 1–8 (1892).

Fieser, L.F., Ardao, M.I.: Investigation of the chemical nature of gonyleptidine. J. Amer. Chem. Soc. **78**, 774–781 (1956).

Gravely, F.H.: Notes on the habits of Indian insects, myriapods and arachnids. Rec. Indian Mus. **11**, 483–539 (1915).

Hansen, N.J., Sørensen, W.: On Two Orders of Arachnida: Opiliones and Ricinulei. Cambridge Univ. Press, 1904.

Howard, L.O.: Note on the vinegarone (Arach., Pedipalpi) Ent. News **30**, 26 (1919).

Immel, V.: Zur Biologie und Physiologie von *Nemastoma quadripunctatum* (Opiliones, Dyspnoi). Zool. Jahrb. Abt. System. **83**, 129–184 (1954).

Irvine, W.J., and Saxby, M.J.: The constituents of certain tobacco types–I. Steam volatile phenols of Latakia. Phytochemistry **7**, 277–281 (1968).

Jones, T.H., Conner, W.E., Kluge, A.F., Eisner, T., and Meinwald, J.: Defensive substances of opilionids. Experientia **32**, 1234–1235 (1976).

Jones, T.H., Meinwald, J., Hicks, K., and Eisner, T.: Characterization and synthesis of volatile compounds from the defensive secretions of some "daddy longlegs" (Arachnida: Opiliones: *Leiobunum* spp.). Proc. Nat. Acad. Sci. **74**, 419–422 (1977).

Juberthie, C.: Structure et fonction des glandes odorantes chez quelques Opilions (Arachnida). Verhandl. Deutsch. Zoologisch. Gesellsch. **1961**, 533–537 (1961a).

Juberthie, C.: Structure des glandes odorantes et modalités d'utilisation de leur sécrétion chez deux opiliones cyphophthalmes. Bull. Soc. Zool. France **86**, 106–116 (1961b).

Kaestner, A.: Invertebrate Zoology. New York: Interscience Publ., 1968, Vol. II.

Krohn, A.: Über die Anwesenheit zweier Drüsensäcke im Cephalotherax [sic.] der Phalangiden. Arch. f. Naturgesch. **33**, 79–83 (1879).

Laurie, M.: On the morphology of the Pedipalpi. J. Linn. Soc. (Zool.) **25**, 20–48 (1894).

Lawrence, R.F.: The odoriferous glands of some South African harvestspiders. Trans. Roy. Soc. South Africa **25**, 333–342 (1938).

Levi, H.W., Levi, L.R.: Spiders and Their Kin. New York: Golden Press, 1968.

McGurk, D.J., Frost, J., Eisenbraun, E.J., Vick, K., Drew, W.A., Young, J.: Volatile compounds in ants: identification of 4-methyl-3-heptanone from *Pogonomyrmex* ants. J. Insect Physiol. **12**, 1435—1441 (1966).

Meinwald, J., Kluge, A.F., Carrel, J.E. and Eisner, T.: Acyclic ketones in the defensive secretion of a "daddy longlegs" (*Leiobunum vittatum*). Proc. Nat. Acad. Sci. **68**, 1467—1468 (1971).

Millot, J.: Ordre des uropyges. In: Traité de Zoologie (Grassé, P.P. ed.) Paris: Masson et Cie., 1949, Vol. VI, 533—562.

Pocock, R.I.: Whip scorpions and their ways. Knowledge **18**, 272—274 (1895).

Sanderson, I.T.: Caribbean Treasure. New York: Viking Press, 1939.

Sankey, J.H.P.: Observations on food, enemies and parasites of British harvest-spiders (Arachnida, Opiliones). Entom. Monthly Magaz. **85**, 246—247 (1949).

Schimkewitsch, W.: Über die Entwicklung von *Thelyphonus caudatus* (L.) verglichen mit derjenigen einiger andrer Arachniden. Z. wiss. Zool. **81**, 1—95 (1906).

Šilhavý, V.: Opiliones. Fauna ČSR 7, Československá Akad. Véd, Prague (1956).

Strubell, A.: *Thelyphonus caudatus* L. Eine biologische Skitze. Verh. naturh. Ver. preuss. Rheinl. **82**, 301—314 (1926).

Vachon, M.: Ordre des Pseudoscorpions. In: Traité de Zoologie (Grassé, P.P. ed.) Paris: Masson et Cie., 1949, Vol. VI, pp. 437—481.

Wasgestian-Schaller, C.: Die Autotomie-Mechanismen an den Laufbeinen der Weberknechte (Arach., Opil.). Thesis, J.W. Goethe University, Frankfurt a.M. (1968).

Werner, F.: Pedipalpen. In: Klassen und Ordnungen des Tierreichs (Bronn, H.G. ed.) Vol. 5(4), pp. 317—490. Leipzig: Akademische Verlagsges., 1935.

Weygoldt, P.: The Biology of Pseudoscorpions. Cambridge: Harvard Univ. Press, 1969.

Weygoldt, P.: Notes on the life history and reproductive biology of the giant whip scorpion, *Mastigoproctus giganteus* (Uropygi, Theliphonidae) from Florida. J. Zool. **164**, 137—147 (1971).

Weygoldt, P.: Geisselskorpione and Geisselspinnen (Uropygi und Amblypygi). Zeitschr. Kölner Zoo **15**, 95—107 (1972a).

Weygoldt, P.: Spermatophorenbau und Samenübertragung bei Uropygen (*Mastigoproctus brasilianus* C.L. Koch) und Amblypygen (*Charinus brasilianus* Weygoldt und *Admetus pumilio* C.L. Koch) (Chelicerata, Arachnida). Zeitschr. Morph. Tiere **71**, 23—51 (1972b).

Wood-Mason, J.: Notes on the anatomy of the scorpion-spiders (*Thelyphonus*) — I. The scent-glands. Proc. Asiat. Soc. Beng. 56—60 (1882).

CHAPTER 6

Review of the Spider Families,
with Notes on the Lesser-Known Poisonous Forms

S. BETTINI* and P.M. BRIGNOLI*

As pointed out in the "Introduction to Venomous Arthropod Systematics", all spiders are, strictly speaking, poisonous, with the sole exception of the small family of Uloboridae, which has secondarily lost its poison; the substitutive glandular apparatus has been studied by GLATZ (1969).

The spiders, as a group, are phylogenetically very old, the first fossil spiders belonging to the Carboniferous period (PETRUNKEVITCH, 1958). As the general morphology of spiders has changed little from the Palaeozoic Era to the present (PETRUNKEVITCH, 1958), it could be inferred that the poison appeared very early.

The Araneae are one of the few groups of animals that employ poison as a tool for aggression. The development of the poisonous apparatus (BRISTOWE, 1939–1941), and the evolution of different types of webs (SAVORY, 1952; KULLMANN, 1975; KULLMANN et al., 1975), have ensured the evolutionary success of the order. However, the fact that the poison is often of the same (or greater) importance to spiders than silk is often overlooked even by arachnologists.

In addition, selection must have had a pronounced influence on the characteristics of toxic or predigestive venom constituents. It has allowed many spiders to develop enzymes that apparently neutralize most of the defensive toxic substances employed, or simply contained, by many other arthropods on which they prey. In fact, though very little is known about the biology of any but a handful of spiders, and practically nothing on their alimentary preferences (BRISTOWE, 1939–1941), it has been proved that at least some species of spiders kill and eat any type of "protected" insect or myriapod (BRISTOWE, 1939–1941).

In strong contrast with many other groups of aggressive Arachnida, the spiders show few morphological features which could help them in subduing preys. They do not possess a defensive tool like the powerful pedipalpi, which are often armed with claws such as those displayed by Scorpionida, Pseudoscorpionida, Uropygi, Amblypygi, or the enormous chelicerae of Solifuga. Their exoskeleton is soft and can be easily pierced, their chelicerae are relatively small and barely mobile, and only in a few groups are the front legs armed with rows of sharp spines. On the other hand, spiders possess venoms of varying degrees of potency, which, when used, reduce the strain of a long and dangerous struggle to subdue the prey. The evolution of silk as a capturing tool has, however, reduced the need of possessing very active paralyzing venoms in some groups. It could thus be inferred that all spiders which actively hunt their victims and fight against them

---

* The authors' names ar placed in alphabetical order. The first is responsible mainly for the toxicological information, the second for that on the systematics and biology of the spider groups.

are selectively advantaged if they possess an active venom. The same is true for those that ambush their prey. In the case of web-builders, on the other hand, things are different. Some groups, for instance, employ their large, bidimensional and relatively fragile orb-webs to capture a large number of small and feeble insects with little effort, so that the poison used on the prey does not necessarily have to possess a high paralyzing activity.

The production of silk is, however, very "expensive", and it would therefore be convenient for the spider to produce also an active venom for blocking the prey's movements before it ruins the web in its efforts to free itself. The fact that some orb-weavers are known to free the larger preys from their net, especially if these struggle very hard, could thus possibly be attributed to a reduction of the venom activity and to the spider's fear of having a large portion of the net damaged by the prey.

In connection with the effects of venoms, we have so far used the general term "active", implying that the target against which venoms are employed is the prey itself. Up to recent times, however, traditional toxicologists have tested the activity of venoms almost exclusively on vertebrates, and only in the last few years have some authors seriously taken into consideration the activity of spider venoms on arthropods (see chapter on Venoms of Theridiidae). A similar investigation has lately been carried out on scorpion venom (see chapter on Venoms of Buthinae). The number of studies in this field is, however, still very low. At this stage, it would therefore be at least incautious to state that venoms of single species show "weak" or "potent" effects on the preys unless the venoms' degree of activity on the spiders' natural targets is definitely known. Further information on this subject through direct field observation and experimental work is much needed. Unfortunately, the many important, recent ethological studies on spiders' web construction have not been associated, nor have they been followed up with investigations on the venoms' activity on the natural preys.

As above mentioned, web evolution might have influenced that of venom. It is difficult, however, to consider the effectiveness of spiders' webs, for these may be of different types, each bound to a particular environment and performing a different function. In addition, other factors make it more difficult to understand venom evolution. Some groups of large wandering spiders, as for instance some *Lycosa* spp., which do not build a net for capturing the prey, possess a strongly proteolytic venom used to predigest the prey while it is vigorously held and macerated by the spider's powerful fangs. On the other hand, other groups of web-builders, as for instance *Latrodectus* spp., possess a typical insect-paralyzing venom, and in addition use silk very efficiently to imprison the prey.

Since venom has evolved over a long period of time, probably many more spiders than supposed feed on selected species. The range of activity of single venoms on species that may be preyed on by spiders is still not known. The recent finding that some venoms contain several components, some of which are active on insects, others on crustaceans and others on vertebrates (see chapter on *Latrodectus* venom), may throw some light on the subject of venom specificity, but it also complicates our understanding of the few simple hypotheses so far accepted on spiders' venom evolution.

The present review treats in taxonomical order all groups of spiders whose venom is known to be more or less toxic to man and animals. Full information on the dangerousness of forms belonging to groups whose toxicology has been less thoroughly studied is also given. For the groups whose venom has been investigated in depth the reader should consult the pertinent chapters.

A. Orthognatha = Theraphosomorphae = Mygalomorphae

This suborder embraces more than 1000 species and includes forms that are considered in many ways as primitive. The members of this group are medium or large in size, and have scarcely mobile chelicera (see Introduction) and simple genitalia. None of them builds a complex web. Several species live more or less permanently in holes dug in the soil, which are often coated with silk, while others live in crevices where they build a simple web. A few are probably wandering forms. Exceptionally, some nocturnal species live among the vegetation, not close to the ground. Except for tropical species, they are rarely found indoors.

Very little is known about most of the species. It is believed that they prey on insects and myriapods, and perhaps on other arachnids that get near their burrows. Occasionally, they may also prey on small vertebrates. VELLARD (1936) reports that in the laboratory some species readily attack reptiles (lizards and snakes) and frogs. It has long been thought that some Orthognatha habitually prey on small birds, but this is still to be proved.

This suborder is usually subdivided by taxonomists into 8 families and a large number of genera, though its systematics has not yet reached a high level.

The venomousness of some species belonging to the largest families (Ctenizidae, Dipluridae, Barychelidae and Theraphosidae) has been studied more or less extensively. From the acquired data it may be inferred that probably almost all species, especially the large ones, possess a venom that is active on vertebrates. Since many of the old identifications of species are incorrect, it would be pointless to list all genera reported as poisonous. Up to now, in fact, not much is known about the venom of the majority of Palaearctic and Oriental genera. All recent studies were carried out on Nearctic, Neotropical, Ethiopian and Australian forms. Several South American species were investigated by VELLARD (1936), whose volume remains practically the only source of information on the older experiments and literature.

However, a list of families that include poisonous forms is given here for general information.

Fam. Ctenizidae: A large family including several hundred species. It is the best represented family of this suborder in Europe (Mediterranean region). Members of this family are distributed all over the world, though they seem to be rare in regions covered by rainy tropical forest. Apparently, almost all species are sedentary, living in soil burrows.

From the few investigations carried out on *Cteniza, Actinopus, Idiops, Pselligmus, Rachias* and *Hermacha,* it appears that their venom shows scant neurotoxicity to vertebrates, has no necrotic effects, and is rarely lethal for laboratory animals. The venom of *Actinopus* produces local pain and temporary contracture in man, but it appears to be inactive in poikylotherms. *Missulena*'s venom (MUS-GRAVE, 1949) seems to be even less active on man.

Fam. Dipluridae: The species belonging to this family (smaller than the Ctenizidae) are especially abundant in the southern hemisphere (Neotropical and Australian regions) while the Palaearctic and North American species are only few. The members of this family are those of the Orthognatha that make more use of the web.

     The genera studied because of their higher toxicity, are few. Among these, *Atrax* and *Trechona* have received most attention (see pertinent chapters).

     The possibility cannot be excluded that the venom of other genera might possess analogous characteristics, though that of *Evagrus* (BAERG, 1929) and of that *Dekana* (MAIN, 1976) appear to be definitely less toxic to vertebrates.

Fam. Barychelidae: This family includes little more than 100 species, almost all of which distributed in the southern hemisphere (a very few, little-known species, are Palaearctic or Nearctic). Little is known about their biology, though on the whole it resembles that of Ctenizidae. Some species are arboricolous. According to VELLARD (1936) the venom of *Neostothis* may be lethal to the pigeon while that of *Trichopelma* seems to be almost inactive.

     In South Africa, the genus *Harpactirella* (one of the local genera whose species are commonly called "baboon spiders") has been reported to cause local pain and even collapse (FINLAYSON and SMITHERS, 1939). In Australia, the only known case of a bite of *Idiommata* sp. was that of a 3-year-old girl bitten in the finger, whose only signs were local redness and edema. It was shown that *Latrodectus indistinctus* antivenin conferred some protection in mice subsequently bitten by *Harpactirella* (FINLAYSON, 1955).

Fam. Theraphosidae: To this family, the largest of the Orthognatha, belong several hundreds of species, distributed all over the world but particularly abundant in South America (a very few are Palaearctic). It is the group to which the name "mygalids" is most appropriate (the name Mygale has since long been abandoned for priority reasons). The family includes some of the largest spiders. All members are "wandering" predatory spiders, though often they dig a very simple burrow.

     From the many experiments carried out on these spiders, it can be assumed that the majority of species possess a rather potent venom. It should be pointed out that, as MAIN (1976) reports, besides the poison secreted by the venomous glands many species of this family possess urticating hairs which, in contact with humans, cause considerable discomfort. It appears also that the hairs may be lethal to small mammals. The only forms of this family with urticating hairs belong to the New World representatives of the subfamilies Ischnocolinae, Grammostolinae, Theraphosinae and Aviculariinae. MAIN (1976) reports that the hairs are essentially a defense against molestation by small mammals and are readily shed if the spiders are provoked or handled. These offensive hairs, whose fine structure and effects on man and small vertebrates have been studied by COOKE (1972) and COOKE et al. (1972) are found in patches on the abdomen dorsum or in clusters of short, dark hairs. BÜCHERL (1971) reported that some genera, especially *Grammostola* and *Lasiodora,* may cause inflammation of the respiratory apparatus and subsequent asphyxia in small rodents.

As reported by MAIN (1976), most North American theraphosids are relatively docile and rarely bite when provoked. However, if annoyed, they indulge in hair-flicking. On the other hand, it appears that urticating hairs are absent in the known African, Asian and Australian genera, though they are particularly aggressive and use their fangs in defense.

Much information on the older studies about the venomosity of this group was summarized by KOBERT (1901), PHISALIX (1922) and VELLARD (1936). Data are more abundant on Neotropical forms, while all that is known about the few Palaearctic species, for instance, that the venom of *Chaetopelma olivaceum* may be lethal to small vertebrates and that North African Arabs fear this species (WILSON, 1901).

The large species of Oriental *Selenocosmia* have long been considered as predators of birds: the Australian species *S. stirlingi* (MAIN, 1976) is known to prey on Anura, and the bite of another species of the same genus from New Guinea (MUSGRAVE, 1949) was reported to have caused muscular spasms followed by collapse in man. As reported by PHISALIX (1922), in South America, the first experimental observations on the toxic effect of Theraphosidae appear to be those of HOUSSAY in Argentina at the beginning of this century. He proved that the venom of *Theraphosa blondii* by direct bite or injected after extraction was highly toxic to rats, mice, guinea pigs, rabbits and pigeons. Dogs, fowls, and frogs seemed to be resistant to the action of the venom. According to VELLARD (1936) the species involved was not *T. blondii* but *Acanthoscurria* sp.

VELLARD (1936) investigated the venom of several genera quite thoroughly. The venom of *Acanthoscurria* especially, and that of the larger species of such other genera as *Phormictopus* was found to be particularly active on laboratory vertebrates, causing curare-like paralysis, icterus, hemoglobinuria and, in some cases, even local necrosis. Similar effects were also ascribed to the venom of *Pamphobeteus.* The venom of *Lasiodora, Grammostola, Eupalaestrus, Eurypelma,* and *Hapalopus* was reported to be less active on birds and mammalians but more dangerous to poikylotherms. According to BAERG (1929) the venom of *Sericopelma* appeared to be also considerably toxic to man, while that of *Dugesiella* and *Psalmopoeus* was less so. VELLARD reports a lethal case of *Phormictopus* bite.

BÜCHERL (1956, 1971) has in part integrated and summarized the information given by VELLARD.

The venom of the tarantula *Aphonopelma* sp. from Central Arizona has been thoroughly studied by STAHNKE and JOHNSON (1967). The venom, collected by electrical stimulation, was centrifuged and lyophilized. Disc electrophoresis with acrylamide gels was used to separate the venom proteins. Preliminary qualitative analysis showed that the venom had protease activity (tested on X-ray film strips) and negligible RNAase but no L-aminoacid oxide or DNAase activities. The venom injected into mice showed an LD_{50} of 14.14 mg/kg. These findings were compared with those obtained in parallel with the venom of the scorpion *Centruroides sculpturatus,* collected in the same region. The authors point out the similarity of syndromes in rats and mice caused by the injection of the venom of the tarantula and of the scorpion. A positive correlation of the two venoms was also shown in the amount of venom protein and in lethality (the tarantula venom was, however, about 12 times less toxic than that of the scorpion), and in the disc electrophoretic distribution of the protein components. Similarities were also found in the enzyme analysis of the two venoms. Gel diffusion-precipitation reactions indicated that venom components were similar in their antigenic properties. Finally, a preliminary test showed that a guinea pig hypersensitized with *C. sculpturatus* venom could be triggered into anaphylaxis by tarantula venom.

Aphonopelma spp. bites have also been recorded in the USA by RUSSELL and WALDRON (1967) and RUSSELL (1969). RUSSELL reports that these species may produce some localized tissue alterations, edema, pain, and lymphadenitis in man. No general symptoms were recorded. There seems to be no specific treatment for these injuries, although some physicians use steroids during the acute stages of the poisoning.

The venom of the Arkansas tarantula, *Dugesiella hentzi,* has been studied by SCHANBACHER et al. (1973a, 1973b). The venom was obtained by electrical stimulation and stored at $-15°$ C, its protein content being 200 µg/µl. The venom showed a high hyaluronidase activity, but no phospholipase A, chitinase, or protease activities were found. Toxicity was tested on adult German cockroaches.

With disc electrophoresis, the authors separated at least 7 anode-migrating protein bands, and gave the densitometric tracing of stained disc gel electrophoresis; hyaluronidase activity coincided with one of the first bands of the electrophoretic pattern.

The chromatographic profile of whole tarantula venom obtained on Sephadex G-100 showed five distinct peaks. Peak 3 contained hyaluronidase, while peak 4 was identified as the primary cockroach toxin of the venom. Peak 5 contained several ninhydrin-positive compounds, including γ-amino butyric, blutamic and aspartic acids.

The molecular weight of peak 3 (hyaluronidase) was 37,000 and that of peak 4 (component toxic to cockroaches) about 7,300.

The LD_{50} of *D. hentzi* whole venom in mice was 0.3 µl/g body weight, while in American cockroaches (6 h) the LD_{50} was 0.31 µl/adult male (BIERY, 1971).

LEE et al. (1974) purified and characterized a necrotoxin from electrically collected venom of *D. hentzi*. The venom was separated through Sephadex and disc gel electrophoresis. Toxicity tests were conducted with white mice (intraperitoneal administration) and in American cockroaches. Three major peaks were obtained by means of chromatography on Sephadex G-25. Only peaks A and B were lethal to mice, while all three peaks killed the injected cockroaches. Further fractionation of peak A, with Sephadex G-100, resulted in four peaks, where peaks 3 and 4 were the major components. Peak 3 had been characterized as hyaluronidase with a molecular weight of 39,000 by SCHANBACHER et al. (1973b). Only peak 4 was found to be toxic to mice and cockroaches. A further purification of this toxin (necrotoxin) through a CM-Sephadex column yielded only one major peak, a protein that retained toxicity to mice and cockroaches. Final purification was achieved by isoelectric focusing. Only one protein peak was evident, with an isoelectric point of 10.0. The molecular weight of the purified necrotoxin was estimated to be 6,500. After injection of the necrotoxin, mice showed an increase of creatine phosphokinase activity, which decreased after 4 h. Histological heart changes in mice injected with the venom had previously been observed by BIERY (1971). Further observations by LEE et al. (1974) showed that the primary lesion consisted in acute focal areas of myocardial necrosis. The results of amino acid analysis of the hydrolized necrotoxin are given. The chemical modification of the tryptophan residue led to loss of toxicity.

CHAN et al. (1975) have recently demonstrated that the venom of *D. hentzi* and *Aphonopelma* sp. are rich in ATP, with levels of 28.1 and 56.6 µg/µl respectively. The toxicity of *D. hentzi* venom was significantly increased when ATP was added. The authors discuss the synergistic toxic effect of ATP which could induce histamine release and cytotoxic effects on most cells of the connective tissues, thus enhancing the venom's necrotoxin activity in mice.

The fine structure of *Aphonopelma chalcodes, A. portala* and *Dugesiella echina* has been studied by RUSSELL et al. (1973). The glandular epithelium is surrounded by a thick muscular layer and is separated from the glandular epithelium by a compact collagenous sheath. The basal region of the epithelium contains a complete system of narrow, interdigitating cell processes. The epithelial cells are innervated by nerves penetrating the collagenous sheath.

In Peru VELLARD described the venomous species *Hapalopus limensis,* which was later studied by de ESPINOZA (1966). The author reports the morphological characteristics and biology, and describes the venom gland histology. The venom's toxic activity was tested on rats, guinea pigs, rabbits, dogs and pigeons through the direct bite of the spider or by injection of macerated glands in saline solution. The symptoms shown by the poisoned animals were substantially similar, whether they had been exposed to the bite or injected. The initial excitatory period was followed in a few minutes by paralysis and death. The approximate minimal lethal dose i.v. was half of one gland for the guinea pig and rabbit, $1^1/_2-2$ glands for the dog and three-quarters of one gland for the pigeon. (One toad injected with 2 glands showed no reaction.) The author compares this symptomatology with that caused by curare, where respiratory paralysis precedes cardiac block. The anatomical lesions of the animals killed by the venom were characterized by intensive visceral congestions and degeneration of liver, kidneys and lungs. No local reactions were observed. The nature and frequency of human accidents is not given.

In the field of tarantulas, the venom of the genus *Pterinochilus* has also been thoroughly investigated. It should be noted that *Pterinochilus,* living in Africa, is the only non-American genus whose venom has been studied.

MARETIĆ (1967) studied the venom obtained by mechanical pressure or by electrical stimulation from specimens of *Pterinochilus* sp. collected in Tanzania. The fresh venom injected i.v. to mice gave an LD_{50} value of about 9 mg per kg body weight. An equivalent activity was obtained with lyophilized venom. The injected mice and guinea pigs soon became highly excited and showed dyspnea, salivation, lacrimation, tetanic convulsions, paretic and paralytic signs.

Intoxicated guinea pigs showed moderate leukocytosis with neutrophilia. The ECG presented flattened or negative T waves in leads I and II. The ECG tracings showed a higher frequency of activity with no changes in form or pattern. It was also demonstrated that the spider toxin penetrates the blood-brain barrier.

When trypan blue solution was injected to the animal together with the venom, sections of the brain were stained.

Histological examination of poisoned animals showed "vacuolar and parenchymatous degeneration of renal tubuli and liver. The brain showed degenerative alterations, and the myocardium less pronounced parenchymatous degeneration. The adrenal cortex, especially the *zonae fasciculata* and *reticularis,* were markedly enlarged. Many cells appeared vacuolated, and contained lipoid granula." With paper electrophoresis strips 5−7 components were detected.

In a subsequent paper Freyvogel et al. (1968) reported in detail on the biology (biotope, mechanisms of preying, food intake, and behavior) of *Pterinochilus* sp. A well documented study was carried out on the anatomy and histology of the venom apparatus. It was found that the regeneration time of an emptied gland was from three to four months. The toxicity of the venom was tested in mice, the LD_{50} values i.v. ranging from 2 to 5 µg/g body weight. The venom lost its activity rapidly unless lyophilized. In contrast to what had been observed with other venomous spiders (see: *Latrodectus*), the hemolymph of *Pterinochilus* was toxic to mice. Injection of the venom to mice resulted in marked neurotoxic symptoms. These symptoms, as well as the ECG, EEG signs, the histologic findings, and the permeability of the brain barrier by injected venom are those previously described by Maretić (1967). The venom was separated electrophoretically on polyacrylamide gel; 8 components with a molecular weight of less than 1,400 and at least 16 components with a molecular weight of over 1,400 were obtained. Four of these components of similar molecular weight proved to be toxic to mice. The authors discuss the low frequency of bites reported in man and correlate it with the spider's behavior, according to which the act of biting is not always accompanied by the injection of venom.

In a more recent paper, Perret and Freyvogel (1973) reported further investigation on the biological activity of the separated venom components of *Pterinochilus* sp. Separation was carried out on a Sephadex G-50 column, followed by disc electrophoresis in acrylamide gel. Mice were used for toxicity tests. Eleven peaks could be distinguished from the venom filtered on Sephadex, while 18 bands could be observed in the venom separated by electrophoresis.

The LD_{50} of the lyophilized crude venom was 3.6 mg/kg body weight. Among the components separated on Sephadex, peaks from 3 to 8 proved to be more toxic to mice than crude venom, the lowest LD_{50} being 0.46 mg/kg, in fraction 6. Neurotoxic effects were found in five components, all of them cathodal proteins. It is interesting to note that no differences could be observed between the venom of males and that of females, with respect to either toxicity or composition.

B. Labidognatha = Araneomorphae

I. Haplogynae

This group, whose systematic position is still not generally agreed, includes about a dozen small families, all of which possess chelicera more mobile than those of Orthognatha, lack a cribellum and have relatively simple genitalia. The members of this group are spiders of small or medium size, often detricolous or cavernicolous. Many of them are wandering predators and some build rather simple webs. The only families of any toxicological importance are Dysderidae, Segestriidae and Scytodidae.

Fam. Dysderidae: This family includes a few hundreds of species, the majority of which are Palaearctic. A few partially synanthropic species, however, have been introduced in various regions of the world. The members of this family are typically lapidicolous spiders that ambush their preys (Isopoda, for instance) and are of small or medium dimensions.

It is very improbable that any *Dysdera* (which include the largest species) has a venom of any significant activity. The old, and dubious, information on the bite effects of members of this genus, as reported by some authors (for instance VELLARD, 1936), probably refer to species of other families.

DUFFEY and GREEN (1975) and MAIN (1976) report two cases of bites from Australian and British *Dysdera*, in which there were no consequences.

Fam. Segestriidae: This is a small family of less than one hundred species with a worldwide distribution, often associated with Dysderidae. More or less all of its species live in fissures of rocks or holes in walls. The large *Segestria florentina*, in particular, is a common synanthropic spider found in most of the world's regions. It is well known (DUGES, 1836) that the bite of this species causes no symptoms in man, except for slight local redness and swelling. However, especially in South America, the bite of several species of this family has been thought to cause severe effects. Without any doubt these spiders were confused with *Loxosceles* species (VELLARD, 1936).

Fam. Scytodidae: This family is distributed all over the world and embraces about two hundred species, all grouped into two genera: *Scytodes* and *Loxosceles* (which were previously considered as members of the Sicariidae, now a dismembered family).

The *Scytodes* "spit" on the prey a sticky substance produced by their modified venom glands and are, therefore, toxicologically less important.

The *Loxosceles,* on the other hand, are much feared for the severe necrotic effects of their venom. In the present text a separate chapter has been devoted to the venom of the better known *Loxosceles* species.

The number of species belonging to the latter genus is the object of debate. The great majority of the species are distributed in America, a few in the Mediterranean region and Africa. Almost all species are lapidicolous and in some cases their dens are provided with a sort of rudimentary web. Various species are more or less synanthropic and, as such, have been scattered to other continents. Due to the extreme uniformity of this genus, it might be inferred that the venom of all species is equally dangerous. It is strange, therefore, that cases of *Loxosceles* bites are unknown outside America.

II. Entelegynae = Trionychae

The majority of spiders belongs to this subdivision: about 20−25 families with several thousands of species. Apart from the absence of a cribellum and of complex genitalia, the characteristic that all members of this group have in common is the presence of three claws on their tarsi. The toxicologically important species belong to the two superfamilies Araneoidea and Lycosoidea.

1. Araneoidea

The members of this group are spiders that have developed their webs to the extreme. The largest forms (Araneidae) often build geometrical and complex webs. Some of the smaller forms build simpler webs and others build tridimensional and apparently irregular ones. The species of this group range from forms bound to vegetation (typical predators of winged insects) to detricolous and lapidicolous forms that build their web in between rocks or under stones. Several species, of all continents, are synanthropic to different degrees.

a) Araneidae = Argiopidae

This is the one family that has developed to the extreme the bidimensional type of web with a logarithmic spiral. Since the web is very fragile, the spider not only bites its prey but also envelops it in silk. From this fact too it may be assumed that the venom of this family is probably not very active. Araneidae include thousands of species, some of which are very common and distributed all over the world.

Several arachnologists (DUGÈS, 1836; GAUBERT, 1892; DENIS, 1947; DUFFEY and GREEN, 1975, etc.) have reported cases of humans bitten by species of *"Epeira"* (now *Araneus*) but showing no serious consequences. The effects of the bite of various members of this genus have recently been studied by different authors. A case of a bite from a spider belonging to a genus very close to *Araneus, Aranea sexpunctata* (= *Nuctenea umbratica*), which is one of the most common European species and is considered harmless for man, was reported by MARETIĆ and MILINA (1976). The symptomatology was characterized by local pain, oppression on the chest and a sense of choking, muscular contracture, weakness and paresthesias in the bitten arm, followed by a similar sensation in all four limbs, and severe pains in the lumbar region and abdomen. The patient also complained of generalized pruritus, moderate sweating, nausea, and hypersalivation. Intense burning of the soles of the feet, deep muscular pain, insomnia, and paresthesias lasted several days. The symptoms as well as some signs (face congestion, sweating) were similar to those caused by latrodectism.

Some species of *Mastophora,* the South American "bolas spiders" are known to be venomous (BÜCHERL, 1971).

In the case of large species it is possible that the effects of the bite may be more evident. In fact, the species *Argiope aurantia* was reported as being venomous in North America (GORHAM and RHENEY, 1968). Immediate local pain, followed by pain in the groin, were the only symptoms suffered by the patient, who recovered in a few hours after symptomatic treatment.

Several South American species were studied by VELLARD (1936). He found that the venom of *Nephila, Argiope* and *Araneus* caused signs in laboratory vertebrates that were similar to, but less severe than, those provoked by *Lycosa, i.e.* necrosis at the bite site. In this case also, due to the large size of the spiders, especially of *Nephila*, it is probable that their venom may have substantial effects.

A particular case is perhaps that of the American species of *Mastophora* (formerly *Glyptocranium*). These forms are known as "bolas spiders" for their peculiar habit of capturing the prey with a sticky droplet hanging at the extremity of a silk thread held by a leg. The bite of *M. gasteracanthoides* was believed in Peru to cause severe effects, and even death (ESCOMEL, 1918). It cannot be excluded that, because of this specialized preying mechanism, its venom might be very active, but a recent confirmation of this hypothesis is lacking. VELLARD (1936), in fact, could not discover any effects due to the bite of a related species.

Cyrtophora citricola has also been reported in Italy to cause local swelling but no general symptoms.

b) Linyphiidae

The members of this family are small or minute spiders, which build non-geometric webs of medium complexity close to the ground. They constitute the majority of spiders, as far as numbers of species and of individuals are concerned, living in the cold regions of the northern hemisphere. The so-called "money spiders" belong to this group. It would be hard to believe that such small spiders could cause any effect on vertebrates. Recently, however, DUFFEY and GREEN (1975) have reported the case of factory laborers working in a sewage-treatment plant being badly affected by the bite of the minute *Leptorhoptrum robustum*. They complained of local redness and swelling. Due to the small size of the members of this group, it is highly improbable that any really dangerous species might exist. This, however, does not imply that the activity of their venom is low.

c) Theridiidae

This is a large family, including thousands of species distributed all over the world. All members build rather simple, tridimensional webs, which are anchored to vegetation and partly hidden under rocks. They capture preys that are usually larger than the spiders themselves.

The two genera *Latrodectus* and *Steatoda* are treated in a separate chapter.

MAIN (1976) was bitten in the finger by the small species *Achaearanea tepidariorum* (a synanthropic and practically cosmopolitan species) but the symptoms were very mild: redness of the bitten finger, mild nausea and headache lasting two days. In another case reported by the same author, the symptoms were more severe and lasted over a longer period.

2. Lycosoidea

Only a few families, including many hundreds of species distributed all over the world, are commonly ascribed to this superfamily. Some of the Agelenidae and Lycosidae build wide, irregular, funnel-shaped webs, which serve more as a support to the spider than as a tool for capturing preys. The other species, of various sizes, include many wandering predators (some of which burrow holes in the soil) and a few detriticolous forms. The few water-spiders also belong to this group.

a) Agelenidae

The members of this family live mainly on webs built on the vegetation or under rocks, or are detriticolous. The family includes the well known large *Tegenaria* found in the European and North American houses. Very little is known, however, about their venom. Duges (1836) and Gaubert (1892) let themselves be bitten by *Tegenaria* without suffering of any serious sign or symptom. Berland (1927) was bitten by the small lapidicolous *Coelotes obesus,* suffering severe local pain and muscular contracture in the injured limb for a few hours. Bonnet (1966) reported a case of a painful bite followed by muscular contracture lasting several hours due to the large *Agelena labyrinthica,* a common spider found on European hedges.

b) Argyronetidae

The bite of the well known European water-spider *Argyroneta aquatica* is apparently not innocuous, but specific data on venom activity are lacking (literature reported by Bonnet, 1945).

c) Pisauridae

Spiders in this family are of average size and they are distributed all over the world; the family includes some rather large species, some of which are wandering predators feeding on vegetation and some semi-aquatic forms that prey on tadpoles or small fish.

The venom of the Holarctic *Dolomedes,* which was proved to be active on fish, does not appear to have a marked effect on man (Bonnet, 1966). Information on *Thaumasia* and *Trechalea* can be found in Vellard's (1936) volume, where it is reported that the venom of these spiders is very active on fish and anura, inducing paralysis, while it causes mild effects on mammalians, birds and reptiles.

(The closely related very small family Desidae, to which belong the only marine spiders of the intercotidal zone, which prey on fish, probably possess a venom of similar activity.)

d) Lycosidae

This large family includes medium or large species, mainly wandering predators. Some of the larger forms burrow a hole in the soil (the "true" tarantulas), while a few build a web. Lycosids are abundant everywhere, in debris as well as in leaves, or even on river banks.

The systematics of this group has not been settled yet, the confusion arising partly from its nomenclature. Only the Holarctic species are relatively well known.

It is also doubtful whether all the so-called *Lycosa* belong to the same genus, and this could explain the difference in effects of the venom between Palaearctic and Neotropical species.

Up to the end of the seventeenth century in Europe the bite of spiders belonging to the genus *Lycosa* was thought to cause a well known somatic and psychic condition called "tarantism" (KOBERT, 1901). The regions where these cases occurred corresponded to some of the distribution areas of *Latrodectus mactans tredecimguttatus*. But not until the middle of the nineteenth century was it demonstrated that hysteria was one of the major factors responsible for this syndrome and that "latrodectism" was to blame only in a few cases. The volume of DE MARTINO (1961) gives a full account of the evolution of this problem. This subject was also treated by MARETIĆ and LEBEZ (1969). PHISALIX (1922) reports some information on different species of *Lycosa*.

The genus *Lycosa* has been treated by BÜCHERL (1971), who reports data on the morphology, biology and habits especially of *L. erythrognatha*. In experiments conducted with venom from electrically milked spiders, the quantity of venom which killed a 20 mg mouse was 0.080 mg i.v. and 1.25 mg s.c.

The venom of *Lycosa tarentula* was studied by LEBEZ (1953) and MARETIĆ and LEBEZ (1969). It was found that the venom, obtained by inducing the spiders to bite a cotton tampon, showed strong hemolytic and proteolytic effects. Polypeptides obtained from venom glands crushed in water had a noxious effect on mice, similar to that of bradykinin. Local effects on experimental animals are characterized by swelling and redness. Salivation and pareses were observed in poisoned cats and mice. The mortality rate was very low. In man, the bite usually provokes only a slight local response. One patient, however, suffered necrosis of the skin, which was confined to the bite site. Necrosis was obtained in experimental animals by injecting the venom intradermally. LEBEZ et al. (1969) separated the venom components of *Hogna* (*Lycosa*) *tarentula* by paper electrophoresis.

Several venomous species of *Lycosa* are found in South America. *Lycosa raptoria* is the most-studied species. VELLARD (1936) gives detailed information on the action of its venom on experimental animals. As in *L. tarentula*, if the venom is injected intradermally, it causes deep necrosis. The s.c. or i.m. injection of even large doses of venom did not provoke death in experimental animals. In man, where the skin is thick and adherent to the deeper layers, the local lesions caused by the bite of this species are very severe, reaching the muscle layer and extending over an areas more than 20 cm in diameter. Marked edema and phlyctenae last for 3–4 days and give place to necrosis, which starts with a whitish plaque near the point of entrance of the venom, turning into an eschar. After 15–20 days, the eschar falls, leaving deep ulceration with irregular and steep borders. It takes 2–4 months for the ulcer to heal into a keloidal scar.

The collagenolytic activity of the venom of *Lycosa erythrognatha* was investigated by KAISER and RAAB (1967). The authors found that at an optimal pH of 9.0 the venom digested azocoll, gelatine and casein but had no lytic action on collagen fibers or collagen powder, even after incubation periods of up to 3 days. However, collagen denatured by heat or urea was also digested by the venom. The mode of action of the venom *in vivo* is discussed.

Unfortunately, apart from the above-mentioned problem concerning the actual taxonomic position of the various Lycosids, too little is known about their biology for us to understand why the South American species have such a potent venom, and why Lycosids of other regions, such as the North American *Lycosa carolinensis* (see KASTON, 1948) and the Australian species (MAIN, 1976), are not dangerous. Nothing is known about the venom of other genera of this family.

e) Oxyopidae

This is a rather small family which includes species of medium or large size, wandering predators living on vegetation. A case of a bite by *Peucetia viridans* that was not followed by serious consequences was reported by HALL and MADON (1973).

III. Entelegynae = Dionychae

This very heterogenous group includes about 15 families with several thousands species. Their only common characteristic is the presence of two tarsal claws. They do not build webs, being wandering predators or living on vegetation or under rocks. The present text follows the traditional, though much discussed, systematics for this group.

1. Gnaphosidae (= Drassodidae = Drassidae)

The Gnaphosidae are a large, rather heterogeneous family of spiders, mainly detriticolous or lapidicolous, also living under bark. Very little is known about their venom. DENIS (1947) reported that the bite of *Gnaphosa* has no effects. On the other hand, MUSGRAVE (1949) and MAIN (1976) observed a few cases of persons bitten by Australian *Megamyrmecion* species who complained of severe pains, and in some cases nausea and headache; in one case, a sore at the site of the bite persisted for some time, with local irritation and pruritus. MAJESKI and DURST (1975) report the bite of *Herpyllus ecclesiasticus* on the left scapula of an adult female. The patient complained of sharp local pain, pruritus, arthralgia, malaise and nausea, which subsided within 48 hours after the bite. DUFFEY and GREEN (1975) suggest that the local effects (permanent scar on the face) thought to be due to the bite of *Herpyllus blackwalli* were probably attributable to another species.

2. Clubionidae

This is also a large family whose members are distributed all over the world. The group is probably heterogeneous, because the true Clubionids are spiders confined to vegetation, where they build their dens with leaves or under bark, while other genera include limitedly synanthropic species.

Toxic effects have been described for *Chiracanthium* only. Spiders belonging to this genus have been reported as venomous since the eighteenth century.

PHISALIX (1922) refers to early reports of FOREL (1876) and BERTKAU (1891), who induced *Chiracanthium punctorium* specimens to bite the authors' fingers. Immediate irradiating pain was followed by cold perspiration, but local signs were slight. It is also reported that SIMON (1886), the famous arachnologist, considered the bite of this species to be very painful to man and lethal to insects.

KOBERT (1901) dedicates four pages of his volume to the description of *C. nutrix* (= *C. punctorium*) and the symptoms caused by its venom in man. The author himself was bitten three times, carefully recording the progression of symptoms. Local swelling and redness were accompanied by pains irradiating from the bitten area and fever.

Data on the venomosity of this species were also reported by MARETIĆ (1962), who described the symptomatology of one of the four patients that he observed. Local pain, necrosis at the bitten area and enlargements of lymph nodes were followed by severe tiredness. The body temperature and routine laboratory findings were within the normal limits.

Cases of arachnidism caused by the bite of *C. inclusum* were reported by FURMAN and REEVES (1957) and GORHAM and RHENEY (1968). The latter authors describe the symptoms of a patient bitten on her left forearm. Immediate local pain was followed by nausea and extension of the pain to muscles of the upper arm around the axilla and chest. The symptoms subsided within the day and no local signs were observed. Treatment was symptomatic.

SPIELMAN and LEVI (1970) report five cases of necrotizing skin lesions attributed to *C. mildei,* which were observed in the vicinity of Boston. "A red wheal developed within minutes of the bite, and a sloughing crust formed one day later. After another day or two, a necrotic area, depressed at its center, formed beneath the eschar. The lesion's margin was usually raised and was surrounded by a zone of induration. The largest lesion was 12 cm in diameter. Lesions healed after 1.5 to 8 weeks. No systemic signs or symptoms were reported." Guinea pigs bitten by the spider showed an erythematous wheal which was replaced by eschars within one day. The largest lesion was 17 mm in diameter. These signs, however, were not consistent.

As reported by MAIN (1976), in accounts of adult humans bitten by the Australian species *C. mordax* and *C. longimanus*, the victims generally related that a burning pain spread rapidly from the site of the bite. Swelling and erytheme followed, this being particularly severe in people bitten on fingers. Systemic symptoms included vague to severe malaise, faintness, dizziness, headache and nausea. Patients were treated with injections and antihistamines and local anesthetics and symptoms subsided within 36 h. From accounts relating to bites of *Chiracanthium* in Australia, the Pacific, Europe, North Africa and North America, it is apparent that all species of *Chiracanthium* are probably venomous to man.

In Japan, ORI (1975) reports five cases of bites from *C. japonicum,* which occurred from 1956 to 1974. The author describes 4 grades of clinical manifestations: grade 1: no general symptoms, only local pain due to the bite; grade 2: mild symptoms and signs consisting of intense pruritus, and often local swelling and redness; grade 3: moderate symptoms, mainly local pain and long-lasting loss of sensitivity; grade 4: general symptoms consisting in nausea, anorexia and mild fever. Recovery takes place within two or several days.

3. Ctenidae

This family is considered by many taxonomists to be close to Clubionidae. It is a family of medium size, distributed mainly in Africa and South America. Only a few species are present in other continents, and rare forms are found in the Holarctic region. Very little is known about the biology of its members, which are wandering predators dwelling largely among vegetation, like Clubionidae. Some are rather large species. The systematics of this family is still unsettled and open to debate. The toxicity of some South American *Ctenus* (see chapter on this group in the present volume) and *Phoneutria* is well known. On the other hand very little is known about species from other regions. MAIN (1976) reports a case of an *Elassoctenus* bite, which caused severe pain followed by headache and impaired vision.

4. Eusparassidae (= Heteropodidae)

The members of this small family are distributed almost exclusively in the tropical regions, Africa in particular. Some species are large with a flattened body and legs extended. Many tropical species are synanthropic: *Heteropoda venatoria* especially, like some of the Ctenids, often reaches other regions hidden in banana bunches. All species are wandering predators; their biology is still little known.

In many countries these spiders are much feared, but apparently with no good reason. VELLARD (1936) studied some "nandu-pés", as the guarani people call these spiders, and in particular *H. venatoria, Polybetes maculatus* and some *Olios*. The venom of *Heteropoda* is not very active on small vertebrates, and causes mild symptoms in man. The venom of *Polybetes,* on the other hand, is definitely more active. BURGHI (1909) reports that a person bitten by a member of this genus suffered high fever, vomiting, land insomnia lasting for a whole week, and even after 45 days the ulcer at the bite site was still unhealed. It appears that the venom of *Olios* is much less active.

As reported by YATES (1968), symptoms similar to those caused by *Polybetes* follow the bite of the South African *Palystes*.

In Australia, MUSGRAVE (1949) ascribed to the bite of *Olios* some effects on man, and MAIN (1976) reports the fear that Australian natives show for *Heteropoda*. The symptoms caused by the venom of this group also seem to be vomiting, headache and insomnia.

According to VELLARD (1936), Selenopidae (a small family related to Eusparassidae) possess a barely active venom, even though they are feared by the indigenous population.

5. Thomisidae

The very numerous members of this family, known as "crab spiders," are distributed all over the world, mostly dwelling on vegetation, where they lie in wait on flowers or wander on bark (several species are, however, detriticolous or lapidicolous). They do not seem to be very dangerous to vetebrates, but their venom is undoubtedly quite active on several insects; even large hymenoptera die immediately if bitten on the head by a spider lying in wait on a flower. Because of the very small size of their chelicera they probably do not succeed in piercing the skin of vetebrates.

The only highly venomous species in this family is *Phrynarachne rugosa,* named "foka" by the people of Madagascar. Of this spider, unfortunately, very little is known. VINSON (1863) reported that the effects of its bite are completely different from those of the bite of the locally most common *Latrodectus* species (*L. menavodi*), the bite of the "foka" causing local swelling extending to the whole body followed by death, while the latter induces the well known neurotoxic symptoms (see chapter on Theridiidae).

6. Salticidae

The very numerous members of this family, which are named "jumping spiders," are abundant in the tropics. Their venom is quite active on several arthropods. These typically wandering predatory spiders capture the prey (at times larger than the spider itself) by jumping on it and inflicting their poisonous bite. Their small size could raise doubts on their ability to cause any serious effect on man. Nevertheless, MAIN (1976) notes one case of poisoning by *Mopsus mormon* in Australia, revealed in painful swelling and erythema lasting for a week.

RUSSELL (1969, 1970) reported the case history of a man bitten twice on the hand by *Phidippus formosus.* (This genus had been previously recorded by WALDRON (1965) and by RUSSELL and WALDRON (1962) as venomous to man.) Several hours later the bite area revealed a 2-mm ulcer, and on the following day the area was swollen. Two days after the bite the swelling involved the entire dorsum of the hand. The swelling and pruritus continued for nine days.

These data lead to the suspicion that there may be some truth in the rumored poisonous effects of two of the so-called "mico-mico" species from Bolivia, *Dendryphantes noxiosus* and *D. sacci.* SACC (in SIMON, 1886) ascribes to their bite such severe effects as intense pain, local inflammation and hematuria, followed by death.

Subsequently, other authors, in particular VELLARD (1939), have expressed doubts about SACC's beliefs. As mentioned in connection with the discussion of other groups, there is no proof that the venom of the many other species of this family is innocuous.

IV. Cribellatae

This group includes a dozen families which, beside the spinnerets, possess another silk-producing organ, the cribellum, whose silk is flocky instead of drop-like. According to some recent authors, this is not a homogeneous group and its members should be distributed among the Entelegynae, Trionychae and Dionychae.

Very little is known about the venom of Cribellatae. VELLARD (1936) dedicated a whole chapter to the Filistatidae, a small family of sedentary spiders living in crevices or holes, like the Segestriidae. From what VELLARD writes one may suspect that in this case also the severe effects observed following bites of South American species should be attributed to *Loxosceles.*

Musgrave (1949) and Main (1976) report some accidents due to the bite of *Ixeuticus* (a genus belonging to the family Amaurobiidae, which includes a few hundreds of species, all web-builders, living under or on top of rocks, or in houses) characterized by severe local pain, diffuse redness, and nausea.

Denis (1947) and Brignoli (unpublished observations) noted that the bite of *Zoropsis* (a genus belonging to the family Zoropsidae, which includes few lapidicolous and very few synanthropic species) has no effect on man.

References

Baerg, W.J.: Some poisonous arthropods of North and Central America. Congr. intern. entomol. **4**, Ithaca, Trans. **2**, 418—438 (1929).

Berland, L.: Contribution à l'étude de la biologie des arachnides (2e mémoire). Arch. Zool. Exp. Gén. **66** (Not. Rév.), 7—29 (1927).

Bertkau, P.: Über das Vorkommen einer Giftspinne in Deutschland. Verh. d. Naturh. Ver. Preuss. Rhein. **48**, 89 (1891).

Biery, T.L.: The biology and venom potential of the Arkansas tarantula *Dugesiella hentzi* (Girard). Ph.D. Thesis, Oklahoma State University, Stillwater, Oklahoma, 1971.

Bonnet, P.: Bibliographia araneorum. Douladoue, Toulouse 1945.

Bonnet, P.: Sur un cas de piqûre venimeuse par une Agélène. Atti Accad. Gioenia Sci. Nat. Catania **18**, 162—164 (1966).

Bristowe, W.S.: The comity of spiders. London: Ray Society 1939—1941.

Bücherl, W.: Südamerikanische Spinnen und ihre Gifte. Arzneim.-Forsch. **6**, 293 (1956).

Bücherl, W.: Venomous animals and their venoms. III. Venomous invertebrates. Eds. W. Bücherl, E. Buckley. New York, London: Academic Press 1971.

Burghi, R.J.: Aracnoidismo. Tesis, Buenos Aires, 27—85, 1909.

Chan, T.K., Geren, C.R., Howell, D.E., Odell, G.V.: Adenosine triphosphate in tarantula spider venoms and its synergistic effect with the venom toxin. Toxicon **13**, 61—66 (1975).

Cooke, J.A.L.: Stinging hairs: A tarantula's defence. Fauna **4**, 4—8 (1972).

Cooke, J.A.L., Roth, V., Miller, F.H.: The urticating hairs of theraphosid spiders. Amer. Museum Novitates **2498**, 43 pp. (1972).

de Espinoza, N.C.: Accion del veneno de *Hapalopus limensis*. Mem. Inst. Butantan, Simp. Internac. **33**, 799—808 (1966).

De Martino, E.: La terra del rimorso. Milano: Saggiatore 1961.

Denis, J.: Le venin des araignées. Bull. Soc. Ent. Nord Fr. **30**, 3—15 (1947).

Duffey, E., Green, M.B.: A linyphiid spider biting workers on a sewage-treatment plant. Bull Brit. Arachn. Soc. **3**, 130—131 (1975).

Dugès, A.: Observations sur les aranéides. Ann. Sci. Nat. Zool. **6**, 159—219 (1836).

Escomel, E.: La *Glyptocranium gasteracanthoides,* araignée venimeuse du Pérou. Etude clinique et expérimental de l'action du venin. Bull. Soc. Path. Exot. **11**, 136—150 (1918).

Finlayson, M.H.: Spider-bite in South Africa. S. Afr. Med. J. **29**, 509—510 (1955).

Finlayson, M.H., Smithers, R.: *Harpactirella lightfooti* as a cause of spider-bite in the Union, with note on biology of *H. lightfooti* (Purcell). S. Afr. Med. J. **13**, 808—810 (1939).

Forel, A.: Une araignée venimeuse (*Chiracanthium nutrix* Walck), dand le canton de Vaud. Bull. Soc. Vaud, Sc. Nat. **14**, 30 (1876).

Freyvogel, T.A., Honegger, C.G., Maretić, Z.: Zur Biologie und Giftigkeit der ostafrikanischen Vogelspinne *Pterinochilus* spec. Acta Tropica **25**, 217—255 (1968).

Furman, D.P., Reeves, W.C.: Toxic bite of spider *Chiracanthium inclusum* (Hentz). Calif. Med. **87**, 114 (1957).

Gaubert, P.: Recherches sur les organes des sens et sur les systèmes tégumentaires, glandulaires et musculaires des appendices des Arachnides. Thèse Fac. Sci. Paris **748**, 31—184 (1892).

Glatz, L.: Corrélations entre la capture de la proie et les structures des pièces buccales chez les Uloboridae. Bull. Muséum Nat. Hist. Natur. **41**, 2e Série, Suppl. 1, 65—69 (1969).

Gorham, J.R., Rheney, T.B.: Envenomation by the spiders *Chiracanthium inclusum* and *Argiope aurantia*. Observations on Arachnidism in the United States. J. Amer. med. Ass. **206**, 1958—1962 (1968).

Hall, R.E., Madon, M.B.: Envenomation by the green lynx spider *Peucetia viridans* (Hentz 1832), in Orange County, California. Toxicon **11**, 197—199 (1973).

Kaiser, E., Raab, W.: Collagenolytic activity of snake and spider venoms. Toxicon **4**, 251—255 (1967).

Kaston, B.J.: Spiders of Connecticut. St. Conn. Geol. Nat. Hist. Surv. Bull. **70**, 1—874 (1948).

Kobert, R.: Beiträge zur Kenntnis der Giftspinnen. Stuttgart: Enke 1901.

Kullmann, E.: Die Produktion von Spinnenfäden und Spinnegeweben. Mitt. Inst. leichte Flächentr. (IL) Stuttgart **8**, 318—378 (1975).

Kullmann, E., Otto, F., Braun, Th., Raccanello, R.: Grundlagen und Ordnungsübersicht der Netzkonstruktionen der Spinnen. Mitt. Inst. leichte Flächentr. (IL) Stuttgart **8**, 304—316 (1975).

Lebez, D.: Prispevki k studiju strupa tarantele. Biol. Vestn. **2**, 27 (1953).

Lebez, D., Kregar, I., Turk, V., Maretić, Z.: Analyse biochimique et biologique de venins d'araignées obtenus par divers procédés. Bull. Mus. Nat. Hist. Natur. (2nd ser.) **41** (Suppl. 1), 255—259 (1969).

Lee, C.K., Chan, T.K., Ward, B.C., Howell, D.E., Odell, G.V.: The purification and characterization of a necrotoxin from tarantula, *Dugesiella hentzi* (Girard) venom. Archs. Biochem. Biophys. **164**, 341 (1974).

Main, B.Y.: Envenomation by Australian spiders of low toxicity. Manuscript (1976).

Majeski, J.A., Durst, G.G.: Bite by the spider *Herpyllus ecclesiasticus* in South Carolina. Toxicon **13**, 377 (1975).

Maretić, Z.: *Chiracanthium punctorium* Villers. Eine europäische Giftspinne. Med. Klinik **57**, 1576—1577 (1962).

Maretić, Z.: Venom of an East African orthognath spider. In: Animal Toxins, Eds. F.E. Russell, P.R. Saunders. Oxford: Pergamon 1967.

Maretić, Z., Lebez, D.: *Lycosa tarentula* in fact and fiction. Bull. Muséum Nat. Hist. Natur. **41** (Suppl. 1), 260—266, 1969 (1970).

Maretić, Z., Milina, O.: A bite by the spider *Aranea sexpunctata* Linné: case report. Toxicon **14**, 392—393 (1976).

Musgrave, A.: Spiders harmful to man. Aust. Museum Magaz. **9**, 411—419 (1949).

Ori, M.: Observations on bites of *Chiracanthium japonicum* Bös. et Str. in Japan. Acta Arachn. Osaka **26**, 64—68 (1975).

Perret, B.A., Freyvogel, T.A.: Further investigations on the venom of the East African orthognath spider, *Pterinochilus* sp. (Preliminary report). In: Animal and Plant Toxins, Ed. E. Kaiser, pp. 23—28. München: Goldmann 1973.

Petrunkevitch, A.: Order Araneida, In: Treatise on Invertebrate Paleontology, Part P, Arthropoda 2 Ed. R.C. Moore, pp. P128—P153. Univ. Kansas Press 1958.

Phisalix, M.: Animaux venimeux et venins. Vol. I, Paris: Masson 1922.

Russell, F.E.: Bites of spiders and other arthropods. In: Current Therapy, Ed. H.F. Conn, pp. 878—879. Philadelphia-London: Saunders 1969.

Russell, F.E.: Bite by the spider *Phidippus formosus:* case history. Toxicon **8**, 193—194 (1970).

Russell, F.E., Järlfors, V., Smith, D.S.: Preliminary report on the fine structure of the venom gland of the tarantula. Toxicon **11**, 439—440 (1973).

Russell, F.E., Waldron, W.G.: Spider bites, tick bites. Calif. Med. **106**, 248—249 (1967).

Savory, Th.H.: The Spider's Web. London: Warne 1952.

Schanbacher, F.L., Lee, C.K., Hall, J.E., Wilson, I.B., Howell, D.E., Odell, G.V.: Composition and properties of tarantula *Dugesiella hentzi* (Girard) venom. Toxicon **11**, 21—29 (1973b).

Schanbacher, F.L., Lee, C.K., Wilson, I.B., Howell, D.E., Odell, G.V.: Purification and characterization of tarantula, *Dugesiella hentzi* (Girard) venom hyaluronidase. Comp. Biochem. Physiol. **44B**, 389—396 (1973a).

Simon, E.: Note sur le Mico (*Dendryphantes noxiosus*) espèce venimeuse de Bolivie. Ann. Soc. Ent. Belg. **30** C.R., 168—172 (1886).

Spielman, A., Levi, H.W.: Probable envenomation by *Chiracanthium mildei;* a spider found in houses. Am. J. trop. Med. Hyg. **19**, 729 (1970).

Stahnke, H.L., Johnson, B.D.: *Aphonopelma* tarantula venom. In: Animal Toxins, Eds. F.E. Russell, P.R. Saunders. Oxford: Pergamon 1967.

Vellard, J.: Le venins des Araignées. Paris: Masson 1936.

Vellard, J.: Le mico-mico, l'araignée venimeuse de Bolivie. Bull. Soc. Zool. Fr. **64**, 70—79 (1939).

Vinson, A.: Aranéides des îles de la Réunion, Maurice et Madagascar. Paris: Roret 1863.

Waldron, W.G.: Observations on spider bites in Southern California. Vector News **12**, 66 (1965).

Wilson, W.H.: On the poison of spiders with especial reference to that of *Chaetopelma olivacea.* Rec. Egypt. Gov. Sch. Med. **1**, 141—150 (1901).

Yates, J.H.: Spiders of Southern Africa. Books of Africa 1968.

CHAPTER 7

Venoms of Dipluridae

M.R. Gray and S.K. Sutherland

Introduction

Scanty research has been carried out on poisonous diplurid genera other than *Atrax* which, because of its venom potency and the occurrence of human envenomations, is the only important genus.

According to Bücherl (1971) the genus *Trechona* from South America includes venomous species which may cause death to man. The description of the genus, its distribution and habits, as well as a description of its venom apparatus are also given. The quantity of venom of *Trechona venosa* which kills a 20 g mouse i.v. is 0.030 mg, and s.c. 0.070 mg. The venom studied was obtained by electrical stimulation.

The South American genus *Pamphobeteus* was also mentioned by Bücherl (1971) as including venomous species. Description of the genus and its behaviour are also reported. The venom quantities which kill a 20 g mouse of four species, *P. roseus, P. sorocabae, P. tetracanthus* and *P. platyomma*, are respectively 0.85, 0.70, 0.60 and 0.80 mg i.v., and 1.7, 1.5, 1.4 and 1.5 mg s.c.

Mebs (1970) investigated the proteolytic activity of the venom of *Pamphobeteus roseus*. The venom's activity tested on casein was very high, comparable to that of venoms of the snakes *Bothrops mummifera* and *Crotalus atrax*. Three proteolytic components were separated from the venom by gel chromatography on Sephadex and Biogel. The optimal pH was found to be 8.5. All three fractions had a molecular weight of about 10,840. The results indicate that the activity is due to an enzyme associated with higher molecular structures. The author assumes that the proteolytic activity of the spider's venom is used in extracorporeal digestion.

A. Systematics and Distribution

M.R. Gray

The genus *Atrax* was erected in 1877 by Cambridge for a female specimen of *A. robustus* from the Sydney region. Since this time a further 8 species have been described. More recently, unpublished work by the author and V.C. Gregg, Associate at The Australian Museum, has resulted in the characterization of 17 additional species. Table 1 provides a summary of the named species and their general distributions.

Table 1

Species	Distribution
A. robustus Cambridge, 1877	New South Wales
A. modestus Simon, 1891	Victoria
A. formidabilis Rainbow, 1914	N. New South Wales, S. Queensland
A. versutus Rainbow, 1914	New South Wales
A. bicolor Rainbow, 1914	New South Wales
A. validus Rainbow and Pulleine, 1918	S. Queensland
A. venenatus Hickman, 1926	Tasmania
A. pulvinator Hickman, 1926	Tasmania
A. infensus Hickman, 1964	N. New South Wales, S. Queensland

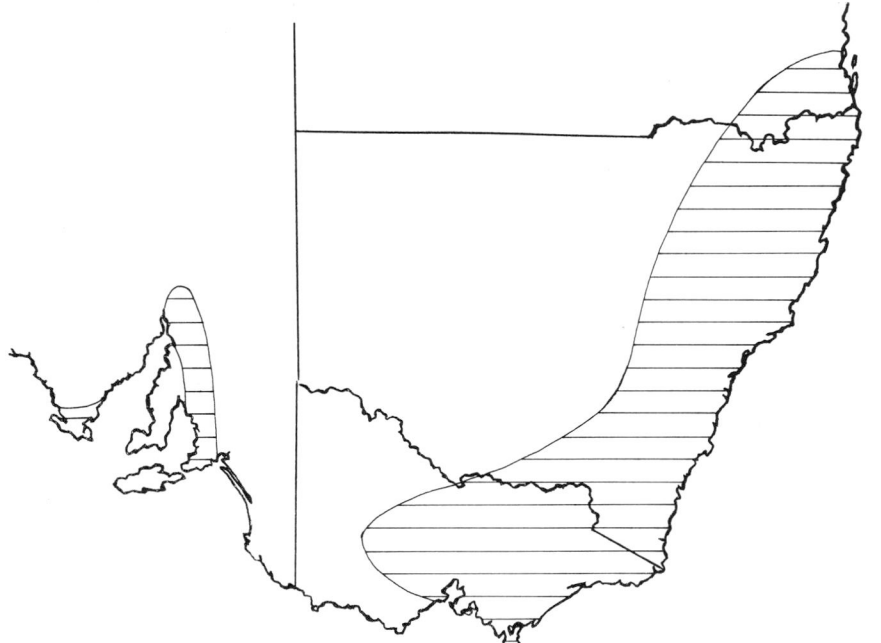

Fig. 1. Distribution of the genus *Atrax* in southeastern Australia (excluding Tasmania)

Funnel-web spiders are confined primarily to southeastern Australia (Fig. 1). Their main geographic range extends from southern Queensland into N.S.W. — Victoria and Tasmania and west to the Eyre Peninsula — Flinders Range regions of South Australia. The genus appears to be rare in central and north Queensland, only a single record being available. Outside Australia *Atrax* has been recorded from Papua, New Guinea and the Solomon Islands.

In general the group is confined to coastal and adjacent mountain regions. This distribution reflects the common preference of funnel-web spiders for moist, relatively cool habitats that are associated with temperate and subtropical forests. Their webs may be found in or under logs, under rocks, at the base of stumps or under thick vegetation (such as tussock grass) and in tree trunks. However, a few species are more dry adapted and their webs can be found in the ground litter of open woodland on the western slopes of the Great Dividing Range and in the Flinders Range of South Australia.

The term 'funnel-web' spider is a little misleading; 'tube-web' spider might be more appropriate. The upper part of the web retreat lies on or is attached to the substrate surface. There are commonly two entrances which are guyed out by radiating trip lines. They lead into wide, semicollapsed tubes which coalesce posteriorly giving the surface part of the web a Y- or T-shaped configuration. A silk-lined burrow of varying depth and complexity descends from this posterior part of the web. Only the juvenile and mature female spiders construct such retreats. The male spiders leave their webs for good on maturation and pursue a vagrant, wandering existence in search of females. This mating activity is evident from October to April by which time most of the relatively short-lived males have died. Whereas male spiders have only one season of reproductive activity, females may have several.

Taxonomically, the genus *Atrax* can be divided into two major groupings, the Robustus Group and the Formidabilis Group. Their distinguishing characteristics are given in Table 2. They involve the dentition of the cheliceral groove and the morphology of the male tibia of the second leg. However, it should be noted that one or two species are not adequately covered by this dichotomy so that some modification may prove necessary.

Table 2

Group	Characteristics
Robustus Group	Intermediate teeth occupy $^1/_3$ to $^1/_2$ of basal part of fang groove. Tibia II of male with pointed, spurlike process
Formidabilis Group	Intermediate teeth occupy full length of fang groove. Tibia II of male with blunt, rounded process or process absent

The Robustus Group consists of a small homogeneous assemblage of species. In fact it is this homogeneity that has made taxonomic decisions in this group rather difficult. At present five species are recognized but only two are named, *A. robustus,* the Sydney funnel-web spider, and *A. pulvinator* from Tasmania.

Robustus Group species are found in southeastern coastal and mountain regions from the Newcastle-Hunter River region in New South Wales to the east Gippsland region of Victoria and the east coastal region of Tasmania. The best known and medically important species, *A. robustus,* occurs in the central coastal region of New South Wales and the adjacent Blue Mountains region to the west. A closely related southern form has a more extensive but mainly coastal distribution in southern New South Wales and Gippsland. This is the species mentioned by WAKE-FIELD (1958) which he refers to *A. robustus,* a placement with which the present author does not concur. Interestingly, yet another undescribed species in the Robustus Group has recently been discovered west of Sydney. At present this is known only from a single very distinctive male specimen. The Tasmanian spider, *A. pulvinator,* has so far been recorded only from the Hobart region and, surprisingly, the male of this species remains unknown.

The Formidabilis Group is both large (20 species) and diverse and occurs over the entire geographic range of the genus. It is convenient to further subdivide this group into two subgroups consisting of those species that possess a male tibial process ('spurred') and those species that lack this process ('spurless'). Of the named species for which the male spider is known, *A. formidabilis* and *A. versutus* possess a tibial spur, while *A. venenatus* and *A. infensus* are spurless. Three of the seven named species, *A. formidabilis, A. infensus,* and *A. validus* are found in the northern New South Wales—southern Queensland area. *A. versutus* (and the dubious *A. bicolor*) is common in the Blue Mountains region west of Sydney. *A. modestus* is recorded from the west Gippsland-Dandenong Range area of Victoria while *A. venenatus* occurs in the north and east of Tasmania.

It is impractical to attempt to go into the details of speciation and distribution in the Formidabilis Group here. A number of species complexes have been determined, based largely on similarities in male palpal morphology, and these generally occupy well-defined geographic regions. The 'versutus' complex is a good example. This contains four species and extends over the central mountains and coastal region of New South Wales. On the tablelands and western slopes of the Great Dividing Range two complexes of 'spurless' species occur in southern ('Oberon' complex) and northern ('infensus' complex) belts. On the coast the large spiders of the 'Port Macquarie' complex contrast markedly with the diminutive spiders of the southern 'Bermagui' complex.

Species related to the 'versutus' complex range south into the eastern and central regions of Victoria. *Atrax* is much less common in western Victoria where dryer conditions predominate; even in the moist Otway Range area the genus is not recorded. The few records available refer to spiders from the Hamilton-Grampian Range area.

At the western limit of the distribution of *Atrax* a very interesting complex occurs as an isolate in the Eyre Peninsula—Adelaide—Flinders Range region. The three species involved are unique in constructing an underground side-chamber which is closed by a heavy pluglike soil door. Interestingly, the young spiders also make a door at the entrance to the burrow, but this behavior is apparently lost as the spider matures, since the adult burrow entrance consists of a simple open silk collar.

Tree dwelling species are confined to the Formidabilis Group. *A. formidabilis,* the tree or Northern Rivers funnel-web spider, was once thought to be unique in its preference for above ground retreats. However, it is now apparent that tree dwelling species are not uncommon. A group of related species on the coast and mountains around Sydney occur in cracks and crevices in rough barked trees such as *Melaleuca* (paper bark), *Banksia* and some *Eucalyptus* species. Their webs are often well disguised by bark debris and lichen.

Systematically, the genus poses a number of problems. Some of these stem from inadequacies or inaccuracies in the descriptions of named specimens. The selection of immature specimens as types has also caused problems. *Aname* (= *Atrax) bicolor* Rainbow is a classic example of such problems to the extent that it has proved impossible to reliably determine the species originally involved. Another major problem with many species of *Atrax* is the similarity of female spiders. Attempts to characterize species satisfactorily on the basis of female characters alone have failed. In contrast, males provide good species characters. It is also often difficult to match male and female specimens collected separately in the field, particularly when up to 3 species may occur in the same geographic region. In this context, it is intersting to note that RAINBOW described the male of *A. robustus* as *Euctimena tibialis* in 1914 some 37 years after CAMBRIDGE had first described *A. robustus* from a female specimen. Several other genera such as *Styphlopis* RAINBOW 1913, *Poikilomorpha* RAINBOW 1914, *Anaepsiada* RAINBOW and PULLEINE 1918 and *Pseudatrax* RAINBOW 1914 are synonomous with *Atrax*.

Even the generic name *Atrax* is not secure. The genus *Hadronyche* was erected by KOCH in 1873 for a spider from the Sydney region (*H. cereberea*) which is undoubtedly a funnel-web spider of the 'versutus' complex. This name therefore precedes the name *Atrax* by some 4 years (CAMBRIDGE, 1877) and so has priority over the latter. However, past usage and current convention should eventually decide this issue officially in favor of the retention of *Atrax* as the valid name of the genus. Only one other Australian *Atrax* species has been referred to *Hadronyche, H. meridiana* HOGG 1902, from Mt. Macedon, Victoria.

A lack of appreciation of the complexity of speciation in *Atrax* and the localized nature of many species distributions has misled some authors. For example, CHISHOLM (1932) records *A. venenatus,* a Tasmanian spider, from the Comboyne Plateau in northern New South Wales. However, spiders from this area in fact belong to the 'New England' species complex which is confined to northern New South Wales. These spiders superficially resemble *A. venenatus* in having spurless males but there the similarity ends.

A number of taxonomic and distributional questions await clarification, particularly with regard to the southern representatives of *Atrax*. However, the data already available is sufficient to allow revision of several major groups in the genus (GRAY and GREGG in prep.).

References

Cambridge, O.P.: On some new genera and species of Araneidea. Ann. Mag. Nat. Hist., **19**, 26−39 (1877).

Chisholm, E.C.: The occurrence of *Atrax venenatus* Hickman on the Comboyne Plateau. Proc. Linn. Soc. N.S.W. **57**, 24−26 (1932).

Hickman, V.V.: Studies in Australian spiders, Part 1. Pap. Roy. Soc. Tas., 52−86 (1926).

Hickman, V.V.: On *Atrax infensus* sp. n. (Araneida: Dipluridae) Its Habits and a method of trapping males. Pap. Roy. Soc. Tas. **98**, 107−112 (1964).

Hogg, H.R.: On Australian and New Zealand spiders of the Suborder Mygalomorphae. Proc. Zool. Soc. Lond. **2**, 218−279 (1901).

Hogg, H.R.: On some additions to the Australian spiders of the Suborder Mygalomorphae. Proc. Zool. Soc. Lond. **2**, 121−142 (1902).

Koch, L.C.: Die Arachniden Australiens nach der Natur beschrieben und abgebildet. Bauer & Raspe. Nurnberg. (1871−1875).

Levitt, V.C.: The funnel web spider in captivity. Proc. Roy. Zool. Soc. N.S.W. 80−84, 1958−1959.

Musgrave, A.: Some poisonous Australian spiders. Rec. Aust. Mus. **16**, 33−46 (1927).

Rainbow, W.J.: Arachnida from the Solomon Islands. Rec. Aust. Mus. **10**, 1−16 (1913).

Rainbow, W.J.: Studies in Australian Araneidae, No. 6. The Territelariae. Rec. Aust. Mus. **10**, 187 – 270 (1914).

Rainbow, W.J. and Pulleine, R.H.: Australian trapdoor spiders. Rec. Aust. Mus. **12**, 81 – 169 (1918).

Rainbow, W.J.: Trapdoor spiders of the "Chevert" Expedition. Rec. Aust. Mus. **13**, 77 – 86 (1920).

Roewer, C.F.: Katalog der Araneae. Volume **1**. Natura. Bremen (1942).

Simon, E.L.: Etudes arachnologiques 23e Memoire XXXVIII. Descriptions d'especes et de genres noveaux de la famille de Aviculariidae. Ann. Soc. ent. Fr. **60** (2 – 3) 300 – 312 (1891).

Simon, E.L.: Histoire naturelle des Araignees. Deuxieme edition. Encyclopedie Roret. Paris (1892 – 1903)

Strand, E.: Mitteilungen aus dem Kgl. Naturalien-Kabinett zu Stuttgart. No. 40. Aviculariidae and Atypidae. Jh. Ver. vaterl. Naturh. Württemb. **63**, 1 – 100 (1907).

Strand, E.: Über einige australische Spinnen des Senckenbergischen Museums. Zool. Jb., Jena, Abt. Syst. **35**, 599 – 624 (1913).

Wakefield, N.A.: The discovery of the Sydney Funnel Web Spider (*Atrax robustus*) in Victoria. Vict. Nat. **74**, 174 – 178 (1958).

B. Biology and Venoms

S.K. Sutherland

I. Introduction

Australia is fortunate in being the only country in the world of large dimensions which has no carnivorous mammals dangerous to man. However, during the 200 years of European settlement an extensive number of terrestrial and marine animals of real or potential lethality to man have been identified (Garnet, 1969). Seven of the 140 species of snake rank amongst the most lethal in the world and constitute a significant environmental hazard as in the sea do the sea wasp (*Chironex fleckeri*) and sharks.

The mode of action of significant Australian venoms has been recently reviewed (Sutherland, 1974) and it is evident that a great deal of research is yet to be done on some aspects of these venoms, many of which appear to be unique in their actions. To date the major research endeavour has been directed at the preparation of effective antivenins and for some time antivenins against the dangerous snakes have been distributed by the health authorities to all major medical centres. A number of human deaths occur following bites or stings by unidentified creatures and because of the relative frequency of such incidents a radioimmunoassay has been developed (Coulter et al., 1974; Sutherland et al., 1975) to detect venom in tissues and tissue fluids. As a rule the venoms of the arthropods in Australia fall into relative insignificance when compared with deaths due to other phyla, and to date it has not been considered necessary to employ such methods in investigating arthropod poisoning.

Australian scorpions rarely cause any significant illness. However, the bush tick (*Ixodes holocyclus*) is of wide distribution and has caused the death of at least 20 individuals this century in one state alone.

The redback spider (*Latrodectus mactans hasseltii*) is found in all Australian states and at least 300 human victims require specific antivenin per annum. No deaths due to redback spiders are known to have occurred since antivenin was made available in 1956.

In 1957 attention was turned in Australian to the venom of the Sydney funnel-web spider *Atrax robustus* Cambr. Extensive studies carried out at the Commonwealth Serum Laboratories in Melbourne by a series of investigators were recently reviewed (SUTHERLAND, 1972a). This spider causes occasional deaths in and around Australia's largest city and is the cause of great public concern, particularly as no specific antivenin or antidote is available. The population of Sydney is over 3 millions and its present radius of some 48 kilometers is well within the known habitat of *A. robustus* which has caused fatalities as far as 160 kilometers from the city center.

II. Notes on Atrax robustus

A. robustus is a large unpleasant spider (Fig. 1) and the sexes are clearly distinguishable in mature specimens. The male is more delicate in build and has a tibial spur on the second pair of legs and markedly modified chelicerae. Like all mygalomorphs they posses four book lungs (Fig. 2). The spinnerets are long with the terminal segment the longest. The fangs are set vertical to the mouth and thus when the spider strikes the fangs thrust downwards inflicting a wound not unlike a snake bite.

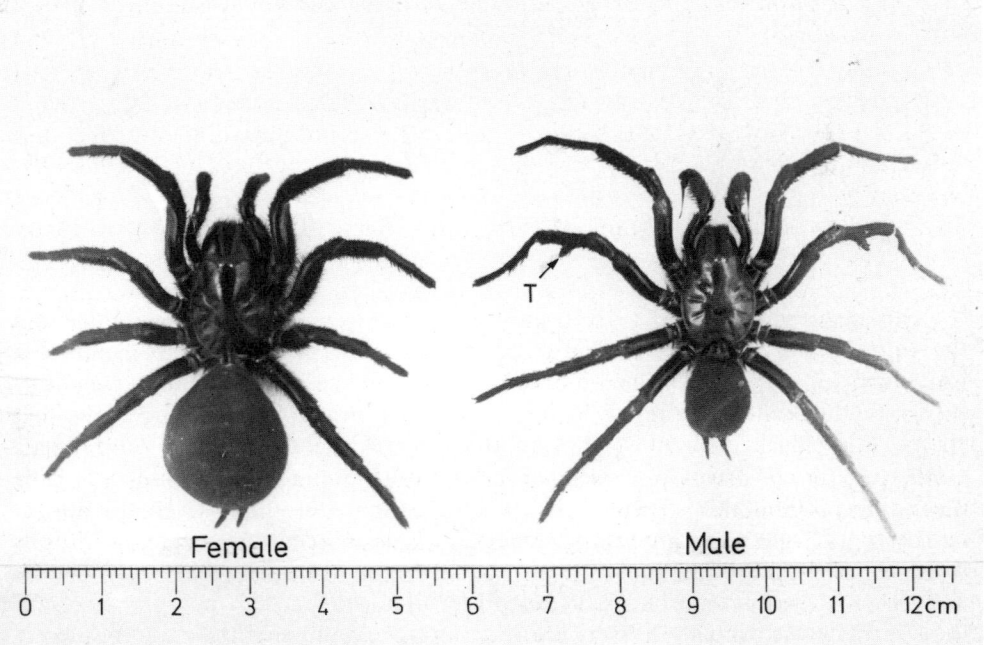

Female   Male

0 1 2 3 4 5 6 7 8 9 10 11 12cm

Fig. 1. Adult female and male Sydney funnel-web spiders (*A. robustus*). Scale in centimeters. Note male's tibial spurs (T) and palpi modified into intromittent sex organs

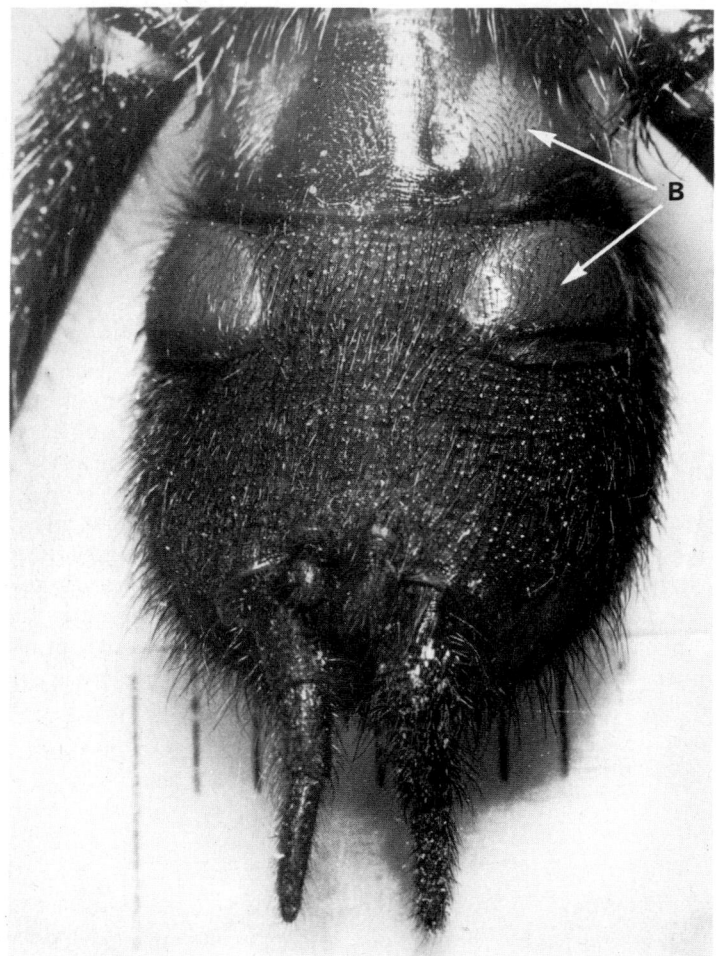

Fig. 2. Abdomen of male *A. robustus* showing four book lungs (B) and long spinnerets

The spider either builds its web in suitable crevices in rock ledges or around the foundations of houses or constructs its own burrow which may be over a foot deep Levitt (1961). The white silken web is usually a roughly woven tube rather than a funnel and is guyed by supporting lines to surrounding rocks and sticks. The spiders like moist cool conditions and the development of housing estates and the construction of rock gardens and swimming pools possibly increases the number of suitable sites for this spider. Colonies of thirty-seven, forty-five, and about one hundred and fifty spiders have been recorded where conditions were very favorable (McKeown, 1963). The diet of the spider is mainly beetles and other large insects which are caught at night and usually not too far from the lair. Whereas the female rarely roams from her chosen area the male frequently may be found in houses and other areas of human habitat. They are particularly common in the summer months which may be the mating season and are often

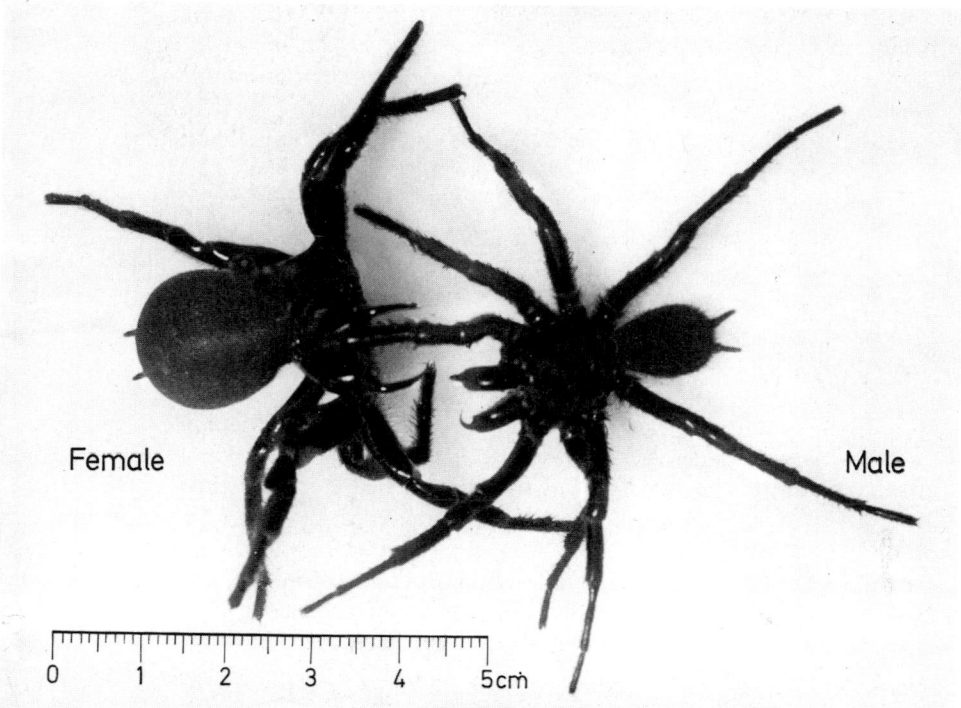

Fig. 3. Confrontation between male and female *A. robustus*. Note size of fangs. Female has reared backwards and has adopted position to strike

found in houses particularly after heavy rain. Little is known about the breeding cycle of these spiders or the average life span in the natural state. Mating is especially dangerous for the male as, prior to pairing, he must lock the females massive fangs with his tibial spurs. The female adopts an aggressive position as he approaches and her fangs are held high in a position to strike (Fig. 3). When he has locked the females' fangs with his spurs and has mated he then has a most precarious retreat to make before the female resumes her normal aversion to him. MCKEOWN (1963) considered that the male always behaves like a perfect gentleman and never strikes back in self defence. The female makes a white silken egg sac 1.5 cm in diameter which contains some one hundred eggs. Nothing is known of the life these spiderlings lead until they are found as immature adults establishing their own webs. Apart from the papers by HICKMAN (1964) and LEVITT (1961) little has been published on the natural history of species *Atrax*.

III. Source of Venom for Experimentation

1. Maintenance of Spiders in the Laboratory

Specimens of *A. robustus* were collected in large numbers in the Sydney area and forwarded in individual containers by air to Melbourne (WIENER, 1957). In captivity the spiders survive for many months in jars kept in a darkened room at a temperature not exceeding 20° C (KAIRE, 1964). Many types of diet have been employed over the years but the most successful and simplest is the common meal worm *T. molitor* which can be maintained conveniently in laboratories (McFERRAN, 1957). The spider jars are 8 cm deep. The bottom is filled with 2 cm of damp soil covered with 1 cm layer of clean coarse sand. The latter is helpful in keeping the spider fangs clean during venom collection. Venom is collected from the spiders the same day each week and after the addition of several meal worms and 5 ml of water to each jar the spiders are left undisturbed for another week. Most spiders spin webs which range from simple carpet to a complex funnel arrangement which may fill the jar. Some female spiders live for at least 2 years under laboratory conditions. Male spiders, however, rarely survive more than 3 months.

2. Collection of Venom and Venom Yields

Both sexes are quite aggressive and when disturbed stand on their rear four legs with their front legs raised high and chelicerae erect. Drops of clear venom are seen on the tips of their large fangs. The spider will strike repeatedly and furiously at any moving object and the tough fangs can penetrate the skulls of small animals or even a human finger nail. Because the spider when captive in a small jar adopts this position it is a simple matter to aspirate the venom from the tip of the fangs. WIENER (1957) compared the venom yield by "milked" venom with that obtained by dissecting out and aspirating the contents of venom glands. The former produced an average of 0.28 mg for females and 0.175 mg for males and the latter process which destroyed the spiders yielded 2.05 mg for females and 0.81 for males. Since the toxicity of the venoms was similar a larger yield of venom was more likely to be obtained by regular milking than by sacrificing the spider. Anesthesia and electrical stimulation as described by MEADOWS and RUSSELL (1970) have not proved worth the effort.

IV. Structure of the Venom Glands in Atrax robustus

The paired venom glands are curved and flask-shaped and measure about 5 mm in length. The venom duct is about 4 mm in length and opens at a small orifice dorsally above the tip of the large and very tough fang. The walls of the venom gland are delicate and translucent. Histologically, a thin spiral of striped muscle surrounds a connective tissue membrane upon which several layers of epithelial cells rest and project into the lumen of gland (WIENER, 1957). The expulsion of venom appears to be under some degree of voluntary control because venom droplets which appear at the tip of a disturbed spider are withdrawn back into the fang if the spider is no longer threatened.

HAMILTON (1975) has studied the microstructure of the venom gland and kindly provided the electronmicrographs (Figs. 4 and 5). The significant features of his studies to date are the extensive innervation of the venom gland and the presence of large amounts of an unidentified crystalline material in both the secretory cells and in the ducts. HAMILTON suggests that the high level of free gamma aminobutyric acid (GABA) in the venom (GILBO and COLES, 1964) may indicate that this is in fact the transmitter substance from the synapses in the venom gland.

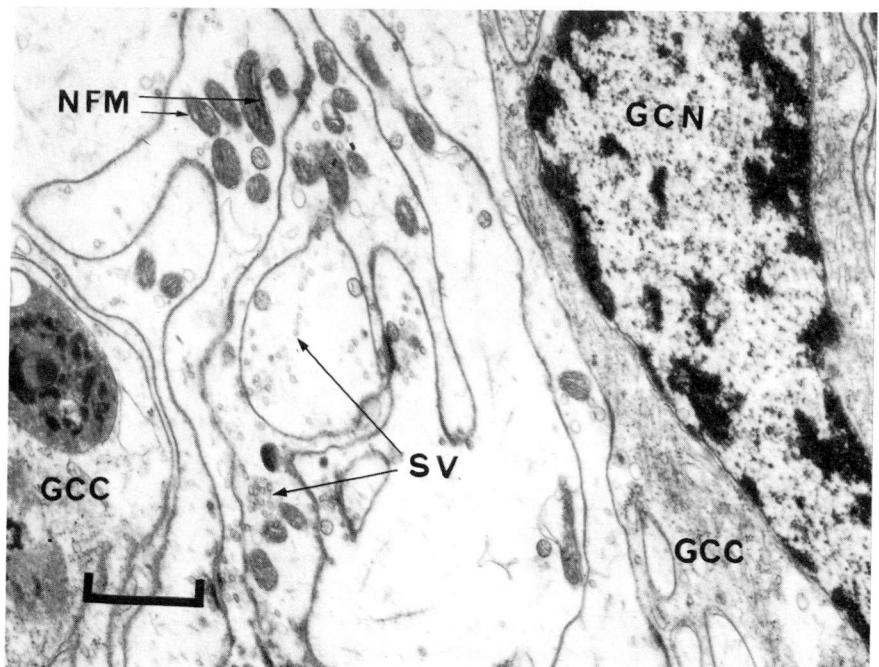

Fig. 4. Electronmicrograph of female *A. robustus* venom gland showing number of nerve fibers between 2 glandular cells. Bar equals 1 μm. *GCN:* glandular cell nucleus *GCC:* glandular cell cytoplasm *NFM:* nerve fibre mitochondria *S.V.:* synaptic vesicles in nerve fibres. (with permission of R.C. Hamilton)

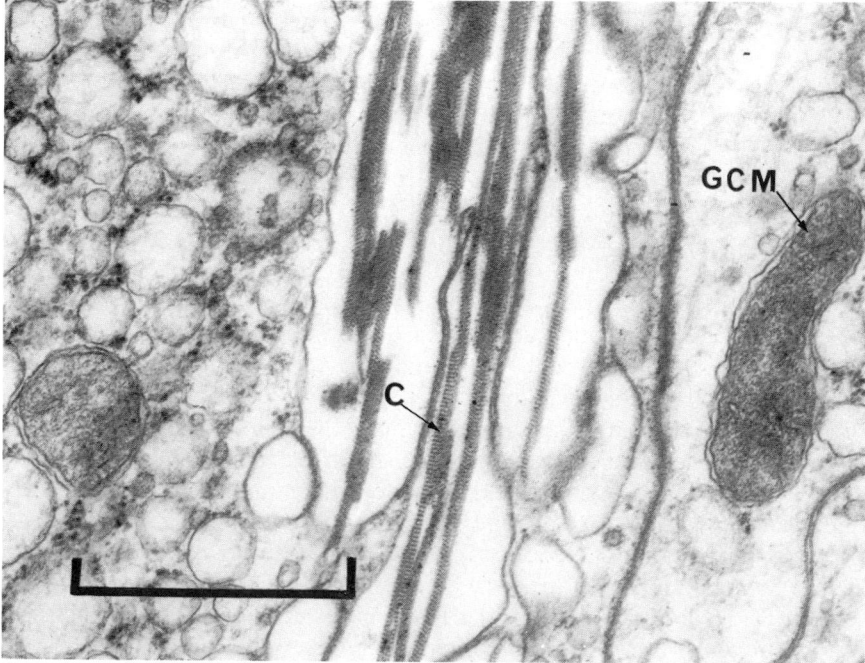

Fig. 5. Crystalline structures (C) in vesicles within glandular cell. These structures also found free in venom ducts. *GCM:* glandular cell mitochondrium. Bar equals 1 μm. (With permission of R.C. Hamilton)

GABA is known to be an inhibitory transmitter in arthropods (TAKEUCHI and TAKEUCHI, 1965).

V. Toxicity of Venom in Various Animal Species

1. Atrax robustus Venom

KELLAWAY (1934) undertook the first scientific study of the venom of the Sydney funnel-web spider and he reported failure to cause death in mice or guinea pigs by inducing female spiders to bite them. He also collected venom directly onto filter paper and eluted the dried venom with distilled water and found that a total dose of 7.3 mg had no effect upon a domestic rabbit of 1.17 kg. In discussing his failure to produce toxic effects in the light of the fact that human fatalities had been recorded, KELLAWAY then speculated that only the higher animals might be susceptible and/or in the case of the rabbit the venom so collected had been fixed or destroyed by the filter paper. Both these hypotheses appear no longer speculative but indeed to be factual. Other workers had difficulty in demonstrating toxicity (WALLACE and STICKA, 1955).

WIENER (1957) found that rabbits were unaffected by subcutaneous doses of whole crude funnel-web spider venom as large as 15 mg. However, he did find that rabbits bitten by male spiders occasionally succumb. In his "biting" experiments WIENER found that rats, large rabbits, and a cat were unaffected by bites by female spiders but that about 20% of mice and guinea pigs died after a bite by a female spider and most died after a male spider bite. Mice and guinea pigs had either died within several hours or completely recovered. After the bite the animal would cry, become restless, and a profuse nasal discharge and salivation would commence. Respiratory distress would develop and incoordination, together with weakness of the extremities, and convulsions. Coma preceded death. Respiratory arrest would be followed a few moments later by cardiac arrest.

Sheep and horses were only slightly affected by massive doses of venom, e.g. 60 mg female venom subcutaneously made a horse go off its food for 24 h and on one occasion some local muscle twitching was noted at the site of the injection (WIENER, 1963).

In a monitored cat a dose of 10 mg/kg i.v. produced a transient mild hypotension and brief apnea but the cat suffered no subsequent ill effects (SUTHERLAND, unpublished) or any of the responses seen in monkeys (see below). In fact one such cat is alive and well some 4 years later.

Toads (*Bufo marinus*) also proved resistant to the venom. Toads of 80 g weight remained symptomless after subcutaneous doses of either 12 mg of female venom or 1 mg of male venom. WIENER (1961a) noted that funnel-web spiders were unaffected when injected with 2 mg of their venom. He did, however, find that Drosophila (WIENER and DRUMMOND, 1956; WIENER, 1957) were susceptible to the venom having an LD_{50} of 0.9×10^{-6} mg.

WIENER (1957, 1959) found that male venom collected by aspiration was about six times more toxic than female venom in both guinea pigs and mice. The M.L.D. in 200 g guinea pigs was 2.4 mg subcutaneously for female venom (0.6 mg for male venom) and 0.9 mg for female venom (0.18 mg for male venom). The intracerebral M.L.D. for mice was $0.003 - 0.006$ mg for female venom and for male venom the dose was $0.00054 - 0.0011$ mg.

The susceptibility of unweaned mice to certain animal viruses has been discussed by SKINNER (1959) and they have proved a very reliable and economic way of assaying venom at these laboratories. A group of mice one or two days old with an average weight of 1.9 g survive 24 h with rarely any one death if kept at room temperature ($22°$ C) in batches of 10 in beakers and lightly covered with cotton wool. Mice are injected subcutaneously using a microliter syringe (Scientific Glass Engineering) with various venom dilutions and are checked 24 h later at which stage (with funnel-web spider venom or fractions) they are either unaffected or dead. The usual volume injected is 25 µl but no deaths are caused with 100 µl volumes of water, saline, or 0.174 M acetic acid. If four or five-day-old mice are selected when their weight has reached 4 g then their susceptibility to funnel-web spider venom decreases by at least fivefold. It is also difficult at this age to obtain mice in a narrow weight range. The subcutaneous LD_{100} for newborn mice (mean weight 1.98 g) is 25 µg for crude female *A. robustus* venom and 5 µg for male venom. Male atraxotoxin (see below) has an LD_{100} of $0.5 - 1.0$ µg (preliminary finding).

Monkeys like man appear to have a particular vulnerability to funnel-web spider venom. In WIENER's biting experiments (1957), two monkeys were bitten by a female spider. One died after developing a syndrome similar to that seen in human cases and the other was unaffected. The author has found that cynomolgus monkeys invariably died within four hours of receiving 3 mg/kg of female venom i.v. and not infrequently would die within eight hours after the same dose injected subcutaneously. A dose of male venom 0.5 mg/kg i.v. or subcutaneously almost invariably resulted in death. Male venom at a dose of 0.2 mg/kg either i.v. or subcutaneously frequently resulted in death making the determination of an accurate monkey LD_{50} difficult and expensive.

Unless the monkey was intubated and the pharynx kept free of secretions the animals sometimes died in the first ten minutes from asphyxia due to laryngospasms and/or inhalation of secretions. In early experiments, it was noted that laryngospasm could occur before the secretory phase had commenced.

2. Venom of Other Species of Atrax

KAIRE (1961) described toxicity studies performed on the venom of *A. formidabilis*. However, subsequently (KAIRE, 1963; HICKMAN, 1964) it was determined that the spider venom under study was a new species (*A. infensus*). KAIRE reported that the LD_{50} in $17 - 20$ g mice was $0.2 - 0.25$ mg intravenously and 0.45 mg when the venom was injected subcutaneously. Venom recently obtained from a small colony of female *A. infensus* was assayed in newborn mice and had an LD_{100} of 5 µg, i.e. it appeared as toxic as male *A. robustus* venom. Small quantities of female *A. versutus* venom that have been assayed have equivalent toxicity. Venom obtained from a new species of *Atrax* collected from Bega (situated 434 kilometers south of Sydney) had a toxicity similar to female *A. robustus* venom. Both *A. infensus* and *A. versutus* cause spontaneous contractions in the chick *biventer cervicis* preparation. Preliminary work suggests that *A. infensus* venom is at least as toxic as *A. robustus* venom in mice.

VI. Chemistry of Sydney Funnel-web Spider (Atrax robustus) Venom

Wiener (1961b) reported that the crude freeze-dried female venom was a slightly hygroscopic white powder which dissolved easily in water forming a solution of pH 4.5 — 5.0. Nontoxic heat coagulable proteins made up 12% — 22% of the venom. Wiener found the toxicity of the venom to be unaffected by heating at 100° C for 1 h with or without the presence of 0.1 M hydrochloric acid. Toxicity was completely destroyed by 0.1 M sodium hydroxide or by heating to 120° C for 20 min. However, using a more sensitive assay (suckling mice) it has been found that the toxicity of the venom can definitely be reduced by about 40% after 1 h at 100° C (Sutherland, unpublished).

Wiener (1961b) demonstrated an 80% reduction in toxicity after dialysis but no fall in toxicity after ether extraction. In crude venom sodium, magnesium, phosphorus, and calcium were detected. Kaire (1963) found that the toxic dialysate prepared from crude venom had an absorption peak at 265 — 270 mμ. Kaire also reported a heat labile protease with optimal activity at pH 7. Curtain electrophoresis of crude venom (Wiener, 1963) resulted in less than a 10% recovery and fractions were of low toxicity. Gilbo and Coles (1964) performed electrophoretic studies on the toxic dialysate and isolated two major ninhydrin-positive substances. One was proven to be gamma aminobutyric acid (GABA) and the other a more basic substance yielding spermine and some unidentified components upon acid hydrolysis. GABA is known to be a not uncommon component in spider venoms (Fischer and Bohn, 1957; McCrone, 1969). Using thin layer chromatographic techniques Birner (1973) has shown that the spermine complex contained indole lactic acid and that the ratio of spermine to this compound was 1:1. This spermine complex was toxic to mice but caused sudden death rather than a slow death with typical symptoms produced by whole venom or the toxic dialysate. A tentative assumption was made that the spermine complex was the active component of the venom and its low molecular weight might explain the failure to produce an effective antivenin. No further investigations were undertaken for 5 years until Sutherland and Telford (1968, unpublished data) endeavoured to make antibodies to the spermine complex by linking it to bovine serum albumin. The low avidity antibodies produced by the spermine complex afforded no protection to mice injected with the spermine complex.

By using ultrafiltration membranes (Sutherland, 1972b) large quantities of the spermine complex as well as four other distinct fractions were obtained. It was found that monkeys which are the only truly susceptible experimental animals (see below) developed no signs or symptoms when injected intravenously with the spermine complex at a dose of 4 mg/kg. There was little loss of total venom or toxicity when a series of ultrafiltration membranes were used. No synergism could be demonstrated when all fractions or combinations of the fractions were tested *in vivo*. The results indicated that 42% of the crude venom had a molecular weight of less than 500 and this material was of low toxicity (M.L.D. adult mouse 3.0 mg subcutaneously). Free GABA was found in this fraction. At least 10%

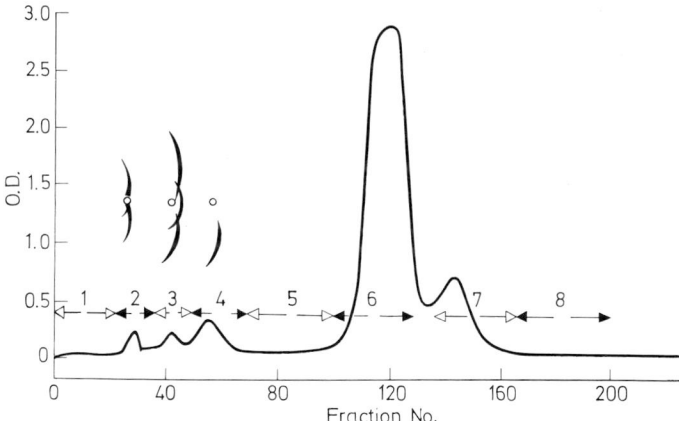

Fig. 6. Elution pattern of 150 mg crude female *A. robustus* venom applied to Biogel P150 in jacketed column (4° C) internal dimensions 80 × 3 cm equilibrated with 0.5 M sodium acetate buffer pH 5.8 with flow rate of 10 ml/h and fraction volumes of 4.5 ml. Immunoelectrophoretic reactions with anti whole funnel-web sera shown above pools 2, 3, and 4. Optical density (*O.D.*) of the eluates monitored at 280 nm

of the venom consisted of an indole lactic acid-spermine complex. High molecular weight heat labile proteins particulary rich in hyaluronidase (see below) made up some 10% of crude female venom. However, interest centered upon the 10% of crude venom which had a molecular weight in the range 15,000—25,000. This fraction, which was relatively free of the spermine complex, produced a syndrome in monkeys at a dose of 1 mg/kg which was undiscernable from that following whole venom. This fraction was the most toxic fraction in mice and caused a slow death whether given intravenously or subcutaneously. Furthermore, this preparation had the strongest pharmacologic activity in isolated nerve-muscle preparations. The active component in this fraction was designated atraxotoxin (SUTHERLAND, 1973a, 1973b).

Preliminary work suggested that the purification of atraxotoxin could be adequately and economically monitored by using suckling mice for in vivo toxicity and chicken biventer cervicis preparations for in vitro activity. Monkeys would be used only on final preparations. Figure 6 shows the elution pattern of crude female funnel-web venom obtained by gel filtration chromatography. Biogel P150 was chosen as it gave the widest separation of the major components. Various eluents were used including 0.1 M sodium formate pH 2.5 and 0.174 M acetic acid. All gave similar results. Pools 1, 2, and 3 contained the immunoreactive proteins and pool 2 was very high in hyaluronidase activity (5700 units/mg, whole crude venom being 160 units/mg). Hyaluronidase activity (BROAD, 1975) was determined by the method of DORFMAN (1955). Pool 6 contained the highly u.v. absorbing spermine-indole lactic acid complex and pool 7 was indole negative but contained some spermine. In calibrating the column, blue dextran (MW 2×10^6) appeared in fraction 20, bovine serum albumin (MW 69,000) in fraction 30, ribonuclease (MW 14,000) in fraction 60 and sodium chloride (MW 58) in fraction 120. However, none of the fractions collected had any significantly enhanced toxicity compared with whole venom and no pharmacologic activity was demonstrated. The only way fractions high in activity could be recovered was using Sephadex G50 and G25 at low pH (see below). It was essential to use siliconized glassware as it was found that atraxotoxin was rapidly adsorbed from solution by paper, cellulose, acetate, agar gel, acrylamide gel, silica, and to a lesser extent glassware. The adsorption of atraxotoxin to paper and cellulose appears irreversible and explains the failure of KELLAWAY (1934) to demonstrate toxicity and also WIENER'S (1963) loss of activity when he used paper electrophoresis. Advantage was taken of the adsorption of atraxotoxin to silica gel when it was found that it could be easily eluted by washing at low pH. Silica gel (Merck) was employed in subsequent fractionation procedures and the atraxotoxin was eluted with 3% acetic acid pH 2.4. Thus as a preliminary step to the purification of atraxotoxin, whole venom was adsorbed by silica gel at the rate of 2 g per 10 mg of venom and silica gel-venom suspensions were washed repeatedly with distilled water. After washing with water the silica gel-venom suspension was washed with 3% acetic acid to elute the adsorbed components. It was found that both high molecular weight proteins and low molecular components were obtained by the water washes and removed from the silica gel. The well-washed silica gel would then release the adsorbed crude atraxotoxin upon acid washing. This method allowed the rapid preparation of crude atraxotoxin with minimal loss of toxicity and recovery of up to 95% of venom components (Table 1). Both female and male crude atraxotoxin have been prepared by this adsorption/elution method. The crude atraxotoxin accounts for at least 80% of the toxicity of crude venom. Preliminary fractionation of the two crude atraxotoxins on Sephadex G25, eluting with 1% acetic acid shows some similarities between venom components obtained from the two sexes.

The first component eluted using Sephadex G25 column chromatography is nontoxic heat stable protein of molecular weight in the range 10,000—15,000. It contains no aromatic aminoacids and to date no biologic activity has been attributed to this component. Precipitating antibodies are easily raised to this protein and the immunoreactivity is similar in both male and female venom. This same protein has electrophoretic characteristics similar to a major protein component of *Atrax* hemolymph (Fig. 9) which is not heat stable.

The second component eluted contains all the toxicity and pharmacologic activity. With male venom the atraxotoxin so obtained is the most toxic isolate to date and the small quantities available have yet to be studied thoroughly. Ultraviolet and infrared spectroscopy findings are inconclusive as are extensive microanalytical studies to date. Female atraxotoxin prepared by the above method is contaminated

Table 1. Preparation of Crude Female Atraxotoxin by Silica Gel Adsorption

	Crude Venom	Aqueous Wash	Acetic Acid Wash 3%	Acetic Acid Wash 6%
%Recovered		77%	9%	5.9%
Certain Lethal Dose (C.L.D.) in Suckling Mice	25 µg	220 µg	4 µg	6 µg
% Total Toxicity		9.7	56	24

by a number of venom components and is of lower toxicity. Until methods are devised to characterize the purified male atraxotoxin it will not be possible to determine the amount of atraxotoxin present in female venom.

VII. Pharmacopathologic Studies with Atrax robustus Venom

1. Intact Animal Experiments

Since the exact mode or modes of action of this interesting and complex venom are as yet speculative it seems reasonable to firstly consider its effect in intact monitored monkeys since they appear to share with man a special susceptibility to the venom.

Cynomolgus monkeys with an average weight of 3 kg were anesthetized initially with phencyclidine hydrochloride 4 mg/kg and after spraying the larynx with xylocaine, intubated with a 2.5 mm endotracheal tube and maintained on minimal halothane anesthesia with spontaneous respiration. If respiratory arrest occurred due to venom, certain animals were artificially ventilated using a self-inflating bag. Carotid or femoral arterial blood pressure was monitored with Statham pressure transducers and pulse rate, respiratory rate, and other signs observed directly. Hypothermia was prevented by a heating box incorporated in the operating table and body temperature monitored with a rectal thermistor. Samples under test were either injected subcutaneously into the forearm or slowly through a femoral vein cannula.

After the intravenous injection of *A. robustus* venom an immediate and profound hypotension occurred which lasted several minutes but was then replaced by marked hypertension for a 10—15 min period. The pupils became unreactive, grossly dilated, and irregular within seconds of the injection. Apnea occurred at the same time but if the airway was kept clear respiration at normal rate usually recommenced within 2—3 min. Usually no further anesthesia was required as the animal was semicomatose.

After about ten minutes generalized muscle fasciculation developed and the hypertension subsided. As the muscle twitching increased, extensive salivation, sweating, and lachrimation occurred, bowel sounds increased and diarrhea was often evident. Over the next two hours a progressive hypotension associated with periods of apnea occurred and the animal usually died despite ventilation with either oxygen or carbogen. Animals receiving doses less than 4 mg/kg could sometimes be salvaged by infusions of metaraminol.

When venom was given subcutaneously an identical syndrome was seen with the exception of the transient hypotension occuring after i.v. injection. Even after the subcutaneous injection there was a delay of only one or two minutes before the systemic effects of the venom were noticed and the syndrome was very similar to that induced by the intravenous route. Figure 7 depicts the syndrome as seen with a small dose of partially purified atraxotoxin. This syndrome was identical to that produced by either large doses of female venom or male venom at a dose of 0.2 mg/kg in monkeys. Atropine sulphate (0.1 mg/kg) decreased the loss of secretions but otherwise did not affect the syndrome. MORGANS et al. (1974) were provided with venom from these laboratories and undertook extensive studies

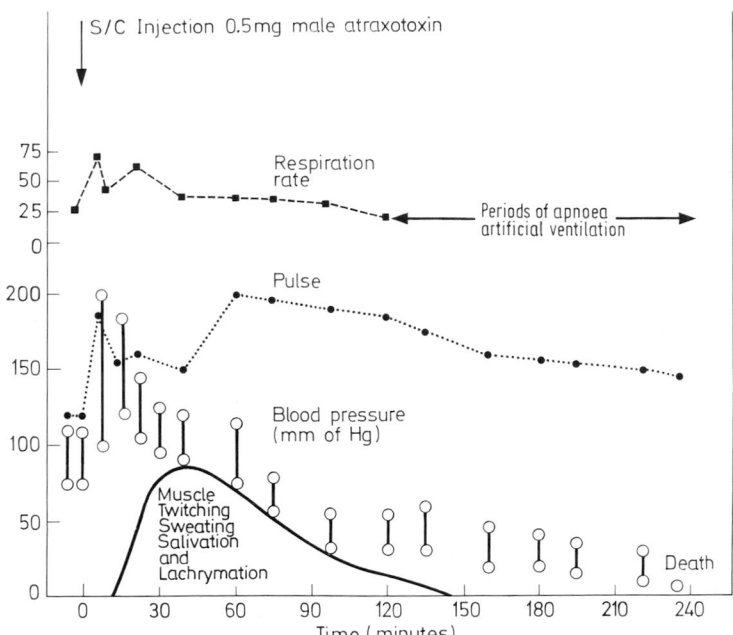

Fig. 7. Response of anesthetized 3 kg Cynomolgus monkey to subcutaneous injection of 0.5 mg of crude male atraxotoxin. Vertical dumbells indicate systolic and diastolic blood pressure

in monkeys to determine whether the cardiovascular changes are secondary to the respiratory disturbances and muscular activity. The monkeys used were either *Macaca nemestrinas* or *Macaca iris*. Ten monkeys were anesthetized with pentobarbitone (30 mg/kg i.v.) and then intubated. Another six monkeys were also given gallamine (4 mg/kg) and artificially ventilated. Venom was infused either intravenously (diluted in 0.9% NaCl) or as was the case in two monkeys via the vertebral artery. Infusion periods were either 5, 10, or 12 min. Recordings were made over a four hour period of the femoral arterial pressure, rectal temperature, endexpiratory CO_2 levels, E.C.G., and E.M.G. (*quadriceps femoris*). New monkeys were used for each infusion experiment.

Male venom (68 µg/kg) was infused for over 5 min in four monkeys and apnea occurred in all within 7 min and artificial ventilation was required for periods of 25–40 min. Initial hypertension (mean+24% at 5–7 min) was seen in 3 animals and all four subsequently developed hypotension (29%) over the next 60–100 min and failed to return to the control level. An infusion of the same dose but administered for over 15 min produced respiratory irregularities but no significant apnea in the four monkeys studied. Again arterial pressure rose (+22%) at 10–15 min and subsequently fell to −23% over 90–170 min. However, by 4 h had approached control levels (−9%). Generalized muscle activity, rectal temperature rise (2–5° C), lachrimation, and salivation were observed in all these animals. These other effects of the venom maximized at about 100–120 min and were no longer evident by 200 min after infusion.

Gallamine-treated monkeys infused with male venom for over 5 min showed even more marked cardiovascular changes. In three monkeys a maximum pressure (+42%) was reached at 7—12 min and fell to −56% over the next 170—200 min with little recovery. In one animal by 8 min the pressure had increased to +85% and 60 min later it was still elevated at +36%. When female venom (2 mg/kg) was infused over 5 min into two monkeys a rise in pressure (+18% and +48%) was followed by a fall of −17% in each animal. All gallamine-treated monkeys remained afebrile with no muscle twitching but lachrimation and salivation occurred. When male venom (21 µg/kg) was injected for over 5 min into the vertebral artery minimal cardiovascular effects were observed but no respiratory irregularities occurred. MORGANS et al. (1974) concluded from these experiments that in the monkey the cardiovascular effects of the venom are not secondary to the changes in respiration or muscular activity.

MORGANS (1975) is currently undertaking studies upon isolated monkey hearts and isolated human intercostal nerve-muscle preparations but no results are as yet available.

2. Studies Upon Isolated Preparations

WIENER (1961 b) reported that crude venom stimulated both the isolated ileum and uterus of guinea pigs. The uterus did not appear to be permanently affected by the venom and it responded to successive doses of the venom with no reduction in reaction to histamine. The addition of atropine and/or an antihistamine did not reduce contractions produced by crude venom. Lysergic acid diethylamide did not alter the response. Temporary cessation of conduction occurred when 2 mg of crude venom were applied directly to the trunk of the rat sciatic nerve. No conduction changes were detected when venom was applied to toad sciatic nerve (longitudinally split) and no alteration was detected in the rate or strength of contraction of an isolated rabbit heart perfused with whole venom (SUTHERLAND, unpublished). Venom applied to the cerebral cortex of the rat caused reduction for some 15 min in the amplitude of fast and slow waves. Using an electro-osmotic technique CURTIS (1973) introduced whole venom into cat spinal dorsal horn interneurones and Renshaw cells. CURTIS found that the responses of both kinds of cells were depressed in a nonspecific fashion similar to that RYALL had found using certain brain extracts (RYALL et al., 1964). WIENER (1961 b) found that the respiratory quotients of brain or liver cells were not affected by the presence of venom nor was the growth of monkey kidney cells in tissue culture altered. The whole crude venom had no anticholinesterase activity in vitro (WIENER, 1961 b).

PARNAS and RUSSELL (1967) found that crayfish deep extensor muscle preparations were blocked presynaptically by *A. robustus* venom but could detect no effect upon rat nerve-muscle preparations. The venom used by these workers may have been of low toxicity or partially adsorbed to glassware as the author has found rat nerve-muscle preparations invariably affected by the venom. Similar effects have been found (SUTHERLAND, 1972 b) using the convenient chicken *biventer cervicis* preparation of GINSBORG and WARRINER (1960). Isolated 10 ml organ baths at 36° C were used and the Krebs solution was of the following composition (mM): NaCl 118; KCl, 4.7, CaCl$_2$ 2.6; KH$_2$PO$_4$, 1.2; MgSO$_4$, 1.2; NaHCO$_3$,

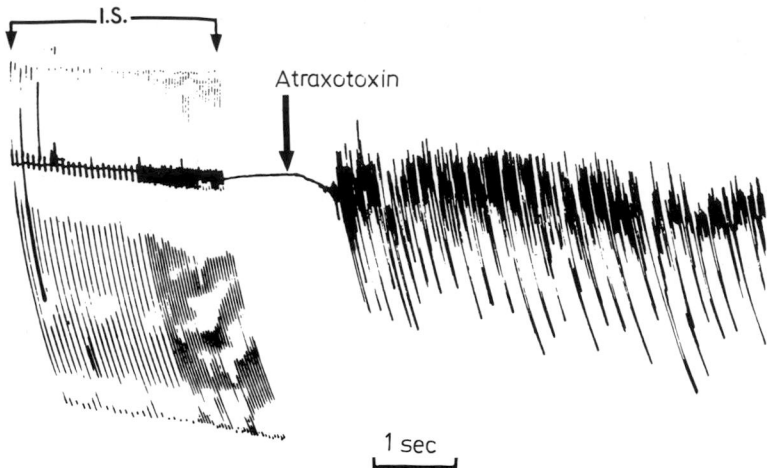

Fig. 8. Effect of 2 µg/ml crude male atraxotoxin upon chicken *biventer cervicis* nerve muscle preparation. I.S.: indirect stimulation. The spontaneous contractions last some 60 min after which preparation gives normal response to indirect stimulation

2.6; and glucose 11.12. The Krebs solution was bubbled with 5% carbon dioxide in oxygen. Indirect stimulation was carried out at a rate of 12 per min with supramaximal rectangular pulses of 0.1 milliseconds duration. Responses were recorded by pen and drum via an isometric transducer and amplifier (Ugo Basile). Uniformity of preparations under test was ensured by discarding any preparation (usually 20%) which failed to give a good response to indirect stimulation with amplitude kept constant.

Figure 8 shows the effect of atraxotoxin on such a nerve-muscle preparation. The remarkable fact is that these contractions persist for 30–90 min and there is no residual loss of function. Indirect stimulation produces an enhanced response during this period. HAMILTON (1972) has found no evidence of any ultrastructural changes in a variety of tissue including rat vas deferens and diaphragm which have been exposed to large quantities of either crude venom or highly toxic atraxotoxin. No suggestion of motor end-plate vesicle degeneration similar to that produced by black widow venom (CLARK et al., 1970) was found. It was found that the effect upon these preparations was directly related to toxicity in suckling mice and thus both an *in vitro* and *in vivo* assay was available for monitoring fractionation procedures. Results of a third assay method, viz. monitored intact monkeys was also directly related to activity found by the above procedures.

The interactions between atraxotoxin and a number of drugs were studied in the chicken nerve-muscle preparation. Both gallamine and suxamethonium prevented any response to atraxotoxin. Lowered calcium (0.1 mM) or elevated magnesium (10 mM) suppressed the response as did tetrodotoxin, lignocaine, and the toxin of the blue-ringed octopus *Hapalochlaena maculosa*. This latter Australian toxin is known to block the movement of sodium ions (DULHUNTY and GAGE, 1971). The effect of the atraxotoxin was not amplified by neostigmine, choline, or acetylcholine but was markedly enhanced by physostigmine (0.1 µg/ml). Levels as low as 0.2 µg/ml of atraxotoxin were easily detected by adding physostigmine either before or after the atraxotoxin. Because of some clinical observations suggesting some beneficial effects of diazepam this drug was investigated. It was found that in the chicken nerve-muscle preparation diazepam (70 µg/ml) rapidly caused loss of indirect response to supramaximal nerve stimulation but this effect was rapidly reversed by a single change of the Krebs solution. If atraxotoxin was added before or after diazepam there was no apparent response until the bath was changed at which stage the preparation responded exactly as if atraxotoxin had just been added. This suggests that atraxotoxin may combine to a specific receptor and is not washed out when the diazepam is removed. BLABER (1973) suggested that the diazepam in these circumstances acts by stabilizing excitable membranes.

Interpretation of the above incomplete findings is difficult and may have been made more complicated by the selection of the chick *biventer cervicis* muscle (CHANG and TANG, 1974). Since atraxotoxin has no anticholinesterase activity the suggestion is made that *in vivo* and *in vitro* it promotes the release of acetylcholine without depletion of the stored transmitter, and the increased release of acetylcholine causes the spontaneous skeletal muscle activity. Prolonged and distressing muscle twitching is induced by a number of arthropod venoms, e.g. *Centruroides* spp. venom (DEL POZO, 1966) however, none show the complete clinical and experimental reversibility that is characteristic of atraxotoxin.

If atraxotoxin produces widespread release of acetylcholine at motor end-plates and at appropriate synapses in both the sympathetic and parasympathetic nervous system then the syndrome as seen in man and monkeys would be superficially explained.

3. Investigation of Antidotes

Since no specific antivenin is available continuing attention has been given to finding a specific pharmacologic or chemical antidote. WIENER (1961 b) suggested that the injection of a 5% potassium permanganate solution into each puncture wound would inactivate any venom still at the site. WIENER also explored a number of therapeutic substances in mice. However, it must be borne in mind that large doses of whole venom are required to kill adult mice and then death is probably due to the large quantities of spermine complex that are injected rather than the atraxotoxin present. WIENER found that antihistamines, atropine, A.C.T.H., mephenesin, and a large number of other drugs failed to alter the time or inevitable death when a mouse lethal dose was employed. A.C.T.H. was also studied by WALLACE and STICKA (1955).

In monkeys the use of diazepam, atropine, and frusemide appear to increase chances of survival (SUTHERLAND, unpublished) but more intensive studies are required. As described above, MORGAN et al. have shown that gallamine-treated monkeys do not develop pyrexia and muscle fasciculation but the cardiovascular effects appear unaltered. In small animals no protection is obtained with either redback spider or tick antivenin (WIENER, 1961 b).

VIII. Immunologic Studies on Atrax Venom

Precipitating antibodies to female *A. robustus* venom were prepared in horses after extensive immunization and a titer of 1:64,000 was obtained (WIENER, 1963). No neutralizing antibodies could be detected in such sera. WIENER injected increasing doses into a sheep over a 3 month period. A total of 147 mg of venom was injected with a first dose of 0.5 mg and a final dose of 60 mg. Precipitating antibodies were detected after two weeks but no neutralizing antibodies developed. Chronic immunization of rabbits and guinea pigs failed to produce neutralizing antibodies. WIENER found that by increasing the dose, venom injected into a guinea pig up to 10.5 mg could be tolerated in an animal of weight 400 g whereas a nonimmunized animal of the same weight would die after an injection of 6 mg. From his experiments WIENER concluded that the main toxin of the venom was either of low antigenicity or was nonantigenic.

Antisera have been raised in rabbits to male and female *A. robustus* venom and female *A. versutus* venom using Freund's complete adjuvant and a variety

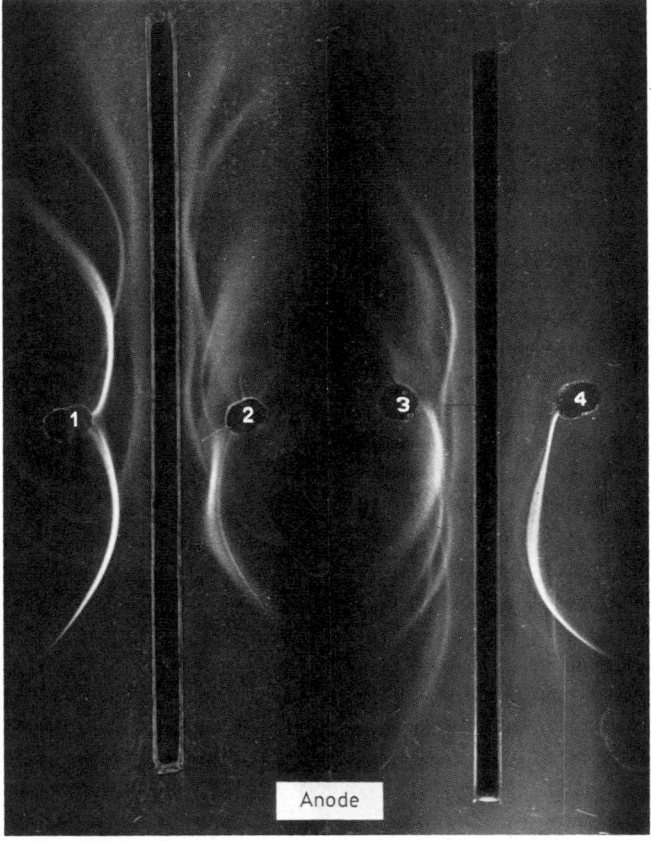

Fig. 9. Microimmunoelectrophoresis of *Atrax* venom and *Atrax* hemolymph. 1. Male *A. robustus* venom 2. Female *A. robustus* venom 3. Female *A. versutus* venom 4. Hemolymph from female *A. robustus* Center Troughs: Anti-female *A. robustus* venom

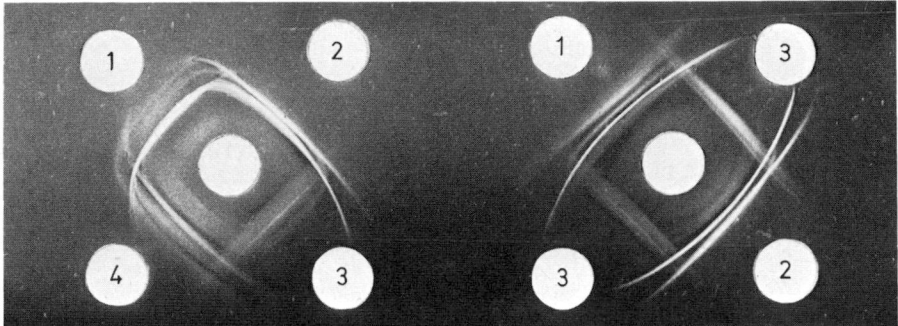

Fig. 10. Gel diffusion against Anti-female *A. robustus* venom (Rabbit IgG) *1.* Male *A robustus* venom *2.* Female *A. robustus* venom *3.* Female *A. robustus* hemolymph *4.* Female *A. infensus* venom

of immunization schedules (Sᴜᴛʜᴇʀʟᴀɴᴅ, unpublished). Hyperimmune rabbit sera was fractionated by ion exchange chromatography to prepare rabbit IgG (Sᴜᴛʜᴇʀ-ʟᴀɴᴅ, 1972b). Although at least five precipitin lines could be obtained by immuno-electrophoresis against the individual venom no *in vivo* or *in vitro* reduction in the toxicity of the venom could be detected.

Figure 9 shows a degree of similarity between male and female *A. robustus* venom in regard to immunoreactive components. A somewhat different pattern of precipitin lines is seen with female *A. infensus* venom. A major line of identity between male and female *A. robustus* venom is seen on gel diffusion (Fig. 10) and another line of identity is also shared with *A. infensus* venom. However, there is clearly no fusion with the hemolymph precipitin line and the venoms studied. Thus, although hemolymph reacts strongly with antibodies prepared to the venom it has immunologic properties distinct from venom components. Wɪᴇɴᴇʀ (1961a) found that hemolymph of *A. robustus* could neutralize the toxic effects of *A. robustus* venom in vitro but not in vivo. The neutralizing factor was heat labile and required a period of at least 10 min to react with the venom. Hemolymph that has been heat-treated no longer reacts with the antisera.

The studies on venoms using gel diffusion are continuing because they have the advantage of allowing the examination of the venom collected from a single spider. However, the current antisera in use may well be criticized in that they have been raised by using pooled venom from a spider colony which may well have harbored unrecognized members of other *Atrax* species, particularly in the case of females.

IX. Human Envenomation by Atrax robustus

1. General

Whereas the data on distribution and likely outcome of a bite by most Australian venomous creatures is well known, information relating to the genus *Atrax* is scanty. All that is certain is that all fatal cases in which the spider has been positively identified have been cases concerning a male *A. robustus*. All fatalities have occurred within a 179 kilometer radius of Sydney. Fortunately no constitutional symptoms develop in the majority of human victims particularly if they have been bitten by female spiders. Information obtained from the medical superintendents of 19 large public hospitals in the state of New South Wales indicate that this is the rule in the majority of cases.

The number of fatalities attributed to this fairly common spider is quite low. At least 11 fatalities have been attributed to *A. robustus* since the first death was reported in 1927 (MUSGRAVE). Until this first recorded fatality the male of the species had been incorrectly designated *Euctimenta tibialis* and thus two species were thought to exist. Naturally the male of one species and the female of the other had never been discovered.

Clinical aspects of envenomation of *A. robustus* have been reviewed by WIENER (1961 b) and SUTHERLAND (1972c, 1974). Most bites occur in the early summer months when the spiders tend to roam into houses and summer camps. The male has a particularly vicious disposition and is extremely aggressive when confronted. A number of fatalities and near fatalities have occurred when the spider has sought refuge in clothing or shoes. Most bites occur on the hands or feet but one fatality resulted by a bite upon the buttock (INGRAM and MUSGRAVE, 1933) and another fatality occurred when a young woman was bitten on her breast when a spider fell upon her as she walked through thick bush country (SUTHERLAND, 1972c). Multiple bites to the hands may occur in children and infants when they accidentally pick up an object that the spider is grasping. Although most cases occur in summer, fatalities have been recorded in both autumn and winter.

2. Signs and Symptoms of Envenomation

Invariably a bite by either a male or female spider is extremely painful because of direct trauma by the large strong fangs and the low pH of the venom. The dimension of this spider and the fact that it is publicly known that no specific antivenin is available produce fear and a variable degree of panic in both the victim and the bystanders. Difficulty is sometimes experienced in removing the spider particularly if the fangs are firmly embedded in the finger nail of a child. As will be discussed later, prompt application of an effective tourniquet may be a life-saving procedure. The bite site may be extremely painful for hours and even days but no local necrosis has been recorded. WIENER (1961 b) studied the local reaction to venom by injecting his own forearm intradermally with 0.05 mg of venom. Intense pain lasted for 30 min and a weal developed at the site of injection and was surrounded by an area of erythema. After 30 min the weal had subsided and localized sweating and erection of hair follicles occurred. Mild erythema persisted for seven days. WIENER suffered no constitutional effects from this small dose of venom at any stage. In clinical cases most envenomation occurs in the subcutaneous tissues and the histology of the bitten area in fatal cases discloses no unusual findings other than tissue damage directly related to trauma caused by the entry of the fangs. Post mortem studies have not to date revealed any significant pathology.

Following envenomation by a spider symptoms of systemic poisoning can develop within 10 min. The early part of the classical syndrome in humans is nausea and vomiting, abdominal pain, diarroea, profuse sweating, brisk salivation, lachrimation and severe dyspnea. Blood pressure may be markedly elevated and although paralysis does not occur, both local and generalized fasciculation of muscles is an invariable feature in severe cases. Muscle twitching may be prolonged and violent and makes the management of the semiconscious patient quite difficult. Spasm of the jaw muscles may make efforts to keep the airway patent quite arduous. Profound coma may last for many hours and appears unaffected by adequate oxygenation and maintenance of blood pressure at a normotensive level. In the second part of the syndrome the generalized muscle activity continues but the production of secretions subsides. Confusion and hypoxia may result in an asphyxial death. Some victims have died from hypotension preceding an irreversible cardiac arrest despite artificial ventilation. Occasionally a relatively symptomless period may occur between the two parts of the syndrome and an uneventful recovery may be incorrectly predicted. In small children in which the dose of venom per body weight may be much higher the whole syndrome may occur much faster and death may occur from 15—90 min after the bite. Adults who have received an effective bite may die up to 30 h or later. No cases of even temporary confusion or coma have been recorded without the victim having some of the characteristic early symptoms of envenomation. Thus a further similarity is found in the way the venom affects humans and monkeys. In some nonfatal cases uncommon signs have been recorded such as urticarial weals (INGRAM and MUSGRAVE, 1933) and hysterical dancing or "tarantulism" as described by WATKINS (1939).

Few clinical reports of envenomation by *A. formidabilis* are available and in some cases the exact identity of the spider (albeit *Atrax*) is uncertain. No fatalities have been reported but cases of extreme severity have occurred. INGRAM and MUSGRAVE (1933) described a case definity attributed to a male *A. formidabilis*. The victim, a strong and healthy timber worker was desperately ill with signs and symptoms similar to that seen after *A. robustus* envenomation. Another severe case was reported by IRWIN (1952) which involved a seven-year-old boy who was fortunate to survive. The infrequency of reported human envenomation by this species, as perhaps with other species of *Atrax,* may be due to merely reduced opportunity of contact with humans rather than any lesser toxicity. With increased settlement of the more remote habitats of species *Atrax* it is inevitable that more human cases will be reported.

3. Treatment of Victims

Prompt application of a tourniquet may prevent the victim from developing severe hypoxia before reaching a center with adequate medical facilities. Since venom probably moves centrally via the lymphatics (BARNES and TRUETA, 1941) immobilization of the limb combined with an adequate broad tourniquet to compress the lymphatics is a very rational procedure in dealing with the type of venom under consideration. Because of the risks involved funnel-web spider bites should be treated with an arterial tourniquet and not a venous tourniquet as suggested for cases of poisoning by Australian snakes (Sutherland, 1975). In cases which have ended fatally no reference has been made to a tourniquet in their clinical notes. There is no place for incision of the peripheral bite or local venesection (Sutherland, 1973a) and the tourniquet should not be released in transit even if there is a risk of ischemic changes as its release may herald the onset of sudden massive systemic envenomation (Sutherland, 1972c).

Clinically atropine, frusemide, and diazepam have proven useful. If hypotension develops plasma volume expanders and perhaps isoprenaline infusion should be commenced (Sutherland, 1974). Since the exact mode of action or actions of the venom is uncertain and the exact cause of death is speculative one cannot be dogmatic about treatment. Intubation and prevention of hypoxia, close monitoring of the patient and dealing with each subsequent event on its merits result in the survival of patients who some years ago most probably would have died. All cases which show any evidence of systemic envenomation should be admitted to an intensive care ward if possible and observed for at least 24 h after the initial symptoms.

Diazepam appears to reduce the gross muscle twitching which is unaffected by infusion of calcium gluconate. Relaxant anesthesia might be considered in cases with severe muscle spasm which make oxygenation difficult, however this has not been tried clinically.

Even if specific antivenin or antidote become available the initial management of cases of severe envenomation by *A. robustus* will still frequently require swift and skilled medical care especially if the victim is a small child.

4. Prognosis

It is impossible to predict which victim will suffer life-threatening systemic effects and when only minor local symptoms will be seen. Provided that first aid is adequate and close monitoring allows the different stages of the syndrome to be treated appropriately then most patients should survive this sudden but critical illness. There are no sequelae once the victim has recovered from the acute effects of the venom.

X. Discussion

There are many unusual features to be found in both the species *Atrax* and their venom. In contrast to the normal situation, the male is far more toxic than the female to humans and susceptible experimental animals. Since the spider's massive fangs can quite adequately deal with its normal prey one wonders why these spiders require such a peculiar and complex venom. Perhaps it is an accident of nature that the higher primates are particularly susceptible to the venom. Possibly the 'milked' venom studied in the laboratory is different in concentration or components to that which the spider injects when enraged and attacking. A monkey may sometimes die after being bitten by a female spider but injecting a monkey with ten times the average yield of female 'milked' venom will rarely kill the monkey. We have seen that the venom glands are highly innervated and venom release may be very accurately controlled according to the spiders assessment of the danger it faces.

With the exception of the enzymes the role of the venom components is quite unknown, as is the interactions between them. Further purification of atraxotoxin may lead to the availability of a unique pharmacologic tool with effects that are apparently reversible.

References

Adams, D.J., Gage, P.W., Spence, I.: Modification of membrane excitability produced by funnel-web spider venom and calcium in aplasia neurones, Proc. Aust. Physiol. Pharmacol. Soc. **7**, 161P (1976).

Barnes, J.M., Trueta, J.: Absorption of Bacteria, Toxins and Snake Venoms from the Tissues. Lancet **1941 I**, 623–626.

Birner, J.: Personal Communication, 1973.

Blaber, L.C.: Personal Communication, 1973.

Broad, A.J.: Personal Communication, 1975.

Carroll, P.R., Glover, W.E., Morgans, D.: Effect of funnel-web spider venom on the isolated ear artery of the rabbit, Proc. Aust. Physiol. Pharmacol. Soc. **4**, 184 (1973)

Carroll, P.R., Morgans, D.: The effect of the venom of the Sydney funnel web spider (*Atrax robustus*) on isolated human intercostal muscles, Toxicon, **14**, 487–492 (1976).

Chang, C.C. and Tang, S.S.: Differentiation between intrinsic and extrinsic acetylcholine. Receptor of the chick *biventer cervicis* muscle. Naunyn Schmiedebergs Arch. Pharmakol. **282**, 379–388 (1974).

Clark, A.W., Mauro, A., Longenecker, H.E., Jr., Hurlbut, W.P.: Effects on the fine structure of the frog neuromuscular junction. Nature (Lond.) **225**, 703–705 (1970).

Coulter, A.R., Sutherland, S.K., Broad, A.J.: Detection of snake venoms in tissue fluids. J. Immunol. Meth. **4**, No. 2, 297–300 (1974).

Curtis, D.R.: Personal communication (1973).

Del Pozo, E.C.: Pharmacology of the venoms of Mexican *Centruroides*. Mem. Inst. Butantan **33**, 615–626 (1966).

Dorfman, A.: Methods in Enzymology. Colowick, S.P., and Kaplan, N.O., (eds.) New York: Academic Press, 1955, Vol. I.

Dulhunty, A., Gage, P.W.: Selecting effect of an octopus toxin on action potential. J. Physiol. **218**, 433–445 (1971).

Fischer, F.G., Bohn, H.: Die Giftsekrete der Vogelspinnen. Liebigs Ann. **603**, 232–250 (1957).

Garnet, J.R.: Venomous Australian Animals Dangerous to Man. Commonwealth Serum Laboratories Publication, Melbourne, 1969.

Gilbo, C.M., Coles, N.W.: An investigation of certain components of the venom of the female Sydney funnel-web spider, *Atrax robustus* Cambr. Aust. J. Biol. Sci. **17**, 758–763 (1964).

Ginsborg, B.L., Warriner, J.: The isolated chick *biventer cervicis* nerve-muscle preparation. Br. J. Pharmacol. **15**, 410–411 (1960).

Hamilton, R.C.: Ultrastructural studies of the action of Australian spider venoms. In: 30th Ann. Proc. Electron Microscopy Soc. Amer., Los Angeles, Calif. Arceneaux, C.J., (ed.) Baton Rouge, Louisiana: Claitor's Publishing Division, 1972.

Hamilton, R.C.: Personal communication, 1975.

Hickman, V.V.: On *Atrax infensus* sp. n. (Araneida: Dipluridae) its habits and a method of trapping the males. Proc. R. Soc. Tasmania **98**, 107–112 (1964).

Ingram, W.W., Musgrave, A.: Spider bite (arachnidism): A survey of its occurrence in Australia, with case histories. Med. J. Aust. **1**,10–15 (1933).

Irwin, R.S.: Funnel-Web Spider Bite. Med. J. Aust. **2**, 342 (1952).

Kaire, G.H.: The north coast funnel-web spider *Atrax formidabilis*. Med. J. Aust. **2**, 450 (1961).

Kaire, G.H.: Observations on some funnel-web spiders (*Atrax* species) and their venoms, with particular reference to *Atrax robustus*. Med. J. Aust. **2**, 307–311 (1963).

Kaire, G.H.: The Sydney funnel-web spider (*Atrax robustus*) in captivity. Vic. Nat. **81**, 38–39 (1964).

Kellaway, C.H.: A note on the venom of the Sydney funnel-web spider *Atrax robustus*. Med. J. Aust. **1**, 678–679 (1934).

Levitt, V.: The funnel-web spider in captivity. Proc. R. Zool. Soc. N. S. W. 80—84 1958—1959 (1961).

McCrone, J.D.: Spider venoms: Biochemical aspects. Am. Zool. **9**, 153—156 (1969).

McFerran, F.: Use of insects for feeding. In: U.F.A.W. Handbook on the Care and Management of Laboratory Animals. 2 nd ed., London: E. and S. Livingstone, 1957.

McKeown, K.: Australian Spiders. Sydney: Angus and Robertson, 1963.

Meadows, P.E., Russell, F.E.: Milking of Arthropods. Toxicon **8**, 311—312 (1970).

Morgans, D.: Personal communication, 1975.

Morgans, D., Carroll, P.R.: A direct acting adrenergic component of the venom of the Sydney funnel-web spider, *Atrax robustus*, Toxicon, **14**, 185—189 (1976).

Morgans, D., Spira, P.J., Myelcharane, E.J., Glover, W.E.: Effect of funnel-web spider venom in the monkey. Proc. Aust. Physiol. Pharmacol. Soc. **5**, 234—235 (1974).

Musgrave, A.: Some poisonous Australian spiders. Rec. Aust. Museum **16**, 33—46 (1927).

Parnas, I., Russell, F.E.: Effects of venoms on nerve, muscle and neuromuscular junction. In: Animal Toxins. Oxford-London-New York-Paris: Pergamon Press, 1967.

Ryall, R.W., Stone, N.E., Curtis, D.R., Watkins, J.C.: Action of acetylcholine extracted from brain on spinal Renshaw cells. Nature (Lond.) **201**, 1034—1035 (1964).

Skinner, H.H.: The use of unweaned mice as experimental animals. In: The U.F.A.W. Handbook on the Care and Management of Laboratory Animals. London: U.F.A.W. 1959.

Spence, I., Adams, D.J., Gage, P.W.: Funnel web spider venom produces spontaneous action potentials in nerve, Life Sciences, **20**, 243—250 (1977).

Sutherland, S.K.: The Sydney funnel-web spider (*Atrax robustus*). A review of published studies on the crude venom. Med. J. Aust. **2**, 528—530 (1972a).

Sutherland, S.K.: The Sydney funnel-web spider (*Atrax robustus*) Fractionation of the female venom into five distinct components. Med. J. Aust. **2**, 593—596 (1972b).

Sutherland, S.K.: The Sydney funnel-web spider (*Atrax robustus*) A review of some clinical records of human envenomation. Med. J. Aust. **2**, 643—646 (1972c).

Sutherland, S.K.: Treatment of funnel-web spider bites. Med. J. Aust. **1**, 1016 (1973a).

Sutherland, S.K.: Isolation, mode of action and properties of the major toxin (Atraxotoxin) in the venom of the Sydney funnel-web spider (*Atrax robustus*). Proc. Aust. Soc. Med. Res. **3**, 172 (1973b).

Sutherland, S.K.: Venomous Australian creatures: the action of their toxins and the care of the envenomated patient. Anaesth. Intens. Care **2**, 316—328 (1974).

Sutherland, S.K.: Treatment of arachnid poisoning in Australia, Aust. Fam. Phycn. **5**, 305—312 (1976).

Sutherland, S.K., Coulter, A.R., Broad, A.J., Hilton, J.M.N., Lane, L.H.D.: Human snake bite victims: the successful detection of circulating snake venom by radioimmunoassay. Med. J. Aust. **1**, 27—29 (1975).

Takeuchi, A., Takeuchi, N.: Localized action of gamma-amino butyric acid on the crayfish muscle. J. physiol. **177**, 225—238 (1965).

Wallace, A.L., Sticka, R.: The effect of ACTH on the toxicity of spider's venom. Med. J. Aust. **1**, 5—6 (1955).

Watkins, A.M.: A bite by *Atrax robustus*. Med. J. Aust. **1**, 710 (1939).

Wiener, S.: The Sydney funnel-web spider (*Atrax robustus*) I. Collection of venom and its toxicity in animals. Med. J. Aust. **2**, 377—382 (1957).

Wiener, S.: The Sydney funnel-web spider (*Atrax robustus*): II. Venom yield and other characteristics of spider in captivity. Med. J. Aust. **2**, 679—682 (1959).

Wiener, S.: The Sydney funnel-web spider (*Atrax robustus*): The neutralization of venom by haemolymph. Med. J. Aust. **1**, 449—450 (1961a).

Wiener, S.: Observations on the venom of the Sydney funnel-web spider (*Atrax robustus*). Med. J. Aust. **2**, 693—699 (1961b).

Wiener, S.: Antigenic and electrophoretic properties of funnel-web spider (*Atrax robustus*) venom. In: Venomous and Poisonous Animals and Noxious Plants of the Pacific Area. Oxford-London-New York-Paris: Pergamon Press, 1963.

Wiener, S., Drummond, F.H.: Assay of spider venom and antivenene in Drosophila. Nature (Lond.) **178**, 267—268 (1956).

Venoms of Theridiidae, Genus Latrodectus

A. Systematics, Distribution and Biology of Species; Chemistry, Pharmacology and Mode of Action of Venom

S. BETTINI and M. MAROLI

I. Systematics and Distribution of Species

The first description of a *Latrodectus* spider is that of ROSSI (1790) at the University of Pisa, who named the species *Aranea 13-guttata;* it was later placed under the genus *Latrodectus* Walckenaer. He was also the first to prove the relationship between the bite of this species and the syndrome of "latrodectism," which had been confused up to that time with the hysteria form known as "tarantism" (see Part B).

The taxonomy of the genus *Latrodectus,* according to workers with a special interest in this group, presents some difficulties, and the vast literature may lead to confusion. Descriptions of *Latrodectus* species have been published in all continents. Thus, until the work of LEVI (1958), the number of species described ran to twenty-one. LEVI suggested that the number of species be confined to five, namely: *L. geometricus* and *L. mactans,* from the warmer regions of America but apparently found also in all continents; *L. curacaviensis,* common in America; *L. hystrix,* from the Yemen; *L. pallidus,* from Palestine, Asia Minor and Russia. On these grounds, LEVI (1959) revised the genus exhaustively, adding one more species, *L. dahli,* from Iran. Synonyms, characteristics, data on variation, habitat, and keys to male and female spiders were also given. The author has overcome the difficulty and confusion that would arise in giving synonyms to some traditionally well-known specific names of what he considers allopatric populations by using trinomials: *L. mactans mactans* of America, *L. mactans tredecimguttatus* (Fig. 1) of Europe and North Africa, *L. mactans menavodi* of Madagascar, *L. mactans hasselti* of India and Australia, etc.

The *L. curacaviensis* group was later reconsidered by MCCRONE and LEVI (1964), who separated it into three species: *L. curacaviensis, L. variolus* and *L. bishopi.* The authors' conclusions were not accepted by GERSCHMAN and SCHIAPELLI (1965), who reiterated their belief that *L. mactans* was synonymous with *L. curacaviensis.*

The taxonomy of the genus, however, did not seem at that stage to be definitely settled. In a small area of the Province of Santiago del Estero (Argentina), ABALOS and BAEZ (1967) carried out an investigation on a very large number of samples, describing five species: *L. geometricus, L. curacaviensis,* and three species belonging

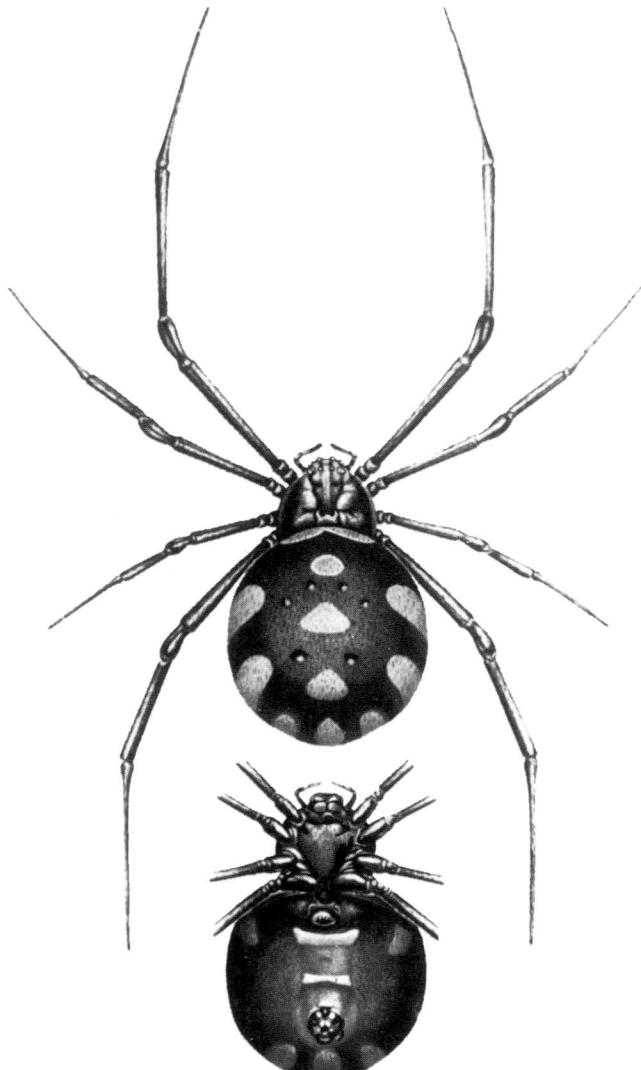

Fig. 1. Female *L. m. tredecimguttatus*

to the *mactans* group but considered as separate taxonomic entities because of their genetic differences and reproductive isolation. This classification was accepted also by Canese (1972), who described two of these forms in Paraguay. Morphological differences had also been found in their egg-sacs (Abalos, 1962). In a subsequent investigation (Barrio, 1966), after double-diffusion tests it appeared that at least two forms of the *mactans* group of Abalos (1962), those indicated as no. 1 and no. 2, showed immunochemical differences, which, together with ecological and ethological characteristics, proved the existence of an isolating mechanism.

On the other hand, immunological and electrophoretical comparison of the venoms of sympatric species such as *L. m. mactans* and *L. variolus* from North America did not show any appreciable differences (McCRONE and NETZLOFF, 1965). Nor were any appreciable differences found by RUSSELL and BUESS (1970) in populations of *L. m. mactans* from different areas of the United States.

SHULOV (1966) reported three species from Israel, *L. mactans, L. pallidus* and *L. revivensis,* the last one described by him (1940), but synonymized by LEVI (1959) in his revision of the genus. SHULOV's conclusions were later also accepted by LEVI (1966).

Differences in the electrophoretic pattern of the hemolymph proteins have been used by McCRONE (1967) as taxanomic characteristics to separate two sibling species, *L. mactans* and *L. variolus.* An accurate morphological and biological study on the North American species, carried out by KASTON (1970) indicated that the species are actually three: *mactans, variolus* and *hesperus.*

It may thus be concluded that the systematics of *Latrodectus* has gone through three phases. The first phase, based mainly on differences of color patterns, led to a considerable increase in the number of species. In the second phase, when the morphology of the genitalia was studied in depth, several species were again classed together. At present, taxonomists are dealing with a third phase, in which biological as well as morphological characteristics are being used; the number of species has slightly increased again.

A full account of the distribution of the five species and of their varieties, taking in the whole genus, was given by LEVI (1959), who included a world map showing the distribution by dorsal abdominal color pattern and setae and body dimensions of *L. mactans* and *L. curacaviensis.*

A list of areas where people have been bitten by *Latrodectus* species is given in Part B of the present text under "Epidemiology of latrodectism." There is obviously overlapping between the distribution of cases and the distribution of spiders, but the contrary may not be true. In the distribution areas of several species whose habits do not lead to a high frequency of man-spider contacts, latrodectism may be absent or very rare, as in Israel (SHULOV, 1966).

Investigations on the distribution of spiders of one or more species in limited areas have been carried out by BAERG (1945) in Jamaica and Haiti (*L. geometricus* and *L. mactans*); by FINLAYSON (1956) in Southern Africa (*L. indistinctus*); by MARIKOVSKJ (1956) in Russia (*L.m. tredecimguttatus*).

An alarming article on the spreading of *Latrodectus* spiders in New England was published by KASTON (1954). BENOIT (1969) discovered four specimens of *L. m. mactans* and one of *L. geometricus* in Belgium respectively during the years 1967 and 1968, which were retained as imported species. Since their whole life cycle was observed by the author under local natural conditions, the possibility of colonization of these species in Northern Europe was also considered.

II. Biology

1. Habitat

Different species and subspecies of *Latrodectus* have adapted themselves to a variety of habitats, whose characteristics greatly influence the frequency of bites to humans or to animals of agricultural interest. Several species live outdoors in cultivated farmland or in wild areas; others are very often found indoors, preferring man-made shelters. Thus *L. m. tredecimguttatus* in Europe prefers wheat fields, or other crop fields, but may also be very abundant on uncultivated land, especially in rocky fields. Consequently, the humans bitten by this species are usually farmers or workers connected with agricultural practice, as in Italy where during the period 1938–1958 74 percent of cases were males (Bettini, 1963).

On the other hand, *L. m. mactans* in North America is found in quite different habitats, choosing cellars, garages, outdoor lavatories and so on to build its web. This species, however, is also found on cultivated land, *e.g.* in vineyards, and in hilly countryside (D'Amour et al., 1936).

2. Habits

The habits of the three sympatric species *L. m. tredecimguttatus, L. pallidus,* and *L. revivensis* in Israel were carefully described by Shulov and Weissman (1959), one of the differential ethological characteristics being their web construction. This function was exhaustively studied by Marikovskj (1956) in *L. m. tredecimguttatus*. In all species the web is decidedly irregular and the silk is very resistant. It has been used for optical apparatuses.

3. Life Cycle

Montgomery (1908) determined the sex ratio in 41,749 newly hatched young and found that there were on average 8.19 males to every female. The sex ratio probably varies according to the nutritional characteristics of immature stages. Monterosso and Floris (1936) showed that *L. m. tredecimguttatus* on a rich diet bore 42 percent males, while on a poor diet the percentage of males was 100. Similar results were obtained by Cantore (1956). The spiderlings usually undergo one molt before emergence, which takes place through an opening in the egg sac. In *L. m. mactans* and in *L. m. tredecimguttatus* the number of molts to reach maturity varies from 4 to 5 for males and from 5 to 8 for females; in *L. variolus,* from 5 to 7 for males and from 7 to 8 for females (Cantore, 1956; McCrone and Levi, 1964). The number of molts varies among species, but is dependent also on environmental factors.

Males reach maturity earlier than females and have a much shorter life span, living only long enough to mate, i.e. one-two months. The life span of females, on the other hand, is several months. Mature and immature females of *L. m. tredecim-guttatus* can be found from May to December, while males are found from May to June. A small number of females, however, probably those that emerge in late summer, survive through the winter (Cantore, 1956). A very similar life cycle has been reported for *L. m. mactans* by D'Amour et al. (1936).

Eggs are laid in late summer. The number of egg sacs averages 3 per female, but twice as many can be easily found; according to Baerg (1945), from 4 to 6. The number of eggs in an egg sac also varies considerably: from 150 to 200 (Rivosecchi and Bettini, 1958) in *L. m. tredecimguttatus;* an average of 174 for *L. pallidus* (Shulov, 1940), an average of 143 in *L. m. mactans* (D'Amour et al.,

1936), and according to BAERG (1945) from none to 700 or 800. A very wide
range was also reported by MARIKOVSKJ (1956).

The parasites of *Latrodectus* egg sacs are considered in a later subchapter, on
epidemiology, by Z. MARETIC. A list of parasites and predators of *L. m. mactans*
is given by JENKINS (1964).

The courtship and mating ritual in *L. m. mactans* has been extensively described
by D'AMOUR et al. (1936) and by CANTORE (1956), and spermatic transmission
with details of copula in *L. mactans, L. curacaviensis* and *L. geometricus* was described by ABALOS and BAEZ (1963).

Males that have fulfilled the act of mating do not survive long. There has
been no confirmation for any species of the popular belief that females kill and
devour their mates. The application of the term "widow" to the females of this
genus is probably due to the fact that only the female is usually found on the
web, the male having died or passing unnoticed because of its small size (Fig. 2).
The females are cannibalistic when confined in a container or when two individuals
are placed on the same web.

The capture of prey has been well described for *L. m. tredecimguttatus* by MON-
TEROSSO and RONSISVALLE (1947). The female ejects a sticky fluid from the tip

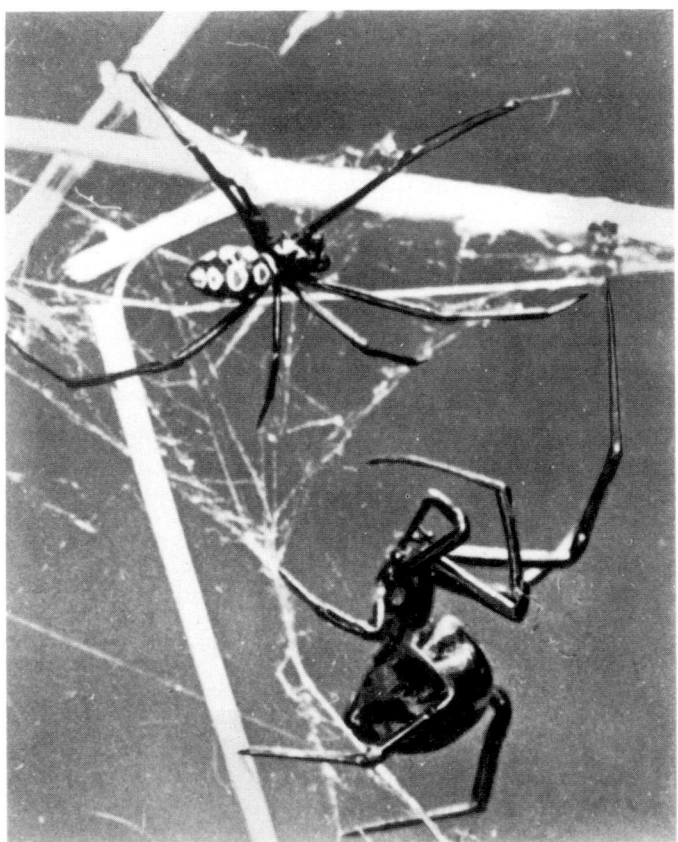

Fig. 2. Male (left) and female *L. m. tredecimguttatus* on web

of its abdomen, thus imprisoning its victim, which is then bitten by the chelicera and paralyzed by the injected venom. *Latrodectus* usually prey on Orthoptera and Coleoptera.

4. Biting Act

Latrodectus females are not aggressive when confronted with large animals. When disturbed (a shadow may be sufficient) they flee from the web to hide about the "nest," which is usually built under a stone or in a crevice, or let themselves drop to the ground. Thus the biting of large vertebrates is only an extreme act of defense. This usually occurs when the spider is pressed accidentally against the skin. Man is bitten most often if a spider is caught between the person's clothes and his skin, or in the case of farmers when picking up wheat bundles, shrubs, or boxes left in the fields, or harvesting various crops, etc. In the case of peridomestic species, such as *L. m. mactans,* which often builds its web in garages and in outdoor toilets, people may be bitten if they accidentally come in contact with the spider. (It is common for man's genitalia to be bitten when the spider's web is built inside the lavatory bowl.)

The act of biting does not have any peculiar characteristics. The fangs are jabbed into the skin and held there for several seconds. If the spider is repeatedly pressed it often bites more than once. When the fangs penetrate the skin, the spider's cephalothoracic musculature contracts so as to compress the venom glands. The muscular layer surrounding the gland concurs in its squeezing and the delivery of the toxic liquid.

Bücherl (1964) measured the distance between the chelicera sting marks of Brazilian *Latrodectus* spp. and compared it with those of other local venomous spiders.

III. Venomous Apparatus

The male's venomous apparatus is much smaller than that of the female, and is inadequate for biting a vertebrate.

The female's venomous apparatus is composed of two main parts, the chelicera and the secreting glands (Fig. 3). The chelicera consist of two basal segments, on each of which a strong sharp fang is articulated. The venom is delivered at its apex, where the gland duct terminates. The two fangs move horizontally so as to constrict the victim.

The venom glands are situated in the cephalothorax: a thin duct from each gland, passing through the whole length of the basal body and chelicerum leads the venom to the fang's apex.

The histology of *Latrodectus* venomous glands has been investigated by many workers (Bordas, 1901, 1905; Ancona, 1931; Millot, 1931; D'Amour et al., 1936; Sampayo, 1942; Reese, 1944; Barth, 1962). Each gland, measuring about 1.4×0.4 mm, is covered by a layer of intrinsic muscles resting on a basal membrane (=extracellular sheath). The extracellular sheath's ultrastructure was studied by Smith and Russell (1967), who found that the sheath contained cross-banded, closely packed collagen-like fibrils exclusively oriented in a circular pattern. Further

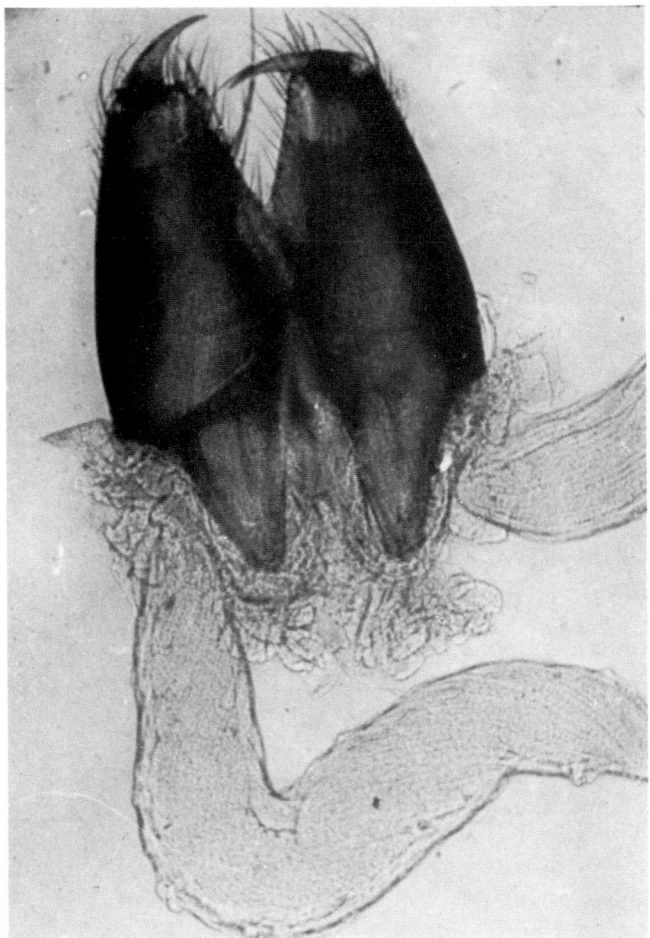

Fig. 3. Chelicera (basal segments and fangs) and venom glands of *L. m. tredecimguttatus*

work (SMITH et al., 1969) showed that the intrinsic gland musculature is mechanically linked to the extracellular sheath. An internal layer constitutes the secretory
epithelium, which is made up of simple but very tall cylindrical cells containing
and excreting a number of morphologically distinct components (SMITH and Rus-
SELL, 1967). (SUOMALAINEN [1964], investigating the histology of the poison gland
in 31 species of spiders belonging to 16 families, has reached the conclusion that
the secretory part of the gland is formed by a syncytium consisting of star-shaped
cells. *Latrodectus* spp. were not represented, the only Theridiid being *Steatoda
bipunctata*.)

In the poison gland, ANCONA (1931) recognizes two kinds, and REESE (1944)
several types of secreting cells, according to differences in cell staining. SMITH
and RUSSELL (1967), found 3 – 4 populations of cells, which differed in their degree
of binding osmium. With the exception of MILLOT (1931) and SAMPAYO (1942),
all authors agree that the secretion of this epithelium is holocrine in type.

With regard to the epithelial-cell secretions, SMITH and RUSSELL (1967), who investigated "milked" and "unmilked" glands, gave a nondefinitive picture of the mechanism of secretion of cell droplets. These authors observed disintegration of the secretory cells, but no replacement cells with mitotic nuclei.

It seems that the droplets of secretion are released during expulsion of the venom through the compression of the extracellular gland sheath effected by the contraction of the intrinsic musculature surrounding the secretory apparatus (JÄRLFORS et al., 1969).

It has been observed (JÄRLFORS et al., 1969) that efferent nerves reach the secretory epithelial cells traversing the extracellular gland sheath. It appears that their axoplasmic content shows a variety of neurosecretory products and electron-lucent vesicles. The authors conclude that "the presence of terminals between *Latrodectus* secretory cells provides strong circumstantial evidence for neural control of some aspect of the cyclic function for the gland."

IV. Venom

The extract of 12 pairs of venom glands from "male" spiders, when injected to a rat, did not evoke any evident alteration of its behavior (D'AMOUR et al., 1936). In discussing the toxicity of the venom we shall, therefore, refer from now on to the effects of the female's venom only.

1. Methods for Obtaining the Venom

The chemical composition of the venom is strictly related to the methods followed in obtaining the venom itself. The venom's toxicity may vary according to the method used (LEBEZ et al., 1969).

Surgical removal of the venom glands followed by homogenization results in forcible contamination of the venom obtained with extracts of foreign tissues (gland muscular layer, nerves, etc.).

"Milking" the spiders by means of electrical stimulation, yields the venom contained in the gland. Even in this case, but to a lesser degree, the venom is not exactly of the same composition as that naturally discharged by the spider. In fact, the expelled venom appears to be relatively homogeneous in comparison with the venom left in the gland lumina of spiders following milking, which is very heterogeneous (MEADOWS and RUSSELL, 1970). The electrically induced stimulation of all the cephalothorax muscles may unnaturally squeeze out from the glands venom fractions that would naturally be retained. This was proven through disc electrophoresis by MEADOWS and RUSSELL (1970).

Another method for obtaining the venom is that of piercing the dissected gland sac with a fine glass capillary, thus obtaining venom from the gland lumen. Impurities can, however, also contaminate the material with this technique (MAJORI et al., 1972).

LEBEZ (1953) has collected venom by absorbing it on a small cotton plug. In this case, as with electrical milking, care should be taken to avoid contamination with foreign substances from the alimentary canal (enzymes, etc.).

Finally, the venom can be obtained by placing the distal portions of the fangs in contact with a pipette, which draws up the venom discharged by the irritated spider by capillyry action (MEADOWS and RUSSELL, 1970; RUSSELL and BUESS, 1970).

The choice of methods obviously depends on the use to be made of the venom. If work is to be carried out on separated venom fractions, whole-gland extracts from large numbers of spiders may be justified.

List of methods for obtaining the venom

a)	Extract of whole homogenized glands	(I)
b)	Electrical milking	(II)
c)	Piercing gland sac with capillary	(III)
d)	Absorbing on cotton plugs	(IV)
e)	Collecting at tip of fangs through capillary pipette	(V)

The above Roman numerals will be used in the text to indicate the method of obtaining the material in each investigation.

2. Chemistry

According to BETTINI and TOSCHI-FRONTALI (1960) at 4° C the venom (I) of *L. m. tredecimguttatus* diluted in saline lost its toxicity slowly with time: in about 35 days the toxicity of the venom decreased to one quarter of its original value. At −15° and at −25° C the toxicity remained constant for at least 35 days. At room temperature, however, the venom lost its activity on the third day. Tests were carried out on house flies.

The venom (I) of *L. m. mactans,* dialyzed against saline solution, showed no decrease in toxicity when assayed on rats (D'AMOUR et al., 1936), and nor did that of *L. m. tredecimguttatus* when tested on guinea pigs (CANTORE and BETTINI, 1958 a) and on insects (BETTINI and TOSCHI-FRONTALI, 1960).

Heating the venom (I) at 75°C for 20 min, or treating it with dilute acid or alkali, or proteolytic enzymes, abolished its toxicity against rats, thus showing the proteinaceous nature of the toxic components (D'AMOUR et al., 1936; CANTORE and BETTINI, 1958 a).

An analysis of the venom (I) of *L. m. trecedimguttatus,* employing ROCKLAND and UNDERWOOD's paper chromatographic method, showed the following free amino acids to be present in higher amounts: taurine, glutamic acid, glutamine, alanine and arginine, followed by glycine, γ-aminobutyric acid, aspartic acid, asparagine, leucine, histidine and lysine (BETTINI and TOSCHI-FRONTALI, 1960). The amino acid composition of a purified neurotoxin from *L. m. tredecimguttatus* venom (I), as recently reported by GRASSO (1976), showed a high content of isoleucine and leucine and a very low content of tyrosine.

A low content of 5-hydroxytryptamine (0.0075−0.015 μg/pair of glands) was found in the venom (I) of *L. m. tredecimguttatus* by PANSA et al. (1972).

LEBEZ (1953) reported "relatively great quantities of lipoids (probably lipoproteins)" to be present in the venom (IV) of *L. m. tredecimguttatus;* however, CANTORE and BETTINI (1958) were unable to detect any lipoproteins in the venom

(I) of the same species when they used a paper electrophoretic method with Sudan-Black B staining.

The presence of proteolytic and glycogenolytic enzymes in the venom (IV) of *L. m. tredecimguttatus* was reported by Lebez (1953, 1954). Cantore and Bettini (1958) observed in the same species, and Kaire (1963) in *L. m. hasselti,* that the venom (I), whether fresh or dry, showed no proteolytic activity, while venom (IV) collected on cotton plugs, or by means of a direct spider bite on gelatine film, showed a marked proteolytic activity. These apparently contradictory results could be explained by contamination of the venom with enzymes from the digestive apparatus. That this inconvenience may actually occur was proven in the case of electrically milked *Ctenus* venom (see: Venoms of Ctenidae).

No proteolytic activity was found by Vicari et al. (1965), working with crude *L. m. tredecimguttatus* venom (I) and fraction LV_1. No glycolytic or proteolytic activity was revealed by Frontali et al. (1976) on a separated fraction consisting of at least four protein components toxic to mice and active on the frog neuromuscular junction.

A hyaluronidase activity of the venom (I) of *L. m. tredecimguttatus* has been shown *in vivo* and *in vitro* (0.070 g/l) by Cantore and Bettini (1958). Since no such activity has been shown in the separated fractions of the venom (I), while the whole venom and the dialyzed venom showed an equal hyaluronidase activity, it appears that this activity is lost during the electrophoretic run or during elution (Bettini and Toschi-Frontali, 1960).

3. Separation of Venom Components

By means of paper electrophoresis, six protein fractions of *L. m. tredecimguttatus* venom were first separated through paper electrophoresis (the spiders were induced to bit the paper strip) by Muic et al. (1956); Cantore and Bettini (1958), also using paper electrophoresis, found five protein components of the venom (I). Bettini and Toschi-Frontali (1960) also obtained five fractions using paper electrophoresis. Successively, Grasso and Toschi-Frontali (1962) and Frontali and Grasso (1964, 1965) separated five protein fractions with column electrophoresis on cellulose powder and three fractions with gel filtration on Sephadex G-200.

McCrone and Netzloff (1965) separated the venom (I) proteins of four *Latrodectus* species by disc electrophoresis: eight major fractions were obtained from *L. m. mactans, L. variolus* and *L. bishopi*, but only six fractions from *L. geometricus*. Each venom showed a distinct electrophoretic pattern.

Seven protein and three nonprotein fractions were isolated from the venom (I) of *L. m. mactans* by McCrone and Hatala (1967) through vertical acrylamide gel electrophoresis and subsequent electrophoresis-convection elution. Russell and Buess (1970) separated a total number of bands varying from 13 to 17 from the venom (V) of the same species from different areas of the United States by electrophoresis. The authors ascribe the difference between their results and those of the previous authors to the different method used in obtaining the venom.

Finally, Ornberg et al. (1976), using a different method, separated electrophoretically *L. m. mactans* venom (I) on acrylamide gel, obtaining 14–15 protein components. This method allowed a better and faster separation, only a few spiders being used.

FRONTALI and GRASSO (1964), experimenting on *L. m. tredecimguttatus* venom (I), estimated the molecular weight of the toxic fractions LV_1, LV_2 and LV_3, as judged by their behavior on Sephadex columns, to be of the same order of that of human hemoglobin. MCCRONE and HATALA (1967) on the other hand, by means of vertical acrylamide gel filtration and subsequent electrophoresis-convection elution, separated a protein fraction from *L. m. mactans* venom (I) which was toxic to mammals and had a light scattering molecular weight of 5000 ± 1000. This was ascribed to a possible complexing of the lethal material with others of high molecular weight (MCCRONE, 1969).

In a subsequent work, FRONTALI et al. (1976) studied a fraction that was separated on a column of Sephadex and proved toxic to mice and active on the frog neuromuscular junction; this fraction consisted of at least four protein components with a similar molecular weight of about 130,000.

About the same time, GRASSO (1976) purified a neurotoxin from *L. m. tredecimguttatus* venom (I); this substance also had a molecular weight of 130,000, and it was active on rat brain synaptosomes and rat iris.

According to the recent publication of ORNBERG et al. (1976), the molecular weight of a fraction active on the cockroach neuromuscular junction obtained by SDS disc electrophoresis was approximately 125,000, while that by analytical centrifugation was $110,000 - 140,000$.

V. Toxicity of Venom in Different Animal Species

1. Whole Venom

The toxic effects of *L. mactans* bites in various animal species belonging to different zoological groups have been reported by many authors since the eighteenth century, and were summarized by SAMPAYO (1942) in his thesis.

The majority of the old authors, however, gave very scanty information on the venom dosage and mortality frequency and, when sublethal doses were administered, limited their observations to the general conditions of the animals. It was reported, for instance (SAMPAYO, 1943), that the dog is highly resistant to the action of the venom, while the cat, the camel, and the horse are very sensitive; fishes and birds also appear to be resistant.

The LD_{50} values of the venom in different species are given in Table 1. The guinea pig is the most susceptible species to the venom, the frog the least. Between the two species there is about a 2000-fold difference in susceptibility. Frog tolerance to the venom was ascribed to its peculiar physiology: its cutaneous respiration, for instance, can overcome any deficiency in pulmonary respiration, such as that produced by the venom (CANTORE and BETTINI, 1958b; BETTINI and CANTORE, 1959; MAROLI et al., 1973).

The LD_{50} in the rat was estimated as 0.032 mg/rat or 0.21 mg/kg (D'AMOUR et al., 1936).

Toxicity tests on insects were first carried out by WIENER and DRUMMOND (1956), who used *Drosophila* flies to assay the activity of *L. m. hasselti* venom (I) and its antivenin. Later, GRASSO and TOSCHI-FRONTALI (1962) and FRONTALI and GRASSO (1964) employed house flies for the same purpose (see: venom components).

Table 1. Toxicity of *Latrodectus mactans tredecimgut-tatus* venom on amphibians, birds, insects and mammals (MAROLI et al., 1973).

Animals	LD$_{50}$ values	
	mg^a/animal	mg^a/kg
Frog	2.18 $\pm$ 0.49	145 $\pm$ 32
Canary	0.085 $\pm$ 0.03	4.7 $\pm$ 1.7
Blackbird	0.42 $\pm$ 0.19	5.9 $\pm$ 2.7
Pigeon	0.11 $\pm$ 0.025	0.36 $\pm$ 0.07
Chick	0.19 $\pm$ 0.04	2.1 $\pm$ 0.57
Cockroach	0.015	2.7
Housefly	0.000013	0.6
Guinea pig	0.028	0.075
Mouse	0.013	0.90

^{a} mg of proteins (LOWRY's method). The results in cockroach, housefly, guinea pig, and mouse are taken from earlier data by BETTINI and TOSCHI-FRONTALI (1960) using dry gland extract.

According to WIENER (1956), at 0° and 37° C the toxicity of *L. m. hasselti* venom (I) to mice is 100 times greater than at 18° to 24°C. These findings were based on the fact that the body temperature of mice varies with that of their external environment.

2. Venom Components

As reported above (see: IV.2. Chemistry), *Latrodectus* venom has been separated by various authors into several components, the number differing according to the separation techniques used. Differences in activity were also observed in relation to the various separation processes. Thus, CANTORE and BETTINI (1958a) reported that only one out of five venom (I) fractions separated electrophoretically on paper showed any toxicity on vertebrates.

Later, BETTINI and TOSCH-FRONTALI (1960) carried out further experiments with venom (I) fractions, using an analogous separation technique, and found that the only component exhibiting toxicity in guinea pig, mouse, and rat was also toxic to the American cockroach *Periplaneta americana*.

GRASSO and TOSCHI-FRONTALI (1962), who used house flies in tests for the toxicity of the venom (I) components, separated through column electrophoresis two components toxic to house flies, one of which (LV$_1$) induced an immediate but reversible paralysis and the other (LV$_2$) a slow but irreversible paralysis as shown by the graph of Figure 4. The LD$_{50}$ at 24 h on house flies for fractions LV$_1$ and LV$_2$ was found to be respectively 24.0 and 12.5 µg/kg.

In a subsequent work, FRONTALI and GRASSO (1964, 1965) used house flies and guinea pigs to test the various venom (I) components obtained by different separation procedures, finding that another component (LV$_3$) was active on guinea pigs.

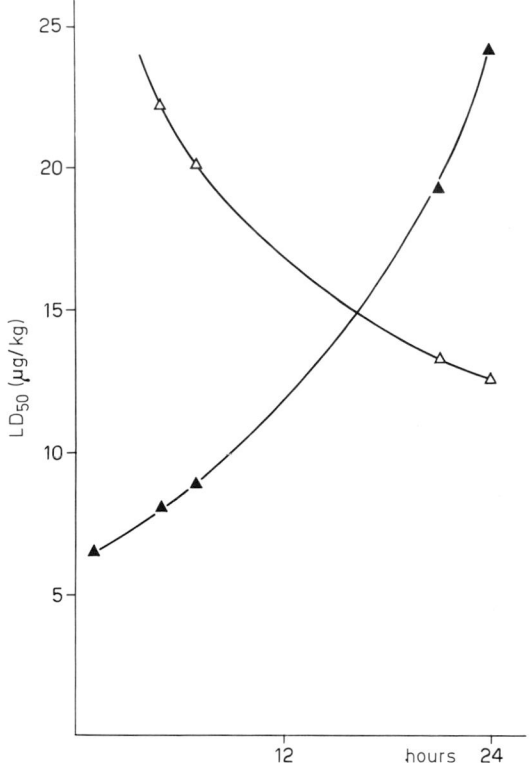

Fig. 4. Groups of houseflies were injected with electrophoretically separated preparations of LV_1 and LV_2 at different dilutions. The LD_{50} values were calculated not only 24 h after injection, but also at different time intervals during the next 24 h. LV_1 (▲▲) produces its maximum effect after one hour, LV_2 (△△) after 24 h. (FRONTALI and GRASSO, 1964)

The inactivation of toxicity by storage of the separated fractions at 26°C for 24 h is shown in the graph of Figure 5. The activity was reduced to zero within 24 h in fraction LV_1, decreased to about 45 percent in fraction LV_2 and unchanged in fraction LV_3 (FRONTALI and GRASSO, 1964).

Treatment with various inactivating or protecting agents was also tested by FRONTALI and GRASSO (1964). Concentrations of 2×10^{-4} and 4×10^4M of mercaptoethanol protected fractions LV_1 and LV_2, respectively, from thermal inactivation (24 h at 26°C).

According to MCCRONE and HATALA (1967), only one protein fraction (B) was lethal to mammals, its LD_{50} for mice being 0.048 mg protein/kg, i.e. 20-fold more toxic than whole venom (I).

In the case of the neurotoxin prepared in a homogeneous form by GRASSO (1976) from L. m. tredecimguttatus venom (I) the LD_{50} in mice was about 49,000 mg pure protein/g body weight, i.e. it was 10—12 times more toxic than the crude venom.

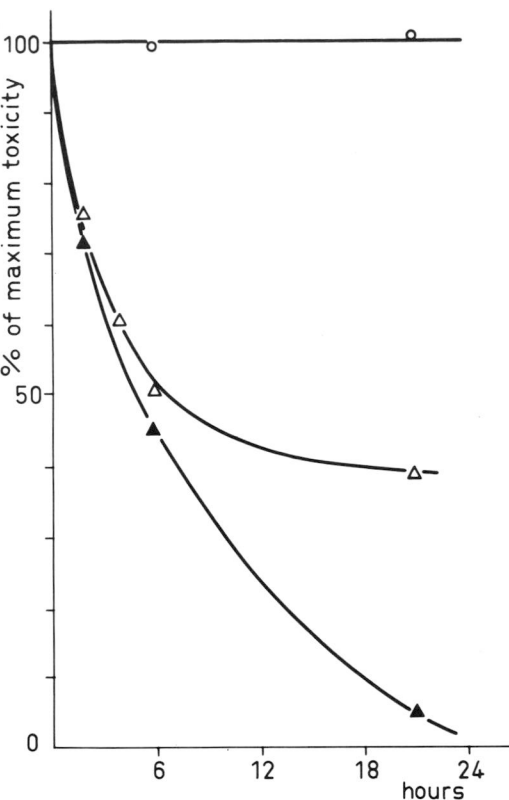

Fig. 5. Effect of storage at 26°C on the toxicity of electrophoretic fractionation preparation of LV$_1$ (▲▲), LV$_2$ (△△), and LV$_3$ (< <). (Frontali and Grasso, 1964.)

VI. Pharmacology and Mode of Action on Different Zoological Groups

For a more useful subdivision of the material, which deals with experiments on different preparations of various animal species, we thought it more practical to group the descriptions of the published works according to the zoological classification of the animal from which the preparation was taken. Within each zoological group, the papers reviewed were ordered chronologically (Table 2).

We deemed it useful to write the following brief introductory account, which offers the reader a chronological overview of the main phases that have characterized the body of research in this particular field.

The first investigation on the mode of action of *Latrodectus* venom dates from 1929, when Troise reported that isolated *sartorius* muscle of toad showed fibrillations if bathed in venom solution.

Extensive works following this initial research were mainly oriented towards finding out whether the venom acted on the peripheral or on the central nervous systems, but the results were contradictory at times.

According to the literature, the period between 1942 and 1958 was marked by any important development in the elucidation of the mode of action of *Latrodectus* venom.

Table 2.

Verte-brates	Animals used	Authors	Preparations used
Pisces	torpedo	GRANATA et al., 1974	electric organ
Amphi-bia	toad	TROISE, 1929 SAMPAYO, 1944	*sartorius* muscle *sartorius* muscle
	frog	D'AMOUR, 1936 LONGENECKER et al., 1970 CLARK et al., 1970 MAROLI and BETTINI, 1971 CLARK et al., 1971 ALKADHI and McISAAC, 1974 DEL CASTILLO et al., 1975 FRONTALI et al., 1976	[a] *sartorius* muscle *cutaneus pectoris* muscle *tibialis anticus longus* muscle *cutaneus pectoris* muscle sympathetic ganglion *sartorius* muscle *cutaneus pectoris* muscle
Aves	chick	MAROLI et al., 1973	*biventer cervicis* muscle
Mam-malia	rabbit	CANTORE, 1958 ALKADHI and McISAAC, 1974	ileum, phrenic-diaphragm, uterus superior cervical ganglion
	guinea-pig	TROISE, 1929 RUSSELL and LONG, 1961 RUSSELL et al., 1961 HAMILTON, 1972 FRONTALI and GRANATA, 1973 EINHORN and HAMILTON, 1974 PINTO et al., 1974	uterus phrenic-diaphragm phrenic-diaphragm ileum mesentery, spleen capsule, inferior vena cava, gut longitudinal muscular layer ileum atria
	rat	PAGGI and ROSSI, 1971 CHMOULIOVSKY et al., 1972 FRONTALI et al., 1972 GRANATA et al., 1972 PAGGI and TOSCHI, 1972 HAMILTON, 1972 FRONTALI, 1972 HAMILTON and ROBINSON, 1973 PALMER, 1975 GRASSO, 1976	superior cervical ganglion superior cervical ganglion cerebral cortex and sup. cerv. ganglia brain cortex, iris, sup. cerv. ganglia superior cervical ganglion phrenic-diaphragm iris *vasa deferentia* phrenic-diaphragm iris
	mice	Maroli and BETTINI, 1971 EINHORN and HAMILTON, 1973	*rectus abdominis* muscle *vasa deferentia*
	cat	OKAMOTO et al., 1971 PINTO et al., 1973 PINTO and ROTHLIN, 1974	*soleus* and *gastrocnemius* strips of spleen strips of spleen
	dog	TROISE, 1929	bronchia

[a] Preparation not reported by the authors.

It was in fact only in 1958 that CANTORE observed that the venom blocked the activity of rabbit phrenic nerve-diagphragm preparation and formulated the hypothesis that this block occurred at the neuromuscular junction level.

The studies on the mode of action of the venom in Arthropods started in 1965 (NERI et al., 1965) and continued in the following years (D'AJELLO et al.,

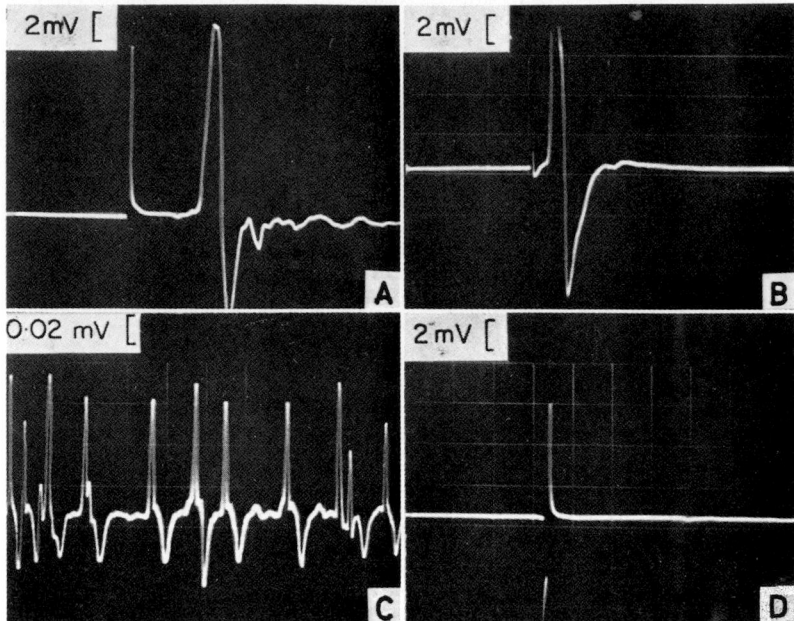

Fig. 6A—D. (A) Response of the giant axons from the region of the third abdominal ganglion to stimulation of the cercal nerve. (B) Response to direct stimulation of the axons. (C) Spontaneous discharges (burst of impulses) before synaptic transmission fails. (D) Disappearance of response to presynaptic stimulation. (D'AJELLO et al., 1969)

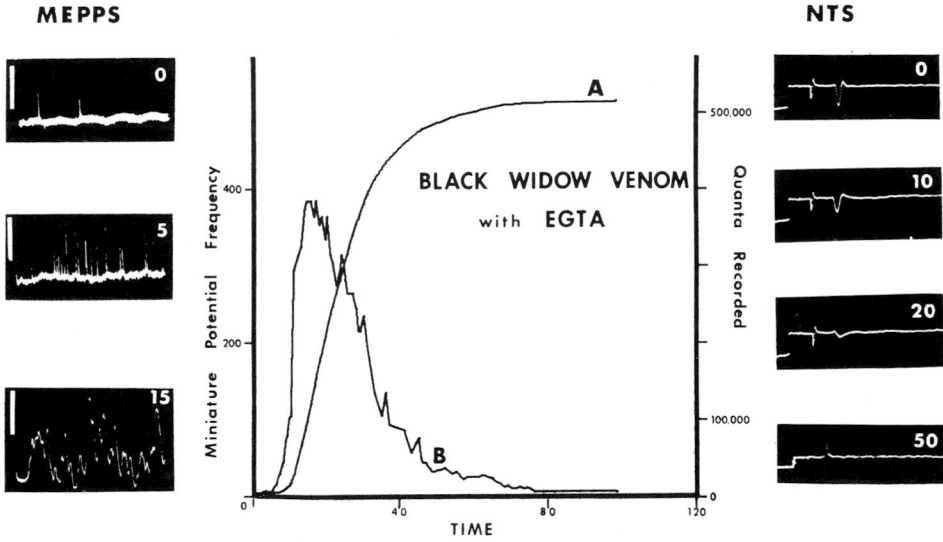

Fig. 7. Effect of BWSV on MEPP frequency and on the NTS in a calcium free solution with EGTA. Numbers in the upper right corner of the left and right columns of pictures are times in minutes after addition of 0.1 ml of BWSV solution to the muscle chamber. Pictures on the left are intracellularly recorded MEPPs. The calibration bar represents 500 μV. Duration of sweeps from top to bottom are 1 s, 1 s, and 0.1 s. Curve B in the central figure is the MEPP frequency per second versus time after addition of BWSV, while curve A represents the total number of MEPPs or quanta recorded. Pictures at the right from a different experiment are computed average (n=20) nerve terminal spikes. The calibration pulse at the left of each record represents 100 μV and 1.7 ms. (LONGENECKER et al., 1970)

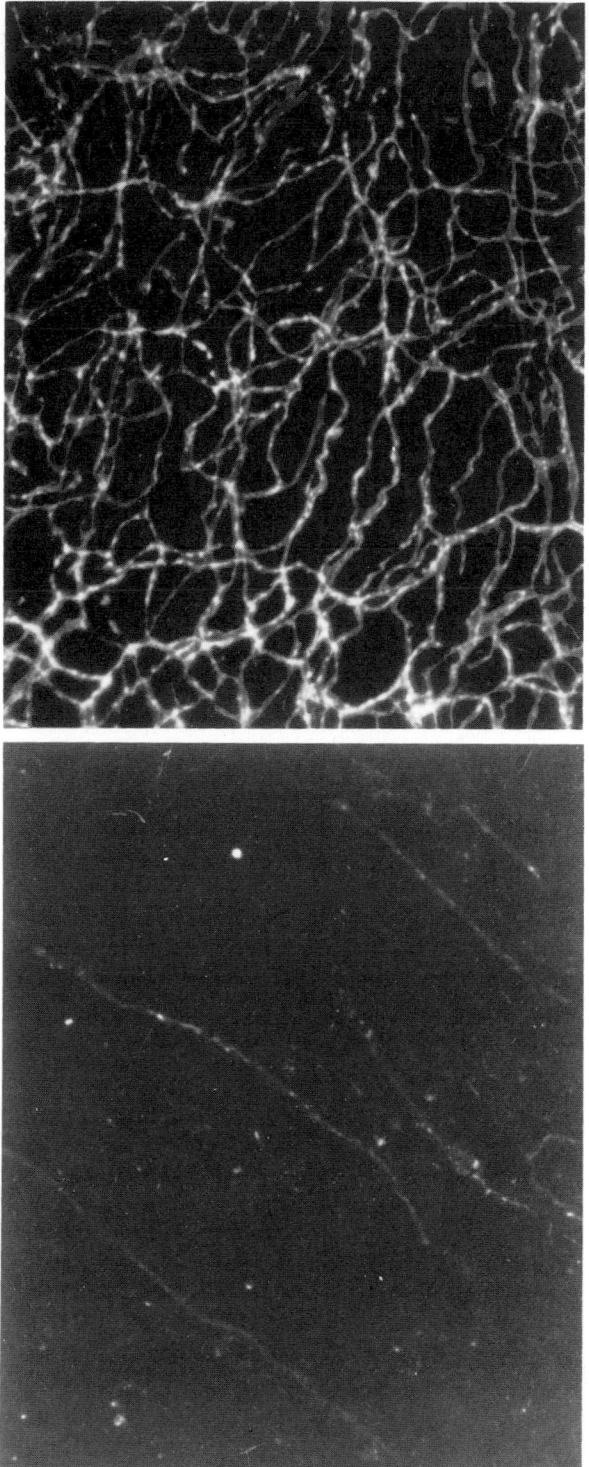

Fig. 8. (A) Yellow-green fluorescence of adrenergic nerve fibers in control rat iris. (B) Residual fluorescence of adrenergic nerve fibers in rat iris incubated with black widow spider venom in low concentration (0.01 couples of glands/ml). (FRONTALI, 1972)

1969) (Fig. 6). While they did not completely elucidate the venom action, they contributed to the development of further research.

The first paper to explain the mode of action of the venom on the vertebrate neuromuscular junction was published in 1970. In that year, Longenecker et al. (1970) demonstrated by refined electrophysiological techniques (intracellular electrodes) that the venom acts at a presynaptic level, causing a massive release of ACh quanta (Fig. 7). This mechanism was confirmed by the ultrastructural electron-microscope study of Clark et al. (1970), who observed that after the application of venom, the nerve endings became completely empty of synaptic vesicles. At this stage of the research the hypothesis that *Latrodectus* venom acted specifically on cholinergic junctions was justified. However, a series of investigations started in 1972 by Frontali (Fig. 8) demonstrated that the venom is also active on adrenergic junctions. These works were then followed by others showing that other types of nerve endings, including the neuromuscular junction of arthropods, are also sensitive to *Latrodectus* venom.

A recent paper by del Castillo and Pumplin (1975) formulates a hypothesis on the intimate mode of action of the venom at the level of the membrane molecular structure.

1. Invertebrates

a) Crustacea

Parnas and Russell (1967) reported that *L. m. mactans* venom (II) had no effect on the nerve-muscle preparation of the crayfish, *Procambarus clarki*.

L. m. tredecimguttatus venom (I) was also tested on the stretch receptor neurone of the crayfish *Astacus astacus* by Grasso and Paggi (1967). The authors showed that the venom affects the frequency of impulses elicited by the orthodromic stimulation and that the cell activity, after a transient increase, is blocked. It was also found that the axonal membrane is unaffected, while the soma and dendrite membrane, where the action potential is generated, are the *locus* of action of the venom.

According to Bettini et al. (1969), only one component of the venom, fraction LV_4, is responsible for the block of the stretch receptor neurone activity.

Kawai et al. (1972) studied the effect of *L. m. mactans* venom (I) on the lobster (*Homarus americanus*) nerve-muscle preparation, which is particularly interesting since it contains both excitatory and inhibitory synapses, neither of which is cholinergic. (Up to 1972 in fact, the effects of venom on invertebrates had been detected only on cholinergic junctions.) After the application of venom, both excitatory and inhibitory postsynaptic potentials were first augmented, then suppressed, and the frequency of miniature potentials was markedly increased. Both excitatory and inhibitory "giant miniature potentials" were evoked in the later stages of venom action. In calcium-free solution the same effects appeared as in normal saline, indicating that the effect of venom is not due to depolarization of the nerve terminals *per se*. The lack of sensitivity of the postsynaptic membrane to venom was shown by measuring the resting potential after the application of GABA, a specific activator of inhibitory membranes in lobster, in preparations treated with venom.

b) Insecta

The mode of action of *Latrodectus* venom was first studied on species belonging to this class of Arthropods. The large cockroach *Periplaneta americana,* whose nervous system, anatomy, and physiology were already well known, was the species of choice.

NERI et al. (1965) studied the effect of the venom (I) on the isolated nerve cord of *P. americana* and showed that the endogenous activity, which has its origin in the nerve cord ganglia, was completely blocked after a transient increase of activity. Each one of the venom protein fractions (LV_1, LV_2, and LV_3) brought about a similar block, which was irreversible after washing, except for fraction LV_3. The blocked cord recovered its endogenous activity completely after bathing with specific antitoxic serum, as prepared by BETTINI et al. (1954).

In a subsequent work, D'AJELLO et al. (1969) studied the effect of the venom (I) on the synaptic transmission of impulses at the level of the sixth abdominal ganglion of *P. americana* and on axonal conduction (giant axons). It was shown that the venom interrupts synaptic transmission but does not modify the axonal conduction of impulses. On the other hand, endogenous activity at the giant axons was temporarily augmented. This was interpreted as an increasing depolarization of the postsynaptic membrane evoked by presynaptic impulses. It was also observed that the time needed for the venom to block endogenous activity as well as the synaptic transmission across the sixth abdominal ganglion was influenced by temperature. The venom's effect on the nerve preparation was not reversed by washing with physiological solution; reversal, however, did occur after treatment with specific antivenin. Although most of the observations were made with crude venom, a few experiments were conducted with the components separated by column electrophoresis, as described by FRONTALI and GRASSO (1964). The results indicated that the fractions designated by them as LV_1 and "Peak 5" were effective in blocking transmission.

A further study on the effect of the venom (I) by intracellular recordings from giant neurones at the sixth abdominal ganglion of *P. americana* was carried out by D'AJELLO et al. (1971). The venom induced: a) a progressive decline of the resting potential of the giant neurones; b) failure of synaptic transmission through a progressive reduction of the evoked presynaptic potentials; c) spontaneous repetitive firing of the giant neurones; d) alterations in the shape and reduction of the propagated action potential. The authors confirm the interpretation given in the previous work, *i.e.* that the venom causes a massive release of transmitter which in turn depolarizes the postsynaptic membrane.

The above results indicate that *Latrodectus* venom has a presynaptic action on nerve-nerve junctions. As demonstrated by several authors, the preparations used had cholinergic junctions, *i.e.* the chemical transmitter was acetylcholine.

MAROLI and BETTINI (1971) obtained negative results from the application of venom (I) to the cockroach *P. americana;* extensor muscles of the trochanter were indirectly stimulated. These results were not surprising since they agreed with those of PARNAS and RUSSELL (1967) obtained on the crayfish neuromuscular junction.

The first demonstration of *L. m. mactans* venom (I) activity on *non-cholinergic junctions* in insects was given by CULL-CANDY et al. (1973), who used intracellular electrodes to record miniature potentials from the metathoracic *extensor tibiae* and *retractor unguis* muscle fibers of the locust *Schistocerca gregaria*. The miniature discharge of these muscle fibers was characterized by periods of high frequency separated by periods of normal frequency. Observation of some venom-treated axon terminals with the electron microscope gave evidence of changes in number and distribution of synaptic vesicles similar to those observed in the spontaneous release of transmitter from these terminals. The results of these studies showed that the venom has qualitatively similar effects on glutamate and acetylcholine synapses.

The above conclusions were confirmed in a subsequent work by GRIFFITHS and SMYTH (1973). These authors, experimenting on *P. americana* metathoracic *flexor tibiae* muscles innervated by both excitatory and inhibitory axons, found that *L. m. mactans* venom (I) induced an increase of miniature excitatory and inhibitory potentials followed by their decrease to zero and finally by junction block.

Recently, ORNBERG et al. (1976) separated a protein that was very active on the cockroach neuromuscular junction from the venom (I) of *L. m. mactans* by electrophoresis.

With regard to a possible action of the venom on postsynaptic membranes, it should be pointed out that D'AJELLO et al. (1971) reported that, following the massive release of transmitter (at cholinergic junctions) and the synaptic block, a subsequent persisting depolarization (a hyperpolarization of 20 mV) of the post-synaptic fibers and a tendency to show spontaneous repetitive firing was observed. This finding was considered by the authors to be a consequence of the massive transmitter release.

Further observations on postsynaptic action were reported by GRIFFITHS and SMYTH (1973), who used a noncholinergic junction. According to these authors, some postsynaptic action did appear within one minute of venom application. The resting potential of the muscle fibers became unstable, fluctuating $1-2$ mV, more often in the hyperpolarizing direction, and after a few minutes the muscle potentials became more stable, usually at a somewhat higher value than before venom application.

ORNBERG et al. (1976), testing the activity of separated venom (I) components of *L. m. mactans* on the cockroach neuromuscular preparation, observed (but only on one fraction) a slow $10-12$ mV depolarizing shift in the postjunctional membrane potential, thought by the authors to be attributable probably to the large amounts of transmitter released. This effect was not induced by the other toxic fraction. No direct effect of venom on postsynaptic membrane was proven by the authors.

The effect of *L. m. tredecimguttatus* venom (I, III) on the heart of the cockroach *P. americana* was studied by MAJORI et al. (1972). The authors used an electrocardiographic method on a semi-isolated heart preparation, and recordings of the heart *in vivo*. It was observed that both forms of the venom (I, III), when injected *in vivo*, showed a selective activity on the heart function compared with the effect on the CNS. The heart function was blocked also by the application of venom on the semi-isolated preparation, the duration of blocking being dependent on venom concentration. The authors suggested that cardiac block is due to impairment of either the cardiac nerve ganglia function (cholinergic) or the myocardial neuromuscular junctions (noncholinergic), or both of them. The blocking effect of the venom on the heart function was reversed by specific antiserum.

Finally, the use of *Latrodectus* venom (I) in insect "immunity" studies should be mentioned. This term has been applied to indicate the peculiar transient state of increased resistance that follows the administration of a sublethal dose of a toxic substance to insects. The work of BETTINI (1965a, 1965b) has shown an increase of resistance to a challenge dose of venom in flies (*Musca domestica*) pretreated with a vaccinating dose. On the other hand, no increase of resistance was obtained in *P. americana*. A positive immune response and partial cross-immunity have been obtained in flies with two toxic fractions of the venom, LV_1 and LV_2 (GATTONE et al., 1966).

An overview of the fraction activities, as reported by BETTINI et al. (1969), is given in Table 3.

Table 3. Activity of electrophoretically separated fractions on different biological systems (BETTINI et al., 1969).

Fraction	house flies (fast knock down)	house flies (slow toxicity)	guinea pigs and mice (toxicity)	cells in culture (cytotoxic effect)	cockroach nerve cord (bock of synaptic transmission)	crayfish stretch receptor (block of activity)	cockroach heart (block of rhythmic contractions)
LV_1	+			+	+		
LV_2		+					+
LV_3			+				
LV_4					+	+	+

Table 4. Qualitative effects of various fractions on different biological systems. (FRONTALI et al., 1976.)

	Frog neuromuscular junction	Mouse toxicity	Housefly toxicity	Cockroach heart beat	Crayfish stretch receptor
Whole extract	+	+	+	+	+
A	−	−	−	−	−
B	+	+	−	−	−
C	+	+	+	+	−
D	−	−	−	−	−
E	−	−	ND	ND	+
B_5	+	+	−	−	−
C_2	−	−	−	−	ND
C_3	−	−	+	+	ND
C_5	+	+	+	−	ND
E_1	−	−	ND	ND	−
E_2	−	−	ND	ND	+

+ = Active. − = Inactive. ND = Not determined.

Another overview has been presented by Frontali et al. (1976), based on the results obtained with venom components separated with a modified technique. In this overview (Table 4), the authors identified the new components with the ones reported in the previous table, as follows. LV_3 contains fraction B_5; LV_1 and LV_2 are probably contained in fraction C; and LV_4 contains fraction E_2.

c) Mollusca

Since some of the preceding studies on the mode of action of *Latrodectus* venom implicated a direct action of the venom on membrane excitability *per se*, Gruener (1973) tested the effect induced by the external and internal application of *L. mactans* venom (I, II) to the squid giant axon. A complete but reversible loss of excitability, with a marked shortening of action potential duration and a consequent reduction in amplitude and eventual failure were observed.

2. Vertebrates [1]

A complete discussion of the literature on the pharmacology of *L. m. mactans* venom was reported by Sampayo (1942). The individual experiments are reported in the present text according to the species tested.

Bettini and Cantore (1959) reviewed all information concerning the clinical signs and symptoms of human latrodectism and the behavior and neuromuscular effects of experimental animals (monkey, dog, cat, sheep, rabbit, guinea pig, rat, mouse, birds, and amphibians).

a) Pisces

Granata et al. (1974) tested the activity of *L. m. tredecimguttatus* venom (I) on *Torpedo* electric tissue. Slices of this tissue were incubated *in vitro* for different time intervals and at different venom concentrations. At the lower concentrations (2 pairs of glands/ml) the venom induced a significant, though not drastic, decrease of ACh content of the tissue, whose ultrastructure, however, did not appear to be altered. At the same venom concentration the ACh content of the subcellular fraction, which is rich in synaptosomes, was similarly decreased, and again the ultrastructure did not appear to be modified.

b) Amphibia

As early as 1929, Troise (1929) studied the effects of *L. mactans* venom (I) on the toad *sartorius* muscle. The author reported that the preparation immersed in a solution of 1:1000 of venom showed fibrillations that were not observed in Ringer solution. A few trials on frog (and dog) led the author to describe the nervous effects as medullary in origin.

D'Amour et al. (1936), in their exhaustive study on the toxicity of *L. mactans* venom (I), also investigated its action on frog neuromuscular preparations (muscle

---

[1] Pathology of *Latrodectus* envenomation in man as well as in experimental animals is reported in Part B by Z. Maretić.

not mentioned). Injection of the venom into the muscle or soaking of the nerve-muscle preparation in venom solution produced no contraction or modification of the impulse conduction or transmission. According to the authors, these findings "supported the view that the action of the venom upon the musculature was by way of the central nervous system rather than peripherally".

SAMPAYO (1944) confirms D'AMOUR's results. Preparations of *sartorius* muscle of toads (*Bufo arenarum*) placed in Ringer's solution containing the venom of *L. mactans* (1 mg of the gland to 10 ml Ringer's) showed no contraction.

LONGENECKER et al. (1970) were the first to study the activity of *L. m. tredecimguttatus* venom (I) on frog nerve-muscle preparation (*m. sartorius*) employing extra- and intracellular electrodes. The authors found that: a) the venom causes an increase in frequency of miniature end-plate potentials which reaches its maximum in 5 min and then decreases; b) this effect takes place even in the absence of calcium ions; c) washing of the preparation does not interrupt the venom action, while the effects are reversed by specific antivenin if this is added in the early stages of the venom action.

As a consequence of the above-mentioned investigation, an electron-microscopic study of the effects of *L. m. tredecimguttatus* venom (I) was carried out by CLARK et al. (1970) on the frog neuromuscular junction (*m. cutaneus pectoris*). In a series of electron micrographs the authors showed that the nerve terminals appear almost completely depleted of ACh vesicles.

MAROLI and BETTINI (1971) investigated the effects of *L. m. tredecimguttatus* (I, III) on the dynamics of frog voluntary muscle. The preparation used was *n. peronierus* connected with the *m. tibialis anticus longus*. The application of both types of the spider's venom induced fibrillation and contracture, varying in intensity according to venom concentration, and the addition of ACh to the venom potentiated its effect. It was also observed that if voluntary muscles isolated from the frog were treated with venom they released a contracture-inducing substance, probably ACh. Denervation and curare neutralized the venom effect; application of antivenin, as opposed to washing, induced complete recovery of the preparation.

CLARK et al. (1972) studied further the changes in the fine structure of frog neuromuscular junctions (*m. cutaneus pectoris*) caused by the action of *L. m. tredecimguttatus* and *L. hasselti* venoms (I), using electrophysiological techniques and electron-microscopic observations. The authors found that the venom induced the synaptic vesicles to fuse with the presynaptic membrane, leading to an increase in both the surface area and the volume of the nerve terminals. An increase in the frequency of miniature end-plate potentials and a reduction in the number of synaptic vesicles of nerve terminals were also observed.

Through intracellular recordings of spontaneous miniature excitatory postsynaptic potentials, from the 10th and 11th ganglion of the paravertebral sympathetic chain isolated from the frog, ALKADHI and MCISAAC (1974) observed that *L. mactans* venom (I) induced a spontaneous release of transmitter.

The venom (I) of the brown widow spider, *L. geometricus,* was studied by DEL CASTILLO and PUMPLIN (1975) on the frog neuromuscular preparation (*m. sartorius*), with the aid of electrophysiological techniques. The authors observed that: a) the venom elicited an increase in the frequency of the miniature end-plate potentials; b) the volleys recur at intervals during the period from 5 to 10 min after the addition of venom; c) the volleys originate at highly localized areas of the nerve terminals; d) in solutions rich in calcium ions, the initial frequency of the miniature potentials in a volley is comparatively higher, declining to one half the volume in a few seconds, after which the volley terminates; e) in solutions poor in calcium ions the volleys of potentials are fewer but much longer in duration. The authors concluded that the action of brown widow spider venom on the motor terminals appeared to be the same as that of *L. mactans*. Finally, the authors discuss the intimate mode of action of the venom on the presynaptic membrane, offering evidence that suggests that the volley of miniature potentials elicited by the brown widow spider venom may be due to temporary formation of channels by penetration of one or several venom molecules into the membrane lipids.

A fraction consisting of at least four proteins was separated by Frontali et al. (1976) from the venom (I) of *L. m. tredecimguttatus* (see: Chemistry of venom) and tested on the excised *cutaneus pectoris* nerve-muscle preparation of frog. The isolated fraction caused a great increase in the frequency of occurrence of miniature end-plate potentials at the neuromuscular junction, and caused swelling of the nerve terminals and depleted them of their vesicles. (The effects of this fraction on other preparations are found in Crustacea and Insecta.)

c) Aves

The venom (I) of *L. m. tredecimguttatus* was tested in different vertebrate species by Maroli et al. (1973). The authors have also investigated the activity of the venom on chick neuromuscular preparation (*m. biventer cervicis*). They reported that a 1 min from venom application (0.5 µl/ml) the muscle showed fibrillation bursts similar to those described by Maroli and Bettini (1971) for the frog neuromuscular preparation. Muscular tension also increased after 1 min, reaching a maximum after 10 min, and disappeared after 30 min.

d) Mammalia

A series of investigations was carried out on different organs of various mammalian species to study the effects of venom on specific functions of the organisms.

Effects of *Latrodectus* venom on the circulatory system were primarily observed on man (see: Part B). Experiments carried out by Troise (1928) in the dog, Shapiro et al. (1939) in the cat, Sampayo (1944) in the dog, cat, and rat, Suarez et al. (1952) in decapitated dogs, Cicardo (1954) also in dogs, and Cantore and Bettini (1958c) in the rabbit, proved that the venom of various *Latrodectus* species induces bradycardia and hypertension. Tachyphylaxis was also evident.

But the greatest evidence of specific toxicity was found on the nervous system of all mammalian species studied. A medullar origin of the nervous symptoms was suggested by Troise (1929), while "a diffused excitatory action throughout the entire central nervous system" involving the autonomic system was the conclusion given by Sampayo (1944).

The employment of new techniques in electrophysiology in recent years has brought fresh impetus to research into the effects of *Latrodectus* venom on the nervous system.

Rabbit. CANTORE (1958) investigated the effects of *L. m. tredecimguttatus* venom (I) on the isolated ileum, uterus and phrenic-diaphragm of rabbit. The venom, even at quite low concentrations, induced a slow but marked contracture of the ileum, similar to that provoked by slow-reacting substances, polypeptide in nature, of the kallidin, bradykinin type. No effect was observed on the uterus. On the other hand, the contractions of the electrically stimulated isolated diaphragm were irreversibly inhibited by the venom, which led the author to assume that neuromuscular junctions were strongly impaired.

The effect of *L. mactans* venom (I) on transmission in the rabbit superior cervical ganglion was studied *in vitro* by ALKADHI and MCISAAC (1974), employing electrophysiological techniques. Stimulation of the preganglionic nerve at supramaximal strength evoked characteristic compound action potentials with two major spikes, S_1 and S_2. When the venom was added to the bath containing the preparation, the S_1 spike often transiently increased above control within 3 min, but the S_2 spike was consistently reduced, decreasing over $20 - 30$ min to a constant value. Increasing the calcium concentration three-fold in the bath transiently stopped the progressive development of block.

Guinea pig. In his pioneer work on *L. mactans* venom (I) TROISE (1929) also included some experiments on the isolated intestine and uterus of guinea pig. The author was unable to detect any effect of the venom on these preparations.

Marked bronchoconstriction with *L. m. mactans* venom (I) was observed by SAMPAYO (1944) in the guinea pig. An analogous effect was shown by CANTORE and BETTINI (1958b) on curarized guinea pigs with venom (I) of *L. m. tredecimguttatus.* It was proven that contraction of thoracic and abdominal muscles has no influence on bronchospasm induced by the venom.

RUSSELL and LONG (1961) obtained contradictory results with the venom of two different species, *L. hasselti* and *L. mactans,* applied to the guinea-pig phrenic-diaphragm preparation. In fact the venom (most probably obtained by electrical extraction) of 40 spiders of the first species produced a gradual depression of the indirectly elicited contractions, leading to a complete neuromuscular block in 56 min. No apparent changes were observed in the directly elicited contractions. On the other hand, 3 mg of the venom of the second species produced no impairment of either the directly or the indirectly elicited contractions.

A depletion of synaptic vesicles from nerve endings in Auerbach's plexus in guinea pig ileum treated with *L. hasselti* venom (I) was shown by HAMILTON (1972).

On the grounds of previous investigations on rat iris (see: rat), FRONTALI et al. (1973) and FRONTALI and GRANATA (1973) carried out more work on adrenergic fibers innervating different guinea pig tissues: iris, fragments of mesentery, spleen capsule, inferior vena cava, gut longitudinal layer. It was found that in all these tissues the venom (I) of *L. m. tredecimguttatus,* at different concentrations, induced a striking decrease of the specific yellow-green fluorescence. It was thus proven that the venom acts on adrenergic nerve fibers and terminals of different mammalian organs, which could explain the origin of latrodectism symptoms.

The effects of *L. hasselti* venom (I) on the guinea pig ileum purinergic nervous system was reported by EINHORN and HAMILTON (1974). Intracellular recordings from venom-treated circular muscle cells showed that the inhibitory junction potentials increased after addition of the venom but were reduced to 20 percent after 20 min. The authors found that all three types of cells with different vesicles observed in the treated tissue (cholinergic, adrenergic and purinergic) were depleted of the vesicles. According to the authors, the venom did not appear to preferentially destroy or spare any particular vesicle type.

The effects of *L. mactans* venom (I) were investigated also on the isolated spontaneously beating guinea-pig atria (Pinto et al., 1974). The venom showed a concentration-dependent positive chronotropic effect, which was antagonized by propranolol and reduced by reserpine pretreatment.

The authors concluded that the venom acting at adrenergic presynaptic sites induced noradrenaline release, which subsequently activates guinea-pig atria's β-adrenoceptors.

Rat. The effect of *L. m. tredecimguttatus* venom (I) was studied by Paggi and Rossi (1970, 1971) on the isolated and desheathed superior cervical ganglion (sympathetic) of the rat. The postganglionic action potentials evoked by preganglionic stimulation was depressed and asynchronous discharges of action potentials were elicited from the unstimulated ganglion. When curare was applied to the preparation, the production of these discharges was greatly diminished (25—30%). Furthermore, the level of labeled ACh was decreased by 50 percent in unstimulated ganglia treated with venom. According to the authors, these findings suggest an indirect depolarization originating at the synaptic level through an enhancement of ACh release at nerve endings.

A further attempt to elucidate the mode of action of *L. m. tredecimguttatus* venom (I) by using the same ganglion preparation and the same technique of extraction and analysis of labeled ACh was carried out by Paggi and Toschi (1970, 1972). The ganglia, however, had been denervated by removal of a tract of the sympathetic trunk 10 days before excision. Calcium-free medium was also employed. In the presence of venom, potentials of minimal amplitude were recorded from the denervated ganglia and ACh release at presynaptic level persisted in the absence of calcium ions.

Direct measurements of ACh content and release from a different section of the nervous system from rat brain cortex slices incubated *in vitro* with *L. m. tredecimguttatus* venom (I) were carried out by Frontali et al. (1972). The slices, incubated in an eserinized low-potassium saline solution, after application of the venom induced a two-fold increase of ACh released in the medium and a corresponding decrease in the ACh content of the tissue. The results indicated that the venom interferes with the distribution of ACh between tissue and medium while it does not affect its synthesis. On the other hand, this synthesis was much reduced by addition of venom to slices incubated in a "high-potassium" medium.

Chmouliovsky et al. (1972a, 1972b) investigated the mode of action of *L. m. tredecimguttatus* venom (I) on the nerve endings by using external electrodes on the isolated rat superior cervical ganglion. It was shown that, after one hour's exposure, the venom caused a complete disappearance of the postganglionic action potential, while the impulse conduction was unaffected. In homogenized ganglia the venom inactivates creatine phosphokinase, measured with an enzymatic fluorimetric method. The authors conclude by suggesting that the action of the venom could be due to a block of SH-containing compounds. One of these could be an enzyme necessary for ACh synthesis or for its metabolism, or could be a compound involved in ACh release or a compound of the ACh receptors.

In order to prove that *L. m. tredecimguttatus* venom (I) was active also on other types of nerve endings besides the cholinergic ones, FRONTALI (1972) used dissected rat iris observed by means of a fluorescence microscope to record the behavior of adrenergic nerve fibers in contact with the venom. The addition of venom to the preparation at a concentration of 0.1 pairs of glands/ml resulted, after one hour's incubation, in total disappearance of the fluorescence, and to a considerable decrease in fluorescence if one-tenth the amount of venom was used. The author suggests that some of the symptoms of latrodectism in vertebrates, such as arterial hypertension, contraction of the nictitating membrane of the cat, and mydriasis, could be due to the release of noradrenaline from peripheral nerves.

In testing separated toxic fractions from *L.m. tredecimguttatus* venom (I) GRA-NATA et al. (1972) found that three protein peaks (two of them in particular) are active *in vitro* on three different preparations from rat which were already known to be affected by the whole venom, i.e. brain cortex slices, which showed an increased release of acetylcholine; iris, whose adrenergic fiber showed disappearance of the histochemical reaction due to catecholamines; and superior cervical ganglion, from which an amplitude decrease of preganglionically evoked action potentials were recorded postganglionically and asynchronous postganglionic action potentials were recorded without stimulating the ganglia. From these results it appears that the toxicity of the three fractions is linked to a common mode of action, affecting neurotransmitter release from cholinergic and possibly adrenergic nerve terminals.

Working with the venom (I) of the Australian red-back spider, *L. m. hasselti,* HAMILTON (1972) observed that the venom had a graded action on the isolated rat diaphragm. In fact, if a diaphragm is fixed when giving a reduced response to nerve stimulation, not all end-plates are affected, while if it is fixed when unable to contract, all end-plates are affected. Preliminary observations on the depletion of nerve endings in rat *vas deferens* were also reported.

Further observations on rat *vasa deferentia* treated with the same venom were given by HAMILTON and ROBINSON (1973). The tissues were fixed when, upon addition of the venom, they no longer responded to stimulation. Demonstration of catecholamines by fluorescence microscopy was carried out in cells from outer, middle, and inner muscle layers. In the cells from the outer and inner layers of venom-treated *vasa,* specific fluorescence disappeared, while in the middle-layer cells nerve endings appeared normal. These cells were the same ones that showed large granular vesicles.

Further investigations on the effect of *L. mactans* venom (I) on rat phrenic nerve — diaphragm preparation was carried out by PALMER (1975). Increased activity of the end-plate, achieved by means of physostigmine, causes slowing of the speed of entry of the venom. Small doses of hemicholium (block of ACh synthesis) can protect the end-plate from the effects of the venom. Low calcium concentrations may also protect the end-plate. The authors concluded that the action of the venom is entirely presynaptic and that in the early stages of envenomation it perhaps acts on the carrier systems within the membrane but with longer contact times it causes complete membrane disruption.

Recently Grasso (1976) prepared in a homogeneous form a neurotoxin from *L. m. tredecimguttatus* venom (I), which released norepinephrine from synaptosomes prepared from rat brain. It was also shown that upon incubation for one hour with the toxin at concentrations of 1 µg/ml rat iris nerve fibers are depleted of catecholamines (fluorescence technique) (see also: Venom Chemistry).

Mouse. Maroli and Bettini (1971) (see: Amphibia) showed that the application of both types of *L. m. tredecimguttatus* venom (I, III) induced fibrillations and contracture varying intensity according to venom concentration, in the isolated *m. rectus abdominis* of mouse. The addition of ACh to the venom potentiated its effects. In the light of the mode of action of the venom, the authors give a tentative explanation of the muscular symptoms in vertebrate envenomation.

The effects on *L. m. hasselti* venom (I) on *vasa deferentia* of adult male mice were reported in detail by Einhorn and Hamilton (1973). The study consisted of intracellular recordings of *vasa deferentia* muscle cells where excitatory junction potentials occur, originating most likely from a purely noradrenergic motor innervation. Following the application of venom, the frequency of spontaneous excitatory junction potentials was greatly increased and the tissue contracted vigorously. After 7 min, neither spontaneous nor evoked potentials could be recorded. Tetrodotoxin did not prevent the discharge of spontaneous potentials evoked by the venom. In the venom-treated tissues examined with the electron microscope, all nerve terminals of surface cell layers were translucent, thus containing practically no transmitter vesicles.

It was also shown by Hamilton and Einhorn (1973) that the release of noradrenaline from nerve terminals was associated with the disappearance of the small, but not the large granular vesicles. The authors concluded that large granular vesicles are not involved in transmitter release from adrenergic nerve terminals.

Cat. The effects of the direct action of *L. m. tredecimguttatus* venom (I) on feline motor nerve endings was investigated by Okamoto et al. (1971) in an electron-microscope study of the nerve terminals. After intra-arterial venom injection and before the onset of block, fasciculation and a slight increase in twitch height were seen. The poisoned nerve-muscle junction showed a sequence of damage to motor nerve endings, which culminated in disruption of the prejunctional membrane and loss of all organelles, including synaptic vesicles. The intra-arterial addition of ACh to the completely poisoned junction showed that the isometric contractile response of the muscle fibers was unaltered if ACh had been administered before the venom, while one hour after the neuromuscular block was complete, *i.e.* when presumably the motor endings were totally destroyed, ACh induced a response that was not only less than in the control but was also less than the contractions normally elicited by single, supramaximal stimulations of the motor nerve.

Pinto et al. (1973) evaluated the possible actions of *L. m. mactans* venom (I) on the peripheral nervous system of cat. The responses of the isolated strip of spleen were recorded on a smoked drum. The venom induced slow and sustained contractions of spleen strips, indicating an agonistic effect on this peripheral adrenergic effector. No response was obtained in spleen strips denervated 6 days before the experiment by removal of both coelic ganglia and of the splenic artery adventitia. No responses were obtained in strips from reserpinized cats, indicating that the presence of the adrenergic transmitter in the nerve terminals is essential for the venom to act.

Further work by the Argentinian authors was carried out on the same preparation (PINTO and ROTHLIN, 1974). It was shown that the venom induced in the spleen strips an irreversible supersensitivity to noradrenaline, of the same magnitude as that produced by denervation and by cocaine. Cocaine failed to potentiate the response to noradrenaline in venom-pretreated strips, indicating that the venom-induced supersensitivity to noradrenaline is the result of a presynaptic action of the venom. Analogous results were obtained by addition of methoxamine to pretreated strips of normal as well as of reserpinized cats.

Dog. Experiments with *Latrodectus* venom on dogs are not numerous. The early work of TROISE (1929) includes some trials on the effect of *L. mactans* venom on decapitated dog with intact vagus. No central or peripheral action on bronchia was observed. Other experiments on the nervous system of dog (and frog) led the author to suggest that the nervous effects were medullary in origin.

3. Toxicity in Cells Cultivated in Vitro

The crude venom (I) of *L. m. tredecimguttatus* and three of its protein fractions were tested by VICARI et al. (1965) in cells cultivated *in vitro,* namely monkey kidney primary cultures (KB line) and amniotic cell cultures (I.S.S. line). It was observed that the crude venom exerts a cytotoxic action on both types of cell cultures. The same type of toxicity was exhibited by one venom component only, fraction LV_1. This protein fraction was shown by other authors (see: 1. Invertebrates) to be toxic to house flies and active on the cockroach nervous tissue, and toxic to mice. According to the authors of this work, tissue cultures provide a more sensitive system of assay than the whole animal for fraction LV_1 and its antibodies. Moreover, tissue cultures act as selective systems when crude preparations of venom are used, as cells react only to one component.

4. Effect of Toxin on Lipid Bilayer Membranes

It appears that morphological changes in tissue cultured neurons are restricted particularly to regions of the neuron with low intramembranous particle density (RUBIN et al., 1975). The possibility that the venom may interact directly with membrane lipids was tested by FINKELSTEIN et al. (1976) on artificial lipid bilayer membranes. It was shown that a purified toxin, fraction B_5 (FRONTALI et al., 1976), interacts irreversibly with the membranes to form cation selective channels. The authors discuss the probable modes of action of the toxin on the nerve membrane *in vivo*. Since the toxin produces morphological changes in several types of neurons, but does not affect non-neuronal cells, it is suggested that specificity of action must reside either in differential toxic binding by specific cell types or in differential responses of cells to uniformily bound toxin.

5. Distribution of Venom in Envenomed Animals

Investigations on the distribution of labeled *L. m. tredecimguttatus* venom in the guinea pig were carried out by Yugoslavian authors. In preliminary experiments

Maretic (1958) showed that homogenates of organs from a severely envenomed rat injected into other experimental animals provoked typical signs of latrodectism.

Inorganic ^{32}P was later used by Lebez et al. (1965) to label the venom *in vivo* by inducing the spiders to drink the isotope. The guinea pigs were then exposed to the bite of the spiders. The ^{32}P activity was evaluated from homogenates of the guinea pig tissues. It appeared that the venom accumulated especially in the CNS and in the peripheral nerves, and to a lesser extent in the lungs, heart, liver and spleen. A large amount of the venom remained around the site of the bite, even up to the death of the animal.

In a subsequent work (Lebez et al., 1968), the venom was labeled with ^{75}S, the same technique being used. The investigation was extended to other spiders. The distribution studies were also carried out on guinea pigs. The results obtained with ^{75}S were consistent with those obtained with ^{32}P.

6. Protective Activity of Venom Against Botulin Toxin

Stern and collaborators have carried out a serie of experiments (Stern and Valjevac, 1972; Stern et al., 1975; Valjevac et al., 1972) designed to test the protective activity of *L. m. tredecimguttatus* venom (I) against botulin toxin. The relatively weak effect of the venom was due most probably to the severe side effects caused in mice. The authors did not succeed in preventing these side effects, mainly bronchospasm, with a β-adrenergic stimulant. The association of venom with different drugs did not lead to any appreciable positive results. Nontheless, according to the authors' experience, *Latrodectus* venom was considered as the most potent antibotulinum agent.

As reported by Pumplin and del Castillo (1975), the interaction between botulin toxin and *L. m. mactans* venom (I) was studied with electrophysiological methods in isolated superior cervical ganglia of rats (Pumplin and McClure, 1972; Pumplin, 1973). While botulin toxin completely suppressed the release of ACh elicited by electrical stimulation of the ganglia, it inhibited only about 45 percent of the ACh release caused by *Latrodectus* venom. The results in rat ganglia suggested to Pumplin and del Castillo that the ACh liberated under these conditions by the venom might be due to the release of the population of vesicles that is not affected by botulin toxin. Since the action of the *L. m. mactans* venom is the same as that exerted by *L. geometricus* at the level of frog neuromuscular junction, the above hypothesis was tested by the same authors by treating frog *sartorius* and *cutaneus pectoris* muscles that had been fully blocked by botulin toxin, with the venom of *L. geometricus*. It was found that two populations of synaptic vesicles exist in motor endings paralyzed by botulin toxin and that both populations appear to be released by *L. geometricus* venom, resulting in a complete depletion of vesicles from the presynaptic endings.

VII. Toxicity of Eggs and Tissue Extracts

This subject has been reviewed by Buffkin et al. (1971). The authors recall the first experiments by Kobert (1888, 1889, 1901), who assumed that *L. m. tredecimguttatus* venom, originally a component of the protoplasm of unhatched eggs, increases in the embryo and as the spider develops is also secreted, but not formed, in the venom glands, for it was found throughout the spider's body. Injection to newborn spiders produced hemolysis and defects in coagulation and severe symptoms such as stupor, dyspnea, and convulsion. Pulmonary edema and congestion of the upper gastrointestinal tract were found on postmortem examination.

ESCOMEL (1919) reported that 60 eggs of *L. mactans* injected subcutaneously were necessary to kill a guinea pig. LEVY (1912a, 1912b) demonstrated that hemolysins were present in high concentrations in *L. m. mactans* eggs. KELLOGG (1915) reported on an experiment conducted by Dr. E.H. COLEMAN, who caused the death of a cat and a rabbit by injecting extracts of *L. m. mactans* eggs. HOUSSAY (1918) found that one egg of *L. m. mactans* provoked lysis of 1 ml of a 5% suspension of rat red cells in 30 min; a five-egg extract given by the intravenous route killed a rabbit with a body weight of 1,500 g.

The toxicity of *L. m. mactans* eggs on rats was also studied by D'AMOUR et al. (1936), who plotted a lethality curve according to which 0.2 mg of fresh egg material killed 100 percent of the animals. The toxicity of crude extracts of eggs and spiderlings of *L. hasselti* was shown by BUFFKIN et al. (1971). The LD_{50} for 1-day- and 4-day-old spiderlings injected i.v. to mice was $0.84 - 4.10$ and $0.90 - 4.50$ mg/kg respectively, that for eggs containing spiders was about 1.70 mg/kg. Death usually occurred within 2 min, preceded by irregular respiration, exophthalmos and ataxia. Injection of crude extracts to cats produced an immediate fall in systemic arterial pressure, changes in venous and cerebrospinal fluid pressures and alterations in the ECG and EEG. Intradermal injection to rabbits caused local hemorrhages. Nine to ten protein components were separated from egg extracts by means of acrylamide gel eletrophoresis.

A detailed discussion on egg and spider lysines in general is given by PHISALIX (1922) (chemical nature, physiological action, general toxicity, hemolytic activity). SAMPAYO (1942, 1943) found that the eggs of *L. m. mactans* induced hemolysis in rabbit red cells but that eggs injected to guinea pigs, horses and humans did not show any hemolytic action.

PARNAS and RUSSELL (1967) could not find any activity of *L. m. mactans* egg sacs on the guinea-pig phrenic nerve-diaphragm preparation.

Several experiments were conducted by KOBERT (1901) with crude extracts of *L. m. tredecimguttatus* injected by various routes in cats, and their toxic signs were recorded. PHISALIX (1922) also reviews lysines extracted from spider tissues. BUFFKIN et al. (1971) found that mice that received (i.v.) extracts prepared from the soft tissues of adult females became somewhat ill, though the syndrome was different from that provoked by the egg-spiderling extracts. The order of lethality of the two preparations was reported as different in different experiments.

References

Abalos, J.W.: The egg-sac in the identification of species of *Latrodectus* (Black-Widow Spiders). Psyche **69**, 268 – 270 (1962).

Abalos, J.W., Baez, E.C.: On spermatic transmission in spiders. Psyche **70**, 197 – 207 (1963).

Abalos, J.W., Baez, E.C.: The Spider Genus *Latrodectus* in Santiago del Estero, Argentina. In: Animal Toxins. Oxford-New York: Pergamon 1967.

Alkadhi, K.A., McIsaac, R.J.: Differential blockade of ganglionic transmission by extract from venom gland of black widow spider (*Latrodectus mactans*). Toxicon **12**, 643–648 (1974).

Ancona, L.: Anatomia e histologia del aparato venenoso de *Latrodectus mactans* o araño capulina. An. Inst. Biol. **2**, 77 (1931).

Baerg, W.J.: The Black Widow and the Tarantula. Trans. Conn. Acad. Arts & Sci. **36**, 99–113 (1945).

Baerg, W.J.: The Brown Widow and the Black Widow Spiders in Jamaica (Araneae, Theridiidae). Ann. Entomol. Soc. Am. **47**, 52–60 (1954).

Barrio, A.: Diferencias immunologicas entre entidades simpatridas de arañas del genero *Latrodectus* Walckenaer. Mem. Inst. Butantan, Simp. Internac. **33**, 865–868 (1966).

Barth, R.: Estudos histologicos sôbre as glândulas peçonhentas da "viuva negra", *Latrodectus mactans* (Fabricius). Mem. Inst. Osw. Cruz **60**, 275 (1962).

Benoit, P.L.G.: Présence et survie d'araignées du genre *Latrodectus* Walck. en Europe occidentale. Bull. Ann. Soc. R. Ent. Belg. **105**, 229–233 (1969).

Bettini, S.: Indagine sui casi di latrodectismo verificatisi negli anni dal 1938 al 1958 in alcune province d'Italia. V. Nota riassuntiva. Riv. Parassit. **24**, 31–43 (1963).

Bettini, S.: *Latrodectus* (Arachnida) venom in insect immunity studies. Proc. XII Int. Congr. Ent. London 1964 p. 230 (1965a).

Bettini, S.: Acquired Immune Response of the House Fly, *Musca domestica* (Linnaeus), to Injected Venom of the Spider *Latrodectus mactans tredecimguttatus* (Rossi). J. Invert. Pathol. **7**, 378–383 (1965b).

Bettini, S., Cantore, G.P.: Quadro clinico del latrodectismo. Riv. Parassit. **20**, 49–72 (1959).

Bettini, S., Frontali, N., Grasso, A.: Recent findings on the biochemistry and toxicology of *Latrodectus mactans tredecimguttatus* venomous gland extract. Bull. Muséum Nat. Hist. Nat. **41**, 251–254 (1969).

Bettini, S., Ravaioli, L., Cantore, G.P.: Nota preliminare sulla preparazione di un siero immune specifico verso il veleno di *Latrodectus 13-guttatus* Rossi. Rend. Ist. Sup. Sanità **17**, 192–199 (1954).

Bettini, S., Toschi-Frontali, N.: Biochemical and toxicological aspects of *Latrodectus tredecimguttatus* venom. (1960) Published for XIth International Congress of Entomology, by Ist. Entomol. Agr. Univ. Pavia (Italy), pp. 115–121.

Bordas, L.M.: Recherches sur les glandes venimeuses ou glandes des chélicères du *Latrodectus 13-guttatus* Rossi ou Malmignatte. Ass. franç. Av. Sci., Ajaccio, **30**, 615 (1901).

Bordas, L.M.: Recherches anatomiques, histologiques et physiologiques sur les glandes venimeuses ou glandes des chélicères des Malmignattes (*Latrodectus 13-guttatus* Rossi). Ann. Sci. Nat. **9**, 147 (1905).

Bücherl, W.: Mecanismo da picada das aranhas peçonhentas perigosas. Mem. Inst. Butantan **31**, 67–76 (1964).

Buffkin, D.C., Russell, F.E., Deshmukh, A.: Preliminary studies on the toxicity of black widow spider eggs. Toxicon **9**, 393–402 (1971).

Canese, A.: *Latrodectus mactans:* variaciones del dibujo y del color. Rev. Parag. de Microb. **7**, 87–89 (1972).

Cantore, G.P.: *Latrodectus tredecimguttatus* Rossi (biologia, caratteristiche e attività del veleno, terapia del latrodectismo). Thesis, University of Rome 1956.

Cantore, G.P.: Contributo allo studio dell'azione farmacologica del veleno di *Latrodectus tredecimguttatus* Rossi. Riv. Parasit. **19**, 158–160 (1958).

Cantore, G.P., Bettini, S.: Contributo allo studio del veleno di *Latrodectus tredecimguttatus* Rossi. Rend. Ist. Sup. Sanità **21**, 794–805 (1958a).

Cantore, G.P., Bettini, S.: Contributo allo studio dell'azione farmacologica del veleno di *Latrodectus tredecimguttatus,* Rossi. II. Azione sulla muscolatura bronchiale. Riv. Parassit. **19**, 297–300 (1958b).

Cantore, G.P., Bettini, S.: Contributo allo studio dell'azione farmacologica del veleno di *Latrodectus tredecimguttatus,* Rossi. III. Azione sul ritmo cardiaco e sul circolo arterioso. Riv. Parassit. **19**, 301–306 (1958c).

Chmouliovsky, M., Dunant, Y., Graf, J., Straub, R.W., Rufener, C.: Inhibition of creatine phosphokinase activity and synaptic transmission by black widow spider venom. Brain Research **44**, 289–293 (1972b).

Chmouliovsky-Moghissi, M., Dunant, Y., Graf, J., Rufener, C., Straub, R.W.: Metabolic and structural lesions of a sympathetic ganglion by black-widow venom. 4th Ann. Meet. Union Swiss Soc. Exp. Biol., Genève 1972a. In: Experientia **28**, 727 (1972a).

Cicardo, V.H.: L'hypertension artérielle produite per le venin de *Latrodectus mactans*. C. R. Soc. Biol. **148**, 1647–1648 (1954).

Clark, A.W., Hurlbut, W.P., Mauro, A.: Changes in the fine structure of the neuromuscular junction of the frog caused by black widow spider venom. J. cell Biol. **52**, 1–14 (1972).

Clark, A.W., Mauro, A., Longenecker, H.E., Jr., Hurlbut, W.P.: Effects of black widow spider venom on the frog neuromuscular junction. II. Effects on the fine structure of the frog neuromuscular Junction. Nature **225**, 703–705 (1970).

Cull-Candy, S.G., Neal, H., Usherwood, P.N.R.: Action of Black Widow Spider Venom on an Aminergic Synapse. Nature **241**, 353–354 (1973).

d'Ajello, V., Magni, F., Bettini, S.: The effect of the venom of the black widow spider *Latrodectus mactans tredecimguttatus* on the giant neurones of *Periplaneta americana*. Toxicon **9**, 103–110 (1971).

d'Ajello, V., Mauro, A., Bettini, S.: Effect of the venom of the black widow spider, *Latrodectus mactans tredecimguttatus,* on evoked action potentials in the isolated nerve cord of *Periplaneta americana*. Toxicon **7**, 139–144 (1969).

D'Amour, F.E., Becker, F.E., van Riper, W.: The black widow spider. Quar. Rev. Biol. **11**, 123–160 (1936).

del Castillo, J., Pumplin, D.W.: Discrete and discontinuous action of brown widow spider venom on the presynaptic nerve terminals of frog muscle. J. Physiol. **252**, 491–508 (1975).

Einhorn, V.F., Hamilton, R.C.: Transmitter release by red-back spider venom. J. Pharm. Pharmacol. **25**, 824–826 (1973).

Einhorn, V.F., Hamilton, R.C.: Red-back spider venom and inhibitory transmission. J. Pharm. Pharmacol. **26**, 748–750 (1974).

Escomel, E.: Le *Latrodectus mactans* ou "Lucacha" au Pérou. Etude clinique et expérimentale de l'action du venin. Bull. Soc. Path. Exot. **12**, 702–720 (1919).

Finkelstein, A., Rubin, L.L., Tzeng Mu-Chin: Black Widow Spider Venom: Effect of Purified Toxin on Lipid Bilayer Membranes. Science, **193**, 1009–1011 (1976).

Finlayson, M.H.: "Knopie-Spider" bite in Southern Africa. Med. Proc. **2**, 634–638 (1956).

Frontali, N.: Catecholamine-depleting effect of black widow spider venom on iris nerve fibres. Brain Research **37**, 146–148 (1972).

Frontali, N., Ceccarelli, B., Gorio, A., Mauro, A., Siekevitz, P., Tzeng, M., Hurlbut, W.P.: Purification from black widow spider venom of a protein factor causing the depletion of synaptic vesicles at neuromuscular junctions. J. Cell Biol. **68**, 462–479 (1976).

Frontali, N., Granata, F.: Neurotransmitter releasing activity of *Latrodectus* venom on mammalian tissue preparations *in vitro*. In: Animal and Plant Toxins, Ed. E. Kaiser. München: W. Goldmann 1973.

Frontali, N., Granata, F., Parisi, P.: Effects of black widow spider venom on acetylcholine release from rat cerebral cortex slices *in vitro*. Biochem. Pharmac. **21**, 969–974 (1972).

Frontali, N., Granata, F., Traina, M.E., Bellino, M.: Catecholamine depleting effect of black widow spider venom on fibres innervating different guinea-pig tissues. Experientia **29**, 1525–1527 (1973).

Frontali, N., Grasso, A.: Separation of Three Toxicologically Different Protein Components from the Venom of the Spider *Latrodectus tredecimguttatus*. Arch. Biochem. Biophys. **106**, 213–218 (1964).

Frontali, N., Grasso, A.: Biochemical and toxicological characteristics of three protein components of the venom of the spider *Latrodectus tredecimguttatus*. Proc. XII Intern. Congr. Entomol. Sect. **3**, 229 (1965).

Gattone, F., Bettini, S., Reali, R.: Specificity of insect immunity to toxic fractions of *Latrodectus tredecimguttatus* venom. First Intern. Congr. Parasit., Rome **1964**, p. 44: Pergamon Press, Oxford; Tamburini Ed., Milan (1966).

Gerschman, B.S., Schiapelli, R.D.: El genero *Latrodectus* Walckenaer, 1805 en la Argentina. Rev. Soc. Ent. Arg. **27**, 51–59 (1965).

Granata, F., Paggi, P., Frontali, N.: Effects of chromatographic fractions of black widow spider venom on *in vitro* biological systems. Toxicon **10**, 551–555 (1972).

Granata, F., Traina, M.E., Frontali, N., Bertolini, B.: Effects of black widow spider venom on acetylcholine release from *Torpedo* electric tissue slices and subcellular fractions *in vitro*. Comp. Biochem. Physiol. **48A**, 1—7 (1974).

Grasso, A.: Preparation and properties of a neurotoxin from the venom of black widow spider (*Latrodectus mactans tredecimguttatus*). Biochim. biophys. Acta (in press).

Grasso, A., Paggi, P.: Effect of *Latrodectus mactans tredecimguttatus* venom on the crayfish stretch receptor neurone. Toxicon **5**, 1—4 (1967).

Grasso, A., Toschi-Frontali, N.: Studi sul veleno del ragno *Latrodectus tredecimguttatus*. Boll. Soc. It. Biol. Sper. **38**, 1814—1816 (1962).

Griffiths, D.J.G., Smyth, T., Jr: Action of black widow spider venom at insect neuromuscular junctions. Toxicon **11**, 369—374 (1973).

Gruener, R.: Excitability blockade of the squid giant axon by the venom of *Latrodectus mactans* (black widow spider). Toxicon **11**, 155—166 (1973).

Hamilton, R.C.: Ultrastructural studies of the action of Australian spider venoms. 30th Ann. Proc. Electron Microscopy Soc. Emer., Ed. C.J. Arceneaux. Los Angeles, California: 1972.

Hamilton, R.C., Einhorn, V.F.: Evidence that large granular vesicles are not involved in transmitter release from adrenergic nerves. J. Anat. **116**, 467 (1973).

Hamilton, R.C., Robinson, P.M.: Disappearance of small vesicles from adrenergic nerve endings in the rat *vas deferens* caused by red back spider venom. J. Neurocytol. **2**, 465—469 (1973).

Houssay, B.A.: Sur les propriétés hémolytiques fermentatives et toxiques des extraits d'araignées. Bull. Soc. Pathol. Exotique **11**, 217 (1918).

Jenkins, D.W.: Pathogens, parasites and predators of medically important arthropods. Bull. World Health Organization, Suppl. **30**, 1—150 (1964).

Järlfors, U., Smith, D.S., Russell, F.E.: Nerve endings in the venom gland of the spider *Latrodectus mactans*. Toxicon **7**, 263—265 (1969).

Kaire, G.H.: Observations on some funnel-web spiders (*Atrax* species) and their venoms, with particular reference to *Atrax robustus*. Med. J. Australia **50**, 307—311 (1963).

Kaston, B.J.: Is the Black Widow spider invading New England? Science, **119**, 192—193 (1954).

Kaston, B.J.: Comparative biology of American Black Widow spiders. Trans. San Diego Soc. Nat. Hist. **16**, 33—82 (1970).

Kawai, N., Mauro, A., Grundfest, H.: Effect of black widow spider venom on the lobster neuromuscular junctions. J. Gen. Physiol. **60**, 650—664 (1972).

Kellogg, V.L.: Spider poison. J. Parasitol. **1**, 107 (1915).

Kobert, R.: Über Spinnengift. Z. Naturf. **61**, 441 (1888).

Kobert, R.: Über die giftigen Spinnen Russlands. Sber. Naturf. Ges. Dorpot. **8**, 340—362 (1889).

Kobert, R.: Beiträge zur Kenntnis der Giftspinnen. Stuttgart: F. Enke 1901.

Lebez, D.: Some biochemical properties of the poison of *Latrodectus tredecimguttatus*. Bull. Scient. Yougoslavie **1**, 74 (1953).

Lebez, D.: Beiträge zum Studium des Giftes von *Latrodectus tredecimguttatus* Rossi. Hoppe-Seyler's Ztschr. f. physiolog. Chem. **298**, 73—76 (1954).

Lebez, D., Kregar, I., Turk, V., Maretić, Z.: Analyse biochimique et biologique de venins d'araignées obtenus par divers procédés. Bull. Mus. Nat. Hist. Natur., 2e Sér. **41** (Suppl. 1), 255—259 (1969).

Lebez, D., Maretić, Z., Kristan, J.: Studies on labeled animal poisons. I. Distribution of P^{32}-labeled *Latrodectus tredecimguttatus* venom in the guinea pig. Toxicon **2**, 251—253 (1965).

Lebez, D., Maretić, Z., Gubensek, F., Kristan, J.: Studies on labeled animal poisons. II. Distribution of the venoms of various spiders labeled with Se^{75} and P^{32} in the guinea pig. Toxicon **5**, 261—262 (1968).

Levi, H.W.: Number of Species of Black-Widow Spiders (Theridiidae: *Latrodectus*). Science **127**, 1055 (1958).

Levi, H.W.: The spider genus *Latrodectus* (Araneae, Theridiidae). Trans. Amer. Microscop. Soc. **78**, 7—43 (1959).

Levi, H.W.: The three species of *Latrodectus* found in Israel. J. Zool. London **150**, 427—432 (1966).

Levy, R.: Relations entre l'arachnolysine et les organes génitaux des femelles des araignées (Epeirides). C. R. Acad. Sc. **154**, 77 (1912a).

Levy, R.: Sur le mécanisme de l'hémolyse par l'arachnolysine. C. R. Acad. Sc. **155**, 233 (1912b).

Longenecker, H.E., Jr, Hurlbut, W.P., Mauro, A., Clark, A.W.: Effects of black widow spider venom on the frog neuromuscular junction. I. Effects on end-plate potential, miniature end-plate potential and nerve terminal spike. Nature **225**, 701−703 (1970).

Majori, G., Bettini, S., Casaglia, O.: Effect of black widow spider venom on the cockroach heart. J. Insect Physiol. **18**, 913−927 (1972).

Maretić, Z.: The health problem of Arachnidi. Thesis Med. Faculty University of Zagreb, 46 pp. (1958).

Marikovskij, P.I.: Tarantola e karakurt. Accad. Sce Rep. Soc. Circassa, Frunze, 1956. (in Russian)

Maroli, M., Bettini, S.: Effects of *Latrodectus mactans tredecimguttatus* venom on the dynamics of vertebrate voluntary muscles. Ann. Ist. Super. Sanità **7**, 44−55 (1971).

Maroli, M., Bettini, S., Panfili, B.: Toxicity of *Latrodectus mactans tredecimguttatus* venom on frog and birds. Toxicon **11**, 203−206 (1973).

McCrone, J.D.: Biochemical differentiation of the sibling black widow spiders, *Latrodectus mactans* and *L. variolus*. Psyche **74**, 212−217 (1967).

McCrone, J.D.: Spider venoms: biochemical aspects. Am. Zoologist **9**, 153−156 (1969).

McCrone, J.D., Hatala, R.J.: Isolation and characterization of a lethal component from the venom of *Latrodectus mactans mactans*. In: Animal Toxins, Eds. F.E. Russell and P.R. Saunders. Oxford, New York: Pergamon 1967.

McCrone, J.D., Levi, H.W.: North American Widow Spiders of the *Latrodectus curacaviensis* Group (Araneae: Theridiidae). Psyche **71**, 12−27 (1964).

McCrone, J.D., Netzloff, M.L.: An immunological and electrophoretical comparison of the venoms of the north American *Latrodectus* spiders. Toxicon **3**, 107−110 (1965).

Meadows, P.E., Russell, F.E.: Milking of arthropods. Toxicon **8**, 311−312 (1970).

Millot, J.: Les glandes venimeuses des Aranéides. Ann. Sci. Nat. Zool. **14**, 113 (1931).

Monterosso, B., Floris, G.: La nutrizione influenza il sesso negli Araneidi? Boll. Zool. **7**, 195−206 (1936).

Monterosso, B., Ronsisvalle, C.: Su la maniera, usata da *Latrodectus tredecimguttatus* Rossi, nel catturare la preda e considerazioni, relative a tale attività nell'ordine degli Araneidi. Rend. Acc. Naz. Lincei, Ser. 8, **3**, 406−410 (1947).

Montgomery, T.H., Jr: The sex ratio and cocooning habits of an aranead and the genesis of sex ratios. J. exp. Zoll. **5**, 429−452 (1908).

Muic, N., Stanic, M., Meniga, A.: Beitrag zur Kenntnis des Spinnengiftes von *Latrodectus tredecimguttatus* Rossi. Ztsch. physiol. Chem. **305**, 70−74 (1956).

Neri, L., Bettini, S., Frank, M.: The effect of *Latrodectus mactans tredecimguttatus* venom on the endogenous activity of *Periplaneta americana* nerve cord. Toxicon **3**, 95−99 (1965).

Okamoto, M., Longenecker, H.E., Jr, Riker, W.F., Jr, Song, S.K.: Destruction of mammalian motor nerve terminals by black widow spider venom. Science **172**, 733−736 (1971).

Ornberg, R.L., Smyth, T., Jr, Benton, A.W.: Isolation of a presynaptic neurotoxin from the venom of *Latrodectus mactans* (Fabr.). Toxicon **14**, 329−333 (1976).

Paggi, P., Rossi, A.: Sintesi e "turnover" di acetilcolina marcata nel ganglio cervicale superiore, isolato *in vitro*. Azione del veleno di *Latrodectus tredecimguttatus,* Rossi. Boll. Soc. It. Biol. Sper. **46**, 966−967 (1970).

Paggi, P., Rossi, A.: Effect of *Latrodectus mactans tredecimguttatus* venom on sympathetic ganglion isolated *in vitro*. Toxicon **9**, 265−269 (1971).

Paggi, P., Toschi, G.: Azione del veleno di *Latrodectus tredecimguttatus,* Rossi, sulla attività funzionale del ganglio cervicale di ratto, isolato *in vitro*. Boll. Soc. It. Biol. Sper. **46**, 965−966 (1970).

Paggi, P., Toschi, G.: Effects of denervation and lack of calcium on the action of *Latrodectus* venom on rat sympathetic ganglion. Life Sciences **11**, 413−417 (1972).

Palmer, M.F.: Aspects of the pharmacology of *Latrodectus mactans* venom. Gen. Pharmac. **6**, 325−331 (1975).

Pansa, M.C., Migliori Natalizi, G., Bettini, S.: 5-Hydroxytryptamine content of *Latrodectus mactans tredecimguttatus* venom from gland extracts. Toxicon **10**, 85−86 (1972).

Parnas, I., Russell, F.E.: Effects of venoms on nerve, muscle and neuromuscular junction. In: Animal Toxins, Eds. F.E. Russell and P.R. Saunders. Oxford, New York: Pergamon Press 1967.

Phisalix, M.: Animaux Venimeux et Venins. Paris: Masson 1922.

Pinto, J.E.B., Rothlin, R.P.: Presynaptic adrenergic supersensitivity induced by crude *Latrodectus mactans* venom. Toxicon **12**, 385—393 (1974).

Pinto, J.E.B., Rothlin, R.P., Dagrosa, E.E.: Noradrenaline release by *Latrodectus mactaus* venom in guinea-pig atria. Toxicon **12**, 385–393 (1974).

Pinto, J.E.B., Rothlin, R.P., Dagrosa, E.E., Barrio, A.: Peripheral adrenergic effect of *Latrodectus mactans* venom. Toxicon **11**, 395—400 (1973).

Pumplin, D.W.: Ph. D. thesis, University of Illinois, 1973. In: Pumplin, D.W., del Castillo, J.: Life Sciences **17**, 137—142 (1975).

Pumplin, D.W., del Castillo, J.: Release of packets of acetylcholine and synaptic vesicles elicited by brown widow spider venom in frog motor nerve endings poisoned by botulinum toxin. Life Sciences **17**, 137—142 (1975).

Pumplin, D.W., McClure, W.O.: 2nd Annual Meet. Soc. for Neurosc., abs. 20.5, 1972. In: Pumplin, D.W., del Castillo, J.: Life Sciences **17**, 137—142 (1975).

Reese, A.M.: The anatomy of the venom glands in the black widow spider, *Latrodectus mactans*. Trans. Am. Micr. Soc. **63**, 170 (1944).

Rivosecchi, L., Bettini, S.: Contributo alla conoscenza dei predatori delle uova di *Latrodectus tredecimguttatus* Rossi. Riv. Parassit. **20**, 249—266 (1958).

Rossi, P.: Fauna Etrusca. Liburnii **2**, 126—138 (1790). (Araneae).

Rubin, L.L., Pfenninger, K.H., Mauro, A.: Abstracts, 5th Annual Meeting, Society for Neuroscience, p. 623 (1975). From: Finkelstein et al. (1976).

Russell, F.E., Buess, F.W.: Gel electrophoresis: a tool in systematics. Studies with *Latrodectus mactans* venom. Toxicon **8**, 81—84 (1970).

Russell, F.E., Long, T.E.: Effects of venoms on neuromuscular transmission. In: Myasthenia Gravis, Ed. H.R. Viets. Springfield, Ill.: Thomas 1961.

Sampayo, R.R.L.: *Latrodectus mactans* y latrodectismo. Estudio Experimental y Clinico. B. Aires: El Ateneo 1942.

Sampayo, R.R.L.: Toxic action of *Latrodectus mactans'* bite and its treatment. Clinical and experimental studies. Am. J. Trop. Med. **23**, 537—543 (1943).

Sampayo, R.R.L.: Pharmacological action of the venom of *Latrodectus mactans* and other *Latrodectus* spiders. J. Pharm. exp. Therap. **80**, 309—322 (1944).

Shapiro, H.A., Sapeike, N., Finlayson, M.H.: Pharmacological actions of the venom of *Latrodectus indistinctus*. S. African J. med. Sci. **4**, 10—17 (1939).

Shulov, A.: On the biology of two *Latrodectus* spiders in Palestine. Proc. Linn. Soc. London, sess. **152**, 309—328 (1940).

Shulov, A.: Biology and ecology of venomous animals in Israel. Mem. Inst. Butantan Simp. Internac. **33**, 93—99 (1966).

Shulov, A., Weissman, A.: Notes on the life habits and potency of the venom of the three *Latrodectus* spider species of Israel. Ecology **40**, 515—518 (1959).

Smith, D.S., Russell, F.E.: Structure of the venom gland of the black widow spider *Latrodectus mactans*. A preliminary light and electron microscopic study. In: Animal Toxins, Eds. F.E. Russell and P.R. Saunders. Oxford, New York: Pergamon 1967.

Smith, D.S., Järlfors, U., Russell, F.E.: The fine structure of muscle attachments in a spider (*Latrodectus mactans*, Fabr.). Tissue & Cell **1**, 673—687 (1969).

Suarez, J.R.E., Albaca, E., Fasciolo, J.C.: Mecanismo de la accion hipertensora del veleno de la araña, *"Latrodectus mactans"*. Cuarto Congreso Interamericano de Cardiologia, B. Aires, **507** (1952).

Suomalainen, K.U.: Histological studies on the poison glands of Araneids. Ann. Zool. Fenn. **1**, 89—93 (1964).

Stern, P., Valjevac, K.: Beitrag zur Therapie der Botulinus-Intoxikation. Arch. Toxikol. **28**, 302—304 (1972).

Stern, P., Valjevac, K., Dursum, K., Dučič, V.: Increased survival time in botulinum toxin poisoning by treatment with a venom gland extract from the black widow spider. Toxicon **13**, 197—198 (1975).

Troise, E.: Action pharmacodynamique du venin de *Latrodectus mactans*. C.R. Soc. Biol. **99**, 1431 – 1433 (1928).

Troise, E.: Action du venin de l'Araignée *Latrodectus mactans*. C. R. Soc. Biol. **102**, 1097 – 1098 (1929).

Valjevac, K., Dučič, V., Stern, P.: Farmakoloska analiza otrova pauka *Latrodectus tredecimguttatus*. Acta med. iug. **26**, 85 – 91 (1972).

Vicari, G., Bettini, S., Collotti, C., Frontali, N.: Action of *Latrodectus mactans tredecimguttatus* venom and fractions on cells cultivated *in vitro*. Toxicon **3**, 101 – 106 (1965).

Wiener, S.: The Australian red back spider (*Latrodectus hasseltii*): II. Effect of temperature on the toxicity of venom. Med. J. Austr. **1**, 331 – 334 (1956).

Wiener, S., Drummond, F.H.: Assay of spider venom and antivenene in *Drosophila*. Nature (Lond.) **178**, 267 – 268 (1956).

B. Epidemiology of Envenomation, Symptomatology, Pathology and Treatment

Z. MARETIĆ

I. Epidemiology

1. Geographical Distribution

Latrodectism, the envenomation due to the bite of spiders of the genus *Latrodectus*, is a cosmopolitan disease which can appear in all areas where these spiders live, i.e., in warm zones of all continents.

a) Europe

In France spider bites were described around Avignon, Vaucluse, Herault, in Corsica, as well as in Brittany around Morbihan and in the Vendée (JUNQUA and VACHON, 1968; KOBERT, 1901).

Latrodectism is known in Portugal as well as in Spain, especially around Tarragona and Barcelona, in the Pyrennées and in the province of Lerida (BONNET, 1945 – 1961; GRAËLLS, 1834; SALEZ VASQUEZ and BIOSCA FLORENSA, 1949).

In Italy latrodectism is known from antiquity. It was already described in works of old authors, such as CELSUS, PLINY, AELIANUS and later BOCCONE (1687), CHELLINI (1728), MARMOCCHI (1800), TOTI (1794), and others. It has been abundant in Volterra, Apulia, Sicilia in Sardinia and especially in the central provinces Grosseto, Viterbo, Roma, and Latina – 492 cases from 1946 to 1950 (BETTINI et al., 1953 – 1964).

In Yugoslavia latrodectism was recorded in Istria (about 200 cases from 1948 to 1965) (MARETIĆ, 1949 – 1971), Croatian littoral, Dalmatia and its islands (DAMIN, 1896a and b, 1900; ŠKARICA, 1949), Herzegowina (GRUJIĆ, 1959; ČUČKOVIĆ, 1973), Montenegro (RAMZIN, 1947), Macedonia (JOVANOVSKI et al., 1956; ORUŠEV, 1958; VANOVSKI, 1962), Kosovo and Metohija, and allegedly in Pomoravlje in Serbia (VANOVSKI, 1962).

In Greece *Latrodectus* and latrodectism were even mentioned by SOCRATES (XENOPHON), ARISTOTLE, NIKANDER and DIOSCORIDES. It is known to occur in the islands of Archipelagos, Peloponnesus, Lemnos, Crete, and Nauplion (Savoura, 1962) and in the Greek part of Macedonia.

Latrodectism was recorded also in Bulgaria in Rumelia and Stara Zagora (Gundrum, 1899; Drensky, 1928), in Rumania in Bessarabia and the delta of Danube (Fuhn, 1966), and allegedly in localities in Hungary (Chyzer and Kulczynski, 1892; Kolosvary, 1935) and Poland (Wagner, 1895).

In the European part of Russia, latrodectism has occurred in Moldavia, in the Ukraine, in the district of Dnjepr, around Molochnaya, Don, and Manich, in Podolia, Powolzhie, the Crimean peninsula, Bessarabia, and in the coastal regions of the Black and Azovian Seas, especially around Odessa, Kherson, and Stavropol, in Tauria, Caucasus, and Ural (Kobert, 1901; Pawlowsky, 1927; Lepilova, 1955; Marikovskij, 1956; Yarovoy and Shewchenko, 1957).

b) Asia

In the Asiatic part of Russia latrodectism exists in Balkash, Astrakhan, Kirghis steppe, near Chokand, Kuldza, Saissan Nor, in Kasakhstan around Alma Ata, in Transcaucasia, Turkestan, Uzbekhistan (Tashkent), in the southern parts of Tadzikhistan, in the Kalmyck Republic, at Kara Bogaz, and in Mongolia (Kobert, 1901; Pawlowsky, 1927; Arustamyan, 1955; Lepilova, 1955; Blagodarny, 1957; Levi, 1959).

Latrodectism occurs also in Asia Minor: in Turkey at Çanakkale (Dardanelles) and in the Taunus Mountains, in Syria, Lebanon, and Israel, in the Arabian Peninsula (Saudi Arabia, Yemen, and Aden) (Levi, 1959; Shulov, 1959), on the island of Sokotra (Persian Gulf), in parts of India, Nepal, Ceylon, on Maladives, the Loyalty Islands, Morotoi, Burma, Indonesia (islands of Timor and Aru), in Borneo, New Guinea, New Hebrides, Marianas, Malayan Archipelago, Polynesia, Bismarck Archipelago, Philippines (Luzon), Hawaii, in the islands of the western Pacific, south of Okinawa, and in the islands of Ryukyu and Ishigaki (Keegan, 1952, 1960; Levi, 1959; Keegan et al., 1964).

c) Africa

Latrodectism is known over the whole of North Africa from Egypt to Lybia, Algeria (Tlemcen), Tunis, and Morocco (Tangier, Fez, Ghart, and Allal Tazi) (Desportes, 1937; Gaud and Delesalle, 1949; Bouisset and Larrouy, 1962), in the Atlantic islands of Madeira, Canary Islands, Porto Santo, St. Helena, on the Gold Coast, Senegal, Congo, Camerun, Togo, Sudan, Abyssinia, Kenya, at the Nyassa Lake, in the area of Shoa, in Zanzibar, along the river Zambezi (Sampayo, 1942; Levi, 1959), in the central parts of the continent in Rhodesia, South African Union (Pretoria, South Rhodesia, Sothwest Africa, Eastern Transvaal, and Natal), and in Madagascar (Finlayson, 1936a, 1936b, 1937, 1956; Finlayson and Hollow, 1945; Levi, 1959; Zumpt, 1968).

d) America

Latrodectism on the North American continent is present from Canada to Patagonia. In Canada it was recorded in the provinces of Ontario, Alberta, British Columbia and Manitoba (THORP and WOODSON, 1945) and in USA in practically in all the states, especially in the South and particularly in California; further it is found in Mexico, Curaçao, Antilles, West Indies (Bahamas, Jamaica, Haiti, Dominican Republic, Cuba, and Portorico), and in Central America. In South America it was recorded in Equador, Bolivia, Peru, Venezuela, Uruguay, Paraguay (Gran Chaco and Mato Grosso), in Argentina, and Chile. In Colombia and Brasil latrodectism is not frequent, being present in the latter only in the southern parts (Rio Grande do Sul) (PUGA-BORNE, 1875; GUZMAN, 1910; ESCOMEL, 1919; SAMPAYO, 1942; THORP and WOODSON, 1945; BAERG, 1954; BÜCHERL, 1965, 1968).

e) Australia

Latrodectism was described in the Northern Territory, in Perth, in Queensland, in Camberra, in the southern part in Adelaide, New South Wales, and in New Zealand, New Caledonia, and Tasmania (KELLAWAY, 1930; THORP and WOODSON, 1945; LEVI, 1959; WIENER, 1961).

In the localities where latrodectism was recorded, as mentioned, the envenomation was provoked by different species or subspecies of the genus *Latrodectus* as listed in the corresponding section.

2. Factors Influencing Number of Spiders and Frequency of Contacts with Man. Epidemics of Latrodectism

Due to various factors described later, the number of spiders increases periodically to a very excessive extent. For example, localities have been noted where during

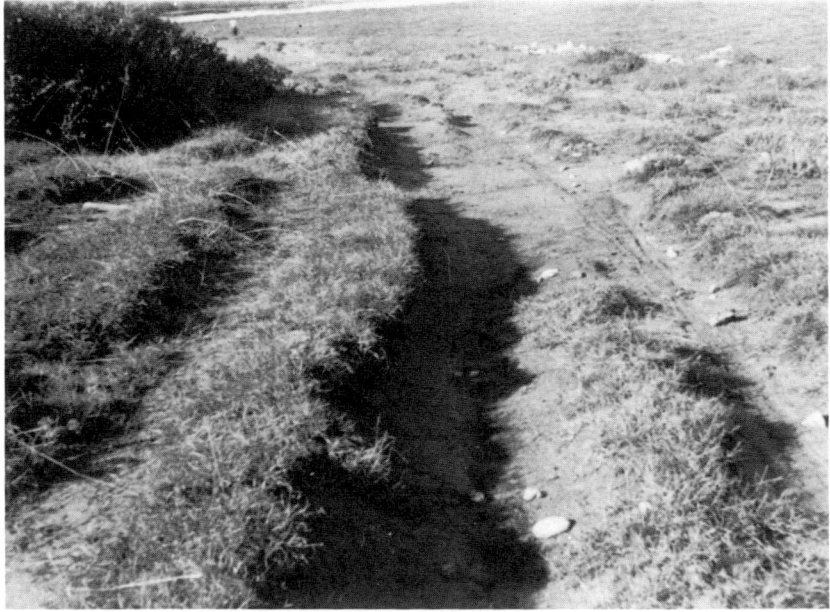

Fig. 1. A Mediterranean scene, a typical biotope of *Latrodectus*. Along the wheal tracks its nests are found next to each other

such periods several specimens could be found per square meter (Maretić, 1959). Since *Latrodectus* species are not aggressive at all, only when the specimens are numerous can their bites have a practical significance or even be so frequent that an epidemic of latrodectism occurs.

After a few years or more, the number of spiders decreases again. The epidemic disappears, the population sometimes forgets it completely, and when eventually latrodectism appears again after many years, people often believe it to be a new illness, or even that it was imported from elsewhere. For instance, during the epidemic of latrodectism in Volterra, Marmocchi (1800) recorded the belief that the spiders were imported with wheat from Sardinia and Africa; similarly when in 1948 the epidemic began in Istria, people in Poreč believed that the spiders came with parcels of UNRRA from America (Maretić, 1951). Even a textbook carried these obviously incorrect data.

With regard to the abundance of spiders, suitable biotopes with a culture that acts favorably on the development of spiders, such as wheat fields, vineyards, cotton, fields, etc., are most important. A good example is given by Popovo polje (Herzegovina, Yugoslavia), where the construction of the hydrosystem on the river Trebišnjica stopped the flooding which used to change this field every autumn into a lake. The population changed to growing wheat and wine grapes instead of the swift-growing varieties of corn. These ecological changes made possible an excessive multiplication of *Latrodectus* and an outbreak of latrodectism in 1971 (Čučković, 1973).

The use of herbicides and insecticides may influence the number of spiders by acting directly on them or indirectly on populations of other insects that represent their prey, predators, or parasites.

Kobert (1901) as well as other Russian, Spanish, and Italian authors (Graëlls, 1834; Kobert, 1901) thought the density of *Latrodectus* to be proportional to that of the grasshopper, *Coloptenus italicus,* which serves as food to the spider. However, according to other observations, a great number of spiders could also be found during years with a low grasshopper density. It is also true that *Latrodectus* feeds on other insects always present in sufficient numbers.

The density of spiders can be decreased by various predators, such as some insects, spiders, lizards, and birds, or by parasites. There are various kinds of wasps that lay their eggs in the coccoons of *L. mactans tredecimguttatus,* such as *Pimpla augens* Grav., *Pimpla oculatoria* Grav., *Pedobius* sp., *Gelis niger* Bris., *Sphex,* and *Pompilus* spp.; the beetle *Malachius* sp. was also described as an egg parasite (Kobert, 1901; Marikovskij, 1956; Rivosecchi and Bettini, 1958). Various authors described and listed other parasites of different *Latrodectus* species. Fungi can also act as enemies of spiders (Bristowe, 1958; Eason et al., 1967).

Although one cannot say today, as some of the old authors did, that high densities of *Latrodectus* are connected with hot dry summers, according to recent investigations (Lebez, unpublished 1973), it seems that there are connections between climatic conditions and the number of spiders. For instance, a sufficient humidity in the microclimate around the nest may determine whether most of the eggs will dry up or not. The drought also may cause the death of embryos or spiderlings within the coccoon, for humidity is necessary for the act of moulting. However, during too humid springs, one can observe mouldy eggs. Bettini (1963) concluded that the oscillations of *Latrodectus* density depend finally on meteorological factors — not quite understandable to us from the available data — which regulate or disturb the equilibrium between *Latrodectus* and its parasites and predators.

In addition to the great abundance of spiders, however, a special condition is necessary for the onset of a latrodectism epidemic, i.e., the increase of man-spider contact frequency. This may occur when man invades for various reasons the biotope of spiders, as in the case of camping, maneuvers, or movements of armies. Such accidents were recorded early by the monks Alberich and Regino in the 9th century in Calabria (KOBERT, 1901); a classical story from Puga Borne (1875) relates that when solders on the eve of the battle at Loncomilla were bitten by spiders, they had to be chloroformed not to betray with their screams the position of the army. *Latrodectus* bites in military personel are also known to have occurred in the USA (FRANK, 1942), Italy (BETTINI, 1963), and Yugoslavia (JOVANOVSKI et al., 1956).

In countries where latrodectism is connected with agricultural practices, especially harvesting and treshing, work in vineyards, in hay and cotton fields, etc., the probability of man-spider contacts increases. A typical "wild species" causing rural latrodectism is *Latrodectus mactans tredecimguttatus*, which is practically never found indoors (MARETIĆ, 1957). The same rural character applies to *L. mactans mactans* in South America (SAMPAYO, 1942) and *L. mactans indistinctus* in South Africa. *L. geometricus* can be found inside buildings, as well as in vineyards of the western provinces in South Africa, where most bites occur during harvesting of grapes (FINLAYSON, 1956).

Table 1. Epidemics of human latrodectism thoughout history (based on BETTINI's list of 1964 and extended)

Year	Locality	No. of cases	*Latrodectus* species	Author
866 — 867	Calabria (Italy)	Troops of Ludwig decimated by spiders	*L.m. tredecim-guttatus*	ALBERICH REGINO
1679	Corsica (France)	"Most venomous spiders of Corsica" (probably epidemic appearance)	*L.m. tredecim-guttatus*	KOBERT
1786 — 1818	Volterra	17 Cases (1 lethal)	*L.m. tredecim-guttatus*	TOTI
	Volterra	30	*L.m. tredecim-guttatus*	MARMOCCHI
	Volterra (Italy)	"Very abundant"	*L.m. tredecim-guttatus*	ROSSI
1830	Tarragona (Spain)	A high number of cases among the harvesters	*L.m. tredecim-guttatus*	GRAËLLS DE LA PAZ
1833	Corsica (France)		*L.m. tredecim-guttatus*	CAURO
1833	Sardinia (Italy)	Epidemic	*L.m. tredecim-guttatus*	KOBERT
1834	Barcelona (Spain)		*L.m. tredecim-guttatus*	GRAËLLS DE LA PAZ

Table 1 (continued)

Year	Locality	No. of cases	*Latrodectus* species	Author
1838—1939	East Russia		*L.m. tredecim-guttatus* var. *erebus*	Motschulsky and Bećker
1839	Sardinia (Italy)	Epidemic		Kobert
1842	New Zealand	Many cases	*L.m. hasselti*	Kobert
1868	Samara (Russia)	43 (2 lethal cases)	*L.m. tredecim-guttatus*	Shchensnowich
1868	Corsica (France)	200 Cases yearly	*L.m. tredecim-guttatus*	Kobert, De Santis
1878—1879	Marseille (France)	"A true epidemic"	*L.m. tredecim-guttatus*	Dax, Rouet, Marignan
1888	Cherson, Berislawov (Russia)	22	*L.m. tredecim-guttatus*	Kobert
1904	Ssir Darja (Russia)		*L.m. tredecim-guttatus*	Rossikov
1910	Uruguay	"An exceptionally high number of cases"	*L.m. mactans*	Phisalix
1925—1926	Bulgaria	87	*L.m. tredecim-guttatus*	Drensky
1926—1927	Dalmatia (Yugoslavia)	Many cases	*L.m. tedecim-guttatus*	Kakuškin
1946—1950	Central Italy	492	*L.m. tredecim-guttatus*	Bettini
1946	Montenegro	Several cases	*L.m. tredecim-guttatus*	Ramzin
1948	Dalmatia	8	*L.m. tredecim-guttatus*	Škarica
1948—1965	Istria (Yugoslavia)	200	*L.m. tredecim-guttatus*	Maretić
1949	Si Allal Tazi (Morocco)	8 Cases	*L.m. tredecim-guttatus*	Gaud and Delesalle
1949—1952	Alma Ata (USSR)	233	*L.m. tredecim-guttatus*	Yarowoy and Shewchenko
1950—1954	Samarkard (USSR)	94	*L.m. tredecim-guttatus*	Arustamyan
1954—1960	Makedonia (Yugoslavia)	31	*L.m. tredecim-guttatus*	Jovanovski et al.; Vanovski and others
1971—1976	Hercegovina (Yugoslavia)	Many cases	*L.m. tredecim-guttatus*	Čučković

On the other hand, *L. mactans mactans* and *L. mactans hesperus* in North America (BOGEN, 1932, 1956; THORP and WOODSON, 1945) as well as *L. mactans hasselti* in Australia are domestic species (KELLAWAY, 1930). They often build their webs in outdoor privies where men are usually bitten on their genitalia. These spiders are also often found in flats, garages, cabins, cellars, dark corners, and even high up in skyscrapers. *L mactans hasselti* can be found around Sydney in gas meters, gratings of ventilators, rubbish boxes, empty tins, etc. When due to various reasons the reproduction rate of these spiders is very high, their bites also can become more frequent and give rise to an epidemic (THORP and WOODSON, 1945).

Most of old epidemics of latrodectism were not recorded and felt into oblivion, Perhaps the first one was recorded by Diodorus Siculus, quoted by Strabo (1st century A.D.), who reported a horrible plague of spiders and scorpions in a region of Abyssinia, where the inhabitants were forced to abandon their rich country. Other epidemics of human latrodectism are listed in Table 1.

3. Other Epidemiological Data

In countries where wild species of *Latrodectus* live, latrodectism occurs among farmers and has quite an *occupational character*. In countries like Argentina, latrodectism is regarded as a professional disease of farm workers (SAMPAYO, 1942). With farmers who harvest with old-fashioned sickles, the bite on the volar side of the left forearm with which they collect the ears or put them on sheaves while binding them is characteristic (MARETIĆ, 1951). With the mechanization of agriculture, this possibility has decreased. In Argentina, bites were most frequent on the thorax, since field laborers carried sacks with hay or corn on their bare shoulders (SAMPAYO, 1942).

In countries where domestic species exist, the victims are of various professions.

Sex incidence depends upon the habits of spiders (wild or domestic species) and the working habits of people. MARETIĆ (1959) reported in Yugoslavia that the proportion between bitten males and females was 101:76; BLAGODARNY (1957) in the USSR reported 116:117; BETTINI (1963) in Italy reported 717:231; BOGEN (1932) in the USA reported 53:7. Similarly, there are variations among age groups in various countries.

The seasonal incidence in countries with rural latrodectism is greatest in summer months, when farming is most intensive. Where domestic species exist, *Latrodectus* bites can also be inflicted during other seasons (BETTINI, 1964).

Bites occur during any time day and night; however, where they are connected with farming, they coincide especially with the daily tempo of field work (MARETIĆ, 1966).

The severity of the clinical picture can also have an epidemiological significance in countries where sympatric species show different toxicity. This occurs, for instance, in South Africa with *L. mactans indistinctus, L. mactans concinnus,* and *L. geometricus* (FINLAYSON, 1956); in Israel it occurs with *L. mactans tredecimguttatus, L. revivensis,* and *L. pallidus* (SHULOV and WEISSMAN, 1959).

The data on latrodectism epidemics in domestic animals are not at all in agreement. Old Russian authors, such as Motshoulsky and Becker, Rossikow, Shchensnowich, and others reported heavy losses in cattle due to latrodectism

(KOBERT, 1901), part of which was perhaps due to other epizootics; fatalities in domestic animals were also recorded by KOLBEN (1719) in South Africa, GRAËLLS (1834) in Spain, by DRENSKY (1928) in Bulgaria, by Puga Borne (1975) in Chile and by ROZA and SOEDIBIO (1950) in Indonesia. No data on latrodectism of such kind are available either from recent North and South American literature or from Yugoslavia and Italy, where recently an increase in density of *Latrodectus* occurred (VELLARD, 1936; BETTINI, 1963, 1964; MARETIĆ, 1966; SAMPAYO, 1942; THORP and WOODSON, 1945).

II. Human Symptomatology

Human latrodectism is a particular clinical entity, a syndrome with very characteristic symptoms. In addition to the specific neurotoxic action, the venom also represents a very potent stress which provokes a series of unspecific reactions (alarm reaction) involving the whole organism into the very dramatic course of intoxication. BLAIR, who in 1933 observed the course of latrodectism on himself, divided the clinical picture into the stages of lymphatic absorption, characterized by local pains, vascular spread, consisting of spread of pains and shock, and the elimination of the venom represented by sweating, hypertension, damage of kidneys, and decrease of muscular pains. The severity of the clinical picture is variable, depending on factors connected with the spider itself, the number of bites, and the act of biting, and on factors connected with the victim, such as the physical condition and age, the site of bite (i.e., if the venom penetrated directly into circulation), and eventually the degree of his immunity, which could be of practical importance in endemic areas where previous bites might have occurred.

The bite itself is usually so slight that, as in 58.2% of MARETIĆ's patients (1966), no pain is recalled from the bite. This is especially true during field work, when the workers are exposed to various microtraumas. Patients bitten during sleep did not awake before the general violent symptoms had appeared.

The latency lasts from 10 min up to 1 h. The first symptom may be the "early pain" in the regional lymphatic nodes. They may appear slightly enlarged (MARETIĆ and JELAŠIĆ, 1953; BETTINI and CANTORE, 1959).

Poor general condition develops soon. In patients with a poor mass of musculature or, according to MILLER (1951), also in alcoholics and luetics, the disease has a more severe course. From the regional lymphatic nodes the pain spreads to the lumbar region, the abdomen, around the waist, the thighs, and the whole lower extremities. With the increase of pain, cramps appear, which from time to time imbue the body of the victim, culminating in true paroxysms. There is also a feeling of tightening and pressure in the chest. Patients experience a tremor of the whole body and complain of arthralgias. The skin of the whole body is hyperesthetic and covered with sweat (BAERG, 1923; BOGEN, 1926; GAJARDO-TOBAR, 1941; MARE-TIĆ, 1951; BETTINI and CANTORE, 1959). The patients are often unable to stand or even sit, and lie helplessly, crying. In the event they succeed in standing up, they have a typical posture of a person suffering from lumbago, and in trying to walk they grope like tabetics or as if they had intermittent claudication (BAERG, 1923; MARETIĆ, 1959). In some patients opisthotonus is marked (GAUD and DELE-SALLE, 1949; MARETIĆ, 1959).

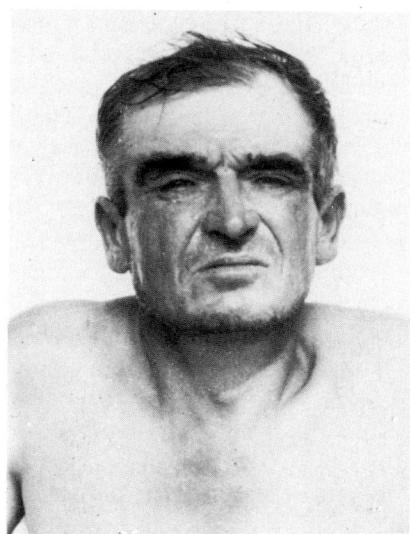

Fig. 2. *Facies latrodectismica*: flushed, sweat-covered, distorted in a painful grimace with blepharo-conjunctivitis and trismus

Patients lose up to 9.1% of their weight (BROWN, 1954) in the first 72 h (MARETIĆ and STANIĆ, 1954). The body temperature is usually slightly elevated (MARETIĆ, 1959). To this characteristic appearance of the patient is added motoric restlessness, muscular contractions, and especially *facies latrodectismica* (MARETIĆ, 1955), i.e., a flushed and sweating face contorted in a painful grimace with swollen eyelids, a strong blepharoconjunctivitis and lacrimation, and often cheilitis, rhinitis, and trism of masseters. Photophobia may be marked (MARETIĆ and STANIĆ, 1954). One often observes miosis at first, which is later followed by midriasis (GAJARDO-TOBAR, 1941). Increased filling of veins of fundus, such as hyperaemia papillae *nerve optici* could be found by ophthalmoscopic examination (MARETIĆ, 1951). Sometimes *tinnitus aurium* can be observed (MARETIĆ, 1959).

Nervous and psychic symptoms. The venom of *Latrodectus* is a neurotoxin that has a strong influence upon the cerebrospinal and vegetative systems, whence a series of neuropsychic symptoms, which dominate the clinical picture, results. The intense muscular pain increases until agony compels the patient to seek medical aid. The pain does not irradiate into the sectors of single nerves. Patients who had previously suffered from other very painful illnesses, operations, or very difficult deliveries, claim that these pains are tolerable when compared with the agony of latrodectism (BOGEN, 1932; THORP and WOODSON, 1945; MARETIĆ, 1959).

In mild cases of latrodectism, patient compared the muscular pains with the muscular soreness after physical exertion (*Muskelfieber*) or after sitting in a draught (BROWN, 1934; MARETIĆ, 1959). The severest pains last about 20 h. The feeling of oppression in the chest, due either to contraction of the thoracic musculature or perhaps to the decreased blood irrigation of the heart, together with the polypnea, dyspnea, and other sensations, brings the bitten person into an intense feeling of anxiety or a state of *pavor mortis* typical of latrodectism (BOGEN, 1926; FRANK,

1942; Sampayo, 1942; Maretić, 1959; Bettini and Cantore, 1959). Robust and healthy men, torn between a feeling of approaching death and unsupportable pains, mad from horror and in a condition of psychomotoric restlessness, throw themselves moaning and lamenting on the bed, roll on the floor, or perform senseless movements, seeking relief. Acute psychoses (Thorp and Woodson, 1945; Bettini and Cantore, 1959) may also develop, and in a few instances it was noted that the family brought such patients first to a psychiatric department in the conviction that they suddenly became mad (Maretić, 1959). Sometimes the psychotic victims tried to escape from the hospital (Bettini and Cantore, 1959; Maretić, 1959). Visual disturbances, hallucinations and deliria were also recorded (Baerg, 1923; Bogen, 1932; Gajardo-Tobar, 1941; Bettini et al., 1954). Xenophon wrote that Socrates discussed a phalangium the size of half an obolos from whose bite one can "lose the mind."

These psychic disorders may last 48–72 h, and the psychomotoric excitation can be followed by a deep torpor (Bettini and Cantore, 1959). Barton (1938) suffered from amnesia 2 months after the bite and did not recognize things and persons. In the case of Baerg (1923), the patient was even in convalescence, unable to follow conversations and understand single words. The characteristic insomnia (Kobert, 1901; Baerg, 1923; Bogen, 1926; Maretić and Stanić, 1954; Pampig-lione, 1958; Bettini and Cantore, 1959) is not based only on pains but also on the action of venom on the hypothalamic centers and can last for some time. After 24–48 h, the pains in the abdomen and the lumbar region mitigate; they become intermittent and appear only by fits with muscle cramps. However, they increase in the thighs, descending also to the calves and soles, where after 48 h the patient feels the most intense pain and burning (Gajardo-Tobar, 1941; Sampayo, 1942; Maretić, 1951). Paresthesia as described by patients in hands and legs is probably due to the toxic neuropathy and hypoxia (Blair, 1934; Bettini et al., 1953).

The muscles of the whole body are hypertonic due to an intense irritation of the neuromuscular apparatus. However, one cannot note a change either in the general sensitivity or in reactivity upon pressure of peripheral nerves. Sometimes one can see fibrillations of adjacent groups of muscle fibers near the site of the bite (Bell and Boone, 1945; Maretić, 1959). Clonic contractions, a fine tremor, such as a tremor of the tongue and jaws, are frequent. Gaud and Delesalle (1949) call all these phenomena the myopathic syndrome of latrodectism.

The knee jerk and other tendom reflexes are increased (Maretić and Stanić, 1954). However, in severe latrodectism Gajardo-Tobar (1941) observed decrease and even the extinction of reflexes. Corresponding to the degree of contracture of abdominal wall, the abdominal reflexes are decreased or even abolished. Generally, pathologic reflexes are not present. In these patients a decrease of rough motor strength and adynamy can be observed (Bell and Boone, 1945), and some authors even recorded pareses and paralyses of lower limbs, sometimes accompanied by loss of sensibility.

Data on encephalograms of patients are not available, but EEG patterns of experimental animals did show a similarity with all states of excitation of the central nervous system, for instance, as in alcalosis or epileptic convulsions or retardation of rhythm with the appearance of points, singly or in groups (Sampayo, 1942; Maretić, 1959).

The toxin has a strong effect on the breaking of the blood-cerebrospinal fluid barrier. This was deduced by experimenting with Goldmann's technique (MARETIĆ and JELAŠIĆ, 1953) which employs intravital staining of the central nervous system with 1% trypan blue in rats and cats. Experiments on intoxicated animals showed that the toxin of *Latrodectus* belongs to those rare substances that possess this type of activity.

Headache, which can be alleviated by lumbar puncture, is frequently present in latrodectism. An increase of intracranial pressure was reported by MARETIĆ and JELAŠIĆ (1953). The examination of cerebrospinal fluid did not reveal abnormalities.

Influence on the vegetative nervous system. An increase of all secretions is characteristic of latrodectism: profuse perspiration, hypo- or hypersalivation, lacrimation, rhinitis, increase of secretions from the gastrointestinal tract, urethra, and bronchi. Therefore, bronchospasm, midriasis, miosis, priapism, ejaculation, vesical and intestinal palsies, and other signs described elsewhere in this chapter should really belong here. Though the venom is a severe neuro-vegetative poison, it also acts directly upon the brain, since some neuro-vegetative signs are partially due to its effect upon subcortical centers. MARETIĆ and JELAŠIĆ (1953) succeeded in interrupting the local sweating in a patient bitten by the spider in the arm through the manchette of a blood pressure apparatus at a pressure of 200 mm of Hg applied to prevent the narcoticum reaching the nerve endings on the site of the bite via the blood. But the toxin acts also peripherally upon the vegetative system, as shown in its effects upon *erectores pilorum* in local latrodectism.

Concluding, one can say that *Latrodectus* venom is mainly neurotoxic involving simultaneously—centrally and peripherally—the cerebrospinal and the vegetative nervous system and provoking both sympathic and parasympathic effects.

Cardiovascular symptoms. Clinically, the main cardiac symptoms are bradycardia (BAERG, 1923; BOGEN, 1932; DE ASIS, 1949; FRANK, 1942) and tachycardia (BELL and BOONE, 1945; GAJARDO-TOBAR, 1941; SAMPAYO, 1942; BETTINI and CALCARA, 1956) as described by many authors who, nevertheless, are not unanimous with regard to their appearance. According to own experience, it seems that a moderate tachycardia (up to 120/min) usually occurs in the first hours of intoxication and that in the later course, especially on the second day, the rhythm changes into a moderate and later into a marked bradycardia (MARETIĆ, 1963). Some authors also mention arrhythmias (BRAUN, 1899; GUZMAN, 1910; BELL and BOONE, 1945; PAMPIGLIONE, 1958), cardiac insufficiency (BARRA, 1957), extrasystoles (BARRA, 1957; PAMPIGLIONE, 1958), and systolic murmurs (BOGEN, 1932; BELL and BOONE, 1945; SCHENONE et al., 1957).

High P_2 and P_3 waves, slurring of the QRS complex, devalation of the ST segment and T waves, and prolonging of the QT interval were registered electrocardiographically (BELL and BOONE, 1945; SCHENONE et al., 1957; MARETIĆ, 1963). In experimental animals Luciani-Wenckebach's period was recorded (MARETIĆ, 1959) such as irregularities of rhythm, cardiac blocks of various degrees, and inversion of T waves (SHAPIRO et al., 1939). Hypertension of the convergent type is typical of latrodectism. In own patients aged 15 — 50, it generally reached 164/108. According to BARKAGAN (1956), the average rise of systolic pressure in his patients ammounted to 27.8% and of diastolic, even 34.3%. In the first phase of intoxication, the state of shock justifies a hypotension, while a rise of blood pressure may later appear (BLAIR, 1934). A rise of venous pressure tentatively explained either by a latent myocardial insufficiency or by a primary venous hypertension was also observed. The toxin has a marked vasoconstrictory action upon the blood vessels in general, except on skin vessels of the head region, where it provokes a strong vasodilation resulting in the above-mentioned facial congestion. According to TROISE (1928), SAMPAYO (1942, 1944) and CICARDO (1954), it seems that hypertension is due to the direct influence of the toxin upon the vasomotor centers in the bulb and spinal medulla which activate the adrenaline of the adrenal glands' medulla and the l-noradrenalin on the *sympathicus* terminations.

In experimental animals treated with equal or increasing doses of toxin, tachyphy-laxia could be observed, i.e., the reduction of the ability of toxin to provoke bradycar-dia and hypertension, which would speak in favor of direct cardiovascular action of the venom (SAMPAYO, 1941; CANTORE and BETTINI, 1958).

Respiratory symptoms. Patients who suffer from bronchospasm have a shallow accelerated breathing, even up to 56 min (MARETIĆ, 1959) and sometimes stridor is heard (SAMPAYO, 1942). Suffocations were also recorded (FINLAYSON, 1956). Tachypnea increases, especially during cramps, when pains also increase, and it is sometimes followed by bradypnea with deeper breathing. Patients sometimes have difficulties in speech and, in single cases, hoarseness or even aphony was observed (KOBERT, 1901). On auscultation, dry or moist bronchitic rhonchi may be heard, since the contracture of the diaphragm (TROISE, 1928) diminishes the amplitudes of respiratory movements. The toxin increases the bronchial secretion and acts on the smooth musculature of the bronchi, provoking bronchoconstriction. Hiccups were also recorded (BOGEN, 1932).

Changes in the digestive functions. Usually hyperfunction, but sometimes also hypofunction, of salivary glands is present. In spite of normacid values of gastric juice, heartburn is often observed. In latrodectism the gastrointestinal secretion is increased. In MARETIĆ's series (1959), about half of the patients had nausea or vomited.

Along with the contracture of the whole musculature, rigidity of the abdominal wall is characteristic (BOGEN, 1926; MARETIĆ, 1951; BETTINI and CANTORE, 1959), which in severe cases becomes hard like a board. The abdomen is on palpation and pressure usually not painful. In some patients one can observe meteorism, an enlarged liver or subicterus (BOGEN, 1932; MARETIĆ, 1959). In single cases, increase of thymol turbidity and flocculation or increase of gammaglobulins in electrophoresis was recorded (MARETIĆ, 1959). HAGAN (1938) described a radiologically evident high position of the left diaphragm due to dilatation of the stomach filled with liquid. There was also an increase in the liver volume which, according to the author, was due to paralysis of the splanchnic system and ingurgitation by the gastrointestinal organs.

Spleen size usually decreases in latrodectism. Fresh ulcerations were found in the stomach and intestines of intoxicated guinea pigs. In cats, MARETIĆ observed a spastic contraction and in guinea pigs a paralytic dilatation of the intestines. In most patients a persistent constipation is characteristic, though in single cases diarrhea was recorded (BLAIR, 1934). Anorexia is typical and sometimes thirst appears (MARETIĆ, 1959).

Urogenital dysfunctions. The majority of patients suffered oliguria or anuria during the first 12 h. This can be ascribed in the case of urine retention (BOGEN,

1932; FINLAYSON, 1936a; GAJARDO-TOBAR, 1941, 1950; MARETIĆ, 1951) to impaired innervation of the bladder sphincter, to a decreased flow of urine into the bladder because of dehydration (BOGEN, 1932; FINLAYSON, 1956a; GAJARDO-TOBAR, 1941; MARETIĆ, 1959) due to intense sweating, salivation and vomiting, to initial shock, or to kidney damage (MARETIĆ and STANIĆ, 1954; SAMPAYO, 1942), nephritis included (GREER, 1942). Paresis, pains, and right colics of the bladder were recorded (BOGEN, 1932; GAJARDO-TOBAR, 1950; GENNARI, 1952). The urine is of high specific gravity, frequently one finds albuminuria and in the sediment leukocytes, erythrocytes, and exceptionally rough and fine granular casts (BOGEN, 1932; SAMPAYO, 1942; CONSTANT and GOUERE, 1949; MILLER, 1951; MARETIĆ and STANIĆ, 1954). The concentration and dilution test, which is not indicative due to the high loss of liquids, shows a decreased secretion and a high specific gravity. In these patients chromocystoscopy revealed a delayed output of stain (MARETIĆ, 1951).

Priapism (BETTINI et al., 1953; BOGEN, 1932; GAJARDO-TOBAR, 1941; VANOVSKI, 1962) described by a number of authors is probably due not only to the action of the toxin upon the vegetative centers but also to the increased blood viscosity. Old authors such as NIKANDROS and AVICENNA, as well as recent ones also reported ejaculation (SAMPAYO, 1942).

Though abortion was observed on intoxicated pregnant white rats and guinea pigs, MARETIĆ (1959) did not observe abortus or *partus praematurus* in any of three women in the second, fourth, and eighth month of pregnancy.

Local latrodectism is characterized by typical, though not severe, signs. A slightly red, goose-flesh area of 0.5 cm in diameter appears immediately at the site of the bite, which increases in size and intensity with time. A bristling of hairs due to irritation of *erectores pilorum* can be observed. Ray-like red beams corresponding to lymphatic pathways may extend from the site of the bite toward the lymphatic nodes. In the middle a slight whitish elevation similar to urtica appears, and around it a local sweating. It is the stage of early erythema (MARETIĆ and JELAŠIĆ, 1953). A few hours later one may see locally a pallid area up to 5 cm in diameter delimited by a reddish, bluish circular border (stage of typical ring) (MARETIĆ and JELAŠIĆ, 1953). Sometimes one can see the pointlike marks of the fangs in the center. Locally, anesthesia, anesthesia dolorosa, hyperpathia (MARETIĆ and JELAŠIĆ, 1953), or itching can develop. Occasionally on the site of the bite, a slight necrosis can be found (MARETIĆ, 1959). According to BOGEN (1956), local necrosis in latrodectism is generally the consequence of excessive local treatment, such as application of chemicals, incision, or scarification.

The stage of early erythema could be due to the local action of the toxin on blood vessel permeability. In the midst of the urtica area, the concentration of the injected venom is greatest, thus paralyzing the secretory nerves and sweat glands, so that the urtica itself remains dry, while the lower concentration of venom in the surrounding tissues provokes an irritation of secretory nerves and, consecutively, an increased sweating. In the stage of typical ring, MARETIĆ and JELAŠIĆ observed a histamine reaction of diminished intensity locally, which could be used in the differential diagnosis (MARETIĆ and JELAŠIĆ, 1953).

A rash appears on about the fourth day in most untreated severe cases of latrodectism (BRAUN, 1899; KELLAWAY, 1930; BROWN, 1934; MARETIĆ, 1951; BETTINI and CANTORE, 1959; VANOVSKI, 1962; TARTAGLIA, 1966). The rash may be scarlatiniform,

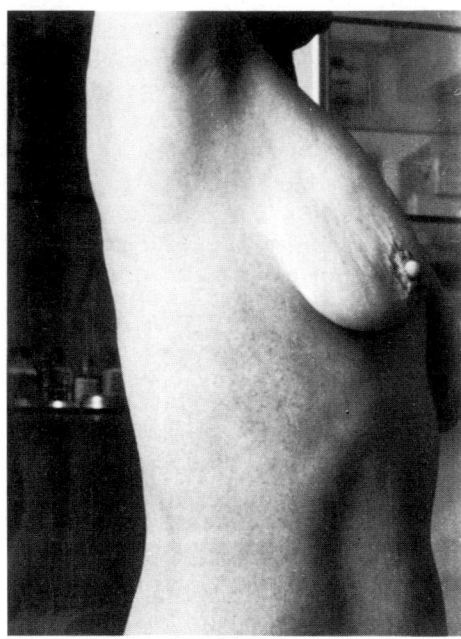

Fig. 3. A generalized minute rash a few days after the bite

morbilliform, or papulous localized around the site of the bite, or generalized. An enanthema may also be observed occasionally. The rash may be accompanied by itching. Due to strong perspiration, *miliaria crystallinia* may also appear (MARE-TIĆ, 1959).

Unspecific signs and reactions in latrodectism. Latrodectism represents a severe and sudden stress for the whole organism, provoking a series of nonspecific system reactions in the sense of a "general syndrome of adaptation," according to SELYE. While in experimental animals which survive in the stage of alarm reaction one can also observe the stages of resistance and of exhaustion, in man only the stage of alarm reaction is present, with eventually the phases of shock and countershock. The syndrome does not usually develop further, since recovery ensues. Signs of shock with pallidness, hypotension, weak filiform pulse, and other characteristic signs of the first phase of latrodectism were observed in a number of instances, and BLAIR experienced it also in his autoexperiment. But mostly one sees the patients only in the phase of countershock. Laboratory findings also speak in favor of alarm reactions. The differential blood count shows aneosinophilia, neutrophilia, and lymphopenia. There is also a moderate leukocytosis varying around 11,400/mm^3, but reaching at times 26,000/mm^3 (BOGEN, 1932). No changes in the erythrocyte sedimentation rate were observed. The number of erythrocytes, as well as values of hemoglobin, color index, and hematocrit are increased due to hemoconcentration (MARETIĆ and STANIĆ, 1954).

Thrombocytes and time of bleeding and clotting are normal (MARETIĆ and STANIĆ, 1954). The values of blood sugar were correspondingly elevated, and in a series of experimental rats in which the blood sugar was determined in various phases of intoxication, the curve showed typical decreases in the phases of shock and exhaustion, as well as an increase in the phase of countershock and resistance (MARETIĆ, 1959).

Increase of blood urea and NPN is also often seen. In regard to electrolytes, one sees in general a slight decrease of sodium and chlorides and a slight increase of potassium and phosphates (MARETIĆ, 1959). According to BOGEN (1932), false positive seroreactions for syphilis may be found.

III. Differential Diagnosis

Though latrodectism in its patent form is so characteristic that any experienced physician would be able to make the diagnosis on first sight, it would cause perplexities to anyone who had never seen a case because of its bizarre and peculiar symptoms and signs. A negative anamnesis with regard to spider bite, as often occurs, represents one of the most serious draw-backs. Differential diagnosis should exclude the following conditions:

Other spiders or insects bites. Even if the patiens know that they were bitten by a spider, they may refer the envenomation to the bite of other nontoxic species (MARETIĆ, 1949). Often the patients indicate *Lycosa tarentula* as the biter instead of *L. mactans tredecimguttatus.* HOUSSAY in South America, where the difficulties are even greater due to a greater number of venomous species, had similar experiences (SAMPAYO, 1942). Other insect bites or stings should be taken into consideration in the differential diagnosis. Inexperienced physicians may suspect that any insect bite could be a *Latrodectus* bite (which occurs especially in endemic areas or during epidemics). The stings of Mutillidae (Hymenoptera) can sometimes be puzzling, since both symptomatologies show severe pains, agitation, anuria, and after 2−3 days of duration of illness, a convalescence characterized by asthenia and neurovegetative dystony (PAMPIGLIONE, 1958).

Acute abdomen conditions. Differential diagnosis should take into consideration all diseases characterized by abrupt onset, severe pain, poor general condition, and eventually shock. If these conditions are accompanied by rigidity of the abdominal wall, leukocytosis, and vomiting, it becomes understandable why latrodectism is oftenly mistaken for acute abdomen due to perforated ulcers, appendicitis, ileus, etc. (HARGRAVES and MACKENZIE, 1942; WILSON, 1943). Unnecessary laparatomies were performed on these grounds (GENNARI, 1952).

Latrodectism can also be wrongly diagnosed as food poisoning or as an exanthematic disease, such as scarlatina. Furthermore, in the literature are listed the diseases where differential diagnosis with latrodectism may be difficult: acute psychoses, tabic crises, meningitis, tetanus, pneumonia, coronary thrombosis, acute renal failure, renal or biliary colics, cerebral hemorrhages, ischias, malarial coma, erysipelas, porphyria, lead poisoning, etc.

Ex juvantibus therapy may be of value in differential diagnosis, i.e., specific antivenin and calcium i.v. The cutaneous histamine test, in which an i.d. injection of histamine at the site of the bite is made, and the usual histamine reaction, i.e., the large, intensively red zone, fails to develop (MARETIĆ and JELAŠIĆ, 1953), can also be used.

Table 2. Differential diagnosis between latrodectism and acute abdomen conditions (Modified from SAMPAYO, 1942)

	Latrodectism	Acute abdomen
1. Anamnesis: report of spider bite; local findings	May be positive	Negative
2. Anamnesis: gastric troubles	Negative except by coincidence	Mostly positive
3. Collapse or shock	Not frequent	Frequent
4. Blood pressure	Increased	Low or normal
5. Facies	*Facies latro-dectismica*	Sometimes *facies abdominalis*
6. Localization of pains in the abdomen	Usually absent	Present
7. Radiologically, air in abdominal cavity	Negative·	May be positive
8. Rigidity of musculature	Positive	Negative
9. Pains in thighs and feet	Positive	Negative
10. Motoric restlessness, anxiety	Positive	Negative

IV. Clinical Course, Duration of Hospitalization, Convalescence, and Complications

1. Course

As mentioned above, the most acute symptoms usually last 24—48 h in untreated patients. Then most of the symptoms are mitigated; the pains appear only in fits, descending to the lower extremities where an intense burning of the soles is felt, as clearly described by GAJARDO-TOBAR (1941).

In untreated patients the illness lasts altogether about a week or even less (KOBERT, 1901; GAJARDO-TOBAR, 1941; SAMPAYO, 1942; MARETIĆ, 1959; SAVOURA, 1962). The duration of hospitalization, however, depends, besides the medical indications, also upon various psychological, socioeconomic and other factors.

Patients treated adequately with antivenin recover rapidly, and for them, as well as for those treated with muscle relaxants, hospitalization may not be needed, or may last only 1—2 days (RUSSELL et al., 1973).

2. Convalescence

In latrodectism convalescence is long and characterized by an asthenic and often neurasthenic syndrome. Patients suffer from a feeling of weakness, fatigue, pains in various parts of body, headache, and sleeplessness. GAUD and DELESALLE (1949) recorded impotence lasting up to 4 months. The duration of the convalescence period, according to various authors, ranges from a fortnight to a few months and in exceptional cases even more than a year.

3. Complications

In latrodectism, complications are not frequent. Single cases of pulmonary edema (GAJARDO-TOBAR, 1950), thrombosis of the popliteal vein (SALEZ VAZQUEZ and BIOSCA FLORENSA, 1949), peripheral polyneuritis, and myositis (JACOBS, 1969) have been noted. Some symptoms of latrodectism itself, if severely accentuated, can be regarded as complications, such as acute psychoses, or they can lead to complications, especially in cases of preexisting illnesses of some organs and systems. Thus, the characteristic hypertension in latrodectism may provoke cerebral insult, failure of an hypertonic heart, or have a negative influence on cardiac lesions or coronary diseases. Furthermore, the toxin may cause complications in an *a priori* damaged kidney, severe emphysema, or poor general conditions.

V. Prognosis

Prognosis in latrodectism is generally good, although according to BOGEN (1932), in the United States of 613 cases reported 38 (6.17%) were fatal. It must by taken into consideration, however, that these statistics certainly did not include all cases with a favorable course which did not attract the attention of reporters, but which, if recorded, would have very significantly lowered the fatality rate. In our 177 patients, there were no deaths (MARETIĆ, 1966).

Fatal cases have been mentioned by old authors, such as CAIUS JULIUS SOLINUS and AVICENNA, and by a number of European, American, and South African authors from the end of 18th to the beginning of the 20th century (KOBERT, 1901; PHISALIX, 1922; PAWLOWSKY, 1923; VELLARD, 1936; THORP and WOODSON, 1945). In the more recent literature, fatalities were described, among others, by INGRAM and MUSGRAVE in Australia (1933), SAMPAYO in Argentina (1942), CONSTANT and GOUERE in Madagascar (1948), GAJARDO-TOBAR in Chile (1950), and BARRA in Italy (1953).

VI. Post-Mortem Findings

Data on post-mortem findings in latrodectism are very scarce. BOGEN (1926) wrote that he was not able to find in the available literature data a single fatal case in the USA in which a post-mortem was performed. The only paper where a more detailed autopsy finding is presented is that of GAJARDO-TOBAR (1950). A severe pulmonary edema, a very marked hyperemia of pia and the brain, edema of medullary pia, and hyperemia of the liver and kidneys, and cortex of the adrenal glands and other organs were found in a 15-is-year-old boy.

The scarce data on post-mortem examinations of human cases can partially and eventually be replaced by histopathologic findings on experimental animals. In guinea pigs and rats there were found subdural hematomas, hyperemia, and edema of the brain; in the lungs edema with emphysema in the early stage and edema with atelectatic zones in the later stage; hyperemia, eventually parenchymatous degeneration of myocardium, fresh ulcerations in the stomach and parenchymatous degeneration and necrotic zones in the liver; hyperemia and edema of kidneys with degeneration and even necrosis of tubular epithelium; pyknosis and karyorrhexis in thymus and decay of lymphocytes in the spleen and lymphatic nodes; signs of exhaustion of the hypophysis but also accumulation of still undifferentiated main cells, indicating a renewal of their function; enlargement of the adrenals with hyperemia of the medulla and an enlarged zona fasciculata and zona reticularis and a thin zona glomerulosa. The pathohistological findings in the thyroid, parathyroids, ovaries, testes, and parotid glands did not show significant alterations (MARŽAN, 1955).

AGOSTINI and CANTORE (1958) described the CNS histopathological picture observed in guinea pigs injected with lethal doses of venom: congestion of all vessels, especially in the pial and choroid plexi, general edema, subarachnoid hemorrhages, acute alterations of the trunc and medullary nerve cells, and ischemic alterations of Purkinje's cells.

The characteristic conjunctivitis which accompanies the symptoms of latrodectism in man and in other mammalians has been studied in the rat by BETTINI and CANTORE (1959) through histological examination of the eye tissues in the various phases of intoxication. No lesions could be observed except *hyperemia* of the conjunctiva.

VII. Aspecific Therapy

The old ideas how to treat latrodectism have been maintained up to the present by popular methods originating from most ancient, times described by the early authors. They are mainly based on inducing physical exertion and on provoking vasodilatation by various means.

The old methods of curing spider bites by physical strain date back from the times of the ancient tarantism and consisted of dancing or swinging on ropes, which was also performed in recent times in Tigrea (Abyssinia). If one eliminates all the superstitions, simulations, and other deformations, these methods also surely have their pathophysiological foundations, as has been discussed by MARETIĆ and LEBEZ (1970).

Vasodilatation also has its justification as retained by old and present folklore medicine. It is provoked either by alcoholic drinks or by heat, such as warm baths or even by heating in ovens or by burning with fire (KOBERT, 1901; VELLARD, 1936; GAUD and DELESALLE, 1949).

Some of the old authors also used opiates to alleviate the pains (KOBERT, 1901).

According to BOGEN (1956), in the more recent medical literature more than 100 different drugs are used for latrodectism. The length of this list points to the little use that most of them have. Some of them, such as caffein, adrenaline and strychnine can even be harmful. Extensive local treatments should especially be avoided, for burning, cutting, or applying various chemicals can be the source of secondary infection, while no medicinal value can be expected due to rapid spreading of the venom.

Morphine is not very efficacious in combating pains in latrodectism, and even to achieve modest results, it must be applied in heavy doses (BOGEN, 1932; KEEGAN, 1958; MARETIĆ, 1959). According to some authors, its depressive action on respiratory centers may be disadvantageous in latrodectism, whose neurotoxic action could eventually have a paralytic effect on respiratory centers. The same applies to barbiturates (SAMPAYO, 1942). For alleviating pains, authors such as RUSSELL et al. (1973) recommend meperidine hydrochloride (Demerol), 50 – 100 mg. SAMPAYO (1942) used chloralhydrate in clysma in cases involving children.

As symptomatic treatment, hot baths, cardiotonics, rehydration diuretics, diaphoretics, and laxatives can be used. Alcohol is contraindicated, and even a fatal termination after its use has been recorded (FINLAYSON, 1937).

Authors are not unanimous in interpreting the effects obtained with antihistamines. BETTINI and CANTORE (1954) obtained a certain protective effect in about 33% of experimental guinea pigs with antihistamines, as well as with Largactil.

Various authors recommended neostigmine methyl sulphate (BELL and BOONE, 1945, physostigmine + atropine = Phyatromine (HOLLOWAY, 1950), or atropine alone (GOTTLIEB and FRIED, 1964), considering the cholinesterase-inhibiting effect of physostigmine and the muscarine-inhibiting effect of atropine as relaxants of the contracted musculature. Specific muscular relaxants, such as D-tubocurarin, Tensilon, and succinylcholine chloride (ALLEN, 1953; TAUSSIG, 1956), used carefully in regard to the side-effects on respiratory musculature, were also recommended. RUSSELL (1962) described favorable results with mephenesin and RUSSELL (1962) and LI (1960) with methocarbamol (Robaxin). In experimental mice, mephenesin and D-tubocurarin decreased the rigidity of musculature but not the fatality rate (VALJEVAC et al., 1972). Procaine used intravenously, as recommended by ARUSTAMYAN (1965), gives a significant but only a very transient relief. However, its local infiltration can be useful in single cases of local pains (MARETIĆ and STANIĆ, 1954).

The idea of application of corticosteroids and ACTH in latrodectism is quite logical. As shown previously, the clinical picture is composed not only of very specific symptoms but also of a series of quite nonspecific signs and symptoms, provoked by the neurotoxin of *Latrodectus* which, like many other toxins, acts as strong stressor. Certain favorable effects of these drugs were described not only on experimental animals (BETTINI and CANTORE, 1954) but also on patients (MARETIĆ, 1953); however, the effect of this treatment falls behind the effect of calcium and still more behind the specific treatment. Observing the treated patients clinically, it seems like the drugs do not act by interrupting the course of latrodectism but by accelerating its course and recovery. On experimental rats the treatment with corticosteroids significantly prolonged the time of survival (MARETIĆ and STANIĆ, 1954).

Magnesium sulphate, if given i.v., causes sweating, flushing, and a feeling of warmth due to cutaneous vasodilation. In high concentrations it provokes a strong depression of all parts of the central nervous system and the neuromuscular apparatus, and by decreasing the muscular spasm, it prevents convulsions, has an antispastic effect upon the smooth musculature of small blood vessels, and decreases the blood pressure. DE ASIS (1934) in the Philippines was the first to use it in latrodectism. As the feeling of warmth progresses, the pains of latrodectism also disappear. The negative side of this treatment is that the symptoms return soon, and the injection of the drug cannot be repeated too often, since the therapeutic doses are close to the toxic. Calcium which is a magnesium antidote, should be held ready when administering this substance.

Calcium, however, has even a stronger effect on latrodectism. It was first used for this purpose in 1935 by GILBERT and STEWART. Calcium decreases the irritability of cells and increases the impermeability of cell membranes. It has a depressive effect on the neuromuscular platelets on which the *Latrodectus* toxin also acts. Calcium activates cholinesterase, hindering the nervous and muscular stimulation. Various salts of calcium, such as chlorate, gluconate, bromate, and Calcihept, were used. The intravenous injection has a much more rapid effect than the intramuscular one. Pains and spasms disappear readily as calcium is injected in the vein, provoking vasodilatation. If pains reappear, the injection can be repeated. Some authors were so impressed with the effect of calcium that they considered it to be a sufficient remedy for latrodectism (Škarica, 1949; Greer, 1949). No doubt calcium is a very valuable drug in combating latrodectism, but specific antivenin remains the drug of choice for inducing an irreversible disappearance of symptoms.

VIII. Specific Therapy

1. Preparation of Sera

Latrodectus venom has antigenic properties to such an extent that antibodies can even be transferred from mother animals to their descendents (Cantore and Bettini, 1957). Though the process is altogether different, an immune response was also shown in insects (Bettini, 1965). However, in rare instances where humans were bitten on two occasions by *Latrodectus,* no immunity could be observed (Maretić, 1959); in one case even an anaphylactic shock developed (Dameski and Massin, 1960). Therapeutic trials with convalescent sera gave no satisfactory results (Bogen, 1932; Maretić, 1951).

As early as 1901, Kobert thought of producing *Latrodectus* antivenin using the whole spider body extract as an antigen, since he believed that the venom spread equally thoughout the whole body.

In 1903, the Russian author Shcherbina immunized camels, first with direct bites and then with extracts of cephalathoraxes of *L. tredecimguttatus*. This antivenin was able to save camels, which are very sensitive towards the venom, intoxicated with doses 13 times higher than the lethal dose. Even better results were obtained by Konstansov in 1904 (Pawlowsky, 1927).

The Argentines Houssay and Negrette (1918) prepared an antivenin from rabbits by direct bites.

In Brasil, Troise (1928) immunized rabbits with the toxin from venomous glands, showing that 0.05 ml of this serum could protect a guinea pig to which an extract of one-third of the venom gland was given intravenously.

Becker and D'Amour (1934) in the USA produced antilatrodectic sera from white rats for experimental purposes. In 1936, D'Amour showed that the protective power of the serum from hyperimmunized white mice was by far higher than that of convalescent serum.

In South Africa, Finlayson (1936b) prepared rabbit and goat sera against the venom of *L. mactans indistinctus, L. mactans concinnus,* and *L. geometricus.* With *L. mactans indistinctus* antivenin, it was possible to treat bites of all three species. One ml of the goat serum was able to protect a 350 g guinea pig from 150 animal lethal doses subcutaneously (1 MLD = 2.0 mg of the venom of *L. geometricus* or 0.5 of *L. indistinctus*). A total of 18 patients treated with this serum were cured within

24 h. A 5 ml dose of antivenin was given i.m. to all patients except one. In 1949, the South African Institute for Medical Research prepared a refined and concentrated *L. indistinctus* and *L. geometricus* antivenin from horses, 1 ml of which could neutralize 400—600 lethal doses for mice.

In 1938, Smith Dorm and D'Amour in the USA prepared an antilatrodectic serum from rabbit by injecting 150 toxic doses during 11 weeks in one animal and 3000 toxic doses during 6 months in another. One ml of these antivenins could protect 50% of the rats from four and five median lethal doses, respectively.

Maxianovich (1939), from Usbekh USSR, prepared an antivenin from horse first using an anatoxin obtained by treating the venom with heat and formaldehyde and then the direct bites of up to 40 spiders simultaneously. With this antivenin he was able to cure guinea pigs bitten by two to three *Latrodectus* (kara kurt) spiders. In 1941—1942 the Argentines Pirosky, Sampayo, and Franceschi produced a purified antivenin by immunizing horses with extracts of cephalothoraxes. One ml was able to protect a guinea pig from 3000 median lethal doses. Following i.m. application of 5 ml, patients recovered within a few hours.

In the USA Sharp and Dohme began in the 1940s to produce Lyovac, a refined and purified lyophilized horse serum using frozen extracts of macerated venom glands as an antigen. One ml contained 4000 units, one unit being the amount which mixed with 1 LD_{50} of venom and able to ensure a survival at least for 72 h for 50% of 11 g mice.

In 1951 in Pula (Yugoslavia), Maretić produced an antivenin from rabbits using direct bites. At the end of immunization the serum animals were able to survive even 120 bites simultaneously. One ml of this serum was able to neutralize in vitro 100 DCL (*dosis certe letalis*) for mice. In 12 patients treated with this serum following i.m. injection of 5—10 ml, a significant amelioration ensued within 4—5 h and a complete recovery within 12 h.

In 1952 at the Central Hygiene Institute of Croatia in Zagreb (Yugoslavia), Stanić prepared an antivenin using macerates of the anterior part of spider cephalothoraxes as an antigen; 0.1 ml of this serum neutralized in vitro 4 DCL for mice. Later, the serum was also prepared from donkeys.

The i.v. injection of this serum in patients provoked a significant relief in 10—20 min and a recovery practically in 2—3 h. The effect of intramuscular application was of course slower.

In 1953 in Rome (Italy), Bettini, Ravaioli, and Cantore produced an antivenin from rabbits and later from sheep. As an antigen they first used homogenates of venomous glands and later of cephalothoraxes: 0.017 ml of the antivenin was able to protect a 250 g guinea pig from 5 ml LD_{50} of venom applied subcutaneously. A patient treated with this antivenom intramuscularly recovered in a few hours (Bettini and Calcara, 1953). Several patients have been treated in Italy with the lyophilized antivenom prepared at the Istituto Superiore di Sanità, Rome, Italy.

In 1956 Wiener in Australia used the venom of *L. mactans hasselti* absorbed on aluminium phosphate at pH 5.0 as an antigen for preparing an antivenin from rabbits. On ml of this serum was able to neutralize 75 LD_{50} for mice intraperitoneally.

The Russian author Chepurov and his collaborators (1959) developed an antivenin against the venom of kara kurt.

At the present time, according to data available, the production of antilatrodectic sera is still maintained in the USA (Lyovac prepared by Merck and Sharp and Dohme Co.), in the South African Union by the Institute for Medical Research in Johannesburg, and in Italy by the Istituto Superiore di Sanità in Rome.

2. Cross Activity of Sera Obtained with Antigens from Different Species of Spiders

It appears that spider venoms and their antivenins are higly specific. For instance, an anti-*Lycosid* or anti-*Ctenus* serum has no effect upon the envenomation of *Latrodectus* and vice versa. There is not even a cross-immunity among toxins of *L. mactans tredecimguttatus* and *Steatoda paykulliana,* though both species not only belong to the same family but also produce signs and symptoms of the same type, although those provoked by *S. paykulliana* are of less intensity (MARETIĆ et al., 1964).

The positive effect of a spider antivenin on a toxin can also be used as a test for the relationship with other species.

It has been shown that a cross-activity between sera and toxins exists within some species and subspecies of the genus *Latrodectus.* The antivenin produced by immunization with the venom of *L. mactans indistinctus,* for instance, also neutralizes the venom of the other species, such as *L. geometricus* (FINLAYSON, 1956). The same experiments on animals, such as therapeutic trials with antivenin produced in different countries with antigens of different subspecies, did show that there exists a cross-immunity among subspecies *L. mactans tredecimguttatus, L. mactans hasselti, L. mactans indistinctus,* and *L. mactans mactans* (MARETIĆ, 1953; KEEGAN, 1955; GAJARDO-TOBAR, 1956; CANTORE and BETTINI, 1957).

3. Time and Dose of Serum Administration

The advantage of anti-latrodectic sera, if compared with some other antivenins, such as the antiophidics, lies in the fact that the response is very prompt, that it ensues a *restitutio ad integrum,* and that the antivenin acts equally efficiently in every phase of the intoxication. As reported in previous chapters, after administration of an effective anti-latrodectic serum a significant relief can be obtained from half an hour to a few hours following intramuscular administration and even in 10 – 20 min following intravenous injection. Complete recovery usually ensues within 12 h. In administrating the serum, especially intravenously, all usual measures of precaution should be followed. The dosage of antivenins should be 2 – 5 ml.

But there is a method, as recommended by D.G. MILLER Jr. (1949), which gives even better results. If one first applies calcium intravenously, the pains disappear almost immediately. If calcium is followed closely by antivenin (especially intravenously) the action of antivenin begins sooner, and the patient shows a dramatic recovery within the short time necessary to manipulate the syringes.

According to RUSSELL et al. (1973), the application of serum intravenously and hospitalization is indicated in all patients below 16 or over 60 years, in those with hypertensive heart disease or in those with symptoms and signs of severe intoxication. In other patients they recommend 10 ml of methocarbamol (Robaxin) i.v. over a 5-min period followed by another 5 or 10 ml in a drip of 250 ml of 5% dextrose in water. If relief ensues, 500 mg of Robaxin every 6 h for 24 h should be given.

In cases of persistent local pains, which is rare, ice (RUSSELL et al., 1973) or infiltration with 1% procaine (MARETIĆ and STANIĆ, 1954) can be applied locally.

If antivenin or Robaxin is not available, treatment with calcium should be considered first.

IX. Prevention of Latrodectism

In countries where latrodectism has a rural character, mechanization of agricultural practices offers the best protection from the bite of these spiders. Suitable protective clothing for farmers should also be taken into consideration (BOGEN and LOOMIS, 1936).

With the disappearence of old-fashioned privies in other countries, for instance, the possibilities of man-spider contacts have decreased. Before the appearence of modern insecticides, physical destruction of spiders and cobwebs was the best method for combating them (BOGEN and LOOMIS, 1936).

Though laboratory trials cannot be compared with field experiments, insecticides exist today which could be used especially in peri-domestic infestations of spiders. DDT, Gammexane, Ethiol, and ortho-Dibrom have been shown to be active, but only at high doses (MARETIĆ and STANIĆ, 1954; MARETIĆ, 1959).

KNOWLTON (1967) recommends the following rules for the control of *L. mactans mactans:* sealing of small openings through which the spider could enter the home, removing the litter in which the black widow could hide, and destroying of individual spiders and coccoons by spraying 18% Dieldrin and 75% Chlordane, one-third pint in each 3 gallons of mixed spray. Lindane is also recommended.

References

Abalos, J.W., Baez, E.C.: The spider genus *Latrodectus* in Santiago dell Estero, Argentina. In: Animal Toxins. Russell, F.E. and Saunders, P.R. (eds.). Oxford-New York: Pergamon Press, 1967.

Agostini, L., Cantore, G.P.: Le alterazioni del sistema nervoso centrale di cavia intossicata col veleno di *Latrodectus tredecimguttatus*-Rossi. Riv. Neurol. **28**, 391−398 (1958).

Allen, G.W.: Black widow poisoning treated with d-tubocurarine chloride. Ann. intern. Med. **39**, 624−628 (1953).

Arustamyan, A.T.: The treatment of patients bitten by kara kurt with procaine intravenously. Med. Paraz. Bol. **24**, 355−357 (1955). In Russian.

Avicenna: Canon medicinae. Basel, 1556.

Baerg, W.J.: Effect of bite of *Latrodectus mactans* (Fabricius). J. Parasit. **9**, 161−169 (1923).

Baerg, W.J.: The brown widow and the black widow spiders in Jamaica. Ann. ent. Soc. Amer. **47**, 52−60 (1954).

Barkagan, Z.S.: On changes in blood pressure and tonus of vessels in patiens bitten by the venomous spider kara kurt. Terap. Arh. **28**, 45−51 (1956). In Russian.

Barra, S.: Su un caso di morte in seguito a morso di *Latrodectus malmignatus*. Boll. Soc. ital. Biol. sper. **33**, 34 (1957).

Barton, Ch.: How it feels to be bitten by a black widow. A case history. Nat. Hist. **42**, 43−44 (1938).

Becker, F.E., D'Amour, F.E.: Anti-serum against black widow spider venom. Proc. Soc. exp. Biol. (N.Y.) **32**, 166−167 (1934).

Bell, J.E., Boone, J.A.: Neostigmine methylsulphate, an apparent specific for arachnidism (black widow spider bite). J. Amer. med. Ass. **129**, 1016−1017 (1945).

Berland, L.: Les arachnides. Encyclopédie Entomologique 1:485. Paris: Lechevalier, P. and Fils (eds.)., 1932.

Bettini, S.: Indagine sui casi di latrodectismo verificatisi negli anni dal 1938 al 1958 in alcune province d'Italia. V. Nota riassuntiva. Riv. Parassit. **24**, 31−43 (1963).

Bettini, S.: Considerazioni su di un fenomeno epidemico di latrodectismo in Italia. Riv. Parassit. **24**, 105−118 (1963).

Bettini, S.: Epidemiology of latrodectism. Toxicon **2**, 93−102 (1964).

Bettini, S.: Acquired immune response of the house fly, *Musca domestica* (Linnaeus) to injected venom of the spider *Latrodectus mactans tredecimguttatus* (Rossi). J. Invertebr. Path. **7** (3), 378−383 (1965).

Bettini, S., Antonini, E., Cantore, G.: La terapia del morso di *Latrodectus 13-guttatus* Rossi. Nota II.−Cinque nuovi casi di latrodectismo trattati con gluconato di calcio endovena. Arch. ital. Soc. Med. Trop. Parassit. **34**, 579−587 (1953).

Bettini, S., Calcara, S.: Terapia del morso di *Latrodectus tredecimguttatus* Rossi. Nota I.−Sul primo caso di latrodectismo trattato con siero immune in Italia. Riv. Parassit. **17**, 186−189 (1956).

Bettini, S., Cantore, G.: Sull azione prottetiva dell'ACTH, del cortisone, del gluconato di calcio, della pirilamina (Neoantergan), della prometiazina (Fargan), dalla cloropromazina (Largactil) nel latrodectismo indotto nella cavia. Riv. Parassit., **15**, 259−265 (1954).

Bettini, S., Cantore, G.: Quadro clinico del latrodectismo. Riv. Parassit. **20**, 49−72 (1959).

Bettini, S., Ravaioli, L., Cantore, G.: Nota preliminare sulla preparazionè di un siero immune specifico verso il veleno di *"Latrodectus 13-guttatus"* Rossi. Rend. Ist. Sup. San. **17**, 192−199 (1954).

Blagodarny, Ya.A.: On clinic and treatment of kara kurt bites. Klin. Med. **35**, 76−79 (1957). In Russian.

Blair, A.W.: Spider poisoning, experimental study of the effect of the bite of the female *Latrodectus mactans* in man. Arch. intern. Med. **54**, 831−834 (1934).

Boccone, S.: Museo di fis. e di esperienze. Venezia, 1687, quoted by Kobert, 1901.

Bogen, E.: Arachnidism. A study in spider poisoning. Arch. intern. Med. **38**, 623−634 (1926).

Bogen, E.: Poisonous spider bites. Ann. intern. Med. **6**, 375−388 (1932).

Bogen, E.: The treatment of spider bite poisoning. In: Venoms. Buckley, E.E. and Porges, N. (eds.). Berkeley: Amer. Ass. Advanc. Sci (1956).

Bogen, E., Loomis, R.N.: Poisoning poisonous spiders. Calif. west. Med. 45:31 (1936).

Bonnet, P.: Bibliographia araneorum (3 Vols.). Toulouse: Les Frères Douladoure, 1945−1961.

Bouisset, L., Larrouy, G.: Envenimation par *Latrodectus tredecimguttatus* Rossi, varieté *lugubris* L. Dufour. Presse méd. **70**, 1019−1020 (1962).

Braun, G.: Über *Latrodectus tredecimguttatus*. Wien. med. Presse No. **6**, 223−224 (1899).

Bristowe, W.S.: The world of spiders. London: Collins (St. James Place), 1958.

Brown, W.L.: Spider bite, case report. Sthwest. Med. **8**, 131−132 (1924).

Bücherl, W.: *Latrodectus* e latrodectismo na America do Sul. Mem. Inst. Butantan **32**, 95−100 (1965).

Bücherl, W.: *Latrodectus* e latrodectismo na America do Sul. Rev. Bras. Pequi. méd. biol. **1**, 83−88 (1968).

Cantore, G.P., Bettini, S.: Preparazione di un siero anti-*Latrodectus*. Riv. Parassit. **18**, 202−206 (1957a).

Cantore, G., Bettini, S.: Transmissione del potere immunitario anti-*Latrodectus* dalla madre al feto. Riv. Parassit. **18**, 206−207 (1957b).

Cantore, G.P., Bettini, S.: Contributo allo studio dell'azione farmacologica del veleno di *Latrodectus tredecimguttatus* Rossi, III. Azione sul ritmo cardiaco e sul circolo arterioso. Riv. Parassit **19**, 301−306, 1958.

Celsus, A.C.: De medicina. Vol. 2. Cambridge: Harvard University Press, 1953, p. 14.

Chellini, 1728; cited by Kobert, 1901.

Chepurov, K.P., Arkhangelski, J.J., Shatokin, N.G., Mnatsakanian, V.B.: Antitoxin against the kara kurt (*Latrodectus lugubris*) poison. Veterin. Moscow. **36**, 55, 1959.

Chyzer and Kulczynski, 1892., 1897., quoted by Bonnet.

Cicardo, V.H.: Mecanismo de la hipertension arterial producida por la ponzona de *Latrodectus mactans*. Rev. Soc. argent. Biol. **30**, 19−24 (1954).

Constant, Y., Gouere, P.: Sur les phénomènes d'aranéisme provoqués par *Latrodectus menavodi*. Bull. Soc. Path. Exot. **41**, 234—237 (1948).

Čučković, S.: Prestanak plavljenja Popovog polja uslovio je pojavu malminjata pjegavog. Priroda **62**, 277—282 (1973).

Dameski, D., Masin, G.: Patogeneza i terapija na šok predizvikan od povtorno kasnuvanje na pajakot — *Latrodectus tredecimguttatus* Rossi. Maked. med. pregl. **15**, 389—392 (1960).

Damin, N.: *Latrodectus 13-guttatus* Rossi. knj. 126, Zagreb: Rad JAZU 1896.

Damin, N.: Prilog fauni dalmatinskih i istarskih pauka. knj. 128, Zagreb: Rad JAZU, 1896.

Damin, N.: Pauci Dalmacije, Hrvatske, Slavonije i Istre. knj. 143, Zagreb: Rad JAZU, 1900.

D'Amour, E.F.: A comparative essay of black widow antisera. Proc. Soc. exp. Biol. (N.Y.) **35**, 262, 1936.

De Asis, C.: Red-back spider bite and magnesium sulfate treatment (A clinical study of four cases). Amer. J. trop. Med. **14**, 13—14 (1934).

De Meillon, B., Gear, J.: A Note on three noxious arthropods occuring on the Witwatersrand. S. Afr. med. J. **21**, 407—411 (1947).

Desportes, C.: "*Latrodectus schuchi*", araignée venimeuse du Maroc. Arch. Inst. Pasteur Maroc **1**, 651—655 (1937).

Dioscorides, Pedanius, quoted by Kobert, 1901.

Drensky, P.: *Latrodectus 13-guttatus*, eine giftige Spinne aus Bulgaria. Mitt. Landw. Min. Bulg., Zbl. Bakt. **17**, 9—11 (1928).

Eason, R.R., Peck, W.B., Whitcomb, W.H.: Notes on spider parasites including of reference list. J. Kansas ent. Soc. **40**, 422—434 (1967).

Escomel, E.: Le *Latrodectus mactans* ou "Lucacha" au Perou. Etude clinique et expérimentale de l'action du venin. Bull. Soc. Path. Exot. **12**, 702—720 (1919).

Finlayson, M.H.: "Knoppie-Spider" bite. S. Afr. med. J. **10**, 43—45 (1936a).

Finlayson, M.H.: "Knoppie-Spider" antivenene. S. Afr. med. J. **10**, 735—736 (1936b).

Finlayson, M.H.: Some properties of the venon and arachnolysin of *Latrodectus indistinctus*. S. Afr. J. med. Sci. **2**, 151—155 (1937).

Finlayson, M.H.: "Knoppie-Spider" bite in Southern Africa, Med. Proc. **2**, 634—638 (1956).

Finlayson, M.H., Hollow, K.: Treatment of spider-bite in South Africa by specific antisera. S. Afr. med. J. **19**, 431—433 (1945).

Frank, L.: The black widow spider syndrome. Mil. Surg. **91**, 329—336 (1942).

Fuhn, J.E.: Vaduva Neagra-*Latrodectus mactans tredecimguttatus* (Rossi, 1790) peinsula Popina (Razelm). Ocrotirea Naturii **10**, 77—81 (1966). In Romanian.

Gajardo-Tobar, R.: El latrodectismo. Prensa Med. **6**, 3—18 (1941).

Gajardo-Tobar, R.: Algo mas sobre latrodectismo. Rev. med. Valparaiso **3**, 150—159 (1950).

Gajardo-Tobar, R.: Die spezifische Natur der Antiseren gegen Spinnengifte. Acta trop. (Basel) **13**, 82—85 (1956).

Gaud, J., Delessale, D.: Aranéisme dû aux morsures de Latrodectes au Maroc. Bull. Inst. Hyg. Maroc. **9**, 233—237 (1949).

Gennari, G.: Sindrome addominale da morso di aracnide simulante l'ulcera gastrica o duodenale perforata. Il Policlinico **59**, 1—9 (1952).

Gilbert, E.W., Stewart, C.M.: Effective treatment of arachnidism with calcium salts; Preliminary report. Amer. J. med. Sci. **189**, 532—536 (1935).

Ginsburg, H.M.: Black widow spider bite, Report of 44 cases. Calif. west. Med. **46**, 381—386 (1937).

Gottlieb, A.F., Fried, A.: A cases of black widow spider bite treated by atropine. Harefuah, J. Israel med. Ass. **68**, 223—224 (1964).

Graëlls de la Paz, M.: Sur les accidents provoqués en Catalogne par le Theridion malmignatte. Ann. Soc. ent. Fr. III, 1834, quoted by Bogen.

Greer, W.E.R.: Arachnidism. New Engl. J. Med., **240**, 5—8 (1949).

Grujić, I.: Otrovni pauci kod nas, Život i zdravlje. **13**, 12—16 (1959).

Gundrum-Oriovčanin, F.S.: Ugriz od pauka. Lij. vj. **21**, 83—84 (1899).

Guzman, C.: Progr. med., 1896 (Chile). An. Admin. Sanit. Asist. Pub. **6**:423 (1910), quoted by Bonnet.

Hagan, H.: Arachnidism (spider poisoning). Kentucky Med., J., 36:120 (1938), quoted by Sampayo, 1942.

Hargraves, W.H., Mackenzie, K.G.F.: Spider bite simulating acute abdomen. J. roy. Army med. Corps. **78**:37 (1942).

Holloway, O.R.: The use of physostigmine in the treatment of the black spider bite. J. Ark. med. Soc. **47**, 75—76 (1950).

Houssay, B.A., Negrete, J.: Estudios esperimentales sobre la accion de los venenos de las arañas. Trab. Soc. Biol. Barc., 4:194 (1918), quoted by Sampayo, 1942.

Ingram, W.W., Musgrave, A.: Spider bite (Arachnidism). Survey of its occurence in Australia with case histories. Med. J. Aust. **2**, 10—15 (1933).

Jacobs, W.: Possible peripheral neuritis following a black widow spider bite. Short communications, Toxicon **6**, 299—230 (1969).

Jovanovski, V., Radojković, M., Niča, K.: Povodom 6 slučajeva neurotoksičnog sindroma izazvanog ujedom insekta. Srp. arh. **84**, 673—677 (1956).

Junqua, C., Vachon, M.: Les arahnides venimeux et leurs venins. Etat actuel des recherches. Bruselles: Acad. roy. Sci. Outre Mer., 1968.

Kakuškin, N.: Otrovni pauci. Priroda **19**, 289—292 (1932).

Keegan, H.L.: Geographic distribution of *Latrodectus hasselti*. Amer. J. trop. Med. Hyg. **1 (8)**, 1043—1046 (1952).

Keegan, H.L.: Effectiveness of *Latrodectus tredecimguttatus* antivenin in protecting laboratory mice against effects of intraperitoneal injections of *Latrodectus mactans* venom. Amer. J. trop. med. Hyg. **4 (4)**, 762—764 (1955).

Keegan, H.L.: Some venomous animals of the Far East. 406th Med. Gen. Lab., Camp Zama, Japan, 7—11 (1958).

Keegan, H.L.: Some venomous and noxious animals of the Far East. 406th Med. Gen. Lab., San Francisco, 10—13 (1960).

Keegan, H.L., Weaver, R.E., Toshioka, S., Matsui, T.: Some venomous and noxious animals of East and Southern Asia. 406th. Med. Labor. Japan (spec. rep.), 1—43 (1964).

Kellaway, C.H.: The venom of *Latrodectus hasselti*. Med. J. Aust. **1**, 41—46 (1930).

Knowlton, G.F.: Black widow spider. Entomol. mimeo ser. No. 78, Utah. St. Univ., Logan, 1967.

Kobert, R.: Beiträge zur Kenntnis der Giftspinnen. Stuttgart: Ferd. Enke Verl., 1901.

Kolben, 1719, quoted by Kobert, 1901.

Kolosvary, 1935, quoted by Bonnet.

Lebez, D., Maretić, Z., Gubenšek, F., Kristan, J.: Studies on labeled animal poisons. IV: Incorporation of SE_{75} and P_{32} in spider venoms. Biološki vestnik **16**, 11—15 (1968).

Lebez, D., Maretić, Z., Kristan, J.: Studies of labeled animal poisons. I: Distribution of P_{32} labeled *Latrodectus tredecimguttatus* venom in guinea-pig. Toxicon **2**, 251—253 (1965).

Leffkowitz, M., Kadish, U., Stern, J.: Spider bite. Dapim Refuiim (special issue), **21**, 4—12 (1962).

Lepilova, A.S.: The clinic of the disease provoked by the bite of kara kurt. Klin. Med. **33**, 80—82 (1955). In Russian.

Levi, H.W.: The spider genus *Latrodectus* (Araneae, Theridiidae). Trans. Amer. micr. Soc. **78 (1)**, 7—43 (1959).

Li, J.R.: Methocarbamol in the treatment of black widow spider poisoning. J. Amer. med. Ass. (1960).

Maretić, Z.: Toksičnost pauka *Tarentula apuliae*. Lij. vj. **71**, 169—172 (1949).

Maretić, Z.: Araneizam u Istri kao praktični problem. Lij. vj. **73**, 203—208 (1951).

Maretić, Z.: Arachnidism treated with cortisone. J. Amer. med. Ass. **152, 169** (1953).

Maretić, Z.: Medicinsko značenje ujeda paukova u našim krajevima. Med. glas. **9**, 159—163 (1955).

Maretić, Z.: Araneizam—sosobitimosvrtom na Istru. Thesis, Med. Faculty Univ. Zagreb, 1959.

Maretić, Z.: Electrocardiographic changes in man and experimental animals provoked by the venom of *Latrodectus tredecimguttatus*. Toxicon **1**, 127—130 (1963).

Maretić, Z.: Latrodectism, Bull. International Yugosl. Acad. Sci. Arts, **17**, 63—87. Zagreb, 1966.

Maretić, Z.: Latrodectism in Mediterranean countries including south Russia, Israel and North Africa, In: Venomous Animals and their venoms. Bücherl, W. and Buckley, E.E. (eds.). Vol. 3., New York-London: Academic Press, 1971.

Maretić, Z., Jelašić, F.: Über den Einfluß des Toxins der Spinne *Latrodectus tredecimguttatus* auf das Nervensystem. Acta trop. (Basel) **10**, 209−224 (1953).

Maretić, Z., Lebez, D.: *Lycosa tarentula* in fact and fiction. Bull. Mus. Nat. Hist. Natur. ser. 2, **41 (1)**, 260−266 (1970).

Maretić, Z., Levi, H.W., Levi, L.R.: The theridiid spider *Steatoda paykulliana* poisonous to mammals. Toxicon **2**, 149−154 (1964).

Maretić, Z., Stanić, M.: The health problem of arachnidism. Bull. Wld Hlth Org. **11**, 1007−1022 (1954).

Marikovskij, P.I.: Tarantula and karakurt, Acad. Sci. Circassian Sov. Soc. Rep., Frunze 1956.

Marmocchi, F.: Memoria sopra il ragno rosso dell'agro Volterrano. Atti Ac. Sci. Siena **8**, 218 (1800).

Maržan, B.: Pathologic reactions associated with bite of *Latrodectus tredecimguttatus*. Observations on experimental animals. Arch. Path. (Chicago) **59**, 727−728 (1955).

Maxianowitch, M.J.: Le venin du kara-kourte, *Latrodectus 13-guttatus* agissant comme antigène, effectivité de l'antitoxine dans les experiences sur les animaux. Med. Parasitol., Parasit. Dis. Moscow, **8**, 51−64 (1939). In Russian.

Miller, D.G., Jr.: Reply to querries and minor notes. J. Amer. med. Ass. **139**, 1238 (1949).

Miller, D.G., Jr.: Bites and stings. G.P., **4**, 35−42 (1951).

Nikandros: Theriaka. In: Poetae bucolici et didactici. Paris: K.F. Ameis, 1851.

Orušev, T.: Lathrodectismus−po povod eden slučaj pri gravidna bolna. Maked. med. pregl. **13 (7−9)**, 40−45 (1958).

Pampiglione, S.: Il latrodectismo nella zona di Cerveteri. Nuov. An. Ig. Microbiol. **9**, 1−11 (1958).

Pampiglione, S.: Sulla "terapia musicale" dell' avvelenamento da puntura di imenotteri (Mutillidae) in Sardegna. Nuov. An. Ig. Microbiol., **9**, 1−2 (1958).

Pawlowsky, E.N.: Gifttiere und ihre Giftigkeit. Jena: G. Fischer Verl. (1927).

Phisalix, M.: Les animaux venimeux et venins. Vol. 1., Paris: Masson & Cie, 1922.

Plinius, Caius Secundus: Naturalis historia, Vol. VI. Leipzig: C. Mayhoff, 1897.

Prince, G.E.: Arachnidism in children. J. Pediat. **49**, 101−108 (1956).

Puga Borne, F.: Sobre la puesta del *Latrodectus formidabilis* de Chile, Act. Soc. Sc. du Chili. **5**, 202 (1875) quoted by Sampayo, 1942.

Ramzin, S.: Otrovni pauk *Latrodectus tredecimguttatus,* Vojnosan. pregl. **4**, 267−268 (1947).

Ravaioli, L., Cantore, G., Bettini, S.: Preparazione di un siero immune anti-*Latrodectus* per uso umano, Riv. Parassit. **18**, 202−206 (1957).

Rindone, G.: Pseudoaddome acuto a tipo appendicolare consequente a morso di aracnidi. Gior. Med., Mil., **2**, 144−150 (1947).

Rivosecchi, L., Bettini, S.: Contributo alla conoscenza dei predatori della ova di *Latrodectus tredecimguttatus* Rossi, Riv. Parassit. **19**, 249−265 (1958).

Roza, M., Soedibio, R.: *Latrodectus hasselti* Thorell, Hemera Zoa, Bogor. **58**, 169 (1950).

Russell, F.E.: Injuries by venomous animals in the United States, J. Amer. med. Ass. **177**, 903−907 (1961).

Russell, F.E.: Muscle relaxants in black widow spider (*Latrodectus mactans*) poisoning. Amer. J. med. Sci. **243**, 81/159, 83/161 (1962).

Russell, F.E., Wainschel, J., Gertsch, W.J.: Bites of spiders and other arthropods. In: Current Therapy. Conn, H.F., (ed.). Philadelphia-London-Toronto: W.B. Saunders Co., 1973.

Russell, F.E., Waldron, W.G.: Spider bites, tick bites. Letters to Editor, Calif. Med. **106**, 248−249 (1967).

Salez Vazquez, M., Biosca Florensa, M.: Contribucion al estudio del araneidismo. Med. clin. **12**, 244−249 (1949).

Sampayo, R.R.L.: *Latrodectus mactans* y latrodectismo. Buenos Aires: El Ateneo, 1942.

Sampayo, R.R.L.T.: Pharamacological action of the venom of *Latrodectus mactans* and other *Latrodectus* spiders. J. Pharmacol. exp. Ther. **80**, 309−322 (1944).

Savoura, A.: Contribution to the study of latrodectism in Greece. Thesis, Univ. of Athens, 1962. In Greek.

Schenone, H., Niedmann, G., Bahamonde, L., Bonnefoy, J.: Algunas alteraciones cardiovasculares observadas en el latrodectismo. Bol. Chil. Paras. **12**, 29−30 (1957).

Selye, H.: Die Entwicklung des Streßkonzeptes. Med. Welt **20**, 915−933 (1969).

Shapiro, H.A., Sapeika, N., Finlayson, M.H.: Pharmacological actions of the venom of *Latrodectus indistinctus*. S. Afr. J. med. Sci. **4**, 10—17 (1939).

Shcherbina (Schtscherbina), A.: Serum als Heilmittel bei den Bisse der Karakurte (*Latrodectus malmignattus*). Arb. d. Entom. Bureau, St. Petersburg, 2, No. 4, (1903), (In Russian), quoted by Pawlowsky, 1927.

Shulov, A., Weissman, A.: Notes on the life habits and potency of the venom of the three *Latrodectus* spider species of Israel. Ecology **40**, 515—518 (1959).

Smith, D., D'Amour, F.E.: Black widow antivenin production in rabbits. Proc. Soc. exp. Biol. (N.Y.) **40**, 686 (1939).

Stanić, M.: Beitrag zur Immunologie des Latrodektismus. Acta trop. (Basel) **10**, 225—232 (1953).

Strabo: Geographica, Vol. 2, Leipzig: A. Meinecke, 1903.

Škarica, M.: Lathrodectismus u Dalmaciji. Zbornik I Kongresa ljekara FNRJ. Beograd **3**, 168—172 (1949).

Tartaglia, P.: Beiträge zur Kenntnis des Latrodectismus. Z. Tropenmed. Parasit. **17**, 36—39 (1966).

Taubenhaus, L.J.: Correspondence, J. Amer. med. Ass. **152**, 1652 (1953).

Taussig, B.L.: Arachnidism. Clin. Med. **3**, 971—974 (1956).

Thorp, R.W., Woodson, W.D.: Black widow, America's most poisonous spider. Chapel Hill: Univ. N. Carol. Press, 1945.

Toti, L.: Memoria fisico-medica sopra il falangio o ragno venefico dell'agro volterrano (I, II parte ed Osserv.). Atti Acc. Sc. Siena Fisiocr. **7**, 244—265 (1794).

Troise, E.: Preparacion de un suero immunizante contra el "*Latrodectus mactans*". Rev. Soc. argent. Biol. **4**, 467—475 (1928).

Troise, E.: Action pharmacodynamique du venin de *Latrodectus mactans*. C. R. Soc. Biol. (Paris) **99**, 1431—1433 (1928).

Valjevac, K., Dučić, V., Stern, P.: Pharmacological analysis of *Latrodectus tredecimguttatus* spider toxin. Acta med. jugoslav. **26**, 85—91 (1972).

Vanovski, B.: Latrodektizam u Jugoslaviji. Lij. vj. **84**, 131—137 (1962).

Vellard, J.: Le venin des araignées, Paris: Masson & Cie, 1936.

Wagner, 1895, quoted by Bonnet.

Wiener, S.: The Australian red black spider (*Latrodectus hasseltii*), preparation of antiserum by the use of venom adsoebed on aluminium phosphate, Med. J. Aust. **1**, 739—742 (1956).

Wiener, S.: Red back spider in Australia, analysis of 167 cases. Med. J. Aust. **2**, 44—49 (1961).

Wilson, H.: Acute abdominal symptoms in arachnidism. Surgery **13**, 924—928 (1943).

Xenophon: Memorabilia Socratis, Lib. I, cap. 3. (Transl. in German by J. Irmscher.) Berlin: Phil. Studientexte, 1955.

Yarovoy, D.V., Shewchenko, M.S.: Disease provoked by the bite of kara kurt in grasslands and cultivated land in Stawropol country. Klin. Med. **35**, 143—144 (1957). In Russian.

Zumpt, F.: Latrodectism in South Africa. S. Afr. med. J. **42**, 385—390 (1968).

CHAPTER 9

Venoms of Theridiidae, Genus Steatoda

Z. Maretić

A. Introduction

The genus *Steatoda* (Sundewall, 1833) is one of the 140 genera belonging to the family Theridiidae (Sundewall, 1833). Some species of this genus, like *S. triangulosa,* are found on all continents. Until recently, however it was not known that some of these species could be regarded as venomous, although the venomous steatods should be considered as animals of minor toxicity and of minor practical importance.

B. Venomous Spiders of the Genus Steatoda

I. Steatoda paykulliana Walckenaer 1805

1. Distribution, Biology, Morphology, and Venomous Apparatus

Though *S. paykulliana* (*Lithyphantes paykulliana*) has been known to zoologists for a long time, its toxicity was not known till 1962 (Maretić et al., 1964). Berland (1932) wrote explicitly that the species was not toxic, and even expressed doubt that the alleged specimen of *Latrodectus,* by which the arachnologist Lucas was bitten without having symptoms of intoxication, was a misidentified *S. paykulliana.* Even when the spider was found in 1962 near Pula, the species was at first mistaken for *Latrodectus,* and only later, after careful examination of the specimens and especially after rearing the males from the eggs, it was identified correctly (Maretić et al., 1964).

 S. paykulliana is found in southern and middle Europe. Walckenaer (1806) found it as far north as near Paris. In Yugoslavia, it was found in the northern part at Postojna (Slovenija), which has an almost middle European climate, and especially in the coastal regions with Mediterranean climate, Dubrovnik and Pula (Croatia) and Trebinje in Herzegovina (Maretić et al., 1964).

 S. paykulliana prefers to build its net in crevices, holes, and recesses, especially on declivious sides of trenches and on the eroded borders of loose earth overhung with roots and other vegetation. There the spider nets its typical irregular theridiid cobweb around the openings of its resort. Near the opening one usually finds the coccoons. The cobweb is similar to that of *Latrodectus,* only it is more delicate with silk-like threads.

 In Pula, adult males and females are found in May, when mating also takes place. Later, in June and July, one can no longer find males which probably, after fulfilling their generative tasks, are subjected to the same fate of *Latrodectus* males.

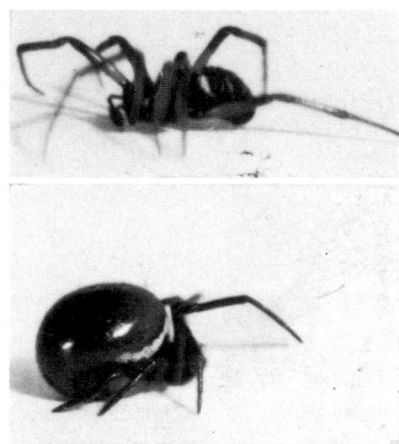

Fig. 1. *Steatoda paykulliana:* male (*above*) and female (*below*). (Magnification 100%)

The eggs are spun in coccoons (smaller than those of *Latrodectus*) of fluffy cotton-like appearence and are rose-colored. The spiderlings emerge from the coccoons by the end of summer, about a hundred from each one. Unlike the *Latrodectus,* young *Steatoda* in this zone hibernate and after several moultings reach the adult stage by the beginning of the following summer. Subadult specimens can be found in late autumn in crevices of grumous plough-fields and during winter inside buildings.

In laboratory conditions it is easier to raise young *Steatodae* than *Latrodectus,* since they are not cannibalistic like the latter, and since they do not have to be fed with living insects but only with freshly killed insects.

The adult female *S. paykulliana* is similar to that of *Latrodectus*, only smaller in size. The body length of the specimens varies from 8 to 12 mm (if pregnant). The abdomen is round-shaped, of shiny black color, and, on the anterior part of the dorsal side, bears a new-moon-shaped mark which in young specimens is of ivory and in elder specimens of orange color. The genitalia are very similar to those of *S. triangulosa* but different from those of *Latrodectus*. Sexual dimorphism, like in *Latrodectus,* is present, though the difference in size of both sexes is not so great. The male is of brighter color and has bunchy palpi. The *Steatoda* are more aggressive than the *Latrodectus,* and in experimental animals show a greater willingness to bite. The bites are mechanically stronger.

The venomous apparatus is composed of venom glands, excretory ducts, and fangs which consist of a cranial and a caudal article. In contrast to *Latrodectus* the cranial article of the *Steatoda* has a tooth on the anterior margin. Through the hollow fangs, the excretory ducts reach their opening at the top of the thorn-like caudal articulation. The anatomy of venom glands was studied by Millot (1931). During the act of biting, the venom is ejected from the venom glands by contraction of the muscular walls.

2. Effects of the Toxin

Only female *Steatoda* are toxic. With one bite, 0.2—0.3 mg of limpid venom are injected (Maretić et al., 1964). Though local signs, i.e., swelling, redness, and small

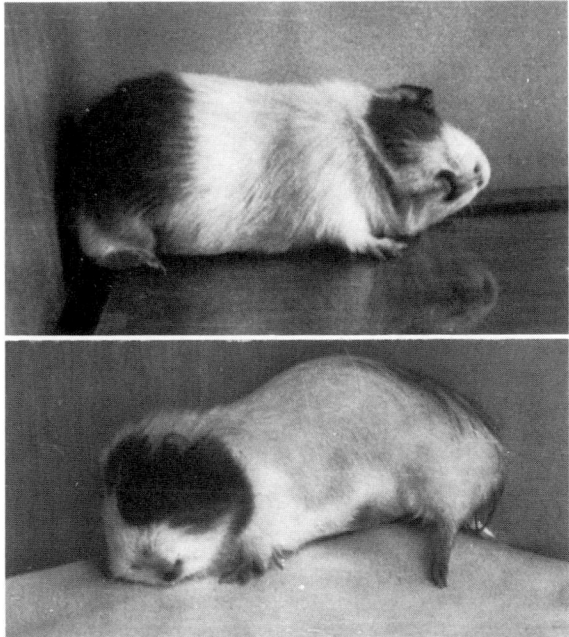

Fig. 2. Steatodism in the guinea pig

necrosis, are more marked than in envenomations due to *Latrodectus* bite, this venom is also a neurotoxin which also affects other organs and systems. Experiments on animals with phosphorus-labeled *Steatoda* venom showed that the greatest part of the toxin, other than at the site of the bite, was directed toward nervous tissues (LEBEZ et al., 1968a and 1968b).

Guinea pigs intoxicated by direct bite showed signs similar to those observed in latrodectism. With a latency period of 5—10 min, the bitten animal rubbed its snout and started to distort its neck; further, motoric restlessness with clonic cramps, curving of the whole body on a side, extension of the hind legs, paretic signs and excessive salivation were observed. In contrast to latrodectism, due to which most the of guinea pigs died, in steatodism most of the animals recovered within 4—5 h; a loss in body weight up to 21.8% could also be registered.

Mice appeared to be more susceptible to the direct bite of *Steatoda,* perhaps due to their smaller body mass. Signs similar to those described in guinea-pigs in the early phase were observed. In a subsequent phase, i.e., after 6—7 h or more, somnolence, dejection, ataxia, tremor, decrease of reactivity to outside stimuli, and paretic and paralytic signs, often followed by death, were recorded. Preliminary experiments performed on single rats and cats showed a higher resistance of these animals to the toxin of *Steatoda.*

The effect of *Steatoda* toxin on human beings has not been recorded.

In intoxicated guinea pigs, leukocytosis with neutrophilia and lymphopenia was observed. Hyperglycemia could also be observed. Penetration of the blood-brain barrier, as well as of the blood—CSF barrier was proven also for the toxin of *Steatoda.*

The ECG on guinea pigs showed depression of final complexes. In EEG, a diffuse or periodical appearance of highly voltaged late waves and of sharp waves in single groups was recorded.

The postmortem of experimental animals revealed edema of the brain and lungs, enlargement of the adrenal cortex, and ulcerations and hemorrhages of the gastric mucosa.

The histological picture showed edema and hyperemia of the adrenal cortex, in single cases lipoid granula in zona fasciculata, decay of lymphocytes in thymus and spleen, dystrophy and necrosis of myocardial fibrils, fatty degeneration and necrotic foci in the liver, and nephrosis.

Large doses of the toxin are necessary to cause death in experimental animals, but the bite of a single spider, even of a subadult specimen caught during hibernation, is sufficient to provoke typical signs and symptoms.

The toxin is highly antigenic. It was possible to immunize guinea pigs and to protect other guinea pigs from intoxication with their sera. But as mentioned previously, due to the high specifity of spider venoms and antisera, it was not possible to protect experimental animals from the venom of *S. paykulliana* with anti-*Latrodectus* serum, nor to prevent *Latrodectus* intoxication with *Steatoda* anti-venin (MARETIĆ et al., 1964).

II. Steatoda grossa WALCKENAER

Steatoda grossa is a cosmopolitan species. In North American literature this spider, called the comb-footed or false black widow, is indicated as a possible cause of arachnidism (HOREN, 1963 and RUSSELL et al., 1973). Its venom, differently than that of *S. paykulliana,* should provoke only local reactions. HOREN (1963) listed this species among the potentially dangerous spiders of United States but was doubtful about the intensity of the reaction.

References

Berland, L.: Les arachnides. Ency. Ent., Paris, **1**, 485 (1932).
Horen, W.P.: Arachnidism in the United States. Amer. J. Med. **185**, 839 – 843 (1963).
Lebez, D., Maretić, Z., Gubenšek, F., Kristan, J.: Studies on labeled animal poisons. II. Distribution of the venoms of various spiders labeled with SE_{75} and P_{32} in the guinea-pig. Toxicon **5**, 261 – 262 (1968a).
Lebez, D., Maretić, Z., Gubenšek, F., Kristan, J.: Studies on labeled animal poisons. IV. Incorporation of SE_{76} and P_{32} in spider venoms. Biološki vestnik. **16**, 11 – 15 (1968b).
Maretić, Z., Levi, H.W., Levi, L.R.: The theridiid spider *Steatoda paykulliana* poisonous to mammals. Toxicon **2**, 149 – 154 (1964).
Millot, J.: Les glandes venimeuses des Aranéides. Ann. Sci. nat. Zool. **14**, 113 – 147 (1931).
Russell, F.E., Wainschel, J., Gertsch, W.J.: Bites of spiders and other arthropods. In: Current Therapy (H.F. Conn ed.), W.B. Saunders Co., p. 868 – 870 1973.
Walckenaer, C.A.: Histoire Naturelle des Aranéides, Paris 1806.

CHAPTER 10

Venoms of Ctenidae

S. Schenberg and F.A. Pereira Lima

A. Introduction

This chapter deals only with the spider *Phoneutria nigriventer* (Keyserling, 1891) and its venom. Also known in Brazil as "aranha armadeira" (spider that assumes an armed display), and wandering or banana spider, it is the most important species of the genus *Phoneutria* (Perty, 1833), and its very toxic venom is the best studied amongst other species from the Ctenidae family.

   P. nigriventer is a species of the family Ctenidae, suborder Labidognatha and order Araneida. It has a geographical distribution ranging from North Argentina to Uruguay, and in Brazil from the states of Rio Grande do Sul to Rio de Janeiro.

   Walckenaer in 1837 synonymyzed the genus *Phoneutria* with the older genus *Ctenus* (Walckenaer, 1805). Other arachnologists also agreed with this synonym: Keyserling (1891); Cambridge (1897); Cambridge (1902, 1892); Simon (1897); Petrunkevitch (1911). The genus *Phoneutria* was reviewed by Koch (1848). Mello-Leitão (1936) differentiated the species *P. nigriventer* and Bonnet (1956) and Bücherl

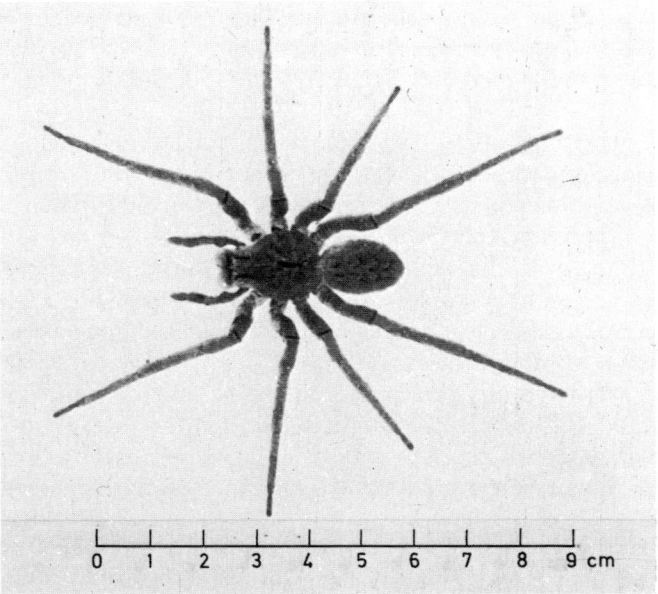

Fig. 1. *P. nigriventer* (female). Female has a larger abdomen and relatively larger cephalothorax than the male, and its color is generally darker

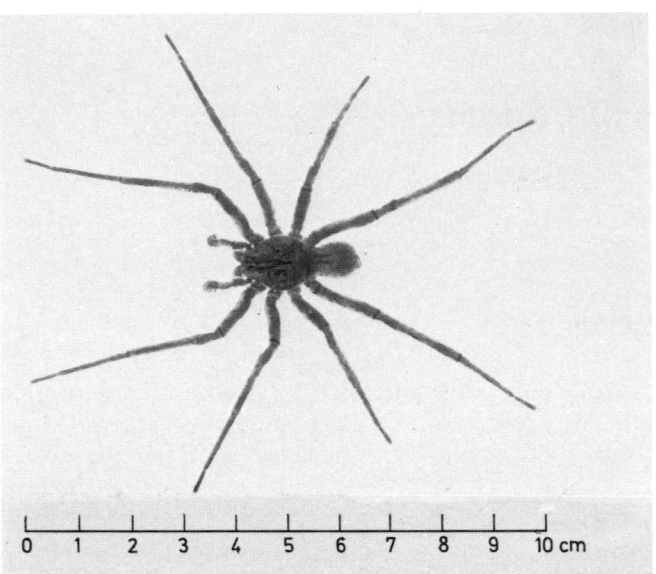

Fig. 2. *P. nigriventer* (male.). Small abdomen and light brown yellowish color, facilitate differentiation from female

(1971) accepted this new species. The various denominations of *C. ferus, C. nigriventer,* probably also *C. medius* and even *P. fera,* used by different authors who worked with spiders taken from the above-mentioned areas, are presumably synonyms of *P. nigriventer,* and this denomination, though not yet well established, must be accepted until a new revision is made.

The adult *P. nigriventer* constructs no web and is the largest true spider of South America; the female body is nearly 3 cm in length (Fig. 1), the male a little less (Fig. 2), and has a leg span of $10-12$ cm. It is grayish to brownish-gray in color with light eyes in three rows$-2-4-2$, the last two being the largest and the two laterals, of the second row, the smallest.

The chelicerae have a red brush of long hairs, a differentiating characteristic of the *Phoneutria* genus, and the dorsal side of the abdomen has whitish marks. It is preferentially nocturnal, but wanders in the shade during daylight. Being aggressive, it assumes a very characteristic defensive-aggressive display (Fig. 3); hence its popular name "aranha armadeira." The female does not kill the male after mating as some believe to occur in other species.

The very small quantity of venom that can be obtained from individual spiders renders it difficult to secure the amounts required for separation and purification of its active components. This is essential for a good approach to their pharmacologic activities, as toxic constituents conceal some activities, and a few of them have predominant antagonistic effects.

The introduction of such a simple technique as electrical stimulation in the process of collecting spider venoms was, however, very important regarding the yield and purity of the venoms. The spiders can be milked several times, and the venoms collected directly from the fangs are free of cellular material from other

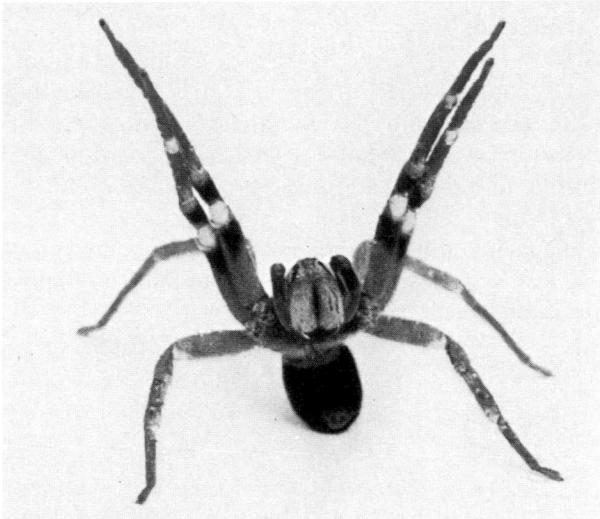

Fig. 3. A *P. nigriventer* female in a characteristic defensive-aggressive display. The two fangs are visible

tissues, as occurs with those obtained by grinding venomous glands. Though electrical stimulation afforded a better yield, the supply of *P. nigriventer* venom continues to be low, and only in the winter months, with the larger quantity of spiders, is more venom available. In spite of these difficulties, some of the venom components have unique pharmacologic and biochemical activities, and will, certainly, be used as new tools for the elucidation of specific biological phenomena.

B. Morphology of the Venomous Apparatus

The *P. nigriventer* venomous apparatus is constituted by one pair of chelicerae, one of venom glands and striated muscles.

The chelicerae are diaxial in relation to the body length, and the fangs move horizontally, a characteristic of the representatives of the suborder Labidognatha.

I. Chelicerae

1. Fangs or Claws

These organs are hollow, hard, and convex chitinous tusks having a small orifice near their tip on the convex (outer) side, through which the venom is expelled. They differ from similar ophidian fangs which have the venom-output orifice in their tip. Their length is 4.2–4.8 mm (BÜCHERL, 1971), and they have a sort of articulation with the basal cylindrical segment.

As can be seen in Figure 3, when the spider is provoked, and assumes a defensive-aggressive display, the fangs are generally distended and become visible.

2. Basal Segment

As Figure 3 shows, the basal segments have a cylindrical form, are articulated to the fangs, and according to Bücherl (1971) have a length of 6.2 – 7.8 mm. Chitinous in nature, the fang muscles and the venomous gland duct are located in their hollow central part. Their walls are sufficiently rigid to support the tensions resulting from contractions of the fang muscles, which have one of their extremities indirectly attached to their inner side.

The basal segments are moved together with the fangs by special muscles which permit the opening distance between the fang tips to increase approximately 17 mm, facilitating the accomplishment of the biting act.

When relaxed, the fangs lie in grooves situated at the inferior extremity of the basal segment.

3. Musculature

The venomous apparatus has muscles, which move the fangs, basal segments, venom canals and glands. All of them are of striated fibers and probably contract under voluntary control.

According to Bücherl (1971) the fang abductor muscle of *P. nigriventer* is formed by four muscle bundles (each one connected to a whitish tendon), which are attached to the fang in its outside posterior border. By their contractions the fangs are opened. From the tendons, the thin white-yellowish muscle fibers expand fanlike, penetrating into the basal segment, and each fiber is attached independently to the *membrana basalis* of its epidermis.

The fang adductor, whose contractions must result in a stronger force for the biting mechanism, has more muscle bundles. Four to six tendons are connected in a nearly quadrangular chitinous sclerite, called the interarticular sclerite, located on the inner side of the fang posterior border. From the interarticular sclerite, the fibers enter into the basal segment, and in a similar way to the abductor muscle they insert independently in the *membrana basalis* of the epidermis on the opposite side of the abductor fibers. The adductor contraction close the fangs; it must be an abrupt movement during the bite act.

Also connected to the fang article is found a powerful tendon which runs along the venom canal in the cheliceral basal segment from where it passes to the cephalothorax. Muscular fibers attached to the *membrana basalis* of the epidermis, and to the venomous canal (both in the chelicerae), join the tendon which also receives muscular fibers connected to the *adventitia* of the muscular fibers on the anterior part of the venom gland, corresponding to the front end of the cephalothorax. This muscle enlarges the venom canal and is a "traction muscle" of the venom gland.

The cheliceral basal segment also has thinner abductor and adductor muscles as compared to that of the fangs. Their tendons are inserted in its posterior border, on the inner face of the dorsal (abductor) and the ventral side (adductor). The abductor is located at the external face of the dorsal border, and the adductor at the internal. By contraction of these muscles the basal segments move laterally. The other extremities of these muscles are inserted at the *membrana basalis* of the cephalothorax epidermis (abductors), and partly on the musculature of the stomach (adductors) according to Bücherl (1971).

The posterior border of the cheliceral basal segment is very constricted, and the venom gland cannot pass through it. In addition, this border is in contact with a circular muscle which, by its contraction, diminishes this opening even more. The contraction of the traction muscle, compresses the venomous gland against this muscular ring, provoking, together with the gland muscles contraction, a rapid ejection of its venom.

II. Venom Glands

The glands are situated inside the cephalothorax, and each one has a nearly cylindrical or, more exactly, a carrot-like shape. At its anterior part the glands are continued by their ducts which, after passing internally through the basal segments and fangs, finish at the venom output orifices near their tips. Together with its ducts, each gland has an ampoule-like shape.

The gland is 7.6 — 10.4 mm long and 2.4 — 2.7 mm wide (BÜCHERL, 1971). Being an appreciable part of the whole spider body volume, the gland seems to indicate the paramount functional importance that this organ must have for the life of the ctenidic spiders.

1. Musculature

The whole gland, in the cephalothorax, is surrounded by bundles of striated muscular fibers which encircle the gland in a serpentine-like form. They run in opposite directions forming, by superposition, two or three muscular layers. Both extremities of the muscular bundles are attached to the gland basement membrane (BRAZIL and VELLARD, 1925; VELLARD, 1936; BÜCHERL, 1971). The gland musculature is covered by a thin *adventitia* which sends filaments into the muscle bundles.

The *adventitia,* in its inner side, is connected to the gland basal membrane giving the impression of a double basement membrane. The *adventitia* binds the muscular bundles in their positions around the basement membrane avoiding them to slip, namely during their contraction.

The glands lie completely free inside the cephalothorax, permitting them to be easily squeezed by contraction of their muscular mantle, by means of which the venom, stored in the gland lumens, is ejected through the venom output-orifices of the fangs.

2. Histology of the Glandular Tissue

The secretory cells are of two types, both epithelial in nature. One is flattened or subcuboidal, the other is high and columnar or cylindrical. They cover the inner side of the sac formed by the thick basal membrane, which is surrounded externally by the muscular mantle and its *adventitia*. The basal membrane sends a sort of fringes, into the gland lumen which are also covered by secretory cells, by means of which the secretory surface is increased.

The subcuboidal cells have an oval nucleus. For BÜCHERL (1971) they may form a continuous layer, generally covering the gland internally; however, they are only seen as islands at the base of the high columnar cells. Also, according to Bücherl (1971), these cells will substitute for the secretory columnar cells after their degeneration, which takes place after secretion, though Bücherl never found intermediary forms indicating the transformation of a subcuboidal cell into a columnar one. He considered these cells as belonging to the apocrine type. For Brazil and Vellard (1925) and Vellard (1936), these cells are all flattened in glands having their lumens filled with venoms, as a consequence of their compression by the venom stored in the gland lumen.

The columnar cells are attached by their base to the basal membrane and its fringes. The subcuboidal and columnar cells are disposed in a serpentine form upon the basement membrane.

At the beginning of the secretory phase, the large oval nuclei of the columnar cells are situated near their basal extremity, and are strongly stained due to their high content of chromatin. Fine well-stained particles are found in the cytoplasm beneath the nucleus. Afterward, the nucleus migrates to the center of the cell and the granules to its lateral sides, the latter increasing their size. Finally, the nucleus moves to the apical cytoplasm and becomes faint in color. The granules are transformed into droplets also suffering a condensation. Vellard (1936) reports that the droplets are extruded together with the nucleus into the lumen, and classifies these cells as belonging to the holocrine type; however, he could not find nuclei in the venom. Bücherl (1971) reports that the droplets are extruded into the lumen but sometimes the nucleus remains in the cell; when extruded together with the droplets the cells degenerate. According to Millot (1931), these cells are of the merocrine type.

Vellard (1936) reports that after the gland is emptied, the subcuboidal cells present a high proliferative process and regenerate the columnar cells. He also observed that it takes almost 6 days for the gland to regenerate its lumen venom.

These reports are based on observations using light microscopes. However, they resemble new findings furnished by electronic microscopy for protein secretion by pancreatic acinar cells. The fine basal granules might represent proteins synthesized by the ribosome of the granular endoplasmatic reticulum, which are then transported to the Golgi region where they are concentrated, and the droplets formed are stored in the apical cytoplasm, and ultimately released at the free surface of the cell in the lumen.

Considering the numerous proteins contained in the venom, it seems more probable that the gland has, independently, subcuboidal and columnar cells. It must also be taken into account that after releasing a large volume of droplets, water vacuoles may not substitute the whole volume from which the cells were deprived, but they will then flatten giving the impression of subcuboidal cells.

C. Methods of Collecting Venoms

The relatively large size of the spider *P. nigriventer,* and also of its glands, makes it easy to handle both of them and to secure their venoms either by extraction from isolated glands or by collecting it from the fangs after electrical stimulation of the spider's cephalothorax.

1. Method of Collecting Venom by its Extraction From the Glands

To remove the glands, the spider is first killed in a closed atmosphere of sulfuric ether or chloroform. The cephalothorax of the dead spider is fixed with the fingers, and by grasping the fangs with a forceps, gentle movements of the fangs are made directed toward the dorsal side of the cephalothorax. The glands become free from their ligaments and are then removed. Lateral movements of the fangs must not be made, nor the fangs pulled, since their attachments to the glands may be ruptured. The *adventitia* and the muscular mantle may be separated from the gland with a small forceps. The glands are ground, with or without the fangs, with washed sand in a small volume of NaCl 0.85% (BRAZIL and VELLARD, 1925).

After centrifugation, the supernatant may be used. Its activity is preserved when dried in a dessicator under vacuum at room temperature or by lyophilization.

Although the oldest method, extraction of the venom by grinding the glands is not the best one to secure this venom. Yet, it is used by those who are not familiar with the handling of venomous spiders regardless of the availability of electrical stimulators.

2. Method of Collecting Venom by Electrical Stimulation

Electrical stimulation must be considered as the choice method for collecting this araneidan venom. Also, the venom collected presents a high degree of purity as it is free from contaminations with cellular material from the neighboring gland tissues.

The spider is taken from its individual cage with a long forceps by delicately grasping the lateral sides of the cephalothorax. Afterward, the spider is laid on a table still immobilized by the forceps. After gently pressing the dorsal cephalothorax

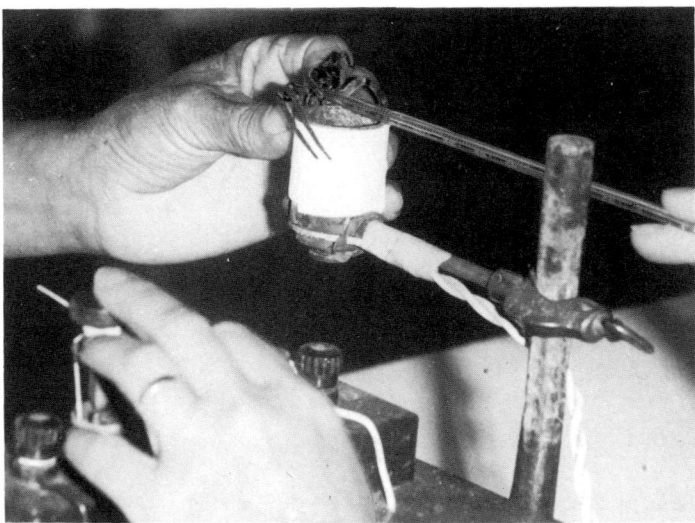

Fig. 4. Venom extraction by electric shocks. The spider is held with the fingers and cephalothorax is in contact with both electrodes. Three or four shocks of 6V are given, and venom is collected by capillarity with a 0.1 ml pipette

against the table with the forefinger, the forceps is taken off, and the cephalothorax is grasped laterally by the thumb and middle finger. The spider's anterior cephalo-thorax, near the fangs, is then brought into contact with the two vertical stainless electrodes as can be seen in Figure 4.

When handling the spiders, care must be taken to avoid their being hurt or killed. Some experience must be acquired so that only the necessary force is applied when grasping the spider.

After electrical stimulation (6V) the venom is collected from the fangs by capillar-ity through a 0.1 ml pipette as is illustrated in Figure 4.

The venom is a colorless, transparent liquid, and it must be discarded when it presents some turbidity since, in these cases, it is contamined with some vomiting, provoked by the electric shocks.

According to BÜCHERL (1953, 1956), the amount of dried venom obtainable from single specimens of *P. nigriventer* may reach 1.8 mg in winter and 2.5 mg in summer.

D. Physiology of Biting

The venomous apparatus serves the spiders for hunting and defense purposes (BRAZIL and VELLARD, 1925). Apparently, the venom is only injected in excessively large preys or when the spider finds no way to escape an attack.

The spider uses its chelicerae to kill small insects by simple traumatism; not allowing the venom to run, but rather keeping it as a last recourse. This independency of functions between the venomous gland and the biting act must be emphasized due to its importance when appreciating the results of direct bitings.

The same authors observed that during bitings the spider brings together the two anterior legs, and by strongly contracting itself over this base, rapidly holds its victim with the fangs. This movement seems to be fundamental to expel the venom since a spider, held by its cephalothorax, can bite a mouse, maintaining its fangs under the animal's skin for a long time without provoking any sign of envenomation.

In the biting mechanism, the spider seems to control the injected venom in a similar manner as do snakes. BRAZIL and VELLARD (1925) report an experiment in which a 20 g white mouse was confined with an adult *P. nigriventer* female. The spider, very agressive, bit the mouse rapidly 5 or 7 times, and after some envenomation manifestations the animal died. All the events took 1 min.

Immediately after, a second mouse was kept with the same spider which, less active, bit the mouse 2 or 3 times (14:13 h). After 1 h, the animal became paralytic and died during night, beyond 17:30 h.

The same spider, maintained at rest for 3 days accumulated enough venom to kill a 48 g guinea pig.

E. Crude Venom Pharmacology

The *P. nigriventer* venom used in the investigations herein reported, was extracted by electrical stimulation of specimens taken predominantly from the city of São

Paulo and environs, where these spiders are relatively common. The venom was dried at room temperature, in a vacuum over $CaCl_2$; its solutions were made at 37° C, and for experimental purposes it was dissolved either with NaCl 0.85%, or distilled water or buffers.

I. Effect on Dogs

The *P. nigriventer* venom, subcutaneously injected in male dogs, in low lethal doses (180 − 200 µg/kg body weight) successively induces: excruciating local pain, violent sneezing, lacrimation, mydriasis, hypersalivation, adynamia, ataxia, prostration, drowsiness, dyspnea, vomiting, erection, ejaculation, sanguinolent feces, and, in some cases, death. Paralysis phenomena are not observed in dogs. Differing from dogs, erection is induced in mice with non-lethal doses. In dogs, when intravenously injected, subcutaneous effective doses provoke a sharp fall of blood pressure, soon followed by death.

Experiments with dogs have the disadvantage of consuming large amounts of venom, but these animals must be used for the study of blood pressure actions, mydriasis, and local pain. On the other hand, a large number of animals are required to study the venom fractions, and this can only be practically achieved with mice.

1. Excruciating Local Pain

The venom, when subcutaneously injected, provokes excruciating local pain; it makes dogs yelp for nearly 1 h and forces them to keep the injected hind leg contracted for periods longer than 1 h (Fig. 5).

The specific antivenin neutralizes the pain-producing component *in vitro*, which excludes the possibility of this effect being caused by histamine or serotonin contained

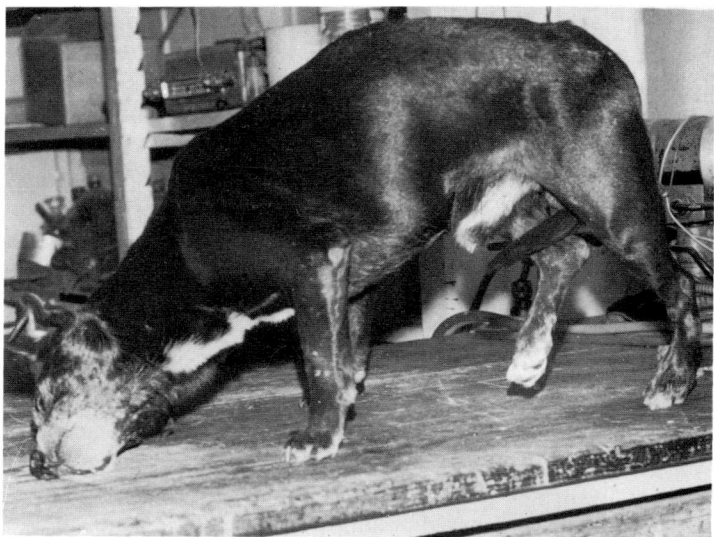

Fig. 5. Mydriasis provokes visual disturbances, and dog rubs its face and eyes on table as to remove foreign bodies. Right hind leg is contracted due to local pain

in the venom. Since the pain factor is dialyzable, its molecule must be relatively small; for this reason it is unlikely that the factor is a bradykinin-releasing enzyme.

Erection in dogs may appear during the pain period with the dog yelping. The local pain is one of the most serious effects in human accidents, and must be treated immediately with locally injected anesthetics, since it commonly provokes a pronounced fall in blood pressure with consequent fainting, and probably shock.

2. Sneezing

In dogs, sneezing is one of the first manifestations of envenomation. The sneezes occur intermittently and are persistent, being observed for more than 24 h. Violent attacks occur within the first 2 h, during which period the animal throws its head violently and uncontrollably toward the floor and, very often, hurts its nose and lips.

3. Lacrimation and Mydriasis

Lacrimation is a constant effect during envenomation, and is also provoked in anesthetized animals. Mydriasis is an early manifestation after venom injection and persists for many hours. The dogs present visual disturbances as a consequence of mydriasis, as exteriorized by characteristic movements of the paws over the eyes and the rubbing of the face against the table (Fig. 5) as if to remove foreign bodies from the eyes.

4. Hypersalivation

As Figure 6 shows, the venom-provoked salivation is abundant, resembling that induced by pilocarpine.

Initially, the saliva must be of the serous type. It is copiously secreted and can be appreciated by constant swallowing movements, or by drops that fall from the animal's mouth. Afterward, the secretion of mucous saliva is increased, and unswallowed saliva drips continuously from the animal's mouth for hours. It is blocked by atropine. Eserine and hexamethonium, though they slightly increase the signs of poisoning, do not seem to interfere with this effect (SCHENBERG and PEREIRA LIMA, 1962). Subcutaneous doses, which provoke hypersalivation, fail to produce it when injected in dogs under chloralose, chloroform, and barbituric anesthesia; however, intravenously, the same doses are effective. This seems to show that hypersalivation results from a direct action of the venom upon the effector organs.

5. Erection

In a similar way to sneezing, the venom-induced erection (SCHENBERG and PEREIRA LIMA, 1962) is also of an intermittent and long-standing character. It occurs repeatedly for hours, very often over 24 h, in which cases, edema is generally formed at the distal penis extremity corresponding to the glans. The erection develops slowly, taking more than 15 min from its beginning (Fig. 7) to its final stage (Fig. 8).

It generally appears at a more advanced envenomation level when the dog has

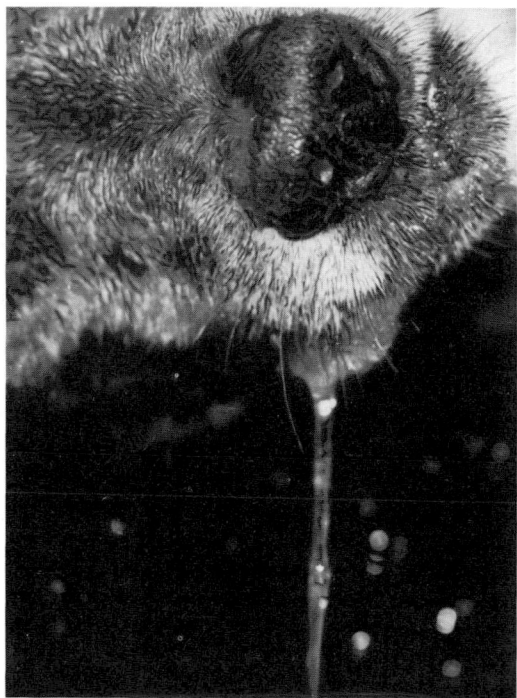

Fig. 6. Hypersalivation is an early manifestation. Prostrated dog lies on table, and a very viscous saliva drops slowly and continuously from its mouth

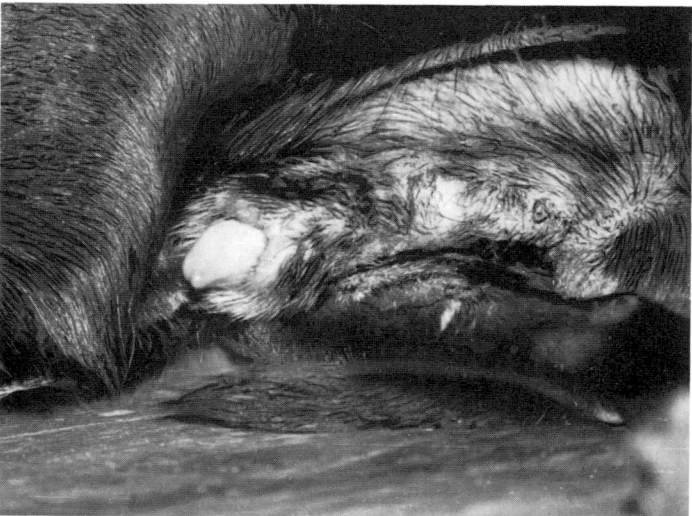

Fig. 7. Erection is induced slowly and can be observed from its beginning

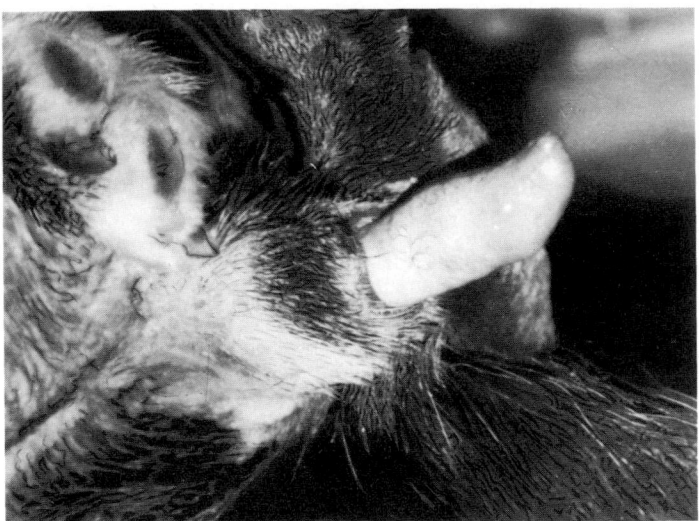

Fig. 8. Erection attains its complete stage around 15 min after its beginning

already displayed sneezing, mydriasis, visual disturbances, adynamia, ataxia, drowsiness, dyspnea, and vomiting. Erection could not be induced in anesthetized dogs, even when the venom was applied intravenously in larger doses than that which are effective subcutaneously. However, this failure does not constitute evidence that erection results from a direct action of the venom upon the central nervous system, since by increasing the venom doses, the frequency of erection decreases, a fact well observed with mice, indicating a dose-effect antagonism probably due to a higher degree of envenomation which is followed by a fall in blood pressure.

Erection induction does not seem to depend on the excitation of higher nervous system centers, since it could be provoked in dogs in which the medulla has been cut at D 12 (SCHENBERG and PEREIRA LIMA, 1963). Unlike cantharidin-induced erection, that seen in araneidan envenomation does not seem to result from reflexes caused by irritation of the urinary tract. In dogs, the venom induces erection before micturition occurs, and erection is seen in animals in which urine flow through the urethra has been prevented by implanting both ureters in the skin; it is not induced by perfusing venom solutions through the urethra into the bladder. Also, the molecular weights of these factors are close to 6000. They are immunogenic and probably cannot pass through the blood-cerebrospinal barrier.

Erection is also induced when the dog is yelping, due to the excruciating local pain.

6. Ejaculation

The *P. nigriventer* venom induces ejaculation in dogs, during or after the onset of erection. A milky liquid drips from the penis or prepuce during short periods. The first drops are free of spermatozoa, as normally occurs with dogs. This effect seems to result from excitation of organs other than the seminal vesicles, since these organs are absent in dogs (SCHENBERG and PEREIRA LIMA, 1963).

7. Toxicity

P. nigriventer venom is approximately 4 times more toxic in dogs than in mice. When 200 µg/kg of venom is injected subcutaneously, some dogs survive for several hours before death, with sneezing, salivation, and erection occuring during the severe intoxication phase.

8. Hypotensive Response

Intravenously injected, small doses of venom provoke a sharp fall in blood pressure. The histamine content of venom at these doses is too low to affect the blood pressure.

9. Tachyphylaxis

The venom of the black widow spider (*Latrodectus mactans*) provokes tachyphylaxis in dogs (SAMPAYO, 1942). Tachyphylaxis phenomena were not observed with *P. nigriventer* venom; neither with those manifestations of short duration nor for long-standing and intermittent effects. The latter effect would probably not be exhibited for hours, if tachyphylaxis was involved. Also, dogs, which had recently recovered from the effects of a venom injection, displayed the same responses to venom when another dose was injected. These facts seem to demonstrate that tachyphylaxis is not a universal characteristic of spider venom constituents; they also point up the different molecular structures of the active principles involved.

II. Guinea Pig Ileum Contraction

Two polypeptides, which contract the guinea pig ileum, were separated from the *P. nigriventer* venom by DINIZ (1963a). According to his findings, the fraction containing one of these polypeptides was also responsible for the toxicity of the venom.

III. Effects on Mice

The erection induced in dogs injected with *P. nigriventer* venom (SCHENBERG and PEREIRA LIMA, 1962) was reproduced in mice by DINIZ (1963b). Except for the excruciating local pain, sneezing, vomiting and blood pressure effects, which are difficult to follow in mice, all the other *P. nigriventer* venom actions can easily be appreciated in these small rodents (SCHENBERG and PEREIRA LIMA, 1963). Mice were shown to be suitable assay animals for this venom investigation, permitting qualitative and quantitative study of the venom effects with low venom consumption. They also present the advantage of being slowly immunized, and the same animal can be used for several assays over a period of 30 days, before immunization may significantly affect quantitative responses, which do not depend on age and body weight. The facility of handling a large number of mice, in addition to their low venom consumption and their capacity to reproduce the venom effects induced in dogs, permitted us to pursue our investigations on a biochemical level. Also, a distensive and a flaccid paralysis, provoked by this araneidan venom, were only revealed by using mice.

Strain and weight control are essential for reprodutive quantitative assays. The best responses from mice of the Instituto Butantan strain (Strain C, Statens Serum-institut, Copenhagen 1956), are obtained by using animals in a 22—25 g weight range. In mice weighing less than 20 g, toxic effects occur more often than erection. The method of Reed and Muench (1938) has been shown to afford a statistically valid estimate of venom-produced erection and of its other effects.

1. Local Pain

Local pain in mice does not display such a dramatic manifestation as in man and dog, and is not well exteriorized. The animal, after the subcutaneous injection, becomes restless, runs agitatedly with or without jumping, and very often it bites the injection area. Very soon, depending on the dose, distensive paralysis takes place and no pain manifestation can be visualized.

2. Hypersalivation

P. nigriventer venom provokes an abundant hypersalivation in mice as Figure 9 illustrates. Initially, small bubbles accumulate at the mouth. Later on, depending on the venom dosage, the animals may have a large part or nearly all of its fur wetted by saliva. Small doses of venom cause hypersalivation without any sign of toxicity. With larger doses, hypersalivation can be seen before toxicity signs

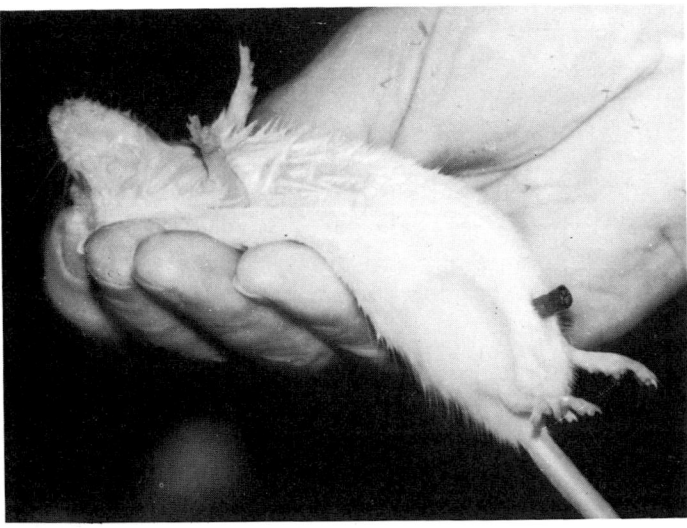

Fig. 9. Hypersalivation and erection in mice. Large area of fur is wet with saliva and erection is of the complete type. Penis ends in a funnel-shaped form

and continues with the appearance of these signs. The venom ED_{50} for hypersalivation is 0.43 mg/kg body weight.

3. Erection

Figure 9 shows a venom-induced erection in a mouse. In mice it is possible to distinguish three forms of erection provoked by the venom (SCHENBERG and PEREIRA LIMA, 1975).

In the first form, which was called by us as "complete erection," the organ attains its maximal tumescence, and its distal part is funnel-shaped with its opening looking outward as can be seen in Figure 9. In a second form, named "semicomplete erection," the organ presents a smaller tumescence and no funnel is formed. In the third form, designated as "incomplete erection," the penis attains the volume and tumescence of the complete or semicomplete form. However, it is not exteriorized, remaining underneath the prepuce skin, which is elevated by its volume. The penis' cyanotic color communicates, by transparency, a bluish-purple color to the elevated prepuce skin. By forcing the prepuce caudally, the erected penis emerges from it. With lethal doses, the penis, after attaining the complete or semicomplete erection, decreases its volume and becomes very thin, without any vasodilatation sign, but is not brought back inside the prepuce, even after death, which simulates a post-mortem erection (SCHENBERG and PEREIRA LIMA, 1975). The penis of mice has a bony structure, and it seems that this particularity affords its ejection from the prepuce by some muscular mechanism that is set in action during erection. This may be a relaxation, similar to that of the bovine retractor penis. Assuming this hypothesis as correct, since we were unable to find any literature regarding this particular point of mice erection, the venom would act in both of these mechanisms, the muscular and the vascular, the latter being successively responsible for the vasodilatation and tumescence. Also strengthening this hypothesis is the fore-mentioned simulated erection which persists after death occurs.

The erection dose-effect relationship in mice, is maintained until a maximum response in a group of animals is attained; thereafter, increasing doses of venom produce a decrease in the number of animals that experience erection, and death supervenes in some of them before this effect appears. Toxicity would thus exert a sort of functional antagonism to erection. Similar to hypersalivation, small doses of venom can induce erection in mice without any toxic manifestations; in this case, mice react differently from dogs. The erection ED_{50} for mice is 0.25 mg/kg body weight.

4. Ejaculation

P. nigriventer venom also provokes ejaculation in mice, which is more easily observed in the prepuce, where small coagulated milky drops can be seen.

5. Toxicity

The severe envenomation pattern in mice is characterized by dyspnea, prostration, and distensive paralysis, which are followed by death. The LD_{50} is 0.76 mg/kg body weight.

6. Distensive Paralysis

As Figure 10 illustrates, the distensive paralysis, or distensive paraplegia, is a characteristic sign of crude venom envenomation in mice. Crotamine also provokes this kind of paralysis in mice.

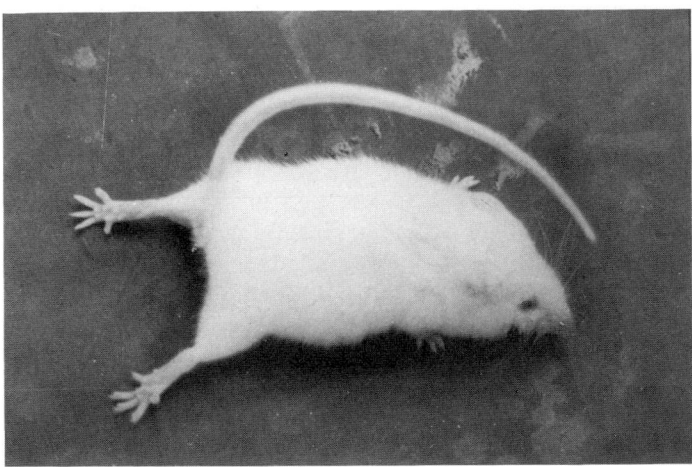

Fig. 10. Distensive paralysis in mice. Hind legs are distended and tail is contracted over the mouse. Soon after death mouse displays *rigor mortis*

After its onset, distensive paralysis is of long duration, and in lethal doses, the animals present a premature sort of *rigor mortis* soon after death. As can be seen in Figure 10, distensive paralysis is accompanied for some time, by a contraction of the mouse tail which is very often maintained bent upon the animal's back for short periods. Distensive paralysis is preceded by hypersalivation and erection. Lethal fractions of the venom which provoke distensive paralysis were obtained, but the animals die without presenting *rigor mortis,* which seems to point out that the latter manifestation is not induced by the distensive paralysis factor.

IV. Effects on Other Animals

BRAZIL and VELLARD (1925) and VELLARD (1936) investigated the effects of *P. nigriventer* venom on mice, rats, guinea pigs, rabbits and pigeons. They observed in these animals a great hypothermia, hypersalivation, lacrimation, diarrhea, and also hematuria when death occurs slowly. Strong local pain in hypodermic and intramuscular injections, muscular trepidation and distensive paralysis of the injected leg, and a generalized violent agitation were also observed. The animals do not present these first symptoms when using the venous route; in this case dyspnea and hypersalivation are the first signs. The same authors observed that pigeons are very resistant to this venom, and that in these animals, the neck is also affected by distensive paralysis. They observed an eye hemorrhage in rabbits. Also, they verified that cold-blooded animals are very resistant to *P. nigriventer* venom. Subcutaneously injected, toads only present local muscular fibrillations. In snakes, the venom injected intracraneally or intracardically provokes no sign of envenomation.

Excepting erection, guinea pigs display nearly all responses to envenomation seen in dogs and mice, but our investigations with these rodents were only superficial due to their larger venom consumption. Nevertheless, the almost solid consistence of their coagulated semen makes them very appropriate for the study of the effect of semen ejaculation (SCHENBERG and PEREIRA LIMA, 1962, 1963). For the purposes of our research, rats and rabbits are very resistant; 500 µg injected in 150 g rats provokes an eye hemorrhage, and 1000 µg injected subcutaneously in 2000 g rabbits induces a moderate hypersalivation and slight intoxication (SCHENBERG and PEREIRA LIMA, 1962).

F. Biochemistry of the Phoneutria Nigriventer Venom, and Procedures for its Fractionation

Neuromuscular and muscular effects induced by electrophoretic fractions of *P. nigriventer* venom were reported by BARRIO (1955). DINIZ (1963) demonstrated, with electrophoretic fractionation, that the venom contains histamine, serotonin and two polypeptides that contract the guinea pig ileum. FISCHER and BOHN (1957) separated its histamine by electrophoresis, demonstrating that the venom also contains free glutamic acid (23.6%), aspartic acid (1.0%), and lysine (0.2%). WELSH and BATTY (1963) studied its serotonin content, while hyaluronidase and a proteolytic enzyme of this venom were reported by KAISER (1953, 1956). The venom histamine content varies, according to different reports, from 0.06 to 1.0%, and serotonin from 0.03 to 0.25%.

I. Immunologic Aspects of the Venom

As Table 1 shows, all the *P. nigriventer* venom-active polypeptides are neutralized by the specific antivenin, excepting the polypeptides which contract the guinea pig ileum (SCHENBERG and PEREIRA LIMA, 1975). These polypeptides, not being neutralized by the antivenin, clearly demonstrate that they are not associated with the venom toxicity. The neutralized constituents show that they are relatively large molecules, probably protein in nature (SCHENBERG and PEREIRA LIMA, 1962). The number of venom antigens, as determined by double-diffusion agar immunoprecipitation (Ouchterlony method), is nearly 15, of which 13 were determined by agar immunoelectrophoresis (PEREIRA LIMA and SCHENBERG, 1964). Thus, the venom might have several distinct components, each associated with one or more of its multiple effects. This also opens possibilities of separating toxic from non-toxic components; other principles could be isolated, and their pharmacological properties better investigated, if freed of the masking effects of toxic components.

II. Enzymic Inactivation

Except for histamine and serotonin, all the other pharmacologically active components of the venom are inactivated by trypsin, chymotrypsin, and pepsin, thus

Table 1. Differentiation of the *P. nigriventer* venom active polypeptides by their immunobioche-mical properties, and by ammonium sulfate, DEAE-Cellulose, CM-Sephadex C-50, and Sephadex G-50 fractionation

Treatment	Activities					
	Ileum Contrac-tion	Erection	Hyper-sali-vation	Toxicity (lethality)	Paralysis	
					Dis-tensive	Flaccid
Antivenin	$++++$ 0	0	0	0	0	0
Trypsin, chymotrypsin, pepsin	0	0	0	0	0	0
0.4% Formaldehyde (2 h)	$+++$	$++$	$++$	$++$	$++$	$-$
Electrophoresis migration (pH 8.6)	$-$	Cathode	Cathode	Cathode	Cathode	Cathode
Electrophoresis migration (pH 5.0)	$-$	Cathode	Cathode	Cathode	Cathode	Cathode (activity disclosed)
$(NH_4)_2\ SO_4$ precipitation (% saturation)	$60-70$	$45-65$	$45-65$	$45-75$	$45-65$	$70-75$ (activity disclosed)
DEAE-cellulose: active peaks	(2)	(4)	(4)	(2)	(1)	(1)
CM-Sephadex C-50: active peaks	(4)	(3)	(4)	(2)	$-$	$-$
Sephadex G-50 (after heating at 100° C for 6 min in phosphate buffer, pH 8.0, 0.05 M): active peaks	(2)	(2)	(2)	(2)	(2)	(1)

demonstrating their protein nature (Table 1) (Schenberg and Pereira Lima, 1971). The proteolytic enzyme of *P. nigriventer* venom only inactivates its guinea pig ileum-contracting polypeptides. The proteolytic enzyme of the venom also degrades casein much more rapidly than it does albumin (Schenberg and Pereira Lima, 1967).

III. Physicochemical Properties of the Active Polypeptides

As can be seen in Table 2, the pharmacologically active components are resistant to heating. Venom solutions in physiologic saline can be heated at 100° C for 20 min without loss of activity. However, inactivation occurs when these solutions are heated at the same temperature for 6 min at pH 8.0 (Schenberg and Pereira Lima, 1971). Under these conditions, the guinea pig ileum-contracting polypeptides prove to be the most heat-resistant of all the components; these polypeptides were 100% active after this treatment, while activity after heating of some of the other components were decreased as follows: erection 39.2%; hypersalivation 24.2%; and toxicity 19.1% (Table 2). These data and others, which will be reported later on, seem to show that the venom has at least two toxic components, which vary in their resistance to heat (Schenberg and Pereira Lima, 1971).

Table 2. Differentiation of *P. nigriventer* venom active polypeptides through their inactivations by heating, acid and alkaline incubations, and solvents

Treatment	Activities					
	Ileum Contrac-tion	Erection	Hyper-sali-vation	Toxicity (lethality)	Paralysis	
					Dis-tensive	Flaccid
Heating (100° C for 6 min, 500 µg/ml, phosphate buffer, pH 8.0, 0.05 M)	++++	++	++	+	++	++++
Heating (100° C for 30 min)	++++	++	++	+	++	−
Concentrated acetic acid (1 h)	−	+	+	+	+	−
0.1 N HCl (2 h)	++++	++++	++++	++++	++++	−
0.1 N HCl (5 min at 100° C)	+++	++	++	++	++	−
0.1 N NaOH (2 h)	I ++	+	+	+	+	−
1.0 N NaOH (2 h)	+	0	0	0	0	0
Sulfuric ether, acetone, chloroform, butanol	++++	++++	++++	++++	++++	−
Ethanol	+++	++	++	++	++	−

Treatment of the venom with concentrated acetic acid for 1 h greatly diminishes its capacity to induce erection, hypersalivation, and death (Table 2). The fractions responsible for these actions and for the guinea pig ileum-contracting effect are more resistant to acids (0.1 N HCl) than to alkalis (0.1 N NaOH); also, they are not completely inactivated by heating at 100° C for 6 min in 0.1 N HCl. Stronger alkaline solutions (1.0 N NaOH), however, inactivate these four components. The ileum-contracting polypeptides are the most resistant, being more resistant than the other four to 0.1 N NaOH, 0.4% formaldehyde, ethanol, and to heat at 100° C for 6 min in 0.1 N HCl (Table 2). Sulfuric ether, acetone, chloroform and butanol do not inactivate any of these components (Table 2), though the first three solvents extract a significant amount of an inactive material from the crude venom, together with some histamine and serotonin (PEREIRA LIMA and SCHENBERG, 1964).

IV. Dialysis

The protein nature of most of the venom-active factors was reported before in some parts of this chapter. Dialysis through Visking tubes could furnish some more information regarding their molecular weight, according to their permeability. The Visking tube 24/32 (impermeable to insulin) is impermeable to all the large active factors of the venom; tube 18/32 (impermeable to insulin) is more permeable to the components which induce erection and hypersalivation than to those that induce intoxication as is illustrated in Table 3. All the active constituents of the venom dialyze rapidly through tube 8/32, while, insulin dialyzes slowly (PEREIRA LIMA and SCHENBERG, 1964; SCHENBERG and PEREIRA LIMA, 1962, 1971). Since these components dialyze through tube 18/32, their molecular weight must be lower than that of insulin, which is 5733. According to these data, the larger pharmacologically active components of the *P. nigriventer* venom can be considered as polypeptides

Table 3. Approximate molecular weight of *P. nigriventer* venom active polypeptides estimated by immunologic, dialysis, and gel filtration procedures

Treatment	Activities					
	Ileum Contraction	Erection	Hyper-salivation	Toxicity (lethality)	Paralysis	
					Distensive	Flaccid
Antivenin	++++	0	0	0	0	0
Dialysis—Visking tubes No. 24/32 (48 h)	—	0	0	0	0	0
Dialysis—Visking tubes No. 18/32 (48 h)	—	+++	+	+	+	—
Dialysis—Visking tubes No. 8/32 (48 h)	—	++++	++++	+++	+++	—
Sephadex G-25	—	Excluded	Excluded	Excluded	Excluded	Excluded
Sephadex G-50	Diffuses	Diffuses	Diffuses	Diffuses	Diffuses	Diffuses

since: (1) they are also hydrolyzed by proteolytic enzymes and (2) they are immunogenic, except for the ileum-contracting polypeptides.

V. Venom Fractionation

1. Ammonium Sulfate, Electrophoresis, Barium Sulfate Adsorption

The venom fractionation, by salting out with ammonium sulfate, did not present satisfatory resolutions. The flaccid paralysis component and the ileum-contracting polypeptides were separated out by 65—75% ammonium sulfate saturation (see Table 1). The flaccid paralysis factor was precipitated either from venom solutions in physiologic saline or from phosphate buffer solutions at pH 7.0, but not from buffer solutions at pH 5.0.

Electrophoresis of the *P. nigriventer* venom was performed with different supporting media: agar plates (immunoelectrophoresis), starch blocks, filter paper, and cellulose acetate strips, the latter gave better resolutions. All active components are positively charged and migrate to the cathode. The flaccid paralysis component was the only one separated by electrophoresis, in agar plates or cellulose acetate strips, in acetic acid ammonium acetate buffer at pH 5.0 (PEREIRA LIMA and SCHENBERG, 1963).

2. Flaccid Paralysis

The venom fractionation by electrophoresis in agar plates at pH 5.0, permitted the obtainment of fractions which injected subcutaneously induced a sort of flaccid paralysis (see Table 1). The same factor was also separated on cellulose acetate strips at pH 5.0 (PEREIRA LIMA and SCHENBERG, 1963) (Table 1). As can be seen in Figure 11, the hind legs are paralyzed and flaccid (not distended), the tail is flaccid, and the animal is motionless; when movement is attempted the forelegs are used

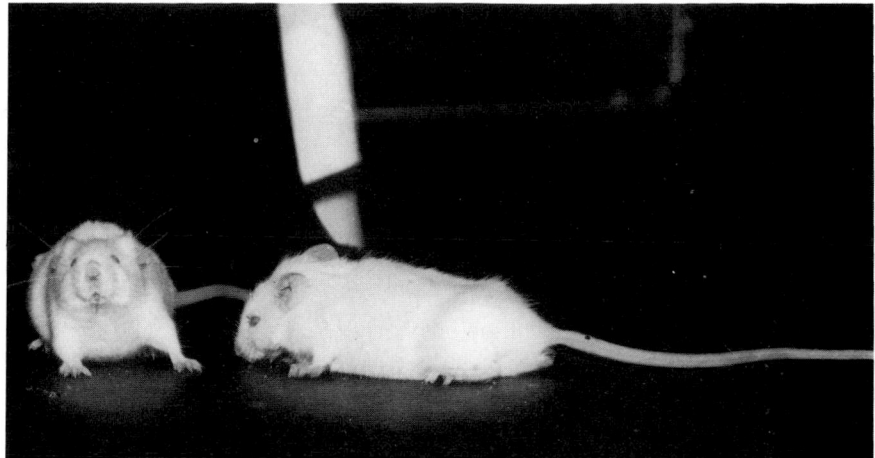

Fig. 11. Flaccid paralysis induced with a fraction of a DEAE-cellulose column. Hind legs are paralyzed in an undistended form, and forelegs are used for slow movements. Fraction is toxic, and after death animals do not diplay *rigor mortis*

to pull the body. This fraction is very toxic, and when death occurs the mice present a flaccid body, as compared to death produced by crude venom by which the animals very soon present *rigor mortis*. Fractions with the factor responsible for this effect can be separated by other methods and will be described later. Flaccid paralysis is probably masked by the dominant distensive paralysis in crude venom assays.

3. Hemorrhagic Effect

Brazil and Vellard (1925), observed eye hemorrhage in rabbits after intravenously injecting the venom. Eye hemorrhage can also be provoked in rats, applying the venom subcutaneously. The venom provokes sanguinolent feces in dogs. Crude venom does not, however, exteriorize any hemorrhagic manifestation in mice. The eluates from crude venom solutions, after adsorption on barium sulfate, induce hemorrhage in the erected penis of mice, and also through their mouths (Schenberg and Pereira Lima, 1975). Apparently, the blood eliminated through the mouth does not originate from the stomach or lungs since no hemorrhagic manifestations were observed in these organs. It is more probable that hemorrhage occurs in some place of the upper respiratory or digestive tract. Crude venom provokes hemorrhagic spots on mice pleura and liver, and also a pink mucoid exudate, which fills the alveoli, is formed. Barium sulfate eluates intensify all these manifestations. No explanation was yet given for the crude venom being ineffective, and its eluates effective. Crude venom incubated for 3 min in a boiling water bath also reproduces these effects of barium eluates.

VI. Gel Chromatography

In columns of Sephadex G-25, all the large molecule components are excluded. The polypeptides, however, diffuse in Sephadex G-50. These data indicate that the molecular weight of these polypeptides are higher than 5000, but less than 30,000; this, in some way, confirms the above mentioned data obtained with dialysis. Both sets of data seem to indicate that the larger pharmacologically active molecules of the *P. nigriventer* venom have a molecular weight between 5000 and 5733. These components are also immunogenic, and subject to hydrolysis by proteolytic enzymes they were inactivated, and were, therefore, considered to be polypeptides.

A chromatogram of a 20 mg *P. nigriventer* venom run in a Sephadex G-50 column (760 × 22 mm), and eluted with phosphate buffer at pH 7.5 (0.05 and 0.1 M NaCl) can be seen in Figure 12 (PEREIRA LIMA and SCHENBERG, 1964). Except for flaccid paralysis, most of the other activities herein reported, are found in the effluent fractions. The activities are distributed in two zones. They are not associated with 280 nm absorption peaks, which can be better seen in Figures 14 and 15, which seems to indicate that the venom-active polypeptides contain little or no tyrosine, tryptophan, and phenylalanine. Some of the same effects are produced by components found in the two activity zones, an indication that they are differentiated by their molecular size. These data show that this particular venom contains components of different molecular weight which have, however, identical pharmacologic activities.

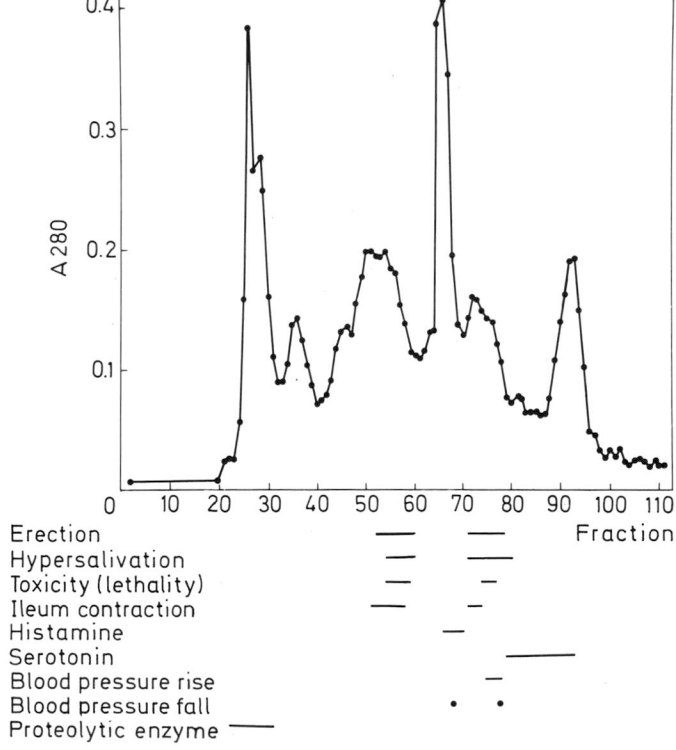

Fig. 12. Chromatogram of *P. nigriventer* venom, fractionated on a Sephadex G-50 column. Thirteen pharmacologically active components are distributed in two zones. The same effect can be provoked by two molecules of different sizes. The proteolytic enzyme was detected in tubes of the first 280 nm peak. Flaccid paralysis remains masked by the dominant distensive paralysis

From the venom constituents, the proteolytic enzyme is easily distinguished from the pharmacologically active polypeptides by its larger molecular weight. The ileum-contracting polypeptides, histamine and serotonin, were obtained, free from other active components in a few fractions; this is considered evidence that toxicity and ileum contraction are produced by different fractions of the venom. The polypeptides responsible for erection, hypersalivation, and toxicity are not separated by Sephadex G-50. Most of the toxic components were not detected in all tubes from the second zone, which contained the hypersalivation and erection polypeptides. Probably, because of their low concentration in the tubes, corresponding to the descending parts of the activity peaks (horizontal lines), and also, because very little solution was left after the other assays, the fraction might not have been present in large enough quantities for a toxicity assay which requires a higher dose.

Fractions of this column do not induce flaccid paralysis, since the polypeptide responsible for this effect, is probably found together in the same tubes with that responsible for the dominant distensive paralysis in mice.

The Sephadex G-50 columns permitted the separation of two other components of this venom. One, administered intravenously in dogs, provoked a rise in blood pressure and the other a fall in blood pressure (SCHENBERG and PEREIRA LIMA, 1966, 1967, 1971). Neither has been well studied, though it has been found that

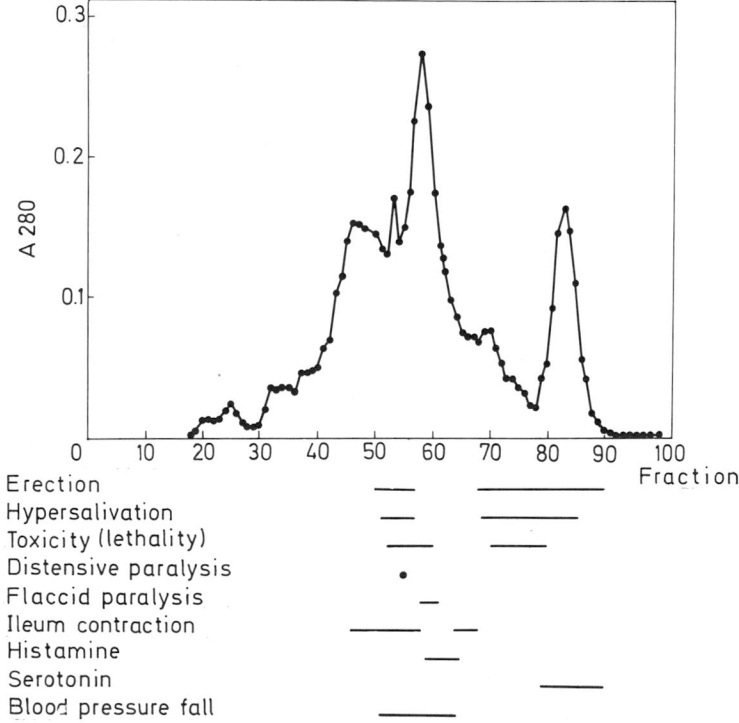

Fig. 13. This chromatogram is similar to that of Figure 12, except for the venom which was submitted to separation after being heated at 100° C for 6 min in 0.05 M phosphate buffer at pH 8.0. Some 280 nm peaks were denatured (proteolytic enzyme). Distensive paralysis was partially inactivated, permitting to detection of flaccid paralysis

some of these fractions contain neither histamine nor serotonin. With crude venom the hypotensive effects dominate and mask the hypertensive ones (SCHENBERG and PEREIRA LIMA, 1966, 1971).

The chromatogram of Figure 13 represents the distribution of the fractions of 20 mg of venom, which had been heated at 100° C for 6 min in 0.005 M phosphate buffer at pH 8.0, and than were made to run on a Sephadex G-50 column.

The first 280 nm absorption peak of Figure 12, represents venom components, which are excluded in Sephadex G-50, including the venom proteolytic enzyme. They were denatured by heating and are absent in Figure 13. The other 280 nm peaks are of components which, by enduring boiling temperature, are probably polypeptides, and maintained their positions. As mentioned before, about 80% of the toxicity is lost by this heat treatment, and this seems to be indicated (Fig. 13) by the absence of the distensive paralysis polypeptides from a large number of tubes. Their absence revealed the flaccid paralysis component, which is also toxic, since the two components ordinarily overlap (SCHENBERG and PEREIRA LIMA, 1971). A third toxic component, not associated with paralysis, seems to be present in the venom.

VII. Ion-Exchange Columns

More data on this spider venom-composition were furnished by ion-exchange columns. Figure 14 shows a chromatogram of 20 mg of venom run on a DEAE-cellulose column (300 × 20 mm), and equilibrated with a 0.005 M glycine buffer at pH 8.35. The same buffer was used to dissolve the venom and also as the first eluent solution; in stepwise elution, its molarity was increased.

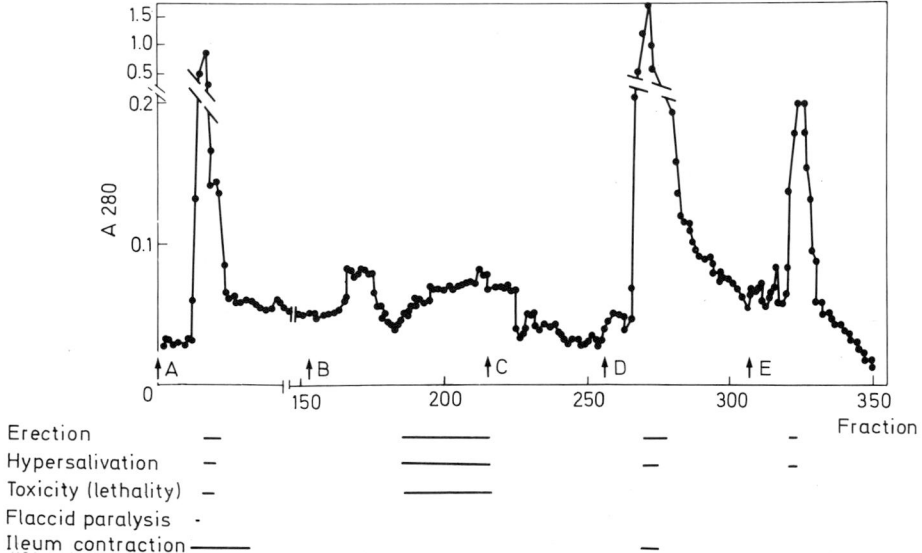

Fig. 14. Chromatogram of *P. nigriventer* venom fractionated on a DEAE-cellulose column. Four components differing in charge can induce the same effect. Two peaks of 280 nm superpose with two activity peaks. Flaccid and distensive paralysis were separated

The pharmacologically active components are distributed in four zones by DEAE-cellulose columns, similar to the two zones reported before by using Sephadex G-50 columns (SCHENBERG and PEREIRA LIMA, 1971). In the fourth zone the 280 nm absorption peak seems to overlap the activity peaks (represented by horizontal lines) associated with erection and hypersalivation fractions. These activities are free of toxic components on the third and fourth zones, which would indicate that toxicity, erection, and hypersalivation are not provoked by a single component. However, these findings are not definitive, since in mice, erection and hypersalivation are both induced by lower doses than is toxicity.

The venom factors, responsible for flaccid and distensive paralysis, are found in independent fractions from DEAE-cellulose columns. Distensive paralysis, not represented in Figure 14, was induced by part of the tubes of the toxicity peak of the first zone, and by all of the second zone. According to these data, the venom would contain 14 pharmacologically active components, including histamine and serotonin, not assayed in the effluent fractions of this column. Two of the three activity peaks attributed to the ileum-contracting effects in Figure 14, probably correspond to these amines.

The chromatogram of Figure 15 represents the fractionation of 20 mg of venom in a CM-Sephadex C-50 column (270 × 10 mm) in gradient and stepwise elutions. The effluent activities do not overlap with the 280 nm, and again, four activity zones were recorded. As in the previous chromatogram, two of the four activity

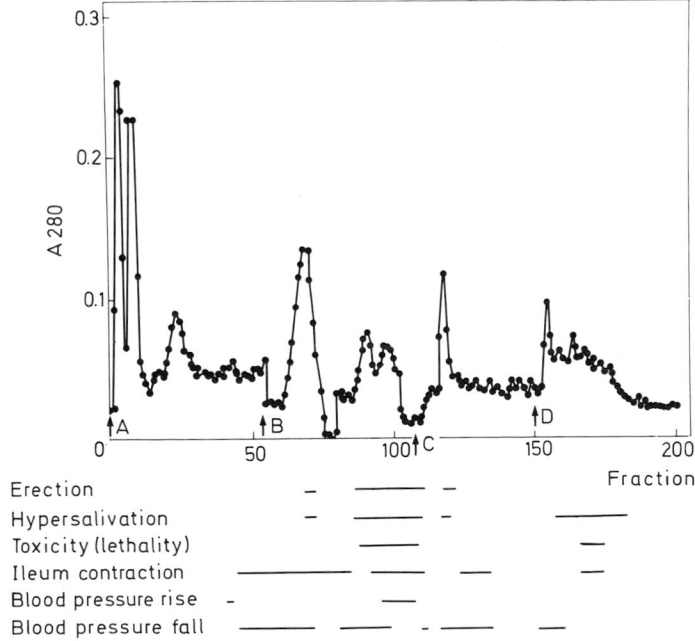

Fig. 15. Chromatogram of *P. nigriventer* venom fractionated in a CM-Sephadex C-50 column by gradient and stepwise elutions. Again, four components differing in charge can induce the same effect. Erection is absent in fourth zone, indicating possibility that molecules might differ from those responsible for hypersalivation and toxicity

peaks assigned to the ileum-contracting effects, are thought to correspond to the histamine and serotonin of the venom, which were not assayed. Flaccid and distensive paralysis were not separated by this column, and the former could not be revealed. Toxicity was not detected together with erection and hypersalivation in the first and third zones; however, as stated before, large volumes are necessary to induce this effect, which does not exclude its presence in both these zones and was not detected in the assays (SCHENBERG and PEREIRA LIMA, 1971).

Erection was not revealed in the fourth zone, constituting a very significant fact, since its minimal effective dose is much smaller than that of toxicity. The tubes containing this fraction killed mice before any sign of erection, a possible indication that erection and toxicity might depend on two distinct polypeptides.

The data reported here furnish evidence which seems to demonstrate that the molecules of each activity-zone differ from those of other zones in weight and electrical charge. The molecules of a single zone also differ from each other by their pharmacologic activities.

The problem increases in complexity when it must be assumed that four different polypeptides can induce the same effect, and that this is extended to several of the venom actions. The individual synthesis of such a large number of polypeptides by a small and hollow gland with pratically only one monocellular layer of secretive cells would represent a tremendous burden.

A better investigation of the venom proteolytic enzyme might give some more information about this apparently paradoxical fact. As was mentioned before, all *P. nigriventer* venom-active polypeptides are inactivated by trypsin, chymotrypsin, and pepsin. The venom's proteolytic enzyme differs in its activity from the former three by its specificity. It only inactivates the ileum-contracting polypeptides. Also, it hydrolyzes casein more rapidly than albumin. Thus, it seems probable that the veneniferous gland would secrete the proteolytic enzyme into its lumen simultaneously with a few large proteins. These will be hydrolyzed by the enzyme. The proteins would act as a kind of precursors of the active polypeptides. The precursors should have one or more specific bonds for the venom's proteolytic enzyme, and according to its cascade hydrolysis, the venom accumulated in the veneniferous gland might contain molecules having the same pharmacologic center but linked to other smaller or larger molecules which would affect their charge and weight. This hypothesis seems to be supported by the presence of free amino acids in the venom, namely glutamic acid (23.6%). They are, probably, residues of proteins hydrolyzed by the venom's proteolytic enzyme. It is reasonable to assume that these amino acids are obligatorily connected to specific bonds of the precursors which will be hydrolyzed. After the bonds rupture, the amino acids are set free.

G. Envenomation in Man

I. Symptomatology

ROSENFELD et al. (1963) report that the bite signal may not be visible or is represented either by a punctiform mark, a small erosion of the skin or a mild erythema. The local pain, which may be very intense, is immediate, irradiating to the entire affected limb and extending to the trunk. The bite provokes hypothermia, sudoresis, tachycardia, and an increase in blood pressure. However, when it acts successfully against local pain, the sedative treatment, rapidly normalizes all these symptoms, since they must represent simple consequences of pain. Death rarely occurs, and is only seen in very weak patients and small children. The venom, though being very toxic, is inoculated in very small doses to have a lethal effect. The peripheral vascular collapse, which sometimes occurs, must also be a consequence of pain (ROSENFELD et al., 1963).

In children with severe envenomation, erection is very often one of the signs of a *P. nigriventer* bite.

II. Frequency of Cases

In the city of São Paulo, the number of human accidents by *P. nigriventer* bites increases during winter. Cold weather makes the spiders invade houses, and leave nearby gardens, small vegetations, outside accumulated stones, bricks or other material where the spiders can find a dark place to hide. Inside the houses, these spiders commonly hide in shoes, clothes, and underneath bedcovers. The accidents occur when using these personal utilities.

A high frequency of accidents is found among professional workers who handle clusters of bananas. This species has a special preference to hide in clusters of bananas, and does not leave the cluster during its transportation from banana plantations, even when shipped to foreign countries. Accidents with these spiders have been reported in Argentina and Switzerland, with a few deaths among workers who handled imported clusters of bananas.

III. Therapy of Envenomation

Local pain is the principal symptom, and must be attacked energetically and promptly with analgesics and sedatives which must act in proportion to the intensity of the symptoms. In severe cases, morphine must be injected intramuscularly, and when necessary, intravenously (ROSENFELD et al., 1963).

Local infiltrations with Novocain of Xylocaine are indicated in mild cases. In the Hospital Vital Brazil of the Instituto Butantan, when pain reappears again after 30 min infiltration with analgesics, one ampoule of the specific antivenin is applied i.m.

Peripheral vasodilatation relieves pain, and can be obtained with warm water or rubefacient ointments. General vasodilatation can be attempted by injecting i.v. an ampoule of nicotinamide, which constitutes an auxilliary medication in severe cases, and is the unique treatment of this symptom when it is not too intense (ROSENFELD et al., 1963).

When respiration is affected with severe tachypnea, and in the case of small children, opium derivatives (morphine, papaverine) must be avoided, since they can potentiate the venom action on respiration. Other analgesics with barbiturics should then be used.

Antihistamines (Phenergan) must be given not only because the *P. nigriventer* venom contains this amine but also due to its tissular liberation by the venom.

Intramuscular injection of antihistamines must precede those of antivenin, since it may minimize serum accidents, which are very rare due to the advances in serum production.

In severe cases, namely in children, from 1 to 5 ampoules of antivenin must be administred intramuscularly, followed by the same quantity intravenously.

Susceptibility to serum anaphylaxis must be checked by dropping one drop of the antivenin on the conjintiva. In cases of susceptibility, the antivenin must be injected in increasing doses following a desensitization method. Fading of pain or erection in children can be taken into consideration to evaluate the antivenin action.

The Instituto Butantan produces the Soro Antiaracnídico Polivalente which is active against the species of *Phoneutria, Lycosa,* and *Loxosceles.*

References

Barrio, A.: Spastic action of the venom of the spider *Phoneutria fera.* Acta physiol. lat.-amer. **5**, 132–143 (1955).

Bonnet, P.: Bibliographia Araneorum, Analyse méthodique de toute la litérature Aranéologique jusqu'en 1939, Tome II. Toulouse 1956.

Brazil, O.V. and Vellard, J.: Contribuição ao estudo de veneno das aranhas. Mem. Inst. Butantan **2**, 1–70 (1925).

Bücherl, W.: Dosagem comparada da atividade dos extratos glandulares e do veneno puro de *Phoneutria nigriventer* (Keyserling), 1891. Mem. Inst. Butantan **25**, No. 2, 1–21 (1953).

Bücherl, W.: Studies on dried venom of *Phoneutria fera* Perty, 1833. In: Venoms. Ed. E.E. Buckley and N. Porges. Washington, D.C.: Amer. Ass. Advanc. Sci. 1956, pp. 95–97.

Bücherl, W.: Spiders. In: Venomous Animals and Their Venoms. Ed. W. Bücherl and E.E. Buckley. New York-London: Academic Press 1971, Vol. III, pp. 197–277.

Cambridge, F.: Ann. Mag. Nat. Hist. [6], 19, 76 (1897), cited by W. Bücherl: Venomous Animals and Their Venoms, Ed. W. Bücherl and E.E. Buckley, New York-London: Academic Press 1971, Vol. III, pp. 197–277.

Cambridge, O.P.: Biol. Centr. Am. **1**, 93 (1892), cited by W. Bücherl: Venomous Animals and Their Venoms, Ed. W. Bücherl and E.E. Buckley, New York-London: Academic Press 1971, Vol. III, pp. 197–277.

Cambridge, O.P.: Proc. Soc. Zool. London **1**, 247 (1902), cited by W. Bücherl: Venomous Animals and Their Venoms, Ed. W. Bücherl and E.E. Buckley, New York-London: Academic Press, 1971, Vol. III, pp. 197–277.

Diniz, C.R.: Separação de proteinas e caracterização de substâncias ativas em venenos de aranhas do Brasil. Anais Acad. bras. Cienc. **35**, 283–291 (1963a).

Diniz, C.R.: Personal communication (1963b).

Fischer, F.G., Bohn, H.: Die Giftsekrete der brasilianischen Tarantel *Lycosa erythrognata* und der Wanderspinne *Phoneutria fera.* Z. Physiol. Chem. **306**, 265–268 (1957).

Kaiser, E.: The enzymatic activity of spider venom. Mem. Inst. Butantan **25**, No. 1, 35–39 (1953).

Kaiser, E.: Enzymatic activity of spider venom. In: Venoms, Ed. E.E. Buckley and N. Porges. Washington, D.C.: Amer. Ass. Advanc. Sci. 1956, pp. 91–93.

Keyserling, G.E.: Brasilanische Spinnen. Nürenberg: Verlag von Bauer & Raspe 1891.

Koch, C.L.: Die Arachniden. Fünfzehnter Band, p. 1–136. Nürenberg 1848.

Mello-Leitão, C.: Contribution à l'étude des Cténides du Brésil, Festschrift für Prof. Dr. Embrik Strand **1**, 1–31 (1936).

Millot, J.: Les glandes venimeuses des aranéides. Ann. Sci. Nat. Zool. **14**, 113–147 (1931) cited by J. Vellard: Le venin des araignées. Paris: Masson 1936.

Pereira Lima, F.A., Schenberg, S.: Separação dos componentes ativos de veneno de *Phoneutria fera* por eletroforese em acetato de celulose (Oxoid). Cienc. e Cult. (São Paulo) **15**, 268 (1963).

Pereira Lima, F.A., Schenberg, S.: Caracteristicas e separação dos componentes do veneno de *Phoneutria fera*. Cienc. e Cult. (São Paulo) **16**, 187 (1964).

Perty, M.: Delectus Animalium, 1833, pp. 197 cited by W. Bücherl: Venomous Animals and Their Venoms. Ed. W. Bücherl and E.E. Buckley. New York-London: Academic Press 1971, Vol. III, pp. 197—277.

Petrunkevitch, A.: Bull. Amer. Mus. Nat. Hist. **29**, 473 (1911), cited by W. Bücherl: Venomous Animals and Their Venoms. Ed. W. Bücherl and E.E. Buckley. New York-London: Academic Press, 1971, Vol. III, pp. 197—277.

Reed, L.J., Muench, H.: A simple method of estimating fifty per cent endpoints. Amer. J. Hyg. **27**, 493—497 (1938).

Rosenfeld, G., Nahas, L., de Cillo, D.M., e Fleury, C.T.: Envenenamentos por serpentes, aranhas e escorpiões. In: Atualização Terapeutica, 5a ed. Rio de Janeiro, Ed. F. Cintra do Prado, J.A. Ramos e J. Ribeiro do Valle, Livraria Luso-Espanhola e Brasileira, 1963, pp. 1148—1160.

Sampayo, R.R.L.: *Latrodectus mactans* y lactrodectismo. Tesis de doctorado en Medicina, Universidad Nacional de Buenos Aires, Buenos Aires, 1942.

Schenberg, S., Pereira Lima, F.A.: Estudo farmacológico do veneno de *Phoneutria fera*. Cienc. e Cult. (São Paulo) **14**, 237 (1962).

Schenberg, S., Pereira Lima, F.A.: Individualização dos componentes ativos do veneno de *Phoneutria fera*. Cienc. e Cult. (São Paulo) **14**, 237—238 (1963).

Schenberg, S., Pereira Lima, F.A.: Priapism, sialorrhea and other toxic effects induced in dogs and mice by polypeptides of spider (*Phoneutria fera*) venom. Abstracts of 3rd Int. Pharmacol. Congr. São Paulo, p. 189 (1966).

Schenberg, S., Pereira Lima, F.A.: Componentes ativos do veneno de *Phoneutria fera*. Cienc. e Cult. (São Paulo) **19**, 456—457 (1967).

Schenberg, S., Pereira Lima, F.A.: *Phoneutria nigriventer* venom—Pharmacology and biochemistry of its components. In: Venomous Animals and Their venoms. Ed. W. Bücherl and E.E. Buckley. New York-London: Academic Press, 1971, Vol. III, pp. 279—297.

Schenberg, S., Pereira Lima, F.A.: Unpublished observation (1975).

Simon, E.: Histoire Naturelle des Araignées, fasc. 1, pp. 1—192, 2. édit., Tome II. Paris 1897.

Vellard, J.: Le vénin des araignées. Paris: Masson 1936.

Walckenaer, C.A.: Ins. Apteres **2**, 211—272 (1837), cited by W. Bücherl: Venomous Animals and Their Venoms. Ed. W. Bücherl and E.E. Buckley. New York-London: Academic Press, 1971, Vol. III, pp. 197—277.

Walckenaer, C.A. (1805), cited by W. Bücherl: Venomous Animals and Their Venoms. Ed. W. Bücherl and E.E. Buckley. New York-London: Academic Press, 1971, Vol. III, pp. 197—277.

Welsh, J.H., Batty, C.S.: 5-Hydroxytryptamine content of some arthropod venoms and venom—containing parts. Toxicon **1**, 165—173 (1963).

CHAPTER 11

Venoms of Scytodidae. Genus Loxosceles

H. Schenone and G. Suarez

A. Distribution and Biology of Venomous Species; Chemistry, Toxicity, Pharmacology, and Mode of Action of Venom

I. Systematics and Distribution of Species

Spiders of the genus *Loxosceles* Heinecken and Lowe belong to the subfamily *Loxoscelinae,* family *Scytodidae,* suborder Araneomorphae.

Willis J. Gertsch (1958, 1967) from the American Museum of Natural History in New York has made important contributions in this field of arachnology and most of the information therefore in this section comes from this source.

These spiders are widely distributed in temperate and tropical regions. Native species are only known from two main centers, Africa and the Americas. About 17 species range from temperate South Africa towards the north through the tropics into the Mediterranean zone and southern Europe. Only 2 species exist in the warmer regions of Europe. Nearly 50 species have been described in the Americas. In other regions *Loxosceles* are represented only by the so-called cosmopolitan *Loxosceles rufescens* (Dufour), which might have been transported by trade and which has apparently settled in numerous countries of the Near East, the Orient, and in parts of the United States.

Regarding their threat to man, all members of the genus *Loxosceles* must be considered "guilty until proved innocent" (Gorham, 1968). Nevertheless, in a general sense, only four species, *L. laeta, L. reclusa, L. rufescens,* and *L. gaucho* have been shown to be the cause of envenomation in man (Gertsch, 1967). In addition, some relatively recent publications have reported that *L. rufipes, L. spadicea, L. unicolor,* and *L. arizonica* produce human pathology (Schenone et al., 1957; Bücherl, 1964a, b; Delgado, 1969; Russell et al., 1969).

The most widespread and important species in different areas of the world are *L. laeta* (Nicolet), *L. reclusa* (Gertsch and Mulaik) and *L. rufescens* (Dufour). *L. laeta* probably originated from west South America, has been verified in Chile, Argentina, Uruguay, Brazil, Ecuador, and Peru, and has spread northward to Guatemala, Honduras, and some parts of the United States and Canada. *L. reclusa,* the brown spider, is native to the United States, the country in which it is principally found in the south and central states. *L. rufescens,* which probably originated from the Mediterranean region of Europe and Africa, has been recorded in Spain, France, Italy, the Balkans, Greece, southern Russia, all the North African countries, Madagascar, Israel, Burma, China, Japan, the eastern United States, Mexico, Brazil, Paraguay, and many islands in the Atlantic Ocean (Bonnet, 1957; Bücherl, 1964a, b;

Levi and Spielman, 1964; Gertsch, 1967; Brignoli, 1969; Efrati, 1969; Canese, 1972; Puffer et al., 1972).

II. Morphology and Biology

Spiders of the genus *Loxosceles* are medium sized: body length 8–15 mm, leg length 18–30 mm. The most common color is brown and varies from deep walnut to pale fawn. The abdomen is darker than the cephalothorax and the legs. On the dorsal surface of the cephalothorax they have six eyes in three diads distributed in a semicircle and they possess a broad and deep median groove. Most of them present a dark mark shaped like a violin with the handle directed posteriorly (Fig. 1). Males are slightly smaller and more slender than the females (Bücherl, 1960–62; Gertsch, 1967).

Both female and male spin a large, irregular web in the dark. The female elaborates cottonlike whitish discoidal egg sacs or ootecae, about 15–20 mm in diameter, containing 22–138 eggs with an average of 88 (Galiano, 1967).

Eggs are pale yellow in color and 1.1–1.2 mm in diameter. After an incubation period of about 13 days the eggs hatch giving rise to small spiderlings. After 9–12 months the adult stage is reached. The average time required to reach adulthood varies between 336 days in *L. reclusa* (Hite et al., 1966) to 315 days for females and 406 days for males in *L. laeta* (Galiano, 1967). Average life span in laboratory colonies is for *L. rufipes* and *L. rufescens* 365–550 days (Bücherl, 1961), for *L. reclusa* 301–796 days for males and 356–894 days for females (Hite et al.,

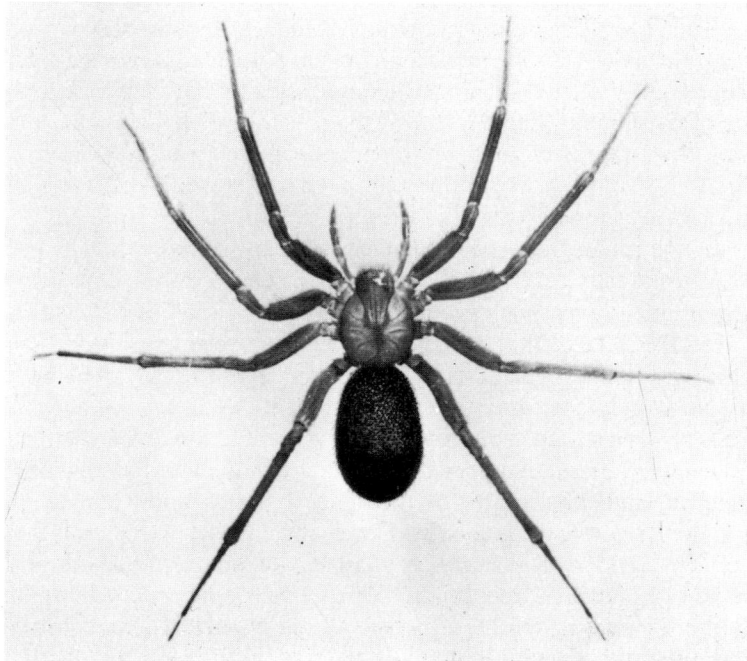

Fig. 1. *L. laeta* adult female

1966), and for *L. laeta* 696, 1155, 1536, and 1894 days for mated males, unmated males, mated females, and unmated females respectively (GALIANO and HALL, 1973).

Loxoscelines feed on flies, moths, beetles, and other small arthropods that become entrapped in the web. But they also forage for food at night (GORHAM, 1968). Among the adults there exists generally one male for every $6-7$ females (BÜCHERL, 1961; SCHENONE et al., 1970; VILLARROEL et al., 1971).

According to GERTSCH (1967) they are shy, solitary, sedentary spiders active mostly at night, and they occupy a great variety of habitats in natural and domestic situations. They prefer the darkness and some live under rocks, loose bark, tree trunks, and ground litter, in holes of trees and natural openings of cliffs. Man provides suitable habitats for them in and around his buildings. The spiders move actively or are passively transported by man within different materials into such outbuildings as garages, cellars, barns, storage sheds, chicken coops, yard walls, and also into his homes. In buildings they are found under furniture and all kinds of objects, behind picture frames and clothing hung against walls. They are also found in closets, drawers, and corners of rooms.

L. laeta has been found both in natural and domestic habitats (MACKINNON and WITKIND, 1953; VELLARD, 1954b; SUAREZ and CASAVILCA, 1967). In Chile, it has been found almost exclusively in domestic habitats and it is called "araña de los rincones" (corner spider) and "araña de detrás de los cuadros" (spider behind the pictures). In a random survey of 2,189 houses of central Chile it was found infesting 40.6% of rural and 24.4% of urban houses (SCHENONE et al., 1970).

The activity of spiders and other similar arthropods, among other factors, depends on the environmental temperature conditions. Winter environment even inside the houses has been a rigorous limiting factor for cold-blooded animals. Winter weather, particularly low temperature, has been therefore an ecologic barrier against the extension of their range, even for domestic, or better, synanthropic species. The use of central heating or other kinds of heating creates a summerlike environment in the house, favorable to the settlement and development of spiders and other arthropods (GORHAM, 1968).

III. Anatomy and Histology of the Venomous Apparatus

Loxoscelids have two-segmented chelicerae which consist of a very short fang attached to a stout basal segment capable of limited lateral motion (GERTSCH, 1967). The fangs are $0.39-0.60$ mm long; the basal segment $1.45-1.71 \times 0.65-0.89$ mm (BÜCHERL, 1964a; DELGADO, 1969; SCHENONE et al., 1975a). The opening of the venom duct is situated on the lateral aspect of the fang (SMITH and MICKS, 1968). Abductory and adductory muscles inserted in the inner parts of the cephalo-thorax move the chelicerae (Figs. 2A and 2B).

The venom glands are endocephalic large sacculate bodies, wide in the center and narrow at the base of the efferent duct. The mean measures of *Loxosceles* glands are $1.7-1.9$ mm long and $0.3-0.8$ mm wide. The efferent duct is 1.5 mm long (Fig. 2A). Externally the glands present a strong striated intrinsic musculature which is distributed in circular and longitudinal layers. Extrinsic musculature main-tains the efferent ducts and the glands in their positions and contributes to the

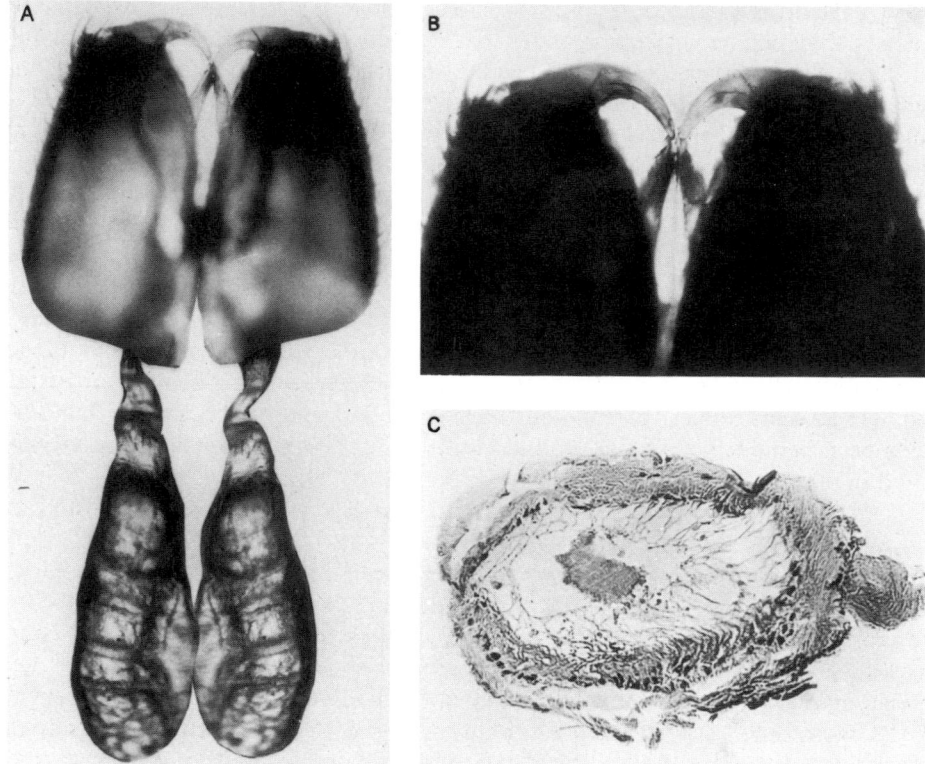

Fig. 2A – C. Venom apparatus of *L. laeta*. (A) Chelicerae (basal segments and fangs) and venom glands. (B) Detail of fangs. (C) Microscopic aspect of transverse section of venom gland

expulsion of the venom at the moment of the bite (BÜCHERL, 1964a; SCHENONE et al., 1975a).

Histologically, the gland presents an external muscularis, a basal membrane, and a venom excretory epithelium. The basal membrane is delicate and lines the muscularis internally. The epithelium is simple and presents three types of cell, which are orientated towards a central space or reservoir for elaborated venom. a) High cylindrical cells, in active process of venom production. b) Cubic cells, attached to the basal membrane, besides the cylindrical ones, and which functionally represent a source of replacement for the constantly degenerating cylindrical cells (Fig. 2C). c) In the neck region also exist cylindrical excretory cells, whose duration and functions are permanent (BÜCHERL, 1964b).

IV. Physiology, in Particular Physiology of the Bite

In nature, biting and feeding are related physiologic actions exerted by the spiders. Frequently the mechanical action of the chelicerae is sufficient to paralyze and kill the prey without participation of the venom. When the spider bites, digestive juices from glands near the mouth may be emptied into the area of the bite (BÜCHERL,

1964; VELLARD, 1966a; GERTSCH, 1967). These juices contain enzymes that digest the prey tissues *in situ*, which are afterward sucked by the spider (DELGADO, 1966).

It is well known that bites of human beings produce no benefit for the spider, they are mere accidents, as when the arachnid comes into direct contact with human skin. This happens when spiders live in relatively close contact with man either in his home or in his varied areas of activity. The loxoscelid frequently crawls into beds and clothing and may become incarcerate either in the folds of garments or between clothes and skin of individuals sleeping or dressing. Thus, when the spider is disturbed or when it is tightly held or crushed, it tries to defend itself by biting. The sharp and short fangs are jabbed into the skin of the victim, and simultaneously in most cases venom is injected.

At the moment of biting both the fangs and basal segments are mobilized into a piercing action by the abductory and adductory muscles. Different muscle bundles produce simultaneously a vigorous contraction of the venom glands, push them forward, and dilate the efferent ducts, and the venom is expelled (BÜCHERL, 1964b).

V. Chemistry of the Venom

Until very recently almost nothing was known about the chemical nature of the venom of spiders of the genus *Loxosceles*. For instance, a recent review on toxicology of arthropods (PAVAN and VALCURONE DAZZINI, 1971) includes the specific comment that studies on this genus are limited to their pathogenic effects on man. The chemical characterization of the venom gland secretion of these spiders has been hampered by the difficulties encountered in obtaining the raw material in preparative amounts. The lack of chemical knowledge about these toxins has not permitted the construction of a satisfactory model concerning their mechanism of action. However, it has been suggested (BIGGEMANN, 1971) that the efforts toward isolating the active components might be facilitated by studies on the mechanism of action using partially purified extracts. It is also important to bear in mind that the venom action could represent the final effect of cooperative interactions between several components of the venom gland secretion. Although similar lesions in man and rabbit have been found to be produced by *L. unicolor, L. arizonica,* and *L. rufescens* (RUSSELL et al., 1969; EFRATI, 1969), biochemical studies seem to be restricted to the venom extracts of the species *L. laeta* and *L. reclusa,* which will be the main subject of this review.

1. Methods of Obtaining the Venom

The techniques which have been used to obtain the venomous secretion from spiders of this genus vary from author to author. MORRIS and RUSSELL (1975) have proposed mild electrical stimulation to elicit the extrusion of venom from the chelicerae to a micromanipulated pipette. This method has the advantage of allowing several extractions from the same specimen since the spider is unharmed. Alternative procedures involve the homogenization of the poison apparatus of *L. reclusa* (GEREN et al., 1973) or the dissected venom glands of *L. laeta* (SUAREZ et al., 1971a). In both methods the initial crude extract is the supernatant fluid obtained after centrifugation. It is claimed that these procedures avoid contamination with stomach contents as would occur with electrical stimulation (Geren et al., 1973).

2. Chemical Composition of Venom Extracts

Using the technique of electrical stimulation Morris and Russell (1975) found in the venom of *L. reclusa* a water content of 82% and a protein concentration of 26%. The volume of the obtained venom fluid is higher for female (0.29 µl) than for male (0.15 µl) specimens. The average amount of venom protein per spider was found to be 68 µg in *L. reclusa* (Berger et al., 1973) and 48.6 µg in *L. laeta* (Suarez et al., unpublished).

The components present in extracts from *L. laeta* venom glands, that possess necrotizing activity on the skin of the rabbit, are proteins since they are nondialyzable, thermolabile, and are inactivated by treatment with trichloroacetic acid or pepsin (Suarez et al., 1971a). The venom proteins apparently do not require essential sulfhydryl groups, for their activity is not influenced after reacting with p-hydroxy-mercuribenzoate. The presence of functionally essential carbohydrates covalently bound to protein constituents is indicated by the disappearance of venom activity after oxidation with periodate and the detection of a positive anthrone reaction in dialyzed crude extracts as well as in partially purified active fractions. These findings suggest a glycoprotein nature for the active components of *L. laeta* venom. Neuraminic acid does not appear to be involved, at least from a functional point of view, since the treatment with neuraminidase has no effect.

3. Fractionation and Characterization of Venom Proteins

The standard techniques for the fractionation of proteins have been applied to venom preparations. In the case of *L. reclusa* the use of gel filtration through Sephadex G-25 allowed the separation of the venom extract into two major components: a high molecular fraction which was lethal to mice and a low molecular fraction which proved to be nontoxic. The high molecular weight material could be further resolved by the sequential use of gel filtration through Sephadex G-100 and preparative gel disc electrophoresis into several components, two of which are endowed with toxic properties (Geren et al., 1973). These protein fractions have been named toxin 1 and toxin 2 by investigators. Their molecular weight is in the range of 24,000 and their isoelectric pH is apparently 8.3. A closer study of these toxins (Odell et al., 1975) revealed that toxin 1 is responsible for the lesions produced in rabbits and is lethal for mice and rabbits, whereas toxin 2 does not produce external lesions and is toxic only to rabbits.

The venom of *L. laeta* has been subjected to gel filtration and a highly purified fraction of molecular weight approximately 20,000 has been obtained (Suarez et al., 1971a). The behavior of this fraction in ion exchange resins suggests the presence of more than one component with very different isoelectric pH's (Biggemann, 1971) and the ability to produce qualitatively different lesions in the rabbit. The active fractions are devoid of the enzyme activities which have been found in the whole extract (see below).

In summary, the data available lead to the view that the active constituents of the venom of the species of the genus *Loxosceles* studied so far are at least two proteins with qualitatively different pathogenicities.

4. Enzymatic Properties of Venom

The most common enzymatic activities which have been described in snake venoms are not found in the toxic secretions of these spiders. Table 1 summarizes the enzymes which have been searched for in the venoms of the species *L. laeta* and *L. reclusa*. None of the phospholipases are present in the extracts of either species. An alkaline phosphatase has been found in the venom of *L. reclusa* which is inactivated by p-hydroxy-mercuribenzoate (HEITZ and NORMENT, 1974). The insensitivity of the venomous activity of *L. laeta* venom toward this reagent makes this enzyme an unlikely participant of the toxic action if both species are biochemically related. Hyaluronidase has been found in the whole extracts of *L. laeta* but not in their active fractions (BIGGEMANN, 1971). The same enzyme has been recognized in *L. reclusa* (HALL, 1970; WRIGHT et al., 1972). Hyaluronidase probably plays the role of a spreading factor, favoring the propagation of the lesions into contiguous areas of the skin by gravitation, although it is not a toxic element per se. Protease was absent in the venom *L. laeta* and the contradictory results obtained in *L. reclusa* might be a reflection of different modes of preparation of the venom. The absence of collagenase (SUAREZ et al., 1971 a; WRIGHT et al., 1972) in these toxins does not explain in enzymatic terms, the histologic alterations of connective tissue found in the lesions (PIZZI, 1975).

Unfractionated extracts of the venom of *L. laeta* inhibit the *in vitro* incorporation of free amino acids into protein in cell-free systems derived from mammalian as well as bacterial sources. However, there is no interference with protein synthesis if it proceeds from aminoacyl transfer ribonucleic acid (SUAREZ et al., 1970, 1971 b). Since the stability to hydrolysis of aminoacyl transfer ribonucleic acid is not in-

Table 1. Enzyme activities of venoms of *Loxosceles* spiders

Enzyme investigated	Species	Result	Reference
Adenosinetriphosphatase	*L. laeta*	+	SUAREZ et al., 1971b
Alkaline phosphatase	*L. reclusa*	+	HEITZ and NORMENT, 1974
Collagenase	*L. laeta*	−	SUAREZ et al., 1971a
Collagenase	*L. reclusa*	−	WRIGHT et al., 1972
Esterase	*L. reclusa*	+	WRIGHT et al., 1972
Hyaluronidase	*L. reclusa*	+	WRIGHT et al., 1972; HALL, 1970
Hyaluronidase	*L. laeta*	+	BIGGEMANN, 1971
Lipase	*L. reclusa*	+	NAZHAT, 1968
Phosphodiesterase	*L. laeta*	−	SUAREZ et al., 1971a
Phospholipase A	*L. laeta*	−	SUAREZ et al., 1971b
Phospholipase A	*L. reclusa*	−	HALL, 1970; WRIGHT et al., 1972
Phospholipase C	*L.laeta*	−	SUAREZ et al., 1971a
Phospholipase C	*L. reclusa*	−	NAZHAT, 1968
Phospholipase D	*L. reclusa*	−	NAZHAT, 1968
Protease	*L. laeta*	−	SUAREZ et al., 1971a
Protease	*L. reclusa*	−	GEREN et al., 1973; NAZHAT, 1968
Protease	*L. reclusa*	+	WRIGHT, 1972

fluenced by the venom, the most plausible explanation of its inhibitory effect is the inactivation of a cofactor or substrate required for amino acid activation. The finding of adenosinetriphosphatase points to the hydrolysis of ATP as the most probable cause of the venom effect on in vitro protein synthesis (Biggemann et al., 1970). Since this enzyme is not present in partially purified active fractions its involvement in the pathogenicity of the venom can be ruled out.

5. Immunogenicity of the Venom

Venom preparations have proved to be very effective antigens. Schenone et al. (1970) were able to induce the resistance of rabbits to venom doses as high as the contents of 64 glands of L. laeta by periodical intradermal inoculations of increasing amounts. Antibodies to venom constituents of the same species have been detected by immunodiffusion technique (Rojas et al., unpublished results). However, it has not been possible to demonstrate antibody response to L. reclusa venom in humans with a history of previous bites (Denny et al., 1964) a fact which has been interpreted in terms of the possible existence of membrane-bound antibodies (Berger et al., 1973). Susceptible species such as rabbit, mouse, and man do not exhibit natural antibodies against L. reclusa in their sera.

Specific antisera to toxin 1 and toxin 2 of L. reclusa have been prepared (Odell et al., 1975).

Cross reactivity in immunodiffusion studies has been found between extracts from L. laeta and L. rufipes (Rojas et al., unpublished results). This would indicate that the protein components of the venom have similar structural features. Similarly, using lymphocyte transformation, Berger et al. (1973) were able to demonstrate immune cross reactivity between the venoms of L. reclusa and L. arizonica. Moreover, the kinetics of the immune response in patients with a history of recent bites by L. reclusa, as monitored by lymphocyte transformation tests, has suggested that this is an example of delayed hypersensitivity.

VI. Toxicity of Venom and Other Components of Loxosceles on Various Animal Species

1. In Vivo Studies

With different species of Loxosceles and using several techniques of injection many authors have produced experimental envenomation on various animal species. The overall results of studies with venom are summarized in Table 2.

Even though some of the authors expressed the doses of venom injected in diverse manners, such as mg of dry content, mg of protein content or simply the content of one gland, in order to have a common element of comparison all the doses used were translated using the gland as a unit. As it may be observed the degree of toxicity varies according to the dose, species, and size of the animal studied.

Whereas some animals are not susceptible to the action of the venom, others are extremely susceptible and therefore suitable to reproduce even local or systemic lesions or both, quite similar to those observed in man. Through the analysis of the results presented in Table 2, according to the weight of the animals and dosages

Table 2. Action of *Loxosceles* venom on various animal species

Animal species	*Loxosceles* species	No. of glands	Route of injection	Effect	References
Guinea pig	*L. laeta*	0.4–1.0	i.d.	Local necrosis	MACCHIAVELLO, 1947b; PIZZI et al., 1957
	L. laeta	0.3–20.0 × kg	i.d.	Death 4–48 h	MACCHIAVELLO, 1947
	L. laeta	0.5–8.0 × kg	p.	Death 4–20 h	VELLARD, 1956
	L. laeta	2.0	i.d.	Death 32–96 h	PIZZI et al., 1957
	L. rufescens and *L. rufipes*	1.1	s.c.	LD 50	FURLANETTO, 1961
Rabbit	*L. laeta*	1.2–2.0	s.c.	LD 50	MACKINNON and WITKIND, 1953
	L. laeta	0.4–1.0 × kg	i.d.	Death 1.3–20 h	VELLARD, 1956
	L. laeta	0.2–6.0 × kg	v.	Death 0.2–24 h	VELLARD, 1956
	L. laeta	1.5	i.d.	LD 50	SCHENONE et al., 1970, 1975a
	L. laeta	3.0–6.0	v.	Death 12–24 h	SCHENONE et al., 1975a
	L. laeta	3.0–9.0	i.d.	Death 12–48 h	SCHENONE et al., 1975a
	L. rufescens and *L. rufipes*	0.7	v	LD$_{50}$	FURLANETTO, 1961
Mouse	*L. laeta*	0.6–1.2	s.c.	LD$_{50}$	MACKINNON and WITKIND, 1953
	L. laeta	0.1–0.3	i.d.	LD$_{50}$	PIZZI et al., 1957
	L. laeta	1.0	i.d.	LD$_{50}$	SCHENONE et al., 1975a
	L. rufescens and *L. rufipes*	0.9	v.	LD$_{50}$	FURLANETTO, 1961
Rat	*L. laeta*	0.25–25.0	i.d.	Not affected	SCHENONE et al., 1975a
Hamster	*L. laeta*	5.0	i.d.	LD$_{50}$	SCHENONE et al., 1975a
Dog	*L. laeta*	1.0–1.5 × kg	v.	Death 1–13 h	VELLARD, 1956
	L. laeta	0.8–2.0 × kg	i.m.	Death 12–30 h	VELLARD, 1956
	L. laeta	3.0–9.0	i.d.	Not affected	SCHENONE et al., 1975a
	L. reclusa	2.0	v.	LD$_{50}$	DENNY et al., 1964
Pigeon	*L. laeta*	1.0–10.0	v.	Death 0.7–12 h	VELLARD, 1956
	L. rufescens and *L. rufipes*	0.3	v.	LD$_{50}$	FURLANETTO, 1961
Chicken	*L. laeta*	1.0–9.0	s.c.	Not affected	SCHENONE et al., 1975a
	L. laeta	11.0–15.0	i.m.	Death 24 h	SCHENONE et al., 1975a
Toad (*Bufo spinulosus*)	*L. laeta*	5.0–10.0	?	Death 24–48 h	VELLARD, 1956
	L. laeta	5.0–15.0	i.m.	Death 96–192 h	SCHENONE et al., 1975a
Frog (*Calyptocephalella gayi*)	*L. laeta*	1.0–13.0	i.m.	Not affected	SCHENONE et al., 1975a
	L. laeta	15.0	i.m.	Death 96 h	SCHENONE et al., 1975a
Fish (*Cyprinus carpio*)	*L. laeta*	5.0–9.0	p.	Not affected	SCHENONE et al., 1975a

i.d. = intradermal; p. = peritoneal; s.c. = subcutaneous; v = venous; i.m. = intramuscular

used, their susceptibility to the venom may be classified as follows: high (rabbit, mouse, guinea pig, dog), moderate (hamster, pigeon, chicken, toad) low (frog) and null (rat, fish).

In spite of the attempt made to present the data, summarized in Table 2, in a simplified and uniform manner, one must keep in mind that results of experimental work may change from one author to another as a consequence of some of the variables. Among these variables are extraction procedures of venom and the resulting product, technique of injection, regional venom activity of different species and strains of *Loxosceles.*

To measure and compare the toxic activity it is advisable to use extracted venom rather than experimental bites where the results are irregular because under experi-

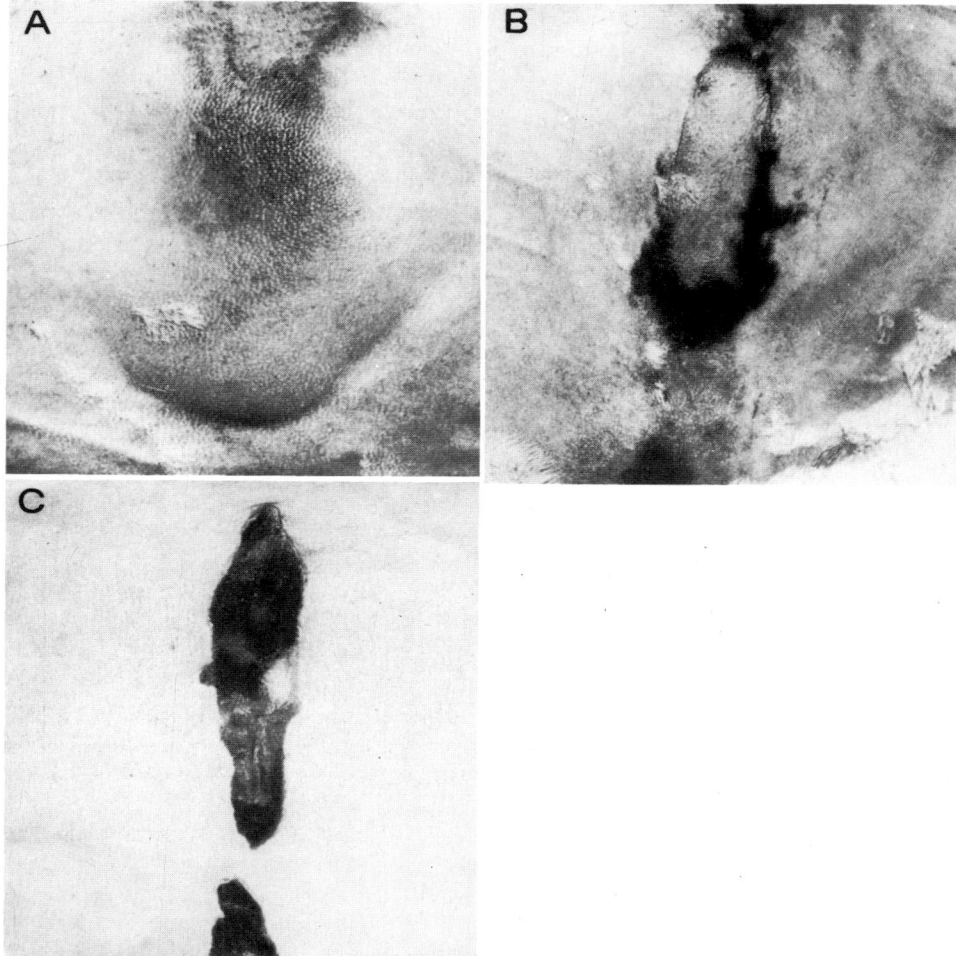

Fig. 3 A — C. Experimental loxoscelism in rabbit. Evolution of local lesions produced by intradermal injection of content of 0.5 venom gland of *L. laeta* (A) 7 h after injection. Echymotic plaque surrounded by an erythematous halo. Intense edema. (B) 48 h. Well-defined necrotic plaque. Erythema persists. Edema decreased. (C) 14 days. Necrotic eschars in process of elimination. Erythema and edema completely disappeared

Table 3. Effects of different components of *Loxosceles* spiders injected into the skin of the rabbit

Component	Effect
Cephalothorax extract (with venomous glands)	General and local necrotic lesions similar to those obtained with venom
Cephalothorax extracts (venomous glands removed)	Minimal edema and necrotic lesion
Abdomen extracts	Erythema and induration without necrosis
Hemolymph	Edema and medium-sized necrotic lesion
Eggs	Edema and local infiltrate

mental conditions the spider does not always bite and also because the amount of venom injected is quite variable (MACKINNON and WITKIND, 1953). Using *L. laeta* and guinea pigs MACCHIAVELLO (1947b) was 37.3% successful in making the spiders bite. But when histopathologic studies on local reactions are desired, without producing important initial skin lesions with needles, sophisticated techniques of induced *Loxosceles* bites may be convenient (HERYFORD, 1970).

Because the rabbit reproduces almost exactly the same lesions as in man, the cutaneous and systemic, it has preferably been used for experiments either with venom or other components of the spider (Fig. 3). SMITH and MICKS (1968) and SCHENONE et al. (1975a) have carried out preliminary studies with some components of *Loxosceles* spiders which are briefly summarized in Table 3.

Studies performed by SCHENONE et al. (1970) with *L. laeta* showed that venom of female spiders had a minimum necrotizing dose of 0.06 gland and an LD_{50} of 1.5 glands on ID injection into rabbits. Venom of male spiders was much weaker and was not used in the experiments dealing with resistance. When increasing doses of venom are given to rabbits on alternate days, tolerance is rapidly established. After 8 injections, the animals can withstand a dose of 64 glands without ill effect other than the production of a local necrotic lesion. This resistance lasts at least 120 days after the last injection. Precipitins were demonstrated in the serum of the rabbits on the sixth day and reached a high titer by the fifteenth day. The resistance of the rabbits is believed to be due to specific antibody response plus increased ability of the animal to detoxify and eliminate the venom.

2. In Vitro Studies

MACCHIAVELLO (1947b), in studying the hemolytic action observed in some cases of human loxoscelism, made some previous experiments and showed that *L. laeta* venom was not capable of producing hemolysis on rabbit and guinea pig erythrocytes, but that cephalothorax extracts of the same spider did produce this phenomenon. These results made other researchers interested in this particular experimental field. This interest increased when severe cases of human loxoscelism with intense hemolysis were observed in different countries (GOTTEN and MACGOWAN, 1940; DROGUET

Table 4. In vitro hemolytic action after 4 and 24 h of the venom and other components of *L. laeta* on human and animal erytrocytes (Knierim et al., 1975)

Species	Venom		Hemolymph		Cephalothorax		Abdominal wall		Abdominal content		Eggs	
	4	24	4	24	4	24	4	24	4	24	4	24
Man												
Group A	−	−	++++	+++++	++	++	+++++	+++++	−	++++	++	++
Group B	−	−	+++++	+++++	+	+	+++++	+++++	+	++++	++++	+++++
Group AB	−	−	++++	+++++	−		++++	++++	−	++++	++++	++++
Group 0	−	−	+++	+++	+	++	+++++	++++	−	+++	+++	+++
Mice	−	−	++++	+++++	+	+++	+++	+++++	++	++++	+++	+++++
Rat	−	−	++++	+++++	++	+++	+++	+++++	+	+++++	+++	+++++
Guinea pig	−	−	++++	+++++	+	++	+++	+++++	+++	+++++	+++	+++++
Hamster	−	−	++++	+++++	−	+++	++++	+++++	+	+++	+++	+++++
Rabbit	−	−	++++	+++++	+	+++	++++	+++++	−	+++	+++	+++++
Cat	−	−	++++	+++++	+	+++	++++	+++++	+	++++	+++	++++
Dog	−	−	++++	+++++	++	+++	++++	+++++	+++	++++	+++	+++++
Sheep	−	−	+++	+++++	++	++	+++	++++	+++	+++	+++	+++++
Chicken	−	−	+++	++	+	+	++	++	+	+++++	++	+
Frog (*Calypto-cephalella gayi*)	−	−	++++	a	+	a	+++	a		a		a
Toad (*Bufo spinulosus*)	−		+++	a	+	a	+++	a	+	a	+++	a
Fish (*Cyprinus carpio*)	−	−	++++	a	++	a	+++	a	+	a	+++	a

a Total hemolysis after 24 h, including the control with saline.

et al., 1951; SCHENONE et al., 1959; WIENER et al., 1960; NANCE, 1961; NICHOLSON and NICHOLSON, 1962; DILLAHA et al., 1964; GAJARDO-TOBAR, 1966; TAYLOR and DENNY, 1966).

Thus, DENNY et al. (1964) using blood from normal persons and *L. reclusa* venom obtained hemolysis whose intensity was proportional to the protein content of the venom. On the other hand, SMITH and MICKS (1968) who used venom and extracts of cephalothorax and abdomen from *L. rufescens, L. reclusa,* and *L. laeta* and human red cells in Ouchterlony immunodiffusion plates observed that although there was no hemolysis with the venoms, there was hemolysis with both cephalothorax and abdominal extracts.

Recently, KNIERIM et al. (1975) made a series of experiments with red blood cells from human (4 blood groupings) and from 12 animal species (mouse, rat, guinea pig, hamster, rabbit, cat, dog, sheep, chicken, toad, frog, and one fresh water fish) which were put in contact with venom and 4 other components of *L. laeta*. The results of these experiments are shown in Table 4.

As shown, the venom caused no hemolytic action on any of the erythrocytes studied, but hemolymph, extracts of abdominal wall, eggs, abdominal content, and cephalothorax did present different degrees of hemolytic activity.

VII. Pharmacology and Mechanism of Action

The paucity of established facts concerning the molecular properties of venoms of *Loxosceles* spiders is reflected in the existence of several hypothesis about their mechanism of action.

In view of the early lesions of the blood vessels which mimic the Arthus phenomenon an anaphylactoid reaction has been invoked. This would be promoted by the products of proteolytic action at the site of inoculation and, through amplification processes, would lead to tissue damage (PIZZI et al., 1957; PIZZI, 1975).

In dogs, the administration of the venom of *L. reclusa* by the intravenous route has been reported to cause marked thrombocytopenia, moderate intravascular hemolysis, and hemolytic anemia (DENNY et al., 1964). In rabbits, it has not been possible to demonstrate lethal effects following the intravenous injections of venom extracts from *L. reclusa*. This fact has been attributed to the inability of transporting the venom in an active form by the blood (GEREN et al., 1973).

A plasma coagulating activity appears to be associated with toxin 1 described for *L. reclusa* (ODELL et al., 1975).

The enzymology of venom extracts does not allow an explanation of the lesions. As was already pointed out, hyaluronidase would play only the role of a cooperative component favoring the dissemination of the tissue damage. In larvae of *Heliothis virescens,* NORMENT and VINSON (1969) have found that the venom of *L. reclusa* has a lytic action on fat body and muscle tissue which they attributed to a potent protease. This enzyme would help the spider to process its food. However, a direct enzymatic assay was not done in the extracts.

The venom of *L. reclusa* is able to produce cytotoxic effects in cell cultures of human epithelial cells (HeLa) and fibroblasts (MORGAN and FELTON, 1965). Also, in HEp-2 cells cultivated *in vitro* extracts from *L. laeta* have shown strong cytophatic effects (Suarez et al., 1975). It is noteworthy that in both cases the sources of the cells tested are susceptible species.

In invertebrates, *L. reclusa* venom extracts have been shown to have a hemolytic effect on hemocytes of *Acheta domesticus* (Norment and Smith, 1968). Hemolytic activity *in vitro* has also been detected in sheep blood cells incubated with concentrated venom preparations of *L. reclusa*, provided that serum is present (Kniker et al., 1969). However, using rabbit (Geren et al., 1973) or sheep (Biggemann, 1971) washed erythrocytes no hemolytic effect has been detected in the venom extracts of *L. reclusa* and *L. laeta*, respectively.

A potent, nondialyzable inhibitor of hemolytic complement activity has been demonstrated in the venom of *L. reclusa*. This factor would interfere with the function of the 3b component of guinea pig complement and the equivalent fifth component of the human system. Apparently the molecular properties of these components remain unchanged and the inhibitory effect can be overcome by increasing their concentration (Kniker and Morgan, 1967; Kniker et al., 1969). A corresponding anticomplementary effect has been observed in the extracts and partially purified fractions of *L. laeta* venom, but, as apposed to the results obtained for the case of *L. reclusa*, only a limited reversal of the effect is attained at higher complement titers. The venom would interfere with receptor sites for complement fractions located at the membrane surface since sensitized sheep erythrocytes preincubated with venom and subsequently washed are not lyzed by the addition of complement (Biggemann et al., 1971). This view gains further support with the direct observation of binding of antivenom fluorescent antibodies to red cells previously treated with the venom (Rojas et al., unpublished results). Accordingly, erythrocytes incubated with venom and then washed several times show necrotizing effects on the skin of the rabbit. These facts substantiate the view that active venom components of *L. laeta* interact strongly with cell membranes. For the same reason, one is tempted to generate the hypothesis that the pathogenic effects of the venom are triggered by an initial disturbance of membrane function.

Not all mammalian species are sensitive to the venom of *L. laeta*. For instance, rats (*Rattus norvegicus*) are not harmed by large doses of venom. In the serum of this species it has not been possible to detect the presence of an inactivator of the venom; neither has a stimulator of the venom in sensitive animals been found (Biggemann, 1971). These results suggest that resistance and susceptibility are the reflection of genetically determined features of target cells rather than humorally mediated processes.

B. Epidemiology, Symptomatology, Pathology, Prognosis, Treatment, and Prevention of Envenomations

I. Epidemiology of Envenomations. Geographic and Temporal Distribution of Cases. Other Epidemiologic Data

Until 1968 a cursory review of the literature on hand on necrotic spiderbites (loxoscelism) made by Gorham (1968) revealed reports of at least 126 cases in the United States and about 400 cases in South America.

Keeping in mind that not all cases are diagnosed and consequently that not all are recorded and published, a careful search in the available literature gave the following lists for several countries.

Chile. A first block of references covers the period from 1873 to 1939 making a total of 70 cases with one fatality (MACCHIAVELLO, 1937, 1947b). Up to 1962 different authors published another 84 cases including 14 deaths (ESCUDERO, 1936; JAEGER, 1941; URETA and ESPINOZA, 1944; DONOSO BARROS, 1948; ROSENBERG, 1948; ESPINOZA, 1949; BERTIN, 1950; DROGUET et al., 1951; KIRBERG et al., 1952; MENEGHELLO and EMPARANZA, 1952; WEINSTEIN et al., 1952; DE BONADONA and BARROS, 1960; DONCKASTER and COHEN, 1960; STEEGER and FUENTEALBA, 1961; VUKUSIC, 1962).

Furthermore, GAJARDO-TOBAR (1966) in Valparaiso and SCHENONE et al. (1975b) in Santiago published 200 and 133 cases with 22 and 19 fatalities respectively.

Argentina. After a review of the literature and his personal observations IBARRA-GRASSO (1944) reports 12 cases of hemolytic anemia and jaundice with a fatal outcome, probably caused by "a mysterious homicidal and small domestic spider". In 1957 in Mendoza a fatal case concerning a 29-year-old woman was reported (SCHENONE et al., 1957). Later, in Buenos Aires 4 severe cases with one death are reported (BARRIO and IBARRA-GRASSO, 1966).

Uruguay. MACKINNON and WITKIND (1953) analyzed the local literature, and together with their personal experience, gathered 29 cases (2 deaths) registered between 1938 and 1953. Twenty years later an additional 3 cases (one fatal) were published (CAMPALANS et al., 1973–1974).

Peru. The most important statistics recorded have been made in Lima (IZU, 1953; DELGADO, 1969) with a total of 83 cases, including 10 fatalities. Another 7 cases, which occurred in Lima and Arequipa, including one death, were recorded by other authors (CUADRA, 1950; PESCE and LUMBRERAS, 1954; NAQUIRA et al., 1962).

Brazil. FURLANETTO (1961) reported 28 cases, one of which was a very severe envenomation.

Bolivia. VELLARD (1954b, 1966b) notes that in Cochabamba and Sucre there exists a domiciliary *Loxosceles* spider which frequently causes severe accidents with local necrosis, hematuria, and even death.

Cuba. Only one presumed case, in a 65 year old man, has already been reported (FERNANDEZ and DIAZ, 1972).

Mexico. BIAGI (1974) has seen some cases of loxoscelism in the states of Veracruz, Puebla, and Morelos.

United States. Human loxoscelism seems to have been recorded since the late 1800s (PRESLEY, 1896) making a total of about 200 known cases with at least 6 deaths (GOTTEN and MACGOWAN, 1940; ATKINS et al., 1958; LESSENDEN and ZIMMER, 1960; WEINER et al., 1960; JAMES et al., 1961; NANCE, 1961; NICHOLSON and NICHOLSON, 1962; DENNY et al., 1964; DILLAHA et al., 1964; MINTON and OLSON, 1964; LEWIS and REGAN, 1966; TAYLOR and DENNY, 1966; GORHAM, 1968; RUSSELL et al., 1969). Almost all the accidents have occurred in Missouri, Kansas, Arkansas, Oklahoma, Tennessee, Texas, Indiana, California, and Arizona.

Epidemiologic studies carried out by DENNY et al. (1964) and RUSSELL et al. (1969) suggest that the incidence of loxoscelism in the United States is considerably higher than previously suspected. As greater attention is given to the rather character-istic clinical syndrome, the number of cases diagnosed should continue to increase.

Israel. Efrati (1969) reported that during 1958—1964, 7 patients were admitted for skin lesions and mild general symptoms following suspected *Loxosceles* spider bites. One of these patients brought the culprit spider which was identified as *L. ru-fescens.* Shulov (1966), who identified the above-mentioned spider, states that several envenomations with quite severe symptoms have been reported in Israel as a result of the bite of this common house spider.

Even though cases of loxoscelism may present themselves all the year round, most of them (70—73%) occur in summer and spring (Macchiavello, 1947a; Schenone and Prats, 1961; Naquira et al., 1962; Barrio and Ibarra-Grasso, 1966; Gajardo-Tobar, 1966; Schenone et al., 1975b).

About 80% of the accidents take place indoors, mostly in bedrooms when the persons are sleeping or dressing (Gajardo-Tobar, 1966; Schenone et al., 1975).

In 60—75% of the cases the person has seen the offending spider and in a lesser proportion the specimen has been undoubtedly identified as a *Loxosceles* (Macchiavello, 1937; Izu, 1953; Mackinnon and Witkind, 1953; Gajardo-Tobar, 1966; Delgado, 1969; Efrati, 1969; Russell et al., 1969; Schenone et al., 1975b).

In a recent paper from Chile (Schenone et al., 1975b) it is reported that in 133 cases of loxoscelism the interval between the time of the bite and medical attention ranged from 10 min to 120 h, with a mean of 19 h. Fifty percent consulted during the first 12 h and 79% during the first 24 h.

II. Human Symptomatology

When a *Loxosceles* spider bites a person almost always a local burning-stinging sensation is the first symptom. The most frequent sites of bites are upper limbs (43%), lower limbs (19%), and face (15%) (Schenone et al., 1975b). The action of the venom may bring about two clinical variants of loxoscelism: 1. The cutaneous form. 2. The viscerocutaneous or systemic form.

1. Cutaneous Form of Loxoscelism

The cutaneous form of loxoscelism is the most commonly seen and may develop either into a local skin necrosis or into a local edema without necrosis. Both lesions are very painful.

The local skin necrosis usually begins with an area of edema which centrally presents a violaceous (livedoid) plaque surrounded by an erythematous halo. This plaque will progress to a darker color, and bleb or blister formations may appear on its surface in 40—41% of the cases (Gajardo-Tobar, 1966; Schenone et al., 1975b). The violaceous plaque, which varies in size from 3 mm to 35 cm, will gra-dually be supplanted by the well-known blackish eschar, which was earlier called the "gangrenous spot of Chile" (Macchiavello, 1937, 1947a) (Fig. 4A — B). Usually this lesion is not accompanied by enlargement of local lymph nodes, and when this happens is due to secondary bacterial infections (Prats and Schenone, 1957; Gajardo-Tobar, 1966; Delgado, 1969). The eschar, accordingly with its size and

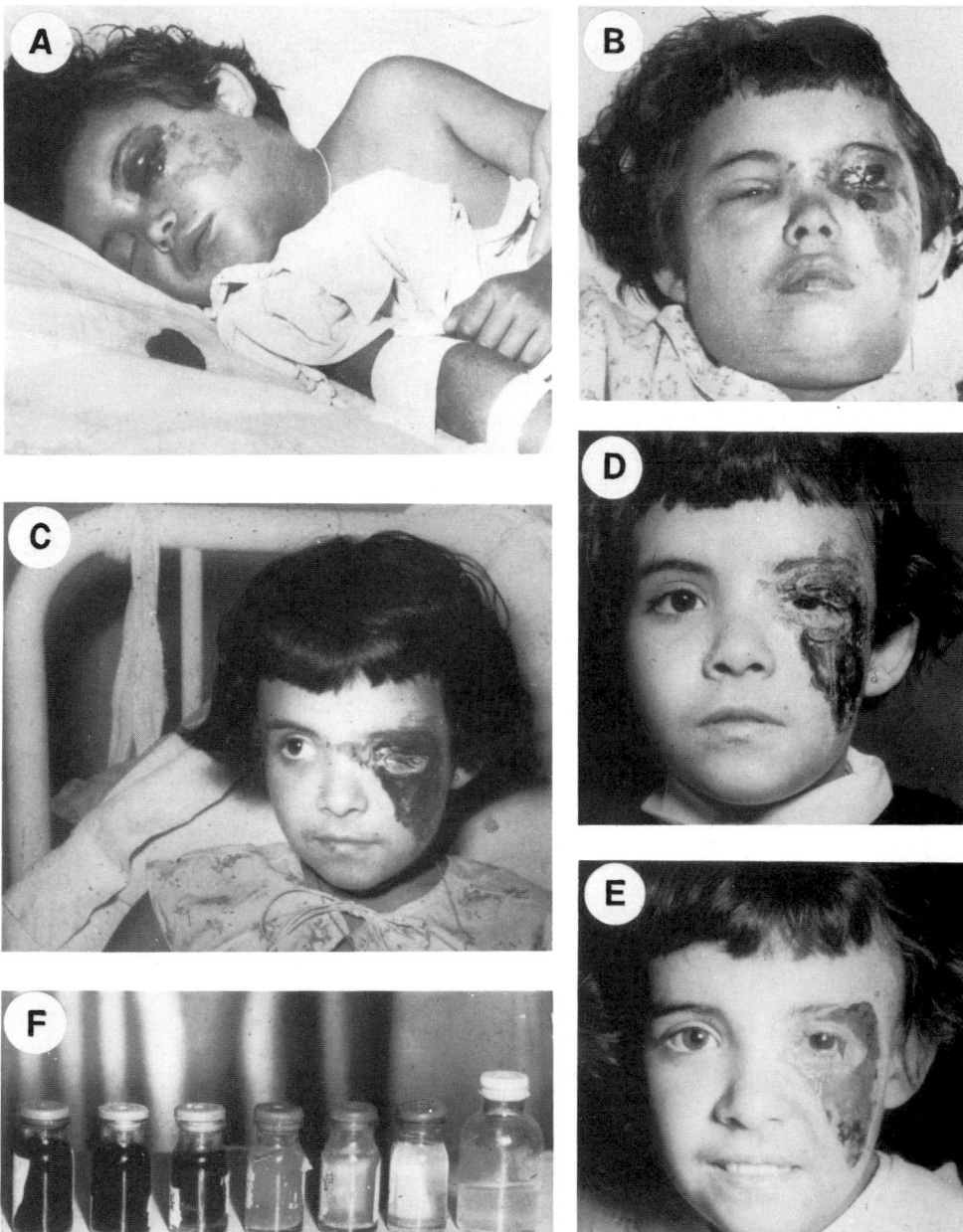

Fig. 4A—F. Viscerocutaneous loxoscelism in 7-year-old girl (temperature 39.6° C, hemoglobinuria, hematuria, jaundice, coma). (A) Large edema of entire face with livedoid plaque on left eyelids and cheek 20 h after bite. (B) Livedoid plaque 48 h after bite. (C) and (D) Necrotic eschar 21 and 40 days later. (E) Large ulcer after surgical abrasion. (F) Evolution of macroscopical aspect of urine 2, 3, 5, 6, 7, 8, and 9 days after bite

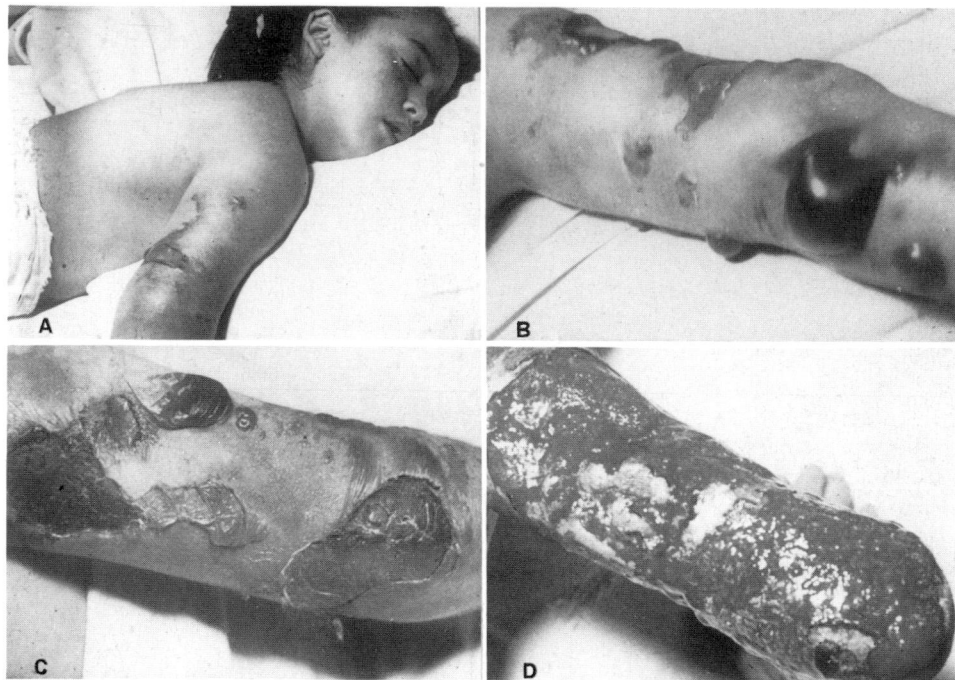

Fig. 5A—D. Viscerocutaneous loxoscelism in a 8 year old girl (temperature 38° C, hemoglobinuria, hematuria, comatous condition). (A) General aspect of patient 24h after bite. Echymotic lesion and edema of the arm. (B) livedoid plaque and serohematic blisters 72 h later. (C) Necrotic eschar on day 14. (D) Large ulcer resulting from surgical removal of the necrotic tissues. Skin graftings were necessary

deepness, will slough within 2—5 weeks, either superficially (67%) or leaving a necrotic ulcer (33%) (Fig. 4C—E). The ulcer may extend to the underlying muscular layers, but without involving them (Fig. 5). The ulceration is frequently slow to heal. Granulation and scarring may take from 3 to 16 weeks (GAJARDO-TOBAR, 1966; SCHENONE et al., 1975b). Secondary violaceous plaque and its subsequent eschar and necrotic ulcer may appear below the primary lesion, perhaps due to a spreading and gravitative process.

The edematous form without necrosis, which occurs in 4.5% of the cases, presents a notably large edema, particularly when the bite is on the face (Fig. 6).

Additionally, 75% of the patients present one or more of the following general symptoms and signs: insomnia, febril sensation, asthenia, restlessness, generalized exanthema and pruritus, nausea, vomiting, and malaise.

2. Viscerocutaneous Form of Loxoscelism

The viscerocutaneous form, is very severe and occurs in an average of 13% of the total number of cases of loxoscelism. In addition to the local manifestations, identical to those observed in the cutaneous form, the main symptoms consist of

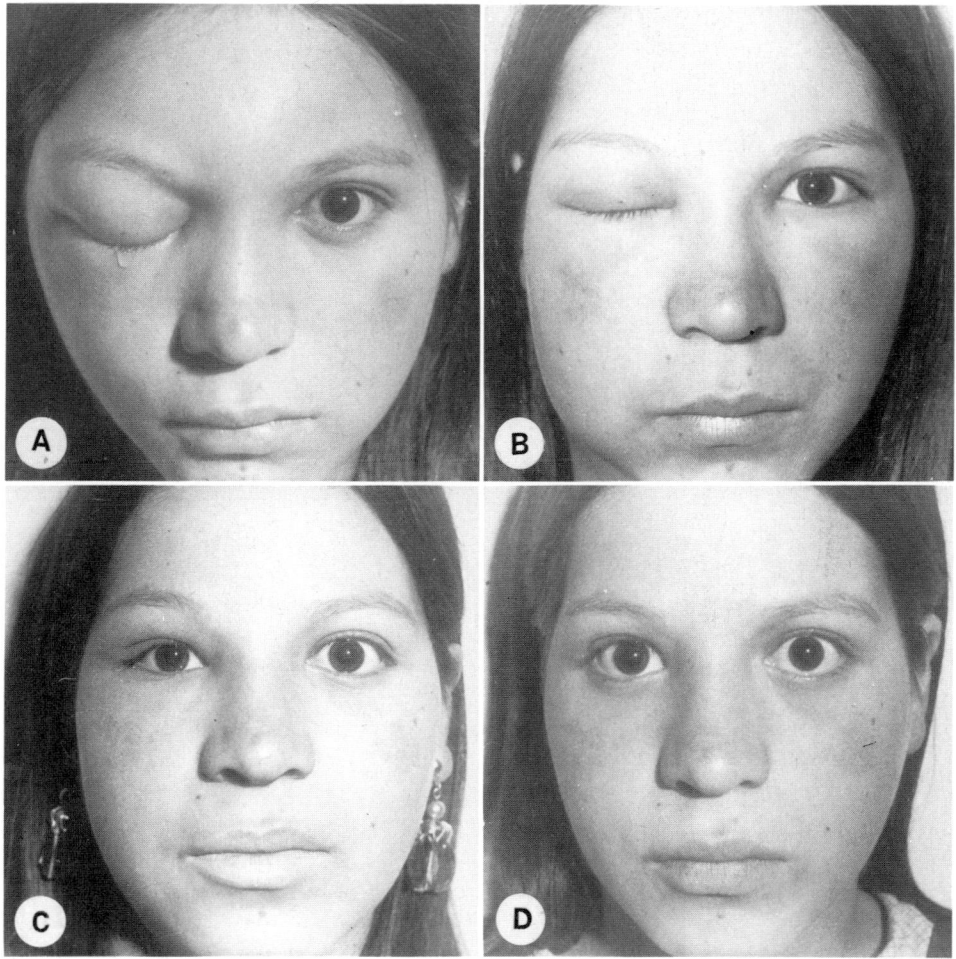

Fig. 6A–D. Edematous form of loxoscelism without necrosis in 17-year-old woman. Large facial edema without necrotic lesion. Evolution 24 (A), 48 (B), 96 (C), and 120 (D) h after bite

hemolytic anemia, hemoglobinuria, hematuria, jaundice, fever and sensorial involvement generally appearing within the first 6—24 h after the bite. The temperature may reach 41° C and the patient may become prostrate, with labored breathing and passing dark, "Coca-cola" colored urine. (Fig. 4F). In the most severe cases the patient may fall in a comatous condition and the hemolytic process, besides conditioning the production of hemoglobinuria and hematuria, may lead to a marked oliguria and even to anuria (NANCE, 1961; GAJARDO TOBAR, 1966; TAYLOR and DENNY, 1966; DELGADO, 1969; REID, 1975; SCHENONE et al., 1975b). The occurence of this syndrome has no relationship to age, sex, season, site of bite, nor size of local lesion.

III. Differential Diagnosis

1. Cutaneous Forms

a) Necrotic. In a first group of conditions it includes anthrax malignant pustule, ecchymosis (traumatic or purpuric), and caustic burning by chemical substances (kerosene). In a second group of conditions are gangrenous erypsipelas, boils, phlegmon, cellulitis, cutaneous leishmaniasis, herpes zoster, local lesions of rat-bite fever (*Streptobacillus moniliformis* and *Spirillum minus*), Nicolau's livedoid gangrenous dermitis, and vascular occlusion. b) *Predominant edematous.* This includes anthrax malignant edema, wasp and bee-stings, kissing bug bites, local syndrome in acute Chagas disease, and angioneurotic edema (MACCHIAVELLO, 1947 a; DONOSO BARROS, 1948; PRATS and SCHENONE, 1957; DILLAHA et al., 1964; RUSSELL et al., 1969).

2. Viscerocutaneous Form

With or without conspicuous local lesions, it includes *Clostridium perfringens* septicotoxemia and other etiologies producing acute hemolytic anemia.

IV. Clinical Course and Duration of Hospitalization

1. Local Necrosis and Ulcer

Regardless of the clinical form of loxoscelism, but according to the extension and deepness of the lesions in 89.6% of the cases they may heal in a very complete and convenient form, within 1—3 weeks. Their location and slowness to cure (up to 16 weeks) make necessary skin grafts in 10.4% of the cases. Pain is the last symptom to disappear (MACCHIAVELLO, 1947a; GAJARDO-TOBAR, 1966).

2. Viscerocutaneous Involvement

Recovers rather rapidly within one to two weeks (NANCE, 1961; GAJARDO-TOBAR, 1966; SCHENONE et al., 1975b).

V. Prognosis and Frequency of Lethal Cases

When a person is bitten by a *Loxosceles* spider a couple of crucial questions arises. Which form of loxoscelism is the victim going to develop? A non life threatening cutaneous form or a highly dangerous, life-threatening one? Frequently both questions may have an answer within the first 24 h after the bite because the most important clinical manifestations of systemic involvement (hemoglobinuria, hematuria, and fever) appear during this term. In other words, if these manifestations do not appear during this period, it is quite possible that the case is going to be a cutaneous one. As it has been expressed, the systemic form only occurs in an average of 13% of the total number of cases of loxoscelism.

In the cutaneous lesions the prognosis depends on the site and extent of the ulcer and the resulting scar which may implicate either the esthetics or the functions of the affected area (e.g. eyelids, joints).

Table 5. Some statistical data on loxoscelism in different countries and periods. Frequency of viscerocutaneous or systemic cases. Lethality rates

Country	Period	No. of systemic cases/ Total No. of cases	Lethality	
			No. of deaths/ Total No. of cases	No. of deaths/ No. of systemic cases
Chile (SCHENONE, 1964)	1873—1962	?/154 —	15/154 (9.7%)	15/? —
Chile (GAJARDO-TOBAR, 1966)	1955—1966	22/200 (11.0%)	7/200 (3.5%)	7/22 (31.8%)
Chile (SCHENONE et al., 1975b)	1955—1974	19/133 (14.3%)	5/133 (3.8%)	5/19 (26.9%)
Uruguay (MACKINNON and WITKIND, 1953)	1938—1953	8/29 (27.6%)	2/29 (6.9%)	2/8 (25.0%)
Peru (IZU, 1953)	1943—1952	?/31 —	5/31 (16.1%)	5/? —
Peru (DELGADO, 1969)	1962—1969	28/52 (53.9%)	5/52 (9.6%)	5/28 (17.9%)
Brasil (FURLANETTO, 1961)	1954—1960	1/28 (3.6%)	0/28 (0.0%)	0/1 (0.0%)
U.S.A. (DENNY et al., 1964; GORHAM, 1968)	1896—1968	18/126 (14.3%)	6/126 (4.8%)	6/18 (33.3%)

In the viscerocutaneous form, as occurs in other similarly severe diseases, the prognosis will depend on the promptness of adequate treatment.

According to different statistics the mean lethality rates for loxoscelism are 5.7 and 29.4%; the 5.7% refers to the number of deaths versus the total number of cases, while the 29.4% refers to the total number of deaths versus the total number of systemic cases. The latter percentage clearly indicates the high lethality rate concomitant with the systemic form of loxoscelism. In Table 5 rates of clinical forms of loxoscelism and lethality are summarized.

Within the general graveness of the systemic involvement, anuria and coma are manifestations that darken the prognosis. Due to the fact that in the majority of the fatal cases death takes place during the first 24—72 h, the patients that surpass this critical term have a good chance of survival and complete recovery (SCHENONE, 1966).

VI. Pathology

Local lesions consisting of inflammation and necrosis of the skin are predominant. Edema, vacuolization, and necrosis of epidermal cells especially those of the *stratum basale,* with accumulation of liquid at the dermoepidermal level, accompanied by a marked vasculitis and thrombosis of small vessels in the dermis, degenerative processes of the connective tissue and focal hemorrhages are the main early pathologic changes. Sometimes the local lesions are deeper and reach the subcutaneous tissue and the muscular layer. Later on the lesion turns into a necrotic eschar that frequently leaves a sharply defined granular area, surrounded by the raised edges of healthy skin (PIZZI, 1975).

Typical local necrotic lesions are rarely seen in autopsies of systemic cases of loxoscelism because the death occurs before they are well developed (GAJARDO-TOBAR, 1966).

In systemic loxoscelism, the most frequent visceral findings apart from jaundice are edema, congestion, hemorrhages, degenerative processes, and even necrosis of different organs (ESPINOZA, 1944; URETA, 1944; ROSENBERG, 1948; WEINSTEIN et al., 1952; SCHENONE et al., 1975b). The heart muscle, liver, lungs, and kidneys are especially affected.

The kidneys appear swollen and dark red in colour, with extensive hemorrhages in cortex and medulla. Intravascular hemolysis leads to hemoglobinemia and consequent hemoglobinuria, giving place to an acute tubular necrosis. The renal tubules are filled with blood casts. The bladder usually holds a dark brown urine that contains erythrocytes and hemoglobin. The brain is edematous with a diffuse and perivascular inflammation. The mucous membranes of the digestive tract present edema, congestion, petechiae, and erosions. In the most severe fatal cases hemorrhages raised extensive cutaneous echymoses and/or hemothorax and hemopericardium (ESPINOZA, 1944; DONOSO-BARROS, 1948; GAJARDO-TOBAR, 1963, 1966; TAYLOR and DENNY, 1966; CAMPALANS et al., 1973–1974; SCHENONE et al., 1957, 1959, 1975b).

VII. Laboratory Findings

A thorough revision of the scores of the available published data, some of which were more relevant (ROSENBERG, 1948; DE BONADONA and BARROS, 1960; NANCE, 1961; DILLAHA et al., 1964; BARRIO and IBARRA-GRASSO, 1966; GAJARDO-TOBAR, 1966; CAMPALANS et al., 1973–1974; SCHENONE et al., 1975b), permitted us to build up Table 6.

Most of the results shown in the table correspond to tests made either at the onset of the clinical picture or within the first 72 h.

While the cutaneous form regularly does not cause blood or urine alterations, the systemic form does. Nevertheless, due to the hemoconcentration produced in the predominantly edematous cutaneous form, an increase of erythrocytes, hemoglobin and hematocrit levels is observed (SCHENONE, 1959; STEEGER and FUENTEALBA, 1961; SCHENONE et al., 1975b).

Some of the extreme values found in the viscerocutaneous form were: erythrocytes 840,000, hemoglobin 17.1%, hematocrit 8.0%, bilirubin 11.5 mg per 100 ml, leukocytes 95,000, thrombocytes 28,000, urea nitrogen in blood 330 mg per 100 ml, albuminuria 4000 mg per 100 ml and a marked hemoglobin reaction and a high number of red blood cells in urine were almost constant. The increasing of serum bilirubin was mainly based on the indirect reacting fraction; in some cases it could not be determined because of the intense degree of hemolysis (NANCE, 1961; MINTON

Table 6. Mean values found in laboratory examinations of blood and urine from patients with cutaneous and viscerocutaneous loxoscelism

Examinations	Cutaneous	Viscerocutaneous
Blood		
Erythrocytes (per cu. mm.)	4,863,330	2,858,000
Hemoglobin (%)	89.3	57.2
Hematocrit (%)	41.6	20.1
Serum bilirubin (mg per 100 ml)	0.85	2.92
Leukocytes (per cu. mm.)	10,075	23,153
Thrombocytes (per cu. mm.)	230,000	96,340
CO_2 combining power (mEq. per 1)	24	15.4
Serum sodium (mEq. per 1)	120	132
Serum potassium (mEq. per 1)	4.5	5.3
Urea nitrogen (mg per 100 ml	32	173
Urine		
Albumin (mg per 100 ml)	traces	1,650
Hemoglobin	−	+ + to + + + +
Erythrocytes	−	+ to + + + +

and OLSON, 1964; TAYLOR and DENNY, 1966). Leukocytosis is usually accompanied by a marked shift to the left.

Normalization of laboratory examinations customarily takes place in the term of 7 — 14 days.

Bacteriologic studies of material taken from the blisters or from the area of ulceration have usually been negative (SCHENONE, 1959; LEWIS and REGAN, 1966).

VIII. Treatment

The effectiveness of any therapeutic measure will depend on the promptness with which its administration begins.

As general clinical procedure, two basic statements must be considered in the treatment of loxoscelism. (a) When organic lesions (local or systemic) are established no medication is going to make them vanish and treatment will only be able to attempt to limit and reduce their consequences. (b) Since the viscerocutaneous form is highly dangerous, rather than worrying about the eventual extent of the local necrosis (in some cases insignificant or almost absent), the primary target of treatment should be the systemic involvement and the use of specific, nonspecific, and supportive treatment measures, or a combination of these depending on the decision of the attending clinician.

Therapy of loxoscelism may be classified into nonspecific and specific.

1. Nonspecific

It is based fundamentally on prompt injection of corticosteroids. The occurrence of important lesions in the mucosa of the digestive tract has made the parenteral route preferable to the oral one (SCHENONE et al., 1959; GAJARDO-TOBAR, 1966).

Although, according to different authors, the clinical results of using corticosteroids are not always satisfactory (De Bonadona and Barros, 1960; Minton and Olson, 1964; Taylor and Denny, 1966), the majority of them agree on their protective capacity from the systemic effects of the venom and they are probably lifesaving in some cases (Kirberg et al., 1952; Meneghello and Emparanza, 1952; Schenone et al., 1959; Dillaha et al., 1964; Gajardo-Tobar, 1966; Campalans et al., 1973—1974; Russell, 1974; Russell et al., 1974). In a very demonstrative experimental work, Dillaha et al. (1964) challenged a series of 10 rabbits with an equal amount of pooled venom. Intravenous methyl prednisolone was seen to protect all 3 rabbits receiving this steroid 6 h following the venom injection. Five out of 6 animals receiving the drug 24—48 h after the challenge died within 3 days, as did the single untreated control.

According to the patient's age and weight, corticosteroids must be given in large doses during the acute phase for 2—4 days (e.g. hydrocortisone 125—200 mg every 6 h; methyl prednisolone or prednisone 15—30 mg every 8—12 h; dexamethasone 1—4 mg every 6—8 h). Afterwards the patient may be placed on a decremental dose of the drug in accordance with standard clinical practices.

Antihistamines, particularly injected, have also been used with some success in the treatment of cutaneous forms of loxoscelism (Schenone, 1959; Naquira et al., 1962; Horen, 1966; Delgado, 1969).

2. Specific

Loxosceles antiserum has been used with a variable success. Some authors claim satisfactory results in some cases (Vellard, 1954b; Furlanetto, 1961; Gajardo-Tobar, 1966). Others obtained poor or dubious results, for the necrotic lesion and for the systemic involvement (Barrio and Ibarra-Grasso, 1966; Delgado, 1969; Schenone et al., 1975b). The results obtained by Smith and Micks (1968) in experimentally poisoned rabbits were no more encouraging. Nevertheless, Gajardo-Tobar (1966) recommends the injection of large doses of antiserum, 2 or more 5 ml ampoules, each containing 50 antitoxic units [1].

In attempting to avoid acute hemolytic renal failure, it may be advisable to administer orally 10—15 g per day of sodium bicarbonate to alkalify the urine, and thus to make the hemoglobin more soluble (Gonzalez, 1970).

General supportive measures such as blood exchange transfusions, repeated

---

[1] *Loxosceles* antiserum for human use has been produced by Vellard (1954) at the Instituto de Higiene in Lima (Peru) and by Furlanetto (1961) at the Instituto Butantan in Sao Paulo (Brazil). For the production of the sera Vellard used the ass and *L. laeta* venom, whereas Furlanetto employed the horse and *L. rufescens* venom. Both immunized the animals by subcutaneous injections of successive and progressively increasing doses of venom for 21 and 9 weeks respectively. The initial doses injected were the equivalent to the venom content of 0.01 and 6 glands, while the final doses corresponded to 106 and 108 glands. For human use it is recommended the injection of a dose of 1—4 (5 ml) ampoules containing 50 antitoxic units each, which may be repeated after 12 h. One antitoxic unit neutralizes the venom activity of the content of one gland. Furlanetto (1961) maintains that serum is useful only within the first 36 h after the bite. To the best of our knowledge, the Instituto Butantan in Sao Paulo, Brazil, is at the present time the only institution producing *Loxoscles* antiserum for medical use.

hemodialysis, or use of antibiotics will depend on the particular conditions and evolution of the patients. These same factors will be considered for deciding excision of the necrotic lesion and/or skin graftings.

IX. Prevention

Prophylactic measures of Loxosceles bites are based principally on the knowledge of the biology of the spider, therefore specific community health education is highly desirable. These measures, that were recommended by SCHENONE and REYES (1963) may be summarized as follows:

1. Thorough house cleaning at least twice a year, paying special attention to dark corners, closets, attics, and the like. Furniture, curtains, pictures, as well as clothes, trunks, and other baggage kept in closets, must be completely removed and thoroughly cleaned.

2. It is advizable to place beds at least 20 cm away from walls. Clothing should not be hung on walls; in any case, it must be carefully inspected and shaken out before being used.

With regard to the use of insecticides as a control measure, the highly qualified opinion of GORHAM (1968) is quoted:

"The brown recluse spider is probably susceptible to every contact or fumigant insecticide on the market. Lindane, chlordane, malathion, dichlorvos (DDVP), and paradichlorobenzene have been recommended. But insecticides are probably not the most efficient means for preventing contact between man and spider. The more toxic fumigants (therefore the most likely to kill brown recluse spiders) are rarely used in houses. In regard to contact insecticides, the toxicant has to touch the spider or the spider has to touch the insecticidal residue. But the brown recluse spider occupies microhabitats that may easily be missed in the routine application of household insecticides. Spiders in small, enclosed spaces such as closets may be adversely affected by paradichlorobenzone or by dichlorvos impregnated plastic strips".

Finally, we are in complete agreement with GORHAM (1968) in the opinion that good housekeeping by creating an unsuitable habitat for the spider, is the best control technique.

References

Atkins, J.A., Wingo, C.W., Sodeman, W.A., Flynn, J.E.: Necrotic arachnidism. Am. J. Trop. Med. Hyg. 7, 165 (1958).

Barrio, A., Ibarra-Grasso, A.: Casos de loxoscelismo grave ocurridos en la ciudad de Buenos Aires y alrededores en los últimos años. Mem. Inst. Butantan. 33, 809 (1966).

Berger, R.S., Millikan, L.E., Conway, F.: An *In Vitro* test for *Loxosceles reclusa* spider bites. Toxicon 11, 465 (1973).

Bertin, V.: Consideraciones sobre aracnoidismo en Chile. Rev. Chil. Hig. 12, 37 (1950).

Biagi, F. Animales venenosos. In: Enfermedades Parasitarias. Mexico. La Prensa Médica Mexicana: Editorial Fournier, S.A., 1974.

Biggemann, U.: Estudios bioquimicos del veneno de la araña *L. laeta* y su mecanismo de acción. Thesis, University of Concepción, Chile, 1971.

Biggemann, U., Socias, T., Suarez, G., Schenone, H.: Actividad adenosintrifosfatásica en veneno de *Loxosceles laeta*. Arch. Biol. Med. Exp. (Chile) 7, R−5 (1970).

Bonnet, P.: Bibliographia araneorum. Imp. Douladoure: Toulouse, 1957, Vol. II, 3.

Brignoli, P.M.: Note sugli Scytodidae d'Italia e Malta (Araneae). Fragmenta Entomologica, **6**, 121 (1969)

Bücherl, W.: Aranhas do género *Loxosceles* e loxoscelismo na America. Cienc. e Cult. **13**, 213 (1961).

Bücherl, W.: Aranhas do género *Loxosceles* e "loxoscelismo" na America do Sul. I Introducao, comentarios bibligraficos, caracterizacao da sub familia Loxoscelinae do genero *Loxosceles* e enumeracao das especies da America do Sul. Mem. Inst. Butantan **30**, 167 (1960 – 1962).

Bücherl, W.: Histologia das glandulas de veneno de algunas aranhas y escorpioes. Mem. Inst. Butantan. **31**, 77 (1964a).

Bücherl, W.: Biología de artropodos peconhentos. Mem. Inst. Butantan. **31**, 85 (1964b).

Campalans, L.A., Rodriguez, L., Llopart, T., Acosta Ferreira, W., Witkind, J., Petrucelli, D., Vila, J.M.: Insuficiencia renal aguda por mordedura de araña (a propósito de tres casos de loxoscelismo). Rev. Uruguaya Pat. Clin. y Microbiol. **11**, 13 (1973 – 1974).

Canese, A.: *Loxosceles rufescens* (Dufour 1820) en Isla Pucú del Departamento de la Cordillera (Paraguay). Rev. Parag. de Microb. **7**, 83 (1972).

Cuadra, M.: Araneismo por *Loxosceles laeta*. Viernes Med. (Lima, Perú) **7**, 141 (1950).

Delgado, A.: Investigación ecológica sobre *Loxosceles rufipes* (Lucas) (1834) en la región costera del Perú. Mem. Inst. Butantan. **33**, 683 (1966).

Delgado, A.: Loxoscelismo. 1. Formas clínicas del sindrome cutáneo. Rev. Soc. Peruana de Dermatol. **3**, 73 (1969).

Dillaha, C.J., Jansen, G.T., Honeycutt, W.M., Hayden, C.R.: North American Loxoscelism. Necrotic Bite of the Brown Recluse Spider. J.A.M.A. **188**, 33 (1964).

Denny, W.F., Dillaha, C.J., Morgan, P.N.: Hemotoxic effect of *Loxosceles reclusa* venom: *in vivo* and *in vitro* studies. J. Lab. Clin. Med. **64**, 291 (1964).

Donoso Barros, R.: Considerationes sobre aracnoidismo cutáneo en Chile. Arch. Uruguayos Med. **33**, 184 (1948).

De Bonadona, S., Barros, M.: Loxoscelismo en niños. Rev. Chil. Pediat. **31**, 180 (1960).

Donckaster, R., Cohen, H.: Un caso de loxoscelismo de difícil diagnóstico. Bol. Chil. Parasit. **15**, 81 (1960).

Droguet, A., Raffo, P., Cabezas, J., Moreno, J.: Anemia hemolitica por picadura de araña. Rev. Med. Chile. **79**, 263 (1951).

Efrati, P.: Bites by *Loxosceles* spiders in Israel. Toxicon **6**, 239 (1969).

Escudero, E.: Un caso de aracnoidismo mortal en Chile. Rev. Chil. Hist. Nat. **39**, 339 (1936).

Espinoza, J.: Intoxicación por aracnoidismo. Rev. Med. **18**, 288 (1944).

Espinoza, J.: Intoxicación por aracnoidismo. Arch. Chil. Morfol. **7**, 222 (1949).

Fernandez, L., Diaz, J.: Necrosis de los dedos de la mano izquierda por picadura de araña. Bol. Hig. Epid. **10**, 103 (1972).

Furlanetto, R.S.: Estudos sobre a preparacao do soro antiloxoscélico. Thesis. Faculdade de Farmacia e Odontología, Universidad de Sao Paulo (1961).

Gajardo-Tobar, R.: La clínica del aracnidismo. Bol. Hosp. de Viña del Mar. **19**, 179 (1963).

Gajardo-Tobar, R.: Mi experiencia sobre loxoscelismo. Mem. Inst. Butantan. **33**, 689 (1966).

Galiano, M.E.: Ciclo biológico y desarrollo de *Loxosceles laeta*. (Nicolet, 1849) (Araneae, Scytodidae) Acta. Zool. Lilloana. **23**, 430 (1967).

Galiano, M.E., Hall, M.: Datos adicionales sobre el ciclo vital de *Loxosceles laeta* (Nicolet) (Araneae). Physis. **32**, 277 (1973).

Geren, C.R., Chan, T.K., Ward, B.C., Howell, D.E., Pinkston, K., Odell, G.V.: Composition and properties of extract of fiddleback (*Loxosceles reclusa*) spider venom apparatus. Toxicon. **11**, 471 (1973).

Gertsch, W.J.: The spider genus *Loxosceles* in North America, Central America and the West Indies. Am. Mus. Novitates No. 1907, 1 – 46 (1958).

Gertsch, W.J.: The Spider Genus *Loxosceles* in South America (Araneae, Scytodidae). Bull. Am. Mus. Nat. Hist. **136**, 121 (1967).

Gonzalez, M.: Loxoscelismo (Mordedura de Araña). Rev. Asist. Publica (Chile) **1**, 25 (1970).

Gorham, J.R.: The Brown Recluse Spider *Loxosceles reclusa* and Necrotic Spiderbite. A New Public Health Problem in the United States. J. Envir. Health **31**, 138 (1968).

Gotten, H.B., Macgowan, J.J.: Blackwater fever (Hemoglobinuria) caused by Spider Bite. J.A.M.A. **114**, 1547 (1940).

Hall, J.E.: A study of protein and peptide components of venoms of *Loxosceles reclusa* (Gertsch and Mulaik) and *Dugesiella hentzi* (Girard). M.S. Thesis, Oklahoma State University, Stillwater, Oklahoma, 1970.

Heitz, J.R., Norment, B.R.: Characteristics of an alkaline phosphatase activity in brown reclusa venom. Toxicon **12**, 181 (1974).

Heryford, N.N.: Techniques for experimental brown spider envenomation. Toxicon **8**, 315 (1970).

Hite, J.M., Gladney, W.J., Lancaster, J.M., Whitcomb, W.H.: Biology of the brown recluse spider. Univ. Arkansas Agric. Exp. Sta. Bull. **711**, 1 (1966).

Horen, W.P.: Arachnidism. Clin. Med. **73**, 41 (1966)

Ibarra-Grasso, A.: Arañas y araneismo. Semana Médica, Buenos Aires. Tomo cincuentenario (2), **763** (1944)

Izu, W.: Aracnoidismo por *Loxosceles laeta* en el Perú. Estudio clínico y experimental. Thesis Bach. Med. No. 2564. Lima, 1953.

Jaeger, H.: Aracnoidismo en Chile. VI J. Traum. (Chile) Dic. (1941).

James, J.A., Sellards, W.A., Austin, O.M., Terril, B.S.: Reactions following suspected spider bite. A form of Loxoscelism. Am. J. Dis. Child. **102**, 395 (1961).

Kirberg, M., Gonzalez, I., Bauza, J.: Loxoscelismo cutáneo visceral y cortisona. Arch. Hosp. Clin. Niños R. del Río. **19**, 112 (1952).

Knierim, F., Letonja, T., Schenone, H.: Actividad *in vitro* del veneno y otros componentes orgánicos de *Loxosceles laeta* sobre eritrocitos humanos y animales. Bol. Chil. Parasit. **30**, 43 (1975).

Kniker, W.T., Morgan, P.N.: An inactivator in spider venom of the fifth component of complement. Fed. Proc. **26**, 362 (1967).

Kniker, W.T., Morgan, P.N., Flanigan, W.J., Reagan, P.W., Dillaha, C.J.: An Inhibitor of Complement in the venom of the Brown Recluse spider, *Loxosceles reclusa*. Proc. Soc. Exp. Biol. Med. **131**, 1432 (1969).

Lessenden, C.M., Zimmer, L.K.: Brown spider bites. A survey of the current problem. J. Kansas. Med. Soc. **61**, 379 (1960).

Levi, H.W., Spielman, A.: The biology and control of the South American brown spider, *Loxosceles laeta* (Nicolet), in a North American focus. Am. J. Trop. Med. Hyg. **13**, 132 (1964).

Lewis, M.I., Regan, J.F.: Necrotic Arachnidism. California Med. **105**, 457 (1966).

Macchiavello, A.: La *Loxosceles laeta,* causa del aracnoidismo cutáneo o mancha gangrenosa de Chile. Rev. Chil. Hist. Nat. **41**, 11 (1937).

Macchiavello, A.: Aracnoidismo cutáneo o mancha gangrenosa de Chile. Puerto Rico J. Publ. Health Trop. Med. **22**, 462 (1947a).

Macchiavello, A.: Aracnoidismo cutáneo experimental con veneno glandular de *Loxosceles laeta*. Puerto Rico J. Publ. Health Trop. Med. **23**, 279 (1947b).

Mackinnon, J.E., Witkind, J.: Aracnoidismo necrótico. An. Fac. Med. Montevideo. **38**, 75 (1953).

Meneghello, J., Emparanza, E.: Loxoscelismo cutaneo-visceral y cortisona (Relato de un caso). Bol. Inf. Paras. Chil. **7**, 9 (1952).

Minton, S.A., Olson, C.: A case of spider bite with severe hemolytic reaction. Pediatrics. **33**, 283 (1964).

Morgan, P.N., Felton, W.W.: Utilization of mammalian cell cultures in spider venom studies. Bacteriol. Proc. 65th Annual Meeting 120 (1965).

Morris, J.J., Russell, R.L.: The venom of the brown recluse spider *Loxosceles reclusa:* composition, properties, and an improved method of procurement. Fed. Proc. **34**, 225 (1975).

Nance, W.E.: Hemolytic anemia of necrotic arachnidism. Am. J. Med. **31**, 801 (1961).

Naquira, F., Montesinos, J., Córdova, E.: Loxoscelismo cutáneo en Arequipa, Perú. Arch. Peruanos Pat. Clin. **16**, 209 (1962).

Nazhat, N.: Venom of *Loxosceles reclusa:* protein components. M.S. Thesis, Oklahoma State University, Stillwater, Oklahoma, 1968.

Nicholson, J.F., Nicholson, B.H.: Hemolytic anemia from brown spider bite (necrotic arachnidism). J. Okla. State Med. Assoc. **55**, 234 (1962).

Norment, B.R., Smith, O.E.: Effect of *Loxosceles reclusa* Gertsch and Mulaik venom against hemocytes of *Acheta domesticus* (L.). Toxicon **6**, 141 (1968).

Norment, B.R., Vinson, S.R.: Effect of *Loxosceles reclusa* Gertsch and Mulaik venom on *Heliothis virescens* (F) larvae. Toxicon **7**, 99 (1969).

Odell, G.V., Chan, T.K., Geren, C.R., Lee, C.K., Ward, B.C., Howell, D.E.: Chemical and biological properties of tarantula and brown recluse venom toxins. Fed. Proc. **34**, 504 (1975).

Pavan, M., Valcurone Dazzini, M.: Toxicology and Pharmacology-Arthropoda. In: Chemical Zoology. Florkin, M. and Sheer, B.T. (eds.) New York: Academic Press, 1971, Vol. VII B, p. 392.

Pesce, H., Lumbreras, H.: Aracnoidismo en Lima por *"Loxosceles laeta"*. Rev. Med. Per. **25**, 3 (1954).

Pizzi, T.: Estudio histopatológico del aracnidismo necrótico por *Loxoscles laeta*. Bol. Chil. Parasit. **30**, 34 (1975).

Pizzi, T., Tacarias, J., Schenone, H.: Estudio histopatológico experimental en el envenenamiento por *Loxosceles laeta*. Biológica **23**, 33 (1957).

Prats, F., Schenone, H.: Mordeduras de arañas. Nuevas consideraciones sobre loxoscelismo. Bol. Chil. Parasit. **12**, 7 (1957).

Presley, T.E.: A case of spider bite. Memphis Med. Monthly J. **16**, 520 (1896).

Puffer, H.W., Parker, J.W., Russell, F.E., Warner, N.E.: Pathology of *Loxosceles laeta* venom poisoning in the rabbit. In: Animal and Plant Toxins. Kaiser, E. (ed.) Darmstadt (Germany) September 11–13 (1972).

Reid, H.A.: Venomous bites and stings. Trop. Doctor **5**, 12 (1975).

Rosenberg, D.: Picaduras de arañas y su tratamiento. Thesis. University of Chile. Escuela Tip. "La Gratitud Nacional" (1948).

Russell, F.E.: Prevention and Treatment of Venomous Animal Injuries. Experientia **30**, 8 (1974).

Russell, F.E., Wainschel, J., Gertsch, W.J.: Bites of spiders and other arthropods. Current Therapy. Conn, H.F. (ed.) Philadelphia: W.B. Saunders Co., 865 (1974).

Russell, F.E., Waldron, W.G., Madon, M.B.: Bites by the brown spiders *Loxosceles unicolor* and *Loxosceles arizonica* in California and Arizona. Toxicon **7**, 109 (1969).

Schenone, H.: Estudio de 27 casos de loxoscelismo. Bol. Chil. Parasit. **14**, 7 (1959).

Schenone, H.: Aracnidismo en el mundo. Proceedings of the Seventh International Congresses on Tropical Medicine and Malaria **4**, 199 (1964).

Schenone, H.: Latrodectismo y loxoscelismo en Chile. Incidencia, características clínicas, pronóstico, tratamiento y prevención. Mem. Inst. Butantan **33**, 207 (1966).

Schenone, H., Courtin, L., Knierim, F.: Resistencia inducida del conejo a dosis elevadas del veneno de *Loxosceles laeta*. Toxicon **8**, 285 (1970).

Schenone, H., Letonja, T., Knierim, F.: Algunos datos sobre el aparato venenoso de *Loxosceles laeta* y toxicidad de su veneno sobre diversas especies animales. Bol. Chil. Parasit. **30**, 37 (1975a).

Schenone, H., Prats, F.: Arachnidism by *Loxosceles laeta*. Report of 40 cases of Necrotic Arachnidism. Arch. Dermatol. **83**, 139 (1961).

Schenone, H., Reyes, H.: Loxoscelismo. Nociones sobre su epidemiología y profilaxis. Bol. Chil. Parasit. **18**, 38 (1963).

Schenone, H., Rojas, A., Reyes, H., Villarroel, F., Suarez, G.: Prevalence of *Loxosceles laeta* in houses in Central Chile. Am. J. Trop. Med. Hyg. **19**, 564 (1970).

Schenone, H., Rosales, S., Garcia, E.M.: Caso de loxoscelismo cutáneo visceral en Mendoza. Bol. Chil. Parasit. **12**, 56 (1957).

Schenone, H., Rubio, S., Villarroel, F., Rojas, A.: Epidemiología y curso clínico del loxoscelismo. Estudio de 133 casos causados por la araña de los rincones (*Loxosceles laeta*). Bol. Chil. Parasit. **30**, 6 (1975b).

Schenone, H., Semprevivo, L., Schirmer, E.: Consideraciones a propósito de dos casos de loxoscelismo cutáneo-visceral. Bol. Chil. Parasit. **14**, 17 (1959).

Shulov, A.: Biology and ecology of venomous animals in Israel. Mem. Inst. Butantan. **33**, 93 (1966).

Smith, C.W., Micks, D.W.: A comparative study of the venom and other components of three species of *Loxosceles*. Am. J. Trop. Med. Hyg. **17**, 651 (1968).

Steeger, A., Fuentealba, G.: Loxoscelismo cutáneo localizado. Rev. Chil. Pediat. **32**, 359 (1961).

Suarez, G., Biggemann, U., Schenone, H.: Estudios bioquímicos del veneno de *Loxosceles laeta* y de sus mecanismos de acción. Bol. Chil. Parasit. **26**, 60 (1971a).

Suarez, G., Casavilca, A.: Arañas venenosas de la Provincia de Trujillo. Rev. Fac. Cienc. Biol. **1**, 45 (1967).

Suarez, G., Contreras, G., Schenone, H.: Effect of *Loxosceles laeta* venom on human cell lines. Toxicon. **14**, 335 (1976).

Suarez, G., Schenone, H., Socias, T., Biggemann, U.: Veneno de *Loxosceles laeta*. Purificación parcial. Arch. Biol. Med. Exp. **7**, R 39 (1970).

Suarez, G., Socias, T., Schenone, H.: *Loxosceles laeta* venom. Partial purification. Toxicon **9**, 291 (1971b).

Taylor, E.H., Denny, W.F.: Hemolysis, renal failure and death, presumed secondary to bite of brown recluse spider. South. Med. J. **59**, 1209 (1966).

Ureta, E.: Latrodectismo, loxoscelismo y aracnoidismo benigno. Rev. Med. Chil. **72**, 694 (1944).

Ureta, E., Espinoza, J.: Aracnoidismo en Chile. Rev. Chil. Pediat. **7**, 489 (1944).

Vellard, J.: Preparation de un sérum contre le venin de *"Loxosceles laeta"*. C. R. Acad. Sci. **238**, 2078 (1954a).

Vellard, J.: L'araneisme au Pérou et dans les régions meridionales de l'Amérique du Sud. Trav. Inst. Franc. Etudes Andines. **4**, 133 (1954b).

Vellard, J.: Etude du venin de l'araignée *Loxosceles laeta* (Nicolet). C. R. Acad. Sci. **243**, 433 (1956).

Vellard, J.: La fonction venimeuse ches les araignées. Mem. Inst. Butantan. **33**, 35 (1966a).

Vellard, J.: El araneismo en Bolivia. Mem. Inst. Butantan **33**, 699 (1966b).

Villarroel, F., Schenone, H., Rojas, A., Sanhueza, H.: Distribución por estado de desarrollo y sexo de *Loxosceles laeta* capturadas en la zona Central de Chile. Bol. Chil. Parasit. **26**, 59 (1971).

Vukusic, A.: Loxoscelismo cutáneo-visceral mortal. Bol. Chil. Parasit. **17**, 25 (1962).

Weinstein, M., Gonzalez-Diaz, I., Alvarez, G., Osorio, A.: Loxoscelismo cutáneovisceral y cutáneo tratados con cortisona y ACTH. Rev. Med. Chil. **80**, 296 (1952).

Wiener, R.G., Stoffer, R.P., Chornock, F.W., Young, R.B.: Massive intravascular hemolysis. J. Kansas. Med. Soc. **61**, 206 (1960).

Wright, R.P.: Antiserum for brown recluse spider. Chem. Eng. News Sept. 11, 21 (1972).

Wright, R.P., Campbell, B.J., Barrett, J.L.: Enzymatic characterization of Missouri brown spider venom. 164th ACS Meeting, New York. (Abstr. SO) (1972).

CHAPTER 12

The Genus Centruroides (Buthidae) and Its Venom

H.L. STAHNKE

In North America scorpions of medical importance belong to the genus *Centruroides* Marx (1889) of the family Buthidae (SIMON, 1879) and the superfamily Buthoidea (BIRULA, 1917). The name *Centururus* is a synonym for *Centruroides* but the latter is correct as explained by POCOCK (1920f), who is also quoted by STAHNKE (1971). The type species is *Centruroides exilicauda* (WOOD) (1863b), one of the species designated by Marx (1889) as a *Centruroides*.

The genus *Centruroides* is principally an American taxon with its center of distribution in Mexico. LAMORAL et al. (1975) report specimens of *C. margaritatus* (Gervais) taken on Cape Verde Islands, Sierra Leone, and Gambia, W. Africa. *Centruroides* are found from the southern half of the United States to Central America and in the West Indies. A few species have invaded South America as far as Argentina, Ecuador, and Chile.

Centruroides scorpions are those members of the Buthidae that possess the following characteristics[1]: Interior and exterior pedal spurs well developed, often bearing a small basal thorn and macrochaetes; tibial spurs lacking; the fixed cheliceral finger bears one large tooth on its interior margin, while that of the movable finger bears two large teeth; mesosomal terga mono- or tri-keeled; subaculear protrusion of telson obsolete to strongly developed, sometimes spinoid; male cauda not broader distad but distinctly longer than that of female, often extremely so; caudal segment V dorsal furrow shallow or absent; sternite III of basilary area smooth, or at most weakly granular, but sometimes weakly furrowed; trichobothrium D_2 more distad than D_3; pedipalp tarsus (movable finger) cutting edge bearing from seven to nine oblique rows of denticles (or granules), sometimes plus a short apical row of three to five denticles; these oblique rows flanked externally and internally by large, dentate, lateral granules; between the lateral granules are one to four granules that are much smaller and referred to as *supernumerary* granules, which serve as a quick reference for identifying a centrurid scorpion. These accessory granules, as a rule, do not appear until about the fourth instar, and therefore juveniles of the larger species, like *C. gracilis*, might be mistaken for an *Isometrus* species if just this characteristic is used to identify the genus, as has frequently been done.

In the history of *Centruroides* systematics, color and color pattern seemed like excellent attributes for the identification of the species. However, STAHNKE (1971) through the use of geographic distribution, electrophoretic comparison of venoms, hybridization, and the serologic studies of POTTER and NORTHEY (1962) proved conclusively that the species *C. gertschi* Stahnke was merely a color phase

---

[1] Nomenclature after that of STAHNKE (1970).

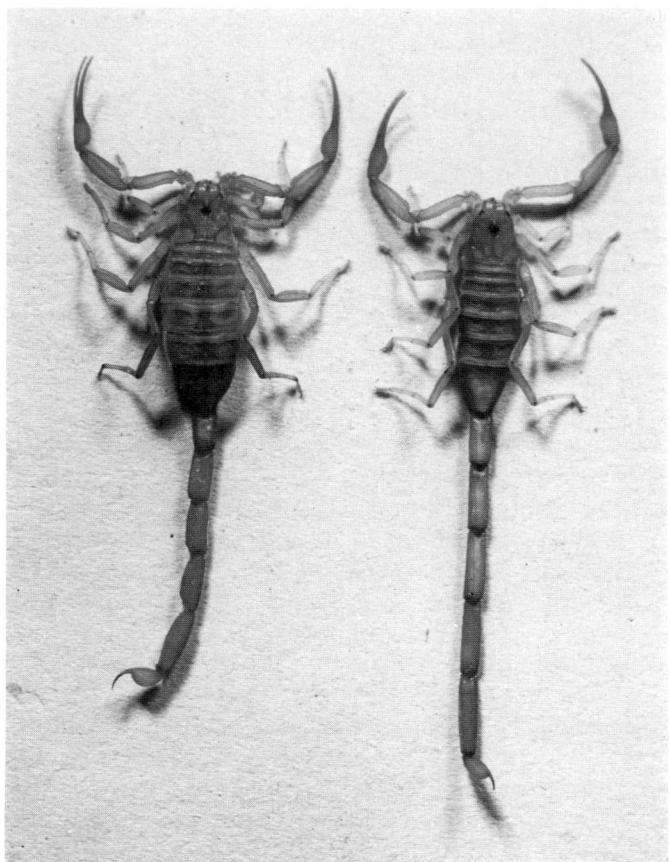

Fig. 1. *Centruroides sculpturatus. Left:* Female *Right:* Male

(principally a pattern of two dorsal black stripes over a straw color) of the concolorous *C. sculpturatus* Ewing (Fig. 1).

A study (unpublished data) of about 50 litters from *C. exilicauda* females captured from a mixed population and born in the laboratory, indicates that the
same condition exists in this species, i.e., it consists of both concolorous and
patterned individuals. This study also revealed that the young all have well-developed subaculear processes — mainly spinoid — and that not all adults have this structure obsolete. To date many writers characterize *C. exilicauda* as lacking a subaculear tooth or tubercle.

From preliminary evidence it appears that *C. chisosarius* Gertsch and *C. pantheriensis* Stahnke are just other color phases of *C. vittatus* (Say).

Hoffman's (1932a) key to the *Centruroides* of Mexico indicates a possible
confusion in our present knowledge of *Centruroides* systematics. His first dichotomy
in this key divides all the Mexican *Centruroides* into "unstriped species" vs. "striped
species." Thus, according to present evidence, he may have unwittingly automatically created a number of artificial species. A study of three litters of *C. hentzi*

(Banks) suggests that it and *C. keysi* Muma may be conspecific. Obviously the genus is in need of serious systematic study. The species mentioned herein are those recognized in the literature.

A. Species and Their Distribution

Centruroides aguayoi Moreno, 1939a: Cuba

C. argentinus Werner, 1939; Campos Santo, Salto Province, Argentina

C. bertholdi (Thorell), 1876b: Central Jalisco, Mexico

C. bicolor (Pocock), 1898: Costa Rica: Panama

C. chisosarius Gertsch, 1939: Chisos Basin, Big Bend National Park, Texas

C. dammanni Stahnke, 1970b: St. John, Virgin Islands

C. danieli (Prado and Rois-Patiño), 1939: Columbia (Andes).

C. dasypus Mello-Leitâo and Araúyo Felio, 1948: Andahuaylas, Peru.

C. elegans (Thorell), 1876b; Jalisco, Guerrero, Michoacán, Nayarit, Mexico, (four subspecies).

C. exilicauda (Wood), 1863b: St. Margarita Island, Cape St. Duras (type locality), Baja California, Mexico. San Diego, California. Reports of finding it on the Mexican mainland have proven to be incorrect determinations.

C. flavopictus (Pocock), 1898: Veracruz, Chipas, and Jalapa, Mexico (three subspecies).

C. fulvipes (Pocock), 1898: Xantipu, Guerrero, Mexico.

C. gracilis (Latreille), 1804: Mexico to northern South America; Antilles; Cuba; Jamaica; Santa Cruz de Tenerife; Florida (five subspecies).

C. hasethi (Pocock), 1902b: Curaçao (West Indies) (two subspecies).

C. hentzi (Banks), 1900: Florida.

C. infamatus (C.L. and L. Koch), 1845: Michoacán, Jalisco, Zacatecas, Durango and Veracruz, Mexico (two subspecies).

C. insulanus (Thorell), 1876: Jamaica; Choco; Brazil (two subspecies).

C. keysi Muma, 1967 (see *C. hentzi*).

C. limbatus (Pocock), 1898: Sirirea in Talamanca, Costa Rica; Chanquinole, Panama; Quezaltenango, Guatemala.

C. limpidus (Karsch), 1879b; Central Guerrero, Morelos, southern Puebla and along western coast, Mexico (two subspecies).

C. margaritatus (Gervais), 1841: Cuba; northern Mexico to northern South America; Cape Verde Islands, Sierra Leone and Gambia, West Africa, (five subspecies).

C. nigrescens (Pocock), 1898: Southern part of Guerrero, Mexico, and mainly in the Pacific coastal region and extending along the coast to Oaxaca.

C. nigrimanus Pocock), 1898: Oaxaca, Mexico; Honduras.

C. nigrovariatus (Pocock), 1898c: Oaxaca, Mexico.

C. nitidus (Thorell), 1876b: Puerto Rico; Haiti; Brazil, (two subspecies).

C. noxius Hoffmann, 1932a: City of Jalisco, Nayarit, and southern Sinaloa, Mexico.

C. ochraceus (Pocock), 1898: Yucatán and Campeche, Mexico.

C. pallidiceps (Pocock) 1902: Presidio, Sinaloa, and parts of Sonora, Mexico.

C. pantheriensis Stahnke, 1956b: Panther Junction, Big Bend National Park, Texas.
C. rubricauda (Pocock), 1898: Costa Rica.
C. sculpturatus Ewing, 1928: Arizona, western New Mexico, and eastern California; northern Mexico.
C. subgranosus (Kraepelin), 1899: Central America.
C. suffusus (Pocock), 1902: central portion of the state of Durango, Mexico (two subspecies).
C. testaceous (Geer) 1778: Montserrat; Haiti (two subspecies).
C. thorelli (Kraepelin), 1891: Cuba; Central Mexico to Central America (two subspecies).
C. vittatus (Say), 1821: South, Central and western United States, and adjacent Mexican states.
C. zweifeli Gertsch 1958: San Martin Island, Baja California, Mexico.

Species synonyms in the genus *Centruroides* and the old *Centrurus* are listed by Stahnke (1977).

B. Some Aspects of Behavior

Centrurid scorpions are often referred to as "bark" scorpions because they are frequently found under the loose bark of trees (e.g., in Arizona that of cottonwood, pepper, eucalyptus trees) and in the crevices at the base of old petiole stubs of palm fronds. These are habitats of choice, especially in the winter months when they may be found literally in clusters of 20–30 animals. In laboratory containers, *Centruroides sculpturatus,* when not active during the day time, will be found stacked in the container corners and, when the numbers are large enough (200–500 specimens), may form a living ramp along which active specimens escape over the edge of the container. When hiding under objects they generally display negative geotaxis. Frequently people are stung while picking up a board or rock because they press a scorpion clinging to the underside.

When inactive, bark scorpions generally rest the curled cauda laterally on the substrate. When crawling leisurely at about 15° C they make a definite "tail-drag" (Brady, 1947) in a fine dry sand substrate.

Most scorpions are vigorous, rapid diggers. If you place them under an inverted beaker on loose sand they will dig under and out in a short time. They dig vigorously with the four front legs while resting on the posterior four. When digging ceases, the hind four are used to kick the soil still farther back. If a centrurid scorpion is placed under the beaker it may wait hours before attempting to escape. Its action is quite different. If it can find a free edge of the beaker, the first three legs on one side are used to scrape out loose sand and then the three opposite legs are used in a similar manner. When a small space is gained under the vessel edge, the pedipalps are pushed through and used in a pulling action while the last pair of legs is used for pushing. Then a pushing, pulling, wriggling action takes place. Even the telson may be used to help in the pushing action. The total activity is not very vigorous and the scorpion may rest frequently for periods of 5–20 min. Once the pedipalps and carapace are under the edge of the beaker a wriggling, pushing action finally makes escape a reality. *Centruroides* scorpions will, likewise, *not dig* under objects to hide. If a slight crevice is made available the wriggling action forces them under.

Centrurid scorpions invade human dwellings frequently. They will crawl on walls and ceilings, often eating prey while in such locations. Occasionally, they lose their "claw hold" and fall; the landing place may be an otherwise occupied human bed.

The use of ultraviolet (UV) detection (STAHNKE, 1972a) of scorpions has given us a much greater insight into their nocturnal activities. Centrurid scorpions not only crawl over the ground but on the side of huge boulders and high into trees looking for prey. People walking through brush unwittingly get stung as they grab a branch to push their way through.

HADLEY and WILLIAMS (1968) studied the surface activities of four vejovid species of scorpions and *C. sculpturatus* using UV light. Two species of vejovid scorpions showed a decrease in surface occurrence as the evening progressed, while *C. sculpturatus* showed a random occupation throughout the night. Increased intensity of moonlight resulted in a significant decrease in surface occurrence in two of the vejovid species but *C. sculpturatus* showed no significant response to increased illumination.

Whereas many vejovid scorpions will seek shelter during a strong wind and rain, *C. sculpturatus* will actually be moving about in search of prey, providing that surface water does not accumulate.

Scorpions feed on a wide variety of prey ranging from spiders, various insects to small reptiles—any animal that they can subdue. STAHNKE (1966) noted that a satiated scorpion may not respond to an insect crawling on it while a hungry scorpion reacts to its presence often without physical contact. A *C. sculpturatus* scorpion, placed in an opaque vessel covered with an opaque piece of cardboard and not fed for 2 weeks, will not react if the cardboard is carefully removed so as not to cause a vibration on the container nor produce even a slight current of air. If, however, a slender, camel's-hair brush is placed, with a slight sideways movement, within an inch or two of the scorpion it will react quickly with out-stretched pedipalps and open chela. If a live scorpion is placed on a wide-field microscope using a cold light, the trichobothria can be observed swaying in even a very slight air movement. (This can sometimes be observed on preserved speci-mens.) If one observes a specimen like *Hadrurus arizonensis* it becomes obvious that the function of the trichobothria cannot be primarily tactile. The macrochaetes on the pedipalps of this genus are very dense and so long that physical contact with the relatively tiny trichobothria could not be made. Air currents must be the external stimulus. These setae with their very slender and mildly tapering shafts seem to be the first receptors of food—not by chemical sense but mechanical movement. The following observation will give further credence to this concept: If a starved *C. sculpturatus* specimen is carefully and gently presented with a sow bug it will grab the Isopod at once but then slowly drop the potential food. Over the past 30 years I have repeatedly offered sow bugs to *C. sculpturatus* many times because of the great abundance of the former. The reaction on the part of the scorpion is always the same: The hungry make a quick grab, only to slowly drop them.

The general rule on the choice of prey seems to be the degree of satiation and the ability to subdue the captive. *C. sculpturatus* will feed on the large, foul-smelling cockroach *Periplaneta americana*. Often after it grabs the large prey, it will in turn be dragged around by the roach until a successful penetration of its aculeus is accomplished.

STAHNKE (1966) described the feeding process in detail and pictures an *H. arizonensis* feeding on an 8-inch *Cnemidophorus* lizard, and in 1943b shows a photograph of a *C. sculpturatus* subduing a *P. americana* considerably larger than itself.

Satiation seems to play an important role in scorpion survival. Scorpions are much more alert when hungry than when satiated, as indicated above. Well-fed *C. sculpturatus* specimens have survived 30 days in glass vials, closed with cork stoppers, without food or water.

C. sculpturatus is able to resist the toxic products of some fumigants. The products of burning formaldehyde or sulfur candles produce no apparent harmful effects on these scorpions. During exposures up to 1 h they were inactive but not incapacitated. Immediately upon release from the test chamber, the test specimens moved about in an apparently normal manner. On the other hand, kerosene solutions of pyrethrum and the chlorinated hydrocarbons are quite effective on scorpions. A 0.15% concentration of pyrethrum will prove lethal in 20 min. A 10% DDT solution placed only on the scorpion pectines by means of a small camel-hair brush will gradually produce the DDT syndrome and prove lethal in approximately 3—5 days. Similar contact on other small areas of the body will prove lethal within 5—8 days. Three-percent chlordane is not only lethal but fast acting.

C. The Prevention and Control of Scorpions

C. sculpturatus is the only scorpion in the United States that has a potentially lethal venom. In Arizona from 1929 to 1965 (STAHNKE, 1966b) this scorpion was responsible for almost twice as many deaths as all other venomous animals, including 17 species or rattlesnake, gila monsters, spiders, insects (mainly bees, wasps, etc.) etc. During these 37 years, deaths occurred every month of the year except November. The greatest number of deaths occurred in June and July. The number of deaths (STAHNKE, 1972) peaked in 1931—1940 when the population of the state was about 5 million. By 1970 the population had increased to 17 million, i.e., a 3.5-fold increase. Since this lethal species of scorpion is a frequent inhabitant of human dwellings—much more so than other species—it is reasonable to assume that an increase in scorpion-human contact would produce a consequent increase in mortality.

The statistics, however, indicate a >3-fold *decrease* in deaths from scorpion stings. From 1950 to 1971, the range was 0—2 deaths *per year,* with an average of 0.35. During 14 of these 21 years, there were no deaths from scorpion stings. The few deaths that have occurred were children living in remote areas away from medical assistance.

The decrease in mortality can be attributed primarily to a) effective control and eradication, something that was not available before 1946, b) improved therapeutic practices, and c) education of the public via special publications, news stories, radio, and a special 3-year weakly half-hour television series.

1. Control and eradication (STAHNKE, 1948a, 1948b, 1948c) were realized through: a) *Cultural techniques:* decreasing the habitats and destroying the food supply. b) *Biologic method:* encouraging their natural enemies, e.g., cats, ducks (not chickens), bats and owls. c) *Mechanical devices:* tight house construction, well-fitted doors, windows, and overhanging roofs; the use of screening on windows and subfloor ventilation openings. MAZZOTTI (1962) suggests "placing a layer or two of tile around the base of the house to prevent access to the walls of the house." Protection of baby cribs or beds can be accomplished by covering the bed with mosquito netting and placing each bed leg in a can of water or kerosene. d) *Chemical control:* the use of residual insecticides in a kerosene solvent, e.g., DDT, chlordane, and other long-lasting hydrocarbons for killing. A 10% creosote oil solution can be poured along the base of the foundation as a repellent.

2. Improved therapeutic practices consisted of four approaches. a) *Prevention*: The public was educated regarding certain behaviors (STAHNKE, 1948, 1960, 1966) of *C. sculpturatus* (e.g., clinging to the underside of objects, etc.) and were impressed with the slogan "do not put your fingers where your eyes cannot see."

b) *First aid:* Again the public was educated in the proper use of cryotherapy (STAHNKE, 1965a) and in the recognition of their reactions (STAHNKE, 1965b).

c) *The medical profession and the public* were presented with the fact that medications like morphine sulfate and its derivatives (STAHNKE and DENGLER, 1964) might increase the toxicity of the venom seven fold. A study of the medications used by physicians (STAHNKE and STAHNKE, 1957c) revealed that some scorpion deaths and severe reactions in adults were apparently induced by morphine sulfate, Demerol, etc. Later research also incriminated Thorazine and Valium (STAHNKE, 1972b). The suggestion was made to physicians that therapeutic agents should not be used for treatment of scorpion stings unless previous laboratory tests indicated their safety and effectiveness.

STAHNKE (1957a) demonstrated that Dihydroergotamine methanesulfate (D.H.E.-45 Sandoz) and Bellafoline (Sandoz) used respectively in a combined dosage of 5 mg/kg plus 2.5 mg/kg, raised the rat LD_{50} of the venom from 0.96 mg/kg, with a 95% confidence interval of $0.85-1.09$ mg/kg, to 1.72 mg/kg, with a confidence interval of $1.17-2.51$ mg/kg.

In another study, STAHNKE (1963) reported the existence of synergism in rats between epinepherine and this venom. It was noted, however, that when 1 cc of epinephrine, at a concentration of 1 mg/cc, is administered in one dose after the injection of the venom, the LD_{50} is not modified, but if a total of 1 cc is given in four equal doses at 10-min intervals, the toxicity of the venom is increased 2.38 times.

Empirically we have learned that a child's death can generally be prevented through the use of heroic dosages of a long-acting barbiturate. Generally Na phenobarbital was administered. Not less than 4 grains was used even for the youngest child suffering severe convulsions. Sufficient barbiturate would be administered to bring about complete relaxation. This has a threefold importance: First, to prevent physical exhaustion; second, to prevent stressing and the concomitant increase in blood epinepherine; third, more time is gained for the proper administration of antivenin.

d) *The development of a species-specific antivenin in* 1947 (STAHNKE, 1972) was the final solution to the medical phase of the scorpion problem. The first product was a liquid serum with the rabbit as the host animal. It was very effective but the high temperatures of July and August prevented mailing the product to other parts of the state.

The first lyophilized antivenin was a cat serum. This host was selected on the basis of economy and excellent immune response. Only cats in excellent health, immunized and held in quarantine for 3 weeks were used. The increased need for antivenin caused a change in 1965 to goats as the host animal. No deaths have occurred with the prescribed use of the antivenin since 1947.

D. Morphology and Function of the Venom Apparatus

All scorpions are venomous. Venom is economically injected by means of a stinger (*aculeus*) (Fig. 2) found at the distal end of the *telson*. The bulbous portion, the *vesicle* (or ampulla), of the telson contains two glands, each surrounded and segregated by a muscle bundle and with a separate duct opening into a laterally placed tear-drop shaped orifice near the tip of the stinger. Thus, there are two large outlets for the venom.

In the act of stinging, the sharp tip of the stinger makes a very small puncture which is spread by the increasing thickness of the stinger shaft. At the termination of the thrust striated muscles medially located, surrounding each gland and attached to the endocuticle of the exoskeleton, contract and thus squeeze the gland against the exoskeleton; an action which forces the venom through the lateral orifices of the stinger. Since the orifices flare more or less funnel-like and the lumen of the venom duct is much smaller in diameter, no back-pressure is built up at the time of injection. When the stinger is withdrawn, the small, stretched wound automatically contracts. In so doing, the victim's tissue squeegees the remaining venom out of the tear-drop shaped orifice just before the wound seals to prevent loss through leakage.

Two histologic studies have been made of centrurid venom glands, both using light and electron microscopy. MAZURKIEWICZ and BERTKE (1972) used *C. sculpturatus* glands. They state:

Each of the paired glands is lined by secretory epithelium made up of a single layer of columnar cells. Extensive folding in the epithelial layer creates a primitive acinar gland. The secretory products are either membrane-bound or unbound vesicles with discrete morphologies and are observed in the extruded venom, within the lumen of the gland, and within single secretory cells. Some cells are seen with their cytoplasm bulging out at the luminal border. The plasma membrane is continuous across the bulge and microvilli are absent. The secretory process was micro-apocrine. The lumen of the gland is suggested to serve as an extracellular storage site for the venom. There is an abundance of membrane bound vesicles within the lumen, segregating the morphologically different secretion products. The various ingredients of the venom are probably mixed upon injection which may rupture these membranes.

KEEGAN and LOCKWOOD (1971) examined the venom glands of *C. vittatus,* a low-toxicity species, and the highly toxic *C. limpidus tecomanus.* They state:

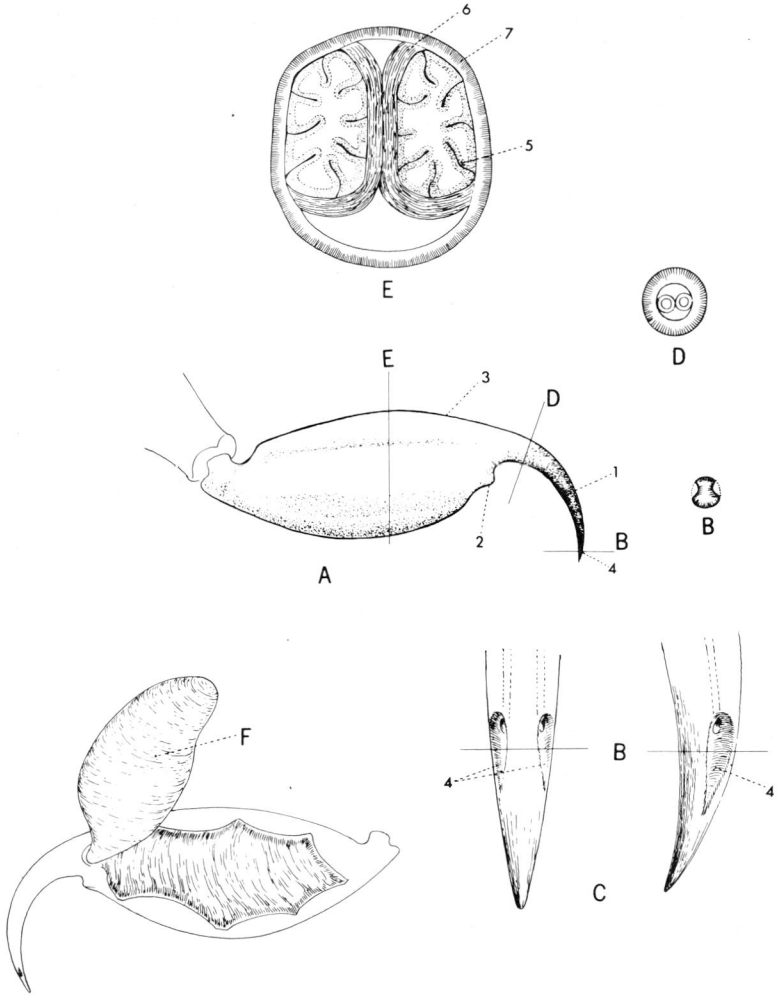

Fig. 2. Scorpion venom apparatus. *A*. Telson, composed of: (*1*) stinger or aculeus; (*2*) subacular tubercle; (*3*) ampulla or vesicle; (*4*) venom aperture. *B*. Cross-section at level of apertures. *C*. Enlarged tip of aculeus. *D*. Cross-section showing both venom ducts. *E*. Cross-section showing both (*5*) venom glands; (*6*) muscles; (*7*) ampulla wall. *F*. Right venom gland removed from telson

In both species the glandular epithelium was thrown into numerous ridges, folds, and irregular finger-like processes. The luminal surface of the epithelium was marked by the presence of closely spaced microvilli, a finding not previously noted. Three types of granule-containing cells, classified by granule size, were present. These granules, fine, medium, and large, stained dark blue with metachromatic dyes in material prepared for light microscopy. Each cell contained granules of only one size. We assumed that the granules were venom particles. Two types of mucous-containing cells were interspersed among the venom cells. In one type the contents were amorphous; in the other, the mucous was contained in globules of various sizes and had either a linear or dotted appearance. Contents of these cells stained pink with toluidine blue. The secretory process was apocrine in both species. Although the species studied differ greatly in their toxicity for man, no differences in morphology of their venom glands were found by light or electron microscopy.

Nerve endings and migratory cells of the leucocytic type, deep within the venom glands of scorpions, had not been reported previously. The high magnification and superior resolution of the electron microscopy were required for their clear demonstration in the scorpion.

The muscles that surround the venom gland are characteristic of smooth muscle found elsewhere.

The findings of the two studies are essentially in agreement. The secretory process is apocrine and each cell seems to specialize in producing only one type of granule. The studies differed in finding microvilli. Also, one study suggests that the secretory products are either membrane bound or unbound vesicles with discrete morphologies. They also disagree on the type of muscle, i.e., smooth or striated, surrounding the two glands.

E. Extracting Venom

The early investigators used venom obtained by grinding dried telsons in a mortar and extracting the "venom" with distilled water, physiologic saline or glycerine. This process is still used by some producers of antivenin. Obviously this technique extracts other soluble products present in the whole telson.

Contemporary methods obtain venom by electric stimulation and collect it in special pipettes. Electrical stimulation causes the telson to move. In order to prevent breaking the aculeus the orifice of the pipette must be great enough to accommodate for this movement.

The type of electric stimulation used is an important factor. An induction coil may produce too high an amperage so as to partially coagulate the inner-telson tissue.

Consequently, the scorpion may not yield venom after about two or three "milkings." If the venom yield is not clear or opalescent, i.e., contains small amounts of mucoid material, the current strength is too great. For each species of scorpion the current must have a given strength. We have found that observing this and milking them weekly, scorpions will produce for many months. We have also observed that if the scorpion is removed from the milking colony at the first indication of diminished yield, after about 1 month's rest the production will become normal.

When producing an antivenin speed of operation is important since thousands of scorpions must be milked for each lot of antivenin. To accomplish this we constructed an electrical conducting forceps approximately 6 in (155 mm) long attached to an electrical cord approximately 3 ft (1 m) in length. The operator, using these forceps, grasps the scorpion by the fifth caudal segment, directs the aculeus into the pipette lumen and turns on the electricity with a knee-operated switch. Several short charges produce more venom, and apparently do less tissue damage, than prolonged charges. The venom is centrifuged at 4000 rpm to bring down cellular debris, and the supernatant is pipetted into a tared vial. The product is frozen quickly at $-60°$ C and lyophilized in a Re PP sublimator. After lyophilization, the remaining moisture is removed in a vacuum oven-desiccator assembly at 37° C and the vials capped. These are now refrigerated until ready for use. We find this procedure gives us more consistent results and gives a truer picture of the venom reaction.

F. Mammalian Physiologic Reaction to the Venom

I. Clinical Observations

1. Symptoms of Severe Envenomization (Children Under 16 Years of Age)

The venom of *C. sculpturatus* does not produce any visible effects at the site of the sting but the patient may experience hyperesthesia and intense local pain. He may also experience difficulty in swallowing, a sensation of "thick tongue," extreme nervousness, respiratory difficulties, alternating emprosthotonic and opisthotonic spasms,[2] excessive salivation, gastric hyperdistention, mydriasis, nystagmus, diplopia, temporary blindness, involuntary micturation and defecation, penile erection, respiratory arrest, hypertension and cardiac failure (STAHNKE, 1950, 1963).

2. Symptoms of Envenomization in Adults

Depending on age and state of health, adults may experience any of the reactions listed above for children. In severe cases they frequently experience diplopia or temporary blurred vision. Deaths have occurred in the elderly having hypertension since the venom is a strongly hypertensive agent.

II. Preclinical Observations

1. Pharmacologic Considerations

PATTERSON (1962b) found that this venom caused stimulation of visceral smooth muscle. Venom, added to isolated gut preparations of the rat ascending colon, rabbit duodenum, and guinea pig ileum, initially caused a reduction in spontaneous activity followed by an increase in tonus. Later, slow rhythmic contraction developed. Atropine sulfate prevented the initial, but not the developed, contractions. Hexamethonium chloride, a ganglionic blocking agent, failed to alter the activity of venom in the guinea pig ileum. Therefore, no ganglionic stimulating action of venom was demonstrated.

PATTERSON (1960) also reported that this venom caused hypertension, respiratory failure and skeletal muscle stimulation in anesthetized dogs, rabbits, and cats. No significant action was found on isolated skeletal muscle preparations. Hypertension resulted in part from release of pressor substance from the adrenal gland, although neither direct action nor action mediated by vasopressor centers can be ruled out. Respiration and skeletal muscle stimulation followed a pattern which

---

[2] At lethal levels, the convulsions are chaotic.

suggests an initial peripheral action followed by an action dependent on the central motor centers.

SWEARINGEN (1962), using rats and cats, investigated the importance of the adrenergic mechanism involved with the actions of $2 \times LD_{50}$ of this venom. He used dibenzyline, an adrenergic blocking agent, and hexamethonium chloride for inhibiting ganglionic function. The ventilatory patterns, blood pressures, and electrocardiograms of rats and cats of the three groups were analyzed through recordings of these activities. Venom alone caused ventilatory inhibition or transitory apnea, either a decrease or an increase in pulse rate, and hypotension followed by hypertension. Animals pretreated with Dibenzyline before infusion of venom developed reduced responses different in sequence but of the same type as those developed by animals treated only with venom. Envenomized animals pretreated with hexamethonium maintained very stable ventilatory patterns, little change in pulse rate, minor increases and decreases in blood pressure, and greater ability to withstand the toxicity of venom through a period of 30 min. These responses, he concluded, indicate: that the initial reactions made to venom probably occur in the peripheral areas of the autonomic nervous system; that venom may have the ability to perform as a sympathomimetic agent or stimulate some sympathetic element which was not inactivated by Dibenzyline; and, finally, that epinepherine may possibly act synergistically with venom in normal animals.

POZO (1968) states: "The pharmacological properties of the venoms of different Mexican *Centruroides* are qualitatively similar. The intensity of the actions vary considerably." This intensity of action is perhaps due to the difference in the protein concentration. STAHNKE and JOHNSON (1967) demonstrated this to be true for the venom of the tarantula *Aphonopelma* sp. versus that of *C. sculpturatus*. Tarantula venom is about 5% protein, while that of the scorpion is 62%. The number of protein fractions, as shown by disc electrophoresis, is 10 for the tarantula venom and 16 for *C. sculpturatus*.

Tarantula natural bite tests produced little, if any, apparent chemical effects. However, when 10 mg of this venom was injected into the right groin of an adult rat it produced, within 20 min, severe convulsions, and death in about an hour. There were no visible reactions at the locus of the injection, but about 10 min after venenation the animal went through almost a typical *C. sculpturatus* venom syndrome, i.e., moving about nervously, patting the front feet on the cage floor and occasionally going through face cleaning movements, followed by chaotic convulsions, copious drooling, and finally death. Postmortem examinations revealed gastric hyperdistention, hepatic and nephric hyperemia, and petechiae on the lungs.

2. Pathologic Effects

BERTKE (1961), using rats made a histopathologic study in which he indicated that "the most significant gross finding was the hypertrophy of the adrenal gland beginning the second day and continuing to the 10th day after administration of venom in a dosage of 0.6 mg/k body weight." These glands were approximately twice the size of the control's adrenals. In general, this histopathologic study of envenomized rats revealed normal brain, spleen, heart, and muscle. The most consistent finding in the kidney was peritubular congestion in the early hours of envenomation and cloudy swelling in the later days. The liver reactions were inconsistent. They varied from normal to hemorrhagic necrosis. The liver of a 2-h rat showed generalized hydropic degeneration extended into the central vein area. The 4-h rat liver appeared normal except for one area of hemorrhagic necrosis. The 24-h rat resembled the 2-h rat with the exception that there was $+2$ to $+3$ necrosis. One 5-day and one 10-day rat revealed one area of hemorrhagic necrosis and also generalized moderate clumping of cytoplasm. The 48-h and 5-day controls showed slight clumping of cytoplasm and dilated congested sinusoids. All other rats had normal livers.

3. Allergic Potentialities

DORO et al. (1957), using guinea pigs, were not able to elicit an allergic response with this scorpion venom, either by means of anaphylaxis experiments or the Schult-Dale tests. Blood counts taken at the time of the latter test indicated no eosinophilia. Later tests (unpublished), using rats and rabbits also failed to provide an allergic response. In contrast to bee venom, this venom has not been observed to produce an allergic response in individuals accidentally stung.

G. Human Behavior and Scorpions

The characteristics of habitats that attract scorpions are that they contain insect and arachnid food. One of the most common is a poorly constructed dwelling place. Earlier, Durango, Mexico had numerous scorpions because of the large numbers of adobe houses and poorly screened windows. Any brick house with poorly pointed mortar provides ideal habitats. If the floor is elevated above the ground scorpions are attracted under it by the hundreds. Seldom disturbed storage rooms, piles of brick or lumber and the crevices around petiole stubs of palm trees, loose bark of trees, etc., are all highly attractive to scorpions.

What do people do to get stung by scorpions? The data in Tables 1−3 were taken from reports filed by the physicians who treated the patients, and reported by STAHNKE (1950).

MAZZOTTI and BRAVO-BECHERELLE (1963) have given an excellent, detailed report on scorpions in the Mexican Republic. Anyone interested in the subject should read this. It is too extensive to summarize in a paper of this type.

H. Venom Chemistry

In its natural condition *C. sculpturatus* venom is a somewhat opalescent, milky, translucent fluid with a pH of 7.12 (STAHNKE, 1963). When the lyophilized venom is reconstituted with water it contains some insoluble material, most of which is cellular debris. The water filtrate of this solution passed through a sterilizing Millipore filter contains the toxic factors and has a mouse LD_{50} about 1.12 mg/kg and a rat LD_{50} of 1.00 mg/kg. In contrast to this the venom of the vejovid scorpion,

Table 1. Data on scorpion sting cases

Age (months)	Sex	Time	Part of body and circumstances when stung
3	m	2 a.m.	Leg. Asleep in crib.
9	f	2 p.m	Abdomen. Lying in bed.
12	f	9 p.m.	Sole of foot. Scorpion in shoe.
14	f	11 p.m.	Hand. Sleeping on floor with mother.
16	f	10 a.m.	Hand. Reached for doll; scorpion under doll's clothes.
18	f	2 a.m.	Leg. Sleeping on floor of jail with mother.
20	m	9 a.m.	Finger. Lifted board in yard.
21	m	2 p.m.	Hand. Picked up damp cloth.

(years)			
2	m	5 p.m.	Thigh. While dressing; scorpion in clothes.
3	m	1 a.m.	Thigh. Scorpion crawled on him while sitting in chair.
4	m	8 a.m.	Leg. Scorpion crawled on leg during breakfast.
4	m	6 p.m.	Hand. Picking bark off tree; scorpion in crevice.
5	m	10 p.m.	Wrist. Playing around rocks in desert.
6	m	2 p.m.	Hand. On school grounds; scorpion hiding in dust rag.
8	f	3 p.m.	Foot. Helping wash dishes; scorpion on towel; mother saw it and tried to brush it off; landed on foot of patient.
10	f	9 p.m.	Foot. Walking barefoot in house.
16	m	3 p.m.	Penis. Putting on swim suit.
21	f	noon	Leg, below knee. Sitting on chair.
27	m	5 p.m.	Hand. While reaching in trash barrel.
31	f	9 a.m.	Finger. Tried to kill scorpion with piece of tissue.
35	m	9 a.m.	Thigh. Lifting flagstones; scorpion crawled up leg.
43	m	9 a.m.	Foot. In shower bath.
44	f	10 a.m.	Breast and chest. Scorpion fell from drapes, down neck and inside brassiere.
45	f	8 a.m.	Finger. Reached into paper sack which had been on ground overnight.
47	f	9 a.m.	Finger. Reached under damp board.
62	f	9 p.m.	Foot. Walking barefoot in grass.
73	f	9 a.m.	Foot and finger. Picked up wash cloth in sink and was stung on finger; threw scorpion to floor and got stung on foot.
75	m	10 a.m.	Toe. Walking barefoot in bathroom.

Table 2. Distribution of scorpion stings by months

Month	Percent
January	3.7
February	2.3
March	2.8
April	5.5
May	11.5
June	17.5
July	17.4
August	14.7
September	9.6
October	8.7
November	3.2
December	3.2

Table 3. Frequency of body part stung

Part of body	%frequency	
1. Trunk		
a) Chest or shoulder	8.5 ⎫	
b) Abdomen	5.6 ⎭	14.1
2. Leg (not including foot)	15.5 ⎫	
a) Foot	15.5 ⎭	31.0
3. Arm (not including hand)	7.0 ⎫	
a) Hand	47.9 ⎭	54.9
	100.	

Table 4. Semiquantitative spectrographic analysis of scorpion venoms

Elements	C. sculpturatus in%	H. arizonensis in%
Calcium	0.29	0.17
Sodium	5.6	4.5
Zinc	0.044	trace less than 0.03
Silicon	0.32	0.080
Aluminium	0.048	0.24
Magnesium	0.15	0.078
Boron	0.0040	0.0020
Iron	0.034	0.040
Manganese	0.020	0.014
Lead	0.013	0.030
Molybdenum	not detected-less than 0.001	not detected-less than 0.003
Lithium	not detected-less than 0.01	trace-less than 0.03
Copper	0.0052	0.035
Silver	not detected-less than 0.0001	not detected-less than 0.0003
Nickel	0.033	not detected-less than 0.003
Potassium	1.7	8.2
Strontium	trace-less than 0.0001	not detected-less than 0.0003
Chromium	0.0056	not detected-less than 0.0001
Phosphorus	0.096	trace-less than 0.10
Tin	0.016	0.20
Tungsten	0.15	not detected-less than 0.10
Cobalt	not detected-less than 0.001	0.0054
Total ash= (as sulfates and oxides)	23.6	33.9

Hadrurus arizonensis, which has a similar physical appearance in the fluid state, has a mouse LD_{50} of about 168 mg/kg.

    C. sculpturatus, which seldom reaches a length of 65 mm, is about 150 times as toxic as this large 110 mm scorpion. Table 4 presents an elemental semiquantitative spectographic analysis of these two species (unpublished data). It is interesting to note that the more toxic venom has a greater quantity of eleven of the detectable elements. It is too soon to speculate as to the role in toxicity played by this imbalance of elements.

At 4° C, in the lyophilized state, the toxicity of the venom is retained indefinitely. Even in the reconstituted condition at 4° C the toxicity has been retained for several years. On the other hand, alternate freezing and thawing of the reconstituted venom significantly reduces the toxicity. In contrast to this the venom is quite thermostable. However, WATT (1964) found that the toxic principle is slowly inactivated by heat. At 92° C the LD_{50} changed from 1.46 to 4.29 mg/kg when heated for 40 min and after 80 min, no toxicity was observable.

Some immunologic studies by POTTER (1961) suggested that a polysaccharide antigen may be present in this venom. WATT (1964) was not able to get a positive test for either monosaccharides or polysaccharides and concludes that the components of the venom are proteins with the possible presence of some free amino acids. Although he obtained positive tests for those amino acids containing an aromatic ring, absorption spectra showed that these structures are present in very low concentrations.

STAHNKE (1966) reported 16 protein fractions for C. sculpturatus and 62% protein. In contrast to this H. arizonensis venom has 14 fractions and 32.9% protein. From this evidence and that reported by STAHNKE and JOHNSON (1967) in which tarantula and C. sculpturatus venoms were compared it becomes clear that the toxic properties are protein. In this case the mouse LD_{50} of the tarantula venom was 14.14 mg/kg and its protein content 5%. The scorpion venom mouse LD_{50} was 1.12 mg/kg and the protein content 62%. The ratios between the percent protein of the two venoms is 12.4 and between the $LD_{50's}$ is 12.6. In the same study an enzyme analysis did not detect L-amino acid oxidase and DNAase activity and only negligible RNAase activity. Protease activity was indicated with an endpoint at 0.625 mg/ml.

An interesting case of intergeneric relationship indicated through venom activity in rats was reported by PALMER (1954). Part of the venom syndrome of C. sculpturatus is the absence of visual symptoms of venom activity at the site of penetration, excessive salivation, nasal secretions, hyperesthesia, severe convulsions, severe local pain and often eyes dull and glassy. The venom of two vejovid scorpions, Vejovis spinigerus (Wood) and H. arizonensis Ewing when introduced by natural sting generally produce only local symptoms in the form of local swelling, a sharp burning pain, redness, and often local numbness. A severe sting by V. spinigerus in man has been known to produce the sensation of formication around the mouth.

PALMER reported that when white rats were given large quantities of these vejovid venoms the rats demonstrated such symptoms as excessive salivation, nasal secretions, lacrimation, and cyanosis of the immediate area of injection. The rats also became hypersensitive so that a slight touch would cause a strong convulsive response. Rats receiving large doses of H. arizonensis demonstrated in addition fibrillation of skeletal muscle and apparent impairment of vision.

These symptoms produced by large quantities of venom are those characteristic of C. sculpturatus venom and that of some other Centruroides. At this point it seems as though the systemic reactions have their origin in the much greater protein concentration of C. sculpturatus and that it is primarily composed of fractions not well represented in the two vejovid venoms. PALMER also was able to produce an antivenin of only low titer with *H. arizonensis* venom.

POTTER and NORTHEY (1962) in an immunologic evaluation of scorpion venoms did not show an intergeneric relationship between *C. sculpturatus* and the above two vejovid venoms. Apparently the toxic fractions involved are either weakly represented or only weakly antigenic.

WATT (1964) concluded that toxicity of *C. sculpturatus* venom, as measured by death, is associated with one (or at most two) components. He states that on the basis of dialyzability the toxin is a peptide of relatively low molecular weight. Dialysis with either water or 0.01 M acetic acid removed about 47% of the solids within 12–24 h and proved highly toxic. After 24–32 h, the residue remaining in the dialysis bag contained little, if any, toxicity measured by the appearance of symptoms, i.e., hyperpnea, hypersensitivity, salivation, and seizure activity.

WATT and McINTOSH (1967) reported indirect evidence that the toxicity of the venom of *C. sculpturatus* may be associated with the formation of acetylcholine. However, this evidence was not supported in potentiation and inhibition studies using chemicals known to effect the acetylcholine transmitter system. They concluded that the toxic portion of the venom is not associated with the acetylcholine destruction.

McINTOSH and WATT (1967) studying the biochemical-immunochemical aspects of this venom conclude that the crude venom is stable to a wide range of pH, i.e., from 7.4 (normal) to 11.1, and to enzymatic digestion. Results indicate that toxicity is dependent on the presence of sulfhydryl groups and that the major components migrate as cations. The toxic component(s) identify with the major electrophoretic bands.

WATT and McINTOSH (1972) report on the effects by group-specific reagents on letality of toxins in *C. sculpturatus* venom. They observed that those reagents which reduce disulfide bonds decrease lethality, as does O-methylisourea, a reagent for ε-amino group. However, reagents which react with sulfhydryl and free carboxyl groups do not affect the venom lethality. In this study, however, their former conclusion with the toxic dependency on the presence of sulfhydryl groups was not substantiated, since effects of other reagents specific for sulfhydryl groups did not reduce lethality.

KATZ and EDWARDS (1972) studied the effect of *C. suffusus suffusus* venom on the neuromuscular junction of the frog. They report that, at the concentrations used, this venom acts on the motor nerves. Their venom source was "the dried scorpion tails" … which "were macerated in Ringer solution and left in the cold overnight." Thus, other products foreign from the venom could be present.

They used the isolated frog *sartorius* nerve-muscle preparation. In the presence of the venom, single shocks applied to the nerve produced repetitive responses in both nerve and muscle. Reduction of the sodium concentration in the bathing medium abolished the repetitive acitvity; addition of calcium had no observed effect. Bathing the nerve in Ringer solution with venom occasionally produced repetitive activity. The authors conclude that the results suggest that the site most accessible to the action of the venom is the exposed area of the axon near its termination.

J. Suggestions for Therapy

Although the *C. sculpturatus* venom syndrome has certain identifying characteristics, other existing conditions may modify the expected clinical picture. In the case of a very small child, the parents are alarmed with its behavior but cannot confirm that the reactions are the result of scorpion sting. Sometimes they will report a scorpion sting but they cannot indicate the species. Diagnosis for determining whether the scorpion was *C. sculpturatus* or one of the other highly toxic *Centruroides* is relatively simple. Since the venom produces extreme hyperesthesia at the site of the sting, a sharp tap with the finger tip on or near the site of penetration will produce sharp pain and cause rapid withdrawl of the stung member or an outburst of crying. No known nonlethal scorpion venom in North America will produce such intense hyperesthesia.

The use of narcotics as analgesic agents is strongly contraindicated. Avoiding stress is important and barbiturates are indicated. Therapeutic agents previously untried with the *Centruroides* venenation should be used with extreme caution.

Incision and suction is of no value and may be harmful. The amount of venom usually injected is very minute and the aculeus puncture so small as to be most generally imperceptible. Thus incision and suction would only be an irritant and hasten absorption.

Antivenins are available for *Centruroides* envenomization from Laboratories Myn, Av. Coyoacan 1707, Mexico 112, D.F. and from the Anti-venin Production Laboratory, Arizona State University, Tempe, Arizona, 85282. The Mexican antivenin is a horse-serum and the Arizona antivenin is a goat serum.

References

Anonymous: Venin de Scorpions, Part I of Chap. 1, Sect. P, Envenimements et intoxications. In: Notice sur l'Institut Pasteur d'Algérie, Tomo II, Alger, Dec. 12, 1949 (Scorpions pp. 277—304.)
    On pp. 295-6: Brief comparison of the venom of scorpions of North Africa and the Mexican scorpions: *Centruroides noxius* and *C. limpidus*.
Altamirano, F.: Algunas observaciones fisiologicas sobre los efectos de la ponzõna del alacràn de Jojutla. Mem. Soc. Cien. "Antonio Alzate" **14**, 327—330 (1900).
    Centrurus mexicanus (Alacràn de Jojutla)=*Centruroides l. limpidus*. Joutla, Mexico is associated with the work of Dr. Amador Espinosa.
Armas, L.F. de: Tipos de las colecciones escorpiològicas P. Franganillo y Universidad de la Habana (Arachnida: Scorpionida). Poeyana (La Habana) **101**, 1—18 (1973)
    Centruroides elegans guanensis (=*C. guanensis guanensis*, n.comb.); *C. gracilis pectinatissimus* (*C. pectinatissimus*, n. comb.); *C. thorelli aguayoi* (=*C. aguayoi*, n. comb.); *C. thorelli cubensis* (=*C. guanensis cubensis*, n. comb.).
Armas, L.F. de: Escorpiones del Archipiélgo Cubano. V. Nuevas especies de *Centruroides* (Scorpionida, Buthidae). Poeyana (La Habana) **145**, 1—55 (1976).
    New taxa: *C. anchorellus*, *C. arctimanus*, *C. a. banensis*, *C. armadai*, *C. baracoae*, *C. cajennensis*, *C. guanensis sanfelipensis*, *C. maisiensis*, *C. robertoi*, *C. zayasi*; in addenda (p. 53—5), *C. antiguensis*, *C. farri*, *C. hummelincki*, *C. underwoodi*, *C. eustatius*. Also discusses systematics of *C. gracilis* (Latreille) relative to Cuban forms.
Baerg, W.J.: Some poisonous arthropods of North and Central America. Trans. 4th Int. Cong. Ent. (Ithaca) **2**, 420—438 (1929).
    Inc. discussion of general physiological effects of venom of five Centruroid species on white rats and man. Considers *C. mexicanus* from Jojutla=*C. suffusus*.

Baggini, A., Pavan, M.: Studi sugli scorpioni. III. Scorpioni ed altri chelicerati esaminati alla luce di Wood per fluorescenza dell' epicuticola. Boll. Zool. **22**, 329—340 (1955).
Inc. *Centrurus infamatus* and *C. margaritatus*.

Banks, N.: Synopses of North-American invertebrates IX. The scorpions, solpugids and pedipalpi. Am. Nat. **34**, 421—427 (1900).
Inc. in key: *Centrurus exilicauda, C. nigrescens, C. margaritatus, C. testaceus, C. gracilis, C. carolinianus, C. hentzi*.

Banks, N.: The arachnida of Florida. Proc. Acad. Nat. Sci. (Philad.) **56**, 120—147 (1904).
Inc. *Centrurus gracilis, C. carolinianus, C. hentzi* n.sp., *C. margaritatus*.

Banks, N.: Arachnida from the Bahamas. Bull. Am. Mus. Nat. Hist. **22**, 185—189 (1906).
Inc. *Centrurus vittatus* Pal. de Beauv.

Banks, N.: The scorpions of California. Pom Col. J. Entomol. **2**, 185—188 (1910).
Inc. in key only *Centrurus californicus, C. exilicauda*.

Banta, B.H.: Lizards eaten by scorpions. Herpetologica **13**, 202 (1957).
Mentions *Centruroides* sp., but is not specific.

Beer, R.E.: A new species of *Pimeliaphilus* (Acarina Pterygosomidae) parasitic on scorpions with discussion of it postembryonic development. J. Parasitol. **46**, 433—440 (1960).
More than 400 mites were recovered from 16 specimens of *Vejovis p. punctatus*. Although this species and *Centruroides thorelli* were often under a single rock none of the mites were found on the *Centruroides* species.

Bender, G.L.: Studies on a synthetic diet for the scorpion, *Centruroides sculpturatus*. Ann. N.Y. Acad. Sci. **77** (2), 262—266 (1959).

Berland, L.: Note sur un scorpion muni de deux queues (Arachn.). Bull. Soc. Entomol. Fr. **10**, 251—252 (1913).
Juv. *Centrurus infamatus*.

Berthold, A.A.: Über drei neue Skorpionarten Neu-Granada's. Nachr. Ges. (Göttingen) **3**, 56—62 (1846).
Of the three, *Scorpio (Atraeus) nigrifrons* = *Centrurus gracilis*.

Bertke, E.M., Atkins, J.H.: Effect of *Centruroides sculpturatus* venom upon rat tissue: a histopathologic study. Toxicon **2**, 205—209 (1961).

Birula, A.: Arachnoides Arthrogastra Caucasica. I. Scorpiones. Mem. Mus. Caucase Tiflis, Series A, No. 5:1—253, (1917a).
Systematics involving *Centrurus* pp. 19, 164, 183, 190.

Birula, A.: Arachnoidea: Scorpions. Fauna of Russia and adjacent countries. **1**, 1—227 (1917b).
Development of scorpion systematics involving *Centrurus:* pp. 39—42, 45—46.

Bishop, A.S., Farris, M.G. De: Estudio morfologico, histologico e histoquimico de la glandula venenosa de algunas especies de alacranes de los generos *Vejovis* C.L. Koch, *Diplocentrus* Peters, *Centruroides* Marx. An. Inst. Biol. (Mex.) **35**, 139—155 (1964).

Borelli, A.: Scorpioni raccolti nel Darien dal Dott. E. Festa. Boll. Mus. Zool. Anat. Comp. (Torino) **14**, 1—3 (1899a).
Inc. *Centrurus margaritatus*.

Borelli, A.: Viaggo del Dr. Enrico Festa nell'Ecuador e regioni vicine. XVIII Scorpioni. Boll. Mus. Zool. Anat. Comp. (Torino) **14**, 1—18 (1899b).
Inc. *Centrurus margaritatus*.

Borelli, A.: Scorpioni raccolti dal Prof. F. Silvestri nell' America settentrionale e alle isole Hawai. Portici Boll. Zool. **3**, 222—227 (1909).
Inc. *Centrurus subgranosus, C. vittatus, C. elegans, C. margaritatus*.

Borelli, A.: Scorpioni nuovi o poco noti del Messico. Boll. Mus. Zool. (Torino) **30**, 1—7 (1915).
Inc. *Centruroides Chiaravigli* nov sp.

Borelli, A., Boush, G.M., Riley, G.B.: Control del alacran *Centruroides limpidus* Karsch. Folleto Tecnico **12**, 5—19 (1954).

Bowerman, R.F.: A muscle receptor organ in the scorpion postabdomen. I. The sensory system. J. comp. Physiol. **81**, 133—146 (1972a).
Study used *Centruroides gracilis*.

Bowerman, R.F.: A muscle receptor organ in the scorpion postabdomen. II. Reflexes evoked by MRO stretch and release. J. comp. Physiol. **81**, 147—157 (1972b).

Bowerman, R.F., Larimer, J.: Structure and physiology of the patella-tibia joint receptors in scorpion pedipalps. Comp. Biochem. Physiol. [A] **46**, 139–151 (1973).
Used *Centruroides vittatus.*

Brady, L.F.: Invertebrate tracks from the Coconino sandstone of Northern Arizona. J. Paleon. **21**, 466–472 (1947).
Living *Centruroides sculpturatus* used to give evidence that tracks in sandstone were scorpionid.

Briseno, C.: Presencia de un ejemplar de alacran, de la especie *Centruroides noxius,* con dos colas. Rev. Inst. Salubr. Enferm. Trop. (Méx.) **23**, 185–186 (1963).

Bücherl, W.: Escorpiões e escorpionism no Brasil. X. Catálogo da coleção escorpiônica do Instituto Butantan. Mem. Inst. Butantan **29**, 255–275 (1959a).
Inc. 15 sp. and ssp. of *Centruroides.*

Bücherl, W.: Distribuição geografica dos araconóides peçonhentos temiveis (Classe *Arachnomorpha,* sub-classe *Arachnoidea,* ordens *Scorpiones* e *Araneida*). Mem. Inst. Butantan **31**, 55–66 (1964b).
Inc. seven *Centruroides* species.

Bücherl, W.: Classification, biology, and venom extraction of scorpions, Chap. 55. In: Venomous Animals and Their Venoms, Vol. III. Venomous Invertebrates. Bücherl, W., Buckley, E.R. (eds.). New York: Academic Press 1971c.
Chap. 55, pp. 317–347. *Centruroides* taxa are briefly mentioned on the following pages: 327, 334, 343–5.

Cahalan, M.: Modification of sodium channel gating in frog myelinated nerve fibers by *Centruroides sculpturatus* scorpion venom. J. Physiol., **244**, 511–534 (1975).

Campos, R.F.: Algunos casos teratologicos obervados en los artropodos. Ann. Entomol. Soc. **11**, 97–98 (1918a).
Inc. bifurcated cauda on *Centrurus margaritatus.*

Campos, R.F.: Notas teratoartropológicas, Caso de un alacrán (*Centrurus margaritatus,* Gerv.). con diartrosis femoro-tibial en un palpo macilar. Rev. Chil. Hist. Nat. **34**, 280–281 (1930).

Caporiacco, L. Di: Aracnidi del Messico, di Guatemala e Honduras Britannico. Atti. Soc. Ital. (Milano) **77**, 251–282 (1938).
Inc. *Centruroides gracilis*

Caporiacco, L. Di: Studi sugli aracnidi del Venezuela raccolti dalla sezione di biologia. Part I. Scorpiones, opiliones, solifuga y chernetes. Acta Biol. Venezuelica **1**, (1951).
Inc. *Centruroides gracilis.*

Castro, H.L.: The venom of certain species of scorpions. J. Am. Inst. Homeopathy **32**, 340–343 (1939).
Inc. interesting folklore on origin of scorpions and mentions the genus *Centruroides* but lists *Centrurus gracilis, C. margaritatus, C. exilicauda, C. infamatus, C. fulvipenis, C. nitidus, Centruroides elegans* and *Centruroides suffusus.*

Cekalovic-K, T.: Contribucion al conocimiento de los escorpiones Chilenos. Mus. Nacion. Hist. Nat. (Santiago) **10**, 1–9 (1966).
Inc. *Centruroides margaritatus, C. gracilis, C. infamatus.*

Cervera, E., Varela, G.: The poison of the scorpion *Centruroides limpidus limpidus* Karsch. [In Spanish] Med. Rev. Mex. **17**, 81–83 (1937).

Chamberlain, R.V., Ivie, W.: Arachnida of the orders Pedipalpi, Scorpionida and Ricinulida. Carnegie Inst. (Washington) **491**, 102–103 (1938).
Inc. *Centrurus yucatanus* n.sp. from Oxkutzcab: Loltus Cave. One adult male and one juvenile.

Cooper, L.H.: The scorpion venoms compared (in relation to their homeopathic use.). J. Am. Inst. Homeopathy **32**, 258–263 (1939).
Inc. the Durango Scorpion but incorrectly refers to it as ("*Centrurus Exilicauda*"). If it is truly the Durango Scorpion, than it is *Centruroides suffusus.*

Crawford, C.S., Krehoff, R.C.: Diel activity in sympatric populations of the scorpions *Centruroides sculpturatus* (Buthidae) and *Diplocentrus spitzeri* (Diplocentridae). J. Arach. **2**, 195–204 (1975).

Dexter, R.W.: Traveling scorpions. Nature **41**, 440 (1940).
Two scorpions (*Centrurus carolinianus* and *C. gracilis*) transported to Akron, Ohio in cotton

shipments from the southern United States and in bananas from Florida. *C. carolinianus* is an incorrect designation. It was either *C. vittatus* or *Vejovis carolinianus*. It was probably the former, since the latter is a ground dwelling form.

Días, E., Libanio, S., Lisboa, M.: Lucta contra os escorpiòes. English version: The struggle against scorpions. Mem. Inst. Oswaldo Cruz **17**, 27—45 (1924).
Inc. *Centrurus gracilis*.

Díaz-Nájera, A.: Alacranes de la Republica Mexicana: Identificacion de ejemplares capturados en 235 localidades. Rev. Inst. Salubr. Enferm. Trop. (Mex.) **24**, 15—30 (1964).
Lists 20 sp. and ssp. of *Centruroides* and gives the localities in which they were taken.

Díaz-Nájera, A.: Alacranes de la Republica Mexicana. Clave para identificar especies de *Centrurus* (Scorpionia: Buthidae). Rev. Invest. Salud Pública **26**(2) 109—122 (1966).
Presents a key to 21 species. Another key and the geographical distribution of the six most toxic species is given.

Díaz-Nájera, A.: Contribution al conocimiento de los alacranes de Mexico (Scorpionida). Rev. Invest. Salud Publica **30**, 111—112 (1970).
Inc. only *Centrurus* in key. Does not mention species.

Díaz-Nájera, A.: Listas y datos de distribución geográfica de los alacranes de Mexico (Scorpionida). Rev. Invest. Salud Publica **35**, 1—36 (1975).
Inc. 29 sp. and ssp. of *Centruroides* and their geographic distribution.

Doro, D.S., Ornelas, E.S., Johnson, R.M.: Failure to induce allergic response in guinea pigs with scorpion venom. J. Allergy Clin. Immunol. **28**, 540—541 (1957).
The venom of *Centruroides sculpturatus* was used.

Duke-Elder, Sir Stewart: System of ophthalmology. Vol. I, The Eye in Evolution. London: Henry Kempton 1958, p. 843.

Espinosa, A.: Estudio sobre los efectos de la ponzoña del alacrán de Mexico. Studio **2**, 65 (1890).
Inc. *Centrurus mexicanus* (Alacran de Jojutla)

Ewing, H.E.: The scorpions of the Western part of the U.S. with notes on those occuring in Northern Mexico. U.S. Natl. Mus. (Washington) **73**, 1—24 (1928).
Provides a key to the following *Centruroides: C. nigrescens, C. margaritatus, C. exilicaudata, C. vittatus, C. californicus, C. sculpturatus* n.sp. Ewing was not aware of the severe toxicity of the last mentioned (personal communication.).

Franco, L.V., Jaime, M.L.: Consideraciones epidemiologicas sobre la picadura por alacran en la cuidad de Durango. Rev. Invest. Salud Publica **26**, 7—21 (1966).
Involves *Centruroides suffusus suffusus*.

Franganillo Balboa, P.: Má arácnidos nuevos de la isla de Cuba. Inst. Nac. Invest. Cient. **1**, 92—97 (1930).
Inc. *Centruroides gracilis, C. subviridis*.

Franganillo Balboa, P.: Excursiones aracnologicas durante el mes de Agosto de 1930. Rev. Belen **4**, 116—120 (1931).
Inc. *Centruroides elegans guanensis* ssp.n., *C. gracilis nigrescens* ssp.n.

Franganillo Balboa, P.: Aracnidos Cubanos estudia dos desde 1930 hasta 1934. Mem. Soc. Poey (Univ. Habana) **8**, 145—168 (1934).
Inc. *Centruroides elegans guanensis, C. gracilis guanensis*.

Franganillo Balboa, P.: Estudio de los arácnidos recogidos durante el verano de 1934. Rev. Belen **9**, (1935).
Inc. *Centruroides gracilis nigrescens, C. elegans guanensis, C. subviridis* sp.n.

Franganillo Balboa, P.: Un monstruo aracnologico. Mem. Soc. Cubana Hist. Nat. **11**, 55—56 (1937).
Anomalous *Centruroides gracilis*.

Gain, D.L.: Extraction and purification of fluorescing organic compounds from *Centruroides sculpturatus* Ewing exoskeletons. John Hopkins Univ. Undergrad. Sci. Bull. **3**, 81—86 (1973).

Geer, C. de: Mem. pour servir a l'hist. de insectes: bibliothèque du museum d'hist. nat. cinquiems memoire. Des Scorpions et Fauxscorpions. (Posthumous publication). Stockholm: Pierre Hesselberg, Vol. VII, pp. 325—350.
Inc. *Scorpio testaceus = Centruroides testaceus* and *Scorpio americanus = Centrurus americanus = Isometerus americanus*.

Gertsch, W.J.: Report on a collection of arachnida from the Chisos Mountains. Baylor Univ.
    Mus. Contrib. 17—26, (1939).
    Inc. *Centruroides chisosarius,* new species.
Gertsch, W.J.: Results of the Puritan-American Museum expedition to Western Mexico. 4.
    The scorpions. Am. Mus. Novitates **1903**, 1—20 (1958).
    Inc. *Centruroides elegans, C. pallidiceps, C. exilicauda; C. zweifeli,* new species.
Gervais, M.P.: Zoologic: arachnides, famille des pedipalpes, genre scorpion-scorpio, linnè.
    In: Eydoux et Souleyet, Voyage du Monde—La Bonité **1**, 281—285 (1841).
    Inc. *Scorpio margeritatus* = *Centruroides margaritatus.*
Gervais, M.P.: Order III. Scorpionides, part II. Scorpions. In: Walckenaer, Histoire Nat.
    des Insectes, Apteres 1844, Vol. III, pp. 7—74.
    Inc. *Scorpio margaritatus* = *Centruroides margaritatus.*
Gervais, M.P.: Remarques sur la famille des scorpions et description de plusieurs espèces
    nouvelles de la collection du muséum. Arch. Mus. Hist. Nat. **4**, 201—240 (1844).
    Inc. *Scorpio (Atreus) margaritatus* = *Centruroides margaritatus.*
Gervais, M.P.: Myriapodes et scorpions. In: Castelnau, F. De: Animaux Nouveaux ou Rares
    Recueillis Pendant L'Expedition Dans les Parties Centrales de l'Amérique du Sud, de
    Rios de Janeiro a Lima, et de Lima au Para. Paris: P. Bertrand 1859.
    "Sur sept espèces de Scorpions Américains". Mentions *Scorpio granosus* = *Centruroides
    elegans.*
Girard, C.: III. Scorpionidae. In: Marcy, Nat. Hist. Red. River, of Louisiana in 1852. Washing-
    ton, pp. 256—260.
    Inc. *Scorpio (Atreus) californicus* = *Centruroides californicus, Scorpio (Atreus) sayi* = *Centru-
    roides vittatus.*
Glenn, W.G., Keegan, H.L.: Intergeneric relationships among various scorpion venoms and
    antivenins. Science **135**, 434—435 (1962).
    Inc. *Centruroides suffusus* and *C. sculpturatus.*
Gungle, E.J.: Cases of scorpion stings. Southwestern Med. **20**, 218—222 (1936).
    Only one species' name is given, i.e. *Centruroides gracilis.* The reactions subscribed to
    this taxon make it obvious that the scorpion was incorrectly identified. Although the
    scorpions involved in the other cases were not named, the reactions indicate *Centruroides
    suffusus* and *C. sculpturatus.*
Hadley, N.F.: The scorpion fauna of Cholla Bay. Cholla Chatter **10**, 4—5 (1967).
    Inc. *Centruroides sculpturatus.*
Hadley, N.F.: Water uptake by drinking in the scorpion,   *Centruroides sculpturatus* (Buthi-
    dae). Southwestern Nat. **15**, 495—505 (1971).
Hadley, N.F.: Adaptational biology of desert scorpions. J. Arach. **2**, 11—23 (1974).
    Inc. *Centruroides sculpturatus.*
Hadley, N.F., Hill, R.D.: Oxygen consumption of the scorpion Centruroides sculpturatus.
    Comp. Biochem. Physiol. **29**, 217—226 (1969).
Hadley, N.F., Williams, S.C.: Surface activities of some North American scorpions in relation
    to feeding. Ecology **49**, 726—734 (1968).
    Inc. *Centruroides sculpturatus.*
Hadzi, J.: Skorpije Schmidtove Zbirke (*Euscorpius italicus polytrichus* n.sp. I Ostale Nove
    Rase). Die Skorpione der Schmidt'schen Sammlung (*Euscorpius italicus polytrichus* n.sp.
    und Andere Neue Rassen). Bull. Ass. Mus. Slovenie Letnik **10**, 39—41 (1929).
    Use *Centrurus* sp.aff. *infamatus* for comparison.
Herrera, M.: Los alacranes de Mexico. Bol. Dir. Estr. Biol. (Mes.) **2**, 265—275 (1917).
    Inc. fifteen *Centruroides* sp., ssp.
Hoffmann, C.: Monografias para la entomologia medica. Monografia Num. 2. Los scorpiones
    de Mexico. part II. Buthidae. An. Inst. Biol. **3**, 243—282 (1932a).
    Centruroides pp. 244—282, key and species descriptions.
Hoffmann, C.: Monografias para la entomologia medica. Monografia Num. 2. Los scorpiones
    de Mexico (conclusion). An. Inst. Biol. **3**, 283—358 (1932b).
    Centruroides keys and species descriptions.
Hoffmann, C.: Nota acerca de los alacranes del Valle de Mezquital, HGO. An. Inst. Biol.
    8, 201—206 (1937).
    Inc. *Centruroides gracilis, C. infamatus infamatus.*

Hoffmann, C.C., Roaro, N.: Segunda contribucion al conocimiento de los alacranes Mexicanos. An. Inst. Biol. Nacion. **10**, 83—92 (1939).
Used the venom of *Centruroides suffusus suffusus, C. limpidus tecomanus* and *C. noxius.*
Hood, R.D., Watson, O.F., Deason, T.R., Benton, Jr., C.L.B.: Ultrastructure of scorpion spermatozoa with atypical axonemes. Cytobios **5**, 167—177 (1972).
Inc. *Centruroides vittatus.*
Horen, W.P.: Insect and scorpion sting. JAMA **221**, 894—898 (1972).
Inc. *Centruroides sculpturatus.*
Horne, F.R.: Purine excretion in five scorpions, a uropygid and a centipede. Biol. Bull. **137**, 155—160 (1969).
Inc. *Centruroides margaritatus, C. vittatus.*
Ingles, L.G.: The seasonal and associational distribution of the fauna of the Upper Santa Ana River (Wash.) J. Entomol. Zool. **21**, 1—48 (1929).
Inc. *Centrurus exilicauda.*
Jackson, H.V.: Preliminar del "alacran ponzoñoso" incluyendo una revista de cierta literatura reciente sobre el asunto, y algunas experiencias personales. Alianza Cient. Univ. **1**, 94—115 (1910).
Scorpion used is identified as *Centrurus exilicauda* Wood. Evidence of venom action indicates the species *Centruroides suffusus* was involved.
Jaume, M.L.: Catalogo de scorpionida de Cuba (arachnida). Circ. Mus. Biblio. Zool. (Habana) **13**, 1085—1902 (1954).
Lists ten *Centruroide* species and subspecies and their Cuban distribution.
Johnson, B.D., Tullar, J.C., Stahnke, H.L.: A quantitative protozoan bio-assay method for determining venom potencies. Toxicon **3**, 297—300 (1966).
Inc. *Centruroides sculpturatus.*
Johnson, J.D., Allred, D.M.: Scorpions of Utah. Great Basin Nat. **32**, 154—170 (1972).
Inc. *Centruroides sculpturatus.*
Johnson, R.M.: Preparation of Scorpion Anavenom. Phoenix: Poisonous Amimals Res. Lab. (Arizona State Univ.) 1959.
Centruroides sculpturatus venom was used.
Johnson, R.M., Stahnke, H.L.: Chromatographic comparison of scorpion venoms. Science **132**, 895—896 (1960).
Inc. *Centruroides sculpturatus, C. gertschi, C. pantheriences, C. vittatus* plus three vejovids.
Karsch, F.: Scorpionologische Beiträge. I. Mitt. Munch. Entomol. Ver. **3**, 6—22 (1879a).
Mentions in key *"Centrurus"* and incorrectly gives *C. gracilis* as the type species.
Karsch, F.: Scorpionologished Beiträge II. Mitt. Munch. Entomol. Ver. **3**, 97—136 (1879b).
Inc. *Centrurus limpidus,* n.sp., *C. testaceo* (Deg.), *C. republicanus,* n.sp., *C. gambienis,* n.sp., *C. princeps,* n.sp., *C. heterurus,* n.sp.
Katz, N.L., Edwards, C.: The effect of scorpion venom on the neuromuscular junction of the frog. Toxicon **10**, 133—137 (1972).
Inc. *C. s. suffusus.*
Keegan, H.L., Lockwood, W.R.: Secretory epithelium in venom glands of two species of scorpion of the genus *Centruroides* Marx. Am. J. Trop. Med. Hyg. **20**, 770—785 (1971).
Inc. *C. vittatus* and *C. limpidus tecomanus.*
Kent, M.L., Stahnke, H.L.: Effect and treatment of Arizona scorpion stings. Southwestern Med. **23**, 120—124 (1939).
The scorpion involved was *Centruroides sculpturatus.*
Koch, C.L.: Übersicht des Arachnidensystems. Nürnberg: 1837, pp. 36—39.
Mentions *Centrurides* and *Centrurus* but no discussion.
Koch, C.L.: Die Arachniden. Nürnberg, 1838, Vol. IV, pp. 1—143.
Centrurus galbineus is described but appears to be a juvenile *Heterometrus longimanus* Hbst.
Koch, C.L.: Die Arachniden. Nürnberg. 1845, Vol. XI, pp. 1—48.
Gives *Tityus infamatus=Centruroides elegans.*
Kopstein, F.: Die Skorpione des Indo-Australischen Archipels. Mit Grundlage der in Holländischen Sammlungen, Vornehmlich der des Rijks-Museums in Leiden, vorhandenen Arten. Leyden: Rijks Museum von Natuurlijke Zoologische Mededelingen 1921, Vol. VI, pp. 115—144.
Introduces the subfamily Centrurinae and gives *"Centrurus infamatus* Koch."

Kraepelin, K.: Revision der Skorpione. I. Die Familie der Androctonidae. Mitt. Nat. Hist.
    Mus. (Hamburg) **8**, 1—139 (1890a).
    Presents key and descriptions to eleven *Centrurus* species and gives *C. thorellii,* n.sp.
Kraepelin, K.: Revision der Skorpione I. Die Familie der Androctonidae. Ham. Wiss. Anst.
    8, 145—281 (1890b).
    Text the same as above but double-paged.
Kraepelin, K.: Die Gattungen der Andrectendae. Nachtrag zu Theil I der Revision der Scor-
    pione. Nat. Hist. Mus. **12**, 75—95 (1894).
    Additional information on genus *Centrurus* and five species.
Kraepelin, K.: Scorpiones and Pedipalpi. Das Tierreich, Lief. 8. Scorpiones und Pedipalpi.
    Berlin: R. Friedländer und Sohn 1899.
    From p. 87 to 95: a key and descriptions of thirteen species *Centrurus.*
Kraepelin, K.: Zur Nomenklatur der Skorpione und Pedipalpen. Zool. Anzeiger **28**, 195—204
    (1904).
    Inc. a discussion of the nomenclature *Centrurus* vs *Centruroides.*
Kraepelin, K.: Neue Beiträge zur Systematik der Gliederspinnen. Mitt. Nat. Mus. (Hamburg)
    28, 59—99 (1910).
    Inc. a discussion of the systematics of seven *Centruroides.* provides a key to these and
    introduces *C. koesteri* n.sp.
Kraepelin, K.: Beitrag zur Kenntnis der Skorpione und Pedipalpen Columbiens. Dr. O. Fuhr-
    mann et Dr. E. Mayor Voyage d'Exploration Scientifique en Colombie. Neuchatel Mem.
    Soc. Sci. Nat. **5**, 15—28 (1914).
    Inc. *Centruroides margaritatus.*
Kraus, O.: Sobretiro de 'communicaciones' del Instituto Tropical de investigaciones cientificas
    de la Universidad de El Salvador. Escorpiones El Salvador **4**, 101—104 (1955).
    Inc. *Centruroides margaritatus.*
Kubota, S.: On the toxicity of the venom of the Mexican (Durango) scorpion as compared
    with that of the Chinese scorpion. J. Pharmacol. Exp. Ther. **11**, 447—489 (1918).
    Name of Mexican species given as "*Centrurus exilicauda,* Wood" or "*Centrurus gracilis,*
    Latreille" The species obviously is *Centruroides suffusus.* The name of the Chinese scorpion
    is not given and, from the evidence, cannot be determined.
La Grange, R.G., Russell, F.E.: Effects of *Centruroides scupturatus* and *C. gertschi* venom
    on the mammalian nerve-muscle preparation: a possible mechanism of action. Proc. West.
    Pharmacol. Soc. **14**, 163—165 (1971).
    It is now known that *C. gertschi* is a patterned phase of *C. sculpturatus.* Thus the results
    are from one species.
La Grange, R.G.: Mode of action of a scorpion neurotoxin. In: Abstracts of Papers Submitted
    to the 1972 General Meeting of the International Society on Toxinology, Darmstadt,
    Germany Sept. 11—13, 1972. Toxicon **10**, 523—558 (1972).
    Lamoral, B.H., Reynders, S.C.: A catalogue of the scorpions described from the Ethiopian
    faunal region up to Dec. 1973. Ann. Natal Mus. (Pietermaritzburg, So. Afr.) **22**, 499—576
    (1975).
    Inc. *Centruroides margaritatus* but incorrectly states that the type-species: *Scorpio margarita-*
    tus.
Latreille, P.A.: Histoire naturelle, general et particulière des crustaces et des insectes. Lectere
    de Buffon, **7**, 110—129, (1804).
    Inc. *Scorpio gracilis* = *Centruroides gracilis, Scorpio punctatus* = *C. punctatus.* Also gives
    Scorpio americanus but gives the locality as Sierra Leona in Africa.
Lincecum, G.: Scorpion of Texas. Am Nat. **1**, 203—205 (1867).
    Scientific name not given but evidence indicates *Centruroides vittatus.*
Lonnberg, E.: Skorpioner och Pedipalper i Upsala Universitets Zoologiska Museum. Ent.
    Tidskr. **18**, 175—192 (1897).
    Inc. *Centrurus infamatus* (C.L. Koch), *C. gracilis* (Latr.) *C. de Gerii* (Gerv.), *C. insulanus*
    Thorell.
Lope, D.V.: Continuación de "El Estudio". Ann. Inst. Med. Natl. **7**, 376—378 (1905).
    Inc. *Centrurus mexicanus* = *C. limpidus;* includes a very brief report on antivenin production.
Lucas, P.H.: Arachnides, myriapodes et thysanoures. Hist. Nat. Iles Canaries. 23—52, (1844).
    Inc. *Androctonus biaculeatus* = *Centruroides biaculeatus.*

Mc Alister, W.H.: The mating behaviour of *Centruroides vittatus* Say (Arachnida : Scorpionida). Texas J. Sci. **17**, 307—312 (1965).

McIntosh, M.E., Watt, D.D.: Biochemical-immunochemical aspects of the venom from the scorpion *Centruroides sculpturatus*. In: Animal Toxins, First International Symposium on Animal Toxins. Atlantic City, New Jersey, April 9—11, 1966, pp. 47—58 (1967).

Machan, L.: Studies on structure and electrophysiology of scorpion eyes—the time course of dark adaptation determined by constant stimulus and constant response methods. So. Afr. J. Sci. **63**, 512—520 (1967).
Inc. *Centruroides sculpturatus*.

Machan, L.: Spectral sensitivity of scorpion eyes and the possible role of shielding pigment effect. J. Exp. Biol. **49**, 95—105 (1968).
Inc. *Centruroides sculpturatus*.

Marinkelle, C.J., Stahnke, H.L.: Toxicological and clinical studies on *Centruroides margaritatus* (Gervais). A common scorpion in Western Colombia. J. Med. Entomol. **2**, 197—199 (1965).

Marx, G.: On the morphology of scorpionidae. Proc. Entomol. Soc. (Wash.) **1**, 108—112 (1888).
Inc. *Centrurus biaculeatus.*

Marx, G.: Arachnida in the Scientific results of explorations by the U.S. Fish Commission Steamer Albatros. Proc. U.S. Natl. Mus. **12**, 207—211 (1889).
Inc. *Centrurus biaculeatus* Luc., *Centruroides exilicauda* Wood, *Centruroides luctifer* sp. nov.

Masi, L.: Note sugli scorpioni appartenenti al R. Museo Zoologico di Roma. Boll. Soc. Zool. Ital. **1**, 188—108 120, 144 (1912).
Inc. *Centrurus margaritatus*.

Masurkiewicz, J., Bertke, E.M.: Ultrastructure of the venom gland of the scorpion *Centruroides sculpturatus*. J. Morphol. **137**, 365—384 (1972).

Maus, L.M.: Report on the scorpion of Durango, Mexico. Rept. Surg. Gen. Army, U.S.A. 126—128 (1896).
Discusses the Durango scorpion (*Centruroides suffusus*) but refers to it as "a variety of the *Ischnurus Mexicanus* of Villada".

Mazzotti, L.: Proteccion mecanica de las casas contra la entrada de alacranes (Escorpiones). Rev. Inst. Salubr. Enferm. Trop. **22**, 183—198 (1962).
Inc. *Centruroides limpidus* and *C. suffusus*.

Mazzotti, L.: Descripcion del esperatoforo de la especie *Centruroides limpidus*. Rev. Inst. Salubr. Enferm. Trop. **22**, 57—59 (1963a).

Mazzotti, L.: Resultados de la aplicacion de corriente electrica alterna en escopiones. Rev. Inst. Salubr. Enferm. Trop. **22**, 61—63 (1963b).

Mazzotti, L.: Resistencia de los alacranes a la sumersion en agua. Rev. Inst. Salubr. Enferm. Trop. **23**, 181—183 (1963c).
Used *Centruroides limpidus*.

Mazzotti, L.: Enemigos de los alacranes: tarantula del genero *Aphonopelma*. Rev. Inst. Salubr. Enferm. Trop. **23**, 9—10 (1964a).
Used *Centruroides limpidus*.

Mazzotti, L.: Medidas complementarias en relacion con la proteccion mecanica de los edificios contra los alacranes. Rev. Inst. Salubr. Enferm. Trop. **24**, 11—14 (1964b).
Used *Centruroides limpidus*.

Mazzotti, L.: Estudio sobre enemigos naturales de los alacranes. Rev. Invest. Salud Publica **26**, 51—55 (1966).
Used *Centruroides limpidus, C. gracilis*.

Mazzotti, L., Bravo-Becherelle, M.A.: Scorpionism in the Mexican Republic. In: Venomous and Poisonoous Animals and Noxious Plants of the Pacific Region. Symposium in the Public Health and Medical Science Division at the Tenth Pacific Science Congress. Keegan, H.L., Mac Farlane, W.V. (eds.). New York: MacMillan 1963, pp. 119—131.

Mazzotti, L., Rhodes, R.H., López, F., Telich, J.: Radiacion con rayos gamma de escorpiones de la especie *Centruroides limpidus*. Rev. Inst. Salubr. Enferm. Trop. **21**, 125—127 (1961).

Mazzotti, L., Palacios, A.M., Ramírez, J.: Ensayo experimental sobre la accion del dieldrin en alacranes de la especie *Centruroides limpidus*. Rev. Inst. Salubr. Enferm. Trop. **22**, 179—182 (1962).

Meise, W.: Scorpiones. NYT Mag. Nat. Christiana **74**, 25—43 (1934).
A systematic study of the genera *Rhopalurus* and *Centruroides*.

Mello-Leitão, C.: Escorpiões Sul-Americanos. Arq. Mus. Nat. (Rio de Janeiro) **40**, 1—468 (1945).
Discusses and provides a key to the following *Centruroides* species: *agrentinus, danieli, exsul, gracilis, margaritatus*.

Mello-Leitão, C., Araújo, J. De: Notas sobre pequena colecção de aracnidos do Peru. Bol Mu. Paraense "Emilio Goeldi" Belen **10**, 313—324 (1950).
Inc. *Centruroides dasypus*, sp. n.

Mills, L.H.: Mexican scorpions and the treatment of scorpion sting. Boston Med. Surg. J. **167**, 183—188 (1912).
Inc. *Centrurus mexicanus = Centruroides suffusus. Centrurus gracilis*.

Mitchell, R.W., Reddell, J.R.: The Invertebrate Fauna of Texas. Caves. Nat. Hist. Tex. 35—90 (1972).
Inc. *Centruroides vittatus*.

Moreno, A.: Contribution al estudio de los escorpionidos Cubanos. Part II. Superfamilia *Buthoides*. Mem. Coc. Cubana Hist. Nat. **13**, 63—75 (1939a).
Inc. *Centruroides gracilis gracilis, C. g. ruber, C. g. pectinatissimus*, subsp. nov., *C. g. johannis* subsp. nov. *C. thorelli thorelli, C. t. aguayoi* subsp. nov.

Muma, M.H.: Scorpions, whip scorpions and wind scorpions of Florida. Arthropods Florida **4**, 1—28 (1967).
Inc. *Centruroides hentzi, C. keysi* n.sp., *C. gracilis, C. biaculeatus, C. margaritatus, C. vittatus*.

Newlands, G.: Zoogeographic factors involved in the trans-Atlantic dispersal pattern of the genus *Opisthacanthus*. Ann. Transvall Mus. **28**, 91—98 (1973).
Briefly discusses the genus *Centruroides*.

Ocaranza, F.: Contribucion experimental para el estudio de la acción fisiologica de la ponzoña de los alacranes de Mexico. 2a Memoria. Ponzona del alacran de Durango (*Centrurus exilicauda*) Rata Blanca. Rev. Mex. Biol. **3**, 201—205 (1922—1923a).
Scorpion involved was obviously *C. suffusus*, not *C. exilicauda*.

Ocaranza, F.: Estudio experimental acerca de la acción fisiológica de la ponzoña de los alacranes de Mexico. 1. Memoria. Veneno del "*Centrurus exilicauda*" inoculacion cuy. *Rev. Mex. Biol.* **3**, 194—200 (1923b).
See remarks above.

Ocaranza, F.: Memoria preliminar acerca de la ponzoña de los alacranes de Mexico. Rev. Mex. Biol. **3**, 179—193 (1923c).

Ocaranza, F.: Contribucion experimental para el estudio de la ponzoña de los alacranes de Mexico. 3a Memoria. Anatomia patológica del envenenamiento por la ponzoña del alacran de Durango. (*Centrurus exilicauda*). Rev. Mex. Biol. **5**, 321—331 (1925).
Should be *C. suffusus*.

Ocaranza, F.: Estudio experimental acerca de la ponzoña de los alacranes de Mexico. 4a Memoria. Alacran de Sonora (*Centruroides thorelli*) Rata Blanca. Rev. Mex. Biol. **6**, 77—80 (1926a).

Ocaranza, F.: Estudio experimental acerca de la ponzõna de los alacranes en Mexico. 5a Memoria. Veneno del "*Centrurus mexicanus*" (Alacran de Manzanillo). Rev. Mex. Biol. **6**, 81—84 (1926b).

Ochoterena, L.: El alacran de Durango (*Centrurus exilicauda*). Mem. Rev. Soc. Cien. Antonio **37**, 215—226 (1910a).
Durango scorpion is *C. suffusus*.

Ochoterena, L.: Estudio sobre el alacran de Durango. Alianza Cien. Univ. **1**, 88—92 (1910b).

Patterson, R.A.: Physiological action of scorpion venom. Am. J. Trop. Med. Hyg. **9**, 400—413 (1960).
Used *Centruroides sculpturatus*.

Patterson, R.A.: Pharmacologic action of scorpion venom on intestinal smooth muscle. Tox. Appl. Pharmacol. **4**, 710—718 (1962).
Used *C. sculpturatus*.

Patterson, R.A.: Effects of venom from the scorpion *Centruroides sculpturatus* on the rat. Toxicon **2**, 167—170 (1964).

Patterson, R.A., Wooley, D.: Effect of scorpion venom of *Centruroides sculpturatus* on the carotid body and superior cervical ganglion of the cat. Tel aviv, Israel Symposium on toxins, Paper IV-10. (1971). In: Toxins of Plant and Animal Origin **2**, 741—748 (1971).

Pavlovsky, E.: Skorpiotomische Mitteilungen. I. Ein Beitrag zur Morphologie der Giftdrüsen der Skorpione. Z. Wiss. Zool. **105**, 157—177 (1913).
Inc. *Centrurus gracilis.*

Pavlovsky, E.: On the morphology of the male genital apparatus in scorpions. Trans. Soc. Nat. (Liningrad) **53**, 17—86 (1924).
Inc. *Centrurus elegans* and *C. margaritatus.*

Pavlovsky, E.N.: Studies on the organization and development of scorpion. 5. Lungs. Q. J. Microsc. Sci. **70**, 135—146 (1926).
Inc. genus *Centrurus.*

Penther, A.: Beitrag zur Kenntnis amerikanischer Skorpione. Ann. K.K. Nat. Hist. Hof. Mus. **27**, 239—252 (1913).
Inc. *Centrurus agamemnon* (C. Koch), *C. bicolor* Poc., *C. gracilis.*

Peters, W.: Vortrag über eine neue Einteilung der Skorpione und über die von ihm im Mossambique gesammelten Arten von Skorpionen, aus welchem hier ein Auszug mitgetheilt wird. Gesamtsitzung, **16**, 507—516 (1861).
Inc. systematics on *Centrurini.*

Petrunkevitch, A.: The shape of the sternum in scorpions as a systematic and phylogenetic character. Am. Nat. **50**, 600—608 (1916).

Pocock, R.I.: A revision of the genera of scorpions of the family *Buthidae*, with descriptions of some South-African species. Zool. Soc. Lond. Trans. **12**, 114—141 (1890).
Discusses genus *Centrurus.*

Pocock, R.I.: Contributions to our knowledge of the scorpion fauna and pedipalpi; with a supplementary note upon freshwater decapoda of St. Vincent. J. Linn. Soc. **24**, 374—404 (1894).
Descriptions and key to: *Centrurus princeps, C. gracilis, C. margaritatus, C. nitidus, C. testaceous, C. insulanus.*

Pocock, R.I.: Descriptions of some new scorpions from Central and South America. Ann. Mag. Nat. Hist. **1**, 384—394 (1898).
Inc. *Centrurus barbudensis, C. ochraceus*, sp.n., *C. nigrovariatus*, sp.n., *C. flavopictus*, sp.n., *C. limbatus*, sp.n. *C. bicolor*, sp.n., *C. nigrimanus*, sp.n., *C. rubricauda*, sp.n., *C. nigrescens*, sp.n., *C. fulvipes*, sp.n.

Pocock, R.I.: On the scorpions, pedipalps and spiders from Tropical West Africa represented in the collection of the British Museum. Zoo.. Soc. Lond. Proc. 833—837 (1899).
Inc. *Centrurus margaritatus.*

Pocock, R.I.: Arachnida, scorpiones, pedipalpi and solifugae. Biol. Centr. Am. 1—71 (1902a).
Centruroides pp. 19—71, key and species descriptions.

Pocock, R.I.: A contribution to the systematics of scorpions. Ann. Mag. Nat. Hist. **10**, 364—379 (1902b).
Inc. *Centruroides Hasethi*, sp.n., *C. exilicauda.*

Potter, J.M.: An antigenic analysis of selected scorpion venoms. Arizona State University, M.S. Thesis, 1961.

Potter, J.M., Northey, W.T.: An immunological evaluation of scorpion venom. Am. J. Trop. Med. Hyg. **2**, 712—716 (1962).
Inc. *Centruroides sculpturatus.*

Pozo, E.C. Del: Los efectos musculares del veneno de escorpiones Mexicanos. Bol. Inst. Est. Med. Biol. **6**, 59—69 (1948a).
Used *C. suffusus suffusus* and *C. noxius.*

Pozo, E.C. Del: The action of the venom of a Mexican scorpion (*Centruroides noxius*, Hoffmann) on cholinesterases. Br. J. Pharmacol. **3**, 219—222 (1948b).

Pozo, E.C. Del: Ressemblances et differences dans les actions physiologiques des venins des scorpions. Arch. Inst. Pasteur Alger. **27**, 35—38 (1949a).

Pozo, E.C. Del: Relaciones entre la activitas anticolinesterasica, las propiedades de activacion muscular y la toxicidad de los venenos de diversos alacranes de Mexico. Rev. Inst. Salubr. Enferm. Trop. **10**, 203—213 (1949b).
Used *Centruroides noxius, C. suffusus suffusus, C. limpidus limpidus, C. l. tecomanus.*

Pozo, E.C. Del: Farmacologia de los venenos de los *Centruroides Mexicanos*. Rev. Invest. Salud Publica. **28**, (1968).
   Used same scorpions as above.
Pozo, E.C. Del, Anguiano, G.: Physiological action of scorpion venom Fed. Proc. **5**, 1 (1946).
   Used *Centruroides suffusus suffusus*.
Pozo, E.C. Del, Anguiano, L.G.: The effects of scorpion venom on striated muscles. Abstr. Commun. 17th Internatl. Physiol. Congress, Oxford, 1947, pp. 1—2.
   Used *Centruroides suffusus suffusus* and *C. noxius*.
Pozo, E.C. Del, Anguiano, G., González, J.: Acciones del veneno de alacran sobre el sistema vaso-motor. Rev. Inst. Salubr. Enferm. Trop. **5**, 227—240 (1944).
   Used *Centruroides suffusus suffusus*.
Randall, W.C.: Microanatomy of the heart and associated structures of two scorpions, *Centruroides sculpturatus* Ewing and *Uroctonus mordax* Thorell. J. Morphol. **119**, 161—180 (1966).
Ridgway, R.L., McGregor, T., Flanigan, J.F.: The effect of residual deposits of insecticides on the scorpion, *Centruroides vittatus*. J. Econ. Entomol. **55**, 1012—1013 (1962a).
Ridgway, R.L.: Laboratory studies of the effect of Dri-Die 67 on the scorpion, *Centruroides vittatus*. J. Econ. Entomol. **55**, 1014 (1962b).
Roewer, C.F.: Über eine neuerworbene Sammlung von Skorpionen des Natur-Museum Senckenberg. Senckenbergiana **26**, 205—244 (1943).
   Inc. nine *Centruroides* species with locality data.
Romero, F.J.: El alacran de las Tierras Calientes. Cronica Medica Mexicana **3**, 157—160 (1900).
Ross, R.H.: Utilization of acetate-1-^{14}c by the tarantula, *Aponeplema* sp., and the scorpion, *Centruroides sculpturatus*, in lipid synthesis. Comp. Biochem. Physiol. **36**, 765—773 (1970).
Russell, F.E.: Phosphodiesterase of some snake and arthropod venoms. Toxicon **4**, 153—154 (1966).
   Scorpion venoms used: *Centruroides sculpturatus* plus three vejovid species.
Sanchez, J.: Arácnidos y insectos. Datos Zool. Med. Mex., 52—79 (1893).
   Inc. *Centrurus mexicanus* = *Centruroides suffusus*. *C. edwardsii* Gerv. = *Centruroides margaritatus, C. gracilis*.
Santacruz, M.A.: Estudio de la sintomalogia por picadura de alacran. Thesis: Dept. Microb. y Parasit. Fac. Med Mexico, DF, 1966, pp. 1—47.
   Inc. ten *Centruroides* species.
Say, T.: An account of the arachnids of the United States. J. Acad. Nat. Sci. (Philad.) **2**, 59—61 (1821).
   Inc. *Buthus vittatus* sp.n. = *Centruroides vittatus*.
Scheuring, L.: Die Augen der Arachnoideen. Zool. Jahrb. Abt. Ont. Tiere **33**, 553—634 (1913).
   Inc. *Centrurus margaritatus*.
Scorza, J.V.: Contribucion al estudio de los escorpiones Venezolanos. Clave para la identificacion de especies y consideraciones generales sobre los escorpiones domicilarios. Arch. Venezol. Patol. Trop. Parasit. **2**, 157—165 (1954a).
   Inc. *Centruroides margaritatus*.
Scorza, J.V.: Sistematica, distribucion geographica y obervaciones ecologicas de algunos alacranes encontrados en Venezuela. Soc. Cien. Nat. (La Salle) **14**, 179—214 (1954b).
   Inc. *Centruroides margaritatus, C. gracilis*.
Sergent, E.: Etude comparative du venin de scorpions Mexicains et de scorpions Nord-Africains. Arch. Inst. Pasteur Alger. **27**, 31—33 (1949).
   Inc. *Centruroides noxius, C. limpidus limpidus*.
Smith, F.: Observations on scorpions. Science **65**, 64 (1927).
   Inc. *Centruroides vittatus*.
Stahnke, H.L.: The venomous effects of some Arizona Scorpions. Science **88** (1938).
   Inc. *Centruroides sculpturatus*.
Stahnke, H.L.: The Scorpions of Arizona. Thesis Abstr. Iowa State College J. Sci. **15**, 101—103 (1940).
   Inc. *C. sculpturatus*.

Stahnke, H.L.: The venomous nature of some arthropods of Arizona. Southwestern Med. **25**, 292–204 (1941).
    Inc. *C. sculpturatus.*
Stahnke, H.L.: First aid for scorpion sting. Pub. Health News **36**, (1943).
Stahnke, H.L.: How deadly is Arizona's public enemy No. 1? Pop. Sci. **142**, 84–87 (1943b).
Stahnke, H.L.: Scorpions of the United States. Turtox News **22**, 20–22 (1944a).
Stahnke, H.L.: Scorpions. Safety Ed., **24**, 1–4, (1944b).
Stahnke, H.L.: Some poisonous animals of the United States. Merck Report **55**, 22–26 (1946).
    Inc. *C. sculpturatus.*
Stahnke, H.L.: Scorpion control. Crop Comments **1**, 4 (1948a).
Stahnke, H.L.: The control of scorpions and the treatment of scorpion poisoning. 24th Annual Mtg. AAAS, Southwestern Division, 1948b, pp. 1–9.
Stahnke, H.L.: Scorpions. Bul. (Arizona State College) **71**, 1–6 (1948c).
Stahnke, H.L.: Scorpions. Booklet, Arizona State College Bookstore, pp. 1–23 (1949).
Stahnke, H.L.: The Arizona scorpion problem. Ariz. Med. **7**, 23–29 (1950).
Stahnke, H.L.: Some scorpion anomalies. J. Colo. Wyom. Acad. Sci. **4**, 104 (1952a). Abstr. Anomalies included the carapace, pedipalps, walking legs, telson vesicle and aculeus. Inc. *Centruroides sculpturatus.*
Stahnke, H.L.: Hypothermia and scorpion venenation. Southwestern Med. **46**, 286–287 (1952b).
Stahnke, H.L.: The L-C treatment of venomous bites and stings. Am. J. Trop. Med. Hyg. **2**, (1953).
Stahnke, H.L.: Demerol® as an anti-scorpion therapeutic agent. Ariz. Med. **11**, 51–52 (1954).
Stahnke, H.L.: Scorpions. Phoenix: Poisonous Animals Research Lab. (Arizona State Univ.) 1956a, pp. 1–36.
Stahnke, H.L.: A new species of scorpion of the Buthidae: *Centruroides pantheriensis.* Entomol. News, **97**, 15–19 (1956b).
Stahnke, H.L.: Synergism between meperidine (Demerol®) and scorpion venom. Ariz. Med. **13**, 225–227 (1956c).
Stahnke, H.L.: The effect of D.H.E.-45 and bellafoline on the LD of *Centruroides sculpturatus* Ewing scorpion venom. Ariz. Med. **14**, 343 (1957a).
Stahnke, H.L.: Scorpions for laboratory study. Am. Biol. Teacher **19**, 75–79 (1957b).
Stahnke, H.L.: How to get stung by a scorpion. Desert Mag. **23**, 19, 19 (1960).
    Inc. discussion of patients age and part of body and circumstances when stung, e.g. Age $1^1/_2$ yrs.—sleeping on floor of jail with mother.
Stahnke, H.L.: Some pharmacological and biochemical characteristics of *Centruroides sculpturatus* venom. 2nd Int. Pharm. Meeting, Prague 1963, pp. 63–70.
Stahnke, H.L.: Stress and the toxicity of venoms. Science **150**, 1456–1457 (1965).
    Inc. *Centruroides sculpturatus.*
Stahnke, H.L.: Some aspects of scorpion behavior. Bull. So. Calif. Acad. Sci. **65**, 65–80 (1966a).
Stahnke, H.L.: The Treatment of Venomous Bites and Stings. Phoenix: Arizona State Univ. 1966, pp. 1–117.
    Inc. *Centruroides sculpturatus.*
Stahnke, H.L.: Lethal time of *Centruroides sculpturatus* venom in rats. J. Ariz. Acad. Sci. **4**, 229–230 (1967a).
Stahnke, H.L.: Lethal time as a measure of venom potency. J. Ariz. Acad. Sci. **4**, 220–221 (1967b).
Stahnke, H.L.: Effect of paraldehyde on scorpion and rattlesnake venom toxicity. Southwestern Med. **48**, 187 (1967c).
Stahnke, H.L.: Scorpion nomenclature and mensuration. Entomol. News **81**, 297–316 (1970a).
Stahnke, H.L.: *Centruroides dammanni,* sp.n. A new Virgin Island buthid scorpion. J. Ariz. Acad. Sci. **6**, 51–55 (1970b).
Stahnke, H.L.: Some observations of the genus *Centruroides* (Buthidae, Scorpionida). Entomol. News **82**, 281–307 (1971).
Stahnke, H.L.: UV light, a useful field tool. Bio sci. **22**, 604–607 (1972a).

Stahnke, H.L.: Effect of thorazine and valium on scorpion venom toxicity. Ariz. Med. **29**, 424 (1972 b).

Stahnke, H.L.: Arizona scorpion antivenin. JAMA **224**, 637 (1973 a).

Stahnke, H.L.: Scorpion venom potency. Insect World **1**, 1—4 (1973 b).

Stahnke, H.L.: Arizona's lethal scorpion. Ariz. Med. **29**, 504—507 (1972 c).

Stahnke, H.L.: An estimate of the number of taxa in the order Scorpionida. Biosci. **24**, 339 (1974).

Stahnke, H.L., Calos, M.: A key to the species of the genus *Centruroides* Marx (Scorpionida: Buthidae). Entomol. News (1977) (in press).

Stahnke, H.L., Dengler, A.H.: The effect of morphine and related substances on the toxicity of venoms. I. *Centruroides sculpturatus* Ewing scorpion venom. Am. J. Trop. Med. Hyg. **13**, 346—351 (1964).

Stahnke, H.L., Johnson, B.D.: *Aphonopelma* Tarantula venom. Animal toxins, Russell, F.E., Saunders, P.R. (eds.). Oxford: Pergamon Press 1967, pp. 35—39 (First International Symposium on Animal Toxins Atlantic City, Ney Jersey, 1966, 1967).
   C. sculpturatus venom is compared with tarantula venom.

Stahnke, H.L., Stahnke, J.: The treatment of scorpion sting. Ariz. Med. **14**, 576—580 (1957 c).

Thorell, T.: On the classification of scorpions. Ann. Mag. Nat. Hist. **17**, 1—15 (1876 a).

Thorell, T.: Études scorpiologiques. Atti. Soc. Ital. Sci. **19**, 75—272 (1876 b).
   Inc. descriptions of eleven species of genus *Centrurus*.

Torres, F., Heatwole, H.: Orientation of some scorpions and tailless whip-scorpions. Z. Tierpsychol. **24**, 546—557 (1967 a).
   Inc. *Centruroides nitidus, C. vittatus.*

Torres, F., Heatwole, H.: Factors influencing behavioral interactions of female parent and offspring in scorpions. Carib. J. Sci. **7**, 19—22 (1967 b).
   Inc. *C. nitidus.*

Vachon, M., Niaussat, P., Ebersole, J.H., Grenot, G.: Sur la radiosensibilité comparée, vis-à-vis du rayonnement de quelques espèces de scorpions. C.R. Acad. Sc. (Paris) **259**, 3389—3391 (1964).
   Inc. *Centruroides sculpturatus.*

Varela, G., Hiranaka, H.: Conservacion del *Toxoplasma Gondi* en el *Centruroides limpidus tecomanus.* Rev. Inst. Salubr. Enferm. Trop. **25**, 182 (1965).

Vyas, A.B., Laliwala, S.M.: Microanatomy of the book lungs of scorpions and the mechanism of respiration. Vidya **15**, 122—128 (1972).
   Inc. *Centruroides* in discussion.

Watt, D.D.: Biochemistry of the venom from the scorpion *Centruroides sculpturatus.* 7th Int. Congress on Trop. Med. and Malaria., 1963, pp. 406—407.

Watt, D.D.: Biochemical studies of the venom from the scorpion, *Centruroides sculpturatus.* Toxicon **2**, 171—180 (1964).

Watt, D.D., McIntosh, M.E.: Molecular aspects of neurotoxic principles in venom of the scorpion *Centruroides sculpturatus.* In: Animal Toxins, First International Symposium on Animal Toxins, Atlantic City, New Jersey, April 9—11, 1966, pp. 41—46, (1967).

Watt, D.D., McIntosh, M.E.: Effects of lethality of toxins in venom from the scorpion *Centruroides sculpturatus* by group specific reagents. Toxicon **10**, 173—181 (1972).

Werner, F.: Die Skorpione, Pedipalpen und Solifugen in der zoologisch-vergleichend-anatomischen Sammlung der Universität Wien. Verhandl. Zool. Bot. Ges. (Wien) pp. 595—608, (1902).
   Inc. five species of *Centrurus.*

Werner, F.: Scorpiones, pedipalpi. In: Bronns Klassen und Ordnungen des Tierreich. 1934, Vol. V, pp. 1—316.
   Gives key to subfamily *Centrurinae* and distribution of species of *Centruroides.*

Werner, F.: Neu-Eingänge von Skorpionen im Zoologischen Museum in Hamburg. Part II. Fest. zum 60 Geb. von Prof. Dr. Embrik Strand, 1939, Vol. V, pp. 351—362.
   Inc. *Centruroides argentinus* n.sp. plus seven older taxa of this genus.

Wheeling, C.H., Keegan, H.L.: Effects of scorpion venom on a tarantula. Toxicon **10**, 305—306 (1972).
   Centruroides limpidus tecomanus involved.

Williams, S.C.: Birth activities of some North American scorpions. Proc. Calif. Acad. Sci. **37**, 1—24 (1969).
Inc. *Centruroides sculpturatus.*
Williams, S.C.: Developmental anomalies in the scorpion *Centruroides sculpturatus* (Scorpionida: Buthidae). Pan-Pacific Entomol. **47**, 76—77 (1971).
Wood, H.C.: On the pedipalpi of North America. J. Acad. Nat. Sci. [New Series] **5**, 359—376 (1863a).
Inc. discussion of *Centrurus.*
Wood, H.C.: Description of new species of North American pedipalpi. Pro. Acad. Nat. Sci. **15**, 107—112 (1863b).
Inc. *Buthus exilicauda = Centruroides exilicauda,* et al.
Woodward, A.: Durango City of Scorpions. Westways, 1954, pp. 24—25.
Yarom, R.: Scorpion venom: a tutorial review of its effects in men and experimental animals. Clin. Toxicol. **3**, 561—569 (1970).
Inc. *Centruroides suffusus.*
Yoshida, Y., Toshioka, S.: Studies on spermatogenesis in scorpions. I. Numbers of chromosomes in male germ-cells of three species of scorpions. Acta Arachnologica **19**, 1—4 (1964).
Inc. *Centruroides vittatus.*
Zahl, P.A.: Scorpions, living fossils of the sands. Natl. Geog. **133**, 435—442 (1967).
Inc. *Centruroides sculpturatus.*

CHAPTER 13

Venoms of Buthinae

A. Systematics and Biology of Buthinae

A. Shulov and G. Levy

The *Buthidae* are the largest family of scorpions with more than 500 species distributed throughout the world. Vachon (1973) lists 42 genera. The systematic position of certain groups is uncertain, therefore, the division into subfamilies is still pending. The Buthids of the Old World, however, are included in *Buthinae*. The diagnostic character of the *Buthinae* is represented by the complement rows of denticles on the cutting edge of the pedipalps movable finger. While the size of most of these scorpions is from 6 to 12 cm, postabdomen included, some are only 1 – 2 cm long. Coloration is yellowish-brown to black. Many species have slender, long pincers, but a few have rather broad ones.

In some species of *Isometrus* (Probst, 1972) there is prominent sexual dimorphism, in others, adult males and females can be differentiated only by observing their genital apertures.

Most species are eremic and inhabit deserts or semiarid biotopes; some, however, prefer moister and colder climate. Many species are found on various types of soil, some on a few types only. Thus all species of *Buthacus* are found on sand dunes and sandy soils, while others, e.g., certain species of *Androctonus, Buthotus,* and *Compsobuthus* are found on terra rossa, basalt, rendzina, and some also in the stony desert and on loesslike soil (Shulov, 1962).

Many species live under large or small stones, or sometimes in stone fences and rock crevices, some occasionally inhabit empty burrows of rodents or isopods. Species of *Buthotus* and *Compsobuthus* are sometimes found under bark of trees. *B. judaicus* and *Leiurus quinquestriatus* at times enter house and tents. Species belonging to the genera *Buthus* and *Leiurus* may dig short burrows oblique to the surface of the ground typical for each species. The scorpions also build small retreats under stones. They prevent the entrance of rain water into the retreat by lifting the edges with pieces of soil. Scorpions usually are solitary, but species of *Compsobuthus* are sometimes found in winter in aggregations of over a dozen specimens under the same stone (Zinner and Amitai, 1969).

In some places the population of scorpions may be extremely dense causing frequent stings and casualties. In a village situated near the Gilboa hills in Israel some 4500 *L. quinquestriatus* scorpions were collected within 2 months on the area of 4000 m². However, the repopulation of the same area is very slow. In consecutive collections within 30 years only few scorpions have been found each time (Shulov, 1962).

On the contrary, Probst (1972), working with *I. maculatus* in Tanzania, came to the conclusion that this scorpion has been able to immigrate and populate vast new areas.

When running, scorpions usually hold the pedipalps ahead, for they apparently orient with the aid of trichobothria sensitive to air currents; the postabdomen (tail) may be arched high above the back, or, as in *Orthochirus* pressed to the back in a curled position with the sting completely hidden (Shulov and Amitai, 1960). In *Compsobuthus* the postabdomen is usually curved laterally.

The period of activity extends throughout the warm season; occasionally they wander on warm nights in winter. Activity on full moon nights is restricted or absent. The preference temperature of *L. quinquestriatus* was determined as 33° C. At 45–48° C individuals belonging to this species enter a kind of heat stupor and at 48.5–50° C they die instantly (Shulov, 1938). Diurnal activity occurs occasionally in early spring or after the first rains in autumn in relation with the sudden appearance of numerous insects and other arthropods which constitute their food (Shulov, unpublished observations). Preying usually takes place on the ground, on the bark of trees or, by burrowing species, even on bushes. Small prey is usually handled by the pedipalps alone, but it may be stung if it struggles; the chelicerae then tear the animal apart and its juices are sucked (Shulov, 1955). The food of scorpions consists of small arthropods including other scorpions; when endevoring to kill or to paralyze the prey they probe its integument with the sting and introduce the sting only into soft intersegmental membrane. Water is taken by crouching over a drop or holding the drop between the fingers of one pedipalp and bringing it to the mouth. Excrements are deposited on surrounding objects, rarely on the ground.

Males usually are more slender and may have a larger number of denticles on the pectines. A spermatophore is formed in the internal paraxial organs. These are paired, complicated, elongated structures investing two parts of the spermatophore, which are pushed outside before copulation through the genital aperture. During expulsion the two parts become sealed together longitudinally. The sclerotized inside of the paraxial organs provides a systematic character of specific importance in males. The details of courtship differ slightly in various genera. Generally, however, the male approaches the female, he may grasp her pedipalps with one or both his pedipalps while the postabdomen of both may be held vertical, jerking. The pair then moves backward and forward and when a suitable firm surface is detected the male deposits the spermatophore, which is glued upright. The male then endevors to pull the female over it in a way that her genital opening will touch the spermatophore which explodes bringing its seminal fluid into the female's genital tract (Shulov and Amitai, 1958). Courting and parturition takes place, generally, in the warmer season.

The period of pregnancy is significantly different in various *Buthinae*: from 42 days in *O. innesi* ssp. *negebensis* (Shulov and Amitai, 1960) to 296 in *B. occitanus* (Auber, 1963). Five gestations were found to be common in *I. maculatus* (Probst, 1972). The number of larvae in one litter is fluctuating from 9 as an average in *Orthochirus* (Shulov and Amitai, 1960), to 30–70 in *B. occitanus* (Auber, 1963). The duration of postembryonal development until adulthood is 7–8 months in *Isometrus* in comparison to some 6 years in *L. quinquestriatus* (Shulov, 1938). The length of adult life fluctuates between 2 years in *Isometrus* to at least 4 years in *Pandinus pallidus* (PROBST, 1972).

At emergence the young are contained in an embryonic envelope from which they escape within several minutes from birth, and soon climb to the mother's back, where they remain for a week or two, accepting no food, and pass through at least one moult. Afterward, they begin their independent life. In a few days, the young scorpions are able to sting and the amount of venom extruded during two stings can kill a white mouse. The amount of venom produced by a scorpion increases with each moult (SHULOV, 1938). This may be correlated with the increase of folds and diverticula of the poisonous glands which occurs at each successive stage (PROBST, 1972; PAWLOWSKY, 1913).

PAWLOWSKY (1913, 1914, 1925) investigated the structure and development of the venomous gland in different species and families of scorpions. PROBST (1972) followed both embryonal and postembryonal development of the venomous gland in *Isometrus*.

The interior part of the gland consists of a lumen formed by a single layer of cylindrical epithelial cells of 100 μ high in average. The connective tissue "basal-membrane" surrounding the epithelial layer is 5 μ high. Among the high epithelial cells are different nonexcreting cells mostly in basal position, described by PAW-LOVSKY (1913) as supporting ones (*Stutzzellen*) and by BÜCHERL (1964) as substitute ones (*Ersatz*). The whole gland is covered by one or several layers of muscles (SHULOV, unpublished results). The lumen of the gland is connected by a duct to an aperture in the aculeate of the telson.

There are two such glands in each telson separated medially by the connective tissue. Each gland has a separate duct leading to a separate aperture. The epithelial layer is smooth, as a rule, in the earliest stages of development. The folds and diverticula develop later increasing gradually in numbers. PAWLOVSKY (1913) describes those glands which, in adult stages, have only few folds as "embryonal" or "primitive" and those with more complicate structure as "definitive." *L. quinquestriatus* has, in its adult stage, very many such folds (ABD-EL-WAHAB, 1952).

The production of venom and the fate of the producing cells was discussed by many authors (KUBOTA, 1918; BÜCHERL, 1964; SAMANO-BISHOP and GOMEZ DE FERRIZ, 1964; and PROBST, 1972). PROBST thinks that the secretion is being formed at the basal part of the cell, moved toward the lumen, and pushed into it after the neighbour cells already have emptied their content. According to him, the same cell is able to produce venom several times, i.e., they are "merokrin."

The scorpions are very resistant against their own venom. The experiments on *L. quinquestriatus* have shown that in order to kill scorpion of this species some 18 stings of the homospecific scorpions are needed. However, when two scorpions fight, the stronger tries to turn the weaker one upside down and to sting it into the middle of the abdomen aiming at the neural abdominal chain. A sting into ganglion causes immediate death (SHULOV, 1955).

It appears that the hemolymph of the scorpion is able to neutralize its venom. This was found experimenting on white mice. Following this finding the hemolymph of some 30 *L. quinquestriatus* were injected into a child who was in such desperate condition that, not having specific antiserum available, it was decided to use scorpion's hemolymph as a last resource. Fortunately the influence of hemolymph was immediate and positive. The child was almost normal after several hours (ADLER et al., 1955).

Predators of scorpions are nocturnal birds, hedgehogs, snakes, skinks, and lizards, solifuges, spiders (*Latrodectus*), and also other scorpions.

References

Abd-el-Wahab, A.: Notes on the morphology of the scorpion *Buthus quinquestriatus* (H.E.). Publ. Fouad I Desert Inst. No. 3, 1—129 (1952).

Adler, S., Berman, S., Shulov, A., Levi, N.: A case of scorpion sting treated by intramuscular injection of haemolymph of *Leiurus* (*Buthus*) *quinquestriatus*. Harefuah, J. med. Ass. Israel, **49**, 215—217 (1955).

Auber, M.: Reproduction et croissance de *Buthus occitanus* Amx. Ann. Sci. nat. Zool. Paris **5**, 273—286 (1963).

Bücherl, W.: Histologia des glândulas de veneno de algunas aranhas e escorpiões. Mem. Inst. Butantan, **31**, 77—84 (1964).

Kubota, S.: An experimental study of the venom of the Manchurian scorpion. J. Pharmacol. exp. Ther. **11**, 379—388 (1918).

Pawlowsky, E.: Scorpiotomische Mitteilungen. I. Ein Beitrag zur Morphologie der Giftdrüsen der Skorpione. Z. wiss. Zool. (Leipzig) **105**, 157—177 (1913).

Pawlowsky, E.: Contribution to the structure and development of the venom glands of scorpions (Russian). Rev. russ. Entomol. (Russk. entomol. obozr.), **14**, 57—71 (1914).

Pawlowsky, E.: Zur Morphologie des weiblichen Genitalapparats und zur Embryologie der Skorpione. Ann. Mus. Zool. Acad. Sci. URSS, **26**, 137—205 (1925).

Probst, P.J.: Zur Fortpflanzungsbiologie und zur Entwicklung der Giftdrüsen beim Skorpion *Isometrus maculatus* (De Geer, 1778) (*Scorpiones: Buthidae*). Acta trop. (Basel) **29**, (1), 1—87 (1972).

Samano-Bishop, A., Gomez-de-Ferriz, M.: Estudio morfologico, histologico e histoquimico de la glandula venenosa de algunas species de alacranes de los generos *Vejovis* C.L. Koch, *Diplocentrus* Peters y *Centruroides* Marx. Ann. Inst. Biol. Univ. Mexico, **35**, 139—155 (1964).

Shulov, A.: On the poison of scorpions in Palestine (I). (Hebrew). Harefuah, J. med. Ass. Israel **15**, 85—86 (1938).

Shulov, A.: On the poison of scorpions in Israel (II). (Hebrew). Harefuah, J. med. Ass. Israel, **49**, 131—133 (1955).

Shulov, A.: On some Israeli scorpions. (Hebrew). Dapim Refuiim (Folia med.), **21** (7), 657—660 (1962).

Shulov, A., Amitai, P.: On mating habits of three scorpions, *Leiurus quinquestriatus* H. et E., *Buthotus judaicus* Simon, and *Nebo hierichonticus* Simon. Arch. Inst. Pasteur Algér. **36** (3), 351—369 (1958).

Shulov, A., Amitai, P.: Observations sur les scorpions. *Orthochirus innesi* Simon, 1910, ssp. *negebensis* nov. Arch. Inst. Pasteur Algér. **38** (1), 117—129 (1960).

Vachon, M.: Étude des caractères utilisés pour classer les familles et les genres de Scorpions (Arachnides). Bull. Mus. nat. Hist. nat. (Paris) (3) No. 140 Zool. **104**, 857—958 (1973).

Zinner, H., Amitai, P.: Observations on hibernation of *Compsobuthus acutecarinatus* Simon and *C. schmiedeknechti* Vachon (Scorpionidea, Arachnida) in Israel. Israel J. Zool., **18**, 41—47 (1969).

B. Epidemiology Symptomatology and Treatment of Buthinae Stings

P. EFRATI

Although stings of scorpions occur frequently in tropical and subtropical countries, there are relatively few investigations in the medical literature dealing with the clinical aspects of these stings. The explanation of this fact is probably that most of the stings occur in geographical regions where medical centers are not abundant. Another cause could be the circumstance that most of the stings occur in adults, in whom usually no signs of general poisoning are present. The main symptoms are local pains which last a few hours. Medical literature published in the first half of the present century dealt usually with case reports and serotherapy while interest in pathogenesis and pathophysiology arose in the decades that followed.

It becomes evident that in spite of the zoological difference between the stinging scorpions signs and symptoms of envenomation are quite similar and concernes mainly the vegetative nervous system.

In the following pages the clinical syndrome of envenomation by Buthinae in different countries will be reviewed with emphasis on pathogenesis and pathophysiology as a possible clue to rational therapy.

The most poisonous scorpions of India belong, according to CAINS and MASHKAR (1932) to the genera *Buthus* and *Palamneus*. Fatalities after scorpion stings were rarely encountered, and then only in children. The commonest signs of envenomation were: hyperreflexia, shivering, tremor, convulsions, excessive lachrymal, nasal and salivary secretion, involuntary urination and defecation, vomiting, diarrhea, disturbances of breathing (terminating sometimes in respiratory paralysis) and at times increased blood pressure was observed.

RASU (1939) in Calcutta, India, described 19 cases, 5 of which died, all of them children. Symptoms of the envenomation were: severe pains at the site of the sting, headache, giddiness, nausea, vomiting, profuse perspiration, chilliness, hypothermia, and tachypnea. At times loss of consciousness was observed.

Recently, SANTHANAKRISHNAN and BALAGOPAL RAJU (1974) reported on 301 cases of scorpion stings in India comprising children admitted to two pediatric institutions in Madras during 1971 — 72, recording 7 deaths. The manifestations of the envenomation were: profuse sweating, restlesness, cold and clammy extremities, cardiovascular disturbances such as myocarditis (diagnosed mainly on electrocardiographic findings) tachycardia, dyspnea, symptoms of heart failure, hyperthermia, and convulsions. Local symptoms were absent conspicuosly at the time of admission of the children. The patients were treated with lytic cocktail (LABORIT and HUGUÉNARD, 1951).

SERGENT of Algeria (1930 — 1946) collected observations on thousands of cases of envenomation by scorpion sting from many physicians in the country. Symptoms recorded in his series were: severe pain at the site of the sting, dizziness, profuse sweating, feeling of chilliness, pallor, cyanosis, severe headache, and sometimes myoclonic twitchings. He observed also, disturbances of the regulation of temperature (hypothermia or pyrexia), as well as tachypnea, pulmonary edema, tachycardia, nausea, vomiting, abdominal pain, excitement or coma, meningismus, and pupillary disturbances. He tried to convince physicians to use serotherapy in treating the patients — demonstrating the effectiveness of it in his observations. The most important scorpions belong to the genera *Prionurus* and *Buthus*.

EFRATI (1949) summarized his observations in 22 cases of stings of scorpions in Israel inflicted mainly by *Leiurus quinquestriatus*. The clinical manifestations presented were in order of their frequency as follows: hyperirritability, vomiting, polypnea, hypersalivation, profuse perspiration, pain at the site of the sting, cyanosis, myoclonic twitchings, flushing of the face, hyperthermia, priapism, thirst, clouding of consciousness, tachycardia, urinary retention, mydriasis, meteorism, disorder of speech, bradycardia, hyperreflexia, abdominal pain, frothing at the mouth, shivering, areflexia, hypertension, ptosis of the lid, shock, pallor, generalized erythema, local hypoesthesia, abdominal tension, hypothermia, rhinorrhea, miosis, pupillary areflexia, involuntary defecation, pollakiuria, piloerection. An interesting laboratory finding was leukocytosis reaching maximal values of 42,000 − 70,000. Six cases terminated fatally. Treatment was symptomatic.

Similar manifestations were described in another series, by Sturman (1962) in the southern part of Israel. In her series of 36 cases there were 13 with general manifestation and 2 fatalities.

In the late 1960s and following years cases were described in the southern part of Israel, concerning children as well as adults, with a quite different symptomatology. The manifestations observed in these cases and the laboratory examinations allowed to work out the pathogenesis of the envenomation and initiated new pharmacologic experiments in Israel and abroad.

I. Pathophysiology of the Envenomation

Ali Hassan and Ahmed Hassan Mohammed (1940) from Egypt already hypothesized in the early 1940 on the pathophysiologic mechanism of the envenomation by scorpion sting. They demonstrated in animal experiments that scorpion venom is a powerful stimulant of the autonomic nervous system. It produces a rise of blood pressure in anesthetized dogs. In the rabbit it produces hyperglycemia lasting 3 or 4 h. In the isolated toad's heart scorpion venom caused acceleration of the beats, etc. As a stimulant of the parasympathetic system it excites salivation and lachrymation, which are characteristic manifestations of the envenomation in some mammals. They tried ergotoxin − a depressor of the sympathetic and atropine as a parasympathicolytic depressor agent in the treatment of experimental envenomation in rat and dog, with considerable success. The present author applied this method of treatment in envenomation of children but had no success at all. The doses were probably inadequate.

Analyzing the manifestations of envenomation in affected children, I came to the conclusion that stimulation of the hypothalamus by scorpion venom could explain more adequately the pathophysiology of the envenomation, as hypothalamic discharge could cause disturbances in sympathetic and parasympathetic systems, as well as some integrative action of the hypothalamic centers resulting in shivering, piloerection, rise of temperature, etc. Polypnea compares well to the rapid breathing following stimulation of some diencephalic regions. Other symptoms such as hyperirritability (sham rage?), leukocytosis, etc., could also be explained as due to hypothalamic discharge (Efrati, 1951).

In the late 1960s clinical reports were published in Israel indicating a single common pathway toward understanding the pathophysiology of scorpion stings − mainly by the yellow scorpion (*L. quinquestriatus*). Most illustrative was the case described by Sklarovsky and Levin (1969) from the Joseftal Medical Center at Eilat, Israel. Their patient, a 27-year-old male, was admitted to the hospital $1^1/_2$ h after having been stung by a yellow scorpion. He was restless, his sensorium clouded, he was perspirating profusely; hypersalivation, lachrymation, vomiting, and priapism were also present. The blood pressure was raising quickly, reaching after a while

260/190, the pulse rate was 150/min. At that time the patient complained of headache and of severe pains in his precordium. The ECG tracing revealed left axis deviation and left heart strain. At this stage an α-blocking agent Regitine was injected i.v. Blood pressure returned to normal values in a few minutes but the tachycardia persisted. Then 4 mg of propranolol were injected i.v. and in a matter of 30 min all the symptoms improved or disappeared and the pathologic changes in the ECG regressed. Laboratory investigations revealed increased SGOT activity and the excretion of a total VMA of 25.5 mg in 24 h, the normal excreted amount being usually less than 6 mg/24 h.

GUERON and YAROM (1970) reported on a series of 82 hospitalized patients stung by scorpions (GUERON et al., 1967) who were treated in the Negev Hospital at Beer Sheva. A total of 34 clinical charts were reviewed. The authors concentrated mainly on cardiovascular disturbances. Hypertension, peripheral vascular collapse, congestive heart failure, and pulmonary edema were observed. In 14 of the 28 electrocardiograms reviewed, "early" myocardial infarction like patterns were observed. Vanilloyl mandelic acid was elevated in 7 of the 34 patients and total free epinephrine and norepinephrine in 8; 9 patients died. Necropsy studies showed degenerative changes and focal necrosis in the muscle fibers, as well as interstitial edema and cellularity. According to the authors' hypothesis, the cardiovascular manifestations and morphologic abnormalities are related to the level of circulating catecholamines and are caused by a direct effect of scorpion venom on the sympathetic system.

Experimental studies on dogs carried out by YAROM and BRAUN (1969, 1971), after injection of different amounts of venom of the scorpion L. quinquestriatus, revealed similar changes in the myocardium.

Further pharmacologic studies elucidated the way of action of the scorpion venom, especially on the cardiovascular system.

MOSS et al. (1973, 1974) reported in several articles on experimental release of catecholamines in rats. They showed that in both normal and adrenalectomized rats in which ganglionic transmission has been blocked by hexamethonium, scorpion venom (of L. quinquestriatus) produces a dramatic increase in blood pressure which is accompanied by a massive discharge of catecholamines into the blood. The increases in serum catecholamines and blood pressure accompanying injections of venom represent the effects of both sympathetic and adrenal discharge. Acutely adrenalectomized animals manifested an increase in serum catecholamines which was about 50% of that found in intact animals and was identical to that found in chronically adrenalectomized animals. Since hexamethonium blocks ganglionic transmission and adrenal medullary response to splanchnic nerve stimulation, the effect of the venom is presumably the result of a direct action on the adrenal medulla and the postganglionic neuron and does not represent the secondary effects of cholinergic discharge.

CHEYMOL et al. (1974) carried out studies on the cardiovascular actions of the venom of North African scorpions (Androctonus australis, L. quinquestriatus and Buthus occitanus). They have shown an action on the sympathetic ganglia. There was a release of catecholamines from nerve endings causing hypertension, peripheral vasoconstriction, lachrymation, salivation, breathing spasms, indirect inotropic effect, and later ganglionic blockade lead to hypotension. There was also direct action on the heart causing direct inotropic effect, bradycardia, arrhythmia, leading to fibrillation, and involvement of intracardiac receptors, particularly of the β-adrenergic receptors.

OSMAN et al. (1973) proposed an explanation of the hyperthermia often encountered in envenomation by scorpion stings. They injected venom from *L. quinquestriatus* intraventricularly into rabbits and produced a pronounced hyperthermia. This effect was not antagonized by the prior intraventricular or intravenous injection of scorpion antiserum. The venom may act by releasing noradrenaline in the anterior hypothalamus or by causing in the posterior hypothalamus a shift in the balance of Na and Ca.

II. Treatment

BALOZET (1956) reported on production of antisera against North African scorpions. MOHAMMED et al. (1975) showed that it is possible to produce potent antivenins against the venoms of *L. quinquestriatus, B. occitanus,* and other Egyptian scorpions. Trials with sera produced in Egypt (Agouza Lab.), in Algeria (Pasteur Institute), and England (Lister Institute) revealed that antiscorpion serum is highly specific and offers weak or no paraspecific action.

A potent antiserum against the sting of *L. quinquestriatus* is being prepared in donkeys by the Department of Entomology and Venomous Animals, the Hebrew University of Jerusalem (SHULOV et al., 1959).

In spite of the progress in serotherapy of envenomation by venomous animals, there is no convincing evidence of the value of serotherapy in envenomation by stings of scorpions. This could be explained by assuming that antisera presently available are not effective. Animal experiments and the experience of some authors, notably SERGENT, contradict this possibility. Animal experiments pointing to the rapid resorption of the scorpion venom could be the result of low molecular weight of the venom (not yet reported) or of the content of hyaluronidase, which has been reported already (JACQUES, 1956). Most probably, the reason of ineffectivity of the serum lays in the inadequate quantity used. Such a change occurred in serotherapy of viper bites when the quantity of serum was increased considerably and the serum was injected intravenously.

I would propose to give specific antiserum intramuscularly — as a preventive measure — to children, in cases not presenting signs of generalized envenomation. When signs of generalized envenomation are present antiserum has to be injected intravenously in quantities of 15—30 ml, and even more, according to the concentration of antitoxin in the serum and the weight of the child. Agents blocking α- and β-receptors have to be used also, according to the symptoms present.

References

Ali Hassan, Ahmed Hassan Mohammed: Atropin and ergotoxin as antidotes to scorpion toxin, Lancet (1940) **1**, 1001—1002 (1940).

Balozet, L.: Scorpion venoms and antiscorpion serum, In: Venoms, Amer. Ass. Advanc. Sci., 141—144 (1956).

Balozet, L.: Scorpionism in the Old World, In: Venomous Animals and their venoms, Vol. III, ch. 56, pp. 349—371. New York, London: Academic Press 1971.

Cainus, J.F., Mhaskar, K.L.: Notes on Indian scorpions, Indian med. Res. Mem. 24, pp. 100—102 (1932).

Cheymol, I., Bourillet, F., Roch-Arveiller, M., Heckle, I.: Action cardiovasculaire de trois venins de scorpions Nord-Africains (*Androctonus australis, Leiurus quinquestriatus, Buthus occitanus*) et deux toxines extraites de l'un d'entre eux, Toxicon, **12**, 241—248 (1974).

Efrati, P.: Poisoning by scorpion stings in Israel, Amer. J. trop. Med., **29**, 249—257 (1949).

Efrati, P.: Acute hypothalamic discharge in man due to scorpion sting. Confin. neurol. (Basel) **11**, 152—167, (1951).

Gueron, M., Stern, I. Cohen, W.: Severe myocardial damage and heart failure in scorpion sting, Report of five cases. Amer. J. Cardiol., **19**, 719—726 (1967).

Gueron, M., Yarom, R.: Cardiovascular manifestations of severe scorpion sting, Clinipathologic correlations Chest, **57**, 156—162 (1970).

Jaques, R.: The hyaluronidase content of animal venoms, In: Venoms, Amer. Ass. Advanc. Sci. 291 (1956)

Laborit, H., Huguénard, P.: L'hibernation artificielle par moyens pharmacodynamiques et physiques, Presse méd., **59**, 1329 (1951).

Mohammed, A.H., Darwish, M.A., Hani Ayobe, M.: Immunological studies on scorpion (*B. quinquestriatus*) antivenin, *Toxicon*, **13**, 67—68 (1975).

Moss, J., Kažič, T., Henry, D.P., Kopin, I.J.: Scorpion venom induced discharge of catecholamines accompanied by hypertension, Brain Res. **54**, 381—385 (1973).

Moss, J., Thoa, N.B., Kopin, I.J.: On the mechanism of scorpion toxin-induced release of norepinephrine from peripheral adrenergic neurons, J. Pharmacol. exp. Ther., **190**, 39—48, (1974).

Osman, O.H., Ismail, M., Wenger, T.: Hyperthermic response to intraventricular injection of scorpion venom. Role of brain monoamines. Toxicon **11**, 361—368 (1973).

Rasu, U.P.: Observations on scorpion sting and snake bite. Amer. J. trop. Med., **19**, 385—391, (1939).

Santhanakrishnan, B.R., Balagopal Raju, V.: Management of scorpion sting in children, Amer. J. trop. Med. Hyg. **77**, 133—135 (1974).

Sergent, E.: Sérotherapie antiscorpionique. Obsérvations médicale recues pendant l'anné 1942., Arch. Inst. Pasteur Algér. **21**, 186—202 (1943).

Sergent, E.: Sérotherapie antiscorpionique. Obsérvations médicale recues pendant l'anné 1943., Arch. Inst. Pasteur Algér. **22**, 18—39 (1944).

Sergent, E.: Sérotherapie antiscorpionique. Obsérvations médicale recues pendant l'anné 1944., Arch. Inst. Pasteur Algér. **23**, 111—114 (1945).

Shulov, A., Flesh, D., Gerichter, Ch., Eshkol, Z., Schillinger, C.: The antiscorpion serum prepared by use of fresh venom and the assessment of the efficacy against scorpion stings, Proc. Fifth Int. Meeting for Biological Standardization, Jerusalem, 1959, pp. 489—492.

Sklarovsky, L., Levin, M.: Alfa and beta receptor blocking agents in a case of yellow scorpion sting with severe cardiovascular effects. Harefuah, **77**, 521—522 (1969). (In Hebrew)

Sturman, N.: Envenomation caused by scorpion stings in the Negev. Dapim Refuiim (Folia Medica), **21**, 661—665 (1962). (In Hebrew)

Yarom, R., Braun, K.: Myocardial pathology following scorpion venom injection, Israel J. med. sci., **5**, 849—852 (1969).

Yarom, R., Braun, K.: Electron microscopic studies of the myocardial changes produced by scorpion venom injections in dogs., Lab. Invest., **24**, 21—30 (1971).

C. Chemistry and Pharmacology of Buthinae Scorpion Venoms

E. Zlotkin[1,2], F. Miranda[2], and H. Rochat[2]

I. Introduction

In the past, the medical aspect of scorpion venoms served not only as the primary motivation but as the sole purpose of scientific research on the subject. In several

[1] Department of Entomology and Venomous Animals, The Hebrew University of Jerusalem, Jerusalem, Israel.
[2] Faculté de Médecine, Secteur Nord, Biochimie, Marseille, France.

regions of the world, such as Mexico (MAZZOTTI and BRAVO-BECHERELLE, 1963), Brazil (BÜCHERL, 1971), North Africa (BALOZET, 1971), and the Middle East (SHU-LOV, 1955), scorpions still represent a medical problem and a life hazard to children. However, it appears that recent rural agricultural developments and improvement of medical services have reduced this health hazard, and will continue do so in the future.

Despite the relative decrease in the medical significance of scorpion venoms, however, it seems that scientific investigation on this subject has been undergoing a constant process of expansion in recent years. This increase in scientific interest follows from certain essential changes in both the theoretical and practical attitudes to the subject. Scorpion venom and toxins may serve as pharmacologic tools and can be applied in the study of physiologic processes where neural excitatory phenomena or induction of chemical transmission are required (Sect. C IV, V). Because of their specific action on axons and their affinity for axonal membranes, scorpion toxins may be employed as useful tools in chemical characterization of the molecules involved in ionic conductance (Secretion C V). It is most fascinating to note that scorpion venoms contain selective toxins, highly specific in their lethal action, which differentiate between toxonomically phylogenetically related groups of arthropods (Sect. C VI). This may allow detection of new essential physiologic processes related to the mechanism of such highly specific intoxication and typical of the respective groups of organisms. Scorpion venoms may be also used in the study of their zooecological relationships and taxonomy (Sects. B II, C VI).

Selectivity and specificity in the action of different components of crude venom strongly encourages investigation of composition and structure, leading to the study of structure function relationships (Sect. B II). The presence of some factors which are not lethal to mammals but still elicit reversible excitatory phenomena in mammalian systems (Sect. VI, 3) may be of immediate pharmaceutic importance and should further encourage chemical investigations. While considering the above-mentioned conceptions in preparation of the present survey, we did not abandon the clinical pathologic aspects which underly and initiate any toxinologic investigation. These also serve as a background and point of departure in the presentation of the pharmacologic aspects. Actually, the study of scorpion venom may serve as an exciting meeting point for the collaborative efforts of the chemist, pharmacologist, and clinician.

The present survey deals mainly with Buthinae scorpion venoms, however, for purpose of comparison and completeness, it also includes basic information about the venoms of the genera *Centruroides* and *Tityus* which all belong to the family of Buthidae (BÜCHERL, 1971) and closely resemble the above in their composition and pharmacologic action.

II. Chemistry

The chemical studies of Buthinae venoms were medically motivated, and dedicated mainly to those few species of scorpions which are dangerous to the human being. Emphasis was placed on the isolation, purification, and characterization of those principles which are toxic to mammals. These cannot be enzymes, since scorpion venoms are most often devoid of or at best very poorly equipped with them (BALOZET, 1971). Enzymatic activities, when present, have generally been demonstrated only on a qualitative level and no attempt was made to purify them, as in the case of phospholipase (IBRAHIM, 1967; MOHAMMED et al., 1969) and hyaluronidase (ZLOTKIN et al., 1972c). Proteolytic and phosphodiesteratic activities were electrophoretically separated from the venom of *Buthus tamulus* (MASTER et al., 1963). The 5-hydroxytryptamine which was found in *Leiurus quinquestriatus* venom (ADAM and WEISS, 1958, 1959a) in a greater amount than in other animal venoms (ZLOTKIN, 1973), does not seem to play any role in actual intoxication. In fact, the lethal and paralytic activity of scorpion venoms is due to their containing neurotoxins which are generally basic proteins of low molecular weight.

1. Isolation and Purification

The history of the study of scorpion venom composition parallels the history of the new concepts and techniques developed in protein chemistry. The proteic low molecular basic nature of toxic principles (histones) had already been assumed by Wilson in 1904, but final purification of scorpion toxins, as indicated by physical and chemical criteria was achieved in our laboratory[1]. The mode of preparations as used by WILSON (1904), based on saline (0.15 M) extraction of telsons and precipitation by ethanol, later adopted with certain modifications by MOHAMMED (1942) and ADAM and WEISS (1959b), did not result in pure products. These were obtained only after introduction of modern column chromatographic techniques based on gel filtration and ion-exchange.

After the first attempts to purify scorpion toxins, using telsons as starting material (MIRANDA and LISSITZKY, 1958), successive improvements were introduced, leading to a general method of animal toxins purification (MIRANDA et al., 1970a, 1970b). Preliminary experiments (LISSITZKY et al., 1956; MIRANDA and LISSITZKY, 1958; MIRANDA et al., 1960, 1961) showed that the toxic principles: (1) migrated toward the cathode when submitted to electrophoresis at pH 8.6; (2) were soluble in pure water; (3) were precipitated from their aqueous solution by acetone between 60 and 80% concentration; (4) partially dialyzed, especially in low pH solutions. This has clearly indicated that these principles might be low molecular weight basic proteins.

These properties served as guidelines for the application of reversible absorption on Sephadex G-25 swollen in water (MIRANDA et al., 1962) and ion-exchange chromatography on Amberlite IRC-50 in ammonium acetate buffer at near neutral pH, in order to obtain the purified mammal toxins (MIRANDA and LISSITZKY, 1958, 1961). Ammonium acetate, due to its volatility, was used as a buffer from the start, and was found perfectly suitable for purification of scorpion as well as snake toxins. In spite of the homogeneity by ultracentrifugation, further studies with starch gel electrophoresis and equilibrium chromatography on Amberlite IRC-50 (MIRANDA et al., 1964a, b, c) showed that the purified proteins were dimers of noncovalent associated monomers or nontoxic material (MIRANDA et al., 1966). Two pure monomeric mammal toxins from the North African scorpion *Androctonus australis Hector* collected in the area of Tozeur (Tunisia) were later obtained

---

[1] Faculté de Médecine, Secteur Nord, Biochimie, Marseille, France.

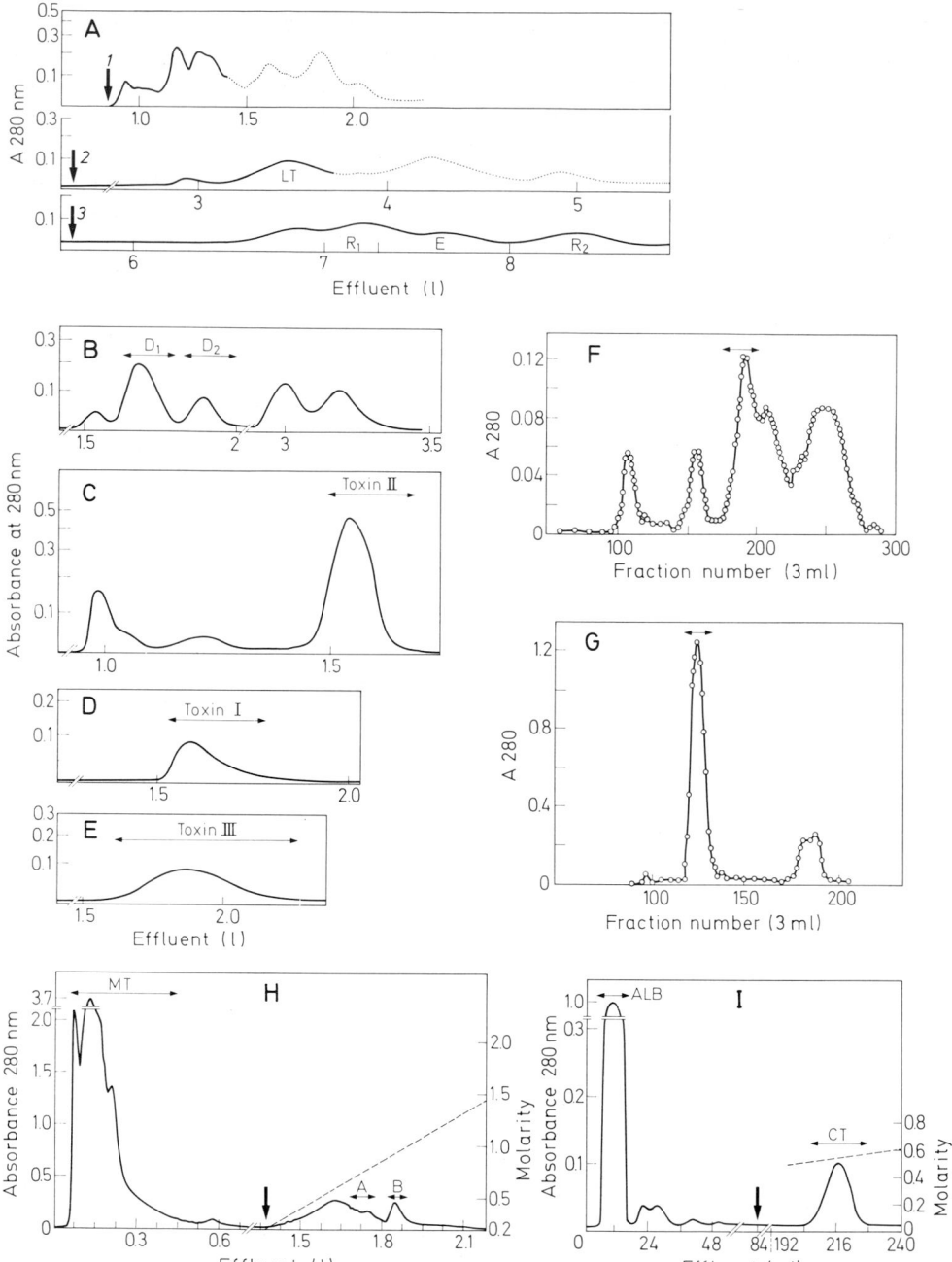

Fig. 1 A−I. Isolation and purification of different toxins from venom of scorpion *A. australis Hector*. (A) Recycling gel filtration on Sephadex G 50: Four columns of 3.2×100 cm in series in 0.1 M ammonium acetate buffer pH 8.5−8.6. Flow rate 60 ml/h Mixture submitted to fractionation is water extract of 2 g of crude venom, *vertical arrows* and *numbers* correspond to beginning of consecutive cycles. Fractions of elution curves indicated by full line are collected. Material marked by *dotted line* is recycled. Toxicity to mice is located in fractions *R1* and

with Sephadex G-50 filtration, chromatography on Amberlite IRC-50 at pH 6.30 and 6.70 and on DEAE Sephadex A-50 at alkaline pH (8.50) in ammonium acetate buffers (ROCHAT et al., 1967). In that study, ultracentrifugation confirmed that the true molecular weight (about 7000) corresponded to the minimum molecular weight estimated from amino acid composition. Further improvement over the preceding method was obtained by introducing recycling gel filtration on Sephadex G-50 and using another cation-exchanger: CM-Sephadex G-50 (MIRANDA et al., 1970a). The latter method is generally applied to venoms which are milked by cycling electrical stimulations of the postabdomen, but it was also found to function in the purification of toxins from homogenates of dried telsons of *B. occitanus tunetanus* and *Centruroides suffusus suffusus* (GARCIA et al., in preparation). However, in those cases, only the toxins present in large amounts could be obtained in a pure form. The absence of proteolytic enzymes in the Buthinae venoms allows column chromatographic separations at room temperature.

A general method for the purification of scorpion toxins composed of several steps has been developed, based on experience accumulated, as described above. The first step consists of an extraction of the venom by distilled water followed

---

R2, toxicity to fly larvae is located in fraction *LT* and toxicity to isopods is located in fractions *E* and *R2* (taken from ZLOTKIN et al., 1972b). (B) Purification of "mammal" toxins: Chromatography on DEAE—Sephadex A50 of fraction *R1* of preceding step obtained from 4 g of crude venom. Column 4 × 200 cm in 0.1 M ammonium acetate buffer pH 8.50, flow rate 4 ml/h. D1 and D2 toxic fractions to mice. (C) Chromatography on Amberlite CG 50 at pH 6.7 of *R2* mice toxic fraction obtained in A from 4 g crude venom, resulting in pure mammal toxin II. Column 4 × 150 cm in 0.2 M ammonium acetate buffer pH 6.70. Flow rate, 48 ml/h. (D) Chromatography on Amberlite CG 50 at pH 6.30 of D1 toxic fraction obtained in B from 2 g of crude venom, resulting in purification of mammal toxin I. Column 4 × 150 cm in 0.2 M ammonium acetate buffer pH 6.30. Flow rate 48 ml/h. (E) Chromatography on Amberlite CG 50 at pH 6.15 of D2 toxic fraction obtained in B from 6 g of crude venom, resulting in final purification of mammal toxin II. Column 4 × 150 cm in 0.2 M ammonium acetate buffer pH 6.15. Flow rate 48 ml/h (taken from MIRANDA et al., 1970a). (F) Purification of "insect" toxin: Chromatography on DEAE Sephadex A-50 of fly larvae toxic fraction (*LT*) obtained in A. from 0.5 g of crude venom. Column 2 × 200 cm in 0.1 M ammonium acetate buffer pH 8.50. Flow rate 12 ml/h. *Horizontal arrow* indicates fractions toxic to fly larvae. (C) Chromatography on Amberlite CG 50 of toxic fractions obtained in F. from 0.5 g of venom. Column 2 × 200 cm in 0.2 M ammonium acetate buffer pH 6.30. Flow rate 12 ml/h. *Horizontal arrow* indicates finally purified insect toxin fraction (taken from ZLOTKIN et al., 1971d, see Section C VI 3). (H) Purification of "crustacean" toxin: Chromatography on Amberlite CG 50 of fraction *R2* obtained in A. from 10 g of crude venom. Column 2.5 × 20 cm. Buffer: ammonium acetate, equilibrium conditions: 0.2 M pH 6.30; linear gradient conditions: up to 2.0 M and pH 7.3. Flow rate 30 ml/h. Fractions of 7.5 ml were collected. Dotted line—linear gradient of buffer concentration. *Vertical arrow* indicates starting of gradient elution. *MT* fraction toxic to mice, which corresponds to "mammal" toxin II. A and B: fractions toxic to isopods. (I) Chromatography on CM-Sephadex of 2.9 OD$_{280}$ units of fraction B obtained in H and mixed with 29 mg of albumin prior to lyophilization in order to preserve its activity. Column 1.4 × 12 cm. Buffer: ammonium acetate 0.2 M pH 7.3 followed by linear gradient of concentration. Flow rate: 5 ml/h in equilibrium conditions and 10 ml/h in gradient elution. Fractions of 2.4 ml were collected. Dotted line: linear gradient of buffer concentration. *Vertical arrow* indicates starting of gradient elution. *ALB*: albumin fraction. *CT*: crustacean toxin (taken from ZLOTKIN et al., 1975, see Section C VI 3)

by a dialysis at 2% of the extract against the same solvent. The toxins are dissolved in pure water in order to eliminate the mucoproteins, present in the venoms in variable amounts, which could render inefficient further ion exchange chromatographies. When the mucoproteins are present in large amounts (as in the venom of *B. occitanus tunetanus*), acetone fractionation is used instead of water extraction. The dried venom is dissolved in 0.15 M NaCl at 0° C. Chilled acetone ($-20°$ C) is added dropwise and the mixture progressively cooled to $-15°$ C. The precipitate obtained between 60% and 80% (v/v) of acetone concentration, contains almost all the toxicity. Recovered by centrifugation, it is rapidly dried in open air, dissolved in water and freeze-dried. An alternative method for removal of mucoproteins is applied following the above water extraction and dialysis, and is based on Sephadex G-50 chromatography (single column, 4×200 cm for 2 g of venom) using 0.5 M acetic acid as solvent. In this solvent, the aqueous extract yields a solution which is much less viscous than that obtained in neutral or alkaline ammonium acetate buffers and the high molecular weight acidic mucoproteins are easily excluded from the gel and separated from the toxins. This method was found to be preferable to the above acetone fractionation when applied on *B. occitanus tunetanus* (Rochat et al., in preparation) and *B. occitanus paris* (Martin, 1974) venoms. Furthermore, the 0.5 M acetic acid solvent was found to be very efficient in obtaining toxins free from molecular associations with other components of the venom.

The second step is a molecular sieving, using Sephadex G-50 in 0.1 M ammonium acetate buffer (pH 8.6), in a recycling system composed of a set of four columns (3.2×100 cm) connected in series with a flow rate of $77-80$ ml/h controlled by a peristatic pump (Fig. 1). The long column allows the maintenance of a large number of proteins in the recycling system, thus enabling their discrimination and isolation. Columns charged with a well-equilibrated and degassed gel can be reused for almost 1 year, since ammonium acetate, generally at pH 8.6, is an unfavorable medium for microorganism growth.

The toxic fractions separated by gel filtration are then subjected to ion-exchange chromatography. In most cases, the toxic extracts are successively filtered on resins of opposite polarity: Amberlite IRC-50 or CM Sephadex G-50 and DEAE Sephadex A-50. Generally, equilibrium chromatography (i.e., the same buffer serves during the whole operation) is preferred to gradient chromatography, since it is considered to be a better criterion of homogeneity. However, in the purification of the crustacean toxin (Fig. 1, Sect. C IV, Zlotkin et al., 1975a) the application of gradient elution with ion exchangers was successful.

The operations are carried out in calibrated glass columns fitted with sintered glass supports, $50-200$ cm in height and 1, 2, 3, or 4 cm width, with a maximum flow rate of 5 ml/cm^2/h. Amberlite is washed and cycled according to Hirs (1955). Sephadex ion-exchange gels are cycled through the Cl$^-$ and OH$^-$ form using HCl and NaOH (0.5 M) as indicated by the supplier. Columns can be used again after exchange of the upper 5 cm with fresh support, to remove absorbed contaminated proteins. Buffers are prepared by adjusting the pH of ammonium acetate solutions with concentrated ammonium hydroxide or acetic acid as required. The concentration of ammonium ions is determined by the Kjeldahl process.

2. Composition and Structure

The venoms of five scorpions belonging to the Buthinae have been studied so far, and 22 toxic proteins were isolated, purified, and characterized on the chemical level, at least by amino acid compositions and/or automatic sequencing of their N- terminal end: 20 are active on mammals, 1 to insects and 1 to crustaceans. Their amino acid compositions, lethal potency to mice and at least partial primary sequences are presented in Tables 1 and 2 and Figure 2, respectively. Additional information concerning the toxins selectively active on arthropods is presented in Section C VI 3.

The venom of the North African scorpion *A. australis Hector*(AaH) served as the main object of our investigation and Figure 1 presents its column chromatographic separation employing Sephadex gel filtration as well as ion exchangers, resulting in the purification of the three mammal toxins, the insect toxin, and the crustacean toxin (Tables 1 and 2, Fig. 2). The structure of the toxins derived from the venom of the scorpion AaH may serve as a typical example of taxonomic implications derived from chemical information. It has been found that venom collected from scorpions originating from two different geographic regions in North Africa contain different toxins. The venom from Tozeur (Tunisia) scorpions contains Toxins I, II, and I' and that from Chellala (Algeria) scorpions contains Toxins I, II, and III (Fig. 2). Toxin I' and III may be considered as isotoxins to AI, the first differing only by a conservative amino acid change in position 17 (AaH I Val, AaH I' Ile, ROCHAT et al., 1970a) and the second by greater number of amino acid residues (MIRANDA et al., 1970a). The subspecies *A. a. Hector* has been considered, from a taxonomic point of view, as being homogenous (VACHON, 1952). However, the interchange between toxins AaH III and AaH I', which must be a genetic characteristic, suggests a taxonomic heterogeneity. Recently, the taxonomy of *A. australis* has been reconsidered and constant morphologic differences between scorpions of both geographic origins were found (Vachon: personal communication).

The complete amino acid sequences of AaH I, AaH I', and AaH II (ROCHAT et al., 1970c, 1972) as well as the first 35 amino residues from the N-terminal end of AaH III (ROCHAT et al., 1975a), have been determined (Fig. 2). The positions of the disulfide bridges of AaH II have been established, using digestion of the native protein by proteolytic enzymes: trypsin, chymotrypsin, papaine, thermolysin. From the study of the cystine-containing peptides, the four disulfide bridges were found to link the half-cystine residues number 12 and 63, 16 and 36, 22 and 48 (KOPEYAN et al., 1974). Two disulfide bridges of AaH I are located in identical positions (ROCHAT et al., 1970a). It is not unlikely that half-cystine residues are actually paired in the same manner in every scorpion mammal toxin. Therefore, the location of the disulfide bonds must play a fundamental role in the structure-activity relationships of these "mini-proteins." The conformation of AaH II has been studied by CHICHEPORTICHE and LAZDUNSKI (1970). Using optical rotatory dispersion and ultraviolet difference spectrophotometry, they found that this toxin can exist in four different molecular forms, depending on pH and temperature. The form which is predominant between pH 4 and 9 is very stable under heat

Table 1. Amino acid composition of some Buthinae neurotoxins

Amino acid	Androctonus australis Hector						Androctonus mauretanicus		Buthus occitanus paris
	I[a]	I′[b]	II[a]	III[a]	IT[c]	CT[d]	I[e]	II[e]	III[f]
Aspartic acid	9	9	8	8	11	6	9	10	9
Threonine	2	2	3	0	4	4	1	1	3
Serine	6	6	2	6	6	4	4	3	2
Glutamic acid	0	0	4	0	3	10	4	4	3
Proline	6	6	3	6	1	2	3	3	2
Glycine	6	6	7	6	4	4	6	7	7
Alanine	1	1	3	3	3	2	3	3	6
Half-cystine	8	8	8	8	8	10	8	8	8
Valine	5	4	4	6	3	4	1	1	1
Methionine	0	0	0	0	0	0	0	0	0
Isoleucine	2	3	1	3	2 – 3	2	3	3	3
Leucine	4	4	2	4	5 – 6	2	3	3	2
Tyrosine	3	3	7	3	5	4	5	6	4
Phenylalanine	1	1	1	1	1	0	2	2	1
Lysine	6	6	5	6	7	4	5	6	4
Histidine	1	1	2	2	1	0	0	0	0
Arginine	2	2	3	1	1	9	2	3	3
Tryptophan	1	1	1	1	1	2	2	2	2
Total	63	63	64	64	66 – 68	69	61	65	60
Molecular weight	6794	6808	7249	6826	7383 – 7609	8104	6898	7430	6574

[a] MIRANDA et al., 1970a; [b] determined from sequence data; [c] ZLOTKIN et al., 1971; [d] ZLOTKIN [h] not determined.

denaturation and treatment with 9.5 M urea; it has a high degree of ordered structure.

Two mammal toxins, Am I and Am II, have been purified from the venom of *A. mauretanicus* (Tables 1 and 2, Fig. 2) collected in Morocco. Their amino acid compositions were determined (ROSSO et al., in preparation) and the amino acid sequence of the N-terminal end of Am II was established (ROCHAT et al., 1975a).

Two toxins active on mammals, Bop I and Bop II, have been purified from the venom of *B. occitanus paris* (see Tables 1 and 2, Fig. 2), collected in the northern part of Morocco. Their amino acid composition was further established (MARTIN, 1974) and they were both characterized by automatic Edman degradation (ROCHAT et al., 1975a).

Three toxins, Bot I, Bot II, and Bot III, have been purified from the venom of *B. occitanus tunetanus* (see Tables 1 and 2, Fig. 2), collected in the area of Mecheria (Algeria). Both their amino acid compositions and their amino acid sequences from the N-terminal end were determined (MIRANDA et al., 1970a; RO-CHAT et al., 1970b). The abundance of mucoproteins in this venom has obliged the employment of acetone fractionation, which has, however, resulted in a poor yield of toxicity. This problem was corrected by using 0.5 M acetic acid in Sephadex

Table 1 (continued)

Buthus occitanus tunetanus							Leiurus quinquestriatus quinquestriatus				
I [a]	I' [g]	I'' [g]	I''' [g]	II [a]	III [a]	III' [g]	I [a]	II [a]	III [a]	IV [a]	V [a]
9	11	8	10	9	9	9	10	10	9	9	10
2	3	3	3	1	3	3	1	2	1	3	1
2	2	3	2	2	2	2	2	4	3	3	3
5	3	3	2	5	4	5	2	2	2	3	4
4	3	4	3	3	3	1	3	4	2	3	2
6	5	5	5	6	7	7	8	5	5	7	7
5	6	4	6	5	3	3	4	2	5 − 6	4	3
8	8	8	8	8	8	8	8	8	8	8	8
2	4	3	4	2	4	5	5	3	3 − 4	3	2
0	0	0	0	0	0	0	0	0	0	0	0
3	2	3	2	4	1	1	4	1	2	4	2
3	2	4	2	3	1	3	3	2 − 3	2	3	2
4	7	7	7	5	7	6	3	5	6	5	6
1	1	0	1	1	1	1	1	0 − 1	1	0	2
4	3	6	4	5	5	4	4	4	4	6	8
1	1	1	1	1	1	1	3	1	1	0	0
2	2	1	2	3	4	5	1	2	3	3	3
2	h	h	h	2	1	1	2	1	2	2	2
63				65	64	65	64	56 − 58	59 − 61	66	65
6980				7539	7270	7395	6928	6211 − 6472	6693 − 6863	7313	7462

et al., 1975; [e] Rosso et al., to be published; [f] MARTIN, 1974; [g] ROCHAT et al., to be published;

G-50 chromatography, enabling the isolation of several other mammal toxins, characterized by their amino acid composition (ROCHAT et al., in preparation) as well as by the N-terminal amino acid sequences (ROCHAT et al., 1975a).

Five toxins active on mammals, Lqq I to Lqq V, have been purified from the venom of *L. quinquestriatus quinquestriatus* (see Tables 1 and 2), collected in the area of Khartom (Sudan) and their amino acid compositions were determined (MIRANDA et al., 1970a). It is likely that isotoxins might be found in Lqq II and Lqq III, where fractional numbers of amino acid residues are observed, i.e., leucine and phenylalanine (Lqq II), alanine and valine (Lqq III). Determination of the sequence will solve this problem, which may be identical with the case of toxin I of *A. australis Hector* collected in Tozeur (Tunisia) (see above). The N-terminal sequences of Lqq III and Lqq V have been determined (ROCHAT et al., 1970b).

For purification of scorpion toxins, the above method (Sect. B I.) was also successfully employed to the venom of the scorpion *C. suffusus suffusus* (GARCIA et al., in preparation, see Fig. 2).

Scorpion toxins are composed of a single polypeptide chain cross-linked by four disulfide bridges. Table 1 presents their amino acid composition. Molecular weight was calculated according to these data, rather than by ultracentrifugation, as had been done previously for AaH I and AaH II, the first two toxins to be

Table 2. Activity of Buthinae mammal neurotoxins

Toxin	Specific activity LD_{50}/absorbance unit at 280 nm	Weight of the LD_{50} per kg mouse μg
AaH	1980	17
AaH I'	1980 [a]	17 [a]
AaH II	2400	9
AaH III	1290	23
Am I	720	29
Am II	1000	19
Bop I	80	[b]
Bop II	100	176
Bot I	205	91
Bot I'	40	[b]
Bot I''	500	[b]
Bot I'''	125	[b]
Bot II	126	144
Bot III	956	21
Bot III'	22	810
Lqq I	375	63
Lqq II	544	47
Lqq III	259	64
Lqq IV	265	70
Lqq V	717	25

[a] AaH I' must have same activity as AaH I since mixture of AaH I and I' purified from venom of animals living in Tunisia shows same activity than pure AaH I from animals living in Algeria.

[b] Not determined.

characterized (Rochat et al., 1967). However, as all these proteins are eluted from columns of Sephadex G-50 in a volume very close to that of AaH I and AaH II, it is evident that the minimum molecular weight of the isolated toxins represents their actual molecular weight. This was entirely confirmed by the amino acid sequence determinations. Figure 2 shows the results obtained so far on 16 toxins from Buthinae, including the insect toxin of *A. australis Hector* and two toxins from a Centrurinae (*C. suffusus suffusus*). Maximum homology in the sequences is obtained when half-cystine residues are placed at identical sequence positions. This result is particularly obvious when considering the N-terminal part: Residue 2 is basic (Lys or Arg); Residue 3 is acidic (Asp or Glu) except in the case of Bop I (where a Gly was found); Residues 4, 6, and 7 are always hydrophobic; Tyr is always found in position 5; Asn is found in position 11 in all Buthinae toxins but Gly exists in the two Centrurinae toxins; Tyr is generally constant in positions 15 (with the exceptions of Lqq V and Am II which contain Phe) and 25 (except when this position corresponds to a deletion as for AaH I, I' and III).

It was claimed previously that scorpion toxins formed a new set of homologous proteins, divided into three groups according to structure similarities (Rochat et al., 1970b). Group 1 would comprise AaH I, I', and III.; Group 2 AaH II, Bot III', III, Lqq V, and Am II; and Group 3 Bot I, I', I'', II, Lqq III, Bop I, and II. However, the last two toxins, which obviously belong to the third group

```
                    10        20        30        40        50        60        70
AaH IT      KKDGYAVDSS-GKAPECLL---SNYCNDZCKTVHYADKGY ...

AaH I       KRDGYIVYPN-NCVYHCVPP-----CDGLCKKN-GGSSGSSCFLV-PSGLACWC-KDLPDNVPIKDTSRKCT
AaH I'      KRDGYIVYPN-NCVYHCIPP-----CDGLCKKN-GGSSGSSCFLV-PSGLACWC-KDLPDNVPIKDTSRKCT
AaH III     VRDGYIVNSK-NCVYHCVPP-----CDGLCKKN-GASSGSSC ...

AaH II      VKDGYIVDDV-NCTYFCGR---NAYCNEECTKL-KGESG-YCQWASPYGNACYCYK-LPDHVRTKGPGR-CH
Bot III'    LKDGYIVDDR-NCTYFCGT---NAYCNEECVKL-KGE ...
Bot III     VKDGYIVDDR-NCTYFCGR---NAYCNEEC ...
Lqq V       LKDGYIVDDK-NCTFFCGR---NAYCNNEC ...
Am  II      LKDGYIIEDI-NCVFFCGR---NAYCDXXC ...

Bop II      GRDAYIADDX-NCAYXCAL---XXYCN ...
Bop I       GRGVYIADIA-NCAY ...
Bot I       GRDAYIAQPE-NCVYECAE---NSYCNDWC ...
Bot I'      VRDAYIAQNY-NCVYTCFK---NEYCNDLCXXN-G ...
Bot I''     GRDAYIAQPE-NCVYECAK ...
Bot II      GRDAYIAQPE-NCVYECAK---NWYCND ...
Lqq III     VRDAYIAKNY-NCVYECFR---DSYCNDLC ...

Css III     -KEGYLVSKSTGCKYECLKLGDNDYCLRECKQQYGKSSGGYCYAF-----ACWC-EALPDHTOVW-VPNKCT
Css I       -KEGYLVSKSTGCKYECLKLGDNDYCL ...
CsE I       -KDGYLVEK-TGCKKTCYKLGENDFCNRECKWKHIGGSYGYCYGF-----GCYC-EGLPDSTQTWPLPNKCT
```

Fig. 2. Primary sequences of some Buthinae and *Centruroides* scorpion toxins. AaH = *Androctonus australis Hector*. Am = *Androctonus mauretanicus*. Bop = *Buthus occitanus paris*. Bot = *Buthus occitanus tunetanus*. CsE = *Centruroides sculpturatus* Ewing. Css = *Centruroides suffusus suffusus*. Lqq = *Leiurus quinquestriatus quinquestriatus*. Different toxins (indicated by roman numbers), were purified according to criterion of mice lethality, and therefore belong to the group of "mammal" toxins. AaH IT represents insect toxin of *A. australis*. (See Sect. C VI 3.) Amino acids were placed in a manner to obtain maximum homology. — : deletion, X : not determined

according to their first seven residues, show in positions 8 (for both) and 9 (for Bop II) amino acids which are found in the same position in toxins of Group 1. To the above three groups of the Buthinae venoms one has now to add a new group characteristic of Centrurinae which includes both toxins I and II of *C. suffusus suffusus*. Neurotoxin I of *C. sculpturatus*. Ewing the amino acid sequence of which has been determined by Babin et al. (1975), obviously belongs to the same group (Fig. 2).

The specific toxicities of scorpion toxins differ considerably (Table 2). Of particular interest is the comparison of AaH II, Bot III, and III'. Taking into account their amino acid compositions (Table 1), and the sequences already established, we may expect that the high degree of homology found in their N-terminal ends will also exist in their C-terminal sequences. Since AaH II is twice as active as Bot III and about 100 times more active than Bot III', the nature of the amino acid residues found in position 10 and 19 might be of importance with regard to the biological activity of these proteins. Thus, the comparative study of primary sequences might yield significant information concerning structure activity relationships of scorpion toxins. Furthermore, since the above three proteins were found to possess common antigenic properties (Delori personal communication), Bot III', which is the least potent, may be considered as a natural anatoxin of AaH I, which might be of great importance in antivenomous serotherapy.

3. Chemical Modifications

Chemical modifications of certain functional amino acid residues in AaH, AaH II and AaH III have been performed (Sampieri and Habersetzer-Rochat, 1975). The results indicate that: (1) One of the four disulfide bridges of AaH II could be selectively reduced; after S-methylation of the cysteine residues thus formed, the toxicity was lost. (2) The only tryptophan residue (position 38) of AaH II is not included in the active site. (3) In the case of AaH II, modification of five carboxylates out of seven (two of them are buried — Chicheportiche and Lazdunski, 1970), suppresses the toxic activity. (4) Acetylation of AaH II results in a nontoxic derivative which does not precipitate with the specific antiserum against native AaH II. Treatment with hydroxylamine, which reverses only the acetylation of phenol groups, recovered the serologic response of the modified protein. It is concluded that at least one tyrosine residue must be involved in an antigenic site. Similar results have been obtained with AaH I, but, in that case, hydroxylamine treatment is unnecessary in order to obtain a serologic response of the modified protein. These results prompted the preparation of an antiserum, employing anatoxins obtained by acetylation of the total toxic fraction separated by the gel filtration of the venom. This resulted in the preparation of a very potent antiserum against the crude venom (Delori, personal communication). (5) Modifications, including acetylation of amino groups, of the mammal toxins led to inactive derivates exept in those modifications which preserve the electrical charge (guanidination). In the case of AaH I, the loss of activity very closely follows the alkylation of one lysine residue.

Iodination of AaH I and AaH II enabled incorporation of 0.6 iodine atom per molecule of protein without loss of activity (Rochat, C. et al., 1972). Using KI at pH 8.0, radioiodinated fully active mammal toxins with specific radioactivities of about 40 Ci/mmole were obtained. The relative reactivities to iodine of the three tyrosine residues of AaH I were determined using automatic Edman degradation of the modified derivatives. It was concluded that tyrosine in position 8 is not directly involved in the activity.

The need for radioiodinated derivatives with very high specific radioactivities in order to study their binding to the receptor sites, demanded the development of a new method. Using lactoperoxydase and hydrogen peroxyde to oxidize $Na^{125}I$, ^{125}I-labeled derivatives of specific radioactivities higher than 2000 Ci/mmole and preserved toxicity were obtained with AaH I and AaH II (Rochat et al., 1975b). Approximately one iodine atom was incorporated per mole of protein. Recovery of the labeled mammal toxins is obtained upon their precipitation with a monospecific antiserum and dissociation of the precipitates by acetic acid. This procedure allows the recovery of the modified protein in a short time (4 h), with a good yield (60—80%) and in a small volume (1 ml). The specific radioactivity is very high and can be easily calculated, since the exact amount of modified mammal toxin recovered is known.

III. Pharmacology

1. Lethal Potency and Symptomatology

It is common in the practice of toxinology that the first acquaintance with the pharmacologic properties of a toxic material is obtained through determination of its lethal potency and the careful observation of the symptoms preceding the relevant organism's death. It may appear perplexing that discrepancies exist among reports of different workers with data concerning the simplest and commonest toxinologic criteria of the 50% lethal dose (LD_{50}) of scorpion venoms, as determined with laboratory mice. These discrepancies follow from certain technical-experimental variables, such as differences in strains of laboratory mice (STAHNKE, 1963; ZLOTKIN et al., 1975b), routes of injection (BÜCHERL, 1953; BÜCHERL and PUCCA, 1956) methods for extraction and treatment of the venom (MIRANDA et al., 1964a; ZLOTKIN and SHULOV, 1969b; BÜCHERL, 1955), the geographic origin of scorpions collected (BALOZET, 1971), and even statistical methods of sampling and manipulation of experimental data, which all may strongly influence the results.

Table 3 presents mice LD_{50} data of 17 electrically milked and lyophilized buthid venoms subcutaneously injected, listed in the order of their toxicity to mice. Of these venoms, 16 were applied in 1 single experiment, using identical methods (ZLOTKIN et al., 1971a), and as such are well comparable. For comparative purposes the reader is also referred to the data of BALOZET (1971) and BÜCHERL (1971). It may be briefly stated that the lethal potency of the dangerous scorpion venoms ranges between 0.3 and 1.0 mg/kg and, as such, these may be classified among the most potent animal venoms (ZLOTKIN, 1973).

There exists a strong resemblance between the symptoms of envenomation

Table 3. The 50% lethal dose to mice (LD_{50}) and the contraction paralysis unit (CPU) to blowfly larvae of different scorpion venoms[a]

Scorpion	[b]LD_{50} mg/kg mice	[c]CPU mg/kg larvae
L. quinquestriatus	0.25	2.2
A. aeneas aeneas	0.31	0.5
A. mauretanicus mauretanicus	0.31	4.7
A. australis	0.32	2.9
C. santa maria	0.39	32.2
A. crassicauda	0.40	6.8
Tityus serrulatus	0.43	21.7
Buthiscus bicalcaratus	0.60	0.7
C. limpidus tecomanus	0.69	2.2
A. amoreuxi	0.75	3.6
Buthacus leptochelis	0.77	0.9
B. occitanus tunetanus	0.90	0.7
B. arenicola	0.99	0.7
C. sculpturatus[d]	1.12	not tested
B. occitanus paris	4.15	0.3
Buthotus minax	4.25	3.0
Parabuthus transvaalicus	4.25	3.5

[a] Taken from ZLOTKIN et al. (1971a). The venoms were obtained by electrical milking followed by lyophilization.
[b] Subcutaneous injection into mice of both sexes weighing about 20 g.
[c] Tested on Sarcophaga argyrystoma larvae weighting about 100 mg. See Section C IV.
[d] Taken from STAHNKE (1963a).

of test animals as induced by different buthid scorpion venoms such as Buthinae (BALOZET, 1971) or those belonging to the genera of *Centruroides* (WATT et al., 1974) as well as *Tityus* (SCHÖTTLER, 1954; BÜCHERL, 1971). The characteristic phenomena generally appear in the following order: (1) Immediate local pain. (2) Hyperexcitability, restlessness, violent jumpings. (3) Salivation and lacryma- tion. (4) Accelerated respiration. (5) Convulsions and contractions and muscle twitchings. (6) Spastic paralysis with tautness of limbs. (7) Death due to respiratory failure may occur from a few minutes to several hours.

General neurotoxicity of an excitatory nature, including the autonomic (para- sympathetic and sympathetic) as well as the skeletal neuromuscular system was indicated also by the symptoms following human envenomation by buthid scor- pions (EFRATI, 1949; BARSOUM et al., 1954; STURMAN, 1962; GUERON and YAROM, 1970; BALOZET, 1971; DINIZ, 1971). The commonest symptoms include parasympa- thetic phenomena such as salivation, lacrymation, sphincter relaxation, gastric hyperdistension, bradycardia and hypotension, as well as typical sympathetic phe- nomena, such as mydriasis, pilo-erection, perspiration, hyperglycemia, tachycardia, and hypertension, accompanied by clear effects on the skeletal musculature expressed in twitching, spasms, and muscle contraction. Lethality to humans is often related to cardiovascular collapse and pulmonary edema (STURMAN, 1962; GUERON et al., 1967; GUERON and YAROM, 1970).

The above symptoms and clinical observations have directed and guided experi- mental investigation of the pharmacologic action of scorpion venoms and toxins. Special emphasis was given to the effect on the cardiovascular, respiratory, and neuromuscular systems, as presented below.

2. Cardiovascular Effects

a) Clinical Investigations

Clinical investigation has indicated that the cardiovascular manifestations and dam- age which are related to general sympathetic involvement, play an important role in the pathology of scorpion envenomation. A survey of 39 patients stung by *L. quinquestriatus* indicated electrocardiographic abnormalities such as hyperten- sion, peripheral vascular collapse, congestive heart failure, pulmonary edema, and morphologic changes in the myocardium (GUERON et al., 1967; GUERON and YA- ROM, 1970). These effects were ascribed to the increase in the level of circulating catecholamines as indicated by the elevation of vanylmandelic acid (VMA), adrena- line, and noradrenaline in the urine of patients with severe scorpion sting (GUERON and WEIZMANN, 1969). Myocarditis was also found in 34 out of 45 patients stung by the scorpion *Tityus trinitatis;* this was considered as a common complication of scorpion sting in Trinidad and a frequent cause of death (POON-KING, 1963). The above clinical findings were subjected to experimental examination with labo- ratory test animals.

b) Histopathologic Changes

The morphologic changes in the myocardium were observed by necropsy studies in fatal scorpion sting, and consist of degenerative muscle fiber changes, local

necrosis, and interstitial edema and cellularity (GUERON and YAROM, 1970). These
were experimentally reproduced in hearts of dogs injected with (i.m. and i.v.)
L. quinquestriatus venom (see Fig. 3, YAROM and BRAUN, 1969, 1970). It has been
indicated that it is unlikely that the myocardial damage is due to ischemia or
anoxia (no changes in coronaries and mild pulmonary pathology); rather, it is
a result of catecholamine overdosage (SCHENK and MOSS, 1966). The presumption
of sympatomimetic overstimulation as the primary cause of myocardial injury
was supported by its diminution following adrenergic blocking agents (YAROM
and BRAUN, 1969, 1970). However, a more careful examination of the ultrastructural

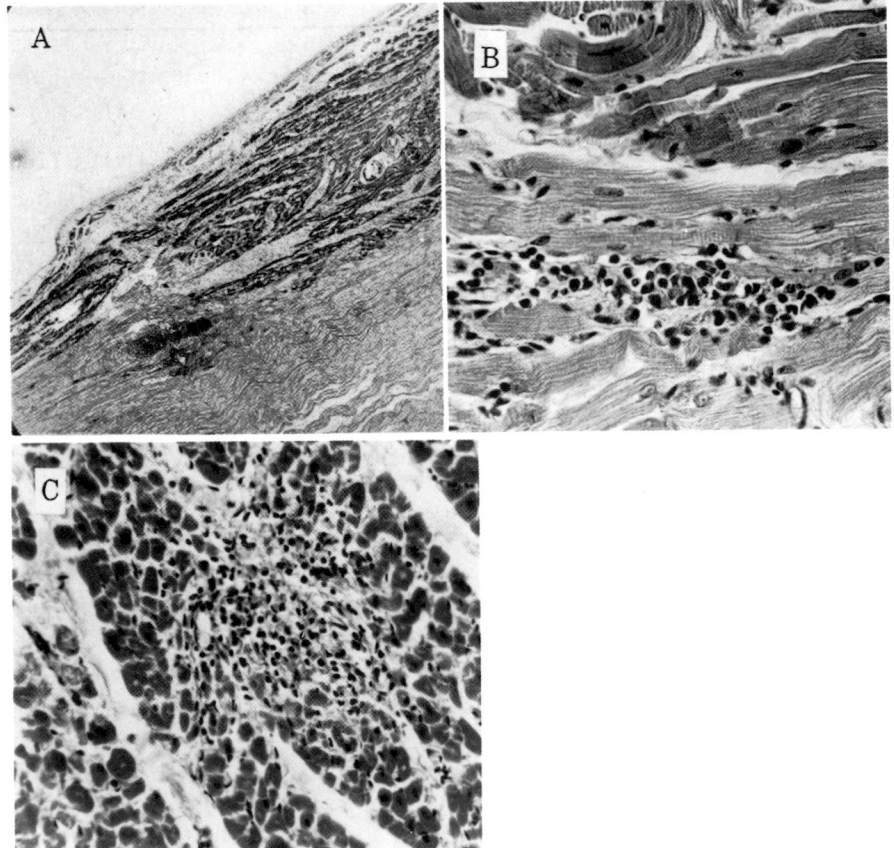

Fig. 3A–C. Histopathologic changes in hearts following treatment with scorpion venom. (A)
Dog's heart injected i.m. with 0.5 mg/kg of wet (unlyophilized) *L. quinquestriatus* venom.
Subendocardial focal necrosis (darker staining) in dog's heart examined 24 h after scorpion
venom injection. Selye's acid fuchsin technique × 42 (taken from YAROM and BRAUN, 1969).
Focal lesions consisted of well-defined areas of exudate containing numerous polymorphonuclear cells as well as lymphocytes accompanied by capillary and venous congestion and interstitial cellularity. (B) As above, magnified view of myocardium demonstrating focal muscle
necrosis and interstitial cellularity (lymphocytes and histiocytes). H & E × 260 (from YAROM,
personal communication) (C) Section of myocardium of 2-year-old child who died about
12 h after *L. quinquestriatus* scorpion sting. There is focal muscle necrosis and marked interstitial
cellularity. H & E × 270. (taken from GUERON and YAROM, 1970)

myocardial changes induced by scorpion venom expressed in intracellular edema, dilation of the tubular system, scattered destruction of I-band, lipid deposition and no changes in mitochondria, nucleus, or sarcolemma (YAROM and BRAUN, 1971 a), indicate that they differ in their severity, kinetics, and in some qualitative features from those caused by massive overdosage or sustained infusion of catecholamines (FERRANS et al., 1969; MOSS et al., 1966). Therefore, it has been concluded that "catecholamine oversecretion alone cannot explain all the cardiovascular changes or the rapid heart failure," emphasizing the complexity of the pathogenesis of the myocardial damage (YAROM and BRAUN, 1971 a, b).

The possibility of a direct effect on the cell membrane, altering its permeability to ions, was hinted at by ultrastructural visualization of calcium ions in myocardial biopsies from dogs intravenously injected with *Leiurus* scorpion venom (YAROM and BRAUN, 1971 b). Assuming that this represents a primary effect of the venom, it might explain the increased contractility of the cardiac muscle. However, the primacy of the effect on calcium displacement and permeability is doubtful and should be supported by experimental evidence (See Sect. C VII.). On the other hand, it has been shown by YAROM and BRAUN (1971 a) that smaller doses of venom (0.15 mg/kg wet venom) introduced directly via a coronary artery and causing an evident positive inotropic effect, produced no ultrastructural changes in the heart muscle. In recent studies YAROM et al. (1974), using rat hearts perfused with various doses of crude *Leiurus* venom, showed that the ultrastructural changes are transient and temporary and that some recovery occurred while the venom was being administered. It is noteworthy that the histologic changes were in accordance with EKG examinations, indicating a typical myocardial infarct pattern, which was reversible. The origin of the transience of the above effects is not clear, but it is reminiscent of the rhythmical changes in contractility which are transmitter-release dependent, observed in smooth muscle preparations subjected to scorpion venom (TAZIEFFE-DEPIERRE, 1972; CUNHA-MELO et al., 1973; TINTPULVER, 1975, see Section C IV.3).

It may be concluded that the above morphologic changes induced by scorpion venom certainly serve as a histopathologic presentation of the myocardial lesion, but it is unlikely that they do indeed represent its primary effect. It appears that they are secondary manifestations which probably follow from a release of pharmacologic substances, either through a systemic effect on the central nervous system and/or by a local transmitter release due to an effect at the postganglionic nerve fiber level or at nerve terminals at the neuromyocardial junctions.

c) Vascular Effects

Attention was directed to the hemodynamic aspects of cardiovascular injury. The initial positive inotropism, tachycardia, and hypertension followed by arrhythmias, bradycardia, and hypotension due to an intravenous application of scorpion venom, was demonstrated with venomous species of all the main dangerous genera of Buthidae, such as *Centruroides* (DEL POZO, 1956; PATTERSON, 1960) *Tityus* (FREIRE-MAIA et al., 1970, 1974) *Leiurus* (BRAUN et al., 1969; CHEYMOL et al., 1974), *Androctonus* and *Buthus* (CHEYMOL et al., 1974). Hypertension may be considered as a very characteristic effect of all buthid venoms and has been observed in a wide variety of test animals (WILSON, 1904; ARTHUS, 1913; HOUSSAY, 1919; PHISALIX, 1922; MOHAMMED, 1942; DEL POZO et al., 1944; RAMOS and CORRADO, 1954; FREIRE-MAIA and FERREIRA, 1961). The administration of *Leiurus* venom into open-chested dogs in doses varying between 0.2 and 0.5 mg/kg evoked a rise in systemic blood pressure accompanied by increased systemic blood flow, augmented myocardial contractility and a rise in pulmonary arterial and venous pressures (BRAUN et al., 1969). It was indicated that the above hemodynamic alternations caused by scorpion venom resembled those observed following infusion of adrenaline or noradrenaline (RAAB, 1960; SARNOFF, 1960). Catecholamines may elevate the blood pressure either by vasoconstriction or increasing the heart output. Release of catecholamines may originate either from sympathetic nerve terminals due to preganglionic, ganglionic, or postganglionic stimulation and/or from the adrenal gland due to a sympathetic stimulation.

Postganglionic activation and adrenal release were suggested as the main causes of hypertension induced by *Centruroides* venom. Hypertension was not influenced by spinal destruction (DEL POZO, 1956) but was strongly affected by ligation or removal of the adrenal glands (PATTERSON, 1960; DEL POZO, 1956). The supposition that scorpion venoms may induce sympathetic release was suggested by the early works of MOHAMMED (1950) and MOHAMMED et al. (1954), indicating the elevation of sugar and potassium concentration and the decrease in sodium concentration in the blood upon injection of sublethal doses of *L. quinquestriatus* venom. The release of catecholamines from the sympathetic postganglionic nerve endings as the main cause of the hypertensive effect of *Tityus* venom and its purified toxin was suggested by RAMOS and CORRADO (1954), FREIRE-MAIA and FERREIRA (1961), CORRADO et al. (1974), and FREIRE-MAIA et al. (1974). It has been found that spinalization adrenalectomy and hexamethonium did not alter the hypertensive response, which was, on the other hand, blocked by alpha-sympatholytic agents, absent in reserpinized animals, and abolished by guanethidine in adrenalectomized animals.

Sympathetic stimulation as a cause of the hypertensive effects of scorpion venom was similarly demonstrated with the venoms of Buthinae such as *L. quinquestriatus* (ISMAIL et al., 1972; CHEYMOL et al., 1974) *B. minax* (ISMAIL et al., 1973); *A. australis* and *B. occitanus* (CHEYMOL et al., 1974). This was indicated by its counteraction by andrenolytic agents (ISMAIL et al., 1972, 1973; CHEYMOL et al., 1974), its absence in reserpinized animals (ISMAIL et al., 1972, 1973). CHEYMOL et al. (1974) suggested that the release of catecholamines originated not only from nerve terminals but also from the adrenal gland. This conclusion was supported by a direct estimation of adrenaline and noradrenaline contents of the blood. The primary site of stimulation was defined as preganglionic since venom-induced contraction of the nictitating membrane (accompanied by a simultaneous hypertension) was blocked by hemicholinium. If this conclusion is true, then the venom-induced hypertension should have been blocked or at least partially affected by a ganglionic blocker such as hexamethonium. The effect of hexamethonium was not indicated in the above investigation (CHEYMOL et al., 1974).

It has been indicated that the brief initial hypotensive effect preceding the hypertension caused by *B. minax* venom in cats and rats was partially blocked by atropine. As such it was defined "to be of a cholinergic nature" (ISMAIL et al.,

1973). However, since there is no parasympathetic innervation of blood vessels, it may be assumed that the above cholinergic action affecting blood pressure was mediated by the heart, decreasing its output. As such, a short lasting hypotension preceding the hypertension has been indicated also with the venom of *Tityus* (Ramos and Corrado, 1954; Freire-Maia and Ferreira, 1961) as well as with that of *A. australis* (Cheymol et al., 1974, Fig. 2c). Freire-Maia et al. (1974) attribute the hypotensive effect of *Tityus* toxin, at least in part, to sinus bradycardia and to sinoatrial and atrioventricular blockade.

d) Cardiac Dynamics

If appears, therefore, that the above hemodynamic changes are partially dependent on, or at least correlated to, the responses of the heart. The electrocardiographic recordings obtained by the application of *Leiurus* venom to dogs (Braun et al., 1969) closely resemble those described for *Tytius* toxin (Freire-Maia, 1974). In both cases sinus tachycardia (higher doses evoked sinus bradycardia), ventricular ectopic beats, widening of QRS complex, atrioventricular block, idioventricular rhythm, atrial fibrillation, and arrhythmias were indicated. The mechanism of these phenomena was clarified in the exhaustive study of Freire-Maia et al. (1974) who found that the bradycardial effect in vagotomized animals was enhanced by physiostigmine, decreased by hexamethonium, and abolished by atropine. Bradycardia was ascribed to the release of acetylcholine by action on vagal ganglia and postganglionic nerve endlings in the heart. Tachycardia was antagonized by propranolol. It has been concluded that arrhythmias are due to the release of catecholamines and acetylcholine. The sinus tachycardia, ventricular ectopic beats and idioventricular rhythm are caused by activation of β-adrenergic receptors. These main conclusions are in general accord with previous and recent investigations with hearts either *in situ* or as isolated perfused preparations. The ability of scorpion venoms to activate both components of the autonomic nervous system at the postganglionic level, resulting in the local release of the corresponding transmitters, was demonstrated by Corrado et al. (1968) applying *Tityus* scorpion venom on the isolated perfused heart of a guinea pig. The action of the venom (10 µg/ml) is expressed in a short transient bradycardia (which is blocked by atropine and potentiated by eserine) followed by a strong and chronotropic response which is abolished by propranolol and is absent in the hearts of reserpine-treated animals. Both the stimulatory and depressory effects of the venom were not affected by hexamethonium.

This fundamental study of Corrado et al., (1968) may serve as a basis for comparing some recent investigations using the same preparation performed with several venoms of Buthinae such as *L. quinquestriatus* (Ismail et al., 1972; Cheymol et al., 1974) *B. minax* (Ismail et al., 1973) *A. australis* and *B. occitanus* (Cheymol et al., 1974). The following main findings were indicated: (1) The dual activation of the sympathetic and parasympathetic fibers has been equally demonstrated with the above Buthinae venoms. (2) Propranolol antagonizes the stimulatory effect whereas atropine antagonizes the depressory effects. (3) The initial cardiac action of the above venoms is stimulatory (and not inhibitory, see Fig. 4) unlike *Tityus* venom (Corrado et al., 1968). It is then followed by bradycardia, negative

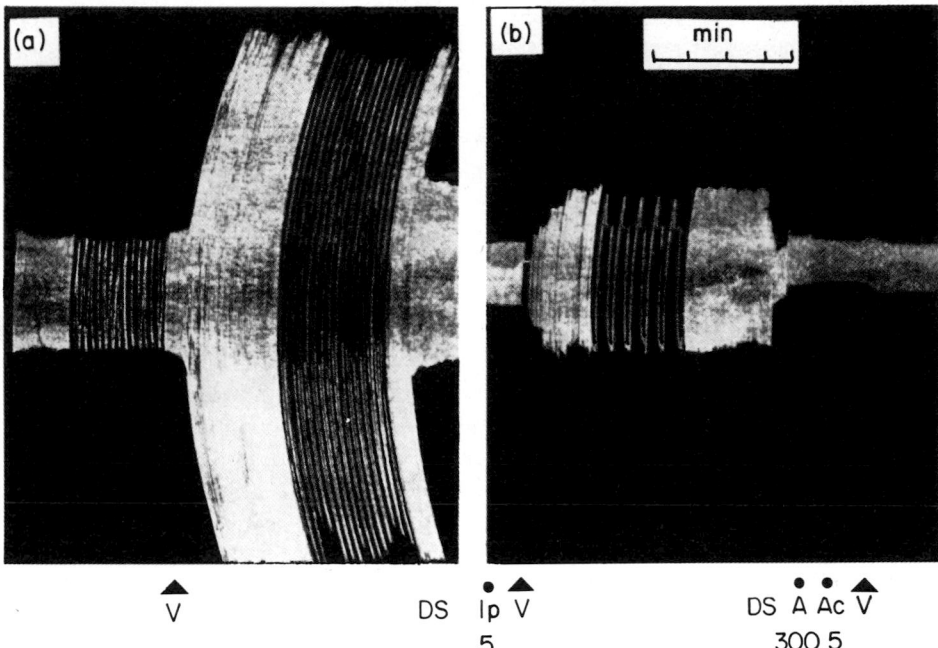

Fig. 4. The Effect of *B. minax* scorpion venom on isolated rabbit's heart. *V*, venom (50 µg); *Ip*, isoprenaline; *A*, atropine; *Ac*, acetylcholine. Numbers indicate total dose in micrograms. At DS, drum was stopped and where individual contractions are clearly seen drum speed was increased to 125 mm/min for 5 s. Between (*a*) and (*b*) propranolol was infused at a rate of 1 µg/min for 30 min. A marked positive inotropic effect, starting immediately after venom application and partly antagonized by propranolol, is indicated. (taken from ISMAIL et al., 1973)

inotropism, arrhythmia, and irreversible blockage. As previously indicated, the above release of autopharmacologic substances not only affects cardiac dynamics but also induces histopathologic changes, resulting in an infarct which certainly contributes to heart failure.

Considering the background of the above information, the recent discovery by FAYET et al. (1974) that scorpion toxin stimulates cultured cardiac cells is highly interesting. It has been found that toxin II of *A. australis* (similar results were obtained using the closely related toxins I and III, MIRANDA et al., 1970a) in concentrations of 0.1 — 1 and 10 µg/ml when applied to a tissue culture of isolated or clustered 11-day-old chick embryo heart cells, caused an apparent positive chronotropic effect and an arrhythmia followed by fibrillation and tetanus, respectively. Since the above tissue culture is considered nerve-free (FAYET et al., 1974), this stimulatory effect should be considered as direct and not mediated by adrenergic transmitter release. This conclusion is strongly supported by the fact that: (1) reserpine-treated (10^{-5} M for 24 h) cells had the same contractive activity and responded to scorpion toxin in the same way as untreated cells. (2) DL-propranolol does not inhibit scorpion toxin action at doses which completely antagonize the effects of adrenergic agonists. These facts stand in a clear contradiction to data concerning scorpion venom and toxin effects on the heart. As stated above, preliminary reserpination, as well as propranolol application, greatly abolish venom-induced stimulatory effects on isolated perfused heart preparation (CORRADO et al., 1968; ISMAIL et al., 1972, 1973; CHEYMOL et al., 1974). Therefore, it may be concluded that there exists an essential difference in the response to scorpion venom between the embryonic heart cells and the heart. This may resemble the phenomenon of extreme differences in sensitivity to tetrodotoxin (TTX) during normal embryonic development of the chick heart, due to the replacement of tetrodotoxin-insensitive slow Na^+ channels by tetrodotoxin-sensitive fast Na^+ channels, or the conversion of the former to the latter (SHIGENOBU and SPERLAKIS, 1971; SPERELAKIS and SHIGENOBU, 1974). The apparent decrease in sensitivity to the direct stimulatory effect of scorpion toxins as demonstrated in the finally differentiated and organized heart tissue when compared to its embryonic stages, may also represent essential structure functional changes. This phenomenon should serve as an object for further investigation.

3. Respiratory Effects

Clinical observation on scorpion-envenomated humans emphasized the typical irregularities in the respiratory movements which are sometimes of the Cheyne-Stokes type (BALOZET, 1971). Death is very often attributed to respiratory paralysis, caused by Buthinae (BALOZET, 1971) Centruroides (DEL POZO, 1956), and Tityus (MAGALHAES, 1928) scorpion envenomations.

Pharmacologic investigations of the respiratory effects of scorpion venom were substantially performed with Tityus and Centruroides venoms, which may serve as a background to the relatively scanty information presented in the Buthinae venom. The injection of crude venom into different test animals resulted in hyperpnea, tachypnea, respiratory paralysis, and periodic respiration (MAGALHAES, 1928; DEL POZO et al., 1945; PATERSON, 1964; STAHNKE, 1966). Bronchiolar obstructions (due to secretions) and laryngeal and bronchiolar muscle contraction, are common manifestations of scorpion envenomation (DEL POZO, 1956; BALOZET, 1971) which certainly contribute to respiratory distress, but are not the main causes of asphyxia.

Respiratory paralysis as caused by Mexican Centruroides envenomation was assumed to originate from an effect of the central nervous system (DEL POZO, 1956). This assumption was supported by the prevention of lethality after paralysis through electrophrenic respiration, following the introduction of minute amounts of venom into the cerebellomedullar cistern (DEL POZO et al., 1945, 1956). On the other hand, PATTERSON and WOOLEY (1970) suggested that respiratory distress may follow from a peripheral afferent discharge due to stimulation of carotid body receptors. This attitude, the possibility of a reflex mechanism as the origin of the respiratory distress caused by scorpion venom envenomation, was supported by recent investigations of FREIRE-MAIA et al. (1970, 1973). It has been found that rats injected with Tityus toxin (5—15 µg/100 g) demonstrated respiratory irregularities expressed in deep respiratory movements of the gasping type, intermingled with irregularities in rate, and amplitude of respiration ("ataxic" rhythm), and accompanied by periods of apnea lasting from 0.5—3 min ("periodic" respiration). Higher doses (20—100 µg/100 g) resulted in respiratory paralysis in the expiratory position. Gaspic, ataxic, and periodic respirations were prevented and the transient periods of apnea were considerably shortened by a bilateral vagotomy and denervation of carotid bodies (FREIRE-MAIA et al., 1973). Respiratory arrhythmias were also abolished by local anesthesia of the cervical vagus nerves and the carotid body regions (FREIRE-MAIA et al., 1974). It has been concluded that the above respiratory disturbances are chiefly due to stimulation of peripheral receptors and may be considered as reflex reactions.

Recent investigation (ISMAIL et al., 1973) with the venom of *B. minax* (Buthinae) is in general accord with the above findings. It has been found that an intravenous injection of this venom into cats and dogs resulted in a decrease in rate and increase in depth of respiration. Repeated injections of the venom produced complete arrest of respiration. Carotid sinus and body denervation in both cats and dogs abolished bradypnea, suggesting that this phenomenon is mediated through chemoreceptors in the carotid body. It has been also suggested that such reflex mechanism from the carotid sinus is secondary to the hypertensive effect of the venom (ISMAIL et al., 1973). On the other hand, FREIRE-MAIA et al. (1973) indicated that the blockade of the hypertensive effect of *Tityus* toxin by sympatholytic drugs did not prevent respiratory irregularities.

4. Muscular Effects

The stimulatory effect of scorpion venom on the skeletal musculature is well known and serves as one of the most typical manifestations in the syndrome of scorpion envenomation (Sect. C I.). Muscle contractions, twitchings, or fibrillations may be due to a direct excitatory effect on the muscle membrane, or mediated through an activation (either direct or central) of motor nerves, resulting in the release of transmitter.

Experimental data as obtained by different workers point to the availability of all the above-mentioned possibilities, emphasizing the role of the peripheral motor nerve ending as the main site of venom action.

The early work of DEL POZO and ANGUIANO (1947) has already manifested the essential elements in scorpion venoms muscular action: (1) Muscular twitchings and fibrillations due to an intravenous injection of *Centruroides* venom disappear upon destruction of the spinal cord or cutting of the motor nerves, thus indicating their central origin. (2) Local application of venom on the muscle or through an interarterial injection results in the above twitchings and fibrillations, indicating the peripheral origin of the muscular action. (3) Local application of the venom to a motor nerve trunk did not produce any effects on the muscles, indicating the relative impermeability of nerve trunks. (4) The venom does not activate denervated muscles. These data emphasize the role of peripheral axonal action in the muscular effects of scorpion venom.

The above conclusion has been strongly supported by the majority of recent investigations, presenting the muscular effects mainly as a consequence of the peripheral presynaptic action of scorpion venoms (Sect. IV 3). On the contrary, however, several investigations suggest that scorpion venom may directly affect skeletal muscles without any neural mediation. This information is presented in the next section.

a) Direct Effects on Skeletal Muscles

ADAM and WEISS (1959b) demonstrated that an application of *L. quinquestriatus* venom (5 — 10 µg/ml) to either a dissected or chemically denervated preparation of a frog sartorius muscle and rat diaphragm resulted in strong contractions which were dosage-dependent and demonstrated tachyphylactic behavior. Additions of sufficient tubocurarine to repress completely the response to acetylcholine did not show any alteration in their responses to venom. Smaller doses of venom (0.5 — 1 µg/ml) increased the direct electrically induced muscle contractions. Under the influences of the venom, resting membrane potential from *sartorius* fibers demonstrated a slow depolarization until action potential was elicited (ADAM and WEISS, 1966). The involvement of calcium ions in the muscular response to scorpion venom was indicated by the fact that the effect of the venom was: (1) antagonized by high calcium concentrations; (2) potentiated by lowering the calcium concentration; (3) mimicked by veratrine (assumed to act by displacing calcium from cell membrane and by increasing its sodium conductivity — FRANK, 1958; NICKERSON, 1971); (4) mimicked by citrate (which binds calcium ions). The similarities in action of the venom and the above substances were explained by the assumption that the stabilizing function of calcium at the muscle membrane is interfered with by the active constituent of venom. It has been suggested that excitatory action of the venom on muscle membrane may be due to the displacement of calcium by venom from the sites that bind calcium at the muscle fiber membrane (ADAM and WEISS, 1959b).

The conception of scorpion venoms' direct muscular effect has recently obtained additional experimental support. It was indicated by CHEYMOL et al. (1973), that the crude venom of *L. quinquestriatus, B. occitanus,* and *A. australis,* and toxins I and II isolated from the latter induce a muscular contraction in denervated and curarized preparations of the isolated and *in situ* preparations of the diaphragm of the rat and in the *rectus abdominis* muscle of the frog. It has been concluded that the above contraction follows from a depolarization of the muscle membrane. The above contractions were also produced by veratrine and antagonized by TTX, suggesting a certain link to calcium ions and sodium permeabilities.

b) Effects Through Neuromuscular Junctions

The main elements of scorpion venom neuromuscular intoxication have been presented in the study by BRAZIL et al. (1973) which will serve herein as a basis for comparison with certain other works, especially those concerning Buthinae venoms. What is most impressive in this investigation is the apparent contradiction to the direct effect on skeletal musculature as obtained by ADAM and WEISS (1959b) (Sect. IV 1). It has been found that *T. serrulatus* venom (20 µg/ml) added to the phrenic nerve-diaphragm preparation elicits: (1) spontaneous twitchings, preceded by a period (30 s — 20 min) of latency; (2) increases the muscular response to indirect stimulation and delays its relaxation; (3) induces a sustained contraction in low calcium. All the above effects are either prevented or abolished by d-tubocurarine. In the chronically denervated rat hemidiaphragm the venom usually does not produce twitches and never increases the amplitude of the twitches obtained by direct stimulation. Incubation of the innervated diaphragm with venom in the presence of eserine results in the appearance of a blood pressure-reducing substance which is readily antagonized by atropine and resists boiling in acidic conditions. This substance, assumed to be acetylcholine, cannot be obtained from a chronically denervated diaphragm otherwise equally treated. The release of acetylcholine is calcium-dependent and is blocked by magnesium, neomycin, and procaine. It has been concluded that scorpion venom acetylcholine release may follow the same mechanism as that caused by the nerve impulse (BRAZIL et al., 1973). In other words, in both cases, the transmitter release is dependent upon primary depolarization of the nerve. This conception was supported by a recent work of KATZ and EDWARDS (1972) who have simultaneously recorded the electrical responses from the muscle and nerve in the isolated sartorius nerve-muscle preparation of a frog when treated by C. suffusus scorpion venom. In the presence of the venom, single shocks applied to the nerve produced repetitive responses in both nerve and muscle. It has been found that: (1) each end-plate potential (EPP) in the train of repetitive responses was preceded by a nerve terminal spike; (2) omission of Ca^{2+} which abolished the EPP (certainly due to a blockage in the release of transmitter from the nerve terminals) did not block or reduce the antidromic discharges recorded from the nerves. Reduction of the sodium concentration in the bathing medium abolished the repetitive activity in the nerve and the muscle. This indicated that the neuromuscular action of the venom is certainly due to primary action on the nerve. However, since the nerve was found to be quite resistent and impermeable to the venom (KATZ and EDWARDS, 1972), it was assumed that the most likely site of venom action is the exposed area of the axon near its termination. The relative resistance and impermeability of intact nerve trunks to different Buthidae scorpion venoms, was indicated by several researchers, dealing either with vertebrate (HOUSSAY, 1919; DEL POZO and ANGUIANO, 1947; ADAM and WEISS, 1959b; LA GRANGE and RUSSELL, 1971) or arthropod preparations (PARNAS and RUSSELL, 1967; ZLOTKIN et al., 1970).

This main conception, the release of transmitter due to a presynaptic excitatory effect of scorpion venom as the cause of the muscular phenomena, was strongly supported by additional experimentation with vertebrate preparations (RUSSELL and LONG, 1961; LA GRANGE and RUSSELL, 1971), as well as with arthropod preparations (PARNAS and RUSSELL, 1967; PARNAS et al., 1970, see Sect. C IV.2). It was also confirmed in several investigations dealing with Buthinae venoms, either on vertebrate or invertebrate preparations (PARNAS et al., 1970, Sect. IV.2). BENOIT and MAMBRINI (1967) have reported that the venom of L. quinquestriatus (0.5−1 µg/ml) produced an increase in the duration of the presynaptic nerve action potential and an increase in the mean number of quanta released by a nerve impulse − when applied at the frog neuromuscular junction. The excitatory effect of A. mauretanicus on neuromuscular junctions was demonstrated in a rat in situ preparation of the diaphragm. The initial increase in the amplitude of the evoked contraction was accompanied by several spontaneous contractions followed by paralysis of decreasing reversibility (CHEYMOL et al., 1973). In a most recent work (LIN et al., 1975) it has been demonstrated that the spontaneous contraction induced by toxin II from the venom of A. australis (MIRANDA et al., 1970a) to the chick biventer cervicis preparation is inhibited by procaine and TTX, increased by addition of Ca^{2+}, inhibited by Mg^{2+} and partly inhibited by addition of bungarotoxin and d-tubocurarine (LIN et al., 1975). This may indicate the presynaptic origin and transmitter-release dependence of the above muscle contracture.

c) Effects on Smooth Muscles

The common preparation of the ileal smooth muscle serves as an useful tool in the study of venoms. It is one of the better understood and thoroughly investigated preparations (BÜLBRING et al., 1970), and, in spite of its technical simplicity, it contains all the basic elements of excitable tissues, including a ganglion nerve end-plate and muscle.

The venom of *A. australis* and its most potent toxin II (MIRANDA et al., 1970), tested on the smooth muscle preparation of the guinea pig ileum, were found to induce qualitatively identical effects (TAZIEFF-DEPIERRE et al., 1972). The most pronounced effect of the venom and toxin was expressed in the induction of strong autorhythmic spasmodic activity (Fig. 5) of the ileum, which was completely blocked by atropine and TTX. Addition of TTX Mg and Mn ions and lowering Ca concentration, which were all found to affect the spontaneous as well as venom induced release of acetylcholine in the ileal segments, concomitantly depressed the contractive response (TAZIEFF-DEPIERRE et al., 1973a, 1973c, 1974). This clearly indicates that the contractive response of the ileal muscles is due to a release of acetylcholine following a presynaptic excitatory action (TAZIEFF-DEPIERRE et al., 1972, 1973a). Using the same preparation, as well as venom and toxin, it has been recently shown (TINTPULVER et al., 1976) that hexamethonium, in doses completely blocking nicotine, was unable to affect the venom or toxin-induced response, thus exluding the possibility of venom's ganglionic stimulation. It has also been demonstrated that the venom and toxins may exert a partially reversible

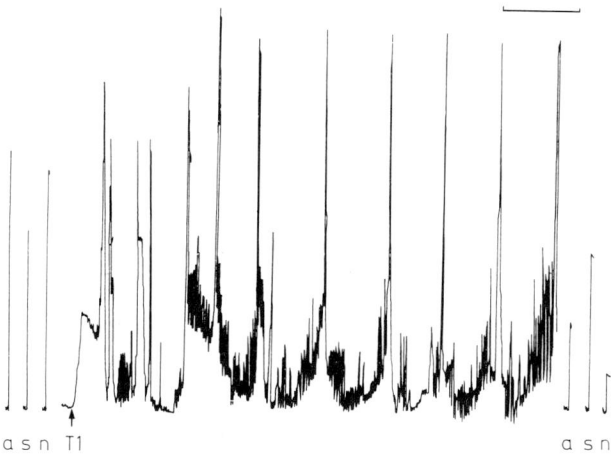

Fig. 5. Effect of mammal toxin I of *A. australis* on guinea pig ileum smooth muscle preparation. The rhythmic spasmodic ileal response is clearly indicated, followed by depressed response to several agonists. $T1 = $ "mammal" toxin I (500 ng/ml), $a = $ acetylcholine (5 ng/ml), $s = $ serotonine (100 ng/ml), $n = $ nicotine (1000 ng/ml). Time base 10 min. (Taken from TINTPULVER et al., 1976)

depressory postsynaptic action, expressed by the apparent decrease of the ileal muscular response to agonists such as acetylcholine, histamine, and especially serotonin, following prolonged (above 30 min) venom of toxin application (TINT-PULVER et al., 1976). The exclusiveness of the cholinergic mechanism in exerting the above spasmodic smooth muscle activity was demonstrated by its complete blockage with atropine (TAZIEFF-DEPIERRE et al., 1972, 1973a; TINTPULVER, 1975) as well as by the inability of additional antagonists (benadryl and methysergide) to affect the action of the venom (TINTPULVER, 1975).

The presynaptic cholinergic origin of ileal venom-induced spasmodic activity was previously demonstrated with the venom of *T. serrulatus* (DINIZ and VALERI, 1959; DINIZ and TORESS, 1968). Recently, the effects of a purified toxin from *T. serrulatus* (Tityutoxin) were examined on an ileal rat preparation (CUNHA-MELO et al., 1973). The involvement of acetylcholine release, due to toxin's postganglionic presynaptic stimulation, in spasmodic rhythmical activity was demonstrated by its depression with atropine, potentiation with eserine, tachyphylactic behavior, and the ineffectiveness of hexamethonium. An increase in tonus, accompanied by fast contractions which were decreased by atropine, potentiated by eserine, and which evinced a tachyphylactic response, were also demonstrated with the venom of *C. sculpturatus* when tested on guinea pig ileal preparation (PATTERSON, 1962). The effects on ileal preparations of Tityutoxin and *C. sculpturatus* venom closely resemble those of *A. australis* venom and its toxin. However, a more careful comparison of the data of CUNHA-MELO et al. (1973) concerning the effect of Tityutoxin on the rat ileum to those concerning the *A. australis* venom and its toxin on the guinea pig ileum (TAZIEFF-DEPIERRE, 1972; TINTPULVER, 1975) may reveal some essential differences: (1) The spasmodic activity induced by Tityutoxin was only partially abolished by atropine, suggesting the participation of additional mediators. (2) On the basis of some indirect evidence, the involvement of substance P in the ileal response to Tityutoxin was postulated. (3) In addition to stimulatory action, Tityutoxin has also elicited a transient ileal relaxatory response blocked by sympatholytic agents, indicating its adrenergic origin. Such an effect was never observed with the venom of *A. australis* and its toxin. It should be noted, however, that the above differences may not only indicate differences in the mode of action of these toxins but they may also partially represent some differences in responsiveness between the rat and guinea pig ilea.

The findings concerning the release and involvement of catecholamines and substance P in the ileal response to Tityutoxin (CUNHA-MELO et al., 1973) were recently supported by ultramicroscopical studies. It has been shown (TAFURI et al., 1974) that the incubation of ileal segments of the rat with Tityutoxin caused a decrease in the number of agranular (dense) vesicles and an increase in the number of granular vesicles of the Auerbach's plexus. It has been suggested that granular vesicles contain catecholamines and substance P, and that scorpion toxin, by releasing both substances, decreases the number of these vesicles.

5. Action on Axonal Membranes

On the basis of the information concerning the pharmacologic action of scorpion venom presented so far (Sect. C. II, III, and IV), it is evident that the above

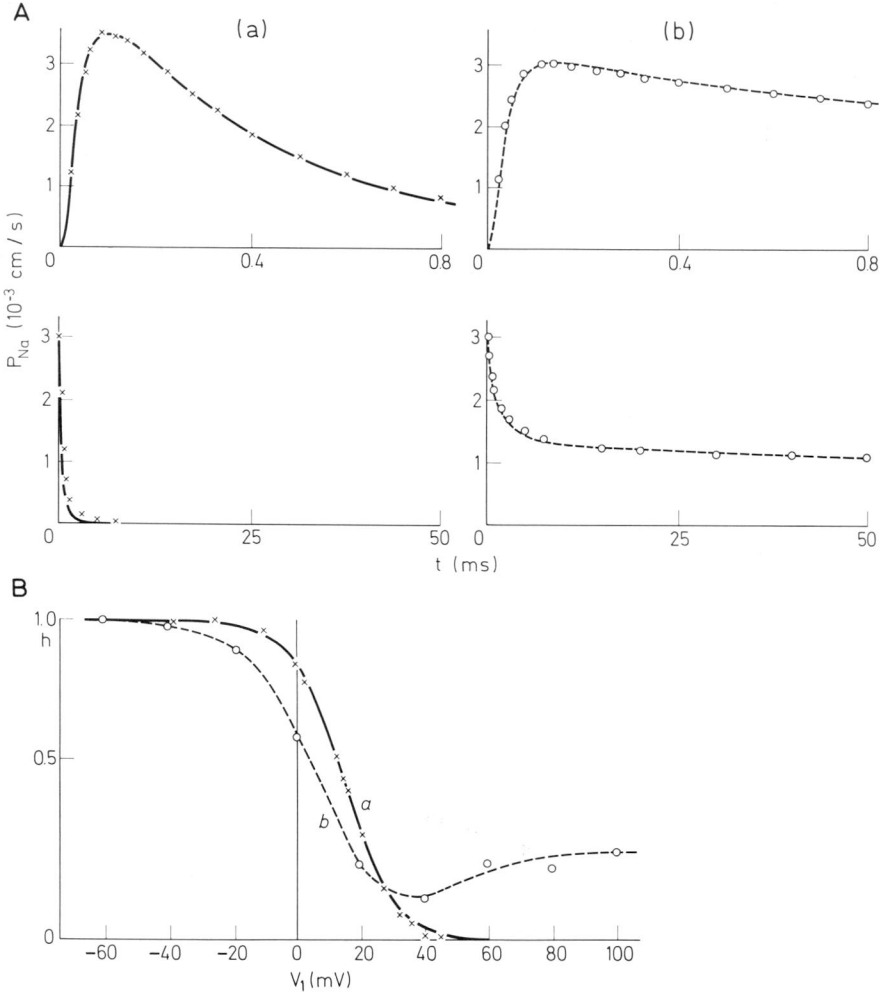

Fig. 6A and B. Effect of scorpion venom on axonal sodium conductance. (A) Time course of sodium permeability (P Na) before (a) and after (b) application of *L. quinquestriatus* venom in nerve fiber. In order to measure time course of sodium permeability (PNa) during long-lasting depolarization of Ranvier node of single myelinated frog nerve fiber, the node was superfused with ringer solution which contained 114.5 m M KCL in addition. The membrane potential was clamped at its normal value (V=0). A test pulse of V=67 mV depolarized membrane to potassium equilibrium potential. Membrane current during pulse consisted of leak and sodium current only. From the latter time course of PNa was calculated. *Ordinates:* PNa during depolarized pulse. *Abscissae:* Duration of pulse. Note different time scales. Filled and open circles are PNa values measured before (a) and after (b) application of venom. While rate of increase of PNa is hardly changed by venom, rate of decrease is considerably reduced, which is mainly due to very slow phase of inactivation (taken from KOPPENHOFER and SCHMIDT, 1968a, c). (B) Steady state activation of sodium conductance as function of transmembrane potential before (*crosses*) and after (*circles*) application of scorpion venom in nerve fibers. Incomplete sodium inactivation is demonstrated where ability of membrane to undergo an increase of PNa is given in terms of variable *h*. Peak value of PNa was determined during test pulse, V2, which was preceded by a conditioning prepulse (V1) of varying amplitude and polarity. Duration of V1 was 50 ms for normal node Ranvier and

action is mainly due to a primary excitatory effect of nerves. This essential point has been given special attention by several workers investigating the direct effects of scorpion venoms and toxins on nerve fibers.

ADAM et al. (1966) have followed up the changes in the resting and action potentials in a Ranvier node from an isolated nerve fiber of a frog, perfused with the venom of the scorpion *L. quinquestriatus* (0.01 – 1.0 µg/ml). The venom was shown to have a depolarizatory effect expressed in the large prolongation (from about 1 ms to more than 1 s) in the duration of the induced or spontaneous action potentials. In the absence of sodium ions in the bathing solution, the above venom effects were abolished. In the presence of scorpion venom, a gradual increase of Ringer's sodium concentration was accompanied by a steep elevation of the membrane resting potential (40 mv per tenfold concentration change as compared to the control), thus indicating that a venom has induced an increase in sodium permeability. Raising the Ca^+ concentration in the Ringer solution has neutralized the above depolarizatory phenomena, paralleling the effect of hyperpolarizing currents.

This avenue of investigation was further developed by KOPPENHÖFER and SCHMIDT (1968a, b, c) applying the voltage clamp technique on a single node of Ranvier in an isolated frog nerve fiber, perfused by the venom of the *L. quinquestriatus* (1 µg/ml). An analysis of the nodal membrane currents has provided a model for the construction of the above-mentioned (ADAM et al., 1966), typically long-lasting, action potentials. It has been found that when a venom-treated node membrane was depolarized, there was no change at the initial of sodium conductance and the rate of increase in sodium permeability was equal to that of the unpoisoned node. However, there was a considerable reduction in the rate of decrease in sodium permeability in the venom-treated node, up to an extreme retardation in phase of sodium inactivation. The time course of sodium permeabilities under various experimental conditions could establish kinetics of sodium inactivation in the form of h-v relations. It has been shown that in contrast to the full inactivation of sodium permeability at a depolarization level of 40 mv in the untreated node, the h value in venom-treated nodes is elevated even in high depolarizations with a tendency to increase at depolarization levels of more than 40 mv.

In conclusion, the venom has affected the sodium permeability by reducing its maximum (Fig. 6, B) and by considerably retarding its inactivation. In addition, scorpion venom has also reduced the maximum potassium permeability to about 35% of its normal value, and slowed down its increase upon depolarization. Both the partial inhibition of sodium inactivation and the depression of potassium permeability may account for the extreme prolongation of the action potential under the influence of scorpion venom.

---

500 ms for poisoned node. *Ordinate:* Peak PNa during test pulse V2 = 50 mv given as fractions of peak PNa which is available at large prepulses V1. *Abscissa:* Amplitude of V1. Curve *a* represents h-v relations of normal node, showing that PNa is fully inactivated at V1 to 40 mV. While at the level of normal resting potential (V=0) scorpion venom (*curve b*) reduces *h* value to about 75% of normal value, in depolarized level of above 40 mv, however, the *h* value has clear tendency to increase (Taken from KOPPENHÖFER and SCHMIDT, 1968b, c)

The above basic findings and conclusions of Koppenhöffer and Schmidt (1968a, b) were strongly supported by Narahashi et al. (1972) who studied the effect of the scorpion *B. tamulus* (applied in relatively high doses of 100 µg/ml) on a squid giant axon preparation employing intracellular electrodes and voltage clamp techniques. External application of the venom caused a gradual depolarization accompanied by spontaneous prolonged discharges. Under voltage clamp conditions, it was shown that the substantial effect of the venom was expressed in a considerable prolongation of the course of the sodium inactivation and the depression of the steady-state potassium outward current. Additional information concerning sodium and potassium conductances in giant axons of a crayfish (*Astacus*) and a lobster (*Homarus*) under voltage clamp conditions, treated by toxin I derived from the venom of the scorpion *A. australis* (Miranda et al., 1970a), was supplied in a most recent investigation by Romey et al. (1975). The prolongation of the action potential with a typical marked plateau, the retardation and partial blockage of the sodium inward current inactivation, as well as the partial depression of potassium permeability (as expressed in the decrease of the outward current), were equally established in the present investigation. The toxin appears to interact with a single type of receptor site in the axonal membrane of the crayfish and the lobster with dissociation constants of the toxin-receptor complexes 0.25 µM and 0.7 µM, respectively.

With the background of the above information, indicating general agreement among scientists using various venoms and preparations (Koppenhöfer and Schmidt, 1958a, b; Narahashi et al., 1972; Romey et al., 1975), recent data concerning the action of *C. sculpturatus* venom on frog nerve fibers are strongly intriguing (Gahalan, 1975). *Centruroides* venom causes evoked and spontaneous repetitive firing leading to an inexcitability of the nerve membrane. When sodium currents through the venom exposed nodal membrane were measured under voltage clamp conditions, then activation and inactivation appeared normal. Venom treatment, however, activates a new sodium current after the termination of each depolarizing pulse, upon repolarization. This current reaches a peak within about 25 ms and then declines over several hundred milliseconds. A depolarizing pulse inactivated the new sodium current, while a hyperpolarizing pulse increased. It appears that under the influence of the venom, the membrane potential-dependent sodium activation in some channels is shifted by some 40—50 mV in the hyperpolarized direction. Thus, the *Centruroides* venom-induced repetitive firing is, actually, not a consèquence of a change in sodium inactivation gating, as previously demonstrated (Koppenhöfer and Schmidt, 1968; Narahashi, 1972; Romey et al., 1975), but rather a shift in sodium activation gating (Cahalan, 1975). An additional different pattern of axonal response to scorpion toxin was demonstrated by a cephalopod (*Sepia*) giant axon when treated by toxin I of *A. australis* (Romey et al., 1975). In contrast to the above-indicated excitatory effect elicited by this toxin in crustacean giant axons, the response of the present preparation was clearly depressive. This was expressed in the decrease of the amplitude and rates of rise and falling of the normal action potential and in the decrease of both the peaks of inward and outward currents by the voltage clamp experiments (Romey et al., 1975).

It may be concluded that affecting axonal sodium conductance appears to be an essential function of scorpion venoms and toxins. However, this basic action may be performed in different manners and mechanisms, either by inhibiting the sodium inactivation (KOPPENHÖFER and SCHMIDT, 1968a, b), or by its reactivation (CAHALAN, 1975) in the case of an excitatory action, or a blockage of sodium conductance in the case of an depressory action (ROMEY et al., 1975). Such a diversity in action may represent not only differences in the composition of the venom or the structure of its toxins but certainly also in the nature of the target tissues.

6. Action on Arthropods

From an ecological point of view an organism's use of chemical means for defense or obtaining food may be considered as an efficient and energy-saving method. The scorpion's venom apparatus serves as a perfect example of this principle. Scorpions feed on freshly killed prey, consisting of arthropods and generally soft-bodied insects. However, as predators, scorpions appear to lack certain essential anatomical and physiologic qualities. They move relatively slowly, are practically blind, and have a rather undeveloped sense of smell. Scorpions actually do not seek their food actively, but rather wait for the prey to approach their lairs (BEARG, 1961; STAHNKE, 1966b). Thus, a device for paralyzing the prey at the earliest moment of contact is essential. This is achieved by the venom which is substantially employed against arthropods and especially insects. As we shall see below, this function is associated with highly specified chemical adaptations.

Lethality and Symptomatology

Sensitivity to crude scorpion venom varies considerably between different insect species, even those which are closely related. In tenebrionid beetles, the LD_{50} of the venom of *L. quinquestriatus* ranged between 12 µg/g for *Blaps sulcata* up to $180-300$ µg/g for *Trachyderma (Ocnera)* sp. (ISRAELI-ZINDEL et al., 1973) which may be compared to 12 µg/g and 1.5 µg/g for the larvae of *Sarcophaga* and *Locusta migratoria,* respectively (KAMON and SHULOV, 1963; ZLOTKIN et al., 1971a). Tarantula spiders (*Aphonopelma smithi*) were found to be practically resistant to the venom of the *C. limpidus tecomanus,* possibly due to a detoxifying effect of their hemolymph (WHEELING and KEEGAN, 1972).

The symptoms of scorpion envenomation in arthropods mainly indicate a stimulatory effect on the skeletal musculature. In the locust, when injected with the venom of *L. quinquestriatus,* this is expressed in uncoordinated leg movements, trembling of hindlegs, and spasmodic contractions of the genital valves (KAMON and SHULOV, 1963). Similarly, injection of 2 LD_{50} (23 µg per 100 mg of body weight) *A. australis* venom into isopods (*Armadillium vulgare,* a terrestrial crustacean) causes a paralysis within $2-3$ min preceded by irregular and uncoordinated movements of the legs and a curvature of the body due to a sustained contracture of the ventral body musculature (Fig. 7B; ZLOTKIN et al., 1972). In blowfly larvae, injection of small amounts of different scorpion venoms (see Table 3) causes an immediate and sustained contraction of body musculature, expressed in drastic thickening and shortening of the body and accompanied by complete paralysis.

The rate and duration of the above contraction-paralysis are dosage-dependent (Fig. 7 A). Injection of scorpion venom into the abdominal region of ligated larvae (thus nullifying the central nervous system, which in fly larvae is located in the thoracic region) resulted in the above-mentioned contraction, thus indicating the peripheral nerve-muscle stimulatory effect of scorpion venom (ZLOTKIN et al., 1971 a). The above venom-induced spastic paralysis, was also demonstrated with other fly larvae (*Calliphora, Lucilia, Musca, Drosophila*) as well as with larvae of the wax moth (*Galleria*) and the grain beetle (*Trogoderma*), all possessing a clear segmental arrangement of their body musculature and a soft, flexible, unsclerotized cuticle (ZLOTKIN et al., 1971 a). The paralytic potency of different scorpion venoms to blowfly larvae compared to their mouse-lethal effect is presented in Table 3.

L. *quinquestriatus* venom, when injected in sublethal doses, strongly accelerated phenomena which are naturally under the control of growth hormones such as puparium formation in blowfly larvae (FRAENKEL and ZLOTKIN, 1970) and supernumerary larval molting in last instar diapausing and nondiapausing *Trogoderma* larvae (ZLOTKIN et al., 1971 c). The above action of scorpion venom was hypothetically attributed to its excitatory effect on neurosecretory systems, resulting in a hormonal release. A release of endocrine secretion due to scorpion venom-induced

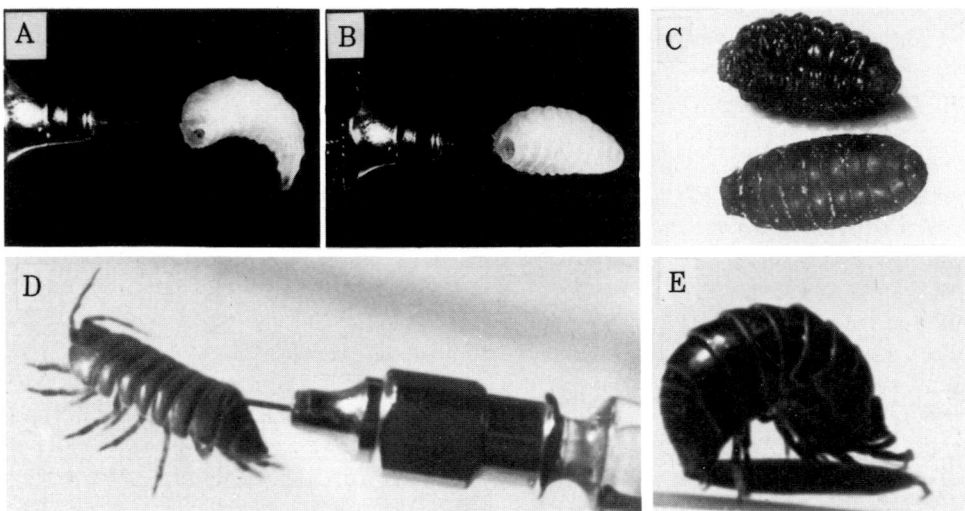

Fig. 7 A–E. Symptoms of scorpion venom paralysis of arthropods. (A) Larva of blowfly (*Sarcophaga*) placed on needle, connected to a micrometrically operated syringe, demonstrating vigorous twisting movements. (B) Same larva immediately following injection of 0.8 µg of *L. quinquestriatus* venom, contracted and completely immobile. (C) Upper figure shows contracted deformed puparium of *Sarcophaga* which has been injected as larva 2 h prior to puparium formation by 0.8 µg of *Leiurus* venom, as compared to normal puparium shown in lower figure. The above contraction-paralysis response was used as bioassay for isolation of "insect toxin" (see next section). (D) Terrestrial crustacean (*A. vulgare*, Isopoda) placed on needle and demonstrating normal appearance. (E) The above 25 s after injection of 30 µg of *A. australis* venom. Body is curved–contracted and immobile, legs exhibit irregular and uncoordinated movements. The above response served as bioassay for isolation of crustacean toxin (see next section). (After ZLOTKIN et al., 1971 a and 1972 b)

neural stimulation was demonstrated in a mammal, expressed by depletion of adrenal catecholamines (CELESTE-HENRIQUES et al., 1968).

Neurophysiologic Investigations

The marked resistance of an intact nerve to scorpion venom as previously shown in vertebrate preparations (see Sect. C IV.) was also demonstrated by the application of concentrated solutions of *L. quinquestriatus* venom to the tympanic nerve (ZLOTKIN et al., 1970) as well as the ventral nerve cord of *Locusta* (PARNAS et al., 1970). Chemical desheathing treatment by pronase enabled the venom to produce a burst of spontaneous activity which gradually decreased up to a complete blockage of the tympanic nerve (ZLOTKIN et al., 1970) and increased by a 1000 times its blocking ability of the ventral nerve cord (PARNAS et al., 1970). It has been found that the quick, complete, and irreversible paralysis of the cockroach *Periplaneta americana,* was induced by amounts (50—100 μg) of *A. australis* crude venom which were much smaller than those necessary to cause an excitatory block of the induced afferent transynaptic response at the sixth abdominal ganglion. The above synaptic blockage-inducing venom concentration (5 mg/ml) only slightly affected the axonal conduction of the connectives and cercal nerves (D'AJELLO et al., 1972), thus further demonstrating the resistance of insects' central nervous system and intact main nerve trunks to scorpion venom.

On this background, one may assume that the excitatory paralysis symptoms of scorpion envenomation in arthropods should represent a peripheral action on the skeletal musculature, either directly or through the neuromuscular junction. The latter point was clarified by PARNAS et al. (1967, 1970) with crustacean and insect neuromuscular preparations. Using the deep extensor abdominal muscle-nerve preparation of the crayfish *Procambarus clarki* and with aid of suitable devices for stimulation and recording from the nerve (externally) as well as from the muscle (internally), it has been found that the venom of *C. sculpturatus* may exert three main effects (PARNAS and RUSSELL, 1967): (1) a blocking action (10 μg/ml) of the indirectly elicited muscle response. The nerve is unaffected and the muscle responds to direct stimulation and to glutamate (a postsynaptic stimulant). It was deduced that the blocking effect was due to an action at the presynaptic terminals. (2) An excitatory effect (100 μg/ml), expressed by a muscle spontaneous activity. When blocked by strychnine (presynaptic blocker of transmitter release), muscle and nerve responded to direct stimulation—again indicating the presynaptic nerve terminals as the site of the above effect. (3) Muscle damage effect, following prolonged exposures of the preparation to high venom concentrations, resulted in the depression of the directly induced muscular response and an anatomical muscular damage.

In an additional investigation employing the same methods, the crude venom of *L. quinquestriatus* was applied to a neuromuscular preparation of locust and crab (PARNAS et al., 1970). In spite of certain differences between the present and previous (PARNAS and RUSSELL, 1967) findings, as expressed in the complete resistance of muscle and the relative increased excitability of the motor nerves in the present work, there still exists a basic similarity. As previously demonstrated, the muscle stimulatory effect of the *Leiurus* venom followed from a presynaptic

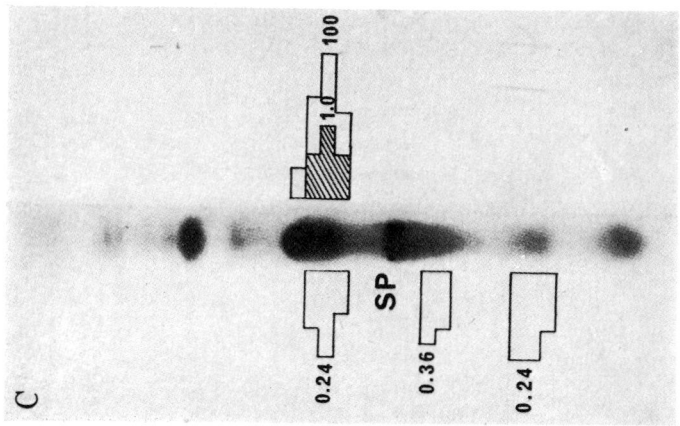

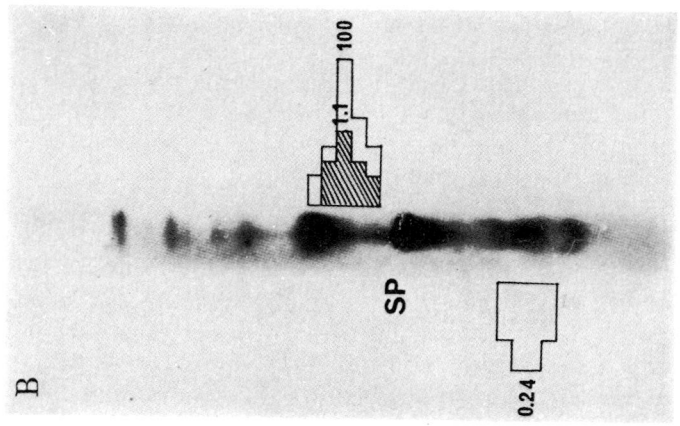

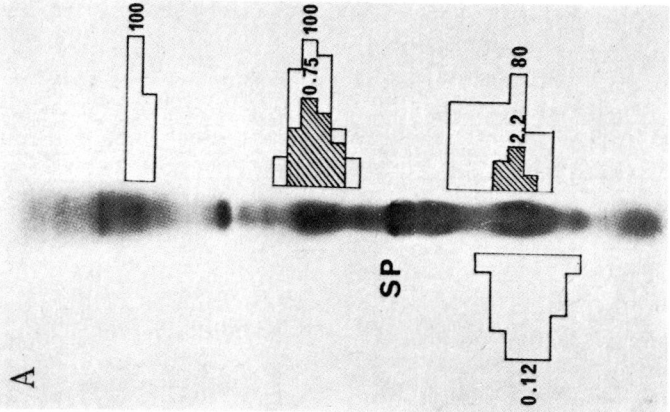

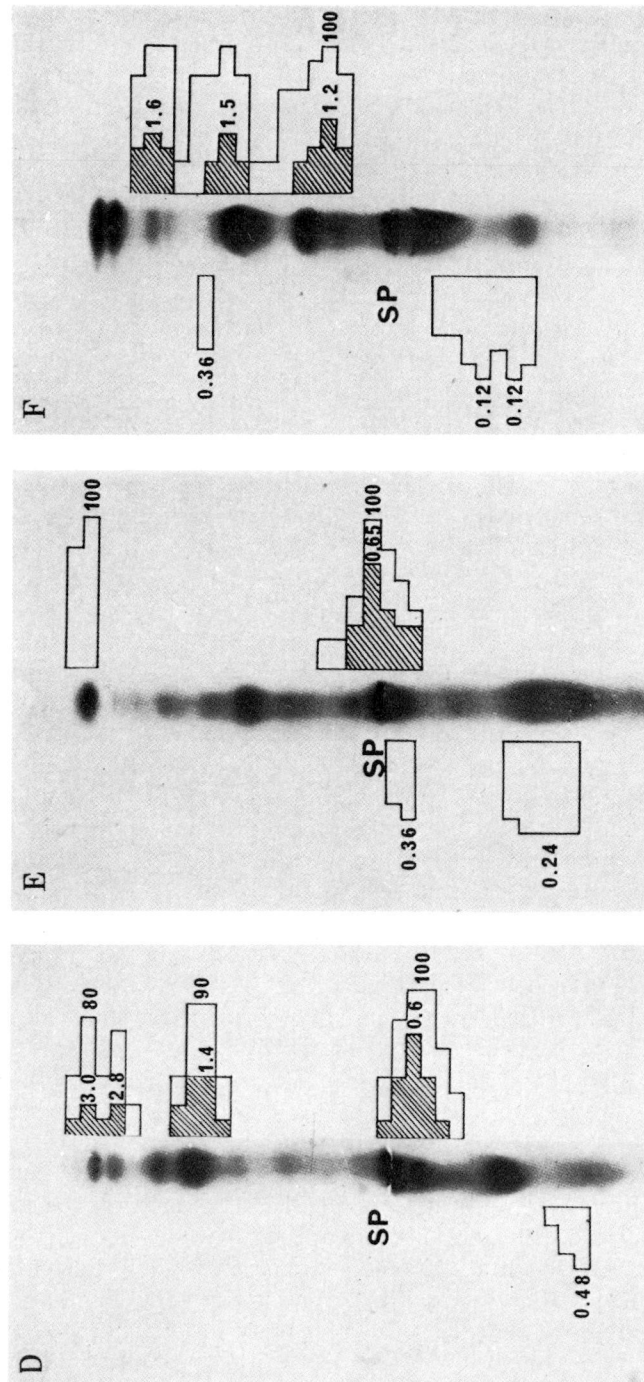

Fig. 8A — F. Starch gel electropherograms of several Buthinae scorpion venoms indicating diversity between mammal and insect toxic fractions. Ten milligrams of crude venom were dissolved in Tris-citric acid buffer pH 8.6 and applied in slot of 23 cm in length. Electrophoresis in 12% gel was performed according to previously described technique (ZLOTKIN et al., 1971 b). After completion of run, starch block was sliced into 40 sections of 0.5 cm width. Following 2 days of storage at −20°C, each section was homogenized in 5 ml 0.14 NaCl and centrifuged. Clear supernatant was used for activity testings. Empty areas on left correspond to mice lethality. Shaded areas on right indicate contraction-paralysis and empty areas on right indicate lethality of larvae. Numbers are related to maximal activities expressed: (1) for contraction-paralysis of larvae as volume (μl) corresponding to one contraction-paralysis unit (ZLOTKIN et al., 1971 a); (2) for larvae lethality as percent death; (3) for mice lethality as minimum volume of eluate (ml) causing death. SP=starting point; Anode at top. Venoms of following scorpions were used: (A) A. aeneas aeneas. (B) A. amoreuxi (C) A. mauretanicus mauretanicus. (D) B. occitanus paris. (E) B. occitanus tunetanus (F) L. quinquestriatus. (Taken from ZLOTKIN et al., 1972a)

origin. This is expressed in the increase of quantal content (0.1 µg/ml, representing an effect on nerve terminals) and in the spontaneous contraction of the muscle caused by repetitive firing from the nerve. Both the axonal excitation and conduction block (10 µg/ml) were assumed to result from the same mechanism, membrane depolarization. The increase in muscle membrane resistance (a postsynamptic action) caused by the venom (0.1 µg/ml), may contribute to the muscle's excitability, but this is only secondary to the axonal presynaptic effects of the envenomation (Parnas et al., 1970).

The most remarkable feature of the effect of scorpion venoms on arthropods is its strong resemblance to action on mammals. This is expressed in the excitatory symptoms of envenomation and is mainly emphasized when comparing the action of scorpion venom on the neuromuscular preparations of an insect, crustacean as well as a mammal. In all the above preparations, the venom exhibited muscular stimulatory effects due to presynaptic excitation, especially at the level of the exposed nerve endings, resulting in the release of the corresponding transmitter. This similarity in action may lead to the assumption that the effect of scorpion venoms on mammals and arthropods results from the same chemical compounds in the crude venom. This basic point is discussed in the next section.

Selective Toxins

Using the contraction paralysis response of blowfly larvae (Fig. 7) as a bioassay for the quantitative estimation of scorpion venom's potency to insects, it has been found that there was no correlation between larvae paralysis and mice lethal potencies of 16 different Buthidae venoms (Zlotkin et al., 1971 a, Table 3), hinting at the possibility that the two toxic activities may result from different factors. This assumption was strongly supported by the finding that the potent toxins I and II of *A. australis* (Fig. 1, Table 1), which are strongly lethal to mice (Table 2), were completely inactive on larvae (Zlotkin et al., 1971 b). The final proof of the diversity among factors affecting mammals and those paralyzing insects in scorpion venoms, was obtained by starch gel electrophoretic separation of the venom of *A. australis* (Zlotkin et al., 1971 b), and six other Buthinae venoms (Fig. 8, Zlotkin et al., 1972). It has been found that three of the above venoms contain more than one larvae contraction paralysis fraction. These fractions, apart from being strongly paralytic to fly larvae (Fig. 8), are equally lethal and readily inactivated by trypsin, thus demonstrating their protein nature (Zlotkin et al., 1972a).

The same method used for purification of the so-called mammal toxins (see Sect. B I), enabled isolation and purification of the insect toxin from the venom of *A. australis*. Following a sequence of steps composed of water-extraction, dialysis, recycling Sephadex G-50 gel filtration, and ion exchangers equilibrium chromatography by DEAE-Sephadex A-50 followed by Amberlite CG-50- (Fig. 1), a final product, 267-fold purified and with a yield of 95% toxicity was obtained (Zlotkin et al., 1971 d). It is a single-chained, low molecular weight, protein composed of 70 amino acids and crosslinked by four disulfide bridges. Its N-terminal primary sequence compared to the scorpion "mammal" toxins is presented in Figure 2.

In contrast to the crude venom of *A. australis,* the "insect" toxin and the so-called mammal toxins I and II (Fig. 1) were unable to affect an isopod (terrestrial crustacean, *Armadillium vulgare*) or a scorpion (*B. occitanus*), suggesting the possibility that the activity of the crude venom on these arthropods is due to discrete new toxins (ZLOTKIN et al., 1972 b). Using a new bioassay, based on paralysis of isopods (Fig. 7) as well as column chromatography by Sephadex G-50 gel filtration (ZLOTKIN et al., 1972 b) and ion exchange gradient chromatography on Amberlite CG 50 followed by CM-Sephadex, a protein specifically toxic to isopods, called the "crustacean" toxin, was isolated and purified from the venom of *A. australis* (Fig. 1, ZLOTKIN et al., 1975). The pure toxin contained about 20% of the crude venom's toxicity to isopods and was 250 times more active. Compared to the insect and mammal toxins derived from the same venom, the crustacean toxin showed a higher content of half cystines (indicating five disulfide bridges instead of four and also more *Glu* plus *Gln* than *Asp* plus *Asn,* which is in contrast to all other toxins obtained until now from Buthinae venoms (Table 2).

Considering the symptomatology, potency, and speed of action of the "insect" as well as "crustacean" toxins, it was assumed that both are basically neurotoxic. Some indirect evidence was recently obtained, suggesting that the specificity or selectivity in the action of these toxins is based on specific affinity to neural systems of the corresponding groups of animals. It has been found that the "insect" toxin is able to duplicate the action of the crude venom in performing an excitatory block of the induced afferent transynaptic response at the sixth abdominal ganglion of the cockroach *P. americana,* in contrast to the complete inactivity of high doses of the "mammal" toxin II (D'AJELLO et al., 1972). Similarly, an isopod toxic fraction obtained by Sephadex G-50 chromatography (ZLOTKIN et al., 1972), was able to mimick the excitatory and blocking action of the crude venom on the crayfish stretch receptor organ, in contrast to the "insect" and "mammal" toxins, which were inactive (PANSA et al., 1973).

These findings have established the conception claiming that scorpion venoms contain different toxins, selectively active on different groups of organisms, which may represent a chemical adaptation of scorpions to changes in food sources during evolution (ZLOTKIN, 1973). In order to test and clarify the above conception of specificity, the action of the different "mammal" as well as arthropod scorpion toxins was recently investigated on mammal as well as arthropod neurophysiologic preparations, as presented in Section D IV.

IV. Action Mechanisms

1. Autopharmacologic Intoxication

On the basis of the above-reviewed information, one may deduce that the cardiovascular respiratory and muscular manifestations of scorpion venom and toxins follow from release of transmitter substances due to their excitatory effect on the nervous system, expressed in increased axonal sodium conductance. This fundamental point, the induction of release of autopharmacologic substances by scorpion venoms, served as the object of several recent investigations.

CELESTE-HENRIQUES et al. (1968) have shown that sublethal doses of *T. serrulatus* venom, when injected into rats, produced a depletion of adrenal gland catecholamines, which was blocked (prevented) upon denervation of the adrenals. Moss et al. (1973) have shown that the strong increase in blood pressure and the massive discharge of catecholamines in rats treated by *L. quinquestriatus* venom followed from both sympathetic and adrenal discharge, presumably due to a direct action on the adrenal medulla and/or the postganglionic neurons. These conclusions were based on the facts that adrenalectomized animals manifested an increase in serum catecholamines which was about 50% of that found in intact animals, and that hexamethonium did not affect the vasopressor, as well as catecholamine release effects of the venom. In accordance with the above, the strong hyperthermic response of rabbits, when injected intraventricularly by *L. quinquestriatus* venom, was supposed to follow either from noradrenaline release or shift in sodium calcium balance in the hypothalamus (Osman et al., 1973).

Transmitter releasing effects of scorpion toxin were also demonstrated on isolated brain tissues. Gomez et al. (1973) have shown that Tityutoxin causes a calcium- and sodium-dependent release of acetylcholine from incubated slices of rat brain, which is completely nullified by EGTA, as well as by TTX. This, together with the most recent finding that Tityutoxin enhances the uptake of Na^{24+} by cortical slices, may suggest that the action of the toxin is mediated through an increase of an inward flux of Na^+ (Gomez et al., 1975). It has been also shown that Tityutoxin has increased the output of acetylcholine from an eserinized longitudinal muscle strip of guinea pig ileum. This effect was clearly counteracted by the removal of sodium and calcium ions or by the addition of TTX (Diniz et al., 1974). Similarly, it has been shown that an isolated fraction from the venom of the scorpion *L. quinquestriatus* releases norepinephrine from synaptosomes prepared from rat brain, and this action is affected by the absence of calcium as well as by the addition of TTX (Moss et al., 1974). Scorpion venom-induced transmitter releasing effect suggests that the venom actually duplicates the effect of nerve stimulation, and, since the intact nerve appears to be relatively resistant to the action of the venom (Parnas and Russell, 1967; Zlotkin, 1970; Katz and Edwards, 1972), the nerve terminal seems to serve as the primary target for venom action.

A hypothetical molecular mechanism of cholinergic release on the nerve terminal level was recently suggested by Smythies et al. (1974). On the basis of the amino acid sequence of toxin II from *A. australis*, the authors have constructed a model of the conformation of this protein, including its pattern of disulfide bond formation, which was to a great extent sterochemically complementary to a stack of nine molecules of CAMP. This is in accordance with their previous hypothesis that the storage and release of acetylcholine from nerve terminals is based on a stack of CAMP molecules which binds acetylcholine in a ratio of 1:1 (Smythies et al., 1974). However, even if the above hypothetical conformation of toxin II would have been experimentally confirmed, the very conception of a nerve terminal as a site of action strongly requires direct experimental support, which is still lacking at the present moment. Furthermore, the blockage of scorpion venom-induced transmitter release by TTX (known to have no direct effect on transmitter release from nerve terminals Elmqvist and Feldman, 1965; Katz und Miledi, 1967), either in brain slices and synaptosomes (Gomez et al., 1973, 1975; Moss et al., 1974) or neuromuscular preparations (Tazieff-Depierre, 1972; Tintpulver, 1975; Cheymol et al., 1974) may suggest that the axons serve as the main target for the action of scorpion venom. On the background of the above information and that presented in the previous sections, it is more probable that the excitatory presynaptic action of scorpion venom is due to action on axons (preferably at their relatively exposed regions at their endings, closer to the synaptic regions; ZLOTKIN and SHULOV, 1969) rather than a direct effect on the nerve terminal. Direct evidence indicating that the peripheral final nerve branches are actually the primary target of scorpion toxins action was obtained most recently. It has been found that the prolonged spontaneous firing induced by the "insect" toxin (see Sect. C VI 4 and Fig. 10d) and recorded from the main trunk of the locusts *extensor tibiae* motor nerve, could have been gradually abolished by a progressive "pruning" of the nerve terminal peripheral side branches. The finally disconnected main nerve trunk, which did not demonstrate any spontaneous activity, responded perfectly to electrical stimulation (WALTHER et al., 1976).

2. Is There a Direct Excitatory Effect on Muscles?

On the background of the heavily accumulated evidence on the presynaptic origin of the muscular action of scorpion venoms and their toxins in vertebrate (Sect. C IV 2) as well as arthropod systems (Sect. C VI 2), the indications of direct muscular effects are perplexing.

Thus, BRAZIL et al. (1973), demonstrating the absence of a direct excitatory effect on skeletal muscles by scorpion venom, in contrast to the previous findings of ADAM and WEISS (1959b), attributed these discrepancies to the very low dose of d-tubocurarine and to a possible incomplete degeneration of nerve terminals in the chronically denervated preparations as employed by the latter. We also feel that an incomplete denervation (either chemical or operative) has influenced the experimental data presented by CHEYMOL et al. (1974) concerning the muscular action of several Buthinae venoms and toxins.

On the other hand, most recently it has been found (WALTHER et al., 1976) that the crude venom of *A. autralis*, when applied on a habrobracon paralyzed (thus blocking the excitatory transmitter release, WALTHER and RATHMAYER, 1974) locust *extensor tibiae* nerve muscle preparation, demonstrated a direct depolarizatory muscular effect. This was expressed in transient fluctuations in the muscle membrane potential up to rhythmic oscillations accompanied by spontaneous muscle twitchings and fibrillations. Such a direct muscular effect was not obtained with the "insect" toxin, which was the most potent in induction of presynaptic excitatory phenomena (see Sect. D IV). It may be assumed that the postsynaptic excitatory muscular effects of scorpion venoms may be due to factors which differ from those responsible for the venom axonal presynaptic effects. This would explain some of the discrepancies among different investigations by different venoms. The assumption should be clarified experimentally.

A clear indication of a direct excitatory action of a scorpion toxin on muscle cells is given by FAYET et al. (1974), expressed in the contractile activity of the anatomically denervated cultured chick embryo heart cells. As previously indicated (see Sect. C II 4), the response of these embryonic cells may represent some specific physiologic properties of this specific preparation and, as such, it may not be representative of other organizations of muscular tissues, such as skeletal or finally differentiated heart muscles.

3. Interactions with Sodium, Calcium and TTX

In contrast to the discrepancies concerning the direct muscular effect of scorpion venoms, there are certainly no such ambiguities with regards to their excitatory action on axonal membranes. This action (as presented in Sect. C V) is expressed in the depolarization of the membrane based on an increase and prolongation of sodium permeability, due either to a delay of sodium inactivation (Koppenhöfer and Schmidt, 1968a; Narahashi et al., 1972; Romey et al., 1975) or induction of the opening of additional sodium channels at the repolarization phase of the action potential (Cahalan, 1975). This basic function of the venom explains the strong dependence of its action on external sodium (Adam et al., 1966; Katz and Edwards, 1972; Gomez et al., 1973, 1975) and its high sensitivity to TTX.

It has been shown in different experimental systems that both the increase and decrease in calcium concentration from normal values may affect the response induced by scorpion venom or toxin. An increase of Ca^{++} from the normal value of 1.8 to 7.2 mM has eliminated the excitatory effects of *L. quinquestriatus* venom on the preparation of single myelinated nerve fibers in a frog (Adam et al., 1966). The membrane was repolarized, action potentials shortened, and the spontaneous activity was blocked. Using voltage clamp experiments on isolated Ranvier nodes in frog axons, it has been demonstrated (Schmitt and Schmidt, 1972) that incomplete sodium inactivation due to scorpion venom is eliminated and the reduced potassium permeability is partially corrected by Ca^{++} addition. Contractive responses of skeletal musculature, which were supposed to indicate a direct effect on scorpion venom, were suppressed by addition of calcium into the bathing solution (Adam and Weiss, 1959b; Tazieff-Depierre, 1968; Cheymol et al., 1974).

It has been assumed by Adam and Weiss (1959b, 1966) that the primary action of the venom is based on the displacement of calcium ions in the muscular as well as axonal membranes, thus modifying the ionic permeabilities to sodium. The strong antagonistic action of TTX to scorpion venom and toxins could have been interpretated as supporting the above conception. It has been claimed (Dettbarn, 1971) that the axonal depressory effect of TTX is based on the binding and fixation of the membranal calcium, thus preventing its displacement, which is necessary for sodium permeability. However, some recent investigations have clearly indicated that TTX does not compete on the same receptors, and the interaction is certainly of an "allosteric" nature. This has been indicated in a recent investigation (Catterall, 1975) of interactions between veratridine, batrochotoxin, aconitine, and *L. quinquestriatus* scorpion venom, all of which increase Na^+ permeability (supposed to reflect ion transport activity of the action potential Na^+ ionophore) in an electrically excitable mouse neuroblastoma cell culture. It has been found that the above toxins interact with two distinct classes of sites, one specific for the alkaloids (which show competitive interaction among them) and the second specific for scorpion toxin (which interacts cooperatively with each of the three alkaloid toxins). The increase rate of sodium uptake ($^{22}Na^+$) caused by scorpion toxin was totally inhibited by TTX. However, 30-fold variations in the concentrations of scorpion venoms did not affect the rate of inhibition of an equal dose of TTX, thus indicating that scorpion venom toxin must bind at sites that are separate from the TTX binding site. These results suggested the existence of three functionally separate components which bind activating neurotoxins and interact allosterically in controlling the activity of a third ion transport component, which binds TTX (CATTERALL, 1975). The clear independence between the binding sites of TTX and scorpion toxin was simply demonstrated by the very fact that TTX nonsusceptible embryonic heart muscle cells are strongly affected by scorpion toxin (FAYET et al., 1974). In a most recent investigation (COURAUD et al., 1976) it has been shown that in the embryonic chick heart cells, binding of scorpion toxin (toxin II of *A. australis*) to its specific sites may unmask latent TTX-sensitive fast channels.

Lowering calcium concentrations from the normal value of 1.4 mM to 0.2 mM has canceled the effects of *A. australis* toxin II on the guinea pig ileum (TAZIEFF-DE-PIERRE, 1972, 1973a). Equally, KATZ and EDWARDS (1972) demonstrated that omission of calcium blocked scorpion venom evoked neuromuscular transmission in frog skeletal muscles, while increase of 8-fold Ca^{++} did not affect its neuromuscular action. Absence of calcium, either by omission or by its specific binding has diminished the scorpion venom-induced release of transmitter substances in brain slices and synaptosomes (GOMEZ et al., 1973, 1975; MOSS et al., 1974). Omission of calcium has also stopped the release of acetylcholine in the phrenic nerve diaphragm preparation (BRAZIL et al., 1973). On the other hand, lowering the calcium level had increased the muscles' sensitivity to transmitter.

In spite of certain controversies and discrepancies among different workers concerning the role of calcium in scorpion envenomation, the majority of data stand in good accordance to certain well-established conceptions concerning the function of calcium in excitable tissues (BAKER and REUTER, 1975). The ability of increased calcium concentration to antagonize the effects of scorpion venom as well as the increased sensitivity to venom at low calcium levels (ADAM and WEISS, 1959a; SCHMITT and SCHMIDT, 1972; BRAZIL et al., 1973; TAZIEFF-DEPIERRE, 1972) may be explained by the stabilizing properties of calcium to excitable membranes. The above effect of divalent cations, particularly calcium, is attributed to their binding affinity to negative fixed charges at membrane surfaces, thus affecting the permeabilities to monovalent cations, which determine the excitability of many biological membranes (FRANKENHAUSER and HODGKIN, 1975; BIANCHI, 1968; GILBERT and EHRENSTEIN, 1969; FISHMAN et al., 1971). On the other hand, the decrease or elimination of scorpion venom-induced responses by lowering or removal of calcium is certainly linked to its function in the excitation secretion coupling (BAKER and REUTER, 1975). The release of neural transmitter substances is dependent on Ca^{++} ions, as calcium entry is the first step of stimulus secretion coupling (DEL CASTILLO and KATZ, 1956; KATZ and MILEDI, 1967; HUBBARD, 1970; RAHAMIMOFF, 1970).

Thus, the possible interaction of scorpion venom and calcium ions may be expressed at least either in its "displacement" in the excitable membrane and/or the increase of its permeability. The latter was clearly indicated in a most recent investigation (COURAUD et al., submitted) indicating that toxin II of *A. australis* has stimulated the passive uptake of Na^+ and Ca^{++} in chick embryo heart cells;

the passive Ca^+ uptake was found to be coupled to a passive Na^+ ionophore. Some previous investigations based on histochemical recognition and localization of calcium in the rat diaphragm (Tazieff-Depierre, 1968) as well as in heart muscles (Yarom and Braun, 1967b) treated by scorpion venom may also supply some indirect evidence supporting the above conception on Ca^{++}-displacement and Ca^{++}-permeability increase by scorpion venom, raising a strong demand for more direct and clear experimental evidence. How far does interaction with calcium serve as the *primary* and essential effect of scorpion toxins? This question should still be considered as a reasonable working hypothesis which deserves further experimental clarification.

4. The Pharmacologic Diversity of Scorpion Toxins

The phenomenon of specificity and selectivity in the action of scorpion toxins (see Sect. C VI 3), which was based mainly on simple bioassays, demanded a further neurophysiologic examination. The crude venom of the North African scorpion *A. autralis Hector* and its derived "mammal" toxins I and II (Sect. B II), "insect," and "crustacean" toxins (Sect. C IV 3), all previously purified according to their mouse lethality and fly larvae and isopod paralysis respectively, were tested on mammal, insect, and crustacean nerve muscle preparations. The choice of such preparations was based on the consideration that they actually represent the true target organ for the paralytic action of scorpion venoms and their toxins.

Due to the accumulated background information concerning the action of scorpion venom on the guinea pig ileal smooth muscle preparation (see Sect. C IV 3) this preparation was chosen to represent a mammalian neuromuscular system. It has been found that the "crustacean" toxin induced a sustained prolonged contraction (Fig. 9 A) in contrast to the rhythmic spasmodic ileal behavior caused by the crude venom and the mammal toxin (Fig. 5). The excitatory effect of the "crustacean" toxin was completely inhibited by atropine, potentiated by eserine, tachyphylactic, blocked by TTX and morphine, and unaffected by hexamethonium. It may be concluded that, as in the case of the crude venom and the "mammal" toxins (see Sect C IV 3), the action of the "crustacean" toxin was due to a postganglionic presynaptic stimulation resulting in the release of a cholinergic transmitter. Prolonged application of the "crustacean" toxin has caused also a depressory postsynaptic action expressed in the reduced ileal response to several agonists (Fig. 9 A). The insect toxin was inactive in the ileum smooth muscle preparation (Fig. 9 B).

The above toxins were applied on the neuromuscular preparations of an insect (the *extensor tibiae* muscle of *Locusta* hind leg, Walther et al., 1976), crustacean (the dactylus opener in the walking leg of the crayfish *Astacus leptodactylus*, Rathmayer et al., in preparation), and arachnid (the claw closer muscle in the leg of the mygalomorph spider *Dugesiella hentzi*, Ruhland et al., 1977). For complementary and comparative purpose, their effect on the crayfish CNS axonal preparation (Rathmayer et al., 1977) as well as their paralytic effect on locusts (Walther et al., 1975) were also tested. In all the above preparations it has been found that muscular effects of the venom and the different toxins, expressed in the augmentation of the recorded junction potentials, evoked

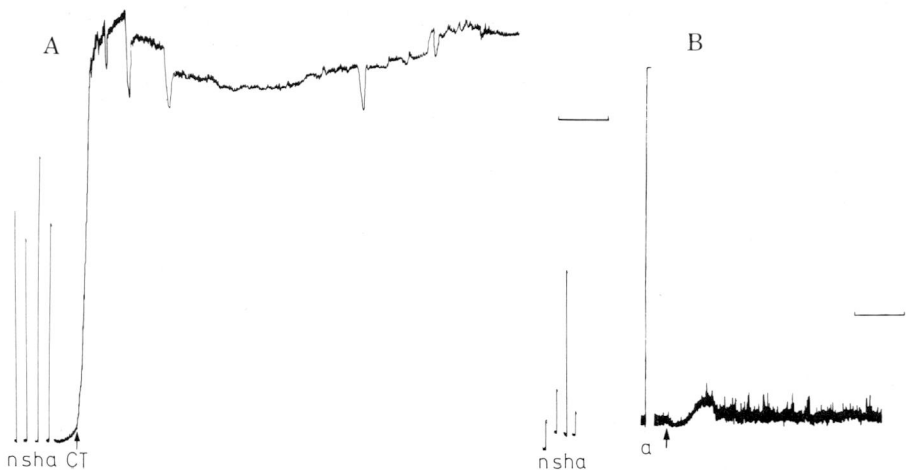

Fig. 9 A and B. Effect of "arthropod" toxins of *A. australis* on guinea pig ileum smooth muscle preparation. (A) Ileal prolonged contractive response to application of "*crustacean*" toxin followed by depressed response to several agonists. *CT*-Crustacean toxin (750 ng/ml) *a*-acetyl-choline (8 ng/ml); *h*-histamine (3 ng/ml); *s*-serotine (50 ng/ml); *n*-nicotine (600 ng/ml). Time base 15 min. (B) Ileal response to application of high dose (*arrow* 20 μg/ml) of insect toxin. *a*-acetylcholine 15 ng/ml. Time base 5 min. Only very small and transient change in muscular tonus was obtained. (A) taken from TINTPULVER et al., 1976)

repetitive firing and spontaneous muscular repetitive firing (Fig. 10), are due to excitatory presynaptic effects (Fig. 10) of the terminal nerve branches. The ability of the different toxins to induce these phenomena in the different preparations were tested.

Using the insect nerve-muscle preparation, it was found that the insect toxin was the most potent in the induction of the above neuromuscular effects as well as in the paralysis of whole insects, about 100 and 25 times stronger than the crude venom, respectively. It was specifically effective in the induction of sponta-neous repetitive firing of the nerve (Fig. 10 D), but did not affect the pattern of the externally recorded nerve action potentials (Fig. 11 B, b, c). The "crustacean" toxin was about 20 times more potent than the crude venom when tested on the insect neuromuscular preparation, but was definitely less active than the latter in inducing paralysis of the insect (locust Table 4). The "mammal" toxin I was about 7 times more potent than the crude venom in the indication of the neuromus-cular effects as well as paralysis of the whole animal. This compound demonstrated a clear prolongation of the evoked and spontaneous externally recorded nerve action potentials (Fig. 11 B, b). The most potent "mammal" toxin II demonstrated only a limited effect on the neuromuscular preparation and a very weak effect (5 times less than the crude venom) on the paralysis of the above animal (Table 4).

When tested on the crustacean nerve-muscle preparation, it was found that the "crustacean" toxin was the most potent in the induction of neuromuscular effects (Fig. 10 A) and was about 125 times stronger than the crude venom. On the axonal preparation it caused an extreme prolongation of the action potential as well as repetitive activity (Fig. 11 A). The "mammal" toxin I, which was about

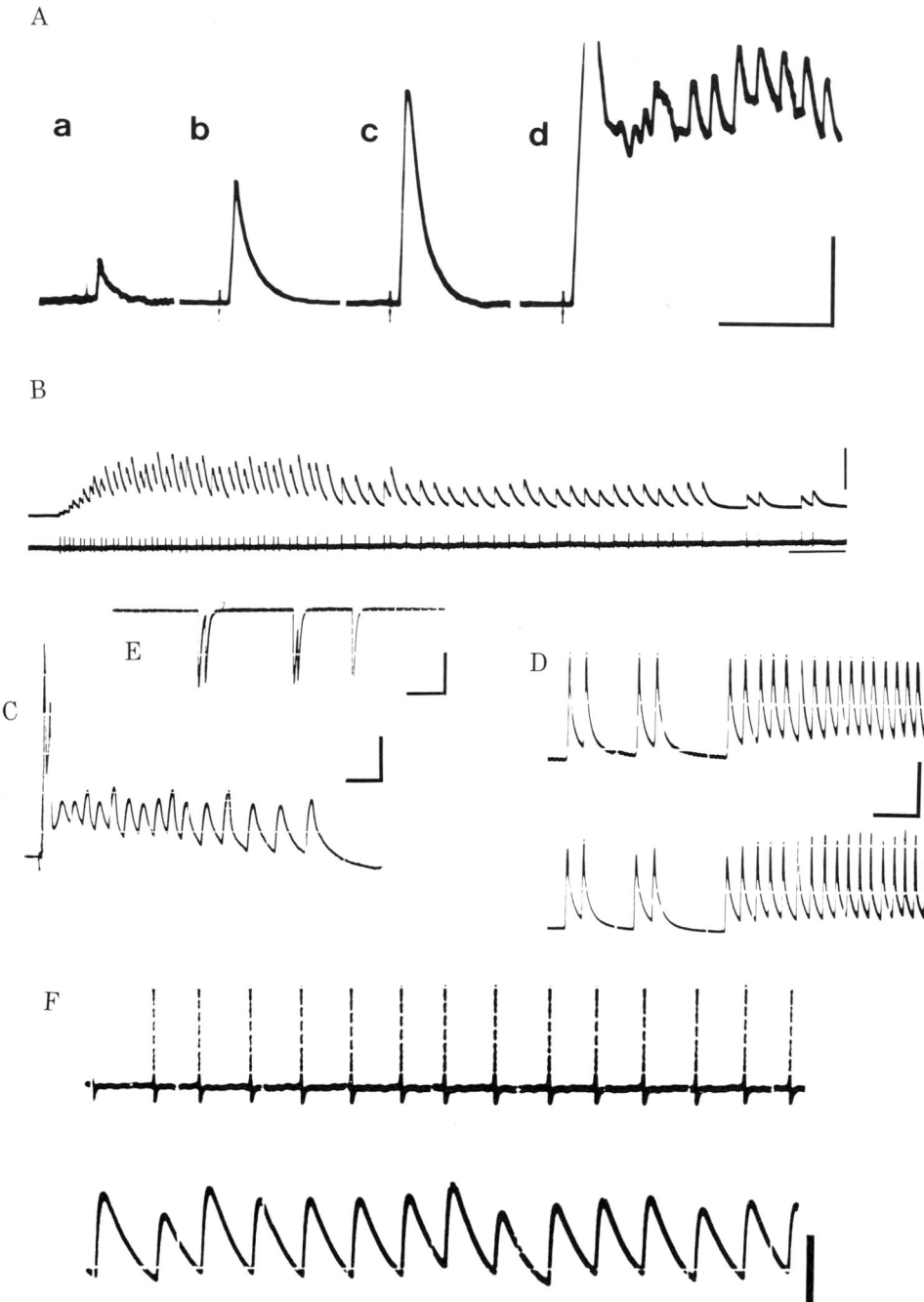

Fig. 10 A – F. Neuromuscular effects of different scorpion toxins on crayfish and locust preparations. (A) different stages of intoxication by 0.026 µg/ml of "crustacean" toxin when applied to dactylus opener muscle and its excitatory motor nerve of walking leg of crayfish *Astacus leptodactylus. a*: normal junction potential before venom, *b* and *c*: 20 and 45 s after application; a strong increase in amplitude, *d*: 50 s after application, strong response to single stimulation

25 times stronger than the crude venom in the induction of repetitive neuromuscular activity, was also effective in inducing the prolonged and spontaneous action potentials in the crayfish axonal preparation. The "mammal" toxin II was only about 4 times stronger than the crude venom in the induction of the neuromuscular effects and was inactive on the axonal preparations. Qualitative differences between "mammal" toxins I and II of *A. australis* were also expressed in their cardiovascular effects. Toxin I, in contrast to II, did not demonstrate any ganglionic blocking effect and its cardiotoxic action was hardly antagonized by propranolol (CHEYMOL et al., 1974).

When tested on the spider nerve muscle preparation, it was found that the "insect" toxin was inactive in contrast to the "crustacean" toxin which was the most potent in the induction of the neuromuscular effects (about 70 times as active as the crude venom). The "mammal" toxins I and II were found to be about 10 and 5 times as active as the crude venom.

The relative activity of the different toxins on the different preparations is summarized in Table 4. From the point of view of specificity and selectivity in the action of the different toxins, the data presented in Table 4 may indicate that: (1) The "crustacean" and the "mammal" toxins should be considered as possessing only a relative affinity or specificity to different organisms. The pharmacologic diversity of these substances may represent either multiplicity of active sites or differential affinities to identical receptor sites in different organisms. It is noteworthy that the presence of a component such as the crustacean toxin, which by itself is nonlethal to mammals but is able to perform an excitatory action in mammalian systems, may possess certain pharmacologic as well as pharmaceutic advantages. (2) The discrepancy between the potency of the "crustacean" and the "mammal" II toxins on the locust nerve muscle preparation, as compared to their locust paralysis activity, may indicate that the specificity of the above toxins may be at least partially attributed to their specific resistance or susceptibility to inactivation processes in the body. (3) There exists a close resemblance between

---

followed by train of repetitive firing. Cal. a 2 mv, b−d 20 mv, 200 ms. (B) Simultaneous recording from muscle (*upper trace*) and its motor nerve (*lower trace*) of same preparation (A) about 3 min after application of 0.2 µg/ml of crustacean toxin. Full synchrony between nerve action potentials and muscle junction potentials clearly indicates axonal origin of muscle response. Calibration 20 mv, 1 s. (C) Single response of "fast" and repetitive response of "slow" ejps in *extenso tibiae* muscle in hindleg of locust *Locusta migratoria* to single synchronous stimulation of two motor axons, 60 min after application of 0.7 µg/ml of crustacean toxin. Calibration: 10 mv, 50 ms. (D) Start of spontaneous train of ejps recorded synchronously from two different bundles of *extensor tibiae,* 50 min after application of 0.15 µg/ml of insect toxin. Clear synchrony between two bundles may indicate a common presynaptic origin of the muscular excitatory response (see F). Calibration: 10 mv, 100 ms. (E) Spontaneous inhibitory junction potentials (ijps) recorded from the *extensor tibiae* preparation 50 min after application of 8 µg/ml of *A. australis* crude venom. Preparation was paralyzed by *Habrobracon* venom (WALTHER and RATHMAYER, 1974) thus blocking the excitatory neuromuscular transmission and enabling full expression of inhibitory response. Calibration: 5 mv, 500 ms. (F) Spontaneous neuromuscular activity caused by insect toxin in above locust preparation: Synchronous recording from "slow" motor axon (*upper trace:* upward going signals, positive) and muscle fibre in main part of *extensor tibiae* (*lower trace*) 65 min after application of 0.4 µg/ml of insect toxin. Calibration: 50 ms: upper 0.5 mv, lower 10 mv (A, B)—taken from RATHMAYER et al., 1977. (C−F) taken from WALTHER et al., 1976

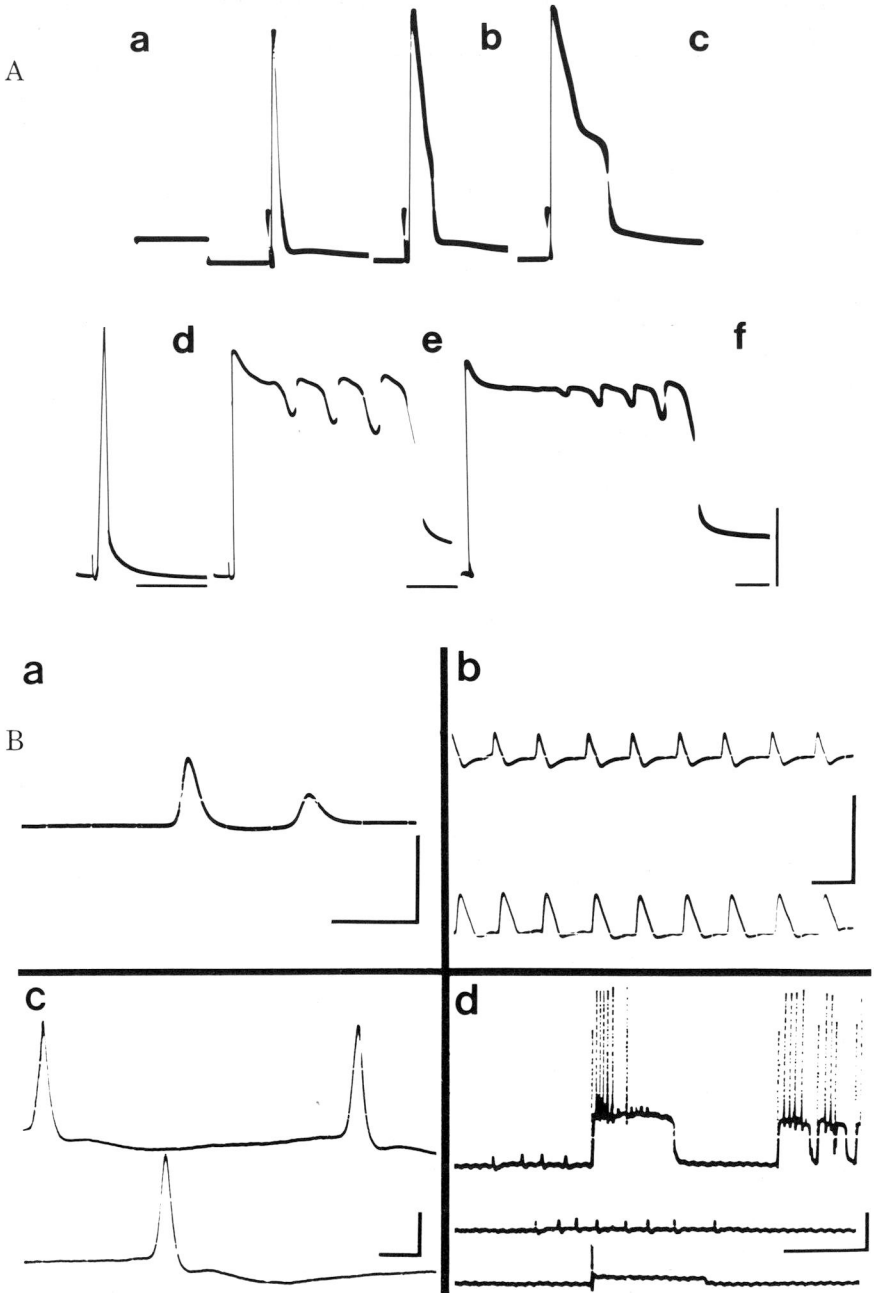

Fig. 11A and B. Effects of toxins on nerve action potentials. (A) Effect of "crustacean" toxin on isolated lateral giant axon from central nervous system of crayfish *A. leptodactylus*. Evoked action potentials were intracellularly recorded. *a*. Before toxin, normal action potential. *b*. Slight prolongation of decay phase obtained 6 min following application of 0.13 µg/ml of crustacean toxin. *c*. Increase in prolongation of action potential 25 min after application of toxin. *d*. New experiment, before toxin. *e*. 8 min following application of 1.3 µg/ml of

Table 4. Relative activity of different scorpion toxins on several nerve muscle preparations[a] as well as insect paralysis

Toxic material[b]	Insect[c]	Crustacean[d]	Arachnid[e]	Mammal[f]	Insects[g] paralysis
Crude venom	1	1	1	1	1
"Insect" toxin	115	No effect	No effect	No effect	25
"Crustacean" toxin	18	127	67	0.7	0.7
"Mammal" toxin I	7	27	11	1	5.7
"Mammal" toxin II	2	4	5	25	0.2

[a] Based on comparison of average minimal doses causing an evoked repetitive muscular response. Numbers express activity in terms of folds of that of crude venom. [b] The different toxins were purified from crude venom of the scorpion *A. australis Hector* (see Sect. B II and C VI 3) [c] Locust leg *extensor tibiae* preparation. [d] Crayfish walking leg dactylus opener preparation. [e] Claw closer muscle preparation in leg of mygalomorph spider. [f] Guinea pig ileum smooth muscle preparation. [g] Determined by injection into body cavity of 2nd and 3rd instar locusts larvae.

the response of the crayfish and the spider nerve-muscle preparation to the different toxins (Table 4). This may indicate certain structural and functional similarities between the neuromuscular systems of these two classes of arthropods, differentiating them from insects. (4) The "insect" toxin represents substances demonstrating a high degree of selectivity being able to diversity between related groups of arthro-

---

"crustacean" toxin. Note large prolongation of action potential accompanied by "oscillations" in membrane potential. *f.* 16 min after above toxin application, additional prolongation of action potential. Such effect, in same preparation, was also obtained by "mammal" toxin I, but not with "insect" as well as "mammal" II toxins. Calibration: a—c calibration pulse 10 mv, 10 ms; d, 20 mv; 20 ms; e and f, 25 mv 20 ms (taken from RATHMAYER et al., 1977) (B) Effects of different toxins on motor nerve to *extensor tibiae* muscle of locust. Recording was performed with specially adapted thin glass suction electodes enabling recording of positively shaped and monophasic action potentials. Their identification as "slow" or "fast" excitatory or inhibitory was obtained by synchronous muscle recording and because this nerve (nerve 3c Hoyle, 1955) contains only axons supplying *extensor tibiae* muscle. a) Control: Action potentials recorded from "slow" (first) and inhibitory axons—simultaneously stimulated. Calibration: 1 mv, 2 ms. b) Application of 8 μg/ml of mammal toxin I. Synchronous recording from both ends of nerve. Spontaneous activity of slow axon. Note prolonged decay phase of action potentials. Calibration 1 mv, 20 ms. c) Successive recording from distal end of nerve, 45 min after application of 2 μg/ml of insect toxin. Spontaneous repetitive activity of "slow." Note late negative after potentials. Calibration: 0.2 mv and 2 ms. d) Spontaneous activity 60 min after application of 0.8 μg/ml crustacean toxin. *Upper trace:* short train of small action potentials in inhibitory axon, followed by "plateaus" with superimposed burst of large action potentials in slow action. *Middle trace:* train of action potentials from inhibitory axon only. *Lower trace:* single action potentials and plateau due to activity of fast excitatory axon. Calibration 0.2 mv, 200 ms. Prolongation of action potentials and "plateau" phenomena appear to be typical quality of scorpion venom (see Section C V). Insect toxin, however, seems not to share this basic property. This toxin in contrast to others, induced long spike trains or even continuous axonal activity, and was most potent with respect to excitatory neuromuscular action as well as paralytic effects. (See Table 4, taken from WALTHER et al., 1976)

pods. As such the "insect" toxin may serve as a pharmacologic tool in the investigation of insect neurons, and the molecular mechanism of its action should be clarified.

Acknowledgement: This work was supported by grant nb. 730 from the United-States-Israel Binational Science Foundation (BSF), Jerusalem, Israel.

References

Adam, K.R., Weiss, C.: The occurence of 5-hydroxytriptamine in scorpion venom. J. exp. Biol., **35**, 39—41 (1958).

Adam, K.R., Weiss, C.: 5-hydroxytryptamine in scorpion venom. Nature (Lond.), **183**, 1398 (1959a).

Adam, K.R., Weiss, C.: Actions of scorpion venom on skeletal muscle. Brit. J. Pharmacol. **14**, 334—339 (1959b).

Adam, K.R., Weiss, C.: Some aspects of the pharmacology of the venoms of african scorpions. Mem. Inst. Butantan. **33**, 603—614 (1966).

Adam, K.R., Schmidt, H., Stampfli, R., Weiss, C.: The effect of scorpion venom on single myelinated nerve fibres of the frog. Brit. J. Pharmacol., **26**, 666—677 (1966).

Arthus, M.: Recherches expérimentales sur le venin de *Buthus quinquestriatus*. C.R. Acad. Sci. (Paris) **156**, 1256—1258 (1913).

Babin, D.R., Watt, D.D., Goos, S.M., Mlejnek, R.V.: Amino acid sequence of neurotoxin I from *Centruroides sculpturatus* Ewing. Arch. Biochem. Biophys., **166**, 125—134 (1975).

Baker, P.F., Reuter, H.: Calcium movement in excitable cells. 1st ed. New York-Toronto-Sydney-Oxford-Braunschweig: Pergamon, 1975.

Balozet, L.: Scorpionism in the old world. In: Venomous animals and their venoms, Bücherl, W., Buckley, E.E. (eds.) vol. III, p. 349, New York-London: Academic Press, 1971.

Barsoum, G.S., Nabavy, M., Salama, S.: Scorpion poisoning—its signs, symptoms and treatment. J. Egypt. med. Ass. **37**, 857—862 (1954).

Bearg, W.J.: Scorpions: Biology and effect of their venom. Agric. exp. Station, Univ. Ankansas Bull. 649 (1961).

Benoit, P.R., Mambrini, J.: Action du venin de scorpion sur la jonction neuromusculaire de la grenouille. J. Physiol. (Paris) **59**, 348 (1967).

Bianchi, C.P.: Cell calcium. London: Butterworths, 1968.

Böhn, G.M., Pompolo, S., Diniz, C.R., Gomez, M.V., Pimenta Aurea, F., Netto, J.C.: Ultrastructural alterations of mouse diaphragm nerve endings induced by purified scorpion venom, tityutoxin. Toxicon, **12**, 509—511 (1974).

Braun, K., Stern, S., Werkson, S.: Sympathomimetic effects of scorpion venom of the cardiovascular system. Israel J. med. Sci. **5**, 853—854 (1969).

Brazil, O.V., Neder, A.C., Corrado, A.P.: Effects and mechanism of action of *Tityus serrulatus* venom on skeletal muscle. Pharmacol. Res. Commun. **5**, 137—150 (1973).

Bücherl, W.: Escorpiones e escorpionismo no Brazil. II. Mem. Inst. Butantan, **25**, 53—82 (1953).

Bücherl, W.: Studien über einige brasilianische Skorpione und ihre Trockengifte. Arzneimittel-Forsch. **5**, 68—71 (1955).

Bücherl, W.: Classification, biology, and venom extraction of scorpions. In: Venomous animals and their venoms. Bücherl, W., Buckley, E.E. (eds.). Vol. III, p. 317, New York, London: Academic Press, 1971.

Bücherl, W., Pucca, N.: Escorpiones e escorpionismo no Brazil. III. Mem Inst. Butantan **27**, 41—50 (1956).

Bülbring, E., Branding, A.F., Jones, A.W., Tomita, I. (eds.): Smooth muscle. 1st ed. London: Arnold, 1970.

Cahalan, M.D.: Modification of sodium channel gating in frog myelinated nerve fibers by *Centruroides sculpturatus* venom. J. Physiol. (Lond.) **244**, 511—534 (1975).

Catterall, W.A.: Cooperative activation of action potential Na ionophore by neurotoxins. Proc. nat. Acad. Sci. (Wash.) **72**, 1782–1786 (1975).

Celeste-Henriques, M., Gazzinelli, G., Diniz, C.R., Gomez, M.V.: Effect of the venom of the scorpion *Tityus serrulatus* on adrenal gland catacholamines. Toxicon, **5**, 175–179 (1968).

Cheymol, J., Bourillet, F., Roch-Arveilier, M., Heckle, J.: Action neuromusculaire de trois venins de scorpions nord-africains (*Leiurus quinquestriatus, Buthus occitanus* et *Androctonus australis*) et de deux toxines extraites de l'un d'entre eux. Toxicon, 277–282 (1973).

Cheymol, J., Bourillet, F., Roch-Arveilier, M., Heckle, J.: Action cardiovasculaire de trois venins de scorpions nord-africains (*Androctonus australis, Leiurus quinquestriatus, Buthus occitanus*) et de deux toxines extraites de l'un d'entre eux. Toxicon, **12**, 241–248 (1974).

Chicheportiche, R., Lazdunski, M.: The conformation of small proteins. The state-diagram of a neurotoxin of *Androctonus australis Hector*. Europ. J. Biochem. **14**, 549–555 (1970).

Corrado, A.P., Antonio, A., Diniz, C.R.: Brazilian scorpion venom (*Tityus serrulatus*) an unusual sympathetic postganglionic stimulant. J. Pharmacol. exp. Ther. **164**, 253–258 (1968).

Corrado, A.P., Riccioppo Neto, F., Antonio, A.: The mechanism of the hypertensive effect of Brazilian scorpion venom (*Tityus serrulatus* Lutz e Mello). Toxicon, **12**, 145–150 (1974).

Couraud, F., Rochat, H., Lissitzky, S.: Stimulation of sodium and calcium uptake by scorpion toxin in chick embryo heart cells. Bioch. Biophys. Acta **433**, 90–100 (1976).

Cunha-Melo, J.R., Freire-Maia, L., Tafuri, W.L., Maria, T.A.: Mechanism of action of purified scorpion toxin on the isolated rat intestine. Toxicon, **11**, 81–84 (1973).

D'Ajello, V., Zlotkin, E., Miranda, F., Lissitzky, S., Bettini, S.: The effect of scorpion venom and pure toxin on the cockroach central nervous system. Toxicon, **10**, 399–404 (1972).

Del Castillo, J., Katz, B.: Biophysical aspects of neuromuscular transmission. Progr. Biophys., **6**, 121–170 (1956).

Del Pozo, E.C.: Mechanism and pharmacological actions of scorpion venoms. In: Venoms. Buckley, E.E., Porges, N. (eds.) Amer. Ass. Advanc. Sci. p. 123, 1956.

Del Pozo, E.C., Anguiano, L.G.: Acciones del veneno de alacran sobre la actividad motora de musculo estriado. Rev. Inst. Salubr. Enferm. trop. (Méx.), **8**, 231–263 (1947).

Del Pozo, E.C., Gonzales, J., Mendez, T.H.: Acciones del veneno de alacran sobre el aparato respiratorio. Rev. Inst. Salubr. Enferm. trop. (Méx.) **6**, 77–84 (1945).

Dettbarn, W.D.: Mechanism of action of Tetrodotoxin and Saxitoxin. In: Neuropoisons. vol. 1. Simpson, L.L. (ed.): New York-London: Plenum Press 1971.

Diniz, C.R.: Chemical and pharmacological properties of *Tityus* venoms. In: Venomous animals and their venoms. Bücherl, W., Buckley, E.E. (eds.). Vol. III p. 311, New York, London: Academic Press, 1971.

Diniz, C.R., Torres, J.M.: Release of an acetylcholine-like substance from guinea pig ileum by scorpion venom. Toxicon, **5**, 277–281 (1968).

Diniz, C.R., Valeri, V.: Effects of a toxin present in a purified extract of telsons from the scorpion *Tityus serrulatus* on smooth muscle preparations and in mice. Arch. int. Pharmacodyn. **121**, 1–9 (1959).

Diniz, C.R., Pimenta, A.F., Netto, J.C., Pompolo, S., Gomez, M.V., Böhn, G.M.: Effect of scorpion toxin from *Tityus serrulatus* (Tityustoxin) on the acetylcholine release and fine structure of the nerve terminals. Experientia (Basel) **30**, 1304–1305 (1974).

Efrati, P.: Poisoning scorpion stings in Israel. Amer. J. trop. med. **29**, 249 (1949).

Elmqvist, D., Feldman, D.S.: Spontaneous activity at a mammalian neuromuscular junction in tetrodotoxin. Acta physiol. scand. **64**, 475–476 (1965).

Fayet, G., Couraud, F., Miranda, F., Lissitzky, S.: Electro-optical system for monitoring activity of heart cells in culture: application to the study of several drugs and scorpion toxins. Europ. J. Pharmacol. **27**, 165–174 (1974).

Ferrans, V.J., Hibbs, R.G., Walsh, J.J., Burch, G.E.: Histochemic and electron microscopic studies on the cardiac necroses produced by sympathomimetic agents. Ann. N.Y. Acad. Sci., **156**, 309–314 (1969).

Fishman, S.N., Khodorov, B.I., Volkenstein, M.V.: Molecular mechanisms of membrane ionic permeability changes. Biochem. biophys. Acta, **225**, 1–10 (1971).

Fraenkel, G., Zlotkin, E.: Acceleration of puparium formation in *Sarcophaga argyrostoma* by electrical stimulation and scorpion venom. J. Insect Physiol., **16**, 1549–1554 (1970).

Frank, G.B.: Effect of veratrine on muscle fibre membrane and on negative after potential. J. Neurophysiol. **21**, 263—278 (1958).

Frankenhauser, B., Hodgkin, A.L.: The action of calcium on the electrical properties of squid axons. J. Physiol. (Lond.) **137**, 218—244 (1975).

Freire-Maia, L., Azevedo, A.D., Costa Val, V.P.: Respiratory arrhythmias produced by purified scorpion toxin. Toxicon, **11**, 255—257 (1973).

Freire-Maia, L., Azevedo, A.D., Lima, E.G., Beirao, P.S.L., Ribeiro, I.A.: Pharmacological blockade of the cardiovascular and respiratory effects produced by tityustoxin in the rat. Toxicon, **13**, 92—93 (1975).

Freire-Maia, L., Diniz, C.R.: Pharmacological action of a purified scorpion toxin in the rat. Toxicon, **8**, 132 (1970).

Freire-Maia, L., Ferreira, M.C.: Estudo do mecanismo da hiperglicemia e da hipertensao arterial, produzidas pelo veneno de escorpiao, no cao. Mem. Inst. Osw. Cruz, **59**, 11—22 (1961).

Freire-Maia, L., Pinto, G.I., Franco, I.: Mechanism of the cardiovascular effects produced by purified scorpion toxin in the rat. J. Pharmacol. exp. Ther. **188**, 207—213 (1974).

Freire-Maia, L., Ribeiro, R.M., Beraldo, W.T.: Effects of purified scorpion toxin on respiratory movements in the rat. Toxicon, **8**, 307—310 (1970).

Garcia, L.G., Garcia, A., Martinez, G., Pakaris, A., Rochat, H., Miranda, F.: Purification of animal toxins: isolation and characterization of three toxins from the venom of the American scorpion *Centruroides suffusus suffusus*. In preparation.

Gilbert, D.L., Ehrenstein, G.: Effect of divalent cations on potassium conductance of squid axons: determination of surface charge. Biophys. J., **9**, 447—464 (1969).

Gomez, M.V., Dai, M.E.M., Diniz, C.R.: Effect of scorpion venom, tityutoxin, on the release of acetylcholine from incubated slices of rat brain. J. Neurochem. **20**, 1051—1061 (1973).

Gomez, V.M., Diniz, C.R., Barbosa, T.S.: A comparison of the effects of scorpion venom tityustoxin and ouabain on the release of acetylcholine from incubated slices of rat brain. J. Neurochem. **24**, 331—336 (1975).

Gueron, M., Stern, J., Cohen, W.: Severe miocardial damage and hearth failure in scorpion sting. Report of five cases. Amer. J. Cardiol. **19**, 719—726 (1967).

Gueron, M., Weizmann, S.: Catecholamine excretion in scorpion sting. Israel J. med. Sci. **5**, 855—857 (1969).

Gueron, M., Yarom, R.: Cardiovascular manifestations of severe scorpion sting. Clinopathologic correlations. Chest, **57**, 156—162 (1970).

Hirs, C.H.W.: Chromatography of enzymes on ion exchange resins. In: Methods in enzymology, vol. I, p. 113. New York: Academic Press, 1955.

Houssay, B.A.: Action physiologique du venin des scorpions (*Buthus quinquestriatus* and *Tityus bahiensis*). J. Physiol. Path. gén. **18**, 305—317 (1919).

Hubbard, J.I.: Mechanism of transmitter release. Progr. Biophys. molec. Biol. **21**, 33—124 (1970).

Ibrahim, S.A.: Phospholipase A in scorpion venoms. Toxicon, **5**, 56—61 (1967).

Ismail, M., Osman, O.H., El-Asmar, M.F.: Pharmacological studies of the venom from the scorpion *Buthus minax* (L. Koch). Toxicon, **11**, 15—20 (1973).

Ismail, M., Osman, O.H., Ibrahim, S.A., El-Asmar, M.F.: Cardiovascular and respiratory responses to the venom from the scorpion *Leiurus quinquestriatus*. E. Afr. med. J., **49**, 279—285 (1972).

Israeli-Zindel, I., Zlotkin, E., Shulov, A.: The resistance of insects to the venom of the yellow scorpion *Leiurus quinquestriatus*. In: Toxins of animal and plant origin. De Vries, A., Kochwa, E. (eds.) New York, London, Paris: Gordon and Breach, vol. 3, p. 933 1973.

Kamon, E., Shulov, A.: Estimation of locust resistance to scorpion venom. J. Insect Path. **5**, 206—214 (1963).

Katz, B., Miledi, R.: Tetrodotoxin and neuromuscular transmission. Proc. roy. Soc. B. **167**, 8—22 (1967a).

Katz, B., Miledi, R.: Ionic requirements of synaptic transmitter release. Nature, Lond. **215**, 651 (1967b).

Katz, N.L., Edwards, Ch.: The effect of scorpion venom on the neuromuscular junction of the frog. Toxicon, **10**, 133—137 (1972).

Kopeyan, C., Martinez, G., Lissitzky, S., Miranda, F., Rochat, H.: Disulfide bonds of toxin II of the scorpion *Androctonus australis* Hector. Europ. J. Biochem. **47**, 483—489 (1974).

Koppenhöfer, E., Schmidt, H.: Die Wirkung von Skorpiongift auf die Ionenströme des Ranvierschen Schnürrings. I. Die Permeabilitäten PNa and Pk. Pflügers Arch. ges. Physiol. **303**, 133—149 (1968a).

Koppenhöfer, E., Schmidt, H.: Die Wirkung von Skorpiongift auf die Ionenströme des Ranvierschen Schnürrings. II. Unvollständige Natrium-Inaktivierung. Pflügers Arch. ges. Physiol. **303**, 150—161 (1968b).

Koppenhöfer, E., Schmidt, H.: Incomplete sodium inactivation in nodes of Ranvier treated with scorpion venom. Experientia (Basel) **24**, 41—42 (1968c).

La Grange, R.G., Russell, F.: Effects of *Centruroides sculpturatus* and *C. gertschi* venom on the mammalian nerve-muscle preparation: a possible mechanism of action. Proc. West. Pharmacol. Soc. **14**, 163—165 (1971).

Lin, S.S., Huang, M., Tseng, W.C., Lee, C.Y.: Comparative studies on the muscular contracture induced by cobra cardiotoxin and scorpion toxin. Communication at 4th International Symposium on Animal, Plant and Microbial Toxins, Tokyo 1974. Toxicon, **13**, 108, (1975) abstract.

Lissitzky, S., Miranda, F., Etzensperger, P., Mercier, J.: Sur la toxicité du venin de deux espèces de scorpions nord-africains. C. R. Soc. Biol. (Paris) **150**, 741—743 (1956).

Magalhaes, O.: Contribucao para o contrecimiento da intoxicao pelo veno dos "escorpiones". Mem. Inst. Osw. Cruz, **21**, 5—159 (1928).

Martin, M.F.: Purification et caractérisation des neurotoxines du venin du scorpion *Buthus B. occitanus paris*. Diplôme d'Etudes Approfondies, Faculté des Sciences, Marseille (1974).

Master, R.W.S., Rao, S., Soman, P.D.: Electrophoretic separation of biologically active constituents of scorpion venom. Biochim. biophys. Acta, **71**, 422 (1963).

Mazzotti, L., Bravo-Becherelle, M.A.: Scorpionism in the Mexican republic. In: Venomous and poisonous animals and noxious plants of the Pacific area. Keegan and MacFarlane (eds.) London, New York, Sydney: Pergamon, pp. 119—131, 1963.

Miranda, F., Kopeyan, C., Rochat, C., Lissitzky, S.: Purification of animal neurotoxins. Isolation and characterization of eleven neurotoxins from the venom of the scorpions *Androctonus australis* Hector, *Buthus occitanus tunetanus* and *Leiurus quinquestriatus quinquestriatus*. Europ. J. Biochem., **16**, 514—523 (1970a).

Miranda, F., Kopeyan, C., Rochat, H., Rochat, C., Lissitzky, S.: Purification of animal neurotoxins. Isolation and characterization of four neurotoxins from two different sources of *Naja haje* venom. Europ. J. Biochem., **17**, 477—484 (1970b).

Miranda, F., Lissitzky, S.: Purification de la toxine du venin de scorpion. Biochim. biophys. Acta, **30**, 217—218 (1958).

Miranda, F., Lissitzky, S.: Scorpamins the toxin proteins of scorpion venoms. Nature (Lond.), **190**, 443—444 (1961).

Miranda, F., Rochat, H., Lissitzky, S.: Sur la neurotoxine du venin de scorpions. I.-Purification à partir du venin de deux espèces de scorpions nord-africains. Bull. Soc. Chim. biol. (Paris) **42**, 379—391 (1960).

Miranda, F., Rochat, H., Lissitzky, S.: Sur la neurotoxine du venin des scorpions. II-Utilisation de l'électrophorèse sur papier pour l'orientation et le contrôle de la purification. Biochimie, **43**, 945—952 (1961).

Miranda, F., Rochat, H., Lissitzky, S.: Propriétés échangeuses d'ions du gel de dextrane (Sephadex). Application à la mise au point d'une technique de rétention réversible des protéins basiques de faible poids moléculaire. J. Chromatogr., **7**, 142—154 (1962).

Miranda, F., Rochat, H., Lissitzky, S.: Sur les neurotoxines de deux espèces de scorpions nord-africains. I-Purification des neurotoxines (scorpamines) d'*Androctonus australis* (L.) et de *Buthus occitanus* (Am.). Toxicon, **2**, 51—69 (1964a).

Miranda, F., Rochat, H., Lissitzky, S.: Sur les neurotoxines de deux espèces de scorpion nord-africains. II-Propriétés des neurotoxines (scorpamines) d'*Androctonus australis* (L.) et de *Buthus occitanus* (Am.). Toxicon, **2**, 113—121 (1964b).

Miranda, F., Rochat, H., Lissitzky, S.: Sur les neurotoxines de deux espèces de scorpions nord-africains. III-Déterminations préliminaires aux études de structure sur les neurotoxines (scorpamines) d'*Androctonus australis* (L.) et de *Buthus occitanus* (Am.). Toxicon, **2**, 123–138 (1964c).

Miranda, F., Rochat, H., Rochat, C., Lissitzky, S.: Complexes moléculaires présentés par les neurotoxines animales. I-Neurotoxines des venins de scorpions (*Androctonus australis Hector* et *Buthus occitanus tunetanus*). Toxicon, **4**, 123–144 (1966).

Mohammed, A.H.: Preparation of antiscorpion serum. Use of atropine and ergotine. Lancet, **2**, 364–365 (1942).

Mohammed, A.H.: Blood sugar response to Egyptian scorpions. Nature (Lond.), **166**, 734–735 (1950).

Mohammed, A.H., Kamel, A., Ayobe, M.H.: Studies of phospholipase A and B activities of egyptian snake venoms and scorpion toxin. Toxicon, **6**, 293–298 (1969).

Mohammed, A.H., Rohayem, H., Zaky, O.: The action of scorpion toxin on blood sodium and potassium. J. trop. Med. Hyg., **57**, 85–87 (1954).

Moss, J., Colburn, R.W., Kopin, I.J.: Scorpion toxin induced catecholamine release from synaptosomes. J. Neurochem. **22**, 217–221 (1974).

Moss, J., Kazic, T., Henry, P., Kopin, I.J.: Scorpion venom induced discharge of catecholamines accompanied by hypertension. Brain Res. **54**, 381–385 (1973).

Moss, A.J., Vittands, I., Schenk, E.A.: Cardiovascular effects of sustained norepinephirine infusions. Circulat. Res. **18**, 596–601 (1966).

Narahashi, T., Shapiro, B.I., Deguchi, T., Scuka, M., Wang, Ch.M.: Effects of scorpion venom on squid axon membranes. Amer. J. Physiol. **222**, 850–857 (1972).

Nickerson, M.: Antihypertensive agents and the drug therapy of hypertension. In: The pharmacological basis of therapeutics. Goodman, L.S., Gilman, A. (eds.) London-Toronto: MacMillan, p. 728, 1971.

Osman, O.H., Ismail, M., Wenger, T.: Hyperthermic response to intraventricular injection of scorpion venom: Role of brain monoamines. Toxicon, **11**, 361–368, (1973).

Pansa, M.C., Migliori-Natalizi, G., Bettini, S.: Effect of scorpion venom and its fractions on the crayfish stretch receptor organ. Toxicon, **11**, 283–286 (1973).

Parnas, I., Avgar, D., Shulov, A.: Physiological effects of venom of *Leiurus quinquestriatus* on neuromuscular systems of locust and crab. Toxicon, **8**, 67–79 (1970).

Parnas, I., Russell, F.E.: Effects of venoms on nerve, muscle and neuromuscular junction. In: Animal toxins. Russell, F.E., Saunders, P.R. (eds.) Oxford, New York, Toronto, Paris: Pergamon, p. 401, 1967.

Patterson, R.A.: Physiological action of scorpion venom. Amer. J. trop. med. Hyg. **9**, 410–414, (1960).

Patterson, R.A.: Pharmacologic action of scorpion venom on intestinal smooth muscle. Toxicol. appl. Pharmacol. **4**, 710–719 (1962).

Patterson, R.A.: Effects of venom from the scorpion *Centruroides sculpturatus* on the rat. Toxicon, **2**, 167–170 (1964).

Patterson, R.A., Wooley, D.: Effect of scorpion venom (*Centruroides sculpturatus*) on the carotid body and superior cervical ganglion of the cat. Toxicon, **8**, 145 (1970) Abstract.

Phisalix, M.: Animaux venimeus et venins. Paris: Masson et Cie, 1922.

Poon-King, T.: Myocarditis from scorpion stings. Brit. med. J., 374–377 (1963).

Raab, W.: Key position of catecholamines in functional and degenerative cardiovascular pathology. Amer. J. Cardiol., **5**, 579–583 (1960).

Rahamimoff, R.: Role of calcium ions in neuromuscular transmission. In: Calcium and cellular function. Cuthbert, A.W. (ed.) MacMillan, 1970.

Ramos, A.O., Corrado, A.P.: Efecto hiperpirético do veneno de escorpiao (*Tityus serrulatus* e *Tityus bahiensis*). An. Fac. Med. S. Paulo, **28**, 81–98 (1954).

Rathmayer, W., Walther, Ch., Zlotkin, E.: The effect of different toxins from scorpion venom on neuromuscular transmission and nerve action potentials in the crayfish. Comp. Biochem. Physiol. **56c**, 35–39 (1977).

Rochat, C., Rochat, H., Miranda, F., Lissitzky, S.: Purification and some properties of the neurotoxins of *Androctonus australis* Hector. Biochemistry, **6**, 578–585 (1967).

Rochat, H., Kopeyan, C., Garcia, L.G., Martinez, G., Rosso, J.P., Pakaris, A., Martin, M.F., Garcia, A., Martin-Moutot, N., Gregoire, J., Miranda, F.: Recent results of the structure of scorpion and snake toxins. Communication at the 4th International Symposium on Animal, Plant and Microbial Toxins, Tokyo, Sept. 1974, Abstract: Toxicon, **13**, 116—117 (1975a).

Rochat, H., Pakaris, A., Martin, M.F., Miranda, F.: Purification of animal toxins: multiplicity of the toxins in the scorpion venom from *Buthus occitanus tunetanus.* In preparation.

Rochat, H., Rochat, C., Kopeyan, C., Lissitzky, S., Miranda, F., Edman, P.: Structure of scorpion neurotoxins. In: Toxins of animals and plant origin, De Vries, A., Kochwa, E. (eds.), vol. 2, p. 525. London: Gordon and Breach, 1972a.

Rochat, H., Rochat, C., Kopeyan, C., Miranda, F., Lissitzky, S., Edman, P.: Scorpion neurotoxins: a family of homologous proteins. F.E.B.S. Lett. **10**, 359—351 (1970b).

Rochat, H., Rochat, C., Miranda, F., Lissitzky, S., Edman, P.: The amino acid sequence of neurotoxin I of *Androctonus australis* Hector. Europ. J. Biochem. **17**, 262—266 (1970c).

Rochat, H., Rochat, C., Sampieri, F., Miranda, F., Lissitzky, S.: The amino acid sequence of neurotoxin II of *Androctonus australis* Hector. Europ. J. Biochem., **28**, 381—388 (1972).

Rochat, C., Sampieri, F., Rochat, H., Miranda, F., Lissitzky, S.: Iodination of neurotoxins I and II of the scorpion *Androctonus australis* Hector. Biochimie, **54**, 445—449 (1972).

Rochat, H., Tessier, M., Miranda, F., Lissitzky, S.: Enzymatic radio-iodination of animal toxins to very high specific radioactivity. Communication at the 4th International Symposium on Animal, Plant and Microbial Toxins, Tokyo, Sept. 1974, Abstract: Toxicon, **13**, 117 (1975b).

Romey, G., Chicheportiche, R., Lazdunski, M., Rochat, H., Miranda, F., Lissitzky, S.: Scorpion neurotoxin: a presynaptic toxin which affects both Na$^+$ and K$^+$ channels in axons. Biochem. biophys. Res. Commun. **64**, 115—121 (1975).

Rosso, J.P., Kopeyan, C., Rochat, H., Miranda, F.: Purification of animal toxins: isolation and characterization of the neurotoxins from the venom of the scorpion *Androctonus mauretanicus.* In preparation.

Ruhland, M., Zlotkin, E., Rathmayer, W.: The effect of toxins from the venom of the scorpion *Androctomis australis* an a spider nerve muscle preparation. Toxicon, **15**, 157—160 (1977).

Russell, F.E., Long, T.E.: Effects of venoms on neuromuscular transmission. In: Myasthenia gravis. Viets, B.A., (ed.) Springfield Ill.: C.C Thomas, p. 101, 1961.

Sampieri, F., Habersetzer-Rochat, C.: Structure function relationship of scorpion neurotoxins. Communication at the 4th International Symposium on Animal, Plant and Microbial Toxins, Tokyo (1974). Abstract: Toxicon, **13**, 120 (1975).

Sarnoff, S.J.: Certain aspects of the role of catecholamines in circulatory regulation. Amer. J. Cardiol., **5**, 579—585 (1960).

Schenk, E.A., Moss, A.Y.: Cardiovascular effects of sustained norepinephrine infusion. Circulat. Res. **18**, 605—609 (1966).

Schmitt, O., Schmidt, H.: Influence of calcium ions on the ionic currents of nodes of Ranvier treated with scorpion venom. Pflügers Arch. ges. Physiol. **333**, 51—61 (1972).

Schöttler, W.H.A.: On the toxicity of scorpion venom. Amer. J. trop. Med. Hyg., **3**, 172—178 (1954).

Shigenobu, K., Sperelakis, N.: Development of sensitivity to tetrodotoxin of chick embryonic hearts with age. J. molec. cell. Cardiol., **3**, 271—286 (1971).

Shulov, A.: On the poison scorpions in Israel. Harefuah, **49**, 1—3 (1955).

Smythies, J.R., Benington, F., Brandey, B.J., Bridgers, W.F., Morin, R.D.: On the mechanism of action of scorpion neurotoxin II from *Androctonus australis* Hector. J. theor. Biol., **43**, 65—72 (1974).

Sperelakis, N., Shigenobu, K.: Organ cultured chick embryonic hearts of various ages. I. Electrophysiology. J. molec. cell. Cardiol. **6**, 449—471 (1974).

Stahnke, H.L.: Variables in venom research. Biosystems **34**, 64—71 (1963a).

Stahnke, H.L.: Some pharmacological characteristics of *Centruroides sculpturatus* Ewing scorpion venom. In: Recent advances in pharmacology of toxins. Proc. 2nd. Int. Pharmacol. Meet., Prague, **9**, 63—70 (1963b).

Stahnke, H.L.: The treatment of venoms bites and stings. Arizona State University, 1966a.

Stahnke, H.L.: Some aspects of scorpion behavior. Bull. Sth Calif. Acad. Sci. **65**, 65—80 (1966b).

Sturman, N.: Scorpion sting poisoning in the Negev. Dapim Refuiim, **21**, 661—665 (1962).

Tafuri, W.L., Maria, T.A., Freire-Maia, L., Cunha-Melo, I.R.: Effect of the scorpion toxin on the granular vesicles in the Aurbach's plexus of the rat ileum. J. neurol. Trans. **35**, 233–240 (1974).

Tazieff-Depierre, F.: Venin de scorpion, calcium et émission d'acetylcholine par les fibres nerveuses dans l'ileon de cobaye. C.R. Acad. Sci. (Paris) D, **275**, 3021–3024 (1972).

Tazieff-Depierre, F., Andrillon, P.: Sécrétion d'acétylcholine provoquée par le venin de scorpion dand l'iléon de cobaye et sa suppression par la tétrodotoxine. C.R. Acad. Sci. (Paris) D, **276**, 1631–1633 (1973b).

Tazieff-Depierre, F., Andrillon, P., Goudou, D.: Calcium et action spasmogène du venin de scorpion sur l'iléon de cobaye. C.R. Acad. Sci. (Paris) D, **276**, 2985–2987 (1973c).

Tazieff-Depierre, F., Goudou, D., Andrillon, P.: Influence du calcium sur la désensibilisation de l'iléon isolé de cobaye au venin de scorpion. C.R. Acad. Sci (Paris) D, **227**, 1089–1092 (1973a).

Tazieff-Depierre, F., Lievremont, M.M., Czajka, M.: Mise en évidence de l'apparition de calcium dans des fibres musculaires par l'action du chlorure de potassium et des toxines du venin de scorpion (*Androctonus australis*). C.R. Acad. Sci. (Paris) D, **267**, 1477–1479 (1968).

Tazieff-Depierre, F., Metezau, Ph., Goudou, D.: Suppression de l'action spasmogène du venin de scorpion sur l'iléon isolé de cobaye par un inhibiteur de la permeabilité membranaire au calcium. C.R. Acad. Sci. (Paris) D, **279**, 1725–1728 (1974).

Tintpulver, M.: The action of different toxins derived from scorpion venom on the ileal smooth muscle preparation. M. Sc. thesis, Hebrew University, Jerusalem, 1975.

Tintpulver, M., Zerachia, T., Zlotkin, E.: The action of different toxins derived from scorpion venom on the ileal smooth muscle preparation. Toxicon. **14**, 371–377 (1976).

Vachon, M.: Etudes sur les scorpions. Alger, Inst. Pasteur 1952.

Walther, Ch., Rathmayer, W.: The effect of *Habrobracon* venom on excitatory neuromuscular transmission in insects. J. comp. Physiol., **89**, 23–38 (1974).

Walther, Ch., Zlotkin, E., Rathmeyer, W.: Action of different toxins from the scorpion *Androctonus australis* an a locust nerve-muscle preparation. J. Insect. Physiol. **22**, 1187–1194 (1976).

Watt, D.D., Babin, D.R., Mlejnek, R.V.: The protein neurotoxins in scorpion and elapid snake venoms. J. Agric. Food Chem., **22**, 43–51 (1974).

Wheeling, C.H., Keegan, H.L.: Effects of a scorpion venom on a tarantula. Toxicon, **10**, 305–306 (1972).

Wilson, W.H.: The physiological action of scorpion venom. J. Physiol. (Lond.) **31**, 48–49 (1904).

Yarom, R., Braun, K.: Myocardial pathology following scorpion venom injection. 4th Asian-Pacific Congr. Cardiol., **5**, 849–851 (1969).

Yarom, R., Braun, K.: Cardiovascular effects of scorpion venom, morphological changes in the myocardium. Toxicon, **8**, 41–46 (1970).

Yarom, R., Braun, K.: Electron microscopic studies of the myocardial changes produced by scorpion venom injections in dogs. Lab. Invest. **24**, 21–30 (1971a).

Yarom, R., Braun, K.: Ca^{24} changes in the myocardium following scorpion venom injections. J. molec. cell. Cardiol., **2**, 177–179 (1971b).

Yarom, R., Yallon, S., Notowitz, F., Braun, K.: Reversible myocardial damage by scorpion venom in perfused rat hearts. Toxicon, **12**, 347–351 (1974).

Zlotkin, E.: Chemistry of animal venoms. Experientia (Basel) **29**, 1453–1466 (1973).

Zlotkin, E., Blondheim, S.A., Shulov, A.: Effect of the venom of the scorpion *Leiurus quinquestriatus* on the tympanic nerve of the locust *Locusta migratoria migratorioides*. Toxicon, **8**, 47–49 (1970).

Zlotkin, E., Fraenkel, G., Miranda, F., Lissitzky, S.: The effect of scorpion venom on blowfly larvae; a new method for the evaluation of scorpion venom potency. Toxicon, **9**, 1–8 (1971a).

Zlotkin, E., Lebovitz, N., Shulov, A.: Toxic effects of the venom of the scorpion *Scorpio maurus palmatus* (Scorpionidae). Riv. Parassit., **33**, 237–243 (1972c).

Zlotkin, E., Martinez, G., Rochat, H., Miranda, F.: A protein toxic to crustacea from the venom of the scorpion *Androctonus australis*. Insect Biochem., **5**, 243–250 (1975a).

Zlotkin, E., Menashe, M., Rochat, H., Miranda, F., Lissitzky, S.: Proteins toxic to arthropods in the venom of elapid snakes. J. Insect Physiol. **21**, 1605—1611 (1975b).

Zlotkin, E., Miranda, F., Kupeyan, C., Lissitzky, S.: A new toxic protein in the venom of the scorpion *Androctonus australis Hector*. Toxicon, **9**, 9—13 (1971b).

Zlotkin, E., Miranda, F., Lissitzky, S.: Proteins toxic to mammals and insects in six scorpion venoms. Toxicon, **10**, 207—210 (1972a).

Zlotkin, E., Miranda, F., Lissitzky, S.: A toxic factor to crustacean in the venom of the scorpion *Androctonus australis Hector*. Toxicon, **10**, 211—216 (1972b).

Zlotkin, E., Rochat, H., Kupeyan, C., Miranda, F., Lissitzky, S.: Purification and properties of the insect toxin from the venom of the scorpion *Androctonus australis Hector*. Biochimie **53**, 1073—1078 (1971d).

Zlotkin, E., Rochat, H., Kupeyan, C., Miranda, F., Lissitzky, S.: Proteins in scorpion venoms specifically toxic to arthropods. In: Animal and plant toxins. Kaiser, E. (ed.): Godman Verlag, p. 29, 1973.

Zlotkin, E., Shulov, A.S.: A simple device for collecting scorpion venom. Toxicon, **7**, 331—332 (1969b).

Zlotkin, E., Shulov, A.: Recent studies on the mode of action of scorpion neurotoxins. Toxicon, **7**, 217—221 (1969a).

Zlotkin, E., Stanic, V., Shulov, A.: The effect of scorpion venom on the moulting activity of larvae of the beetle *Trogoderma granarium*. Entomol. exp. appl., **14**, 175—178 (1971c).

CHAPTER 14

Venoms of Tityinae

A. Systematics, Distribution, Biology, Venomous Apparatus, etc. of Tityinae; Venom Collection, Toxicity, Human Accidents and Treatment of Stings

W. BÜCHERL

1. The Venomous Species and Their Geographical Distribution

The venomous scorpions of the subfamily Tityinae from the family Buthidae (SIMON, 1880) differ from the representatives of the other families by virtue of: a sternum longer than broad, narrow in front, nearly triangular, with anteriorly converging sides; movable finger of pedipalps with more than seven rows of granules obliquely positioned, largely overlapping each other.

The most important genus of this subfamily is the neotropical *Tityus* (KOCH, 1836), with the typespecies *T. bahiensis,* characterized as follows: tergites with only one longitudinal median keel; inferior face of immobile finger of the chelicerae with only one tooth; inner side of the movable finger of the pedipalps generally with 11−22 oblique rows of granules, without secundary granular rows, but with one lateral granule; hand with several distinct keels; telson with a spine at the ventral base of the stinger, compressed laterally, and often with two smaller protuberances on each side. Combs with 11−24 teeth, the mesal portion of the lamella intermediaria in females often vesicularly enlarges. The tail in adults is always longer than the cephalothorax and preabdomen, in the males of many species significantly longer than in females; the hands of pedipalpi in females are often smaller than in the males.

This genus actually includes 63 species with 21 subspecies (DE MELLO-LEITÃO, 1945), confined to the tropical, subtropical, and temperate climates of South America.

In Argentina: *Tityus mazzai* (MELLO-LEITÃO, 1935) male; the following species are found Jujuy, *bolivianus argentinus* (BORELLI, 1899) San Lorenço, Jujuy, Tucuman, Cordoba, Santiago, and Misiones, *carinatoides* (MELLO-LEITÃO, 1945) female, *sectus* (MELLO-LEITÃO, 1934) male, both from Santa Fé, and *trivittatus confluens* (BORELLI, 1900) Chaco. [1;2]

T. bolivianus uruguayensis (BORELLI, 1900) has been described from Salto, Uruguay.

---

[1] If sex is indicated, only the holotype specimen is known.
[2] All references before 1945 may be seen under MELLO-LEITÃO (1945).

T. paraguayensis (KRAEPELIN, 1895) and *trivittatus trivittatus* (KRAEPELIN, 1898) are from Asuncion and San Salvador, Paraguay, ranging from the south of Brazil to the north of Argentina to the province of Buenos Aires.

T. bocki (KRAEPELIN, 1912) female, is from Yungas, *bolivianus bolivianus* (KRAEPELIN, 1895) from Tipuani and *b. andinus* (KRAEPELIN, 1912) from Coxabamba and La Paz, Bolivia; the last was also found near Arequipa, Peru. *Metuendus* (POCOCK, 1897) is from Iquitos, *b. soratensis* (KRAEPELIN, 1912) from Sorata near Lake Titicaca, and *footei* (CHAMBERLIN, 1911) female, from Andes, Peru.

The following species have been described from Ecuador: *T. intermedius* (BORELLI, 1899) from Ibana, *bolivianus ecuadorensis* (KRAEPELIN, 1895) and *b. simonsi* (POCOCK, 1900) male, from Loja, *kraepelini* (BORELLI, 1899) from Ibarra, *forcipula spinatus* (POCOCK, 1898) male, from Cuenca, *kraepelinianus* (MELLO-LEITÃO, 1931). The *pugilator,* female; *rosenbergi,* female; and *timendus,* male—all found by POCOCK (1898) in Cachavi.

Those found in Columbia are *T. parvulus,* female, and *fuhrmanni* (KRAEPELIN, 1914) in Angelopolis, *charalaensis* (MELLO-LEITÃO, 1940) in Charala, *engelkei* (POCOCK, 1902) *macrochirus* (POCOCK, 1897) and *pachyurus* (POCOCK, 1897) are from Bogota, the last was also found in the west of Venezuela; *festae* (BORELLI, 1899) is from Danan, *forcipula forcipula* (GERVAIS, 1844) from Popahan, and *nematochirus* (MELLO-LEITÃO, 1940) male, from Villavicencio. The most frequent in Bogota is *T. colombianus* (THORELL, 1876) found also in La Pedreira, Sarrina, San Mateo.

SCORZA (1954b) describes the following species from *Venezuela: Clathratus* (KOCH, 1846) Caracas, Los Rosales, Los Chorros, Valera, Charallave, San Cristobal, Nirgua; *flavostictus* Schenkel 1932, Merida, Tabay, San Cristobal, Valera; *melanostictus* (POCOCK 1893) Caracas: Los Venados, university city (Trinidad?); *spinipalpis* (LUTZ, 1932) male, Los Teques, *androcottoides* (KARSCH, 1879) delta of Orinoco (Colombia, Panama, Britisch Guayana: Demerara); *dasyurus fulvipes* (MELLO-LEITÃO, 1945) Caracas: on old houses; *discrepans* (KARSCH, 1879) Caracas: Los Chorros, Country Club, Los Teques, Rancho Grande); *funestus* (HIRST, 1911) *magnimanus interstitialis* (MELLO-LEITÃO, 1939) female, and *magnimanus rugosus* (SCHENKEL, 1932) Merida; *urbinai* (SCORZA, 1952) Alto Orinoco: Mawari-Anejidi; *valerae* (SCORZA, 1954) Valera, at 1604 meters (SCORZA, 1952, 1954a).

T. trinitatis (POCOCK, 1897) is the common venomous scorpion in Trinidad—Tobago. SCORZA (1954b) studied two females from Nueva Esperta, *Venezuela.*

T. dasyurus dasyurus (POCOCK, 1897) female, is from *Portorico* and *marmoratus* (WERNER, 1939) from *Surinam:* Cotica, Marwine, Paramaribo (WERNER, 1939).

The following species are from *Brazil:*

a) *Amazonas (AM), Marajó, and Pará (PA):*

Strandi (WERNER, 1939) female, Sacambu, AM; *amazonicus* (GILTAY, 1928) Óbidos, *carvalhoi* (MELLO-LEITÃO, 1945) female, Tapirapés, *sampaiocrulsi* (MELLO-LEITÃO, 1951) male, Cuminá river, *evandroi* (MELLO-LEITÃO, 1945) female, Piratuba, *rufofuscus* (POCOCK, 1897) (distribution not known), *bispinosus* (PESSOA, 1934) male, and *silvestris* (POCOCK, 1897) both from Santarém, *duckei* (BORELLI, 1910) male, *paraensis* (KRAEPELIN, 1896) and *asthenes* (POCOCK, 1893) are from Belém, PA; *T. cambridgei* (POCOCK, 1897) may be considered as the "most common black scorpion from the lower and higher Amazonas, from PA, Marajó, to AM, Ecuador, the northern regions from Goiás" (MELLO-LEITÃO, 1945).

b) Rio Grande do Norte, Paraíba and Pernambuco:

T. neglecíus (MELLO-LEITÃO, 1932) female, RN; *pusillus* (POCOCK, 1893), Iguaraçú, PE; *stigmurus* (THORELL, 1877): common in PE and Paraíba, east of the Borborema mountains (MELLO-LEITÃO, 1945).

c) Goiás (GO) and Mato Grosso (MT):

T. blaseri (MELLO-LEITÃO, 1931) female, Veadeiros, GO; *trivittatus charreyroni* (VELLARD, 1932) Leopoldina; *acutidens* (MELLO-LEITÃN, 1933) female, Bananál Island, *bahiensis uniformis* (MELLO-LEITÃO, 1931) Veadeiros, and *serrulatus vellardi* (MELLO-LEITÃO, 1939) male, Catalão, GO. — *T. lutzi* (GILTAY, 1928) female, Cuiabá, *mattogrossensis* (BORELLI, 1901) *indecisus* (MELLO-LEITÃO, 1934) female, Campo Grande, MT.

d) Minas Gerais (MG):

T. microcystis (LUTZ and MELLO, 1922) female, Mariana.

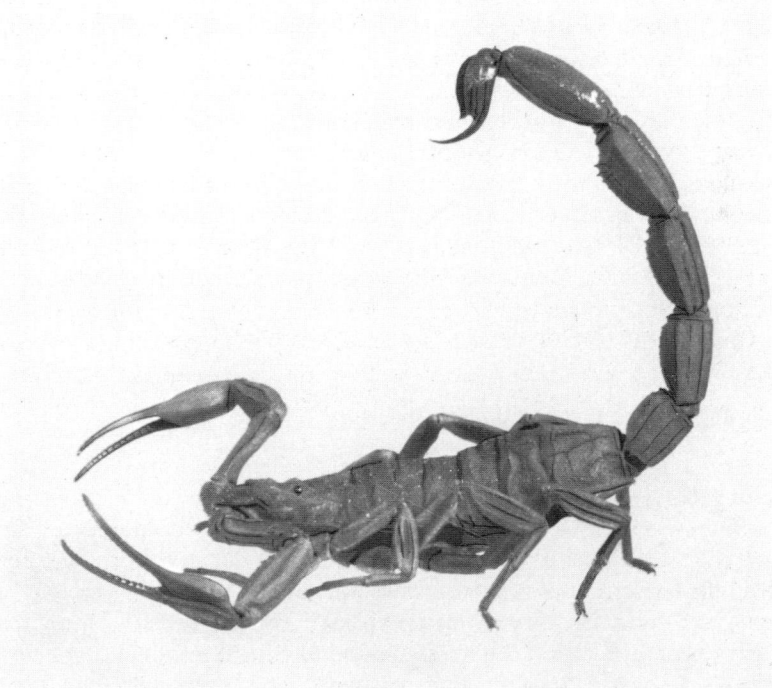

Fig. 1. *Tityus s. serrulatus*, female (note the larger granules on the third and fourth dorsal keels of the tail)

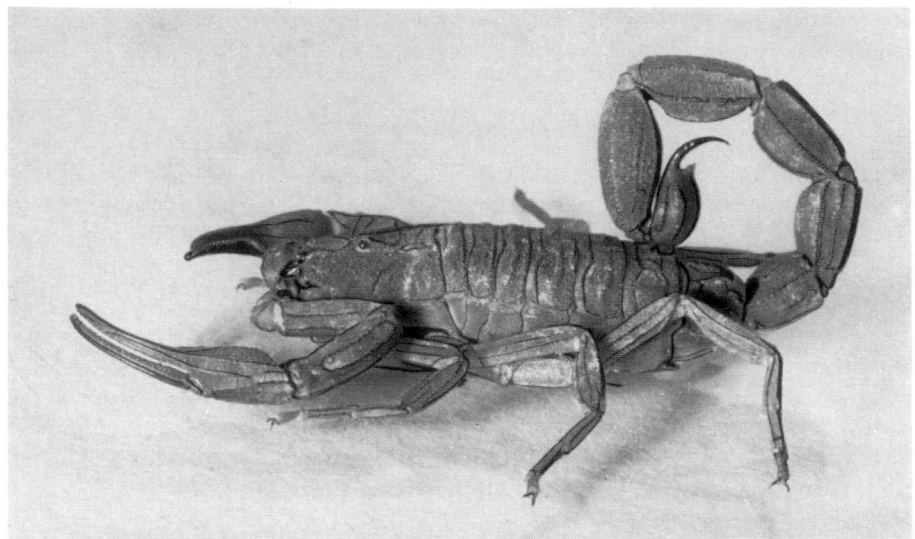

Fig. 2. *Tityus b. bahiensis, male*

e) Distributed over several central states:

T. trivittatus dorsomaculatus (Lutz and Mello, 1922): MG: Viçosa, Belo Horizonte; Rio de Janeiro; GO: Rodeio. *T. bahiensis bahiensis* (Perty, 1834) Type
locality: Salvador, BA; from Bahia to Sta. Catarina in the south and MT as
for as Paraguay in the southwest. It is frequently found in and around the São
Paulo City area, in older houses, gardens, under stones, also in Ouro Preto, Bar-
bacena, MG.

    T. serrulatus serrulatus (Lutz and Mello, 1922) type locality: Belo Horizonte.
The most common scorpion in Belo Horizonte, Betim, Sabará, Mariana, Passagem, Sta. Bárbara, Nova Era, Bom Jesus, Montes Claros, MG; Osasco, São José
dos Campos, Aparecida, Bananál, Roseira, Atibaia, Serra Negra, near Campinas,
Ribeirão Preto, SP; Goiânia, GO.

    Only Chile seems to be free of representatives of this genus.

2. Description of the Most Venomous Species

T. s. serrulatus: From about 17 mm in length. Cephalothorax and the six first
tergites are yellowish brown; the last tergite and caudal segments, legs, pedipalps,
and mandibles are pale yellow. The underside of the fifth caudal segment from
the middle to the posterior border, fingers and stinger are blackish; telson and
pincers reddish; dorsal paramedian keels of caudal segments two to four with
bigger posterior granules, very distinct, especially on the fourth segment (nomen);
inferior paramedian keels of the same caudal segments parallel; anterior median
keel of the tibia of palps irregularly denticulated.

    T. b. bahiensis: Total length of about 70 mm. Uniformly brown on the upper
side of the trunk, legs brown-reddish, tail reddish brown, more blackish behind;

dorsal paramedian keels of the caudal segments two to four without bigger hind denticles. Males with bigger hands than the females and with a basal lobe between the fingers.

T. trinitatis: About 70 mm long, males often 90 mm. Carapace and cauda yellowish to blackish brown, pedipalps and legs reddish-yellow, in juveniles often with blackish spots, finger deeper brown, sternites yellowish, finely punctured and densely granular; sternite four with one median keel and two lateral keels, sternite five with four granulated keels; first caudal segment with ten keels, the two inferior, paramedian, being parallel in the first two segments, united distad on the third and in their posterior half in the fourth. Cauda in males seven times longer than the third caudal segment; caudal segments between the keels granulated. Type locality: Trinidad.

T. trivittatus dorsomaculatus: from about 70 mm; cephalothorax yellowish brown, with blackish spots; tergites with three longitudinal blackish bands, the median larger, divided by a small median yellow line; sternites pale yellowish; tail of the female yellowish brown, the last two segments blackish; tail of the male yellowish, the third segment reddish, segments four and five blackish. Legs pale yellowish with blackish spots, irregularly distributed. Coxa of pedipalps yellow, trochanter pale yellow, femur with two larger brownish spots, tibia pale yellowish, hand yellowish or blackish.

3. Frequency of the Most Venomous Species

The Instituto Butantan received, from 1956 to 1974, about 425,000 *T. s. serrulatus* (BÜCHERL, 1969, 1971), chiefly from Nova Era, Passagem, Bom Jesus, Roseira, Aparecida, and Ribeirão Preto, and about 40,000 *T. b. bahiensis* (BÜCHERL, 1969, 1971) from the São Paulo City area (cemeteries, Pacaembu, Pacaembuzinho, Lapa, in old houses along the Pinheiros river), Pindamonhangaba, and Ouro Preto.

They are found under stones, rocks, along rivers, in logs, and loose bark of trees, in gardens, older buildings, garages, cellars, washhouses; entire streets in the older parts of cities have formerly been invaded, the silent "invaders" bearing true "domiciliary habits" and living in all darker places in the houses (BÜCHERL, 1971; MAGALHÃES DE, 1935).

4. Food and Life Habits

They feed on other scorpions, even of their own species, spiders, mealworms, cockroaches, grasshoppers, eggs of ants and termites (Nova Era, MG), and other soft-bodied insects. The mother will often eat her young on her back. They can live for several months without any food. Yet they must always have water, especially during dry seasons.

T. s. serrulatus is *parthenogenetic* (MATTHIESEN, 1962, 1971a, 1971b), while *bahiensis, trivittatus,* and *trinitatis* are bisexual. We observed the mating habits of *trivittatus* and *bahiensis,* in the years 1953 — 1954 (BÜCHERL, 1955/56b). The female never killed the male; the latter has a great number of spermatophores which allow him to mate successively with other females. After a single insemination the females can have two or more parturitions at intervals of 6 — 11 months (MAT-

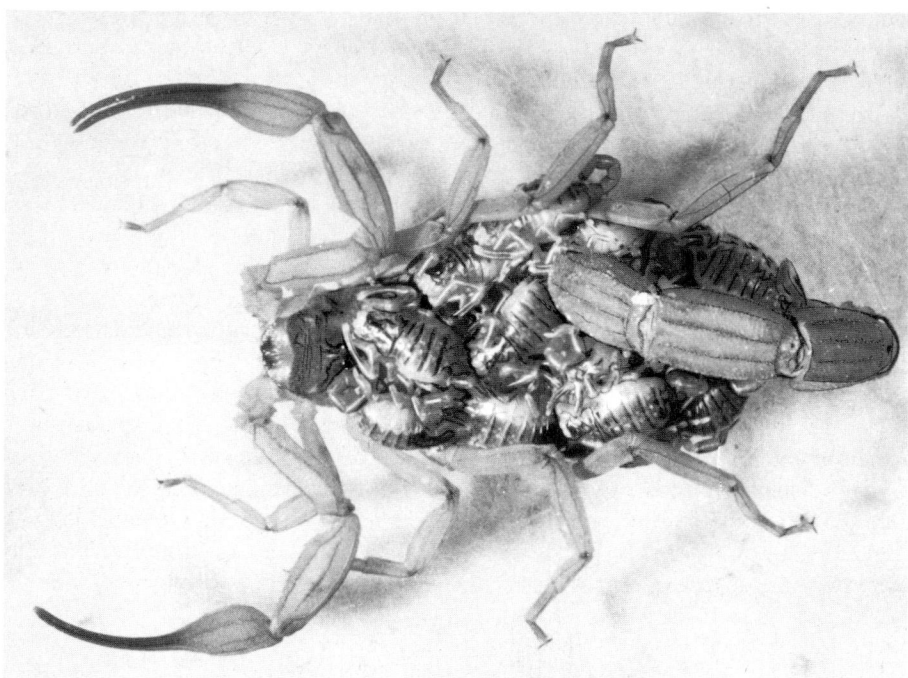

Fig. 3. *Tityus s. serrulatus,* female, with young on her back

THIESEN, 1971 b). The duration of life may be from 1365—1565 days for *serrulatus* (MATTHIESEN, 1971 b).

5. Venom Glands

The venom is secreted by a pair of ampullated glands, both located in the last caudal segment, the telson, each one measuring about 3.5×2.0 cm (in *serrulatus* and *bahiensis*) and each one with its own efferent duct, extending along the curved sting, and opening separately on each side, near the tip of the aculeus (BÜCHERL, 1969, 1971). In both species, studied by us, longitudinal, tangential, and cross sections, stained with hematoxylin-eosin, show an external muscularis, the basement membrane, and the venom-excreting epithelial cell layer.

The muscularis forms a double layer, separated by a sheet of connective tissue, and covers the whole venom gland, except the efferent duct. The external layer is circular, three to four muscle bundles encircling the gland body, while the internal layer is longitudinal, showing about 50 muscle bundles, with the nuclei more or less centrally positioned. All the fibrils are cross-striated.

The thin basement membrane forms a continuous layer inside the muscularis.

Two kinds of epithelial cells are present: very small subcuboidal cells attached to the basement membrane, with small elliptic nuclei in a rest stage. Obviously, these cells will substitute the destroyed venom-secreting cells. These form the true functional epithelial cells, 5—8 times larger than the substituting elements, and of a high columnar type. Cell walls, nuclei, cytoplasma, and venom granules are visible. These granules are fine or agglutinated to droplets at the center of the cell. In the final stages of venom production, thick droplets break off the apical portion of the cell wall, the venomous elements being extruded into the central lumen (apocrine type). The cell produces venom as long as its nuclear and cytoplasmatic substances remain vital; then the cell degenerates, its inert material being extruded into the central lumen of the gland.

The excretory duct shows a small central lumen, a chitinous internal layer, small cuboidal epidermal cells, and a thin basement membrane, without a proper muscularis (BÜCHERL, 1971).

All parts of the venom glands as well as the cells of the excretory duct are generously innervated from a conspicuous nerve originating from the double postabdominal ganglion (LUCAS et al., 1965). The venom ejection is violent and rapid, conditioned by the voluntary contraction of the muscles of the gland, favored especially by the very rapid movements of the telson and the whole tail. In soft-bodied arthropods, the aculeus will penetrate to the deeper subcuticular epithelium.

6. Quantities and Storage of the Venom

To obtain scorpion venom in sufficient quantities for immunologic or pharmacologic purposes, these arachnids must be kept in the laboratory (BÜCHERL, 1953a). The venom may be extracted every 3 or 4 weeks by a proper manual technique or with electric stimulus (BÜCHERL, 1971). From 1951 until June 1953 we collected 309 mg of dry *T. serrulatus* venom, obtained from 4105 electric extractions of several hundred specimens, kept alive in captivity; and 697 mg of *T. bahiensis* venom from 6148 extractions of 1112 specimens. 141,285 and 45,900 electric extractions of *serrulatus* and *bahiensis*, respectively, made in the Butantan Institute from 1953 to 1963, gave 87,805 and 17,849 mg of whitish-grayish, hygroscopic, vacuum-dried venom; it was stored in the dark in a vacuum dessicator over calcium chloride at room temperature. In 1953 the mean yield per individual was about 0.075 mg from *serrulatus* and 0.113 mg from *bahiensis* and in 1963 0.062 mg from *serrulatus* and 0.39 mg from *bahiensis*. The maximum yield of dry venom from *serrulatus*, *bahiensis*, and *t. dorsomaculatus* may be 3.0 mg.

7. Toxicity and Human Accidents

LD$_{50}$ values of dry venom from Tityinae scorpions on white rats (wt = 20 g)

Species	Intravenously	Subcutaneously
T. serrulatus	0.016 mg	0.022 mg (BÜCHERL, 1953b)
T. bahiensis	0.022 mg	0.045 to 0.140 mg (BÜCHERL, 1953b)
T. costatus	0.200 mg	1.100 mg (BÜCHERL and PUCCA, 1956a)
T. t. dorsomaculatus	0.014 mg	0.059 mg (BÜCHERL and PUCCA, 1956a)

Tityus venom causes in man a rapid and transient burning sensation around the site of the sting (probably true of more than 80% of the species), a sharper and intensive local pain, which may last from a few minutes to several hours (15%), or an intensive and immediate local burning (3%). An individual sting on a finger may feel pain throughout the whole arm. Under normal conditions, or if the scorpion has not injected all of its venom, all of these local symptoms are transient, disappearing after 15—24 h, with no serious danger.

However, the venoms of *serrulatus, trinitatis,* rarely of *trivittatus,* and more rarely of *bahiensis* may produce intensive local pain and systemic *neurotropical* actions, with progressive numbness, tightness in the throat, difficulty in speaking, restlessness, involuntary twitching of the muscles. Some victims, especially babies and young children, may have sneezing spasms, which develop into a serious convulsive condition. In severe cases they undergo labored breathing, severe respiratory difficulties, and finally death caused by respiratory paralysis (MAGALHÃES, 1935).

In all those who recover, these symptoms disappear completely.

WATERMAN (1957) reports 698 human accidents in Trinidad from 1929 to 1933 with a mortality rate for children under five years of about 25%; DE MAGALHÃES (1935) 2449 cases in Belo Horizonte with 145 deaths; Tito Lopes da Silva, 985 accidents in the city of Ribeirão Preto from 1945 to 1950. The statistics from the Municipal Hospital of the same city show 300 accidents from 1951 to 1952 (BÜCHERL, 1969). It seems to us to be correct to state that in Brazil the *T. serrulatus* may cause the death of 0.8—1.4% of the adults, 3—5% of the school children, and 15—20% of the babies and young children (BÜCHERL, 1971). This dramatic scorpionism occurs in Brazil only with *serrulatus,* and in Trinidad only with *trinitatis.* The statistics from 1954 to 1965 of the hospital Vital Brazil at the Butantan Institute, compiled by Dr. G. Rosenfeld, include 1277 patients stung by scorpions around the city of São Paulo: 701 of these by *T. bahiensis,* with only two deaths; 36 by *serrulatus,* 6 by *Bothriurus* sp.; and 534 by unidentified scorpions (ROSENFELD, personal communication).

8. Treatment of Scorpion Envenomation

All severe cases of envenomation by scorpion sting must be treated with *antiscorpion serum,* produced by the Butantan Institute. Two to five ampules are administered i.v., and the same quantity is injected subcutaneously as early as possible after the sting, to neutralize in any case the maximum venom quantity, possibly inoculated by the sting. If there is an interval of 2 h after the sting the success of serum treatment can become questionable. From the 985 cases in Ribeirão Preto, 64 have been very severe and were treated with antiserum; only 7 deaths, in children of 3 months to 7 years, resulted, i.e., a mortality rate of about 0.7% which shows the unquestionable value of the serum treatment.

References

Bücherl, W.: Manutenção de escorpiões em viveiros e extração do veneno. Mem. Inst. Butantan **25** (1), 53—82 (1953a).
Bücherl, W.: Atividade das peçonhas de *Tityus serrulatus* e *bahiensis* sobre camundongos. Mem. Inst. Butantan **25** (1), 83—108 (1953b).

Bücherl, W.: Observações sobre o eparelho reprodutor masculino e o acasalamento de *Tityus trivittatus* e *bahiensis*, Mem. Inst. Butantan **27**, 121—155 (1955/56b).

Bücherl, W.: Escorpionismo no Brasil. Mem. Inst. Butantan **34**, 9—24 (1969).

Bücherl, W.: Classification and biology of scorpions, In: Venomous animals and their venoms 3, Venomous invertebrates, pp. 339—342 (Bücherl, W. and Buckley, E.D., eds.). New York: Academic Press 1971.

Bücherl, W., Pucca, N.: Titulação em camundongos das peçonhas de *Tityus costatus, trivittatus* e *Bothriurus bonariensis*. Mem. Inst. Butantan **27**, 41—50 (1955/56a).

Giltay, A.: Arachnides nouveaux du Brésil. Ann. Bull. Soc. Ent. Belg. **68**, 79—82 (1928).

Koch, C.L.: Arachniden **3**, 33 (1836).

Lucas, S., Eichstedt, V.D., von, Bücherl, W.: Sobre o sistema nervoso de *Tityus serrulatus*. Mem. Inst. Butantan **32**, 15—26 (1965).

Magalhães, O. de: Contribuição para o conhecimento do mecanismo da intoxicação pelo veneno dos escorpiões. Ann. Fac. Med. Belo Horizonte **1(1)**, 3—52 (1935).

Matthiesen, F.A.: Parthenogenesis in scorpions. Evolution **16**, 255—256 (1962).

Matthiesen, F.A.: The breeding of *Tityus serrulatus* in captivity. Rev. bras. Pesq. med. Biol. **4** (4—5), 299—300 (1971a).

Matthiesen, F.A.: Observations on four species of Brazilian scorpions in captivity. Rev. bras. Pesq. med. Biol. **4** (4—5), 301—302 (1971b).

Mello-Leitão, C. de: Escorpiões Sulamericanos. Arq. Mus. Nac. Rio de J. **40**, 298—434 (1945).

Scorza, J.V.: Contribución al estudio de los alacranes venezolanos. Nov. Cient. Mus. Hist. Nat. La Salle, ser. Zool. **8**, 15 (1952).

Scorza, J.V.: Dos especies nuevas de alacranes de Venezuela. Nov. Cient. Mus. Mist. Nat. La Salle, ser. Zool. **12**, 9—12 (1954a).

Scorza, J.V.: Observationes ecologicas de algunos alacranes. Mem. Soc. Ci. Nat. La Salle **14(38)**, 204—210 (1954b).

Simon, E.: Descriptions de genres et espèces de l'ordres des Scorpions. Ann. Soc. Ent. France 376—398 (1880).

Waterman, J.A.: Some notes on scorpions: poisoning in Trinidad. Caribean med. J. **19** (1—2), 113—128 (1957).

Werner, F.: Neueingänge von Skorpionen in das Zoologische Museum Hamburg. Festschr. E. Strand **5**, 351—360 (1939).

B. Chemical and Pharmacologic Aspects of Tityinae Venoms

C.R. DINIZ

Introduction

Interest in the study of scorpions from the Tityinae subfamily was initiated because of the high frequency, in some populated areas of South America, of stings inflicted in humans by three species of *Tityus* scorpions: *T. serrulatus* (LUTZ and MELLO, 1922), *T. bahiensis* (PERTY, 1834), and *T. trinitatis* (POCOCK, 1897). VITAL BRAZIL (1909), who started studies on venoms at the Instituto Butantan, São Paulo, was one of the first to describe scorpion poisoning in Brazil, followed by MAURANO (1915) in Rio de Janeiro. HOUSSAY (1919) in Buenos Aires, Argentina, initiated experimental studies on the mechanism of action of venoms from South American scorpion. It is interesting to note, however, that the most dangerous scorpion of the Tityinae subfamily, *T. serrulatus,* a brown-yellow scorpion indigenous to the Brazilian territory, was described only in 1922 by Lutz and Mello, 1922 (Mello Campos, 1924). This species of scorpion is widespread in the southeastern region of Brazil, and in some towns such as Belo Horizonte, the planned capital of the State of Minas Gerais and Ribeirão Preto in the state of São Paulo, scorpionism became a health problem for many years (Magalhães, 1938; Lopes da Silva, 1960). Magalhães delved into studies of clinical and experimental intoxication induced by *Tityus* venoms from 1925 to 1946. He made an extensive description of the effects of scorpion poisoning in man and animals, and his work attained a distinct scientific value for the understanding of several aspects of *Tityus*-venom intoxication (Magalhães, 1925, 1928, 1938, 1939, 1946).

The description of clinical manifestations caused by stings of *T. trinitatis* (Waterman, 1938, 1957) also aroused interest in the study of this species as it occurs in the northern part of South America (Bartholomew, 1970).

I. Chemical Properties of Tityinae Venoms

Studies on the chemical properties of venoms from the Tityinae subfamily have been confined to the secretions of *T. serrulatus* and *T. bahiensis,* obtained mostly by electrical or manual stimulation. The venom secured by these methods is a mixture of proteins, associated with a small proportions of free amino acids and salts (Diniz and Gonçalves, 1956, 1960; Fisher and Bohn, 1957). Scorpion venom is secreted in microgram quantities. Microtechniques in the separation and identification procedures, coupled with sensitive biological assays are important tools in the study of scorpion venoms. So far, the chemical studies of venoms from the Tityinae subfamily have been centered on the isolation and characterization of toxic substances active on vertebrate organisms. However, sensitive enzymatic assays demonstrated that *T. serrulatus* and *T. bahiensis* venoms are devoid of proteolytic, fibrinogen clotting, cholinesterase, cholinesterase inhibition, phospholipase, and hemolytic activities. Hyaluronic-acid depolymerizing activity (hyaluronidase) was found in relatively high proportion (11.0 and 2.3 viscosity reduction units/mg of dry venoms of *T. bahiensis* and *T. serrulatus,* respectively). Histamine, acetylcholine, serotonin, catecholamines, and kinins were not detected by bioassays in these crude venom preparations. Substances with an influence on capillary permeability, probably due to histamine release, were detected in small amounts (Diniz and Gonçalves, 1960; Beraldo and Dias da Silva, 1966).

1. Purification of Toxic Components from Tityinae Venoms

In some rural areas of the state of Minas Gerais in Brazil, *Tityus serrulatus* scorpions are found living in the mounds of termite colonies (Isoptera). They can be captured in large numbers and kept in the laboratory for months to produce venom for limited chemical studies. In spite of the small amount of venom obtainable from each scorpion by electric stimulus (ca. 0.3 mg), in the author's laboratory and at the Instituto Butantan it has been possible to accumulate venom in gram quantities, thanks to the dedication and patience of able technicians. To date, only one highly purified toxin, Tityustoxin (TsTx), from *T. serrulatus* venom has been separated (Gomez and Diniz, 1966; Coutinho Netto and Diniz, 1975), whereas the venoms of several African species of scorpions have been extensively studied under several chemical and physicochemical aspects, including the amino acid sequence of different insect and vertebrate toxins (ROCHAT et al., 1971, 1972; MIRANDA et al., 1970; SLOTKIN, 1973). Paper and starch gel electrophoresis in the earlier work of DINIZ and GONÇALVES (1956) showed that the venoms of *T. bahiensis* and *T. serrulatus* are formed mainly from basic proteins. Besides the toxic properties, the eluted material from the electropherograms contracted the smooth muscle of guinea pig ileum. These activities were destroyed by trypsin and chymotrypsin, demonstrating their polypeptide nature. A suggestion that one component active upon the smooth muscle could be similar to the kinin polypeptides was not supported by later pharmacologic and chemical work.

GOMEZ and DINIZ (1966) and GOMEZ (1967) purified a toxic component from *T. serrulatus* venom using a combination of column chromatography procedures to reach homogeneity by criteria of zone electrophoresis (polyacrylamide and cellogel). In a first step the toxin was retained in a Sephadex G-25 column according to the method of GELOTTE (1960) and MIRANDA et al. (1960) with slight modifications, and later eluted using ammonium acetate buffer 0.5 M, pH 9.0. Two peaks of active material were separated. For further purification only one peak was used. The toxic eluates were concentrated and submitted to chromatography in a CM-cellulose column. Stepwise elution employing ammonium acetate released the toxic component in a single peak, which displayed a constant toxic activity (LD_{50} 90.0 µg/kg mice, i.p.) and showed a single band in polyacrylamide (12%) gel electrophoresis (GOMEZ and DINIZ, 1966). MIRANDA et al. (1966) fractionated *T. serrulatus* venom also by a similar procedure except that a carboxylic resin (Amberlite CG-50) was used as the second step of column purification. Two toxic components were separated.

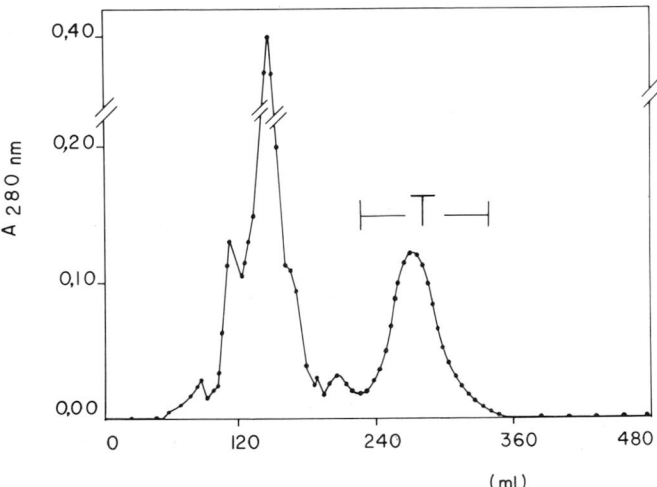

Fig. 1. CM-cellulose equilibrium chromatography of toxic fraction eluted from Sephadex G-50 columns CM cellulose. Columns 117 × 1.1 cm equilibrated with 0.15 M ammonium acetate buffer, pH 8.5. Toxic peak (T) showed constant specific activity and a single band in polyacrylamide gel electrophoresis at pH 4.3 and 8.2

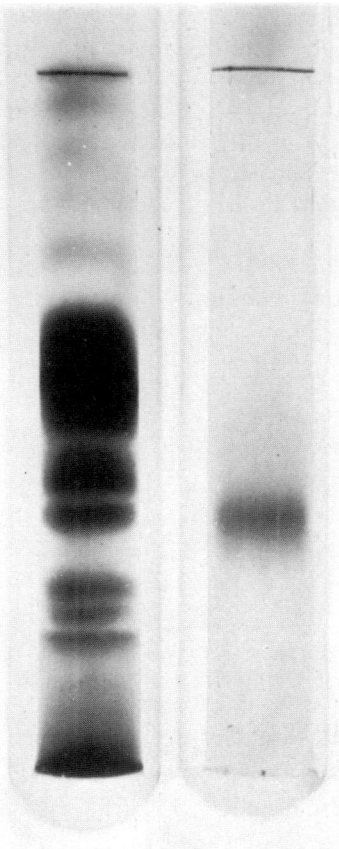

Fig. 2. Polyacrylamide gel electropherogram of 500 μg of whole scorpion venom compared with 100 μg of tityustoxin obtained from CM cellulose columns. Gel concentration 12%, β-alanine buffer pH 4.3

More recently, COUTINHO NETTO (1975) developed in a new method of TsTx purification in the author's laboratory, employing gel permeation in Sephadex G-50. The toxin was found among the components of lower molecular weight in a single peak. Further purification of the toxin component was achieved by equilibrium chromatography in CM-cellulose-W-52 columns at pH 8.5 and elution with 0.15 M ammonium acetate buffer (Fig. 1). This procedure leads to the isolation of a basic protein (pHi 8.25) homogeneous in polyacrylamide gel and immunoelectrophoresis (Fig. 2). The LD_{50} i.p. was a constant 15.0 μg/kg mice. The recovery of toxicity was high (ca. 80%) and indicated that the content of TsTx in the venom reaches at most 1.0% of the total proteins of the venom. The aminoacid composition of TsTx showed the following proportions: Lys_7, His_1, Arg_1, Cys_6, Asp_9, $Meth_0$, Thn_2, Ser_3, Gly_4, Pro_3, Gly_5, Ala_4, Val_2, Ile_2, Leu_3, Tyr_6, Phe_1, Trp_2. The minimum chemical molecular weight calculated on the basis of 61 amino acid residues was 6.996. Lysine was the only amino acid found at the N terminal position, which is suggestive of a single-chained polypeptide. A diversity of isotoxins was found by ROCHAT et al. (1972) in the venoms of several African species of scorpions. This apparently was not the rule in the venom of the *T. serrulatus* population of scorpions living in a very restricted area of the state of Minas Gerais in Brasil. In amino acid composition of venom, however, the Brazilian species have several features in common with the African scorpions: absence of methionine, low histidine and phenylalanine content, and a predominance of hydrophobic aromatic and basic amino acids.

II. Pharmacology of Tityus Venom Intoxication

The symptoms of acute intoxication by scorpion venom differ from that of snake venoms by a lack of intense local reaction or dramatic muscular effects. Pain is always referred to in human incidents. In animals, or even in man, injection of the venom is followed by cries, agitation, excitation, hair-bristling, accelerated respiration, mydriasis, salivation, lacrymation, and sphincter relaxation. Respiration later becomes short and in animals the posterior limbs often extended backward. A short-lived hypotension is usually observed, followed by a prolonged increase in blood pressure. Arrhythmias and a slowing of heart frequency is seen during the hypertension effect (MAURANO, 1915; MAGALHÃES, 1939; RAMOS and CORRADO, 1954; FREIRE MAIA, 1974). Metabolic disturbances such as hyperglycemia and glucosuria are constant features of *Tityus* venom intoxication (MAGALHÃES, 1939; FREIRE MAIA and FERREIRA, 1961). MAGALHÃES (1946) concluded from his clinical and experimental observations that a selective action of the venom on the sympathetic- and parasympathetic-autonomic centers of the medulla would explain most of the effects of the *Tityus* venom in vertebrates. This interpretation was supported by the description of macroscopic lesions in the central nervous system (CNS) as cerebral congestions and hematomas, in addition to findings of microscopic alterations of nervous cells in the medulla (BARROS, 1936, 1938). Therefore, the neurotoxic nature of *Tityus* venom was apparent to the first investigators. The sites of action of the venom, however, are not confined to the CNS. Most of the effects of this venom are also observed in isolated organs, neuromuscular preparations, and in animals after spinalectomy (DINIZ and VALERI, 1959; RAMOS and CORRADO, 1956).

1. Release of Neurotransmitters by Tityus Venom

a) Acetylcholine

CARVALHO (1938) made the important observation that the extract from the telson of the black scorpion *T. bahiensis* contracted isolated preparations of cat and rabbit duodenum in vitro. This effect was antagonized by atropine, and the author concluded that the telson extract contained an active parasympathomimetic substance.

Trying to identify biologically active components from *Tityus* venoms, DINIZ and GONÇALVES (1956, 1960) used paper and starch electrophoresis to separate toxic components of a polypeptide nature, which after a latency period also induced a slow contraction of the smooth muscle of the guinea pig ileum. The effect on the smooth muscle was antagonized by atropine. A correlation was found between the smooth muscle activity and the toxicity of the venom in mice. Both the muscular and the toxic effects of the purified extract were potentiated by eserine, a cholinesterase inhibitor, and antagonized by atropine. Hexamathonium did not affect the smooth muscle contraction induced by the venom. Morphine, which prevents the release of acetylcholine from myenteric plexuses (SCHAUMAN and SCHAUMAN, 1957) depressed the spasmogenic effect of the venom in guinea pig ileum. It was suggested that the toxic and smooth muscle activities were caused by the same protein. The smooth muscle contraction and several toxic effects were indirect and imputed to the release of acetylcholine from the nervous structures by action of the venom (DINIZ and VALERI, 1959).

The ability of the *Tityus* venoms to release acetylcholine was later documented by experimental demonstration. A substance not distinguishable pharmacologically from acetylcholine, and which also shared several chemical properties of this neuro-transmitter, accumulated in the suspending media when guinea pig ilea strips, *in vitro,* were incubated in the presence of *Tityus* venom (TORRES and DINIZ, 1964; DINIZ and TORRES, 1968; DINIZ and CORRADO, 1971). This effect is pH- and dose-dependent, and displays a saturation type of curve at higher concentrations of venom. Acetylcholine is also released from rat brain slices by TsTx (GOMEZ et al., 1971, 1973) and from rat diaphragm by the crude venom extract (VITAL BRASIL, et al., 1973). These results demonstrated that the cholinergic effect of *Tityus* venom or TsTx was not due to a direct action on the cholinergic receptors in the muscle but probably to a prejunctional effect in the nerves that leads to the release of acetylcholine. Investigations of the conditions by which the venom affects the physiologic processes of release contributed to a better understanding of the interaction of the toxin with the neural tissues (GOMEZ et al., 1973; DINIZ et al., 1974).

The increased output of acetylcholine from brain slices and myenteric plexus with TsTx is likely coupled with a corresponding acceleration of acetylcholine synthesis, since the content of acetylcholine in these tissues remains constant or slightly below the resting levels, although the output stays above the level of controls. At a concentration of 10^{-6}M, hemicholinium, a compound known to interfere with Ach synthesis, reduces to a low level the acetylcholine production elicited by TsTx. It was observed that Ca^{++} and Na^+ in the external medium are necessary for the release of AcCh, either by *Tityus* venom or the purified TsTx. In the absence of these ions the enhanced release of acetylcholine induced by the venom is not observed (GOMEZ et al., 1971, 1973; DINIZ et al., 1974). In cortical slices exposed to TsTx, the uptake of $^{45}Ca^{2+}$ follows a time course similar to the uptake of $^{24}Na^+$ (GOMEZ et al., 1975). The puffer fish poison tetrodo-toxin, a compound that selectively blocks axonal conductions by preventing the increase in the permeability to sodium ions associated with the raising phase of action potentials (KAO, 1966), abolishes entirely the release of Ach induced by TsTx. K^+ does not effect the process, and excess of Ca^{++} or Mg^{++} inhibits the output of the mediator (GOMEZ et al., 1973; DINIZ et al., 1974) (Fig. 3). In absence of oxygen and metabolic energy, TsTx does not stimulate AcCh production (Fig. 4). It was concluded that TsTx probably changes the permeability properties of the neural membranes to the ions in a way very similar to the action potential.

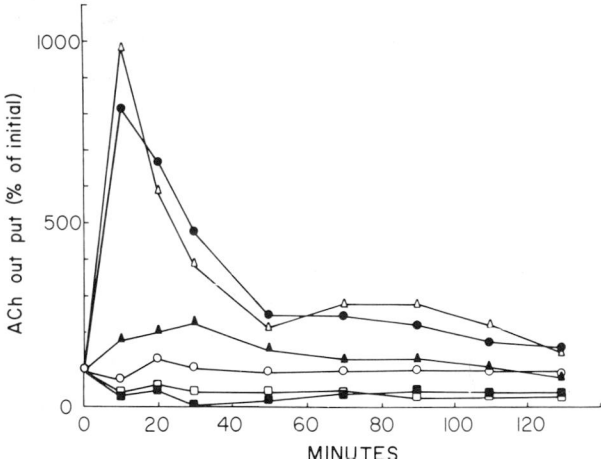

Fig. 3. Effect of TsTx on acetylcholine (*ACh*) output from eserinized longitudinal muscle strip of guinea pig ileum. Initial rate of ACh output in presence of normal Krebs solution, 0.23 ± 0.03 nmoles/g/min taken as 100%. TsTx added as indicated in text to reach a concentration of 12 μg/ml. ●——●, ACh release of strip exposed continuously to TsTx in normal Krebs solution. △——△, Strip incubated only in first 10 min with TsTx; during subsequent periods strip was suspended in normal Krebs solution. ▲——▲, Rate of ACh release in a strip treated with TsTx in a Na-free solution, sucrose substitution. □——□, Output of ACh produced by TsTx in strips bathed in a Ca-free Krebs solution. ■——■, TTx and TsTx added simultaneously to normal bathing Krebs solution. ○——○, Output of ACh of control strips suspended in normal Krebs solution in absence of TsTx. Output of control strips in Na-free and Ca-free solutions or exposed to TTx in absence of TsTx are not shown and did not differ significantly from the TsTx-exposed strips in these conditions. Each point represents ACh output during preceding period and was mean of two experiments on same schedule (A.F. PIMENTA and C.R. DINIZ, unpublished results)

T. serrulatus venom added to the rat phrenic nerve diaphragm preparation elicits spontaneous twitches, potentiates the maximum twitch, and causes a delay in its relaxation. In the chronically denervated rat diaphragm these effects are not observed. The venom causes acetylcholine release from the innervated but not from the denervated rat diaphragm (VITAL BRASIL et al., 1973).

Electrophysiologic observations have shown that surface muscular fibers in rat diaphragm were depolarized by 30%, and miniature end plate potential (mepp) frequency transiently increased from 5 to 500/sec with TsTx. Repetitive end-plate potentials summated and consequently triggered an action potential and muscle twitch: during repetitive stimulation, the falling phase of the directly elicited action potential was prolonged and the half decay time was longer than 5 msec. Tetrodotoxin or reduction of $(Na^+)_0$ to 5 mM of less blocked the action of TsTx. In the presence of EGTA (10 mM), TsTx had little effect on mepp frequency, but when Ca^{++} was microiontophoretically applied to end-plates of these muscles, mepp frequency increased to 500/sec or higher. The increase in mepp frequency produced by TsTx is probably related to a partial depolarization of the nerve terminal with simultaneous $(Ca^{2+})_0$ mobilization (Figs. 5 and 6). The membrane depolarization caused by toxin may be due to the appearance of a new or delayed sodium component (WARNICK et al., 1976).

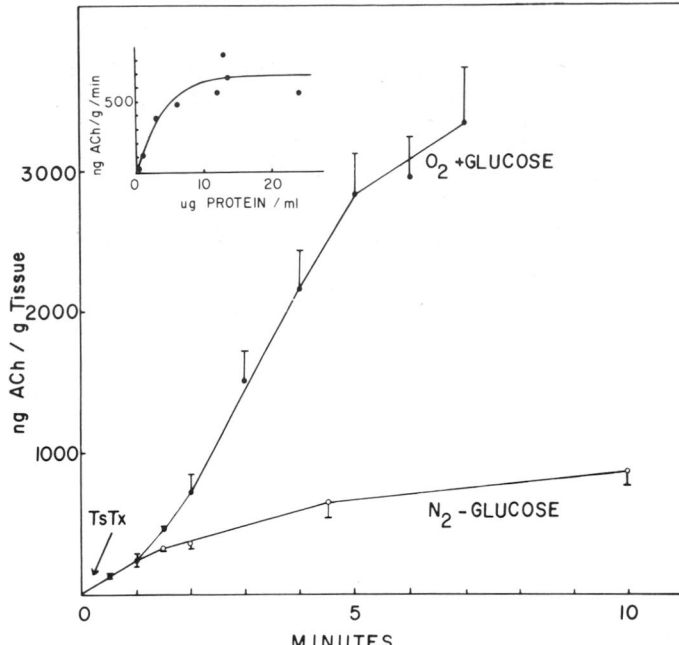

Fig. 4. The Release of Ach into incubation bath by longitudinal muscle from guinea pig ileum plotted against time of incubation with 13 μg/ml TsTx, in presence and absence of glucose and O_2. Upper left-hand insert plots steady rate of AcCh release observed in the first 2—5 min in presence of increasing concentration of TsTx. In absence of glucose and with replacement of O_2 by N_2, TsTx-stimulated release of AcCh is inhibited. (From DINIZ et al., 1975)

Electron microscopy of the neuromuscular junction of diaphragm from a mouse injected with TsTx displays striking morphological changes in the nerve terminals, such as swelling of mitochondria, abnormalities in size and distribution of synaptic vesicles (BÖHM et al., 1974; DINIZ et al., 1974).

The possibility that the liberation of AcCh induced by TsTx in rat brain slices originated because of an inhibition of the activity of Na^+- plus K^+-dependent ATPase was discarded on the grounds that TsTx, as opposed to ouabain did not affect this enzyme in rat brain homogenate in vitro. In addition, in brain slices the enhanced release of AcCh by TsTx, and not by oubain, is dependent on the presence of Ca^{2+} ions in the incubation media. The uptake of $^{24}Na^+$ and $^{45}Ca^{2+}$ by the slices was enhanced by TsTx in contrast to TsTx-free controls. It was suggested, however, that moderate inhibition of Na^+, K^+. ATPase as a consequence of TsTx-facilitated influx of Ca^{++}, would explain the release AcCh by TsTx (GOMEZ et al., 1975).

b) Epinephrine and Norepinephrine

The initial rise of blood pressure following the injection of *Tityus* venom remains unaltered in spinal and adrenalectomized animals and is not affected by hexametho-

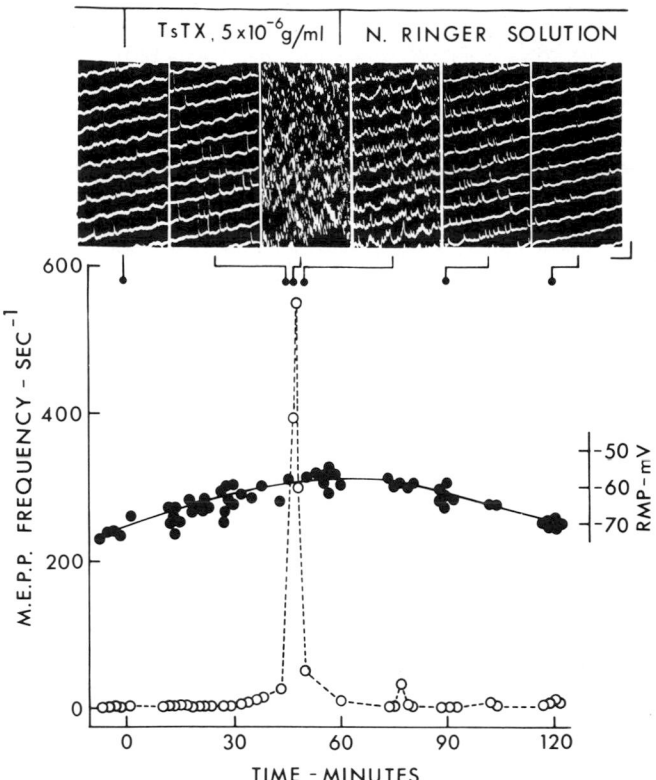

Fig. 5. Time course of tityustoxin (TsTx)—induced increase in miniature end plate potential (*m.e.p.p.*) frequency (*o*) and on resting membrane potential (*RMP; o*). The upper records show the mepps at the time indicated by the dot under each record and correspond to the time on the abcissa. After 60 min preparation was washed with normal Ringer's (*N. Ringer*) solution. Calibration 1,0 mV and 50 ms Temp: 23° C. (From WARNICK et al., 1976)

nium. On the other hand, dibenamine, an alpha-adrenergic blocking agent, avoids completely the increased blood pressure elicited by the venom (RAMOS and COR-RADO, 1954; FREIRE MAIA and FERREIRA, 1961). These results suggested that the venom action is indirect and is due to release of catecholamines from the sympathetic post-ganglionic nerve endings.

Perfusion of isolated guinea pig heart with *T. serrulatus* venom extracts or with a highly purified TsTx preparation disclosed adrenergic and cholinergic effects of the venom and indicated that the same substance affects the two major components of the autonomic nervous system (CORRADO et al., 1966, 1968). The characteristic effect of the venom on the isolated heart is a short-lived bradycardia, followed by an increase in heart rate and force of contraction; these effects are seen in a concentration of 2×10^{-6} to 4×10^{-5} g/ml of venom. The bradycardia was blocked by atropine and potentiated by neostigmine. The positive inotropic effect was very resistant to tachyphylaxis and completely blocked when the heart was infused with propanolol, a beta-sympatholytic, or bretylium. The positive inotropic effect of the venom is absent in the hearts of reserpinized animals.

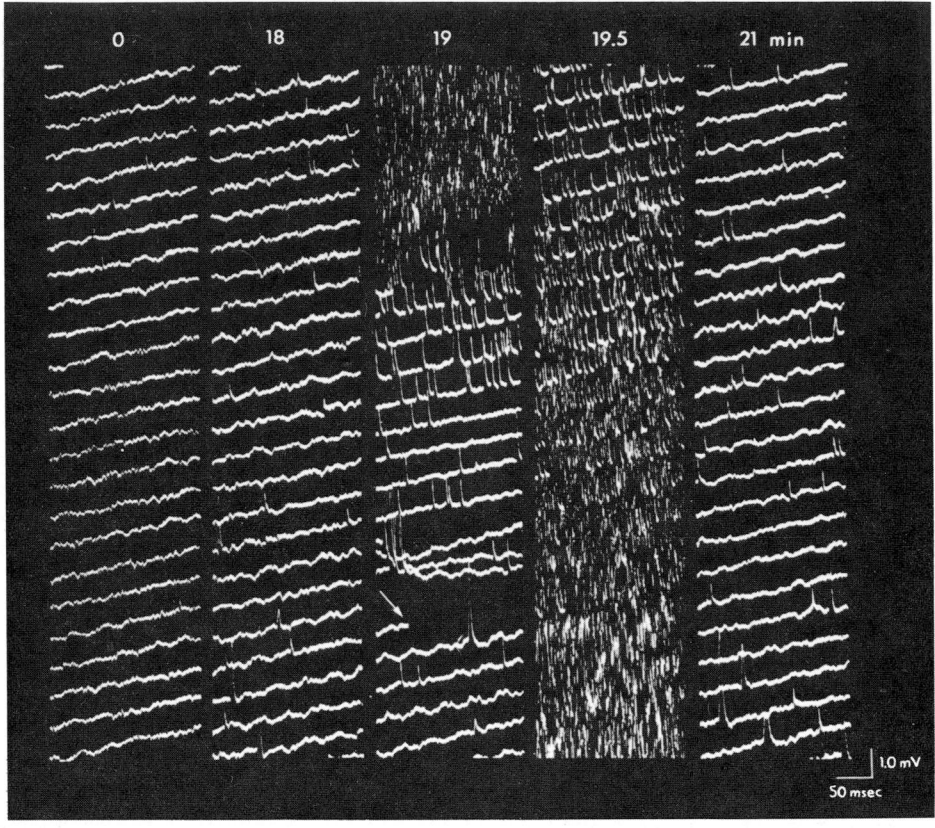

Fig. 6. Facilitation of transmitter release by microiontophoretically applied calcium in a rat diaphragm muscle preteated for 60 min with calcium-free Ringer's solution containing EGTA (10 mM) and then exposed to TsTx (10^{-5} g/ml). Arrow in the third panel at 19 min after addition of TsTx indicates time at which calcium was applied to the end-plate region by passing a 50 msec pulse through the 2M $CaCl_2$ pipette. Temp: 23° C. (According to Warnick et al., 1976)

The venom also produces a marked rise in the phosphorylase *a* activity of the perfused heart. Hexamethonium, in doses that abolished the effects of nicotine, did not affect the cardiac actions of the venom (Fig. 7). These results also indicated an indirect action of the venom on the heart through the release of catecholamines and acetylcholine. The site of action of the venom is probably the postganglionic nerve endings of both the sympathetic and parasympathetic systems and, like guanethidine, mimicks the action potential (Corrado et al., 1968).

Depletion of adrenal catecholamines in venom-treated rats was observed only when innervation was intact (Henriques et al., 1968). Rossi et al. (1974) also showed depletion of catecholamines by use of fluorescence microscopy of catecholamines in heart valves of rats injected with *T. serrulatus* venom. Tafuri et al. (1971, 1974) observed a depletion in the number of granular vesicles in the myenteric plexus of rats injected with TsTx that could be related to the release of catecholamines or other active substances like substance P.

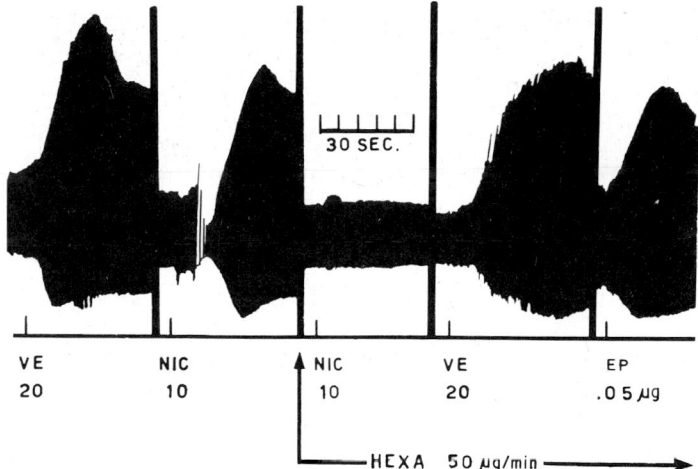

Fig. 7. Isotonic contractions of isolated heart of normal guinea pig. Numbers represent total dose in micrograms. Infusion of hexamethonium (*HEXA*), starting at arrow, blocks both effects of nicotine (*NIC*) but not cardiac stimulation by venom (*VE*) or epinephrine (*EP*). After effect of each drug, kimograph was stopped for 20 min (*vertical bars*) (CORRADO et al., 1975)

A more direct demonstration of the neurotransmitter-releasing properties of TsTx on the adrenergic nerve terminals has been done by LANGER et al. (1975). Exposure to the scorpion toxin of isolated guinea pig atria, previously labeled with ^{3}H-noradrenaline, enhances the spontaneous outflow of radioactivity. This effect coincides with the increase in atrial rate. Analysis of the radioactive products indicate that ^{3}H-noradrenaline accounted for 60% of the total increase in outflow of radioactivity elicited by TsTx (Fig. 8). The ^{3}H-deaminated glycol (3,4 dihydroxy-phenylglycol) represents the main metabolite formed. The increase in atrial rate evoked by TsTx is concentration-dependent and the positive chronotropic effect persisted for several minutes after the toxin has removed from the bath. Other than the selective increase in the release of ^{3}H-noradrenaline and ^{3}H-deaminated glycol, no labeled substances were found in the perfusates. The pattern of release is similar to that obtained by nerve stimulation (LANGER et al., 1975).

In addition to releasing noradrenaline the venom also enhances transmitter overflow elicited by nerve stimulation through a prejunctional effect that in several respects differs from the known mechanisms of action of adrenergic substances. After 20 min of incubation, if the venom is removed from the incubation media, stimulation of the accelerans nerve increases the transmitter overflow approximately eight-fold compared with controls stimulated without any contact with the toxin. The increase in transmitter overflow obtained after exposure to the venom could be due either to an actual increase in transmitter release or to inhibition of sites of transmitter loss, such as neuronal or extraneuronal uptake of noradrenaline (LANGER et al., 1975). Neither inhibition of neuronal nor that of extraneuronal uptake appear to be involved. It is likely that the enhancement in transmitter release by nerve stimulation evoked by TsTx is related to the ability of this toxin

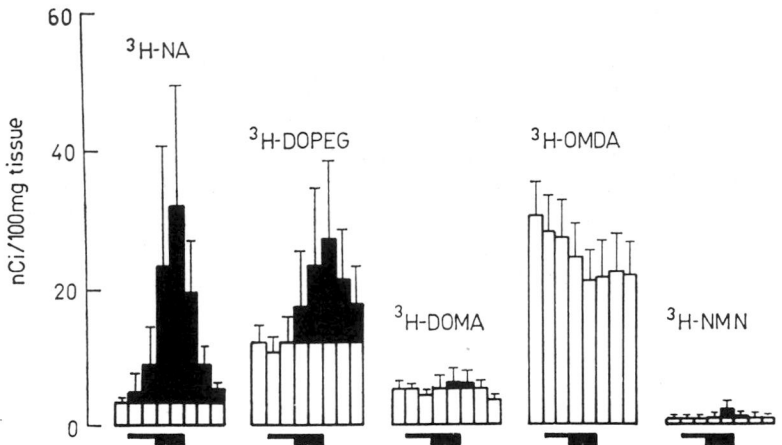

Fig. 8. Release of radioactive products elicited by scorpion venom tityustoxin (TsTX) from spontaneously beating guinea pig atria. Locke's solution, 37° C. Ordinate: nc/100 mg of tissue. Open bars represent spontaneous outflow in consecutive 5-min samples, collection of which started 70 min after end of incubation with ^{3}H-noradrenaline (*NA*). Period of exposure to 0.3 μg/ml TsTX is shown by thin black rectangle, and exposure to 1.0 μg/ml TsTX is shown by thick black rectangle. Dark areas indicate increase in release induced by exposure to TsTX. Note selective increase in release of ^{3}H-NA and ^{3}H-DOPEG (3,4-dihydroxyphenylglycol) during exposure to TsTX and the persistance of releasing effects after the scorpion venom has been washed out. ^{3}H-DOMA 3,4-dihydroxymandelic acid; ^{3}H-OMDA O-methylated de-aminated metabolites; ^{3}H-N M N normetanephrine. Shown are mean values ± S.E.M. of four experiments. (According to Langer et al., 1975)

and other scorpion venoms to elicit a prolongation of the duration of the action potential (Warnick et al., 1976; Kopenhöfer and Schmidt, 1968).

The enhancement of noradrenaline release by TsTx after nerve stimulation might be responsible for the potentiation of hypertensive response to carotid artery occlusion observed after intravenous administration of *Tityus* venom (Corrado et al., 1975).

The selective stimulation of *T. serrulatus* venom caused a discharge of neuro-transmitters probably by depolarization of prejunctional structures of the nerve fibers. In addition, the nerve fiber apparently remains sensitized for a long period of time. The response to a second stimulus after a previous exposure to the venom is probably amplified several-fold, leading again to an abnormally elevated discharge of chemical mediators. Hence, the response of *Tityus* venom in the whole animal or in an innervated tissues should be the summation of a variety of direct and indirect effects of the venom and also of the released neurotransmitters.

The site of action of the venom, however, is probably the external membrane of excitable tissues, mainly the nerve structures. A strong binding to specific sites, followed by a long-lasting modification in the membranes of these tissues, is suggested as an explanation for the observed changes in the permeability to ions (Gomez et al., 1975; Diniz et al., 1975) and in the electrical properties of the membranes (Warnick et al., 1976).

III. General Effects

A large variety of physiologic and pathologic alterations in cardiovascular, respiratory, digestive, and nervous systems are induced in animals by *Tityus* venoms. The proper use of neurotransmitter antagonists and of substances that affect their metabolism demonstrated that several effects of the venom are indirect and might be of physiopathologic significance (DINIZ and VALERI, 1959; CORRADO et al., 1968; FREIRE MAIA et al., 1970, 1973, 1974; ROSSI et al., 1973, 1974; BARTHOLOMEW, 1970; CUNHA MELLO et al., 1973; MACHADO and SILVEIRA, 1974).

Myonecrosis induced by the injection of *T. serrulatus* venom in cockroaches suggests that toxins active on insects might also be present in these venoms (ROSSI et al., 1973).

The basic knowledge accumulated in recent years in an attempt to determine the mechanism of action of scorpion venoms has been useful in formulating new approaches for the treatment of patients stung by scorpions. From 1972 to 1974, 122 children envenomated by scorpions of the genus *Tityus* were treated at the John XXIII Hospital at Belo Horizonte. Each child received specific serum therapy; however, 18 presented serious cardiovascular complications (arrhythmias, hypertension, heart failure, shock, acute lung edema) and were removed to the local Medical School Hospital for intensive care. In spite of this care one child ($1^1/_2$ years old) died. In the others, the sinus rhythm returned to normal only after 2 or 3 days (CAMPOS et al., 1975; CAMPOS, 1975).

IV. Conclusion

Scorpion venom is a promising tool for the study of essential physiologic processes controlled by the nervous system. Highly purified and potent toxins isolated from these venoms and active upon excitable tissues could be used to investigate molecular changes responsible for important functions such as the synthesis, storage, and release of neurotransmitters. In addition, the study of the interaction of scorpion venom with terrestrial invertebrate organisms may constitute an interesting model of biological interaction. Efforts in these directions are worth pursuing.

Acknowledgement: This work was supported in part by the State of São Paulo Research Foundation (Grant Biol. 12/1341) and the Brazilian Research Council (Grant TC−10.580).

References

Bartholomew, C.: Acute scorpion pancreatitis in Trinidad. Brit. med. J. **1**, 668−670 (1970).

Barros, E.F.: Beitrag zur Kenntnis der Skorpionvergiftung. Virchows Arch. path. Anat. **304**, 371−396 (1936).

Barros, E.F.: O quadro clínico da intoxicação escorpiônica. Hospital (Rio de J.) **14**, 1−25 (1938).

Beraldo, W.T., Dias da Silva, W.: Release of histamine by animal venoms and bacterial toxin. In: Handbuch der experimentellen Pharmakologie, Vol. XVIII. Histamine and antihistaminics, Part 1. Edit. by M. Rocha e Silva, Berlin-Heidelberg-New York: Springer 1966.

Böhm, G.M., Pompolo, Sueli, Diniz, C.R., Gomez, M.V., Pimenta Aurea, F., Netto, J.C.: Ultrastructural alterations of mouse diaphragm nerve endings induced by purified scorpion venom, tityustoxin. Toxicon **12**, 509 – 511 (1974).

Campos, J.A.: Aumento da amilase sanguinea em crianças picadas por *Tityus serrulatus*. Ann. Cong. Panan Pediat. (1975).

Campos, J.A., Silva, O.A., Guimaraês, P.V., Lopez, M., Maia, L.F.: Manifestações cardiovasculares nos acidentes por picada de escorpião. Ann. Congr. Panan. Pediat. (1975).

Carvalho, P.: Ação da peçonha de escorpiões brasileiros sobre o sistema nervoso. Arq. Inst. Benj. Baptista **4**, 21 – 45 (1938).

Corrado, A.P., Antonio, A., Diniz, C.R.: Recent advances on the mechanism of action of Brazilian scorpion venom (*Tityus serrulatus*). Mem. Inst. Butantan **33**, 957 – 960 (1966).

Corrado, A.P., Antonio, A., Diniz, C.R.: Brazilian scorpion venom (*Tityus serrulatus*) an unusual sympathetic postganglionic stimulant. J. Pharmacol. exp. Ther. **164**, 253 – 258 (1968).

Corrado, A.P., Diniz, C.R., Antonio, A.: Neurotransmitter release by the toxin of Brazilian scorpion (*Tityus serrulatus* Lutz e Mello). In: Concepts of membranes in regulation and excitation, pp. 193 – 199. Ed. by M. Rocha e Silva and G. Suarez Kurtz. New York: Raven Press 1975.

Corrado, A.P., Riccioppo Neto, F., Antonio, A.: The mechanism of the hypertensive effect of Brazilian scorpion venom (*Tityus serrulatus*, Lutz e Mello). Toxicon **12**, 145 – 150 (1974).

Coutinho Netto, J., Diniz, C.R.: A new method of purification of Tityustoxin. Ann. Acad. Bras. Cienc., in press (1975).

Cunha Mello, J.R., Freire Maia, L., Tafuri, W.L., Maria, T.A.: Mechanism of action of purified scorpion toxin on the isolated rat intestine. Toxicon **11**, 81 – 84 (1973).

Diniz, C.R., Corrado, A.P.: Venoms of insects and arachnids. In: International Encyclopedia of Pharmacology and Therapeutics. Sect. 71, pp. 117 – 139. Ed. by H. Raskova. Oxford-New York: Pergamon Press 1971.

Diniz, C.R., Coutinho Netto, J., Pimenta, A.F., Larson, R.E.: Biochemical properties of Tityustoxin. In: Concepts of membranes in regulation and excitation, pp. 217 – 221. Ed. by M. Rocha e Silva and G. Suarez Kurtz. New York: Raven Press 1975.

Diniz, C.R., Gonçalves, J.M.: Some chemical and pharmacological properties of Brazilian scorpion venoms. In: Venoms. Publ. No. 44, pp. 131 – 139. Am. Assoc. Adv. Scienc. Washington, D.C. (Buckley, E., and Porges, N. eds.). Washington: A.A.A.S. Press 1956.

Diniz, C.R., Gonçalves, J.M.: Separation of biologically active components from scorpion venom by zone electrophoresis. Biochim. biophys. Acta (Amst.) **41**, 470 – 477 (1960).

Diniz, C.R., Pimenta, A.F., Coutinho Netto, J., Pompolo, S., Gomez, M.V., Böhm, G.M.: Effect of scorpion venom from *Tityus serrulatus* (Tityustoxin) on the acetylcholine release and fine structure of the nerve terminals. Experientia (Basel) **30**, 1304 – 1305 (1974).

Diniz, C.R., Torres, J.M.: Release of an acetylcholine-like substance from guinea-pig ileum by scorpion venom. Toxicon **5**, 227 – 236 (1968).

Diniz, C.R., Valeri, V.: Effects of a toxin present in a purified extract of telson from the scorpion, *Tityus serrulatus* on smooth muscle preparations and in mice. Arch. int. Pharmacodyn. **71**, 1 – 12 (1959).

Fisher, F.G., Böhn, H.: The toxins of the Brasilian scorpion *Tityus serrulatus* and *Tityus bahiensis*. Hoppe-Seylers Z. physiol. Chem. **306**, 269 – 272 (1957).

Freire Maia, L., Azevedo, A.P., Costa Val, V.P.: Respiratory arrythmias produced by purified scorpion toxin. Toxicon **11**, 225 – 257 (1973).

Freire Maia, L., Azevedo, A.D., Lima, E.G.: Pharmacological blockade of the cardiovascular and respiratory effects produced by Tityustoxin – Comn. Soc. Int. Toxin. Japan, 1973.

Freire Maia, L., Ferreira, M., Carvalho, P.: Estudo do mecanismo da da hiperglicemia e da hipertensão arterial produzidas pelo veneno de escorpião no cão. Mem. Inst. Osw. Cruz **59**, 11 – 22 (1961).

Freire Maia, L., Pinto, G.J., Franco, I.: Mechanism of cardiovascular effects produced by purified scorpion toxin in the rat. J. Pharmacol. exp. Ther. **188**, 207 – 212 (1974).

Freire Maia, L., Ribeiro, R.M., Beraldo, W.T.: Effect of a purified scorpion toxin on respiratory movements in the rat. Toxicon **8**, 307 – 312 (1970).

Gelotte, B.: Studies on gel filtrations sorption properties of the bed material Sephadex. J. Chromatogr. Sci. **3**, 330 – 342 (1960).

Gomez, M.V.: Purificação e caracterização da toxina do escorpião *Tityus serrulatus*. Tese de Doutoramento. Universidade de Minas Gerais, Belo Horizonte (1967).

Gomez, M.V., Dai, M.E.M., Diniz, C.R.: Release of acetylcholine by Tityustoxin in brain slices. Acta cient. venez. 22-R.32 (1971).

Gomez, M.V., Dai, M.E.M., Diniz, C.R.: Effect of scorpion venom Tityustoxin on the release of acetylcholine from incubated slices of rat brain. J. Neurochem. **20**, 1051—1061 (1973).

Gomez, M.V., Diniz, C.R.: Separation of toxic components from the Brazilian scorpion — *Tityus serrulatus* — venom. Mem. Inst. Butantan **33**, 899—902 (1966).

Gomez, M.V., Diniz, C.R., Barbosa, T.S.: A comparison of the effects of scorpion venom Tityustoxin and ouabain on the release of acetylcholine from incubated slices of rat brain. J. Neurochem. **24**, 331—336 (1975).

Henriques, M.C., Gazzinelli, G., Diniz, C.R., Gomez, M.V.: Effect of the venom of the scorpion *Tityus serrulatus* on adrenal gland catecholamines. Toxicon **5**, 175—179 (1968).

Houssay, B.A.: Action physiologique du venin des corpions *Buthus quinquestriatus* et *Tityus bahiensis*. J. Physiol. Path. gén. **18**, 305—317 (1919).

Kao, C.Y.: Tetrodotoxin, saxitoxin and their significance in the study of excitation phenomena. Pharmacol. Rev. **18**, 007—1048 (1966).

Kopenhöfer, E., Schmidt, H.: Die Wirkung von Skorpiongift auf die Ionesmstrom des Ranvierischen Schurrig II—Unvollständige Natrium—Inaktivierung. Pflügers Arch. ges. Physiol. **303**, 150—161 (1968).

Langer, S.Z., Adler-Grachinsky, E., Almeida, A.P., Diniz, C.R.: Prejunctional effects of a purified toxin from the scorpion *Tityus serrulatus*. Release of ³H-noradrenaline and enhancement of transmitter overflow elicited by nerve stimulation. Naunyn-Schmiedeberg's Arch. Pharmacol. **287**, 243—259 (1975).

Lopes da Silva, T.: Escorpionismo em Ribeirão Preto. Notas sobre epidemiologia e profilaxia. Arch. Hig. (S. Paulo) **15**, 79—90 (1950).

Lutz, A., Mello, O.: Descripção de 5 espécies brasileiras dos generos *Tityus* e *Rhopalurus*. Folha méd. **4**, 25—26 (1922).

Machado, J.C., Silveira, J.F.: Obtenção do quadro anátomo-patológico da pancreatite hemorrágica aguda no cão pela inoculação de venenos de *Tityus serrulatus*. Mem. Inst. Butantan **35**, 159—162 (1974).

Magalhães, O.: Contribution à la connoissance de l'action du venin des scorpions. C.R. Soc. Biol. (Paris) **93**, 35—37 (1925).

Magalhães, O.: Contribuição para o conhecimento da intoxicação veneno dos escorpiões. Mem. Inst. Osw. Cruz **21**, 5—139 (1928).

Magalhães, O.: Scorpionism. J. trop. Med. Hyg. **41**, 393—399 (1938).

Magalhães, O.: The scorpionic syndrome. J. trop. Med. Hyg. **42**, 1—5 (1939).

Magalhães, O.: Escorpionismo. IV Memoria-Monografias do Inst. Osw. Cruz—Imprensa Nacional, Rio (1946).

Maurano, H.R.: Do escorpionismo. Tese—Faculdade de Medicina do Rio de Janeiro, Rodrigues & Cia (Jornal do Comercio) Rio de Janeiro (1915).

Mello-Campos, O.: Os escorpiões brasileiros. Mem. Inst. Osw. Cruz **17**, 237—363 (1924).

Miranda, F., Kupeyan, H., Rochat, H., Rochat, C., Lissitzki, S.: Purification of animal neurotoxins. Isolation and characterization of eleven neurotoxins from the venoms of the scorpions *Androctonus australis Hector, Buthus occitanus tunetanus, Leiurus quinquestriatus quinquestriatus*. Europ. J. Biochem. **16**, 514—523 (1970).

Miranda, F., Rochat, H., Lissitzki, S.: Sur la neurotoxine du venin de deux espèces de scorpions nord-africains. Bull. Soc. Chim. biol. (Paris) **42**, 379—391 (1960).

Miranda, F., Rochat, H., Lissitzki, S.: Essais de purification des neurotoxines du venin d'un scorpion d'Amérique du Sud (*Tityus serrulatus L* e *M*) par des methods chromatographiques. Toxicon **4**, 145—152 (1966).

Ramos, A.O., Corrado, A.P.: Efeito hiperpiretico do veneno de escorpião (*T. serrulatus* e *T. bahiensis*). An. Fac. Med. Univ. S. Paulo **28**, 81—98 (1954).

Rochat, H., Rochat, C., Miranda, F., Lissitzki, S., Edman, P.: The amino acid sequence of neurotoxin I of *Androctonus australis Hector*. Europ. J. Biochem. **17**, 262—269 (1971).

Rochat, H., Rochat, C., Sampieri, F., Miranda, F.: The aminoacid sequence of Neurotoxin II of *Androctonus australis Hector*. Europ. J. Biochem. **28**, 381—392 (1972).

Rossi, M.A., Ferreira, A.C., Santos, J.C.M.: Catecholamine repleting effect of Brazilian scorpion (*Tityus serrulatus*) venom on adrenergic nerves of rat atrioventricular valves. Experientia (Basel) **30**, 513—514 (1974).

Rossi, M.A., Ferreira, A.L., Paiva, S.M.: Fine structure of pulmonary changes induced by Brazilian scorpion venom. Arch. Path. (Chicago) **97**, 284—288 (1974).

Rossi, M.A., Ferreira, A.L., Paiva, S.M., Santos, J.C.M.: Myonecrosis induced by scorpion venom. Experientia (Basel) **29**, 1271—1274 (1973).

Schaumann, W.: Inhibition by morphine of the release of acetylcholine from the intestine of the guinea pig. Brit. J. Pharmacol. **12**, 115—118 (1957).

Slotkin, E.: Chemistry of animal venoms. Experientia (Basel) **29**, 1453—1488 (1973).

Tafuri, W.L., Maria, T.A., Freire Maia, L., Cunha Mello, B.: Effect of the scorpion toxin on the granular vesicles in the Auerbach's plexus of the rat ileum. J. Neural. Transm. **35**, 233—240 (1974).

Tafuri, W.L., Maria, T.A., Freire Maia, R., Cunha Mello, J.R.: Effect of purified scorpion toxin on vesicles components in the myenteric plexus of the rat. Toxicon **9**, 427—428 (1971).

Torres, J.M., Diniz, C.R.: Release of acetylcholine by scorpion venom. Cienc. Cult. S. Paulo **16**, 197 (1964).

Vital Brasil: Contribuicão ao estudo do envenenamento pela picada do escorpião e seu tratamento. Coletanea de trabalhos do Instituo Butantan, pp. 69—81. Inst. Butantan São Paulo (1909).

Vital Brasil, O., Neder, A.C., Corrado, A.P.: Effects and mechanism of action of *Tityus serrulatus* venom on skeletal muscle. Pharmacol. Res. Commun. **5**, 137—150 (1973).

Warnick, J.E., Albuquerque, E.X., Diniz, C.R.: Electrophysiological observations on the action of purified scorpion venom, Tityustoxin on nerve and skeletal muscle of the rat. J. Pharmacol. Exp. Ther. **198**, 155—167 (1976).

Waterman, J.A.: Some notes on scorpion poisoning in Trinidad. Trans. roy. Soc. trop. Med. Hyg. **31**, 607—624 (1938).

Waterman, J.A.: Some notes on scorpion poisoning in Trinidad. Caribbean med. J. **19**, 113—128 (1957).

CHAPTER 15

Chactoid Venoms

M. GOYFFON and J. KOVOOR

I. Introduction

As stated by VACHON (1952), numerous morphologic characteristics serve to divide the order of scorpions into two groups, the buthoids and the chactoids, without, however, designating them as suborders. The buthoids consist of a single family, the Buthidae, while the chactoids include five others. Both of these groups are widely represented on the surface of the earth.

A characteristic biochemical feature may be added to the classical differences between these groups. Indeed, the taxonomic importance of polyacrylamide gel electrophoregrams of hemolymph proteins has been pointed out already (GOYFFON et al., 1970, 1973). An analysis of the proteins of about fifty species from both groups has shown that one of the bands, the slowest of the migrating fractions, is typical of the Buthidae (Fig. 1). This argues in favor of retaining KRAEPELIN'S (1905) terminology which, in the present case, has the further merit of being convenient. Thus, when we refer to chactoids and their venoms we include the families Chactidae, Scorpionidae, Diplocentridae, Bothriuridae, and Vejovidae.

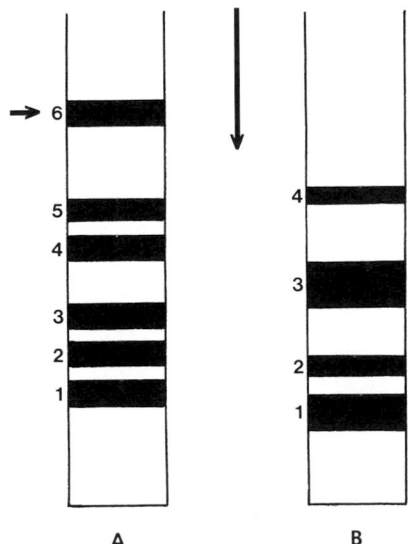

Fig. 1. Disc-electrophoregram of hemolymph proteins of *Androctonus amoreuxi* (A) and *Scorpio maurus* (B). Band 6 is the "Buthid band"

These five families comprise about 60% of the species of scorpions described up to now. However, biochemical and physiologic studies of the venoms of the chactoids are far fewer than those devoted to the buthoids. Representatives of only a few genera, seven in all, consisting of four Scorpionidae, a Diplocentridae, and two Vejovidae, have been investigated in detail. Nothing in fact is known of the chemical composition and the physiologic effects of the venoms of the Chactidae and the Bothriuridae since the members of these two groups have the reputation of being not very dangerous or even quite harmless to man. The anatomic and histologic study of venom glands, which ought to properly precede or at least accompany other investigations, has hardly progressed, however, since the works of PAVLOVSKY (1913, 1914, 1918, 1924). Some histochemical data on the secretory products of the venom glands of a *Vejovis* and a *Diplocentrus* appear in the article of SAMANO-BISHOP and GOMEZ DE FERRIZ (1964). Some of the first results of a histochemical study of the same glands in the Scorpionidae, *Pandinus imperator,* are given in the following pages (KOVOOR, unpublished).

II. Morphology of the Telson in Chactoids

The sixth and last segment of the metasoma of scorpions often shows anatomic characteristics used by taxonomists. For this reason both classical and modern works on systematics carry descriptions with illustrations of the telson sometimes extremely precise in details (e.g. KRAEPELIN, 1899; MELLO CAMPOS, 1925; VACHON, 1952). The color, form, ornamentation, and size of the vesicle and the aculeus are much more varied in the chactoids than in the buthoids. It would therefore appear useful to recall here, with the help of some examples, certain important anatomic features of the telson which can have a bearing on those of the enclosed glands.

The anatomic characteristics of the telson may be related according to the family, subfamily, or genus to which a particular scorpion belongs, as well as according to its sex. The telson of the Diplocentridae shows a tubercle under the aculeus at the distal end of the vesicle. The telson is smooth and without any tubercle in the Euscorpiinae (Chactidae) and many Vejovidae. The telson of the Uroctoninae is often much shorter and narrower than the articles of the tail. On the other hand, in the Scorpioninae of the genera *Heterometrus, Pandinus* (VACHON, 1953), and *Scorpio,* the vesicle is swollen and generally wider than the caudal segments, while its thick and hard wall is granulous both ventrally and laterally.

Sex-linked characteristics are the most interesting since they often influence the form of the glands. They might also very well affect the quality of venom although, to the best of our knowledge, no author has yet reported any difference in the composition or physiologic effect between venoms obtained from male and female scorpions of the same species. KRAEPELIN (1899) has observed that the male vesicle is larger and more swollen than the female one in the genus *Euscorpius,* except for *E. flavicaudis* where the sex-linked difference concerns only the aculeus which is more curved in the male than in the female (VACHON, 1952). PAVLOVSKY (1913) has shown that the different external aspect of telsons of both sexes corresponds to a bigger size of the male venom glands. It is also well known that the vesicle of the male *Hemiscorpion* (Scorpionidae), elongated and with two small tubercles under the very short aculeus, differs from that of the female which is oval and without a tubercle. As in the case of *Euscorpius,* PAVLOVSKY (1913) has established that the venom gland of the male fills the whole internal cavity of the vesicle as well as inside the tubercles. In other cases, differences in size, if not in shape, are noticed. Among the Chaerilinae (Chactidae), for example, the telson of the male *Calchas nordmanni* is smaller than that of the female. The precise measurements of the female telson made by WILLIAMS (1968) in several species of *Vejovis* (Vejovidae) show that it is always bigger than that of the male, even after accounting for the generally bigger size of the whole female scorpion. Among the Bothriuridae, in certain species of the genera *Urophonius* (KRAEPELIN, 1899) and *Bothriurus* (KRAEPELIN, 1899; PAVLOVSKY, 1918, 1924; SAN MARTIN, 1968), the vesicle of the male telson is provided with a scutelliform depression on its dorsal surface which does not exist in the female. While studying this feature in *Bothriurus vittatus* Guer., PAVLOVSKY found underneath the epiderm of the depressed region a special pleated epithelium which appeared to be glandular and which the author named *glandula plicata;* the function of this organ still remains unknown. The pleated epithelium occupies more than a quarter of the vesicle and, consequently, the volume of the venom glands is reduced.

III. Anatomy and Development of the Venom Glands

The venom glands of chactoids, as those of buthoids, are long twin sacs, parallel to the axis of the vesicle. Each gland is provided with an excretory duct which runs along the aculeus and opens into it laterally, at a short distance from the blind end. Glands are bordered on the external lateral surface and ventrally by the telson cuticle, and covered dorsally and on their lateral internal surface by a thick sheath of muscular fibers.

According to LAURIE's observations (1894) on *Euscorpius italicus* (Chactidae), the venom gland arises in the last segment of the body as two epidermal buds during the fifth embryonic phase, which lasts from the formation of the appendages to the hatching of the embryo. PAVLOVSKY (1913, 1914), studying the structure of the gland of a new-born *Euscorpius mingrelicus* and three young specimens of *E. germanus,* observed that on hatching, each gland of the scorpion consists of a compact group of non-functional cells, covered with several layers of muscular cells, and a well-differentiated duct provided with a cuticular intima. After the first moult, the size of the glands increases and cells are arranged in a thick and regular epithelium surrounding a median tubular and narrow lumen. The first granules of secretion, staining with safranin and iron hematoxylin, appear in the cytoplasm. Some connective cells can be detected between the glandular cells. PAVLOVSKY (1913) also noted that in young individuals of *Palamnaeus indicus* L. (= *Heterometrus cyaneus* C.L.K.) (Scorpionidae) the glands of which show the same structural characteristics as that of the Chactidae, the glandular epithelium forms a thick but regular and unfolded sheath around a narrow lumen.

By studying adult scorpions belonging to different families, we know, however, that a complex structure of the venom glands appears in families other than the Chactidae; greatest complexity is observed in the Buthidae and the Diplocentridae. The first detailed investigations are again those of PAVLOVSKY (1913, 1914, 1924). They led to a classification of the venom glands based on the several categories of forms of the secretory epithelium. Venom glands of the Chactidae, of which the genera *Euscorpius, Teuthraustes, Chaerilus,* and *Calchas* have been investigated, are the most "primitive". The epithelial layer without folds, like those of early juvenile scorpions, comprises either columnar cells of equal size, arranged regularly (Type IA) or cells of different height which render the lumen border irregular (Type I A1). Among the Vejovidae, glands of the simple type are found in *Uroctonus mordax* and in the genera *Scorpiops* and *Vejovis* (RUIZ LUGA, 1963; SAMANO-BISHOP and GOMEZ DE FERRIZ, 1964). On the other hand, the complex type is exhibited with different degrees of complexity in the venom glands of the genera *Hadruroides, Iurus,* and *Hadrurus,* where the glandular epithelium forms true folds which can even exceed five in number, and comprise both glandular cells and underlying connective tissue (Type IIB2). Venom glands of the Scorpionidae are also of several types. The epithelium is smooth in the Homurinae and slightly irregular in *Opisthocentrus madagascariensis* (=*Opisthacanthus madagascariensis* Kraepelin). It forms false folds in *Opisthacanthus elatus* (Type IA2) but the genera *Hemiscorpion* and *Urodacus,* as also the Scorpioninae, are provided with glands of complex structure (Type IIB, B1 or B2). An even more complex structure is observed in the venom glands of *Nebo hierichonticus* (Diplocentridae) studied by ROSIN (1965, 1972). In fact, the venom gland is divided longitudinally into two different parts by a septum which arises in the distal portion from the lateral internal wall of the gland along which it extends, fused with the dorsal and ventral walls. This septum which consists of two epithelial layers separated by connective tissue terminates freely in the proximal part of the gland, that is, not far from the beginning of the excretory duct. The gland is thus divided into two distinct lobes converging in the proximal region: a lateral internal and a lateral external lobe. Apart from the septum, other folds extend into the lumen, especially arising from the lateral internal wall of the gland; these folds may have secondary branchings. In *Diplocentrus keyserlingi tehuacanus* Hoffmann, the only other Diplocentrid which has been studied up to now (SAMANO-BISHOP and GOMEZ DE FERRIZ, 1964) the venom glands have not been shown to be provided with such a complex structure as in *Nebo hierichonticus.*

The structural complexity of the venom glands is acquired progressively during the successive stages of post-embryonic development. VACHON (JUNQUA and VACHON, 1968) therefore put forward the hypothesis according to which the different structural aspects of the venom glands would appear as a consequence of a neotenic process that stabilizes the glands in a certain stage of the development. The question then arises as to how the anatomic complexity of the glands is correlated with their secretory activity as revealed by their histochemistry in adult scorpions.

IV. Comparative Histology and Histochemistry of the Venom Glands in Adults

Until ROSIN' studies (1965, 1972), it seemed established that the histologic structure of the venom glands was uniform throughout the whole order of scorpions. Apart from the thick muscular layer surrounding the glands and the connective tissue limiting the glandular epithelium, a single type of glandular cells had been described (BÜCHERL, 1971; JUNQUA and VACHON, 1968) for all the different stages of the secretory process. SAMANO-BISHOP and GOMEZ DE FERRIZ (1964) detected myoepithelial cells inserted between glandular cells in the glands of *Vejovis* and *Diplocentrus;* these particular cells would act directly on the neighboring venom cells to facilitate venom extrusion which is initiated by the contraction of the external muscular layer. The secretion is of the apocrine type; glandular cells are therefore able to accomplish several secretory cycles before their elimination into the lumen of the gland, though the existence of substitution cells is still a matter of controversy.

According to ROSIN (1965), however, two types of glandular cells can be distinguished in the venom gland of *Nebo hierichonticus*. They produce two distinct secretory products, one in the form of small highly eosinophilic granules and the other as globules, which with the hematoxylin-eosin technique take on various shades from pink to light blue. Each secretory product is proper to each one of the two particular lobes of the glands. The characterization of these two products is, however, based only on a single general stain (hematoxylin-eosin), and precise histochemical tests would be required to disprove, if at all, JUNQUA's interpretation (JUNQUA and VACHON, 1968), i.e., that the clearly different appearance of the two lobes of the gland described by ROSIN (1965) is due to a difference in the stages of maturation of a single product during the secretory process and not to the elaboration of two distinct products. Indeed JUNQUA reports that when Heidenhain's azan is applied at the beginning of the secretory cycle, the secretory product shows an affinity for azocarmine, while at the end of the cycle or during storage it takes on anilin blue. Maturation of the secretory product has also been demonstrated in certain cells of the venom glands of buthids (KOVOOR, 1973) and also in a Scorpionid (*Pandinus imperator*) (KOVOOR, unpublished). However, it likely does not concern *all* the cells which elaborate several distinct products, as may be the case in *Nebo hierichonticus*.

Some histochemical data are given by SAMANO-BISHOP and GOMEZ DE FERRIZ (1964) on the venom glands of several *Vejovis,* a *Diplocentrus,* and *Centruroides* (Buthidae). These authors do not specify whether the different compounds are located in every glandular cell or confined to certain ones. However, for the first time, it is shown that the epithelial layer contains polysaccharides and acidic mucosubstances besides proteins. These compounds have been detected in the venom glands of all the species studied. But it has been noted in these Mexican specimens that polysaccharides which strongly react with periodic acid-Schiff (P.A.S.) are more abundant in the more dangerous scorpions, such as *Diplocentrus* and *Centruroides,* than in *Vejovis,* the venom of which causes much less harm to man.

A histochemical study has been made recently (KOVOOR, unpublished) of the venom glands of two adults of *Pandinus imperator* C.L.K. which were kept in the laboratory without stinging for several days. Although the results have yet to be verified over a number of individuals, some preliminary conclusions are given below. The venom gland of *Pandinus imperator* is of a complex type (Type IIB2 of PAVLOVSKY). The folds of the epithelial layer are numerous and deep, thus reducing, the space in the lumen. Secreting cells are about 250 μ long and 20—50 μ broad according to their shape. Some cells are bottle-shaped, basally

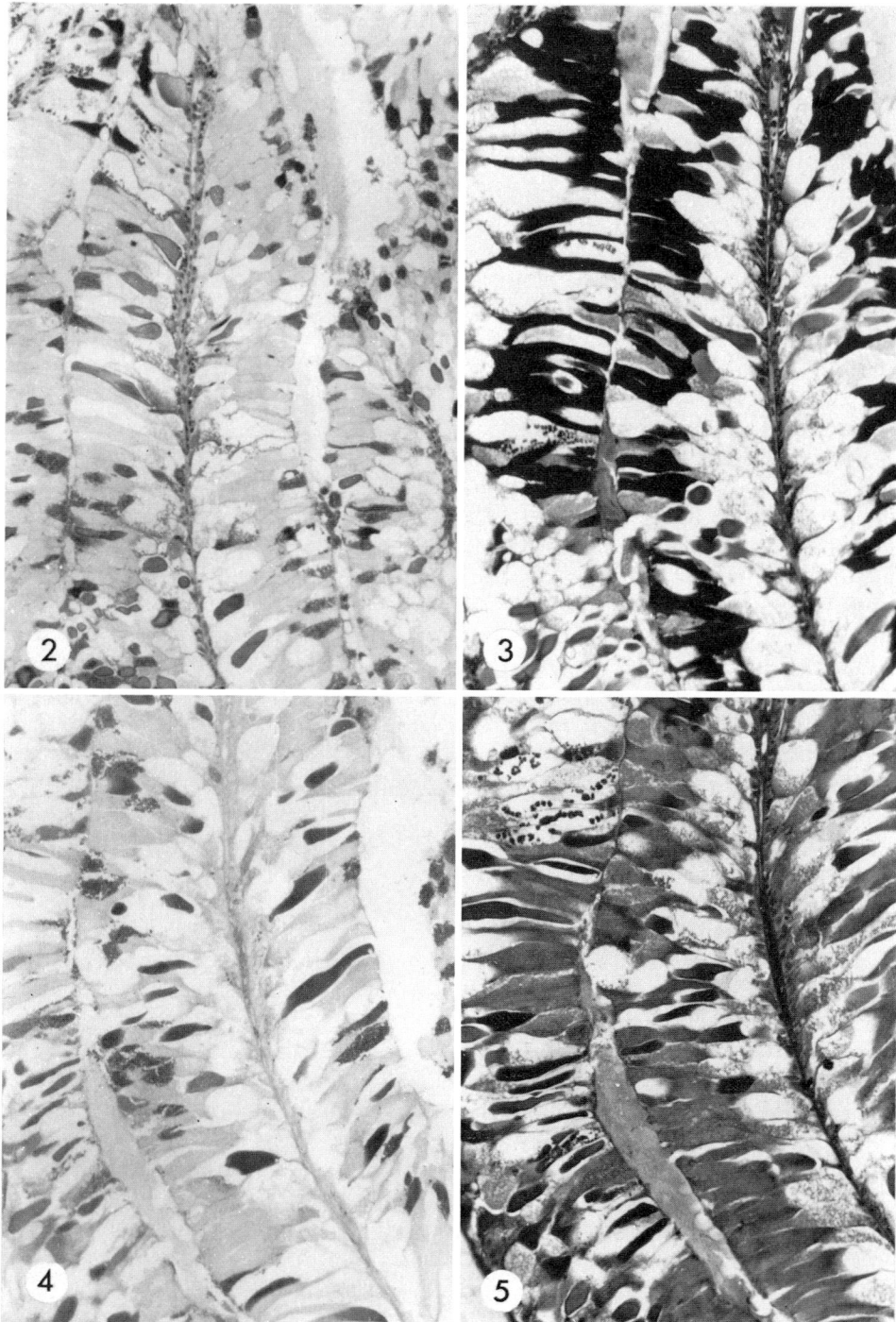

Figs. 2—5. Some histochemical features of the venom gland of *Pandinus imperator* C.L.K. (Scorpionidae) (Kovoor, unpublished)

wide and apically narrow, or vice versa, while others are columnar. These various shapes are associated with different aspects, tinctorial affinities, and histochemical characters of the secretory products. These characters are detectable not only inside the cells, but also in the lumen of the gland; we are, therefore, inclined to regard them as indicative of distinct cellular categories. Following these histologic and histochemical criteria, at least five categories of glandular cells may be recognized in the different lobes of the gland. They contain complex compounds in the form of granules, beads or patches, that are cyanophilic or erythrophilic (Fig. 2) and all are more or less rich in proteins (Fig. 5). Those secretory cells which are not very rich in proteins, contain in addition a polysaccharidic compound, strongly reactive to the PAS reaction, and very acidic mucosubstances. These cells are missing in the ventral part of the proximal three-quarters of the gland which is closer to the aculeus. On the other hand, this region shows another type of cell which is absent elsewhere in the gland. It produces a strongly PAS-positive product which is devoid of acidic mucosubstances but very rich in proteins as shown by a positive reaction to all the tests for the latter. Three kinds of cells secrete only proteins which can be distinguished histochemically. Abundant indole derivatives are detected in the three secretory products; one of them only contains tyrosine and reducing groups. These three types of cells are uniformly distributed in all the glandular lobes.

Unfortunately these results cannot be compared with any available biochemical data on the venom of *Pandinus imperator*. ISMAIL et al. (1974), however, have isolated from the venom of *Pandinus exitialis* 16 protein fractions of possibly the same variety as the proteins produced from the 5 kinds of cells in the gland of *Pandinus imperator*. The plurality of the indole derivatives may also be indicated by their localization in three different types of cells. BHASKARAN NAIR et al. (1973) have in fact identified four indole derivatives (tryptophan, 5-hydroxytryptophan, serotonin and tryptamine) in venom of another Scorpionid, *Heterometrus scaber*. On the other hand, the occurrence of strongly acidic mucosubstances, the role of which still remains unknown, does not seem to be an exception since the same authors (BHASKARAN et al., 1973a) have determined significant quantities of chondroitin sulphate A, B, and C, heparin sulphate and hyaluronic acid in the venom of *Heterometrus scaber*. Mucosubstances have been detected through histochemical tests in the venom glands of the Buthidae (KOVOOR, 1973), but their acidity is weak compared to that of the venoms of *Pandinus imperator* and *Heterometrus scaber*.

---

(2) View of epithelial lobe of the venom gland. The secretory product in certain cells is erythrophilic (*black*) and cyanophilic in others. Bouin, one-step trichrome, green filter. ×95. (3) Polysaccharides and mucosubstances in a dorsal lobe of the same gland as Fig. 2. Mucins appear black; a certain number of cells are completely devoid of these compounds. Bouin, PAS-haematoxylin, green filter. ×110. (4) Indole derivatives in the same lobe of the gland. Cf. with Fig. 3. Cells which are rich in indole derivatives (*black*) are devoid of mucins. Bouin, post-coupled benzylidene reaction, orange filter. ×110. (5) Proteins in the same lobe of the gland. Cells of all types contain proteins which react more or less to Danielli's coupled tetrazonium reaction. Bouin, green filter. ×110

Histochemical studies on chactoid venom glands are still only in the initial stages, and no general conclusion can be drawn until modern techniques have been applied in thorough studies of a large number of species representing every family.

V. Chemical Composition of Chactoid Venoms

The chemical composition of chactoid venoms is still not fully understood. Various methods are employed for the extraction of the venom, and their effect on the composition and toxicity of the venom have not been taken into account. These methods are as follows:

Maceration of the telsa in distilled water or in a physiologic saline solution.

Pipetting the venom after removing the sting.

Compression of the telson with forceps when the cuticle is soft (GRASSET et al., 1946).

The scorpion is made to sting a sheet of soft plastic covering a receptacle that catches the venom.

Manual excitation of the cephalothorax or the postabdomen. The venom thus obtained is clear, transparent, and of low viscosity.

Electrical stimulation of the telson (first described by CHARNOT and FAURE, 1934, and since redescribed many times with numerous variations) with a Ruhm-korff coil or a transformer giving voltages of 80–300 V. The venom thus obtained is whitish, thicker, and more viscous than the manual venom, and forms a white sediment after centrifugation.

After collection, the venom is kept in closed tubes, fresh, lyophilized or dessicated on $CaCl_2$ without loss of activity for several months.

Despite the fact that MIRANDA et al. (1964) have demonstrated in their studies of buthoid venoms the differences between the manual venom which he calls "physiologic venom" and the electric venom, these two most commonly used processes of extraction are sometimes employed indiscriminantly by the same author without investigating the effect of the extraction method.

A first analysis of a chactoid venom was performed by CHARNOT and FAURE (1934). According to them, the venom of *Scorpio maurus* was found to contain 75–78% water and a dry residue containing mineral salts, lipids, small quantities of pigments and albuminoid compounds. Its density was 1.05, it had a pH between 6 and 7.2 and its viscosity was not constant. When fresh, it contained 5.57% NaCl, 0.83% cholesterol, and 8.97% proteins. Since the work by CHARNOT and FAURE, electrophoresis and chromatography have accounted for great progress in the analysis of the venoms.

Protein fractions were obtained by starch-gel electrophoresis at pH 8.6 of the venom of *Heterometrus* (= *Palamnaeus*) *gravimanus*, five of which fractions have been distinguished migrating to the cathode side and three to the anode side. A 5′-nucleotidase, two proteases, and a guinea-pig ileum contracting factor were identified but none of these fractions had a lethal effect on mice. Phospholipase A, cholinesterase and L-amino-acid oxidase were not detected (MASTER et al., 1963). In the venom of the related species *Heterometrus scaber* which contains 39.04% protein when dry and 5.86% protein when fresh (BHASKARAN NAIR and KURUP,

1973b), OOMEN and KURUP (1963) have separated two anodic fractions and three cathodic fractions by paper electrophoresis at pH 8.6. At pH between 6.4 and 7.4 three anodic fractions and four cathodic fractions were obtained and at pH 5.9 as well as pH 8.6, two anodic fractions and three cathodic fractions. At pH 8.6, two glycoprotein fractions with low electrophoretic mobility were observed, one anodic and the other cathodic. No lipoprotein could be detected. The venom of *Heterometrus fulvipes* showed analogous characteristics (BABU et al., 1970). The venom of the Diplocentrid *Nebo hierichonticus* seemed to be poor in proteins. Paper electrophoresis showed the presence of a very fast anodic fraction, possibly a large polypeptide, an important nonmigrating fraction (33%) and a cathodic fraction (33.4%) (ROSIN, 1973). The venom of the Vejovid *Vejovis spinigerus* contains 51.4 mg protein per 100 mg lyophilized matter. Disc electrophoresis of this venom (RUSSELL, 1967; RUSSELL and ALENDER, 1967; RUSSELL et al., 1968) and the venom of *Hadrurus hirsutus* (MCINTOSH et al., 1970) gave 10 to 15 distinct bands. Using cellulose acetate membranes at pH 8.6, the venom of *Pandinus exitialis* was fractionated into 16 bands, 4 of which exhibited a cathodic mobility (ISMAIL et al., 1974).

To summarize, electrophoresis has shown the presence of 6–16 protein fractions in chactoid venoms, depending on the species and the separating power of the support used. Basic proteins were always found which migrated towards the cathode at pHs of about 8.

By fractional precipitation of the venom of *Heterometrus scaber* with ammonium sulphate, OOMEN and KURUP (1964) separated four protein fractions at 0.3, 0.5, 0.7, and 0.9 saturation. Three of these fractions, which all appeared heterogenous, were toxic for mice. Further chromatographic separation was performed following this fractionation in order to isolate the enzyme activities (KURUP, 1966). In the venom of 7 species of scorpions, six major components were defined by two-dimensional paper chromatographic analysis, some of which were common to all species, others were common to related species only (JOHNSON and STAHNKE, 1960). On Sephadex G-50, four major peaks were obtained from the venom of *Vejovis spinigerus* and the lethal activity was associated with the second peak (RUSSELL, 1967; RUSSELL et al., 1968). On carboxymethylcellulose, the same venom was fractionated into five components, the last peak only being toxic. The venom of *Hadrurus hirsutus* when chromatographed on carboxymethylcellulose using a discontinuous gradient was separated into six major components, the first and the last peak being lethal for mice. The same venom when subjected to gel filtration on Sephadex G-25 was resolved into 4 peaks, peaks 2 and 3 being lethal for mice. Molecular weight of lethal fractions was estimated to be approximatively 15.000 for *V. spinigerus* and *H. hirsutus* (MC INTOSH et al., 1970). Using Biogel P 100, the venom of *Pandinus exitialis* was fractionated into 6 fractions (ISMAIL et al., 1974). Thus the separating power of chromatography is not so good as electrophoresis, but the localization and isolation of toxic fractions is easier by this method.

Immunologic techniques have been used to define interspecific affinities of these proteic fractions. Using the Ouchterlony gel diffusion technique, POTTER and NORTHEY (1962) studied antigenic interrelationships between the venom of 8 species, 3 Vejovids and 5 Buthids in homologous and heterologous antigen-antibody systems. The total number of antigenic fractions in the homologous venom antivenom system varied from 3 precipitating bands for *Vejovis flavus* to 5 precipitating bands for *V. spinigerus* and *Hadrurus arizonensis*. In experiments involving heterologous systems, the number of precipitating bands is generally higher when the species are related; however, *H. arizonensis* which shared 5 precipitating bands with *Buthus occitanus* antivenom is an exception. By the same method, Kapadia et al. (1964) proved the existence of a common antigen in the venom of *Heterometrus* (= *Palamnaeus*) *gravimanus* and two buthids, *Leiurus* (= *Buthus*) *quinquestriatus* and *Buthus tamulus*. Using the Scheidegger gelose microimmuno-electrophoresis technique, Irunberry and Pilo-Moron (1965) have studied the antigenic fractions of the buthid *Androctonus australis* venom and the venom of 6 other species of scorpions, 5 of which were Buthids and one Scorpionid. It was found that the number of fractions common to both groups diminished as a function of the phylogenic distance: *Scorpio maurus* had only one common antigenic fraction whereas a species of the same genus, *Androctonus mauretanicus* possessed eleven common antigenic fractions out of the sixteen precipitation lines existing in the homologous system. These observations of paraspecifity of venoms are very interesting in view of the preparation and use of antivenoms (Whittemore et al., 1961).

Enzyme activities: it is generally considered that the venoms of scorpions contain few enzymes (Junqua and Vachon, 1968). This point of view merits further investigation especially regarding chactoids. The existence of hemolytic activity in the venom of various scorpionids has been known for a long time. This activity is weak in the venom of *Hadogenes* (Grasset et al., 1946) whereas it is very marked in the venom of *Heterometrus scaber* (Oomen and Kurup, 1963) and *Scorpio maurus*. The hemolytic properties of the venom of *S. maurus* first noted by Levy (1924) were described by Balozet (1951 and 1952) and have since been confirmed many times (Rosin, 1968; Zlotkin et al., 1972a, b). This hemolytic action appeared only in the presence of exogenic or endogenic lecithin for the venoms of *S. maurus* and *H. scaber* (Bhaskaran Nair and Kurup, 1973b). Hemolysis caused by the Diplocentrid *Nebo hierichonticus* has a different aspect: it had the characteristic appearance of α-hemolysis produced by certain bacteria (Rosin, 1968). According to Zlotkin et al. (1972b), the crude venom of *S. maurus palmatus* was able to hemolyze washed human erythrocytes but was ineffective in the presence of the serum. The phenomenon is inverse with horse erythrocytes. With the aid of starch-gel electrophoresis it was shown that there are two different thermostable factors acting on human and horse erythrocytes. The hemolytic action of this venom may resemble that of snake venoms in the presence of two hemolytic factors, one with a phospholipase A-like activity and the other with a direct lytic activity. The presence of a spherogenic factor on horse erythrocytes in the venom of *S. maurus* could be related to its hemolytic action (Balozet, 1962).

A phospholipase A activity was found in the venom of *H. scaber*. This activity, which is concentrated in the fraction of the venom obtained by 55% saturation with ammonium sulphate, has a slight toxicity, whereas the highly toxic fraction obtained by 90% saturation with ammonium sulphate possesses very little enzyme activity. The phospholipase A of *H. scaber* is not inhibited by iodoacetate which could mean the probable absence of a thiol group. It readily hydrolyses the phospholipids of the red cell ghosts but is inactive against the phospholipids of the intact erythrocytes (KURUP, 1966). The enzyme make-up of this strongly hemolytic venom was determined. Besides the phospholipase A activity, acid phosphatase, ribonuclease, 5'-nucleotidase, hyaluronidase, and acetylcholinesterase were found. There was no DNase nor alkaline phosphatase (BHASKARAN NAIR and KURUP, 1973b). As the enzyme activities of electrically obtained venoms were studied, it is possible that some of these enzyme activities do not exist in the "physiologic venom" but result from more or less damaged cells of the sediment. In the venom of a related species, *Heterometrus* (=*Palamnaeus*) *gravimanus,* proteases, and 5'-nucleotidase were found on starch-gel electrophoregrams but phospholipase A, cholinesterase, and L-amino-acid oxidase were not detected (MASTER et al., 1963).

The venom of *Vejovis spinigerus* exhibited an acetylcholinesterase activity but no proteolytic, amylase, phosphodiesterase, or L amino acid oxidase activity (RUSSELL, 1967 and 1968). An acetylcholinesterase was found in the venom of another Vejovid, *Hadrurus arizonensis* (SAUNDERS and JOHNSON, 1970).

The proteolytic activities are variable. A hyaluronidase activity which plays the role of a spreading factor was observed in the venom of *Scorpio maurus palmatus* but it is probably common to all scorpion venoms and more generally to most animal venoms (BALOZET, 1971). Proteolytic activity *sensu stricto* of the venom of *S. maurus* was first described by BAILLY (1949) who observed and related the proteolytic effect to the inactivation of the rabid virus incubating in dilutions of the venom. The venom of *S. maurus* is particularly rich in enzymes since it possesses a gelatinase activity (ZLOTKIN et al., 1972a) and a mild coagulase activity (BALOZET, 1952 and 1955) but no anticoagulase activity (ZLOTKIN et al., 1972a). These two last enzyme activities are both present in the venom of a related species, *Heterometrus* (=*Palamnaeus*) *gravimanus.* These procoagulant and anticoagulant properties were not completely separated by DEAE-Sephadex chromatography (HAMILTON et al., 1974).

To summarize, enzyme activities of only a few chactoid venoms were investigated. Hemolytic and hyaluronidase activities are generally present. Proteolytic activities are more contingent, and acetylcholinesterase activity is perhaps not limited to Vejovids. A systematic study revealed the existence of ribonuclease, 5'-nucleotidase and acid phosphatase in the venom of a *Heterometrus,* however these enzymes are probably more widespread.

Biogenic amines. Since the work of ADAM and WEISS (1956) the pain provoked by a scorpion sting has been attributed to the serotonin. First identified in the venom of the buthid *Leiurus quinquestriatus,* 5-hydroxytryptamine (5 HT) has been found in some other species. RUSSELL et al. (1968) indicated its presence in the venom of *V. spinigerus* at a concentration of 4.0 µg per mg of dried venom. It was found in the venom of *Heterometrus scaber* at a lower concentration, 2.8 mg per g of dried venom together with numerous indole compounds some of which were identified by thin layer chromatography: 5-hydroxytryptophan, tryptophan, and tryptamine at concentrations of 2.45 mg/g, 4.20 mg/g, and 3.85 mg/g respectively, expressed as tryptophan per g of dry venom (BHASKARAN NAIR et al., 1973).

Recently, the presence of histamine was found in the venom of *Heterometrus* (=*Palamnaeus*) *gravimanus* (ISMAIL et al., 1975).

Other components. The venom of scorpions contains numerous free aminoacids.

Sixteen free amino-acids were identified in the venom of *Heterometrus scaber* among which the most abundant were glycine and aspartic acid (18.85 mg/g dry venom), alanine (15.39 mg/g), cysteine (15.20 mg/g), tryptophan (12.87 mg/g), glutamic acid (11.95 mg/g), and arginine (10.42 mg/g). More than fifty amino-acids were present in the venom of *Vejovis* (Russell, 1967a and b). In the venom of *Pandinus exitialis* eight amino-acids were identified by two-dimensional chromatography: aspartic acid, serine, glycine, alanine, lysine, norvaline, leucine, and phenylalanine (Ismail et al., 1974).

The venom of *H. scaber* also contains glycosaminoglycans sulphated such as hyaluronic acid or sulphated such as chondroitin sulphate A, B, C. Free hexosamines were found and were estimated at 47.9 µg/g wet venom or 466.5 µg/g dry venom (Bhaskaran Nair and Kurup, 1973a).

The venom of *V. spinigerus* per 100 mg of lyophilized product was found to contain 51.4 mg protein and 1.5 mg carbohydrates but results are not concordant for nonprotein nitrogen, sodium, potassium, and calcium (Russell, 1967a; Russell and Alender, 1967; Russell et al., 1968).

Pearce (1973) was unable to detect any nerve growth factor in the venom of *Heterometrus* (= *Palamnaeus*) *gravimanus*.

VI. Pharmacology of Chactoid Venoms

According to Cheymol (1974) the principal symptoms of scorpionism result from neuromuscular and cardiovascular effects for all species.

Neuromuscular effects. Del Pozo (1949) has described the occurence of fibrillations and clonic contractions when putting the venom on the surface of an innervated muscle, but the application of the venom on the nerve did not provoke any effect on the corresponding muscle. The excitation of the nerve of a muscle treated by the venom produced contractions much more intense than those of an untreated muscle. High doses of the venom blocked muscular responses to the nervous stimulation. To summarize, the scorpion venoms were believed to have decurarisant and anticholinesterase properties. No difference was made between buthoid and chactoid venoms.

Master et al. (1963) have identified a guinea pig ileum-contracting factor in the venoms of *Buthus tamulus* and *Heterometrus* (= *Palamnaeus*) *gravimanus* which is more potent in the venom of the buthid. In the venom of *Pandinus exitialis* a rabbit intestine contracting factor was also found but intestine contractions were preceded by an initial relaxation, in contrast to the effects of the venom from some buthids which only caused contractions. The powerful contraction of the rat uterus provoked by this venom could not only be attributed to the serotonine content but also to the release of kinins, prostaglandins, and slow-reacting substances (Ismail et al., 1974). In this case it was found, with the exception of the degree of intensity, that the effects of the venoms of *Pandinus exitialis* and the buthids *Leiurus quinquestriatus* and *Buthotus* (*Buthus*) *minax* were the same.

Parnas and Russell (1967) have compared the effects of six scorpion venoms, one buthid venom, and five vejovid venoms on the classic phrenic nerve-diaphragm preparation and on the deep extensor abdominal muscles (DEAM) of the crayfish.

Three effects were thus observed according to the dose of the venom. First, a blocking activity of the muscle response to stimulation through the nerve was manifested with a concentration of 10 μg of venom per ml saline solution. Nerve conduction was not affected even when there was a complete block of the indirectly stimulated muscle which would indicate that the venom probably exerts its deleterious effects at the neuromuscular junction. The excitatory activity was induced for a minimal dose of 100 μg/ml only for the most potent venoms, those of the buthid *Centruroides sculpturatus* and of the chactoids *Hadrurus arizonensis* and *Paruroctonus mesaensis*. The lytic activity was induced for a minimal dose of 500 to 1000 μg/ml (PARNAS et al., 1970). The venom produced membrane damage and altered the muscle. The degree of these irreversible damages appeared to be directly related to the concentration of the venom and the time of exposure, but this effect was only seen with those venoms which provoked the excitatory activity. In fact, the actions of these scorpion venoms also differ more in intensity than in the nature of their effects. In this case, only the venoms of *H. arizonensis* and *P. mesaensis,* with the venom of the buthid *C. sculpturatus* could warrant being called "potent neurotoxins" for humans. However, on the basis of the observations recorded, it may be concluded that the six scorpion venoms studied produced similar neuromuscular effects in the crayfish, guinea pig, rat, and human (PARNAS and RUSSELL, 1967). The venom of *V. spinigerus* which is much less potent, approximately one hundred times less than that of the buthid *Centruroides sculpturatus* (RUSSELL et al., 1968) had some effect on neuromuscular transmission, but did not significantly shift the reflex discharge nor the antidromic inhibition curve (RUSSELL and ALENDER, 1967).

The effects of chactoid venoms on invertebrates are also powerful. The venom of *Heterometrus fulvipes* stopped the muscular contractions, heart beat, spontaneous electrical activity of the nerve cord, and blocked synaptic transmission of the cockroach *Periplaneta americana* (BABU et al., 1971). The ciliary activity of the fresh water mussel *Lamellideus marginalis* was inhibited by small quantities of the venom of *Heterometrus scaber* (CHENGAL RAJU et al., 1971). The venom of the scorpionid *Heterometrus* (= *Palamnaeus*) *gravimanus* as well as the venom of *Buthus tamulus* when applied externally caused a gradual depolarization of the nerve membrane of the squid giant axon, but had no effect on the resting potential when applied internally (NARAHASHI et al., 1972). A slow depolarization was also observed on the muscular fibers of the two classical muscular preparations, isolated rat diaphragm and frog *rectus abdominis* with the venom of *Heterometrus caesar* (CHEYMOL et al., 1973).

There is not as yet agreement on the action site of the venoms. According to PARNAS and RUSSELL (1967) the venom toxins act on the neuromuscular junction. However, CHEYMOL (1974) believes that they directly affect the muscular fibers since they do not modify the contracturing action of acetylcholine. Moreover, because of the disturbances of the ionic exchanges which were observed at the level of the nerve cells or muscular cell membranes (NARAHASHI et al., 1972) the contracting properties of the venoms were found to be comparable with those of veratrin (CHEYMOL, 1974).

Cardiovascular effects. These effects were observed chiefly on mammals. The injection of the venom generally provoked an increase in the systemic arterial pressure, but this action has been rarely investigated with chactoid venoms. The venom of *Vejovis spinigerus* injected into a cat caused an immediate fall in the blood pressure, followed by a rise within two minutes of the injection. This elevated arterial pressure was maintained or sometimes increased for several hours after the injection (RUSSELL et al., 1968). Comparing the venoms of the buthid *Androctonus mauretanicus* and of the scorpionid *Heterometrus caesar,* CHEYMOL et al. (1973) observed a rise in the blood pressure of rats, transient but reproducible for the venom of *H. caesar,* which was more durable for the venom of *A. mauretanicus.* In these two cases, this hypertensive effect was followed by a bradycardia evoking the vaso-vagal reflex caused by catecholamines. The hypertensive effect of the venom of *Pandinus exitialis* was attributed to the stimulation of both parts of the autonomic nervous system and the release of tissue catecholamines as is the case with the venom of the buthids *Leiurus quinquestriatus* and *Buthus minax.* However, the positive inotropic effect of the venom of *P. exitialis* was not accompanied by a chronotropic effect (ISMAIL et al., 1974). The increase in the urinary excretion of vanillyl-mandelic acid observed in rabbits injected with the venom of *Heterometrus scaber* proved that there was an increase in catecholamines released (BHASKARAN NAIR and KURUP, 1973c).

Other effects a) The hyperglycemia produced by the injection of the venom *of H. scaber* (as with the venom of all scorpions) is linked to the release of catecholamines (BHASKARAN NAIR and KURUP, 1973c). b) The profuse salivation is one of the most prominent symptoms of a scorpion sting. This effect may be due to a nicotine-like action for massive doses of scorpion toxins while the small doses may possess an excitatory effect on the central and peripheric nervous system (SAMAAN and IBRAHIM, 1959). The cerebral intraventricular injection of the venom of *Vejovis spinigerus* and the venom of the buthid *Centruroides sculpturatus* provoked a hypersalivation which accompanied severe motor and respiratory disturbances resulting in death (RUSSELL and BOHR, 1962). c) The venom of scorpion can inhibit the activity of certain enzymes. The venom of *Heterometrus scaber* was found to strongly inhibit citric, lactic, and succinic dehydrogenases of frog muscles, and this effect may be the cause of the inflammatory action of the scorpion sting (OOMEN and KURUP, 1966). Succinate, lactate dehydrogenases, and acetylcholinesterase activities were completely or partially inhibited in the muscle of the cockroach *Periplaneta americana* by the venom of *Heterometrus fulvipes* but the decrease of these activities in the nerve cord was not significant (BABU et al., 1971). Lastly, SELVARAJAN et al. (1972) have shown that the venom of *H. fulvipes* had no influence on the activity of succinate dehydrogenase of the hepatopancreas of the same species but inhibited it in the cephalothoracic neuronal mass while it elevated glutamate dehydrogenase activity in these two tissues. This caused a shift in the ratio NADH/NAD, and thus in the nergy charge of the cell.

VII. Experimental Toxicity

Acute toxicity. Mice are generally employed for the study of scorpion venom toxicity, and the toxicity was sometimes given in "telsa" or in "fractions of telsa" needed to kill a mouse weighing 20 g. In order to eliminate individual variations, it was necessary to use a large number of macerated or pounded telsa, from 40 to 100 or more telsa (SERGENT, 1946). Hence, the lethal dose of *Scorpio maurus* venom is 7 telsa. In comparison, the lethal doses of some buthid venoms are: 1/20 telson for *Androctonus* (= *Prionurus*) *australis*, and 1/2 telson for *Buthus occitanus*. Thus *Scorpio maurus* venom is not very toxic. The fact that the chactoid venoms are less well known than the buthid venoms is explained by their weaker toxicity is a general observation. *Scorpio maurus* venom may be much more toxic for sparrows (NICOLLE and CATOUILLARD, 1905) and is very deleterious when injected through an intracerebral or transorbital route in rabbits (BLANC and DELAGE).

More often, the toxic doses of the venoms were expressed in mg of dry matter per mouse of 20 g or per kg/body weight mice. Thus the lyophilized venom of *Scorpio maurus palmatus* possessed a LD_{50} (the lethal dose of 50% animals injected with venom) of 11 mg/kg when injected intraveneously (ZLOTKIN et al., 1972). The minimal lethal dose of the dry venom of *Heterometrus scaber* is 115 mg/kg body weight mice when injected subcutaneously (OOMEN and KURUP, 1966). The intravenous LD_{50} of the crude lyophilized venom of *Vejovis spinigerus* was found to be 8.87 mg/kg (RUSSELL and ALENDER, 1967) to 4.87 mg/kg body weight mice (RUSSELL et al., 1968). The venom of the scorpionid *Heterometrus caesar* is weakly toxic: the intravenous LD_{50} was found to be 22 mg/kg body weight mice (CHEYMOL et al., 1973). The intraperitoneal LD_{50} of the lyophilized venom of *Pandinus exitialis* was 40 mg/kg body weight mice (ISMAIL et al., 1974). Finally, there is little data concerning the lethal doses of chactoid venoms. As experimental procedures often vary, comparisons are unreliable.

Experimental envenomation. The envenomation signs are quite similar for all species. They were studied chiefly on mice in which they appear rapidly following the venom injection. According to SERGENT (1946) *Scorpio maurus* venom causes torpor and immobilization resulting in the death of the animal and not agitation and convulsions as found with most buthid venoms. On the other hand, after the injection of *Scorpio maurus palmatus* venom, restlessness, salivation, arhythmic tachypnea followed by complete paralysis were observed on mice, and death occured accompanied by lacrimation and diuresis (ZLOTKIN et al., 1972). When rabbits were injected intraveneously with the venom of *S. maurus* no effect was observed, however when injected via a transorbital or intracerebral route, it caused many disorders similar to herpetic encephalitis, resulting in death in extension (BLANC and DELAGE, 1947). Identical symptoms were observed in mice after an intraperitoneal injection of lethal doses of the venom of *Pandinus exitialis* (ISMAIL et al., 1974). Injection of 115 mg/kg of dry venom of *Heterometrus scaber* caused the death of mice after a period of restlessness and dyspnea which lasted from 2–18 h (OOMEN and KURUP, 1966). The symptoms of the envenomation of the venoms of the buthid *Androctonus mauretanicus* and the scorpionid *Heterometrus caesar* are identical but the former is much more powerful. For both venoms agitation, contractures, dyspnea, lacrimation, salivation were observed, however only *H. caesar* venom caused hematuria and convulsions. Death was caused by pulmonary oedema (CHEYMOL et al., 1973). The venom of *Nebo hierichonticus* when injected into mice caused paralysis of the limbs, hiccupping, and spasms of the trunk. Mice died with extended limbs and hemorrhagic diuresis (ROSIN, 1969).

The contractions, salivation, lacrimation, loss of urines, and feces are similar to the effects of cholinergic or anticholinesterasic drugs. Hematurias were observed with the venoms which had a hemolytic action *in vitro*. Generally, the autopsy did not show any characteristic sign except for oedema which was sometimes hemorrhagic at the site of the sting and promoted due to the presence of spreading factor. Congestion of the viscera (CILLI and CORAZZI, 1946) also occurred with occasional extensive hemorrhagias as caused by the venom of *Nebo hierichonticus* (ROSIN, 1969).

Experimental toxicity for invertebrates or even protists was also investigated. The venom of *Nebo hierichonticus* caused complete and rapid cessation of motion of the ciliate *Paramecium caudatum* when introduced in the culture medium. The protoplasmic material was then seen to swell gradually and with the weaker solutions the trichocyts were expelled (ROSIN, 1969a). Besides stopping the heart beat, a loss of body tonus and normal leg movements followed by complete immobilization, a decrease in body temperature and oxygen consumption were observed in the cockroach *Periplaneta americana* after injection of the venom of *Heterometrus fulvipes* (BABU et al., 1971). The effects of the venom of 18 scorpions, 16 buthids and 2 chactoids on the larvae of the blowfly *Sarcophaga argyrostoma* were compared (ZLOTKIN et al., 1971). The buthid venoms caused an immediate contraction and paralysis, the duration of which was dependant on dosage. This response enabled a "contraction paralysis unit" or C.P.U. to be defined. The C.P.U. did not correlate with LD_{50} for mice, which implies the existence of different toxic factors for mammals and insects. It was not possible to determine a LD_{50} for mice or a C.P.U. for *S. argyrostoma* with the two chactoid venoms, *Scorpio maurus* and *Opisthophthalmus glabifrons*. However, the venom of *S. maurus palmatus* was effective on the larvae of insects such as *Sarcophaga falculata, Calliphora erythrocephala* and *Locusta migratoria migratorioides* but it induced a relaxatory flaccid paralysis as opposed to the strong contraction caused by buthid venom. The effects of the buthid venoms and the venom of *S. maurus palmatus* on mice were similar except for the dosage used. This fact confirmed the existence of different toxins acting on mammals and insects (ZLOTKIN et al., 1972).

As for the effect of the scorpion venoms on scorpion themselves, it appears that scorpions are not very sensitive to their own venoms (NICOLLE and CATOUILLARD, 1905) and they are only slightly more sensitive to the venoms of other species (GRASSET et al., 1946). However, when eighteen *Leiurus quinquestriatus* were stung by *Nebo hierichanticus,* eight died within several days (ROSIN, 1969a).

VIII. Toxicity for Humans

Scorpions have always been feared; however, they are not aggressive animals. Accidents often occur when scorpions have taken shelter in clothes or shoes of careless people or when they are disturbed in their refuges by children when playing. Most accidents occur during summer as scorpions hibernate. In Algeria, 50% of the stings occur during the months of July and August, 80% of the stings during the months of June, July, August, and September. The stings are often localized on the extremities of the limbs; feet, ankles, hands, and wrists are stung in 70% of the cases (SERGENT, 1942). Stings on the trunk or face and multiple stings are rare. Only in exceptional cases will the same scorpion sting two different persons such as a mother and her child (SERGENT, 1942). The scorpion causing the sting is identified only in about 10% of the cases.

Chactoid venoms are generally less toxic than buthid venoms. Since the largest scorpions (genus *Pandinus, Heterometrus, Nebo*) however, are chactoids, they are capable of injecting large quantities of venom. Some of them are greatly feared. Their stings which are always very painful because of their serotonin content, can be dangerous. Out of 75 cases of envenomation seen in India during 14 years, MUNDLE (1961) observed 23 deaths including 9 adults. Although no details are given concerning the identity of the species concerned, it is likely that some were *Heterometrus*. JUNQUA and VACHON (1968) have given a list of the species whose stings have caused or could cause death. These included Scorpionids (*Heterometrus, Pandinus, Scorpio, Urodacus*) Vejovids (*Hadrurus*) and Bothriurids (*Bothriurus*). Even the sting of *Euscorpius flavicaudis* or of the related species *E. italicus* normally considered as harmless, occasionally provoked severe symptoms (JUNQUA and VACHON, 1968; MARETIC and ZUNIC, 1970).

FLORES-PEREZ (1963) distinguished five clinical types of envenomation based on general symptomatology, local signs being identical, severe pain and sensation of burning in all cases. The first type is a mild form of envenomation with some local paresthesia or dysesthesia following the sting. The symptoms of the second type are more varied: nose itching, salivation, paresthesia, dyspnea; but the symptoms are not severe. The third type is more serious: besides the above symptoms, local edema, hemorrhagia, and paralysis of some muscles can be observed. The fourth type corresponds to the characteristic envenomation of dangerous buthids: venoms and cardiovascular symptoms are predominant, and dyspnea and pulmonary edema aggravate the prognosis. The fifth type is a very particular envenomation: the symptomatology is reduced to a flaccid paralysis of the legs, and a hypertonicity of the sphincters which disappear quite rapidly. The etiologic diagnosis is difficult especially if the patient does not know that the sting was caused by a scorpion.

In practice, the clinical symptomatology of chactoid envenomation is seldom serious. The local signs always present are sometimes discrete, even insignificant when caused by the sting of a small species, for example *Euscorpius,* or immature subjects. The pain is transient and weak, like the prick of a needle. More often, the local signs are important: burning pain and cutaneous hyperesthesia are intense. The local edema is variable and limited and sometimes accompanied by hitching as after the sting of the diplocentrid *Nebo hierichonticus* (ROSIN, 1969), or extensive, reaching the forearm when a finger is stung and hindering use of the hand for 24 h as with the sting of *Vejovis confusus* according to the observation of WILLIAMS (1970). The sting of *Vejovis spinigerus* which is not a dangerous species causes a transient pain with local cutaneous swelling and hyperesthesia which disappear after 24 h (ENNIK, 1972). The general symptoms, rarely marked, are transient and can be constituted by a slight fever or mild asthenia. The signs of envenomation which usually are present immediately after the sting can sometimes be delayed a few hours (YAROM, 1973) but this is observed more often with buthid venoms.

In rare cases the envenomation of chactoid venoms is very serious and even dramatic. Local necrosis, gangrene of a finger, have been observed. In a case recorded by ANSARI (1948), the species of the scorpion concerned was unknown. The sting of *Euscorpius italicus* may have severe consequences such as violent generalized pain, restlessness, profuse perspiration, nausea, hematuria (MARETIC and ZUNIC, 1970). The case of hemiplegia with motor aphasia following a scorpion sting, which was reported by JAMMIHAL and SRINIVAS (1972), was probably due to a *Heterometrus* according to the description of the animal. All these disorders can be related to the hemolytic and coagulant activities of the venoms. According to their experiments, HAMILTON et al. (1974) have evoked the possibilities of diffuse intravascular coagulation following the inoculation of a chactoid venom. But deaths definitely caused by chactoid venoms are very rare.

IX. Treatment and Prophylaxis of Scorpion Poisoning

Because of the rarity of serious accidents, there is no specific treatment for chactoid stings, that is there is no specific antivenomous serum. Thus the treatment will be symptomatic. A local disinfection and the prevention of tetanus are recommended (JOUGLARD et al., 1970) though no case of tetanus was described after a scorpion sting. The treatment has the purpose of soothing the pain, restlessness and swelling. Some pharmacodynamic drugs such as dihydroergotamine and atropine were recommended (MOHAMMED and EL KAREMI, 1953). The effectiveness of cryotherapy, the "L.C. treatment" of STAHNKE (1953) that is ligature cryotherapy is certain (JACQUEMIN, 1954). The diffusion and the absorption of the venom throughout the organism is slackened. Morphine, atropine, corticoids were largely employed but for some authors morphine is contraindicated because of its inhibitory effect on the bulbar respiratory centers (BALOZET, 1971). To relieve pain the injection *loco dolenti* of procaine (QUINN, 1963) or local electroshock therapy from an automobile spark plug wire (DEN HARTOG, 1973) were recommended. When the symptoms of cardiovascular failure are present, artificial hibernation with a lytic cocktail has given good results (SANTHANAKRISHNAN et al., 1972). Despite the fact the chactoid venoms are generally not dangerous, 12 or 24 h observation is advisable for children because of their greater sensibility to scorpion venoms.

Practically, speaking according to RUSSELL (1974), there are no first aid measures to recommend other than rest, assurance, maintenance of body warmth. The "L.C. treatment" must not be omitted when the sting site makes it possible (finger, toe). No other therapeutic measures have appeared of value in controlled studies. The superior treatment of "lethal" scorpion stings (of which all are buthids) is the antivenin serum, hence, the identification of the scorpion concerned is very important. When in doubt, a proper antivenin must be used, that is the antibuthid serum of the lethal species known in the country where the patient was. JUNQUA and VACHON (1968) have given the repartition of the dangerous species and the list of antivenins prepared in the world.

The prophylaxis of the envenomations is founded on the destruction of scorpions (descorpionization) and on some precautions related to the ethology of these Arachnids. Scorpions are nocturnal animals, rarely seen, since they spend the daylight hours hidden in shelters. They usually emerge at night and often climb walls, which is easy for them due to the claws of their ambulatory legs, provided that the wall is not too smooth. In this way scorpions enter indoors and during the day they keep themselves hidden in some clinks of the walls, in clothes, or clung to the underside of objects. They sting when they are disturbed. The most important

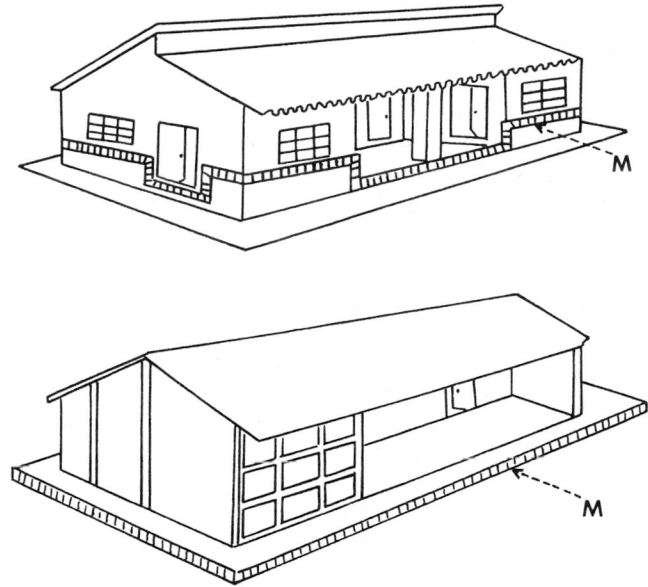

Fig. 6. Houses protected against entering of Scorpions by a mosaic flooring (*M*) (according to MAZZOTTI, 1962)

precaution, then, consists in hindering the entrance of scorpions into houses. MAZZOTTI (1962) has given several effective rules, easy to follow, in order to protect the house against scorpions entering (Fig. 6).

The natural enemies of scorpions are more numerous than is generally believed. Many mammals, birds, reptiles do not scorn scorpions in their alimentation. Among the mammals, there are in America the coati, *Nasua narica,* and the kinkajou, *Potos flavus* (MAZZOTTI, 1966); in Africa monkeys such as Cercopithecidae, the baboon, *Papio papio* (VACHON, 1952), or the chimpanzee, *Pan troglodytes* (HLADIK, 1973). In the Sahara, several reptiles eat a great number of scorpions, such as the "fish sand" *Scincus scincus,* or the monitor-lizard *Varanus griseus,* the largest terrestrial predator in the saharan erg (VERNET and GRENOT, 1973). However, the most active among the predatory animals are the birds, Gallinaceous, diurnal, and nocturnal rapacious crows (VACHON, 1954; MAZZOTTI, 1973). The detection of the remains of scorpions in the excreta of predators is very easy because of the fluorescence of their integument in ultraviolet radiation, which is not altered by the chemical processes of digestion (PAVAN and VACHON, 1954). In fact, the greatest enemy of scorpions is man, who limits or reduces their population by capturing and effectively destroying them with common insecticides. JUNQUA and VACHON (1968) have compiled a list of the most common insecticides employed against scorpions.

References

Adam, K.R., Weiss, C.: Five-hydroxytryptamin in scorpion venom. Nature, **178**, pp. 421—422 (1956).

Ansari, M.Y.: Gangrene after scorpion sting. Brit. Med. J., **2**, pp. 388 (1948).

Babu, K.S., Murali Krishna Dass, K.P., Venkatachari, S.A.T.: Effects of scorpion venom on some physiologic processes in cockroach. Toxicon, **9**, pp. 119–124 (1971)

Bailly, J.: Action du venin de scorpion sur le virus rabique. Arch. Inst. Pasteur Algérie, **27**, pp. 310–311 (1949)

Balozet, L.: Propriétés hémolytiques des venins de scorpions. Arch. Inst. Pasteur Algérie, **29**, pp. 200–207 (1951)

Balozet, L.: Propriétés diastasiques des venins de scorpions. Arch. Inst. Pasteur Algérie, **30**, pp. 1–10 (1952).

Balozet, L.: Venins de scorpions et sérum antiscorpionique. Arch. Inst. Pasteur Algérie, **33**, pp. 90–100 (1955).

Balozet, L.: Les venins, la sphérocytose des hématies et leur sédimentation. Arch. Inst. Pasteur Algérie, **40**, pp. 149–178 (1962).

Balozet, L.: Le Scorpionisme en Afrique du Nord. Bull. Soc. Pathol. Exot., **57**, pp. 33–38 (1964).

Balozet, L.: Scorpionism in the Old World. In: Venomous animals and their venoms, **3**, Bücherl, W., and Buckley, E.D. New York: Academic Press pp. 349–371 (1971).

Bhaskaran Nair, R., Kurup, P.A.: Glycosaminoglycans in the venom of the South Indian Scorpion, *Heterometrus scaber*. Ind. J. Biochem. Biophys., **10**, pp. 133–134 (1973a).

Bhaskaran Nair, R., Kurup, P.A.: Enzyme make-up of the venom of the South Indian Scorpion, *Heterometrus scaber*. Ind. J. Biochem. Biophys., **10**, pp. 230–231 (1973b).

Bhaskaran Nair, R., Kurup, P.A.: Hyperglycaemia produced by the venom of the South Indian Scorpion, *Heterometrus scaber*. Ind. J. Biochem. Biophys., **10**, pp. 232 (1973c).

Bhaskaran Nair, R., Kaleysa Raj, R., Kurup, P.A.: Indole compounds of the venom of the South Indian Scorpion, *Heterometrus scaber*. Ind. J. Biochem. Biophys., **10**, pp. 231 (1973).

Blanc, G., Delage, B.: Contribution à l'étude du venin de *Scorpio (Heterometrus) maurus* Lin. Test de toxicité par voie nerveuse. C.R. Soc. Biol., **141**, pp. 322–324 (1947).

Bouisset, L., Larrouy, G.: Envenimation par *Scorpio maurus* et *Buthus occitanus* dans le département de Tlemcen. Bull. Soc. Pathol. Exot., **55**, pp. 139–146 (1962).

Bücherl, W.: Biologia de Artropodes peçonhentos. Mem. Inst. Butantan, **31**, pp. 85–94 (1964).

Bücherl, W.: Classification, biology and venom extraction of Scorpions. In: Venomous animals and their venoms, 3. Bücherl, W. and Buckley, E.D.: New York, Academic Press, pp. 317–347 (1971).

Bücherl, W., Buckley, E.E.: Venomous animals and their venoms. **3**, 357 p. New York, Academic Press (1971).

Chaix, E.: Les envenimements par piqûre de Scorpions dans l'annexe de Touggourt. Intérêt de la sérothérapie. Thèse-Fac. Méd. Alger, p. 46 (1940).

Charnot, A., Faure, L.: Les Scorpions du Maroc, leur venin; leur danger pour l'homme et les animaux. Bull. Inst. Hyg. Maroc **4**, pp. 1–72 (1934).

Chengal Raju, D., Krishna Moorthy, R.V., Subbarami Reddi, A.: Effect of Scorpion venom on the ciliary activity of fresh water mussel. Veliger **14**, pp. 192–194 (1971).

Cheymol, J., Bourillet, F., Roch-Arveiller, M.: Venins et toxines de scorpions. Effets neuro-musculaires. Actual. pharmacolog. Masson édit., pp. 241–258, Paris (1972).

Cheymol, J., Bourillet, F., Roch-Arveiller, M., Heckle, J.: Etude comparative de différents effets périphériques produits par le venin de scorpion indien *Heterometrus caesar* et par le venin de scorpion marocain *Androctonus mauretanicus mauretanicus*. C.R. Soc. Biol. **167**, pp. 1574–1579 (1973).

Cheymol, J.: Envenimation par les Scorpions. Mécanisme d'action. Rev. Palais Découverte **2**, pp. 18–40 (1974).

Cilli, V., Corazzi, G.: Ricerche sul veleno di alcuni scorpioni eritrei (*Parabuthus liosoma abyssinicus* e *Pandinus magrettii*) e sulla preparazione di un antisiero specifico. Boll. Soc. Ital. Med. Hig. Trop. **6**, pp. 397–406 (1946).

Del Pozo, E.C.: Ressemblances et différences dans les actions physiologiques des venins des Scorpions. Arch. Inst. Pasteur Algérie **27**, pp. 35–38 (1949).

Den Hartog, J.G.: Scorpion stings. J.A.M.A. **223**, p. 693 (1973).

Deoras, P.J.: Studies on Bombay Scorpions. I. Collection of, rearing and a method for the electrical extraction of venom. J. Univ. Bombay **29**, pp. 179−192 (1960).

Deoras, P.J., Vad, N.E.: The milking of Scorpions. Toxicon **1**, p. 41 (1962).

Deoras, P.J.: Handling of Scorpions. Proc. 3rd internat. Symp. on Lab. animals, Academic Press, NewYork, 17−20 (1967).

Ennik, F.: A short review of Scorpion biology, management of stings and control. Calif. Vector Views **19**, pp. 69−80 (1972).

Flores-Perez, R.: Observaciones sobre sintomatologia y tratamiento de la intoxicacion por picadura de alacran. Rev. Inst. Salubr. Enferm. trop. **23**, pp. 175−179 (1963).

Gentilini, M.: Animaux venimeux terrestres. Encycl. Méd. Chir. **16078**, A10, pp. 1−2 (1966).

Goyffon, M., Lamy, J., Vachon, M.: Identification de trois espèces de Scorpions du genre *Androctonus* à l'aide du protéinogramme de leur hémolymphe en gel de polyacrylamide. C.R. Acad. Sc., **D**, **270**, pp. 3315−3317 (1970).

Goyffon, M., Le Fichoux, Y., Deloince, R., Niaussat, P.: L'arachnidisme. I. Le Scorpionisme. Rev. Corps Lanté Arm. **12**, pp. 345−356 (1971).

Goyffon, M., Stockmann, R., Lamy, J.: Valeur taxonomique de l'électrophorèse en disques des protéines de l'hémolymphe chez le Scorpion: étude du genre *Buthotus* (Buthidae). C.R. Acad. Sc., **D**, **277**, pp. 61−63 (1973).

Grasset, E., Schaafsma, A., Hodgson, J.A.: Immunological studies on scorpions. J. Immunol. **51**, pp. 231−248 (1945).

Hamilton, P.J., Ogston, D., Douglas, A.S.: Coagulant activity of the Scorpion venoms *Palamneus gravimanus* and *Leiurus quinquestriatus*. Toxicon **12**, pp. 291−296 (1974).

Hladik, C.M.: Alimentation et activité d'un groupe de chimpanzés réintroduits en forêt gabonaise. La Terre et la Vie **27**, pp. 343−413 (1973).

Horen, W.P.: Insect and Scorpion sting. J.A.M.A. **221**, pp. 894−898 (1972).

Irunberry, J., Pilo-Moron, E.: Etude antigénique de quelques venins de Scorpions du bassin méditerranéen. Arch. Inst. Pasteur Algérie **43**, pp. 123−128 (1965).

Ismail, M., Osman, O.H., Ibrahim, S.A., El-Asmar, M.F.: Cardiovascular and respiratory responses to the venom from the Scorpion *Leiurus quinquestriatus*. East Afr. Med. J. **49**, pp. 273−281 (1972).

Ismail, M., Osman, O.H., El-Asmar, M.F.: Pharmacological studies of the venom from the Scorpion *Buthus minax* (L. Koch), Toxicon **2**, pp. 15−20 (1973).

Ismail, M., Osman, O.H., Gumaa, K.A., Karrar, M.A.: Some pharmacological studies with Scorpion (*Pandinus exitialis*) venom. Toxicon **12**, pp. 75−82 (1974).

Ismail, M., El-Asmar, M.F., Osman, O.H.: Pharmacological studies with Scorpion (*Palamnaeus gravimanus*) venom: evidence for the presence of histamine. Toxicon **13**, pp. 49−56 (1975).

Jacquemin, P.: La cryothérapie des envenimations dues aux piqûres de Scorpion. Auto-observation. Bull. Soc. Hist. nat. Afr. Nord **45**, pp. 378−382 (1954).

Jammihal, J.H., Srinivas, H.V.: Hemiplegia following Scorpion sting. A case report. Indian Pediatr. **10**, pp. 337−338 (1973).

Johnson, R.M., Stahnke, H.L.: Chromatographic comparison of Scorpion venoms. Science **132**, pp. 895−896 (1960).

Jouglard, J., Imbert, M., Poyen, D., Frappa, G.: La piqûre de Scorpion dans la région marseillaise. Marseille Méd. **107**, pp. 1−3.

Junqua, C., Vachon, M.: Les Arachnides venimeux et leurs venins. Etat actuel des recherches. Ac. Roy. Sc. Outre mer, Cl. Sci. Nat. **17**, pp. 1−136 (1968).

Kapadia, Z.S., Master, R.W.P., Rao, S.: Immunological studies in telson extracts of Indian and Egyptian Scorpions venoms. Indian J. exp. Biol. **2**, pp. 75−77 (1964).

Keegan, H.L., Lockwood, W.R.: Secretory epithelium in venom glands of two species of Scorpion of the genus *Centruroides* Marx. Am. J. Trop. Med. Hyg. **20**, pp. 770−785 (1971).

Kovoor, J.: Etude histochimique des glandes à venin des *Buthidae* (Arachnida, Scorpiones). Ann. Sc. Nat. Zool. **15**, pp. 201−220 (1973).

Kraepelin, K.: Scorpiones und Pedipalpi. In: Das Tierreich, Berlin, **8**, pp. 1−265 (1899).

Kraepelin, K.: Die geographische Verbreitung der Scorpionen. Zool. Jb. Abt. Syst. **22**, pp. 321−364 (1905).

Kurup, P.A.: Studies on the venom of the South Indian Scorpion *Heterometrus scaber*. Phospholipase A from the venom. Naturwissensch. **52**, pp. 478 (1965).

Kurup, P.A.: Phospholipase A of the venom of South Indian Scorpion, *Heterometrus scaber*. Ind. J. Biochem. **3**, pp. 164—168 (1966).

Kurup, P.A.: Action of phospholipase A of the venom of *Heterometrus scaber* on human red cell ghosts and intact erythrocytes. Naturwissensch. **53**, pp. 84—85 (1966).

Laurie, M.: The embryology of a scorpion (*Euscorpius italicus*). Quart. J. micr. Sci. **31**, pp. 105—141 (1890).

Levy, R.: Sur le mécanisme de l'hémolyse par le venin de Scorpion. C.R. Acad. Sc. **179**, pp. 1093—1095 (1924).

McIntosh, M.E., Watt, D.D.: Biochemical-immunochemical aspects of the venom from the scorpion *Centruroides sculpturatus*. In: Animal Toxins. Collect. Papers 1st internat. Symp. Atlantic City, N.J. 1966, Braunschweig symp. Pergamon Press, 1967, pp. 47—58.

McIntosh, M.E., Puffer, H.W., Russel, F.E.: Preliminary studies on venoms from *Hadrurus hirsutus* and *Vejovis spinigerus*. Proceed. West. Pharmacol. Soc. **13**, pp. 114—120 (1970).

Magalhaes, O. de: Escorpionismo. Monogr. Inst. Oswaldo Cruz. **3**, pp. 220 (1946).

Maretic, Z., Zunic, I.: O Otrov nosti naših škorpiona (On venimosity of our Scorpions). Med. Jad. **2**, pp. 3—12 (1970).

Master, R., Rao, S., Soman, P.: Electrophoretic separation of biologically active constituents of Scorpion venoms. Bioch. Biophys. Acta, **71**, pp. 422—428 (1963).

Mazzotti, L.: Proteccion mecanica de las casas contra la entrada de alacranes (escorpiones). Rev. Int. salubr. Enferm. trop. **22**, pp. 183—198 (1962).

Mazzotti, L.: Medidas complementarias en relacion con la proteccion mecanica de los edificos contra los alacranes. Rev. Inst. Salubr. Enferm. trop. **24**, pp. 11—14 (1964).

Mazzotti, L.: Estudio sobre enemigos naturales de los alacranes. Rev. Invest. Salud. Publ. **26**, pp. 51—55 (1966).

Mazzotti, L.: Enemigos de los escorpiones: dos especies de aves de la America tropical (Tucanes). Ann. Parasit. hum. comp. **48**, pp. 351—353 (1973).

Mello Campos, O.: Os escorpioes brasileiros. Mem. Inst. Oswaldo Cruz **17**, pp. 237—365 (1925).

Miranda, F., Rochat, H., Lissitzky, S.: Sur les neurotoxines de deux espèces de scorpions nord-africains. I. Purification des neurotoxines (scorpamines) d'*Androctonus australis* (L.) et de *Buthus occitanus* Am. Toxicon **2**, pp. 51—69 (1964).

Mohammed, A.H., El Karemi, M.: An antidote to scorpion toxin. J. Trop. Med. Hyg. **56**, pp. 58—59 (1953).

Mundle, P.M.: Scorpion stings. Brit. Med. J. **1**, pp. 1042 (1961).

Narahashi, T., Shapiro, B.I., Deguchi, T., Scuka, M., Wang, C.M.: Effects of scorpion venom on squid axon membranes. Am. J. Physiol. **222**, pp. 850—857 (1972).

Nicolle, C., Catouillard, G.: Sur le venin d'un scorpion commun de Tunisie (*Heterometrus maurus*). C.R. Soc. Biol. **57**, pp. 100—102 (1905).

Nitzan (Tischler), M., Shulov, A.: Electrophoretic patterns of the venom of six species of Israeli scorpions. Toxicon **4**, pp. 17—23 (1966).

Nitzan Tischler, M.: Thermostability of the venom of the scorpion *Leiurus quinquestriatus* (H. et E.). Toxicon **8**, pp. 245—246 (1970).

Oomen, P.K., Kurup, P.A.: Protein and amino acid contents and physiological properties of the venom of the South Indian Scorpion, *Heterometrus scaber*. Ind. J. Exp. Biol. **2**, pp. 78—80 (1964).

Parnas, I. and Russell, F.E.: Effects of venoms on nerve, muscle and neuromuscular junction. In Animal Toxins (Russell, F.E., and Saunders, P.R., eds.), Oxford Pergamon Press. pp. 404—415 (1963).

Parnas, I., Avgar, D., Shulov, A.: Physiological effects of venom of *Leiurus quinquestriatus* on neuromuscular system of locust and crab. Toxicon **8**, pp. 67—69 (1970).

Pavan, M., Vachon, M.: Sur l'existence d'une substance fluorescente dans les téguments de scorpions (Arachnides). C.R. Ac. Sc. **239**, pp. 1700—1702 (1954).

Pavlovsky, E.N.: Skorpiotomische Mitteilungen. I Ein Beitrag zur Morphologie der Giftdrüsen der Skorpione. Z. Wiss. Zool. **105**, pp. 157—177 (1913).

Pavlovsky, E.N.: Contribution à la structure et le développement des glandes venimeuses des Scorpions. Rev. Russe Ent. St Pétersbourg **14**, pp. 57—71 (1914).

Pavlovsky, E.N.: *Glandula plicata*, nouvel organe chez le mâle de *Bothriurus vittatus*. Bull. Mus. Natl. Hist. Nat. Paris **24**, pp. 19—21 (1918).

Pavlovsky, E.N.: Studies on the organization and development of scorpions. Quart. J. micr. Sci. **68**, pp. 615—640 (1924).

Pearce, F.L.: Absence of nerve growth factor in the venoms of bees, scorpions, spiders and toads. Toxicon **11**, pp. 309—310 (1973).

Pene, P., Gastaut, J.A.: Le traitement des envenimations. Med. Afrique Noire **20**, pp. 7—13 (1973).

Potter, J.M., Northey, W.T.: An immunological evaluation of scorpions venoms. Amer. J. Trop. Med. Hyg. **11**, pp. 712—716 (1962).

Quinn, W.M.: Scorpionism. Canad. Med. Ass. J. **88**, pp. 493 (1963).

Rolli, K.: Essais de différents insecticides dans la destruction des Scorpions. Arch. Inst. Pasteur Tunis **49**, pp. 267—274 (1972).

Rosenfeld, G. and Kelen, E.M.A.: Bibliography of animal venoms, envenomation and treatments (Period 1500—1968). Saõ Paulo, Brazil: Industria Grafica Saraiva, pp. 583 (1969).

Rosin, R., Shulov, A.: Studies on the scorpion *Nebo hierichonticus*. Proc. Zool. Soc. (Lond). **140**, pp. 547—575 (1963).

Rosin, R.: A new type of poison gland found in the scorpion *Nebo hierichonticus* (E. Sim.) (Diplocentridae, Scorpiones). Riv. Parassitol. **26**, pp. 111—122 (1965).

Rosin, R.: Note on the α-hemolytic effect of the venom of the scorpion *Nebo hierichonticus*. Toxicon **6**, pp. 225—226 (1968).

Rosin, R.: Effects of the venom of the scorpion *Nebo hierichonticus* on white mice, other scorpions and paramecia. Toxicon **7**, pp. 71—73 (1969a).

Rosin, R.: Sting of the scorpion *Nebo hierichonticus* in man. Toxicon **7**, pp. 75 (1969b).

Rosin, R.: Venom, venom effects and poison gland of the scorpion *Nebo hierichonticus* (Diplocentridae). Ciencia e Cultura **24**, pp. 246—249 (1972).

Rosin, R.: Paper electrophoresis of the venom of the scorpion *Nebo hierichonticus* (Diplocentridae). Toxicon **11**, pp. 107—108 (1973).

Ruiz Luga, M.F.: Morfologia e histologia de la glandula venenosa de *Vejovis mexicanus mexicanus* C.L. Koch (Arachnida, Scorpionide). Thesis 1963, *cited by* Samano-Bishop and Gomez De Ferriz (1964).

Russell, F.E., Bohr, V.C.: Intraventricular injection of venom. Toxicol. appl. Pharmacol. **4**, pp. 165—173 (1962).

Russell, F.E.: Pharmacology of animal venoms. Clin. Pharmacol. Therapeut. **8**, pp. 849—873 (1967a).

Russell, F.E.: Comparative pharmacology of some animal toxins. Feder. Proceed. **26**, pp. 1206—1224 (1967b).

Russell, F.E., Alender, C.B.: Properties of the venom of the scorpion *Vejovis spinigerus*. Feder. Proceed. **26**, pp. 521 (1967).

Russell, F.E., Alender, C.B., Buess, F.W.: Venom of the scorpion *Vejovis spinigerus*. Science **159**, pp. 90—91 (1968).

Russell, F.E., Wainschel, J., Madon, M.B., Ennik, F.: Insect and scorpion bites and stings. J.A.M.A. **224**, pp. 131 (1973).

Russell, F.E.: Prevention and treatment of venomous animal injuries. Experientia **30**, pp. 8—12 (1974).

Samaan, A., Ibrahim, H.H.: The effects of scorpion venom on salivary secretion. Arch. internat. Pharmacodyn. **72**, pp. 249—264 (1959).

Samano Bishop, A., Gomez de Ferriz, M.: Estudio morfologico e histoquimico de la glandula venenosa de algunas especies de alacrances de los generos *Vejovis* C.L. Koch, *Diplocentrus* Peters y *Centruroides* Marx. An. Inst. Biol. Mex. **35**, pp. 139—155 (1964).

San Martin, P.R.: *Bothriurus vachoni* n.sp. del Brasil (Scorpionida, Bothriuridae). Acta Biol. Venez. **6**, pp. 38—51 (1968).

Santhanakrishnan, B.R., Sundaravalli, N., Raju, V.B.: Artificial hibernation with lytic cocktail in management of peripheral failure due to scorpion sting. Indian Pediatr. **9**, pp. 23—25 (1972).

Saunders, J., Johnson, B.D.: *Hadrurus arizonensis* venom: a new source of acetylcholinesterase. Am. J. Trop. Med. Hyg. **19**, pp. 345—348 (1970).

Selvarajan, V.R., Radakrishna Murthy, C., Swami, K.S.: Influence of scorpion venom on enzyme systems of scorpion *Heterometrus fulvipes*. Curr. Sc. **43**, pp. 272—274 (1974).

Sergent, E.: Quelques observations épidémiologiques et cliniques sur les piqûres de Scorpions. Arch. Inst. Pasteur Algérie **20**, pp. 130—134 (1942).

Sergent, E.: Venin de *Scorpio maurus* L. (=*Heterometrus maurus*). Arch. Inst. Pasteur Alger. **24**, pp. 301—303 (1946).

Sergent, E.: Sur le venin des scorpions *Prionurus australis* L. et *Prionurus aeneas* C. Koch. Arch. Inst. Pasteur Alger. **26**, pp. 21—23 (1948).

Sergent, E.: Etude comparative du venin de scorpions mexicains et de scorpions nord-africains. Arch. Inst. Pasteur Algér. **27**, pp. 31—34 (1949).

Stahnke, H.L.: The L.C. treatment of venomous bites or stings. Am. J. Tr. Med. **2**, pp. 142—143 (1953).

Stahnke, H.L., Stahnke, J.: The treatment of scorpion sting. Arizona Med. **14**, pp. 576—580 (1957).

Stahnke, H.L.: The treatment of venomous bites and stings. Arizona State Univ., Tempe, Arizona, U.S.A., pp. 117 (1966).

Stahnke, H.L.: Scorpions. Poisonous Animals Research Laboratory, Tempe, Arizona, U.S.A. pp. 36 (1966).

Stahnke, H.L.: A review of *Hadrurus* scorpions (Vejovidae). Entom. News **80**, pp. 57—65 (1969).

Stahnke, H.L.: Effect of thorazine and valium on scorpion venom toxicity. Arizona Med. **29**, pp. 424 (1972).

Stahnke, H.L.: Arizona scorpion antivenin. J.A.M.A. **224**, pp. 637 (1973).

Strassberg, J., Russel, F.E.: The milking of scorpions. Toxicon **1**, pp. 41 (1962).

Vachon, M.: Etudes sur les scorpions. Institut Pasteur d'Algérie pp. 483 (1952).

Vachon, M.: Quelques aspects de la biologie des scorpions. Endeavour **12**, pp. 80—89 (1953).

Vachon, M.: Remarques sur les ennemis des scorpions. A propos de la présence de restes de scorpions dans l'estomac de la Chouette *Athene noctua*. L'Oiseau et R.F.O. **24**, pp. 171—174 (1954).

Vachon, M.: Quelques remarques sur les scorpions, hôtes indésirables des lieux habités. Trav. Centre Biol. Ind. Agr. C.N.A.M. **1**, pp. 3—7 (1963).

Vernet, R., Grenot, C.: Etude du milieu et structure trophique du peuplement reptilien dans le Grand Erg Occidental (Sahara algérien). C.R. Soc. Biogéogr. **433**, pp. 112—123 (1972).

Watt, D.D., Babin, D.R., Mlejnek, R.V.: The protein neurotoxins in scorpions and elapid snake venoms. Agric. Food. Chem. **22**, pp. 43—51 (1974).

Whittemore, F.W. Jr, Keegan, H.L., Borowitz, J.L.: Studies of scorpions antivenins. I. Paraspecificity. Bull. Org. mond. Santé **25**, pp. 185—188 (1961).

Whittemore, F.W. Jr, Keegan, H.L., Fitzgerald, C.M., Bryant, H.A., Flanigan, J.F.: Studies of scorpion antivenins. 2. Venom collection and Scorpion colony maintenance. Bull. Org. mond. Santé **28**, pp. 505—511 (1963).

Williams, S.C.: Scorpions from Northern Mexico; five new species of *Vejovis* from Coahuila, Mexico. Occ. Pap. Calif. Acad. Sci. **68**, pp. 1—24 (1968).

Williams, S.C.: The effects on man of a natural sting by the scorpion *Vejovis confusus* Stahnke. Pan Pacif. Ent. **46**, pp. 77—78 (1970).

Yarom, R.: Scorpion venom: a tutorial review of its effect in man and experimental animals. Clin. Toxicol. **3**, pp. 561—569 (1970).

Zlotkin, E., Shulov, A.S.: A simple device for collecting scorpion venom. Toxicon **7**, pp. 331—332 (1969).

Zlotkin, E., Fraenkel, G., Miranda, F., Lissitzky, S.: The effect of scorpion venom on blowfly larvae. A new method for the evaluation of scorpion venoms potency. Toxicon **9**, pp. 1—8 (1971).

Zlotkin, E., Lebovits, N., Shulov, A.: Toxic effects of the venom of the scorpion *Scorpio maurus palmatus* (Scorpionidae). Riv. Parassitol. **33**, pp. 237—243 (1972a).

Zlotkin, E., Lebovits, N. and Shulov, A.: Hemolytic action of the venom of the scorpion *Scorpio maurus palmatus*. Toxicon **10**, pp. 537 (1972b).

CHAPTER 16

Tick Paralysis

M.F. Murnaghan and F.J. O'Rourke

A. Introduction

The history of tick paralysis as a disease of man and domestic animals has not yet been written, nor will it be easy to write, since it is often difficult to be sure that the disease being described is in fact tick paralysis as defined in Section IV. The best approach would be to work out the distribution of ticks known to secrete potent venom and cause paralysis and then work on the earlier reports, paying careful attention to the present known distribution of tick paralysis and to the symptomatology of the disease being described. The area of distribution of the disease has no doubt changed and is changing, and there are reports of the virulence of the tick venom increasing in some places.

Bearing these factors in mind we may look at the records currently available. Gregson (1973), in his comprehensive review of tick paralysis, regards the first known reference to the disease to be in the diary kept by William Hovell in 1824, while travelling from Lake George to Port Phillip with his friend Hume. He wrote about a tick "which buries itself in the flesh and would in the end destroy either man or beast if not removed in time" (Scott, 1921). This is not a clear-cut reference to tick paralysis, although it is a very probable one. More satisfactory is the work of Backhouse in 1843 (cited by Stanbury and Huyck, 1945, and by Gregson, 1973), again carried out in Australia where typical paralysis of sheep and calves was related to the attachment of the hard tick *Ixodes holocyclus*. Leclercq (1969) says: "since 1843, an acute ascending paralysis, caused by the bites of certain ticks, has been reported from certain regions". However, he gives no reference for the 1843 record. Anderson Stuart (1894) referred to hundreds of cases in dogs and suggested that ticks were involved, but Bancroft (1884) had earlier described cases in dogs where "death appears to reside in the salivary secretions of the tick". The disease was first recognized in man by Cleland (1912). The extensive studies of Ross (1926) gave strong evidence that the condition was due to a toxin in the saliva.

Although most of the work on tick paralysis has been carried out in North America, the first mention of the disease in that continent was not recorded until Todd (1912) published a preliminary note on the condition in British Columbia. In the United States, Temple (1912) described 12 human cases with a 25-percent mortality from Oregon and Idaho, under the very significant title of "Acute Ascending Paralysis or Tick Paralysis". Stanbury and Huyck (1945) maintain that the earliest case occurred in 1898.

In South Africa the disease was reported in 1890 (Neitz, 1962) and again in 1893, when sheep farmers reported "paralysis of sort among their stock". Hellier (NEITZ, 1962) in 1893 was the next to report cases. MALLY (1904) showed that ticks were responsible in all cases which occurred in sheep. BORTHWICK (1905) described the symptoms and signs in sheep, and he showed that dipping of sheep, which killed off the ticks, prevented the outbreak of tick paralysis.

By far the greatest majority of human cases have been caused by three species of hard tick, *Ixodes holocyclus,* found in Australia, *Dermacentor andersoni* in Western North America, and *Dermacentor variablis* in the eastern United States. Most cases in large domestic animals and dogs have been caused by *the first two* species. Other species of hard ticks have been implicated from time to time in various parts of the world. A similar condition caused by soft ticks is apparently not unusual in poultry and there are occasional reports of the condition recurring in mammals including, very rarely, man. Paralysis caused by soft ticks differs from hard-tick paralysis in a number of ways, perhaps most notably in that the paralysis is caused not by an adult female, as with hard ticks, but by immature stages of soft tick. Recent physiological studies (discussed below) suggest that similar but different mechanisms are involved in the production of paralysis by the two types of tick.

It seems clear that considerably more work is required on tick paralysis before we can be sure of any broad generalizations made about the global status of the disease; it is a dramatic disease which is known from North America, Australia, South Africa and Europe (sporadic cases) and there have been occasional reports from many other tick-infested areas. Removal of the tick even at a stage of very advanced paralysis generally results in rapid and complete recovery. The Australian disease is sometimes an exception to this rule and death may occur even after the tick has been removed.

B. Ticks

I. The Biology of Ixodid Ticks

Ticks are arthropods that belong to the class Arachnida, which are characterized by possessing four pairs of walking legs and no antennae. With the mites, they comprise the subclass Acari, although they form a sharply distinct grouping. EVANS et al. (1961) include all the ticks within the order Mesostigmata, whereas the mites are divided into six distinct orders. The possession of an elongate, medial, heavily armed hypostoma (Fig. 1), together with the occurrence of Haller's organ on tarsus I, are diagnostic features of ticks, all 800 species of which are ecto-parasites of warm-blooded vertebrates (occasional species attack reptiles).

All but a single species of tick (*Nuttalliellia*) fall into two families, the Hard Ticks (so-called because of the tough cuticle) and the Soft Ticks, whose cuticle is of a pliable leathery kind. The Ixodidae and Argasidae, as they are properly called, are found throughout the world but are more abundant in the tropics and subtropics. There are 644 known species of Ixodid tick and 149 of soft tick.

The hard ticks have throughout life a rigid cuticle, with a well developed dorsal scutum. The mouth-parts are anterior and easily visible from above, and

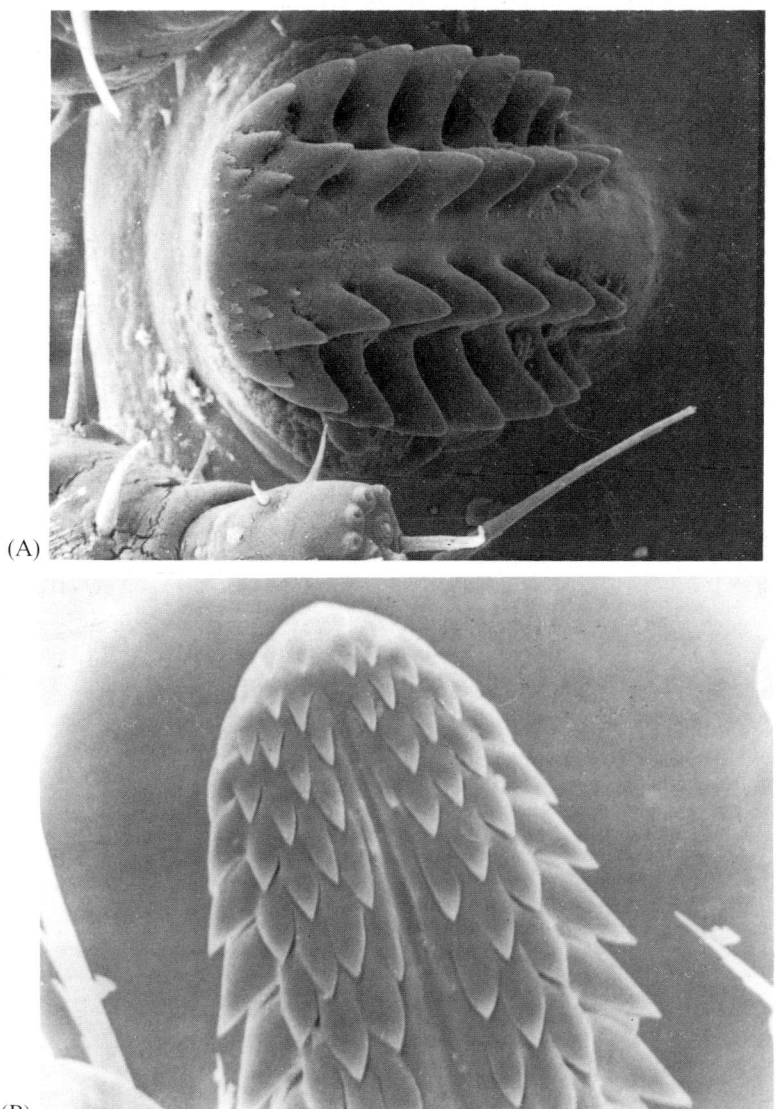

(A)

(B)

Fig. 1A and B. Hypostome of *Ixodes uriae* Mag. × 640 (A). Hypostome of larval *Ornithodorus maritimus* Mag. × 800 (B)

blood meals are taken only three times during life. The soft ticks have a leathery type of cuticle, which in most species is covered with fine mamillae. The mouthparts are ventral and cannot be seen from above. Blood meals are taken rapidly and often frequently.

The Ixodidae have a larval, a nymphal, and an adult stage and before the completion of each stage a blood meal must be taken. In the case of the female, the final meal, taking 11—12 days, may increase the tick's weight by a factor of several hundreds. Typically, therefore, each tick attacks three different hosts and such typical (like *I. ricinus*) ticks are called three-host ticks.

Some species only require one host during their life cycle and all three stages, larva, nymph, and adult feed on the one host and moult on that host. Such species include the economically important *Boophilus decoloratus*. Other species, the two-host ticks, feed as larvae on the host, moult and feed again as nymphs which drop off the host, moult on the ground and then as adults feed on a second host. *Rhipicephalus evertsi* is an example of such a tick.

Mating takes place mainly on the last host, and, while the female drops off after the meal, the males may remain attached for some time. The female lays her eggs in one batch (up to about 20000) and then dies. The seed ticks (=larvae) climb to the top of the vegetation in search of hosts.

Unlike the Ixodids the Argasids are generally associated with the den or nest of the host. Thus *Argas persicus* lays its eggs in batches of 20—100 in the crevices of fowl houses. The larvae feed for about five days. The adults and two nymphal stages feed nocturnally for about two hours. The females lay eggs after each feed and live for about five years.

II. Classification of Ticks

Table 1. Classification of Ixodidae (after STARKOFF, 1958) listing only the genera known to cause tick paralysis

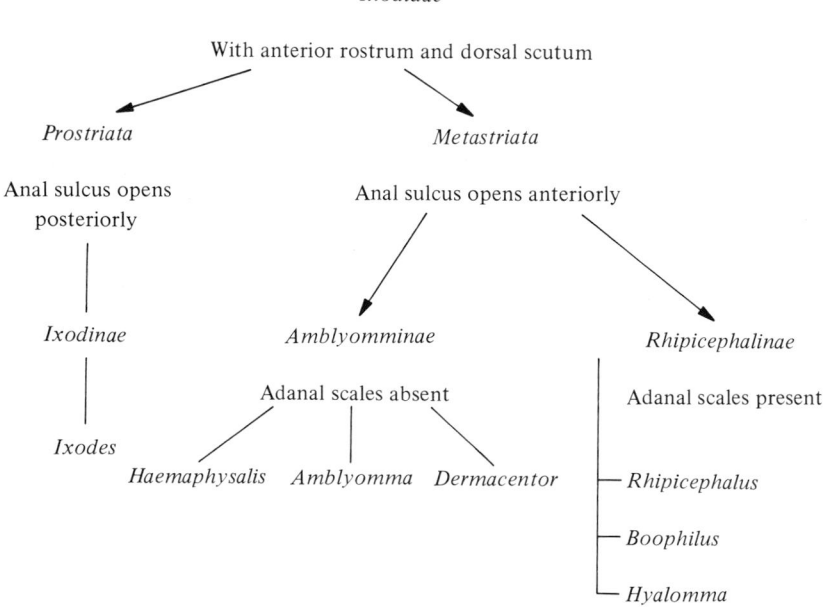

Table 2. List of Ixodid ticks implicated in tick paralysis, together with the geographical areas in which they cause the disease

Sub-family Ixodinae

Ixodes brunneus	Southern States of N. America
cornuatus	Australia (Tasmania)
crenulatus Koch	Eastern Europe
hexagonus Leach	England and France
hirtsi Hassall	Australia
++ holocyclus Neumann	Australia
ricinus (L.)	Eastern Europe
rubicundus Koch	Eastern Europe
scapularis (Say)	N. America
? tancitarius Cooley and Kohls	Mexico

Sub-family Amblyomminae

Haemaphysalis cinnabarina Packard	N.W. America
inermis Birula	Eastern Europe
kutchensis Hoogstraal and Trapida	India
punctata Can and Fran	Crete, Macadonia, Bulgaria
Amblyomma americanum (L.)	Southern States of N. America
maculatum Koch	Southern States of N. America, Uruguay
++ *Dermacentor andersoni* (Stiles)	N.W. America
* auratus Supino	India
? marginatus Sulz.	Italy
occidentalis Marx	N. America
variabilis (Say)	E. and S. of North America

Sub-family Rhipicephalinae

Rhipicentor nuttalli Cooper and Robinson	S. Africa
Hyalomma aegyptum (L)	Yugoslavia
scupense Sch.	Russia
truncatum Koch	S. Africa
transiens	S. Africa
Rhipicephalus evertsi Neum.	S. Africa
sanguineus (Latr)	S. America
simus Koch	Europe, S. Africa
tricuspis Donitz	
Boophilus annulatus (Say) (=calcaratus)	Yugoslavia

++ Indicates the most important ticks in the causation of tick paralysis.
? Species doubtfully implicated.
* Referred to by HOOGSTRAAL (1973) as "the so-called *D. auratus* group (which) I am revising".

Table 3. Genera of ixodidae in relation to tick paralysis

Genus[a]	No. of Spp.[a]	No. of Spp. causing tick paralysis	Percentage of Spp. causing tick paralysis
Ixodes	250	11	4.4
Haemaphysalis	150	4	2.7
Aponomma	26	0	0
Amblyomma	100	2	2.0
Dermacentor	31	5	16.1
Rhipicentor	2	0	0
Cosmiomma	1	0	0
Hyalomma	21	4	19.0
Nosomma	1	0	0
Rhipicephalus	63	4	6.3
Anomalohimalaya	1	0	0
Boophilus	5	1	20.0
Margaropus	3	0	0

[a] Listed after Hoogstraal (1973).

Table 4. List of Argasid ticks associated with tick paralysis-type conditions, together with the geographical areas in which they occur

Argas persicus (Oken)	Africa, Kashmir
arboreus	used experimentally
walkerae	used experimentally
Ornithodorus lahorensis Neum.	Kazakhstan, Russia
savigny Audouin	Nigeria
Otobius megnini (Duges)	Brit. Columbia, S. Africa

III. Feeding in Ixodid Ticks

Once an Ixodid tick is on the host it may either attack almost at once or move about until it finds a suitable spot. The tick then uses the chelicerae and hypostoma (Fig. 1) to cut into the epidermis. The process takes 3—5 min (Balashov, 1968). The chelicerae cut in by moving from side to side; they are armed with cutting teeth. The salivary glands then secrete a cement which hardens within 15 min and fixes the mouth parts to the skin, forming a cylindrical sheath around the wound and the mouth parts. Moorhouse (1969) showed that not all species of *Ixodes* formed cement; in three of the four species he studied cement was not produced. However, six other genera were found to form cement. Where the cement does not occur the mouth parts are inserted into the tissues. Tatchell (1969) says of the Ixodids that: "In all other genera the mouthparts are enveloped in cement which has a characteristic form for each genus; the depths to which the mouthparts are inserted into the host is also characteristic of each genus". *I. holocyclus* and *I. ricinus,* the two main causes of tick paralysis, do not produce cement. This may be significant, although *Rhipicephalus,* which scarcely reaches the epidermis with its mouthparts, has been implicated in the occurrence of tick paralysis. Clearly this line of research has considerable implications for those interested in tick paralysis.

Blood is then sucked into the oral chamber due to the sucking action of the pharynx. The saliva usually contains anticoagulant and other antigenic materials which stimulate antibody production in the host, as was first shown by TRAGER (1939). More recent work by ALLEN (1973) showed that immunosuppressive drugs such as methotrexate prevent the host's (guinea pig) response to the feeding of larval *D. andersoni*. The saliva of *D. andersoni* has no anticoagulant (TATCHELL, 1969), nor are there any active constituents (such as cytolysins), although it does have marked antigenic properties despite the extremely low protein content. The same is true of saliva produced by Gregson's (1957) method, which marked a major advance in the methodology available for the study of tick saliva. The same is true of the finding by TATCHELL (1967) that injection to the tick (*B. microplus*) of 0.01 ml of 10% saline solution of pilocarpine increased the amount of saliva obtained by tactile means by a factor of six. For *D. andersoni* GREGSON (1973) later abandoned the pilocarpine for the simpler technique described fully in the appendix to his 1973 review.

Any further advances in the study of tick paralysis will surely depend on these or similar techniques, which have so far scarcely been exploited for research into the source and nature of the toxin. Recent studies by MEREDITH and KAUFMAN (1973) and COONS and ROSHDY (1973) on the fine structure and histochemistry of a number of Ixodid and of one Argasid tick (*O. moubata*) have indicated that there is a general similarity between all the genera studied. To date these researchers have not thrown any new light on the formation of the toxin. MEREDITH and KAUFMAN (1973), in their detailed work on the histology and ultrastructure of the salivary gland of *D. andersoni,* provide the basis for future localization of the origin of the toxin produced by this species.

IV. Virulence

The existence of apparently marked variation in the ability of ticks to produce paralysis has long been known to those interested in the disease. The two most important causal ticks, *D. andersoni* and *I. holocyclus,* both demonstrate the phenomenon which is perhaps best documented for the American species, as can be seen in later sections of this paper. Although it would appear to be less well studied in the Australian species, recent surveys indicate that in New South Wales there is appreciable loss of cattle in a relatively small proportion of holdings. The campaigns against predators there and in Queensland have led to such a reduction of foxes and dingos that bandicoots, the main natural hosts of the tick, have so increased as to give rise to a tick paralysis problem. Other work showed that "prior exposure of cattle to adult female *I. holocyclus* infestations induces a high degree of immunity to subsequent feeding of female ticks. This resistance may provide a way of protecting cattle from paralysis" (BAGNALL and DOUBE, 1975).

Of course these data are essentially epizootiological although they do point to the complexity of factors, biochemical and ecological, that may lead to fluctuations in what might appear to be tick virulence. Virulence must be tested for against individual species of host; thus, using *D. andersoni* from the Kamloops area Gregson (1973) had varying results with dogs, whereas O'Rourke and Murnaghan (1954), using the same strain of ticks, airmailed by Gregson, produced paralysis in all seven long-haired mongrels infested with from one to nine ticks in Ottawa. In subsequent studies, Murnaghan (1958a, 1960b, 1961) produced paralysis in 95 percent of dogs, using 10–20 female ticks per animal. Gregson (1973) later showed that the toxin was virulent to marmots and to hamsters, which proved very suitable experimental animals although what appears to be the development of immunity, possibly to the bite, made it desirable to use the hamster once only.

Gregson's work on tick virulence in hamsters appears to be the most extensive ever done, and he gives an account of it in his 1973 paper, which must be read in the original. His main conclusions are that "it appears that the ticks reared from selected paralysing females are more virulent, and that further selection might increase their potency". When ticks failed to produce paralysis on first feeding, "26 transfers of 13 initially non-paralysing ticks yielded no positive cases". He further stated that these experiments "dispelled doubt of there being an intrinsic and inheritable susceptibility to the disease".

For a variety of reasons Gregson's experimental work on the tick toxin virulence to cattle was limited, but 27 cattle were used by Doube and Kemp (1975) in Queensland. Two- to three-week old calves were paralyzed by 10 female *I. holocyclus*. Calves weighing 80–160 kg were not paralyzed by up to nine ticks, but 20 ticks caused paralysis and nine out of ten paralyzed calves died. Eleven calves which recovered were infested with at least 25 ticks. No calves in this group died and only two were paralyzed.

C. Hosts

I. Humans

1. Distribution

The incidence of tick paralysis in humans is greatest in North America and Australia, occasional cases being recorded from Africa and some European, Mediterranean and other countries. Since tick paralysis in northwestern America is caused exclusively by *D. andersoni* Stiles, with the exception of one fatal case attributed to *Haemaphysalis cinnabarina* by Todd (1919), one would logically assume that the geographical distribution of the disease would coincide with the geographical distribution of the tick. As indicated below this does not necessarily occur. In northwestern America the highest incidence of the disease is in Western Canada, predominantly southern British Columbia (Todd, 1912; McCaffrey, 1916; Mail and Gregson, 1938; Phillips and Murphy, 1950; Hopkyns, 1953; Rose, 1954; Schmitt et al., 1969) with a few cases recorded from Alberta (Bow and Brown, 1945; Adler, 1966) and Sasketchewan (Bow and Brown, 1945). It has never been reported from the other provinces. Schmitt et al. (1969) have listed 305 cases as occurring in British Columbia between 1900 and 1968, and these are on record at the Entomology Laboratory at Kamloops, British Columbia. Approximately 180 cases were recorded for the first 27 years, the remainder being for the subsequent

41 years. The case fatality rate was about 10 percent. Nearly all the British Columbia cases have occurred between the costal range and the Rocky mountains in the valleys of the Frazer, North Thompson, Okanagan, Columbia and Kootenay rivers from 49–53° latitude to 115–124° longitude. The most northern case was at Barkerville, about 300 miles north of the Canadian-USA border, which is probably near the northern limit of distribution of the wood tick. Three cases have been reported by TODD (1912, 1914) west of the costal range at Bella Coola, Rosedale and Vancouver, which are well beyond the known range of the tick. It is possible that the ticks in some cases were acquired elsewhere due to travel by the host.

In the United States of America, although *D. andersoni* is distributed throughout the western states of Washington, Montana, Oregon, Idaho, Wyoming, Nevada, Utah, Colorado and the northern parts of Arizona, New Mexico and California, human cases of paralysis due to this species of tick have been confined to the northwestern Rocky mountain states, *i.e.* the eastern areas of Washington (TEMPLE, 1912; McCORNACK, 1921), western Montana (McCORNACK, 1921), northeastern Oregon (TEMPLE, 1912; RICE, 1949) and northern Idaho (McCORNACK, 1921; BARNETT, 1937), with a few cases in Wyoming and Colorado (BASSOE, 1924; JEFFREY, 1929; AMESSE and LYDAY, 1939; CHERINGTON and SNYDER, 1968). To date the respective numbers of cases recorded in each of the six states are 14, 52, 15, 23, 4 and 6, giving a total of 114. They are on file at the Rocky Mountain Laboratory of the United States Public Health Service at Hamilton, Montana. Although one case of paralysis is recorded by a Californian paediatrician (DONOVAN and FELDMAN, 1960), it was evidently acquired while the child was on a trip to Oregon. No human cases of paralysis have been recorded as due to the western *D. occidentalis* species, which has on occasions paralyzed livestock and wildlife. Two enigmas are apparent here—the scarcity of tick paralysis in regions where ticks are plentiful cannot be attributed to lack of tick bites, and there is no correlation between the distribution of tick paralysis and that of Rocky mountain spotted fever, which is spread by the same species of tick. About two-thirds of Colorado is within the range of the tick but only six cases of paralysis have ever been recorded and they were from the northern counties. In Oregon cases have been reported only in the northeastern counties and in Washington they have been distributed mainly along the eastern boundary. While ticks are abundant in Idaho the greatest incidence of spotted fever is in the southern part of the state but paralysis has been reported only from the northern counties. While spotted fever cases have been widely distributed throughout Montana, paralysis cases have been more numerous in the northwestern counties. Finally, although more cases of paralysis due to *D. andersoni* have been recorded in southern British Columbia than in all the northwestern United States, only two cases of spotted fever have been recorded from that province, and they were from near the southern boundary.

While *D. variablis* Say, the dog tick, is distributed in the central and eastern United States and in the central and eastern provinces of Canada from the southern area of Saskatchewan to Nova Scotia, *i.e.* essentially excluding the States and provinces enumerated for the distribution of *D. andersoni,* cases of paralysis due to *D. variablis* have only been recorded from the eastern and southern United States and none have been recorded in Canada. The published cases of paralysis identified as definitely or probably due to *D. variablis* occurred in the following states: New York (DeSanctis and de Sant'Agnese, 1943; Costa, 1952), Pennsylvania (Dawson et al., 1950), Virginia (Stiller, 1946; Randolph, 1947; McCue et al., 1948), North Carolina (Townsend and Nash, 1940; Perry and Ragland, 1949; Renuart and De Maria, 1961; Roddey and McAlister, 1962; Zanzenbacher and Conrad, 1968), South Carolina (Gibbes, 1938; Beach and Ravenel, 1941; Ryan and Canning, 1944), Georgia (Robinow and Carroll, 1938; Mulherin, 1940; Harper, 1942; Ransmeier, 1949; Coggins and Derivaux, 1952; Wilkes, 1957), Kentucky (Prince et al., 1946), Tennessee (Kittrell, 1951; Chesney, 1955), Missouri (McDermott, 1957), Alabama (Bashinsky and Little, 1949), Texas Bloxsom and Chandler, 1944) and Florida (Heidt, 1954; Jaffe and Perlmutter, 1954). While at least 40 cases due to *D. variablis* have been reported, only a few due to other species of ticks have been recorded: for example Paffenbarger (1951) described a case in Lousiana due to *Amblyomma maculatum,* and Swartzwelder and Seabury (1947) published a case in a young boy, in whom paralysis was due to the nymph stage of this species of tick. In addition, Henderson (1961) recorded a case in Florida due to *Amblyomma americanum.* Due apparently to early diagnosis, all of these cases recovered except two, one being in Florida in which the species of tick was not identified (Alexander, 1952).

Although an earlier reference had been made to the occurrence of human tick paralysis in Australia (Bancroft, 1884), it was not until 1912 that Cleland published the first detailed account of two human cases of the disease. It was in the same year that Todd reported the occurrence of human tick paralysis in British Columbia and Temple described 12 human cases which occurred in the northwestern United States.

Undoubtedly cases occurred before and after this date but were not diagnosed as due to ticks. From 1912 to 1940 a total of 21 human cases with ten deaths have been reported in Australia (Cleland, 1912; Eaton, 1913; Strickland, 1915; Ferguson, 1924; Moss, 1924; Sinclair, 1930; Foster, 1931; Crossle, 1932; Hamilton, 1940). The species of tick which causes paralysis in Australia, *Ixodes holocyclus* Neumann, which is commonly called the 'dog tick' in New South Wales and the 'scrub tick' in Queensland, occurs throughout the costal areas of eastern Australia, extending from north Queensland to Victoria. In these areas several species of native animals, such as the bandicoots (*Peramales* spp.), are found, which are the normal hosts for the tick.

In South Africa tick paralysis in humans is uncommon. Zumpt and Glajchen (1950) reported a case of generalized paresis in an adult male due to a single tick identified as *Rhipicephalus simus* Koch, and Erasmus (1952) described three cases of localized paresis in two adult males and a child, the former due to *Hyalomma transiens* and the latter to *Ixodes rubicundus* Neumann. In one of the former the tick was identified as a male. In addition Swanepoel (1959) reported regional paralysis due to *Hyalomma truncatum* Koch. Death did not occur in any of these cases. Reports of paralysis have been recorded from Algeria (Martin, 1944) and Lorenço Marquez (Sant'Anna, 1911).

Occasional human cases of tick paralysis have occurred in England (Neitz, 1962) and France (Garin and Bujadoux, 1923), caused by *I. hexagonus* Leach or an unidentified tick (Lechevailer et al., 1974), and in Spain (Beato Gonzales, 1947), in Greece (Tzortzakis and Papadakis, 1936), in Somalia (Veneroni, 1928) by *R. simus,* in Israel (BEN-BASSAT, 1962) in which the species of tick was not identified, in Mexico (HOFFMANN, 1969), caused by *I. tancitarius* Cooley and Kohls, and rarely in other countries. Paralysis caused by Argasid larval ticks is rare in humans. In South Africa an infantile case due to *Otobius megnini* has been described by PEACOCK (1958), and in Russia cases due to infestation with large numbers of *Ornithodoros lahorensis* have been documented.

2. Seasonal Incidence

The occurrence of tick paralysis is related to the seasonal activity of the ticks. Temperature, humidity, and the duration of daylight and whether it is increasing or decreasing influence the feeding rate of ticks and consequently their degree of engorgement (GREGSON, 1943). Paralysis due to *D. andersoni* Stiles occurs in British Columbia and the northwestern United States in April, May, and June when the ticks are most prevelant, while poliomyelitis, with which it might be confused, is a summer and autumn disease. In the southeastern United States most of the cases of paralysis produced by *D. variablis* Say occur in June and July, but the period of tick activity can extend from March until August, so that the incidence of paralysis overlaps that of poliomyelitis in this area.

In Australia paralysis is most common in the costal scrubs in spring and summer. In the more northerly parts of eastern Australia, *i.e.* costal parts of Queensland, where the winters are seldom cold enough to arrest the life cycle of the tick, paralysis may occur at any time. In South Africa the disease occurs from May to July.

3. Age

Tick paralysis is most prevelant in children, and by far the greatest number of deaths recorded have been in this age group. Out of 166 cases due to *D. andersoni* Stiles in British Columbia and the northwestern United States in which the influence of age was studied (JELLISON and GREGSON, 1950), 139 occurred in children (less than 16 years of age, including infants) and the remainder in adults. The majority of cases were in children 1 to 7 years of age. About 12 percent of the children but none of the adults died. Only two deaths occurred in about 40 cases in the southeastern United States, because of early removal of the tick, and in one of these deaths the subject was an adult male and the tick(s) remained unidentified (ALEXANDER, 1952). In Australia, out of 21 cases of paralysis due to *I. holocyclus* 18 were in children, 10 of whom died. Of five cases in South Africa, three occurred in adult males and all recovered.

4. Sex

Female children have a higher incidence of paralysis caused by *D. andersoni* and *D. variablis* in North America than male children. No difference in incidence has been recorded between male and female children paralyzed by *I. holocyclus* in Australia. Paralysis in adults occurs about 4—5 times more frequently in males because of their greater occupational exposure.

II. Livestock

1. Natural Occurrence

Over the years, particularly since records have been kept, it is clear that tick paralysis in cattle and sheep has resulted in loss of livestock, often considerable on occasions, in British Columbia, Canada and the north western United States due to *Dermacentor andersoni* (BRUCE, 1925; MOILLIET, 1937; DAVIDSON, 1941; MUTH, 1945; EMMINGER,1951; JELLISON et al., 1951; GREGSON, 1966; RICH, 1971). Horses have not been commonly affected there but can be paralyzed by even one female tick (GREGSON, 1973). In California paralysis has been produced in cattle, ponies and deer by *Dermacentor occidentalis* (LOOMIS and BUSHNELL, 1968; BRUNETTI, 1965). Paralysis due to *D. andersoni* occurs in the spring months, while that caused by *D. occidentalis* is in the late autumn and winter, these being the respective seasons of activity of the two species of tick.

In Australia paralysis of sheep, cattle, goats, pigs and horses is produced by *Ixodes holocyclus* (SEDDON, 1951; KNOTT, 1961; BOOTES, 1962; SLOAN, 1968).

In South Africa *Ixodes rubicundus* has paralysed sheep, cattle and goats (STAMPA, 1959). This paralysis is commonly referred to as 'Karoo paralysis' as it occurs over wide expanses of the Karoo, consisting of the southern parts of the Orange Free State and a restricted area in the eastern Transvaal. 'Karoo paralysis' is essentially a winter occurrence because of this seasonal activity of *I. rubicundus*. In addition *Hyalomma truncatum* Koch paralyses sheep and lambs (THEILER, 1949) and *Rhipicephalus evertsi* affects spring lambs (CLARK, 1938; STAMPA, 1959) and calves (NEITZ, 1962).

Tick paralysis has also been recorded in livestock in Europe and Asia. MLINAC and OSWALD (1936) showed that the paralytic condition of "Shimterra" in sheep in Yugoslavia was transmitted by *Hyalomma aegyptium (savigni)* and by representatives of the genera *Rhipicephalus* and *Boophilus*. Sheep, cattle, and goat paralysis by *Ixodes ricinus* has been recorded in Yugoslavia (CVJETANOVIC, 1956) and Turkey (KURTPINAR, 1960), by *Haemaphysalis punctata* in Macedonia and Bulgaria (PAVLOV and MILJOWSKI, 1942) and by Dermacentor ticks in Italy (TASSELLI, 1958). Sheep paralysis has also been reported in Crete due to *I. ricinus* and *H. punctata* (BLANC and CAMINOPETROS, 1924) and in the Ukraine, Moldavia and Transcarpathia by *Ixodes crenulatus* (POMERANTZEV, 1950). Paralysis of foals by *I. ricinus* in Russia (BALABEKIAN, 1954), of domestic animals by *Dermacentor auratus* in India (HOOGSTRAAL, 1970) and of poultry by *H. punctata* in Bulgaria and Macedonia (PAVLOV, 1963) have been noted. Paralysis by soft ticks, of sheep by *Ornithodorus lahorensis* Neumann in the U.S.S.R. (JURAVLEV, 1936; MAMIKONJAN, 1946) and Yugoslavia (MIKAILOV, 1954), and of fowl by *Argas persicus* in Africa (STAMPA, 1959) and in India (MEHTA and SHAH, 1971) has also been described.

2. Experimentally Induced

Cattle: Because of the cost and the emphasis placed on adequate control of infestation with acaricides cattle have not usually been used as experimental animals. However in 1968—70 tests were carried out using *D. andersoni* in British Columbia, Canada (GREGSON, 1973). Six animals were each infested with 100—200 female ticks, prefed males being added on the fifth day. Paralysis occurred in three animals where the numbers of engorged ticks were 72, 73 and 73. In the other three animals the numbers of engorging ticks were 0, 28 and 55. In six further trials where feeding of the ticks was poor paralysis did not occur. Repetition with unmated females lowered the number of engorging ticks required to produce paralysis to 29. Long storage and geographic site of origin appeared to influence the tick virulence.

Sheep: HADWEN (1913) applied 8—11 female *D. andersoni* with several accompanying male ticks to each of three lambs; paralysis occurred in all three lambs in 6—7 days. GREGSON (1944) infested a sheep with 32 female and 9 male *D. andersoni* and a mild paralysis occurred. The susceptibility of lambs to tick paralysis by *D. andersoni* was examined later (1952) by the same author. The ticks were applied under dome-shaped capsules, which were placed over a clipped and washed area and were anchored to the surrounding wool with linen threads. In 38 infestations of 18 lambs with 1—10 female ticks, with or without accompanying males, paralysis occurred eight times. The paralysis was slight in five cases (one female tick feeding in three of these, two in one and eight in one). In one trial paralysis was moderate (two female ticks feeding) and in two it was severe (five and seven female ticks feeding). Infestation of 3 lambs with 4, 12 and 20 male ticks failed to produce paralysis. As a result of these studies the author concluded that 1) paralysis is caused only by the female tick, 2) mated, rapidly-feeding ticks are more likely to cause paralysis than slower-feeding ones, and 3) the general incidence of the paralysis was increased in proportion to the number of ticks feeding. The success rate in experimental induction of paralysis was not as great as has been obtained with dogs (*vide infra*); the overall MPD_{50} (minimum paralyzing dose) for lambs appeared to require infestations of 30—40 ticks. In humans a single slow-feeding female commonly causes paralysis, so that sheep can be considered to be only moderately susceptible to *D. andersoni* when compared with man. As with adults or children, age and size did not appear to influence susceptibility to paralysis in sheep.

Pigs: GREGSON (1973) reported that paralysis occurred when 30 previously unfed female *D. andersoni* were applied to one pig but that six pairs of ticks failed to paralyze a second pig. However, pigs are not normally exposed to tick infestation and have not been reported in North America to be accidentally affected by *D. andersoni,* but KNOTT (1968) states that they can be paralyzed by *I. holocyclus* in Australia.

III. Wildlife

Tick paralysis of wildlife is apparently uncommon. The mule deer (*Odocoileus hemionus hemionus*) has never been observed to be paralyzed by *Dermacentor andersoni* in its natural habitat in Canada. However a fawn and buck have been experimentally paralyzed (WILKINSON, 1965, 1970) with 20 and 29 engorging mated female ticks respectively. Blacktail deer (*O.h. columbianus*) and California mule deer (*O.h. californicus*) have been paralyzed in the wild by *Dermacentor occidentalis* in California (BRUNETTI, 1965). An outbreak of paralysis in six head of American buffalo *Bison bison* (L.) has been recorded by Kohls and Kramis (1952). A bear cub was paralyzed by a single female tick in British Columbia (Abel, quoted by Gregson, 1973). A muskrat, a pheasant, and a heavily infested porcupine were unaffected by *D. andersoni* (Gregson, 1973), but Marsh (1929) records the paralysis of a fox in Montana. Marmots (*Marmora flaviventris avara*) have never been observed to be affected in their natural habitat, but paralysis has been produced in the laboratory over 160 times, with a success rate of over 90 percent, with *D. andersoni*. Gregson (1973) has found marmots a reliable test animal because of their susceptibility. However, difficulty in obtaining an adequate supply, their ferocity, and their short period of activity due to hibernation limit their usefulness. Paralysis has been experimentally induced in the laboratory in coyote (*Canis latrans*) and skunk (*Mephitis mephitis*) (Wilkinson, 1970) and in 13 out of 15 ground squirrels (*Citellus c. columbianus*) with four female ticks (Hughes and Philip, 1958). Three pack rats *(Neotoma cinerea occidentalis)* died when infested with four pairs of *D. andersoni* (Hughes and Philip, 1958). In Australia bandicoots, the natural reservoir for feeding by *Ixodes holocyclus,* are paralyzed on rare occasions (Stanbury and Huyck, 1945). In Africa wild rhebuck (*Pelea capreolus* Bechst.) are reported to be paralyzed by ticks (Van Rensburg, 1928). Occasionally paralysis by ticks in bird life has been reported. A waxwing (*Bombycilla* sp.) and goldfinch (*Astragalinus* sp.) have been mentioned to be paralyzed by *Ixodes brunneus* (M.N. Kaiser quoted by Gregson, 1973) in Georgia, U.S.A., and a crow was paralyzed by *I. holocyclus* in Australia (Ranby, 1960).

IV. Pets

1. Natural Occurrence

Tick paralysis in dogs in North America is largely due to *Dermacentor andersoni,* and the greatest incidence occurs in the Pacific northwest, *i.e.* British Columbia, Southern Alberta, Montana, Oregon, Wyoming, Idaho, Colorado and Washington. Infestation by *Dermacentor variablis* has been recorded as accountable for cases in California (Loomis and Bushnell, 1968) and in the southeastern United States. Cases have been reported as far north as New York (Costa, 1952) and as far south as Florida (Heidt, 1954). *Rhipicephalus sanguineus* (Wells, 1934) and *Ixodes scapularis* (Dr. Rogers, quoted by Gregson, 1973) have also been implicated in rare cases in Florida. Although *D. variablis* is the common tick in the eastern provinces of Canada, cases of paralysis in dogs have not been recorded.

    Ixodes holocyclus, which is responsible for cases of tick paralysis in dogs in Australia, is found along the eastern coastline from north Queensland to Victoria. In Queensland it is known as the 'scrub tick' and in New South Wales as the 'dog tick' or 'bottle tick'. Hundreds of dogs have become paralyzed (Reid and Marbach, 1961). In many of the naturally occurring cases in dogs the paralysis was produced by a single tick *i.e.* in at least 10 out of 23 cases due to *D. andersoni* in British Columbia (Gregson, 1973), and in 3 out of 4 due to *Ixodes holocyclus* in Australia (Hindmarsh and Purcell, 1935). It has been recently reported that tick paralysis in dogs and cats in Tasmania is due to *Ixodes cornuatus* (Mason et al., 1974).

In South Africa dogs have been paralyzed by *Rhipicephalus evertsi* (NEITZ, 1962), *Rhipicentor nuttalli* (THEILER, 1949), *Hyalomma transiens* (Dr. G.H. ROUX quoted by ERASMUS, 1952) and rarely by *Ixodes rubicundus* (STAMPA, 1959), in Crete by *Ixodes ricinus* and *Haemaphysalis punctata* (BLANC and CAMINOPETROS, 1924), in Venezuela by *Rhipicephalus sanguineus* (VILORIA, 1954), in Uruguay by *Amblyomma maculatum* (VOGELSANG, 1925) and in Mexico probably by *Ixodes tancitarius* (HOFFMANN, 1969).

Cats in North America appear to be resistant to tick paralysis by *D. andersoni* and *D. variablis,* and although in Australia they are susceptible to *Ixodes holocyclus,* a greater percentage of cats than dogs survive paralysis due to this species of tick and they tend to develop a better immunity on recovery (KNOTT, 1968). ROBERTS (1961) observed two cats, each of which was paralyzed by a single female of *Ixodes hirsti.* In Crete cats have been paralyzed by *Ixodes ricinus* and *Haemaphysalis punctata* (BLANC and CAMINOPETROS, 1924).

2. Experimentally Induced

Probably the earliest case of tick paralysis produced experimentally in the laboratory was reported by HADWEN and NUTTALL (1913) in Cambridge, England. They applied to a dog a single female *D. andersoni,* wrongly called *D. venustus,* which was collected in British Columbia one month previously. Paralysis appeared eight days later and the dog recovered fully by the fifteenth day. The tick was two-thirds engorged.

At Kamloops in British Columbia, Canada, the incidence of tick paralysis was studied between 1949 and 1954 by applying *D. andersoni* to dogs of varying ages (GREGSON, 1973). Of six pups three became paralyzed with 2—4 feeding female ticks, and eight of 16 adult dogs became paralyzed with 12—54 feeding female ticks. In 1958 HUGHES and PHILIP in Montana, U.S.A. failed to produce paralysis in two dogs after applying to each one female *D. andersoni* which had already produced paralysis in humans, but they obtained paralysis in seven out of 11 dogs infested with 4—14 'wild' female ticks from British Columbia each. It was concluded that while pups and small dogs could be paralyzed with two or more female feeding ticks, large dogs were not susceptible to less than 10 mated ticks. However, field records indicate only two test series in which dogs infested with engorging ticks did not become paralyzed, and in at least 10 of these 23 cases they were infested with solitary females (GREGSON, 1973).

In 1954 O'ROURKE and MURNAGHAN produced paralysis seven times in seven trials on four mongrel dogs, using 1—9 female *D. andersoni* with accompanying males obtained in the wild from British Columbia and posted air-mail to Ottawa, Ontario. In these cases the hair was cut over an area approximately 3 cm in diameter on the back of the dog, the ticks were applied and the surrounding hairs were then tied over the ticks to form a tent. In a further trial by MURNAGHAN (1954, unreported) four pairs of cultured ticks were applied five times on each of two dogs without producing paralysis. In all subsequent trials by MURNAGHAN only wild ticks collected in British Columbia and posted air-mail were used. In 1955—56 the ticks were applied under a dome-shaped wire-net capsule which was fixed to the surrounding hairs with an adhesive cement. In 25 trials on 16 dogs with 10 pairs (*i.e.* male and female) of ticks, paralysis only occurred nine times (2 mild, 3 moderate and 4 severe). This low incidence of paralysis was largely due to failure of the ticks to feed because the dog scratched off the capsule. In all subsequent studies an adhesive (Elastoplast) bandage was wrapped around the chest of the dog to hold the capsule firmly in place on its back—a small hole was cut in the bandage over the capsule to permit adequate ventilation. From 1957 to 1964 (Murnaghan 1958a, 1958b, 1960a, 1960b, 1961; Murnaghan and MacConaill, 1967) in 70 trials conducted on 68 mongrel dogs 3.2—11.8 kg in weight (Mean ± S.E.M. 5.7 ± 0.19) and using 10—20 (18.9 ± 0.36) female ticks per animal, paralysis occurred 68 times (10 mild, 23 moderate and 35 severe), and in each of these cases 5—20 (15 ± 0.6) female ticks were engorged. In the first 47 trials, 5—10 (9.38 ± 0.23) male ticks were included because mating had been claimed to increase the female feeding rate (Gregson, 1944); in the remaining 23 trials only female ticks were applied. Paralysis invariably occurred within 6—8 days (7.0 ± 0.12) after application of the ticks. Six trials in which the dogs died within 1—6 (4.3 ± 1.0) days are excluded because of uncertainty of the cause of death; diarrhoea occurred in three animals. Apparently when an adequate number of ticks (20 females) are applied and precautions are taken to prevent the dog from removing them before they become engorged paralysis can be produced in over 95 percent of trials. Furthermore, mating of the ticks is not essential for a high incidence of paralysis. This investigation was concerned with producing paralysis for experimental physiological study in as high a proportion of animals as possible and consequently the minimal number of ticks required to produce paralysis in the laboratory was not under investigation. Table 5 shows that paralysis did not occur when only about three female ticks per dog became engorged (0.39 per kg of dog weight). Although neither the weight of the engorged ticks nor

Table 5. Effect of dogs weight, the number of engorged female *D. andersoni* per animal and their weight on the degree of paralysis (Mean ± S.E.M.)

	Paralysis				No Paralysis
	Severe	Moderate	Slight	Combined	
No. of dogs	39	26	13	78	12
Dogs' body weight (kg)	5.85 ± 0.26[1]	5.79 ± 0.29[1]	6.73 ± 0.73	5.97 ± 0.20[1]	8.98 ± 0.91
No. of ticks	15.11 ± 0.77 (38)[1]	14.15 ± 1.02[1]	11.27 ± 1.68 (11)[1]	14.21 ± 0.59 (75)[1]	3.20 ± 0.81 (10)
No. of ticks/ dog weight	2.77 ± 0.18[1]	2.71 ± 0.26[1]	2.02 ± 0.39[2]	2.65 ± 0.14[1]	0.39 ± 0.10
Tick weight (g)	3.10 ± 0.33 (27)	2.79 ± 0.37 (16)	3.03 ± 0.69 (6)	2.99 ± 0.23 (49)	1.53 ± 0.16 (3)
Tick weight/ dog weight	0.57 ± 0.06	0.53 ± 0.06	0.47 ± 0.10	0.54 ± 0.04	0.23 ± 0.04

Significant difference between paralysis and no paralysis. $P < 0.001$ [1], 0.01 [2]. Where the number of female ticks or their engorged weight was not recorded, the remaining number of values is in parenthesis.

their weight divided by the dog weight varied significantly between the paralyzed and nonparalyzed dogs, the weight of the dog, the number of ticks and their number divided by the dog weight clearly did. Analysis of Variance indicated that the values for the five parameters studied were not significantly different for the three degrees of paralysis.

Apart from DODD (1921), who produced a fatal paralysis in a dog by applying a single female tick, and ROSS (1926), who produced paralysis in 8 out of 12 trials in dogs (5 being due to a single tick) in Australia, little experimental work has been carried out with *Ixodes holocyclus*. BRUMPT (1933) produced paralysis in one dog with two female ticks, and ROSS (1934) showed that the time before the appearance of the paralysis could be shortened from the usual 5—6 days to 4 days if a large number (30) of ticks was applied.

Like man, dog is highly susceptible to paralysis produced by *Ixodes holocyclus* and *D. andersoni* insofar as one female tick may suffice in both cases, particularly with *I. holocyclus*.

To date female *D. andersoni* have failed to produce paralysis when applied experimentally to cats. Four infestations with 12 pairs of ticks and one with 10 females was made on four young cats and a kitten but paralysis did not occur (KMR, April 1956, 1957). HUGHES and PHILIP (1958), also using wild *D. andersoni* from British Columbia, failed to produce paralysis in six cats when four female ticks were applied to each. In 1957, Murnaghan (unreported) applied five female *D. andersoni* to one cat and 20 to another cat with accompaning male ticks. None of the five female ticks engorged on the first cat; 18 became engorged on the second cat but paralysis did not occur.

V. Laboratory Animals

Rabbits: Rabbits appear to be quite resistant to paralysis by *D. andersoni*. HUGHES and PHILIP (1958) report only occasional paralysis despite the use of a large number of animals. Philip (quoted by GREGSON, 1973) mentioned that 100—150 *D. andersoni* ticks per rabbit were applied on hundreds of occasions but only rarely did a rabbit become paralyzed. In India SINGH (1963) paralyzed rabbits with 10 or more adults of *Haemaphysalis kutchensis*.

Guinea-pigs: McCORNACK (1921) recorded that a guinea-pig was experimentally paralyzed by a female *D. andersoni* removed from a paralyzed girl from Washington State, U.S.A. HUGHES and PHILIP (1958) found that 16 out of 23 guinea-pigs were paralyzed when 1—6 'wild' female ticks from British Columbia were applied, but only one out of six were paralyzed when four 'wild' female ticks from western Montana were applied. GREGSON (1973) records that at Kamloops in British Columbia 35 out of 44 animals were paralyzed by 4—10 female ticks. DODD (1921) produced paralysis in a guinea-pig with *Ixodes holocyclus* (1 female).

Hamsters: Experimentally produced paralysis has been recorded by HUGHES and PHILIP (1958). Of 39 hamsters, 37 were paralyzed with 1—4 'wild' female British Columbia ticks and 18 of 54 when 'wild' ticks from western Montana were used. GREGSON (1973) has described 34 out of 79 cases of paralysis that occurred when

1—6 cultured British Columbia ticks which produced paralysis when they were repeatedly transferred to other hamsters in an attempt to assess tick virulence.

White mice: No paralysis occurred when 26 mice were infested with 1—5 female *D. andersoni*. When 18 mice were infested with mating ticks 10 died and eight became sluggish after engorgement of the ticks: however, death was believed to be due to exsanguination (Gregson, 1973).

White rats: Hughes and Philip (1958) failed to produce paralysis in seven white rats infested with 1—3 female British Columbia *D. andersoni*.

Monkey: Six female *D. andersoni* from British Columbia paralyzed a monkey (Hughes and Philip, 1958).

D. Symptomology

I. Humans

The clinical picture of tick paralysis produced in humans in North America by *Dermacentor andersoni* Stiles (wood tick) and *Dermacentor variablis* Say (common dog tick) has been described by Abbott (1944) and that of tick pralysis produced in humans in Australia by *Ixodes holocyclus* Neumann by Hamilton (1940); other descriptions are found in the many case reports published by various authors in these and other countries. The symptoms and signs of tick paralysis are very similar in the different geographical areas with minor variations; however, the syndrome produced has commonly been confused with other neurological diseases, *e.g.* poliomyelitis, Landry's ascending paralysis, etc., with disastrous consequences. It is imperative that the medical profession be acquainted with the existence of the condition so that if the patient has come from a tick-infested area, a search will be made for the engorging tick to allow it to be removed as early as possible. Unfortunately in the past this has not always been the case, with tragic results, because if an intensive search for the tick is not made it can easily be missed as it is commonly attached to the scalp and consequently hidden by long hair, particularly in young girls. Indeed, ticks have on occasion only been discovered during a post-mortem examination or when the body was being prepared for burial. Preventing ticks from attaching is not a simple problem, although some repellants work very satisfactorily in some people. The wearing of knee-length boots reduces the ability of the ticks to attach.

The disease consists of a widespread lower motor neurone paralysis, which commences after the tick has been feeding for about 5—6 days and gradually increases in severity. The victim, often a child and in North America commonly a female, is frequently irritable for 12 or 24 hours preceding the onset of the paralysis, and may experience numbness or tingling in the extremities, lips, throat or face. The onset of the paralysis is generally in the legs. The child is initially noticed to be unsteady in walking; this is commonly seen when the child first gets out of bed in the morning, the gait being first ataxic rather than weak. In a short time weakness becomes apparent; when she attempts to walk she staggers a few steps and her legs then give way under her. Having fallen she has difficulty in rising. The weakness increases and spreads so that the child can neither walk nor stand. Within a day or two the paralysis spreads to involve the upper extremities and trunk. In the early stages of upper limb involvement the parents of the child find that she cannot feed herself because of incoordination (dysmetria and asynergia) and will feed her and put her to bed. By this stage the lower limbs exhibit a flaccid paralysis and an increasing weakness becomes evident in the upper limbs. The trunk muscles become limp, so that the child has difficulty in sitting up and constipation may be severe. Further headward spread of the disease process gives the symptoms and signs of bulbar involvement. As the cranial nerves become involved the sternocleidomastoid, trapezius, tongue and pharyngeal muscles become affected first, then the facial and extra-ocular muscles and finally respiratory paralysis, and death results, sometimes preceded by convulsions. The neck becomes limp and the child has difficulty in holding up her head; she suffers from dysphagia and dysarthia so that she not only has difficulty in swallowing but may regurgitate food through the limp mouth and fluids through the nose; the voice becomes thick and indistinct, and also nasal if the palatal muscles are involved. Weakness of the extrinsic eye muscles may produce a transient squint or diplopia if muscle imbalance exists. Usually, however, there is no squint, but if the eye is turned to one side a nystagmus may appear. Weakness of the intrinsic eye muscles produces blurring of near vision and dilated pupils. As the respiratory muscles become involved the respiratory rate becomes increased, the breathing laboured and the child restless and anxious. The alae nasi become distended and cyanosis develops. The voice and cough become feeble. The expansion of the chest from intercostal muscle action becomes noticeably lessened and the bulge of the epigastrium from the downward movement of the diaphragm during inspiration disappears. As the child's restlessness increases the pulse becomes increasingly rapid and feeble and the body temperature may rise. Death is due to respiratory failure or aspiration pneumonia. Pain, dizziness, myoclonic jerks, choreiform movements, nuchal rigidity, vertigo, photophobia, nausea and vomiting, and urinary retention may occur, but these are rare. Heart failure (FERGUSON, 1924; PEARN, 1966) has been described in Australia. There may be local skin changes round the bite and morbilliform rashes (TAYLOR, 1966) have been reported.

Neurological examination confirms the symptomatic evidence of a widespread paralysis due to involvement of the lower motor neurons. The tendon reflexes are absent and the superficial abdominal reflexes are diminished or absent. The plantar response if present remains flexor in type. The reaction of the pupil to light and accommodation may be diminished. Muscle wasting is only slight for the disease is of short duration. Sensory changes such as hyperaesthesia, anaesthesia or dysaethesia may or may not be present, singly or in combination, but are uncommon. The cerebrospinal fluid is normal and no significant changes in blood or urine chemistry or blood culture have been detected.

Provided the paralysis is not too far advanced recovery is usually complete in 3—4 days following removal of the tick in the North American disease, though it may take more than a week. In at least one of the cases reported, however, the child died two days after removal of the tick (PRINCE et al., 1946). Thus a thorough search for the tick and its early removal are mandatory. The paralysis usually recedes in the reverse order of its progression.

The disease in Australia due to *Ixodes holocyclus* tends to be more acute than the American and Canadian version; vomiting is more common, and the height of the illness is commonly not reached until 48 h after the tick has been extracted, so that death may not be prevented by tick removal and recovery may be protracted. Removal of the tick must be complete, because EATON (1913) described a case in Australia where removal of all but the mouth parts in the preparalytic stage did not prevent the onset of severe paralysis within the next 24 h and clinical recovery only occurred on removal of the remainder of the tick.

The tick is commonly located on the scalp or neck, in or around the ear, under the breasts, in the groin, axilla, perineum and genitalia. Various means of removal of the tick have been employed: the application of petroleum jelly or oil which interfers with the air exchange of the arthropod, the application of ether, chloroform, paraffin, petrol or heat to encourage withdrawal, lifting off with a hypodermic needle or dagger-pointed scalpel or, where necessary, excision of the skin to which the tick is attached. Apart from tick removal the treatment is symptomatic. In Australia, however, canine immune serum in doses of 20—30 ml intramuscularly is used to treat small children and babies paralyzed by *I. holocyclus*. Where the bulbar type of paralysis is present a respirator may be needed as well as mechanical suction to clear the airway. Such treatment can be life-saving even when the paralysis is severly advanced.

Occasionally only a localized paralysis may occur in the region of the attached tick. MCKAY (1933) has suggested that this may be due to a local oedema, probably allergic in type, causing pressure on the regional nerve. An alternative explanation is that the toxin is neurotrophic and is absorbed by the peripheral nerves where it blocks their conduction. These localized paralyses are uncommon in North America but have been recorded in Australia and South Africa. Such isolated nerve palsies have been described involving the facial muscles due to attachment of *I. holocyclus* in the external auditory meatus (FOSTER, 1931; CROSSLE, 1932) or on the right temple (HAMILTON, 1940), and involving the upper extremity where the tick, located in the axilla, was probably either *I. holocyclus* (HAMILTON, 1940) or *Hyalomma transiens* (ERASMUS, 1952). Localized paralyses with paraesthesias, often bilateral, and associated with bilateral facial palsies have been described in France by BOUDIN et al. (1974). Male ticks have occasionally caused localized paralysis, *e.g.* in the upper limb where the tick was located in the axilla (BEN-BASSAT, 1962), or on the arm (BROWN, 1952).

II. Animals

The symptoms and signs in animals are similarly that of an ascending flaccid paralysis due to involvement of the lower motor neurons by the tick toxin. They consist of lack of coordination in the hind limbs followed by paralysis which spreads to involve the forelimbs and chest and neck muscles, and may proceed to a bulbar palsy. The first indication of the condition in cattle is a weaving gait; the animals spread their hind legs wide apart to prevent swaying of the hind quarters. They become apprehensive, fall often and as the paralysis progresses are unable to sit up or raise their heads. They struggle, may fall into a gully, and sometimes drown in streams. In the initial stages sheep and lambs are generally restless, stagger and bump against obstacles, and occasionally fall when trying to stop; later they fall down but cannot rise and consequently struggle. In both cattle and sheep the head may be bent against the body as it lies on the ground. In addition, keratitis commonly develops in paralyzed sheep. In dogs, lack of appetite and stretching and yawning may precede the onset of paralysis. Grunting and wheezing noises are heard during breathing, and a change in the bark to a gruff cough occurs. As with other animals the hind limbs are affected first but the tail movements usually remain. In Australia vomiting and keratitis are common in dogs, and puppies have been said to travel away and never be seen alive again. Death may be due to heart failure (BANCROFT, 1884). The first symptom of the paralysis in marmots is that their shrill whistle becomes husky and eventually develops into a sharp coughlike expulsion of air. The hind legs adopt a splayed appearance and as they become more flaccid they make a lateral swimming motion. Like guinea-pigs they exhibit keratitis.

If the ticks are removed from the animal, particularly a farm animal, in the early stages of paralysis rapid recovery is likely. However the mortality rate due to *I. holocyclus* is as high as 50 percent in dogs, but is usually much lower in farm animals. As laboratory animals marmots and hamsters appear to be particularly susceptible. Prevention of the disease and of others spread by ticks is a major problem of veterinary epidemiology and must take into account the economics of ecological intervention or the use of acaricides on a major scale, whether on the ground or in the form of animal dipping or spraying. ARTHUR (1962) and others have reviewed the techniques and problems involved, and different approaches may be required for each species or even for the same species in different areas. The injection of hyperimmune serum can be used to mitigate the severity of the disease in dogs in Australia.

E. Mechanism of the Paralysis

1. Physiology and Pharmacology of Paralysis due to D. andersoni

1. Neuromuscular Transmission

In 1955 MURNAGHAN found that the anterior tibial muscle in the dog paralyzed by *Dermacentor andersoni* responded to direct electrical stimulation but failed to contract when stimulated through the peroneal nerve. This finding, which was reproduced in numerous experiments, was the first significant experimental observation concerning the mechanism of tick paralysis, because it indicated either that the motor nerve fibres could not conduct a nerve impulse or that there was a block at the neuromuscular junction. The anterior tibial muscle was selected for study because it was found to be involved early in the paralysis and its degree of contraction could be readily measured in the anaesthetized animal by cutting its tendon and connecting it to a mechanical lever, and fixing the knee-joint by inserting a drill-bit into the upper end of the tibia. ROSE and GREGSON (1956) confirmed that indirect peroneal nerve stimulation failed to contract the muscles supplied by it in two paralyzed dogs and a lamb. ROSE had previously found in 1954 (unpublished) that the thigh muscles of a 3-year-old child who was completely paralyzed responded to galvanic stimulation.

MURNAGHAN (1958 a) then found in the tick-paralyzed dog that when a mixed nerve (sciatic-peroneal) was stimulated electrically action potentials could be recorded from it. Furthermore, when the animal was lightly anaesthetized it whined during application of the stimulus, indicating that the sensory fibres were conducting the nerve impulse. He also exposed the 6th lumbar ventral root in a paralyzed dog, stimulated it and recorded the conducted electrical activity further down (160–180 mm) on the peroneal nerve. An action potential was obtained for each stimulus applied, suggesting that the motor nerve fibres were conducting 'normally'. However, the recorded action potential was a single biphasic one and its probably small amplitude was not recognized at that stage due to a calibration fault in the amplifier. Exposure of the 7th lumbar dorsal root permitted demonstration of conduction in sensory nerve fibres, but in retrospect with similar reservations. These findings at that time consequently led to the assumption that the defect in tick paralysis lay primarily at the neuromuscular junction. The next series of studies was consequently directed towards an understanding of the mechanism involved at this site.

At this stage therefore, the possibility of a curare-type paralysis had to be envisaged. An isolated rat phrenic nerve-diaphragm preparation was immersed in heparinized plasma from a paralyzed dog and stimulated indirectly through the nerve (MURNAGHAN, 1955). Good contractions of the muscle were obtained during the several hours of investigation. However rats have never been paralyzed by *D. andersoni,* and even if a toxin was present in the plasma it might not have acted within the period of study. The following findings (MURNAGHAN, 1958 a) precluded the possibility that the toxin acted in the same way as curare: a) when acetylcholine was injected intra-arterially by the method described by BROWN (1938) into the paralyzed anterior tibial muscle in doses of 2.5, 10 and 40 µg it caused contractions approximately as large as that in the normal muscle. If the paralysis had been due to a curare-like substance the response to injected acetylcholine would have been abolished or reduced; b) application of a direct cathodal current to the muscle failed to facilitate neuromuscular transmission during nerve stimulation; c) tetanus was moderately well maintained and only slightly potentiated subsequent twitch contractions; and d) neostigmine (Prostigmine) given intra-arterially and intravenously increased muscular contractions only slightly.

The fact that the paralysis could not have been due to a depolarizing blocking agent was confirmed by the findings that pentamethonium, an antagonist to depolarizing blocking agents, when given intra-arterially and intravenously failed to improve the paralysis, application of a direct anodal current to the muscle failed to improve neuro-muscular transmission, and the administration of curare intensified the paralysis while neostigmine did not.

The normal response to intra-arterially applied acetylcholine, the fact that neostigmine did not decrease the contractions, and the moderately well-maintained tetanus also excluded the possibility of the toxin acting as an anticholinesterase. Furthermore, an intravenous injection of acetylcholinesterase 0.3 mg/kg and of diisonitrosoacetone 40 mg/kg (an anticholinesterase antagonist) failed to improve muscular contractions. Other workers have shown that Prostigmine failed to overcome the paralysis in a lamb (ROSE and GREGSON, 1956) or in a child (WEBB and EARNEST, 1963) and that Protopam chloride (anticholinesterase antagonist) was ineffective in a paralyzed marmot (KMR, August 1967).

The study was next logically directed towards a study of the muscle end-plates (MURNAGHAN, 1957, 1958b). That they were functioning adequately in the paralyzed dog was indicated by a) the contraction of the anterior tibial muscle following intra-arterial injections of acetylcholine, and b) the demonstration that the endplates were depolarized by succinylcholine. Table 6 shows the response of the normal, partially and completely paralyzed anterior tibial muscle to intra-arterial injections of acetylcholine. Increasing paralysis apparently produced increasing sensitivity of the muscle to acetylcholine, the paralyzed muscle behaving as a denervated one. This 'denervation' sensitization to acetylcholine was not confirmed by EMMONS and McLENNAN (1959) in paralyzed ground-hogs (marmots). However, in their experiments paralysis was induced in 18—36 h, instead of 6—8 days as in the dogs, by the application of partially engorged female D. andersoni, which may have resulted in a shorter 'denervation' period before testing. End-plates could be located in the paralyzed anterior tibial muscle by sweeping its undersurface with a wick electrode after an injection of succinylcholine, the technique being similar to that described by BURNS and PATON (1951). Usually four or more endplate regions could be located in this way. The depolarizing effect of the succinylcholine was then allowed to wear off. In an apparently completely paralyzed muscle, one or more small bundles of muscle fibres usually contracted on nerve stimulation and the site of minimum latency of the action potential corresponded to only one of the located end-plate regions. Neither action nor end-plate potentials could be detected at the other located end-plate regions. These two findings suggested that the probable mechanism of the paralysis was due to failure in the liberation and/or synthesis of acetylcholine at the nerve terminals.

In order to prove conclusively that tick paralysis was due to failure in the release of acetylcholine, paralyzed and normal anterior tibial muscles were perfused with oxygenated eserinized (10^{-5} g/ml) Locke-Ringer solution which was maintained at 37°C and the amount of acetylcholine liberated into the perfusion solution was measured (MURNAGHAN, 1959, 1960b). The isolated muscle, maintained at 37°C in a moist chamber, was perfused with 15 ml of the Locke solution, which was continuously recycled and filtered for 30 min. At the end of that time the solution was collected in addition to a further 5 ml of fresh solution which

Table 6. Sensitivity of anterior tibial muscle to rapid close intra-arterial injection of acetylcholine

Anterior tibial muscle	No. of experiments	Approximate average dose (µg) of acetylcholine to produce	
		Threshold contraction	Contraction = maximal muscle twitch
Normal	4	5	50
Partially paralyzed	3	1	15
Fully paralyzed	1	?	1

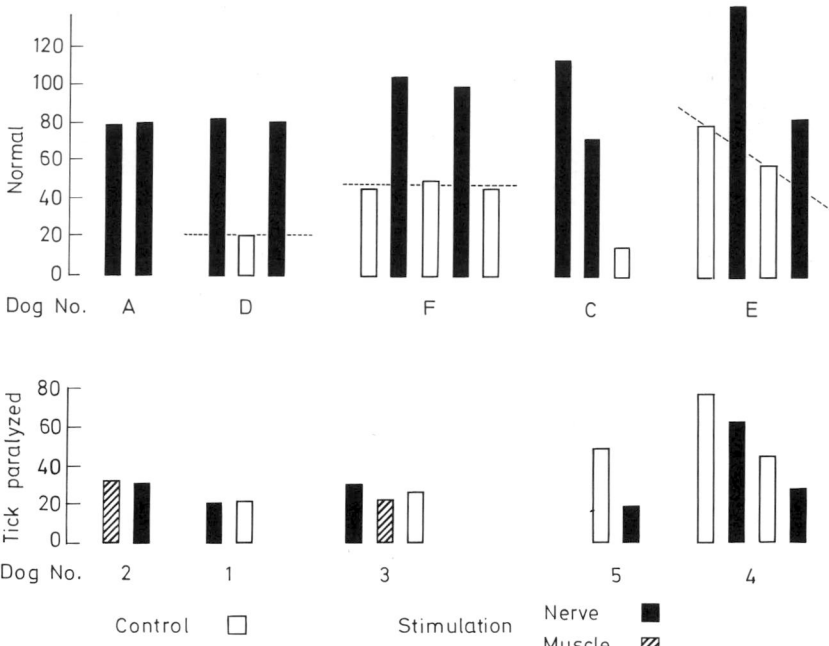

Fig. 2. Acetylcholine output (mμg) per 30-min period of perfused anterior tibial muscle of dog

was used to wash out the apparatus. A further 15 ml of solution was then added and recycled as before. Two to five such 30-minute recirculation periods were used. During the 30-minute perfusion either the muscle was stimulated indirectly through the peroneal nerve (1-4 V, 0.2 msec, 5 Hz) or directly (150 V, 2 msec, 5 Hz) or it was not stimulated (Control). Because the peroneal nerve contains some adrenergic nerve fibres which on stimulation release noradrenaline, the vasodilator response in the eserinized-eviscerated cat could not be used to estimate the amount of acetylcholine in the perfusate. Consequently the morphinized-eserinized leech muscle was developed at this time as a suitable assay object for acetylcholine (Murnaghan, 1958c). Figure 2 shows the results in five normal and five severely paralyzed anterior tibial muscles. The results indicate that some acetylcholine is liberated from both normal and paralyzed muscles during a control perfusion. However, while peroneal nerve stimulation in the normal muscle increased significantly ($P < 0.001$) the output of acetylcholine from 45 ± 8.2 to 94.6 ± 7.3 ng per 30-minute perfusion period (6.0 pg per nerve volley), neither nerve nor direct stimulation of the paralyzed muscle significantly ($P > 0.2$) altered the acetylcholine output (30.5 ± 4.9 ng) against that of the control (43.2 ± 9.9). Emmons and McLennan (1959) similarly showed that the muscles of the perfused hind leg of the ground-hog paralyzed by *D. andersoni* also failed to release acetylcholine when the sciatic nerve was stimulated.

The next questions to be answered were whether the failure in the release of acetylcholine by nerve stimulation was due to a) failure in the synthesis of acetylcholine, b) inability to store the acetylcholine, or c) a defect in the release mechanism itself. Acetylcholine is synthesized by the enzyme choline acetylase which requires as substrates choline and acetylcoenzyme A to supply active acetate. Due to the low choline acetylase activity and acetylcholine concentration in muscle, and the fact that these substances are synthesized in the neuron and migrate down the axon, they were estimated in the lower lumbar ventral roots and the (sciatic) peroneal nerves. The choline acetylase activity was measured in prepared acetone powders of these. The acetylcholine produced per gram of acetone powder per hour for ventral roots was 15.6 ± 0.7 mg in five normal and 13.6 ± 1.8 in nine paralyzed dogs. The respective values for peroneal nerves were 1.3 ± 0.15 and 1.2 ± 0.2. The mean acetylcholine content of ventral roots was 8.4 ± 0.9 µg/g in 4 normal and 12.2 ± 3.3 in three paralyzed dogs. The respective values for the sciatic-peroneal nerves was 2.0 ± 0.3 and 2.5 ± 0.7. No significant difference existed between normal and paralyzed dogs either for choline acetylase activity or for acetylcholine content. In the method used for estimating choline acetylase activity excess choline and acetylcoenzyme A were included; the latter was supplied by its synthesis from coenzyme A and acetylphosphate with the aid of phosphotrans-acetylase. Choline deficiency as a cause of the paralysis is very probably excluded because the mean choline outputs in the 30-minute perfusions of the normal and paralyzed anterior tibial muscles were similar, 3.74 ± 0.33 and 3.86 ± 0.5 µg respectively. Furthermore an intravenous injection of 20 mg/kg choline chloride to a paralyzed anaesthetized dog in which the mechanical response of the anterior tibial muscle was recorded during peroneal nerve stimulation produced no apparent beneficial effect on neuromuscular transmission (MURNAGHAN, 1960b). DESMEDT (1958) developed a sensitive test for measuring inadequate acetylcholine synthesis by using hemicholinium which interfers with the uptake of choline by the neuron. When a train of seven electrical pulses was applied at a rate of 3 Hz each minute to a motor nerve, the fifth electromyographic response was reduced in magnitude in respect to the first. In one moderately paralyzed dog the 5th electromyographic response of the anterior tibial muscle to peroneal nerve stimulation was not reduced (MURNAGHAN, 1960b).

In order to exclude deficiency of acetylcoenzyme A as a cause of the paralysis, a preparation of it prepared either by enzymic or chemical synthesis was (a) added to the Locke solution during perfusion of a paralyzed muscle, (b) injected intra-arterially into the anterior tibial muscle and intravenously in anaesthetized par-alyzed dogs during recording of the mechanical response of the anterior tibial muscle when the exposed unligated peroneal nerve was stimulated, and (c) injected intravenously to unanaesthetized paralyzed dogs. The approximate amounts of acetylcoenzyme A administered were in a) 60 µg, in b) and c) 2 mg. In all cases no lessening in the paralysis occurred and in the unanaesthetized dog the paralysis was still present 24 h after the injection. To date the results indicated that in the paralyzed animal there was no apparent disturbance in the mechanism for synthesis of acetylcholine and the stores of the latter were adequate. However the stores of acetylcholine were measured in the anterior roots and peroneal nerves and not in the small nerve terminals from which it is released. In order to do this the anterior tibial muscle was perfused with eserine-Locke solution containing four times (23 mM) the normal concentration of potassium and the acetylcholine released by the depolarizing action of the high potassium was measured in the eserinized-eviscerated cat (MURNAGHAN, 1960b). The morphinized-eserinized leech muscle could not be used as the assay object because the high concentration of potassium in the perfusate caused it to contract. Previous reserpinization of the paralyzed dog to deplete the stores of noradrenaline prevented the latter's appearance in the perfusate because high potassium releases noradrenaline as well as acetylcholine. In both normal and paralyzed muscles the high-potassium Locke solution caused a marked release of acetylcholine compared with the small amount present in the normal Locke perfusate indicating that the stores of acetylcholine are adequate in the paralyzed animal. MacIntosh (1959) has emphasized the importance of the calcium ion, carbon dioxide and a chloroform-soluble dialyzable plasma factor for acetylcholine release. When the mechanical response of the anterior tibial muscle was recorded during peroneal nerve stimulation in the paralyzed anaesthetized dog (an intravenous injection of calcium chloride 30 mg/kg), an increase in the carbon dioxide tension in the blood by the induction of asphyxia by tracheal occlusion and replacement of part (100 ml) of the animal's plasma by that from a normal dog failed to produce any beneficial effect on neuromuscular transmission (Murnaghan, 1960b). A disturbance of magnesium metabolism in tick paralysis was considered a possibility because excess magnesium interferes with the release of acetylcholine during nerve stimulation. However, the inability of the intravenously administered calcium chloride mentioned above to overcome the paralysis probably excludes this mechanism. An intravenous injection of ephedrine (1 mg/kg), potassium chloride (20 mg/kg), and 1 mg/kg eserine or neostigmine as mentioned earlier were tested because of their beneficial effect in myasthenia gravis; they failed to improve neuromuscular transmission significantly in the paralyzed dog.

2. Nerve Conduction

All evidence to date indicated that tick paralysis is due neither to defective synthesis or storage of acetylcholine nor to the absence of essential release factors in the paralyzed animal and consequently must be due to inability of the nerve impulse to traverse the terminal motor nerve fibres. Consequently, at this stage it was decided to reinvestigate conduction in motor nerve fibres because in the initial study (Murnaghan, 1958a), although conduction had been demonstrated to be present, neither measurement of the magnitude of the action potential nor a comparison with that in normal dogs was carried out, due to inadequate calibration of the amplifier in use at that time.

In the reinvestigation (Murnaghan, 1960a, 1960c, 1961) the sixth lumbar ventral root was stimulated and the nerve action potentials were recorded with silver-silver chloride surface electrodes at three sites. The sciatic-peroneal nerve in the thigh was laid on a triple-pole electrode, the sciatic lying on the uppermost pole and the peroneal on the lower two. The recording from the upper two poles was designated S-P, and that from the lower two P_t. The part of the peroneal nerve where it winds round the neck of the fibula was laid on a double-pole electrode and the recording site was designated P_f. In six normal dogs the potentials recorded at any one of the three sites consisted of an initial biphasic component of small amplitude and short latency followed by a multiple complex consisting invariably in three large overlapping potentials in turn succeeded by two small ones (Fig. 3). The initial biphasic component was evidently due to a small homegeneous population of rapidly conducting, large-diameter fibres and the multiple complex to a large heterogeneous population of fibres of varying, slower, conduction rates and varying smaller diameters. As bipolar recording was used it was not possible to measure the amplitude or latency of the individual components in the multiple complex. The amplitude recorded for the multiple complex was from the highest to the lowest peak; the latency was to the commencement of this complex.

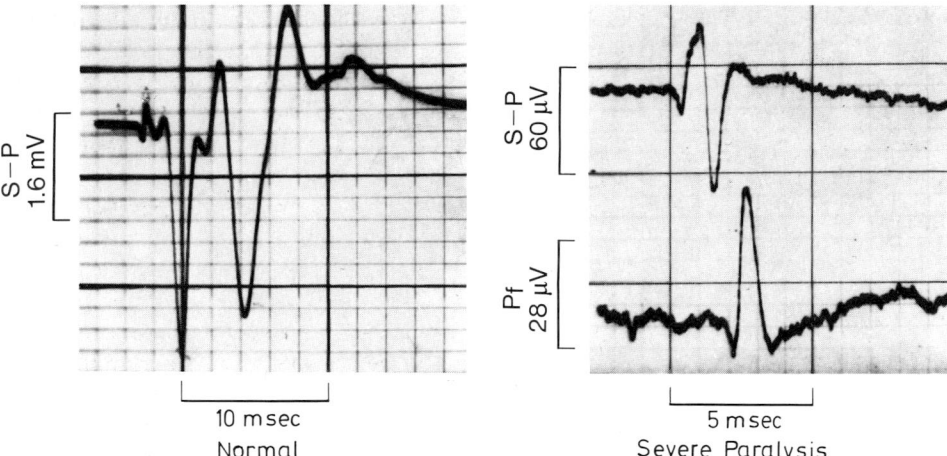

Fig. 3. Nerve action potentials recorded in normal dog (left) at sciatic-peroneal nerve and in severely paralyzed dog (right) at sciatic-peroneal nerve (above) and peroneal nerve at fibula (below). Note difference in calibration between normal and paralyzed

The arithmetic mean $\pm$ S.E.M. values for amplitude and conduction velocity of the initial biphasic potential and the subsequent multiple complex at the three recording sites in six normal and four moderately paralyzed dogs are given in Table 7. While the amplitude of the initial potential originating from the more rapidly conducting fibres was only reduced by a factor of 3 in moderate paralysis, that of the subsequent multiple complex originating from slower-conducting fibres was reduced by approximately 14 times. Furthermore, analysis of variance demonstrated that moderate paralysis did not influence the rate of decrease in potential size as recorded at the three successively more peripheral sites, i.e. S-P, P_t and P_f, respectively. A comparison of the conduction velocity of the pooled data at the three sites of recording indicated that moderate paralysis significantly ($P < 0.01$) reduced the conduction velocity. In contrast to the normal and moderately paralyzed cases only a single biphasic potential of small amplitude was recorded at each of the three sites and the conduction velocity was reduced in four severely paralyzed dogs (at site S-P 0.07 ± 0.02 mV and 52 ± 14 m/sec respectively). Although it was not realized at the time, it was now apparent that a marked conduction block was present in the motor nerve fibres of the severely paralyzed dog in the earlier study because only a single biphasic potential of probably small amplitude was present (see Fig. 1a, MURNAGHAN, 1958a). In one normal and one moderately paralyzed dog sensory nerve conduction was also investigated by stimulating the sixth lumbar dorsal root. The initial biphasic potential was not much affected by the tick 'toxin', i.e. 1.2 mV in the normal, 0.8 mV in the paralyzed dog; on the other hand the subsequent multiple complex was markedly reduced, e.g. from 4 mV to 80 µV.

Because of the laborious procedure involved in dissecting and exposing the lumbar nerve roots it was decided at this stage to investigate whether a disturbance in conduction could be demonstrated in a shorter stretch of a mixed nerve (MURNAGHAN and MacCONAILL, 1967).

Table 7. Mean $\pm$ S.E.M. of amplitude (mV) and conduction velocity (m/sec) of potentials recorded at three sites in 6 normal and 4 moderately paralyzed dogs

Dog	Recording site	Amplitude mV		Conduction velocity m/sec	
		Initial biphasic	Subsequent multiple complex	Initial biphasic	Subsequent multiple complex
Normal	S-P	0.94 ± 0.4	4.48 ± 1.2	105 ± 6.2	60 ± 3.2
	P_t	0.29 ± 0.09	2.14 ± 0.33	110 ± 4.1	61 ± 2.7
	P_f	0.16 ± 0.08	1.83 ± 0.57	91 ± 3.8	56 ± 5.0
Moderately paralyzed	S-P	0.25 ± 0.11	0.37 ± 0.21	100 ± 3.8	50 ± 3.8
	P_t	0.17 ± 0.08	0.15 ± 0.12	100 ± 6.0	48 ± 5.5
	P_f	0.04 ± 0.015	0.10 ± 0.045	91 ± 8.3	50 ± 5.1

Two procedures were adopted: 1) sciatic-peroneal nerves were removed from the dog and laid on electrodes in a moist chamber; 2) electrodes were applied *in situ* to the sciatic and peroneal nerves. In the former the distance between the stimulating and the first recording electrode was 30 mm, in the latter 60 mm. While no significant difference could be detected in the amplitude of the action potentials between two normal and six paralyzed (4 severe and 2 moderately) animals when the shorter stretch of isolated nerve was tested, a just significant reduction by a factor of 2 was noted in four cases of paralysis (3 severe and 1 moderate) compared with 2 normal dogs when the longer stretch of nerve was tested *in situ*. Removal of the nerve from the body into a Locke solution did not appear to influence the response. This reduction in amplitude by the paralysis for the nerve *in situ* was very much smaller than that obtained when conduction was measured from the motor and sensory roots to the peroneal nerve (14 times and greater) where the approximate distance was 160 to 240 mm according to the position of the recording site.

Emmons and McLennan (1960) had reported a decrease in amplitude of action potentials recorded from the sciatic nerve *in situ* of tick-paralyzed marmots, but they did not state the electrode distance used. Cherington and Snyder (1968) measured the rate of conduction in the median nerve of a 5-year-old girl from Coloroda, U.S.A., who was paralyzed by an engorging tick, most probably a female *D. andersoni*. They stimulated the median nerve at the wrist and elbow and recorded the muscle action potentials with surface electrodes at the motor end point of the right thenar muscles. The potentials were markedly reduced but assumed normal values on recovery from the paralysis. The nerve conduction velocity was calculated from the differences in the times required for the appearance of the electromyographic response when the nerve was stimulated close to and distal from the muscle. The velocity of nerve conduction was reduced by the paralysis from about 50 to 43 m/sec.

In tick paralysis a progressive block in conduction of motor and sensory nerve fibres occurs, probably due to suppression of an increasing number of nodes of Ranvier because of a statistical distribution in their sensitivity to the action of the 'toxin'. Consequently the greater the length of the single nerve fibre examined, the greater would be the likelihood of the impulse meeting a depressed node. Furthermore, due to the random distribution of the depressed nodes an increasing number of fibres should show a block in conduction as the length of the nerve trunk examined is increased. This hypothesis could explain, in part, why the longer nerves to the lower limbs are usually involved early during the development of the paralysis. Associated with this conduction block is a decrease in the conduction velocity. The smaller-diameter fibres with slower conduction rates are affected to a greater extent than the largest-diameter, faster-conducting fibres in the early stages of the paralysis; in severely paralyzed animals the slower-conducting fibres appear to be completely blocked, and when the paralysis becomes total, conduction in all motor, and possibly sensory, fibres would probably be completely abolished. As the tick 'toxin' evidently exhibits a predilection for smaller-diameter fibres one would expect that the terminal motor nerve fibres would be affected at an early stage of the paralysis. The fact that direct muscle stimulation failed to liberate acetylcholine in the tick-paralyzed muscle, as mentioned earlier, indicates not only that the conduction block in the terminal motor fibres was complete but also that the block must have extended to the terminal end. Due to the relatively smaller size of the terminal motor fibres it is possible that they are affected to a greater extent than their parent motor fibre in the early stages of the paralysis. This, however, does not imply that the block in tick paralysis spreads from the tip of the terminal fibre centripetally up along the parent fibre, as in this case the rate of fall-off in potential size recorded from S-P, P_t and P_f would presumably have been increased by the paralysis, which in fact did not occur. As the parent fibre does not appreciably change in diameter throughout its length, impairment of conduction, from its inception, probably involves the whole fibre.

While the tick toxin interferes with conduction in somatic nerve fibres one might also expect it to interfere with conduction in autonomic nerve fibres, particularly the preganglionic ones which resemble somatic motor nerve fibres in that they are medullated and they release acetylcholine at their nerve terminals. However stimulation of the cervical sympathetic nerve in the neck proximal to the superior cervical ganglion resulted in normal dilatation of the pupil and retraction of the nictitating membrane in a paralyzed dog, and stimulation of the peripheral end of the vagus in the neck caused normal cardiac slowing (MURNAGHAN, 1958 b). In addition, if acetylcholine liberation in sympathetic ganglia was depressed due to diminished conduction in the preganglionic fibres in a paralyzed animal one might have expected to find low blood pressure. The blood pressure in five paralyzed dogs was within normal limits (148 ± 15.6 mm Hg). It would appear therefore that the tick toxin exhibits a predilection for somatic nerve fibres; however, a failure to demonstrate a conduction block in the autonomic nerves may have been due to the inadequate length of nerve tested. Dilated pupils and cycloplegia have been recorded during severe paralysis in humans.

3. Central Nervous Transmission

At an early stage in this investigation it had been noted that not only was there a peripheral component to account for the paralysis, but also a defect in transmission in the central nervous system appeared to be involved (MURNAGHAN, 1955, 1958a). In one completely paralyzed dog, when a stimulus was applied to the posterior tibial nerve, no reflex potentials could be recorded from the ipsilateral peroneal nerve. In a less severely paralyzed dog the potentials, after a single stimulus to the posterior tibial nerve, consisted of multiple monosynaptic and polysynaptic forms which lasted several seconds instead of the normal polysynaptic pattern lasting approximately 10 msec. In a third slightly paralyzed dog the reflex action potentials were normal in character. These findings were interpreted as follows. In the completely paralyzed dog reflex potentials could not be obtained because of a conduction block in the small-diameter terminal sensory fibres synapsing in the spinal cord. It could have been due, however, to a block in peripheral nerve conduction. It was suggested at that time that since the toxin blocked the release of acetylcholine at the termination of the peripheral motor fibres it would also block its release at the termination of its intraspinal collateral fibre which synapses with the Renshaw cell. As the Renshaw cell exerts an inhibitory action on the anterior horn cell, absence of this inhibitory mechanism could lead to repetitive discharge in the motor nerve fibres arising from these anterior horn cells. It is of interest to note that occasionally myoclonic jerks have been noted in moderate cases of paralysis. The studies of ESPLIN et al. (1960) give some support to the concept of a central nervous transmission disturbance in the mechanism of tick paralysis. These authors observed that the stretch reflexes of paralyzed dogs and marmots were absent even though neuromuscular transmission was often only partly reduced. They suggested that the early incoordination seen in the paralysis before the muscular power is markedly affected may be attributable to impairment of the monosynaptic pathways by a block in the fine terminal sensory nerve fibres. LAGOS and THIES (1969) supported this hypothesis because a patient of theirs suffered ataxia without muscular weakness. Ataxia is very commonly the first sign noted in most cases of tick paralysis.

4. Miscellaneous Agents

A number of materials have been tried, often on an empirical basis, in attempts to alleviate the paralysis. A vitamin-B preparation (Beminol, B-plex etc.), because of the anti-neuritic effect of thiamine, was tested by a variety of workers during paralysis in dogs (MURNAGHAN, 1961) and in man (ROSE, 1958, quoted by GREGSON, 1973), without any beneficial effect. Other investigators (quoted by GREGSON, 1973) have claimed occasional apparent success with intravenous injections of calcium gluconate in dogs and a lamb. As intravenous injections of calcium chloride, as indicated earlier, failed to improve neuromuscular transmission in paralyzed dogs such claims should be considered with circumspection. Neither hydrocortisone 2 mg/kg in dogs (MURNAGHAN, 1960b) nor 1 – 10 mg prednisolone in divided doses in marmots (KMR, June 1963) altered the course of the paralysis.

Because an increased extracellular concentration of sodium partially antagonizes nerve conduction block produced by local anaesthetics (POSTERNAK and ARNOLD, 1954), it was tried in tick paralysis (MURNAGHAN, 1962, unpublished). Immersion of an isolated sciatic-peroneal nerve from a paralyzed dog in high-sodium Ringer solution failed to improve nerve conduction. When 5 ml/kg of 5 M sodium chloride was given by slow intravenous injection to a slightly paralyzed dog it failed to improve muscular power; after 30 min convulsions occurred, probably due to cerebral dehydration. Only one substance was noted to improve nerve conduction on one occasion (MURNAGHAN, 1959, unpublished). When 25 ml of 56 mM potassium chloride was injected intravenously to a paralyzed dog the amplitude of the initial action potential, recorded at S-P during ventral root stimulation, was increased about 5 times. Unfortunately, due to a defect in the shutter mechanism of the camera the slower-conducting potentials were not recorded. Finally atropine 1, phenoxybenzamine 8, procaine 50, ethylenediamine-tetraacetic acid 30, lecithin 80 (doses mg/kg) by intravenous injection and hypothermia failed to overcome the paralysis (MURNAGHAN, 1961).

II. Experimental Physiological Findings with Other Ticks Species

1. Ixodes holocyclus

Only one experiment, by Ross (1926), is recorded where an attempt was made to identify the physiological basis of the paralysis produced by *I. holocyclus*. He stimulated the common peroneal, femoral and median nerves in an anaesthetized paralyzed dog and obtained normal and powerful contractions of the muscles supplied by these nerves. Because sensation is present but there is loss of voluntary and reflex muscular movements in tick paralysis he concluded that the toxin did not act peripherally but on the motor neurons in the anterior horn cells and in the nerve cells of the cranial nuclei.

2. Argas (Persicargas) persicus

KUNZE and GOTHE (1971) have demonstrated in fowl paralyzed by larvae of *Argas (Persicargas) persicus* that the amplitudes of the evoked compound muscle action potentials were decreased to 15—30 percent of the initial value in severely paralyzed animals and to a lesser degree in moderately paralyzed ones. In addition they showed that motor nerve fibre conduction velocity was reduced to 55 percent and 70 percent of the initial value in severely and moderately paralyzed animals respectively. The faster-conduction fibres were affected more than the slower ones, which is the opposite finding to that obtained with adult *D. andersoni*. Motor nerve fibres were affected more than sensory fibres (GOTHE and KUNZE, 1971). In addition, they (GOTHE and KUNZE, 1974) obtained evidence which they suggest indicates that the toxin may also produce a post-synaptic defect at the neuromuscular junction, possibly through an altered sensitivity of the postsynaptic receptor.

III. Identification of the Presence and Removal of the Toxin

The first attempt to identify that there was a toxin was probably by SABBATINI (1898), who claimed that intravenous injection to dogs and cats of an emulsion of *Ixodes ricinus* caused the signs of paralysis during the course of the injection with recovery within a few hours. MURNAGHAN (1958b) prepared a saline extract (1 g/ml) by homogenizing 128 (28 g) engorged female *D. andersoni* which were removed from paralyzed dogs. The extract was filtered and injected intra-arterially (3 × 1 ml) and intravenously (1, 10 and 10 ml) to a normal anaesthetized dog to see whether it possessed curare-like properties. It produced no detectable effect on the mechanical response of the anterior tibial muscle during stimulation of the peroneal nerve within a period of two hours. As the toxin appears to take a considerable time before it exerts its effect (*vide infra*) the duration of this and subsequent tests for identification of the presence of the toxin were clearly too short. Kaire (1966) in Australia was apparently successful in isolating a toxin which is believed to be similar to that causing natural tick paralysis. Engorged *Ixodes holocyclus* were homogenized in saline, the proteins were precipitated by acetone, redissolved, dialyzed and fractionated on DEAE cellulose columns. Fraction 2, containing the active component, was non-dialyzable; it contained globins, but was not destroyed by pepsin, trypsin or papain. In dogs paralysis occurred in 48 h after injection of fraction 2; mice were affected in 6−8 h. Both animals were protected from the fraction by dog anti-tick serum, and immunization of dogs with fraction 2 protected them from paralysis by live ticks. Currently attempts are being made to purify the toxin by means of chromatographic and electrophoretic techniques. At present the toxin is believed to be a protein of high molecular weight. It is hoped to develop a radio-immune assay (Bagnall and Doube, 1975).

Attempts were made to duplicate the procedure in British Columbia, Canada, with *D. andersoni* (KMR, June 1967). Despite the use of large doses of fractions prepared from this species of tick, 12 marmots and 8 mice remained unaffected; marmots are highly susceptible to live *D. andersoni* collected in British Columbia.

At an early stage in the search for the toxin, Regendanz and Reichenow (1931) noted that tick paralysis in animals and humans did not occur until egg development started in the causative female tick. They proposed that the toxin was formed during egg development and was secreted by the salivary glands. Consequently emulsions of eggs of a variety of ticks were tested on various animals by a large number of investigators. Regendanz and Reichenow used egg extracts of *Rhipicephalus sanguineus* and *Dermacentor reticulatus* on dogs, guinea-pigs, rats, mice, rabbits and canaries and Mlinac and Oswald (1936), using eggs of *Hyalomma* and *Boophilus* ticks on guinea-pigs, claimed that paralysis could be induced in the experimental animal after 1 or more days. Oswald (1938), who also obtained similar results with eggs of *R. bursa* and *R. sanguineus,* then questioned whether this 'ixovotoxin' was identical to that secreted by the salivary glands, because while ticks containing toxic eggs can be found infesting animals throughout the year, paralysis tends to occur at certain seasons. Other workers, including Hoeppli and Feng (1933) using eggs of *D. sinicus, Haemaphysalis campanulata hoeppliama* and *Hyalomma detritum* on dogs, guinea-pigs, rats and hamsters, de Meillon (1942) using eggs of *R. evertsi, B. decoloratus* and *Haemophysalis leachi* on guinea-pigs, Purvis (KMR, July 1960) using eggs of *D. andersoni* and *D. albipictus* on guinea-pigs and marmots, Steinhaus (1942) using eggs of *D. andersoni* on guinea-pigs, and Riek (1957), who used the eggs of various species of ticks in Australia, induced toxic symptoms and often death in the animals when an extract of the eggs of the tick was injected. The symptoms and signs apparently were not closely similar to those of tick paralysis.

Irrespective of where the toxin is produced in the tick's body, it must be secreted by the salivary gland in order to reach the host. Initially interest was concentrated on identification of the presence of an anticoagulating factor in the ticks's salivary glands because it was felt that the paralysis toxin could be associated with it. This factor was shown to be present in the salivary glands of *Ixodes ricinus* (SABBATINI, 1898; MARKWARDT, 1963), *Argas persicus* (NUTTALL and STRICKLAND, 1908; CORNWALL and PATTEN, 1914), *D. simus* and *Hyalomma detritum peritrigatum* (HOEPPLI and FENG, 1933), *D. andersoni* (PRESSESKY, 1952, quoted by GREGSON, 1973) and *Ixodes holocyclus* (ROSS, 1926; MARKWARDT, 1963; KAIRE, 1966). TATCHELL (1969) failed to demonstrate the presence of anticoagulants in the saliva and salivary glands of *B. microplus*. However, KAIRE (1966) showed that the anticoagulant prepared from *I. holocyclus* was not identical with his fraction 2, which produced symptoms of paralysis.

It was hoped that the salivary glands of engorging ticks would contain a sufficient amount of the toxin to produce symptoms resembling tick paralysis. ROSS (1926) produced vomiting and fever in a dog with an intravenous injection of emulsified salivary glands from engorged *I. holocyclus* which had produced paralysis in another dog. He induced lethal symptoms in mice with such an emulsion when it was injected intravenously. He claimed that the symptoms resembled tick paralysis, but this was questioned by STANBURY and HUYCK (1945); many of the effects were probably due to the injection of a foreign protein. Injection of an emulsion of the salivary glands of *D. andersoni* failed to produce paralysis in mice, marmots, a pup and a lamb (GREGSON, 1973).

When the collection of salivary secretion from ticks in capillary tubes had been developed, injection of it to animals was tried, as it was considered that it might be a better and more logical source of the toxin. Salivary secretion collected from engorged *D. andersoni* was injected subcutaneously to two lambs, a dog and two mice without producing any effects (GREGSON, 1957). At a later date, when it was possible to collect larger amounts of salivary secretion, it was administered by continuous subcutaneous infusion, in order to simulate the natural secretion of the tick more closely. Furthermore, marmots and hamsters were used as the test animals, as they had been shown to be capable of being paralyzed within 24 h by infestation with *D. andersoni* females prefed for 5—6 days on other animals. In one trial, when a 530 g marmot received 7 ml of salivary secretion by infusion over 24 h, the result was equivocal; in the second marmot, which weighed 510 g, infusion of the same volume in 8 h did not cause paralysis. The salivary secretion was then infused to young hamsters weighing 35—40 g. Infusion of 0.5 ml over 8 h had no effect on one hamster, but in a second hamster infusion of 1 ml over 16 h produced symptoms apparently similar to those of tick paralysis in this species, *i.e.* splayed-out hind legs and erect mobile tail. In two other hamsters treated similarly to the latter paralysis did not occur. A final hamster infused for 24 h died, but not due to paralysis (GREGSON, 1973).

As a further step in the search for the toxin, cross-circulation experiments were carried out between tick-paralyzed and normal marmots. Groups of 9—45 female *D. andersoni,* prefed for 5—6 days on sheep, were applied to 12 marmots. When paralysis occurred the circulation of each marmot was connected to that of a second, normal, marmot and the cross-perfusion maintained for $6^{1}/_{2}$—32 h. The muscle response to sciatic nerve stimulation was recorded in both animals. There was no indication that the toxin was transferred from the donor to cause paralysis in the recipient animal (GREGSON, 1973). In order to reduce possible loss of toxin by dilution and metabolism, tick-infested isolated ears of rabbits were substituted for donor tick-infested marmots. One day before the perfusion experiment, 15—25 ticks prefed for 5—6 days on another animal were applied to a rabbit ear *in situ*. The rabbit was killed and the infested ear perfused for 3—14 h by the recipient marmot. In three out of 11 marmots symptoms similar to those of tick paralysis occurred. However, after careful consideration, the author (Gregson, 1973) decided that despite these symptoms, the deaths could well have been due to a reaction to a foreign protein.

A series of isolated tissues were tested to attempt to identify the presence of the toxin of *D. andersoni*. Murnaghan (1955) immersed the isolated phrenic nerve-diaphragm preparation of the rat in heparinized plasma from a paralyzed dog but neuromuscular transmission was not affected over several hours. Lumbrical muscles with their nerves attached (Jenden et al., 1951) from a rabbit and a marmot gave no indication of the presence of a blocking agent over 4 h after the application of tick saliva. A salivary gland emulsion from ticks was applied to crayfish stretch receptors with negative results (Gregson, 1973). Immersion of the isolated sciatic-peroneal nerve of a normal dog for several hours in plasma from a tick-paralyzed dog failed to alter its conduction (Murnaghan, 1963, unpublished). However, as mentioned previously, conduction in nerves from normal and paralyzed dogs was similar when they were measured in the isolated state and were short. None of these tests would appear to be relevant because of the short duration of the test and of the nonsusceptibility of the test object or animal to tick paralysis in some cases.

In an attempt to determine whether the spleen or liver of the host animal played a significant role in the modification or detoxification of the tick toxin, ticks prefed on a sheep for five days were applied to 17 previously splenectomized and 15 splenectomized plus four-fifths hepatectomized marmots (Gregson, 1973). Each marmot was infested with five or 10 *D. andersoni*. When the marmots were infested with five prefed ticks paralysis occurred in five normal animals in 34 ± 5 h, in eight splenectomized animals in 34 ± 3.4 h, and in four splenectomized plus 4/5 hepatectomized animals in 27 ± 5.4 h. When 10 prefed ticks were applied paralysis occurred in nine splenectomized marmots in 26 ± 3.4 h and in nine splenectomized plus four-fifths hepatectomized marmots in 32.4 ± 5.7 h.

Attempts have been made to remove the toxin from the animal or tissue being studied. In two paralyzed dogs a Ringer solution preparation (Inperinol, Abbott) was run into the peritoneal cavity via a cannula with tubing and then replaced with approximately 100 ml of fresh warmed solution each hour. The first dog with a moderate degree of paralysis did not improve after nine hours, and died of respiratory failure. The second dog did not show much improvement after 5 h despite the removal of the ticks at the commencement of the peritoneal dialysis; it had recovered the next day but this apparently was not related to the dialysis treatment. In two other dogs suffering from severe paralysis where about 200 ml of fluid was exchanged per hour, death occurred in $2^1/_2$ and 3 h (Murnaghan, 1962, unpublished). Gregson (1973) reported the use of peritoneal dialysis in five paralyzed marmots, using Dupernal solution; 400—950 ml was exchanged every 1—2 h for 4—12 h. The body temperature of the animals decreased progressively and they died in 12 h without having shown any decrease in the degree of the paralysis.

In one moderately paralysed dog weighing 4.5 kg, 1,800 ml of warmed Ringer solution (Abbott) was given by intravenous drip over 2 h and 100 mg of chlorothiazide was incorporated in the infusion. Large amounts of urine were secreted but the degree of paralysis was not altered (MURNAGHAN, 1962, unpublished). In a paralyzed marmot 30 ml of an intravenous drip of mannitol-NaHCO$_3$-NaCl solution given over $1^1/_2$ h produced no beneficial effect, and the animal died 24 h later (GREGSON, 1973). These results suggest that the tick toxin cannot readily be removed by peritoneal dialysis or diuresis. During the removal of the sciatic-peroneal nerve in the dog for conduction studies it was thought that moistening the nerve with Ringer solution during removal to avoid dessication and its immersion in the bath of Ringer before recording conduction could have resulted in washing out the toxin and so account for the absence of difference in conduction between nerves from normal and paralyzed animals. This appeared not to be the case, however, as moistening the 'paralyzed nerve' with, and immersing it in, plasma from a normal or paralyzed dog made no difference to the result (MURNAGHAN and MacCONAILL, 1967).

There is some evidence to indicate that the toxin of *Ixodes holocyclus* is protein in nature if we accept that fraction 2 isolated by KAIRE (1966) is identical to the toxin from this species of tick. On the other hand, GREGSON (1973) failed to isolate a 'toxin' from *D. andersoni* when he prepared an extract in a similar manner to that used by KAIRE. However, if the toxin was not protein in nature it could have been discarded in the isolation of a protein fraction. This toxin might resemble tetrodotoxin because of the similar effects on nerve conduction. The fact that paralysis usually abates when *D. andersoni* is removed from the animal or man but often progresses even to a fatal outcome despite the removal of *Ixodes holocyclus*, as well as the lack of proof that conduction in motor nerve fibres is depressed in paralysis due to *Ixodes holocyclus*, suggests that the toxins differ in nature.

IV. Immunity

As has recently bee pointed out (BAGNALL and DOUBE, 1975) by M.D. MURRAY in Australia, immunity may mean immunity to the toxin of the tick or to the attachment and feeding of the ticks.

Of the two best known and commonest forms of tick paralysis, the toxin secreted by *I. holocyclus* in Australia readily induces immunity, whereas that produced by *D. andersoni* in the Pacific Northwest of North America does not do so. GREGSON (1973), in his recent review, discussed the evidence available concerning *D. andersoni*. Some of the data he produces had not previously been published and cover experimental work with man, rabbits and marmots. The marmot is especially sensitive and should prove to be a useful model. GREGSON (1973) also showed that work at Kamloops demonstrated that experimentally induced anaphylaxis does not produce the same symptoms as tick paralysis in marmots. It had been suggested that tick paralysis due to *D. andersoni* was an allergic response to tick feeding. It now seems certain that the cause of the paralysis is a toxin in the tick's saliva.

In Australia it has been established for some time (ROSS, 1935) that dogs become immune to tick paralysis and that the transfer of serum from an immune dog can protect another and can cure tick paralysis in both dogs and children. Canine immune serum is available from the Australian Commonwealth Serum Laboratories, Melbourne, and is regularly used to treat human cases in doses of 20–30 ml for small children and babies. C.B. Philip (Gregson, 1973) tried the anti-*holocyclus* serum in a case of *andersoni* tick paralysis at Hamilton, Montana. It was not effective.

It must be remembered that animals develop immunity to the saliva of the tick and that this may prevent the tick from completing its blood meal. This could produce the picture of immunity to the toxin although no such immunity might exist.

While for some decades past more work on the disease was carried out in North America than elsewhere the attendance of about 30 workers at a one-day workshop on the problem in Queensland augurs well for future reports from Australia (Bagnall and Doube, 1975).

V. Autopsy Findings

Pathological lesions involving neurons which could account for the symptoms and signs of the paralysis have not been clearly detectable. Dodd (1921) found no abnormal findings in the brain and spinal cord, apart from an abnormal quantity of cerebrospinal fluid in one case, in dogs paralyzed by *Ixodes holocyclus*. Ross (1926) studied sections of the cord and medulla stained by Nissle's haematoxylin and eosin method from dogs also paralyzed by *I. holocyclus*. He stated

"such sections showed congestion of both anterior and posterior horns and in some cases numerous capillary haemorrhages both into the adventitial sheath, and around the nerve cells, accompanied by excess of mononuclear cells, with some perivascular infiltration. Distinct neurophagia may be present. On the whole the nerve cells appear healthy and undistorted, though the borders of some were ill defined and others stained imperfectly".

Ferguson (1924) has described changes in the brain and spinal cord in a boy of 16 months (Auburn case) who died due to paralysis by *I. holocyclus*.

"All portions of the brain showed intense engorgement of the vessels with the presence of numerous small newly formed capillaries, in places diffuse infiltration with small round cells apparently plasma cells was noted; there were however no perivascular sheaths or cuffs of small round cells. Some of the vessels contained polymorphonuclear leucocytes. In the spinal cord similar congestion was present with some small haemorrhages".

Similarly, histological examination of the brain in animals dying from Karoo paralysis due to *Ixodes rubicundus* showed localized hyperaemia and focal hae-morrhages (Arthur, 1962). In two cases of paralysis in sheep due to *D. andersoni* the coverings of the brain were congested and a fibrinous exudate was present in the ventricles in one of the animals (Hadwen, 1913). Murnaghan (1958a) reported that no pathological changes could be detected in the anterior horn cells but that the terminal boutons appeared to be enlarged in the lumbar region of the spinal cord in two dogs paralyzed with *D. andersoni*.

Gothe et al. (1971) could detect no lesion in the parenchyma of peripheral nerve fibres in fowl paralyzed by *Argas (Persicargas) persicus*. In contradistinction to these minimal pathological findings Regendanz and Reichenow (1931) showed that the injection of an emulsion of a large number of eggs of *Rhipicephalus sanguineus* and *Dermacentor reticulatus* into dogs caused extensive degeneration

(Marchi staining) in all parts of the spinal cord. However it is doubtful whether the effects of this ixovotoxin are identical to that produced by the toxin secreted by the salivary glands of the tick.

F. Summary

While the first reference to the condition of tick paralysis is attributed to WILLIAM HOVELL in 1824 in Australia, subsequent reports in the latter half of that century refer to paralysis in livestock and other animals on that continent and in South Africa. Although BANCROFT in 1884 referred to cases in humans in Australia, the first description of the disease in man was published in 1912 by CLELAND in Australia, TODD in British Columbia, Canada and TEMPLE in the United States of America. Subsequently paralysis by ticks in animals and occasionally in humans has been reported also from other countries.

Most cases of tick paralysis are due to the hard ticks, *Ixodidae,* belonging to the subfamilies *Ixodinae, Amblyomminae* and *Rhipicephalinae,* and are restricted not only to certain genera but also to a limited number of species. The great majority of cases of tick paralysis, particularly in humans, are due to *Dermacentor andersoni* Stiles and to a lesser extent *Dermacentor variabilis* Say on the north American continent and to *Ixodes holocyclus* Neumann in Australia. Most of our knowledge about tick paralysis is due to case reports and experimental studies involving these species of ticks. Reference however is made in this report to the soft argasid ticks, although they differ considerably from the *Ixodidae,* because recent studies of paralysis in fowl with the argasid ticks indicate that there is a similarity in the type of paralysis produced by both types.

The Ixodid tick attaches to its host by cutting into the epidermis with its chelicerae, which are armed with cutting teeth; some genera also secrete a cement from their salivary glands which aids fixing the mouth parts to the skin. Blood is sucked into the oral cavity by the suction action of the pharynx. The salivary gland secretion usually contains antigenic material which may produce allergic reactions in the host and may contain an anticoagulant substance. Because of the characteristics of the paralysis produced in the host the saliva is thought to contain a toxin which acts on neurons.

Virulence of the tick to induce paralysis is dependent not only on the species of tick, but also on the type of host and whether immunity develops to the secretion of the tick. The most virulent species of tick are *I. holocyclus* and *D. andersoni.* Livestock, dogs and humans are the most susceptible hosts. While immunity has been shown to develop in dogs, cattle and particularly in cats to *I. holocyclus* it does not readily occur to *D. andersoni,* except probably in hamsters. Failure of a tick to engorge adequately because of host immunity to its saliva will give rise to an apparent reduction in virulence. Studies on tick virulence in hamsters indicates that ticks reared from selected paralyzing females are more virulent, so that further selection might increase their potency. There is apparently no intrinsic and inheritable susceptibility to tick paralysis.

Tick paralysis in humans occurs on the North American continent, in Australia and South Africa, and occasionally in Europe and Asia. By far the greatest number of cases in North America have been due to *D. andersoni* Stiles; about three-quarters of the approximately 420 recorded have been in southern British Columbia, Canada, the remainder being in the north-western Rocky mountain states in the U.S.A. Approximately 45 cases due to *D. variablis* Say have been reported in the literature from the southeastern United States, particularly in the states along the Atlantic seaboard. *Amblyomma maculatum* and *A. americanum* have occasionally caused paralysis in states bordering the Gulf of Mexico. Paralysis in Australia is due to *Ixodes holocyclus* Neumann and is confined to the eastern coastal areas. Most of the cases in humans in South Africa have consisted of localized paresis; the ticks responsible were *I. rubicundus, Rhipicephalus simus* Koch, *Hyalomma transiens* and *H. truncatum.*

Paralysis occurs only occasionally in wild animals which appear to be naturally resistant to the disease. Animals which have been affected in North America have been deer, buffalo, a bear cub, a fox and birds, in Australia bandicoots (*Peramales* spp.) and a crow, and in South Africa the rhebuck. Experimental paralysis has been produced with *D. andersoni* in marmots, a coyote, a skunk, ground squirrels and pack rats.

Paralyses in livestock in British Columbia and the north western United States is due to *Dermacentor andersoni,* in California to *Dermacentor occidentalis,* in Australia to *Ixodes holocyclus,* in South Africa to *Ixodes rubicundus, Hyalomma truncatum* and *Rhipicephalus evertsi,* and in Europe to *Hyalomma aegyptum, Ixodes ricinus, Ixodes crenulatus* and representatives of the genera *Dermacentor, Rhipicephalus* and *Boophilus.*

Pets have been frequently affected. Dogs have been paralyzed by *D. andersoni* in British Columbia and in the northwestern United States and by *D. variablis* in the southeastern United States. Paralysis in dogs in Australia is due to *I. holocyclus.* Rarely, cases in dogs due to *Rhipicephalus sanguineus* have been reported in Florida and Venezuela, to *I. scapularis* in Florida, *I. tancitarius* in Mexico, *Amblyomma maculatum* in Uruguay, *I. rubicundus, Rhipicephalus evertsi, Rhipicentor nuttalli* and *Hyalomma transiens* in South Africa and *I. ricinus* and *Haemaphysalis puctata* in Crete. Paralysis can be induced experimentally in a high proportion of dogs when infested with *D. andersoni;* they are a very suitable test animal for investigations into the mechanism of tick paralysis. Cats are highly resistant to paralysis. Paralysis by *D. andersoni* has been induced experimentally in hamsters, guinea-pigs, marmots and a monkey.

Tick paralysis in animals and humans usually presents itself as an ascending paralysis involving the lower motor neurons, which commences after the tick has been feeding for 5—6 days and gradually increases in severity. Starting in the lower limbs, the flaccid paralysis spreads to involve the trunk and upper limbs and finally the head and neck; death is due to paralysis of the respiratory muscles. Occasionally in humans the paralysis may be limited to a localized part of the body in the vicinity of the attachment of the tick; localized paraesthesias are also often present.

Tick paralysis due to *D. andersoni* has been shown to be due to a presynaptic involvement of the neuromuscular junction. Post-synaptic involvement has been excluded because the paralysis is not similar to that due to a competitive inhibitor or depolarizing blocking agent or an overdose of an anticholinesterase substance. Furthermore, the end-plates respond to acetylcholine but neither action nor end-plate potentials can be detected in a fully paralyzed muscle when the nerve is stimulated, indicating that there is a failure in the liberation of acetylcholine at the neuromuscular junction. This was confirmed by showing that excess acetylcholine is released into the eserinized-Ringer perfusate of the isolated anterior tibial muscle during stimulation of a peroneal nerve from a normal dog but not of a peroneal nerve from a completely paralyzed one. This absence in the liberation of acetylcholine is not due to failure in synthesis or storage, or to the absence of release factors; choline and choline acetylase are present in adequate amounts in the nerves, and choline and acetylcoenzyme A fail to overcome the paralysis; the stores of acetylcholine within the nerves are within normal limits, and a high-potassium Ringer solution releases large amounts of acetylcholine from the isolated perfused paralyzed anterior tibial muscle; and excess calcium and carbon dioxide and the injection of plasma from a normal dog failed to overcome the paralysis. This failure in the liberation of acetylcholine at the neuromuscular junction has been demonstrated to be due to a disturbance in conduction in nerve fibres in the paralyzed dog, the fastest-conducting fibres apparently being least affected. This block in conduction involves the small-diameter terminal motor nerve fibres to their extremity because direct electrical stimulation of the perfused anterior tibial muscle fails to release acetylcholine into the perfusate. However, the block in conduction does not appear to spread centripetally up along the parent fibre from the terminal fibres, but rather involves the whole fibre from its inception. Due to the probably varying sensitivity of the nodes of Ranvier to the tick toxin and the random distribution of those affected, the longer the nerve fibre the greater the likelihood of the nerve impulse meeting a depressed node and the greater the number of fibres to show a block in conduction. Although the study showed that a small population of very fast-conducting fibres appear to be least affected, the fact that slowing in conduction occurs in efferent fibres when studied in the whole nerve suggests that the faster of the slower-conducting motor fibres may be involved earlier, which would account for the apparent discrepancy in the results in conduction between those obtained with adult *D. andersoni* and *Argas (Persicargas) persicus* larvae. Consequently the mechanism of the paralysis due to both of these species of ticks appears to be similar.

While a disturbance of conduction in peripheral motor nerve fibres resulting in inadequate neuromuscular transmission would account for the paralysis, some workers have suggested that inadequate transmission in the central neurons may contribute towards the paralysis induced by *D. andersoni,* because in moderate paralysis in marmots the stretch reflex was abolished while neuromuscular transmission was only slightly reduced and in humans ataxia in the absence of muscular weakness may be noted. Paralysis due to *I. holocyclus* is probably due to a disturbance in central nervous transmission.

Attempts to show that the toxin of *D. andersoni* is circulating in the blood and consequently to demonstrate its transfer from a paralyzed marmot to a non-paralyzed one or from a rabbit tick-infested ear to a normal marmot by cross-circulation experiments have not been successful. Furthermore, the use of isolated tissues, *e.g.* nerve-muscle preparation etc. for the demonstration of the presence of the tick toxin have failed, probably because of the inadequate period of exposure to fluid containing the toxin, *i.e.* plasma, salivary secretion etc. Our knowledge about the fate of the toxin in the body is sparse. Apparently the toxin of *D. andersoni* is destroyed neither by the liver nor by the spleen and it is not readily removed from the body by a marked diuresis or by peritoneal dialysis.

The results of attempts at the identification of the tick toxin remain equivocal. The claims of some authors that extracts of emulsified tick eggs and salivary glands produce effects similar to tick paralysis are questionable; they are more probably due to the injection of a foreign protein. The findings obtained by infusing large amounts of tick saliva into a small susceptible animal such as a hamster, where paralysis probably occurred in one out of four trials, suggest that this method merits further investigation. The isolation procedures used by Kaire (1966) suggests that the toxin of *I. holocyclus* is protein in nature; Gregson's (1973) failure to isolate the toxin from *D. andersoni* by the same isolation method suggests that the toxin in this species may not be a protein. The development of immunity to *I. holocyclus* but not to *D. andersoni* appears to confirm this. Indeed, because of the effect of *D. andersoni* toxin on nerve conduction it may resemble tetrodotoxin in some respects. Furthermore, the fact that early removal of *I. holocyclus* may not prevent the progression in the degree of paralysis but usually does so with *D. andersoni* suggests that the toxin of the former fixes more firmly to the tissue.

The absence in post-mortem material of characteristic neuropathological lesions apart from some congestion in the central nervous system and the transitory nature of the disease suggest that the lesion produced by the tick toxin is a functional (biochemical) rather than a structural one.

Addendum: B.J. Cooper and I. Spence (Temperature-dependent inhibition of evoked acetylcholine release in tick paralysis. Nature 263, 693–695, 1976) have shown that when the hemidiaphragm of mice paralysed with 10 nymphal Ixodes holocyclus is stimulated through its phrenic nerve that it contracts and end-plate potentials can be recorded at low temperatures but not when above 30° C. They suggest that the toxin blocks the intermediate step between depolarization and release of acetylcholine because they recorded normal action potentials from the phrenic nerve. However the studies on isolated nerve mentioned on page 446 in the text suggest that a reduction in amplitude of the action potential would not be expected over such a short stretch of nerve from a paralysed animal.

References

Abbott, K.H.: Tick-borne diseases (with particular reference to tick paralysis). Dis. nerv. Syst. **5**, 19—21 (1944).

Adler, K.: Tick paralysis. Canad. med. Ass. J. **94**, 550—551 (1966).

Alexander, R.M.: Tick paralysis: report of a case in Florida. J. Amer. med. Ass. **149**, 931—932 (1952).

Allen, J.R.: Tick resistance: basophils in skin reactions of resistant guinea pigs. Int. J. Parasitol. **3**, 195—200 (1973).

Amesse, J.W., Lyday, J.H.: Tick paralysis in Colorado. Rocky Mountain med. J. **36**, 640—641 (1939).

Anderson Stuart, T.P.: Poison of the Australian Bush-tick. Part of Presidential address Roy. Soc. New South Wales. J. roy. Soc. N.S.W. **28**, 10—12 (1894).

Arthur, D.R.: Ticks and Disease. Oxford, London, New York, Paris: Pergamon 1962.

Bagnall, B.G., Doube, B.M.: The Australian paralysis tick *Ixodes holocyclus*. Aust. vet. J. **51**, 159—160 (1975).

Balabekian, T.P.: Tick paralysis in foals. Veterinariya (Moscow) **31**, 44 (1954).

Balashov, Y.S.: Blood sucking ticks (Ixodoidea): vectors of diseases to man and animals (English translation). Mix. Pub. Ent. Soc. Amer. **8**, 161—376 (1968).

Bancroft, J.: Queensland ticks and tick blindness. Aust. med. Gaz. **4**, 37—38 (1884).

Barnett, E.J.: Wood tick paralysis in children. J. Amer. med. Ass. **109**, 846—848 (1937).

Bashinsky, L.M., Little, S.C.: Tick paralysis, discussion and case report. J. med. Ass. Alabama **18**, 276—278 (1949).

Bassoe, P.: Paralysis of ascending type in an adult due to a bite of a wood tick. Arch. Neurol. Psychiat. (Chicago) **11**, 564—567 (1924).

Beach, M.W., Ravenel, B.O.: Tick paralysis in South Carolina. J. Sth. Carolina med. Ass. **37**, 323—325 (1941).

Beato Gonzalez, F.: Paralysis in man due to tick bite, with report of cases. Med. colon. Madrid **9**, 235—258 (1947).

Ben-Bassat, Y.: Paralysis due to tick bite. Harefuah **63**, 134—135 (1962).

Blanc, G., Caminopetros, J.: La tick paralysis observée sur les moutons de la region di Sitra (Crete). Bull. Soc. Pathol. exot. **27**, 378—380 (1924).

Bloxsom, A., Chandler, A.C.: Transient paralysis due to bite of American dog tick (*Dermacentor variablis* Say). Amer. J. Dis. Childh. **67**, 126—127 (1944).

Bootes, B.W.: A fatal paralysis in foals from *Ixodes holòcyclus* Neumann infestations. Aust. vet. J. **38**, 68—69 (1962).

Borthwick, J.D.: Tick paralysis affecting sheep and lambs. Vet. J. (London) **12**, 33—35 (1905).

Boudin, G., Vernant, J.C., Lanoé, Y., Vojir.: Les paralysies par morsure de tiques: arbovirose ou origine toxinique? Ann. Méd. interne (Paris) **125**, 55—60 (1974).

Bow, M.R., Brown, J.H.: Tick-borne disease of man in Alberta (including tick paralysis). Canad. med. Ass. J. **53**, 459—465 (1945).

Brown, G.L.: The preparation of the tibialis anterior (cat) for close-arterial injections. J. Physiol. **92**, 22P—23P (1938).

Brown, J.H.: Tick paralysis: a note on a human case caused by a male tick. J. Econ. Entomol. **45**, 737—738 (1952).

Bruce, E.A.: Tick paralysis. J. Amer. vet. med. Ass. **68**, 147—161 (1925).

Brumpt, E.: Paralysis produced experimentally in a dog by the bite of the Australian tick, *Ixodes holocyclus*. C.R. Acad. Sci. Paris **197**, 1358—1361 (1933).

Brunetti, O.A.: Tick paralysis in California deer. Calif. Fish and Game **51**, 208—210 (1965).

Burns, B.D., Paton, W.D.M.: Depolarization of the motor end-plate by decamethonium and acetylcholine. J. Physiol. **115**, 41—73 (1951).

Cherington, M., Snyder, R.D.: Tick paralysis: neurophysiologic studies. New Engl. J. Med. **278**, 95—97 (1968).

Chesney, J.: Paralysis due to the bite of a tick. J. Tenness. med. Ass. **48**, 77—80 (1955).

Clark, R.: Note on paralysis in lambs caused apparently by *Rhipicephalus evertsi*. J.S. Afr. vet. med. Ass. **9**, 143—145 (1938).

Cleland, J.B.: Injuries and diseases of man in Australia attributable to animals. Aust. med. Gaz. **32**, 295—299 (1912).

Coggins, R.P., Derivaux, J.H.: Tick paralysis. J. med. Ass. Georgia. **41**, 136—137 (1952).

Coons, L.B., Roshdy, M.A.: Fine structure of the salivary glands of unfed male *Dermacentor variabilis* (Say). J. Parasitol. **59**, 900—912 (1973).

Cornwall, J.W., Patten, W.S.: Some observations on the salivary secretion of the commoner blood sucking insects and ticks. Indian J. med. Res. **2**, 569—593 (1914).

Costa, J.A.: Tick paralysis on the Atlantic seaboard. Amer. J. Dis. Childh. **83**, 336—347 (1952).

Crossle, F.C.: Facial paralysis following tick bite. Med. J. Aust. **2**, 764 (1932).

Cvjetanovic, U.: On the species, distribution and seasonal incidence of ticks in Dalmatia with the reference to the occurence of tick paralysis. Veterinaria (Sarajevo) **5**, 589—595 (1956).

Davidson, W.B.: The Rocky Mountain wood tick and tick borne diseases. Canad. J. Comp. med. vet. Sci. **5**, 123—137 (1941).

Dawson, K.E., Sherman, A.J., La Broccetta, A.C.: Tick paralysis; case in Philadelphia. Amer. J. Dis. Childh. **79**, 491—494 (1950).

De Meillon, B.: A toxin from the eggs of South African ticks. S. Afr. J. med. Sci. **7**, 226—235 (1942).

De Sanctis, A.G., di Sant'Agnese, P.A.: Tick paralysis (Report of a case in New York). J. Amer. med. Ass. **122**, 86—88 (1943).

Desmedt, J.E.: Myasthenic-like features of neuromuscular transmission after administration of an inhibitor of acetylcholine synthesis. Nature (Lond.) **192**, 1673—1674 (1958).

Dodd, S.: Tick paralysis. Agric. Gaz. N.S.W. Misc. Publ. **2**, 342: 1—15 (1921).

Donovan, W.B., Feldman, D.: Tick paralysis. Marquette med. Rev. **26**, 8—10 (1960).
Doube, B.M., Kemp, D.H.: Paralysis of cattle by *Ixodes holocyclus* Neumann. Aust. J. agric. Res. **26**, 635—640 (1975).
Eaton, E.M.: A case of tick-bite followed by widespread transitory muscular paralysis. Aust. med. Gaz. **33**, 391 (1913).
Emminger, A.C.: Tick paralysis in cattle—case report. Calif. Vet. **5**, 26 (1951).
Emmons, P., McLennan, H.: Failure of acetylcholine release in tick paralysis. Nature (Lond.) **183**, 474—475 (1959).
Emmons, P., McLennan, H.: Some observations on tick paralysis in marmots. J. exp. Biol. **37**, 355—362 (1960).
Erasmus, L.D.: Regional tick paralysis. S. Afr. med. J. **26**, 985—987 (1952).
Esplin, D.W., Philip, C.B., Hughes, L.E.: Impairment of muscle stretch reflexes in tick paralysis. Science (Washington) **132**, 958—959 (1960).
Evans, G.O., Sheals, J.G., Macfarlane, D.: The terrestrial acari of the British Isles, Vol. 1. London: British Museum (Natural History) 1961.
Ferguson, E.W.: A case of tick paralysis. Med. J. Aust. **2**, 346—348 (1924).
Foster, B.: A tick in the auditory meatus. Med. J. Aust. **1**, 15 (1931).
Garin, M.M., Bujadoux, O.: Un cas de tick paralysis. Lyon Med. **132**, 160 (1923).
Gibbes, J.H.: Tick paralysis in South Carolina. J. Amer. med. Ass. **111**, 1008—1009 (1938).
Gothe, R., Hager, H., Jehn, E., Kunze, K., Thoenes, W.: Pathologisch-anatomische Untersuchungen an peripheren Nerven bei der durch *Argas* (*Persicargas*) *persicus*-Larven bedingten Zeckenparalyse der Hühner. Z. Tropenmed. Parasitol. **22**, 285—291 (1971).
Gothe, R., Kunze, K.: Zu Erregungsleitungen von efferenten und afferenten peripheren Nervenfasern bei der durch *Argas* (*Persicargas*) *persicus*-Larven bedingten Zeckenparalyse der Hühner. Z. Tropenmed. Parasitol. **2**, 292—296 (1971).
Gothe, R., Kunze, K.: Neuropharmacological investigations on tick paralysis of chickens induced by larvae of *Argas* (*Persicargas*) Walkerae. In: Parasitic Zoonoses; Clinical and Experimental Studies (Ed. E.S. Soulshy.) London: Academic 1974, pp. 369—382.
Gregson, J.D.: The enigma of tick paralysis. Proc. Entomol. Soc. Brit. Columbia **40**, 19—23 (1943).
Gregson, J.D.: The influence of fertility on the feeding rate of the female of the wood tick, *Dermacentor andersoni* Stiles. Rep. Entomol. Soc. Ontario **74**, 46—47 (1944).
Gregson, J.D.: Further studies on tick paralysis. Proc. Entomol. Soc. Brit. Columbia **48**, 54—59 (1952).
Gregson, J.D.: Experiments on oral secretion of the Rocky Mountain wood tick *Dermacentor andersoni* Stiles. Canad. Entomol. **89**, 1—5 (1957).
Gregson, J.D.: Records of tick paralysis in livestock in British Columbia. Proc. Entomol. Soc. Brit. Columbia **63**, 13—18 (1966).
Gregson, J.D.: Tick paralysis: an appraisal of natural and experimental data. Canad. Dept. Agric. Monogr. 9, (1973).
Hadwen, S.: On tick paralysis in sheep and man following the bite of *D. venustus*. Parasitology **6**, 283—297 (1913).
Hadwen, S., Nuttall, G.H.F.: Experimental "tick paralysis" in the dog. Parasitology **6**, 298—301 (1913).
Hamilton, D.G.: Tick paralysis: a dangerous disease in children. Med. J. Aust. **1**, 759—765 (1940).
Harper, A.: Tick paralysis—report of a case in Florida. J. med. Ass. Georgia **31**, 442 (1942).
Heidt, J.H.: A report on a case of tick paralysis in Dade county, Florida. Florida Entomologist **27**, 149—150 (1954).
Henderson, F.W.: Tick paralysis: report of a case in Florida. J. Amer. med. Ass. **175**, 615—617 (1961).
Hindmarsh, W.L., Purcell, R.T.: Tick paralysis in dogs. Mortality after serum treatment. Aust. vet. J. **11**, 229—234 (1935).
Hoeppli, R., Feng, L.C.: Experimental studies on ticks. Chinese med. J. (Peking) **47**, 29—43 (1933).
Hoffmann, A.: Un caso de parálisis por picadura de garrapata. Rev. Latino Amer. Microbiol. Parasitol. **11**, 75—77 (1969).

Hoogstraal, H.: Human infestation by ticks (Ixodidae) in the Himalaya. In: Commemorative volume for H.D. Srivastava. Cairo, U.A.R.: U.S. Naval Med. Res. Unit 3 1970, pp. 75−89.

Hoogstraal, H.: Acarina (Ticks) in viruses and invertebrates (Ed. A.J. Gibbs. North Holland 1973.

Hopkyns, J.: Wood tick paralysis. Alberta med. Bull. **18**, 40−41 (1953).

Hughes, L.E., Philip, C.B.: Experimental tick paralysis in laboratory animals and native rodents. Proc. Soc. exp. Biol. Med. **99**, 316−319 (1958).

Jaffe, E., Perlmutter, I.: Tick paralysis (successfully treated in the stage of ataxia). J. Pediat. **45**, 98−100 (1954).

Jeffrey, C.W.: Tick toxemia. Colorado Medicine **26**, 326 (1929).

Jellison, W., Gregson, J.D.: Tick paralysis in northwestern United States and British Columbia. Rocky Mountain med. J. **47**, 28−32 (1950).

Jellison, W.L., Stoenner, H.G., Kramis, N.J., Beardmore, H.F.: An outbreak of tick paralysis in cattle in western Montana. Vet. Med. **46**, 163−166 (1951).

Jenden, D.J., Kamijo, K., Taylor, D.B.: The rabbit lumbrical: a new isolated mammalian nerve-muscle preparation. Nature (Lond.) **168**, 880−881 (1951).

Juravlev, M.S.: Tick paralysis in sheep caused by *Ornithodorus lahorensis*. Sovyet. Med. **5**, 78−82 (1936).

Kaire, G.H.: Isolation of tick paralysis toxin from *Ixodes holocyclus*. Toxicon **4**, 91−97 (1966).

Kittrell, B.M.: Tick paralysis; a case. J. Amer. med. Ass. **147**, 1561−1562 (1951).

KMR (Kamloops Monthly Report): Reports of data and experiments by personnel of the Veterinary-Medical Entomology Section, Research Station, C.D.S., Kamloops, B.C., 1956, 1957.

Knott, S.G.: Scrub tick paralysis. Queensland agric. J. **87**, 41−46 (1961).

Knott, S.G.: Scrub tick paralysis in farm animals. Queensland agric. J. **94**, 470−474 (1968).

Kohls, G.M., Kramis, N.J.: Tick paralysis in the American buffalo, *Bison bison* (Linn.). Northwest Sci. **26**, 61−64 (1952).

Kunze, K., Gothe, R.: Die durch *Argas* (*Persicargas*) *persicus* Larven bedingte Paralyse der Hühner. III. Neurophysiologische Untersuchungen. Z. Parasit. Kunde **36**, 251−264 (1971).

Kurtpinar, H.: Türkiye kene felci (Tick paralysis) üzerinde arastirmalar. Turk. Vet. Hek. Derm. Derg. **39**, 737−745 (1960)

Lagos, J.C., Thies, R.E.: Tick paralysis without muscle weakness. Arch. Neurol. **21**, 471−474 (1969).

Lechevailer, B., Houtteville, J.P., Beet, J.N.: Ocular paralysis after tick sting of the lower eye lid (Correspondence). Nouvelle Presse méd. **3**, 456 (1974)

Leclercq, M.: Entomological parasitology. The relations between entomology and the medical sciences. Oxford: Pergamon 1969.

Loomis, E.C., Bushnell, R.B.: Tick paralysis in California livestock. Amer. J. Vet. Res. **29**, 1089−1093 (1968).

MacIntosh, F.C.: Formation, storage, and release of acetylcholine at nerve endings. Canad. J. Biochem. Physiol. **37**, 343−356 (1959).

Mail, G.A., Gregson, J.D.: Tick paralysis in British Columbia. Canad. med. Ass. J. **39**, 532−537 (1938).

Mally, C.W.: Notes on the so-called paralysis tick *Ixodes pilolus*. Agr. J. Cape Good Hope **25**, 291−296 (1904).

Mamikonjan, M.M.: Les tiques *Ornithodorus lahorensis* et la paralyse du mouton provoquée par cette tique. XXVᵉ Plenum de la Section Vétérinaire d'Agriculture en U.R.S.S., 1946, p. 18.

Markwardt, F.: Blutgerinnungshemmende Wirkstoffe aus blutsaugenden Tieren. Jena: Fisher 1963, pp. 88−92.

Martin, R.: Pathogenesis of ascending paralysis due to ticks. Arch. Inst. Pasteur d'Algérie **22**, 125−130 (1944).

Marsh, H.: Some obscure diseases of sheep; tick paralysis. J. Amer. vet. med. Ass. **74**, 724−735 (1929).

Mason, J., Kemp, D.H., King, S.J.: *Ixodes cornuatus* and tick paralysis. Aust. vet. J. **50**, 580 (1974).

McCaffrey, D.: Effect of tick bites on man. J. Parasitology **2**, 193–194 (1916).

McCornack, P.D.: Paralysis in children due to the bite of wood ticks. J. Amer. med. Ass. **77**, 260–263 (1921).

McCue, C.M., Stone, J.B., Sutton, L.E., Jr.: Tick paralysis; 3 cases of tick (*Dermacentor variabilis* Say) paralysis in Virginia with summary of all cases reported in Eastern United States. Pediatrics **1**, 174–180 (1948).

McDermott, A.E.: Tick paralysis. Report of a case. Missouri Med. J. **54**, 1054 (1957).

McKay, W.J.S.: Facial paralysis following tick bite. Med. J. Aust. **1**, 204 (1933).

Mehta, M.L., Shah, H.L.: Tick paralysis due to *Argas persicus* in the fowl. Indian vet. J. **48**, 204–206 (1971).

Meredith, J., Kaufman, W.R.: A proposed site of fluid secretion in the salivary gland of the Ixodid tick *Dermacentor andersoni*. Parasitology **67**, 205–217 (1973).

Mikailov, M.: Incidence of *Ornithodorus lahorensis* and tick paralysis in Bitola, Yugoslavia. Vet. Glasn. **2**, 814–818 (1954).

Mlinac, F., Oswald, B.: Preliminary studies on the poisonous properties of the species of ticks occurring in Yugoslavia. Yugosl. Vet. Glasn. **16**, 415–421 (1936); (Rev. Appl. Entomol. B, **24**, 246 (1936).

Moilliet, T.K.: A review of tick paralysis in cattle in British Columbia with notes on several new cases. Proc. Soc. Entomol. Brit. Columbia **33**, 35–39 (1937).

Moorhouse, D.E.: The attachment of some Ixodid ticks to their natural hosts. 2nd International Congress on Acarology, 1967. Budapest: Akademiai Kiado 1969.

Moss, H.St. Leger.: A case of tick paralysis. Med. J. Aust. **2**, 556 (1924).

Mulherin, P.A.: Ataxia due to bite of American dog tick (*Dermacentor variablis* Say). J. Pediat. **16**, 86–88 (1940).

Murnaghan, M.F.: Tick Paralysis. Rev. Canad. Biol. **14**, 273–274 (1955).

Murnaghan, M.F.: Neuroanatomical site of tick paralysis. Rev. Canad. Biol. **15**, 270–271 (1957).

Murnaghan, M.F.: Tick Paralysis in the dog: a neurophysiological study. 10th Internat. Cong. Entomology, Montreal, August 1956. Proceedings, Vol. 3, pp. 841–847. 1958a.

Murnaghan, M.F.: Neuroanatomical site in tick paralysis. Nature (Lond.) **181**, 131 (1958b).

Murnaghan, M.F.: The morphinized eserinized leech muscle in the assay of acetylcholine. Nature (Lond.) **182**, 317 (1958c).

Murnaghan, M.F.: A defect in the release mechanism of acetylcholine caused by tick paralysis. Proc. Canad. Fed. Biol. Soc. **2**, 48–49 (1959).

Murnaghan, M.F.: Site and mechanism of tick paralysis. Science (Washington) **131**, 418–419 (1960a).

Murnaghan, M.F.: Conduction block of terminal somatic motor nerve fibres in tick paralysis. Canad. J. Biochem. Physiol. **38**, 287–295 (1960b).

Murnaghan, M.F.: Motor nerve fibre conduction in tick paralysis. Fed. Proc. **19**, 298 (1960c).

Murnaghan, M.F.: Nerve fibre conduction block in tick paralysis. Rev. Canad. Biol. **20**, 19–24 (1961).

Murnaghan, M.F., MacConaill, M.: Peroneal nerve conduction in tick paralysis. Irish J. Med. Sci. 6th Series **502**, 473–477 (1967).

Muth, O.H.: Tick paralysis in beef cattle due to *Dermacentor andersoni*. North Amer. Vet. **26**, 668 (1945).

Neitz, W.O.: The different forms of tick toxicosis: a review. 2nd meeting FAO/OIE expert panel of tick-borne diseases of livestock. Cairo, U.A.R.: FAO/OIE 1962 (Dec. Working paper No. 2).

Nuttall, G.H.F., Strickland, C.: On the presence of an anticoagulin in the salivary glands and the intestine of *Argas persicus*. Parasitology **1**, 302–310 (1908).

O'Rourke, F., Murnaghan, M.F.: Tick paralysis in the dog. Nature (Lond.) **173**, 131 (1954).

Oswald, B.: Review of work published in Yugoslavia on the tick problem and research on toxins in the eggs of ticks. Ann. Parasitol. Hum. Comp. **16**, 548–559 (1938).

Paffenbargar, R.S.: Tick paralysis: implicating *Amblyomma maculatum*. New Orleans Med. Surg. J. **103**, 329–332 (1951).

Pavlov, P.: Research on "Tick Paralysis" observed in chickens in Bulgaria and caused by nymphs of *Haemaphysalis punctata* Can. and Franz. Ann. Parasitol. Hum. Comp. **38**, 459–461 (1963).

Pavlov, P., Miljowski, K.: Investigations on tick paralysis in Bulgaria. Dtsch. Österr. Tierärztl. Wschr. **50**, 529–542 (1942).

Peacock, P.B.: Tick paralysis or polio-myelitis. S. Afr. med. J. **32**, 201–202 (1958).

Pearn, J.H.: A case of tick paralysis with myocarditis. Med. J. Aust. **53**, 629–630 (1966).

Perry, W.J., Ragland, R.B.: Tick paralysis: Report of 2 cases in North Carolina. North Carolina med. J. **10**, 133–136 (1949).

Phillips, P., Murphy, M.A.: Tick paralysis. Canad. med. Ass. J. **63**, 38–39 (1950).

Pomerantzev, B.I.: Fauna of the U.S.S.R. Arachnida. Akad. Sci. USSR **4**, 1–224 (1950).

Posternak, J., Arnold, E.: Action de l'anélectrotonus et d'une solution hypersodique sur la conduction dans un nerf narcotisé. J. Physiol. (Paris) **46**, 502–505 (1954).

Prince, G.E., Keeley, J.C., Scott, E.P.: Tick paralysis in children. J. Pediat. **28**, 597–601 (1946).

Ranby, P.D.: Scrub tick paralysis in a crow. Queensland agric. J. **86**, 28 (1960).

Randolph, M.F.: Tick paralysis: Clin. Proc. Child. Hosp. **3**, 278–282 (1947).

Ransmeier, J.C.: Tick paralysis in Eastern United States: summary with report of 4 new cases from Georgia. J. Pediat. **34**, 299–308 (1949).

Regendanz, P., Reichenow, E.: Über Zeckengift und Zeckenparalyse. Arch. Schiff. Trop. Hyg. **35**, 255–273 (1931).

Reid, E.M., Marbach, W.: The paralysis tick (on dog and cat – Ed.), 2nd ed. Sydney: N.S.W. Dept. Agric. 1961, p. 9.

Renuart, A.W., De Maria, W.J.A.: Tick paralysis. A report of eight cases. Medical Times **89**, 1010–1016 (1961).

Rice, D.B.: Botulism and tick paralysis. J. Pediat. **34**, 716–719 (1949).

Rich, G.B.: Disease transmittance by the Rocky Mountain wood tick *Dermacentor andersoni* Stiles, with particular reference to tick paralysis in Canada. Vet. med. Rev. No. 1, 3–26 (1971).

Riek, R.F.: Studies on the reactions of animals to infestation with ticks. Aust. J. agric. Res. **8**, 215–223 (1957).

Roberts, F.H.S.: Tick paralysis in South Australia. Aust. Vet. J. **37**, 440 (1961).

Robinow, H., Carroll, T.B.: Tick paralysis due to bite of American dog tick; case observed in Georgia. J. Amer. med. Ass. **111**, 1093–1094 (1938).

Roddey, O.F., McAlister, J.C.: Tick paralysis – a report of a case. North Carolina med. J. **23**, 295–296 (1962).

Rose, I.: A review of tick paralysis. Canad. med. Ass. J. **70**, 175–176 (1954).

Rose, I., Gregson, J.D.: Evidence of a neuromuscular block in tick paralysis. Nature (Lond.) **178**, 95–96 (1956).

Ross, I.C.: An experimental study of tick paralysis in Australia. Parasitology **18**, 410–429 (1926).

Ross, I.C.: Tick paralysis in the dog. Aust. Vet. J. **10**, 182–183 (1934).

Ross, I.C.: A fatal disease of dogs and other animals in eastern Australia. J. Coun. scient. ind. Res. Aust. **8**, 8–13 (1935).

Ryan, C.P., Canning, H.B.: Paralysis resulting from infestation with *Dermacentor andersoni* of Stiles, common Rocky Mountain wood tick. J. South Carolina med. Ass. **40**, 229 (1944).

Sabbatini, L.: Fermento Anticoagulante dell'*Ixodes ricinus*. Arch. Ital. Biol. Turin. **31**, 37–53 (1898).

Sant'Anna, J.F.: On a disease in man following tick-bites and occurring in Lorenço Marquez. Parasitology **4**, 87–88 (1911).

Schmitt, N., Bowmer, E.J., Gregson, J.D.: Tick paralysis in British Columbia. Canad. med. Ass. J. **100**, 417–421 (1969).

Scott, E.: Hume and Hovell's journey to Port Phillip. Roy. Aust. Hist. Soc. **7**, Pt6: 289–380 (1921).

Seddon, H.R.: Diseases of domestic animals in Australia. Part 3: Tick and mite infestation. Commonw. Aust. Dep. Health Serv. Publ. No. 7, 1951.

Sinclair, C.W.: A fatal tick bite. Med. J. Aust. **1**, 554 (1930).

Singh, K.R.P.: A note on tick paralysis in rabbits. Curr. Sci. **32**, 116 (1963).

Sloan, C.A.: Mortality in sheep due to *Ixodes* species. Aust. Vet. J. **44**, 527 (1968).

Stampa, S.: Tick paralysis in the Karoo areas of South Africa. Onderstepoort J. vet. Res. **28**, 169—227 (1959).

Stanbury, J.B., Huyck, J.H.: Tick paralysis: a critical review. Medicine (Baltimore) **24**, 219—242 (1945).

Starkoff, A.: Ixodoidea d'Italia. Rome: Il Pensiero Scientifico 1958.

Steinhaus, E.A.: Note on a toxic principle in eggs of the tick, *Dermacentor andersoni* Stiles. U.S. Pub. Health Rep. **57**, 1310—1312 (1942).

Stiller, R.: Tick paralysis: Case report. Clin. Proc. Child. Hosp. **2**, 266—268 (1946).

Strickland, C.: Note on a case of tick paralysis in Australia. Parasitology **7**, 379 (1915).

Swanepoel, A.: Tick paralysis: regional neurological involvement caused by *Hyalomma truncatum*. S. Afr. med. J. **33**, 909—911 (1959).

Swartzwelder, J.C., Seabury, J.H.: Bite of *Amblyomma americanum* associated with possible tick paralysis. J. Parasitol. **33**, 22—23 (1947).

Tasselli, E.: Paralysis due to ticks (?) in the province of Matera. Vet. Ital. **9**, 909—912 (1958).

Tatchell, R.J.: A modified method for obtaining tick oral secretions. J. Parasitol. **53**, 1106—1107 (1967).

Tatchell, R.J.: The significance of host-parasite relationships in the feeding of the cattle tick *Boophilus microplus* (Canestrini). Proc. 2nd International Congress on Acarology, 1967. Budapest: Akademiai Kiado 1969, pp. 341—345.

Taylor, C.W.: Tick paralysis. Canad. med. Ass. J. **95**, 125 (1966).

Temple, I.U.: Acute ascending paralysis, or tick paralysis. Med. Sentinel **20**, 509—514 (1912).

Theiler, G.: Ticks. Presidential address to S. Afr. Biol. Soc. Pamphlet No. 14. Pretoria: Caxton 1949.

Todd, J.L.: Tick bite in British Columbia. J. Canad. med. Ass. **2**, 1118—1119 (1912).

Todd, J.L.: Tick paralysis. J. Parasitol. **1**, 55—64 (1914).

Todd, J.L.: Tick-caused paralysis. J. Canad. vet. med. Ass. **9**, 994—995 (1919).

Townsend, R.G., Nash, J.F.: On certain diseases from the Fields and Woods. South. Med. Surg. **102**, 386 (1940).

Trager, W.: Acquired immunity to ticks. J. Parasitol. **25**, 57—81 (1939).

Tzortzakis, W., Papadakis, G.: La paralysie à tiques chez l'homme et chez les animaux domestiques. N. Comm. à 3e Congrès Internat. de Pathologie Comparée, Athènes, tome 2. Athènes: Eleftheroudakis 1936, pp. 449—452.

Van Rensburg, S.: Tick paralysis in sheep. Farming in South Africa, **18**, 661 (1928).

Veneroni, C.: Le paralisi da zecchi in Somalia. Arch. Ital. Sci. Med. Colon. **9**, 405—406 (1928).

Viloria, D.: Paralasis por garrapatas en caninos. Rev. Med. Vet. Parasitol. (Maracay) **13**, 67—70 (1954).

Vogelsang, E.G.: Existe la tick paralysis en el Uruguay? Bol. Inst. Bacteriol. Escuela Vet. **1**, 6—7 (1925).

Webb, J.H., Earnest, F.: Tick paralysis; a case report. Ohio med. J. **59**, 395 (1963).

Wells, J.: Canine tick paralysis produced by *Dermacentor variablis*. North Amer. Vet. **19**, 41—42 (1934).

Wilkes, W.A.: Tick paralysis (Correspondence). J. Amer. med. Ass. **165**, 874 (1957).

Wilkinson, P.R.: *Dermacentor* ticks on wildlife and new records of paralysis. Proc. Entomol. Soc. Brit. Columbia **67**, 24—29 (1970).

Wilkinson, P.R.: A first record of paralysis of a deer by *Dermacentor andersoni* Stiles and notes on the 'host potential' of deer in British Columbia. Proc. Entomol. Soc. Brit. Columbia **62**, 28—30 (1965).

Zanzenbacher, K.E., Conrad, E.: Tick paralysis—a treatable killer neuropathy. Southern med. J. **61**, 674—676 (1968).

Zumpt, F., Glajchen, D.: Tick paralysis in man. S. Afr. med. J. **24**, 1092—1094 (1950).

CHAPTER 17

Toxins of Blattaria

L.M. Roth and D.W. Alsop

Cockroaches are probably the most pervasive of all insect domiciliary pests. As invaders of the environments we have created for our own comfort, they have established themselves in our homes, businesses, hospitals, places of food storage and preparation, transportation systems, and underground utility networks. Although the number of species involved is not great — less than 10 are true cosmopolitan pests, with some 40 others of greater or lesser local importance — the population densities these insects can attain is enormous, with the result that in many parts of the world it is virtually impossible to avoid contact with cockroaches or their products.

A. Systematics

Cockroach taxonomy began with LINNAEUS, who in 1758 established the genus *Blatta* and named nine species. Today more than 3500 species of cockroaches belonging to over 400 genera have been described, and collectively they are regarded as the Blattaria, a suborder of the Dictyoptera. The earlier classifications of SAUSSURE (1864), BRUNNER DE WATTENWYL (1865), KIRBY (1904), KARNY (1921), HANDLIRSCH (1925, 1930), BRUES and MELANDER (1932), CHOPARD (1949), BEY-BIENKO (1950), and J.W.H. REHN (1951) are reviewed by PRINCIS (1960), who presents a system that is basically an extension and modification of that of HANDLIRSCH's (1930). Using the morphology of the wings, legs, head, and male subgenital plate as his principal taxonomic characters, PRINCIS (1960) divides the cockroaches into 4 suborders and 28 families.

More recently, MC KITTRICK (1964) has presented a quite different classification in which the cockroaches form a single suborder with only 5 families and 21 subfamilies (Table 1). This system is based upon whether or not a group is oviparous or ovoviviparous as its principal unifying character, and is based on a comparative study of (1) female genitalia and their musculature, (2) male genitalia, (3) morphology of the proventriculus, and (4) oviposition behavior. Support for this classification is widespread (ROTH, 1970), and has been reported in comparative studies of malpighian tubules (LECONTE et al., 1967), oviposition behavior (ROTH, 1967a), water changes in oöthecae (ROTH, 1967b), oöthecal structure (ROTH, 1968a, 1971), ovarioles (ROTH, 1968b, 1971), male tergal glands (ROTH, 1969, 1971), spermatophores (GRAVES, 1969), proventriculi (MILLER and FISK, 1971), cephalic glands (BROSSUT, 1973) and, to some extent, by the numerical taxonomic study of HUBER (1974).

Table 1. Classification of the Blattaria. [After McKittrick, 1964; the Tryonicinae were added by McKittrick and Mackerras (1965). The genera shown in parentheses are those mentioned in this chapter.]

Order: Dictyoptera
  Suborder: Blattaria
    Superfamily: Blattoidea
      Family: Cryptocercidae
        Subfamily: Cryptocercinae
      Family: Blattidae
        Subfamilies: Lamproblattinae
                      Tryonicinae
                      Blattinae (*Periplaneta, Blatta, Neostylopyga, Deropeltis,*
                          Pseudoderopeltis)
                      Polyzosteriinae (*Pelmatosilpha, Eurycotis, Cutilia, Platyzosteria,*
                          Polyzosteria, Zonioploca, Megazosteria, Desmozosteria,
                          Drymaplaneta, Euzosteria)
    Superfamily: Blaberoidea
      Family: Polyphagidae (*Ergaula*)
        Subfamilies: Polyphaginae
                      Holocompsinae
      Family: Blattellidae
        Subfamilies: Anaplectinae
                      Plectopterinae (*Supella*)
                      Blattellinae (*Blattella, Parcoblatta, Loboptera*)
                      Nyctiborinae (*Megaloblatta, Nyctibora*)
                      Ectobiinae (*Ectobius*)
      Family: Blaberidae
        Subfamilies: Panesthiinae
                      Blaberinae (*Byrsotria, Blaberus*)
                      Zetoborinae
                      Perisphaerinae
                      Epilamprinae
                      Oxyhaloinae (*Leucophaea, Nauphoeta, Gromphadorhina*)
                      Panchlorinae (*Panchlora*)
                      Diplopterinae (*Diploptera*)
                      Pycnoscelinae (*Pycnoscelus*)

B. Biology

Cockroaches have long been used as experimental animals and a considerable body of biological information concerning them has been amassed. Detailed knowledge, however, is restricted to a very few species, principally those such as *Periplaneta americana* (L.) and *Blattella germanica* (L.) which are household or industrial pests. The biology of cockroaches is reviewed in recent books by Cornwell (1968), Guthrie and Tindall (1968) and a monograph by Beier (1974). Roth and Willis (1957) have monographed the medical and veterinary importance of cockroaches, as well as the associations of these insects with plants and animals (Roth and Willis, 1960). Princis (1962–1970), in the Orthopterorum Catalogus, gives a detailed catalog of cockroach species, together with a comprehensive, systematically arranged bibliography containing references to the economic importance and general biology of these insects, together with extensive data on their systematics and distribution.

C. Allergy Caused by Cockroaches

Cockroaches, as a part of our immediate environment, must be considered as a potentially important source of allergens. In the temperate zone and throughout much of the world the domiciliary pest species (e.g., *P. americana, B. germanica, Blatta orientalis* L.) normally live and reproduce indoors, even though in warmer areas, especially the tropics and subtropics, they can survive outdoors. Since these insects can occur in enormous numbers, direct exposure to them or their products often becomes unavoidable wherever people are crowded together under substandard or unsanitary conditions. Indirect or unknowing exposure to these insects is also common, since cockroaches commonly inhabit kitchens and other food-handling establishments, places where food can be contaminated with their excrement, vomitus, and bodies or parts of bodies (ROTH and WILLIS, 1957).

Although the evidence for cockroach allergenicity was scant and circumstantial at the time of ROTH and WILLIS's (1957) review, considerable information has since been accumulated to indicate that these insects are the sources of 4 classes of allergens—contactants, inhalants, injectants, and ingestants (BERNTON and BROWN, 1969).

1. Contactant Allergens

References to bodily contact with cockroaches are numerous and were summarized by ROTH and WILLIS (1957). BERNTON and BROWN (1969) and BERNTON et al. (1972) describe the following cases of allergic responses to cockroaches. A zoology professor who had worked with cockroaches for 8 years reported that contact with certain species resulted in symptoms of hay fever, asthma, and dermatitis after handling the insects. Other workers in his laboratory developed similar symptoms. Another zoologist developed an eye irritation resulting in conjunctival edema while dissecting *Leucophaea maderae* (F.). If he touched the skin of his neck after handling these cockroaches, an inflamed area would develop. In another laboratory in which many species of cockroaches were bred, two workers became sensitized to the insects, and showed symptoms of itching hands and eruption of papules on the dorsal aspect of their hands and arms. A zoologist working with *Gromphadorhina brunneri* (BUTLER) developed local itching eruptions, sneezing, and asthma. We know of several individuals in our laboratories and elsewhere who were highly allergic to certain species of cockroaches and developed asthmatic and dermatologic symptoms after handling individuals of, or cleaning the cages of one or more of the following: *Nauphoeta cinerea* (OLIVIER), *Gromphadorhina* spp., *L. maderae, Byrsotria fumigata* (GUÉRIN), and *P. americana*. This was not a reaction to cockroaches in general; sensitivity to the first three species (all members of the Oxyhaloinae) was shown by laboratory workers who also handled but were not affected by a number of other cockroach species being cultured in the same place.

To identify more closely the effect of cockroaches as allergen sources, BERNTON et al. (1964, 1969, 1970a, 1970b) prepared extracts of the domiciliary pests *P. americana, B. orientalis, B. germanica,* and *L. maderae* for use in skin (cutaneous and intracutaneous) and inhalation tests by the following procedure: dried, frozen insects were first defatted in 3—4 changes of ether, redried, then crushed and homogenized in Coca's solution. The resulting suspensions were then refrigerated with frequent shaking for a week, filtered, and the filtrates dialysed in 3 times their volume of water, changed several times over a 72-hour period. Extracts for testing consisted of the dialyzed residues, sterilized by filtration.

Using these extracts, skin-sensitizing antibodies were found in the sera of positive cockroach reactors (BERNTON and BROWN, 1964), and peripheral leukocytes from these individuals released histamine when it was added *in vitro* (MAY *in* CHOOVIVATHANAVANICH et al., 1971). However, according to BERNTON and BROWN (1970a), allergens obtained by this method of extraction act primarily as inhalants, and only secondarily as contactants.

2. Inhalant Allergens

The fact that the handling of certain species of cockroaches causes asthmatic symptoms indicates that some of the allergens act through inhalation. BERNTON and BROWN (1969) describe the case of a laboratory worker who reared *L. maderae* in trays stored in a closed cabinet and had to use an inhalation mask covering her nose and mouth to prevent an asthmatic attack whenever a tray containing the insects was exposed; without the mask an attack could occur even if a tray more than 6 feet away was uncovered without her knowledge. Trays containing other species of cockroaches did not induce asthma. This is further evidence (as are the above cases) that the specific inhalant allergens are not the same for every individual.

BERNTON et al. (1972) have found that inhalation of the extract of the German cockroach (*B. germanica*) produces asthmatic attacks in subjects with skin hypersensitivity to both cockroach extract and other noncockroach allergens, but will not do so in asthmatics lacking skin hypersensitivity to cockroach extract. According to SCHULANER (1970) the tendency for allergenic children exposed to cockroaches to develop an allergy to them, as shown by positive skin reactions to extracts of *B. germanica,* suggests that this tendency may play a role in perpetuating allergic symptoms in some children. A number of studies indicate that about one-third of the allergenic child population is sensitive to cockroaches; BERNTON and BROWN (1970b), SCHULANER (1970), and MENDOZA and SNYDER (1970) have found that 38%, 40%, and 30%, respectively, of asthmatic children are positive reactors to cockroach antigen, with the youngest positive reactor (BERNTON and BROWN, 1970b) being a 4-year old asthmatic.

In Thailand, CHOOVIVANATHANAVICH et al. (1970, 1971) have found a significant correlation (61% of allergic patients, ages 6—69) between dermal reactions to house dust extract and cockroach extract (from "different species" found in dwellings of the patients), suggesting that house dust contaminated by cockroach emanations or disintegrating parts is an important source of cockroach antigens. That cockroach feces could be a source of inhalant allergens in the environment has been shown by BERNTON and BROWN (1970a), who demonstrated that in sensitive individuals an extract of feces from *B. germanica* produces positive cutaneous reactions equal in intensity to those produced by whole body extracts in sensitive individuals. These results have been challenged by UY et al. (1973), who, using aerosolized cockroach antigen in bronchial challenge studies on 13 asymptomatic asthmatic children, concluded that cockroaches, as a component of house dust, may not be important in triggering attacks in asthmatic children.

3. Injectant Allergens

Records of cockroaches biting humans, especially sleeping individuals (ROTH and WILLIS, 1957) raises the possibility of introduction of allergens by injection into wounds. PAVLOVSKI and SHTEIN (1931) studied the effect of experimentally induced bites by *B. orientalis* on human skin and noted a resultant degeneration of epithelial cells, necrosis, and inflammation. They attributed this response to a toxic effect of the insect's saliva, since they found that an emulsion of salivary glands, when rubbed into skin with a sterile needle, produced symptoms similar to the bites of the cockroaches. BERNTON and BROWN (1969) have described a case illustrating that the reactions to cockroach bites can be both localized and general: a 25 year-old woman with a 4-year history of asthma, positive to cutaneous tests with cockroach extracts, was awakened one night by the bites of 2 cockroaches on her wrist. Itching at the sites of the bites ensued. Returning to sleep, she was again awakened by continued itching and a marked wheezing attack, presumably a delayed effect of the injection of an allergen.

4. Ingestant Allergens

Because of the varied symptoms of food allergy (gastric, intestinal, respiratory, and dermatologic), diagnosis of the causitive factor may be difficult. However, cockroach contamination should be given consideration in cases where the individuals showing symptoms of food allergy can be shown to have come from cockroach-infested domiciles, or to have obtained food from places where these insects are common (BERNTON and BROWN, 1969). It has been shown that people allergic to cockroaches will react positively to extracts of food partially consumed by cockroaches, and that this allergen is thermostable, not being affected by a temperature of 100°C for 1 h (BERNTON and BROWN, 1964).

BERNTON and BROWN (1967) stress the necessity of including an extract of cockroach allergen among the routine diagnostic allergens. "The possible desensitization with cockroach extract as the sole therapeutic measure, or as an adjunct, may reduce the number of refractory allergic patients, especially of those living in an insect-infested environment." In Puerto Rico, MARCHAND (1966) reported encouraging results in a desensitization program using *B. germanica* extract. CHOOVIVANATHANAVICH et al. (1971) also suggested the supplementary use of cockroach antigen for hyposensitization therapy in people who are refractory to house dust injections alone, and recommended cockroach eradication in the homes of allergic individuals. The latter could be as difficult to achieve as the elimination of house dust.

D. Defensive Glands

Certain cockroaches produce glandular secretions which adversely affect other animals and serve as a means of chemical defense. These secretions are the products of special "defensive" glands and are of two types: a) active chemical defenses, usually effective against both vertebrate and invertebrate predators. These are liquid secretions that act as contact irritants (e.g., aldehydes, quinones) and are discharged only in response to predatory attacks, and b) passive chemical defenses, usually effective only against small invertebrate predators. These are viscid, glue-like secretions that accumulate on the surface of certain body regions and when contacted by small invertebrates, adhere to their mouth parts, antennae, etc., thus serving as mechanical deterrents.

Defensive glands are usually not externally visible and, when present, are either always possessed by both adult sexes and sometimes the nymphs, or are present in one of the adult sexes and both nymphal sexes. These glands should not be confused with a number of other exocrine glands which are not present in nymphs and found in only one of the adult sexes. For example, many male cockroaches have dorsal (tergal) glands which are not found in females and were thought at one time to be defense glands (Oettinger, 1906; Konček, 1924). These readily visible specializations are involved in sexual behavior; they apparently produce a secretion which helps to maneuver the female into the proper precopulatory position during courtship behavior, and arrest her movement so that the male can achieve copulatory connection (Roth, 1969). Similarly, the phallic glands of male *P. americana* and *B. orientalis* considered by Bordas (1901, 1908) to have a defensive function, have been shown by Gupta (1947) to produce the outermost covering of the spermatophore.

Alsop (1970), principally on a basis of their location in the insect, distinguished four morphologically distinct defensive glandular systems, all located in the abdomen (Fig. 1):

Type I.   Paired eversible pleural glands
Type II.   Single ventral intersternal gland
Type III. Paired dorsal intertergal glands
Type IV.   Paired tracheal glands

To this, we add:

Type V.   Hypodermal tergal glands on the terminal abdominal segments.

In the first four types of the above classification, the defensive secretion is stored in cuticle-lined reservoirs and is deployed either by eversion of the reservoirs, or oozes, or is sprayed from uneverted reservoirs. In the fifth type, a viscous proteinaceous material that deters predators mechanically is secreted on to the dorsal surface of the segments.

Secretions from all but the first gland type have been identified. Most commonly, this has first involved obtaining the secretion discharged by traumatized insects (gland types II, III, IV) either directly by collecting the discharge on filter paper (Takahashi and Kitamura, 1972), in a solvent (Chadha et al., 1961; Blum, 1964;

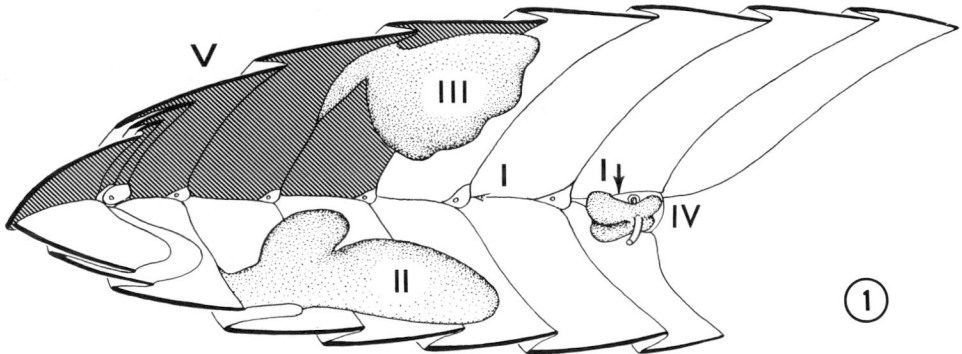

Fig. 1. Diagrammatic sagittal section of a cockroach abdomen, showing relative shapes and opening positions of Gland Types I—IV, and location of secretory fields for Gland Type V. The first of the two Type I glands has been omitted, and its position indicated by an arrow. Note that only one-half of the medially opening Type III gland is shown (Modified from ALSOP, 1970)

DATEO and ROTH, 1967a, 1967b), in capillary tubes (WATERHOUSE and WALLBANK, · 1967; WALLBANK and WATERHOUSE, 1970; TAKAHASHI and KITAMURA, 1972), or indirectly, by collecting it in a dry ice trap from air that has been passed over discharging insects (ROTH and STAY, 1958). In a few cases secretions have been collected by dissecting out entire glands and either opening them in a solvent (ROTH et al., 1956; ROTH and STAY, 1958), or directly in the inlet of an analysis system (ROTH et al., 1956). Secretions from type V glands have been obtained by simply scraping the exudates from the surface of the individuals and placing them in appropriate solvents (ROTH and STAHL, 1956; PLATTNER et al., 1972).

Identification procedures for the liquid secretions have included gas-liquid chromatography, IR, UV, PMR, and mass spectroscopy, and paper and thin-layer chromatography of the secretions and certain of their chemical derivatives (see the above citations). The gland type V secretions have been identified by means of colorimetric tests, paper and thin-layer chromatography, disc electrophoresis, and automated amino acid analysis (ROTH and STAHL, 1956; PLATTNER et al., 1972).

1. Type I Glands

Eversible glands have been reported only in certain members of the polyphagid genus *Ergaula* (GERSTAECKER, 1861). Adults of *Ergaula capucina* (BRUNNER) have two pairs of light yellow sac-like glands which they evert through lateral openings in the pleural membranes between the second and third, and third and fourth abdominal spiracles (Fig. 1) when traumatized. GERSTAECKER (1861) and HAASE (1889), possibly in error, reported that in *E. carunculigera* (GERSTAECKER) the openings are located between the first and second, and second and third abdominal spiracles. When everted the glands are pear-shaped and densely covered with circumferential rows of chitinous spines, the latter presumably being an adaptation for greatly increasing the surface area on which a film of secretion can be held.

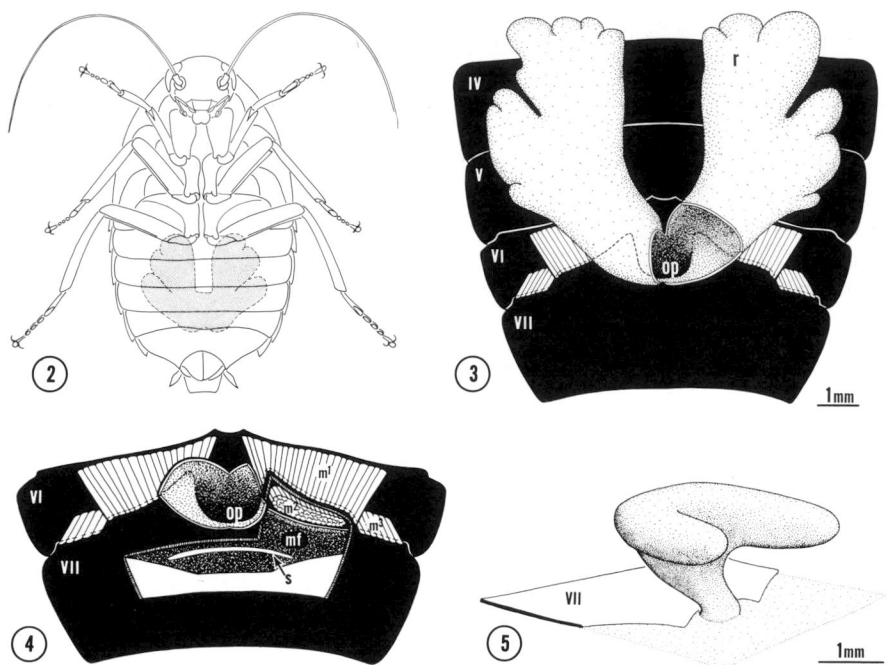

Figs. 2–5. Blattarid type II glands (From Alsop, 1970). (2) *Eurycotis floridana*. Ventral view. Glands stippled. (3) *E. floridana*. Entire gland with small cutaway to show constricted opening (*op*) formed by U-shaped anterior edge of abdominal sternite VI. (4) *E. floridana*. View of sternites VI and VII with most of reservoir cut away and a large opening made in sternite VII, showing the 3 pairs of intersegmental muscles (m^1, m^2, m^3), the great width of the external opening, and the narrow crescentric sclerite (*s*) that stiffens its membranous floor (*mf*). (5) *Periplaneta americana*. Small sternal gland with a portion of sternite VII

The secretory cells lie directly beneath the spines, and are covered by an inner layer of circumferential muscles and an outer layer of longitudinal muscles (Gerstaecker, 1861). Eversion is most probably accomplished by hemolymph pressure, and reinvagination by the longitudinal muscles, together with contraction of the circumferential muscles to drive blood from the gland (Alsop, 1970). Although the secretion produced by these glands has not been identified, it is presumed to be defensive in function since the glands are present in both adult sexes and everted only in response to a traumatic attack.

2. Type II Glands

Unpaired abdominal glands that open midventrally between the sixth and seventh sternites have been found in adults of all species of Blattidae so far examined. Although present in older nymphs of many species, the nymphal glands, with the exception of those of *Methana convexa* (Wallbank and Waterhouse, 1970), do not appear to be functional. This type of gland is not present in *Cryptocercus punctulata* Scudder, a member of the closely related (and more primitive) Cryptocercidae (Alsop, 1970).

There is some doubt as to whether all glands of this type produce defensive secretions. While many species, especially those belonging to the Polyzosteriinae, produce secretions of undoubted defensive effectiveness (Tables 2 and 3), some (e.g., *Drymaplaneta variegata* (SHELFORD) and *Scabina antipoda* (KIRBY)) produce essentially aqueous solutions (WALLBANK and WATERHOUSE, 1970). This is also true of most of the blattine species, only one of which, *Neostylopyga rhombifolia* (STOLL) has been shown to produce a secretion effective in repelling an array of predators (EISNER et al., 1959).

The ventral glands of the following species have been described: *Eurycotis floridana* (STAY, 1957; ALSOP, 1970); *Platyzosteria soror* (CHADHA et al., 1961);

Table 2. Occurrence of *trans*-2-hexenal as the major component of the defensive secretion in Blattaria (Blattidae: Polyzosteriinae)

	References[a]
Eurycotis floridana (Walker)[b]	1, 2, 3
E. biolleyi Rehn[b]	2, 3
E. decipiens Kirby[b]	2, 3
Pelmatosilpha coriacea Rehn	4
Euzosteria nobilis (Brunner)	3, 5
Polyzosteria limbata Burmeister[b, c]	5
P. viridissima Shelford[b, c]	5
P. oculata Tepper[c]	5
P. cuprea Saussure[c, d]	5
P. pulchra Mackerras[c, d]	5
P. mitchelli (Angas)[e]	5
Zonioploca pallida (Brunner)	5
Z. bicolor Shaw	5
Megazosteria patula (Walker)	5
Desmozosteria scripta Mackerras	5
Platyzosteria novaeseelandiae (Brunner)	6
P. soror (Brunner)	7
P. coolgardiensis Tepper	5
P. scabra (Brunner)	5
P. scabrella Tepper	5
P. stradbrokensis Mackerras	5
P. nitidella (Shaw)[f]	5
P. sp.[f, g]	5
Drymaplaneta semivitta (Walker)	5
D. shelfordi (Princis)	5
D. communis Tepper	5

[a] 1) ROTH et al., 1956; 2) DATEO and ROTH, 1967a; 3) ROTH and DATEO, 1967b; 4) BLUM, 1964; 5) WALLBANK and WATERHOUSE, 1970; 6) ROTH and WILLIS, 1960; 7) CHADHA et al., 1961.
[b] plus gluconic acid and its lactones.
[c] plus traces of hexanal, hexenal isomer, 2-hexenol, and *trans*-2-hexenoic acid.
[d] plus traces of octanal, and *trans*-2-octenal.
[e] plus traces of hexenal isomer.
[f] plus oct-2-enal.
[g] plus a trace of dec-2-enal.

Table 3. Aliphatic compounds, other than *trans*-2-hexenal, produced as defensive secretions by polyzosteriine cockroaches (from WATERHOUSE and WALLBANK, 1967, and WALLBANK and WATERHOUSE, 1970)

Species	Compounds produced
Methana convexa (Walker)	2-methylene butanal, 2-methylene pentanal
Platyzosteria armata Tepper	2-pentanol, 2-heptanone, 2-haptanol
P. sp. near *montana*	Octenal, 2-methylene butanal and its dimer
P. occidentalis Mackerras	2-methylene butanal and its dimer
P. castanea Brunner, *P. jungii* (Tepper), *P. morosa* Shelford, *P. ruficeps* Shelford	2-methylene butanal and its dimer, methylene butanol, and 2-methylene propanal, 2-methyl butanol, 2-methyl butanal, 2-methylene butyric acid, and 2-methylene pentanal

Platyzosteria spp. (WATERHOUSE and WALLBANK, 1967); *Periplaneta americana* (LIANG, 1956; ALSOP, 1970); *Blatta orientalis* (HARRISON, 1906; QADRI, 1938; ALSOP, 1970); *Duchailluia* sp. (ALSOP, 1970); and *Deropeltis* sp. (ALSOP, 1970). They also occur in *Periplaneta australasiae* (F.) and *Periplaneta brunnea* Burm. (ROTH and WILLIS, 1960). Nothing is known of the nature of the secretion or its function in these two species nor in *B. orientalis, Deropeltis,* or *Duchailluia.*

There is considerable variation in size and form of the gland reservoirs (Figs. 7—9), although not in gland openings. In all cases, the posterior edge of the opening is formed by a medial indentation in the anteriorly prolonged leading edge of sternite 7, and the anterior edge merges with the intersegmental membrane connecting sternites 6 and 7 (Figs. 3—5).

However, in the polyzosteriines *Eurycotis* and *Platyzosteria* the reservoirs are very large, extending up to, or beyond the anterior edge of sternite 4, and consist of two large lobes, each subdivided into a number of smaller lobules (Figs. 2, 3 and 5), while in the blattines the reservoirs are much smaller, rarely reaching the anterior edge of sternite 6, and consist of two small anteriorly directed lobes (*Periplaneta, Blatta, Deropeltis*) or four small subequal lobes (*Duchailluia*) (Figs. 7—9). In all cases the median portion of the reservoir lies directly beneath the ventral nerve cord, and the lobes are bound to the sternites by numerous tracheal branches.

In *E. floridana* the secretion is produced by tall columnar secretory cells which cover the surface of the reservoir in a discontinuous pattern. Each cell has a large, oval, basal nucleus, granular cytoplasm, and a cylindrical, striated secretory vesicle. Secretion collects within a chitinous organelle situated within the secretory apparatus and is drained away by a cuticular tubule, continuous with the organelle. The draining tubules pass up through the secretory cells, along the surface of other cells, and open, sometimes in clusters of 25 or 30, into the reservoir. Histochemical tests of the glands in *E. floridana* indicate the presence of glycogen and other periodic acid Schiff-positive material in the secretory cells and a high level of alkaline phosphatase activity around the secretory apparatus (STAY, 1957). The gland structure in the Blattinae is basically similar to that in the Polyzosteriinae,

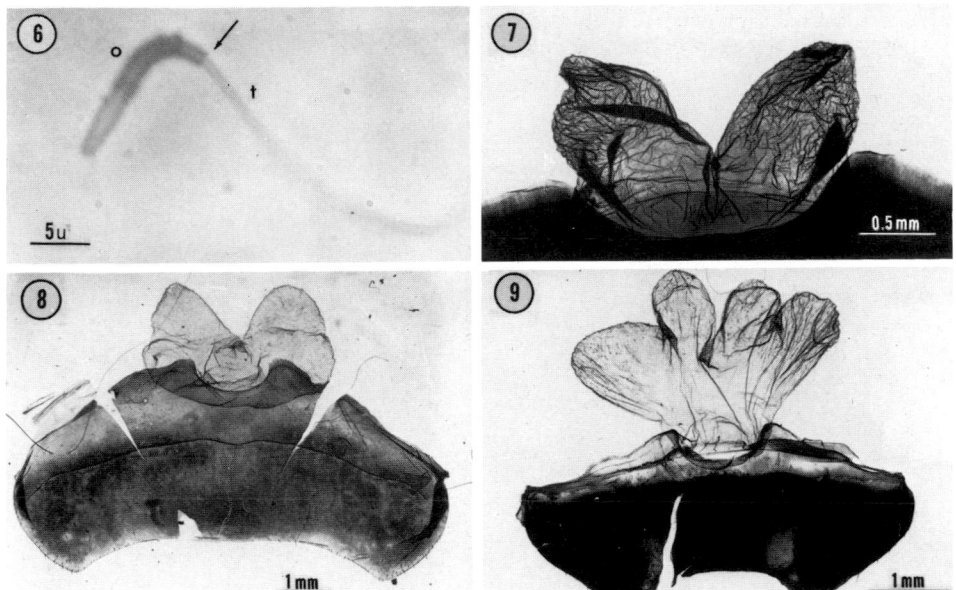

Figs. 6–9. Blattarid type II glands (KOH-digested, Chlorazol black, whole mount, phase) (From ALSOP, 1970). (6) *E. floridana*. Organelle. Arrow indicates junction between organelle (*o*) and draining tubule (*t*). (7) *Deropeltis wahlbergi*. Sternal gland with portion of sternite VII. (8) *Blatta orientalis*. Sternal gland with all of sternite VII. (9) *Duchailluia* sp. Sternal gland with all of sternite VII. Black spots on lobes are clusters of draining tubules

the main differences being in size of the reservoirs, arrangement of the secretory cells, and shape and number of tubule clusters.

All of the polyzosteriine species and *Neostylopyga rhombifolia* (Blattinae) forcibly spray the secretion from their glands when disturbed. Since the reservoirs lack an intrinsic musculature, the force for this expulsion is probably supplied by a rise in hemolymph pressure. Although there are no valves to prevent a loss of secretion, the gland orifice is normally sealed shut against the intersegmental membrane by the tension of two large muscles (m^1; Fig. 4) inserting on the leading edges of sternites 6 and 7. When secretion is to be expelled, the orifice is opened by the action of two pairs of muscles (m^2; m^3; Fig. 4) which simultaneously protract sternites 6 and 7 and bow sternite 6 down, away from sternite 7.

The amount of secretion that can be sprayed is variable and depends on the age of the insect, the size of the reservoir, and the time elapsed since the previous discharge. *Polyzosteria limbata* produced an average of 25 µl (one individual contained 70 µl) and a male of *Polyzosteria pulchra* contained 90 µl (WALLBANK and WATERHOUSE, 1970). Five *Eurycotis floridana* produced 46 µl and two *E. biolleyi*, 29 µl of secretion (DATEO and ROTH, 1967b).

Aliphatic compounds are the most common defensive secretions found in cockroaches, so far investigated, possessing Type II glands. In many of the polyzosteriine species the major component of the secretion is *trans*-2-hexenal (Table 2). A number of members of this group synthesize compounds other than *trans*-2-hexenal

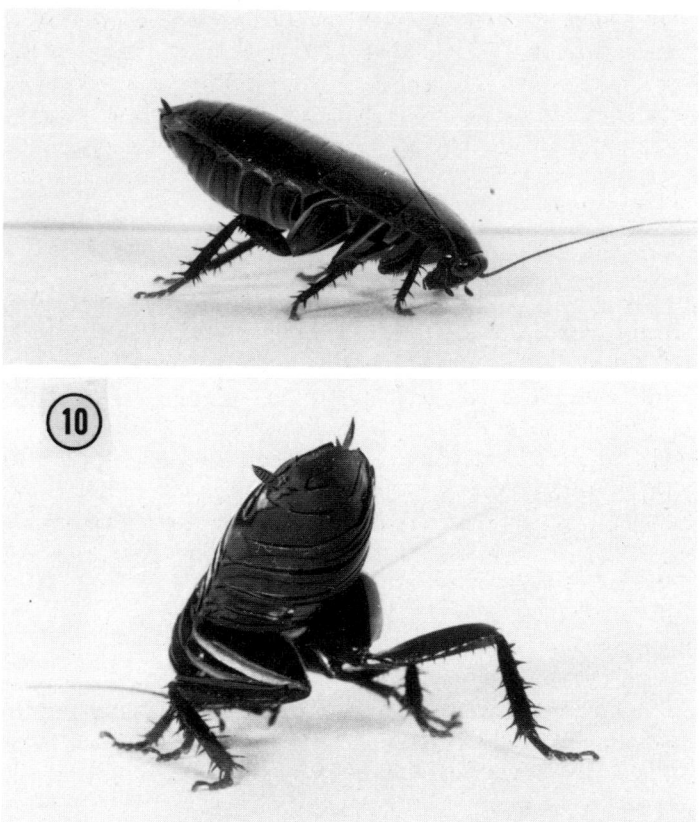

Fig. 10. Warning stance assumed by adult *Platyzosteria castanea* when disturbed. (Bottom figure from Waterhouse and Wallbank, 1967; courtesy of Dr. Douglas Waterhouse, CSIRO, Canberra, Australia)

(Table 3). In almost all cases these polyzosteriine secretions appear to consist of two phases, a volatile phase containing the active defensive compounds, and a nonvolatile aqueous phase containing a glucose derivative such as gluconic acid or δ-gluconolactone (Dateo and Roth, 1967a, 1967b; Wallbank and Water-house, 1970). The function of these latter compounds in the secretions, if any, is not known.

Most of the information regarding the effectiveness of cockroach defensive secretions containing carbonyl compounds has come from laboratory studies in which it has been demonstrated that the repellent value of the secretion depends largely on the species of predator involved. *Trans*-2-hexenal from *Eurycotis decipiens* causes vertigo and nausea in man (Bunting in: Roth and Willis, 1957) and is an effective repellent against the fire ant, *Solenopsis saevissima* (F. Smith), in the laboratory (Dateo and Roth, 1967b). The secretion from *Eurycotis floridana,* which the insect can spray as far as 3 feet, repels small arthropod predators and larger vertebrates such as birds, lizards, and frogs, especially if it strikes them in the eyes (Eisner et al., 1959). Blum (1964) observed that in nature, the ants *Iridomyrmex melleus* WALKER and *Myrmelachista ramulorum* WHEELER were effectively repelled by the *trans*-2-hexenal secretion of *Pelmatosilpha coriacea,* but that the cockroaches were readily eaten by the lizard *Anolis cristatellus* DUMERIL and BIBRON even though they discharged their secretion. When sprayed, the ants hit by the secretion walked abnormally and exhibited tremors, and would not attack the cockroach again for periods as long as 3 minutes, thereby allowing it enough time to escape.

Adults of *Platyzosteria castanea* and *P. ruficeps* move about during the day, sometimes in exposed locations. When disturbed, they assume a characteristic warning stance (Fig. 10) in which the head is held near or touching the ground and the abdomen is flexed upward at a sharp angle, revealing bright orange-yellow markings on their coxae and venters. The gland opening is pointed toward the disturbance, and continued irritation results in the discharge of a secretion containing 90—97 percent methylene butanal. Bulldog ants, *Myrmecia nigriceps,* were effectively repelled in the laboratory by both species, the cockroaches first assuming the warning stance and presenting the posterior end of their abdomens to the ants jaws. Ants that were sprayed became disoriented and were temporarily incoordinated (WATERHOUSE and WALLBANK, 1967). *P. castanea* is capable of spraying 6 or 7 inches (SHAW, 1914).

Aposematic coloring combined with the defensive secretion would aid the predator in learning to avoid the prey after being traumatized by the spray. Adults and nymphs (except young stages) of *Eurycotis decipiens* possess warning coloration (Fig. 11) and although the nymphs do not have defense glands, they would benefit from the coloration once predators learned to avoid the adults, which produce *trans*-2-hexenal (DATEO and ROTH, 1967b). Similarly, nymphs of *Platyzosteria ruficeps,* where the coloration of the late instars resembles that of the adults (MACKERRAS, 1968), also assume a warning stance when disturbed, even though they do not manufacture a defensive secretion (WATERHOUSE and WALLBANK, 1967).

The only blattine species to have its secretion characterized, *Periplaneta americana,* produces a dilute mixture of *p*-cresol and *p*-ethyl phenol (TAKAHASHI and

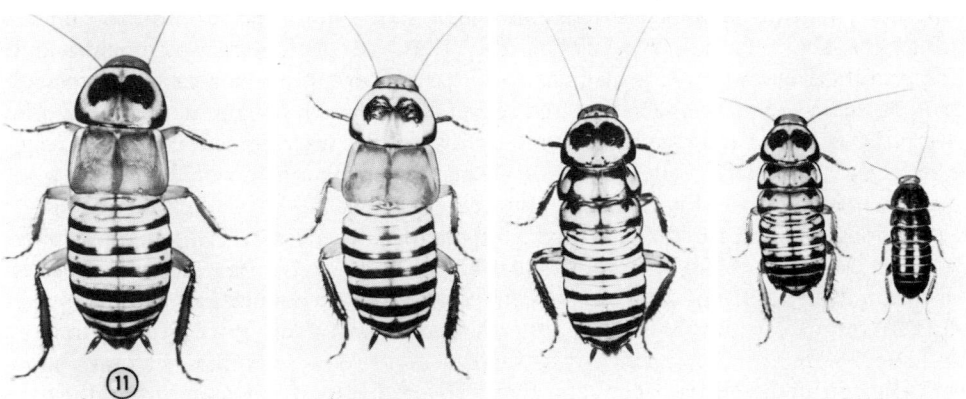

Fig. 11. Habitus illustrations of *Eurycotis decipiens* showing warning coloration of adults and nymphs. From left to right, adult ♀, adult ♂, and 3 nymphs (the smallest has no aposematic markings). (From DATEO and ROTH, 1967b)

KITAMURA, 1972). Their experimental data indicate that this secretion is repellent to nymphs of *P. americana,* but its effectiveness against possible predators has not been determined, nor has the circumstances in which it is discharged been determined. However, phenolic compounds produced by some invertebrates are particularly effective repellents against ants and less so to vertebrate predators (EISNER et al., 1963). TAKAHASHI and KITAMURA further suggest that the phenols produced by this species may also serve as an intraspecific "alarm" substance, or possibly as a defense against microorganisms, since the phenols could be isolated from feces (which showed relatively little fungal growth) and filter paper in the containers housing the insects.

The Malayan cockroach *Archiblatta hoevenii* VOLLENHOVEN, another blattine species, produces a strong phenolic odor when handled (VARLEY, 1964), but the source and chemical composition of the secretion have not been determined.

3. Type III Glands

Paired glands opening between the fifth and sixth abdominal tergites are present in a number of species belonging to the blattid subfamily Blattinae. Glands of this type have not been found in members of the Polyzosteriinae, nor in the closely related Cryptocercidae.

Of all the species so far examined, only two, *Deropeltis erythrocephala* (F.) and *D. wahlbergi* (STÅL), have glands that are demonstrably defensive in function (ALSOP and EISNER, unpubl.). In the others (*Periplaneta americana, Blatta orientalis,* and *Neostylopyga rhombifolia* (= *Periplaneta decorata*), described by MINCHIN, 1888, 1890; HAASE, 1889; KUL'VETS, 1898; OETTINGER, 1906; KONČEK, 1924; LIANG, 1956) the reservoirs are very small (Fig. 15) and produce secretions of unknown nature and function.

In *Deropeltis* the glands consist of two large anteriorly directed reservoirs which open through narrow slits in the intersegmental membrane into a large intersegmental pocket between tergites 5 and 6 (Figs. 12–13). Although there are no specialized valves, loss of secretion is prevented by stretching shut the slitlike openings within the intersegmental membrane. The hind edge of tergite 5 and the anterior border of tergite 6 are modified in such a way that the pocket can be opened, and the secretion permitted to exit posteriorly, or the posterior border of the pocket can be sealed, and the secretion redirected and forced to emerge laterally. The secretion is forced from each reservoir by 3 straplike intersegmental muscles originating on the anterior edge of tergite 5 and inserting on the desclerotized front margin of tergite 6 (Fig. 14). The two tergites are held together by a pair of muscles inserted on apodemes arising from the top of a median sclerotized protuberance in tergite 6, and by several short laterally placed intersegmental muscles. The tergites are separated by intersegmental muscles connecting tergites 4 and 5, and tergites 6 and 7, and by two pairs of short laterally placed protractors (ALSOP, 1970).

The chitinous intima of the reservoir is covered by a thin squamous epithelium. The secretory cells are flat, and form a second layer across the ventral surface of the reservoir, become discontinuous along the edges, and disappear on the dorsal surface. Individual secretory cells have an irregular ameboid shape (Fig. 17).

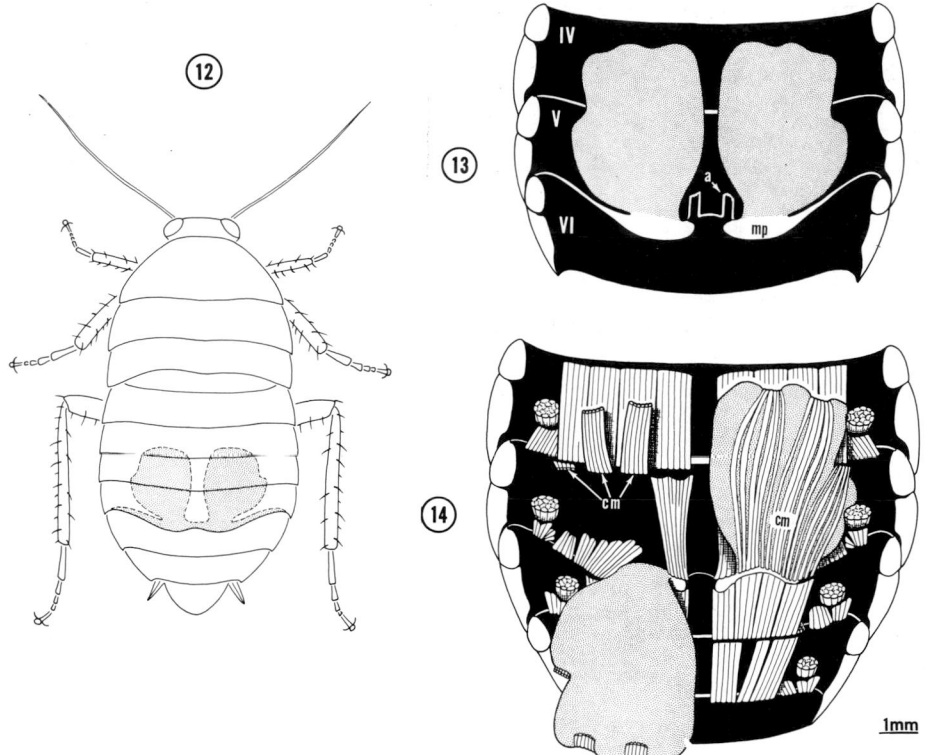

Figs. 12—14. Blattarid type II glands (*Deropeltis wahlbergi*) (From ALSOP, 1970). (12) Glands stippled. (13) View of glands and abdominal tergites IV, V, and VI, with all muscles removed, to show paired apodemes (*a*) on which large tergal retractor muscles insert, and the membranous pockets (*mp*) formed by partial desclerotization of anterior edge of tergite VI. (14) Same as Fig. 13 (with tergite VII), but with all muscles in place. The straplike compressor muscles (*cm*) partially encircling the left hand gland have been cut and the gland folded posteriorly to reveal muscles inserting on tergite V

Each cell has a large ovoid nucleus and a long irregular curving secretory vesicle containing a tapering axial organelle. The organelles (Fig. 18) are drained by long tubules (average length 800 μ) which loop and coil (Figs. 16 and 17) between the secretory cells and epithelial layer, and finally open in pairs into the lumen of the reservoir.

The secretion produced by *D. wahlbergi* is a mixture of benzoquinone, toluquinone, α terpineol, and sugar (MEINWALD, KLUGE, and EISNER, unpubl.). The secretion will ooze out or, more usually, be sprayed from the side being stimulated and can be directed forward, around, and under the anterior parts of the body, as well as posteriorly. "When disturbed, *Deropeltis* assumes a defensive stance in which its body is strongly arched with the posterior part of the thorax elevated and the head and abdominal tip almost touching the substrate. As soon as one side is touched, the side of the thorax closest to the stimulus is lowered and the abdomen twisted in an arc toward it. At the moment of spraying a contractive

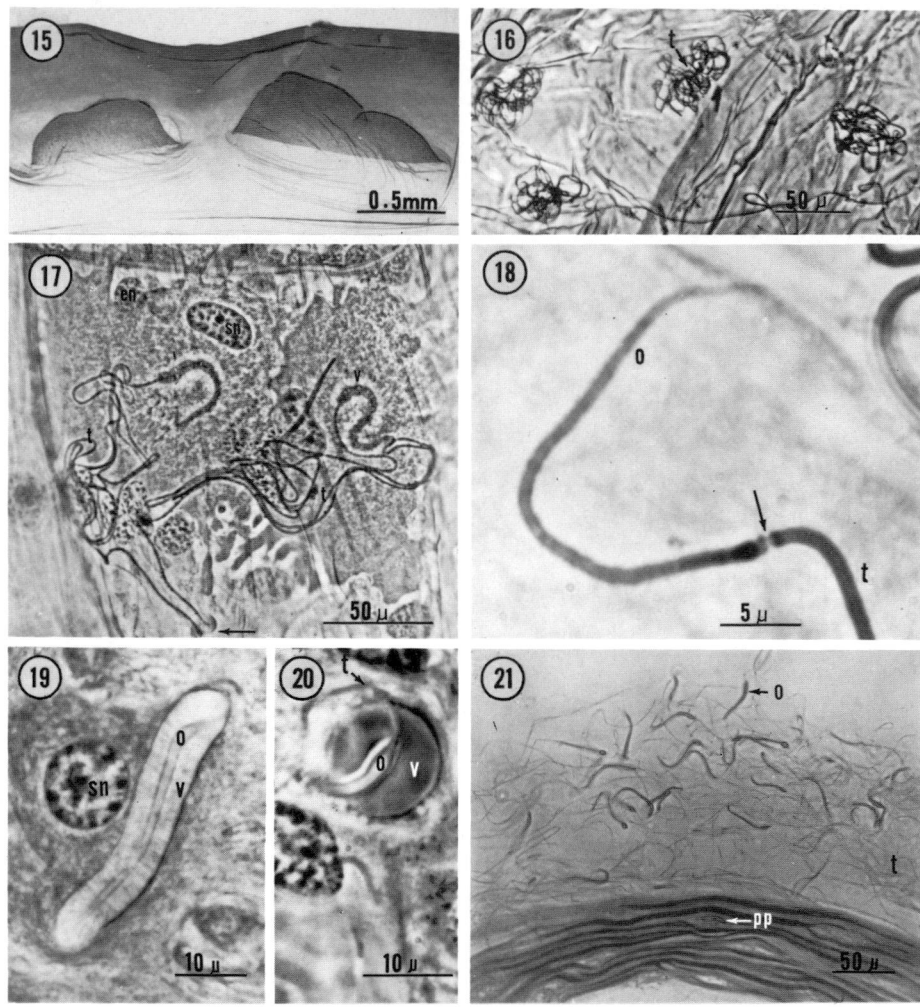

Figs. 15–21. Blattarid defensive glands. (From ALSOP, 1970). (15–18) Type III glands. (15) *Blatta orientalis*. Tergal glands. Field of view includes the full anterior-posterior extent of the intersegmental membrane connecting abdominal tergites V and VI. (KOH-digested, Chlorazol black, whole mount, phase). (16–18) *Deropeltis wahlbergi*. (16) Surface view of lining of gland obtained from the cast skin of a newly moulted cockroach. Note tight clusters of evenly spaced draining tubules. (Chlorazol black, whole mount, phase). (17) Surface view of a pair of secretory cells. Arrow points to paired tubule openings. Note the relatively great size of the secretory nucleus (*sn*) compared to that of a nonsecretory epithelial nucleus (*en*). (Heidenhain's SUSA, hematoxylin and fast green, whole mount, phase). (18) Organelle. Arrow indicates junction between tubule (*t*) and organelle (*o*). (19–21) Type IV glands. (*Diploptera punctata*, (19) Secretory cell with cylindrical secretory vesicle. (20) Portion of secretory cell in which secretory vesicle has a dilated, nearly spherical basal end. (Figs. 19–20, Heidenhain's SUSA, hematoxylin and eosin, whole mount, phase). (21) Organelles and draining tubules. The slender tubules (*t*) end in small pore plates (*pp*) located between the tracheal taenidia

twitch abruptly tightens the arc, causing the laterally emerging secretion to be
flicked forward across the point of disturbance (ALSOP, 1970)." EISNER (1970, Figs.
4G, H) illustrates a tethered *D. wahlbergi* discharging its quinonoid secretion and
the retention of residual secretion on the tergites; the vapors from this residue
presumably are capable of repelling predators and preventing them from resuming
their attack.

Benzoquinones are highly effective in repelling both vertebrate and invertebrate
predators (EISNER, 1970). As parts of defensive secretions, they have been isolated
from more than 50 species in at least 7 orders of Arachnida, Diplopoda, and
Insecta (WEATHERSTON and PERCY, 1970). Only two genera of cockroaches, *Deropeltis* (Gland type III) and *Diploptera* (Gland type IV, below) produce secretions
containing these compounds.

4. Type IV Glands

Adults and nymphs of *Diploptera punctata* (ESCHSCHOLTZ) have rigid sac-like
swellings in the spiracular trunks leading to the second abdominal spiracles (Fig. 22) in
which a mixture of *p*-benzoquinone, 2-methyl-1,4-quinone, and 2-ethyl-1,4-quinone
(plus an unidentified component in nymphs) is produced and stored (ROTH and
STAY, 1958; ALSOP, 1970). The sac is connected with the lateral tracheal trunk
through a long, narrow, coiled trachea (Fig. 23). Secretion is retained within the
gland by the second abdominal spiracular valve, which is opened by a large muscle
extending anteriorly from the valve to the spiracular plate, and closed by a small
muscle extending between conical processes on the rigid portion of the valve.
There are no muscles associated with the reservoirs and no valvular system between
the sac and the rest of the tracheal system. Despite the lack of valves, secretion
apparently does not leak back into the respiratory system. The spiracular valves
of the second abdominal segment are controlled independently of those of other
segments, remaining closed during the normal respiratory cycle, and when opening,
doing so only during the expiratory portion of the cycle, so that the secretion
is expelled by air pressure.

The reservoir is composed of thickened, rigidified taenidia and covered with
a thin nonsecretory epithelium. The secretory cells are tightly packed, mostly in
columnar arrays over the epithelium and confined for the most part to a broad,
multilayered band along the anterior and medial portions of the reservoir (Fig. 23).
The secretory cells have large nuclei with conspicuous nucleoli and cylindrical-
striated secretory vesicles (Fig. 19) often with enlarged, almost spherical basal
ends (Fig. 20). The axial organelles within the secretory vesicle are complex, with
dilated basal ends, and much larger in diameter than their draining tubules which
come together in groups to open through special pore plates interspersed between
the taenidia of the reservoir lining (Fig. 21). Histochemical reactions of secretion
granules surrounding the secretory vesicles suggest that these granules are phenolic
compounds and thus possible precursors of the quinones in the secretion (ROTH
and STAY, 1957; ALSOP, 1970).

Diploptera can control whether secretion is to be sprayed from the left or
right spiracle, or both spiracles, depending on the intensity and point of application
of the traumatic stimulus. The secretion is highly effective against ants, carabid

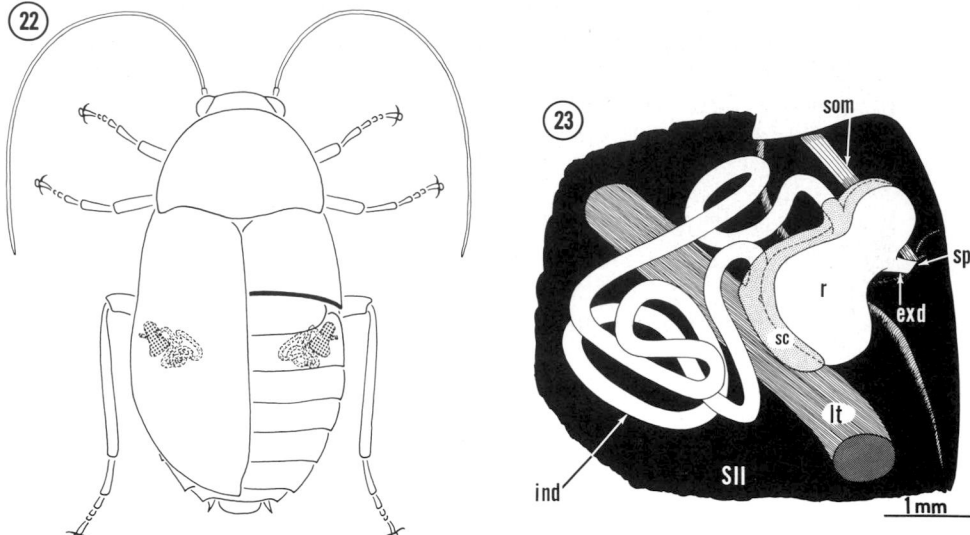

Figs. 22–23. Blattarid Type IV glands (*Diploptera punctata*). (From ALSOP, 1970). (22) Glandular bulbous expansions in tracheae heavily stippled; incurrent ducts lightly stippled. (23) Dorsal
view of the right tracheal gland showing: the lateral tracheal trunk (*lt*), the slender incurrent
duct (*ind*) which arises from the lateral trunk directly under the hardened bulbous reservoir
(*r*), the mass of secretory cells (*sc,* stippled) adhering to the anterior and medial surfaces
of the reservoir, the short excurrent duct (*exd*) leading to the spiracle (*sp*), and the spiracle
opening muscle (*som*), which runs through a deep cleft in the anterolateral surface of the reservoir

beetles, and spiders, the predators releasing the cockroach and retreating upon
being sprayed. Ants and beetles show discoordinated leg movements and impaired
locomotion. Although the affected predators recover completely after a few minutes,
this is sufficient time for the cockroach to escape (EISNER, 1958; EISNER et al.,
1959).

Several species of Blaberidae also possess swollen tracheae leading to the second
abdominal spiracle [*Blaberus craniifer* BURM., *B. giganteus* (L.), *Byrsotria fumigata,
Pycnoscelus surinamensis* (L.)], and sometimes also near the sixth and seventh
abdominal spiracles [*Panchlora nivea* (L.)]. In *Leucophaea maderae,* the tracheae
near the second abdominal spiracles are not modified in shape, but the cells in
this region are whiter than ordinary tracheal epithelium and produce a characteristic
disagreeable odor which is emitted through the second abdominal spiracles when
the species is roughly handled (ROTH and STAY, 1958). Nothing is known of
the chemistry of the secretions produced, if any, nor their roles in the biology
of these species.

5. Type V Glands

Nymphs of both sexes and some adult females of a number of oviparous cockroaches belonging to the Blattidae and Blattellidae often accumulate large amounts
of a grayish, viscous, proteinaceous secretion on tergites 6 and 7, and lesser amounts

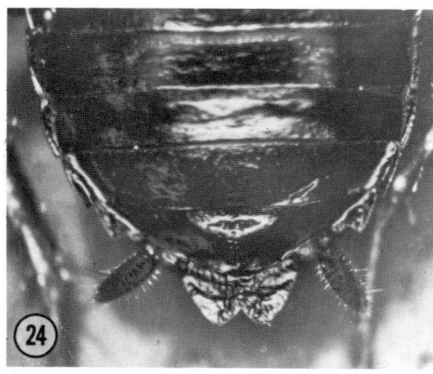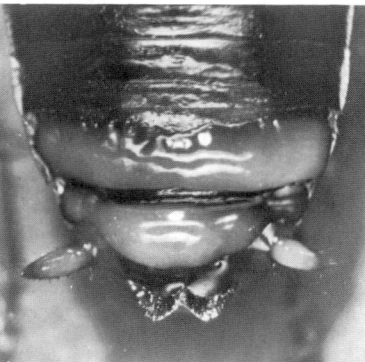

Fig. 24. Terminal, dorsal abdominal segments of adult females of *Blatta orientalis*. (From ROTH and STAHL, 1956). *Left.* Specimen from a crowded culture showing very little secretion on the tergites and cerci. *Right.* Isolated female 2 weeks old, showing accumulation of large amount of proteinaceous secretion on terminal segments and cerci

on segment 10 (segments 8 and 9 are telescoped and hidden) and on the cerci (Fig. 24). According to PLATTNER et al. (1972), a two-layered glandular tissue on tergites 5—10 and on the cerci secrete this material in *Blatta orientalis*. NAYLER (1964) found similar cells only on tergites 6 and 7 in *Pseudoderopeltis bicolor* (THUNB.). In *Blatta orientalis* this secretion is about 90 percent protein, consisting of aspartic and glutamic acids, serine, glycine, tyrosine, alanine, methionine, leucine, proline, and lysine (ROTH and STAHL, 1956). PLATTNER et al. (1972) also found oligo- and polypeptides, in addition to water and free amino acids in this secretion and described the fine structure of the glandular epithelium which secretes the material.

Secretions of similar appearance have been found on the backs of nymphs of *Periplaneta australasiae, P. brunnea, Supella longipalpa* (F.), *Parcoblatta pensylvanica* (DE GEER), *Neostylopyga rhombifolia, Eurycotis floridana, Ectobius livens* (TURT.) (ROTH and STAHL, 1956); *Nyctibora lutze* REHN and HEBARD (WOLCOTT, 1950); *Blatella germanica* (STOCK and O'FARRELL, 1954); *Loboptera decipiens* GERM. (LE-FEUVRE, 1966); *Pseudoderopeltis bicolor* (NAYLOR, 1964); and *Megaloblatta blaberoides* (WALKER) (R. SILBERGLIED, personal communication).

Although these glands have secretory cells similar in structure to those of the other types (i.e., with secretory vesicles, organelles, and chitinous draining tubules), they differ from the others in two important respects. Firstly, there are no reservoirs; secretion flows directly from the secretory cells through the draining tubules to the surface of the tergites without being stored. Secondly, and more distinctively, there appear to be two distinct populations of secretory cells, each producing a different part of the secretion. According to PLATTNER et al. (1972) one population, consisting of the "normal" secretory cells has abundant rough endoplasmic reticulum, numerous mitochondria, golgi apparatuses, and large amorphous secretion granules, and presumably secretes the amino acids and proteinaceous portions of the secretion, whereas the other population of cells has numerous mitochondria, golgi apparatuses, and small clear vesicles, but sparse endoplasmic reticulum, and presumably produces a fluid which dilutes and adjusts the viscosity of already elaborated secretion.

STOCK and O'FARRELL (1954) thought that in *B. germanica* this secretion might help keep nymphs together in loose aggregations, but aggregation in this species is accomplished principally by a pheromone produced by rectal pad cells (ISHII and KUWAHARA, 1967, 1968). ROTH and STAHL (1956) suggested that the material on the backs of the nymphs might be eaten off one another and serve as a supplement food. However, more recently, NAYLOR (1964) found that in *Pseudoderopeltis bicolor* the secretion functions as a mechanical deterrent to invertebrate predators. When ants, carabid beetles, or chilopods seized the posterior end of this cockroach and got some of the secretion on their mouthparts, they often released it and cleaned themselves, thus giving the cockroach an opportunity to escape. The secretion did not deter frogs, geckos, and skinks, nor invertebrate predators that seized the prey at the anterior end of the body. In *Blatta orientalis* the secretion, which is adjusted by the animal to the proper viscosity by dilution, also has a defensive function and mechanically impairs smaller predatory arthropods (PLATTNER et al., 1972). When ants touched the secretion, they pulled away, struggling, and as the material hardened became stuck to one another and the substrate (EISNER, 1972). It is interesting to note that a newly emerged adult of *B. orientalis* was observed to eat its own exuvium and the secretion which had accumulated on it without becoming stuck in the viscous material (ROTH and STAHL, 1956).

References

Alsop, D.W.: Defensive glands of arthropods: Comparative morphology of selected types. Ph.D. thesis, Cornell University 1970.

Beier, M.: Blattariae (Schaben). In: Handbuch der Zool. 1974, Vol. IV, pp. 1–127.

Bernton, H.S., Brown, H.: Insect Allergy–Preliminary studies of the cockroach. J. Allergy **35**, 506–513 (1964).

Bernton, H.S., Brown, H.: Cockroach Allergy II. The relation of infestation to sensitization. South. Med. J. Nashville **60**, 852–855 (1967).

Bernton, H.S., Brown, H.: Insect Allergy: The allergenic potentials of the cockroach. South. Med. J., Nashville **62**, 1207–1210 (1969).

Bernton, H.S., Brown, H.: Insect Allergy: The allergenicity of the excrement of the cockroach. Ann. Allergy **28**, 543–547 (1970a).

Bernton, H.S., Brown, H.: Cockroach Allergy: Age of onset of skin reactivity. Ann. Allergy **28**, 420–422 (1970b).

Bernton, H.S., McMahon, T.F., Brown, H.: Cockroach asthma. British J. Dis. Chest **66**, 61–66 (1972).

Bey-Bienko, G.: Fauna of the U.S.S.R. Insects. Blattodea (In Russian). Zool. Inst. Akad. Nauk, S.S.S.R., Moscow n.s. **40**, 1–343 (1950).

Blum, M.S.: Insect defensive secretions: hex-2-enal-1 in *Pelmatosilpha coriacea* (Blattaria) and its repellent value under natural conditions. Ann. Entomol. Soc. Amer. **57**, 600–602 (1964).

Bordas, L.: Les glandes défensives ou odorantes des blattes. Compt. Rend. Acad. Sci., Paris **132**, 1352–1354 (1901).

Bordas, L.: Produit de sécrétion de la glande odorante des blattes. Bull. Soc. Zool. France **33**, 31–32 (1908).

Brossut, R.: Evolution du système glandulaire exocrine cephalique des Blattaria et des Isoptera. Int. J. Insect. Morphol. and Embryol. **2**, 35–54 (1973).

Brues, C.T., Melander, A.L.: Classification of insects. Bull. Mus. Comp. Zool. Harvard, Cambridge, Mass. **73**, (1932).

Brunner de Wattenwyl, C.: Nouveau système des Blattaires. Vienna-Paris: Brockhaus, 1865.

Chadha, M.S., Eisner, T., Meinwald, J.: Defense mechanisms of arthropods. III. Secretion of 2-hexenal by adults of the cockroach *Cutilia soror* (Brunner). Ann. Entomol. Soc. Amer. **54**, 642—643 (1961).

Choovivathanavanich, P., Suwanprateep, P., Kanthavichitra, N.: Cockroach sensitivity in allergic Thais. Lancet **2**, 1362—1363 (1970).

Choovivathanavanich, P., Suwanprateep, P., Kanthavichitra, N.: House dust and cockroach sensitivity in allergic Thais. J. Med. Assoc. Thailand **54**, 476—481 (1971).

Chopard, L.: Orthoptères. In: Traité de Zoologie. Paris: Grassé, 1949, Vol IX.

Cornwell, P.B.: The Cockroach. A Laboratory Insect and an Industrial Pest. London: Hutchinson, 1968, Vol. I.

Dateo, G.P., Roth, L.M.: D-Gluconic acid: Isolation from the defensive secretion of the cockroach *Eurycotis decipiens*. Science **155**, 88—89 (1967a).

Dateo, G.P., Roth, L.M.: Occurrence of gluconic acid and 2-hexenal in the defensive secretions of three species of *Eurycotis* (Blattaria: Blattidae: Polyzosteriinae). Ann. Entomol. Soc. Amer. **60**, 1025—1030 (1967b).

Eisner, T.: Spray mechanism of the cockroach *Diploptera punctata*. Science **128**, 148—149 (1958).

Eisner, T.: Chemical defense against predation in arthropods. In: Chemical Ecology. New York: Academic Press 1970, Chap. 8.

Eisner, T.: Chemical ecology: On arthropods and how they live as chemists. Verhandl. Deuts. Zool. Gesell. **65**, 123—137 (1972).

Eisner, T., Hurst, J.J., Meinwald, J.: Defense mechanisms of arthropods. XI. The structure, function, and phenolic secretions of the glands of a Chordeumoid millipede and a carabid beetle. Psyche **70**, 94—116 (1963).

Eisner, T., McKittrick, F., Payne, R.: Defense sprays of roaches. Could this be a reason for resistance, a new source for insect repellents? Pest Control **27**, 11—12, 44—45 (1959).

Gerstaecker, A.: Über das Vorkommen von ausstülpbaren Hautanhängen am Hinterleibe an Schaben. Arch. Naturg. **27**, 107—115 (1861).

Graves, P.N.: Spermatophores of the Blattaria. Ann. Entomol. Soc. Amer. **62**, 595—602 (1969).

Gupta, P.O.: On the structure and formation of spermatophore in the cockroach, *Periplaneta americana* L. Indian J. Entomol. **8**, 79—84 (1947).

Guthrie, D.M., Tindall, A.R.: The Biology of the Cockroach. London: Edward Arnold Ltd. 1968.

Haase, E.: Zur Anatomie der Blattiden. Zool. Anz. **5**, 169—172 (1889).

Handlirsch, A.: Geschichte, Literatur, Technik, Paläontologie, Systematik. In: Handbuch der Entomologie, Schröder, Chr. (eds.). Jena: 1925, Vol. III.

Handlirsch, A.: Insecta. In: Handbuch der Zoologie. Kükenthal, W. and Krumbach, Th. (eds.). Berlin: 1930, Vol. IV.

Harrison, R.M.: Preliminary account of a new organ in *Periplaneta orientalis*. Quart. J. Micr. Sci. **50**, 377—382 (1906).

Huber, I.: Taxonomic and ontogenetic studies of cockroaches (Blattaria), Univ. Kansas Sci. Bull. **50**, 233—332 (1974).

Ishii, S.: An aggregation pheromone of the German cockroach, *Blattella germanica* (L.). 2. Species specificity of the pheromone. App. Entomol. Zool. **5**, 33—41 (1970).

Ishii, S., and Kuwahara, Y.: An aggregation pheromone of the German cockroach, *Blatella germanica* L. (Orthoptera: Blattellidae). 1. Site of the pheromone production. Appl. Entomol. Zool. **2**, 203—217 (1967).

Karny, H.: Zur Systematik der Orthopteroiden Insekten. Treubia., I. G. Koleff and Co. Weltevreden, 1921, 269 pp.

Kirby, W.F.: A synonymic catalogue of Orthoptera. London: 1904, Vol. I.

Konček, S.K.: Zur Histologie der Rückendrüse unserer einheimischen Blattiden. Z. wissen. Zool. **122**, 310—322 (1924).

Kul'vets, K.V.: The cuticular glands of Orthoptera and Hemiptera-Heteroptera. (In Russian). Raboty iz Lab. Zool. Kab. Imper. Varshanskago Univ., 1897, 49—82 (1898) [also published in Zool. Anz. **21**, pp. 66—70 (1898), and Zool. Centralbl. **6**, 90 (1899)].

Leconte, O., Lefeuvre, J.C., Razet, P.: Un nouveau critère taxonomique chez les Blattes; l'insertion des tubes de Malpighi. Ct. R. Acad. Sci. (Paris) **265**, 1397–1400 (1967).

Lefeuvre, J.C.: Contribution à l'étude de la biologie de *Loboptera decipiens* Germ. Cahier Natural. **22**, 25–34 (1966).

Liang, C.: The dorsal and ventral glands of *Periplaneta americana* (L.). Ann. Entomol. Soc. Amer. **49**, 548–551 (1956).

Linnaeus, C. von: Systema naturae, I. Ed. decima. Holmiae, 1758.

Mackerras, M.J.: Australian Blattidae (Blattodea). VIII. The *Platyzosteria* Group; Subgenus *Melanozosteria* Stål. Aust. J. Zool. **16**, pp. 237–331 (1968).

Marchand, A.M.: Allergy to cockroaches. Boletin Associacion Medica de P. R. **58**, 49–53 (1966).

McKittrick, F.A.: Evolutionary studies of cockroaches. Cornell Univ. Agr. Expt. Sta., Mem. U.S.A. **389**, 1–197 (1964).

McKittrick, F.A., Mackerras, M.J.: Phyletic relationships within the Blattidae. Ann. Entomol. Soc. Amer. **58**, 224–230 (1965).

Mendoza, J., Snyder, R.D.: Cockroach sensitivity in children with bronchial asthma. Ann. Allergy **28**, 159–163 (1970).

Miller, H.K., Fisk, F.W.: Taxonomic implications of the comparative morphology of cockroach proventriculi. Ann. Entomol. Soc. Amer. **64**, 671–687 (1971).

Minchin, E.A.: Note on a new organ, and on the structure of the hypodermis in *Periplaneta orientalis*. Quart. J. Micr. Soc. (Lond.) **29**, 229–233 (1888).

Minchin, E.A.: Further observations on the dorsal gland in the abdomen of *Periplaneta* and its allies. Zool. Anz. **13**, 41–44 (1890).

Nayler, L.S.: The structure and function of the posterior abdominal glands of the cockroach *Pseudoderopeltis bicolor* (Thunb.). J. Entomol. Soc. S. Africa **27**, 62–66 (1964).

Oettinger, R.: Über die Drüsentaschen am Abdomen von *Periplaneta orientalis* und *Phyllodromia germanica*. Zool. Anz. **30**, 338–349 (1906).

Pavlovskii, E.N., Shtein, A.K.: Experimentelle Untersuchung über die Wirkung des Bisses von *Periplaneta orientalis* auf die Menschenhaut. Arch. Dermat. u. Syph. **162**, 611–620 (1931). [Also published in Russian In: Mag. Parasitol. Musée Zool. Acad. Sci. U.R.S.S. **2**, pp. 263–272 (1931)].

Plattner, H., Salpeter, M., Carrel, J.E., Eisner, T.: Struktur und Funktion des Drüsenepithels der postabdominalen Tergite von *Blatta orientalis*. Z. Zellforsch. **125**, 45–87 (1972).

Princis, K.: Zur Systematik der Blattarien. Eos. **36**, 427–449 (1960).

Princis, K.: Orthopterorum Catalogus. Beier, M. (ed.). Netherlands: Dr. W. Junk, N.V., 13, van Stolkweg 1962–1970, Parts 3, 4, 6, 7, 8, 11, 13, 14. Blattariae.

Qadri, M.A.H.: The life history and growth of the cockroach *Blatta orientalis* L. Bull. Entomol. Res. **29**, 263–276 (1938).

Rehn, J.W.H.: Classification of the Blattaria as indicated by their wings. Mem. Amer. Entomol. Soc. Phil. **14**, 1–134 (1951).

Roth, L.M.: The evolutionary significance of rotation of the oötheca in the Blattaria. Psyche **74**, 85–103 (1967a).

Roth, L.M.: Water changes in cockroach oöthecae in relation to the evolution of ovoviviparity and viviparity. Ann. Entomol. Soc. Amer. **60**, 928–946 (1967b).

Roth, L.M.: Oöthecae of the Blattaria. Ann. Entomol. Soc. Amer. **61**, 83–111 (1968a).

Roth, L.M.: Ovarioles of the Blattaria. Ann. Entomol. Soc. Amer. **61**, 132–140 (1968b).

Roth, L.M.: The evolution of male tergal glands in the Blattaria. Ann. Entomol. Soc. Amer. **62**, 176–208 (1969).

Roth, L.M.: Evolution and taxonomic significance of reproduction in Blattaria. Annu. Rev. Entomol. **15**, 75–96 (1970).

Roth, L.M.: Additions to the oöthecae, uricose glands, ovarioles, and tergal glands of Blattaria. Ann. Entomol. Soc. Amer. **64**, 127–141 (1971).

Roth, L.M., Niegisch, W.D., Stahl, W.H.: Occurrence of 2-hexenal in the cockroach *Eurycotis floridana*. Science **123**, 670–671 (1956).

Roth, L.M., Stahl, W.H.: Tergal and cercal secretion of *Blatta orientalis*. Science **123**, 798–799 (1956).

Roth, L.M., Stay, B.: The occurrence of paraquinones in some arthropods, with emphasis on the quinone-secreting tracheal glands of *Diploptera punctata* (Blattaria). J. Insect Physiol. **1**, 305—318 (1958).

Roth, L.M., Willis, E.R.: The medical and veterinary importance of cockroaches. Smithsonian Misc. Coll. **134**, 1—47 (1957). Ann. Arbor, Mich.: Edwards Brothers, Inc., 1967.

Roth, L.M., Willis, E.R.: The biotic associations of cockroaches. Smithsonian Misc. Coll. **141**, 1—470 (1960).

Saussure, H. de: Mémoires pour servir à l'histoire naturelle du Mexique, des Antilles et des Etats Unies. Geneva-Paris, 1864. IIIme et IVme livraisons, Orthoptères Blattides.

Schulaner, F.A.: Sensitivity to the cockroach in three groups of allergic children. Pediatrics **45**, 465—466 (1970).

Shaw, E.: Australian Blattidae. Part I. Notes and preliminary descriptions of new species. Victorian Natur. **31**, 103—108 (1914).

Stay, B.: The sternal scent gland of *Eurycotis floridana* (Blattaria: Blattidae). Ann. Entomol. Soc. Amer. **50**, 514—519 (1957).

Stock, A., O'Farrell, A.F.: Cercal spinning glands in the cockroach, *Blattella germanica*. Aust. J. Sci. **17**, 64 (1954).

Takahashi, S., Kitamura, C.: Occurrence of phenols in the ventral glands of the American cockroach, *Periplaneta americana* (L.) (Orthoptera: Blattidae). Appl. Ent. Zool. **7**, 199—206 (1972).

Uy, C.G., Young, R.C. Jr., Chehreh, M.N., Scott, R.B.: Bronchial challenge studies with cockroach antigen in asthmatic children. Ann. Allergy **31**, 407—412 (1973).

Varley, G.: [No title.] Proc. R. Entomol. Soc. Lond. (C) **29**, 6 (1964).

Wallbank, B.E., Waterhouse, D.F.: The defensive secretions of *Polyzosteria* and related cockroaches. J. Insect Physiol. **16**, 2081—2096 (1970).

Waterhouse, D.F., Wallbank, B.E.: 2-Methylene butanal and related compounds in the defensive scent of *Platyzosteria* cockroaches (Blattidae: Polyzosteriinae). J. Insect Physiol. **13**, 1657—1669 (1967).

Weatherston, J., Percy, J.E.: Arthropod defensive secretions. In: Chemicals Controlling Insect Behavior. Beroza, M. (ed.). New York: Academic Press, 1970.

Wolcott, G.N.: The insects of Puerto Rico. J. Agr. Univ. P.R. 1948, **32**, 1—224 (1950).

CHAPTER 18

Venoms of Rhyncota (Hemiptera)

J. Weatherston and J.E. Percy

A. Introduction

The Hemiptera are a large group of insects with representative species in abundance throughout the world, there being more than 55,000 known species. Many of these species have made their presence felt by man, some by being serious plant pests, some through transmission of plant viruses, and yet others by being disease vectors of man and other animals. The Hemiptera are not the only insects with a haustellum, but they are the only ones in which this beak is derived from the elongated labium. The haustellum constitutes a sheath for the stylet-like maxillae and mandibles: when the beak pierces plant or animal tissue, salivary fluids are forced into the tissue along one tube and the partially digested materials are withdrawn through the other.

The Hemiptera are divided into two sub-orders, the Heteroptera and the Homoptera, which may be differentiated by their wing structure. In Heteroptera the basal portion of the forewing is thickened and leathery, only the apical portion is membranous. The hindwings are entirely membranous and usually shorter than the forewings; both pairs of wings lie flat over the abdomen. The homopterous insects, on the other hand, have uniformly textured membranous wings.

The majority of heteropterous insects are terrestrial although a large number are aquatic. Many of the terrestrial species are phytophagous although the suborder contains a large number of species which prey on other insects and their eggs. A number of others feed on the blood of man and animals. The aquatic families are all predatory, feeding on other insects, small amphibians, and fish. Almost every heteropteran species has specialized glands which emit pungent protective odors that are usually obnoxious to man.

The Homoptera consist of widely divergent groups, some of which are among the most common and abundant of all insects. They have completely membranous forewings; no aquatic or blood-sucking species are known; all are phytophagous, and many are formidable economic pests. Homopterous insects lack scent glands but specialized wax glands are often present.

The taxonomy of the Homoptera will not be discussed since considerations of homopterous toxins are restricted to the isolates from the species *Aphis nerii* of the family Aphidae (Rothschild et al., 1970).

The taxonomy of the Heteroptera is apparently in a state of flux, there being between 10 and 22 families variously described. In this report it is deemed sufficient to introduce only those families in which the species have been examined with regard to the chemistry of their venoms. The discussion is restricted to five families of aquatic bugs and nine families of terrestrial bugs.

I. Aquatic Heteroptera

1. Belastomatidae or giant water bugs are the largest representatives of the order Hemiptera, some of the *Lethocerus* species attaining a length of 10 cm. The belastomatids have the forelegs modified like a pair of pincers. They are ferocious hunters and prey on other insects, tadpoles, and even fish larger than themselves.

2. Corixidae or water-boatmen are common in still, shallow ponds and are the only aquatic bugs that are not totally predacious. There are about 300 species and their distribution is world-wide.

3. Gelastocoridae or toad bugs are shore-dwelling bugs living on the edge of ponds. These small insects, usually less than 10 mm, are squat, have protuberant eyes, and hop like toads.

4. Naucoridae or creeping water bugs are small bugs, which, as the name implies, creep in submerged vegetation hunting small insects. *Ilyocoris cimicoides* or the "saucer bug" measures about 15 mm. When handled it can deliver a painful stab which has resulted in it being called the "water bee" in many localities.

5. Notonectidae or backswimmers grow to a length of about 20 mm. A representative species, *Notonecta glauca,* is widely distributed in Europe and the New World. It is a voracious predator, using a powerful sting to kill its prey, the body juices of which are then sucked up. The sting is also painful to man.

II. Terrestrial Heteroptera

1. Cimicidae or bed bugs are a family comprised of about 30 species. The most notorious is *Cimex lectularius,* which is widely distributed in temperate regions.

2. Coreidae or squash bugs, of which there are at least 2000 species, are known in Europe as "seam bugs." Some species are predators, while some are plant-eaters and much feared agricultural pests, especially curcubites.

3. Cydnidae or black burrowing bugs resemble members of the Pentatomidae and have a large U-shaped scutellum. They are usually found living beneath rocks and debris.

4. Lygaeidae or seed bugs all feed on the juices of plants or seeds. It is a large family but the insects are small, usually 2—18 mm in length. In North America there are over 200 species, the most well-known being the chinch bug *Blissus leucopterus leucopterus,* an economic pest of various grains and cereals.

5. Miridae or plant bugs; this is the largest family in the order Hemiptera, there being more than 1500 species in the United States and Canada alone. The majority of species are phytophagous and some are known to spread plant diseases. Of economic importance are: *Lygus lineolaris,* which feeds on nursery stocks of dahlias, chrysanthemums, etc., *Poecilocapsus lineatus,* a pest of gooseberries and various currants, and the forest pest *Tropidostreptes amoenus.*

6. *Pentatomidae or stink bugs* derive their common name because of the disagreeable odor which they emit when disturbed. Some species like *Brochymena quadripustulata* feed on elm, willow, and oak, others feed on plants, while yet others are predators, e.g., *Stinetus anchorago,* which feeds on lepidopteran larvae including the pests *Porthetria dispar* and *Malacosoma disstria.*

7. *Plataspidae*

8. *Pyrrhocoridae or fire-bugs or stainers* are fairly large insects, usually brown and red, or black and red in color. Several species are economically important due to the damage they cause to crops such as cotton, citrus fruits, and grapes.

9. *Reduviidae or assassin bugs,* a family consisting of species, mostly predacious, which can inflict a painful sting when handled. A few species are bloodsuckers which often attack man; in tropical regions several species are especially dangerous since they are vectors of *Trypanosoma cruzi.*

B. Morphology and Histology of the Scent Glands

I. Adult Insects

In adult Hemiptera the defensive gland system is located ventrally and consists of paired glands connected to a sac-like reservoir which usually opens laterally in the vicinity of the metathorax. In the Corixidae the ostioles are on the metacoxa and possess a brush of setae (BRINDLEY, 1930); in the Notonectidae they are on the boundary between the metathoracic epimeran and the metathoracic episternum (STADDON and THORNE, 1974). In the Coreidae the ostioles are on the boundary of the sternal and pleural plates of the metathorax (BLUM et al., 1961); in the Cydnidae they are on each metapleuran (ROTH, 1961); and in the Pyrrhocoridae they are on appendages between the meso- and metacoxa (SCHUMACHER, 1971a, b; SCHUMACHER and STEIN, 1971). In the Gerridae there is a single orifice located on the midline near the posterior margin of the metasternum (BRINDLEY, 1930); it is surrounded by many setae which have been described as "hair pile" (BRINKHURST, 1960).

The secretion from the defensive glands of Hemiptera is not usually forcibly discharged, but oozes onto the surface of the insect's cuticle from which it evaporates. This evaporative area has many cuticular projections of various shapes to aid in reducing the rate of evaporation and increase the efficiency of the deterrent (SCHAEFER, 1972).

The reservoir is usually ventrally situated in the concavity of the metasternum posterior to the thoracic ganglion, and may extend as in the coreid *Acanthocephala femorata* from the metathoracic and first abdominal segments to the second abdominal segment (BLUM et al., 1961). The pyrrhocorids *Dysdercus intermedius* and *Pyrrhocoris apterus* have paired reservoirs (YOUDEOWEI and CALAM, 1969; SCHUMACHER, 1971a, b; SCHUMACHER and STEIN, 1971). In *D. intermedius* they are in each metacoxa while in *P. apterus* they are situated behind the metacoxa in the thoracic segment. Reservoirs in the various families are usually oval, cuticle-lined sacs, and sometimes brightly pigmented. Exceptions are found in the Anthocoridae (BRINDLEY, 1930) and the Cimicidae (BRINDLEY, 1930), where the reservoirs are bilobed; and in the Reduviidae (BRINDLEY, 1930) and Belastomatidae (BRINDLEY, 1933) where they are absent. Usually there is no sexual dimorphism with regard to reservoir size; however, in the Lygaeidae (CARAYON, 1948; GRAHAM and STADDON, 1974) the whole gland complex is much larger in the male than in the female. In *D. intermedius* a secondary reservoir is formed by a furca which is directly connected to the ostiole (SCHUMACHER and STEIN, 1971); otherwise short efferent ducts lead from the reservoirs to the external surface. The opening and closing of the ducts are controlled by a chitinous rod on which a large muscle is inserted. In the Naucoridae the muscle has been shown to be innervated from the posterior ganglion (STADDON and THORNE, 1973).

The secretory glands are paired and may be tubular, lobed, racemose, branched, or flattened. Each secretory gland is connected to the reservoir by a collecting duct. The walls of the reservoir are thin. In some families, there is a thickening located at various different positions on its surface which has been called an accessory gland. The location of the accessory gland within the various families is as follows: in the Corixidae it is located dorsally (BRINDLEY, 1930) in the Acanthiidae ventrally (BRINDLEY, 1930), in the Cydnidae posteriorly (ROTH, 1961), and in the Anthocoridae and Cimicidae between the lobes of the gland. In the Pentatomidae it is a narrow band running from one efferent duct to the other (BRINDLEY, 1930). In the pyrrhocorid *D. intermedius* the gland is kidney-shaped (SCHUMACHER and STEIN, 1971) while in another species, *D. howardii,* it is round (BRINDLEY, 1930). Although generalizations on the accessory glands in the above families have been made, there will undoubtedly be variations in development as more representative species are studied. This is exemplified by the Coreidae (MILES, 1972) where the accessory glands are all knob-like and found near the efferent ducts. In the subfamilies Colpurinae and Agriopocorinae, the glands are well developed. In the tribes Amorbini and Mictini of the sub-family Coreinae, the accessory gland is poorly developed, while in the Dasynini it is completely absent. In a closely related family, the Hyocephalidae, there are two accessory glands, both of which are knob-like.

There have been very few histologic studies of the secretory cells of hemipteran defensive glands. The basic structure has become evident from studies of the Corididae (BRINDLEY, 1930), Cydnidae (ROTH, 1961), and ultrastructural studies of the Pyrrhocoridae (SCHUMACHER, 1971a, b; SCHUMACHER and STEIN, 1971), Naucoridae (STADDON and THORNE, 1973), Notonectidae (STADDON and THORNE, 1974), and Pentatomidae (FILSHIE and WATERHOUSE, 1968). The secretory apparatus consists of a secretory cell and a cuticular lined ductule, which carries the secretion from the cell to the reservoir, and is formed by an invagination of its surface. The cuticle of the ductule is secreted by one or two epithelial duct cells. The bases of the duct cells are closely opposed to the secretory cell, which has an enlarged invaginated apical surface completely surrounding the duct cell. On leaving the base of the duct cell, the ductule cuticle is slightly enlarged within the invaginated portion of the secretory cell and closely resembles a funnel. This whole specialized secretory structure has been termed "end apparatus"; it is very commonly encountered in insect secretory cells and has been more completely described by PERCY and WEATHERSTON (1974).

There have been no ultrastructural studies nor indeed accurate histologic studies of the accessory gland cells, however it has been reported that such cells contain a ductule in the families Pentatomidae (BRINDLEY, 1930) and Cydnidae (ROTH, 1961). It is likely that such studies would reveal structure similar to those described above for the secretory apparatus.

Within the gland cells of the pentatomid *Nezara viridula,* many lipid droplets and deposits of glycogen near the base of the cells have been observed (FILSHIE and WATERHOUSE, 1968). Both smooth and rough endoplasmic reticulum are prevalent, but the smooth variety predominates in the vicinity of the lipid droplets and glycogen. As reported by PERCY (1974), smooth endoplasmic reticulum is usually indicative of extensive lipid synthesis. Membrane-bound vesicles, similar in appearance to those seen outside the cell and within the end apparatus, containing a poorly stained fibrillar material have been observed. These were termed "secretory vesicles" by FILSHIE and WATERHOUSE (1968), and are infrequently encountered during nonsecretory cycles of the cell. Lipid droplets and glycogen are also present throughout the cell at this time. In the notonectid *Notonecta glauca,* STADDON and THORNE (1974) reported that "secretory vacuoles" up to 4 μ in diameter containing electro-lucent material were located near the Golgi bodies. The apical portion of the glands cells of both species contain microvilli. From the photomicrographs it is suggested that the contents of the vesicles or vacuoles may be released at the base of and between the microvilli.

The Hemipteran species in which the scent gland morphology has been studied are listed in Table 1.

Table 1. Species and families of hemipteran insects, the adults of which have been studied with regard to the morphology of specialized scent glands

Family	Species	Reference	Remarks
Anthocoridae	*Anthocoris nemoralis*	BRINDLEY, 1930	
Belastomatidae	*Lethocerus medius*	PATTENDEN and STADDON, 1970; STADDON, 1971	
	L. griseus	PATTENDEN and STADDON, 1970; STADDON, 1971	
	L. cordofanus	PATTENDEN and STADDON, 1970; STADDON, 1971	
Cimicidae	*Cimex lectularius*	BRINDLEY, 1930	
Coreidae	*Amorbus rubiginosus*	BRINDLEY, 1930	
	A. alternatus	MILES, 1972	
	Mictis profana	MILES, 1972	
	Aulacosternum nigrorubrum	MILES, 1972	
	Pachycolpura manca	MILES, 1972	
	Agriopocoris froggatti	MILES, 1972	
	Acanthocephala femorata	BLUM et al., 1961	
Corixidae	*Corixa fossorum*	BRINDLEY, 1930	
	C. striata	BRINDLEY, 1930	
	Macrocorixa geoffreyi	BRINDLEY, 1930	

Table 1 (continued)

Family	Species	Reference	Remarks
Cydnidae	*Scaptocoris divergens*	ROTH, 1961	
Gerridae	*Limnotrechus thoracicus*	BRINDLEY, 1930; BRINKHURST, 1960	
Hyodrometridae	*Hydrometra stagnorum*	BRINDLEY, 1930	No scent apparatus
Hycephalidae	*Hyocephalus* spp.	MILES, 1972	
Lygaeidae	*Oncopeltus fasciatus*	GRAHAM and STADDON, 1974	
	Scolopostethus affinis	BRINDLEY, 1930	
Miridae	*Calonis* spp.	BRINDLEY, 1930	
	Phytocoris spp.	BRINDLEY, 1930	
	Rhopalotomus sp.	BRINDLEY, 1930	
Nabidae	*Nabis lativentris*	BRINDLEY, 1930	
	N. limbatus	BRINDLEY, 1930	
Naucoridae	*Naucoris (Ilyocoris) cimicoides*	BRINDLEY, 1930; STADDON and THORNE, 1973	
Nepidae	*Nepa cinerea*	BRINDLEY, 1930	No scent glands
	Rahotra linearis	BRINDLEY, 1930	No scent glands
Notonectidae	*Notonecta glauca*	BRINDLEY, 1930; STADDON and THORNE, 1974	
Pentatomidae	*Palomena prasina*	BRINDLEY, 1930	
	Elasmostethus griseus	BRINDLEY, 1930	
	Nezara viridula	FILSHIE and WATERHOUSE, 1968	
Piesmidae	*Piesma quadrata*	BRINDLEY, 1930	
Pyrrhocoridae	*Dysdercus howardi*	BRINDLEY, 1930	
	D. intermedius	YOUDEOWEI and CALAM, 1969; SCHUMACHER and STEIN, 1971	
	Pyrrhocoris apterus	SCHUMACHER, 1971a, 1971b	
Reduviidae	*Triatoma rubrofasciata*	BRINDLEY, 1930	
	Rhodnius prolixus	BRINDLEY, 1930	
Saldidae (Acanthiidae)	*Salda littoralis*	BRINDLEY, 1930	
	S. pilosa	BRINDLEY, 1930	
Tingidae	*Monanthia cardui*	BRINDLEY, 1930	

II. Larvae

The larval scent glands of the Hemiptera are located dorsally in the abdominal segments. Two or three glands are located between segments 3/4, 4/5, and/or 5/6. The medially located reservoir is lined with cuticle and contains gland cells

Table 2. Hemipteran species for which larval scent glands are described

Family	Species	Location of the gland (between abdominal segments)	Reference
Anthocoridae	*Anthocoris antevolans*	3/4, 4/5, and 5/6	BRINDLEY, 1930
	A. dimorphicus	3/4, 4/5, and 5/6	BRINDLEY, 1930
	A. melanocerus	3/4, 4/5, and 5/6	BRINDLEY, 1930
	Acompocoris lepidus	3/4, 4/5, and 5/6	BRINDLEY, 1930
	Tetraphleps latipennis	3/4, 4/5, and 5/6	BRINDLEY, 1930
Cimicidae	*Cimex lectularius*	3/4, 4/5, and 5/6	BRINDLEY, 1929
Coreidae	*Spathophora clavata*	4/5 and 5/6	MILES, 1972
	Hyalmenus pulcher	4/5 and 5/6	MILES, 1972
Corixidae	*Corixa fossorum*	4/5 and 5/6	BRINDLEY, 1929
	C. striata	4/5 and 5/6	BRINDLEY, 1929
	Macrocorixa geoffreyi	4/5 and 5/6	BRINDLEY, 1929
Cydnidae	*Scaptocoris divergens*	3/4, 4/5, and 5/6	ROTH, 1961
Miridae	*Distantiella theobroma*	4/5 and 5/6	ARYEETEY and KUMAR, 1973
	Sahlbugella singularis	4/5	ARYEETEY and KUMAR, 1973
	Bryocoropsis laticollis	4/5	ARYEETEY and KUMAR, 1973
	Hilopeltis corbisieri	4/5	ARYEETEY and KUMAR, 1973
	Miris laevigatus	4/5 and 5/6	BRINDLEY, 1929
	Rhopalotomus ater	4/5	BRINDLEY, 1929
Pyrrhocoridae	*Dysdercus intermedius*	5/6	STEIN, 1969
Reduviidae	*Apimerus hirtipes*	3/4, 4/5, and 5/6	BRINDLEY, 1929
	Zelus spp.	3/4, 4/5, and 5/6	BRINDLEY, 1929

on the lateral walls. Each gland opens posteriorly via two pores located on or near the intersegmental membranes. As with the adult hemipterans, there have been very few detailed studies of the glands. There are no muscles directly associated with the gland or reservoir but, at least in the Cydnidae, muscles regulate the emission of the fluid (ROTH, 1961). ROTH also reported histologic studies on the secretory cells of a cydnid species. The cells contain a clear vesicle and end apparatus. Collecting ducts lead from the cells to the reservoir. Electron microscopy of the gland cells of a pyrrhocorid support this observation (STEIN, 1969).

Families in which larval scent glands have been found are listed in Table 2.

C. Chemistry of the Secretions

I. Structure of Secretion Components

As with the biological aspects of the glands which produce the venoms and toxins of Ryncota there is a great dearth of knowledge on the chemistry of the toxins themselves. To date toxins of only one homopterous species have been studied. Within the Heteroptera, species from 14 families have been studied, but species representation within these families is generally poor. With the exception of the

Table 3. Distribution, within hemipteran families, of various classes of organic compounds found in their defensive secretions

Ryncota	No. of species examined	Alkanes	Alkanals	Alkenals	Alkanones	Alkenones	Alkanols	Alkanol esters	Alkenol esters	Dicarbonyl compounds	Carboxylic acids	Steroids	Aromatic compounds	Miscellaneous compounds
Heteroptera														
Belastomatidae	2									×				
Cimicidae	1		×	×	×									
Coreidae	23		×	×				×	×		×	×		
Corixidae	2									×				
Cydnidae	2	×	×	×					×	×				×
Gelastocoridae	1									×				
Lygaeidae	3			×					×	×		×		
Miridae	1		×	×									×	
Naucoridae	1												×	
Notonectidae	1													
Pentatomidae	25	×	×	×	×	×				×	×			
Plataspidae	1	×												
Pyrrhocoridae	1	×	×	×						×				×
Reduviidae	3										×			
Homoptera														
Aphidae	1											×		

Coreidae, in which 23 species have been studied, and the Pentatomidae, in which 25 species have been investigated, no other family is represented by more than 3 species.

1. Types of Compounds

The distribution of toxic compounds, according to type of organic compound, among the hemipteran families is given in Table 3.

As can be seen from Table 3, Ryncota toxins are comprised of fairly simple compounds with the exception of the aphid and lygaeid steroids and one as yet uncharacterized pyrrhocorid terpene. Alkanals (saturated aldehydes), alkenals (unsaturated aldehydes), and dicarbonyl compounds are the three classes of compounds most frequently utilized. As will be seen shortly, none of these carbonyl compounds possess more than 12 carbon atoms and usually either 6 or 8 carbon atoms predominate.

Although the significance is not known, it should be noted that each family of aquatic heteroptera apparently depends only on one class of compound for protection.

Table 4. Compounds used for defense by aquatic hemipteran species

Family, genus and species	Compound	Reference
Belastomatidae		
Lethocerus cordofanus	*Trans*-hex-2-enyl acetate	PATTENDEN and STADDON, 1970
L. indicus	*Trans*-hex-2-enyl acetate } *Trans*-hex-2-enyl butyrate }	BUTENANDT and TAM, 1957; DEVAKUL and MAARSE, 1964
Corixidae		
Corixa dentipes	*Trans*-4-oxo-hex-2-enal	PINDER and STADDON, 1965a
Sigara falleni	*Trans*-4-oxo-hex-2-enal	PINDER and STADDON, 1965a, b
Gelastocoridae		
Gelastocoris oculatus	*Trans*-4-oxo-hex-2-enal	STADDON, 1973
Naucoridae		
Ilyocoris cimicoides	*p*-Hydroxybenzaldehyde } Methyl-*p*-hydroxybenzoate }	STADDON and WEATHERSTON, 1967
Notonectidae		
Notonecta glauca	*p*-Hydroxybenzaldehyde } Methyl-*p*-hydroxybenzoate }	PATTENDEN and STADDON, 1968

2. Toxins of Aquatic Heteroptera

The toxins isolated from species of the five families of aquatic Hemiptera, so far examined, are listed in Table 4.

3. Toxins Isolated from Terrestrial Heteroptera

The defensive toxins from the 64 species of terrestrial bugs which have been examined thus far are listed in Table 5.

4. Toxins Isolated from Homoptera

Only one species of the family Aphidae, *Aphis nerii*, has been chemically investigated with regard to toxins. As mentioned above, this insect has been shown to contain steroidal compounds. Although the food plant *Nerium oleander* is known to contain several cardiac glycosides, the aphid apparently sequesters only three: adynerin, odoroside H, and strospeside (ROTHSCHILD et al., 1970).

II. Extraction Methods

The toxins are most commonly obtained by anesthetizing the insects with carbon dioxide or by chilling, then, either by decapitation to expose the glands or by dissecting out the gland reservoirs and collecting the contents by piercing the reservoir with a capillary. This method is exemplified in the work of WATERHOUSE and GILBY (1964) on the scent of members of the super-family Coreidae, and in the reports of McCULLOUGH (1966, 1967) working with *Acanthocephala* species. A rather elaborate refinement of this method was reported by CALAM and SCOTT (1969). To obtain the contents of the thoracic glands of adult *Dysdercus intermedius*,

Table 5. Compounds used for defense by terrestrial hemipteran species

Family, genus, and species	Compound	Reference
Cimicidae		
Cimex lectularius	Acetaldehyde, *trans*-hex-2-enal, *trans*-oct-2-enal, butan-2-one	Schildknecht, 1964; Collins, 1968
Coreidae		
Acanthocephala declivis	*Trans*-hex-2-enal, acetic acid	McCullough, 1967, 1970
A. femorata	*Trans*-hex-2-enal, acetic acid	Blum et al., 1961; McCullough, 1970
A. granulosa	*Trans*-hex-2-enal, acetic acid	McCullough, 1966, 1967, 1970
Acanthocoris sordidus	Hexanal, *Trans*-hex-2-enal	Tsuyuki et al., 1965
Agriopocoris frogatti	Hexanal, hexyl acetate	Waterhouse and Gilby, 1964
Amorbus alternatus	Hexanal, hexyl acetate, hexanol, acetic acid	Waterhouse and Gilby, 1964
A. rhombifer	Butanal, hexanal, butyl butyrate, hexyl acetate, acetic acid	Waterhouse and Gilby, 1964
A. rubiginosus	Hexanal, hexyl acetate, hexanol, acetic acid	Waterhouse et al., 1961; Waterhouse and Gilby, 1964
Aulacosternum nigro- rubrum	Hexanal, hexyl acetate, hexanol, acetic acid	Waterhouse and Gilby, 1964
Chelinidea vittiger	Hexanal, hexyl acetate	McCullough, 1974(a)
Hyocephalus spp.	Hexanal, hexanol	Waterhouse and Gilby, 1964
Hygia opaca	Hexanal	Tsuyuki et al., 1965
Leptoglossus clypeatus	Hexanal, acetic acid	McCullough, 1969
L. oppositus	Hexanal, acetic acid	McCullough, 1968
Libyaspis angolensis	Propanal, butanal, *trans*-dec-2-enal, *trans*-hex-2-enal, *trans*-4-oxo-hex-2-enal	Cmelik, 1969
Mictis caja	Hexanal, butyl butyrate, hexyl acetate, hexanol, acetic acid	Waterhouse and Gilby, 1964
M. profana	Hexanal, hexyl acetate, hexanol, acetic acid	Waterouse et al., 1961; Waterhouse and Gilby, 1964
Mozena lunata	Hexanol, hexyl acetate, acetic acid	McCullough, 1974(b)
M. obtusa	Hexanal, hexyl acetate, acetic acid	McCullough, 1973
Pachycolpuva manca	Hexanal, hexyl acetate, hexanol, acetic acid	Waterhouse and Gilby, 1964
Plinachtus bicoloripes	Hexanal	Tsuyuki et al., 1965

Table 5 (continued)

Family, genus, and species	Compound	Reference
Pternistria bispina (adult)	Butanal, hexanol, hexyl acetate, hexyl butyrate	BAKER and KEMBALL, 1967
(larvae)	*Trans*-hex-2-enal, *trans*-oct-2-enal, *trans*-4-oxo-hex-2-enal	BAKER and JONES, 1969
Stenocoris apicales	Hexanal, *trans*-oct-2-enal, *trans*-dec-2-enal, octyl acetate	BAGGINI et al., 1966
Cydnidae *Macroscytus* sp.	Dodecane, tridecane, *trans*-4-oxo-hex-2-enal, *trans*-oct-2-enyl acetate, *trans*-dec-2-enyl acetate	BAGGINI et al., 1966
Scaptocoris divergens	Propanal, propenal, butenal, pentenal, hex-2-enal, heptenal, octenal, furan, methyl furan, toluquinone	ROTH, 1961
Lygaeidae *Caenocoris nerii*	Adigoside, nerigoside, neritaloside, odoroside A, strospeside	VON EUW et al., 1971
Oncopeltus fasciatus (adult)	Hex-2-enal, oct-2-enal, hexa-2,4-dienal, oct-2,4-dienal, hex-2-enyl acetate, oct-2-enyl acetate, hexa-2,4-dienyl acetate, oct-2,4-dienyl acetate	GAMES and STADDON, 1973(a)
(larvae)	Hex-2-enal, hept-2-enal, oct-2-enal, 4-oxo-hex-2- enal, 4-oxo-oct-2-enal	GAMES and STADDON, 1973(b)
Spilostethus pandurus	Nerigoside, odoroside H	VON EUW et al., 1971
Miridae *Leptopterna dolabrata*	Acetaldehyde, *trans*-oct-2-enal	COLLINS and DRAKE, 1965
Pentatomidae *Aelia fieberi*	*Trans*-oct-2-enal, *trans*-dec-2-enal	TSUYUKI et al., 1965
Apodiphus amygadi	Dodecane, tridecane, hexanal, octanal, decanal, hexenal, 4-oxo-hex-2-enal, 4-oxo-oct-2-enal	EVERTON et al., 1974

Table 5 (continued)

Family, genus, and species	Compound	References
Biprorulus bibax	Undecane, dodecane, tridecane, pentadecane, *trans*-hex-2-enal, *trans*-dec-2-enal, *trans*-hex-2-enyl acetate, *trans*-dec-2-enyl acetate	PARK and SUTHERLAND, 1962; MAC-LEOD et al., 1975
Brochymena quadripustulata	*Trans*-hex-2-enal	BLUM, 1961
Carpocoris purpureipennis	Tridecane	REMOLD, 1963
Commius elegans	Decenal, decenyl acetate	GILBY and WATERHOUSE, 1967
Dolycoris baccarum	*Trans*-hex-2-enal, *trans*-oct-2-enal, *trans*-dec-2-enal	SCHILDKNECHT et al., 1962; SCHILDKNECHT, 1964
Eurydema rugosa	Tridecane, *trans*-hex-2-enal	ISHIWATANI, 1974
E. pulchra	Tridecane, *trans*-hex-2-enal	ISHIWATANI, 1974
Eurygaster spp.	*Trans*-hex-2-enal, *trans*-oct-2-enal	SCHILDKNECHT et al., 1962
Euschistus servus	Tridecane, *trans*-2-hexenal	BLUM, 1960
Graphosoma rubrolineatum	Hexane, *trans*-dec-2-enal	TSUYUKI et al., 1965
Halys dentata	Hexanal, octanal, dec-2-enal, butan-2-one	CHOUDHURI and DAS, 1970
Menida scotti	*Trans*-dec-2-enal	TSUYUKI et al., 1965
Musgraveia sulciventris	Undecane, dodecane, tridecane, pentadecane, *trans*-hex-2-enal, *trans*-oct-2-enal, *trans*-dec-2-enal *trans*-4-oxo-hex-2-enal, *trans*-4-oxo-oct-2-enal, *trans*-oct-2-enyl acetate tridecenyl butyrate, tetradecenyl butyrate	WATERHOUSE et al., 1961; PARK and SUTHERLAND, 1962; GILBY and WATERHOUSE, 1967; MACLEOD et al., 1975
Nezara antennata	*Trans*-dec-2-enal	TSUYUKI et al., 1965;
Nezara viridula	Tridecane, *trans*-hex-2-enal, *trans*-dec-2-enal	WATERHOUSE et al., 1961; TSUYUKI et al., 1965; ISHIWATANI, 1974
Nezara viridula var *smaragdula*	Undecane, dodecane, tridecane, *trans*-prop-2-enal, *trans*-but-2-enal, *trans*-hex-2-enal, *trans*-oct-2-enal, *trans*-dec-2-enal, *cis*-dec-2-enal, butan-2-one, hexan-2-one, octan-2-one, hex-2-en-4-one, *trans*-4-oxo-hex-2-enal,	GILBY and WATERHOUSE, 1963; GORDON et al., 1963; GILBY and WATERHOUSE, 1967

Table 5 (continued)

Family, genus, and species	Compound	Reference
	trans-4-oxo-oct-2-enal, trans-hex-2-enyl acetate, trans-oct-2-enyl acetate, trans-dec-2-enyl acetate	
Oebalus pugnax	Tridecane, trans-hept-2-enal	BLUM et al., 1960; BLUM, 1960
Palomena viridissima	Trans-dec-2-enal	SCHILDKNECHT, 1964
Piezodorus teretipes	Trans-hex-2-enal	GILCHRIST et al., 1966
Poecilometis strigatus	Trans-hex-2-enal, trans-oct-2-enal	WATERHOUSE et al., 1961
Scotinophora lurida	Trans-dec-2-enal	TSUYUKI et al., 1965
Tessaratoma aethiops (adult)	Tridecane, trans-hex-2-enal, trans-oct-2-enal, trans-4-oxo-hex-2-enal, trans-oct-2-enyl acetate	BAGGINI et al., 1966
(larvae)	Tridecane, trans-oct-2-enal, trans-4-oxo-hex-2-enal	BAGGINI et al., 1966
Vitellus insulanis	Undecane, dodecane, tri-decane, trans-dec-2-enal, trans-4-oxo-hex-2-enal	SMITH, 1974
Plataspidae Ceratocoris cephalicus	Tridecane	BAGGINI et al., 1966
Pyrrhocoridae Dysdercus intermedius (adult)	Acetaldehyde, octanal, trans-hex-2-enal, trans-oct-2-enal, terpene hydrocarbon	CALAM and SCOTT, 1969
(larvae)	Dodecane, tridecane, pentadecane, hexanal, trans-hex-2-enal, trans-oct-2-enal, trans-4-oxo-hex-2-enal, trans-4-oxo-oct-2-enal	CALAM and YOUDEOWEI, 1968; CALAM and SCOTT, 1969
Reduviidae Panstrangylus megistus	Isobutyric acid	GAMES et al., 1974
Rhodnius prolixus	Isobutyric acid	PATTENDEN and STADDON, 1972
Triatoma phyllosoma	Isobutyric acid	GAMES et al., 1974

the insects were anesthetized with carbon dioxide, the hind legs and wings removed, and the body embedded in wax. The wax was cut away until the glands were exposed, and the contents drawn out into a capillary.

Homogenization of whole insects is another method that is frequently used; however, this procedure can be criticized from the point of view that the source of the secretion cannot be ascertained. Among reports on the use of this method are those by COLLINS and DRAKE (1965) for the mirid *Leptopterna dolabrata;* COLLINS (1968) to isolate the carbonyl components of the bed bug *Cimex lectularius;* and by ROTHSCHILD et al. (1970) and VON EUW et al. (1971) for the isolation of the steroids sequestered by *Aphis nerii, Caenocoris nerii,* and *Spilostethus pandurus* from oleander. A second extraction stage frequently used with the homogenization method is steam distillation; this latter technique has been employed as the premier extraction method in the case of *Libyaspis angolensis* (CMELIK, 1969) and in the work of PARK and SUTHERLAND (1962) with *Musgraveia sulciventris* and *Biprorulus bibax.*

The most acceptable method of toxin collection is to induce the insects to secrete the material which can be taken up in capillaries or absorbed on to filter paper. Carbon dioxide anesthetization of the aquatic bugs *Ilyocoris cimicoides* and *Notonecta glauca* causes them to secrete the toxin which may be collected in capillaries (STADDON and WEATHERSTON, 1967; PATTENDEN and STADDON, 1968). GORDON et al. (1963) used electric stimulation to obtain the secretion from *Nezara viridula;* a simpler procedure, exemplified by GAMES and STADDON (1973a, b) when working with *Oncopeltus fasciatus,* involves squeezing the insect until the secretion is exuded.

III. Methods of Purification and Structural Elucidation

1. Gas Liquid Chromatography

Since the great majority of defensive compounds are volatile, much use has been made of gas liquid chromatography in the purification and identification of secretion components. Table 6 summarizes the liquid phases and supports which have been used, and the types of compounds analyzed.

Table 6. Liquid phases and supports used in gas chromatographic analysis of heteropteran defensive secretions

Liquid phase	Support	Types of Compounds analyzed	Reference
Apiezon L		Unsaturated esters	PATTENDEN and STADDON, 1970
20% Apiezon L	Celite	Saturated aldehydes, alcohols and esters	PINDER and STADDON, 1965(b); WATERHOUSE and GILBY, 1964; GILBY and WATERHOUSE, 1967
5% Apiezon L	Washed Celite	Hydrocarbons, saturated and unsaturated carbonyl compounds	GILBY and WATERHOUSE, 1963
10% Apiezon L	Celite	Hydrocarbons, aldehydes, and esters	GORDON et al., 1963
5% Apiezon L		Isobutyric acid	PATTENDEN and STADDON, 1972

Table 6 (continued)

Liquid phase	Support	Types of Compounds analyzed	Reference
10% Apiezon L	Universal B	Unsaturated aldehydes and esters	GAMES and STADDON, 1973(b)
Apiezon M	DMCS Embacel	Hydrocarbons, unsaturated aldehydes and esters	PARK and SUTHERLAND, 1962
3% SE 30	Varaport	Hydrocarbons, unsaturated aldehydes and esters	MacLEOD et al., 1975
5% SE 30		Aromatic esters and aldehydes	PATTENDEN and STADDON, 1968
3% OV-1	Gaschrom Q	Hydrocarbons, saturated and unsaturated aldehydes and esters	MacLEOD et al., 1975
3% OV-225	Gaschrom Q	Unsaturated aldehydes and esters	GAMES and STADDON, 1973(a)
10% Silicone UCW 98	Chromosorb W-AW	2,4-Dinitrophenyl-hydrazones	COLLINS, 1968
8% Silicone fluid MS 200/12500	Chromosorb W-AW-DMCS	Hydrocarbons and aldehydes	SMITH, 1974
2.5% XE -60	Chromosorb G-AW-DMCS	Hydrocarbons and aldehydes	SMITH, 1974
1.5% E-301 (Silicone rubber)	Chromosorb W-AW-DMCS	Hydrocarbons and aldehydes	CALAM and YOUDEOWEI, 1968; CALAM and SCOTT, 1969
10% FFAP	Gaschrom Q	Hydrocarbons, aldehydes and esters	MacLEOD et al., 1975
UCON		Unsaturated aldehydes	BLUM, 1961
15% Carbowax 1000		Hydrocarbons and aldehydes	CALAM and YOUDEOWEI, 1968
15% Poly-ethylene Glycol succinate	Chromosorb W	Saturated and unsaturated aldehydes	CMELIK, 1969
10% Didecyl-phthalate		Saturated aldehydes, alcohols, and esters	WATERHOUSE and GILBY, 1964; GILBY and WATERHOUSE, 1963, 1967
5% Diethylene glycol succinate	Chromosorb P-AW	Unsaturated aldehydes	BAKER and JONES, 1969
20% Diethylene glycol succinate		Hydrocarbons, aldehydes	CALAM and YOUDEOWEI, 1968

Table 7. Systems used in TLC analysis of 2,4-dinitrophenylhydrazone derivatives of carbonyl components of defensive secretions

Support	Solvent system	Reference
Silica gel G.	Pet-ether:ether:ethyl acetate (90:5:5)	COLLINS and DRAKE, 1965; COLLINS, 1968
Silica gel G.	Benzene:pet-ether (75:25)	CMELIK, 1969
Silica gel G.	Benzene:ethyl acetate (95:5), benzene:methanol (9:1)	STADDON and WEATHERSTON, 1967
Silica gel H	Benzene	MCCULLOUGH, 1966, 1973
Silica gel H	Benzene:cyclohexane (5:2)	MCCULLOUGH, 1968
Magnesia	Chloroform:hexane (85:15)	COLLINS and DRAKE, 1965; COLLINS, 1968
Neutral alumina	hexane:ethyl acetate (9:1)	MCCULLOUGH, 1966, 1973
Alumina G	*1) 4% Ether in light petrol 2) Light petrol	GILBY and WATERHOUSE, 1963
Alumina G impregnated with phenoxyethanal	Light petrol	GILBY and WATERHOUSE, 1963
Alumina G, 25% AgNO$_3$	Cyclohexane	GILBY and WATERHOUSE, 1963
Alumina G	4% Ether in hexane	CALAM and SCOTT, 1969

*double development.

2. Thin-Layer Chromatography

This separation and identification technique has been almost exclusively used, with respect to insect secretions, in analyses of the 2,4-dinitrophenylhydrazone derivatives of carbonyl compounds. The supports and solvent elution systems are given in Table 7.

The method of SCHWARTZ (1963) for the separation of aliphatic carbonyl compounds into their classes is noteworthy. The 2,4-dinitrophenylhydrazone derivatives of the carbonyl compounds are spotted on a magnesia layer and eluted with a chloroform:hexane (85:15) solvent system. After drying, the colors of the spots are noted: a yellow spot is indicative of a saturated aldehyde; rust red, of 2-enals; lavender of 2,4-dienals; and grey, of methyl ketones.

In a few instances, paper chromatography has been used for identification. The steroid glycosides isolated from the insects associated with oleander were subjected to paper chromatography on five different systems utilizing Whatman's No. 1 paper impregnated with water, propylene glycol, or formamide (VON EUW et al., 1971). MCCULLOUGH (1966, 1970, 1973) used four solvent systems, namely (a) phenol saturated with water, (b) dioxan:t-butanol:water (4:4:3), (c) 75% aqueous t-butanol, and (d) 80% phenol:methyl acetate:water (30:10:3), in his identification of the sodium and potassium salts of carboxylic acids. GILBY and WATERHOUSE (1963), in addition to thin layer chromatography, also chromatographed the 2,4-dinitrophenylhydrazone derivatives from *Nezara viridula* secretion on adiponitrile-impregnated Whatman's No. 1 paper, and eluted with cyclohexane.

3. Spectroscopic Methods

Infrared and ultraviolet spectroscopy and mass spectrometry have been widely used in structural elucidation; however, it is felt sufficient to refer the reader to the excellent paper of GILBY and WATERHOUSE (1965). This paper is a model on the use of gas-liquid chromatography, thin-layer chromatography, and spectroscopic methods in structural elucidation.

D. Function of Hemipteran Secretions

PARK and SUTHERLAND (1962) and MacCONNELL and SILVERSTEIN (1973) speculated that trans-oct-2-enyl acetate and trans-dec-2-enyl acetate may function as sex attractants for the pentatomids Musgraveia sulciventris and Biprorulus bibax respectively. The former authors drew an analogy from the work of BUTENANDT and TAM (1957) with the belastomatid Lethocerus indicus where trans-hex-2-enyl acetate was reputed to function as a sex attractant. Recently, PATTENDEN and STADDON (1970) have shown that both male and female Lethocerus indicus possess trans-hex-2-enyl acetate. Using olfactometer tests MacLEOD et al. (1975) did not observe any attraction between male and female Musgraveia sulciventris, nor was either sex attracted to trans-oct-2-enyl acetate.

It is generally accepted that the secretions of the Heteroptera have a defensive function. This also applies to the toxins of the homopteran Aphis nerii and the lygaeids Caenocoris nerii and Spilostethus pandurus. The aposematic bugs were rejected when offered to bird predators, although the beetle Hippodamia convergens is known to feed on the eggs of Caenocoris nerii and most probably on small larvae as well (VON EUW et al., 1971).

Once again lack of sufficient studies precludes generalizations; however, WATERHOUSE and GILBY (1964) stated that the scent reservoirs of pentatomids contain a two-phase system while the contents of coreid reservoirs are in a single-phase system. The same authors (GILBY and WATERHOUSE, 1967) further reported that the presence of an aldehyde in the scent almost invariably means that the acetate of the corresponding alcohol is also present.

Although the toxins are usually merely exuded by the insects, several examples of spraying have been recorded. Acanthocephala femorata is reputed to be able to spray up to a distance of 8 in. and effectively repel the fire ant Solenopsis saevissima var richteri (BLUM et al., 1961). The pentatomid Brochymena quadripustulata has a range of 6 in. and can discharge for up to 30 sec (BLUM, 1961). This secretion is also effective against the fire ant and the myrmicine Poyomyrmex badius. Earlier workers demonstrated that Anasa tristis has a 5 in. range (MOODY, 1930) and effective repellancy against ants amphibia, birds, and mice (MALOUF, 1933).

The function of the secretion in the Corixidae has not been investigated, but there is some evidence (PINDER and STADDON, 1965a) that fish tend to avoid corixids; however, the function may be bactericidal or fungicidal as was hypothesized for the naucorid *Ilyocoris cimicoides* (STADDON and WEATHERSTON, 1967). The secretion of the cydnid *Scaptocoris divergens* is fungicidal or fungistatic to *Fusarium axysporium f. cubense,* the causative agent of *Fusarium* wilt of bananas, in Petri dishes but it is still unknown whether *Scaptocoris* affects *Fusarium* populations in the field.

CALAM and YOUDOEWEI (1968) suggested that the secretion from the larvae of *Dysdercus intermedius* has at least two functions, firstly defensive and secondly as an alerting pheromone causing aggregations of the larvae to disperse. Although the adults of the same species possess a similar secretion, they lack the hydrocarbons. CALAM and SCOTT (1969) opined that this is because the adults can fly, and the functions of the hydrocarbons are to serve as a wetting agent and to act as a nonvolatile solvent for the active aldehydes, thus reducing the rate of evaporation (REMOLD, 1963). The secretion of the larvae acts as a contact poison requiring the hydrocarbons. Similar reasoning has also been put forward by GAMES and STADDON (1973) who mention that insects which spray do not need hydrocarbons, but those which exude their secretions require them.

E. Other Glands and Secretions

As early as 1922 the effects of bites from assassin bugs (Reduviidae) were reviewed by PHISALIX. More recently there was a report on the assassin bug, *Platymeris rhadamanthus,* concerning its defensive secretion and toxic effects (EDWARDS, 1960). When disturbed the bug ejaculates saliva which can be aimed very accurately. Ejaculation is accomplished by the use of the salivary pump which is enlarged at the expense of the salivary canal. The saliva stops the action of the heart of *Periplaneta* within 60 sec when placed on a dissected preparation. There is no effect when topically applied to the insects. Vertebrates, however, are very sensitive to the toxin contained in the saliva. Topical application results in pain, blisters, paralysis, necrosis and has been shown to cause cell lysis. The toxic activity is contained in the non-dialyzable fraction of the saliva and resembles snake venom in protein and enzyme composition. The active components are secreted by the anterior and posterior lobes of the salivary gland.

PHISALIX also reviewed reports on bites of bed bugs in the genus *Cimex* (Cimicidae). When these insects bite the victims they deposits a drop of liquid on the skin. There is an urticating effect from the liquid not only in the bitten areas but also on other parts of the body (PHISALIX, 1922). One of the compounds contained in the toxic salivary secretion of the bedbugs is hyaluronidase (KAISER and MICHEL, 1958).

References

Aryeetey, E.A., Kumar, R.: Structure and function of the dorsal abdominal gland and defence mechanism in cocoa-capsids (Miridae: Heteroptera) [Hem.]. J. Entomol. A **47**(2), 181—189 (1973).

Baggini, A., Bernardi, R., Casnati, G., Pavan, M., Ricca, A.: Richerche sulle secrezioni difensive di insetti *Emitteri eterotteri.* Rev. esp. Entomol. **42**, 7—26 (1966).

Baker, J.T., Jones, P.A.: Volatile constituents of the scent gland reservoir of the nymph of the coreoid *Pternistria bispina* Stal. Austr. J. Chem. **22**, 1793—1796 (1969).

Baker, J.T., Kemball, P.A.: Volatile constituents of the scent gland reservoir of the coreoid *Pternistria bispina* Stal. Aust. J. Chem. **20**, 395—398 (1967).

Blum, M.S.: The presence of 2-hexenal in the scent of the pentatomid *Brochymena quadripustulata*. Ann. entomol. Soc. Amer. **54**, 410 (1961).

Blum, M.S., Crain, R.D., Chidester, J.B.: *Trans*-2-Hexenal in the scent of the Hemiptera, *Acanthocephala femorata*. Nature (Lond.) **189**, 245 (1961).

Blum, M.S., Traynham, J.G.: The chemistry of the pentatomid scent gland. 11th Int. Congr. Ent. Vienna, Verh. **3**, 48—53 (1960).

Blum, M.S., Traynham, J.G., Boggus, J.D., Chidester, J.B.: *n*-Tridecane and *trans*-2-heptenal in the scent gland of the rice stink bug *Oebalus pugnax*. Science **132**, 1480 (1960).

Brindley, M.D.: On the repugnatorial glands of *Corixa*. Trans. entomol. Soc. Lond. **77**, 7—13 (1929).

Brindley, M.D.: On the metasternal scent-glands of certain Heteroptera. Trans. entomol. Soc. Lond. **78**, 199—207 (1930).

Brindley, M.D.: The development of the thoracic stink-glands in Heteroptera. Proc. roy. entomol. Soc. (Lond.) **8**, 1—2 (1933).

Brinkhurst, R.O.: Studies on the functional morphology of *Gerris najus* (Hem. Het. Gerridae). Proc. zool. Soc. Lond. **133**, 531—559 (1960).

Butenandt, A., Tam, N.: Über einen geschlechtsspezifischen Duftstoff der Wasserwanze *Belostoma indica* Vitalis (*Lethocerus indicus* Lep.). Hoppe-Seylers Z. physiol. Chem. **308**, 277—283 (1957).

Calam, D.H., Scott, G.C.: The scent gland complex of the adult cotton stainer bug *Dysdercus intermedius*. J. Insect Physiol. **15**, 1695—1703 (1969).

Calam, D.H., Youdeowei, A.: Identification and functions of the secretion from the posterior scent gland of fifth instar larvae of the bug *Dystercus intermedius*. J. Insect Physiol. **14**, 1147—1158 (1968).

Carayon, J.: Dimorphisme sexuel des glandes adorantes metathoraciques chez quelques Hémiptères. C. R. **227**, 303—305 (1948).

Choudhuri, D.K., Das, K.K.: The stink apparatus of the pentatomid bug, *Halys dentata* (F.), and its stink components (Hem.: Het.). Proc. zool. Soc. Calcutta **23**(2), 213—221 (1970).

Cmelik, S.: Volatile aldehydes in the odoriferous secretion of the stink bug *Libyaspis angolensis*. Hoppe-Seylers Z. physiol. Chem. **350**, 1076—1080 (1969).

Collins, R.P.: Carbonyl compounds produced by the bug *Cimex lectularius*. Ann. entomol. Soc. Amer. **61**, 1338—1340 (1968a).

Collins, R.P., Drake, T.H.: Carbonyl compounds produced by the meadow plant bug, *Leptopterna dolabrata* (Hemiptera: Miridae). Ann. entomol. Soc. Amer. **58**, 764—765 (1965).

Devakul, V., Maarse, H.: A second compound in the odorous gland liquid of the giant water bug *Lethocerus indicus*. Analyt. Biochem. **7**, 269 (1964).

Edwards, J.S.: Spitting as a defensive mechanism in a predatory reduviid. XI Internat. Kongr. f. Entomol., Wien, Symposium IV, Publ.: Isti. Entomol. Agr. Univ. Pavia, Italy, **3**, 259—263 (1960)

Euw, J. von, Reichstein, T., Rothschild, M.: Heart poisons in the lygaeid bugs *Caenocoris nerii* and *Spilostethus pandurus*. Insect Biochem. **1**(4), 373—384 (1971).

Everton, I.J., Games, D.E., Staddon, B.W.: Composition of scents from *Apodiphus amygdali* (Het.: Pentatomidae). Ann. entomol. Soc. Amer. **67**(5), 815—816 (1974).

Filshie, B.K., Waterhouse, D.F.: The fine structure of the lateral scent glands of the green vegetable bug, *Nezara viridula*. J. Microsc. **7**(2), 231—244 (1968).

Games, D.E., Schofield, C.J., Staddon, B.W.: The secretion from Brindley's scent glands in Triatominae (Het.: Reduviidae). Ann. entomol. Soc. Amer. **67**(5), 820 (1974).

Games, D.E., Staddon, B.W.: Chemical expression of sexual dimorphism in the milkweed bug *Oncopeltus fasciatus* (Dallas) (Heteroptera: Lygaeidae) [Hem.]. Experientia (Basel) **29**(5), 532—533 (1973a).

Games, D.E., Staddon, B.W.: Composition of scents from the larva of the milkweed bug *Oncopeltus fasciatus* (Hem. Het. Lygaeidae). J. Insect Physiol. **19**(8), 1527—1532 (1973b).

Gilby, A.R., Waterhouse, D.F.: Composition of the scent of the green vegetable bug *Nezara viridula*. Proc. roy. Soc. B **162**, 105—120 (1963).

Gilby, A.R., Waterhouse, D.F.: Secretions from the lateral scent glands of the green vegetable bug, *Nezara viridula*. Nature (Lond.) **216**, 90 (1967).

Gilchrist, T.L., Stansfield, F., Cloudsley-Thompson, J.L.: The odoriferous principle of *Piezodorus teretipes* (Stal) (Hemiptera: Pentatomoidae). Proc. roy. entomol. Soc. Lond. A**41**, 55—56 (1966).

Gordon, H.T., Waterhouse, D.F., Gilby, A.R.: Incorporation of ^{14}C acetate into scent constituents by green vegetable bug. Nature (Lond.) **197**, 818 (1963).

Graham, J.D.P., Staddon, B.W.: Pharmacological observations on body fluids from the milkweed bug, *Oncopeltus fasciatus* (Dallas) (Heteroptera: Lygaeidae). J. Entomol. A**48**, 177—183 (1974).

Ishiwatani, I.: Studies on the scent of stink bugs (Hemiptera: Pentatomidae) I. Alarm pheromone activity. Appl. Entomol. Zool. **9** (3), 153—158 (1974).

Kaiser, E., Michel, H.: Die Biochemie der tierischen Gifte (20—21) Wien: Franz Deuticke 1958.

MacConnell, J.G., Silverstein, R.M.: Recent results in pheromone chemistry, references to Cimicidae, Lygaeidae, Miridae, Pyrrhocoridae and Reduviidae. Angew. Chem. (Engl.) **12**, 644—654 (1973).

MacLeod, J.K., Howe, I., Cable, J., Blake, J.D., Baker, J.T., Smith, D.: Volatile scent gland components of some tropical Hemiptera. J. Insect Physiol. **21**(6), 1219—1224 (1975).

Malouf, N.S.R.: Studies on the internal anatomy of the "stink bug" *Nezara viridula* L. Bull. Soc. Entomol. Égypte **17**, 96—119 (1933).

McCullough, T.: Carbonyl and acid compounds produced by *Acanthocephala granulosa* (Hemiptera: Coreidae). Ann. entomol. Soc. Amer. **59**, 410 (1966).

McCullough, T.: Quantitative determination of *trans*-2-hexenal in *Acanthocephala declivis* and *A. granulosa*. Ann. entomol. Soc. Amer. **60**, 862 (1967).

McCullough, T.: Acid and aldehyde compounds in the scent fluid of *Leptoglossus oppositus*. Ann. entomol. Soc. Amer. **61**, 1044 (1968).

McCullough, T.: Chemical analysis of the scent fluid of *Leptoglossus clypeatus*. Ann. entomol. Soc. Amer. **62**, 673 (1969).

McCullough, T.: Acid content of scent fluid from *Acanthocephala femorata, A. declivis* and *A. granulosa* (Hemiptera: Coreidae). Ann. entomol. Soc. Amer. **63**(4), 1199 (1970).

McCullough, T.: Chemical analysis of the defensive scent fluid from the bug *Mozena obtusa* (Hemiptera: Coreidae) [Het.]. Ann. entomol. Soc. Amer. **66**(1), 231—232 (1973).

McCullough, T.: Chemical analysis of the defensive scent fluid of the cactus bug *Chelinidea vittiger* (Het.: Coreidae). Ann. entomol. Soc. Amer. **67**(2), 300 (1974a).

McCullough, T.: Chemical analysis of the defensive scent fluid produced by *Mozena lunata* (Hemiptera: Coreidae) [Het.]. Ann. entomol. Soc. Amer. **67**(2), 298 (1974b).

Miles, P.W.: The saliva of Hemiptera. Advanc. Insect Physiol. **9**, 183—255 (1972).

Moody, D.L.: The morphology of the repugnatory glands of *Anasa tristis*. Ann. entomol. Soc. Amer. **23**, 81—104 (1930).

Park, R.J., Sutherland, M.D.: Volatile constituents of the bronze orange bug, *Rhoecoris sulciventris*. Aust. J. Chem. **15**, 172 (1962).

Pattenden, G., Staddon, B.W.: Secretion of the metathoracic glands of the water bug *Notonecta glauca* (Heteroptera: Notonectidae). Experientia (Basel) **24**, 1092 (1968).

Pattenden, G., Staddon, B.W.: Observations of the metasternal scent glands of *Lethocerus* spp. (Hem.: Het.: Belostomatidae). Ann. entomol. Soc. Amer. **63**, 900—901 (1970).

Pattenden, G., Staddon, B.W.: Identification of iso-butyric acid in secretion from Brindley's scent glands in *Rhodnius prolixus* (Heteroptera: Reduviidae) [Hem.]. Ann. entomol. Soc. Amer. **65**(5), 1240—1241 (1972).

Percy, J.E.: Ultrastructure of sex-pheromone gland cells and cuticle before and during release of pheromone in female eastern spruce budworm, *Choristoneura fumiferana* (Clem.) (Lepidoptera: Tortricidae). Canad. J. Zool. **52**(6), 695—705 (1974).

Percy, J.E., Weatherston, J.: Pheromones: Gland structure and pheromone production in insects, Chapt. 1. Ed. M. Firch. Amsterdam-London-New York: North-Holland 1974.

Phisalix, M.: Animaux venimeux et venins (336—340) Paris: Masson 1922.

Pinder, A.R., Staddon, B.W.: *Trans*-4-oxohexen-2-al in the odoriferous secretion of *Sigara falleni* (Hemiptera: Heteroptera). Nature (Lond.) **205**, 106 (1965a).

Pinder, A.R., Staddon, B.W.: Odoriferous secretion of the water bug *Sigara falleni* (Fieb). J. chem. Soc. **530**, 2955—2958 (1965b).

Remold, H.: Scent-glands of land-bugs, their physiology and biological function. Nature (Lond.) **198**, 764—768 (1963).

Roth, L.M.: A study of the odoriferous glands of *Scaptocoris divergens* (Fruesch). Ann. entomol. Soc. Amer. **54**, 900 (1961).

Rothschild, M., Euw, J. von, Reichstein, T.: Cardiac glycosides in the oleander aphid, *Aphis nerii*. J. Insect Physiol. **16**, 1141—1145 (1970).

Schaefer, C.W.: Degree of metathoracic scent gland development in the trichophorous Heteroptera (Hem.). Ann. entomol. Soc. Amer. **65**, 810—821 (1972).

Schildknecht, H., Holoubek, K., Weis, K.H., Kramer, H.: Defensive substances of the arthropods, their isolation and identification. Angew. Chemie **3**, 73—82 (1964).

Schildknecht, H., Kramer, H.: XC Mitteilung über Insektenabwehrstoffe, XC Zum Nachweis von Hydrochinon neben Chinon in der Abwehrblasen von Arthropoden. Z. Naturforsch. **17**b(11), 701—702 (1962b).

Schildknecht, H., Weis, K.H., Vetter, H.: Mitteilung über Insektenabwehrstoffe. XI—Ungesättigte Aldehyde als Inhaltsstoffe der Stinkblasen der Blattwanze *Dolycoris baccarum* L. Z. Naturforsch. **17**b, 350—351 (1962a).

Schumacher, R.: Zur funktionellen Morphologie der imaginalen Duftdrüsen zweier Landwanzen: 3. Die Drüsenzelle des imaginalen Duftdrüsenkomplexes der Feuerwanze *Pyrrhocoris apterus* L. (Geocorisae, Fam.: Pyrrhocoridae). Z. wiss. Zool. **183**, 71—82 (1971a).

Schumacher, R.: Zur funktionellen Morphologie der imaginalen Duftdrüsen zweier Landwanzen: 4. Das ableitende Kanalsystem und das Reservoir des imaginalen Duftdrüsenkomplexes der Feuerwanze *Pyrrhocoris apterus* L. (Geocorisae, Fam.: Pyrrhocoridae). Z. wiss. Zool. **183**, 83—96 (1971b).

Schumacher, R., Stein, G.: Zur funktionellen Morphologie der imaginalen Duftdrüsen zweier Landwanzen: 1. Mitteilung: Drüsenzellen und ableitendes Kanalsystem des imaginalen Duftdrüsenkomplexes der Baumwollwanze *Dysdercus intermedius* Dist. Z. wiss. Zool. **182**, 395—410 (1971).

Schwartz, D.P.: Thin layer chromatography of carbonyl compounds. Separation of aliphatic carbonyl compounds into classes. Microchem. J. **7**, 403—406 (1963).

Smith, R.M.: The defensive secretion of *Vitellus insularis* (Heteroptera: Pentatomidae). N.Z. J. Zool. **1**(3), 375—376 (1974).

Staddon, B.W.: Metasternal scent glands in Belastomatidae (Heteroptera). J. Entomol. **A46**(1), 69—71 (1971).

Staddon, B.W.: A note on the composition of the scent from metathoracic scent glands of *Gelastocoris oculatus* (F.) (Heteroptera: Gelastocoridae). Entomologist **106**(1326), 253—255 (1973).

Staddon, B.W., Thorne, M.J.: The structure of the metathoracic scent gland system of the water bug *Ilyocoris cimicoides* (L.) (Heteroptera: Naucoridae) [Hem.]. Trans. roy. entomol. Soc. Lond. **124**(4), 343—363 (1973).

Staddon, B.W., Thorne, M.J.: Observations on the metathoracic scent gland system of the back swimmer, *Notonecta glauca* L. (Heteroptera: Notonectidae). J. Entomol. (A) **48**(2), 223—227 (1974).

Staddon, B.W., Weatherston, J.: Constituents of the stink glands of *Ilyocoris cimicoides* (Heteroptera: Naucoridae). Tetra. Letters No. 46, 4567—4571 (1967).

Stein, G.: Über den Feinbau der Duftdrüsen von Heteropteren die hintere larvale Abdominaldrüse der Baumwollwanze *Dysdercus intermedius* (Dist.) (Insecta: Heteroptera). Z. Morph. Tiere **65**, 374—391 (1969).

Tsuyuki, T., Ogata, Y., Yamamoto, I., Shimi, K.: Stink-bug aldehydes. Agric. biol. Chem. (Japan) **29**(5), 419—427 (1965).

Waterhouse, D.F., Foss, D.A., Hackmann, R.H.: Characteristic odour components of the scent of stink bugs. J. Insect Physiol. **6**, 113 (1961).

Waterhouse, D.F., Gilby, A.R.: The adult scent glands and scent of nine bugs of the superfamily *Coridea*. J. Insect Physiol. **10**, 977—987 (1964).

Youdeowei, A., Calam, D.H.: The morphology of the scentglands of *Dysdercus intermedius* Distant (Hem., Het., Pyrrhocoridae) and a preliminary analysis of the scent-gland secretions of the fifth-instar larvae. Proc. roy. entomol. Soc. **A44**, 38—44 (1969).

CHAPTER 19

Venoms of Coleoptera

J. Weatherston and J.E. Percy

A. Introduction

The order Coleoptera contains more than a quarter of a million species divided amongst about 200 families. The members of this order undergo a complete meta-morphosis. Species are known that live on the ground, on plants, in wood, on flowers, in carrion, etc., and in and on water. As will be seen below only 12 families have been studied regarding toxins.

1. Alleculidae: The biology of this family of beetles is not well documented. The species size ranges from 4—19 mm. The larvae live in rotting wood, while the adults are to be found on flowers or under the bark of trees.

2. Cantharidae (solidier beetles): The species of this family are soft-bodies, elongate insects. They are carnivorous, live on flowers preying on other flower-dwelling insects.

3. Carabidae (ground beetles): This family, one of the largest, comprises about 25,000 species of predaceous beetles usually 2—3 cm in length, although certain tropical species attain a length of 6 cm.

4. Cerambycidae (longhorn beetles): There are more than 20,000 species of longhorn beetles, usually cylindrical in shape, measuring anywhere from a few millimeters to 15 cm, as is the case of the South American *Titanus giganteus.* Several species are injurious to trees and cut timber.

5. Chrysomelidae (leaf beetles): This family is comprised of more than 25,000 species, including the well-known agricultural and garden pests, the asparagus beetle, and the Colorado potato beetle.

6. Coccinellidae (ladybird beetles): This family comprised of 3,400 species, is cosmo-politan and usually beneficial to man. They are well known for their voracity in consuming aphids. Certain *Epilachua* species are pests in the southern United States and Central America.

7. Dytiscidae (diving beetles): A family of strong swimmers whose 4,000 species are distributed throughout the world. All dytiscid species are predatory. The larvae, in some parts of the world known as water tigers, are also predatory.

8. Gyrinidae (whirligig bettles): A relatively small family of about 400 species, Gyrinids are aquatic and feed on insects caught on the surface of the water.

9. Meloidae (blister beetles): There are 2,300 species; the most infamous is *Lytta vesicatoria,* the "Spanish fly". The usual egg, larval, pupal, adult development is replaced by hypermetamorphosis, a process in which there is a three-stage larval development dependent on the factor of parasitism on other species.

10. Silphidae (carrion beetles): A family of 2,000 species, both larvae and adults feed on fungi and decaying plant and animal matter.

11. Staphylinidae (rove beetles): A large family of 20,000 species, all are predaceous.

12. Tenebrionidae (darkling beetles): A family of about 17,000 species, nearly all are plant feeders or scavengers in decomposing wood.

B. Morphology and Histology of the Scent Glands

In adult Coleoptera the defensive gland system is usually located dorsally in the abdomen. Often there is a second system located in the prothorax. The abdominal (pygidial) gland consists of a reservoir and associated secretory area and opens on the membranous cuticle of the eighth tergum (Table 1).

In the Carabidae the gland opens on the membranous area posterolateral to the eighth tergite (FORSYTH, 1972), in the Gyrinidae on the pleural region of the eigth segment (BARTH, 1960), and in the Dytiscidae behind the eighth tergite (FORSYTH, 1968). In the Tenebrionidae it opens ventrally or ventrolaterally between segments 7 and 8 (ROTH, 1945), in the Alleculidae on the posterior margin of sternite 7 (KENDALL, 1968), and in the Staphylinidae on the eighth abdominal segment near the edge of the ninth sternite (ARAUJO, 1973).

Prothoracic glands have been described for the Tenebrionidae (ROTH, 1943, 1945; PALM, 1946), the Dytiscidae (FORSYTH, 1968), and the Alleculidae (KENDALL, 1968, 1974). They open on the dorsolateral margin of the prothorax on either side of the head capsule. In some Cerambycidae the gland openings are located in the metasternum near the articulation of the coxa of the hind legs (VIDARI et al., 1973), and in others the glands are located in the head and open at the base of the mandibles (MOORE and BROWN, 1971).

In the Chrysomelidae and the Cantharidae there are several pairs of glands which in the former open dorsally on the meso- and metathorax and the first seven abdominal segments (BLUM et al., 1972) and in the latter open on the first to eighth abdominal tergites (SULC, 1949).

I. Pygidial Gland

1. Reservoir

The reservoir may be muscular or consist of a very thin layer of epithelial cells lined with cuticle. In the Alleculidae, Tenebrionidae, and many species of Carabidae, the reservoir has no muscle layer (PALM, 1946; BLUMBERG, 1961; CASNATI et al., 1965; EISNER et al., 1968; KENDALL, 1968; TSENG et al., 1971; FORSYTH, 1970a and b, 1972). In the carabid genus *Chlaenius* and the tenebrionids *Tenebrio molitor,*

Table 1. Location of toxin producing glands in Coleoptera

	Pygidial gland	Accessory pygidial gland	Thoracic gland	Tergal gland	♂ accessory gland	Mandibular gland	
Alleculidae							
Cteniopus sulphureus	×						KENDALL, 1968
Gonodera murina	×		×				KENDALL, 1968
Cantharidae							
Cantharis rustica				×			SULC, 1949
(adult and larva)							
Carabidae							
Abax ater	×	a					FORSYTH, 1972
Aepopsis robini	×	—					FORSYTH, 1972
Aepus marinus	×						FORSYTH, 1972
Agonum dorsale	×	—					FORSYTH, 1972
A. helmsi	×	—					FORSYTH, 1972
A. ruficornis	×						FORSYTH, 1972
Amara aenea	×	—					FORSYTH, 1972
Anthia artemis	×	—					FORSYTH, 1972
A. thoracica	×						SCOTT et al., 1975
Aptinus displosor	×	×					FORSYTH, 1972
Badister bipustulatus	×	—					FORSYTH, 1972
Bembidion lampros	×	—					FORSYTH, 1972
B. rupestre	×	—					FORSYTH, 1972
B. sp.	×						FORSYTH, 1972
Blethisa multipunctata	×	—					FORSYTH, 1972
Brachinus crepitans	×	—					SCHILDKNECHT, 1970
B. exhalens	×	—					SCHILDKNECHT, 1970
B. explodens	×						SCHILDKNECHT, 1970
B. ganglbaueri	×						SCHILDKNECHT, 1970
B. immacullicornis	×						SCHILDKNECHT, 1970
B. italicus	×						SCHILDKNECHT, 1970
B. plagiatus	×						SCHILDKNECHT, 1970
B. sclopeta	×						SCHILDKNECHT, 1970
Bradycellus harpalinus	×	—					FORSYTH, 1972
Broscus cephalotes	×	—					FORSYTH, 1972
Calathus ambiquus	×	—					FORSYTH, 1972
C. fuscipes	×	—					FORSYTH, 1972
C. mollis	×	—					FORSYTH, 1972
Calosoma senegalense	×	×					FORSYTH, 1972
C. sycophanta	×	×					CASNATI et al., 1965
Carabus arvensis	×	×					FORSYTH, 1972
C. granulatus	×						COLOMBINI, 1935a
C. nemoralis	×	×					FORSYTH, 1972
C. problematicus	×	×					FORSYTH, 1972
C. violaceus	×	×					FORSYTH, 1972
C. sp.	×						BEAMS and ANDERSON, 1961

Table 1 (continued)

	Pygidial gland	Acessory pygidial gland	Thoracic gland	Tergal gland	♂ accessory gland	Mandibular gland	
Carabidae							
Chlaenius cumatilis	×	–					FORSYTH, 1972
C. prasimus	×						HAYES and CHU, 1947
C. rufipes	×						COLOMBINI, 1935a
C. sericeus	×						HAYES and CHU, 1947
C. vestitus	×	–					FORSYTH, 1972
Clivina collaris	×	–					FORSYTH, 1972
C. fossor	×	–					FORSYTH, 1972
Colliaris melanura	×	–					FORSYTH, 1972
Cychrus caraboides rostratus	×	×					FORSYTH, 1972
Cyrtonotus fulvus	×	–					FORSYTH, 1972
Dicheirotrichus gustavi	×	–					FORSYTH, 1972
Dromius linearis	×	–					FORSYTH, 1972
Drypta dentata	×	–					FORSYTH, 1972
Dyschirius globosus	×	–					FORSYTH, 1972
Elaphrus cupreus	×	–					FORSYTH, 1972
Eurynebria complanata	×	–					FORSYTH, 1972
Harpalus aeneus	×	–					FORSYTH, 1972
H. cupreus	×						COLOMBINI, 1935a
H. dimidiatus	×	–					SCHILDKNECHT, 1970
H. rufipes	×	–					FORSYTH, 1972
Hellumorphoides ferrugineus	×						EISNER et al., 1968
H. latitarsus	×						EISNER et al., 1968
Heteropaussus jeanneli	×	×					FORSYTH, 1972
Idiochroma dorsalis	×						SCHILDKNECHT, 1970
Lebia chlorocephalus	×	–					FORSYTH, 1972
Leistus ferrugineus	×	–					FORSYTH, 1972
Licinus depressus	×	–					FORSYTH, 1972
L. silphoides	×						COLOMBINI, 1935a
Loricera pilicornis	×	–					FORSYTH, 1972
Masoreus wetterhalii	×	–					FORSYTH, 1972
Metabletus foveatus	×	–					FORSYTH, 1972
Metrius contractus	×	–					FORSYTH, 1972
Mormolyce phyllodes	×	–					FORSYTH, 1972
Nebria brevicollis	×	–					FORSYTH, 1972
Notiophilus substriatus	×	?					FORSYTH, 1972
Omophron dentatum	×	–					FORSYTH, 1972
Oodes helopioides	×	–					FORSYTH, 1972
Pachyteles marginicollus	×	×					FORSYTH, 1972

Table 1 (continued)

	Pygidial gland	Accessory pygidial gland	Thoracic gland	Tergal gland	♂ accessory gland	Mandibular gland	
Carabidae							
Panagaeus crux-major	×	−					FORSYTH, 1972
Pasimachus elongatus	×	−					FORSYTH, 1972
Patrobus septentrionis	×	−					FORSYTH, 1972
Paussus laevifrons	×	×					FORSYTH, 1972
Pheropsophus lissoderus	×	×					FORSYTH, 1972
Poecilus cupreus	×						FORSYTH, 1972
Pristonychus terricola	×	−					FORSYTH, 1972
Psecadius eustalactus	×	−					FORSYTH, 1972
Pseudozaena orientalis	×	×					FORSYTH, 1972
Pterostichus madidus	×	−					FORSYTH, 1970; 1972
P. melanarius	×	−					FORSYTH, 1972
P. niger	×	−					FORSYTH, 1972
Rhysodes arcuatus	×	−					FORSYTH, 1972
Rhytisternus miser	×						FORSYTH, 1972
Tefflus sp.	×	−					FORSYTH, 1972
Thalassotrechus barbarae	×	−					FORSYTH, 1972
Thermophilum burchelli	×						SCOTT et al., 1975
T. homoplatum	×						SCOTT et al., 1975
T. gibbsi	×	−					FORSYTH, 1972
Trechus obtusus	×	−					FORSYTH, 1972
Zabrus tenebrioides	×	−					FORSYTH, 1972
Cerambycidae							
Stenocentrus ostricilla						×	MOORE and BROWN, 1971
Syllitus grammicus						×	MOORE and BROWN, 1971
Chrysomelidae							
Chrysomela interrupta (larva)				×			BLUM et al., 1972
C. tremula (larva)				×			HINTON, 1951
Melasoma lapponica (larva)				×			GARB, 1915
Dytiscidae							
Acilius sulcatus	×		×				SCHILDKNECHT et al., 1967a
Colymbetes fuscus	×		×				SCHILDKNECHT and TACHECI, 1971
Cybister lateralimarginalis	×		×				SCHILDKNECHT et al., 1967b
C. roeselii	×						COLOMBINI, 1935b
Deronectes duodecimpustulatus	×	×	×				FORSYTH, 1968
Hyphydrus ovatus	×	×	×				FORSYTH, 1968
Ilybius ater	×	−	×				FORSYTH, 1968
I. fenestratus	×		×				SCHILDKNECHT, 1968

Table 1 (continued)

	Pygidial gland	Acessory pygidial gland	Thoracic gland	Tergal gland	♂ accessory gland	Mandibular gland	
Laccophilus minutus	×	−	×				FORSYTH, 1968
Platambus maculatus	×		×				SCHILDKNECHT et al., 1969
Gyrinidae							
Enhydrus sulcatus	×	b					BARTH, 1960
Gyrinus capsius	×	−	−				FORSYTH, 1968
Haliplidae							
Haliplus ruficollis	×	−	−				FORSYTH, 1968
Lagriidae							
Lagria hirta		×					KENDALL, 1968
Meloidae							
Lytta vesicatoria					×		SIERRA et al., 1976
Noteridae							
Noterus capricornis	×	−	−				FORSYTH, 1968
Staphylinidae							
Bledius mandibularis	×						HAPP and HAPP, 1973
B. spectabilis	×						ARAUJO, 1973
Tenebrionidae							
Alphitobius diaperinus	×						TSENG et al., 1971
Blaps gigas	×						MOREAU, 1931
Diaperis maculata	×		×				ROTH, 1945
Eleodes acuta	×						BLUMBERG, 1961
E. dentipes	×						BLUMBERG, 1961
E. extrica	×						BLUMBERG, 1961
E. giganti	×						BLUMBERG, 1961
E. hispilabris	×						BLUMBERG, 1961
E. longicollis	×						BLUMBERG, 1961; EISNER et al., 1964; HAPP, 1968
E. obsoleta	×						BLUMBERG, 1961
E. randykei	×						BLUMBERG, 1961
E. suturalis	×						BLUMBERG, 1961
E. tricostata	×						BLUMBERG, 1961
Gnathocerus cornutus	×						ROTH, 1945

Table 1 (continued)

	Pygidial gland	Accessory pygidial gland	Thoracic gland	Tergal gland	♂ accessory gland	Mandibular gland	
Palorus sp.	×						ROTH, 1945
Tenebrio molitor	×						ROTH, 1945
T. obscurus	×						ROTH, 1945
Tribolium castaneum	×						HAPP, 1968
T. confusum	×				×		ROTH, 1946
T. destructor	×				×		PALM, 1946

[a] Gland not found in this insect.
[b] Gland not separate but located in wall of reservoir.

T. obscurus, and *Alphitobius diaperinus,* the reservoir is eversible (ROTH, 1945; HAYES and CHU, 1947). The Dytiscidae and Gyrinidae have a thin muscular coat (BARTH, 1960; FORSYTH, 1968). In some of the Carabidae there is a thick muscular coat, and when this occurs the beetles can usually spray their secretion and can sometimes aim it rather accurately (FORSYTH, 1970b, 1972). On the other hand, the tenebrionid *Eleodes longicollis* has no muscular coat, but the beetle is capable of spraying up to 50 cm (EISNER et al., 1964).

The shapes and sizes of the reservoirs are very variable. In the carabids, for example, they can be ovoid, pyriform, reniform, globular, constricted, or coiled. Perhaps the most carefully studied carabid beetles have been those belonging to the genus *Brachynus.* In this genus the reservoir is bilobed; the larger vestibule contains the precursors to the final secretion, whereas the smaller vestibule contains the enzymes catalase and peroxidase which are involved in the final biosynthesis of the secretion (SCHILDKNECHT, 1970a and b). Other carabids have reservoirs of the same shapes but do not secrete similar chemicals. In fact, in an exhaustive survey, MOORE and WALLBANK (1968) have shown there is no relationship between the shape and chemical constituents. However, within the Carabidae there does appear to be a phylogenetic relationship between the various morphological characteristics of the reservoir which indicates a parallel evolution of the tribes Ozaenini and Paussini on one line and the Brachini on the other (FORSYTH, 1972).

Except in those insects where the reservoir is eversible, the emission of the secretion is effected through a duct whose opening and closing is controlled by muscles.

2. Secretory Cells

In many families there is one gland consisting of aggregates of several secretory cells. The aggregates may be definite lobes or loose conglomerates. The ductules from the secretory cells may join to form a common collecting canal as in the Carabidae (EISNER et al., 1968; FORSYTH, 1972), the Gyrinidae (BARTH, 1960; FORSYTH, 1968), some Alleculidae (KENDALL, 1968), the Dytiscidae, Noteridae, and Halplidae (FORSYTH, 1968), and the Staphylinidae (ARAUJO, 1973). In the Carabidae there is an annular thickening of the cuticle in the collecting canal (FORSYTH, 1972), and in the Staphylinidae a tracheole enters the single collecting canal (ARAUJO, 1973). The collecting canal enters the reservoir proper or at various spots in the efferent duct (COLOMBINI, 1935a; KENDALL, 1968; FORSYTH, 1970, 1972; HAPP and HAPP, 1973; SCOTT et al., 1975). In the carabid tribe Brachini, which spray a mixture of hydroquinone and H_2O_2 and which have two distinct, but joined chambers in the reservoir, the duct enters the reservoir proper. Only the antichamber which contains the enzymes has a very muscular wall (SCHILDKNECHT et al., 1970). In the latter area the secretory cells are scattered in the cell wall (SCHILDKNECHT, 1970).

In addition to a separate gland in the Gyrinidae (BREGA et al., 1968) and the Alleculidae (KENDALL, 1968), there are individual secretory cells scattered over the surface of the reservoir. The Tenebrionidae do not have glands which are separate from the reservoir (ROTH, 1945; PALM, 1946; BLUMBERG, 1961; EISNER et al., 1964). The cells are located on the surface of the reservoir and may open separately or in groups. In *Eleodes longicollis* there are two distinct groups of these cells called C_1 and C_2 (EISNER et al., 1964; HAPP, 1968). The C_1 cells are located on the upper anterior and distal face of the reservoir. These are individual secretory cells where the cuticular ductule originates in the tubule carrying cell, but the head and body of the organelle are located in a single cell. The ductules enter the reservoir singly. In the C_2 cell the ductule again originates in the tubule carrying cell, but the head of the organelle is located in cell 2a, while the body (bulb and bellows) is located in cell 2b. The ductules from this cell type enter the reservoir in groups at sieve plates. Although there are separate glands in the Alleculidae, there are, in addition, cells similar to those of *Eleodes* scattered on the surface of the reservoir (KENDALL, 1968).

3. Fine Structure of Cells

There have been very few ultrastructural studies of the secretory cells. These include three carabid beetles, *Carabus* sp. (BEAMS and ANDERSON, 1961), *Brachynus crepitans* (SCHNEPF et al., 1969), and *Pterostichus madidus* (FORSYTH, 1970). In these three insects there is only one secretory cell associated with the cuticular ductule. In all cases the cells are gobletshaped with the inverted plasma membrane containing many microvilli. Mitochondria, lysosomes, Golgi complexes, and smooth endoplasmic reticulum are characteristic of the cells, although rough endoplasmic reticulum predominates in *P. madidus*. The ductule forms an 'end apparatus' in the inverted portion of the secretory cell and has the same relationship to the cell and collecting tubule as has been described for the Homoptera (WEATHERSTON and PERCY, see Chapter 18, this volume).

The C_1 cells of the tenebrionid *E. longicollis* have basically the same structure as the carabids (EISNER et al., 1964). The main difference is in the structure of the ductule. There is a distinct 'head' which is located within the inverted portion of the cell. The head is made up of thick porous epicuticle and is surrounded by many fine fibrils.

The C_2 cell unit of *E. longicollis* and the secretory unit of the staphylinid *Bledius mandibularis* are very similar (HAPP and HAPP, 1973). Cell C_{2a} and C_{2b} in *E. longicollis* correspond respectively to the cortical and medullary cells in *B. mandibularis*. In C_{2a} and the cortical cells there are abundant smooth endoplasmic reticulum, dense bodies, mitochondria, and tightly packed microvilli. In C_{2b} and the medullary cells the microvilli are very short and the mitochondria are larger. In C_{2b} there is abundant rough endoplasmic reticulum, while in the medullary cell tubular smooth endoplasmic reticulum predominates. The head of the ductule is similar in both, while there are slight structural differences in the part which passes through the second cell.

Only in *E. longicollis* have extensive histochemical tests been carried out to determine the function of the cell types. It has been shown that cell type C_2 is responsible for the production of hydroquinones and contains the appropriate precursors and enzymes to make this possible (HAPP, 1968). The elaborate organelles found in these cells indicate the capability of the organism to protect itself from the toxicity of the compounds the cells produce.

4. Accessory Gland

In some of the beetles an accessory gland is associated with the pygidial gland. It is present in the Carabini, Cychrini, Paussini, and Brachini of the Carabidae (CASNATI et al., 1965; FORSYTH, 1972); and the Dytiscidae (FORSYTH, 1968). The glands are usually located near the opening valve, and ducts from the secretory cells enter the efferent duct of the pygidial gland except in the Cychrini and Paussini, where they open separately to the cuticle. In the dytiscid, *Hyphydrus ovatus* there is a small integumental gland as well as an accessory gland (FORSYTH, 1968).

II. Thoracic Glands

These glands are located in the dorsal anterior angles of the prothorax and open on either side of the head capsule. They have been studied only in the Alleculidae, Dytiscidae, and Tenebrionidae (ROTH, 1943, 1945; PALM, 1946; FORSYTH, 1968; KENDALL, 1968, 1974). The reservoir is very shallow, and there are no muscles in its walls.

In all, the gland is not a distinct structure, but the secretory cells are scattered on the surface of the reservoir wall. At least in the Tenebrionidae the closing mechanism characteristic of the pygidial glands is absent.

III. Other Glands

It has recently been reported that in at least one species of blister beetles of the family Meloidae, cantharidin is synthesized by the males only and is transferred to the females during copulation. It is synthesized in the accessory glands of the male sex organs (SIERRA et al., 1976).

In two species of cerambycids the defensive secretion is synthesized by modified mandibular glands (MOORE and BROWN, 1971).

Larvae of the Chrysomelidae have defensive glands situated in large conical tubercles located dorsally on the meso and metathorax and several abdominal segments (GARB, 1915; HINTON, 1951; BLUM et al., 1972). The larvae can discharge five or six droplets in succession. Each gland consists of a thin-walled reservoir with glandular cells scattered on its surface. The whole reservoir is everted during secretion. Some of the secretion is retained in the reservoirs of the last larval stages. The cast skin remains attached to the pupae, which can discharge the fluid by a series of jerks so that the insect is protected even in this stage.

Larvae of the carabids *Chlaenius prasimus* and *C. sericeus* have been reported to have defensive glands located on the metapimera of the metathorax (HAYES and CHU, 1947).

C. Chemistry of the Secretions

I. Structure of Secretion Components

Within the Coleoptera only 12 families have been studied with regard to the chemistry of their defensive toxins. Species representation within the families is generally poor (one to ten species), although many meloid species, 108 tenebrionid species and more than one 150 species of the Carabidae have been examined.

1. Types of Compounds

Table 2 gives the distribution within coleopteran families of the various classes of organic compounds present in their defence toxins.

Table 2. Distribution within coleopteran families of various classes of organic compounds present in their defence toxins

Coleoptera	No. of species examined	Aliphatic acids	Aliphatic aldehydes	Aliphatic esters	Hydrocarbons	Aromatic acids	Aromatic aldehydes	Aromatic esters	Quinonoid compounds	Steroidal compounds	Terpenoid compounds	Alkaloids	Miscellaneous
Alleculidae	1								×				
Cantharidae	1	×											
Carabidae	153	×	×	×	×	×	×		×				×
Cerambycidae	4				×		×				×		×
Chrysomelidae	4						×	×					
Coccinellidae	14											×	
Dytiscidae	20				×	×	×			×			×
Gyrinidae	9		×								×		×
Meloidae	?										×		
Silphidae	3												×
Staphylinidae	14	×	×		×				×		×	×	×
Tenebrionidae	108	×	×		×				×				×

The toxins, with very few exceptions, are multicomponent system and usually consist of compounds of different organic types. Quinonoid compounds, which are the most common compounds found in arthropod defensive toxins, have been isolated from four coleopteran families: Alleculidae, Carabidae, Staphylinidae, and Tenebrionidae. In the tenebrionid beetles various quinones, usually accompanied by monounsaturated hydrocarbons, occur in over 100 species.

The complexity of the toxin components varies from ammonia and formic acid, through aromatic aldehydes, acids and esters, to benzoquinones and naphthoquinones, to terpenoids such as iridodial, gyrinidal, and cantharidin, to the steroids testosterone and cortexone, to the alkaloids actinidine, coccinelline, and pederin. The complexity of the molecules is greater amongst the nonexocrine defensive substances than in the glandular-produced materials.

2. Toxins of the Alleculidae

Prionychus ater is the only alleculid species whose defensive secretion has been analyzed (SCHILDKNECHT et al., 1964). The secretion contains ρ-toluquinone and p-ethylquinone.

3. Toxins of the Cantharidae

Although the plant family Compositae is well known as a source of acetylenic compounds, no such compounds were known from insect sources until MEINWALD et al. (1968) reported the isolation and characterization of *cis*-8-dihydromatricaria acid (*cis*-8-decene-4,6-diynoic acid) from the soldier beetle *Chauliognathus lecontei*.

4. Toxins of the Carabidae

The toxins from this important family of predatory beetles, 153 species of which have been studied, are presented in tabular form (Table 3).

Table 3. Defensive toxins of the Carabidae

Carabidae	Components identified in the secretion	References
Abacomorphus asperulus	Angelic acid; formic acid; methacrylic acid; tiglic acid	MOORE and WALLBANK, 1968
Abax ater	Methacrylic acid; tiglic acid	SCHILDKNECHT, 1959, 1970; SCHILDKNECHT and WEIS, 1962
A. ovalis	Methacrylic acid; tiglic acid	SCHILDKNECHT, 1959, 1970; SCHILDKNECHT and WEIS, 1962; SCHILDKNECHT et al., 1968b
A. parallelus	Methacrylic acid; tiglic acid	SCHILDKNECHT, 1959, 1970; SCHILDKNECHT and WEIS, 1962; SCHILDKNECHT et al., 1968b
Acinopus sp.	Formic acid	SCHILDKNECHT, 1964
Agonum assimilis	Formic acid	SCHILDKNECHT et al., 1968b, e

Table 3 (continued)

Carabidae	Components identified in the secretion	References
A. (Idiochroma) dorsalis	Decane; formic acid; salicylic acid methyl ester, undecane	SCHILDKNECHT, 1970; SCHILDKNECHT et al., 1968 b, e
A. marginatum	Formic acid	SCHILDKNECHT et al., 1968 b, e
A. mostum	Formic acid	SCHILDKNECHT et al., 1968 b, e
A. sexpunctatum	Formic acid	SCHILDKNECHT et al., 1968 b, e
A. viduum	Formic acid	SCHILDKNECHT et al., 1968 b, e
Amara familaris	Decane; methacrylic acid; tiglic acid; tridecane; undecane	SCHILDKNECHT, 1970; SCHILDKNECHT et al., 1968 b
A. similata	Decane; methacrylic acid; tiglic acid; tridecane; undecane	SCHILDKNECHT, 1970; SCHILDKNECHT et al., 1968 b
Amblytelus curtus	Formic acid	MOORE and WALLBANK, 1968
Anisodactylus binotatus	Formic acid	SCHILDKNECHT, 1968; SCHILDKNECHT et al., 1968 b, e
Anthia thoracica	Acetic acid; formic acid; tiglic acid; isovaleraldehyde	SCOTT et al., 1975
Arthropterus sp.	p-ethylquinone; p-toluquinone	MOORE and WALLBANK, 1968
Asaphidion flavipes	Salicylaldehyde; valeric acid	SCHILDKNECHT, 1970
Badister bipustulatus	Formic acid	SCHILDKNECHT et al., 1968 b, e
Bembidion andreae	isobutyric acid; isovaleric acid	SCHILDKNECHT et al., 1968 b, e
B. lampros	isobutyric acid; isovaleric acid	SCHILDKNECHT et al., 1968 b, e
B. quadrigottatum	Salicylaldehyde; valeric acid	SCHILDKNECHT, 1970; SCHILDKNECHT et al., 1968 b, e
B. quadrimagulatum	m-cresol.	SCHILDKNECHT et al., 1968 b, e
Brachynus crepitans	p-benzoquinone; p-toluquinone	SCHILDKNECHT, 1957
B. explodens	p-benzoquinone; p-toluquinone	SCHILDKNECHT, 1957
B. sclopeta	p-benzoquinone; p-toluquinone	SCHILDKNECHT, 1957
Broscus cephalotes	isobutyric acid; isovaleric acid	SCHILDKNECHT et al., 1968 b, e
Calathus fuscipes	Formic acid	SCHILDKNECHT et al., 1968 b, e
C. melanocephalus	Formic acid	SCHILDKNECHT, 1964; SCHILDKNECHT et al., 1968 b, e
Callisthenes luxatus	Methacrylic acid; salicylaldehyde	MCCULLOUGH, 1972a
Callistus lunatus	p-benzoquinone; p-ethylquinone; p-toluquinone	SCHILDKNECHT et al., 1968 b, e
Calosoma affini	Salicylaldehyde	MCCULLOUGH, 1966a
C. alternans sayi	Salicylaldehyde	MCCULLOUGH, 1966a
C. externum	Methacrylic acid; salicylic acid	MCCULLOUGH and WEINHEIMER, 1966
C. macrum	Salicylaldehyde	MCCULLOUGH, 1966a
C. marginalis	Methacrylic acid; salicylaldehyde	MCCULLOUGH and WEINHEIMER, 1966
C. oceanicum	Caproic acid; methacrylic acid; salicylaldehyde	MOORE and WALLBANK, 1968

Table 3 (continued)

Carabidae	Components identified in the secretion	References
C. parvicollis	Salicylaldehyde	McCullough, 1966a
C. peregrinator	Methacrylic acid; salicylaldehyde	McCullough, 1969a
C. prominens	Salicylaldehyde	Eisner et al., 1963a
C. schayeri	Caproic acid; methacrylic acid; salicylaldehyde	Moore and Wallbank, 1968
C. scrutator	Methacrylic acid; salicylic acid	McCullough and Weinheimer, 1966
C. sycophanta	Methacrylic acid; salicylaldehyde; tiglic acid	Casnati et al., 1965
Carabus auratus	Methacrylic acid; tiglic acid	Schildknecht, 1970; Schildknecht and Weis, 1962; Schildknecht et al., 1968e
C. auronitens	Methacrylic acid; tiglic acid	Schildknecht, 1970
C. cansellatus	Methacrylic acid; tiglic acid	Schildknecht, 1970
C. convexus	Methacrylic acid; tiglic acid	Schildknecht, 1970
C. granulatus	Methacrylic acid; tiglic acid	Schildknecht and Weis, 1962; Schildknecht et al., 1968b, e
C. problematicus	Methacrylic acid; tiglic acid	Schildknecht, 1970; Schildknecht and Weis, 1962; Schildknecht et al., 1968e
C. taedatus	Ethacrylic acid; methacrylic acid	Benn et al., 1973
Carenum bonelli	Angelic acid; isocrotonic acid; hexenoic acid; methacrylic acid	Moore and Wallbank, 1968
C. interruptum	Angelic acid; isocrotonic acid; methacrylic acid	Moore and Wallbank, 1968
C. tinctillatum	Angelic acid; isocrotonic acid; methacrylic acid; tiglic acid	Moore and Wallbank, 1968
Castelnaudia superba	Acetic acid; methacrylic acid, tiglic acid	Moore and Wallbank, 1968
Chlaenius australis	*m*-cresol	Moore and Wallbank, 1968
C. bipunctatus	*m*-cresol	Schildknecht, 1970
C. chrysocephalus	*m*-cresol	Schildknecht et al., 1968b, e
C. cordicollis	*m*-cresol	Eisner et al., 1963b
C. festivus	*m*-cresol	Schildknecht et al., 1968b, e
C. tristus	*m*-cresol	Schildknecht et al., 1968b, e
C. vestitus	*p*-benzoquinone; *p*-ethylquinone; *p*-toluquinone	Schildknecht et al., 1968b
Clivina basalis	*p*-benzoquinone; *p*-toluquinone	Moore and Wallbank, 1968
C. fossor	*p*-benzoquinone; 2-methoxy-3-methyl-quinone; *p*-toluquinone	Schildknecht et al., 1968b, e
Craspedophorus sp.	*m*-cresol; tridecane	Moore and Wallbank, 1968
Cratoferonia phylarchus	Methacrylic acid; tiglic acid	Moore and Wallbank, 1968

Table 3 (continued)

Carabidae	Components identified in the secretion	References
Cratogaster melas	Methacrylic acid; tiglic acid	MOORE and WALLBANK, 1968
Cychrus rostratus	Tiglic acid	SCHILDKNECHT and WEIS, 1962
Diachromus germanus	Formic acid	SCHILDKNECHT et al., 1968b, e
Diaphoromenus edwardsi	Formic acid	MOORE and WALLBANK, 1968
Dicaelus dilatatus	Formic acid	MCCULLOUGH, 1967
D. purpuratus	Formic acid	MCCULLOUGH, 1969b
D. splendidus	Formic acid	MCCULLOUGH, 1967
Dichirotrichus obsoletus	Formic acid	SCHILDKNECHT et al., 1968b, e
Dicrochile brevicollis	Formic acid	MOORE and WALLBANK, 1968
D. goryi	Formic acid	MOORE and WALLBANK, 1968
Drypta dentata	Formic acid	SCHILDKNECHT et al., 1968b, e
Elaphrus ripareus	isobutyric acid; isovaleric acid	SCHILDKNECHT et al., 1968b, e
Eudalia macleayi	Formic acid	MOORE and WALLBANK, 1968
Eurylychnus blagravei	Methacrylic acid; tiglic acid	MOORE and WALLBANK, 1968
E. olliffi	Methacrylic acid; tiglic acid; isovaleric acid	MOORE and WALLBANK, 1968
Harpalus atratus	Formic acid	SCHILDKNECHT et al., 1968b, e
H. azurus	Formic acid	SCHILDKNECHT et al., 1968e
H. caliginosus	Formic acid	MCCULLOUGH, 1966b
H. dimidiatus	Formic acid	SCHILDKNECHT, 1964; SCHILDKNECHT et al., 1968b, e
H. distinguendus	Formic acid	SCHILDKNECHT, 1964; SCHILDKNECHT et al., 1968b, e
H. griseus	Formic acid	SCHILDKNECHT and WEIS, 1960b; SCHILDKNECHT et al., 1968b, e
H. luteicornis	Formic acid	SCHILDKNECHT et al., 1968b, e
H. pubescens	Formic acid	SCHILDKNECHT and WEIS, 1960b; SCHILDKNECHT et al., 1968b, e
H. tardus	Formic acid	SCHILDKNECHT et al., 1968b, e
Helluo costatus	Formic acid; *n*-nonyl acetate; *n*-nonyl formate	MOORE and WALLBANK, 1968
Hellumorphoides ferrugineus	Formic acid; *n*-nonyl acetate	EISNER et al., 1968
H. latitarsis	Formic acid; *n*-nonyl acetate	EISNER et al., 1968
Laccopterum foveigerum	Ethacrylic acid; hexenoic acid; methacrylic acid; tiglic acid; *n*-caproic acid; crotonic acid; isocrotonic acid	MOORE and WALLBANK, 1968
Lebia chlorocephala	Formic acid	SCHILDKNECHT et al., 1968b, e
Leistus ferrugineus	Methacrylic acid; tiglic acid	SCHILDKNECHT, 1970; SCHILDKNECHT et al., 1968e

Table 3 (continued)

Carabidae	Components identified in the secretion	References
Licenus nitidor	Formic acid	SCHILDKNECHT et al., 1968b, e
Loricera pilicornis	isobutyric acid; isovaleric acid	SCHILDKNECHT et al., 1968e
Loxandrus longiformis	Salicylaldehyde	MOORE and WALLBANK, 1968
Loxodactylus carinulatus	Methacrylic acid	MOORE and WALLBANK, 1968
Megacephala australis	Benzaldehyde	MOORE and BROWN, 1971b
Molops elatus	Methacrylic acid; tiglic acid	SCHILDKNECHT et al., 1968e
Mystropomus regularis	*p*-benzoquinone; *p*-ethylquinone; *p*-toluquinone	MOORE and WALLBANK, 1968
Nebria livida	Methacrylic acid; tiglic acid	SCHILDKNECHT, 1970; SCHILDKNECHT et al., 1968e
Notiophilus biguttatus	isobutyric acid; isovaleric acid	SCHILDKNECHT et al., 1968e
Notonomus angustibasis	Formic acid	MOORE and WALLBANK, 1968
N. crenulatus	Formic acid	MOORE and WALLBANK, 1968
N. miles	Formic acid	MOORE and WALLBANK, 1968
N. muelleri	Formic acid	MOORE and WALLBANK, 1968
N. opulentus	Formic acid	MOORE and WALLBANK, 1968
N. rainbowi	Formic acid	MOORE and WALLBANK, 1968
N. scotti	Formic acid	MOORE and WALLBANK, 1968
N. triplogenioides	Formic acid	MOORE and WALLBANK, 1968
N. variicollis	Formic acid	MOORE and WALLBANK, 1968
Odacantha melanura	Formic acid	SCHILDKNECHT et al., 1968b, e
Omophron limbatum	isobutyric acid; isovaleric acid	SCHILDKNECHT et al., 1968b, e
Pamborus alternans	Ethacrylic acid; methacrylic acid	MOORE and WALLBANK, 1968
P. guerini	Ethacrylic acid; methacrylic acid	MOORE and WALLBANK, 1968
P. pradieri	Ethacrylic acid; methacrylic acid	MOORE and WALLBANK, 1968
P. viridis	Ethacrylic acid; methacrylic acid	MOORE and WALLBANK, 1968
Panagaeus bipistulatus	*m*-cresol	SCHILDKNECHT et al., 1968b, e
Pasimachus californicus	Methacrylic acid	McCULLOUGH, 1969c
P. duplicatus	Methacrylic acid	McCULLOUGH, 1969c
P. elongatus	Methacrylic acid	McCULLOUGH, 1972b
Paussus favieri	*p*-benzoquinone; *p*-toluquinone	SCHILDKNECHT and KOOB, 1969
Philophloeus tuberculatus	Crotonic acid; isocrotonic acid; methacrylic acid; 4-methylvaleric acid; tiglic acid	MOORE and WALLBANK, 1968
Polystichus connexus	Formic acid	SCHILDKNECHT et al., 1968e
Progaleritina mexicana	Formic acid	McCULLOUGH, 1971
Promecoderus spp.	*n*-butyric acid; caproic acid; isovaleric acid	MOORE and WALLBANK, 1968
Prosopognus harpaloides	Methacrylic acid	MOORE and WALLBANK, 1968
Pseudoceneus iridescens	Methacrylic acid; tiglic acid	MOORE and WALLBANK, 1968

Table 3 (continued)

Carabidae	Components identified in the secretion	References
Pterostichus cupreus	Decane; methacrylic acid; tiglic acid; tridecane; undecane	Schildknecht, 1970 Schildknecht et al., 1968e
P. macer	decane; methacrylic acid; tiglic acid; tridecane; undecane	Schildknecht, 1970; Schildknecht et al., 1968e
P. melas	Decane; methacrylic acid; tiglic acid; tridecane; undecane	Schildknecht, 1970; Schildknecht et al., 1968e
P. metallicus	Decane; methacrylic acid; tiglic acid; tridecane; undecane	Schildknecht, 1970; Schildknecht and Weis, 1962; Schildknecht et al., 1968e
P. niger	Decane; methacrylic acid; tiglic acid; tridecane; undecane	Schildknecht, 1970; Schildknecht and Weis, 1962; Schildknecht et al., 1968e
P. vulgaris	Decane; methacrylic acid; tiglic acid; tridecane; undecane	Schildknecht, 1970; Schildknecht et al., 1968e
Rhytisternus laevilaterus	Methacrylic acid; tiglic acid	Moore and Wallbank, 1968
Sarticus cyaneocinctus	Formic acid	Moore and Wallbank, 1968
Scaphinotus andrewsi germari	Methacrylic acid; tiglic acid	Wheeler et al., 1970
S. adrewsi montana	Methacrylic acid; tiglic acid	Wheeler et al., 1970
S. viduus	Methacrylic acid; tiglic acid	Wheeler et al., 1970
S. webbi	Methacrylic acid; tiglic acid	Wheeler et al., 1970
Siagonyx blackburni	Formic acid	Moore and Wallbank, 1968
Sphallomorpha colymbetoides	Formic acid	Moore and Wallbank, 1968
Sphodrosomus saisseti	Formic acid	Moore and Wallbank, 1968
Stenaptinus catoirei	*p*-benzoquinone; *p*-toluquinone	Schildknecht and Holoubek, 1961
S. verticalis	*p*-benzoquinone; *p*-toluquinone	Moore and Wallbank, 1968
Stenolophus mixtus	Formic acid	Schildknecht et al., 1968b, e
Thermophilum burchelli	Acetic acid; formic acid; tiglic acid; isovaleraldehyde	Scott et al., 1975
T. homoplatum	Acetic acid; formic acid; tiglic acid; isovaleraldehyde	Scott et al., 1975
Trichosternus nudipes	Methacrylic acid; tiglic acid	Moore and Wallbank, 1968

5. Toxins of the Cerambycidae

Four species of this family have been studied. *Stenocentrus ostricilla* and *Syllitus grammicus* both utilize *o*-cresol and toluene (Moore and Brown, 1971a). An early investigation of the thoracic gland secretion of the willow beetle *Aromia moschata* indicated the presence of salicylaldehyde (Hollande, 1909). A recent reinvestigation of this cerambycid's secretion (Vidari et al., 1973) has shown that it consists largely of four monoterpenes, namely *cis*- and *trans*-rose oxide, and two isomers of iridodial.

cis—Rose oxide   trans—Rose oxide

δ—Iridodial   γ—Iridodial

Whereas iridodial has been identified in several ant species (CAVILL, 1960) and in four staphylinid species (ABOUDONIA et al., 1971; BELLAS et al., 1974; FISH and PATTENDEN, 1975), rose oxide has never previously been reported in arthropod secretions. This is the first report (VIDARI et al., 1973) that a monoterpene containing a tetrahydropyran ring has been isolated from an insect.

The fourth cerambycid species to have been examined is the common eucalypt longicorn *Phoracantha semipunctata*. The secretion of this Australian beetle contains five components (MOORE and BROWN, 1972), the most abundant of which is 2-hydroxy-6-methylbenzaldehyde. Only two of the remaining four components have been fully characterized, although all four are biosynthetically related. Spectroscopic and synthetic studies have resulted in the structures illustrated below being postulated for the components provisionally named 'phoracanthol' and 'phoracanthal'.

Phoracanthal   Phoracanthol

6. Toxins of the Chrysomelidae

This family is one of the larger coleopteran families; there are over 1,400 species in North America, yet only five species have been studied. The larvae of *Melasoma populi* and an unknown *Plagiodera* species have been reported to secrete salicylaldehyde (HOLLANDE, 1909). WAIN (1943) has also reported the same defensive toxins in larvae of the brassy willow beetle *Phyllodecta vitellinae,* while WALLACE and BLUM (1969) describe this aromatic aldehyde as the primary constituent in the larval defensive secretion of *Chrysomela scripta*. In contrast, *C. interrupta* larvae produce a mixture of the aromatic esters, β-phenethyl-2-methylbutyrate and β-phenethyl isobutyrate in the ratio 4:1 (BLUM et al., 1972).

7. Toxins of the Coccinellidae

Members of the Coccinellidae utilize for their defence a mechanism known as reflex bleeding (HAPP and EISNER, 1961). The haemolymph droplets which form

Table 4. Distribution of alkaloid toxins in the Coccinellidae

Species	Alkaloid							References
	Coccinelline	Precoccinelline	Convergine	Hippodamine	Myrrhine	Propyleine	Adaline	
Adalia bipunctata							×	TURSCH et al., 1973 b
A. 10-punctata							×	TURSCH et al., 1973 a, 1975
Anisosticta 19-punctata				×				TURSCH et al., 1973 a
Cheilomenes propinqua	×	×						TURSCH et al., 1975
(var. *4 lineata*)								
Coccinella californica	×							TURSCH et al., 1975
C. 7-punctata	×	×						TURSCH et al., 1971 a, b
C. 5-punctata	×	×						TURSCH et al., 1973 a, 1975
C. 11-punctata	×							TURSCH et al., 1973 a, 1975
C. 14-punctata	×	×						TURSCH et al., 1973 a, 1975
Coleomegilla maculata[a]		× ?			× ?			HENSON et al., 1975
Hippodamia convergens			×	×				TURSCH et al., 1972 a, 1974
Micraspis 16-punctata		×						TURSCH et al., 1975
Myrrha 18-punctata					×			TURSCH et al., 1975
Propylaea 14-punctata						×		TURSCH et al., 1972 b

[a] HENSON et al. (1975), mainly on the basis of mass spectral evidence, postulated the presence of precoccinelline in this insect. TURSCH et al. (1976) suggest that the infrared spectra are more consistent with the alkaloid being myrrhine.

at the leg joints have a bitter taste, and analysis has shown that the active materials are alkaloidal in nature.

A recent report (TURSCH et al., 1972 b) indicates that in a survey of 30 species of ladybugs, 23 were shown to contain alkaloids. At the present time the chemical structure of seven coccinellid alkaloids are known (TURSCH et al., 1975). Their distribution is given in Table 4.

Coccinelline   Precoccinelline   Convergine

Hippodamine   Myrrhine   Propyleine

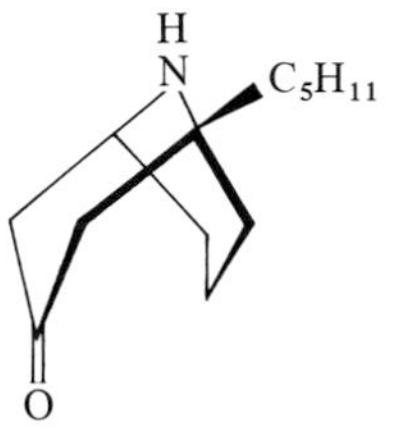

Adaline

The total synthesis of coccinelline, myrrhine, DL-convergine (AYER and DAWES, in press) and DL-adaline (TURSCH et al., 1973a) have been published.

8. Toxins of the Dytiscidae

Members of the Dytiscidae, the predaceous diving beetles, possess two types of toxin-producing glands (see above), the pygidial glands which secrete aromatic aldehydes, acids, esters, and in one instance, a benzofuranone, marginalin, and the prothoracic glands which secrete steroidal compounds. Special mention is made

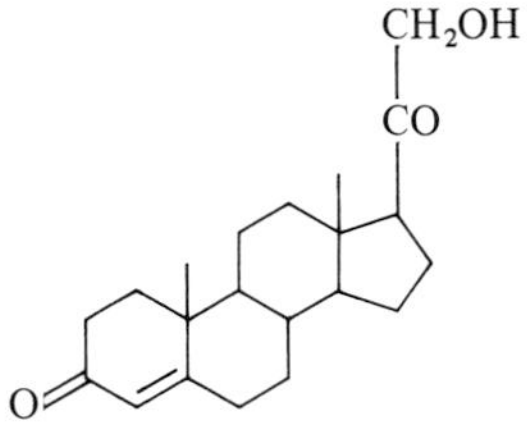

4–Pregnen –21–ol–3,20–dione

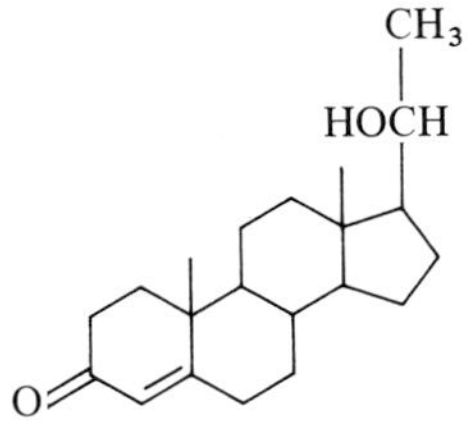

4–Pregnen –20β–ol–3–one

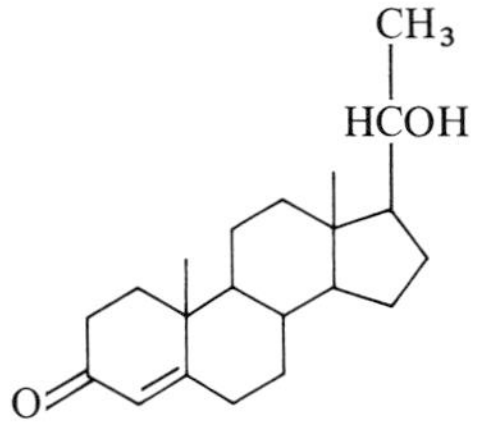

4–Pregnen –20α–ol–3–one

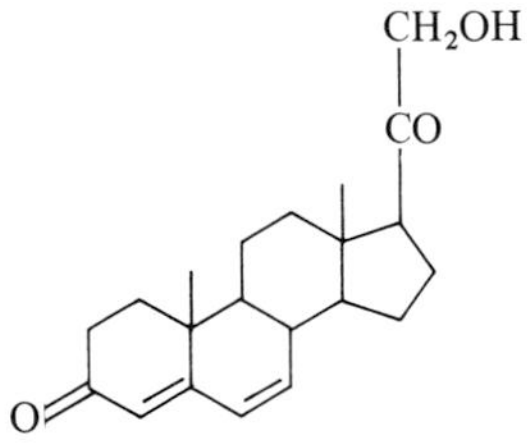

4,6–Pregnadien –21–ol–
3,20–dione

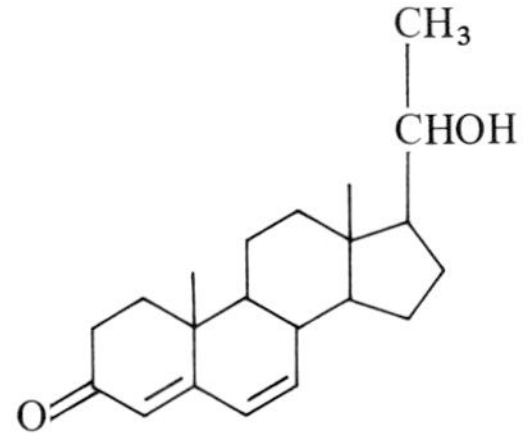

4,6–Pregnadien–20α–ol–3–one

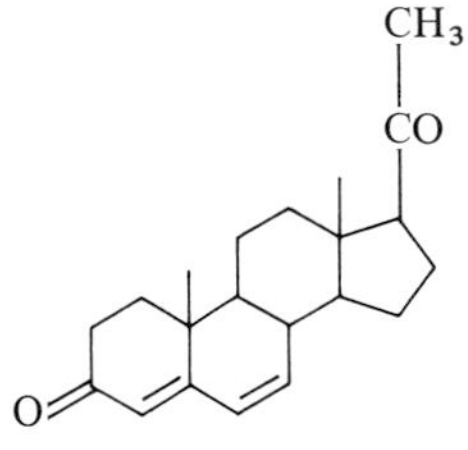

4,6–Pregnadien –3,20–dione

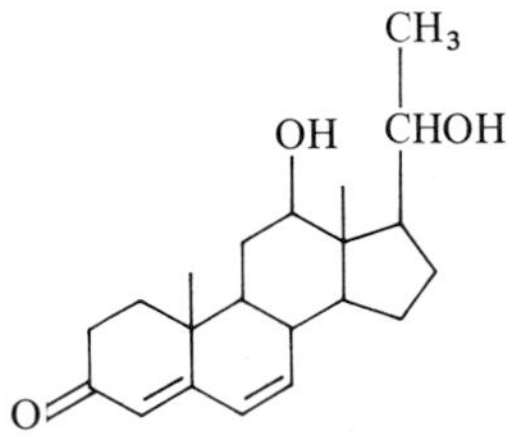

4,6–Pregnadien –12β, 20β–
diol–3–one

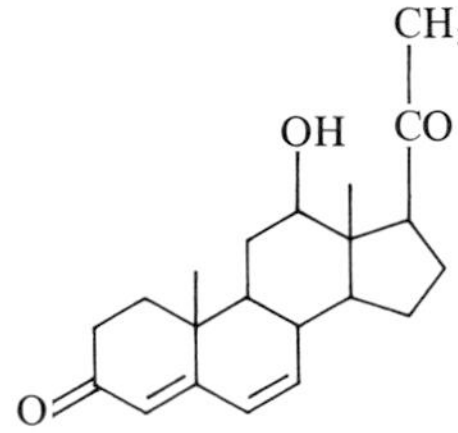

4,6–Pregnadien–12β–ol–
3,20–dione

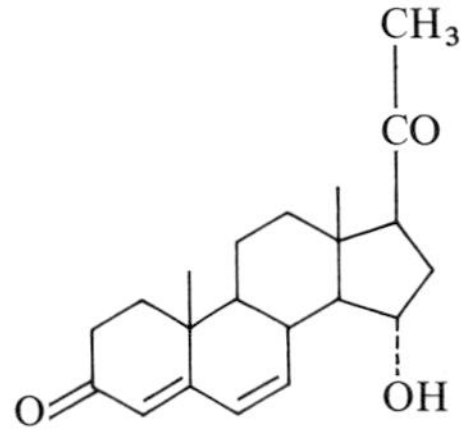

4,6–Pregnadien–15α–ol–
3,20–dione

CH₃

CH_3

CO

$COOCH(CH_3)_2$

$CHOH$

$COOCH(CH_3)_2$

OH

OH

4,6–Pregnadien–3,20–dione–
isobutyrate

4,6–Pregnadien–15α–ol–3–
one–isobutyrate

4–Pregnen–15α, 20β–diol–
3–one

OH

OH

Testosterone

1,2–Dehydrotestosterone

O

OH

HO

HO

Estrone

17β–Estradiol

$COOCH_3$

OH

HO

OH

O

Methyl 8–hydroxyquinoline–
2–carboxylate

Marginalin

of *Ilybius fenestratus* whose prothoracic secretion, in addition to steroids, contains methyl-8-hydroxyquinoline-2-carboxylate.

A complete listing of the dytiscid toxins is presented in Table 5.

9. Toxins of the Gyrinidae

Norsesquiterpenoid compounds dominate the pygidial gland compounds of the Gyrinidae, occurring in all nine species so far studied. SCHILDKNECHT et al. (1976) reported that *Gyrinus natator* also contains 3-methylbutan-1-ol and the corresponding aldehyde. Table 6 gives the distribution of the terpenoid compounds.

Table 5. Dytiscid toxins

Dytiscidae	Components identified in the secretion	References
Acilius sulcatus	Benzoic acid; *p*-hydroxybenzaldehyde; *p*-hydroxybenzoic acid methyl ester; 4,6-pregnadien-3,20-dione; 4,6-pregnadien-20α-ol-3-one; 4,6-pregnadien-21-ol-3,20-dione; 4-pregnen-20α-ol-3-one; pregnen-21-ol-3,20-dione	SCHILDKNECHT, 1968, 1970; SCHILDKNECHT et al., 1967a
Agabus bipustulatus	3,4-dihydroxybenzoic acid methyl ester; *p*-hydroxybenzaldehyde; *p*-hydroxybenzoic acid methyl ester; 4-pregnen-21-ol-3,20-dione	SCHILDKNECHT, 1968, 1970
A. seriatus	*p*-hydroxybenzaldehyde; 4-pregnen-21-ol-3,20-dione	MILLER and MUMMA, 1973
A. sturmi	Benzoic acid; *p*-hydroxybenzaldehyde; *p*-hydroxybenzoic acid methyl ester; 4,6-pregnadien-15α,20β-diol-3-one isobutyrate; 4,6-pregnadien-15α-3,20-dione; 4,6-pregnadien-15α-3,20-dione isobutyrate	SCHILDKNECHT, 1968, 1970
Colymbetes fuscus	Benzoic acid; 3,4-dihydroxybenzoic acid methyl ester; hydroquinone; *p*-hydroxybenzaldehyde; *p*-hydroxybenzoic acid; *p*-hydroxybenzoic acid methyl ester	SCHILDKNECHT, 1970
Copelatus ruficollis	*p*-hydroxybenzaldehyde; *p*-hydroxybenzoic acid methyl ester	SCHILDKNECHT, 1970
Cybister confusus	4-pregnen-21-ol-3,20-dione	CHADHA et al., 1970
C. lateralimarginalis	Benzoic acid; 3,4-dihydroxybenzoic acid ethyl ester; 3,4-dihydroxybenzoic acid methyl ester; *p*-hydroxybenzoic acid methyl ester; 4,6-pregnadien-12β,20α-diol-3-one; 4,6-pregnadien-3,20-dione; 4,6-pregnadien-20α-ol-3-one; 4,6-pregnadien-21-ol-3,20-dione	SCHILDKNECHT, 1964, 1968, 1970; SCHILDKNECHT et al., 1968f
C. limatus	4,6-pregnadien-20α-ol-3-one; 4,6-pregnadien-21-ol-3,20-dione; 4,6-pregnadien-12β-ol-3,20-dione; 4-pregnen-20α-ol-3-one; 4-pregnen-21-ol-3,20-dione; 4-pregnen-12β-ol-3,20-dione	CHADHA et al., 1970; SIPAHIMALANI et al., 1970
C. tripunctatus	Benzoic acid; *p*-hydroxybenzaldehyde; *p*-hydroxybenzoic acid methyl ester; 4,6-pregnadien-12β-ol-3,20-dione; 4,6-pregnadien-20α-ol-3-one; 4-pregnen-20β-ol-3-one; 4-pregnen-21-ol-3,20-dione	SCHILDKNECHT, 1968, 1970; CHADHA et al., 1970; SCHILDKNECHT and KORNIG, 1968a
C. spp.	4,6-pregnadien-12β-ol-3,20-dione; 4,6-pregnadien-21-ol-3,20-dione	SCHILDKNECHT and KORNIG, 1968a

Table 5 (continued)

Dytiscidae	Components identified in the secretion	References
Dytiscus *latissimus*	Benzoic acid; *p*-hydroxybenzaldehyde; *p*-hydroxybenzoic acid methyl ester	SCHILDKNECHT, 1964; SCHILDKNECHT et al., 1968f
P. marginalis	Benzoic acid; 3,5-dihydroxyphenylacetic acid methyl ester; *p*-hydroxybenzaldehyde; *p*-hydroxybenzoic acid methyl ester; 3-(*p*-hydroxyphenylmethylene)-5-hydroxy- benzo [b]furan-2-one; 4,6-pregnadien-20α-ol-3-one; 4-pregen-21-ol-3,20-dione; 4-pregen-20α-ol-3-one	SCHILDKNECHT, 1964, 1968, 1970; SCHILDKNECHT and MASCHWITZ, 1966; SCHILDKNECHT and HOTZ, 1967; SCHILDKNECHT et al., 1968f
Graphoderus *cinereus*	Benzoic acid; 3,4-dihydroxybenzoic acid methyl ester; *p*-hydroxybenzaldehyde; *p*-hydroxybenzoic acid; *p*-hydroxybenzoic acid methyl ester	SCHILDKNECHT, 1970
G. lyberus	*p*-hydroxybenzaldehyde; 4-pregnen-21-ol-3-one	MILLER and MUMMA, 1973
Hydroporus *pallustris*	*p*-hydroxybenzaldehyde	SCHILDKNECHT, 1964; SCHILDKNECHT, 1968f
Ilybius *fenestratus*	1,4-androstadien-17β-ol-3-one; 4-androsten-17β-ol-3-one; benzoic acid; 1,3,5-estratrien-3-ol-17-one; 1,3,5-estratrien-3, 17β-diol; hydroquinone; *p*-hydroxybenzaldehyde; *p*-hydroxybenzoic acid; *p*-hydroxybenzoic acid methyl ester; 8-hydroxyquinoline carboxylic acid methyl ester; 4-pregnen-20β-ol-3-one	SCHILDKNECHT, 1968, 1970; SCHILDKNECHT and BIRRINGER, 1969; SCHILDNECHT et al., 1967c, 1969b
I. fuliginosus	Testosterone	SCHILDKNECHT, 1967c
Platambus *maculatus*	4-pregnen-15α, 20β-diol-3-one	SCHILDKNECHT et al., 1969a
Rhantus *exsoletus*	Benzoic acid; hydroquinone; *p*-hydroxy- benzaldehyde; *p*-hydroxybenzoic acid; *p*-hydroxybenzoic acid methyl ester	SCHILDKNECHT, 1970

Gyrinidal   Isogyrinidal

Gyrinidone   Gyrinidione

Table 6. Compounds isolated from Gyrinid pygidial glands

Gyrinidae	Components identified in the secretion	References
Dineutus assimilis	Gyrinidal; isogyrinidal; gyrinidione; gyrinidone	MILLER et al., 1975
D. discolor	Gyrinidone	WHEELER et al., 1972b
D. horneii	Gyrinidal	MEINWALD et al., 1972
D. nigrior	Gyrinidal; isogyrinidal; gyrinidione; gyrinidone	MILLER et al., 1975
D. serrulates	Gyrinidal	MEINWALD et al., 1972
Gyrinus minutus	Gyrinidal	SCHILDKNECHT et al., 1976
G. natator	Gyrinidal; 3-methylbutan-1-ol; 3-methylbutanal	SCHILDKNECHT et al., 1976
G. substriatus	Gyrinidal	SCHILDKNECHT et al., 1976
G. ventralis	Gyrinidal	MEINWALD et al., 1972

10. Toxins of the Meloidae

The nonexocrine defensive agent of many species of blister beetles has been widely investigated (WALTER and COLE, 1967 and references therein). The toxic principle cantharidin has received much attention since its isolation by ROBIQUET (1810), no doubt due to its notoriety as a supposed aphrodisiac known as 'Spanish fly'.

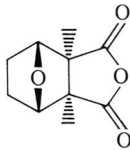

Cantharidin

The above structure was proposed independently by GADAMER (1914) and RU-DOLPH (1916) and later substantiated by the synthesis of desoxycantharidin (WOOD-WARD and LOFTFIELD, 1941). Cantharidin was first synthesized by SCHENK and ZIEGLER (1942), but their extremely low yield prompted STORK and his coworkers (1953) to evolve a more rewarding stereospecific total synthesis.

11. Toxins of the Silphidae

Three species of carrion beetles have been examined: *Oecoptoma thorica, Phospuga etrata,* and *Silpha obscura.* All have been shown to produce ammonia as a defensive agent (SCHILDKNECHT, 1970).

12. Toxins of the Staphylinidae

A total of 14 species of staphylinid beetles have been subjected to chemical analysis of their toxins; 13 species produce exocrine secretions while the 14th, *Paederus fuscipes,* contains, as a non exocrine toxin, the most complex of all insect defensive substances, pederin.

Pederin   R=CH₃; R′=H; R″=OH
Pseudopederin R=H; R′=H; R″=OH
Pederone   R=CH₃; R′+R″=O

The exocrine defensive substances of the Staphylinidae are the most diverse of all coleopteran toxins and include benzoquinones, mono- and di-unsaturated hydrocarbons and aldehydes, terpenes, and alkaloids.

Citronellal   Neral   Geranial   Isopiperitenol

Actinidine   1,8—Cineole   N—Ethyl−3−(2−methylbutyl)
                                           −piperidine

The components which have been identified in staphylinid secretions are given in Table 7.

Table 7. The components of Staphylinid toxins

Staphylinidae	Components identified in the secretion	References
Bledius mandibularis	γ-dodecalactone; geranial; neral; p-toluquinone; 1-undecene	WHEELER et al., 1972a
B. spectablis	γ-dodecalactone; geranial; methyl benzoquinone; neral; 1-undecene	WHEELER et al., 1972a
Creophilus erythro-cephalus	Iridodial	BELLAS et al., 1974
Drusilla canaliculata	dodecanal; hydroquinone; 2-hydroxy-3-methylhydroquinone; 2-methoxy-3-methylhydroquinone; 3-methoxy-p-toluquinone; 2-methylhydroquinone; tetradec-5-enal; tetradeca-5,8-dienal; tetradecanal; p-toluquinone; tridec-4,7-diene; tridec-4-ene; tridecane; undecane	BRAND et al., 1973
Eulissus orthodoxus	Citronellal; iridodial; isovaleraldehyde	BELLAS et al., 1974
Hesperus semirufus	Actinidine	BELLAS et al., 1974
Lomechusa strumosa	p-benzoquinone; p-ethylquinone; p-toluquinone; tridecane; 1-tridecene	BLUM et al., 1971
Paedenus fuscipes	Pederin, pederone and pseudo-pederin	CARDANI et al., 1965a, 1965b, 1967
Philonthus politus	Actinidine	BELLAS et al., 1974
Staphylinus olens	Iridodial; 4-methylhexan-3-one	ABOU-DONIA et al., 1971; FISH and PATTENDEN, 1975
Stenus bipunctatus	1,8-cineole; 6-methylhept-5-en-2-one; isopiperitenol	SCHILDKNECHT, 1970
S. comma	1,8-cineole; N-ethyl-3-(2-methyl-butyl)-piperidine; 6-methylhept-5-en-2-one; isopiperitenol	SCHILDKNECHT et al., 1975, 1976
Thyreocephalus lorquini	Citronellal; iridodial; isovaleraldehyde	BELLAS et al., 1974
Zyras humeralis	isovaleric acid	KOLBE and PROSKE, 1973

13. Toxins of the Tenebrionidae

A total of 108 species from this family have been examined, and the quinonoid compounds dominate in almost all of the species. Table 8 summarizes the data on the components of tenebrionid secretions.

Table 8. The distribution of defensive secretions within the Tenebrionidae

Tenebrionidae	Components identified in the secretion	References
Alphitobius diaperinus	*p*-ethylquinone; *p*-methylquinone	Tseng et al., 1971
Amphidora littoralis	*p*-ethylquinone; 2-methoxy-3-methylquinone; *p*-toluquinone; 1-tridecene	Tschinkel, 1975a
A. nigropylosa	*p*-ethylquinone; 2-methoxy-3-methylquinone; 1-pentadecene; *p*-toluquinone; 1-tridecene	Tschinkel, 1975a
Anomalipus variolosus	*p*-ethylquinone; *p*-toluquinone; 1-undecene	Tschinkel, 1975a
Argoporis alutacea	*p*-benzoquinone; 6-butyl-1,4-naphthoquinone; 6-ethyl-1,4-naphthoquinone; *p*-ethylquinone; 6-methyl-1,4-naphthoquinone; 6-propyl-1,4-naphthoquinone; *p*-toluquinone	Tschinkel, 1972, 1975a
A. bicolor	6-butyl-1,4-naphthoquinone; 6-ethyl-1,4-naphthoquinone; *p*-ethylquinone; 6-methyl-1,4-naphthoquinone; 6-propyl-1,4-naphthoquinone	Tschinkel, 1975a
A. rufipes	6-butyl-1,4-naphthoquinone; 6-ethyl-1,4-naphthoquinone; *p*-ethylquinone; 6-methyl-1,4-naphthoquinone; 6-propyl-1,4-naphthoquinone; *p*-toluquinone	Tschinkel, 1975a
Blaps approximans	*p*-benzoquinone; *p*-ethylquinone; *p*-toluquinone; 1-tridecene	Tschinkel, 1975a
B. gigas	*p*-benzoquinone; *p*-ethylquinone; *p*-toluquinone	Schildknecht, 1964
B. juliae	*p*-benzoquinone; *p*-ethylquinone; *p*-toluquinone; 1-tridecene	Tschinkel, 1975a
B. lethifera	*p*-benzoquinone; *p*-ethylquinone; *p*-toluquinone; 1-tridecene	Schildknecht, 1964; Schildknecht and Weis, 1960a; Tschinkel, 1975a
B. mortisaga	*p*-ethylquinone; *p*-toluquinone	Schildknecht, 1964; Schildknecht and Weis, 1960a
B. mucronata	*p*-ethylquinone; *p*-toluquinone	Schildknecht, 1964; Schildknecht and Weis, 1960a
B. polycresta	*p*-benzoquinone; *p*-ethylquinone; *p*-toluquinone	Tschinkel, 1975a
B. proheta	*p*-ethylquinone; *p*-toluquinone; 1-tridecene	Tschinkel, 1975a

Table 8 (continued)

Tenebrionidae	Components identified in the secretion	References
B. requienii	*p*-ethylquinone; *p*-toluquinone	SCHILDKNECHT, 1964; SCHILDKNECHT and WEIS, 1960a
B. stranchi	*p*-ethylquinone; *p*-toluquinone; 1-tridecene	TSCHINKEL, 1975a
B. sulcata	*p*-benzoquinone; 2-ethylhydro-quinone; *p*-ethylquinone; hydroquinone; 2-methylhydro-quinone; *p*-toluquinone; 1-tridecene	IKAN et al., 1970; TSCHINKEL, 1975a
B. wiedermanni	*p*-benzoquinone; 2-ethylhydro-quinonc; *p*-cthylquinone; hydroquinone; 2-methylhydro-quinone; *p*-toluquinone; 1-tridecene	IKAN et al., 1970
Bolitotherus cornutus	*p*-ethylquinone; *p*-toluquinone	TSCHINKEL, 1975a
Cratidus osculans	*p*-ethylquinone; 1-heptadecene; 1-nonene; *p*-toluquinone; 1-tridecene; 1-undecene	TSCHINKEL, 1975a
Diaperis boleti	*p*-ethylquinone; *p*-toluquinone	SCHILDKNECHT, 1964
D. maculata	*p*-ethylquinone; *p*-toluquinone	SCHILDKNECHT, 1964
Eleates occidentalis	*p*-ethylquinone; 1-heptadecene; *p*-toluquinone	TSCHINKEL, 1975a
Eleodes acuta	*p*-ethylquinone; 1-nonene; *p*-toluquinone; 1-tridecene; 1-undecene	TSCHINKEL, 1975a
E. acuticauda	*p*-benzoquinone; *p*-ethylquinone; 1-nonene; octanoic acid; *p*-toluquinone; 1-tridecene; 1-undecene	TSCHINKEL, 1975a
E. armata	*p*-ethylquinone; 1-nonene; *p*-toluquinone; 1-tridecene; 1-undecene	TSCHINKEL, 1975a
E. aristatus	*p*-ethylquinone; 2-methyl-3-methoxybenzoquinone; 1-pentadecene; *p*-toluquinone; 1-tridecene	TSCHINKEL, 1975a
E. beameri	*trans*-2-decenal; *n*-heptanal; *trans*-2-heptenal; *n*-hexanal; *trans*-2-hexenal; 1-hexanol; *n*-3-nonanone; 1-nonen-3-one; *trans*-2-nonenal; 1-nonene; *n*-octanal; toluquinone; 1-undecene	TSCHINKEL, 1975b
E. blanchardi	*p*-ethylquinone; 2-methoxy-3-methylbenzoquinone; 1-nonene; *p*-toluquinone; 1-tridecene; 1-undecene	TSCHINKEL, 1975a

Table 8 (continued)

Tenebrionidae	Components identified in the secretion	References
E. carbonaria	*p*-ethylquinone; 1-pentadecene; *p*-toluquinone; 1-tridecene; 1-undecene	TSCHINKEL, 1975a
E. caudifera	*p*-benzoquinone; *p*-ethylquinone; 1-heptadecene; *p*-toluquinone; 1-tridecene; 1-undecene	TSCHINKEL, 1975a
E. consobrinus	*p*-ethylquinone; 1-nonene; *p*-toluquinone; 1-tridecene; 1-undecene	TSCHINKEL, 1975a
E. constrictus	*p*-ethylquinone; 2-methoxy-3-methylbenzoquinone; *p*-toluquinone; 1-tridecene	TSCHINKEL, 1975a
E. cordatus	*p*-ethylquinone; 2-methoxy-3-methylbenzoquinone; 1-nonene; *p*-toluquinone; 1-tridecene; 1-undecene	TSCHINKEL, 1975a
E. dentipes	*p*-ethylquinone; 1-nonene; *p*-toluquinone; 1-tridecene; 1-undecene	TSCHINKEL, 1975a
E. dissimilis	*p*-benzoquinone; *p*-ethylquinone; 1-nonene; octanoic acid; *p*-toluquinone; 1-tridecene; 1-undecene	TSCHINKEL, 1975a
E. extricata	*p*-benzoquinone; *p*-ethylquinone; 1-nonene; *p*-toluquinone; 1-tridecene; 1-undecene	TSCHINKEL, 1975a
E. femorata	*p*-ethylquinone; octanoic acid; *p*-toluquinone; 1-tridecene; 1-undecene	TSCHINKEL, 1975a
E. gigantea	*p*-ethylquinone; 1-nonene; *p*-toluquinone; 1-tridecene; 1-undecene	TSCHINKEL, 1975a
E. goryi	*p*-ethylquinone; 1-heptadecene; 1-pentadecene; *p*-toluquinone; 1-tridecene; 1-undecene	TSCHINKEL, 1975a
E. gracilis	*p*-ethylquinone; 1-nonene; octanoic acid; *p*-toluquinone; 1-tridecene; 1-undecene	TSCHINKEL, 1975a
E. grandicollis	*p*-ethylquinone; 2-methoxy-3-methylbenzoquinone; 1-nonene; octanoic acid; *p*-toluquinone; 1-tridecene; 1-undecene	TSCHINKEL, 1975a
E. hispilabris	*p*-ethylquinone; 1-nonene; octanoic acid; *p*-toluquinone; 1-tridecene; 1-undecene	BLUM and CRAIN, 1961; TSCHINKEL, 1975a

Table 8 (continued)

Tenebrionidae	Components identified in the secretion	References
E. incultis	*p*-ethylquinone; 2-methoxy-3-methylbenzoquinone; *p*-toluquinone; 1-tridecene	TSCHINKEL, 1975a
E. knullorum	*p*-ethylquinone; 1-nonene; 1-pentadecene; *p*-toluquinone; 1-tridecene; 1-undecene	TSCHINKEL, 1975a
E. laticollis	*p*-ethylquinone; 1-nonene; octanoic acid; *p*-toluquinone; 1-tridecene; 1-undecene	TSCHINKEL, 1975a
E. longicollis	*p*-benzoquinone; *p*-ethylquinone; *p*-methylquinone; octanoic acid; 1-tridecene; 1-undccenc	CHADHA et al., 1961; MEINWALD and EISNER, 1964; HURST et al., 1964; TSCHINKEL, 1975a
E. longipilosa	*p*-ethylquinone; *p*-toluquinone; 1-tridecene	TSCHINKEL, 1975a
E. neotomae	*p*-ethylquinone; 2-methoxy-3-methylbenzoquinone; 1-nonene; *p*-toluquinone; 1-tridecene; 1-undecene	TSCHINKEL, 1975a
E. nigrina	*p*-ethylquinone; 1-nonene; *p*-toluquinone; 1-tridecene; 1-undecene	TSCHINKEL, 1975a
E. obsoleta	*p*-benzoquinone; *p*-ethylquinone; 2-methoxy-2-methylbenzoquinone; 1-nonene; 1-pentadecene; *p*-toluquinone; 1-tridecene; 1-undecene	TSCHINKEL, 1975a
E. omissa	*p*-ethylquinone; *p*-toluquinone; 1-tridecene; 1-undecene	TSCHINKEL, 1975a
E. parowana	*p*-ethylquinone; *p*-toluquinone; 1-tridecene; 1-undecene	TSCHINKEL, 1975a
E. pimelioides	*p*-ethylquinone; 2-methoxy-3-methylbenzoquinone; 1-nonene; *p*-toluquinone; 1-tridecene	TSCHINKEL, 1975a
E. sponsa	*p*-benzoquinone; *p*-ethylquinone; 1-nonene; octanoic acid; *p*-toluquinone; 1-tridecene; 1-undecene	TSCHINKEL, 1975a
E. subnitens	*p*-ethylquinone; 1-pentadecene; *p*-toluquinone; 1-tridecene; 1-undecene	TSCHINKEL, 1975a
E. tenebrosus	*p*-ethylquinone; 2-methoxy-3-methylbenzoquinone; *p*-toluquinone; 1-tridecene; 1-undecene	TSCHINKEL, 1975a

Table 8 (continued)

Tenebrionidae	Components identified in the secretion	References
E. tenuipes	*p*-ethylquinone; 1-nonene; *p*-toluquinone; 1-tridecene; 1-undecene	Tschinkel, 1975a
E. tricostata	*p*-benzoquinone; *p*-ethylquinone; *p*-toluquinone; 1-undecene	Tschinkel, 1975a
E. obscura	*p*-ethylquinone; 1-heptadecene; 1-nonene; octanoic acid; *p*-toluquinone; 1-tridecene; 1-undecene	Tschinkel, 1975a
E. ventricosa	*p*-ethylquinone; 1-nonene; 1-pentadecene; *p*-toluquinone; 1-tridecene; 1-undecene	Tschinkel, 1975a
Embaphrion muricatum	*p*-benzoquinone; caprylic acid; *p*-ethylquinone; 1-nonene; *p*-toluquinone; 1-tridecene; 1-undecene	Tschinkel, 1975a
Epanitus obscurus	*p*-ethylquinone; *p*-toluquinone	Tschinkel, 1975a
Eurynotus capensis	*p*-ethylquinone; 1-heptadecene; *p*-toluquinone; 1-tridecene	Tschinkel, 1975a
Gnaptor spinimanus	*p*-ethylquinone; *p*-toluquinone	Tschinkel, 1975a
Gnathocerus cornutus	*p*-ethylquinone; *p*-toluquinone; 1-tridecene	Tschinkel, 1975a
Gonocephalum arenarium	*p*-ethylquinone; *p*-toluquinone; 1-tridecene	Tschinkel, 1975a
G. kolbi	*p*-ethylquinone; *p*-toluquinone; 1-tridecene; 1-undecene	Tschinkel, 1975a
Gonopus agrestis	*p*-ethylquinone; *p*-toluquinone; 1-undecene	Tschinkel, 1975a
G. tibialis	*p*-ethylquinone; 1-heptadecene; 1-nonene; 1-pentadecene; *p*-toluquinone; 1-undecene	Tschinkel, 1975a
Helops aenus	*p*-ethylquinone; *p*-toluquinone	Schildknecht, 1964
H. quisquilus	*p*-ethylquinone; *p*-toluquinone	Schildknecht, 1964
Iphthimus laevissimus	*p*-benzoquinone; *p*-ethylquinone; *p*-toluquinone	Tschinkel, 1975a
I. serratus	*p*-benzoquinone; *p*-ethylquinone; *p*-toluquinone	Tschinkel, 1975a
Latheticus oryzae	2-ethylquinone; 2-methylquinone	Loconti and Roth, 1953
Leichenum canaliculatum variegatum	*p*-benzoquinone; *p*-ethylquinone; *p*-toluquinone	Happ, 1967
Melanopterus marginicollis	*p*-ethylquinone; 1-nonene; 1-pentadecene; *p*-toluquinone; 1-undecene	Tschinkel, 1975a
M. porcus	1-nonene; *p*-toluquinone; 1-undecene	Tschinkel, 1975a

Table 8 (continued)

Tenebrionidae	Components identified in the secretion	References
Mercantha contracta	*p*-benzoquinone; *p*-ethylquinone; 1-heptadecene; 1-nonene; 1-pentadecene; *p*-toluquinone	TSCHINKEL, 1975a
Morisisa planta tingitiana	*p*-toluquinone	SCHILDKNECHT and WEIS, 1960a
Opatroides punctulatus	*p*-ethylquinone; *p*-toluquinone	SCHILDKNECHT, 1964
Parastizopus balneorum	*p*-ethylquinone; 1-heptadecene; 1-nonene; 1-pentadecene; *p*-toluquinone; 1-undecene	TSCHINKEL, 1975a
Phaleria rotundata	*p*-ethylquinone; 1-heptadecene; 1-pentadecene; *p*-toluquinone	TSCHINKEL, 1975a
P. testacea	*p*-ethylquinone; 1-heptadecene; 1-pentadecene; *p*-toluquinone	TSCHINKEL, 1975a
Pimelia confusa	*p*-toluquinone	SCHILDKNECHT and WEIS, 1960a
Platydema americanum	*p*-ethylquinone; *p*-toluquinone; 1-tridecene; 1-undecene	TSCHINKEL, 1975a
P. flavipes	*p*-ethylquinone; 1-pentadecene; *p*-toluquinone; 1-tridecene	TSCHINKEL, 1975a
P. oregonense	*p*-ethylquinone; *p*-toluquinone; 1-tridecene	TSCHINKEL, 1975a
P. ruficorne	*p*-ethylquinone; 1-pentadecene; *p*-toluquinone; 1-tridecene	TSCHINKEL, 1975a
P. subcostatum	*p*-ethylquinone; *p*-toluquinone; 1-tridecene	TSCHINKEL, 1975a
Psorodes calcaratus	*p*-ethylquinone; 1-nonene; 1-pentadecene; *p*-toluquinone 1-undecene	TSCHINKEL, 1975a
P. gratilla	*p*-ethylquinone; 1-heptadecene; 1-nonene; *p*-toluquinone 1-undecene	TSCHINKEL, 1975a
Pyanisia tristis	*p*-ethylquinone; 1-pentadecene; *p*-toluquinone	TSCHINKEL, 1975a
Scaurus aegytiacus	*p*-ethylquinone; *p*-toluquinone; 1-tridecene; 1-undecene	TSCHINKEL, 1975a
S. uncinus	*p*-benzoquinone; *p*-ethylquinone; *p*-toluquinone	SCHILDKNECHT, 1964
Schelodontes sp.	*p*-ethylquinone; 1-nonene; 1-pentadecene; *p*-toluquinone; 1-undecene	TSCHINKEL, 1975a
Tenebrio molitor	*p*-toluquinone	SCHILDKNECHT, 1959, 1964
T. obscurus	*p*-benzoquinone	SCHILDKNECHT and WEIS, 1960a

Table 8 (continued)

Tenebrionidae	Components identified in the secretion	References
Tribolium brevicornis	*p*-ethylquinone; 1-pentadecene; *p*-toluquinone	TSCHINKEL, 1975a
T. castaneum	*p*-ethylquinone; 2-hydroxy-4-methoxypropiophenone; *p*-methoxyquinone; *p*-toluquinone	BARTON and ALEXANDER, 1943; LOCONTI and ROTH, 1953; ROTH and STAY, 1958; SUZUKI et al., 1975
T. confusum	*p*-ethylquinone; 2-hydroxy-4-methoxypropiophenone; 1-pentadecene; *p*-toluquinone	ROTH, 1943; ROTH and HOWLAND, 1941; ENGELHARDT et al., 1965; ENDT and WHEELER, 1971; SUZUKI et al., 1975
T. destructor	*p*-ethylquinone; 1-pentadecene; *p*-toluquinone	LOCONTI and ROTH, 1953; TSCHINKEL, 1975a
Trigonopus capicola	*p*-ethylquinone; *p*-toluquinone	TSCHINKEL, 1975a
Zadenos delandei	*p*-ethylquinone; 1-heptadecene; 1-nonene; *p*-toluquinone; 1-tridecene	TSCHINKEL, 1975a
Z. longipalpus	*p*-ethylquinone; 1-heptadecene; 1-nonene; *p*-toluquinone; 1-tridecene	TSCHINKEL, 1975a
Z. mulsanti	*p*-ethylquinone; 1-heptadecene; 1-nonene; *p*-toluquinone; 1-tridecene; 1-undecene	TSCHINKEL, 1975a
Zophobas rugipes	*p*-benzoquinone; *m*-cresol; *m*-ethylphenol; *p*-ethylquinone; phenol; *p*-toluquinone	TSCHINKEL, 1969

II. Extraction Methods

The methods utilized in obtaining the coleopteran toxins are almost as varied as the types of compounds comprising the toxins. Considering that over 300 species of Coleoptera have been subjected to various extraction procedures, a detailed discussion of extraction methods is not within the scope of this report. Among the methods most commonly used are:

1. Dissecting out the glands after killing the beetles by freezing (BENN et al., 1973) or with potassium cyanide (McCULLOUGH, 1971), or after anethetizing them (WHEELER et al., 1972a).

2. Causing the insects to squirt the defensive secretion into vials. HURST et al. (1964) used this method with *Eleodes longicollis,* while SCOTT et al. (1975), working with carabids, added the refinement of first cooling the vials.

3. Causing the insect to discharge its secretion on to filter paper (CHADHA et al., 1961) or by wiping extruded glands with filter paper, such as was done with a tenebrionid by TSENG et al. (1971), and the tergal gland secretion of the staphylinid *Drusilla canaliculata* (BRAND et al., 1973). The filter paper is then extracted with a suitable solvent.

4. Employing capillaries to collect the secretion as it exudes from the glands. This is the method most often used to collect the prothoracic gland steroids from the Dytiscidae (SIPAHIMALANI et al., 1970; SCHILDKNECHT and KORIG, 1968a; and SCHILDKNECHT et al., 1969). It has also been used by MOORE and BROWN (1972) to obtain the metasternal gland secretion from the cerambycid *Phoracantha semipunctata*.

5. Dipping beetles directly into solvent. BELLAS et al., (1974) and MOORE and BROWN (1971a) preferred carbon disulphide.

6. Warming large numbers of insects while evacuating the container so that the volatiles may be passed through a cold trap (BLUM and CRAIN, 1961). Adaptations of this method were employed by ENGELHARDT et al. (1965) who alternately heated the vessel containing *Tribolium confusum* with a hair drier and cooled it in ice water, as they cold-trapped the volatiles. EISNER et al. (1963) substituted shaking for warming. They placed about a hundred *Calosoma prominens* in a flask which was connected in a closed system to a mechanical pump and a methylene chloride solvent trap. The flask was shaken to induce the insects to spray, and the gas in the system continuously bubbled through the solvent for 30 minutes. SCHILDKNECHT (1959a), in his work with *Tenebrio molitor,* employed a simple system in which air was drawn over a stimulated insect and through a solvent or reagent solution.

7. Passing several 1-s pulses of electrical current through water containing beetles (MILLER and MUMMA, 1973).

The above methods have been used to obtain exocrine secretions. The extraction procedures for the nonexocrine materials, such as cantharidin, coccinelline, and pederin involve the maceration of large numbers of whole insects in a suitable solvent; this crude extract is then further purified by soxhlet extraction (WALTER and COLE, 1967), solvent partition (TURSCH et al., 1971a; CARDANI et al., 1966), or column chromatography (CARDANI et al., 1973).

III. Methods of Purification and Structural Elucidation

1. Gas Liquid Chromatography

The compounds in coleopteran secretions are generally of the same type as those found in hemipteran toxins; the reader is referred to Table 6 of the chapter on Rhyncota.

In his mammoth paper reporting the chemical composition of 147 tenebrionid defensive secretions, TSCHINKEL (1975a) employed four stationary phases, all on Chromosorb W AW (DMCS) 80/100 mesh. These phases were 5% SE-30, 5% NPGS, 10% FFAP, and 3% Carbowax 20M.

Short-chain carboxylic acids, such as propionic, valeric, tiglic, etc., are very prevalent in the coleopteran secretions. MOORE and WALLBANK (1968), using 25%

Carbowax 4000 on Gaschrom P at 125° C, tabulated the retention times of 19 such acids. For analyses of the same compounds SCOTT et al. (1975) used packed columns employing stationary phase of 10% FFAP, 10% Hi-eff 1-BP and 10% Carbowax 20M; in addition, they used 50-ft SCOT columns with DEGS and Carbowax 20M as liquid phases. Details of the analyses of acids and alkanes on seven columns are reported for carabid secretions by SCHILDKNECHT et al. (1960b).

The norsesquiterpenoids from gyrinids were analysed on glass columns of 2% OV-1 on Supelcoport (100/120 mesh) at 170° C, metal columns being avoided since they catalysed isomerisations (MILLER et al., 1975). For their gyrinid work MEIN-WALD et al. (1972) used 5% OV-1 on 60/80 mesh Gaschrom Q. The terpenoids rose oxide and iridodial from *Aromia moschata* were separated by a 5° C per min programme between $50-170$° C on 5% SF-96 (VIDARI et al., 1973).

The acetylenic acids from the cantharid *Chauliognathus lecontei* (MEINWALD et al., 1968) were analysed as the methyl esters on 8% SE-30 at 140°. Synthetic and natural adaline were compared by chromatography on 4% OV-1, 5% SE-30 and 10% Carbowax 20M (TURSCH et al., 1973a).

The use of reaction loops (BIERL et al., 1969) has been made to good effect by MOORE and BROWN (1971a) and BELLAS et al. (1974) in their work with cerambycid and staphylinid secretions.

2. Thin-Layer and Paper Chromatography

As was the case with the hemipteran defensive secretions, thin-layer chromatography has been extensively used in the isolation and identification of carbonyl and quinonoid compounds as their 2,4-dinitrophenylhydrazones. Examples of this technique applied to quinone 2,4-dinitrophenylhydrazones are to be found in the reports of MOORE and WALLBANK (1968) [carabids], BLUM et al. (1971) [staphylinids], IKAN et al. (1970), and HAPP (1967) [tenebrionids]. HAPP (1967) separated the derivatives of benzoquinone, toluquinone, and ethylbenzoquinone on precoated sheets with multiple developments of ethylene dichloride:hexane (1:1). On exposure to ammonia vapour the compounds exhibited characteristic colours. For the identification of salicylaldehyde, as its 2,4-dinitrophenylhydrazone derivative, in *Calosoma* species MCCULLOGH (1966a) used silica gel H eluting with benzene, while MOORE and WALLBANK (1968) preferred silica gel G eluting with benzene:ethyl acetate (95:5). Paper chromatography of the benzoquinone 2,4-dinitrophenylhydrazones from *Brachynus* species has been reported on both untreated and formamide-impregnated paper (SCHILDKNECHT, 1957).

Formic acid, which is poorly detected by flame-ionization detectors in gas chromatography, can be readily identified by thin-layer chromatography on silica gel eluting with ethanol:ammonium hydroxide:water (80:16:4) (SCOTT et al., 1975) or on microcrystalline cellulose with tertiary butanol:water:saturated ammonia (80:16:4) as the mobile phase (MOORE and WALLBANK, 1968). Detection may be achieved with ammoniacal silver nitrate or Universal indicator at pH 8 followed by heating. MCCULLOUGH has frequently employed paper chromatography in the identification of carboxylic acids as their salts; one example is the identification of methacrylic acid in *Callisthenes luxatus* (MCCULLOUGH, 1972a).

The first stage in the purification of the dytiscid steroids is usually thin-layer chromatography. The excellent review paper on the defensive chemistry of land and water beetles by SCHILDKNECHT (1970) contains the literature citations to the use of kieselgel plates with ethyl acetate:cyclohexane (1:1). Four C-21 steroids were isolated from Indian dytiscids by thin-layer chromatography (CHADHA et al., 1970). These authors used a (1:1) mixture of silica gels G and H, prewashed the plates with methanol, and activated them at 100° C prior to use. Multiple elutions were then carried out with ethyl acetate:cyclohexane (1:1).

3. Spectroscopic Methods

Spectroscopic methods have been widely used in the structural elucidation of co-leopteran toxins. It is sufficient at this time to list some examples of their use in the identification of the various types of organic structures. The use of infrared (IR), ultraviolet (UV), and nuclear magnetic resonance (NMR) techniques for benzoquinones and hydrocarbons is given by TSCHINKEL (1975a). In IR, UV, NMR, and mass spectrometry (MS), data for carboxylic acids, phenols, aromatic aldehydes, acids, and esters have been published by MOORE and BROWN (1972), MOORE and WALLBANK (1968), SCHILDKNECHT et al. (1968b, c), and SCOTT et al. (1975).

Most of the work on dytiscid steroids has come from the Heidelberg group of SCHILDKNECHT, which has made full use of spectroscopic data in their reports on the steroids of *Ilybius fenestratus* (1969a), *Acilius sulcatus* (1967a), and *Cybister lateralimarginalis* (1967b).

Terpenoid compounds, such as the gyrinid toxins, staphylinid monoterpenes, and cerambycid secretion components, have been adequately covered by MEINWALD et al. (1972), MILLER et al. (1975), BELLAS et al. (1974), and VIDARI et al. (1973).

Spectroscopic methods played an important role in the elucidation of complex nonexocrine coleopteran toxins. TURSCH et al. (1971b, 1973a, b) reported IR, UV, MS, and NMR data for the coccinellid alkaloids, and CARDANI et al. (1965, 1966) and MATSUMOTO et al. (1968) published the spectroscopic data for pederin. X-ray crystallographic data for pederin di-*p*-bromobenzoate has been published (FURU-SAKI et al., 1968).

IV. Biosynthesis

As noted by WEATHERSTON and PERCY (1970), the study of the biosynthesis of arthropod secretions is still in its infancy. Within the Coleoptera the biosynthetic studies carried out to date are summarized below.

Although HACKMAN et al. (1948) proposed that the quinonoid toxins of *Tribolium* species were derived from phenylalanine or tyrosine, attempts at experimental verification were not forthcoming until the middle 1960's. In preliminary screening experiments using ^{14}C-labelled tyrosine, phenylalanine, sodium acetate, sodium propionate, and sodium malonate, MEINWALD et al. (1966) showed that in *E. longicollis* the preferred pathway to benzoquinone utilized the preformed ring of tyrosine or phenylalanine. The two alkylated quinones synthesized by the beetle appeared, from degradative evidence, to arise via the acetate pathway to aromatic compounds.

Several Coleoptera have been shown to possess quinols. SCHILDKNECHT and KRAMER (1962) and HURST et al. (1964) found glucose, probably derived from the cleavage of quinol glucosides, in *Eleodes* secretion. Glucose has also been detected in the secretion of *Blaps* species (IKAN et al., 1970). HAPP (1968) has indicated the presence of quinols and their glucosides together with β-glucosidase and oxidases in the secretory cells of *E. longicollis* and *Tribolium castaneum*. A special case of quinone production, the explosive discharge of the bombardier beetles, has been well investigated by the Heidelberg group of SCHILDKNECHT (SCHILDKNECHT et al., 1968d, 1970) and the Cornell group (ANESHAMSLEY et al., 1969). Both groups envisage the gland as a two-compartment structure; the larger, the reservoir, contains an aqueous solution of hydroquinones and hydrogen peroxide. The smaller compartment contains a mixture of enzymes. The Heidelberg group (SCHILDKNECHT et al., 1970) report the isolation of four catalases and three polyphenol peroxidases. During the discharge, reservoir fluid flowing through the smaller compartment causes decomposition of the hydrogen peroxide by the catalases, while the peroxidases produce the quinones from hydroquinones. Under pressure from the free oxygen, the defensive spray is discharged with an audible detonation. ANESHANSLEY et al. (1969) have measured the discharge temperature at 100° C.

PAVAN (1959) suggested that salicylaldehyde produced by certain herbivorous chrysomelids and one cerambycid beetle might be of plant origin. In the case of *Melasoma populi* it was proposed that the beetle ingested salicin or populin. After enzymatic hydrolysis and oxidation, the resultant salicylaldehyde could be stored. This route if it is operative in the above families is certainly not the mode of synthesis in the carnivorous members of the Carabidae, a family several of whose species make salicylaldehyde.

BENN et al. (1973) have shown that DL-valine-4-^{14}C is incorporated into methacrylic acid, one of the components of *Carabus taedatus* toxin. The authors did not confirm any of the intermediates of the pathway, which is analogous to the synthesis of angelic or tiglic acids from isoleucine (LEETE and MURRILL, 1967); however, the carbon of formaldehyde derived from the methylene group of methacrylic acid contained activity concomitant with it having originated as one of the valine methyl groups. The report also speculates that ethacrylic acid is derived from isoleucine.

Amongst the compounds which BELLAS et al. (1974) isolated from rove beetles are citronellal, iridodial, and actinidine. They suggest that these components form a graded series reflecting the biosynthetic pathway. Normal terpenoid synthesis would be operative to citronellal, which could, as postulated by CAVILL (1960), be transformed into iridodial via 2,6-dimethyloct-2-en-1,8-dial. Actinidine is facilely formed from iridodial by ammoniation (CAVILL and ZEITLIN, 1967). The alkaloid coccinelline obtained from *Coccinella septempunctata* after feeding with both 1 and 2 ^{14}C sodium acetate possessed incorporated radioactivity (TURSCH et al., 1975). Degradation of the active alkaloid yielded results consistent with a β-polyketoacid from the linear combination of seven acetate units being an intermediate in the synthesis. Preliminary radiotracer work by CARDANI et al. (1973) has shown that the alkaloid pederin is also biosynthesized by the polyketide route.

Males of the meloid *Lytta vesicatoria,* but not females, can incorporate ^{14}C acetate, mevalonate, and farnesol into the toxin cantharidin (SCHLATTER et al., 1968). Continuing this work SIERRA et al. (1976) report a most elegant study using doubly labelled precursors. Their conclusions include (1) that cantharidin is transferred to the female insects during copulation, (2) that 93—98% of the male-produced cantharidin may be transferred, (3) that copulation stimulates the production of the toxin, (4) male *Lytta vesicatoria* continue to produce cantharidin after mating.

The biosynthesis of the dytiscid steroid toxins has still to receive the attention it deserves; however, SCHILDKNECHT (1970) reports that *Acilius sulcatus* incorporated ^{14}C cholesterol and progesterone into its steroid toxins but not ^{14}C mevalono-lactone.

D. Biological and Physiological Effects of the Toxins

The toxins produced by coleopteran species are used for their defence against predators. Several compounds, however, deserve further discussion.

In addition to its well-known properties as a vessicant and its use in veterinary medicine, cantharidin has been shown (CARREL and EISNER, 1974) to be a powerful feeding deterrent to some predaceous insects such as *Pogonomyrmex occidentalis* and *Calosoma prominens*. The terpene at a concentration of 10^{-5} mol in 0.1 M glucose solution effectively deterred feeding by a *Formica* species.

Pederin, the staphylinid alkaloid, causes widespread cutaneous necrotization and acts as a stimulant to tissue development. The biological and pharmacological activity has been summarized (PAVAN and DAZZINI, 1971). The mode of action and cytological effects have been investigated by BREGA et al. (1968), and HISADA and EMURA (1965), respectively. Twenty-five years of investigation by PAVAN into pederin and its physiological effects on animals and plants in vivo and in vitro has recently been reviewed (PAVAN, 1975).

The secretions produced by the prothoracic glands of dytiscid beetles contain steroids, such as testosterone, cortexone, estrone, etc., which are used for protection against fish and amphibians. The most abundant component in the arsenal of *Ilybius fenestratus* is not a steroid but the alkaloid 2-carbomethoxy-8-hydroxyqui-noline (SCHILDKNECHT and TACHECI, 1971). This alkaloid has no effect on amphibians but is poisonous to small mammals, causing clonic spasms in mice. Colymbetin (SCHILDKNECHT and TACHECI, 1971), a component of the prothoracic gland secretion of *Colymbetes fuscus,* has been shown to cause blood pressure lowering in mammals. MILLER and MUMMA (1973) have demonstrated that 11-deoxycorticosterone from certain American water beetles rapidly inactivated and killed minnows. MILLER et al. (1975) have also shown that the terpenoid secretions from the gyrinid beetles *Dineutes assimilis* and *Dineutes nigrior* possess narcotic and toxic activity in a bioassay against minnows, similar to that of the dytiscid toxins. Continuing this work, MILLER and MUMMA (1976a, b) compared the anesthetic and toxic properties of the dytiscid and gyrinid secretions with standard steroids. Results indicated that, in the minnow bioassay, activity of a steroid was related to the degree of oxygenation. Both the terpenes and the steroids exerted their effects at similar concentrations, $10^{-6} - 10^{-5}$ mol, causing anesthesia, with death occurring at $10^{-4} - 10^{-3}$ mol concentrations. The authors (MILLER and MUMMA, 1976b) propose that these compounds act via membrane stabilization and lysis.

Hemolymph from all stages of the Colorado potato beetle (*Leptinotarsa decemlineata*) contains a compound which is lethal when injected into white mice and species from the orders Orthoptera, Hemiptera, Lepidoptera, Coleoptera, and Diptera. No toxic effects are evident when hemolymph is injected into other Colorado potato beetles. The toxic compound, synthesized within the insects, is an acidic protein with a molecular weight about 50,000 and is named leptinotarsin. The site of its action within the insects has not been located; it affects neither the CNS, nor the neuromuscular junctions, nor the cholinergic system (HSIAO and FRAENKEL, 1969). A similar compound has also been isolated from another species, *Leptinotarsa juncta* (PARKER, 1972).

References

Abou-Donia, S.A., Fish, L.J., Pattenden, G.: Iridodial from the odoriferous glands of *Staphylinus olens* (Col. Staphylinidae). Tetra. Lett. No. 43, 4037–4038 (1971).

Alexander, P., Barton, D.H.P.: The excretion of ethylquinone from a flour beetle. Biochem. J. **37**, 463–465 (1943).

Aneshansley, D.J., Eisner, T., Widom, T.A., Widom, B.: Biochemistry at 100° C: Explosive secretory discharge of bombardier beetles (*Brachinus*). Science **165**, 61–63 (1969).

Arara, G.L., Rai, D.: Pygidial glands in *Pherosophus* sp. (Carabidae: Coleoptera). Curr. Sci. **28**, 379–380 (1959).

Araujo, J.: Morphologie et histologie de la glande pygidiale défensive de *Bledius spectablis* Kr. (Staphylinidae-Oxytelinae). C.R. Acad. Sci. (Paris) **D276**, 2713–2716 (1973).

Ayer, W., Dawes, R.: –Canad. J. Chem. *in press*.

Barth, R.: Ueber die Pygidialdruese von *Enhydrus sulcatus* (Wied. 1821) (Coleoptera, Grynidae). Mem. Inst. Osw. Cruz. **58**, 135–147 (1960).

Beams, H.W., Anderson, E.: Fine structure of "intracellular ductules" in certain glands of the carabid beetle. J. Morph. **109**, 159–171 (1961).

Bellas, T.E., Brown, W.V., Moore, B.P.: The alkaloid actinidine and plausible precrusors in defensive secretions of rove beetles. J. Insect Physiol. **20**, 277–280 (1974).

Benn, M.H., Lencucha, A., Maxie, S., Telang, S.A.: The pygidial defence secretion of *Carabus taedatus* (Col. Carabidae). J. Insect Physiol. **19**, 2173–2176 (1973).

Bierl, B.A., Beroza, M., Ashton, W.T.: Reaction Loops for Reaction Gas Chromatography. Subtraction of Alcohols, Aldehydes, Ketones, Epoxides, and Acids and Carbon-Skeleton Chromatography of Polar Compounds. Mikrochim. Acta **3**, 637–653 (1969).

Blum, M.S., Brand, J.M., Wallace, J.B., Foles, H.M.: Chemical characterization of the defensive secretion of a chrysomelid larva (*Chrysomela interrupta*). Life Sci. **11**, 525–531 (1972).

Blum, M.S., Crain, R.D.: The occurrence of *p*-quinones in the abdominal secretion of *Eleodes hispilabris*. Ann. entomol. Soc. Amer. **54**, 474 (1961).

Blum, M.S., Crewe, R.M., Pasteels, J.M.: Defensive secretion of *Lomechusa strumosa*, a myrmecophilous beetle (Coleoptera: Staphylinidae). Ann. entomol. Soc. Amer. **64**, 975–976 (1971).

Blumberg, D.: The repugnatorial glands of the tenebrionid beetle (Coleoptera) *Eleodes obsoleta* (Say.). Trans. Amer. entomol. Soc. **88**, 45–55 (1961).

Brand, J.M., Blum, M.S., Foles, H.M., Pasteels, J.M.: The chemistry of the defensive secretion of the beetle *Drusilla canaliculata* (Col. Staphylinidae). J. Insect Physiol. **19**, 369–382 (1973).

Brega, A., Falaschi, A., de Carli, L., Pavan, M.: Studies on the mechanism of action of pederin. J. Cell Biol. **36**, 485–496 (1968).

Cardani, C., Fuganti, C., Ghiringhelli, D., Grassell, P., Pavan, M., Valcurone, M.D.: The biosynthesis of pederin. Tetra. Lett. No. 30, 2815–2818 (1973).

Cardani, C., Ghiringhelli, D., Mondelli, R., Pavan, M., Quilico, A.: Propriétés biologiques et composition chimique de la Pédérine. Ann. Soc. entomol. Fr. **1**, 813–816 (1965b).

Cardani, C., Ghiringhelli, D., Mondelli, R., Quilico, A.: The structure of pederin. Tetra. Lett. No. 29, 2537–2545 (1965a).

Cardani, C., Ghiringhelli, D., Mondelli, R., Quilico, A.: Strutta della pederina. Gazz. chim. Ital. **96**, 3–38 (1966).

Cardani, C., Ghiringhelli, D., Quilico, A., Selva, A.: The structure of pederone, a novel substance from *Paederus* spp. (Coleoptera: Staphylinidae). Tetra. Lett. No. 41, 4023–4025 (1967).

Carrel, J.E., Eisner, T.: Cantharidin: potent feeding deterrent to insects. Science, **183**, 755–757 (1974).

Casnati, G., Pavan, M., Ricca, A.: Sulla costituzione del veleno dell' insetto *Calosoma sychophanta* L. [Coleoptera Carabidae]. Ann. Soc. entomol. Fr. **1**, 705–710 (1965).

Cavill, G.W.K.: The cyclopentanoid monoterpenes. Rev. pure appl. Chem. **10**, 169–183 (1960).

Cavill, G.W.K., Zeitlin, A.: Synthesis of D-(4)-tecostidine and related actinidine derivatives. Aust. J. Chem. **20**, 349–357 (1967).

Chadha, M.S., Eisner, T., Meinwald, J.: Defense mechanisms of arthropods. IV. *p*-Benzoquinones in the secretion of *Eleodes longicollis* Lec. (Coleoptera: Tenebrionidae). J. Insect Physiol. **7**, 46–50 (1961).

Chadha, M.S., Joshi, N.K., Mamdapur, V.R., Sipahimalani, A.T.: C-21 steroids in the defensive secretions of some Indian water beetles. Tetrahedron **26**, 2061–2064 (1970).

Colombini, N.: Osservazioni sulla struttura delle ghiandole pigidiali di *Cybister roeselii* Fabr. Soc. toscana Sci. Nat. Pisa **45**, 153–162 (1935b).

Colombini, N.: Osservazioni sulla morfologia delle ghiandole pigidiali dei Carabidi. Soc. toscana Sci. Nat. Pisa **45**, 271–281 (1935a).

Edwards, J.S.: Spitting as a defensive mechanism in a predatory reduviid. Eleventh Intern. Cong. Ent. Vienna, Verhandlungen **3**, 259–263 (1960).

Eisner, T., Hurst, J.J., Meinwald, J.: Defense mechanisms of arthropods. XI. The structure, function, and phenolic secretions of the glands of a chordeumoid millipede and carabid beetle. Psyche **70**, 94–116 (1963b).

Eisner, T., McHenry, F., Salpeter, M.M.: Defense mechanisms of arthropods. XV. Morphology of the quinone-producing glands of a tenebrionid beetle (*Eleodes longicollis* Lec.). J. Morph. **115**, 335–400 (1964).

Eisner, T., Meinwald, Y.C., Alsop, D.W., Carrel, J.E.: Defense mechanisms of arthropods. XXI. Formic acid and *n*-nonyl acetate in the defensive spray of two species of *Helluomorphoides*. Ann. entomol. Soc. Amer. **61**, 610–613 (1968).

Eisner, T., Swithenbank, C., Meinwald, J.: Defense mechanisms of arthropods. VIII. Secretion of salicylaldehyde by a carabid beetle. Ann. entomol. Soc. Amer. **56**, 37–41 (1963a).

Endt, D.W.V., Wheeler, J.W.: 1-Pentadecene production in *Tribolium confusum*. Sci. **172**, 60–61 (1971).

Engelhardt, M., Rapaport, H., Sokoloff, A.: Odourous secretion from normal and mutant *Tribolium confusum*. Sci. **150**, 632–633 (1965).

Fish, L.J., Pattenden, G.: Iridodial and a new alkanone, 4-methylhexan-3-one, in the defensive secretion of the beetle *Staphylinus olens*. J. Insect Physiol. **21**, 741–744 (1975).

Forsyth, D.J.: The structure of the defence glands in the Dytiscidae, Noteridae, Haliplidae and Gyrinidae (Coleoptera). Trans. roy. entomol. Soc. (Lond.) **120**, 159–182 (1968).

Forsyth, D.J.: The ultrastructure of the pygidial defence glands of the carabid *Pterostichus madidus* F. J. Morph. **131**, 397–416 (1970a).

Forsyth, D.J.: The structure of the defence glands of the Cirindelidae, Amphizoidae and Hygrobiidae (Coleoptera). J. Zool. (Lond.) **160**, 51–69 (1970b).

Forsyth, D.J.: The structure of the pygidial defence glands of Carabidae (Coleoptera). Trans. zool. Soc. Lond. **32**, 249–309 (1972).

Furusaki, A., Watanabe, T.: The crystal and molecular structure of pederin di-*p*-bromobenzoate. Tetra. Lett. No. 60, 6301–6304 (1968).

Gadamer, J.: The constitution of cantharidin. Arch. Pharm. (Weinheim) **252**, 609 (1914).

Garb, G.: The eversible glands of a chrysomelid larva, *Melasoma lapponica*. J. entomol. Zool. **7**, 88–95 (1915).

Hackmann, R.H., Pryor, M.G.M., Todd, A.R.: The occurrence of phenolic substances in arthropods. Biochem. J. **43**, 474—477 (1948).

Happ, G.M.: Benzoquinones in the defenisve secretion of *Leichenum canaliculatum variegatum* (Coleoptera: Tenebrionidae). Ann. entomol. Soc. Amer. **60**, 279 (1967).

Happ, G.M.: Quinone and hydrocarbon production in the defensive glands of *Eleodes longicollis* and *Tribolium castaneum* (Coleoptera: Tenebrionidae). J. Insect Physiol. **14**, 1821—1837 (1968).

Happ, G.M., Eisner, T.: Haemorrhage in a coccinellid beetle and its repellant effect on ants. Science **134**, 329—331 (1961).

Happ, G.M., Happ, C.M.: Fine structure of the pygidial glands of *Bledius mandibularis* (Coleoptera: Staphylinidae). Tissue Cell **5**, 215—231 (1973).

Hayes, W.P., Chu, H.F.: An undescribed eversible gland in the larvae of *Chlaenius* (Coleoptera: Carabidae). J. Kans. entomol. Soc. **20**, 142—145 (1947).

Henson, R.D., Thompson, A.C., Hedin, P.A., Nichols, P.R., Neel, W.W.: Identification of precoccinellin in the ladybird beetle, *Coleomegilla maculata.* Experientia (Basel) **31**, 145 (1975).

Hinton, H.E.: On a little known protective device of some chrysomelid pupae (Coleoptera). Proc. roy. entomol. Soc. (Lond.) (A). **26**, 69—73 (1951).

Hisada, Y., Emura, M.: Cytological effects of chemicals on tumors. XXVIII. Notes on the effects of extract from *Paederus fuscipes* on a transplantable rat ascites tumor. J. Fac. Sci., Haikkaido Univ. Ser. VI **15**, 684—692 (1965).

Hollande, M.A.Ch.: Sur la fonction d'excrétion chez les insectes salicioles et un particular sur l'existence des derivées salicyles. Ann. Univ. Grenoble Sect. Sci. med. **21**, 459 (1909).

Hsiao, T.H. and Fraenkel, G.: Properties of leptinotarsin, a toxic hemolymph protein from the Colorado potato beetle. Toxicon **7**, 119—130 (1969).

Hurst, J.J., Meinwald, J., Eisner, T.: Defense mechanisms of arthropods. II. Glucose and hydrocarbons in the quinone containing secretion of *Eleodes longicollis*. Ann. entomol. Soc. Amer. **57**, 44—46 (1964).

Ikan, R., Cohen, E., Shulov, A.: Benzo- and hydroquinones in the defensive secretions of *Blaps sulcata* and *B. wiedermanni*. J. Insect Physiol. **16**, 2201—2206 (1970).

Kendall, D.A.: The structure of the defence glands in Alleculidae and Lagriidae (Coleoptera). Trans. roy entomol. Soc. (Lond.) **120**, 139—156 (1968).

Kendall, D.A.: The dermal glands of some adult beetles. J. Entomol. **A46**, 153—159 (1972).

Kendall, D.A.: The structure of defence glands in some Tenebrionidae and Nilionidae (Coleoptera). Trans. roy. entomol. Soc. (Lond.) **125**, 437—487 (1974).

Kolbe, W., Proske, M.G.: Iso-valeriansäure im Abwehrsekret von *Zyras humeralis* Grav. (Coleoptera, Staphylinidae). Entomol. Bl. Biol. Syst. Käfer **69**, 57—60 (1973).

Leete, E., Murvill, J.B.: Biosynthesis of the tiglic acid moiety of metaloidine in *Datura meteloides*. Tetra. Lett. No. 18, 1727—1730 (1967).

Loconti, J.D., Roth, L.M.: Composition of odorous secretion of *Tribolium castaneum*. Ann. entomol. Soc. Amer. **46**, 281—289 (1953).

Matsumoto, T., Yanagiya, M., Maeno, S., Yasuda, S.: A revised structure of pederin. Tetra. Lett. **60**, 6297—6300 (1968).

McCullough, T.: Quantitative determination of salicylaldehyde in the scent fluid of *Calosoma macrum, C. alternans sayi, C. affini* and *C. parvicollis*. Ann. entomol. Soc. Amer. **59**, 1018 (1966a).

McCullough, T.: Compounds in the defensive scent glands of *Harpalus caliginosus* (Coleoptera: Carabidae). Ann. entomol. Soc. Amer. **59**, 1020 (1966b).

McCullough, T.: Compounds found in the defensive scent fluid of *Dicaelus splendidus* and *D. dilatatus*. Ann. entomol. Soc. Amer. **60**, 861 (1967).

McCullough, T.: Chemical analysis of the defensive scent fluid produced by the ground beetle *Calosoma peregrinator* (Coleoptera: Carabidae). Ann. entomol. Soc. Amer. **62**, 1498—1499 (1969a).

McCullough, T.: Chemical analysis of the scent fluid of *Dicaelus pupuratus*. Ann. entomol. Soc. Amer. **62**, 1493—1494 (1969b).

McCullough, T.: Chemical analysis of the scent fluid of *Pasimachus californicus* and *P. duplicatus*. Ann. entomol. Soc. Amer. **62**, 1492 (1969c).

McCullough, T.: Chemical analysis of the defensive scent fluid from *Progaleritina mexicana* (Coleoptera: Carabidae). Ann. entomol. Soc. Amer. **64**, 1191 (1971).

McCullough, T.: Defensive chemistry of the ground beetle *Callisthenes luxatus* (Coleoptera: Carabidae). Ann. entomol. Soc. Amer. **65**, 275 (1972a).

McCullough, T.: Analysis of the defensive scent fluid of *Pasimachus elongatus* (Coleoptera: Carabidae). Ann. entomol. Soc. Amer. **65**, 772 (1972b).

McCullough, T., Weinheimer, A.J.: Compounds found in the defensive scent fluids of *Calosoma marginalis, C. externum* and *C. scrutator*. Ann. entomol. Soc. Amer. **59**, 410 (1966).

Meinwald, J., Koch, K.F., Rogers, J.E., Eisner, T.: Biosynthesis of Arthropod Secretions. III. Synthesis of simple p-benzoquinones in a beetle (*Eleodes longicollis*). J. Amer. chem. Soc. **88**, 1590 – 1592 (1966).

Meinwald, J., Meinwald, Y.C., Chalmers, A.M.: Dihydromatricaria acid: acetylenic acid secreted by a soldier beetle. Science **160**, 890 (1968).

Meinwald, J., Opheim, K., Eisner, T.: Gyrinidal: a sesqeuterpenoid aldehyde from the defensive glands of gyrinid beetles (Coleoptera). Proc. nat. Acad. Sci. (Wash.) **69**, 1208 – 1210 (1972).

Meinwald, Y.C., Eisner, T.: Defense mechanisms of arthropods. XIV. Caprylic acid: an accessory component of the secretion of *Eleodes longicollis*. Ann. entomol. Soc. Amer. **57**, 513 (1964).

Miller, J.R., Hendry, L.B., Mumma, R.O.: Norsesquic terpenes as defensive toxins of whirligig beetles (Coleoptera: Gyrinidae). J. Chem. Ecol. **1**, 59 – 82 (1975).

Miller, J.R., Mumma, R.O.: Defensive agents of the American water beetles *Agabus seriatus* and *Graphoderus liberus* (Coleoptera: Dytiscidae). J. Insect Physiol. **19**, 917 – 925 (1973).

Miller, J.R., Mumma, R.O.: Seasonal quantification of the defensive steroid titer in *Agabus seriatus* (Coleoptera: Dytiscidae). Ann. entomol. Soc. Amer. **67**, 850 – 852 (1974).

Miller, J.R., Mumma, R.O.: Physiological activity of water beetle defensive agents, I. Toxicity and anesthetic of steroids and norsesquiterpenes administered in solution to the minnow *Pimephales promelas* Raf. J. Chem. Ecol. **2**, 115 – 130 (1976a).

Miller, J.R., Mumma, R.O.: Physiological activity of water beetle defensive agents. II. Absorption of selected anesthetic steroids and norsesquiterpenes across the gill membranes of the minnow *Pimephales promelas* Raf. J. Chem. Ecol. **2**, 130 – 146 (1976b).

Moore, B.P., Brown, W.V.: Chemical defence in longhorn beetles of the genera *Stenocentrus* and *Syllitus* (Coleoptera: Cerambycidae). J. Aust. entomol. Soc. **10**, 230 – 232 (1971a).

Moore, B.P., Brown, W.V.: Benzaldehyde in the defensive secretion of a tiger beetle (Coleoptera: Carabidae). J. Aust. entomol. Soc. **10**, 142 – 143 (1971b).

Moore, B.P., Brown, W.V.: The chemistry of the metasternal gland secretion of the common eucalyt longicorn *Phoracantha semipunctata* (Coleoptera: Cerambycidae). Aust. J. Chem. **25**, 591 – 598 (1972).

Moore, B.P., Wallbank, B.E.: Chemical composition of the defensive secretion in carabid beetles and its importance as a taxonomic character. Proc. roy. entomol. Soc. (Lond.) B, **37**, 62 – 72 (1968).

Moreau, L.: La secrétion du *Blaps gigas*. Soc. Linnéene de Province, Marseille Bull. **5**, 34 – 37 (1931).

Palm, N.: Structure and physiology of the stink glands in *Tribolium destructor* Uytt (Coleoptera). Opusc. entomol. **11**, 119 – 132 (1946).

Parker, R.: A comparison of the toxic protein in two species of *Leptinotarsa*. Toxicon **10**, 79 – 80 (1972).

Pasteels, J.M., Deroe, C., Tursch, B., Braekman, J.C., Daloze, D., Hootele, C.: Distribution et activités des alcoloïdes défensifs des Coccinellidae. J. Insect Physiol. **19**, 1771 – 1784 (1973).

Pavan, M.: Biochemical aspects of insect poisons. Int. Congr. Biochem., 4th Meeting, Vienna **12**, 15 – 36 (1959).

Pavan, M.: Sunto delle attuali conoscenze sulla pederina. Publ. Ist. Entomol. agr. Univ. Pavia, 1 – 35 (1975).

Pavan, M., Dazzini, M.V.: Toxicology and Pharmacology – Arthropoda. Chem. Zool. **6**, 365 – 409 (1971).

Robiquet, M.: (1810) from Weatherston, J.: The Chemistry of Arthropod Defensive Substances. Quart. Rev. **21** (1967).

Roth, L.M.: Studies on the gaseous secretion of *Tribolium confusum*. Ann. entomol. Soc. Amer. **36**, 397—424 (1943).

Roth, L.M.: Odoriferous glands in the Tenebrionidae. Ann. Entomol. Soc. Amer. **38**, 77—87 (1945).

Roth, L.M., Howland, R.B.: Studies on the gaseous secretion of *Tribolium confusum* (Duval). Ann. entomol. Soc. Amer. **34**, 151—175 (1941).

Roth, L.M., Stay, B.: The occurrence of paraquinones in some arthropods, with emphasis on the quinone-secreting tracheal glands of *Diploptera punctata* (Blattaria). J. Insect Physiol. **1**, 305—318 (1958).

Rudolph, W.: Cantharidin. Arch. Pharm. (Weinheim) **254**, 423 (1916).

Schildknecht, H.: Zur Chemie des Bombardierkäfers. Angew. Chemie **69**, 62 (1957).

Schildknecht, H.: Über das flüchtige Sekret vom gemeinen Mehlkäfer. Angew. Chemie **71**, 524 (1959).

Schildknecht, H.: Defensive substances of the arthropods, their isolation and identification. Angew. Chemie (Int. Ed.) **3**, 73—84 (1964).

Schildknecht, H.: Das Arsenal der Schwimmkäfer: Sexualhormon und Antibiotica. Chemie Technik 18, 311—312 (1968).

Schildknecht, H.: The defensive chemistry of land and water beetles. Angew. Chemie (Int. Ed.) **9**, 1—9 (1970).

Schildknecht, H., Berger, D., Krauss, D., Connert, J., Gehlhaus, J., Essenbreis, H.: Defense chemistry of *Stennus comma* (Coleoptera: Staphylinidae). LXI. J. Chem. Ecol. **2**, 1—23 (1976).

Schildknecht, H., Birringer, H.: Die Steroide des Schlammschwimmers *Ilybius fenestratus*. Z. Naturforsch. **24**b, 1529—1534 (1969).

Schildknecht, H., Birringer, H., Krauss, D.: Über Arthropodenabwehrstoffe, XXXVI. Aufklärung des gelben Prothorakabwehrdrüsen-farbstoffes aus *Ilybius fenestratus*. Z. Naturforsch. **24**b, 38—47 (1969b).

Schildknecht, H., Birringer, H., Maschwitz, U.: Testosterone as a protective agent of the water beetle *Ilybius*. Angew. Chemie (Int. Ed.) **6**, 558—559 (1967c).

Schildknecht, H., Buhner, R.: Über Arthropodenabwehrstoffe. XXXIII. Über ein Glykoproteid in der Pygidialwehrblasen des Gelbrandkäfers. Z. Naturforsch. **23**b, 1209—1213 (1968).

Schildknecht, H., Holubek, K.: Über einen Inhaltsstoff der Wehrdrüsen des Gelbrandkäfers. Angew. Chemie **71**, 524 (1959).

Schildknecht, H., Holoubek, K.: Die Bombardierkäfer und ihre Explosionschemie, V. Mitteilung über Insektenabwehrstoffe. Angew. Chemie **73**, 1—7 (1961).

Schildknecht, H., Hotz, D.: Identifizierung der Nebensteroide des Prothorakabwehrdrüsen Systems des Gelbrandkäfers *Dytiscus marginalis*. Angew. Chemie (Int. Ed.) **6**, 881—882 (1967).

Schildknecht, H., Hotz, D., Maschwitz, U.: Über Arthropodenabwehrstoffe. XXVII. Die C_{21}-Steroides der Prothorakabwehrdrüsen von *Acilius sulcatus*. Z. Naturforsch. **22**b, 938—944 (1967a).

Schildknecht, H., Koob, K.: Zur Explosionschemie der Bombardierkäfer. Naturwissenschaften **56**, 328 (1969).

Schildknecht, H., Kornig, E.: Protective material from the prothoracic gland of a Mexican *Cybister* species. Angew. Chemie (Int. Ed.) **7**, 62 (1968a).

Schildknecht, H., Krämer, H.: Zum Nachweis von Hydrochinonen neben Chinonen in den Abwehrblasen von Arthropoden—XV. Mitt. über Insektenabwehrstoffe. Z. Naturforsch. **17**b, 701—702 (1962).

Schildknecht, H., Krauss, D., Connert, J., Essenbreis, H., Orfanides, N.: Spreading alkaloid stenusin from the brachypterous insect *Stennus comma* (Coleoptera: Staphylinidae). Angew. Chemie **87**, 421—422 (1975).

Schildknecht, H., Maschwitz, E., Maschwitz, U.: Die Explosionschemie der Bombardierkäfer (Coleoptera: Carabidae). III. Isolierung und Charakterisierung der Explosionskatalysatoren. Z. Naturforsch. **23**b, 1213—1218 (1968d).

Schildknecht, H., Maschwitz, E., Maschwitz, U.: Die Explosionschemie der Bombardierkäfer: Struktur und Eigenschaften der Brennkammerenzyme. J. Insect Physiol. **16**, 749—789 (1970).

Schildknecht, H., Maschwitz, U.: A vertebrate hormone as the defensive substance of the water beetle *Dytiscus marginalis*. Angew. Chemie (Int. Ed.) **5**, 421—422 (1966).

Schildknecht, H., Maschwitz, U., Winkler, H.: Zur Evolution der Carabiden-Wehrdrüsensekret. Naturwissenschaften **55**, 112 – 117 (1968 e).

Schildknecht, H., Maschwitz, U., Krauss, D.: Blausäure im Wehrsekret des Erdläufers *Pachymerium ferrugineum*. Naturwissenschaften **55**, 230 (1968 f).

Schildknecht, H., Siewerdt, R., Maschwitz, U.: Über Arthropoden Abwehrstoffe. XXIII. Cybisteron, ein neues Arthropoden Steroid. Justus Liebigs Ann. Chem. **703**, 182 – 189 (1967 b).

Schildknecht, H., Tacheci, H.: Colymbetin, a new defensive substance of the water beetle *Colymbetes fuscus* (Coleoptera: Dytiscidae) that lowers blood pressure. J. Insect Physiol. **17**, 1889 – 1896 (1971).

Schildknecht, H., Tacheci, H., Maschwitz, U.: 4-Pregnen-15α,20β-diol-3-on im Wehrsekret eines Schwimmkäfers. Naturwissenschaften **56**, 37 – 38 (1969 a).

Schildknecht, H., Weis, K.H.: Über die Tenebrioniden-chinon bei lebendem und totem Untersuchungsmaterial. Z. Naturforsch. **15**b, 757 – 758 (1960 a).

Schildknecht, H., Weis, K.H.: Über das flüchtige Sekret von Totenkäfer *Blaps mortisaga*. Z. Naturforsch. **15**b, 200 (1960 b).

Schildknecht, H., Weis, K.H.: Die Abwehrstoffe einiger Carabiden, insbesondere von *Abax ater*. XII. Mitteilung über Insektenabwehrstoffe. Z. Naturforsch. **17**b, 439 – 447 (1962).

Schildknecht, H., Winkler, H., Krauss, D., Maschwitz, U.: Über Arthropodenabwehrstoffe. XXVIII. Über das Abwehrsekret von *Idiochroma dorsalis*. Z. Naturforsch. **23**b, 46 – 49 (1968 c).

Schildknecht, H., Winkler, H., Maschwitz, U.: Über Arthropodenabwehrstoffe. XXXI. Vergleichend chemische Untersuchungen der Inhaltsstoffe der Pygidialwehrblasen von Carabiden. Z. Naturforsch. **23**b, 637 – 644 (1968 b).

Schlatter, Ch., Waldner, E.E., Schmid, H.: Biosynthesis of cantharidin. I. Experientia (Basel) **24**, 994 – 995 (1968).

Schnepf, E., Wenneis, W., Schildknecht, H.: Über Arthropoden-Abwehrstoffe. XLI. Zur Explosionschemie der Bombardierkäfer (Coleoptera: Carabidae). IV. Zur Feinstruktur der Pygidialabwehrdrüsen des Bombardierkäfers (*Brachynus crepitans* L.). Z. Zellforsch. **96**, 582 – 599 (1969).

Scott, P.D., Hepburn, H.R., Crewe, R.M.: Pygidial defensive secretions of some carabid beetles. Insect Biochem. **5**, 805 – 811 (1975).

Sierra, J.R., Woggon, W.D., Schmid, H.: Transfer of cantharidin during copulation from adult male to the female *Lytta vesicatoria* (Spanish Flies). Experientia (Basel) **32**, 142 – 144 (1976).

Sipahimalani, A.T., Mamdapur, V.R., Joshi, N.K., Chadha, M.S.: Steroids in the defensive secretion of the water beetle *Cybister limbatus*. Naturwissenschaften **57**, 40 (1970).

Stork, G., von Tamelin, E.E., Friedman, L.J., Burgstahler, A.W.: A stereospecific synthesis of cantharidin. J. Amer. chem. Soc. **75**, 384 – 392 (1953).

Sulc, K.: On the repugnatorial stink glands in the beetles of the genus *Cantharis*, Coleoptera. Ceska Akad. ved. a umeni v Praze Bull. Int. **50**, 79 – 100 (1949).

Suzuki, T., Suzuki, T., Huynh, V., Moto, T.: Isolation of 2-hydroxy-4-methoxypropiophenone from *Tribolium castaneum* and *T. confusum*. Agric. biol. Chem. **39**, 1687 – 1688 (1975).

Tschinkel, W.R.: Phenols and quinones from the defensive secretion of the tenebrionid beetle *Zophobas rugipes*. J. Insect Physiol. **15**, 191 – 200 (1969).

Tursch, B., Braekman, J.C., Daloze, D.: Arthropod alkaloids. Experientia (Basel) **32**, 401 – 407 (1976).

Tursch, B., Braekman, J.C., Daloze, D., Hootele, C., Losman, D., Karlsson, R., Pasteels, J.M.: Chemical ecology of arthropods. VI. Adaline, a novel alkaloid from *Adalia bipunctata* L. (Coleoptera: Coccinellidae). Tetra. Lett. No. 3, 201 – 202 (1973 b).

Tursch, B., Chome, C., Braekman, J.C., Daloze, D.: Chemical ecology of arthropods. VIII. Synthesis and absolute configuration of adaline. Bull. Soc. chim. Belg. **82**, 699 – 703 (1973 a).

Tursch, B., Daloze, D., Braekman, J.C., Hootele, C., Cravador, A.: Chemical ecology of arthropods. IX. Structure and absolute configuration of hippodamine and convergine, two novel alkaloids from the American ladybug *Hippodamia convergens* (Coleoptera). Tetra. Lett. No. 5, 409 – 412 (1974).

Tursch, B., Daloze, D., Brakman, J.C., Hootele, C., Pasteels, J.M.: Chemical ecology of arthropods. X. The structure of myrrhine and the biosynthesis of coccinelline. Tetrahedron **31**, 1541 – 1543 (1975).

Tursch, B., Daloze, D., Dupont, M., Hootele, C., Kaisin, M., Pasteels, J.M., Zimmermann, D.: Coccinellin, the defensive alkaloid of the beetle, *Coccinella septempunctata*. Chimia **25**, 307 (1971 b).

Tursch, B., Daloze, D., Dupont, M., Pasteels, J.M. and Tricot, M.C.: A defensive alkaloid in a carnivorous beetle. Experientia (Basel) **27**, 1380—1381 (1971 a).

Tursch, B., Daloze, D., Hootele, C.: The alkaloid of *Propylaea quatuordecimpunctata* L. (Coleoptera, Coccinellidae). Chimia **26**, 74 (1972 b).

Tursch, B., Daloze, D., Pasteels, J.M., Cravador, A., Braekman, J.C., Hootele, C., Zimmermann, D.: Two novel alkaloids from the American ladybug *Hippodamia convergens* (Coleoptera: Coccinellidae). Bull. Soc. chim. Belg. **81**, 649—650 (1972 a).

Tschinkel, W.R.: 6-Alkyl-1,4-naphthoquinones from the defensive secretion of the tenebrionid beetle *Argoporis alutacea* (Coleoptera). J. Insect Physiol. **18**, 711—722 (1972).

Tschinkel, W.R.: A comparative study of the chemical defense system of tenebrionid beetles: chemistry of the secretions. J. Insect Physiol. **21**, 753—783 (1975 a).

Tschinkel, W.R.: Unusual occurrence of aldehydes and ketones in the defensive secretion of the tenebrionid beetle *Eleodes beamri*. J. Insect Physiol. **21**, 659—672 (1975 b).

Tseng, Y.C.L., Davidson, J.A., Menzer, R.E.: Morphology and chemistry of the odoriferous gland of the lesser mealworm. Ann. entomol. Soc. Amer. **64**, 425—430 (1971).

Vidari, G., DeBernardi, M., Pavan, M., Ragozzino, L.: Rose oxide and iridodial from *Aromia moschata* L. (Coleoptera: Cerambycidae). Tetra. Lett. No. 41, 4065—4068 (1973).

Wain, R.L.: The secretion of salicylaldehyde by the larvae of the brassy willow beetle, *Phylodecta vittelinae*. Ann. Rep. Agric. Hort. Station, Long Ashton, Bristol 108—110 (1943).

Wallace, T.B., Blum, M.S.: Refined defensive mechanisms in *Chrysomela scripta*. Ann. entomol. Soc. Amer. **62**, 503—506 (1969).

Wallace, J.B., Blum, M.S.: Reflex bleeding: a highly defined mechanism in *Diabrotica* larvae (Coleoptera: Chrysomelidae). Ann. entomol. Soc. Amer. **64**, 1021—1024 (1971).

Walter, W.G., Cole, J.F.: Isolation of cantharidin in *Epicauta pestifera*. J. pharm. Sci. **56**, 174—176 (1967).

Weatherston, J., Percy, J.E.: Arthropod defensive secretions in Chemicals Controlling Insect Behaviour (Ed. M. Beroza). Acad. Press, N.Y. pp. 95—144 (1970).

Wheeler, J.W., Araujo, J., Happ, G.M., Pasteels, J.W.: γ-Dodecalactone from rove beetles. Tetra. Lett. No. 46, 4635—4638 (1972 a).

Wheeler, J.W., Chung, R.H., Oh, S.K., Benfield, E.F., Neff, S.E.: Defensive secretions of cychrine beetles (Coleoptera: Carabidae). Ann. entomol. Soc. Amer. **63**, 469—471 (1970).

Wheeler, J.W., Oh, S.K., Benfield, E.F., Neff, S.E.: Cyclopentanoid norsesquiterpenes from gyrinid beetles (Coleoptera). J. Amer. chem. Soc. **94**, 7589—7590 (1972 b).

Woodward, R.B., Loftfield, R.B.: Structure of cantharidin and the synthesis of desoxycantharidin. J. Amer. chem. Soc. **63**, 3167—3171 (1941).

CHAPTER 20

Venoms of Lepidoptera

A. Delgado Quiroz

A. Introduction

Lepidoptera may accidentally affect man's health by means of specialized scales and toxic substances, as they use these in both active and passive defence against predatory animal species which compete for their territory (Mooren, 1848; Schroeder, 1896).

Bearing in mind the presence or absence of a specialized poison apparatus, and the way the poison makes pathogenic contact with man and other animals, we have differentiated between two large groups of anthropotoxic lepidoptera (Delgado, 1967).

The first group, that of *phanerotoxic exogenous lepidoptera,* is represented by adult moths and by the larval forms called *erucae* (from the Latin *eruca* = caterpillar); the anthropotoxic erucae are provided with specialized glands which eject their contents (Poulton, 1887; Riley, 1888).

In active defense the primarily defensive role of the poison apparatus shows itself in the victim by its painful, toxic effects. This active defense protects both the individual and the species, and while it does not eliminate enemies, it at least limits their number. The poison acts by direct or indirect contact, producing in man dermic illness and a general symptomatology which has been given the convenient name of *Erucism* (Pesce and Delgado, 1966).

Four super-families of Lepidoptera have erucae with urticating hairs: Papilionida, Zygaenoidea, Noctuoidea, and Bombycoidea (Schroeder, 1925; Riley, 1938; Da Costa Lima, 1945, 1950).

In passive or reflex defense, the exocrinal poison acts by direct contact, as in the case of some adult lepidoptera that have no urticating hairs but possess special glands that produce a golden nauseous secretion. The smell they give off, even from some distance, has a repellent effect on small birds and other anthropods. An example is *Zygaena* spp., which was studied by Rocci (1917). The individual "dose" of poison is, to a certain extent, harmless to man and other domestic animals.

Occasionally harmful in the same way as those already mentioned, are phanerotoxic lepidoptera, but in these the pathogenesis stems from hairs and scales which are shed, temporarily polluting the atmosphere. The minute hairs and scales are foreign bodies which act by contact, and casually penetrate the tegument. They may also be inhaled by man and animals. Leger and Mouzels (1918) proved that the adult moth of the genus *Hylesia* (Saturniidae) has a dermatoxic effect. This satuniid has its abdomen covered with large numbers of scales of a different morphology, among which are found setae modified to the shape of "flechettes," which contain toxic substances. These "flechettes" are easily shed in the air, and casually penetrate the epidermis of the uncovered parts of man and also of animals with epidemic characteristics. The dermic reaction, and also the general symptomatology which occurs, are called *Lepidopterism* (PESCE and DELGADO, 1966; PICARELLI and VALLE, 1971; ROTBERG, 1971).

VIANA and AZEVEDO (1967) reported clinical observations on the painful effects and deformation of the fingers of 24 Brazilian rubber workers, caused by accidental contact with hairy erucae, cocoons and even with the adult of the Artiid *Premolis semirrufa,* WALKER, 1856, HAMPSON, 1901. This illness, which is characterized by a chronic evolution and is contracted during work on *Hevea brasiliensis* rubber trees, is called *Granulomatouse erucism* or *pararama* (DIAS and AZEVEDO, 1973).

Cryptotoxic endogenous lepidoptera. Though they have no specialized apparatus for secreting poison, these are nonetheless toxicopherous, since venomous principles are present in their tissues and body fluids. Their toxicity is related to the individual animal physiology, food specialization etc., as in the case of some Pierids, which have a reputation for possessing poisonous body liquids that produce intestinal inflammation and even death in cattle which eat them accidentally in their larval, and especially in the pupal state along with their fodder. This food intoxication observed in animals is called *erucic gastroenterocolitis.*

B. Erucism

I. Description

Erucism is an intoxication resulting from contact with poisonous larval and pupal forms of ten families of Lepidoptera. It mainly affects the tegument, producing inflammatory reactions and alterations in the vascular wall, at the place where casual contact is made (Fig. 1). It can produce general symptomats of an histaminic and hemorrhagic type, on rare occasions affecting the nervous system. The setae which manage to introduce themselves into the skin, mucous membranes, and underlying tissues produce granuloma of the foreign-body type, frequently found in the fingers and on very rare occasions in the eyeball.

This illness has also been called *erucic dermatitis, nodal erucic ophthalmia, pararama, erucic rash, caterpillar dermatitis,* etc.

The poisonous properties of the erucae (=caterpillars) were topics of study, and the toxic principles derived from them were used, in Graeco-Roman times (PHISALIX, 1922). In South America the erucae were used by the natives in libidinous ceremonies and for the poisoning of arrows, according to reports by Portuguese and Spanish colonists (ANCHIETA, 1960; COBO, 1639−1653; BOSO, 1816). Von IHRING (1914) in his "Historia naturalis Brasiliae" states that Margrave and Piso in 1648 made observations on the dermic reactions caused by the Tatorana (=urticating erucae).

Also in modern times erucic poisoning in men and animals and the different etiological agents of erucism have been topics of study. GEER (1750) gives an account of some of the exogenic properties of erucae. KARSTEN (1848) identified urticating hairs in various Lepidoptera larvae. MOOREN (1848) observed the etiology of erucic illness. There have been attempts to explain the poisonous function of erucae as a means of defense (BURNETT, 1854; SCHROEDER, 1896), and also to explain the effect of erucic poisons (BONNET, 1875; BALDING, 1884; ALTUM, 1896; LONG, 1886).

A clinical account of erucic incidents in horses was published by POURQUIER (1877). The exocrinal gland of the erucae described in the literature (KLEMENSICWICZ, 1882; DIMMOCK, 1883, 1884). Clinical observations have appeared about the signs and symptoms produced in man by erucae poisoning (PERNOT, 1884; RENDALL, 1884; SHARP, 1885; JENKINS, 1886). Attention is given to the study of the dermic effects of the urticating hairs of erucae (SOUTH, 1885; MANDERS, 1887), Emphasis is also laid on the study of the glandular secretions of larval forms of Lepidoptera in the works of SCUDDER (1888), RILEY (1888), DENHAM (1888) and PATTON (1891). The anatomy of the urticating apparatus has also been studied (BEILLE, 1896; PACKARD, 1893−1898).

In this century the etiology and the allergic and occupational character of erucic incidents in different parts of the world have been studied, and it has been discovered that anthropotoxic erucae exist in two families of the suborder Rhopalocera and in eight families of the suborder Heterocera. The symptoms and signs of erucism have also been described more clearly.

ROHR (1900), MEGNIN (1901) and ARTAULT DE VEVEY (1901) studied erucic stomatitis in herbivores. FERTON (1901) observed that erucae have a means of protection which they employ against predatory Hymenoptera.

BORDAS (1902, 1903) carried out a study of the mandibular glands of erucae, SERRÉ (1904) found that the pupal state retains the poisonous properties of the larval state (eruca).

TYSSER (1907b) described the dermatitis produced in Europe by the Lymantriidae caterpillars: *Porthetria dispar* and *Nygmia phaerrohea* DON. [=*Euproctis chrysorrhoea* (L)]. ELTRINGHAM (1913) also studied the urticating properties of the Lymantriid *Porthesia similis* FUESSLY and KEPHART (1914) the poison glands of *Euproctis chrysorrhoea* (L). HASHIMOTO and HAGIWARA (1922) and MILLS (1923) described the erucic dermatitis produced in Japan and China by the Lymantriid *Euproctis flava*. KNIGHT (1922) remarked on the poisonous nature of the North American Lymantriid *Hemerocampa leucostigma,* while GILMER (1928) studied its venom and poison apparatus. CAFFREY (1918) studied the urticating bristles of the United States saturniid, *Hemileuca olivieae*. FOOT (1922) and BISHOPP (1923) describe the dermatitis caused by the most commonly found Megalopygid of the American continent, *Megalopyge opercularis*.

LAPIE (1923) investigated erucic incidents and poisonous caterpillars; MILLS (1925) studied the irritant properties of the erucae Cochlidiid (=limacodid), *Parasa hilarata*.

RANDOLPH (1934) studied the allergic reactions to insect dust made up of Lepidoptera scales. Finally, WEIDNER (1936) enumerates the contributions made to the study of phanerotoxic exogenous erucae. ANDRADE (1940) mentions the ocular pathology produced by Lepidoptera. KATZENELLENBOGEN (1954) considers the forms of erucic dermatitis as an occupational illness.

RANDEL and DOAN (1956) describe erucic dermatitis in the Panama Canal.

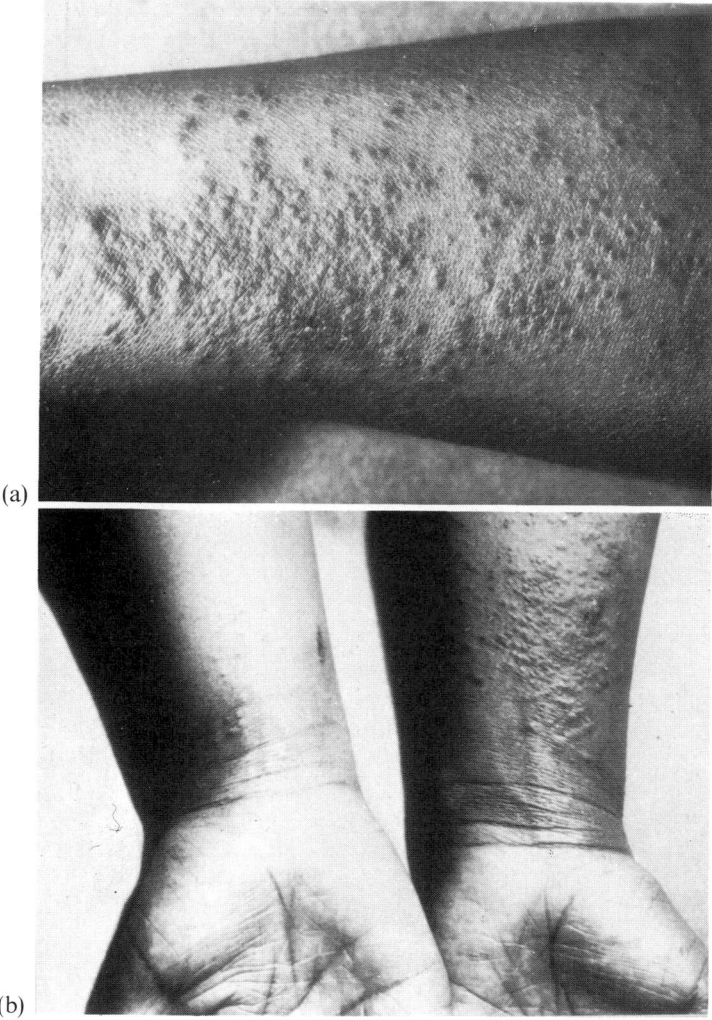

(a)

(b)

Fig. 1a–d. Signs of erucism: Dermic lesions caused by erucae. (a) Papular erythematous reaction produced by *Megalopyge* spp. on the flexure surface of the forearm. (b) Reaction spread over the flexure surface of the forearm. In comparison, on the other arm there are only isolated papules. Both types of lesions caused by *Podalia* spp. (c) Erythematous-vesiculous reaction with a crust formed on the palm of a hand, caused by *Premolis semirrufa*. Note the juxtarticular nodules at the roots of the fingers. (d) Giant vesicle-papule in an experiment using a patch with dry extract from *Dirphia* spp

II. Pathology

The local skin injury caused by contact with the poisonous hairs of erucae seems basically to affect the capillary blood vessels. The skin or mucous membrane display macroscopically the cardinal signs of inflammation, such as redness, heat, and swelling, and urgent pain is felt by the victim.

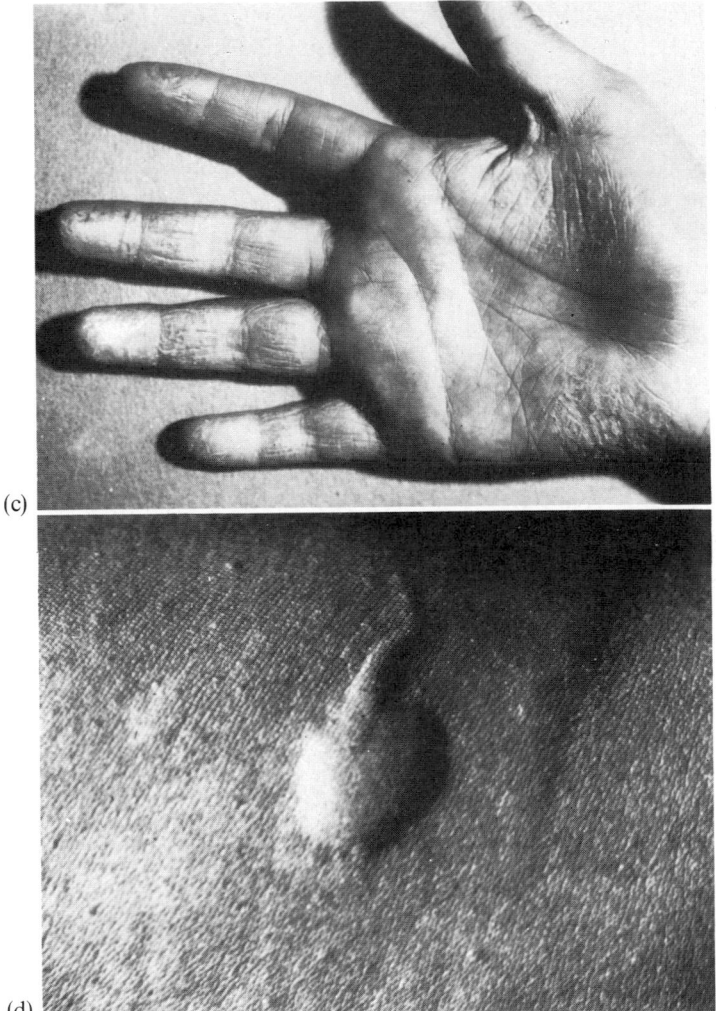

(c)

(d)

Fig. 1c and d

The initial microscopic reactions in the epidermis are intercellular edema and sometimes spongiosis, which leads to the formation of phlyctenae and vesicles containing fibrins, leucocytes and sometimes fragments of erucae hairs. In the dermis there occurs perivascular exudation with lymphocytes, some eosinophils, polymorphonuclear leucocytes and histiocytes. Lymphocytes and eosinophils are sometimes observed in the lymphatic spaces and also in the lumen of the affected capillaries (ROTBERG, 1971).

In very severe cases hemorrhagia is encountered in the dermis, and the epidermis in which the urticating hair has lodged itself reveals bruising and necrosis, while the corium shows perivascular inlammation. In the case of bulbous conjunctiva, DE SCHWEINITZ and SHUMWAY (1904), according to RILEY and JOHANNSEN (1938)

describe erucic nodal ophthalmia, the essential characteristic of which is pseudotu-
bercular conjunctivitis, which on histologic examination is diagnosed by the presence of lepidoptera setae. Macroscopically there appear yellowish-gray nodules,
among which there is marked congestion of the conjunctival and episcleral vessels.

Microscopically the nodules are composed of a layer of spindle cells with
round cells outside. The interior consists of epithelioid cells, between which is
a considerable volume of intercellular substance. In the case described in these
articles the section of a hair was found in the middle of the nodules. The setae
probably come from caterpillars of the arctiid *Spilosoma virginica*. Other cases
have been caused by the hairs of the larvae of *Lasiocampa rubi, L. pini, Porthetria
dispar, Psilura monacha* and *Thaumetopoea* spp. Edematous and fibrous periarticular lesions have been found on the hands of many workers who tap latex from
the rubber tree *Hevea brasiliensis*, when these trees have been infested with bristles
from the *Premolis semirrufa* erucae (Walker, 1956; Hampson, 1901). Dias and
Acevedo (1973) demonstrated in experiments on white mice that the setae of
the *Premolis semirrufa* erucae penetrate the skin and underlying tissues. At the
point where 2-mm-long setae have penetrated there is infiltration by eosinophilic
leucocytes. In the course of time fibrosis develops, along with the formation of
foreing-body granulomas. These granulomas of the foreign-body type have been
discovered in the skin, tendons, sheaths, periosta, bone marrow and lungs in
laboratory white mice.

In general terms the principal cytopathologic changes produced in human beings
and animals by *phanerotoxic exogenous Lepidoptera* with urticating larval forms
are as follows.

In the tegument, congestion, basal infiltration and edema (Foot, 1922; Matta,
1922).

In the dermis, infiltration of eosinophilic cells. In some cases the epidermis
shows evidence of vesicles and necrosis (Foot, 1922).

Hemolysis *in vitro* (Tysser, 1907a) in the blood of guinea-pigs, rats, horses,
and human beings, lecithin being used as a complement (Gaminara, 1928b).

III. Symptomatology

1. Pathogenesis

The pathogenic effects produced by *phanerotoxic exogenous Lepidoptera* with urticating erucae which directly or indirectly effect human beings and animals are
the result of four syndromes in evolutionary sequence, although they may often
occur in parallel.

a) Foreign-Body Syndrome

α) *Immediate*. The immediate effects are lesions that result from a mechanical
trauma, consisting of a small or large number of micropunctures made in the
tegument by the caterpillar's hairs (Fig. 2).

The extent of the lesion will depend on the size of the caterpillar, the nature
of the urticating hair, and also the way in which the victim has touched the

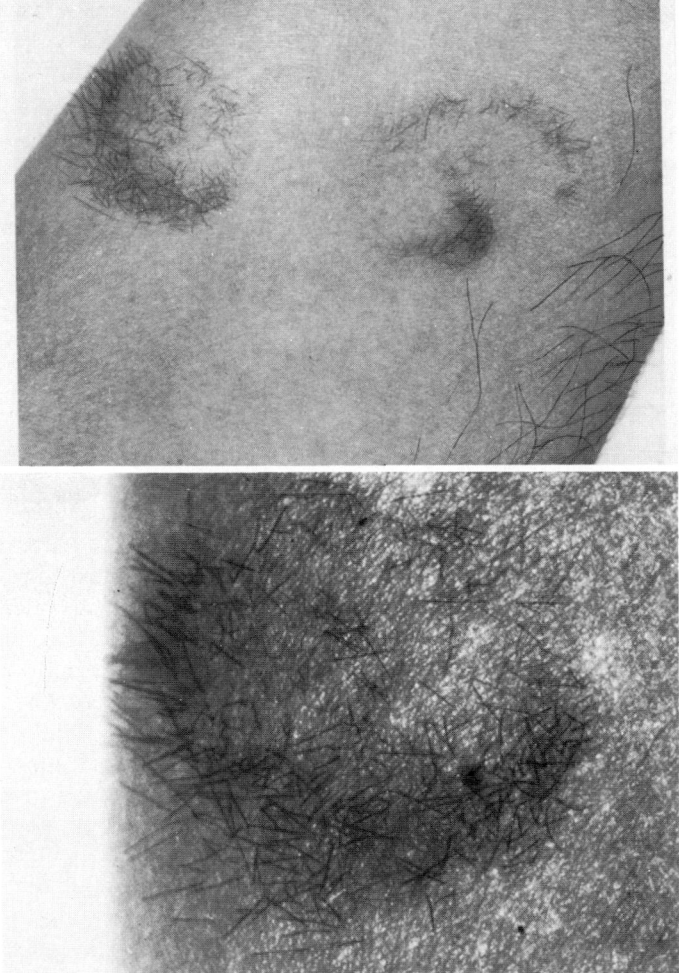

Fig. 2. Pathogenesis: urticating acicular hairs of erucae have penetrated the skin

caterpillar. As a result, the large caterpillars of the genus *Megalopyge* tend to produce more extensive dermatitis (PESCE and DELGADO, 1963). The immediate mechanical traumatism caused by the "nettling" hairs coming in contact with the skin produces irritation and pain which on rare occasions is severe enough to affect the person's general health.

β) Chronic. In addition to the immediate effects described above, experiments on white mice have proved that when the setae of the larva of the arctiid *P. semirrufa* penetrate the skin, they cause granuloma of the foreign-body type, particularly in the peripheral connecting tissues of the joints, which is similar to the clinical and radiological syndrome observed on the hands of forest workers in the state of Para-Brazil (DIAS and ACEVEDO, 1973).

The 2-mm-long setae cause itching, hyperemia and edema of the hands. As well as these immediate results, later ones of a chronic nature have been recorded, which eventually lead to the functional impotence of one of more phalanges, resulting in clinical terms in ankylosis. Radiological examination reveals periarticular edematous and fibrous changes in patients who show articular tumefaction and functional phalangeal impotence (Fig. 1).

On the other hand, the hairs of other arctiid caterpillars may occasionally enter the conjuctiva, cornea or iris, causing chronic nodular conjuctivitis similar to ocular conjunctive tuberculosis.

b) Toxic Syndrome

This refers to lesions caused by the injection of exocrinal substances produced by the caterpillar. It generally includes local and regional symptoms and only rarely is a general symptomatology observable.

α) Locally the poison makes its presence felt in itching, erythematous blotches and weals at the area of contact (McMillan and Durcell, 1964). However, the signs and symptoms vary greatly, since they depend on the nature and quality of the poisonous substance, on the duration and degree of the pressure accidentally exercised by the urticating larva against the skin and mucous membranes, on the body topography and on the victim's state of immunity.

Ocular reactions have been recorded, characterized by photophobia, erythema and giant edema of the eyelids with conjunctivitis and phlyctenular keratitis (Natansen, 1897; Cheverton, 1936; Andrade, 1940).

It has been observed that the mucous membrane of the upper respiratory apparatus, the nasal passages, and the oropharynx reveal varying degrees of hyperemia, after air contaminated by the hairs of urticating caterpillars has been inhaled. These are accompanied by bouts of coughing and rhinorrhea. If fruit contaminated by the dust of urticating hairs of the lymantriid *Liparis chrysorrhoea* is ingested, it produces hyperemic edema of the lips, papular erythema of the oral mucosae, palatine and gingival mucous membrane with sialorrhea (Artault de Vevey, 1901).

Locally, in the human skin, the urticating dust, or direct contact with the poisonous caterpillar produces an immediate, urgent, burning sensation with or without itching, which may last for hours. Objectively, at the point of contact, papular erythema appears, groups of edematous ischemic lesions 2—3 mm in diameter, which as they evolve may coalesce to form urticarial weals, vesicles and bullae (Fig. 1). These primary dermatological lesions are the result of secondary weals caused by the scales and pigmentation, which take 7—15 days to form.

Edematous deformity has been observed in large areas of the body, affecting a whole extremity or the segment of the head, with regional lymphangitis and adenitis (Pesce and Delgado, 1963). Generalized dermatitis has also been noted, when the poisonous hairs have accidentally been picked up on underwear laid out to dry on grass infested with urticating pupae and caterpillars.

In animals, erucic stomatitis has been observed in cattle grazing in regions infested with urticating pupae and caterpillars. Megnin (1901) recorded cases of severe stomatitis in dogs that had eaten leaves infested with hairs of the thaumetopid, *Cnetocampa pityocampa,* and Pourquier (1877) observed that this caterpillar caused urticaria in horses.

β) The symptoms of general toxic syndromes are: fever, general malaise, muscular spasms, nausea and vomiting; also local or regional neuritis of very brief duration, which shows itself in paresthesias, paresis and even paralysis.

The nature and quality of the exocrinal substances that cause these syndromes have not yet been adequately analyzed (VALETTE, 1954). It is known, however, that erucic poisoning is responsible for the immediate reaction and also in certain cases for the delayed reactions that are discovered in human beings and animals.

c) Infectious Syndrome

An infectious syndrome can be caused by bacteria invading the lesion caused by the hairy caterpillar, or to scratching. Pruritus, impetigo, cellulite, eczema, and septicemia of many different bacterial etiologies have been noted (DELGADO and PESCE, 1964).

d) Allergic Syndromes

These result from a previous sensitization of the patient to the setae and subtances present in the urticating caterpillars. These products act as allergens when they make contact with the skin, and may produce what is known as allergic contact dermatitis (RANDOLPH, 1934).

The erucic sensitizer does not normally bring about obvious changes at first contact, but it may produce specific changes in the skin after 5 or more days, when the patient is again exposed to the erucic product (DELGADO, 1971).

It seems reasonable to us to conclude that some of the severe immediate reactions, along with the majority of the delayed reactions associated with the caterpillar's contact with the skin, are due to an anaphylactic-type response such as the one described by SCHMITZ (1917), who records cases of severe hemorrhagic nephritis coinciding with an outbreak of erucic urticaria in Germany. As a result of investigations we know that with neotropical caterpillars there are few cases of sensitization, as shown by studies carried out in 433 cases of erucism in Peru (PESCE and DELGADO, 1963).

2. Evolution

The local or regional toxic syndrome always develops into erythema, frequently accompanied by ischemic erymatous papules. The symptoms are itching. These dermic lesions are produced by all the urticating caterpillars referred to in this study, and last about 24 h, leaving no sequelae. The vesicular bruises and weals, which are less common signs, last from 4 to 7 days, if they are not accompanied by septic syndromes. The symptom is urgent pain, which lasts from 24 to 48 h. The mechanical and particularly the toxic syndrome progresses in a similar way to the histamine, histaminoid and proteolytic type, which in addition to affecting the skin as a result of the trauma, includes important inflammatory signs in the lymphatic systems (lymphatic vessels and ganglions) next to the point where erucic contact is made. Neural involvement is common: urgent pains are almost always superficial and diffuse, and are sometimes accompanied by neuralgia and articular pain.

The proteolytic factor shows itself in the hemorrhagic phlyctenes and superficial necrosis that leave sequelae of residual hyperchromia, especially if there has been bacterial invasion. This development of erucism is frequently noted when it is provoked by Megalopygids, Thaumetopoeids, Lymantriids and some Arctiids and Lasiocampids. The general toxic syndrome involves general malaise, chills, sensation of high temperature, nausea, vomiting and diarrhea, and on rare occasions an urticarian-type exanthema.

The involvement of the nervous system takes the form of confusion and dromophilia. Signs of collapse are also found, such as adynamia, exhaustion and lypothymia (Pesce and Delgado, 1971).

3. Immunity

Between 1958 and 1962, in 14 districts of the Peruvian jungle, we observed closely 433 cases of individual erucic incidents. We noted that rather more than 10 percent of these cases showed a marked attenuation of the symptomatology in the case of further erucic incidents (Pesce and Delgado, 1963). In other places extensively infested by urticating caterpillars, it has been observed that regular and repeated exposure often causes a diminishing of the reaction when the same species of urticating caterpillar is involved.

It may therefore be concluded that the development of resistance to the same noxa is of an immunological nature, which, as we have noted, is not permanent.

The attenuation of the symptomatology may also be interpreted as a process of desensitization, which unfortunately is also not permanent, since we have observed that after some time patients who were formerly resistant to erucic incidents develop serious reactions. As long as we do not have at our disposal specific immunological proofs, having studied typical cases of specific resistance to erucic poisoning and also anomalous reactions in clinics, we may accept that a specific immunity does exist, which is, however, temporary.

IV. Diagnosis

The diagnosis of erucism by means of the identification of the eruca and the cocoon, and the obtaining of the imago which is the carrier of urticating setae from the larval state, have made it possible to list 61 genera that have caused poisoning in different parts of the world; these are classified in two families of the sub-order Rhopalocera (butterflies) and 8 families of the sub-order Heterocera (moths). The recurrence of erucic incidents in human beings and animals, the ecological conditions in the geographical areas infested by Lepidoptera erucae, the study of air and dust contaminated by urticating setae, have all confirmed the clinical diagnosis based on the dermatological lesion and auxiliary examinations. The clinical diagnosis, in addition to providing anamnestic information about the circumstances in which the erucism takes place, and about the evolution and appearance of the lesions, allows differential diagnosis against other exanthematic illnesses.

Examination of the urine and the blood makes it possible to determine the extent to which the system is involved in the development of the erucic process.

The adult Lepidoptera are easily recognizable since they have two pairs of membranous wings covered with overlapping scales. These show a remarkable uniformity in their fundamental structure, which makes it very difficult for lepidopterologists to establish a satisfactory system of classification. However, they are commonly known as moths and butterflies.

The moths are easily distinguished by their large bodies and their filamentous or feathery antennae. They are night fliers (Fig. 17).

The butterflies have slender bodies; the antennae are threadlike, and the tip is enlarged in the form of a knob. They are day fliers. Both moths and butterflies feed on vegetal liquids, mainly nectar.

The young Lepidoptera, the erucae, are vegetarian, so the adults lay their eggs on the appropriate host.

All the erucae have a clearly differentiated head with a masticating buccal apparatus. The thorax and abdomen of the urticating erucae may be hairy or spiny. Each thoracic segment has a pair of short legs. The abdomen presents membranous prolegs (Fig. 3). The salivary glands are silk glands. In moths the silk is used in the spinning of the cocoon within which pupation occurs. The anthropotoxic erucae of butterflies do not spin cocoons.

1. Super-Family Papilionoidea (DYAR, 1902)

These are very large, bright-colored butterflies. Two families of the sub-order Rhopalocera have been noted with urticating caterpillars.

a) Morphidae (KOLLAR, 1850)

These are neotropical Lepidoptera, bright blue in color and iridescent. They change color according to the position in which they are examined. The urticating erucae of this family have been found feeding on the Leguminosae and Menispermaceae: *Morpho achillaena; M. anaxibia,* ESPER, 1798; *M. cypris,* WESTWOOD; *M. hercules* DALM., *M. laertes* DRURY, 1872; *M. menelaus,* LINNAEUS, 1758, and *M. rhetenoi.*

b) Nymphalidae (SWAINSON, 1872)

This family includes the great majority of North American butterflies, which are commonly known as angle-wings. The commonest in the United States are Mourning cloak, *Euvanessa antiopa* [=*Hamadryas antiopa* (L)]. The spiny urticating caterpillar may pierce the skin. Another species with spiny erucae is: *Nymphalis io* (=*Vanessa io* [L]), which is found in Europe and also scattered throughout the Ethiopian and Paleoarctic regions (Fig. 4).

2. Super-Family Bombycoidea (DYAR, 1902)

This super-family is made up of medium-sized moths similar to the silk moths *Bombyx mori.* Three families have urticating erucae.

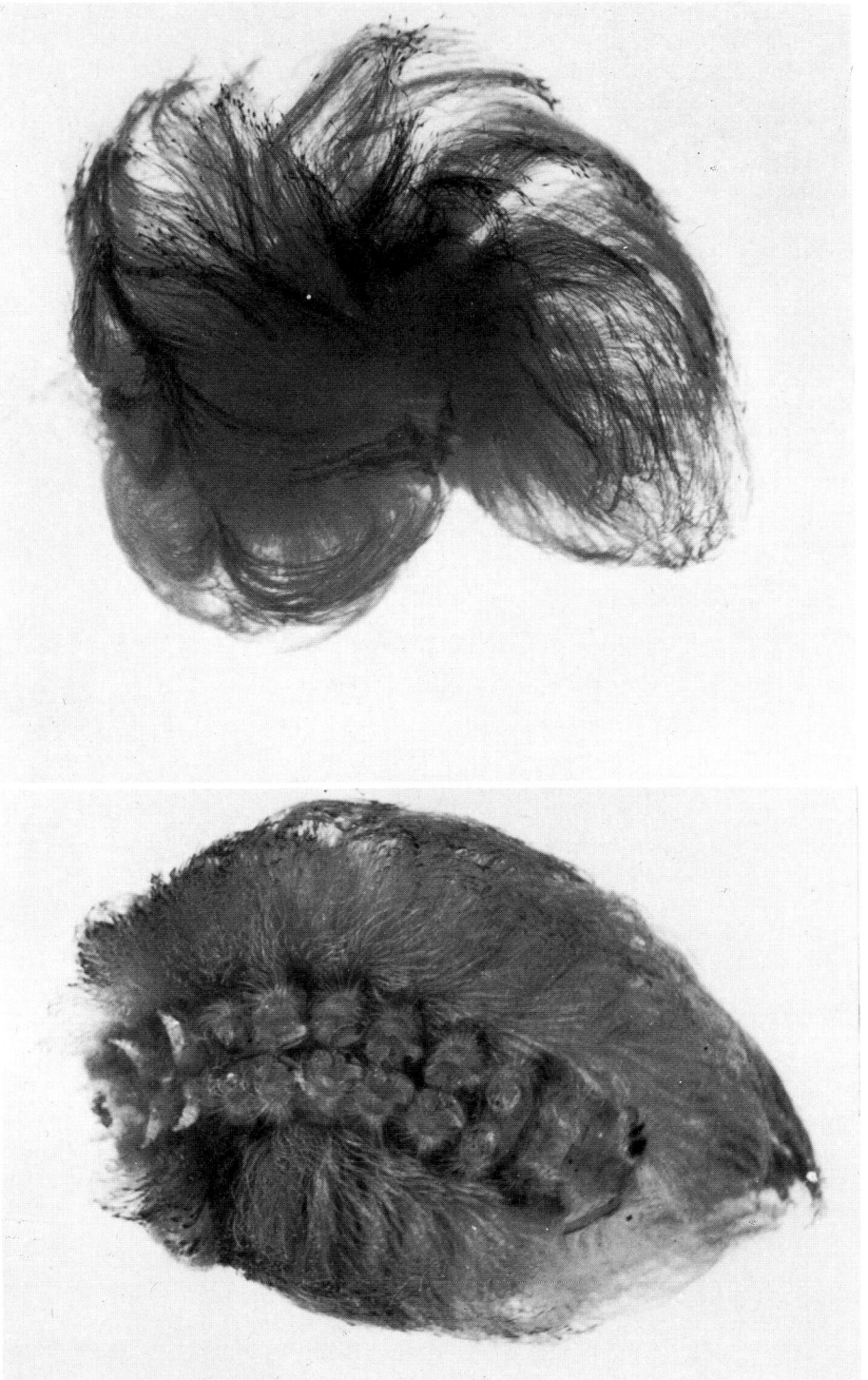

Fig. 3. *Megalopyge* spp. from Rioja, San Martín, Peru. Side view in a defensive attitude. It forms its body into the shape of a ring. Ventral view

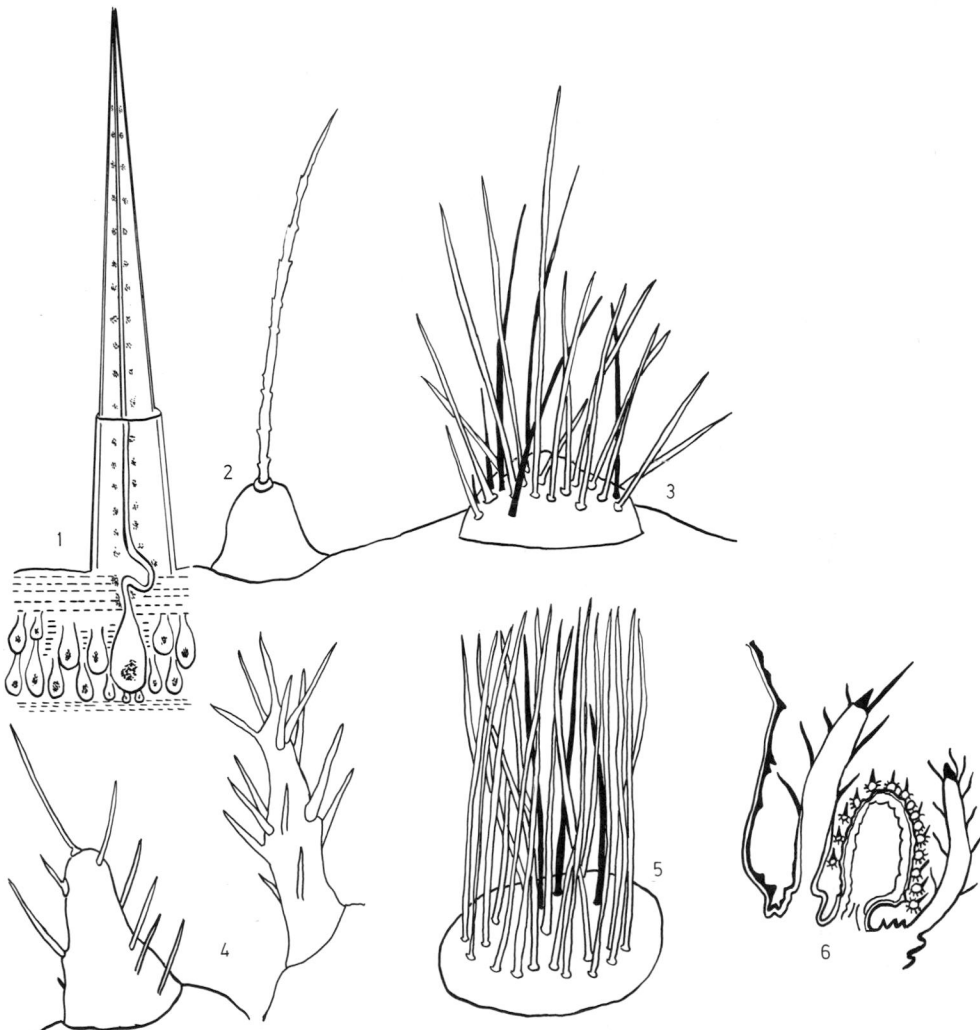

Fig. 4. Explantation of the principal types of the poison apparatus of erucae. 1. Primitive type according to Beyer (1922). 2. Chalaza (Arctiidae) projecting tubercle. 3. Verruca (Arctiidae) elevation of the tegument (Papilla). 4. Verricula (Noctuidae) thick tufts of bristles. 5. Scolii (Nymphalidae) tegumentary processes armed with spiny bristles. 6. Starlike prickles in Cochlidiidae. (According to Weidner, 1936). Adapted from FRACKER (1915), BEYER (1922) and WEIDNER (1936)

a) *Lasiocampidae* (HARRIS, 1841)

This family is found in the Palearctic, Nearctic and Australian regions. The urticating erucae are very hairy. Some of them are gregarious. When they spin their cocoons they strengthen them with urticating hairs from the larval state, which makes the cocoons poisonous too. Very common in North America is the apple-tree tent caterpillary *Malacosoma americana,* which can be found feeding on apple, cherry, wild cherry, choke-cherry and related trees.

The lappet caterpillar, *Tolype* spp. is another North American species, whose urticating larvae are characterized by their flattened appearance and by having a lappet or flat lobe on each side of each segment. Long hairs stem from these lobes, forming a fringe.

In Europe urticating caterpillars of *Cosmotriche* spp. *Gastropacha quercifolia, Lasiocampa quercus* and *Macrothylacia rubi* have been discovered.
Urticating caterpillars of *Taragama igniflua* have been discovered in the Philippines.

In South America, particularly Brazil and Peru, caterpillars of the following species have been observed: *Arctacea cribaria* LYUNG, 1825; *Euglyphes ornata* STOLL, *Macromphalia lignosa* WALKER, 1855; *Tityia proxima* BURMEISTER, 1878 and *Tolype undulosa* WALKER, 1855.

b) *Thaumetopoeidae* (= *Notodontidae*)

These are found in Palearctic, Oriental and Ethiopian regions. The *Anaphe* and *Thaumetopoea* (= *Cnetocampa*) erucae are hairy and spiny. They feed on the foliage of cultivated and coniferous plants. The *Anaphe infracta* erucae are greatly feared in Europe. Also considered dangerous are the processionary erucae, so called because of their way of walking one behind the other, forming double rows which march in orderly fashion, infesting pine, oak and cedar trees. Very common in France are *Thaumetopoea processionea* LINNAEUS 1758 and *T. pityo-campa* SCHIFF, *T. pinnivora*, which reaches as far north in Europe as Germany, Sweden and Russia. *T. wilkinsoni* which has been reported in Europe, Africa and Madagascar (CHEVERTON, 1936) is also common.

c) *Saturniidae* (= *Hemileucidae*) (WALKER, 1855)

These are found in the Palearctic, Neotropical, Ethiopian and Indo-Australian regions. Many species possess spiny urticating erucae, which feed on hickories, oaks, maples and some shrubs (Fig. 14).

The best known nettling erucae in the U.S.A. is the *Automeris io,* which can attain a length of 8 cm. It is a pale yellow color, with sublateral strips of cream and red, and has some black spines among many green ones. The green spines come out of tubercles, which gives the eruca a mossy appearance. The functional venomous hair has a short, stout, peg-like tip, connected with a poison-producing gland. The sharp-pointed, free end of the poisonous hair breaks easily, for example when it makes contact with objects, the skin thus allowing the poisonous secretions to enter the wound easily. In South America, especially in Brazil and Peru, the following anthropotoxic Saturniids are found: *Automeris aurantiaca* WEYMER, 1907; *A. ilustris* WALKER, 1865; *A. melanops* WALKER, 1865; *A. incisa* and *A. complicata.*

In North America the caterpillars of *Cricula* spp. are known to be poisonous, as are those of *Hemileuca lucina, H. maia, H. nevadensi, H. oliviae, Pseudohazis eglanterina, P. hera* and *Samia* spp. They have poisonous spines, and some of them are numerous enough to present a threat to cattle and cattle-breeders (CAFFREY, 1918).

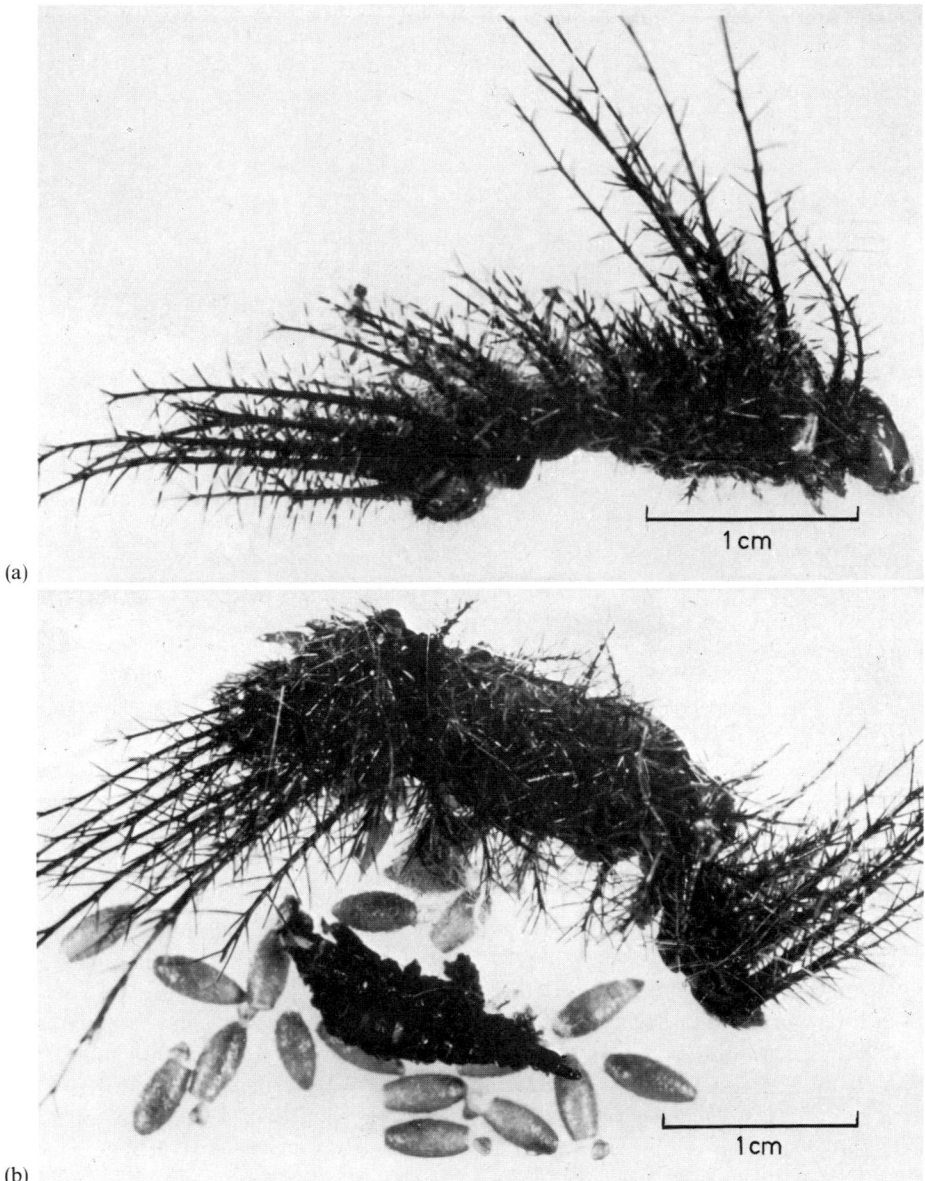

(a)

(b)

Fig. 5a and b. *Dirphia* spp. (a) The spines are similar to pine needles. They are distributed over the dorsal and lateral tubercules. (b) *Dirphia* spp. with Tachinidae parasites (*Diptera*). Myasis Note the pupae

In Brazil and Peru some species of *Dirphia*, such as *D. sabina* and *D. multicolor*, have spine-clad caterpillars shaped like pine branches. These spines are found on dorsal and lateral tubercles (Fig. 5).

3. Super-Family Noctuoidea (Mösher, 1916)

These moths are medium-sized and have nocturnal habits. Three-families have been discovered with species that possess urticating erucae. They are herbivorous, but rarely feed on trees.

a) *Arctiidae* (Stephens, 1829)

The tiger moths are cosmopolitan, but are found most frequently in the Neotropical and Oriental regions.

The erucae of the poisonous species are covered with thick growth of hairs, among which are sharp-pointed and hard ones. They feed on all kinds of herbaceous plants. The following North American genera have species with poisonous erucae: *Adolia* spp., *Callimorpha* spp., *Euchaetia egle, Halysidota caryae* and *Parasemia* spp. Those in Europe that are known to have urticating erucae are: *Arctia caja, Lithosia caniola*, which is often found in people's gardens in France, and *Lithosia griseola*, which lives off the foliage of ornamental plants in Italy, especially in Venice and Padua.

In South America, mainly in Brazil, can be found: *Antarctica fusca, Utheteisa ornatrix, U. pulchela* and *Ecpantheria orsa, Eupseudosoma aberrans, E. involutum, Premolis semirrufa* (Walker, 1856; Hampson, 1901). The last is the one that, produces the so-called occupational erucism.

b) *Lymantriidae (= Liparidae)* (Hampson, 1892)

The tussock moths are cosmopolitan, but are mainly found in the Palearctic, Nearctic and Indo-Australian regions. The poisonous caterpillars are brightly-colored and covered with tufts of hair (Spiegelhaare). The head and the other segments of the body are red, black and yellow. Some are gregarious and feed on the leaves of forest and fruit trees. The cocoons have larval urticating hairs. The adult female does not fly, having smaller wings than the male or none at all. The *Hemerocampa leucostigma* is found in the United States. The wingless adult female oviposits near the cocoons from which it emerges, and covers its eggs with a white froth. The erucae are hairy. *Porthetria dispar* Linnaeus, a native of Europe, is now very common in North America, where it has established itself thanks to its ability to feed on any deciduous tree. The eruca can be up to 6 cm long. It is hairy, and has a pair of blue tubercles on each of the first five segments behind the head and a pair of red tubercles on each of the next six segments.

The brown-tail moth, *Euproctis phaeorrhoea* (= E. chrysorrhoea) is another European species that is now very common in North America. The erucae are found in the tender shoots of trees. When fully grown the eruca attains a length of 37 mm. It is covered with long hairs and has a row of white tufts on each side of the body. Among these hairs there are barbed hairs borne by special tubercles and connected with poison glands. *Euproctis similis* is found in Canada and Europe.

Stillpnotia salicis, which also comes from Europe, is now found all over North America. The erucae have a black head, while the body is bluish-gray with white spots on the back. They are provided with tubercles from which sprout tufts of hairs. They feed on willow and poplar.

Greatly feared in Europe are the erucae of: *Dasychira pudibunda, Lymantria monacha* (= *Liparis monacha*), *Liparis chrysorrhoea, Ocneria* spp. *Orgyia* spp., and *Porthesia similis.*

Euproctis flava, BREMER, has been indicated as the main etiological agent of erucism in Asia, chiefly in Japan (HASHIMOTO and HAGIWARA, 1922) and in China (MILLS, 1923).

c) Noctuidae (STEPHENS, 1829)

Although they are cosmopolitan, the owlet moths are found very frequently in the Nearctic and Neotropical regions. They are strong-bodied and medium-sized. Their habits are nocturnal, and being greatly attracted to light, they invade houses in large numbers. The erucae feed on all kinds of plants, and many of them are glabrous (bare). The urticating ones have sharp-pointed hairs which branch out and form brushes (Bürstenhaare) (Fig. 4).

In North America the following species with poisonous erucae have been identified: *Acronycta oblinita, A. lepusculina, Apateta americana, Catocala* spp.

4. Super-Family Zygaenoidae (GRAVENHORST, 1843)

These moths are of variable size. There are two families containing species with poisonous erucae.

a) Cochlidiidae (= Eucleidae) (DYAR, 1898)

These are found in the Indo-Australian, Ethiopian, — Neotropical and Palearctic regions. The urticating erucae are slug-like, flattened on the ventral surface, with spiny warts and a small retractile head. The back of the *Sibine stimulea* "saddleback" caterpillar of North America is armed with urticating bristles. It has a wide green patch on the middle of its back resembling a saddle cloth, and a dark oval patch surrounded by white, which represents the saddle.

Phobetron pithecium, also from North America, and *P. hipparchia* CRAMER 1777, from South America, have their backs covered with hairs, and are also provided with lateral fleshy processes, which give the erucae the appearance of spiders.

In North America, especially in the United States, the following species have been identified as possessing urticating caterpillars: *Adoneta spinuloides, Natada* spp., *Parasa chloris, P. indetermina* and *Sisyrosea textula.*

In China and Korea, *Parasa hilarata* is known to have urticating erucae (MILLS, 1925); and in the Transvaal, *Parasa latistigra.*

b) Megalopigydae (BERG, 1882)

These are the flannel moths, with poisonous species in the Paleoarctic, Nearctic and Neotropical regions. The greatest concentration of species of this family is found in the West Indies and in the American continent. All the flannel moth erucae investigated possess similar nettling properties and are provided with long, fairly dense, bright-colored hairs. In South America they are known as "Tatorana,"

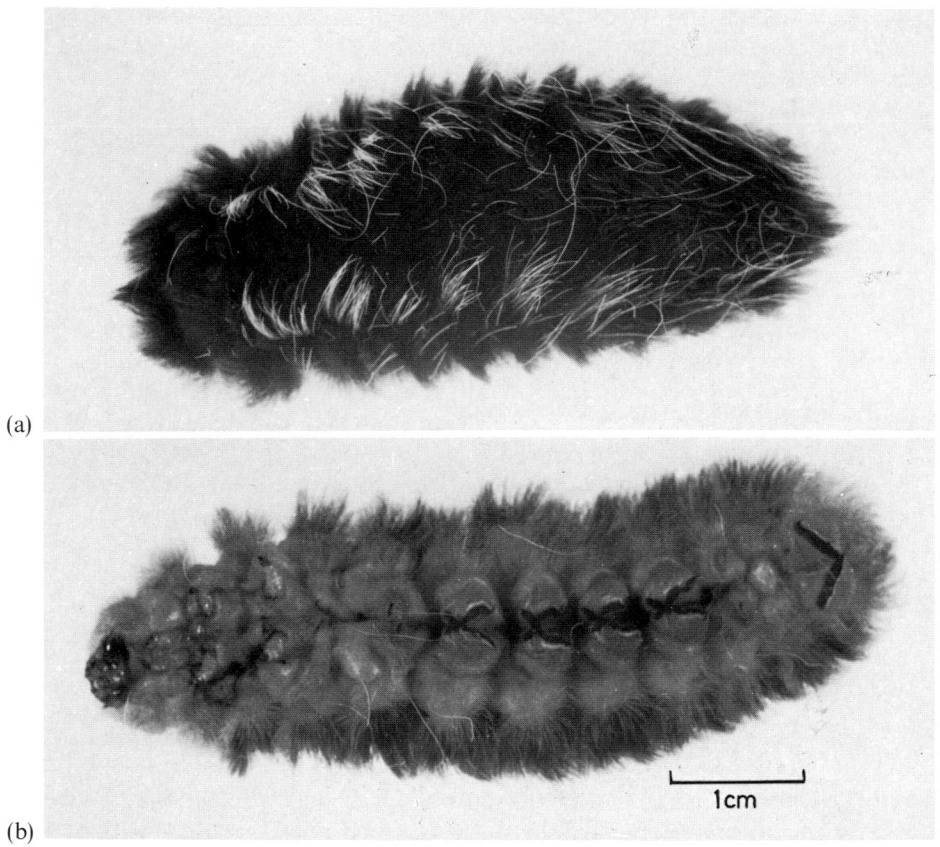

(a)

(b)

1cm

Fig. 6a—d. *Megalopyge* spp. from Tingo María, Perú. (a) dorsal view. (b) ventral view. (c) defensive attitude, the bare (glabrous) ventral area being hidden. (d) Cocoon, dorsal view

"cuy machucuy," "fire caterpillars," etc. Some of the hairs are connected to glands which secrete urticating substances located in the cuticle and sub-cuticle. They are omnivorous, feeding chiefly on the foliage of fruit trees. In tropical America they bear Tachinids (Diptera) as parasites (Fig. 6).

In the south of the United States *Megalopyge opercularis* abounds, the erucae of which are known as "puss caterpillars." They prove very annoying on account of their urticating properties (BISHOPP, 1923; LUCAS, 1942).

The erucism they provoke is characterized by a feeling of numbness, which may even be generalized and is often accompanied by nausea and vomiting. Stings by *M. opercularis* on the wrist have been followed by swelling of the entire arm to almost double its normal size. Children often develop considerable fever and nervous symptoms.

Common in the north of the United States are: *Lagoa crispata* PACKARD, *L. pyxi-difera* in Georgia and neighboring Atlantic states. *Norape* spp. and, in Puerto Rico, *Megalopyge krugii* also produce caterpillar dermatitis.

In South America erucism is known to be caused in Brazil by: *Aidos amanda* HÜBNER, 1816; *Carama* spp., *Megalopyge superba* EDWARDS, 1884. When the erucae

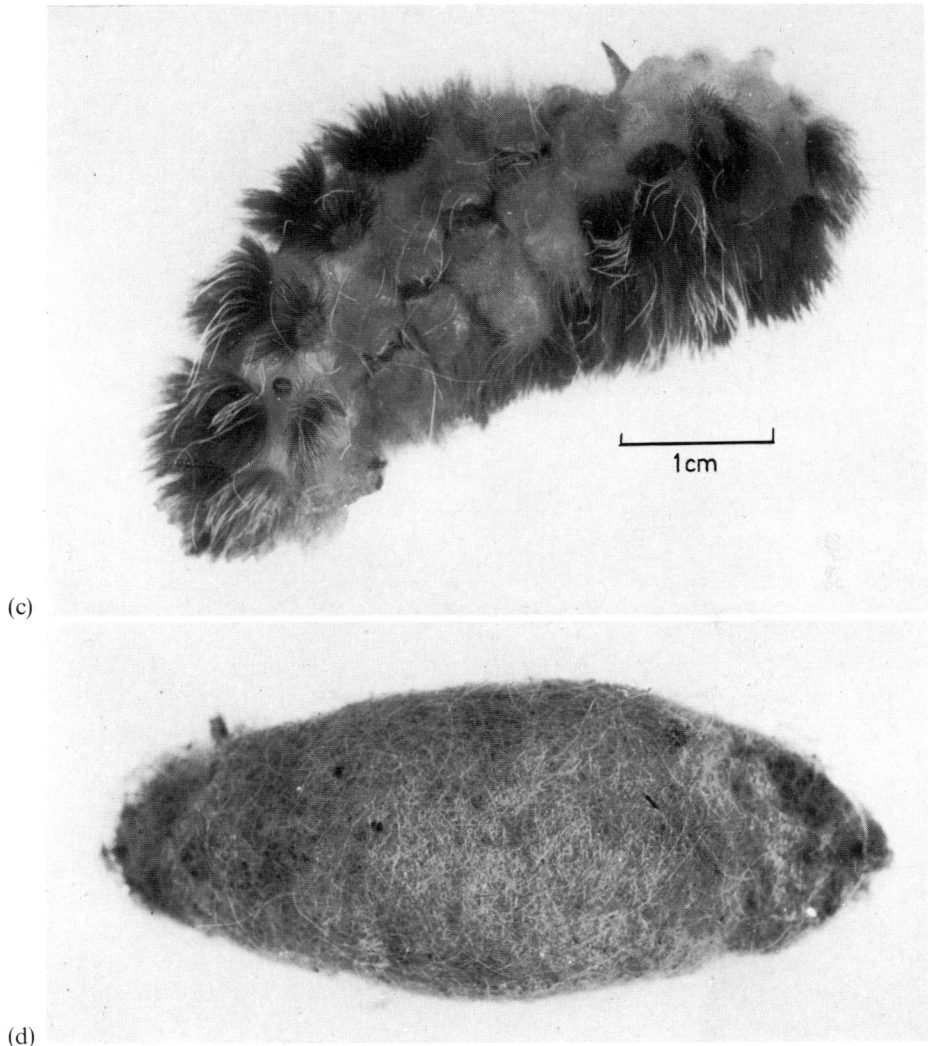

1cm

(c)

(d)

Fig. 6c and d

of the species are fully developed they spin an elongated cocoon covered with red hairs, which has holes at the tips, looking like eyes (Fig. 7).

Megalopyge lanata STOLL-CRAMER, 1780, *M. radiata, M. undulata, Podalia albescens* SCHAUS 1900; *P. chrysocoma* HERRICK-SCHÄFER, 1856; *P. orsilochus* CRAMER, 1775; *P. radiata* SCHAUS, 1792 and *Trosia fallax* FELDER, 1874 are also known to have urticating erucae.

Erucism in Argentina and Uruguay is produced mainly by *Megalopyge urens*.

5. The Poison Apparatus

The production of toxic exocrinal substances fulfills a defensive function in Lepidoptera. The glands are hypodermic, specially adapted for ejecting the poison

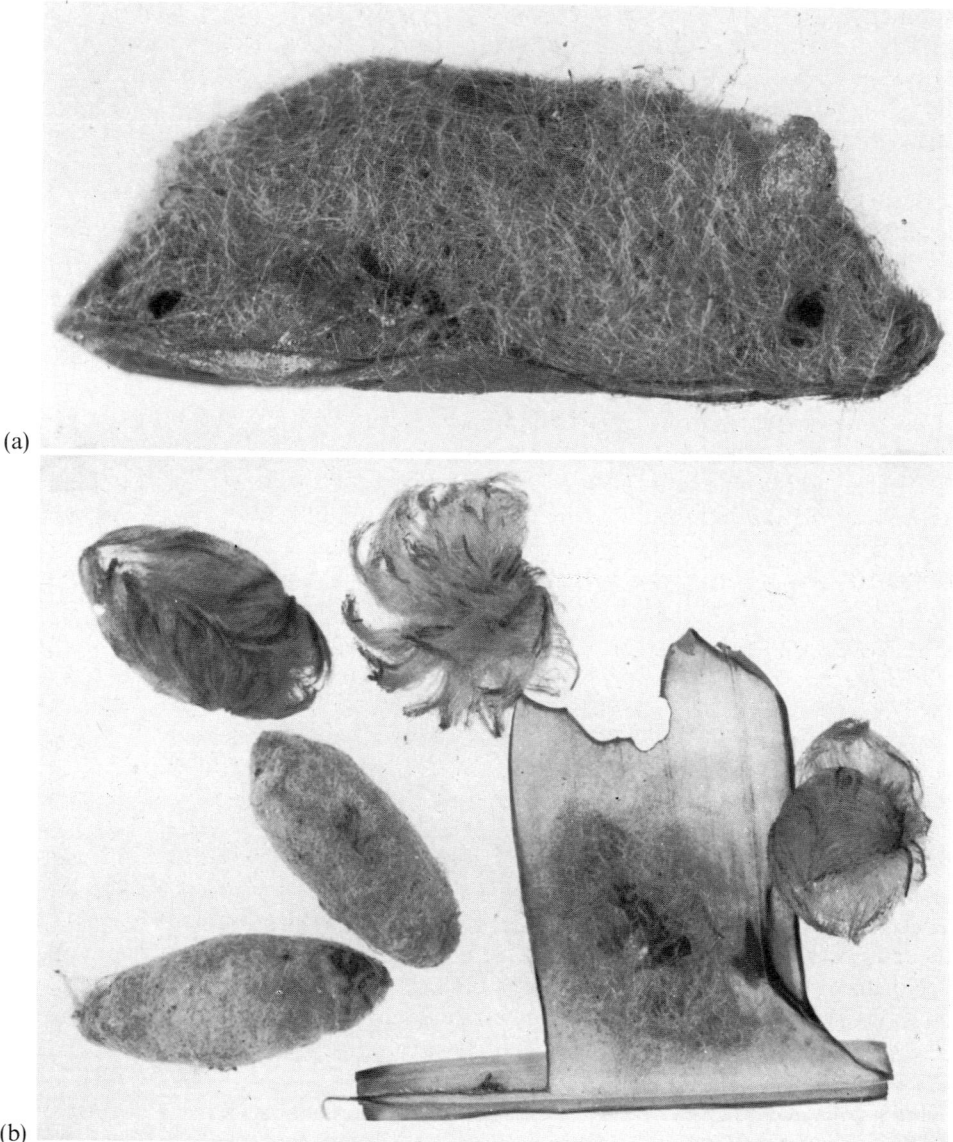

Fig. 7a and b. *Megalopyge superba* from Satipo, Junín, Peru. Top left, erucae: (a) At rest. (b) Irritated. Bottom left, Cocoons. Top right, empty cocoons and ecdysis. Cocoons, side view

by reflex action, by means of a primitive inoculating organ, a hollow hair which articulates in the cuticle of the urticating erucae of Arctiids, Lasiocampids, Lymatriids, Thaumetopoids, and some Noctuids, Morphids and Nymphalids. The most developed inoculating organ, like the most primitive one, has as its primary purpose, the conservation of the individual. The poisonous caterpillar uses it for defence, injecting the toxic substance intradermically to the victim.

Finally, in other Lepidoptera, the poison apparatus lacks an inoculating organ, but has a poison-secreting organ which evaginates like a tentacle. In this case the poison acts mainly through contact with the skin and mucous membranes. The poison apparatus has no fixed position, nor is it permanent in all the larval stages of the erucae; however, it is nearly always found in the dorsal region (POULTON, 1886).

SCUDDER (1888) observed secreting extensible organs in the erucae of *Cyaniris pseudargiolus*. This organ is placed symmetrically on the eleventh post-cephalic ring behind the last pair of stigmata.

For passive defence *Papilio asteria* everts a fleshy gland or osmetrium, which secretes an evil-smelling liquid with a strong acidic reaction BURNETT (1854). This organ is also found in *Orgya* spp. (PACKARD, 1886), *Thais* spp. (PACKARD, 1898), *Papilio crephontes* (CHU, 1949).

The erucae of *Cossus ligniperda* have a pair of glandular tubes that store up the toxic secretion, and can eject it onto the inner edge of the mandible (BORDAS, 1902). This secretion produces a burning sensation on human skin, and can be lethal for small vermivorous birds like the sparrow. The same thing happens with *Cerura* spp. (PACKARD, 1898), *Cossus cossus* of Europe, and *Prionoxystus robinae* of North America (CHU, 1949).

There are erucae that are apparently glabrous (bare) or covered with a soft pubescence; however, nearly all the erucae with urticating properties are more or less hairy or spiny. The hairs and spines are symmetrically arranged in groups, or form tufts. In the poisonous species some of these hairs or spines are related to poison-secreting glands.

a) Primitive-Type Poison Apparatus (BEYER, 1922)

The injury-provoking organ, which inoculates the victim with the toxic secretion, is a hallow aciculate hair, barbed or finely serrated; these hairs may be irregularly distributed over the body and hidden among the harmless, ornamental hairs, or they may be grouped in tussocks.

Normally each hair is planted in a small papilla on the cuticle of the eruca's body, or on slightly protruding cuticles called *chalazas* (Fig. 4). Finally, the primitive-type urticating hairs may be found in tufts growing on raised parts of the cuticle verrucae (FRACKER, 1915).

Each of these acicular urticating hairs is supplied by a single-cell hypodermic gland in direct contact with its lumen (Fig. 8).

Liparis chrysorrhoea has two round, reddish patches in the middle of which grow large numbers of tubercles; from these the gland's excreting duct opens out (GOOSSENS, 1881, 1886). When the eruca of this lymmantriid is excited, the round patches project outwards, and from the glandular area oozes out a pearly secretion that dries quickly, forming a powdery coating. This powder, deposited along with the acicular hairs that make accidental contact with the skin of human beings, causes a very intense pruriginous erythema.

On the eruca of the Lymantriid *Euproctis flava* tubercles are found, which bear the nettling hairs that are hidden in bunches of 36—37 among dark violet-colored, ornamental hairs (MORISITA et al., 1955).

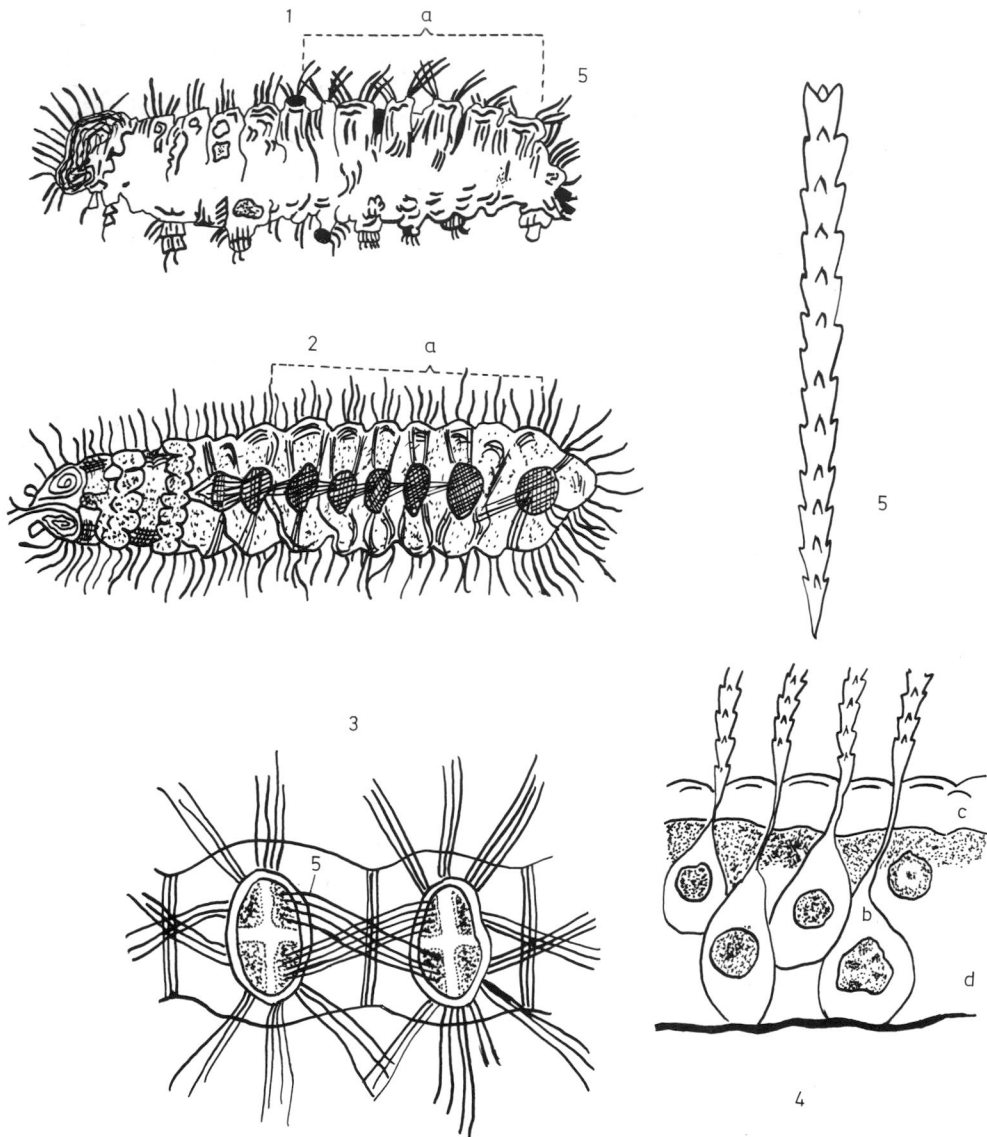

Fig. 8. Poison apparatus of Thaumetopoeidae. *Cnetocampa pityocampa*. 1. Lateral surface. 2. Dorsal surface. 3. Types of urticating hairs on the glandular surface, or Spiegelhaare. 4. Vertical cross-section of the tegument at the level of the glandular surface or Spiegelhaare. 5. Poisonous hairs. a. Glandular area. b. Poisonous glands. c. Cuticle. d. hypodermis. Adapted according to BEILLE (1905) and WEIDNER (1936)

On the cuticle of the eruca of *Euproctis chrysorrhoea,* papillas or cup-like structures are found, closely crowded together, each of them containing 3 to 12 finely barbed acicular urticating hairs, 7 to 10 mm long (KEPHART, 1914; TONKES, 1933) (Fig. 9).

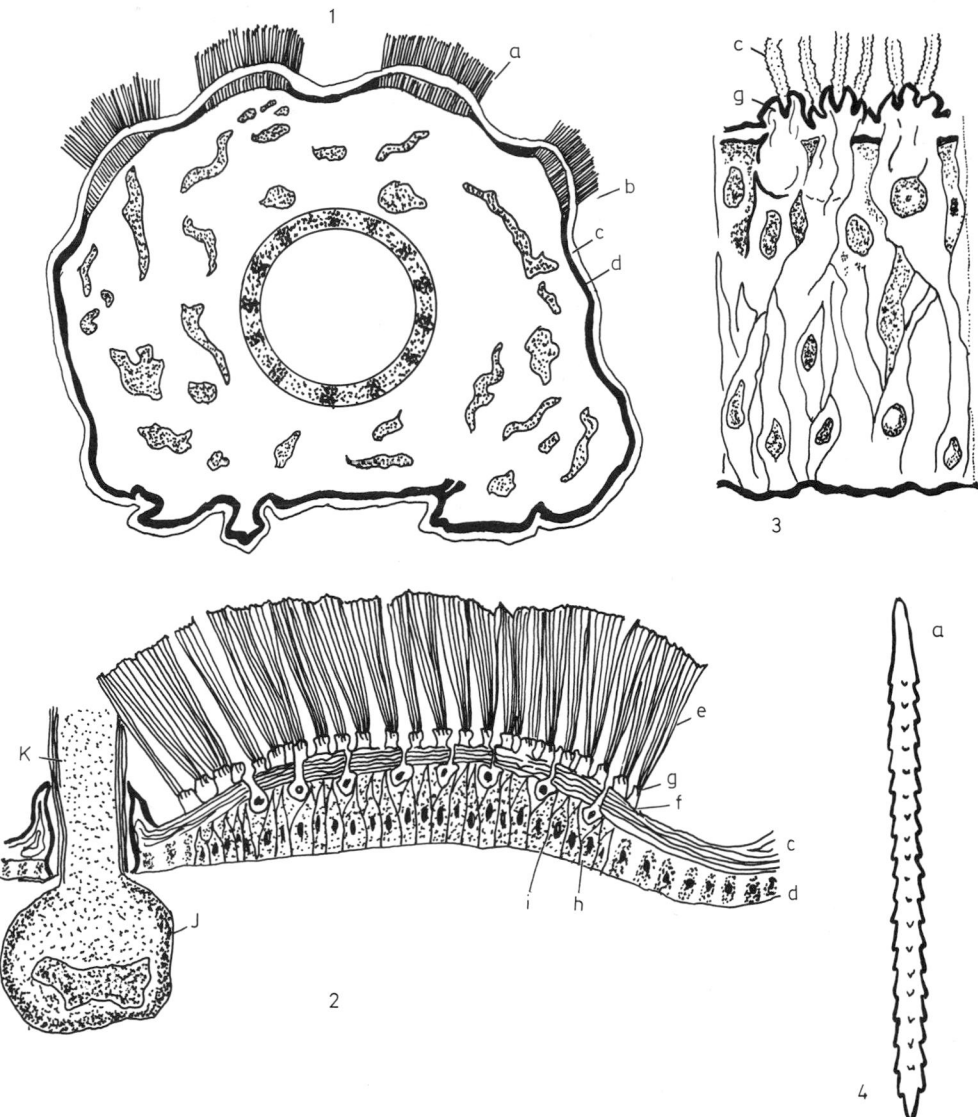

Fig. 9. Poison apparatus of Lymantriidae. *Euproctis chrysorrhoea*. 1. Schematic transversal cross-section of an abdominal segment. 2. Vertical cross-section of the tegument at the level of the tubercle. 3. Cross-section of the hypodermic and cuticular area. 4. Poisonous hair. a. Subdorsal tubercle. b. Lateral tubercle. c. Cuticle. d. Hypodermis. e. Poisonous hairs. f. Duct. g. Papilla. h. hypodermic cells. j. Poisonous cells. k. Trichogynes. l. Chitin. Adapted according to KEPHART (1915) and TONKES (1933)

Some erucae of Arctiidae, Lymantridae and Noctuidae have urticating hairs, grouped together in thick bunches. In this way, in the erucae of the lymantriid *Dasichyra pudibunda,* each of the brushes contains nearly 2,000 bright yellow or grayish yellow hairs. All these hairs are about 4 mm long, have a sharp-pointed base, are barbed and are also spun into the pupal cocoon.

In the eruca of *Thaumetopoea pityocampa,* on the dorsal surface of each of the last eight segments of the body, there is a dark yellow, oval-shaped glandular plate, bearing the hairs known as Spiegelhaare. When the caterpillar is at rest, this glandular plate does not stick out, since it is kept in position at both the front and the back by a fold of the tegument. When the eruca is irritated, the Spiegelhaare rise up noticeably. This glandular plate has 10 fascicles of urticating hairs growing in a chitinous area. The hairs are hollow, acicular and superficially barbed. A duct passes through the centre, linked at its base with a single-cell gland in the hypodermis (GILMER, 1925). Measuring $0.2-0.3$ mm in length, they are stiff and brittle (LAUDON, 1891).

In the eruca of *Thaumetopoea pityocampa* the surface of the glandular plate (Spiegelhaare) is divided into four sections by two perpendicular glabrous bands. Thousands of the primitive-type hairs are inserted into each of the four sections (BEILLE, 1896). Each hair is closed at its distal end, and connects at its proximal end with pyriform hypodermic glandular cells (Fig. 8).

Every time the skin is sloughed off, the hairs of the glandular plate are also discarded, so that the places where the ecdysis of these erucae occurs retain their urticating properties for a long time. On the other hand, when pressure is exerted on the folds of the glandular plate, they prolapse, and thousands of short urticating hairs fall out. As in the case of other poisonous erucae, these primitive-type poisonous hairs are woven into the cocoon of the processionaries.

b) Developed-Type Poison Apparatus (FOOT, 1922)

The organ used for inoculating the poison is a highly chitinous tubular spine with an inner lining of hypodermic cells responsible for the production of the toxic substances. The cells that form the hypodermic lining do not reach to the free distal end. The spine reach to the free distal end. The spine may have lateral ramifications. Both in the simple and in the ramified spine, the free end breaks when it penetrates the skin of the victim, thus enabling the poison to be ejected.

The basal end is fixed into cuticular processes called scolii and verriculae (Fig. 4). The organ responsible for storing the poison is a bulbar evagination of the body wall. Both in length and in diameter these spines vary greatly. When growing from verriculae they are found grouped in the shape of rosettes.

In the eruca of the cochlidiid *Parasa vivida,* the urticating spines are planted together irregularly in scolii, while in the eruca of *Sibine stimulea,* the tubular spines articulate to dorsal, sub-dorsal or lateral tubercles.

The spines end in a point, sealed off distally. They have an inner lining of flattened hypodermic cells, except at the most distal end, where a small duct forms.

Similarly they have a cuticular duct, lined with hypodermic cells, which in this way connect the spine's bulbar cavity to the hypodermis. The bulbar cavity contains the poisonous secretion (Fig. 10).

In addition to the venomous apparatus described in Cochlidiidae, the erucae are provided with urticating hairs and scales in the shape of stars.

The star-shaped scales are grouped into a central cone (Fig. 4) (WEIDNER, 1936). They separate easily from the cone and break when pressed against the skin.

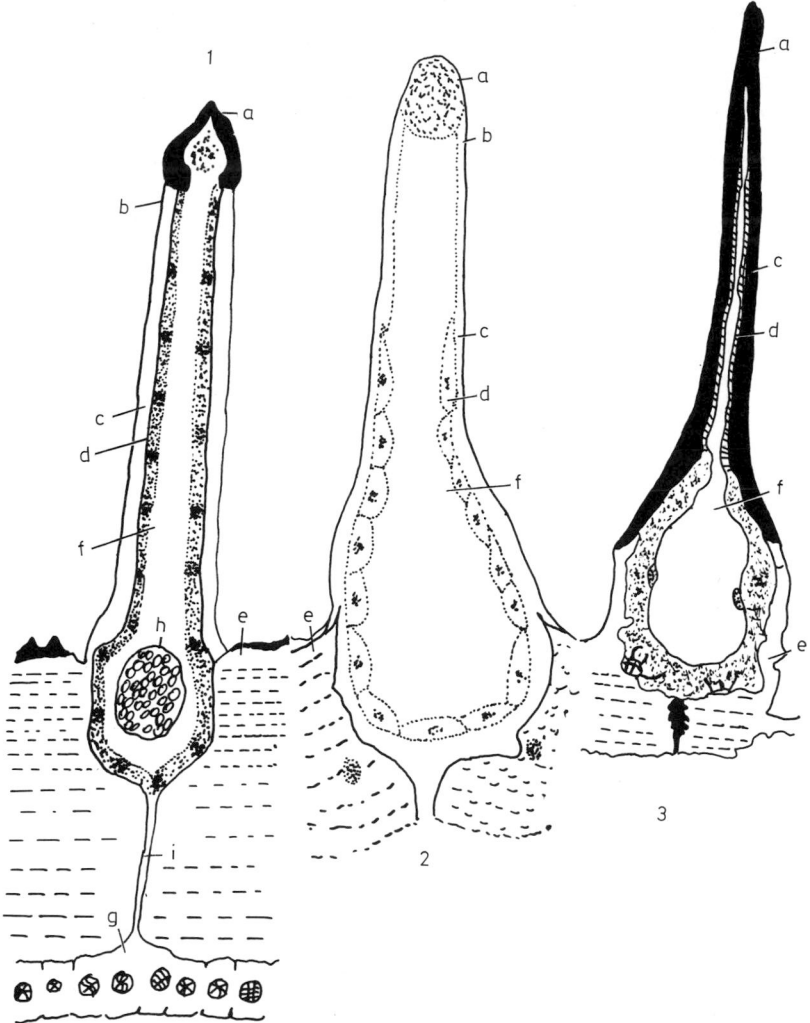

Fig. 10. Developed type of poison apparatus in Cochlidiidae and Megalopygidae. 1. Chitinous covering of the spine. 2. Chitinous tubular spine of Megalopygidae. 3. Chitinous tubular spine of *Megalopyge opercularis*. a. Apical duct. b. Chitinous covering of the spine. d. Hypodermic coating. e. Cuticle. f. Bulbar cavity. g. Hypodermis. h. Poisonous glandular cells. j. cuticular duct. Adapted according to FOOT (1922), WEIDNER (1936)

In the eruca of the saturniid *Dirphia sabina* the urticating spines grow out of an oval cavity located in the cuticle of the body wall, while the distal end is fragile. It breaks easily on entering the victim's skin.

The erucae of the megalopygid, *M. opercularis,* have a similar poison apparatus, but one that has lost its connection with the hypodermis. However, it is easy to detect the joining link, which looks like a radix (Figs. 10, 11, 12). The basal end of the spine is soft and elastic, not very sclerotic, while the distal end is hard and very sclerotic, with the result that the spine can bend without breaking.

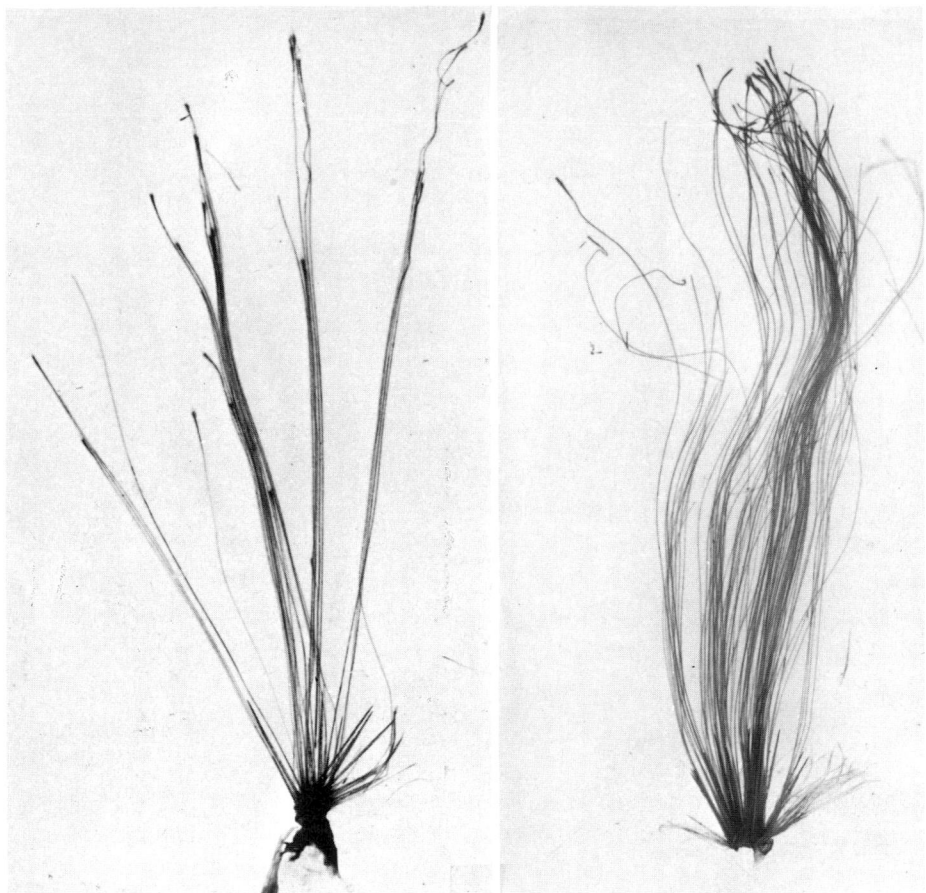

Fig. 11. Tufts of hairs of *Megalopyge* spp. from Rioja, San Martín, Peru. Note the ornamental hairs, spatulated and barbed at the distal end. At the base of the tuft note the poisonous spines implanted into the verruca

6. Toxicology

There is no doubt that the majority of the symptoms and signs observable in the skin of human beings and of animals used for experiments, and also the systemic reactions in erucism, are attributable to the substances produced by the hypodermic glands of poisonous erucae.

In order to gain an understanding of the physicochemical nature of erucic poison, different authors have carried out experiments with extracts from the tegument and hairs of erucae of different families of moths. In spite of their using very varied scientific methods, little is known as yet of the chemical composition of the poison of any of the species of the ten families of poisonous Lepidoptera.

a) Obtaining the Poison

In the case of lymantriid *Euproctis phaerrhoea* (=*Nygmia phaerrhoea*), Tizzer (1970b) obtained strong evidence that the hairs were carriers of the poison. It

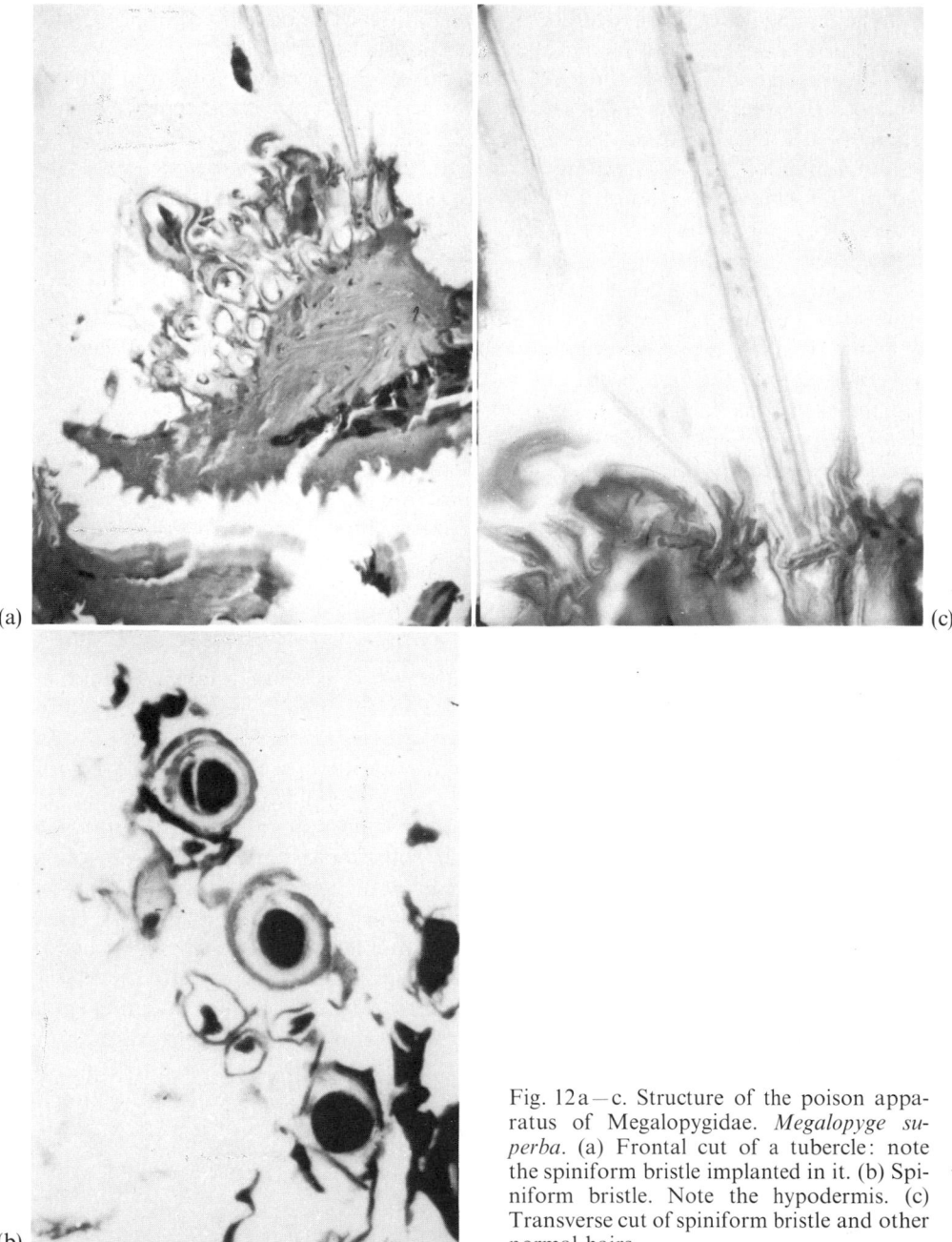

(a)

(c)

(b)

Fig. 12a—c. Structure of the poison apparatus of Megalopygidae. *Megalopyge superba*. (a) Frontal cut of a tubercle: note the spiniform bristle implanted in it. (b) Spiniform bristle. Note the hypodermis. (c) Transverse cut of spiniform bristle and other normal hairs

is true that the urticating hairs are hollow and they contain a definite poisonous principle that when injected into the skin produces a rash (PAWLOWSKY and STEIN, 1927).

The poison is thermolabile, being destroyed by baking for one hour at 110°C or by warming to 60°C in distilled water. It loses its poisonous qualities when soaked in 1% or 0.1% potassium hydrate or sodium hydrate.

The poison contained in the hairs, when mixed with human blood, immediately produces pathologic changes in the red corpuscles *in vitro*. In the processionary erucae of the Thaumetopoeidae family there have been attempts, to identify the poison contained in the urticating hairs, with cantaridine (Goossens, 1881, 1886) and with formic acid (Laudon, 1891). Bleyer (1909) observed a strong smell coming from the broken hairs of the processionary erucae. The crude extract he obtained was alkaline.

The liquid obtained as a result of mechanical stimulation of the urticating spine of the erucae of the saturniid *Automeris ilustris* is as clear and transparent as water. It does, however, contain small, microscopic, green drops. When this secretion reaches the free distal end of the spine, it becomes greenish-blue and acquires a viscous consistency (Weidner, 1936).

From the poisonous spines of another saturniid, *Dirphia* spp., Picarelli and Valle (1971) managed to obtain a crude extract by means of which they calculated that these erucae contain $0.1-0.2$ µg histamine/mg dry tissue. The poisonous spines weigh on average 0.86 mg, which means that each of the urticating spines may contain $0.08-0.17$ µg histamine.

Foot (1922) studied the dermatitis caused by *Megalopyge opercularis,* whose symptomatology is similar to that observed in the South American erucism caused by *M. urens,* particularly in Uruguay. This symptomatology is probably produced by a proteinaceous complex contained in the aqueous extract taken from these erucae (Gaminara, 1928a). Mazzella and Patteta (1928) prepared an extract very sensitive to heat, and a powder from the tegument of the eruca, which conserved its toxic activity for several months. Estable et al. (1966) proved that the poison of *M. urens* from crude extract is of a globuline nature with necrotic, hemolytic and immunological properties. Finally, Ardao et al. (1966), cited by Picarelli and Valle (1971), separated the constituent parts of the poison by means of paper electrophoresis: one fraction with hemolytic activity, a second with hyaluronidase activity, a third with proteolytic activity and a very low hemolytic activity. It was not possible to determine the activity of the fourth fraction.

Picarelli and Valle (1971) used pharmacological methods to study the toxicity of the Brazilian eruca *Megalopyge* spp., obtaining extract from the urticating spines in which there was no evidence of histamine, acetylcholine or 5-hydroxytryptamine. The toxicity of the extract to dogs and guinea-pigs, the hypotensor effect in dogs and cats, and the cutaneous reactions observable in human beings and other animals suggest the existence in the poison of bioamines and fractions of a proteic nature.

b) Conserving the Poison

The live erucae are submerged for 10 to 15 minutes in a sterile physiological solution or sterile distilled water and the whole is stirred slowly with a glass rod in order to stimulate the secretion of the glandular poison. The liquid then contains a solution of the toxic principle of the eruca. The liquid obtained usually changes color according to the erucae and the hydrosolubility of the glandular secretion. It is filtered and tested on experimental animals to see whether it produces in them the same dermic and systemic symptoms that the urticating hairs of the erucae under study produce on the animals affected by them.

When dead specimens are used the dorsal tegument, which is normally rich in urticating hairs, is carefully cut; the ecdysis and cases of the cocoon are also used. This material is dried in a vacuum over Cl_2Ca. It is then kept in amber-colored jars in a nitrogen atmosphere. These jars can be kept in the freezer, maintaining the dry extract unchanged for years. The dry material is crushed with china mortars. This powder is employed in the preparation of aqueous extracts, using distilled water or a saline solution whose pH is then raised to levels fluctuating from 5.6 to 10, adding 0.1 N of Na Cl, using Buffer phosphate. The filtered substance is useful for experiments and can be kept for weeks under refrigeration. The crude extracts obtained in this way are considered high-quality samples of the glandular secretion.

To obtain pure toxin, the aqueous extract is treated by physicochemical methods which make it possible to obtain the poison in a solid state, causing the solvent to evaporate. Recourse may be had to fractioning, either by chromatographic methods or by means of electrophoresis. The dry extracts can be kept indefinitely, whereas the aqueous extracts show lability to the chemical action of alkali.

c) Pharmacology of the Extracts of Erucic Poisoning

The dry or liquid extracts obtained and conserved as described above using Peruvian erucae of *Podalia* spp. and *Megalopyge* spp. were inoculated into the tegument of dogs, guinea-pigs and rabbits. Experimental erucism was produced with constant inflammatory signs in all of them—high blood pressure in the dog's carotid; equimosis and necrosis at the point of injection in dogs and guinea-pigs. Hemolysis was obtained *in vitro* in washed red corpuscles of human and rabbit blood (PESCE and DELGADO, 1963).

Employing pharmacological methods, VALLE et al. (1954), in Brazil, made use of extracts from the poisonous spines of *Megalopyge* spp. to induce slow contractions in isolated guinea-pig ileum and in rabbit duodenum. The extract injected into rats and dogs raised the carotid blood pressure, and this was followed by persistent hypotension. All these reactions were undoubtedly due to the poisonous extract of *Megalopyge* spp. and were not eliminated or affected by antihistamines, atropine or lysergic acid diethylamide. It may therefore be inferred that the effects of the poison of this megalopygid are not due to histamine or acetylcholine or 5-hydroxytryptamine. In rats which have previously received intravenous injections of Evan's blue, the intradermic inoculation of extract from the poisonous spines produces extravasion of the coloring agent.

The extravasation of the Evan's blue also takes place in rats to which antihistaminic drugs or lysergic acid have previously been administered. Finally, the extract showed hemolytic activity on red corpuscles, whether washed or not, of dogs, cats and man.

The extract of *Megalopyge* spp. venomous spines is not dialyzable, nor is it soluble in ethyl ether acetone or ethanol. It is thermolabile, being inactivated by 30 min warming at 45°C or even 2 min warming at 60°C.

The maximum activity is reached at pH 6, and activity ceases at pH 2 or

10. On precipitation it saturates the extract with 75% ammonium sulphate. It is digested by incubation of the extract with trypsin, pepsin or chymotrypsin. PICARELLI and VALLE (1971), using extract from the saturniid *Dirphia* spp., produced contractions in isolated guinea-pig ileum. This effect was totally eliminated by pyrilamine, but not by atropine or lysergic acid diethylamide. In this extract it was not possible to detect acetylcholine even when the most sensitive pharmacological preparation, such as the toad *rectus abdominis* muscle, was used.

However, the histamine-like effects produced by the poisonous setae extracts or *Dirphia* spp. did not run parallel with those resulting from equivalent quantities of histamine.

These results seem to indicate that the effects observed in the pharmacological experiments would depend on the presence or liberation of other pharmacologically active substances besides histamine.

V. Treatment

The aims of treatment are preventing the toxins from spreading over a wider skin surface, counteracting the effect of the toxins by pharmacological means, avoiding secondary infections, and forestalling the appearance of sequelae.

a) Immediate Treatment

At the onset of the erucic incident, care must be taken to prevent sweat, whether scratched or rubbed, from spreading the urticating hairs and causing the toxic products to enter the skin. This is a valuable procedure and proves effective when it is carried out in good time. The following should be included:

α) Removing as many urticating hairs as possible from the skin by submerging the whole body or the part affected in water. This procedure is based on the hydrosolubility of the erucic poison, and also on the minimal weight of the eruca hairs. As a result, the hairs that have stuck to the pores of the skin and those that have penetrated the tegument only superficially come loose, and the erucic poison is then diluted in the water.

β) Painting the site of the sting with iodine tincture, which, judging by the cases we have dealt with, appears to control the erythema and burning pain.

b) Symptomatic and Preventive Treatment

This tends to re-establish the normal tissue functions which have been altered by the intoxication. It also prevents or minimizes the appearance of lesions or sequelae. In these attacks there is generally prompt swelling at the site of the sting. The scratching may result in leaving some of the noxious hairs in contact with the skin and thus prolonging the reaction. The cells destroyed by the erucic toxins liberate cytotoxic lysosome enzymes. These attack healthy cells and liberate more cytotoxins. The damaged cells also liberate histamine, serotonin and heparin. Histamine has a deleterious effect on the capillary structure, causing dilatation and increasing permeability, with exudation into the tissues of neutrophils, lymphocytes and plasma.

In some cases antihistaminics have interrupted the local toxic syndrome, reducing the edema and pruritus within two or three days. They are administered orally every 8 h for 4 to 7 days.

For the treatment of the general toxic syndrome and the allergic syndrome, steroids are used for their anti-inflammatory effect, which prevents or modifies many of the manifestations of hypersensitivity.

Steroids are thought to stabilize lysosome and cell membranes, preventing the release of cytotoxic enzymes into the cytoplasm or past the cell wall into the intercellular fluid. They act directly on the morphology of the fibroblasts, which take on a stable round shape, that makes them resistant to cytotoxins. They stabilize the mast cells, and prevent the explosive liberation of histamine and histaminoid substances (DOUGHERTY, 1961). Steroids have proved very effective in the treatment of both local and generalized reactions to urticating erucae. Edema, burning sensations, redness, and pain usually disappear within 72 h.

It should be borne in mind that when the local reaction is slight and produces no discomfort, it can be ignored. Treatment with a steroid varies in its length and dosage, depending on the severity, course, and duration of the erucism. The substance is normally administered orally, bearing in mind the process the physiological production of the cortisol. Depending on how urgent the case is, the drug can be administered parenterally, using the following steroids or others, according to the practitioner's experience in handling them: hydrocortisone sodium succinate or dexamethasone phosphate.

The treatment for people who cannot be given steroids even for short periods, especially patients with gastric ulcers or possibly tuberculosis, should be limited to aqueous epinephrine 1:1000, 0.2—0.5 ml, given by deep subcutaneous injection and massaged thoroughly. Quick-acting oral antihistamines and sympathomimetic amines such as ephedrine may be of value in hastening relief (FRAZIER, 1966). When the reaction is one of anaphylaxis and death is feared possible, intravenous steroid can be life-saving, as can aqueous epinephrine chloride 1:1000.

If cellulite, lymphangitis or other bacterial conditions result from the scratching, these should be treated with a systemic antibiotic.

c) Treatment of Foreign-Body Syndrome

The formation of foreign-body granuloma, especially in the eyeball and the juxta-articular regions of the hand, necessitates surgical removal.

VI. Epidemiology

The incompleteness of the records of cases of poisoning caused accidentally throughout the world by venomous erucae makes it impossible to carry out a study of the epidemiological characteristics of erucism in each of the continents where poisonous erucae are known to exist.

However, we can study these characteristics on the basis of information scattered throughout scientific publications. On the other hand the means for an etiological diagnosis of erucism are not yet available, as in other cases of arthropod poisoning (DYAR, 1913).

This being so, the epidemiology of crucism has so far been studied on the basis of the incidence of isolated cases or collective outbreaks recorded since the last decades of last century (Bleyer, 1909; Goeldi, 1913; Matta, 1922; Mazza and Frias, 1926; Lucas, 1942; Steele, 1944).

1. Erucism on the American Continent

American medical, entomological and agricultural literature has an abundance of publications dealing with erucic accidents. This information leads the medical practitioner to suspect, according to the latitudes and places in America that are involved, that many of the so-called summer urticarias and morbilliform exanthemas that occur, particularly in outdoor workers in rural areas, are really caterpillar dermatitis (Delgado, 1969).

In this huge continent 9 families of Lepidoptera have 42 genera with urticating species.

The zoogeography of the poisonous species is governed by the characteristics of the surrounding area. The size, and the form of the dispersion area of each of the species with urticating erucae depend mainly on the distribution of the habitats where the vegetal and faunistic associations, including man, cause the occurrence of erucism.

In the tropical, subtropical and temperate regions of America there exist poisonous Lepidoptera; however, each species of Lepidoptera, in keeping with its adaptations, corresponds to a particular environment.

a) In Central and North America, poisonous species of the following families are found:

Cochlidiidae: *Sibine stimulea* is not a very pletiful species, but its reputation as a poisonous one is very widespread in the United States. It is found in the central and southern states.

In the eastern United States are found: *Phobetron pithecium, Adoneta spinuloides, Sisyrosea textula, Parasa chloris, P. indetermina* and *Natada* spp.

Megalopygidae: *Megalopyge opercularis* is a species which in certain seasons of the year is found in great quantities in the southern states of the United States. In one city in Texas, there were so many of these erucae that they caused hundreds of cases of erucism among children. The public schools were closed while the "puss caterpillars" were destroyed from the shade-giving trees (Bishopp, 1922). *Lagoa crispata* is very numerous in the northern United States. *L. pixidifera* is common in Georgia and the Atlantic states, *Norape* spp. and *Carama* spp. are also found in North America (Baerg, 1924).

Nymphalidae: Poisonous examples in this family are the species *Euvanessa antiopa* and *Nymphalis io.*

Saturniidae: *Automeris io*, the best-known uritcating eruca in the United States, is found in all the central and eastern states, reaching as fas as Mexico.

Hemileuca maia is common in the central and eastern states of the United States, while *H. nevadensis* is found in the west and south-west. *H. oliviae* is found more frequently in New Mexico, while *Colorada pandora* appears in the west. *Cricula* spp., *Hemileuca lucina, Samia* spp. *Pseudohazis eglanterina* and *P. hera* have also been recorded in the United States.

Lymantriidae: *Euproctis chrysorrhoea* occurs in the eastern states of the United States, especially in New England. *E. similis* is found throughout Canada. *Hemerocampa leucostigma* and *Stilpnotia salisis* occur all over North America.

Arctiidae: The following species have been recorded in North America: *Adolia* spp., *Callimorpha* spp., *Euchaetia egle*, *Halysidota caryae* and *Parasemia* spp.

Noctuidae: In various state of the United States, as also in Canada, the erucae of *Acronycta oblinita*, *A. lepusculina*, *Apateta americana* and *Catocala* spp. are known to cause erucism.

The Lymantriids, Arctiids and Noctuids often greatly contaminate the atmosphere where the pupae and eggs covered with primitive-type urticating hairs are found. Wind-borne hairs have caused painful conjuctivitis, and, when inhaled, severe inflammation of the upper respiratory tract.

b) Erucism in South America stems from species of 5 families of moths and of one family of butterflies:

Arctiidac: The erucae are very hairy, their hairs normally being long with some stiff and sharp-pointed ones among them. In Brazil and the Amazon basin of Peru the following species with urticating erucae have been recorded: *Antarctia caja*, *A. fusca*, *Ecpantheria orsa*, *Eupseudosoma aberrans*, *E. involutulum*, *Premolis semirrufa*, *Utheteisa ornatrix*, *H. pulchella*.

Cochlidiidae: The poisonous species look like spiders. *Phobetron hipparchia* and *Eurida variolarus*, which are common species in Brazil, have been identified.

Megalopygidae: The species belonging to this family are the ones most feared in South America, particularly: *Megalopyge lanata*, *M. albicollis superba*, *M. radiata* and *M. undulata* (ALVARENGA, 1912). In Uruguay and Argentina *M. urens* is greatly feared. In the tropical regions of South America, the following have been recorded: *Aidos* spp., *Podalia albescens*, *P. crysocoma*, *P. orsilochus*, *P. radiata* and *Trosia fallax* (Fig. 13). Morphidae: The genus *Morpho* Fabricius is typical of those found in the neotropical regions. The following species are known to be poisonous: *Morpho anaxibia*, *M. cypris*, *M. hercules*, *M. laertes*, *M. menelaus*, and *M. rhetenor*. In Amazonian regions, isolated cases occur at any time of the year, but there is an increase in the summer, which is the time when most eggs are produced and consequently the plants are full of larvae.

Lasiocampidae: There are no poisonous examples of this family in North America; however, in South America the following poisonous species occur; their larvae have gregarious habits: *Arctacea cribaria*, *Euglyphes ornata*, *Macromphalia lignosa*, *Titya proxima* and *Tolype undulosa*.

Saturniidae: These are very harmful. The erucae have poisonous spines. Two genera with poisonous species are found in tropical South America: *Dirphia sabina*, *D. multicolor*, *Automeris acuminata*, *A. melanops*, *A. illustris*, *A. aurantiaca*, *A. incisa*, *A. complicata*, and *A. verisdescens*.

On the American continent there are more than 60 indigenous poisonous species, four species of Lymantriidae and one species of Nymphalidae, which come from Europe.

The Nymphalids, Lymantriids and Noctuids are restricted to North America, while the Morphids and Laiocampids are limited to South America. The Saturniids, Arctiids, Cochlidiids and Megalopygids are widely distributed throughout the whole American continent. However, the species mentioned in this work are distributed

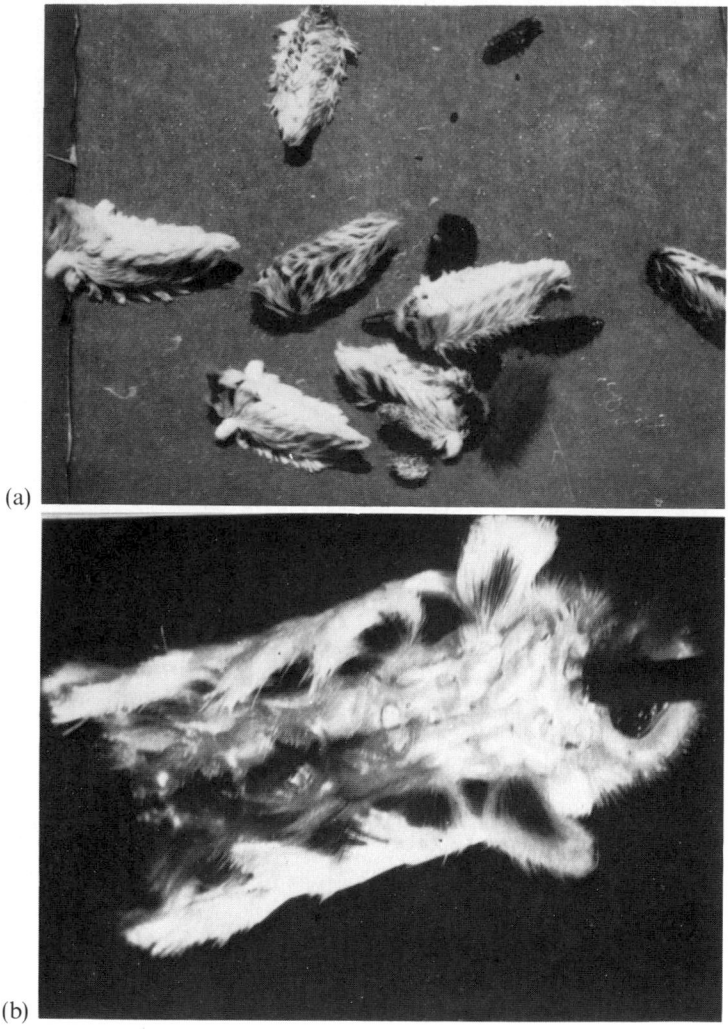

(a)

(b)

Fig. 13a–d. Some poisonous South America erucae. (a) A colony of poisonous erucae of Megalopygidae with two hairy erucae of Sphingidae. (b) *Megalopyge* spp. climbing a stalk. Ventral view. The eruca is clinging to the stalk, hiding its uncovered surfaces. (c) *Dirphia* spp. (Saturniidae). (d) *Automeris* spp. (Saturniidae)

very irregularly and discontinuously, though their greatest concentration is in tropical America.

2. Erucism on the Continent of Europe

In Europe erucism is caused by five families which have species with urticating erucae:

Arctiidae has two genera with poisonous species: *Arctia caja, Lithosia caniola* and *L. griseola.*

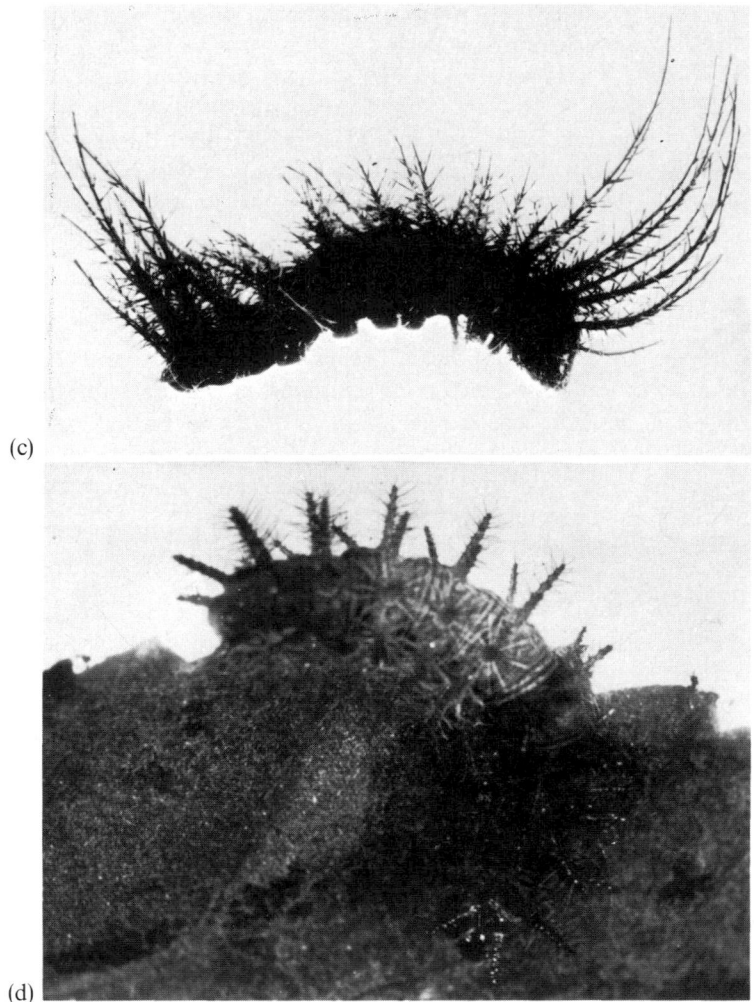

(c)

(d)

Fig. 13c and d

The last two species are common in private and public gardens, in spite of their reputation for being very urticating.

Lasiocampidae: The poisonous erucae of this family are found in the following species: *Cosmotriche* spp., *Dendrolimus pini*, *Gastropacha quercifolia*, *Lasiocampa quercus* and *Macrothylacia rubi*. The last two species roll up into a ball and wriggle their way through the foliage when irritated. On account of their very obvious caustic properties when they fall on uncovered human skin, they have been popularly called "Devil's ring."

Lymantriidae: These are found feeding on the foliage of fruit and forest trees: *Dasichyra pudibunda, Euproctis chrysorrhoea, E. similis, Lymantria monacha, Liparis chrysorrhoea, Ocneria* spp., *Orgya* spp., *Porthetria dispar, Porthesia similis, Stilpnotia salicis*.

Nymphalidae: The adults are butterflies. In their larval state, *Euvannessa antiopa* and *Nymphalis io* have urticating properties.

Thaumetopoeidae: Certain cuticular areas of the urticating caterpillars of this family produce short hairs which are highly urticating. These are the ones most feared in Europe, especially in France, and also in Northern Europe, in Germany, Sweden and Russia. The ones pinpointed as chiefly responsible for European erucism are: *Anaphe infracta, Thaumetopoea pinivora, T. processionea* and *T. wilkinsoni.*

3. Erucism in Africa, Asia and Australia

In Africa there are the Thaumetopoids, *Thaumetopoea pinivora* and *T. wilkinsoni,* but there are many others for which a complete taxonomical description is lacking.

Present in Asia are the cochlidiids: *Parasa hilarata* and *P. latistigra,* the lymantriid *Euproctis flava,* and the thaumetopoiid, *Thaumetopoea* spp.

In Australia are found the lasiocampid *Taragama igniflua*, and others whose taxonomy has been incompletely described.

4. Epidemiological Structure of Erucism

The occurrence of erucic incidents is influenced by many variable factors, such as the poisonous erucae themselves, the urban and rural habitat, the lepidopterian form of dispersion, the place where the phanerotoxic secretion enters the skin of the human beings and animals affected by it, the work habits of the population; in short, all these factors combined, influenced in their turn by the physical and biological environmental factors.

a) Factors Relating to the Aetiological Agent

Erucism usually affects individuals in the neighborhood of their homes, and only in rare cases does it affect groups. It occurs in gardens and orchards, mainly in rural areas and while agricultural work is being carried on. The potential pathogenicity of the erucae of Nymphalids, Morphids, Megalopygids and Saturniids nearly always shows itself when human make real contact with the poison apparatus of the erucae. The result of this incident is erucism, the severity of the outbreak being in direct proportion to the surface area and topography of the skin, and the quantity and quality of the poison injected into the tegument of the victim. The erucism by Thaumetopoids, Saturniids, Lymantriids and Noctuids acquires epidemic proportions, when large areas of wooded and arable land are infested with erucic hairs which are then wind-borne to populated areas, whose inhabitants as a result suffer an epidemic of inflammation of the upper respiratory passages and the ocular conjunctivas, with dermic rash.

Finally, the severity and extent of the illness that can be caused by the erucic toxins depend also on the stage of development of the erucae, pupae and pseudo-ooteca protected by urticating hairs, and in addition, of course, on the victim's age, resistance or immunity, the force with which he crushes the caterpillar, and his proximity to the primary source of erucic intoxication.

b) Factors Relating to Erucic Intoxication

In centers of vegetation such as gardens, orchards, and wooded or arable land, the larval forms can be found eating the foliage, while the adult forms of poisonous Lepidoptera feed on vegetal juices, mainly nectar. Since the larval forms—erucae— are exclusively vegetarian, the adults have to lay their eggs on appropriate host plants. The larval life-span is comparatively short, not usually exceeding 10 months. When the larval state has been completed, the poisonous erucae use their salivary glands to spin the cocoon within which pupation occurs. The poisonous hairs remain woven into the cocoon shells.

The plants infested with the poisonous erucae and cocoons thus become a potential primary source of intoxication or storage center of the etiological agent of epidemic or individual erucism. In this way, woods of *Hevea brasiliensis* constitute the primary source of granulomatous erucism in tropical South America. Pine oak and poplar woods are the primary source of European erucism, in France, Italy, and Germany.

c) Factors Relating to the Environment

The density of the poisonous erucae in cultivated, forest, and industrial plants is a factor that conditions the appearance and distribution of erucic incidents in human beings (Fig. 14).

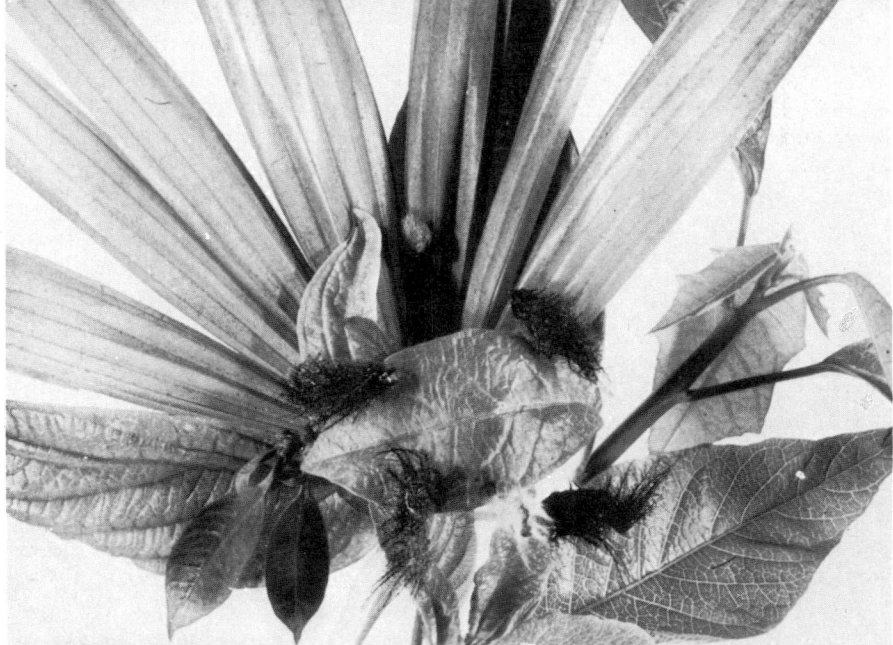

Fig. 14. *Dirphia* spp. erucae infesting vegetation

Many circumstances suggest that the dispersion of anthropotoxic Lepidoptera depends on a combination of favorable or unfavorable factors related to the geographical latitude and landscape, temperature, rainfall, soil relief, etc.

In the Palearctic and Nearctic regions, the life cycle of the Lepidoptera is usually annual. The weather at the end of the spring and beginning of the summer offers the best conditions for laying the Lepidoptera's eggs, so that simultaneously with the greater biological activity of the adult forms, a large quantity or larval forms infest the vegetation used by humans. As a result, the poisonous hairs that break off from the erucae of, mainly, Arctiids, Cochlidiids, Lasiocampids, Lymantriids, Thaumetopoids, and some megalopygids are accidentally wind-borne towards towns, causing epidemic erucic dermatitis. Outbreaks of collective erucism have been reported in Europe, Korea, Japan and the United States.

In the Neotropical, Ethiopian, and Oriental regions, the life cycle of the Lepi-doptera does not seem to experience any delays, since there is no limiting action such as that of the winter temperature and humidity, or any absence of foliage as in the deciduous plants that grow in temperate zones.

Erucae of Cochlidiids, Lasiocampids, Morphids, Saturniids and Thaumetopoids can be seen moving around ar any time in tropical forests and in regions of dense vegetation and heavy rainfall.

These erucae in their turn have to face competition, as they look for their nutrition in the substratum, from numerous other species which feed on the foliage. They also suffer from the predatory action of vermivores (Coleoptera, Avis, Lacer-tilia) and the parasitic action of pathogens (Icheumonids [Hymenoptera], Tachinids [Diptera]) (Fig. 5) (Potton, 1853). The vegetation is periodically infested with urticating hairs which break off the ecdyces, cocoons and pseudo-ooteca, but it is effectively rid of them by the rains which wash the foliage polluted by poisonous hairs and dilute the toxic principles.

On the other hand, there are few winds, and this part of the world is sparsely populated. This means that epidemic erucism is a rare event in these zoogeographic regions, but it has occurred during months of low rainfall. All this goes to show that erucism is an individual accident.

These factors that have been mentioned, and others stemming from the action of human beings, all play their part, though varying constantly in their intensity. In view of this, the epidemiological structure of erucism in the world is variable both in time and space. The favorable and unfavorable factors combine, making the incidence of erucism in human beings the result of this algebraic equation.

5. Epidemiological Characteristics of Erucism

It is not easy to quantify the incidence of erucism according to age and sex with precision at any given time, since it is a frequently repeated, almost always benign occurrence among the inhabitants of rural areas. The erucae and their poisonous hairs can make contact with the skin of any part of the body, which thus becomes the point of entry of the toxin. The parts of the body most affected, in both individual and collective cases, are the head and upper limbs. The poisoning takes place during the day, usually at work, at sport or at leisure. If the skin is covered by clothing, it is difficult for it to be affected. Finally, erucism is more common in natural and rural surroundings because of the existence of conditions appropriate for establishing a biocenosis which leads humans to be in closer contact with Lepidoptera.

6. Prevention of Erucism

Prevention depends on a knowledge of the ecology and all the biological processes of the poisonous Lepidoptera. This knowledge is essential for learning more about the clinical treatment and epidemiology, and especially for controlling the urticating erucae which also prove to be pests for crops (POTTON, 1853; BOURQUIN, 1936, 1939, 1942; BREYER and ORFILA, 1945).

The prophylaxis of erucism aims at making use of a series of measures which would prevent human beings from coming in contact with erucae and their poisonous hairs, or which would eliminate or diminish the effects of erucism.

a) Measures Directed Against the Primary Source

The most radical measure is to attack the Lepidoptera at every stage of their development in the host plants during the favorable season. The following pesticides have been used: chloric hydrocarbons such as: DDT 10%, Dieldrin 3%, Hexachloride of benzene (Gamexano), Lindane 1%. Each of these insecticides or other pesticides reduces the amount of urticating larvae in commercially productive plants.

b) Measures Directed Against the Means of Transmitting the Poisonous Hairs

Thanks to programmes of health education, people exposed to the risk of intoxication come to appreciate that areas infested with poisonous caterpillars are dangerous, and that they should not go into them until after the rains have passed or other processes of natural self-cleansing have taken place. Rooms should be washed with water, especially the floors and walls. Bedclothes, underclothes and clothes used for working in the infested areas should be thoroughly washed for a long time in running water. People who work in contact with the primary source of intoxication should wear gloves and have the uncovered parts of their skin protected.

c) Immunization or Desensitization

In persons subject to sensitization reactions to caterpillar toxin, desensitization or a state of immunological resistance can be achieved by prolonged treatment with small doses of the specific erucic antigen.

C. Lepidopterism

I. Description

The local and general toxic manifestations produced in man by adult of the family Lepidoptera are referred to as lepidopterism. This is an exanthematic epidemic intoxication resulting from contact with toxic substances which have penetrated the skin and are contained in the acicular scales of some Lepidoptera of the genus *Hylesia*. It normally brings about generalized dermatitis and can also affect the mucous membranes of the eye, the upper respiratory system, and the oropharynx. It is also called moth dermatitis or lepidopteran dermatitis.

Lepidopterism seems to be limited exclusively to South America. LÉGER and MOUZELS (1918) were the first, in Cayenne, French Guiana, to offer convincing experimental evidence of the pruriginous dermatitis which occurred periodically among the natives of Cayenne, and which they attributed to contact with certain harmful moths. The dermatitis was obviously due to indirect contact with species of the saturniid *Hylesia* spp. This is the first recorded case in medical literature of lepidopteran dermatitis in South America. The authors describe three cases, characterized by pruriginous erythematous patches that developed papules and vesicles. They proved that the sickness is a result of indirect contact with the harmful moths.

These observations were later verified, also in Cayenne, by BOYE (1932) and TISSEUIL (1935). Following on that, FLOCH and ABONNENC (1944) described the etiological agent of lepidopterism, called *Hylesia urticans,* also in French Guiana. Individual cases have also been recorded in Uruguay and Argentina, in addition to various epidemic outbreaks on a small scale in Argentina and the Caribbean region. More extensive outbreaks affecting more than 40 percent of the population have been recorded in Brazil (GUSMÃO et al., 1961) and Peru (ALLARD and ALLARD, 1958; PESCE and DELGADO, 1966). FLOCH and CONSTANT (1954) describe rhinopharyngitis and tracheitis with obvious respiratory symptoms of whooping cough and fever.

II. Pathology

Macroscopically, erythematous lesions are found, constituting large areas of phlogosis on the skin and mucous membranes. Lesions from scratching also occur, and hemorrhagic suffusions, which are sometimes phlyctenulous.

Microscopically, edematous infiltration and dilatation of the vessels take place, and there is also perivascular and periglandular infiltration with eosinophils and histiocytes.

In some cases giant cells are found containing fragments of setae surrounded by epitheloid cells. Finally, necrosis has been discovered round the poisonous acicular setae.

III. Symptomatology

1. Pathogenesis

It is rare for the female moth to come into direct contact with the victim, but has happened that human beings have brushed against the moth and accidentally rubbed it against their skin. What usually happens is that the female adult forms of the genus *Hylesia,* which have acicular setae, contaminate the atmosphere in and around houses with a vast number of poisonous setae which break off their bodies. When they fall on human tegument they produce the syndromes detailed below.

a) Foreign-Body Syndrome

This marks the beginning of lepidopterism. It is characterized by an itchy sensation due to thousands of acicular setae penetrating the skin and sticking there. As in the case of other non-poison-bearing setae, when they injure the tegument mechanically they cause histaminoid substances to be liberated.

The surface area inoculated in this way is usually very extensive, covering large segments of the uncovered skin of the face, neck and upper limbs. After a few hours the pruritus resulting from the histamine causes scratching, which breaks the poison-bearing setae. This in turn leads to erythema, the intensity of which is in direct proportion to the violence of the scratching.

In people who have been subject to repeated attacks of lepidopterism, small nodules have been found which turn pruriginous when they are touched. When scratched they form ulcers. Microscopically, giant foreign-body cells have been found in them.

b) Toxic Syndrome

This marks the developed stage of lepidopterism which is reached after 6 to 12 h. The signs and symptoms of this syndrome are exclusively due to the toxic substances which enter the tegument when the scratching breaks the poison-bearing setae which had fastened themselves onto the skin and mucous membranes of the head, neck and upper extremities, and, less often, the trunk and lower limbs.

The prime symptom is pruritus, which occurs first of all in the uncovered areas of the skin, but then spreads and becomes more intense on those skin areas where bending takes place—wrists, elbows, axillae, waist and perineum.

Scratching on the one hand, and sweat on the other, spread and aggravate the pruriginous erythema. The characteristic sign is the formation of papulous erythematous patches. Scratching breaks the poison-bearing setae, and sweat dissolves the toxins, which in this way and through the action of gravity succeed in reaching the surface area of the trunk (Fig. 15).

In the covered parts of the body a greater concentration is found where the clothes rub against the skin. At that point papulous erythema usually presents phlyctenes. After a week, as a rule, the papulous-pruriginous eruption subsides. However, the toxic syndrome can increase as long as the same clothes are worn, or the same bed, contaminated with the poison-bearing setae, is slept in. In cases where large quantities have been injected, erythematous rings form on the surface of the flexures, with confluent papules in the center, crowned with equimotic pricks. The papulous surface usually has phlyctenes containing a clear liquid, similar to the vesicular lesions of chicken-pox.

Micropapular erythema is found spread over the skin of the trunk, and within 72 h it becomes generalized. The urticariform rash makes itself very clearly felt

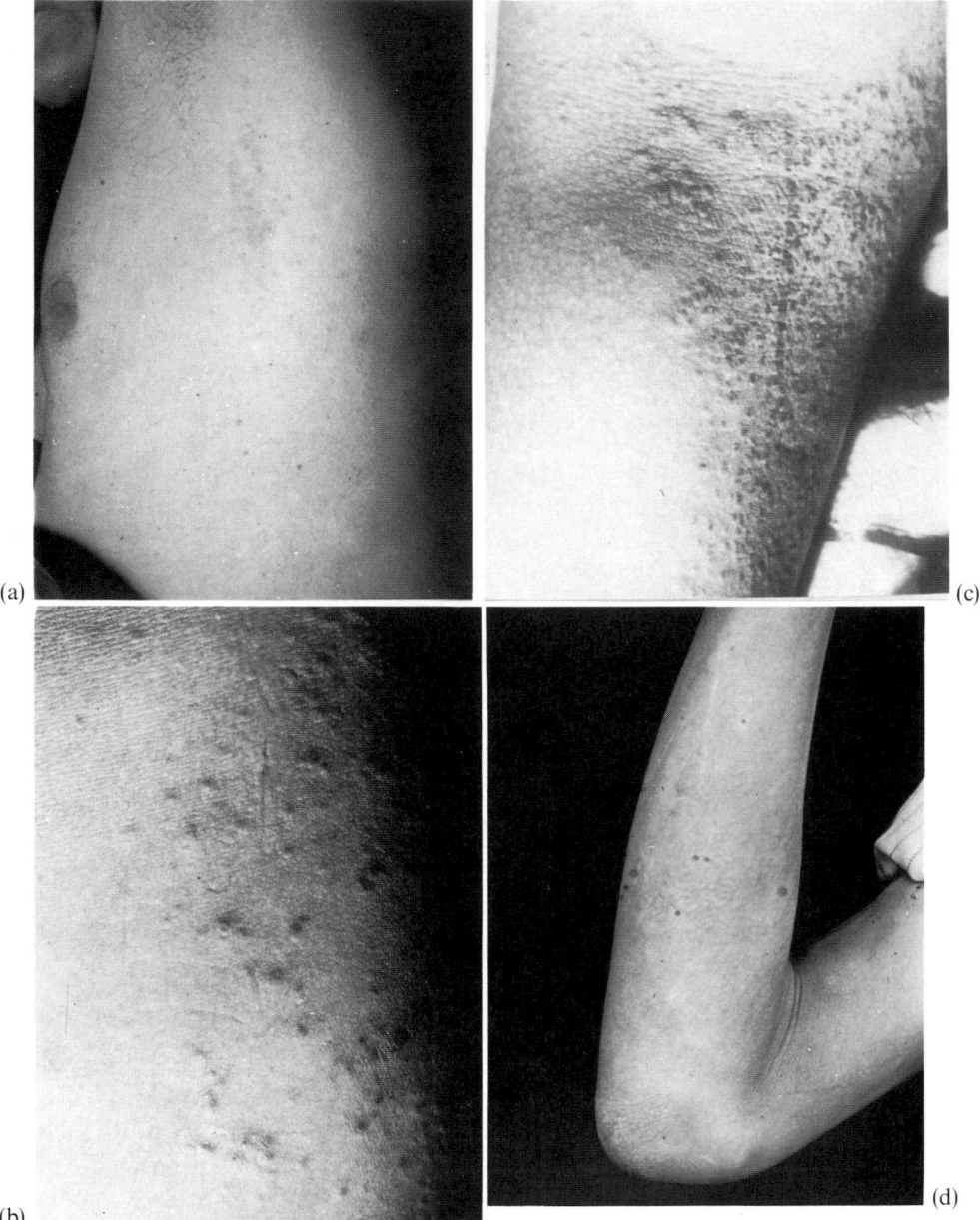

Fig. 15a–d. Clinical description of the lepidopterism caused by *Hylesia* spp. (a) Papular-erythematous reaction spreading to the covered surface of the axillary region. (b) Papular-erythematous lesions grouped together, and lesions caused by itching on the flexure surface of the elbow. (c) Isolated papular-erythematous lesions on the laterodorsal surface of a human being. (d) Papular-erythematous reaction produced by application on a patch of dust taken from the ventral surface of the moth *Hylesia valvex*. Note the hemorrhagic signs

in the axillae, waist, neck and other parts where there has been itching. On the second or third day of the exanthema the patient experiences a general malaise, fever, nausea, vomiting and muscular spasms. The generalized pruritus causes insomnia, general malaise, and a decreased capacity for work; painful conjunctivitis and inflammation of the upper respiratory tract have also been recorded. FLOCH and ABONNENC (1944) describe intense stomatitis in a cat that had eaten a *Hylesia* spp.

c) Infectious Syndrome

Scratching opens the door to secondary infections, whose bacterial etiology is multiple. The predominant features sometimes are impetigo, prurigo and suppurating pustules.

d) Allergic Syndrome

In a small number of people in areas where lepidopterism is endemic it has been possible to record a special sensitivity to the toxins at the third or fourth exposure to the poison-bearing setae of *Hylesia* spp. The patient shows alarming features of polymorphous erythema, giant edema and hemorrhagiparous exanthema with a tendency to shock, when other individuals exposed to the same urticating dust under the same conditions only show the toxic syndrome (PESCE and DELGADO, 1966).

GUSMAO et al. (1961) establish the possibility of some patients becoming sensitive and later falling victim to allergic conditions which coexist with the lesions resulting from the toxin.

2. Evolution

If there are no complications and the bacterial component is not important, the period of regression begins on the eighth day, but in a limited number of cases it takes up to 20 days. The pruritus precedes the erythema. The dermic symptoms are the most important features during the development of the illness. Initially the papules are edematous isquemics with a diameter of 1—2 mm. They are found in small clusters on uncovered parts of the skin. They can be so numerous on the neck that they coalesce to form urticarian patches. These patches feel rough to the touch. The pruritus gets worse when the area is rubbed. Pruriginous erythematous blotches tend to form after 48 h in the areas where they make contact with clothing. These present vesicles and phlyctenes which break when scratched, leading the skin to burst open and hematic scabs to form. After about 8 days the lesions peel off, leaving hyperpigmentation of the skin. In severe cases purple-colored petechiae are sometimes observed (Fig. 15).

The signs and symptoms may reappear if the patient insists on using the same clothes on which the moths deposited their poison-bearing setae.

3. Immunity

It is very obvious in endemic lepidopterism that some people tend to display progressively less symptoms as they experience further exposure to the lepidopterian dust. However, there is always some reaction to the wound, although it is comparatively less severe than that observed under the same conditions in other people (Pesce and Delgado, 1966).

JÖRG (1939) observes the building up of a certain immunity or resistance in people who have suffered successive attacks of lepidopterism. He also notes that the dermic reactions are more severe in foreigners than in natives.

IV. Diagnosis

In epidemic lepidopterism there is no real contact between the moths and the people exposed to them. The patients complain of: pruritus, insomnia, malaise, fever, weakness and even collapse. The rash may be generalized. When the epidemiological characteristics of the illness are not borne in mind, it is very difficult to effect a diagnosis on a clinical basis. It has been confused with measles, chickenpox and other exanthemous illnesses. But the lesions are concentrated mainly on the uncovered surfaces and aroung the waist or at flexures. The pruritus becomes unbearable once the patient starts to scratch. On other occasions allergic symptoms show themselves, including urticarial weals.

Diagnosis is greatly aided by considering the existence of other cases of illness with the same clinical characteristics, the absence of rainfall, occupation, recent activity, the presence of moths in the home or place of work, especially at dusk. The following families have been identified as responsible for one or other of the various forms of lepidopterism.

1. Families with Poisonous Erucae

The intoxication produced by the adult lepidopter is due to poisonous setae coming from the larval state. The setae are taken up by the imago at the moment it bursts out of the pupa. It keeps these setae for some time, during which the adult state also displays toxic properties (Fig. 16).

2. Zygaenidae Family

This includes small fine-bodied moths. Rocci (1917), in Italy, demonstrated that the *Zygaena* spp., which exists in great numbers in the Ligurian region, secretes a yellow liquid with a sour, sickly smell, which has proved fatal in experiments on rats and frogs.

3. Saturniidae Family (= Hemileucidae) (Walker, 1855)

These are woolly-bodied moths. The antennae of the male are doubly pectinated. The legs are short, and the hind tibiae do not have spurs.

The first pair of wings have from 10 to 12 veins without accessory cells. The

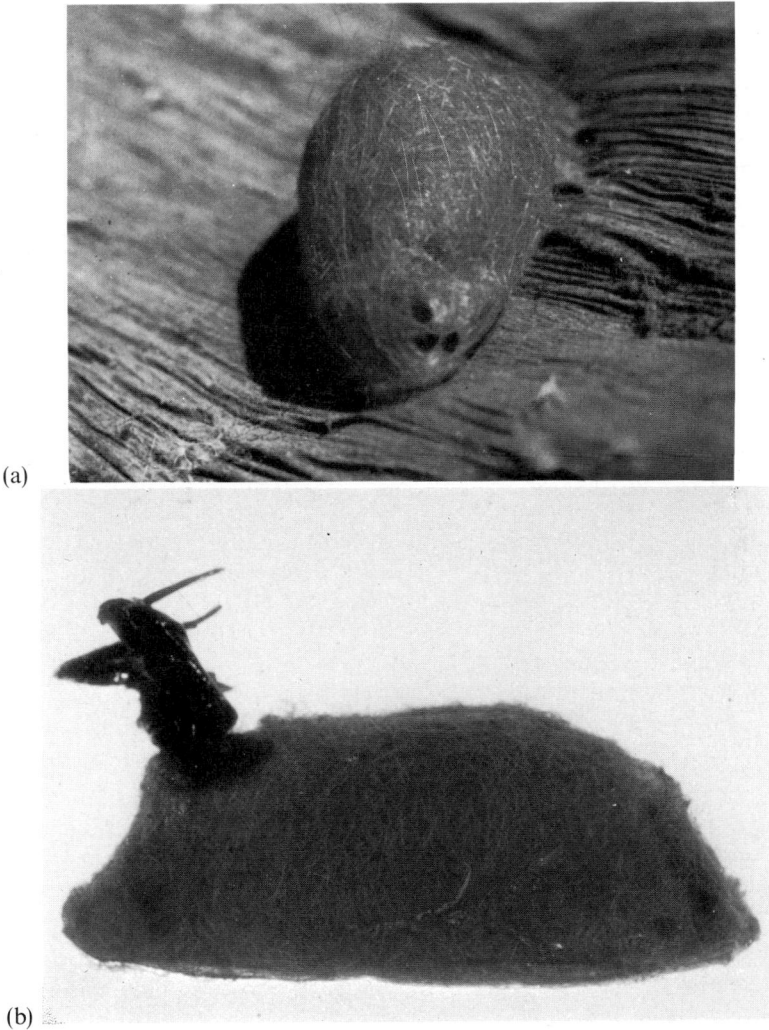

(a)

(b)

Fig. 16a and b. Probability of pseudo-lepidopterism caused by retained larval hairs. (a) Pupa of *Podalia* spp. showing larval urticating hairs. (b) Chrysalis coming out of the cocoon. As it emerges it is contaminated with larval urticating hairs

second pair of wings are broad; they lack a frenulum and possess only one internal marginal vein. The genus *Hylesia* HUBNER includes more than 130 species, morphologically closely related, whose taxonomic position is based fundamentally on the morphological characteristics of the terminalia (Fig. 17).

The poisonous species are grayish-brown in color, except on the terminal part of the abdomen where there are long, clear bristles, reddish or yellowish-brown in color. The body is covered with scales and setae of different morphological types and sizes. On the ventral and lateral surfaces of the final abdominal segments of the female, there are thousands of microscopic setae very similar to flechettes,

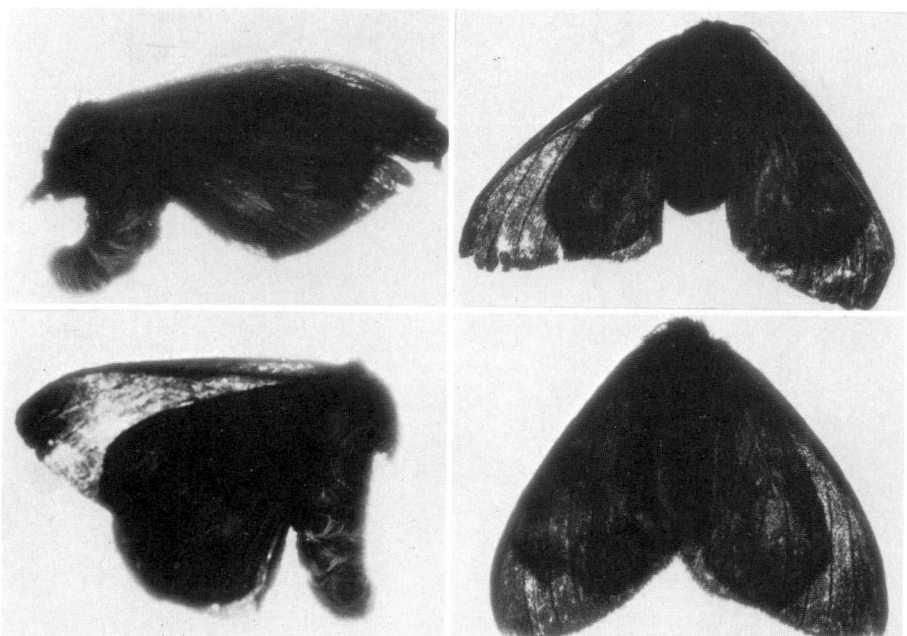

Fig. 17. Saturniidae. *Hylesia* spp. Female specimens. In the lateral view note the hairy abdomen. The final abdominal segments give off urticating dust easily

about 150 μm long and 3 – 5 μm in diameter (Fig. 18). The following species are known to be anthropotoxic: *Hylesia continua, H. canitia, H. fulviventris* Berg, 1883, *H. imbrata* Schauss, 1911, *H. irritans, H. lilex* Dognen, 1923, *H. nigricans, H. urticans* Floch and Abonnenc, 1944 and *H. volvex* Dyar, 1913.

Neither the erucae nor the male moths are armed with these microscopic flechettes. Nevertheless Tisseuil (1935) observed that when these specimens rub against the skin, they cause the formation of short-lived, urticariform erythematous patches.

4. The Poison Apparatus

The presence of sting weapons filled with poison in some species of the genus *Hylesia* has been confirmed by various authors. Léger and Mouzels (1918) discovered in *Hylesia urticans* Floch and Abonnenc, 1944 tiny barbed spines on the venomous function. Boye (1932) called them "flechettes". Tisseuil (1935) noted that only the adult female possesses the flechettes.

In the Peruvian species, *Hylesia volvex, H. irritans* and *Hylesia* spp. the poisonous flechettes are clustered together among the other types of bristles and scales on the ventral and lateral surface of the final abdominal segments. They vary in length, but more so at the distal end. Under the microscope they are easily distinguished from other modified setae (Fig. 18).

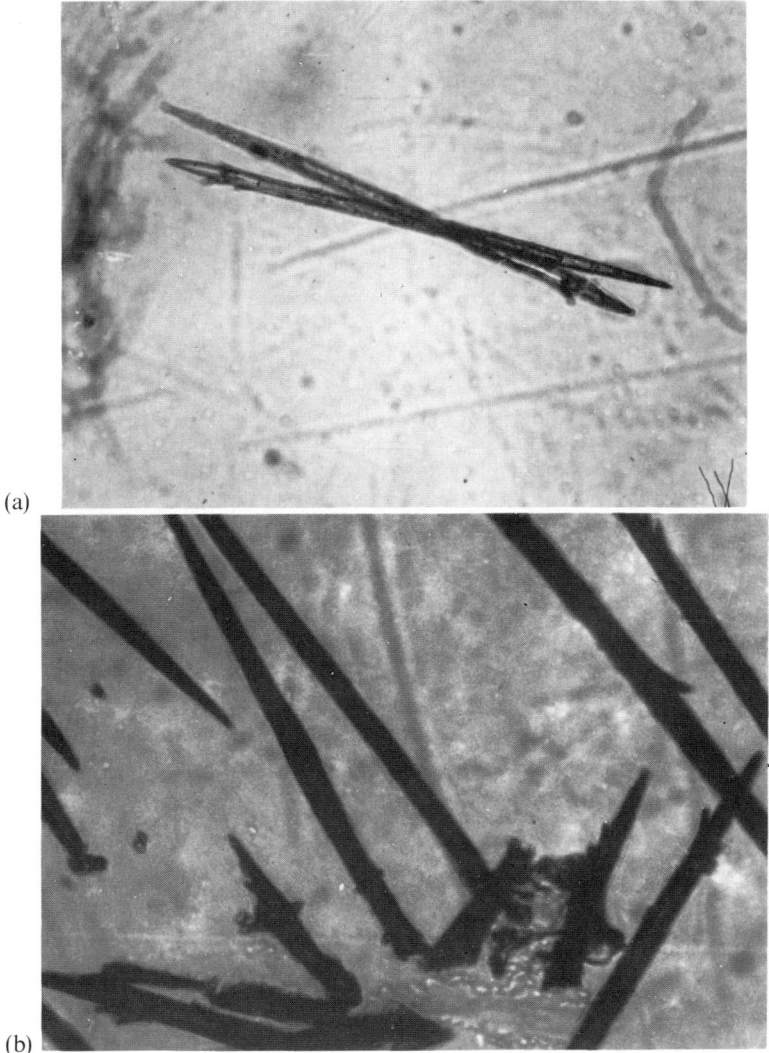

(a)

(b)

Fig. 18a and b. Poison apparatus of *Hylesia* spp. (Saturniidae). Micrograph: (a) Poisonous setae 145 µm long. (b) The poisonous setae have broken under the microscope to allow the poisonous contents of the flechettes to escape

5. Toxicology

a) Extraction of the Poison

From the articulations and antennae of the moth *Zygaena* spp., ROCCI (1917) obtained a sour, sickly-smelling yellow liquid with a slightly acid reaction. By pressing them softly he obtained a sufficiently large amount of the poisonous liquid to study its toxic properties. He inoculated mice and frogs with this liquid, observing subsequent paralysis and, shortly afterwards, death. Through hydrolysis the yellow liquid decomposes into a fixed nontoxic part and a volatile toxic part of a ketonic or aldehydic nature.

To obtain crude extracts of *Hylesia* spp. poison, the female specimens are anesthetized. Using scissors and pincers the tegument of the final body segment is cut. The same procedure is followed with the dead specimens. This material is dried in a vacuum over Cl_2Ca.

To obtain aqueous extracts, the dry extract is used, being placed in sterile physiological serum or distilled water. It is centrifuged at 3000 r.p.m. with glass pearls, so as to break the setae and achieve a greater solubility of the toxin in the solvent. It is then filtered and the aqueous extract obtained in this way is tested on laboratory animals in order to verify its toxic properties.

b) Conservation of the Poison

The crude extracts are kept in amber-colored glass jars in a nitrogen atmosphere. After being kept for 8 years like this the toxic properties are as pronounced as those of poison extracted from recently prepared specimens.

The aqueous extracts are kept for months in the freezer without any alteration in their toxic properties. Rotberg and Boerner (1963), cited by Rotberg (1971), reported that after 3 years the setae of *Hylesia* spp. kept at room temperature without any preservatives were still able to produce intense dermic reactions in volunteer subjects.

c) Pharmacology

Léger and Mouzels (1918) demonstrated that the poison of *Hylesia urticans* is soluble in water and insoluble in alcohol, since the centrifuged aqueous substance had the same toxic properties as the setae. This discovery was also confirmed by Jörg (1933) in *H. nigricans*. Gusmao et al. (1961) proved that the poison was not soluble in ether or olive oil.

The crude dry extract of the poison of *Hylesia* spp. applied with sticking plaster to the skin of laboratory animals and human volunteers invariably produces papulous-pruriginous erythema (Fig. 15). Rotberg (1971) indicated that if the inoculated substance is kept on the skin for several hours the volunteers experience urgent pain. On the affected part, papulous vesicles and superficial necrosis are evident. The toxic nature of *Hylesia* spp. has also been experimentally confirmed by Allard and Allard (1958). These authors used the substance obtained from Peruvian *Hylesia* to rub the skin of volunteer subjects. Similar experiments were carried out by Gusmao et al. (1961).

V. Treatment

This follows the same general lines as the treatment of erucism.

a) Immediate

Avoid scratching and submerge the whole body in water as soon as possible to enable the poisonous flechettes that may have stuck to the skin to come loose, and to dilute the toxins spread by sweat. Change clothing and bedclothes in order to interrupt the toxic process.

b) Symptomatic and Preventive

Apply corticosteroid lotions or creams locally, according to the extent of the lesions.

In order to prevent and modify the hypersensitivity reactions, quick-acting oral antihistamines can be administered; oral or parenteral corticosteroid can be given, according to the severity of the clinical condition.

Antibiotic creams, lotions or powders can be applied if secondary infection is suspected.

A wide spectrum of antibiotics should be administered whenever there are signs of adenitis and lymphangitis, as these are forerunners of septicemic infection.

VI. Epidemiology and Prevention

1. South American Lepidopterism

The lepidopteran dermatitis caused by species of the genus *Hylesia* has only been identified in South America. The majority of the descriptions refer to collective outbreaks (LÉGER and MOUZELS, 1918; BOYE, 1932; DALLAS, 1933; JÖRG, 1933; TISSEUIL, 1935; FLOCH and ABONNENC, 1944; FLOCH and CONSTANT, 1954; ALLARD and ALLARD, 1958; GUSMÃO et al., 1961; PESCE and DELGADO, 1966; DELGADO, 1968).

a) In the Guianas and Venezuela

Lepidopteran dermatitis has been known in French Guiana since LÉGER and MOU-ZELS (1918) described the dermic lesions and established the etiology which was later confirmed by BOYE (1932). FLOCH and ABONNENC (1944) point out that pruriginous dermatitis is localized in the uncovered parts of the body, and occurs at the end of the rainy season. ANDUZE, cited by FLOCH and ABONNENC (1914) told of many cases of lepidopterism in Caracas, Venezuela.

b) In Peru

ALLARD and ALLARD (1958) reported that in Tingo Maria, a small town in the department of Huánuco, epidemic lepidopterism affected between 70 and 80 percent of the population in 1952. That is to say that about 3000 people suffered from lepidopteran dermatitis.

Between 1963 and 1965 we noted and experimented on three epidemic outbreaks of lepidopterism in Rioja, in the department of San Martin. Clouds of moths of the genus *Hylesia* invaded the town for 10 to 13 days consecutively. *Hylesia* was especially active during the hours of dusk, when it was attracted by the light from bulbs and candles. So long as there was light they flew in confusion, bumping against windowpanes and metal shutters. Each time they did so, they let fall a cloud of dust which obviously makes the air a source of stings. In some houses the great quantity of urticating dust made the epidemiological diagnosis of lepidopterism easy. The three outbreaks took place during the months of light rainfall.

c) In Brazil

GUSMÃO et al. (1961) reported that on outbreak of dermatitis caused by the dust of Lepidoptera of the genus *Hylesia* took place in Serra do navio, a town in the state of Amapá, in the Brazialian Amazonian region. Clouds of these moths invaded the town for two weeks on end; 40 percent of the local population were affected, making a total of 707 cases, distributed irrespective of age or sex.

As the days passed the moths gradually disappeared, and new cases of lepidopterism become more rare.

d) In Argentina

KOEHELER (1931) studied the genus *Hylesia* in Argentina, and DALLAS (1933) records two cases of lepidopteran dermatitis in Buenos Aires, Argentina. JÖRG (1935) reports a small epidemic outbreak of lepidopterism in the locality of Entre Rios.

2. Epidemiological Structure of Lepidopterism

Many factors influence the natural occurrence of lepidopterism in America. As a result of studies of the general pattern of the occurrence of lepidopterism, the ecology of the main places where it happens, numerous clinical observations, and experiments on animals and human beings, it has been clearly proved that the genus *Hylesia* HUBNER has anthropotoxic species. The structural adaptation and the behavior of the moths with positive phototropism periodically threaten the inhabitants of the Amazonian regions with dermatitis.

a) Factors Relating to the Anthropotoxic Species
of the Genus Hylesia

The erucae develop in all kinds of vegetation, not showing any preference for one particular kind. The eggs are laid together and covered with various layers of bristles which the female removes from her own abdominal covering while laying her eggs. The poisonous flechettes also find their way into these protective coverings of the eggs. The pseudo-ootecas are therefore toxipherous (Fig. 19).

In French Guiana BOYE (1932) established that the biological cycle of *Hylesia urticans* is repeated every three months.

Each adult female is a carrier of tens of thousands of poison-bearing flechettes which it is constantly shedding. The moths fly in great confusion and bump against metal shutters and window panes, giving off a cloud of dust consisting mainly of acicular setae. The dust inevitably settles on clothes, furniture, floors and the skin, and is also inhaled, producing dermatitis, rhinitis and other toxic upsets.

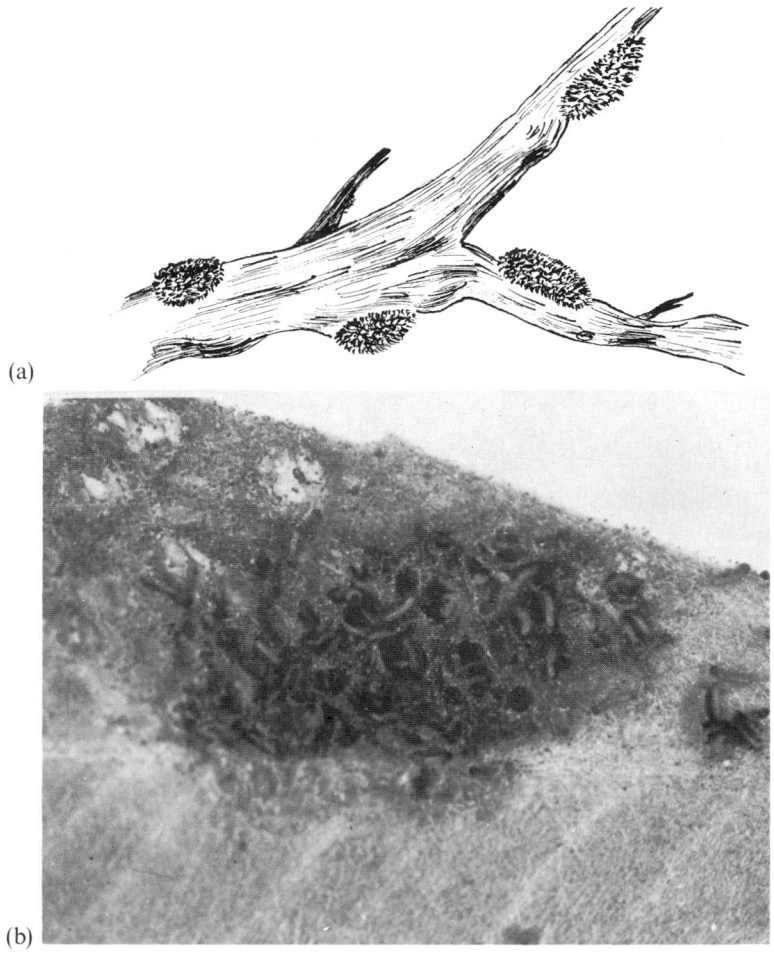

(a)

(b)

Fig. 19a and b. Factors of the anthropotoxic species of the genus *Hylesia* HUBNER. (a) Pseudo-ootecas protected by poisonous setae. (b) Larvae emerging and immediately contaminated by the urticating setae of the pseudo-ooteca

In the Peruvian Amazonian region the adult moths of *Hylesia* spp. appear every three months in short broods of 2 to 4 weeks' duration.

In Argentina, where the seasons are clearly marked, the brood is annual (DALLAS, 1933) and occurs during the first three hottest months of the year (JÖRG, 1933).

b) Factors Relating to the Source of Lepidopteran Intoxication

The anthropotoxic species of *Hylesia* have seldom made direct contact with the victim. The setae come away from the body in great quantities when moths bump against objects. The poison is conveyed through the microscopic acicular setae (Fig. 18).

When the moths are drawn by the light they bump against translucent and transparent objects which come between them and the source of light. On these occasions the cloud of dust is clearly observed, and the poison-bearing flechettes are easily encountered in it.

The dust deposits itself on bedclothes, utensils, furniture, walls and floors, forming the primary source of intoxication for several days.

Another source of lepidopteran intoxication has proved to be utensils, and also tree-trunks, infested with *Hylesia* pseudo-ootecas, which have been stored in sawmills. In addition the poison-bearing particles of *Hylesia* retained in bedding and clothing serve to harbor injurious weapons. The active offensive mechanism of moths does not intervene in the process, but the injurious action takes place accidentally.

c) Factors Relating to the Environment

The epidemiological study of individual cases and of epidemic outbreaks of lepidopterism confirms that phototropism and the absence of rain are factors that condition the appearance and distribution of lepidopteran dermatitis in South America.

Many circumstances show that rains fulfill the function of purifying the environment that has been contaminated by poison-bearing setae.

In this way the moths which are active in the evening and at night are powerfully attracted by light. When there is a lack of rain, the air that has been polluted by poison-bearing flechettes is retained by the plants where the *Hylesia* spp. congregate. When human beings enter the areas infested with these moths, or when the moths invade towns in large numbers, the poison-bearing flechettes invitably fall on uncovered skin surfaces and on articles that people use.

3. Prevention of Lepidopterism

The idea of prophylactic programs is to employ a series of measures aimed at preventing anthropotoxic species of *Hylesia* from making indirect contact with human beings, eliminating or at least minimizing the complications and sequelae which result from the tegument being contaminated.

a) Measures Against the Primary Source of Intoxication

It is possible to apply chemical and biological measures once it is known what host plants contain large numbers of egg-clusters or pseudo-ootecas, cocoons, larvae and adult moths. During the seasons of low rainfall, which are the potentially dangerous ones, epidemic outbreaks have been controlled with DDT and chlordane with no need for taking precautions.

When Dieldrin, Thiocianates and Parathion, which are very effective against erucae, are used, special protection must be provided for human beings and domestic animals in the area that is to be disinfeted. The dead insect should be removed immediately and placed in hermetically sealed jars to prevent their polluting the air if they are swept and shaken.

b) Measures Against the Means of Transmission of the Poison-Bearing Flechettes

Bearing in mind that the *Hylesia* poisonous species are evening fliers and that they are powerfully attracted by lights, it is good to employ the measures adopted in Cayenne (BOYE, 1932), namely, extinguishing lights and fires at nightfall, for one to three hours each evening.

Another preventive measure observed in Rioja, Peru, and in Serra do navio, Brazil (GUSMAO et al., 1961), consists of keeping bedclothes safe from contamination until the very moment of going to sleep. These precautions should continue as long as the *Hylesia* invasion is known to last. Daily washing of contaminated bed-linen should also be carried out.

During and after infestation, lamps, light fittings and other objects that the moths may have knocked against should be wiped with a damp cloth so as to remove lepidopteran dust. Finally attempts may be made to immunize or desensitize people who have become sensitive to lepidopteran toxin and who have to stay in the region where lepidoperism is endemic. If the causal agent is known and poison extracts are available, it is worthwhile making attempts to use a minimal progressive dose for a certain length of time.

References

Allard, R.F., Allard, H.A.: Venomous moths and butterflies. J. Wash. Acad. Sci. **48**, No. 1, 18–21 (1958).

Altum: Neuere Beobachtungen über die Kiefernprozession spinner *Cnethocampa pinivora*. Leitsch. Forst. Jagdwesen Jahrb. 649–662 (1896).

Alvarenga, Z. De. A tatorana: Ann. VII Congr. Bras. Med. Cir., Bello Horizonte 1912.

Anchieta, J.: Carta fazendo a descripção das innumeras coisas naturaes que se encontram na provincia de S. Vicente, hoje São Paulo. Translated from Latin by J. V. Almeida, Casa Eclectica, São Paulo, Brazil, 1900. 26. (1960).

Andrade, C.: Oftalmologia tropical sudamericana. Rio de Janeiro, Brazil: Rodríguez 1940.

Artault de Vevey, S.: Trois observations de stomatite érucique. provoquée par les chenilles du *Liparis chrysorrhroea*. C.R. Soc. Biol. (Paris) **53**, 103 (1901).

Baerg, W.J.: On the life history and the poison apparatus of the white flannel moth, *Lagoa crispata Packard*. Ann. ent. Soc. Amer. **17**, 403–415 (1924).

Balding, G.: On the urticating properties of the hair of *Liparis chrysorrhoea*. Entomologist **17**, 256 (1884).

Beille, L.: Etude anatomique de l'appareil urticant des chenilles processionnaires du pin maritime *Cnethocampus pityiocampa* Borowski. C.R. Soc. Biol. (Paris) **48**, 545–547 (1896).

Beyer, G.E.: Urticating and poisonous caterpillar. Quart. Bull. State Board Health **13**, 161–168 (1922).

Bleyer, J.A.C.: Ein Beitrag zum Studien brasilianischer Nesselraupen und durch ihre Berührung auftretenden Krankheit beim Menschen (Urticaria). Arch. Schiffs- u. Tropenhyg. **13**, 73–83 (1909).

Bishopp, F.C.: The puss caterpillar and the effects of its sting on man. Washington, D.C.: Dept. Agric., in Dept. Circ. No. 288, 14 (1923).

Bonnet, C.: Mémoire sur la grande chenille à queue fourchue du saule dans lequel on prouve que la liqueur que cette chenille fait jaillir est un véritable acide trés actif. Mém. math des Savants étrangers. Paris, II. 267–282. Collection Comp. des oeuvres de C. Bonnet, II, 17–24 (1875).

Bordas, L.: Les glandes mandibulaires et les glandes labiales des larves de *Cossus ligniperda*, C.R. Soc. Biol. (Paris) **54** (1902).

Bordas, L.: Les glandes mandibulaires des larves de Lépidoptéres. C.R. Acad. Sci. (Paris) **134**, 1273 (1903).

Boso, J.M. In: Viaje a las montañas de Yucaraes, Chap. IV. Valdizán & Maldonado. In: La medicina popular peruana. **3**, 348 – 388, vide pp. 369 – 372. Lima-Perú, 1922 (1816).

Bourquin, F.: Notas biológicas sobre *Megalopyge urens*. Rev. Soc. Entomol. Arg. **8**, 125 – 132 (1936).

Bourquin, F.: Metamorfosis de *Podalia nigrocostata* (Lep. *Megalopygidae*). Physis (Paris **17**, 431 – 441 (1939).

Bourquin, F.: Metamorfosis de *Megalopyge albicollus* Walker. Rev. Soc. Entomol. Arg. **11**, 22 – 30 (1941).

Bourquin, F.: Metamorfosis de *Megalopyge albicollus* Walker, Rev. Soc. Entomol. Arg. **11**, 305 – 316 (1942).

Boye, R.: La Papillonite guvanaise. Bull. Soc. Path. exot. **25**, 1099 – 1107 (1932).

Breyer, A., Orfila, R.N.: Las especies del género *Rothschildia* en Tucuman (Argentina) con aclaraciones sobre *R. maura* (Burmeister) y *R. Schreiteriana* nom. nov. (Lep. Saturn.) Rev. Soc. Entomol. Arg. **12**, 299 – 304 (1945).

Burnett, W.I.: Note on the osmeteria of Papilio asterias which he regards as an odoriferous and defensive, rather than tactile organ. Translation of Siebold's Anatomy of the invertebrates, p. 415 (1854).

Caffrey, D.J.: Notes on the poisonous urticating spines of *Hemileuca oliviae* larvae. J. Econ. Entomol. **11**, 363 – 367 (1918).

Cheverton, R.L.: Irritation caused by contact with the processionary caterpillar (Larva of *Thaumetopoea Wilinsoni* tams and its nest). Trans. roy. Soc. trop. Med. Hyg. **29**, 555–557 (1936).

Chu, H.F.: In: How to know the inmature insects, pp. 149 – 189. Dubuque, Iowa: Brown, 1949.

Clifford, J.R.S.: The urticating properties of the hair of *Porthesia chrysorrhoea*. Entomologist **18**, 22 (1885).

Cobo, B.: Historia del nuevo mundo (1639 – 1653), Vol. 2. Ed. I, Sevilla, 273 (1890).

Da Costa Lima, A.: In: Insetos do Brasil. Rio de Janeiro, Brasil, Vol. V., pp. 164 – 180. Dept. Impr. Nacl. (1945).

Da Costa Lima, A.: In: Insetos do Brasil. Rio de Janeiro, Brasil, Vol., p. VI. 260 – 274. Dept. Impr. Nacl. (1950).

Dallas, E.D.: Otro caso de dermitis extendida producida por un lepidóptero y notas sobre *Hylesia nigricans* Berg (Lep. Bombycidae). 8th Reunion Soc. Arg. Patol. Reg. Norte 2, 469 – 474 (1933).

Delgado, A.: La Fauna ponzoñoza del Valle del Rimac. An. Fac. Medicina, Lima **50**, 125 – 170 (1967).

Delgado, A.: Lepidopterismo por *Hylesia* spp (Lepidoptera). 1. Observaciones biocenóticas en la región de Rupa rupa. Dpt. Huánuco – Perú. XIII Convención de la Soc. Entomol. del Perú, Lima 1968.

Delgado, A.: Formas inmaduras urticantes de Lepidóptera. Observaciones biocenóticas en la Selva alta del Perú. XIV convención Nacional de Entomología. Trujillo – Perú. (1969).

Delgado, A.: Lepidopterismo alérgico. I. Congreso Panamericano de asma bronquial. III. Congreso peruano de Alergia (1971).

Delgado, A., Pesche, H.: Erucismo directo en la Selva peruana: 621 observaciones. Resumen del I. Congr. Nac. de Microbiología y Parasitología. 151. Arquipa – Perú (1964).

Denham, C.S.: The acid secretion of *Notodonta concinna*. Insect Live 147 (1888).

Dias, L.B., Azevedo, M.C.: Pararama doenca causada por larvas de Lepidóptero: Aspectos Ecperimentais. Bol. Ofic. sanit. panamer. **75**, 3 (1973).

Dimmock, G.: On some glands which open externally on Insect. Psyche 387 – 389 (1883).

Dimmock, G.: Closed poison-glands of caterpillars. Amer. Nat. **18**, 535 (1884).

Dourgherty, T.F.: Role of steroids in regulation of inflammation. In: Inflammation and Disease of Connective Tissue, pp. 449 – 459. Philadelphia: Saunders 1961.

Dyar, H.J.: Results of the Yale Peruvian Expedition of 1911. Lepidoptera. Washington (1913).

Eltringham, H.: On the urticating properties of *Porthesia similis* Fuess. Trans. entomol. Soc. 423 (1913).

Estable, C., Ferreira-Berruti, P., Ardao, M.I.: Contribución al conocimiento de la toxina de *Megalopyge urens* y de su acción farmacodinámica. Arch. Soc. Biol. Montevideo **12**, No. 3, 186—198 (1945).

Ferton: Sur les Moyens de protection de certaines chenilles contre les Hyménoptères ravisseurs. Ann Soc. Ent. France **70**, 139 (1901).

Floch, H.: Lépidoptère. Arch. Inst. Pasteur Guy Inini., Publ. 262, pp. 297—298 (1952).

Floch, H.: Papillonite. Arch. Inst. Pasteur Guy Inini., Publ. 326, p. 105 (1954).

Floch, H., Abonnenc, E.: Sur la papillonite guyanaise: description du papillon pathogène, *Hyglesia urticans*. Inst. Pasteur Guy & Terr. Inini. Publ. N. 89 (1944).

Floch, H., Constant, Y.: Sur la papillonite guyanaise provoquée par *Hylesia urticans* Floch & Abonnec, 1944. Bol. Entomol. Venezolana **9**, 9—12 (1954).

Foot, N.C.: Pathology of the dermatitis caused by *Megalopyge opercularis,* a Texan caterpillar. J. exp. Med. **35**, 737—753 (1922).

Fracker, S.B.: The classification of Lepidopterous larvae. Illin. Biol. Monogr. **2**, 1915.

Frazier, C.A.: Insect sting allergy and its management. W. Virginia med. J. **62**, 99 (1966).

Gaminara, A.: La acción del veneno de la larva de *Megalopyge urens*. Arch. Trab. 3er. Congr. Nac. Med. Arg. **7**, 968—975 (1928a).

Gaminara, A.: Le venin de la larve de *Megalopyge urens*. Bull. Soc. Pathol. Exotique **21**, 656—662 (1928b).

Geer, C. de.: Observations sur la propriété singulière qu'ont les grandes chenilles à quatorze jambes et à double queue du saule, de seringuer de la liqueur. Mém. des Savants étrangers. Paris II. 530—531 (1750).

Gilmer, P.M.: A comparative study of the poison apparatus of certain Lepidopterous larvae. Ann. entomol. Soc. Amer. **18**, 203—239 (1925).

Gilmer, P.M.: The poison and poison apparatus of the whitemarked tussock moth *Hemerocampa leucostigma* Smith and Abbot. J. Parasit. **10**, 80—86 (1928).

Goeldi, E.A.: Die sanitarische-pathologische Bedeutung der Insekten und verwandten Gliedertiere. Berlin: Friedländer & Sohn 1913.

Goossens, T.: Des chenilles urticantes. Ann. Soc. Entomol. France **1**, 231—236 (1881).

Goossens, T.: Des chenilles vésicantes. Ann. Soc. Entomol. France **6**, 461—464 (1886).

Gusmao, H.H., Forattini, O.P., Rotberg, A.: Dermatite provocada por lepidopteros do gênero *Hylesia*. Rev. Inst. Med. Trop., Sao Paulo 33 **3**, 114—120 (1961).

Hashimoto, T., Hagiwara, H.: The poisonous moth *Euproctis flava* Bren., and the dermatitis caused by it. Japan, Z. Derm. & Urol. **22**, 475 (1922).

Jenkins, M.S.: Urtication by *Bombix rubi*. Entomologist **42** (1886).

Jörg, M.E.: Nota previa sobre el principio activo urticante de *Hylesia nigricans* (Lepidoptera, Hemileucidae) y las dermitis provocades por el mismo. 8th Reunion Soc. Arg. Patol. Reg. Norte **2**, 482—495 (1933).

Jörg, M.E.: Dermatosis lepidopterianas (Segunda nota). 9th Reunion Soc. Arg. Patol. Reg. Norte **3**, 1617—1635 (1939).

Karsten, H.: Bemerkungen über einige scharfe und brennende Absonderungen verschiedener Raupen. Müllers Arch. Anat. Phys. u. vis. med. 375—382, pl. II—12 (1848).

Katzenellenbogen, I.: "Caterpillar dermatitis" as an occupational disease. Trop. Dis. Bull. **51**, 1292—1293 (1954).

Kephart, C.: The poison glands of the larva of the browntail moth. *Euproctis chrysorrhoea* Linn. J. Parasit. **1**, 95—103 (1914).

Kiemensicwicz, St.: Zur näheren Kenntnis der Hautdrüsen bei den Raupen und bei malachius. Verh. K.K. Zool. Bot. Ges. Wien **32**, 459 (1882).

Knight, H.H.: Observation on the poisonous nature of the white-marked tussock moth. J. Parasit. **8**, 133 (1922).

Koehler, P.: El género *Hylesia* en la Argentina. Rev. Soc. Entomol. Arg. **6**, 305—308 (1931).

Lapie, G.: Les chenilles venimeuses et les accidents éruciques. Paris: 1923.

Laudon: Einige Bemerkungen über die Prozessionsraupen und die Ätiologie der Urticaria endemica. Virchows Arch. path. Anat. **125**, 220—238 (1891).

Leger, M., Mouzels, P.: Dermatose prurigeneuse déterminée par des papillons Saturnidés du genre *Hylesia,* Bull. Soc. Path. exot. **11**, 104—107 (1918).

Long, F.R.T.: Urticating by larvae of *Bombix rubi*. Entomologist. **19**, 45 (1886).

Lucas, T.A.: Poisoning by *Megalopyge opercularis* ("Puss caterpillar"). J. Amer. med. Ass. **119**, 877—880 (1942).

Manders, N.: The urticating properties of certain larvae. Ent. Mothly Mag. **29**, 118 (1887).

Matta, A. da: Dermatose vesico-urticante produzida por larvas de lepidopteros. Amazonas médico **16**, 167—170 (1922).

Mazza, S., Frias, D.: Nota sobre accidentes producidos por larvas de *Hyperchiria coraesus* (rupa chico). 2nd Reunion Soc. Arg. Patol. Reg. Norte 293—295 (1926).

Mazzella, H., Patteta, M.A.: Estudio experimental de la acción local de la toxina del *Megalopyge urens* Berg. Arch. Soc. Bio.. Montevideo **13**, 131—136 (1946).

McMillan, C.W., Durcell, W.R.: Health hazard from caterpillars. New Engl. J. Med. **271**, 147—149 (1964).

Megnin, P.: A propos de la stomatite érucique chez les animaux. C.R. Soc. Biol. (Paris) **53**, 129 (1901).

Mills, R.G.: Observations on a series of cases of dermatitis caused by a liparid moth *Euproctis flava* Bremer. China med. J. **37**, 351—371 (1923).

Mills, R.G.: Some observations and experiments on the irritating properties of the larvae of *Parasa hilarata* Staudinger. Amer. J. Hyg. **5**, 342—363 (1925).

Mooren, C.: Observation sur les moeurs de la processionnaire et sur les maladies qu'occasionne cet insecte malfaisant. Bull. Acad. roy. Belg. **15**, 132—144 (1848).

Morisita, T. et al.: On dermatitis due to yellow moth. Acta Sch. med. Gifu. **2**, 347—354 and 471 (1955).

Natansen: Influence pernicieuse de la Chenille velue sur l'oeil humain. Ind. Med. 4 March, 1897.

Packard, A.S.: The fluid ejected by Notodontian caterpillars. Amer. Nat. **20**, 811—812 (1886).

Packard, A.S.: A study of the transformation and anatomy of *Lagoa crispata,* a bombycine moth. Proc. Amer. phil. Soc. **32**, 275—292 (1893).

Packard, A.S.: A textbook of entomology, pp. 187—201 and 375—396. New York: Macmillan 1898.

Patton, W.H.: Scent glands in the larva of Limacodes. (Possédant 8 paries de glandes latérales.) Canad. Entomol. **23**, 42—43 (1891).

Pawlowsky, E.N., Stein, A.K.: Experimentelle Untersuchungen über die Wirkung der überwinternden Goldafterraupen (*Euproctis chrysorrhoea*) auf die Menschenhaut. Z. Morph. Ökol. Tiere **9**, 616—637 (1927).

Pernot: Observations cliniques sur le venin des chenilles Processionaires. Lyon Méd. **45**, 486 (1884).

Pesce, H., Delgado, A.: Observaciones sobre orugas ponzoñosas del Perú, 433 casos. VII. Congr. Internac. Med. Trop. and Mal. Rio de Janeiro **4**, 211—212 (1963).

Pesce, H., Delgado, A.: Lepidopterismo y erucismo. Epidemiología y aspectos clínicos en el Perú. Men. Inst. Butantan. **33**, 3, 829—834 (1966).

Pesce, H., Delgado, A.: Poisoning from adult moths and caterpillars. In: Venomous Animals and their Venoms, Vol. 3, pp. 119—156. New York: Academic Press 1971.

Phisalix, M.: Animaux Venimeux et Venins, Vol. 1, pp. 343—356. Paris: Masson 1922.

Picarelli, L.P., Valle, U.R.: Pharmacological studies on caterpillar venoms. In: Venomous Animals and their Venoms, Vol. 3, pp. 103—118. New York: Academic Press 1971.

Potton: Recherches et observations sur le mal de ver, ou mal de bassine, éruption vesico-pustuleuse qui attaque exclusiment les fileuses de cocon de ver á soie. Ann. d' Hyg. **49**, 245—255 (1853).

Poulton, E.B.: The fluid ejected by Notondontian caterpillars. Ann. Nat. **20**, 811 (1886).

Poulton, E.B.: The secretion of pure aqueous formic acid by Lepidopterous larvae for the purpose of defense. Nature (Lond.) **36**, 593 (1887).

Pourquier: Urticaire du cheval produite par les poils du Bombyx processionnaire du pin. Rec. Vétér. **51**, 1877.

Randel, H.W., Doan, G.B.: Caterpillar urticaria in the Panama Canal Zone. Report of 5 cases. In: Venoms, Publ. No. 44, A.A.A. Sci., pp. 11—116. Washington, D.C.: 1956.

Randolph, H.: Allergic response to dust of insect origin. J. Amer. med. Ass. **103**, 560—562 (1934).

Rendall, P.: Urticating by *Liparis chrysorrhoea*. Entomologist **17**, 275 (1884).

Riley, C.: Notes on the eversible glands of larvae of *Orgya* and *Parorgya leucophoea* and *P. Clintonii* (Achatina). 5th. Rep. U.S. Ent. Comm. **137** (1888).

Riley, W.A., Johannsen, O.A.: In: Medical Entomology, pp. 173—188. New York: 1938.

Rocci, U.: Sur une substance vénéneuse contenue dans les Zygènes. Arch. ital. Biol. **64**, 73—96 (1917).

Rohr: Stomatitis erythemateuse et érysipéle de la face chez le cheval déterminés par les chenilles processionnaires. Assoc. Franç. pour. Avanc. des Sc. Paris (1900).

Rotberg, A.: Lepidopterism in Brazil. In: Venomous Animals and their Venoms, Vol. 3, pp. 157—168. New York: Academic Press 1971.

Rotberg, A., Boerner, A.: 20th. Meeting Brazilian Dermatologists. Porto Alegre, Brazil (1963).

Schmitz, F.: Akute hämorrhagische Nephritis nach Raupenurtikaria. Münch. med. Wschr. 1558 (1917).

Schroeder, C.: Moyens de défense de certaines chenilles en particulier contre les oiseaux et les lézards. Wchr. Entom. **1**, 70–75ff., et Ann. Biol. Delage (1896).

Schroeder, C.: Handbuch der Entomologie, Vol. 3, pp. 852—941. Jena: Fischer 1925.

Scudder, S., H.: Glands and extensile organs of larvae of blue butterflies. Proc. Bos. Soc. Nat. Hist. **33**, 357—358 (1888)

Sharp, H.: Urtication by larvac of *Bombyx rubi*. Entomologist **18**, 324 (1885).

Serre, P.: Venin des cocons de *Cricula trifenestrata*. Bull. Soc. Entomol. France. 254 (1904).

South, R.: On the urticating hairs of some Lepidoptera. Entomologist **18**, 3 (1885).

Steele, C.W., Sawyer, W.H.: The brown tail moth. J. Maine med. Ass. **35**, 157 (1944).

Tisseuil, J.: Contribution à l'étude de la papillonite guyanaise. Bull. Soc. Path. exot. **28**, 719—721 (1935).

Tonkes, P.R.: Recherches sur les poils urticants des chenilles. Bull. Biol. France-Belg. **67**, 44—99 (1933).

Tyzzer, E.E.: The pathology of the browntail moth dermatitis. J. exp. Med. Res. **16**, 43—64 (1907a).

Tyzzer, E.E.: The pathology of the browntail moth dermatitis. Second Report, supt. for Suppressing the Gypsy and Brown-tail Moths, pp. 154—168 (1907b).

Valette, G., Huidobro, H.: Pouvoir histaminoliberateur du venin de la chenille processionnaire du pin (*Thaumetopoea pityocampa* Schiff). C.R. Soc. Biol. (Paris) **148**, 1605—1607 (1954).

Valle, J.R., Picarelli, Z.P., Prado, J.L.: Histamine content and pharmacological properties of crude extracts from setae of urticating caterpillars. Arch. int. Pharmacodyn. **98**, 3: 324—334 (1954).

Viana, C.M., Azavedo, M.C.: Pararama, doenca dos Siringais. Primer congreso de la Sociedad Medico-quirúrgica de Pará. Belem, Brasil (1967).

Von Gorka, V.: Giftige Raupenhaare. Math-natur. Ber. Ungarn **21**, 233 (1907).

Von Ihring, R.: Estudo biologico des lagartas urticante ou tatoranas. Ann. Paulistas Med. Cir. **3**, 129—139 (1914).

Weidner, H.: Beiträge zu einer Monographie der Raupen mit Gifthaaren. Z. angew. Entomol. **23**, 432—484 (1936).

Wilkinson, D.S.: The Cyprus processionary caterpillar (*Thaumetopoea wilkinsoni*). Tams. Bull. Entom. Res. **26**, 163 (1926).

Zaias, N.: Ioannides, G., Taplin, D.: Dermatitis from contact with moth (Genus *Hylesia*) J. Amer. med. Ass. **207**, 525 (1969).

CHAPTER 21

Venoms of Apidae

R. O'CONNOR and M.L. PECK

Introduction

Of the multitude of *Hymenoptera,* the one which has always held man's greatest fascination is the common honey bee[1] (*Apis mellifera* L.). Noted from antiquity as a model of industrious activity and the producer of a delectable honey, this insect has also gained notoriety as a fierce and savage defender of its hive. The venom injected by the stinging honey bee has been the subject of some of the most exhaustive and extensive research activities in the entire field of insect biochemistry.

The social *Apidae* are classified in three main categories: *Apini* (typified by the honey bee), *Bombini* (the bumble bees), and *Meliponini* (the "stingless" bees). Of the last group, whose workers have no stings, only one of the five or more genera (the *Trigona*) exhibits any venomous activity. Poison glands are found at the base of the mandibles of *Trigona* (*Oxytrigona*) *tataira* (KERR and CRUZ, 1961), but the composition of the venom has not been studied. It has been suggested (KERR and DE LELLO, 1962) that the "stingless" bees represent evolutionary development of alternative protection mechanisms, and this postulate is supported by the observation of vestigial venom glands in certain of the *Meliponini*. Little is known of the venoms of *Bombini* or of *Apini* other than *Apis mellifera,* so the major part of the following discussion is concerned with honey bee venom.

From ancient times, bee venom has held a dual interest for man. While the painful, and sometimes fatal, reactions to bee sting have resulted in the development of a healthy respect for the bee as an adversary, potential therapeutic uses for the venom were apparently recognized even in very early civilizations (BARKER et al., 1967). Scientific investigations, beginning with the study of the venom apparatus in 1841 (KERR and DE LELLO, 1962), have increased exponentially as more sophisticated experimental techniques have developed, while each new piece of information has stimulated scientific interest in completing the puzzle of the complex natural venom.

The first chemical investigation of honey bee venom, a crude procedure at best, led to the reporting of formic acid as the main component (LANGER, 1897). Although more careful studies (MERL, 1921; ELSER, 1924) led to the repudiation of this claim, it is not uncommon even today to encounter the belief that bee venom consists of formic acid. A careful vapor-phase chromatographic study has

---

[1] Although both the two-word and single-word (honeybee) forms are in common usage, it has been suggested (SNODGRASS, 1956) that separate words best comply with accepted nomenclature practice in entomology.

established that no detectable amount of formic acid is present in the natural venom (O'Connor et al., 1965). Rather the venom consists of a highly complex mixture of enzymes, peptides, and smaller molecules, many of which exhibit potent physiologic activity (Peck and O'Connor, 1974). The present intensity of bee venom research results from three stimuli: the desire to reduce the incidence of fatal and near-fatal reactions to honey bee sting, the interest in developing potential therapeutic uses of honey bee venom or some of its components, and the natural scientific curiosity concerning the chemistry and pharmacology of venoms. A comparison of some sequential reviews (Tetsch and Wolff, 1936; Neumann and Habermann, 1954a; Kaiser and Michl, 1958; Beard, 1963; O'Connor et al., 1967; Habermann, 1972) with the most recent work described in the following sections readily indicates the burgeoning character of bee venom research.

The reactions of humans to stings of the *Apidae* vary widely, depending on the particular insect involved, the number of stings, the location of sting sites on the body, and the general health and antibody characteristics of the individual stung. Beekeepers appear to suffer the least discomfort from stings, possibly because of the presence in the serum of the beekeeper of antibodies specific to venom antigens (Mohammed and El Karemi, 1961; Barker et al., 1967). In particular, the antihyaluronidase developed against honey bee venom may afford added protection against other stinging insects, since venoms appear to depend on the action of their hyaluronidase enzyme systems to facilitate spreading of the venom through tissue by degradation of the hyaluronic acid intercellular cement (Zlotkin, 1973). The responses of nonprotected individuals to bee sting may be considered in five basic categories: (1) the normal response to one, or a few, stings; (2) a local reaction in the vicinity of sting sites; (3) a toxic reaction to a large number of stings; (4) delayed physiologic response; (5) the generalized reaction, most frequently associated with hypersensitivity to venom components.

The normal response to a bee sting is characterized by sharp, but rarely severe, localized pain. This may result, at least in part, from 5-hydroxytryptamine in the venom (Welsh and Batty, 1963), although the contribution of other components or of component interactions should not be overlooked (Habermann, 1972). The pain usually subsides within a few minutes, but a feverish, itching wheal often remains for several hours. The somewhat more severe local reaction, typified by unusual or prolonged localized edema, commonly associated with heat and itching, is seldom dangerous unless near the eyes or throat. Such a reaction might, however, be an early warning of a developing sensitivity that could lead to increasingly severe responses to subsequent stings (Perlman, 1955). First aid recommended for normal or local responses is generally a simple cold pack, following careful removal of the stinger in such a way as to avoid squeezing additional venom from the attached sac into the wound (Pursley, 1973).

Toxic reactions, while relatively rare, are considered possible in cases of multiple sting, although the survival of a thirty-year-old male of 2243 stings over a 4.5 h period has been reported (Pursley, 1973). The toxicity of bee venom is significantly higher with intravenous injection than with subcutaneous injection (Brooks and Vick, 1972), so in terms of venom toxicity, stings in areas where major blood vessels are susceptible to penetration are most dangerous. In addition, it appears that dermal mast cells may afford protection against subcutaneous envenomation

(HIGGINBOTHAM and KARNELLA, 1970). Calcium gluconate may help in counteracting toxic reactions (PURSLEY, 1973).

Little is known about the so-called "delayed physiological response," although cases of sting fatality several hours after the sting incident have been reported (BARNARD, 1967; PARRISH, 1963). If a bee sting is to cause death, the time between the sting and the fatal response is most often less than 30 min, so delayed fatalities are relatively rare (PARRISH, 1963).

Generalized reactions to bee sting appear to be associated with allergic response to venom antigens and may vary in severity from mild discomfort to anaphylactic shock, often resulting in death. Four stages of the general allergic response are recognized (PURSLEY, 1973): (1) the "slight" reaction, manifested by itching, widespread red blotches, and malaise; (2) the "general" reaction, in which the preceding symptoms are accompanied by wide-spread edema, wheezing, chest constriction, abdominal cramps, nausea, vertigo, and/or vomiting; (3) the "severe general" reaction with additional symptoms such as difficulty in swallowing or breathing, significant weakness, and/or psychologic disorders; (4) the "shock" reaction, typified by a marked decrease in blood pressure, collapse, cyanosis, and unconsiousness. The "shock" reaction, if not treated quickly, may prove fatal. The use of some pressor amine, such as epinephrine, at the onset of a "shock" reaction may prove life-saving (O'CONNOR et al., 1964b). Insect sting fatality has been the subject of investigation for many years (WEGELIN, 1948), and the allergic involvement in many of the cases of death from sting has been thoroughly established (ANTON, 1945; LOMER et al., 1958; PARRISH, 1963; BARNARD, 1967; SHKENDEROV, 1974). Persons of known hypersensitivity, which should be suspected in the event of any general reaction to a bee sting (and considered possible in the case of severe local reactions), may profit from hyposensitization treatments using appropriate allergen preparations. Even so, protection is less than absolute, and emergency first aid kits should be kept available (O'CONNOR et al., 1964b). Sadly enough, the wives of many beekeepers seem unusually susceptible to venom allergy, possibly by the development of an inhalant sensitivity to the particulates adhering to the husband's working clothes (PECK and O'CONNOR, 1974).

The venom of the honey bee, *Apis mellifera,* has long been considered a potentially valuable therapeutic system, either as the whole natural venom (BECK, 1935) or as the source of useful components (HABERMANN, 1972) that could be isolated or synthetically reproduced (PECK and O'CONNOR, 1974). Historically, the greatest interest has been displayed in the possibility of using honey bee venom in the treatment of rheumatoid arthritis (HOLLANDER, 1941; NEUMANN and STRACKE, 1951; BROADMAN, 1962; KATZ and PILIERO, 1969; LORENZETTI et al., 1972). Although the injection of reconstituted venom or the use of live stinging honey bees is accepted medical practice in many countries, the technique has not found universal acceptance in arthritis therapy (COUCH and BENTON, 1972). This is largely due to a feeling that there is, as yet, insufficient information on either the effectiveness of the treatment or the possibilities of adverse side-effects. There is, too, a certain reluctance in some medical circles to adopt a "folk remedy" using a natural mixture whose composition is not yet fully known, whose purity is difficult to determine, and whose dosage might be hard to quantify. The experimental evidence is, however, generally considered sufficient to warrant even more intensive investigation of this possible "natural curative" (Lorenzetti et al., 1972). Additional interest in potential therapeutic uses of bee venom, or of certain of its components, has been stimulated by reports of radioprotective properties of the venom (Shipman and Cole, 1967) and of the isolation of components having potentially valuable medical applications (Vick et al., 1974). One of the more promising uses of the pure venom is in the hyposensitization of persons having an allergic response to honey bee sting (O'Connor et al., 1964b). The physiologic activities of honey bee venom, and of many of the compounds isolated from the venom, are discussed in detail in later sections.

Apis mellifera venom is an exceedingly complex mixture, difficult to obtain in pure natural form. As a result, studies of the chemical composition of the venom and of the pharmacologic properties of venom components have been difficult. All too often, published reports have been inconclusive or erroneous. Cross-references have frequently perpetuated earlier errors, adding to the confusion of the literature. The simplest example is the case of the formic acid report described earlier, but problems have not been limited to inexperienced investigators with primitive equipment. Some of the most experienced modern research teams have discovered the frustration of learning that apparently valid experiments have produced results that have been proved wrong, often in their own laboratories, by later and more sophisticated investigations. At times it almost seems that the honey bee has a perverse desire to maintain its own "military secrets."

Much of the work prior to 1963 was complicated by the use of venom sac extracts rather than pure natural venom (O'Connor et al., 1963). Even with the development of a method for securing "natural" venom in large quantities (Benton et al., 1963), the problem of venom purity was not fully solved (Benton and Morse, 1966), since the "1963 Benton venom" was slightly contaminated by pollen and other materials.

Other classic examples of difficulties encountered are illustrative of the inherent problems of this complex research area. Melittin, the principal component of the dried venom, was "fully characterized" (Habermann and Jentsch, 1967), but five years later the "compound" was shown to be not a pure single substance but a mixture of at least three closely related peptides (Jentsch, 1972). Phospholipase A, like melittin, had been intensively studied by a number of research groups (Neumann and Habermann, 1954a, b; Cole and Shibman, 1970; Rothschild, 1965; Barker et al., 1966; Munjal and Elliott, 1971b; Shipolini, 1971a, b), but improved separation techniques subsequently showed the "original" enzyme to be separable into at least two components of similar activity (Jentsch and Dielenberg, 1972).

Lest it appears that the authors of this discussion are enjoying the discomfiture of other investigators, it must be admitted that the report of antigenic characteristics of *Hymenoptera* venoms (O'Connor and Erickson, 1965) has been partly invalidated by the recent observations of nonimmunochemical complexing between *Hymenoptera* venoms and rabbit sera (Dirks and Sternburg, 1972; Franklin and Baer, 1974).

Every attempt has been made in the following detailed discussions to provide the most critical and current evaluation of the literature. Nevertheless, it is apparent that the subject is not simple, and it is probable that increasingly sophisticated

investigations will change, to some extent, the descriptions of chemical and pharmacologic properties of honey bee venom. It may well be many more years before
the honey bee has yielded the last of its secrets.

A. Venom Apparatus, Sting Mechanism, and Venom Collection

I. Venom Apparatus

1. Apini

The sting accessories of the *Apini* (show schematically in Fig. 1) consist essentially
of a glandular system, a venom sac (reservoir), the sting shaft used for penetration
of the host for venom injection, and associated tissue.

Detailed discussions of the venom apparatus and the mechanisms of its action
are given by SNODGRASS (1956). The wall of the venom sac is a thick, laminated,
cuticular intima. Since it contains no known secretory cells and its walls do not

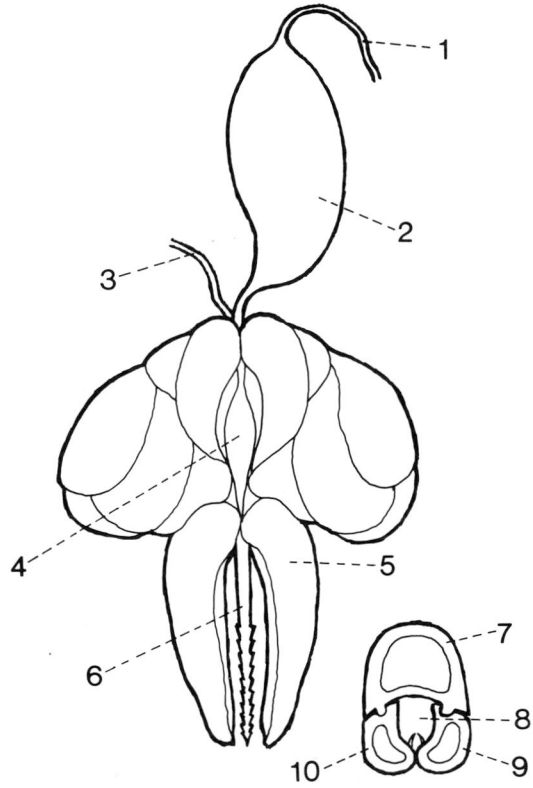

Fig. 1. Schematic representation of venom apparatus of *Apini* (KERR and DE LELLO, 1962;
SNODGRASS, 1956). (*1*) tubule connection to so-called acid gland, (*2*) venom sac, (*3*) tubule
connection to Dufour gland, (*4*) stylet bulb, open on side of poison canal, (*5*) sheath enclosing
retracted sting shaft, (*6*) barbed sting shaft; (cross section, lower right): (*7*) stylet, (*8*) poison
canal, (*9, 10*) barbed lancets

contain muscles capable of aiding in the expelling of the venom, it is believed that the venom sac functions only as a reservoir for the secretions of the attached acid gland.

The so-called "acid" gland appears to be the source of all venom components. This gland is a highly convoluted, branched gland varying in length and complexity among the different members of the genus *Apis* (MAA, 1953). The acid gland is typically shorter in queens than in workers. Histologically, the gland is composed of secretory cells around canaliculi. The secretions of the cells are collected in the numerous canaliculi and released into a membrane-lined central canal. The cells probably secrete in a merocrine way.

A second gland, the Dufour (sometimes referred to as the "alkaline") gland, does not empty its secretion directly into either the venom sac or the poison canal. Thus, the role of the Dufour gland is still something of a mystery (SNODGRASS, 1956; KERR and DE LELLO, 1962).

The sting shaft is normally retracted into the lower abdomen of the bee, being protruded for the act of stinging by a complex plate-and-musculature action. An interesting mechanism is involved in "pumping" the venom into the bee's victim after prenetration of the host by the sting shaft. The shaft consists of four segments (Fig. 1, *lower right*), which taper together to form a sharp, hollow point. Venom is injected through the poison canal, located near the center of the shaft. The two lancets slide back and forth, alternately, along a track-and-groove connection to the stylet. As the lancets move rapidly back and forth, they perform two functions. The barbs on the undersides of the lancets prevent their retraction from the wound, so that each successive lancet penetration drives the sting shaft deeper. At the same time, venom pouring from the sac into the cavity of the stylet bulb, open on the side adjoining the poison canal, is pumped through the poison canal by a successive valve action of lobes at the lancet bases.

Since the barbed lancets hold the stinger tightly in animal skin, the struggles of the bee to escape normally rip the entire venom apparatus from the bee's abdomen. The damaged bee soon dies, while the removed stinger continues its function of penetration and envenomation of the host. Contrary to popular belief, venom is not continuously "squeezed" from the sac by contraction of surrounding muscles, although the sac may be squeezed by the victim in an attempt to withdraw the imbedded stinger. It is the continuing action of muscles controlling the lancet movements that maintain the normal pumping of the venom and the ever-deeper penetration of the sting shaft, even after the sting apparatus is detached from the bee. In stinging other insects, the bee may be able to withdraw the sting shaft (PURSLEY, 1973), and the venom used may be regenerated (O'CONNOR et al., 1963).

While the venom apparatus is essentially the same in each of the four commonly recognized species of *Apis* (*A. mellifera, A. dorsata, A. florea,* and *A. indica*[2]), some differences of possible significance have been noted (KERR and DE LELLO, 1962). As previously mentioned, differences exist in the size and branching of the "acid" glands, while the Dufour gland in *A. dorsata* and *A. florea* is more highly developed than in *A. mellifera*. The consequences of these differences in terms of venom

---

[2] Sometimes referred to as *A. cerana indica,* or *A. cerana.*

composition are largely unknown, since most investigations have concentrated on *Apis mellifera* venom. Preliminary studies suggest that differences in composition do exist (MORSE et al., 1967; BENTON and MORSE, 1968; KREIL, 1973a).

The venom apparatus may also serve as a source of alarm and attack pheromones (BOCH et al., 1962; MORSE et al., 1967). These volatile substances may provide chemical communication among bees in requesting assistance against enemies of the colony. The source of pheromones associated with the venom apparatus has not yet been identified. It is conceivable that future studies may relate some or all of the pheromones to the Dufour gland, whose function is now so uncertain. This is, however, purely speculative as no such relationship has yet been reported.

2. Bombini

Although many of the features of the venom apparatus of *Apis* are preserved in the *Bombini*, major differences in functional details are observed (BORDAS, 1895; KERR and DE LELLO, 1962). The venom sac and glands are appreciably larger and more complex in the *Bombini* and the sting shaft is barbless. Branching characteristics of the "acid" gland in *Bombini* vary appreciably. The first junction in the glandular tubules occurs about 3—4 mm from the venom sac in *Bombus lapidarius, B. hypnorum, B. muscorum*, and *B. sylvarum*. Branching of this gland starts 10—20 mm from the sac in the more highly developed *B. hortorum, B. pratorum*, and *B. pomorum*.

3. Meliponini

There are more than 300 species of the stingless bees. Many contain vestigial venom sacs, often quite large, and some possess vestigial venom gland systems. It has been suggested that the stingless bees represent evolutionary progress in the development of protective mechanisms not requiring a stinging defense (KERR and DE LELLO, 1962).

II. Venom Formation

1. Apini

As mentioned earlier, the Dufour gland appears not to contribute to the venom itself, nor does the poison sac contain secretory cells (KERR and DE LELLO, 1962). Thus, the venom appears to be generated entirely by the "acid" glands (SNODGRASS, 1956), apparently so named because of the early suggestion of formic acid as the venomous component. The "acid" gland extends from its tubular connection with the sac through a series of convolutions, branching into two smaller tubules, each ending in slight glandular enlargements. The principal variation among members of the genus *Apis* is the distance from the sac to the bifurcation. This distance is longest in workers of the *Apis mellifera*.

Venom glands appear to begin functioning soon after the emergence of the new adult bee. Venom is detected by about the third day (PURSLEY, 1973), with full venom sac capacity reached within two to three weeks (KAISER and MICHL,

1958). Protein food appears essential to venom formation (Pursley, 1973). The principal toxin of *Apis mellifera* venom, melittin, is formed slowly in workers. During the first two days following emergence, no melittin is detected in the venom gland, although its precursor (promelittin) was observed (Bachmayer et al., 1972). The venom of *A. mellifera* queens, on the other hand, appears complete on emergence of the insect, possibly because of the immediate need for venom in the battles between newly hatched queens. The formation of histamine and histidine appears to follow a similar age-dependence in worker bees (Owen and Braidwood, 1974).

Although 5-hydroxytryptamine has been reported in extracts of the venom apparatus of *Apis mellifera* in relatively high concentrations, only trace amounts have been claimed for the venom itself (Welsh and Batty, 1963; Grzycki and Czerny, 1973). Whether this substance is actually part of the "acid" gland secretion must still be considered uncertain.

2. Bombini

The Dufour gland in *Bombini* is significantly larger and more complex than in the *Apini,* while the "acid" gland in *Bombini* is more highly branched (Kerr and De Lello, 1962). In addition, secretory cells are observed in a villous epithelium of the venom sac in *Bombini*.

The differences in the mechanisms of venom formation appear to be reflected in different venom compositions of *Bombini* and *Apini* (O'Connor et al., 1964a; Mello, 1970).

3. Meliponini

The possible functions of venom glands in the stingless bees are explored in detail by Kerr and De Lello (1962). Since our interest is primarily in bees having stinging workers, we shall limit further discussions to the venoms of *Apini* and *Bombini*.

III. Venom Collection

1. Venom Sac and Gland Extraction

Most of the early work on the composition of *Apis mellifera* venom was based on studies of the aqueous extracts of extirpated venom sacs and glands. While this method can certainly be used for isolation of some of the components of the natural venom, it is generally unsatisfactory for analytical work, since sac and gland extracts differ significantly from the pure venom (O'Connor et al., 1964a).

Recently, ether extraction has been employed for the isolation of pheromones from the venom apparatus of various bees (Morse et al., 1967). While ether is certainly a reasonably selective solvent for this purpose, there is no assurance that substances extracted from venom apparatus are actually components of the venom itself.

2. Electrical Excitation of Groups of Bees

The original techniques for obtaining honey bee venom by electrical excitation devices, a major step in solving the problems of venom analysis, should be credited to MARKOVIC and MOLNAR (1954). Subsequent modifications of the method (PALMER, 1961; BENTON et al., 1963; BENTON and MORSE, 1966; GUNNISON, 1966) have resulted in significant improvement of the purity of the collected venom.

The improved Cornell Venom Collector (BENTON and MORSE, 1966) utilizes the installation in a bee hive of a frame over which steel wires are stretched at 0.25-in. intervals. The wires are alternately grounded and charged (BENTON et al., 1963). A sheet of nylon parchment taffeta, above two sheets of thin polyethylene, stretched over the collection frame provides a surface through which the shocked bees can sting, depositing venom droplets on the underside of the lower polyethylene sheet. The addition of a cooling coil (GUNNISON, 1966) provides a way of preserving much of the liquid fraction of the venom and probably minimizes any denaturation of venom components. It is estimated that about a gram of venom can be collected by this device from twenty hives over a 2-h period[3].

Honey bee venom collected by "hive excitation" methods may be purchased commercially from various sources[4], but the investigator should attempt to obtain from the supplier a description of methods used to ensure minimum contamination of the venom sample.

It should be mentioned that hives used for venom collection are best located in isolated areas and attended by persons wearing protective hoods and clothing. The bees become quite excited during the electrical shocking and, possibly by pheromone communication (GUNNISON, 1966), alarm other bees outside the hive so that persons in the vicinity may be attacked.

3. Pure Venom from Individual Hymenoptera

Two methods are available for obtaining pure venom samples from single insects. The most satisfactory involves the use of an electrical excitation device (O'CONNOR et al., 1963), as illustrated in Fig. 2, to collect the venom droplets in a microscope well-slide. Insects used are first put to sleep by carbon dioxide or, better, by chilling at $5-10°$ C. The insect is then placed in the holding clamp and excited by an electrical shock as it begins to revive. Careful work permits the collection of pure natural venom from $15-20$ insects per hour by this method. Although slow and tedious, the technique is quite valuable when ultra-pure samples are required. Most of the *Hymenoptera* tested can be "milked" of venom by this method, although it has not proved satisfactory with bumble bees.

For insects, such as the bumble bee, not amenable to electrical excitation, or for studies requiring the complete liquid venom, it is possible to remove the contents of the venom sac by the careful insertion of a very fine needle attached to a microsyringe (O'CONNOR et al., 1967; MELLO, 1970). To minimize possibilities

---

[3] There is a significant variation in the quantity of venom collected as a function of the age of the bees (GALUSZKA, 1972).

[4] For example, Sigma Chemical Co., P.O. Box 14508, St. Louis, Mo., 63178.

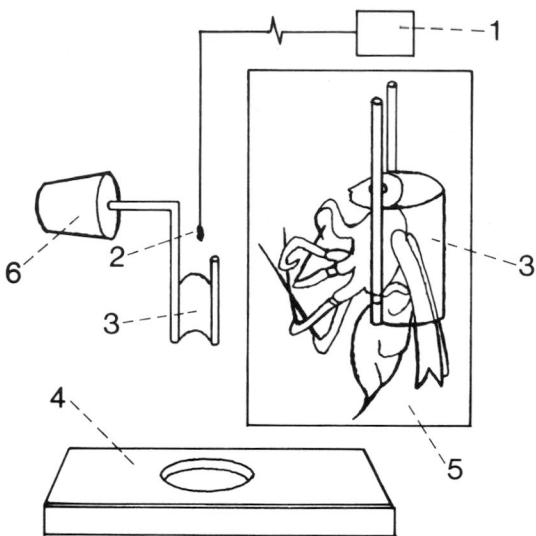

Fig. 2. Electrical exciter (O'Connor et al., 1963). (*1*) spark coil with 6-volt d-c power supply, (*2*) nichrome wire, (*3*) brass mesh half-cylinder, (*4*) microscope well-slide, (*5*) [insert] insect mounted in half-cylinder prior to wrapping with aluminum ribbon, (*6*) insulated handle

of contamination, only freshly extirpated sacs should be used, and the surface of the sac should be blotted on clean filter paper just prior to puncture by the syringe needle.

B. Composition of Apis mellifera Venom

I. Venom Quantity and Purity

The amount of venom produced by worker bees increases with their age, reaching a maximum around 2 or 3 weeks after emergence (KAISER and MICHL, 1958; PURSLEY, 1973). This has been confirmed both by studies of total venom production as a function of age (MÜLLER, 1939) and of various components such as isoamyl acetate (MORSE et al., 1967), histamine (OWEN and BRAIDWOOD, 1974), and melittin (BACHMAYER et al., 1972). Evidence suggests that older bees may have a diminished capability for regenerating venom (GALUSZKA, 1972).

The quantity of venom produced has been estimated by various techniques. In the earliest studies, using venom sac extracts (MÜLLER, 1939), the amount of dried venom from the adult worker was reported as about 0.10 mg. This is in surprisingly close agreement with more recent quantitative studies using venom from electrical excitation of single insects (O'CONNOR et al., 1967), giving the value as 0.07 ± 0.03 mg per "sting." From the weight of dried venom and the percentage of water in the natural venom, it is possible to estimate that the average adult worker bee carries at least 0.6 mg of the liquid venom. Since these studies were made under conditions such that the venom sac was rarely emptied completely, it is estimated that the full sac might contain as much as $3-4$ mg of the liquid venom. It should be noted that *Apis dorsata* produces a significantly larger quantity of venom than does *Apis mellifera* (BENTON and MORSE, 1968).

In addition to the age-dependence of venom production, a seasonal variation has been noted (GALUSZKA, 1972). Venom quantity in worker bees appears to be highest during the summer months while the hive is at its peak of activity and relatively young bees are serving as hive guards.

The problem of venom purity is a serous one. While it is obvious that quantitative studies of venom composition cannot be made with contaminated samples such as sac extracts (O'CONNOR et al., 1964a) or venoms containing extraneous material (BENTON and MORSE, 1966), a more subtle difficulty exists. Because of age and seasonal variations in the venom, any description of "pure honey bee venom" must be considered, at least to some extent, as an oversimplification. Since it is obviously not feasible to determine the full extent of these variations, we shall have to be content with what appears to be a reasonable approximation of the venom composition of the "typical adult worker bee."

II. Water Content

Three independent assays of water content have been made, using venom samples withdrawn by microsyringe from freshly extirpated venom sacs (O'CONNOR et al., 1967). Loss of weight on drying is the least reliable method since there are other volatile components in the venom (GUNNISON, 1966). The gravimetric assay, cross-checked by measuring weight gain by a silica gel desiccant, indicated 86 ± 6 percent water. A second technique, involving vapor phase chromatography of the hydrolysis products of 2, 2-dibutoxypropane by venom moisture, gave more precise results. These were subsequently confirmed as 88.3 ± 0.2 percent water by a third assay method—a vapor phase chromatography system for direct water analysis.

III. Volatile Components

It has been known for some time that social bees utilize complex communication systems (LINDAUER, 1957; MASCHWITZ, 1964), including volatile chemicals called pheromones. Among the alarm pheromones of the honey bee are isoamyl acetate (BOCH et al., 1962) and 2-heptanone (SHEARER and BOCH, 1965). Although the 2-heptanone is a mandibular gland secretion (BUTLER, 1966) that may play more than one role in the chemical communication system (SIMPSON, 1966), the isoamyl acetate appears to be a component of the venom itself (GUNNISON, 1966).

Isoamyl acetate content of *Apis mellifera* venom varies with the age of the bee and, apparently, with the role of the bee in the activities of the colony. It has been estimated as $1-5$ µg in adult worker bees (BOCH and SHEARER, 1966). This pheromone is common to the four species of *Apis,* the largest amount per bee occurring in *Apis dorsata* (MORSE et al., 1967).

As many as thirteen volatile components may be present in *Apis mellifera* venom, although only the isoamyl acetate has been fully characterized as yet (GUNNISON, 1966). If we compare the data on weight loss by drying with the percentage water in the venom (O'CONNOR et al., 1967), then volatile components other than water may account for as much as $4-8$ percent (by weight) of the natural liquid venom.

IV. General Composition

The venom of *Apis mellifera* is a very complex mixture of enzymes, polypeptides, and various smaller molecules (Table 1). Because of the problems in obtaining pure venom for analysis, the age and seasonal variations in venom composition, and the difficulties in isolation and purification of single components, our present picture of venom composition must be considered only partially complete. As has been mentioned earlier, much of the work prior to the 1970's must be reviewed carefully in light of more recent investigations. Of particular importance in this respect are the reports that such "completely characterized" components as "melittin" and "phospholipase A" are separable by sophisticated techniques into additional, but closely related, components (Jentsch, 1972; Jentsch and Dielenberg, 1972).

The complexity of this venom is readily apparent from the information in Table 1. While it is entirely possible that other components will be identified in the course of further study of honey bee venom, it is unlikely that any new

Table 1. General character of *Apis mellifera* venom

Type of component	% of Venom[a]	Selected references	Comments
Water	88(l)	O'Connor et al., 1967	from venom sac contents
Volatile compounds (pheromones?) possibly 13 compounds	4—8(l)	Gunnison, 1966	from modified "Cornell Venom Collector"
isoamyl acetate	~0.1(l)	Boch and Shearer, 1966	from ether extract of sac and glands
Enzymes	13—15(s)	Habermann, 1972	review, prior to report of phospholipase A multiplicity
hyaluronidase	1—3(s)	Barker et al., 1966; Kristeva et al., 1973	enzyme primarily responsible for spreading of venom through tissue
phospholipase A *system*	12(s)	Jentsch and Dielenberg, 1972	careful separations reveal two, possibly three, active fractions
[b] phospholipase B	?	Doery and Pearson, 1964	based on studies of "freeze-dried preparation of bee stings" (not confirmed in natural venom)
[b] "esterases and phosphatases"	?	Benton, 1967	suggests an α esterase, a β esterase, two alkaline phosphatases, three acid phosphatases, and possibly two additional phosphatases in natural venom (neither confirmed nor disputed by later studies)

Table 1 (continued)

Large peptides	50–60(s)	PECK and O'CONNOR, 1974	review of basic peptides
melittin (family)	~50(s)	JENTSCH, 1972	separation of "original melittin" into 3 components
mast cell degranulating (MCD) peptide	~2(s)	HANSON et al., 1974	structure determined and activity characterized
apamin	~2(s)	SHIPOLINI et al., 1967; HAUX et al., 1967	a neurotoxin; structure partially determined
minimine	~3(s)	LOWY et al., 1971	acts on *Drosophila* larvae to reduce size of adult; partially characterized
cardiopep[c]	~0.7(s)	VICK et al., 1974	a cardioactive polypeptide; partially characterized (?)
protease inhibitor	?	SHKENDEROV, 1973	partially characterized
Small molecules	~24(s)	PECK and O'CONNOR, 1974	mostly small peptides
histamine-terminal peptide	~1(s)	NELSON and O'CONNOR, 1968	first such compounds definitely characterized from natural source
procamine	~1(s)	PECK and O'CONNOR, 1974	
seven small peptides	~13(s)	REXOVA and MARKOVIC, 1963	amino acid content determined; some may contain histamine
nineteen free amino acids	~1(s)	NELSON and O'CONNOR, 1968	from individual bees
histamine	~1(s)	MARKOVIC and REXOVA, 1963; OWEN and BRAIDWOOD, 1974	age and seasonal variation studied
[b] 5-hydroxytryptamine	?	GRZYCKI and CZERNY, 1973	detected in venom glands, not confirmed in venom itself
[b] dopamine and noradrenaline	?	OWEN, 1971	isolated from punctured venom sacs, not detected in dried venom
[b] vanilmandelic acid	?	SHEPHERD et al., 1974	reported without information on detection method employed
[b] simple sugars	~2(s)	O'CONNOR et al., 1967	glucose and fructose, by chromatographic assay
[b] six phospholipids	~5(s)	O'CONNOR et al., 1967	by colorimetric reagent

[a]   (l)=% of natural liquid venom, (s)=% of dried venom solids.

[b]   Unconfirmed reports.

[c]   Cardiopep, according to a "note added in proof" by the investigators (VICK et al., 1974), is not a polypeptide. At present, this compound must be considered something of a mystery.

substance will be found in significant amounts. The quantitative assays made so far account for most of the dried venom, and the number of enzymes and polypeptides characterized corresponds to the maximum number of "protein" bands observed in electrophoretic separations (BENTON and PATTON, 1965). Further elucidations of the venom composition will probably concentrate on identification of volatile components and more detailed characterization of nonvolatile compounds of physiologic interest.

The following sections provide a more detailed discussion of venom composition.

V. Enzymes

1. Hyaluronidase

The hyaluronidase enzyme systems are found in a wide variety of venoms (HABERMANN, 1972), providing a mechanism for the spreading of venom through tissue by degradation of the hyaluronic acid polymers of the intercellular cement. Hyaluronidase was first detected in the venom of *Apis mellifera* by NEUMANN and HABERMANN (1954a). The enzyme has, as yet, been only partially characterized (Table 2), but it appears to be a β-hexosaminidase with the rather specific activity of releasing from hyaluronic acid only a hexasaccharide, a tetrasaccharide, and a disaccharide (BARKER et al., 1963). Unlike many of the other natural hyaluronidase systems, the enzyme from honey bee venom (about 2 percent of the dry venom) exhibits optimum activity in the pH range of 4—5 (HABERMANN, 1957).

Hyaluronidase is one of the components of the venom that is difficult to isolate in a pure form in significant amounts (BARKER et al., 1966; IVANOV et al.,

Table 2. Studies of *Apis mellifera* venom hyaluronidase and phospholipase A

	Investigators	Information
Hyaluronidase	NEUMANN and HABERMANN, 1954a	first characterization in honey bee venom
	HABERMANN and EL KAREMI, 1956	first report of antigenic character (in rabbit)
	HABERMANN, 1957	optimum activity at pH 4—5
	LOMER et al., 1958	confirmation of antigenic character
	BARKER et al., 1963	products of action on hyaluronic acid
	HABERMANN and REIZ, 1956b	improved isolation and purification methods
	BARKER et al., 1966	antihyaluronidase in γ-globulin from bee keepers
	BARKER et al., 1967	specificity of bee keeper antihyaluronidase to the venom enzyme
	IVANOV et al., 1972	further improvements in isolation and purification methods

Table 2 (continued)

	Investigators	Information
	KRISTEVA et al., 1973	partial characterization
	SHKENDEROV, 1974	mol. wt. ~38,000; anaphylactogenic properties
Phospholipase A	NEUMANN and HABERMANN, 1954b	first characterization in honey bee venom
	HABERMANN and EL KAREMI, 1956	first report of antigenic character (in rabbit)
	LOMER et al., 1958	confirmation of antigenic character
	COLE and SHIPMAN, 1970	radioprotective activity
	MOHAMMED and EL KAREMI, 1961	antiphospholipase in bee keeper serum (not confirmed by studies of BARKER et al., 1966)
	HABERMANN and REIZ, 1965b	improved isolation and purification methods
	VAZQUEZ-COLON and ELLIOTT, 1966	suggested role in action of venom on mitochondria
	BARKER et al., 1966	unable to detect antiphospholipase A in bee keeper serum
	BENTON, 1967	evidence for multiplicity of enzyme system
	FREDHOLM and HAEGERMARK, 1967a, b, 1969	suggested role in histamine-release mechanism
	VOGT et al., 1970	combined activity with melittin in attacking cell membranes
	MUNJAL and ELLIOTT, 1971a, b	further information on antigenic properties; approx. mol. wt (18,000−19,000); activation by Ca^{2+}
	SHIPOLINI et al., 1971a, b	optimum activity at pH ~8.0; amino acid content and sequence suggestions; mol. wt. $> 14,600$, but $< 18,500$; bound carbohydrates
	JENTSCH and DIELENBERG, 1972	at least 2 (possibly 3) components of similar activity; isoelectric point pH 10.0; mol. wt. ~10,900; amino acid composition
	MUNJAL and ELLIOTT, 1972	optimum activity around 50° C, alternative mol. wt. and composition
	MOLLAY and KREIL, 1974	synergistic action with melittin
	SHEPHERD et al., 1974	antigenic properties confirmed
	SHKENDEROV, 1974	anaphylactogenic properties; mol. wt. ~19,000

1972). As a result, little is known about its structure. Arginine appears to be the N-terminal amino acid of the enzyme (KRISTEVA et al., 1973), and four mannose residues were isolated from the hydrolysis products. No free sulfhydryl groups were detected. The molecular weight of the enzyme is reported to be around 38,000 (SHKENDEROV, 1974).

Hyaluronidase has been identified as one of the antigenic components of honey bee venom (HABERMANN and EL KAREMI, 1956; LOMER et al., 1958; SHKENDEROV, 1974). The sera of beekeepers contain antibodies capable of neutralizing bee venom hyaluronidase (BARKER et al., 1967), and this neutralization undoubtedly accounts, to a significant extent, for the immunity of beekeepers to bee sting.

2. Phospholipase A System

The phospholipase A system of *Apis mellifera* venom is classified as phosphatide acyl hydrolase EC 3.1.1.4 on the basis of activity, similar to that of many other venom phospholipases (CONDREA and DE VRIES, 1965). Although this enzyme system has been studied extensively and a partial structure (Fig. 3) has been proposed, there are serious conflicts among recent reports (Table 2) with respect to such fundamental information as molecular weight and amino acid composition. The suggestion of enzyme multiplicity (BENTON, 1967) seems to have been largely ignored by most subsequent investigators, but the evidence that the phospholipase A in honey bee venom is not a single compound is now substantial (JENTSCH and DIELENBERG, 1972). As a result, any attempt to summarize the accumulated body

H_2N–Ile –Ile –Tyr–Pro–Gly–Thr–Leu–Trp–Cys–Gly–His –Gly–Asn
|
Thr –His –Lys –Phe–Arg–Gly–Leu–Glu–Asn–Pro–Gly–Ser –Ser –Lys
|
Asp –Ala–Cys–Cys–Arg–Thr–His –Asp–Met–Cys–Pro–Asn–Val –Met
|
Ser –Ala–Thr–Asp–Thr–Leu–Gly–His –Lys –Ser –Glu–Gly–Ala –Ser
|
Arg –Leu–Ser –Cys–Asn–Asp–Asn–Asp–Leu–Phe–Tyr–Lys–Asp–Ser
|
Phe –Tyr–Met–Lys–Gly–Val –Phe–Tyr–Ser –Ser –Ile –Thr–Asp–Ala
|
Asn –Leu–Ile –Asn–Thr–Lys–Cys–Tyr–Lys –Leu–Glu–His –Pro–Val
|
Tyr –His –Leu–Cys–Arg–Gly –Glu–Thr–Arg–Glu–Gly–Cys–Gly –Thr
|
Thr –Val–Asp–Lys –Ser –Lys –Pro–Lys–Val –Tyr–Gln–Trp–Phe–Asp
|
Tyr–Lys –Arg–Leu

(C-terminal)

Fig. 3. Proposed amino acid sequence for honey bee venom phospholipase A (SHIPOLINI et al., 1971 b). In light of evidence suggesting enzyme multiplicity (JENTSCH and DIELENBERG, 1972), this sequence must be considered as uncertain at present. The strongly basic character suggests that there are few free carboxyl groups. Binding sites of carbohydrate moieties have not been identified

of knowledge concerning bee venom phospholipase A must contain significant uncertainties.

JENTSCH and DIELENBERG (1972) have described the "total phospholipase A" system as having a "molecular weight of 10,900" and as containing 100—102 amino acids, with isoleucine as the N-terminal unit. Other investigators, apparently working with essentially the same fraction of the venom, have claimed molecular weights and amino acid contents, respectively, ranging from ∼15,000 with 129 amino acids (SHIPOLINI et al., 1971a)[5] to 18,000—19,000 with 183 amino acids (MUNJAL and ELLIOTT, 1972). It is generally agreed that the enzyme system is quite basic, having an isoelectric point around pH 10. Some of the problems in molecular weight determination may arise from covalently bound carbohydrate (SHIPOLINI et al., 1971a)[5] and differences in amino acid analyses may reflect varying degrees of inhomogeneity of samples isolated in slightly different ways. In any event, no structural information can be properly evaluated until the problem of enzyme multiplicity is resolved and careful investigations can be made of pure single substances. Until such studies are completed, we shall have to be content with some relatively general descriptions of the phospholipase A "system".

It has long been recognized that bee venom has certain similarities to various snake venoms (TETSCH and WOLF, 1936; GRASSMAN and HANNIG, 1954). An important aspect of this similarity is in the phospholipase A content (CONDREA and DE VRIES, 1965). Like other venom phospholipase A systems, that of the honey bee is fairly stable to heat and is activated by Ca^{2+} ion (MUNJAL and ELLIOTT, 1972). The honey bee enzyme is reported to contain covalently bound glucosamine, mannose, galactose, and fucose (SHIPOLINI et al., 1971b)[5].

Bee venom phospholipase A has been associated with a number of pharmacologic effects (CONDREA and DE VRIES, 1965; HABERMANN, 1972). The most obvious, of course, is its potent attack on structural phospholipids, in which A_2-type activity is exhibited (SHIPOLINI et al., 1971a)[5]. Although the purified enzyme system alone has no effect on cell membranes, it undoubtedly contributes to the hemolytic properties of whole bee venom via a synergistic action with melittin (VOGT et al., 1970; MOLLAY and KREIL, 1974). The role of this enzyme system in allergic response to insect sting is also indicated (MUNJAL and ELLIOTT, 1971a; SHKENDEROV, 1974; SHEPHERD et al., 1974), although the formation of protective antibodies in bee-keepers, unlike the case of hyaluronidase, is uncertain (MOHAMMED and EL KAREMI, 1961; BARKER et al., 1966).

Although bee venom phospholipase A is reported to have a significant action as a radioprotective system (COLE and SHIPMAN, 1970), the mechanism of this activity is unknown.

3. Other Enzyme Studies

The number of different "protein" components of bee venom is still uncertain. While incomplete separations obviously reveal too few components, it is equally probable that studies of "pooled" venoms from bees of varying ages would suggest more components than are present in the venom of the "typical adult worker

---

[5] SHIPOLINI refers in his papers to the European honey bee as *Apis mellifaca*. This is an older nomenclature, and Systematic Entomology has replaced *mellifaca* with *mellifera*.

bee," since transient precursors to certain components have been identified in the venoms of immature insects (BACHMEYER et al., 1972). If we accept a figure of twelve (BENTON and PATTON, 1965) for the number of "protein" components of the venom, then eleven of these are accounted for by well-characterized components (Table 1). This is inconsistent with the report of a number of additional enzymes (BENTON, 1967). It is, of course, possible that there are more than twelve "protein" components in the venom. It is, perhaps, more likely that some of the components observed in developed zymograms are artifacts of the experimental techniques employed. In the absence of confirming investigations, the reported 2 esterases and 5 — 7 phosphatases must be considered as still open to question.

A phospholipase B activity has been reported (DOERY and PEARSON, 1964), but the source of the enzyme ("freeze-dried preparation of bee stings") and the failure of subsequent investigations to detect this enzyme have led to the general conclusion that its presence in pure venom is doubtful (HABERMANN, 1972).

Bee venom reportedly contains no proteolytic enzymes, while the presence of a protease inhibitor in the venom apparently serves to protect certain venom components from the protease systems of sting victims (SHKENDEROV, 1973).

Although investigations of enzymatic activity of honey bee venom have been underway for many years (TETSCH and WOLFF, 1936; SCHOENTENSACK, 1953), there are still many unanswered questions. It is apparent that the problems of enzyme multiplicity, structure, and activity will require extensive further research.

VI. Large Peptides

1. General Characteristics

The larger peptides characterized in honey bee venom are in the molecular weight range of 2000 — 6000 (PECK and O'CONNOR, 1974) and are strongly basic (Table 3). All have potent physiologic activities. These peptides account for 50 — 60 percent of the dry venom.

The melittin family, constituting the major polypeptide fraction, consists of at least three closely related peptides. This family exhibits pronounced surfactant properties and potent hemolytic activity. Apamin is a powerful neurotoxin, and the mast cell degranulating (MCD) peptide plays a role in the release of histamine from mast cells. Another peptide acts as a protease inhibitor, apparently to protect

Table 3. Studies of larger polypeptides from *Apis mellifera* venom

	Investigators	Information
"Melittin"	MOLLAY and KREIL, 1974	synergistic action with phospholipase A
	SHKENDEROV, 1974	lack of anaphylactogenic properties
	OLSON et al., 1974	effects on mitochondria
	SHEPHERD et al., 1974	antigenic properties
	VYATCHANNIKOV, 1973	effect on central nervous system
	KREIL, 1973a	comparisons among species of bees

Table 3 (continued)

	Investigators	Information
	KREIL, 1973b	biosynthesis and precursor structure
	HEGNER et al., 1973	mechanism of attack on cell membranes
	BACHMAYER et al., 1972	biosynthesis during maturation
	JENTSCH, 1972	separation of "original melittin" into three components
	VICK et al., 1972; VICK and SHIPMAN, 1972	effect on plasma cortisol
	HABERMANN, 1972	review, through 1971
	DIRKS and STERNBURG, 1972	non-immunochemical complexing with rabbit sera
	MIURA et al., 1972	synthesis of 19-tyrosine melittin
	BROOKS and VICK, 1972	toxicity studies
	KREIL and BACHMAYER, 1971	biosynthesis and precursor detection
	MITCHELL et al., 1971	toxicity to *Drosophila* and inhibition of acetylcholinesterase
	LOWY et al., 1971	separation of two "melittin" components
	SCHRÖDER et al., 1971	hemolytic and surfactant properties
	LÜBKE et al., 1971	natural formyl derivative identified
	MUNJAL and ELLIOTT, 1971a	antigenic properties
	HABERMANN and KOWALLEK, 1970	structure modifications and activity
	HABERMANN and ZEUNER, 1970	comparison of possible members of the "melittins group"
	VOGT et al., 1970	synergistic action with phospholipase A
	BHARGAVA et al., 1970	possible association with hemorrhagic action of the venom
	JENTSCH, 1969	conformation in an aqueous medium
	SESSA et al., 1969	interaction with lipid membrane systems
	SHIPMAN and COLE, 1969	improved separations and surfactant character
	GINSBERG et al., 1968	radioprotective activity
	HEGNER and SCHNORR, 1968	action on membranes
	HABERMANN, 1968	review, through 1967
	KREIL and KREIL-KISS, 1967	evidence for natural formyl derivative
	HABERMANN and JENTSCH, 1967 and 1966	amino acid sequence studies
	KREIL, 1965	partial characterization
	HABERMANN and REIZ, 1965a	biochemical studies

Table 3 (continued)

	Investigators	Information
	HABERMANN, 1955	membrane permeability studies
	HABERMANN, 1954; NEUMANN and HABERMANN, 1954a	initial studies
Apamin	SHKENDEROV, 1974	lack of anaphylactogenic properties
	SHEPHERD et al., 1974	antigenic properties
	SPOERRI et al., 1973	neurotoxic effects
	HABERMANN, 1972	review and suggestion of possible substituted form
	VICK and SHIPMAN, 1972	effect on plasma cortisol
	BROOKS and VICK, 1972	toxicity in mice, dogs, and monkeys
	MUNJAL and ELLIOTT, 1971a	apparent lack of antigenic properties
	VOGT et al., 1970	synergistic action with phospholipase A
	WELLHÖNER, 1969	studies of neurotoxic mechanism
	CALLEWAERT et al., 1968	structural information
	SHIPOLINI et al., 1967	partial structure determination
	HAUX et al., 1967	amino acid sequence
	HABERMANN and REIZ, 1965b	improved isolation procedure
	NEUMANN and HABERMANN, 1954a	initial studies
MCD Peptide	HANSON et al., 1974	anti-inflammatory properties
	BILLINGHAM et al., 1973	anti-inflammatory properties
	HABERMANN, 1972	review
	HIGGENBOTHAM and KARNELLA, 1970	possible role in protecting against venom action by heparin release
	HAUX, 1969	amino acid sequence
	FREDHOLM and HAEGERMARK, 1967a, b, 1969	histamine release from mast cells
	BREITHAUPT and HABERMANN, 1968	improved isolation and study of properties
	FREDHOLM, 1966	first isolation
Minimine	HABERMANN, 1972	suggestion of possible contamination by phospholipase A
	LOWY et al., 1971	isolation, amino acid content, action in producing miniature adult *Drosophila*
Protease inhibitor	SHKENDEROV, 1973	isolation, mol. wt., properties

A report of a cardioactive peptide, "Cardiopep" (VICK et al., 1974), concludes with the rather unusual "note added in proof" that "cardiopep is not a polypeptide". Thus, the nature of this substance is as yet unknown.

certain venom components from the action of proteolytic enzymes. All of these compounds can be recognized as contributing significantly to the normal properties of a defensive venom. Minimine, on the other hand, has not been associated with such "typical" activity. The unusual attribute of minimine is its effect on the development of *Drosophila*. An injection of minimine into the larvae results in the production of miniature adult *Drosophila,* many as small as one-fourth normal size.

It is possible that additional polypeptides, not yet characterized, may be present in the venom, since not all the bands observed in electrophoretic separations are yet accounted for. It is also possible that some of the peptides studied thus far are not chemically homogeneous. Further investigations of these pharmacologically interesting compounds will undoubtedly shed more light on the problems still unresolved.

2. The Melittin Family

About half of the dry weight of the venom consists of a family of closely related peptides, the melittins (JENTSCH, 1972; HABERMANN, 1972). When first identified (NEUMANN and HABERMANN, 1954a), this fraction of the venom was believed to be a single compound, and the initial chemical characterizations were made under this assumption (KREIL, 1965; HABERMANN and JENTSCH, 1966). Later studies revealed a second natural component of the melittin fraction, the N_α-formyl derivative (KREIL and KREIL-KISS, 1967), and recent investigations indicate at least one more component (JENTSCH, 1972). In addition, studies of the biosynthesis of melittins indicate a precursor, promelittin (KREIL and BACHMAYER, 1971; BACHMAYER et al., 1972; KREIL, 1973b). Although promelittin appears to be converted into melittin during maturation, significant amounts of the precursor peptide are still present in the venom of young bees (BACHMAYER et al., 1972).

The principal component of this peptide family, melittin I, and the natural N_α-formyl melittin I have been prepared synthetically (LÜBKE et al., 1971). The proposed amino acid sequence (Figure 4) is consistent with the known surfactant properties of the melittins (HABERMANN, 1972), with a basic hydrophilic region (positions 21—26) connected to a generally hydrophobic region (positions 1—20). Optical rotatory dispersion studies suggest a random conformation of the peptide chain in an aqueous medium (JENTSCH, 1969).

Although the melittins are not apparently associated with the anaphylactogenic properties of bee venom (SHKENDEROV, 1974), they may be among the antigenic components (SHEPHERD et al., 1974; MUNJAL and ELLIOTT, 1971a). However, it has been suggested that their apparent antigenicity may, in fact, involve a nonimmunochemical complexing (DIRKS and STERNBURG, 1972).

The melittins form one of the more toxic fractions of honey bee venom (BENTON and MORSE, 1968; BROOKS and VICK, 1972), having a toxicity of about 4 mg/kg for intravenous injection in mice (HABERMANN, 1972). The pronounced surfactant properties of the melittins undoubtedly contribute to their potent direct hemolytic activity (HABERMANN and REIZ, 1965a; SHIPMAN and COLE, 1969; HABERMANN and KOWALLEK, 1970; SCHRÖDER et al., 1971). In addition, a synergism with phospholipase A has been demonstrated (VOGT et al., 1970; MOLLAY and KREIL, 1974).

[position of formyl substitution in N_α-formyl derivative]
↓
H₂N–Gly –Ile –Gly–Ala–Val–Leu
     1   2   3   4   5   6
                                                |
Leu –Gly –Thr–Thr–Leu–Val –Lys
13   12   11   10   9   8   7
  |
Pro –Ala –Leu–Ile –Ser –Trp–Ile
14   15   16   17   18   19   20
                                          |
    Gln –Gln–Arg–Lys–Arg–Lys
    26   25   24   23   22   21
     |
    NH₂

[C-terminal]

Fig. 4. Proposed structures of melittin I and N_α-formyl melittin I (HABERMANN and JENTSCH, 1967; LÜBKE et al., 1971). Note basic hydrophilic character of positions 21—26

Other physiologic effects of the melittin family include attack on mitochondria (OLSON et al., 1974); interference with the central nervous system as shown by its inhibition of the general behavior, exploratory activities, and emotional response of mice (VYATCHANNIKOV and SINKA, 1973); noncompetitive inhibition of acetylcholinesterase (MITCHELL et al., 1971); elevation of plasma cortisol levels (VICK et al., 1972; VICK and SHIPMAN, 1972); and protective action against radiation damage (GINSBERG et al., 1968). Since melittin significantly decreases the interfacial tension between air and salt solutions, it is generally believed that melittin increases the permeability of erythrocytes by physicochemical action (HEGNER et al., 1973; HABERMANN, 1972). The structure—surface activity relationship of this family of compounds has been the object of extensive investigations (HABERMANN and KOWALLEK, 1970).

The melittin family is not unique to *Apis mellifera*. Similar peptides are found in other *Apis* venoms (KREIL, 1973a).

3. Apamin, a Neurotoxin[6]

Like "melittin", "apamin" may be more than a single compound, possibly varying by a single substitution as in the N_α-formyl melittin (HABERMANN, 1972). Although the apamin fraction of bee venom constitutes only about 2 percent of the dry venom, it is of considerable interest as the smallest known peptide(s) having neurotoxic activity.

The apamin fraction of *Apis mellifera* venom was first studied by NEUMANN and HABERMANN (1954a). Later improvements in isolation and purification techniques (HABERMANN and REIZ, 1965b) facilitated pharmacologic and chemical

[6] For an interesting suggestion of structures for apamin and the MCD peptide, see: WARNER, D.T.: Additional application of the hexagonal conformation of calcitonin, myoglobin and other proteins of known sequence. J. Theor. Biol. **46**, 329—351 (1974)

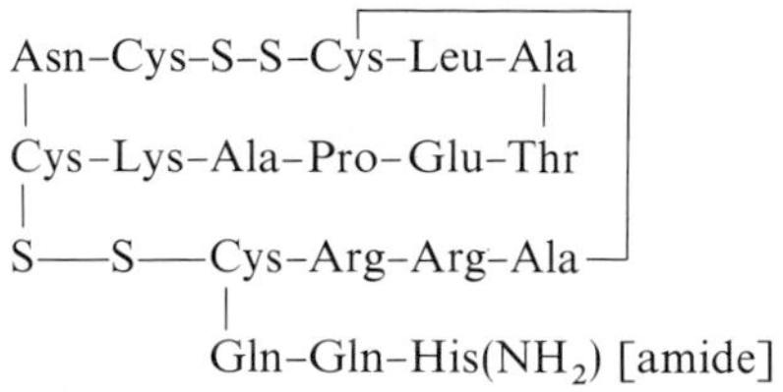

Asn–Cys–S–S–Cys–Leu–Ala
 |
Cys–Lys–Ala–Pro–Glu–Thr
 |
S——S——Cys–Arg–Arg–Ala
                |
     Gln–Gln–His(NH$_2$) [amide]

Fig. 5. Proposed structure of apamin (CALLEWAERT et al., 1968; SHIPOLINI et al., 1967; HAUX et al., 1967). Possible sites of substitution for alternate natural form are uncertain

studies, and a structure has now been proposed (Figure 5). Like melittin, the apamin fraction is quite basic.

Although antigenic properties have been claimed for the apamin fraction (SHEP-HERD et al., 1974), these were not found by MUNJAL and ELLIOTT (1971a), and the lack of anaphylactogenicity has been demonstrated (SHKENDEROV, 1974).

Similarities between melittin and apamin fractions of bee venom are observed in terms of toxicity (HABERMANN, 1972; BROOKS and VICK, 1972), effects on plasma cortisol levels (VICK and SHIPMAN, 1972), and a possible synergism with phospholipase A (VOGT et al., 1970). Possibly because of its more compact structure, due to the disulfide linkages, apamin lacks the surfactant character of melittin.

From studies of apamin's activity on the spinal cord, it has been found that apamin augments polysynaptic reflexes and that it causes excitatory polysynaptic pathways to become more effective than inhibitory polysynaptic mechanisms (WELLHÖNER, 1969).

4. The Mast Cell Degranulating (MCD) Peptide[6]

The role of histamine in honey bee envenomation has long been recognized (NAGA-MITU, 1935). Although the venom itself contains a small amount of histamine (MARKOVIC and REXOVA, 1963), this is insufficient to account for the physiologic effects of the whole venom. Both the melittin and phospholipase A fractions of the venom are capable of releasing histamine by destruction of mast cells (HABER-MANN, 1972), but careful studies (FREDHOLM, 1966) indicated a third, more powerful, mast cell degranulating agent. This so-called MCD peptide has been isolated (BREIT-

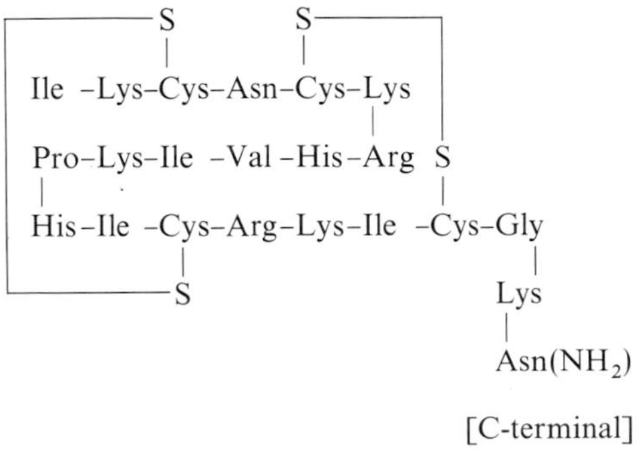

```
        ┌──────S        S──────┐
        │      │        │      │
       Ile –Lys–Cys–Asn–Cys–Lys │
        │                │      │
       Pro–Lys–Ile –Val –His–Arg  S
        │                       │
       His–Ile –Cys–Arg–Lys–Ile –Cys–Gly
        │        │               │
        └────────S        S      Lys
                                  │
                              Asn(NH₂)
```

Asn(NH$_2$)

[C-terminal]

Fig. 6. Proposed structure of the MCD peptide (HAUX, 1969; VERNON et al., 1969)

HAUPT and HABERMANN, 1968), and its role in histamine release has been extensively investigated (FREDHOLM and HAEGERMARK, 1967a, b, 1969). An amino acid sequence has been proposed (Fig. 6).

The MCD peptide has been associated with anti-inflammatory properties (HANSON et al., 1974; BILLINGHAM et al., 1973) and with a possible mechanism of venom resistance by heparin released by disruption of dermal mast cells (HIGGENBOTHAM and KARNELLA, 1970). Although the MCD peptide is a minor component (about 2 percent) of the dry venom, its pharmacologic activity certainly justifies continued investigation.

5. Other Active Peptides

During studies of the effects of bee venom on larvae of *Drosophila melanogaster,* a venom fraction was observed to have a most unusual activity (LOWY et al., 1971). When injected at moderate concentrations into the *Drosophila* larvae, this fraction stopped larval growth without preventing metamorphosis. The developing adults were miniature, some as small as one-fourth normal size. Progeny of the miniature flies appeared normal in all respects. In the belief that the growth-retarding agent was a single peptide, the investigators determined an apparent molecular weight of around 6000, corresponding to 48 — 52 amino acids. The amino acid content of their substance, termed "minimine," is different from that of melittin. However, in light of HABERMANN'S (1972) suggestion of possible contamination of the "minimine" fraction by phospholipase A, it is important to note that all of the amino acids reported for "minimine" are found in phospholipase A. Further studies of the "minimine" fraction will be necessary before we may safely conclude that "minimine" is, indeed, a unique peptide.

SHENDEROV (1973) has recently reported the isolation from *Apis mellifera* venom of a new peptide having a pronounced activity as a protease inhibitor. A molecular weight in the 8000 — 10,000 range is indicated, along with evidence for disulfide (but no sulfhydryl) groups. Additional information awaits further investigation.

The report of a cardioactive compound, "cardiopep," capable of increasing heart rate, aortic blood, and right ventricular force, and of restoring normal cardiac rhythm in arrhythmic hearts without significant changes in arterial blood pressure, central venous pressure or cortical activity (VICK et al., 1974), concludes with a "note added in proof" that the substance is "not a polypeptide." Further in investigations are being conducted on this mysterious and intriguing material.

VII. Small Molecules

1. Some General Considerations

The smaller molecules found in bee venom (Table 4) have received relatively little attention as compared to the pharmacologically active polypeptides and enzymes. In fact, the identification in the venom of small peptides, histamine, and free amino acids, for example, raises some significant questions which have not really been explored. What role, if any, do these compounds play in the action of the venom? Histamine, of course, has a potent activity, but it is not present in a

Table 4. Small molecules in *Apis mellifera* venom

Compounds	% of Venom[a]	Investigators	Comments
Small peptides	~15(s) %	NELSON and O'CONNOR, 1968	
seven small peptides, yielding on hydrolysis: (1) Ala, Asp (2) Ala, Asp, Pro (3) Ala, Glu, Val (4) Asp, Val (5) Ala, Glu, Pro (6) Arg, Glu, Lys (7) Glu, Lys, Val		REXOVA and MARKOVIC, 1963	from "native venom", isolated by electrophoresis and chromatography; possible indication of some histamine-containing peptides
seven additonal peptides, including: Ala-Gly-Pro-Ala-Gln — Histamine	~1(s) %	NELSON and O'CONNOR, 1968	first characterization of a histamine-containing peptide from a natural source
procamine: Ala-Gly-Gln-Gly — Histamine	~1(s) %	PECK and O'CONNOR, 1974	first synthesis of a natural histamine-peptide
Free amino acids			
nineteen: Ala, Arg, Asp, Cys, Glu, Gly, His, Ile, Leu, Lys, Orn, Phe, Pro, Ser, Thr, Tyr, Val, γ-aminobutyric acid and β-aminoisobutyric acid	~1(s) %	NELSON and O'CONNOR, 1968	quantitative assay, using venom from individually excited bees
Biogenic amines			
histamine	~1%(s)	NAGAMITU, 1935	first suggestion of histamine in bee venom
		WERLE and GLEISSNER, 1951	detection in sac extract
		MARKOVIC and MOLNAR, 1954	first quantitative study
		MARKOVIC and REXOVA, 1963	histamine variation with time and location of venom collection
		OWEN and BRAIDWOOD, 1974	histamine variation with age of bee
5-hydroxytryptamine	(?)	WELSH and MOORHEAD, 1960; CRZYCKI and CZERNY, 1973	detected in venom apparatus; *not reported in venom itself*
dopamine and noradrenaline	(?)	OWEN, 1971	reported in venom reservoir, *not identified in venom itself*

Table 4 (continued)

Compounds	% of Venom[a]	Investigators	Comments
Non-nitrogenous compounds			
glucose and fructose	~2% (s)	O'CONNOR et al., 1967	detected by chromato-
lipids (unidentified)	~5% (s)		graphic and colorimetric assay only; not reported by other investigators
vanilmandelic acid	(?)	SHEPHERD et al., 1974	detection method employed not specific: possibly a contaminant rather than part of the venom
thirteen "volatile compounds", including:	4–8% (1)	GUNNISON, 1966 BOCH and SHEARER,	% uncertain an alarm pheromone
isoamyl acetate	~0.1% (1)	1966; MORSE et al., 1967	

[a] (1) = % of natural liquid venom, (s) = % of dried venom solids.

significant amount. Do these small molecules help in controlling the pH of the venom? Do they, in some way, enhance the activity of other components, or are they present just as the result of some "biological accident"? Might some, or all, of the small peptides have significant biological activity, either alone or in synergism with other components? These are some of the questions that may prove difficult to answer, but that should prove stimulating to further investigation.

Of additional interest are questions relating to the origin of the small molecules in the venom. Studies of the biosynthesis of melittin (KREIL, 1973b) indicate a rather unusual phenomenon. Precursors, mainly "promelittin", contain more amino acids than does melittin itself. Somehow these are removed during the course of melittin formation, and the resulting fragments may account for some of the small peptides and free amino acids found in the venom. Studies of biosynthetic mechanisms for production of other venom components may indicate similar phenomena. However, quantitative investigations reveal much lower concentrations of amino acids and small peptides than would be expected from complete melittin production via cleavage of larger precursors. In addition, the mechanism of precursor cleavage is of interest. If, as has been reported, the venom contains a protease inhibitor (SHKENDEROV, 1973) and lacks proteolytic enzymes (SHKENDEROV, 1973; NELSON and O'CONNOR, 1968), then it seems unlikely that precursor cleavage occurs in the aqueous medium of the venom itself. The alternative possibility of some reabsorption of precursor molecules by specialized cells in the venom gland is an interesting speculation and could account for the differences between melittin content and "fragment content" of the venom.

Volatile components, at least one of which has been characterized as an alarm pheromone (GUNNISON, 1966; BOCH and SHEARER, 1966; MORSE et al., 1967), pose additional questions. If, indeed, such components are part of the venom actually injected during stinging, how are they released to the atmosphere to serve as chemical communicating agents to other bees? If, on the other hand, these volatile

agents are somehow released around, rather than through, the inserted sting shaft
or, perhaps, secreted prior to actual stinging, what are the chemical agents involved
and how do they act to transmit a message? The whole subject of honey bee
pheromones poses a rich field for further research.

Of particular interest, in connection with the early reports of formic acid,
is the identification of N_α-formyl melittin (KREIL and KREIL-KISS, 1967). This
may account for the detection of traces of formic acid in venom gland extracts
(ELSER, 1924) and the apparent absence of formic acid from the venom itself
(O'CONNOR et al., 1965).

It is apparent that the questions posed by small molecules reported in honey
bee venom could justify considerable further study.

2. Small Peptides and Free Amino Acids

A series of apparent melittin-precursors have been described (BACHMEYER et al.,
1972; KREIL, 1973b). These appear to fragment by loss of C-terminal amino acids
during the formation of melittin, and this fragmentation might account for some
of the small peptides and free amino acids found in the venom. Although proteolytic
enzymes have not been detected in the venom, fragmentation of precursor polypeptides might involve proteases in the glandular cells. On the other hand, promelittin
is reported to be highly resistant to all proteases except pronase (KREIL, 1973b),
and this particular enzyme may have been undetected by the general protease
assay employed (NELSON and O'CONNOR, 1968) and unaffected by the protease
inhibitor in the venom (SHKENDEROV, 1973), whose activity has been demonstrated
only against trypsin. In any event, all of the amino acids suggested for melittin
precursor fragments are found free in the venom and, in fact, one of the peptides
described by REXOVA and MARKOVIC (1963) is consistent with a tripeptide segment
of promelittin (Fig. 7). Others of the small peptides and free amino acids might

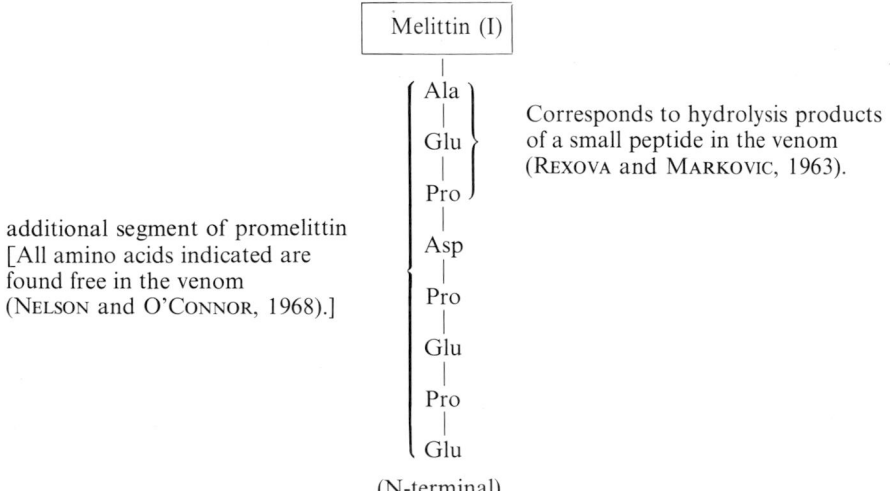

Fig. 7. Promelittin (BACHMEYER et al., 1972; KREIL, 1973), a possible source of amino acids
and small peptides in *Apis mellifera* venom

conceivably originate by similar precursor fragmentation during biosynthesis of other venom polypeptides.

Of particular interest are small peptides containing histamine in lieu of a C-terminal amino acid. The presence in honey bee venom of such compounds, never before detected in nature, was suggested by the early investigations of REXOVA and MARKOVIC (1963). Two histamine-peptides have now been completely characterized (NELSON and O'CONNOR, 1968) and one, procamine, has been produced synthetically (PECK and O'CONNOR, 1974). Little is known yet of the pharmacology of compounds of this type (AROLD and RIETSCHEL, 1969; ROCHA E SILVA, 1943, 1944), and it is hoped that investigations now in progress (PECK et al., 1975) will reveal information of interest about histamine-terminal peptides.

3. Biogenic Amines

Four nitrogenous bases have been reported as associated with *Apis mellifera* venom. Of these, only histamine has been detected in the venom itself (MARKOVIC and MOLNAR, 1954). Dopamine and noradrenaline (OWEN, 1971) and 5-hydroxytryptamine (WELSH and MOORHEAD, 1960; GRZYCKI and CZERNY, 1973) have been reported only in studies of venom glands and sacs.

Like other venom components, histamine content of the venom shows both seasonal (MARKOVIC and REXOVA, 1963) and age variations (OWEN and BRAIDWOOD, 1974). Histamine appears to be first detectable in week-old bees, after which concentrations peak around three to four weeks after emergence and drop off in older bees. Although histamine could account for some of the physiologic response to bee sting, the low histamine content of the venom is probably insignificant when compared to the histamine released during mast cell destruction by melittin, phospholipase A, and the MCD peptide.

4. Non-Nitrogenous Compounds

Among the small molecules reported as present in honey bee venom are a series of lipids and simple sugars (O'CONNOR et al., 1967), vanilmandelic acid (SHEPHERD et al., 1974), and a number of volatile compounds (GUNNISON, 1966). Only one of the volatile substances, isoamyl acetate, has been identified (BOCH and SHEARER, 1966; MORSE et al., 1967). The other reports have not been verified by independent investigation and are based on rather sketchy evidence, at best. For the present, it is safest to assume that a knowledge of the non-nitrogenous compounds in honey bee venom must await more definitive studies.

VIII. Compounds Shown to be Absent

Venoms exhibit a broad spectrum of chemical compositions (MEBS, 1973; ZLOTKIN, 1973), so evidence of the absence of certain compounds or types of compounds is important to the characterization of a unique venom.

If nothing else, it is devoutly to be hoped that the extensive studies of bee venom will finally lay to rest the ancient, but oft repeated, idea that honey bee venom is mainly formic acid (LANGER, 1897). However, the myth may be perpetuated for a few more generations by introductory textbooks of organic chemistry, which sometimes appear to contain sections derived by a process of nonselective plagiarism from nineteenth-century texts.

Among the compounds found in venoms of various snakes, but demonstrated to be absent from honey bee venom are the common proteolytic enzymes (O'CONNOR et al., 1967; SHKENDEROV, 1973) and "nerve growth factor" (PEARCE, 1973). It is perhaps more meaningful to compare honey bee venom with those of other *Hymenoptera*. In this respect, it is noteworthy that the pain-producing kinin peptides and acetylcholine of wasp and hornet venoms are absent from the venom of *Apis mellifera* (HABERMANN, 1972).

IX. Summary of Unresolved Questions on Venom Composition

The fundamental questions of how the venom is produced biosynthetically and of what importance the various components have to the natural function of the total venom system have only begun to be explored. Of smaller scope, but still important, is the necessity to confirm or refute reports of components such as phospholipase B (DOERY and PEARSON, 1964), non-nitrogenous small molecules and some biogenic amines (Table 4), and possible additional enzymes (BENTON, 1967) and proteins (BENTON and PATTON, 1965; MELLO, 1970). The questions of possible contamination (HABERMANN, 1972) of minimine (LOWY et al., 1971) and the strange case of the "nonpeptide" cardiopep (VICK et al., 1974) have still to be resolved, as do the special problems of apparent multiplicity in some of the more extensively studied components (HABERMANN, 1972; JENTSCH, 1972; JENTSCH and DIELENBERG, 1972).

The venom of the honey bee is a very complex mixture and the ultimate determination of its origin, composition, and function will not be an easy task. It is, however, this very complexity that makes further research in this field both challenging and exciting.

C. Physiologic Activity of Apis mellifera Venom

I. Direct and Indirect Activity

Most of the pharmacology of honey bee venom is based on studies of the whole venom, single major components, or pairs of major components. As a result, little is known of the biological activity of the numerous minor components of the venom or of the roles these might play in affecting the activities of other components. In addition, many of the studies have employed incompletely purified fractions of the venom, so that some of the reports of biological activity may have involved the actions of component mixtures, rather than of the single compounds believed under investigation.

The net effects of bee venom on an organism depend upon both direct and indirect activities of venom components (HABERMANN, 1972). Direct activities in terms of toxicity, antigenicity, and cellular rupture have been related to certain specific components (Table 5), but this should not be interpreted as ruling out

Table 5. Some direct activities of *Apis mellifera* venom and known component contributions

Activity	Whole venom or component	Investigators	Comments
Toxicity	whole venom	BROOKS and VICK, 1972	LD$_{50}$ for mice: 1.75 mg/kg (iv), 3.5 mg/kg (sc); LD$_{100}$ for dogs: 5 mg/kg (iv), 200 mg/kg (sc).
		BENTON and MORSE, 1968	*Apis dorsata* venom about as toxic as that of *A. mellifera*; *A. indica* about twice as toxic
		BENTON et al., 1966	mortality reduced by lowering body temperature
	melittin	HABERMANN, 1972	in mice (iv): 4 mg/kg
	apamin		4 mg/kg
	MCD peptide		> 40 mg/kg
	phospholipase A		7.5 mg/kg
Antigenicity	whole venom	CHRISTY, 1967	involved in sting fatalities
	whole venom phospholipase A hyaluronidase	SHKENDEROV, 1974	anaphylactogenicity demonstrated with guinea pigs
	melittin apamin MCD peptide		not anaphylactogenic with guinea pigs
	whole venom	O'CONNOR and ERICKSON, 1965	some common antigenicity with venoms of other Hymenoptera
	hyaluronidase	BARKER et al., 1967	antihyaluronidase in bee keeper serum
	phospholipase A	SHEPHERD et al., 1974; MUNJAL and ELLIOTT, 1971a	antibodies detected in mice and rabbits
	melittin apamin	SHEPHERD et al., 1974	suggested antigenicity, but observations might have involved nonimmunochemical complexing (DIRKS and STERNBURG, 1972)
Localized pain and itching	whole venom	PURSLEY, 1973	reactions of increasing severity also described

Table 5 (continued)

Activity	Whole venom or component	Investigators	Comments
	histamine melittin	HABERMANN, 1972	other components may contribute
Spreading through tissue	hyaluronidase	BARKER et al., 1963; HABERMANN, 1957	selective attack on tissue hyaluronic acid polymers
Direct hemolysis	whole venom	VINCENT et al., 1972	inhibited by heparin
	melittin	HABERMANN, 1972; SCHRÖDER et al., 1971; HABERMANN and KOWALLEK, 1970	hemolytic activity apparently associated with surfactant character of the molecule
Mastocytolysis (see also Table 6)	melittin	HABERMANN, 1972	review
	MCD peptide	BREITHAUPT and HABERMANN, 1968	shown to be much more potent than melittin
		HIGGENBOTHAM and KARNELLA, 1971	possible role in counteraction of envenomation
Neurotoxicity	whole venom	HAHN and OSTERMAYER, 1936	first evidence of a neurotoxin in bee venom
	apamin	WELLHÖNER, 1969	demonstrated attack on spinal cord
Anti-inflammatory properties	whole venom	BECK, 1935	suggested applications in treatment of rheumatoid arthritis
	MCD peptide	HANSON et al., 1974; BILLINGHAM et al., 1973	apparent function involves vascular endothelium
Enzyme inhibition or destruction	protease inhibitor	SHKENDEROV, 1973	trypsin inhibition
	melittin	MITCHELL et al., 1971	antiacetylcholinesterase activity
	phospholipase A	HABERMANN, 1972	modifications of structurebound enzymes
Radioprotection	whole venom	SHIPMAN and COLE, 1967	best protection (for mice) when injected (sc) 24 hours prior to exposure
	melittin	GINSBERG et al., 1968	more effective than whole venom

Table 5 (continued)

Activity	Whole venom or component	Investigators	Comments
	phospholipase A	Cole and Shipman, 1970	first report of radioprotective properties
Elevation of plasma cortisol levels	whole venom melittin apamin	Vick and Shipman, 1972; Vick et al., 1972	suggest stimulation of adrenal cortex
Inhibition of mito-chondrial function	whole venom	Vazquez-Colon and Elliott, 1966	apparently affects oxidative phosphor-ylation
	melittin	Olson et al., 1974	prevents phosphate acceptor control at low concentrations; blocks mitochondrial respiration at higher concen-trations
Other Activities		Habermann, 1972	review

the possibility that other components, not yet fully investigated, may have similar activities or may act in the natural venom to alter the activities of compounds such as melittin or phospholipase A.

Indirect activity (Table 6) refers to the release of chemicals within the envenom-ated organism, as initiated by venom components. Both histamine release by mast cell degranulation and hemolysis by lysophospholipids released by action of phospholipase A are examples of indirect activity of venom components.

Table 6. Some indirect activities of components of *Apis mellifera* venom

Histamine release via mastocytolysis		Indirect hemolysis	
Review of factors involved in hist-amine release	Habermann, 1972	Review of factors involved in hemo-lytic activity	Habermann, 1972
Detailed studies of mechanism of histamine release	Fredholm and Haegermark, 1967a, b; 1969; Fredholm, 1966	Resistance of cellular lipids to phospholipase alone; cytolytic activity of lysolecithins produced by phospho-lipase A	Shipolini et al., 1971; Neumann and Haber-mann, 1954b; Habermann, 1958
Selectivity of the MCD peptide ("MCL peptide")	Habermann and Breithaupt, 1968	Synergism of phospholipase A with melittin	Mollay and Kreil 1974

The hemolytic activity of bee venom has been definitely related to the synergism of melittin and phospholipase A (MOLLAY and KREIL, 1974), and a similar relationship has been suggested with apamin and phospholipase A (VOGT et al., 1970). It is to be expected that additional cooperative effects of venom components will be discovered as studies of the venom continue.

II. Toxicity Studies

Although the toxicity of whole honey bee venom poses no really significant problems to humans stung accidentally, as demonstrated by cases of survival of multiple stings (PURSLEY, 1973), the toxicity of certain components is of concern in connection with potential therapeutic uses of the venom or specific components. Various studies (Table 7) suggest that melittin, apamin, and phospholipase A are the most toxic of the major components of the venom.

Although bees account for a significant number of sting fatalities (PARRISH, 1963; CHRISTY, 1967; PURSLEY, 1973), most of the fatal reactions appear to result from anaphylactic shock rather than from toxicity. Bee venom is, in fact, appreciably less toxic than many of the other venoms (ZLOTKIN, 1973).

Toxic reaction to honey bee venom appears to involve a number of complex physiologic events effecting significant cardiovascular and respiratory alterations

Table 7. Toxicity studies of *Apis mellifera* venom

Substance tested	LD$_{50}$	Method[a]	Investigators	Comments
Crude cobra venom (*Naja naja atra*)	0.4 mg/kg	mice (ip)	ZLOTKIN, 1973	for comparisons
Whole *A. mellifera* venom	1.75 mg/kg 3.5 mg/kg	mice (iv) mice (sc)	BROOKS and VICK, 1972	respiratory and cardiovascular alteration
		mice (iv)	HIGGENBOTHAM and KARNELLA, 1970	lethality reduced by heparin
Melittin I	~3.5 mg/kg	mice (iv)	HABERMANN and ZEUNER, 1970	synthetic melittins about as toxic as natural melittin
N$_\alpha$-formyl-melittin I	~5 mg/kg	mice (iv)		
Apamin	~4 mg/kg	mice (iv)	HABERMANN and REIZ, 1965a, b	death from lack of coordinated respiration
MCD peptide	~40 mg/kg	mice (iv)	BREITHAUPT and HABERMANN, 1968	extreme cyanosis after 0.5 mg/kg
Phospholipase A	~7.5 mg/kg	mice (iv)	HABERMANN, 1972	death by hemolysis and microembolic blood changes

[a] (sc) = subcutaneous, (iv) = intravenous, (ip) = intraperitoneal.

(BROOKS and VICK, 1972). It has been suggested that the protease inhibitor in the venom helps protect toxic components against rapid destruction by proteolytic enzymes of the sting victim (SHKENDEROV, 1973).

Animals appear to have at least two mechanisms for protection against honey bee venom—a drop in body temperature (BENTON et al., 1966) and the reaction of dermal mast cells (HIGGENBOTHAM and KARNELLA, 1970), probably by a mechanism involving heparin (VINCENT et al., 1972).

III. Antigenic Character

1. Venom Hypersensitivity and Immunity

The evidence is overwhelming that humans may develop hypersensitivity to *Hymenoptera* venoms and that severe allergic reactions to insect stings may prove fatal (WEGELIN, 1948; PARRISH, 1963; O'CONNOR et al., 1964b; BARNARD, 1967; CHRISTY, 1967; PURSLEY, 1973). In such cases, death usually results from respiratory tract angioedema or vascular, cerebral or anaphylactic reactions. At least two components of *Apis mellifera* venom, hyaluronidase and phospholipase A, have been demonstrated as being anaphylactogenic (SHKENDEROV, 1974) and at least three additional components produce precipitin bands against human sera (O'CONNOR et al., 1967). In the light of evidence suggesting some nonimmunochemical complexing for certain venom components (DIRKS and STERNBURG, 1972), the roles of melittin, the MCD peptide, and apamin in bee venom allergies are uncertain.

Emergency treatment for severe allergic reactions, necessary within a few minutes of the onset of the reaction, appears most effective with some pressor amine, such as epinephrine (O'CONNOR et al., 1964b). It is possible to develop immunity to venom antigens, and specific antihyaluronidase activity has been detected in the sera of immune individuals (BARKER et al., 1966, 1967). A similar immunity to venom phospholipase A has been suggested (MOHAMMED and EL KAREMI, 1961), although this was not confirmed by the studies of BARKER's group (1966). Use of venom, or of various insect extracts, for clinical hyposensitization of allergic individuals has proved reasonably satisfactory (PURSLEY, 1973), but there have been some questions on the use of whole-insect or venom sac extracts. Both preparations, now commonly used in hyposensitization treatments, contain antigenic substances not present in the venom and appear to be missing some of the venom antigens themselves (O'CONNOR and ERICKSON, 1965; O'CONNOR et al., 1964a; BENTON and PATTON, 1965; SHULMAN et al., 1966).

The complete physiologic pictures of venom hypersensitivity and immunity are complex (ANTON, 1945; LOMER et al., 1958; ROTHENBACHER and BENTON, 1972). The question of how many of the venom proteins are actually antigenic has not been fully resolved (HABERMANN and EL KAREMI, 1956; O'CONNOR and ERICKSON, 1965; MUNJAL and ELLIOTT, 1971a; SHEPHERD et al., 1974; DIRKS and STERNBURG, 1972). In addition, it is difficult to distinguish between some of the pathologic features of immunochemical response to the challenge of venom antigens and certain indirect activities of venom components, such as histamine release by action of melittin, phospholipase A, and the MCD peptide (BLOOM and HAEGERMARK, 1967; FREDHOLM and HAEGERMARK, 1967a, b, 1969). The problem is further complicated by difficulties in distinguishing between a true immune defense mechanism and the "local resistance" by dermal mast cell response to envenomation (HIGGIN-BOTHAM and KARNELLA, 1970).

In any event, hypersensitivity to honey bee venom is a significant problem, probably involving a higher percentage of the population than is commonly recognized (CHRISTY, 1967).

2. Antigenic Comparisons Among Various Venoms

Little is known of the antigenic character of *Apidae* venoms, other than that of *Apis mellifera*. Similarities in protein content of various *Apis* venoms (BENTON and MORSE, 1968) do suggest the probability of a considerable degree of common antigenicity, while *Bombus* venoms (sac contents) exhibit protein patterns significantly different from those of *Apis* venoms (MELLO, 1970; O'CONNOR et al., 1964a).

Antigenic relationships have been suggested between *Apis mellifera* venom and the venoms of many of the other *Hymenoptera* (FOUBERT and STIER, 1958; O'CONNOR and ERICKSON, 1965; LANGLOIS et al., 1965; ARBESMAN et al., 1965). These studies indicate the possibility of hypersensitivity to *Apidae* venoms developed as a result of stings from other *Hymenoptera*. Such a possibility must be considered, at present, as only a tentative conclusion, since many of the studies utilized venom sac extracts rather than pure venoms, and all of the studies were concluded prior to the reports of nonimmunochemical complexing (DIRKS and STERNBURG, 1972).

IV. The Arthritis Question

1. General Considerations

Seldom has a "folk remedy" been so persistently and conscientiously investigated as has the potential use of bee venom in the therapy of rheumatoid arthritis. Claims for the successful use of bee venom, often employing stings from live bees, in the treatment of arthritic conditions have persisted for many years (BECK, 1935; HOLLANDER, 1941; BROADMAN, 1962). HABERMANN (1972) states: "The therapeutic value of the venoms when applied to individual cases is not convincing; it has never been proved by unbiased trial." However, other investigators are convinced that a sufficient therapeutic potential exists to warrant at least further study of the whole venom or its components (VICK et al., 1972; LORENZETTI et al., 1972).

2. Possible Mechanisms

While recognizing that the evidence is insufficient to establish bee venom as a fully accepted therapeutic agent, numerous studies have attempted to establish possible biochemical explanations for the many case history reports of successful use of the venom with arthritic individuals.

One of the earliest investigations (NEUMANN and STRACKE, 1951) concentrated on the role of histamine, as a known effect of honey bee envenomation, against formaldehyde-induced arthritis in the rat. It was soon apparent that more complex mechanisms were involved, and a number of these were explored. Since severe arthritic conditions appeared to be associated with hyaluronic acid degradation, the possibility that antibodies formed against bee venom hyaluronidase could afford protection against human hyaluronidase systems was investigated (BARKER et al., 1967). However, such antibodies proved specific to the venom hyaluronidase and, thus, failed to offer the general protection postulated. In fact, the role of immuno-chemical events in arthritic conditions is less simple than might have been expected (KATZ and PILIERO, 1969).

Recent investigations have concentrated on anti-inflammatory properties of venom components (LORENZETTI et al., 1972; BILLINGHAM et al., 1973; HANSON et al., 1974) and on the effects of whole venom and various components on plasma cortisol levels (COUCH and BENTON, 1972; VICK and SHIPMAN, 1972; VICK et al., 1972; ALFANO et al., 1973). These studies appear to offer substantial promise in elucidating possible mechanisms associated with reported therapeutic activity of bee venom.

3. Potentially Interesting Components

The pronounced activity of honey bee venom in elevation of serum cortisol levels appears to be associated with pituitary function (ALFANO et al., 1973; VICK et al., 1972). Although the exact mechanism of this activity is still uncertain, both apamin and melittin have demonstrable potency in producing significant and sustained elevations of plasma cortisol levels (VICK and SHIPMAN, 1972). Melittin itself appears some ten times as effective as the whole venom (VICK et al., 1972). The toxicities and side effects (Tables 5 and 6) of apamin and melittin make these compounds rather unlikely candidates as therapeutic agents, although structure-function studies might lead to synthesis of compounds having more specific activity of a useful type.

Of greater promise is the less toxic MCD peptide ("401"). This substance appears to be the principal anti-inflammatory agent of bee venom (BILLINGHAM et al., 1973), and its function is not, apparently, dependent on cortico-steroid release (HANSON et al., 1974).

4. Speculations

It seems doubtful, at present, that whole honey bee venom will become a universally accepted therapeutic agent. The complex character of the venom, the difficulties of obtaining consistent supplies of uniform composition and purity, and the potential for systemic or allergic reactions all pose major problems. There is, however, such a wide-spread belief in the value of bee venom therapy that continued investigations seem fully justified. While the bee itself may not supply the ultimate treatment for rheumatoid arthritis, studies of the venom may well point the way to significant advances in chemotherapy.

V. Radioprotective Properties

One of the more novel properties of honey bee venom is its action in affording protection against radiation damage in test animals (SHIPMAN and COLE, 1967).

If this property could be exploited for applications in human subjects, it might offer a means of protecting patients undergoing radiation therapy from some of the adverse effects of radiation.

Two components of the venom have been individually demonstrated to have radioprotective activity, phospholipase A (COLE and SHIPMAN, 1970) and melittin (GINSBERG et al., 1968). Melittin is significantly more effective than whole bee venom.

A number of mechanisms have been postulated for chemical radioprotective activity (BACQ, 1965), but no unique mechanism has been established. One possible explanation for the activity of honey bee venom involves the radioprotective function of histamine (BACQ, 1973), since its release during tissue envenomation is well established. Alternative suggestions have included a "stressor-like action", alteration of the hematopoietic system, or simply an antibacterial activity (SHIPMAN and COLE, 1967).

It would be interesting to determine the radioprotective characteristics of some of the less toxic components of the venom, since these would seem to have the best potential for human applications.

VI. Other Physiologic Properties

The spectrum of physiologic and pharmacologic activities (Table 8) attributed to honey bee venom or to specific venom components reads like the table of contents

Table 8. Summary of known properties of *Apis mellifera* venom and its components

Property	Associated with	Selected references
Acetylcholinesterase inhibition	melittin	MITCHELL et al., 1971
Antibacterial and antifungal activity	whole venom melittin	ORTEL and MARKWARDT, 1955 DORMAN and MARKLEY, 1971
Anaphylactogenicity	whole venom, hyaluronidase, phospholipase A (?)	see Sect. C. III
Antigenicity	whole venom, hyaluronidase, phospholipase A, melittin (?), apamin (?)	see Table 5 and Sect. C. III
Anti-inflammatory activity	whole venom, melittin, apamin, MCD peptide	see Sect C. IV
Blood pressure depression	MCD peptide phospholipase A	HABERMANN and BREITHAUPT, 1968 HABERMANN, 1972
Cardiac anti-arrhythmic effects	cardiopep (?)	VICK et al., 1974
Central nervous system excitation	whole venom, apamin	HABERMANN and REIZ, 1965a, b; SHIPOLINI et al., 1967
Central nervous system inhibition	melittin	VYATCHANNIKOV and SINKA, 1973
Growth retardation of *Drosophila*	"minimine"	LOWY et al., 1971

Table 8 (continued)

Property	Associated with	Selected references
Hemolysis		
— direct	whole venom, melittin	SCHRÖDER et al., 1971
— indirect	phospholipase A	HABERMANN, 1972
— synergistic	phospholipase A with melittin	MOLLAY and KREIL, 1972
Hemorrhagic activity	whole venom, basic components of mol. wt. < 10,000	BHARGAVA et al., 1970
Heparin-release from tissue mast cells	whole venom	HIGGENBOTHAM and KARNELLA 1970
Histamine-release	whole venom, melittin, phospholipase A, MCD peptide	see Table 6
Immune response	hyaluronidase, phospholipase A (?)	see Sect. C. III
Mastocytolysis	whole venom, melittin, phospholipase A, MCD peptide	see Tables 5 and 6
Mitochondrial membrane lysis	phospholipase A, melittin	OLSON et al., 1974
Mitochondrial respiration inhibiton	whole venom, melittin, phospholipase A (?)	VAZQUEZ-COLON and ELLIOTT, 1966; HABERMANN, 1954
Nonimmunochemical complexing	low mol. wt. basic peptides	see Sect. C. III
Pain and itching	whole venom, melittin, histamine	see Table 5
Radioprotection	whole venom, melittin, phospholipase A	see Sect. C.V
Serum cortisol increase	whole venom, various components	ALFANO et al., 1973; see also Sect. C. IV
Spreading through tissue	hyaluronidase	see Table 5
Surfactant properties	melittin	SHIPMAN and COLE, 1969; HABERMANN and KOWALLEK, 1970; SCHRÖDER et al., 1971
Systemic changes in lymph node, liver, spleen, and adrenal gland	whole venom	ROTHENBACHER and BENTON, 1972
Therapeutic potential	whole venom, melittin, apamin, MCD peptide	see Sect. C. IV
Thrombocyte lysis, with serotonin release	melittin	HEGNER and SCHNORR, 1968
Toxicity	whole venom, melittin, apamin, phospholipase A	see Table 7
Trypsin inhibition	"protease inhibitor"	SCHKENDEROV, 1973
Vascular permeability increase	melittin, MCD peptide, phospholipase A	HABERMANN, 1972

of an advanced textbook in the field. Even so, it is probable that there are many properties of the venom still unrecognized. We know so little, as yet, in the area broadly described as "molecular biology", that it is sometimes surprising that the activity of honey bee venom is as well characterized as it is. It may truthfully be said that living systems are probably more complex than we now imagine, and possibly more complex than we *can* imagine.

D. Venoms of Other Apidae

I. Other Apini

Most of the major studies of *Apidae* venoms have been concentrated on the common honey bee, *Apis mellifera*. As a result, our knowledge of other *Apidae* venoms is slight. Even the reports that are available (Table 9) may be less than definitive, since age and seasonal variations in *Apis mellifera* venoms (BENTON and PATTON, 1965; BOCH and SHEARER, 1966; BACHMAYER et al., 1972) are almost as significant as some of the species variations observed. Appreciable differences also appear in comparisons of venoms from queen and worker bees (BACHMAYER et al., 1972).

Table 9. Some comparisons of *Apini* venoms

Comparisons	Investigators	Comments
Venom glands and sacs	KERR and DE LELLO, 1962	In addition to taxonomic variations, note is made of unusual appearance of *A. dorsata* venom and of more painful sting of *A. dorsata*
Protein patterns	BENTON and MORSE, 1968; MELLO, 1970	Although only minor differences were noted between *A. m. adansonii* and *A. m. ligustica,* significant differences appear among *A. mellifera, A. dorsata, A. florea,* and *A. indica (cerana).* [see Fig. 8]
Toxicity	BENTON and MORSE, 1968	*A. florea* venom appears much less toxic than venoms of *A. mellifera* and *A. dorsata* (essentially equivalent in toxicity), while *A. indica* venom is about twice as toxic as that of *A. mellifera.*
Melittins	KREIL, 1973a	Melittins from *A. cerana (indica)* and *A. mellifera carnica* appear identical, while melittin from *A. florea* showed variation in five amino acid units
Isoamyl acetate	MORSE et al., 1967	Differences among *A. mellifera, A. indica (cerana),* and *A. florea* were not significantly greater than variations within a single species. However, *A. dorsata* venom appears to contain 10—20 times as much isoamyl acetate as other *Apis* venoms

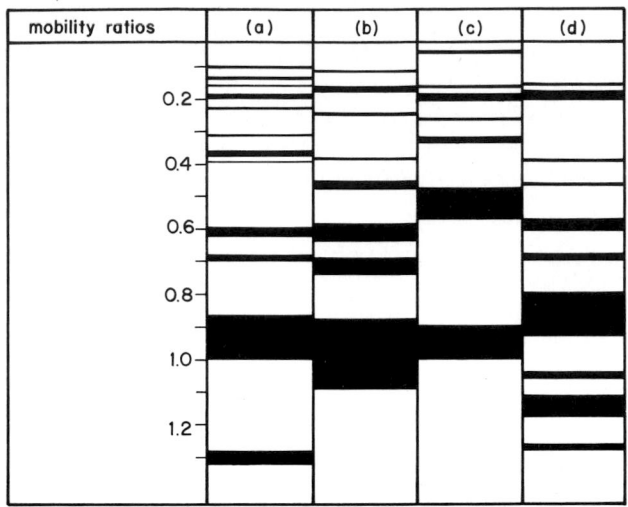

Fig. 8. Electrophoretic patterns of some *Apini* venoms (BENTON and MORSE, 1968) (a) *A. mellifera* [Italy], (b) *A. indica (cerana)* [Thailand], (c) *A. florea* [Thailand], (d) *A. dorsata* [Thailand]

The most significant variations have been reported for protein contents of the venoms (Fig. 8). These are consistent with the observations of melittins from various bees (KREIL, 1973a) and suggest that antigenic character may also vary widely. How these differences correlate with variations in pain from sting (KERR and DE LELLO, 1962) and toxic character (BENTON and MORSE, 1968) are still undetermined.

Table 10. Some studies of *Bombini* venoms (sac contents or extracts)

Information	Investigators	Comments
Venom apparatus description	KERR and DE LELLO, 1962	apparently more "primitive" than in *Apini*
Protein content	O'CONNOR et al., 1964a	four proteins detected in sac extracts from *Bombus huntii* and *Bombus occidentalis*, by electrophoresis at pH 8.3
	MELLO, 1970	nine proteins detected in sac contents from *Bombus atratus*, by electrophoresis at acidic pH
Antigenicity	O'CONNOR and ERICKSON, 1965	possibly five antigenic components in *B. huntii, B. occidentalis* sac extracts
5-Hydroxytryptamine	WELSH and BATTY, 1963	0.02 µg 5-HT per "sting apparatus", compared to 0.0005 for *Apis mellifera*

II. Bombini

Pure bumble bee venom is difficult to obtain, since these bees are not very suscepti-ble to electrical excitation (O'CONNOR et al., 1964a). As a result, our knowledge of bumble bee venoms is very slight and is based entirely on studies of venom sac contents or extracts (Table 10). It would appear that the venoms of *Bombini*, in terms of protein content, are somewhat less complex than those of *Apini*.

Summary

Although our understanding of the complex *Apidae* venoms has increased exponen-tially over the past twenty years, there are still significant gaps in our knowledge of their composition and pharmacology. Throughout this discussion we have repeat-edly stressed the need for further research in the many areas of still unresolved problems. It is important, also, to recognize that *in vitro* studies of pharmacologic activities yield, at best, only tentative understanding of the more complex *in vivo* events (HABERMANN, 1972). There is still much to learn about the *Apidae* venoms that should prove stimulating to further research. These complex natural mixtures are, beyond question, among the most interesting biochemical systems yet investi-gated.

Acknowledgements: Sincere appreciation is expressed to MARK O'CONNOR for the typing of this manuscript, to PAUL GLENN for the technical illustrations, to TIMOTHY JOHNSON for assistance in the literature survey, and to CANDY GONZALES for manuscript assembly.

References

Alfano, J.A., Elliott, W.B., Brownie, A.C.: The effect of bee venom on serum corticosterone levels and adrenal mitochondrial cytochrome P-450 in intact and hypophysectomized rats. Toxicon **11**, 101—102 (1973).

Anton, H.: Bienengift und Immunität. Z. Immunitätforsch. **105**, 241—271 (1945).

Arbesman, C.E., Langlois, C., Shulman, S.: The allergic response to stinging insects: IV. Cross-reactions between bee, wasp, and yellow jacket. J. Allergy Clin. Immunol. **36**, 147—157 (1965).

Arold, H., Rietschel, L.: Synthese einiger Aminoacyl-histamine und -tryptamine. Z. Chem. **9**, 144 (1969).

Bachmayer, H., Kreil, G., Suchanek, G.: Synthesis of promelittin and melittin in the venom gland of queen and worker bees: patterns observed during maturation. J. Insect Physiol. **18**, 1515—1521 (1972).

Bacq, Z.M.: Chemical Protection against Ionizing Radiation. Springfield, Ill.: Charles C Thomas 1965.

Bacq, Z.M.: Histamine as protector against ionizing radiation. Int. Encycl. Pharmacol. Ther. **74**, 109—125 (1973).

Barker, S.A., Bayyuk, S.I., Brimacombe, J.S., Palmer, D.J.: Characterization of the products of the action of bee venom hyaluronidase. Nature **199**, 693—694 (1963).

Barker, S.A., Mitchell, A.W., Walton, K.W., Weston, P.D.: Separation and isolation of the hyaluronidase and phospholipase components of bee venom and investigation of bee ve-nom—human serum interaction. Clin. Chim. Acta **13**, 582—596 (1966).

Barker, S.A., Walton, K.W., Weston, P.D.: The specificity of the anti-hyaluronidase developed in beekeepers serum against bee venom hyaluronidase. Clin. Chim. Acta **17**, 119—123 (1967).

Barnard, J.H.: Allergic and pathologic findings in fifty insect-sting fatalities. J. Allergy Clin. Immunol. **40**, 107—114 (1967).

Beard, A.: Insect toxins and venoms. Ann. Rev. Entomol. **8**, 1—18 (1963).

Beck, B.: Bee Venom Therapy. New York: Appleton-Century, 1935.

Benton, A.W.: Esterases and phosphatases of honeybee venom. J. Apic. Res. **6**, 91—94 (1967).

Benton, A.W., Heckman, R.A., Morse, R.A.: Environmental effects on venom toxicity in rodents. J. Appl. Physiol. **21**, 1228—1230 (1966).

Benton, A.W., Morse, R.A.: Collection of the liquid fraction of bee venom. Nature **210**, 652—653 (1966).

Benton, A.W., Morse, R.A.: Venom toxicity and proteins of the genus *Apis*. J. Apic. Res. **7**, 113—118 (1968).

Benton, A.W., Morse, R.A., Stewart, J.B.: A method of collecting honeybee venom. Science **142**, 228—230 (1963).

Benton, A.W., Patton, R.L.: A qualitative comparison of the proteins in the venom of honey bees. J. Insect Physiol. **11**, 1359—1364 (1965).

Bhargava, N., Zirinis, P., Bonta, I.L., Vargaftig, B.B.: Comparison of hemorrhagic factors of the venoms of *Naja naja, Agkistrodon piscivorus* and *Apis mellifera*. Biochem. Pharmacol. **19**, 2405—2412 (1970).

Billingham, M.E.J., Morley, J., Hanson, J.M., Shipolini, R.A., Vernon, C.A.: An anti-inflammatory peptide from bee venom. Nature **245**, 163—164 (1973).

Bloom, G.D., Haegermark, O.: Studies on morphological changes and histamine release by bee venom, n-decylamine and hypotonic solutions in rat peritoneal mast cells. Acta Physiol. Scand. **71**, 257—269 (1967).

Boch, R., Shearer, D.A.: Iso-pentyl acetate in stings of honeybees of different ages. J. Apic. Res. **5**, 65—70 (1966).

Boch, R., Shearer, D.A., Stone, B.C.: Identification of iso-amyl acetate as an active component in the sting pheromone of the honeybee. Nature **195**, 1018—1020 (1962).

Bordas, J.L.: Appareil glandulaire des *Hyménoptères*. Ann. Sc. Nat. Zool. **19**, 1—362 (1895).

Breithaupt, H., Habermann, E.: Mastzelldegranulierendes Peptid (MCD-Peptid) aus Bienengift: Isolierung, biochemische und pharmakologische Eigenschaften. Naunyn Schmiedebergs Arch. Pharmacol. **261**, 252—270 (1968).

Broadman, J.: Bee Venom—the Natural Curative for Arthritis and Rheumatism. New York: Putnam 1962.

Brooks, R.B., Jr., Vick, J.A.: Toxicological studies of bee venom in mice, dogs, and monkeys. Am. Bee J., 250—251 (July 1972).

Butler, C.G.: Mandibular gland pheromone of worker honeybees. Nature **212**, 530 (1966).

Callewaert, G.L., Shipolini, R., Vernon, C.A.: The disulfide bridges of apamin. FEBS Letters **1**, 111—113 (1968).

Christy, N.P. (ed.): Poisoning by venomous animals. Amer. J. Med. **42**, 107—128 (1967).

Cole, L.J., Shipman, W.H.: A novel mode of chemical radioprotection in mice: Injection of bee venom phospholipase A. Fed. Proc. **29**, 451 (1970).

Condrea, E., De Vries, A.: Venom phospholipase A; a review. Toxicon **2**, 261—273 (1965).

Couch, T.L., Benton, A.W.: The effect of the venom of the honeybee, *Apis mellifera* L., on the adrenocortical response of the adult male rat. Toxicon **10**, 55—62 (1972).

Dirks, T.F., Sternburg, J.O.: Non-immunochemical complexing between *hymenopteran* venoms and rabbit sera. Toxicon **10**, 381—384 (1972).

Doery, H.M., Pearson, J.E.: Phospholipase B in snake venoms and bee venom. Biochem. J. **92**, 599—602 (1964).

Dorman, L.C., Markley, L.D.: Solid phase synthesis and antibacterial activity of N-terminal sequences of melittin. J. Med. Chem. **14**, 5—9 (1971).

Elser, E.: Microchemical recognition of formic acid in the alimentary canal and in the poison sac of bees. Mitt. Lebensm. Hyg. **15**, 28—32 (1924).

Foubert, E.L., Stier, R.A.: Antigenic relationships between honeybees, wasps, yellow hornets, black hornets and yellow jackets. J. Allergy Clin. Immunol. **29**, 13—23 (1958).

Franklin, R., Baer, H.: Immune and nonimmune gel precipitates produced by honey bee venom and its components. Proc. Soc. Exp. Biol. Med. **147**, 585—588 (1974).

Fredholm, B.: Studies on a mast cell degranulating factor in bee venom. Biochem. Pharmac. **15**, 2037 — 2043 (1966).

Fredholm, B., Haegermark, O.: Histamine release from rat mast cells induced by a mast cell degranulating fraction in bee venom. Acta Physiol. Scand. **69**, 304 — 312 (1967 a).

Fredholm, B., Haegermark, O.: Histamine release from rat mast cell granules induced by bee venom fractions. Acta Physiol. Scand. **71**, 357 — 367 (1967 b).

Fredholm, B., Haegermark, O.: Studies on the histamine release effect of bee venom fractions and compound 48/80 on skin and lung tissue of the rat. Acta Physiol. Scand. **76**, 288 — 298 (1969).

Galuszka, H.: The research on a most effective method of the collection of bee venom by means of electric current. Zool. Pol. **22**, 53 — 69 (1972).

Ginsberg, N.J., Dauer, M., Slotta, K.H.: Melittin used as a protective agent against x-irradiation. Nature **220**, 1334 (1968).

Grassmann, W., Hannig, K.: Elektrophoretische Untersuchungen an Schlangen- und Insektentoxinen. Z. physiol. Chem. **296**, 30 — 44 (1954).

Grzycki, S., Czerny, K.: Cytochemical studies on the poison gland of honey-bee sting. Acta Anat. **82**, 91 — 96 (1973).

Gunnison, A.G.: An improved method for collecting the liquid fraction of bee venom. J. Apic. Res. **5**, 33 — 36 (1966).

Habermann, E.: Zur Pharmakologie der Melittin. Naunyn Schmiedebergs Arch. Pharmacol. **222**, 173 — 175 (1954).

Habermann, E.: Über Permeabilitätsänderungen durch tierische Gifte. Naunyn Schmiedebergs Arch. Pharmacol. **225**, 158 — 160 (1955).

Habermann, E.: Eigenschaften und Anreicherung der Hyaluronidase von Bienengift. Biochem. Z. **329**, 1 — 10 (1957).

Habermann, E.: Zur Wirkung tierischer Gifte und von Lysocithin auf Grenzflächen. Z. Gesamte Exp. Med. **130**, 19 — 23 (1958).

Habermann, E.: Biochemie, Pharmakologie und Toxikologie der Inhaltsstoffe von Hymenopterengiften. Ergeb. Physiol. **60**, 220 — 325 (1968).

Habermann, E.: Bee and wasp venoms. Science **177**, 314 — 322 (1972).

Habermann, E., Breithaupt, H.: MCL-peptide, a selectively mastocytolytic factor isolated from bee venom. Naunyn Schmiedebergs Arch. Pharmacol. **260**, 127 — 128 (1968).

Habermann, E., El Karemi, M.M.A.: Antibody formation by protein components of bee venom. Nature **178**, 1349 (1956).

Habermann, E., Jentsch, J.: Über die Struktur des toxischen Bienengiftpeptides Melittin und deren Beziehung zur pharmakologischen Wirkung. Naunyn Schmiedebergs Arch. Pharmacol. **253**, 40 — 41 (1966).

Habermann, E., Jentsch, J.: Sequenzanalyse des Melittins aus den tryptischen und peptischen Spaltstücken. Z. Physiol. Chem. **348**, 37 — 50 (1967).

Habermann, E., Kowallek, H.: Modifikationen der Aminogruppen und des Tryptophans im Melittin als Mittel zur Erkennung von Struktur-Wirkungs-Beziehungen. Z. Physiol. Chem. **351**, 884 — 890 (1970).

Habermann, E., Reiz, K.G.: Zur Biochemie der Bienengiftpeptide Melittin und Apamin. Biochem. Z. **343**, 192 — 203 (1965 a).

Habermann, E., Reiz, K.G.: Ein neues Verfahren zur Gewinnung der Komponenten von Bienengift, insbesondere des zentral wirksamen Peptids Apamin. Biochem. Z. **341**, 451 — 466 (1965 b).

Habermann, E., Zeuner, G.: Comparative studies of native and synthetic melittins. Naunyn Schmiedebergs Arch. Pharmacol. **270**, 1 — 9 (1970).

Hahn, G., Ostermayer, H.: Über das Bienengift (I. Mitteil). Ber. deutsch. Chem. Ges. **69 B**, 2407 — 2419 (1936).

Hanson, J.M., Morley, J., Soria-Herrera, C.: Anti-inflammatory property of 401 (MCD-Peptide), a peptide from the venom of the bee *Apis mellifera* (L.) Brit. J. Pharmacol. **50**, 383 — 392 (1974).

Haux, P.: Die Aminosäurensequenz von MCD-Peptid, einem spezifisch mastzellendegranulierenden Peptid aus Bienengift. Z. Physiol. Chem. **350**, 536 — 546 (1969).

Haux, P., Sawerthal, H., Habermann, E.: Sequenzanalyse des Bienengift-Neurotoxins (Apamin) aus seinen tryptischen und chymotryptischen Spaltstücken. Z. Physiol. Chem. **348**, 737—738 (1967).

Hegner, D., Schnorr, B.: Die Wirkung von Melittin und einigen basischen Polymeren auf lysosomale Membranen. Naunyn Schmiedebergs Arch. Pharmacol. **260**, 135—136 (1968).

Hegner, D., Schummer, U., Schnepel, G.H.: The interaction of a lytic peptide, melittin, with spin-labeled membranes. Biochim. Biophys. Acta **291**, 15—22 (1973).

Higgenbotham, R.D., Karnella, S.: The significance of the mast cell response to bee venom. J. Immunol. **106**, 233—240 (1970).

Hollander, J.L.: Bee venom in the treatment of chronic arthritis. Amer. J. Med. Sci. **201**, 796—801 (1941).

Ivanov, C.P., Shkenderov, S., Krysteva, M.A.: Isolation and purification of hyaluronidase from bee venom. Tr. Acad. Bulg. Sci. **25**, 2—7 (1972).

Jentsch, J.: Weitere Untersuchungen zur Aminosäuresequenz des Melittins. IV: Messung der optischen Rotationsdispersion. Z. Naturforsch. **24**, 33—35 (1969).

Jentsch, J.: Drei Melittine im Bienengift. Liebigs Ann. Chem. **757**, 193—195 (1972).

Jentsch, J., Dielenberg, D.: Mindestens zwei Phospholipasen A im Bienengift. Liebigs Ann. Chem. **757**, 187—192 (1972).

Kaiser, E., Michl, H.: Die Biochemie der tierischen Gifte. Vienna: Franz Deuticke 1958.

Katz, L., Piliero, S.J.: A study of adjuvant-induced polyarthritis in the rat with special reference to associated immunological phenomena. Ann. N.Y. Acad. Sci. **147**, 517—536 (1969).

Kerr, W.E., Cruz, C.: Funcóes diferentes tomadas pela glândula mandibular na evolucão des abelhas em geral e em *Trigona (Oxytrigona) tataira* em especial. Rev. Bras. Biol. **21**, 1—16 (1961).

Kerr, W.E., De Lello, E.: Sting glands in stingless bees—a vestigial character (*Hymenoptera: Apidae*). N.Y. Entomol. Soc. *LXX*, 190—243 (1962).

Kreil, G.: Isolierung und Charakterisierung von Melittin, dem Haupttoxin des Bienengiftes. Monatsch. Chem. **96**, 2061—2063 (1965).

Kreil, G.: Structure of melittin isolated from two species of honey bees. FEBS Letters **33**, 241—243 (1973a).

Kreil, G.: Biosynthesis of melittin, a toxic peptide from bee venom: amino acid sequence of the precursor. Europ. J. Biochem. **33**, 558—566 (1973b).

Kreil, G., Bachmayer, H.: Biosynthesis of melittin, a toxic peptide from bee venom: detection of a possible precursor. Europ. J. Biochem. **20**, 344—350 (1971).

Kreil, G., Kreil-Kiss, G.: The isolation of N-formylglycine from a polypeptide present in bee venom. Biochem. Biophys. Res. Commun. **27**, 275—280 (1967).

Kristeva, M., Mesrob, B., Ivanov, C., Shkenderov, S.: Partial characterization of hyaluronidase from bee venom. Dokl. Bolg. Akad. Nauk **26**, 917—918 (1973).

Langer, J.: Über das Gift unserer Honigbiene. Arch. Exp. Path. Pharmak. Leipz. **38**, 381—396 (1897).

Langlois, C., Shulman, S., Arbesman, C.E.: The allergic response to stinging insects: III. The specificity of venom sac antigens [rabbit]. J. Allergy Clin. Immunol. **36**, 109—120 (1965).

Lindauer, M.: Communication among the honeybees and stingless bees of India. Bee World **38**, 3—14; 34—39 (1957).

Lomer, R., Boguet, P., Izard, Y.: Sensibilité et hypersensibilité aux venins des *Hyménoptéres*. Presse Méd. **66**, 1887—1890 (1958).

Lorenzetti, O.J., Fortenberry, B., Busby, E.: Influence of bee venom in the adjuvant-induced arthritic rat model. Res. Commun. Chem. Pathol. Pharmacol. **4**, 339—352 (1972).

Lowy, P.H., Sarmiento, L., Mitchell, H.K.: Polypeptides minimine and melittin from bee venom: Effects on *Drosophila*. Arch. Biochem. Biophys. **145**, 338—343 (1971).

Lübke, K., Matthes, S., Kloss, G.: Isolation and structure of N_α-formyl melittin. Experientia (Basel) **27**, 765—767 (1971).

Maa, T.C.: An enquiry into the systematics of the tribus *Apidini* or honey bees (*Hymenoptera*). Treubia **21**, 525—640 (1953).

Markovic, O., Molnar, L.: Isolation and determination of honeybee poison. Chem. Zvesti **8**, 80—90 (1954).

Markovic, O., Rexova, L.: The components of various types of honeybee venoms. Chem. Zvesti **17**, 767—684 (1963).

Maschwitz, U.W.: Alarm substances and alarm behavior in social *Hymenoptera*. Nature **204**, 324—327 (1964).

Mebs, D.: Chemistry of animal venoms, poisons, and toxins. Experientia **29**, 1328—1334 (1973).

Mello, M.L.S.: A qualitative analysis of the proteins in venoms from *Apis mellifera* (including *A.m. adansonii*) and *Bombus atratus*. J. Apic. Res. **9**, 113—120 (1970).

Merl, T.: The bodies of bees as formic acid carriers. Z. Nahr Genussm. **42**, 250—251 (1921).

Mitchell, H.K., Lowy, P.H., Sarmiento, L., Dickson, L.: Melittin: Toxicity to *Drosophila* and inhibition of acetylcholinesterase. Arch. Biochem. Biophys. **145**, 344—348 (1971).

Miura, Y., Sugiyama, H., Maki, Y., Seto, S.: The solid phase synthesis of 19-tyrosine melittin. Chem. Pharm. Bull. **20**, 215—218 (1972).

Mohammed, A.H., El Karemi, M.M.A.: Immunity of beekeepers to some constituents of bee venom: phospholipase A antibodies. Nature **189**, 837—838 (1961).

Mollay, C., Kreil, G.: Enhancement of bee venom phospholipase A$_2$ activity by melittin, direct lytic factor from cobra venom and polymixin B. FEBS Letters **46**, 141—144 (1974).

Morse, R.A., Shearer, D.A., Boch, R., Benton, A.W.: Observations on alarm substances in the genus *Apis*. J. Apic. Res. **6**, 113—118 (1967).

Müller, E.: Die Giftproduktion der Honigbiene. VII Int. Congr. Ent. **3**, 1857—1864 (1939).

Munjal, D., Elliott, W.B.: Studies of antigenic fractions in honeybee (*Apis mellifera*) venom. Toxicon **9**, 229—236 (1971a).

Munjal, D., Elliott, W.B.: A simple method for the isolation of a phospholipase A from honeybee (*Apis mellifera*) venom. Toxicon **9**, 403—409 (1971b).

Munjal, D., Elliot, W.B.: Further studies on the properties of phospholipase A from honeybee (*Apis mellifera*) venom. Toxicon **10**, 367—375 (1972).

Nagamitu, G.: Beiträge zur physiologischen Wirkung des Histamins: Über das Gift der Honigbienen. Okayama-Igakkai-Zasshi **47**, 3005—3012 (1935).

Nelson, D.A., O'Connor, R.: The venom of the honeybee (*Apis mellifera*): Free amino acids and peptides. Can. J. Biochem. **46**, 1221—1226 (1968).

Neumann, W., Habermann, E.: Beiträge zur Charakterisierung der Wirkstoffe des Bienengiftes. Naunyn Schmiedebergs Arch. Pharmacol. **222**, 367—387 (1954a).

Neumann, W., Habermann, E.: Über die Phospholipase A des Bienengiftes. Z. Phys. Chem. **296**, 166—179 (1954b).

Neumann, W., Stracke, A.: Untersuchungen mit Bienengift und Histamin an der Formaldehydearthritis der Ratte. Naunyn Schmiedebergs Arch. Pharmacol. **213**, 8—17 (1951).

O'Connor, R., Erickson, R.: *Hymenoptera* antigens: an immunological comparison of venoms, venom sac extracts and whole insect extracts. Ann. Allergy **23**, 151—157 (1965).

O'Connor, R., Henderson, G., Moran, M., Nelson, D., Peck, M.L.: The quantitative investigation of wasp, hornet, and bee venoms. Abstr. Papers of 150th Meeting Am. Chem. Soc., 10 (Sept. 1965).

O'Connor, R., Henderson, G., Nelson, D., Parker, R., Peck, M.L.: The venom of the honeybee (*Apis mellifera*): general character. in Animal Toxins. New York: Pergamon Press, 1967, pp. 17—22.

O'Connor, R., Rosenbrook, W., Erickson, R.: *Hymenoptera:* Pure venom from bees, wasps and hornets. Science **139**, 420 (1963).

O'Connor, R., Rosenbrook, W., Erickson, R.: Disc electrophoresis of *Hymenoptera* venoms and body proteins. Science **145**, 1320—1321 (1964a).

O'Connor, R., Stier, R.A., Rosenbrook, W., Erickson, R.W.: Death from "wasp" sting. Ann. Allergy **22**, 385—393 (1964b).

Olson, F.C., Munjal, D., Malviya, A.N.: Structural and respiratory effects of melittin (*Apis mellifera*) on rat liver mitochondria. Toxicon **12**, 419—425 (1974).

Ortel, S., Markwardt, F.: Untersuchungen über die antibakteriellen Eigenschaften des Bienengiftes. Pharmazie **10**, 743—746 (1955).

Owen, M.D.: Insect venoms: Identification of dopamine and noradrenaline in wasp and bee stings. Experientia **27**, 544—545 (1971).

Owen, M.D., Braidwood, J.L.: A quantitative and temporal study of histamine and histidine in honey bee (*Apis mellifera L.*) venom. Can. J. Zool. **52**, 387—392 (1974).

Palmer, D.J.: Extraction of bee venom for research. Bee World **42**, 225–226 (1961).

Parrish, H.M.: Analysis of 460 fatalities from venomous animals in the United States. Am. J. Med. Sci. **245**, 129–141 (1963).

Pearce, F.L.: Absence of nerve growth factor in the venoms of bees, scorpions, spiders and toads. Toxicon **11**, 309–310 (1973).

Peck, M.L., O'Connor, R.: Procamine and other basic peptides in the venom of the honeybee (*Apis mellifera*). J. Agric. Food Chem. **22**, 51–53 (1974).

Peck, M.L., O'Connor, R., Johnson, T.: Investigations of histamine-terminal peptides (1975).

Perlman, E.: Near fatal reactions to bee and wasp stings: a review and report of seven cases. J. Mt. Sinai Hosp. **22**, 336–341 (1955).

Pursley, R.E.: Stinging *Hymenoptera*. Am. Bee J. **113**, 131–132; 135 (1973).

Rexova, L., Markovic, O.: Chemical characterization of some low-molecular components of honeybee poison. Chem. Zvesti **17**, 884–890 (1963).

Rocha e Silva, M.: Pharmacological properties of simple compounds of histamine with amino acids. J. Pharmacol. **77**, 198–205 (1943).

Rocha e Silva, M.: Inhibition of histamine effects by compounds of histamine, histidine, and arginine. J. Pharmacol. **80**, 399–408 (1944).

Rothenbacher, H., Benton, A.W.: Pathologic features in mice hyposensitized to bee venom. Am. J. Vet. Res. **33**, 1867–1874 (1972).

Rothschild, A.M.: Histamine release by bee venom phospholipase A and melittin in the rat. Brit. J. Pharmacol. Chemother. **25**, 59–66 (1965).

Schoetensack, W.: Bienengift und Bernsteinsäuredehydrierung. Naunyn Schmiedebergs Arch. Pharmacol. **218**, 107–108 (1953).

Schröder, E., Lübke, K., Lehmann, M., Beetz, I.: Haemolytic activity and action on the surface tension of aqueous solutions of synthetic melittins and their derivatives. Experientia **27**, 764–765 (1971).

Sessa, G., Freer, J.G., Colacicco, G., Weismann, G.: Interaction of a lytic polypeptide, melittin, with lipid membrane systems. J. Biol. Chem. **244**, 3575–3582 (1969).

Shearer, D.A., Boch, R.: 2-Heptanone in the mandibular gland secretion of the honey-bee. Nature **206**, 530 (1965).

Shepherd, G.W., Elliott, W.B., Arbesman, C.E.: Fractionation of bee venom. I. Preparation and characterization of four antigenic components. Prep. Biochem. **4**, 71–88 (1974).

Shipman, W., Cole, L.J.: Increased resistance of mice to x-irradiation after the injection of bee venom. Nature **215**, 311–312 (1967).

Shipman, W.H., Cole, L.J.: A surfactant bee venom fraction. Anal. Biochem. **29**, 490–497 (1969).

Shipolini, R., Bradbury, A.F., Callewaert, G.L., Vernon, C.A.: The structure of apamin. Chem. Commun., 679–680 (1967).

Shipolini, R., Callewaert, C.L., Cottrell, R.C., Doonan, S., Vernon, C.A., Banks, E.C.: Phospholipase A from bee venom. Europ. J. Biochem. **20**, 459–468 (1971a).

Shipolini, R.A., Callewaert, G.L., Cottrell, R.C., Vernon, C.A.: The primary sequence of phospholipase A from bee venom. FEBS Letters **17**, 39–40 (1971b).

Shkenderov, S.: A protease inhibitor in bee venom. FEBS Letters **33**, 343–347 (1973).

Shkenderov, S.: Anaphylactogenic properties of bee venom and its fractions. Toxicon **12**, 529–534 (1974).

Shulman, S., Langlois, C., Miller, J.B., Arbesman, C.E.: The allergic response to stinging insects: V. Fractionation of whole body and venom sac extracts of bee. J. Allergy Clin. Immunol. **37**, 350–358 (1966).

Simpson, J.: Repellancy of the mandibular gland scent of worker honeybees. Nature **209**, 531–532 (1966).

Snodgrass, R.E.: Anatomy of the Honeybee. Ithaca, N.Y.: Comstock 1956.

Spoerri, P.E., Jentsch, J., Glees, P.: Apamin from bee venom: Effects of the neurotoxin on cultures of the embryonic mouse cortex. Neurobiol. **3**, 207–214 (1973).

Tetsch, C., Wolff, K.: Untersuchungen über Analogien zwischen Bienen- und Schlangen- (*Crotalus*) Gift. Biochem. Z. **288**, 126–136 (1936).

Vazquez-Colon, L., Elliott, W.B.: On the response of rat liver mitochondria to treatment with bee venom. Toxicon **4**, 61–63 (1966).

Vernon, C.A., Hanson, J.M., Brimblecombe, R.W.: Peptides. British Patent No. 1324823 (1969).

Vick, J.A., Mehlman, B., Brooks, R., Phillips, S.J., Shipman, W.: Effect of bee venom and melittin on plasma cortisol in the unanesthetized monkey. Toxicon 10, 581—586 (1972).

Vick, J.A., Shipman, W.H.: Effects of whole bee venom and its fractions (apamin and melittin) on plasma cortisol levels in the dog. Toxicon 10, 377—380 (1972).

Vick, J.A., Shipman, W.H., Brooks, R.: Beta adrenergic and anti-arrhythmic effects of cardio-pep, a newly isolated substance from whole bee venom. Toxicon 12, 139—144 (1974).

Vincent, J.E., Bonta, I.L., Noordhoek, J.: Some effects of guinea pig serum and heparin on hemolysis induced by *Naja naja, Agkistrodon piscivorus* and *Apis mellifera* venom. Toxicon 10, 415—417 (1972).

Vogt, W., Patzer, P., Lege, L., Oldigs, H., Wille, G.: Synergism between phospholipase A and various peptides and SH-reagents in causing haemolysis. Naunyn Schmiedebergs Arch. Pharmacol. 265, 442—454 (1970).

Vyatchannikov, N.K., Sinka, A.Y.: Effect of melittin, the major constituent of bee venom, on the central nervous system. Farmakol. Toksikol. (Moscow) 36, 526—530 (1973).

Wegelin, C.: Anatomic findings in patients dying of bee and wasp stings. Schweiz. Med. Wochenschr. 78, 1253—1261 (1948).

Wellhöner, H.-H.: Spinale Wirkungen von Apamin. Naunyn Schmiedebergs Arch. Pharmacol. 262, 29—41 (1969).

Welsh, J.H., Batty, C.S.: 5-Hydroxytryptamine content of some arthropod venoms and venom-containing parts. Toxicon 1, 165—173 (1963).

Welsh, J.H., Moorhead, M.: The quantitative distribution of 5-hydroxytryptamine in the invertebrates, especially in their nervous systems. J. Neurochem. 6, 146—169 (1960).

Werle, E., Gleissner, R.: Über die Herkunft des Histamins der Bienen. Z. Vitamin Hormon Fermentforsch. 4, 450—455 (1951).

Zlotkin, E.: Chemistry of animal toxins. Experientia 29, 1453—1588 (1973).

CHAPTER 22

Venoms of Sphecidae, Pompilidae, Mutillidae, and Bethylidae

W. RATHMAYER

A. Introduction

Studies dealing with hymenopteran venoms are almost exclusively concerned with the venoms of the honey bee (*Apis mellifera*) or, to a minor extent, of wasps belonging to the family Vespidae (HABERMANN, 1968, 1971, 1972). Although the sphecid and pompilid wasps possess paralyzing venoms of great pharmacologic and physiologic interest, they have attracted only very few research groups to study their intriguing effects. In a recent, most comprehensive survey on the biochemistry, pharmacology and toxicology of the constituents of hymenopteran venoms (HABERMANN, 1968) only half a page is devoted to the paralyzing venoms of Sphecidae. A somewhat more lengthy treatment of paralyzing venoms of solitary wasps is to be found in the reviews of BEARD (1963), and PIEK and SIMON THOMAS (1969).

B. Venoms of Sphecidae

I. General Aspects

1. Biological Notes

Wasps of the family Sphecidae exist throughout the world. Usually, members of this family are seasonal, spending the cooler periods of the year as diapausing larvae in nests provided by the mother wasp. Wherever field studies have been performed they show that, with a few exceptions of cleptoparasitism, the adult females prey upon other insects and spiders for provisioning their nests to care for the offspring. In most cases the prey is more or less deeply paralyzed by injection of venom into the body through the modified ovipositor, the sting apparatus. The immobilized prey is then carried to crevices or specially prepared nests in wood or soil where the egg is laid on the prey and larval development of a new generation takes place.

For details of the biology and ethology of Sphecidae the reader is referred to the books of G. and E. PECKHAM (1898), P. and N. RAU (1918), BISCHOFF (1927), NIELSEN (1933), CLAUSEN (1940), OLBERG (1959), EVANS (1966a), and KROMBEIN (1967b) and to the review article (mainly on Japanese species) of IWATA (1942). Detailed references of the older literature on European species are contained in BERLAND (1925). The synoptic catalogue of the *Hymenoptera of America North of Mexico* (MUESEBECK et al., 1951), together with its two supplements (KROMBEIN,

1958, 1967a) represents a most comprehensive source for the literature on the North American species.

2. Sting Apparatus and Venom Glands

Anatomical studies of the sting apparatus and the venom glands in Sphecidae (BORDAS, 1895; PAWLOWSKY, 1927; RATHMAYER, 1962b) bear a close resemblance to the situation in other aculeate Hymenoptera, in particular to the Apidae, which have been studied in far greater detail (PAWLOWSKY, 1927; FLEMMING, 1957; MASCHWITZ and KLOFT, 1971).

The sting apparatus of Sphecidae lies within the posterior end of the abdomen and is covered by the seventh abdominal tergite and sternite. The modified tergites and sternites of segments 8, 9 and 10, together with their appendices, form the sting apparatus which is phylogenetically derived from the ovipositor. The sting apparatus can be divided into two functionally different parts: a chitinous and muscular part which serves in the insertion of the sting and the injection of venom into the prey, and a glandular part consisting of several glands, one of which produces the venom.

Details of the skeletal parts of the sting have been described in particular

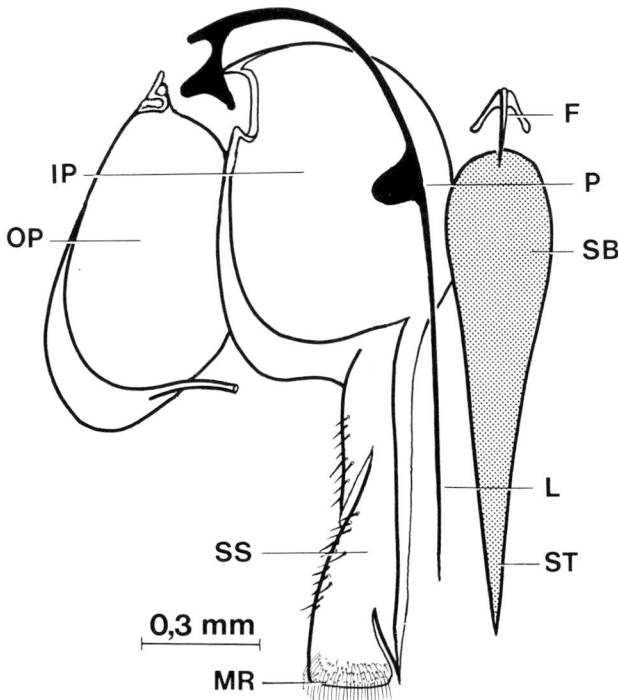

Fig. 1. Skeletal parts of the sting apparatus of a sphecid wasp (*Philanthus*). Only left half is shown, the connection of the two outer plates has been cut at midline. Parts have been folded apart for clarity. Abbreviations: *F*=furcula; *IP*=inner plate; *L*=lancet; *OP*=outer plate; *P*=chitinous pouch; *SB*=stylet bulbus; *SS*=sting sheath; *ST*=stylet. (Modified from RATHMAYER, 1962b)

for *Apis* and *Vespa* (for references, see MASCHWITZ and KLOFT, 1971). The few anatomical investigations on the sting apparatus of sphecid wasps (OESER, 1961; RATHMAYER, 1962b) are in general agreement with studies on other Aculeata. Figure 1 shows the typical skeletal parts of a sphecid sting apparatus. A system of plates (outer and inner plate), derived from tergite 9, and the furcula serve as attachment sites for the muscles which move and protrude the long and pointed sting (aculeus). The sting consists of two pairs of rami the first of which is long and thin and called the lancets. These are not attached to each other and can be moved independently. They slide along tracklike ridges on the fused second pair of rami, the stylet (see Fig. 4b). The stylet is hollow and usually shows a bulbous enlargement at its base. Between the stylet and the two lancets a tube is formed (venom canal) in which the venom is transported outward during stinging (see also Sect. B, II, 1., b, α). The pouches on the lancets may play a role in venom expulsion.

Of the several glands associated with the sting apparatus of aculeate Hymenoptera three are usually present in sphecid wasps (Fig. 2): the proper venom gland, also called the acid gland, and two smaller accessory glands (Bordas' gland and Dufour's gland) which probably do not make contributions to the secreted venom. From analogy with other Aculeata we infer that the venom is produced in the secretory epithelia lining the walls of tubular structures which extend in pairs, often branching diffusely, into the abdominal body cavity. The tubular glands empty into the lumen of an unpaired reservoir of different form and size. From there the venom can be ejected through a single duct which leads into the venom canal formed by the stylet and the two lancets. The mechanism by which the venom actually is expelled is not clear. Examples of the sting apparatus and the venom gland of Sphecidae can be found in PAWLOWSKY (1927) for *Sphex flavipennis,* in RATHMAYER (1962b) for *Ammophila heydeni, Philanthus triangulum* (see also Sect. B, II, 1., b, α) and *Tachysphex nitidus.* The sting apparatus of *Bembex rostrata* is depicted in OESER (1961).

Neither ultrastructure nor histochemistry of venom glands of sphecid wasps have been studied. No data exists on the biochemistry of venom production, on the question of whether the venom secreted in the tubulus is already active, or on the importance of the epithelia of the reservoir. With the exception of the venom of *Sceliphron caementarium* (see Sect. B, II, 1) neither composition nor biochemistry of any of the sphecid venoms have been investigated.

3. Stinging of the Prey

During hunting for the prey optical cues, for prey identification odor stimuli probably play the most important roles. Once the wasp has grasped the prey with its legs it immediately tries to insert the sting. Observational data indicate that there are species which insert the sting only once and others which apply several stings (EVANS, 1966b). The ventral side of the prey is invariably preferred for the insertion of the sting.

Many wasps which prey upon Hemiptera or on adult holometabolous insects apply typically only one sting through the thin intersegmental membranes on the base of the legs or the ventral skin between head and prothorax (neck). Sphecids preying upon Orthoptera or larval insects, in particular caterpillars, typi-

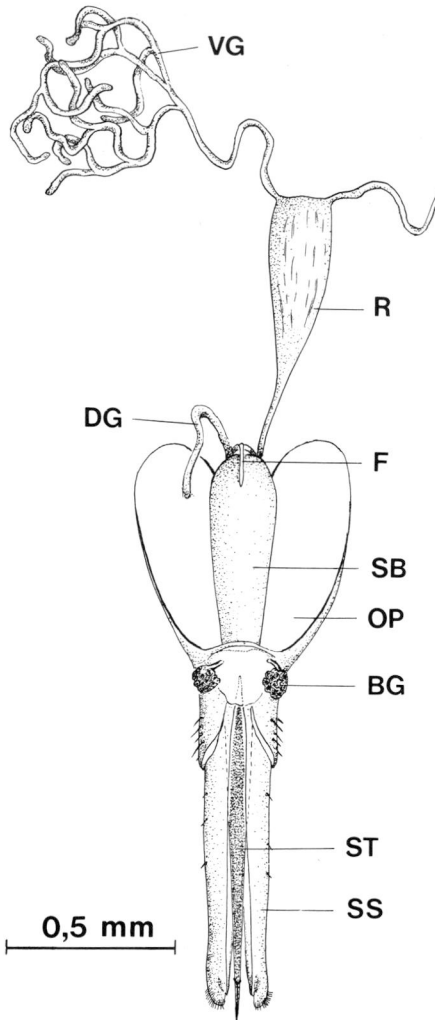

Fig. 2. Sting apparatus and venom gland of digger wasp *Ammophila heydeni*. Only left venom gland is depicted. Inner plates and lancets not shown. Abbreviations: *BG* = Bordas' gland; *DG* = Dufour's gland; *F* = furcula; *OP* = outer plate; *R* = reservoir; *SB* = stylet bulbus; *SS* = sting sheath; *ST* = stylet; *VG* = venom gland. (After RATHMAYER, 1962b)

cally sting several times (MOLITOR, 1939; EVANS, 1966b). STEINER has shown for *Liris nigra* (1958a, b; 1962) and for two nearctic species of *Liris* (1976) that the first sting applied to the captured cricket is always placed at the base of the jumping legs. This is usually followed by three additional stings, always at the base of the front legs, middle legs and in the ventral neck region, in that order. The sting is directed toward the ganglia in the thorax and the subesophageal ganglion. Although STEINER writes (1958b, 1962) that the sting hits these ganglia, this has not been substantiated through histologic investigations. The recovery of the cricket, which has been observed under certain conditions, makes destruction of parts of the ganglia by the sting also unlikely. Stinging of caterpillars by *Ammophila* and *Podalonia* has been described among others by MOLITOR (1939), BAERENDS (1941), OLBERG (1959), GERVET and FULCRAND (1967). *A. heydeni* stings noctuid caterpillars in varying sequences into all segments (MOLITOR, 1939). In *P. hirsuta* paralysis of caterpillars of the noctuid moth *Agrotis* is achieved by a varying number of stings which are placed according to a certain sequence (GERVET and FULCRAND, 1968). The precision of the first sting is greater than that of the consecutive ones.

The insertion of the sting is guided by tactile stimuli as has been shown for *Liris* by STEINER (1962). On the sting sheaths of those sphecid wasps which have been investigated under this aspect, groups of mechanoreceptors of the Sensilla chaetica-type have always been found (RATHMAYER, 1962b), (Fig. 4) which may play an important role in localization of the proper point of insertion.

4. Venom Actions

To make statements on the mechanism of action of the venoms of Sphecidae, one has to rely almost exclusively on observations of more or less qualitative character because quantitative physiological studies employing modern techniques have so far been only performed with the venom of *P. triangulum* (see Sect. B, II, 1., b, α).

The venom of Sphecidae immobilizes the prey at different speeds and to different degrees (see Sect. B, II, 1., b, β). In most cases, paralysis starts within the first min. Even in cases of deep and permanent paralysis the palpi and the tarsi of the prey show trembling movements for a long time (up to 2 days) after the stinging. The venom apparently impairs only the locomotion of the prey. There are several reports that the functions of the gut and the heart continue for many days in a paralyzed prey (PAWLOWSKY, 1927; NIELSEN, 1935; RATHMAYER, 1962b, 1966; PIEK and SIMON THOMAS, 1969). A delayed onset in the action of the venom has been reported for species of *Halictus* (Apidae), paralyzed by *Cerceris rybiensis* (MOLITOR, 1939; unpublished own observations), for beetles taken by *Eucerceris ruficeps* (LINSLEY and MACSWAIN, 1954) and for buprestid beetles captured by *C. californica* (LINSLEY and MACSWAIN, 1956). The early controversy whether the injection of venom directly into the central nervous system of the prey is a prerequisite for paralysis has been discussed by NIELSEN (1935). The observations of PECKHAM and PECKHAM (1898) and RABAUD (1917), however, suggest that in order to obtain paralysis it is sufficient that the venom is injected into the body of the prey. From the point of puncture it will be distributed by the hemolymph to the sites of action. The experiments on braconid paralyzing venoms (BEARD, 1952; PIEK, 1966; PIEK and ENGELS, 1969; WALTHER and RATHMAYER, 1974) and on the venom of *Philanthus triangulum* (RATHMAYER, 1962b; PIEK et al., 1971; see also Sect. B, II, 1., b, β) contribute to the principal sources of information on the action of paralyzing venoms. In both cases it could be shown that these venoms block neuromuscular transmission presynaptically. It has yet to be proven whether this is also the case with the paralyzing venoms of other solitary wasps.

NIELSEN (1935) investigated the metabolism of normal and paralyzed caterpillars by measuring oxygen consumption. The metabolism of caterpillars paralyzed by *Ammophila campestris* showed a steady decline over 140 h which was only slightly less than that of unparalyzed but starving caterpillars of the same species (Fig. 3).

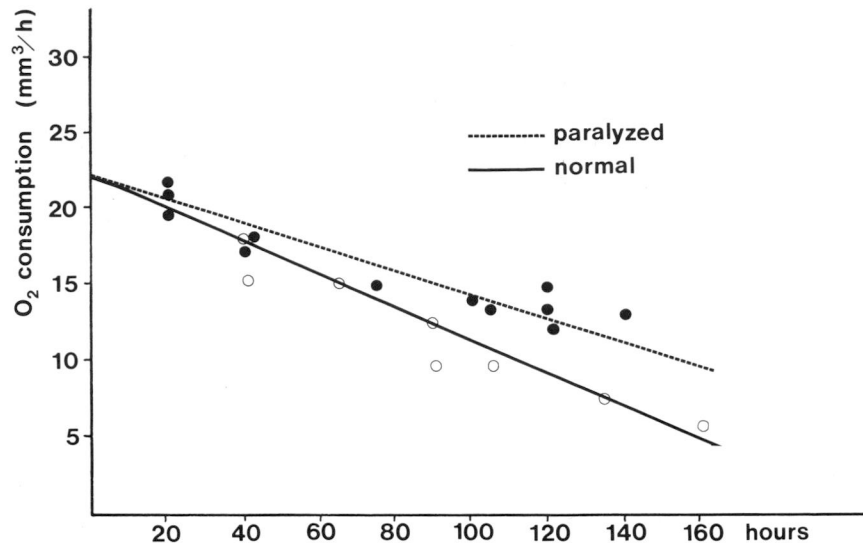

Fig. 3. Metabolism of noctuid caterpillar paralysed by digger wasp *Ammophila campestris.* As a control, values of a normal but starving caterpillar of the same species are shown. (From NIELSEN, 1935)

NIELSEN (1935) also reported heavy lesions in the central nervous system of one caterpillar paralyzed by *A. campestris.* Degeneration had also spread to the supraesophageal ganglion which lies in a segment which was not stung. This observation led NIELSEN to the conclusion that the venom of *Ammophila* acts as a neurotoxin which diffuses from the point of puncture to the ganglia where it exerts its blocking effects by producing lesions. This view has been criticized by RATHMAYER (1962b) although central effects at later stages of intoxication have not completely been ruled out. Lesions within the central nervous system (brain, subesophageal ganglion, thoracic ganglia) have also been reported by HARTZELL (1935) for cicadas (*Tibicen pruinosa*) paralyzed by *Sphecius speciosus.* It is surprising that there are no recent histologic reinvestigations to bring this problem to clarification.

With regard to the effects of the venom of Sphecidae on man only little data exist. Even with large specimens, the sting usually cannot pierce the human skin. Whenever it happened that the wasp was forced to sting into the soft skin, only slight pain was felt. This might be due to the lack of 5-hydroxytryptamine in the venom of Sphecidae as has been shown for *Bembex texana* and *Stictia carolina* by WELSH and BATTY (1963), for *P. triangulum* by PIEK et al. (1971) and for *S. caementarium* by O'Connor and ROSENBROOK (1963).

5. Effectiveness of Paralysis

The venom injected through the sting into the prey results in various degrees of paralysis. According to a classification proposed by LECLERCQ (1954) five stages of paralysis can be distinguished:

a) Temporary paralysis which is more or less incomplete. This is regarded as a primitive form of paralysis. It is found among the lower subfamilies as Ampulicinae, Sphecinae, and Larrinae. For example, mole crickets paralyzed by *Larra analis* recover within 5 – 10 min after the sting (SMITH, 1935).

b) Permanent but local paralysis so that the prey can partially move is again to be found among the Ampulicinae, Sphecinae, and Larrinae. In crickets (*Acheta domesticus*) paralysis resulting from stings of *L. nigra* (Larrinae) is the sum of stings applied. If stings out of the typical sequence (see Sect. B, I, 2) are omitted, the extremities next to the place where no venom has been injected can be moved normally (STEINER, 1958b). STEINER's experiments (1963, 1976) also show with *Liris* that the degree of paralysis depends on the dose of venom injected.

c) Permanent local paralysis in which the prey is unable to move away. This form of paralysis is widespread among Sphecinae, Trypoxylinae, Stizinae, Bembecinae, Astatinae, and some Larrinae. STEINER (1958b) describes this state of paralysis among crickets which have been paralyzed by *Liris nigra* with a complete series of stings. He observed partial molting of the paralyzed cricket. The abdomen and the antennae were free to move, the legs however, were paralyzed so the animal could not leave its exuvia.

d) Permanent and complete paralysis. The prey is completely immobilized and its metabolism reduced (NIELSEN, 1935). Normally there is no recovery and the prey remains in flaccid paralysis for at least 1 week. This is the most common form of paralysis within the subfamilies regarded as highest in evolutionary rank (see App.) such as Philanthinae, Crabroninae, Pemphredoninae, and Nyssoninae. Some members of subfamilies belonging to category c are also to be found in this group.

e) Death of the prey. This is the case in many Pemphredoninae and also with the genus *Glenostictia* and *Steniolia* (EVANS, 1966a). In some *Bembex* species the pedestal fly is apparently killed by the wasp. Subsequent flies are merely weakly paralyzed living up to 9 days (EVANS, 1966a). In other species of *Bembex* all the flies appear to be killed. Many bugs caught by *Astata* also seem to be killed by the sting (PECKHAM and PECKHAM, 1898; EVANS, 1957).

From these field observations, however, one cannot yet decide whether in these instances death of the prey is actually caused by the venom or rather by external mechanical destructions (pinching of the thorax with the mandibles has been reported for *Pemphredon* preying upon aphids: JANVIER, 1955) or internal destructions by the sting.

IWATA (1942) has reported that temporary paralysis (type a) mainly occurs with orthopteran prey. Local and incomplete paralysis (type b) has been again observed with Orthoptera, and in addition with larvae of Lepidoptera and Heteroptera. It has to be borne in mind that this is also the type of prey which is usually treated by the wasps with several stings instead of a single stroke (see Sect. B, I, 3). Complete permanent paralysis is generally prominent among prey-insects belonging to the orders Coleoptera, Hymenoptera, Homoptera, and Diptera as well as spiders.

It is not clear as to what mechanisms cause these differences in paralysis. Differences in accessibility of the neuromuscular system to the venom, or partial immunity and rapid inactivation of the venoms, i.e. factors within the prey itself, probably play a more important role than peculiarities of the individual venoms. To clarify these points, experiments employing modern techniques are necessary. They will certainly open a valuable field for future research.

6. Specificity of Venoms

Since there is almost a total lack of experimental data on the specificity of sphecid venoms, we have to rely profusely on prey records from field studies because they at least yield indirect information on venom specificities. Table 1 lists insect orders used as prey mainly by European and North American genera of Sphecidae. In the compilation of this table, data from the summarizing work of Berland (1925), Muesebeck et al., (1951), Leclercq (1954), and Evans (1966) have been used to a large extent. It was beyond the scope of the present review to go into the vast original literature on the reproductive biology and nesting behavior, although these papers often contain interspersed prey records. This list is by no means complete but it shows, nevertheless, that adult and immature insects of almost all orders as well as springtails and many families of spiders appear as prey. The table indicates (a) that sphecid venoms in general are broadly effective among insects and arachnids, (b) that, although there are sphecids which prey upon one genus only, there is a tendency for predation upon members of genera within one or related families of one or sometimes several (*Cerceris, Ectemnius, Glenostictia*) orders.

The prey of sphecid wasps of the tribe Gorytini, for example, usually consists of either adults or nymphs of small Homoptera of several families. There is little tendency of one genus to restrict itself to one family of prey (Evans, 1966a). A relatively high degree of specificity, however, is exhibited within this tribe by genera like *Sphecius* and *Exeirus* which are specialists on cicadas, or like *Argogorytes* which captures spittle insects (Cercopidae) from their masses of froth (Evans, 1966a).

Table 1

List

Order	Family	Genera Sphecidae
Aphidina	Aphididae	*Diodontus*[1, 9]*; Nitela*[1]*; Passaloecus*[1, 9]*; Pemphredon*[4]*; Pysen*[1]*; Rhopalum*[1, 6]*; Spilomena*[1]*; Stigmus*[1, 4]*; Xylocelia*[4]
	Psyllidae	*Crossocerus*[6]*; Diodontus*[1]*; Glenostictia*[8]*; Gorytes* s.l.[8]*; Rhopalum*[8]*; Stizus*[7]
Coleoptera	Bruchidae	*Cerceris*[1,4,12]
	Buprestidae	*Cerceris*[1,12]
	Chrysomelidae	*Cerceris*[4,12,15]*; Entomognathus*[1,6]
	Curculionidae	*Cerceris*[1,4,12]
	Nitidulidae	*Cerceris*[12]
	Phalacridae	*Cerceris*[12]
	Scarabaeidae	*Cerceris*[15]
	Tenebrionidae	*Cerceris*[4,12]
Collembola	Entomobyidae	*Microstigmus*[10]
	Sminthuridae	*Microstigmus*[10]

Order	Family	Genera of Sphecidae
Diptera	Many families, among others:	
	Anisopodidae	*Crossocerus*[6]
	Anthomyidae	*Crabro*[6]; *Crossocerus*[6]; *Glenostictia*[8]; *Mellinus*[1]; *Oxybelus*[1,21]
	Agromyzidae	*Crossocerus*[6]; *Dasyproctus*[6]; *Oxybelus*[21]
	Bibionidae	*Crabro* s. l.[6]
	Bombyliidae	*Bembex*[1,8]; *Ectemnius*[6]; *Glenostictia*[8]; *Mellinus*[17]; *Oxybelus*[21]; *Rhopalum*[6]
	Calliphoridae	*Bembex*[1,8]; *Crabro*[1,6]; *Crossocerus*[6]; *Ectemnius*[6]; *Mellinus*[17]; *Oxybelus*[1,21]; *Podagritus*[6]; *Rhopalum*[6]; *Steniolia*[2]; *Stictia*[8]; *Stictiella*[4]
	Cecidomyidae	*Oxybelus*[21]
	Ceratopogonidae	*Crossocerus*[6]; *Lindenius*[6]
	Chironomidae	*Crossocerus*[6]; *Glenostictia*[8]; *Oxybelus*[11]; *Rhopalum*[6]
	Chloropidae	*Crossocerus*[6]; *Glenostictia*[8]; *Lindenius*[6]; *Oxybelus*[11,21]; *Rhopalum*[6]
	Culicidae	*Crossocerus*[6]; *Rhopalum*[6]; *Stictia*[8]
	Cyrtidae	*Ectemnius*[6]
	Dolichopodidae	*Crabro*[6]; *Crossocerus*[6]; *Dasyproctus*[6]; *Ectemnius*[6]; *Lindenius*[6]; *Rhopalum*[6]
	Drosophilidae	*Crossocerus*[6]; *Piyuma*[6]; *Rhopalum*[6]
	Empididae	*Crabro*[6]; *Crossocerus*[6]; *Ectemnius*[6]; *Lindenius*[6]; *Rhopalum*[6]
	Ephydridae	*Crabro*[6]; *Crossocerus*[6]; *Oxybelus*[21]
	Heleidae	*Crabro* s. l.[6]
	Helomyzidae	*Crossocerus*[6]; *Ectemnius*[6]; *Podagritus*[6]; *Rhopalum*[6]
	Hippoboscidae	*Bembex*[1]
	Itonididae	*Crossocerus*[6]; *Rhopalum*[6]
	Larvaevoridae	*Crabro*[6]; *Crossocerus*[6]; *Ectemnius*[6]
	Lauxaniidae	*Crossocerus*[6]; *Lindenius*[6]; *Mellinus*[17]; *Oxybelus*[1,21]; *Rhopalum*[6]
	Lonchaeidae	*Crossocerus*[6]; *Oxybelus*[21]
	Lycoriidae	*Crossocerus*[6]; *Lindenius*[6]
	Milichiidae	*Oxybelus*[21]
	Muscidae	*Bembex*[1,8]; *Crabro*[1,4,6]; *Crossocerus*[6]; *Ectemnius*[6]; *Glenostictia*[8]; *Mellinus*[1]; *Oxybelus*[4,21]; *Podagritus*[6]; *Steniolia*[8]; *Stictia*[4,8]
	Mycetophilidae	*Crossocerus*[6]; *Rhopalum*[6]
	Neriidae	*Rhopalum*[6]
	Otidae	*Oxybelus*[21]
	Phoridae	*Crossocerus*[6]
	Pipunculidae	*Crabro* s. l.[26]; *Oxybelus*[21]
	Platypezidae	*Crabro* s. l.[26]; *Oxybelus*[21]
	Platystomatidae	*Crabro* s. l.[26]; *Oxybelus*[21]
	Psychodidae	*Rhopalum*[6]
	Rhagionidae	*Crabro*[6]; *Crossocerus*[6]; *Ectemnius*[6]; *Oxybelus*[21]
	Sarcophagidae	*Bembex*[8]; *Glenostictia*[8]; *Oxybelus*[4,21]; *Stictia*[4,8]
	Scatophagidae	*Mellinus*[1]; *Oxybelus*[1]
	Scatopsidae	*Crossocerus*[6]
	Sepsidae	*Crossocerus*[6]
	Simuliidae	*Crabro* s. l.[1,6]; *Crossocerus*[6]; *Lindenius*[6]; *Oxybelus*[11]
	Sphaeroceridae	*Oxybelus*[21]

Order	Family	Genera of Sphecidae
	Stratiomyidae	*Bembex*[1,8]; *Crabro*[6]; *Crossocerus*[6]; *Ectemnius*[6]; *Glenostictia*[8]; *Mellinus*[1]; *Oxybelus*[11]; *Piyuma*[6]; *Stictia*[4,8]
	Syrphidae	*Bembex*[1,6]; *Crabro*[6]; *Crossocerus*[6]; *Ectemnius*[6]; *Glenostictia*[8]; *Mellinus*[1]; *Oxybelus*[21]; *Podagritus*[6]; *Steniolia*[8]; *Stictia*[8]
	Tabanidae	*Bembex*[1,8]; *Crabro*[6]; *Ectemnius*[6]; *Glenostictia*[8]; *Stictia*[4,8]
	Tachinidae	*Bembex*[8]; *Crabro* s. l.[1,6]; *Glenostictia*[8]; *Mellinus*[17]; *Oxybelus*[21]; *Stictia*[4,8]
	Tephrididae	*Oxybelus*[21]
	Therevidae	*Crabro*[6]; *Crossocerus*[6]; *Ectemnius*[6]
	Thrypetidae	*Crossocerus*[6]; *Ectemnius*[6]; *Lindenius*[6]; *Piyuma*[6]; *Podagritus*[6]; *Rhopalum*[6]
	Tipulidae	*Crossocerus*[6]; *Rhopalum*[6]
	Trichoceridae	*Crossocerus*[6]
Ephemeroptera	Baëtidae *(Chloëon dipterum)*	*Crossocerus walkeri*[1,6]
Heteroptera	Coreidae	*Astata*[1]; *Bicyrtes*[4,8]; *Crabro* s. l.[1]; *Plenoculus*[4]; *Solierella*[5]
	Cydnidae	*Astata*[1]; *Bicyrtes*[8]; *Dryudella*[4,20]
	Lygaeidae	*Astata*[1,4]; *Bicyrtes*[8]; *Solierella*[1,4,5]
	Miridae	*Anacrabro*[6]; *Belomicrus*[22]; *Crossocerus*[6]; *Glenostictia*[8]; *Lindenius*[6]; *Plenoculus*[4]
	Nabidae	*Dinetus*[1]; *Solierella*[5]
	Pentatomidae	*Astata*[1,4]; *Bicyrtes*[4,8]; *Dryudella*[20]; *Solierella*[5]
	Reduviidae	*Bicyrtes*[4,8]; *Dinetus*[1]; *Dryudella*[4,20]; *Solierella*[5]
	Scutelleridae	*Astata*[20]
Homoptera	Cercopidae	*Alysson*[8]; *Bembecinus*[8]; *Didineis*[1]; *Gorytes* s. l.[1,8]; *Psen*[4]; *Stizus*[1]
	Cicadidae	*Exeirus*[8]; *Sphecius*[8]
	Delphacidae	*Alysson*[1,8]; *Didineis*[1]; *Mimesa*[1,4]
	Fulgoroidea	*Bembecinus*[8]; *Didineis*[8]; *Gorytes* s. l.[1,8]
	Issididae	*Alysson*[1]; *Gorytes* s. l.[1]; *Stizus*[1]
	Jassidae	*Alysson*[1]
	Membracidae	*Bembecinus*[8]; *Gorytes* s. l.[1,8]; *Psammaecius*[4]; *Psen*[1]
	Typhlocybidae	*Crossocerus*[6]
Hymenoptera	Apidae	*Bembex* (Australia)[24]; *Cerceris*[1]; *Glenostictia*[8]; *Palarus*[1]; *Philanthus*[1,4,19]; *Trachypus*[23]
	Braconidae	*Glenostictia scitula*[8]; *Lindenius pygmaeus*[6]
	Chalcididae	*Lindenius pygmaeus*[1,6]
	Formicidae	*Aphilanthops*[4]; *Clypeadon*[4]; *Encopognathus*[6]; *Glenostictia*[8]; *Lindenius*[6]; *Rhopalum*[6]; *Tracheliodes*[9]
	Ichneumonidae	*Palarus variegatus*[1]; *Philanthus*[19]
	Mutillidae	*Palarus variegatus*[1]
	Ophionidae	*Lindenius pygmaeus*[1,6]; *Palarus variegatus*[1]
	Pteromalidae	*Lindenius pygmaeus*[6]
	Scoliidae	*Palarus variegatus*[1]
	Sphecidae	*Glenostictia scitula*[7]; *Palarus variegatus*[1]; *Philanthus*[19]; *Trachypus*[23]
	Tenthredinidae (larvae)	*Ammophila*[3,7]

Order	Family	Genera of Sphecidae
	Tiphiidae	*Palarus variegatus*[1]
	Torymidae	*Glenostictia scitula*[8]
	Vespidae	*Palarus variegatus*[1]; *Philanthus*[19]; *Trachypus*[23]
Lepidoptera	Caterpillars, among others of	
	Gelechiidae	*Ammophila*[7]
	Geometridae	*Ammophila*[18]
	Hesperiidae	*Ammophila*[18]
	Noctuidae	*Ammophila*[1,4,18]; *Podalonia*
	Adults, among others of	
	Crambidae	*Lestica*[1,6]; *Stictiella*[6]
	Drepanidae	*Ectemnius*[6]
	Geometridae	*Lestica*[1,6]; *Ectemnius*[6]
	Hesperiidae	*Stictiella*[4,7]
	Lycaenidae	*Ectemnius*[6]; *Stictiella*[4]
	Noctuidae	*Ectemnius*[6]; *Stictiella*[4,8]
	Nymphalidae	*Stictiella*[4,8]
	Pyralidae	*Ectemnius*[6]; *Lestica*[1,6]
	Torticidae	*Ectemnius*[6]; *Lestica*[1,6]
Neuroptera	Myrmeleonidae	*Bembex wilcannia* (Australia)[24]
Odonata		*Bembex* (Australia)[8,24]
Orthoptera	Many families, among others	
	Acrididae	*Solierella*[4,5]; *Sphex*[1,4]; *Stizus*[1]; *Tachysphex*[2,4]; *Tachytes*[1,4]
	Catantopidae	*Sphex*[1]; *Stizus*[1]
	Gryllidae	*Larra*[4]; *Larropsis*[4]; *Lyroda*[16]; *Motes*[16]; *Notogonia*[1]; *Sphex*[1,4]; *Tachysphex*[1];
	Gryllotalpidae	*Larra*[1,6]; *Tachytes*[4]
	Tetrigidae	*Tachysphex*[4]; *Tachytes*[4]
	Tettigoniidae	*Ectemnius furuchii*[6]; *Moniaecera*[9]; *Sphex*[1,4]; *Stizus*[8]; *Tacysphex*[1]; *Tachytes*[4]
Blattodea	Blattidae	*Ampulex*[2,4]; *Podium*[4,9]
	Pseudomopidae	*Ampulex*[1]; *Dolichurus*[1,4]; *Tachysphex*[1,4]
Mantodea	Mantidae	*Chlorion*[2]; *Stizus*[1]; *Tachysphex*[1,4]
Psocoptera		*Rhopalum*[4,6]
Thysanoptera	Thripidae	*Ammoplanus*[2]; *Microstigmus thripoctenus*[14]; *Spilomena*[1]; *Xysma*[4]
Arachnida	Various families of Araneae	*Miscophus*[1,13]; *Nitelopterus*[4,13]; *Pison*[1]; *Pisonopsis*[22]; *Sceliphron*[1,4]; *Trypoxylon*[1]

Sources
[1]BERLAND (1925); [2]BISCHOFF (1927); [3]ADRIAANSE (1947); [4]MUSEBECK et al. (1951); [5]WILLIAMS (1950), Kurczewski (1967); [6]LECLERCQ (1954); [7]EVANS (1965); [8]EVANS (1966a); [9]KROMBEIN (1967); [10]MATTHEWS (1968); [11]SNODDY (1968); [12]SCULLEN and WOLD (1969), EVANS (1971); [13]KURCZEWSKI (1969); [14]MATTHEWS (1970); [15]EVANS and MATTHEWS (1971); [16]KURCZEWSKI and KURCZEWSKI (1971); [17]HUBER (1961); [18]EVANS (1959a); [19]EVANS and LIN (1959), EVANS (1966c); [20]PARKER (1962, 1969); [21]PECKHAM et al. (1973); [22]EVANS (1969); [23]EVANS and MATTHEWS (1973); [24]EVANS and MATTHEWS (1975); [25]HAMM and RICHARDS (1926); [26]BRISTOWE (1948).

A few species of wasps prey only upon one species: *Clypeadon (Aphilanthops)* *laticinctus* is specialized on worker ants of *Pogonomyrmex occidentalis; A. frigidus* preys almost exclusively upon queens of the ant *Formica fusca* during their nuptial flights (Wheeler, 1913; Evans, 1962); or *Cerceris tuberculata* hunts selectively for one species of curculionid beetles (*Cleopus ophthalmicus*) (Berland, 1925; Pawlowsky, 1927).

Host specificity, however, does not imply that the venom is specific for this species of insect (see Sect. B, II, 1., b, δ). That some sphecid venoms exhibit considerable nonspecificity can be inferred from prey records for *Palarus variegatus* which in Southern Europe paralyzes members of such different hymenopteran families as Ichneumonidae, Tiphiidae, Scoliidae, Sphecidae, Apidae, and Vespidae (Berland, 1925). The North American *Glenostictia scitula* prey upon different Hemiptera and Heteroptera, and in addition on many species of various families of Diptera and Hymenoptera including sphecid wasps (Evans, 1966a). *Ammophila azteca* prey upon caterpillars of various Lepidoptera and upon two genera of sawflies (Tenthredinidae, Hymenoptera) simultaneously (Evans, 1965).

These observations together with the prey records for many species suggest that the venoms of sphecid wasps generally do not exhibit great species specificity in their effects (see also Sect. B, II, 1, b, δ). They seem to be effective in a large number of insects from different orders and in addition also on arachnids. It has not been shown whether this holds true for arthropods in general since no experiments of injecting venom, for example into isopods (Crustacea), have been performed.

II. Venoms of Specific Genera

1. Genus Philanthus

a) Aspects of Biology and Preying

The genus *Philanthus* occurs with about 135 species in the holartic, Ethiopian, and oriental regions. The systematics of the European and North African species have been worked out by Kohl (1891), de Beaumont (1949, 1951, 1960) and Mochi (1939), that of the American species by Strandtmann (1946) and Bohart (1972).

All species construct burrows in the soil and in general stock them with bees of many genera, sometimes with wasps (Vespidae, Sphecidae, Chrysididae, Ichneumonidae; Evans and Lin, 1959; Evans, 1966c, 1975). Prey selection seems to depend on the abundance of a particular prey in an area. At least three species have specialized on the honey bee, *Apis mellifera:* the North American *Philanthus flavifrons* (=*crabroniformis*) (Bohart, 1954) and *P. sanbornii* (Evans, 1955) and the European *P. triangulum* (Berland, 1925; Bischoff, 1927; Rathmayer, 1962b). The prey is paralyzed at the site of capture and carried to the nest in swift flight beneath the body of the wasps (see photographs in Olberg, 1953, 1959).

Usually several bees are piled venter up in a cell and the egg is laid on the top bee once the cell is fully provisioned. The larva hatches within a few days and feeds from the stored prey. Five to 8 days after hatching, it spins an ovoid cocoon in which it hibernates as prepupa.

Further observations on the biology of different species are contained in PECK-HAM and PECKHAM (1898), RAU and RAU (1918), REINHARD (1924), HAMM and RICHARDS (1930), GRANDI (1931), VERGNE (1931), TINBERGEN (1932, 1935), MOLITOR (1939), OLBERG (1953, 1959), EVANS and LIN (1959), POWELL and CHEMSACK (1959), EVANS (1964), ARMITAGE (1965), EVANS (1966c, 1973), SIMON THOMAS and SIMON THOMAS (1972), and ALCOCK (1974). EVANS (1966c) regards *Philanthus* as one of the most interesting and rewarding genera of digger wasps for comparative ethological studies.

b) Philanthus triangulum

α) *Anatomy of the Sting Apparatus.* The sting apparatus of *P. triangulum* has been described by BORDAS (1895) and RATHMAYER (1962b). The skeletal part consists of a pair each of outer and inner plates which serve as attachments for an elaborate musculature. The aculeus is formed by three parts, the unpaired stylet and the paired lancets. The lancets can be moved alternately through movements of the outer plates, over a ridge along the proximal edge of the inner plates. Within the stylet, the lancets glide on its ventral side over tracklike ridges (Fig. 4b and c). Movements of the outer plates finally will result in alternating protrusion and retraction of the lancets at the tip of the stylet. The stylet itself can also be protruded by muscles inserting at the furcula. The lancets pierce the wound through which the venom, flowing in a canal formed by the stylet and the two lancets, is injected into the prey.

The venom is most probably produced in the tubular venom gland (Fig. 4a) and stored in the reservoir until use. For paralysis, only the contents of the reservoir are essential (RATHMAYER, 1962b). The function of the two accessory glands (Bordas and Dufour glands), both of which do not open into the venom canal, is uncertain.

β) *Stinging of the Bee and Action of the Venom.* The bees captured by *P. triangulum* are invariably stung only once into the soft membrane behind one of the front coxae (Fig. 5). The point of puncture can be easily identified in paralyzed bees even many days after the stinging by its blackish appearance which is probably due to oxidation of tyrosine within the hemolymph. Histologic serial sections of bees stung by *Philanthus* showed that, in general, the central nervous system, in particular the prothoracic ganglion, was not reached by the sting. The track taken by the sting within the bee could be traced in histologic sections in several instances (RATHMAYER, 1962b). It ended within the intrinsic muscles of the front legs in the vicinity of the first thoracic ganglion but without injuring the sheath surrounding it. However, in 2 out of 12 cases investigated, the perilemma of the prothoracic ganglion was injured by the sting.

When *Philanthus*-wasps were forced to sting bees experimentally at various points (ventral side of the neck, mesonotum, episternum, tip of the abdomen) paralysis could always be achieved. This is clear evidence that all that is necessary in order to immobilize the bee is to bring the venom into the hemolymph (RATH-MAYER, 1962b; PIEK et al., 1971). The point of stinging bears no importance in this respect. In a different context, however, it is of great importance: the closer the point of venom to the main centers of locomotion, i.e. the leg muscles in

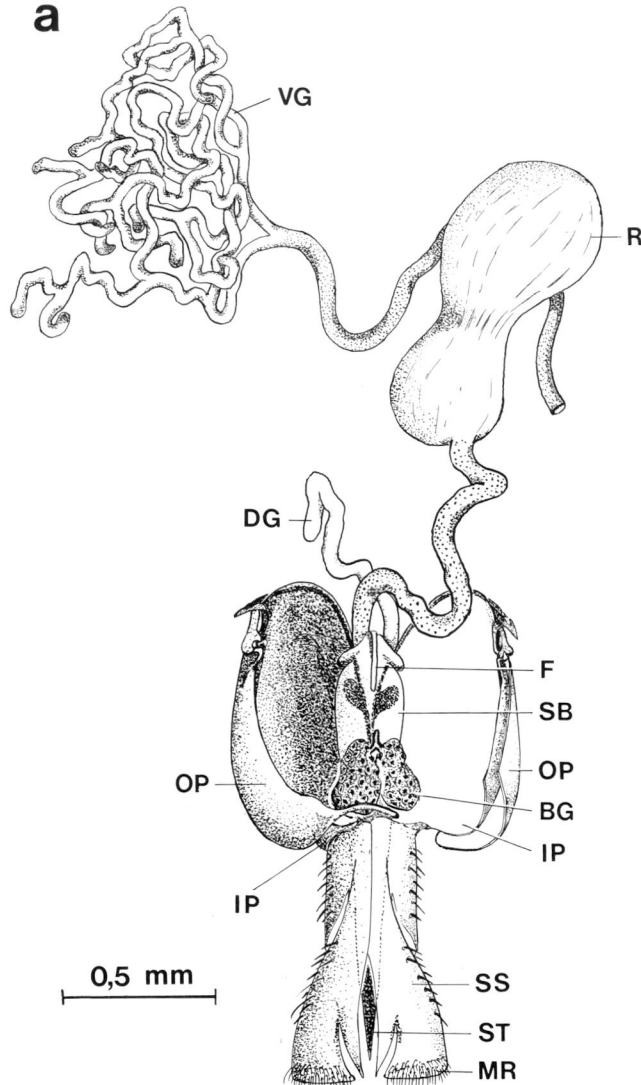

Fig. 4a−c. Sting apparatus of bee wolf wasp *Philanthus triangulum*. (a) Total view. At right side venom gland is omitted and outer and inner plates have been cut open for clarity. (b) and (c) opposite page. Cross section through region of sting sheaths at a proximal and very distal point to show relation of sting sheaths to aculeus and formation of the venom canal respectively. Abbreviations: BG=Bordas' gland; DG=Dufour's gland; F=furcula; IP=inner plate; L=lancet; MR=mechanoreceptors; N=afferent nerve from mechanoreceptors; OP= outer plate; R=reservoir; SB=stylet bulbus; SS=sting sheath; ST=stylet; VC=venom canal; VG=venom gland

the thorax, the quicker the onset of paralysis (Rathmayer, 1962b). A summary of 26 experiments is depicted in Figure 6.

The point of entry of the sting under natural conditions behind the first pair of legs guarantees the quickest onset of immobilization. Observations of many stinging acts exerted by *P. triangulum* showed that immediately after the stinging,

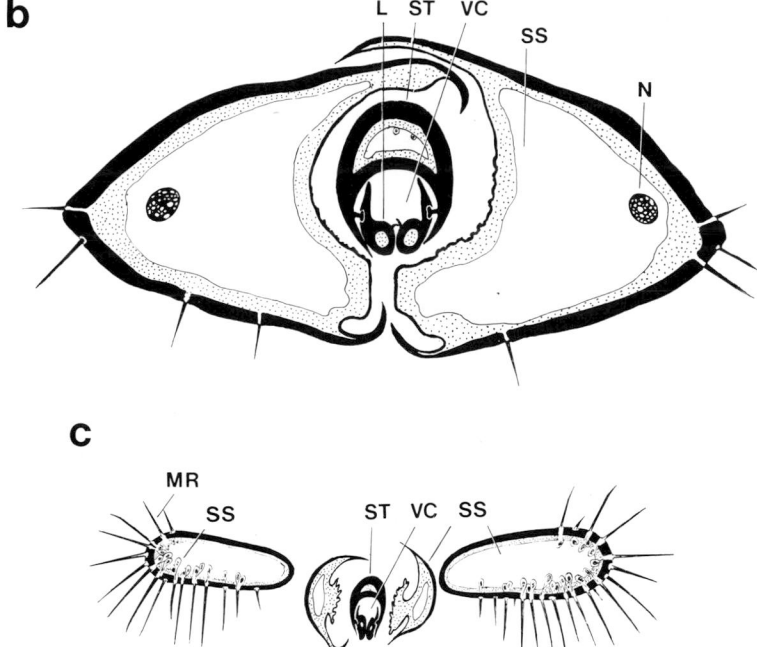

Fig. 4b and c (see text opposite page)

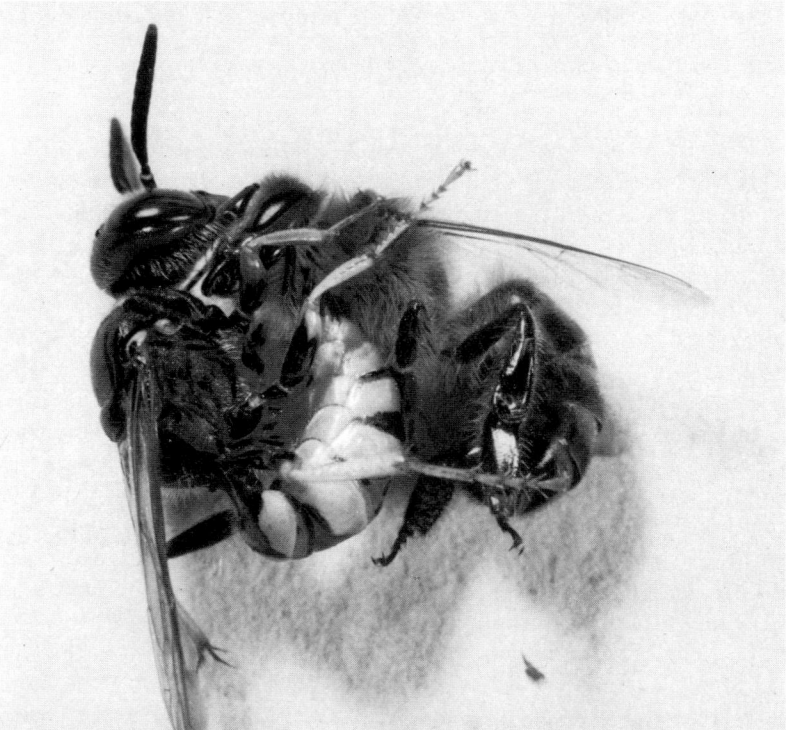

Fig. 5. *Philanthus triangulum* stinging its prey, the honey bee, *Apis mellifica*. Bee is held with the front and middle legs. Sting is inserted behind front legs

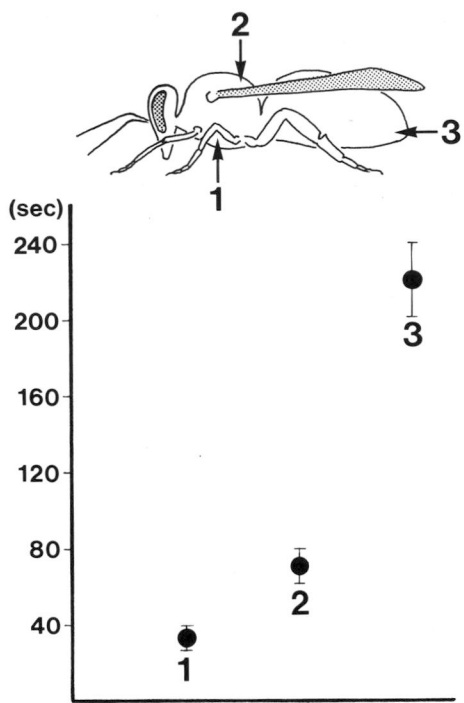

Fig. 6. Dependence of time of onset of paralysis in honey bee *Apis mellifera* from point of venom injection through stings of *Philanthus triangulum*. 1 = mesosternum; n 11; 2 = scutellum; n 8; 3 = tip of abdomen between tergite 6 and 5; n 7. The bars represent standard error. (Modified from RATHMAYER, 1966)

which lasted for approximately 30 s, front and middle legs cannot be moved any more. Paralysis spreads to the hind legs which start to become immobilized after another min. There is also a spread of paralysis within a given leg, progressing from the coxa toward the tibia. Metatarsus and tarsi can still be moved 30—40 min after the other parts of the leg have become completely paralyzed.

There is some indication that newly hatched wasps possess less venom in their reservoir than adults, so paralysis performed by young *Philanthus* wasps usually is not permanent and the bees recover within some hours. The reservoir of adult wasps contains enough venom to deeply paralyze up to four bees within 30 min permanently.

PIEK et al. (1971) have tested the activity of the venom of *P. triangulum* extracted from reservoirs on bees by injecting small venom-containing samples of 10 µl into the thorax. The pharmacologic activity of the venom was expressed in bee units (B.U.): one B.U. was defined as that quantity of venom which produced paralysis of more than 1 h duration in 5 out of 10 bees. The bee unit is comparable to an ED_{50}. The time to obtain an ED_{50} depended linearly on the amount of venom injected. Testing venom solutions of highest activity, PIEK et al. (1971) could show that the venom contents of the reservoir of one wasp corresponded to 1 or 1.25 B.U. In other words, this means that the venom present in the reservoir of one *Philanthus* is enough to paralyze 5 to 6 bees at least for 1 h.

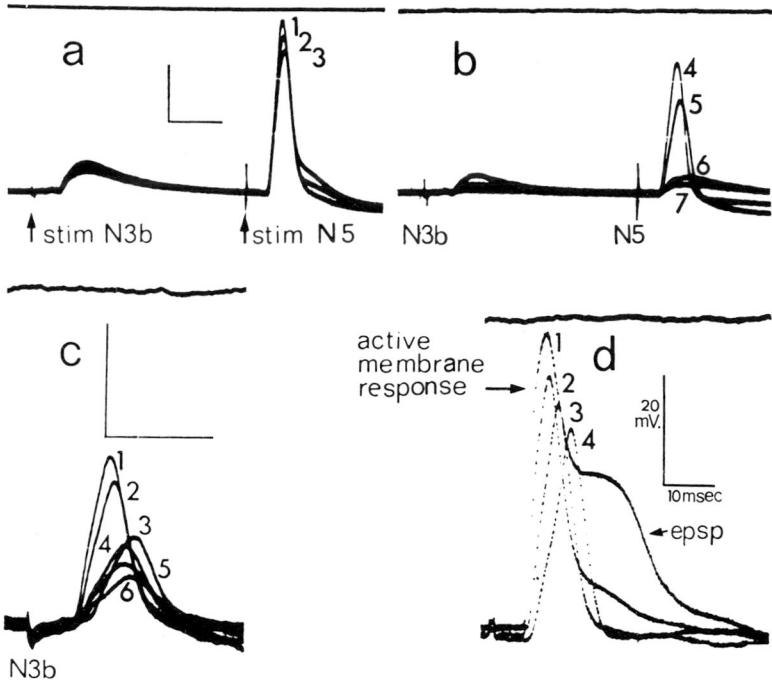

Fig. 7. Effect of venom of *Philanthus triangulum* on excitatory postsynaptic potentials (epsp's) in *Extensor tibiae*-muscle (a to c) and *Retractor unguis*-muscle (d) of locust *Schistocerca gregaria*. Stimulation of nerve 3b resulted in epsp's produced by "slow" motoraxon, stimulation of nerve 5 in epsp's elicited by "fast" motoraxon. a. Venom application in concentration of 3 B.U./ml and, b. of 6 B.U./ml. c. Effect of 5 B.U./ml on "slow" epsp's in a different (proximal) part of same muscle. d. Effect of 3 B.U./ml on active membrane responses. The numbers represent consecutive records taken every 30 s. Upper lines indicate zero potential. Calibration bars: 20 mV, 10 ms throughout. (From PIEK et al., 1971)

γ) Mechanism of Action of the Venom. From a series of observations and experiments (RATHMAYER, 1962a, b) it was concluded that the venom of *P. triangulum* exerts its paralyzing effects not through an action on the central nervous system but through a peripheral block of neuromuscular activity. PIEK et al. (1971) have performed electrophysiologic investigations on the mechanism of action of this venom on nerve-muscle preparations. They confirmed the conclusions reached by RATHMAYER (1962b) on different experimental evidence. The experiments of PIEK et al. (1971) show that application of *Philanthus* venom with a concentration of 3 B.U./ml (see Sect. B, II, 1., b, *β*) to a nerve-muscle preparation (*extensor tibiae*) of the locust *Schistocerca gregaria* caused a decline of the amplitude of the excitatory postsynaptic potentials (epsp's) which had been evoked by stimulation of the "fast" and "slow" motor axons. At a venom concentration of 6 B.U. both types of epsp's disappeared (Fig. 7). In cases where the "fast" epsp reached threshold depolarization for eliciting an electrically excitable response at the muscle fibre membrane (Fig. 7c and d), both rate of rise and amplitude of the active component declined. This probably reflects the effect of the venom on the epsp. These results of PIEK et al. (1971) on the one hand correct some earlier conclusions (PIEK, 1966a, b) from experiments which had suffered from several technical difficulties, and on the other hand they confirm the general view on the mode of action of *Philanthus* venom. Electrical responses of the muscle fiber evoked by direct stimulation as well as nervous activity in afferent systems and within the central nervous system (PIEK et al., 1971) were not affected by the venom even at high doses (50 B.U.).

PIEK et al. (1971) reported also that the electrical responses of the muscle fibers of the *adductor coxae* in *Schistocerca,* evoked by stimulation of the inhibitory axon, are blocked by the venom. In some cases block of the inhibitory postsynaptic potentials (ipsp's), however, needed higher venom concentrations and longer time of exposure to the venom.

A study of spontaneous transmitter release at neuromuscular endings at the adductor coxae of *Schistocerca* (PIEK et al., 1971) revealed that the amplitude of both inhibitory and excitatory miniature potentials (mipsp's and mepsp's) remained fairly constant under the influence of *Philanthus* venom (Fig. 8). The frequency, however, of mepsp's and mipsp's started to decrease between 1 and 3 min after venom application reaching zero after 7 to 10 min. In some cases an initial increase in frequency of mepsp's was seen immediately after venom application, similar to that shown in Figure 8 for the mipsp's. This effect of the venom on the frequency of the mepsp's without a major change in their amplitude has been observed by PIEK et al. (1971) in several nerve-muscle preparations of different test insects including the flight muscles of the honey bee (PIEK and NJIO, 1975).

These experiments show that paralysis by the venom of *P. triangulum* is caused by a block of neuromuscular transmission. The analysis of the miniature potentials proves that this effect is produced presynaptically. The venom progressively reduces the amount of transmitter released by the presynaptic nerve-action potential until it stops both evoked and spontaneous release. In a first electronmicroscopic investigation of flight muscles of paralyzed bees PIEK and NJIO (1975) could detect no difference in the number and distribution of synaptic vesicles within the terminals. The question whether central synapses and other structures are also affected after some time has not been settled. There are indications that there are secondary effects of the venom on the central nervous system also. This has been discussed by RATHMAYER (1962b) and PIEK et al. (1971) but awaits further experimental clarification.

The observations on the mode of action of *P. triangulum* venom are in close agreement with the mechanism of action of another paralyzing venom, that of the braconid wasp *Habrobracon* (*Microbracon*) where the analysis of its pharmacologic effects has been recently carried even further (PIEK, 1966c; PIEK and ENGELS, 1969; PIEK and MANTEL, 1970; WALTHER and RATHMAYER, 1974; RATHMAYER and WALTHER, 1976; WALTHER and REINECKE, 1976).

Since much of the observational data on prey paralyzed by other solitary wasps fit with the experimental evidence obtained for the venom of *P. triangulum* and *Habrobracon* one might assume that this mechanism of presynaptic action is a general feature of the venoms of paralyzing wasps.

δ) *Specificity of the Venom.* Although *P. triangulum* preys exclusively upon honey bees, its venom is highly unspecific. It paralyzes practically all other insects which have been tested (37 genera from 15 families out of 7 orders) as well

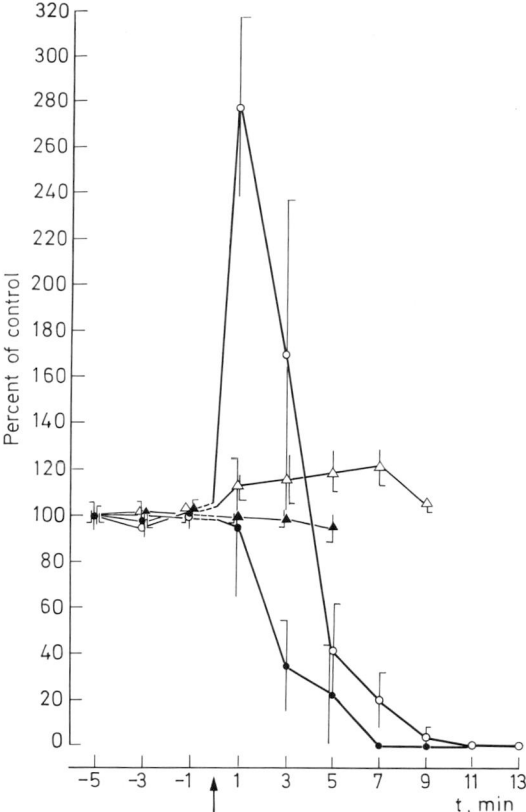

- frequency of mepsp
○ frequency of mipsp
▲ amplitude of mepsp
△ amplitude of mipsp
↑ time of venom application

Fig. 8. Effect of *Philanthus triangulum* venom (3 B.U./ml) on the frequency and amplitude of excitatory (mepsp's) and inhibitory (mipsp's) miniature potentials of *Adductor coxae*-muscle of locust *Schistocerca gregaria*. Vertical bars represent standard error of the mean (n = 5) (From PIEK et al., 1971)

as spiders. The results of experiments in which *Philanthus* was forced to sting other insects into the mesonotum are summarized in Table 2. PIEK et al. (1971) have also shown that venom extracted from *P. triangulum* is active on neuromuscular preparations of several insects.

Two species, however, have proven to be insensitive to the venom of *P. triangulum*: *Philanthus* itself is immune against its own venom, and *Palarus variegatus* which also preys upon *P. triangulum* among other digger wasps, showed no effects upon injection of *Philanthus*-venom (RATHMAYER, 1962b).

The chemical composition of the venom is unknown. Preliminary experiments (VISSER and SPANJER, 1969) suggesting that the active compound probably has a molecular weight of less than 700 have not been completed to date.

Table 2. Effect of venom of *Philanthus triangulum* on different arthropods. (Data compiled from RATHMAYER, 1962b)

Order	No of families tested	No of genera tested	No of species tested	Effect
Insecta				
Hymenoptera	5	25	33	dp
Lepidoptera (caterpillars)	2	4	4	dp
Coleoptera	1	1	1	dp
Orthoptera	2	2	2	wp
Hemiptera	2	2	2	dp
Odonata	1	1	1	pd
Diptera	2	2	2	pd
Arachnida	1	1	1	dp

dp = deep paralysis; wp = weak paralysis; pd = dead after initial paralysis.

2. Genus Sceliphron

a) Composition of the Venom

The only experiments on the chemistry of sphecid venoms have been performed on the venom of the mud-dauber *S. caementarium* (O'CONNOR and ROSENBROOK, 1963; ROSENBROOK and O'CONNOR, 1964a, b). The species of *Sceliphron* prey exclusively on different spiders which are deeply paralyzed by the sting. The biology of this group is treated by SCHAFER (1949) and EBERHARD (1970).

The venom was obtained by electrically "milking" the wasps. No 5-hydroxy-tryptamine, histamine, acetylcholine or small peptides (kinins) could be detected (O'CONNOR and ROSENBROOK, 1963) which are, for example, prominent constituents in venoms of vespid wasps (HABERMANN, 1968). The maximum protein content of the dried venom amounting to only $25 \pm 3\%$ is unexpectedly low (ROSENBROOK and O'CONNOR, 1964a). It consists of at least five different proteins. By further chromatographic separation-techniques additionally 17 non-protein constituents have been found: free amino acids (histidine 1%, methionine 1%), free pipecolic acid (0.1%), lecithin (6%), salt of a hydroxy acid, partially with a steroid character (58%), and six or seven unidentified components (11%). It is unlikely that a single component of this venom produces paralysis but rather a co-operative action of several substances will be effective (ROSENBROOK and O'CONNOR, 1964b).

A comparison of the venom obtained by electrically milking the wasps with that from extracts of the whole sting apparatus showed that in the latter an additional 15 compounds, not present in the pure venom, could be detected. This emphasizes the necessity to work with pure venoms (ROSENBROOK and O'CONNOR, 1964b).

C. Venoms of Pompilidae

I. General Aspects

The time is simply not yet ripe to review the venoms of Pompilidae, not to speak of Mutillidae and Bethylidae. Virtually no quantitative data exists on the venoms of these families. They are nevertheless included within this chapter to summarize observational data on the state of paralysis elicited by these venoms.

Wasps of the family Pompilidae occur all over the globe. They are regarded as phylogenetically older than the Sphecidae. All species prey exclusively upon spiders, the size of which is approximately that of the hunting wasp. All pompilids provision their brood cells with a single spider only. Although there is generally a considerable degree of host specificity among spider wasps (EVANS and YOSHIMOTO, 1962; KURCZEWSKI and KURCZEWSKI, 1968) many species do show a broad spectrum of prey records (RICHARDS and HAMM, 1939). *Priocnemis cornica* for example, virtually preys upon any errant spider of proper size (EVANS, 1953).

For details of the preying behavior as well as for prey records the reader is referred to the work of PECKHAM and PECKHAM (1898), BISCHOFF (1927), NIELSEN (1932), RICHARDS and HAMM (1939), IWATA (1942), EVANS and YOSHIMOTO (1962) and (particularly) KURCZEWSKI and KURCZEWSKI (1968).

II. Stinging and Effects of the Venom on Locomotion

The procedure of stinging seems to differ little within the whole family. Many spider wasps sting the prey several times rapidly into any part of the body, usually into the abdomen. If this first sequence of stings was successful, a final slower sting is applied into the venter of the cephalothorax as has been described for *Anoplius autumnalis* (EVANS and YOSHIMOTO, 1962) for example. The venom paralyzes the spider completely although for different periods of time. Stings into the cephalothorax alone have also been reported for many species.

The effect of the venom on the spiders is quite different within different genera of pompilid wasps. Although deep paralysis is usually present immediately after the stings, many spiders recover partially or completely. This is the case in particular within the genus *Anoplius*. Also, spiders stung by *Homonotus* recover very quickly from paralysis and take up their normal activities until the wasp larva, developing like an ectoparasite on the abdomen, finally kills the spider (RICHARDS and HAMM, 1939).

In other cases, however, paralysis is profound and of long duration (*Priocnemis, Aupoplus, Dipogon, Episyron* and others). Three spiders taken, for example from *Sericopompilus apicalis* before oviposition, remained alive, though immobilized for 18, 44, and 46 days (EVANS, 1953).

It is not clear what facts determine whether paralysis is temporary or permanent. This is not only a question of different genera of spider wasps or prey. The published accounts on the state of paralysis of spiders captured by a given species of pompilid indicate much variation already. EVANS and YOSHIMOTO (1962) found, for example, with *Anoplius marginatus* several spiders to be deeply paralyzed which even died after several days. On the other hand, they also obtained spiders which recovered after several days and one spider recovered fully after 24 h. Similar results are known in other species, too.

From the observational data it is likely that the venom exerts a similar blocking action in most cases as has been found for other paralyzing hymenopteran venoms (see Sect. B, II, 1., b, γ). Stinging right into the central nervous system, as has been claimed in the older literature, is certainly not necessary for immobilization since stings into the abdomen, which is devoid of ganglia, are fully effective.

Rabaud (1917) also denied for anatomical reasons that stings which are placed into the ventral side of the cephalothorax penetrate the ganglia. It could be shown experimentally (Rabaud, 1917) that for paralysis of a spider it is sufficient if the venom of the wasp is brought into the hemolymph independent of the point of administration: Rabaud forced pompilid wasps of six species to sting 40 spiders of 17 genera into the tip of the abdomen and achieved paralysis in every single instance. The venom of pompilid wasps can also paralyze young crickets and caterpillars (Rabaud, 1917). This might be taken as evidence that these venoms, as those of Sphecidae, are not very specific.

There must, however, be differences in the composition of pompilid and sphecid venoms. This is simply demonstrated by the fact that, in contrast to the venoms of Sphecidae, pompilid venoms always inflict heavy and burning pain when the sting pierces the human skin.

D. Venoms of Mutillidae

The Mutillidae comprise a large family of more than 2000 species which is most numerous in Australia, Central and South America. Very little is known about the habits of these wasps and on the use of the venom. The biology of some North American species is treated by Mickel (1928). All mutillids are parasites on larvae of other Hymenoptera, such as Apidae, Vespidae, Sphecidae, Pompilidae and, as reported recently (Mickel, 1974), also Evaniidae. But also larvae of Coleoptera, Lepidoptera and Diptera have been reported as prey. An annotated bibliography on mutillid research has been compiled by Mickel (1970).

The females, always apterous, run on the ground in search of their host's nest, where they deposit their eggs in the cocoons. They possess a sting apparatus which they use fiercely for defense but apparently (Herman, 1968) not for paralysis of the host's larvae. The venom apparatus of some species has been described by Pawlowsky (1927), Oeser (1961) and Herman (1968, 1975). The venom of mutillid wasps produces heavy burning pain, in particular that of *Dasymutilla occidentalis* (Mickel, 1928) and that of the large species living in tropical forests. Stings into the sole of the foot, occurring frequently among natives of South America, are very painful for more than 24 h (Baer, 1901).

The chemistry and pharmacologic actions of the venoms are unknown. Welsh and Batty (1963) failed to detect 5-hydroxytryptamine in the venom of the mutillid *Dasymutilla* spec.

E. Venoms of Bethylidae

The Bethylidae are a cosmopolitan family of some 500 species of very small size. They are considered as the most primitive of existant Hymenoptera. Details of the biology of some species as well as prey records can be found in Voukassovitch (1924), Bischoff (1927), van Emden (1931), Nielsen (1932), Kearns (1934), Powell (1938), Finlayson (1950a, b), Evans (1964b), Yamada (1955) and Gordh (1976). Almost all members prey on the larvae of Coleoptera or Lepidoptera. The females do not construct brood cells. They hunt for hosts living in cryptic habitats (wood, stems, galls, fruits, seeds, leaf-rolls, etc.), usually sting the prey several times and in general attach several eggs to its outside. The development of the larvae is external. The prey is sometimes transported to new places, such as crevices, and sometimes it is left where it has been attacked.

Bethylids show various degrees of host specificity among the coleopterous and lepidopterous hosts. Under experimental conditions, however, the venom also paralyzes hymenopterous larvae and even termites (BRIDWELL, 1920). The genus *Pseudisobrachium* has switched from coleopterous prey to ants: they live as myrmecophiles among ants of various subfamilies and prey upon their larvae (EVANS, 1961).

Bethylid wasps sting the prey many times and into many parts of the body without great precision, sometimes over a period of days, until movements cease. The anatomy of the sting apparatus of one species has been described (*Cephalonomia*: VAN EMDEN, 1931; OESER, 1961). BRIDWELL (1920) described paralysis exerted by *Scleroderma immigrans*: depending on the size of the beetle larvae (Cerambycidae) a different number of stings is inflicted. The first stings are usually applied to the region of the head, probably to immobilize the dangerous mandibles of the prey. *Goniozus gallicola* stings the prey (moth larvae of the family Gelechiidae) at frequent intervals over a period of 2 or 3 days. The venom is injected near the host's ventral nerve cord usually posterior to the gula (GORDH, 1976). The venom apparently spreads from the point of sting insertion to the centres of locomotion and produces rapid, but incomplete immobilization. The ganglia are not reached by the sting. Permanent paralysis of the prey is normal, though there are many reports of full recovery (cf. CLAUSEN, 1940).

Nothing is known about the venom itself. Stings of bethylid wasps have, however, received special attention because of their effects on man (VAN EMDEN, 1931; BERNARD and JACQUEMIN, 1948; WALTON, 1948; DISS and TIMON-DAVID, 1951; FUCHS, 1952; JACQUEMIN and VAISSIERE, 1952; THEODORIDES, 1955; NICOLI and ERLANDE-BRANDENBURG, 1957; GUIGLIA, 1958). The minute wasps of the genus *Scleroderma* inflict 4 to 5 very painful stings usually when trapped between clothing and skin. The pain persists for many hours. In a case report given by NICOLI and ERLANDE-BRANDENBURG (1957) symptoms such as oscillations in body temperature and painful swellings in the vicinity of the stinging are mentioned. Treatment with antihistamines was without success.

Appendix 1: Classification of the Family Sphecidae

The following classification lists the subfamilies, tribes, and genera of sphecid wasps mentioned in the present text showing their systematic relationships (based on MUESEBECK et al., 1951; LECLERCQ, 1954; DE BEAUMONT, 1964)

Family Sphecidae	
Subfamily: Ampulicinae	*Ampulex, Dolichurus*
Subfamily: Astatinae	*Astata, Dryudella*
Subfamily: Larrinae	
Tribe: Miscophini	*Lyroda, Plenoculus, Solierella, Miscophus, Nitelopterus, Nitela*
Tribe: Dinetini	*Dinetus*
Tribe: Tachytini	*Tachytes, Larropsis, Tachysphex*
Tribe: Larrini	*Larra, Motes, Notogonia*
Tribe: Palarini	*Palarus*
Subfamily: Trypoxylinae	*Pison, Trypoxylon*

Subfamily: Pemphredoninae
   Tribe: Psenini   *Diodontus, Psen, Mimesa*
   Tribe: Pemphredonini   *Pemphredon, Stigmus, Microstigmus, Passaloecus, Spilomena,*
                                   Xysma, Ammoplanus, Xylocelia

Subfamily: Sphecinae
   Tribe: Sphecini   *Sphex*
   Tribe: Ammophilini   *Ammophila, Podalonia*
   Tribe: Sceliphronini   *Sceliphron, Podium, Chlorion*
Subfamily: Mellininae   *Mellinus*
Subfamily: Nyssoninae
   Tribe: Alyssonini   *Alysson, Didineis*
   Tribe: Gorytini   *Argogorytes, Exeirus, Gorytes, Ochleroptera, Psammaecius,*
                                   Sphecius
   Tribe: Stizini   *Bembecinus, Stizoides, Stizus*
   Tribe: Bembecini   *Bembex, Bicyrtes, Steniolia, Stictia, Stictiella*
Subfamily: Philanthinae
   Tribe: Philanthini   *Aphilanthops (Clypeadon), Philanthus, Trachypus*
   Tribe: Cercerini   *Cerceris, Eucerceris*
Subfamily: Crabroninae
   Tribe: Crabronini   *Anacrabro, Crabro, Crossocerus, Encopognathus, Ectemnius,*
                                 Entomognathus, Lestica, Lindenius, Moniaecera, Dasyproctus,
                                 Piyuma, Podagritus, Rhopalum, Tracheliodes
   Tribe: Oxybelini   *Belomicrus, Oxybelus*

The following dendrogram shows the phylogenetic relationships of the subfamilies of diggerwasps mentioned in the present text (according to LECLERCQ, 1954).

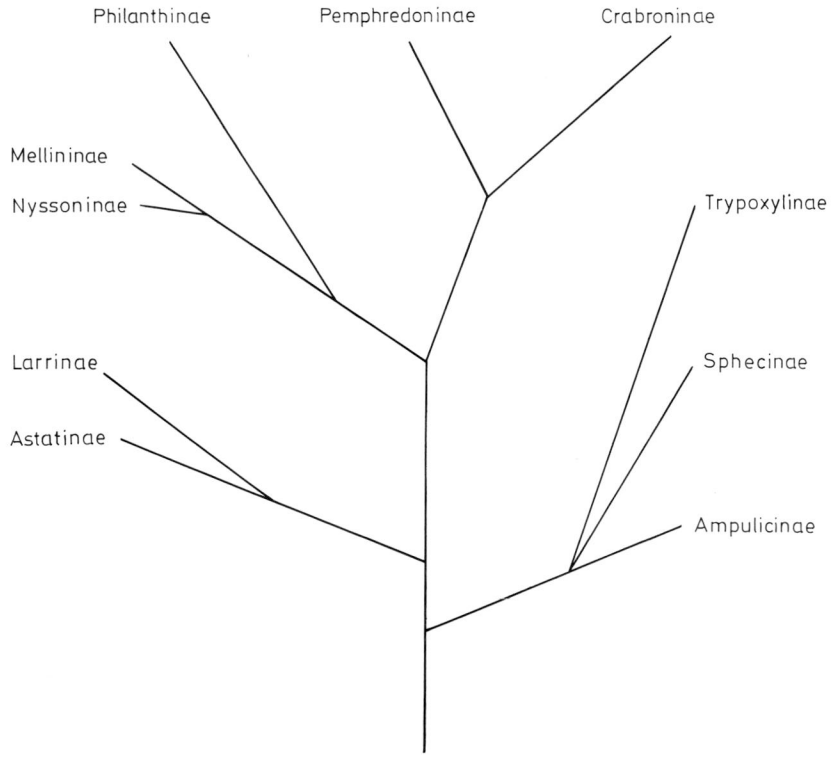

Note added in proof: After completion of the manuscript two important books have been published: one on the comparative ethology of solitary wasps (K. IWATA: Evolution of Instinct. Comparative Ethology of Hymenoptera. 535 p. New Delhi: Amerind Publ. Co. 1976) containing numerous prey records of mainly Japanese species. The other book deals with the systematics of the sphecids of the world (R.M. BOHART and A.S. MENKE: Sphecid Wasps of the World. A Generic Revision. 695 p. Berkeley: Univ. of California Press 1976).

References

Adriaanse, A.: *Ammophila campestris* Latr. und *Ammophila adriaansei* Wilcke. Ein Beitrag zur vergleichenden Verhaltensforschung. Behaviour **1**, 1—34 (1947).

Alcock, J.: The behavior of *Philanthus crabroniformis* (Hymenoptera: Sphecidae). J. Zool. (London) **173**, 233—246 (1974).

Armitage, K.: Notes on the biology of *Philanthus bicinctus* (Hymenoptera: Sphecidae). J. Kans. entomol. Soc. **38**, 89—100 (1965).

Baer, G.A.: Note sur le venin de divers arthropodes du Perou. Bull. Soc. entomol. France **180**—181 (1901).

Baerends, G.P.: Fortpflanzungsverhalten und Orientierung der Grabwespe *Ammophila campestris* Jur. T. entomol. **84**, 68—275 (1941).

Beard, R.L.: The toxicology of *Habrobracon* venom: A study of natural insecticide. Conn. Agr. Exp. Sta. Bull. No 562, 3—27 (1952).

Beard, R.L.: Insect toxins and venoms. Ann. Rev. Entomol. **8**, 1—18 (1963).

Beaumont, J. de: Les *Philanthus* et *Philoponidea* de l'Afrique du N.-O. (Hym. Sphec.). Mitt. schweiz. entomol. Ges. **22**, 173—216 (1949).

Beaumont, J. de: Les espèces européene du genre *Philanthus* (Hym. Sphecid.). Mitt. schweiz. entomol. Ges. **24**, 299—315 (1951).

Beaumont, J. de: Notes sur les *Philanthus* paléarctiques. (Hym. Sphec.). Mitt. schweiz entomol. Ges. **33**, 201—212 (1960).

Beaumont, J. de: Hymenoptera: Sphecidae. In: Insecta Helvetica. Fauna. Lausanne: Imprimerie la Concorde 1964.

Berland, L.: Hymenoptera vespiformes I. (Sphecidae, Pompilidae, Scoliidae, Sapygidae, Mutillidae). In: Faune de France, t. 10. Paris: P. Lechevalier 1925.

Bernard, F., Jacquemin, P.: Effects de piqures de *Scleroderma* (Hymenoptéres Bethylidae) et revision des espèces nordafricains. Bull. Soc. Hist. Nat. Afr. N. **39**, 160—167 (1948).

Bischoff, H.: Biologie der Hymenopteren. Berlin: Springer 1927.

Bohart, G.E.: Honey bees attacked at their hive entrance by the wasp *Philanthus flavifrons* Cresson. Proc. entomol. Soc. Wash. **56**, 26—27 (1954).

Bohart, R.: New North American *Philanthus*. Proc. entomol. Soc. Washington **74**, 397—403 (1972).

Bordas, L.: Appareil glandulaire des Hyménoptères. Ann. Sci. nat. Zool. **7**, Ser. 19, 1—362 (1895).

Bridwell, J.C.: Some notes of Hawaian and other Bethylidae with a description of a new genus and species. 2nd paper. Proc. Hawai. entomol. Soc. **4**, 291—314 (1920).

Bristowe, W.S.: Notes on the habits and prey of twenty species of British huntings wasps. Proc. Linnaean Soc. Zool. (Lond.) **160**, 12—37 (1948).

Clausen, C.: Entomophagous Insects. New York: McGraw Hill 1940.

Diss, A., Timon-David, J.: Accidents provoqués en France par un insecte piqueur, *Scleroderma domestica*. Bull. Soc. Derm. Syph. **58**, 35—36 (1951).

Eberhard, W.G.: The natural history and behaviour of the wasp *Trigonopsis cameronii* Kohl (Sphecidae). Trans. roy. entomol. Soc. Lond. **125**, 295—328 (1974).

Eberhard, W.G.: The predatory behaviour of two wasps, *Sceliphron caementarium* (Sphecidae) and *Agenoidens humilis* (Pompilidae) on the orb weaving spider *Araneus cornutus* (Araneidae). Psyche (Camb.) **77**, 243—251 (1970).

Emden, F. van: Zur Kenntnis der Morphologie und Ökologie des Brotkäferparasiten *Cephalonomia quadridentata* Duchussoy. Z. Morph. Ökol. Tiere **23**, 425—574 (1931).

Evans, H.E.: Comparative ethology and the systematics of spider wasps. Syst. Zool. **2**, 155 – 172 (1953).

Evans, H.E.: *Philanthus sanbornii* Cresson as a predator on honeybees. Bull. Brooklyn entomol. Soc. **50**, 47 (1955).

Evans, H.E.: Ethological studies on digger wasps of the genus *Astata* (Hymenoptera, Sphecidae). J. N.Y. entomol. Soc. **65**, 159 – 185 (1957).

Evans, H.E.: Observations on the nesting behaviour of digger wasps of the genus *Ammophila*. Amer. Midland Nat. **62**, 449 – 473 (1959a).

Evans, H.E.: Biological observations on digger wasps of the genus *Philanthus* (Hymenoptera: Sphecidae). Wasmann J. Biol. **17**, 115 – 132 (1959b).

Evans, H.E.: A revision of the genus *Pseudisobrachium* in North and Central America. (Hymenoptera, Bethylidae.) Bull. Mus. comp. Zool. (Harvard) **126**, 211 – 318 (1961).

Evans, H.E.: A review of nesting behavior of digger wasps of the genus *Aphilanthops,* with special attention to the mechanics of prey carriage. Behaviour **19**, 239 – 260 (1962).

Evans, H.E.: Notes on the nesting behaviour of *Philanthus lepidus* Cresson (Hymenoptera, Sphecidae). Psyche (Camb.) **71**, 142 – 149 (1964a).

Evans, H.E.: A synopsis of the American Bethylidae (Hymenoptera, Aculeata). Bull. Mus. comp. Zool. (Harvard) **132**, 1 – 222 (1964b).

Evans, H.E.: Simultaneous care of more than one nest by *Ammophila asteca* Cameron (Hymenoptera, Sphecidae). Psyche (Camb.) **72**, 8 – 23 (1965).

Evans, H.E.: The Comparative Ethology and Evolution of the Sand Wasps. Cambridge: Harvard University Press, 1966a.

Evans, H.E.: The behavior patterns of solitary wasps. Ann. Rev. Entomol. **11**, 123 – 154 (1966b).

Evans, H.E.: Nests and prey of two species of *Philanthus* in Jackson Hole, Wyoming (Hymenoptera, Sphecidae). Great Basin Natural. **26**, 35 – 40 (1966c).

Evans, H.E.: Notes on the nesting behavior of *Pisonopsis clypeata* and *Belomicrus forbesii* (Hymenoptera, Sphecidae) J. Kans. ent. Soc. **42**, 117 – 125 (1969).

Evans, H.E.: Observations on the nesting behavior of wasps of the tribe Cercerini. J. Kans. entomol. Soc. **44**, 500 – 523 (1971).

Evans, H.E.: Burrow sharing and nest transfer in the digger wasp *Philanthus gibbosus* (Fabricius) Anim. Behav. **21**, 302 – 308 (1973).

Evans, H.E.: Nesting behavior of *Philanthus albopilosus* with comparisons between two widely separated populations. Ann. entomol. Soc. Amer. **68**, 888 – 892 (1975).

Evans, H.E., Lin, Ch.S.: Biological observations on digger wasps of the genus *Philanthus* (Hymenoptera, Sphecidae). Wasmann J. Biol. **17**, 115 – 132 (1959).

Evans, H.E., Lin, Ch.S., Yoshimoto, C.M.: A biological study of *Anoplius apiculatus autumnalis* (Banks) and its parasite, *Evagetes mohave* (Banks) (Hym.: Pompilidae). J. N.Y. entomol. Soc. **61**, 61 – 78 (1953).

Evans, H.E., Matthews, R.W.: Notes on the nest and prey of Australian wasps of the genus *Cerceris*. J. Aust. entomol Soc. **9**, 153 – 156 (1971).

Evans, H.E., Matthews, R.W.: Observations on the nesting behavior of *Trachypus petiolatus* (Spin.) in Colombia and Argentina. J. Kans. ent. Soc. **46**, 165 – 175 (1973).

Evans, H.E., Matthews, R.W.: The sand wasps of Australia. Sci. Amer. **223**, 108 – 115 (1975).

Evans, H.E., Yoshimoto, C.M.: The ecology and nesting behavior of the Pompilidae (Hymenoptera) of the Northeastern United States. Misc. Publ. entomol. Soc. Amer. **3**, 67 – 119 (1962).

Ferton, Ch.: La vie des abeilles et des guêpes. (Oevres choisies, groupées et annotées par E. Raubaud et F. Picard.) Paris: Chiron 1923.

Finlayson, L.H.: The biology of *Cephalonomia waterstoni* Gahan (Hym., Bethylidae), a parasite of *Laemophloeus* (Col., Cucujidae). Bull. Ent. Res. **41**, 79 – 97 (1950a).

Finlayson, L.H.: Host preference of *Cephalonomia waterstoni* Gahan, a bethylid parasitoid of *Laemophloeus* species. Behaviour **2**, 275 – 316 (1950b).

Flemming, H.: Die Muskulatur und Innervierung des Wehrstachelapparates von Aculeaten. Z. Morph. Ökol. Tiere, **46**, 321 – 341 (1957).

Fuchs, H.: Urticaria papulosa durch Stiche von *Scleroderma domestica*. Dermatologica **55**, 215 – 216 (1952).

Gervet, J., Fulcrand, J.: Le thème de piqure dans la paralysation de sa proie par l'ammophile *Podalonia hirsuta* Scopoli (Hymen. Sphec.). Z. Tierpsych. **27**, 82—97 (1969).

Gordh, G.: *Goniozus gallicola* Fouts, a parasite of moth larvae, with notes on other bethylids (Hymenoptera: Bethylidae. Lepidoptera: Gelechiidae). U.S. Dept. Agricult. Techn. Bull. **1524**, 27 p. (1976).

Grandi, G.: Contributi alla conoscenza della biologìa e della morfologìa degli imenotteri melliferi e predatori. (XII). Boll. entomol. Bologna **4**, 19—72 (1931).

Guiglia, D.: Les sclerodermines par rapport à l'homme. Proc. 10. Int. Congr. Entomol. Montreal 1956, **3**, 883—887 (1958).

Habermann, E.: Biochemie, Pharmakologie und Toxikologie der Inhaltsstoffe von Hymenopterengiften. Rev. Physiol. Biochem. Pharmacol. **60**, 220—325 (1968).

Habermann, E.: Chemistry, pharmacology and toxicology of bee, wasp, and hornet venoms. In: Venomous Animals and Their Venoms. W. Bücherl, E. Buckley (eds.). New York: Academic Press, 1971, Vol. 3, pp. 61—93.

Habermann, E.: Bee and wasp venoms. Science **177**, 314—322 (1972).

Hamm, A.M., Richards, D.W.: The biology of British fossorial wasps of the families Mellinidae, Gorytidae, Philanthidae, Oxybelidae and Trypoxylidae. Trans. entomol. Soc. Lond. **78**, 75—131 (1930).

Hamm, A.H., Richards, O.W.: The biology of British Crabronidae. Trans. entomol. Soc. London **74**, 297—333 (1926).

Hartzell, A.: Histopathology of nerve lesions of cicada after paralysis by the killer-wasp. Contr. Boyce Thompson Inst. **7**, 421—425 (1935).

Hermann, H.R.: The hymenopterous poison apparatus IV. *Dasymutilla occidentalis* (Hymenoptera: Mutillidae). J. Ga. entomol. Soc. **3**, 1—10 (1968).

Hermann, H.R.: The ant-like venom apparatus of *Typhoctes peculiaris,* a primitive mutillid wasp. Ann. entomol. Soc. Amer. **68**, 882—884 (1975).

Huber, A.: Zur Biologie von *Mellinus arvensis* L. (Hym. Sphec.) Zool. Jb. Syst. **89**, 43—118 (1961).

Iwata, K.: Comparative studies on the habits of solitary wasps. Tenthredo **4**, 1—146 (1942).

Jacquemin, P., Vaissiere, R.: Un cas de piqures par *Scleroderma domestica*. Bull. Soc. Hist. Nat. Afr. N. **41**, 49—50 (1952).

Janvier, H.: Paralysie des pucerons par constriction thoracique. C.R. Acad. Sci. (Paris) **241**, 608—609 (1955).

Kearns, C.W.: A hymenopterous parasite (*Cephalonomia gallicola* Ash.) new to the cigarette beetle (*Lasioderma serricorne* Fab.). J. econ. Entomol. **27**, 801—806 (1934).

Kohl, F.F.: Zur Kenntnis der Hymenopteren-Gattung *Philanthus* Fabr. Ann. k. k. Nat. hist. Mus. (Wien) **6**, 345—370 (1891).

Krombein, K.V. (ed.): Hymenoptera of America North of Mexico. Synoptic Catalog. First Supplement., Washington, U.S. Govt Printing Office 1958.

Krombein, K.V. (ed.): Hymenoptera of America North of Mexico. Synoptic Catalog. Second Supplement. Washington, U.S. Govt Printing Office 1967a.

Krombein, K.V.: Trap-nesting Wasps and Bees. Life Histories, Nests and Associates. Washington, Smithsonian Press 1967b.

Kurczewski, F.E.: A note on the nesting behavior of *Solierella inermis* (Hymenoptera: Sphecidae, Larrinae). J. Kans. entomol. Soc. **40**, 203—208 (1967).

Kurczewski, F.E.: Comparative ethology of female digger wasps in the genera *Miscophus* and *Nitelopterus*. (Hymenoptera: Sphecidae, Larrinae.) J. Kans. entomol. Soc. **42**, 470—509 (1969).

Kurczewski, F.E., Kurczweski, E.J.: Host records for some North American Pompilidae with a discussion of factors in prey selection. J. Kans. entomol. Soc. **41**, 1—33 (1968).

Kurczwski, F.E., Kurczewski, E.J.: Host records for some species of *Tachytes* and other *Larrinae*. J. Kans. entomol. Soc. **44**, 131—136 (1971).

Leclercq, J.: Monographie systématique phylogénétique et zoogéographique des Hyménoptères crabroniens. 371 p., Liège, Lejeunia 1954.

Linsley, E.G., MacSwain, J.W.: Observations on the habits and prey of *Eucerceris ruficeps* Scullen. Pan-Pacific Entomol. **30**, 11—14 (1954).

Linsley, E.G., MacSwain, J.W.: Some observations on the nesting habits and prey of *Cerceris californica* Cresson (Hymenopt. Sphecidae). Ann. entomol. Soc. Amer. **49**, 71—84 (1956).

Maschwitz, U., Kloft, W.: Morphology and function of the venom apparatus of insects: bees, wasps, ants, and caterpillars. In: Venomous Animals and Their Venoms. W. Bücherl, E. Buckley (eds.). New York: Academic Press (1971), Vol. 3, pp. 1—60.

Matthews, R.W.: Nesting biology of the social wasp *Microstigmus comes* (Hymenoptera: Sphecidae, Pemphredoninae). Psyche (Camb.) **75**, 24—45 (1968).

Matthews, R.W.: A new *Thrips*-hunting *Microstigmus* from Costa Rica. Psyche (Camb.) **77**, 120—126 (1970).

Mickel, C.E.: Biological and taxonomic investigations on the mutillid wasps. Bull. U.S. nat. Mus. **143**, 1—351 (1928).

Mickel, C.E.: Two hundred years of mutillid research. An annotated bibliography. Tech. Bull. Agric. Exp. Stn. Univ. Minnesota, Nr. 271, 77 p. (1970).

Mickel, C.E.: Mutillidae miscellanea: taxonomy and distribution. Ann. entomol. Soc. Amer. **67**, 461—471 (1974).

Mochi, A.: Revisione delle specie egiziane dei generi *Philanthus* Fab. e *Nectanebus* Spin. Bull. Soc. Fouad 1ᵉʳ entomol. **23**, 86—138 (1939).

Molitor, A.: Das Verhalten der Raubwespen. Z. Tierpsych. **3**, 60—74 (1939).

Muesebeck, D.F.W., Krombein, K.V., Townes, H.K. (eds.): Hymenoptera of America North of Mexico. Synoptic Catalog. 1420 p., Washington, U.S. Govt Printing Office (1951).

Nicoli, R.M., Erlande-Brandenburg, G.: L'envenomation par piqure de *Scleroderma*. Ann. parasit. hum. comp. **32**, 551—562 (1957).

Nielsen, E.T.: Sur les habitudes de hyménoptères aculéates solitaires (Bethylidae, Scoliidae, Cleptidae, Psammocharidae). Entomol. Meddel. Kbh. **18**, 1—57 (1932).

Nielsen, E.T.: Sur les habitudes des hyménoptères aculéates solitaires. III. Sphecidae. Entomol. Meddel. Kbh. **18**, 259—348 (1933).

Nielsen, E.T.: Über den Stoffwechsel der von Grabwespen paralysierten Tiere. Vedensk. Medd. Naturhist. Foren. **99**, 149—231 (1935).

O'Connor, R., Rosenbrook, Wm., Jr: The venom of the mud-dauber wasp. I. *Sceliphron caementarium:* preliminary separation and free amino acid content. Canad. J. Biochem. Physiol. **41**, 1943—1948 (1963).

Oeser, R.: Vergleichend-morphologische Untersuchungen über den Ovipositor der Hymenopteren. Mitt. zool. Mus. Berl. **37**, 3—119 (1961).

Olberg, G.: Bienenfeind *Philanthus* (Bienenwolf). Neue Brehmbücherei. Nr. 94. Wittenberg: Ziemsen 1953.

Olberg, G.: Das Verhalten der solitären Wespen Mitteleuropas. (Vespidae, Pompilidae, Sphecidae) Berlin: Deutscher Verlag der Wissenschaften 1959.

Parker, F.D.: On the subfamily Astatinae, with a systematic study of the genus *Astata* of America North of Mexico (Hymenoptera: Sphecidae). Ann. entomol. Soc. Amer. **55**, 643—659 (1962).

Parker, F.D.: On the subfamily Astatinae. Part VI. The American species in the genus *Dryudella* Spinola (Hymenoptera: Sphecidae.) Ann. entomol. Soc. Amer. **62**, 963—976 (1969).

Pawlowsky, E.N.: Gifttiere und ihre Giftigkeit. 516p., Jena: G. Fischer Verlag 1927.

Peckham, D.J., Kurczewski, F.E., Peckham, D.B.: Nesting behavior of nearctic species of *Oxybelus* (Hymenoptera: Sphecidae Ann. entomol. Soc. Amer. **66**, 647—661 (1973).

Peckham, G., Peckham, E.: On the instincts and habits of the solitary wasps. Wisconsin Geol. Nat. Hist. Surv. Bull. **2**, 1—245 (1898).

Piek, T.: Site of action of the venom of the digger wasp *Philanthus triangulum* F. on the fast neuromuscular system of the locust. Toxicon **4**, 191—198 (1966a).

Piek, T.: The effect of the venom of the digger wasp *Philanthus* on the fast and slow excitatory and inhibitory system in the locust muscle. Experientia (Basel) **22**, 462—463 (1966b).

Piek, T.: Site of action of venom of *Microbracon hebetor* Say (Braconidae, Hymenoptera). J. Insect Physiol. **12**, 561—568 (1966c).

Piek, T., Engels, E.: Action of the venom of *Microbracon hebetor* Say on larvae and adults of *Philosamia cynthia* Hübn. Comp. Biochem. Physiol. **28**, 603—618 (1969).

Piek, T., Mantel, P.: The effect of the venom of *Microbracon hebetor* (Say) on the hyperpolarizing potentials in a skeletal muscle of *Philosamia cynthia* Hübn. Comp. gen. Pharmacol. **1**, 87—92 (1970).

Piek, T., Mantel, P., Engels, E.: Neuromuscular block in insects caused by the venom of the digger wasp *Philanthus triangulum* L. Comp. gen. Pharmacol. **2**, 317—331 (1971).

Piek, T., Nijo, K.D.: Neuromuscular block in honey bees by the venom of the bee wolf wasp (*Philanthus triangulum* F.). Toxicon **13**, 199—201 (1975).

Piek, T., Simon Thomas, R.T.: Paralysing venoms of solitary wasps. Comp. Biochem. Physiol. **30**, 13—31 (1969).

Powell, D.: The biology of *Cephalonomia tarsalis* (Ash.), a vespoid wasp (Bethylidae: Hymenoptera) parasite on the sawtoothed grain beetle. Ann. entomol. Soc. Amer. **31**, 44—49 (1938).

Powell, J.A., Chemsak, J.A.: Some biological observations on *Philanthus politus pacificus* Cresson (Hymenoptera: Sphecidae). J. Kans. entomol. Soc. **32**, 115—120 (1959).

Rabaud, E.: L'instinct paralyseur des hyménoptères vulnérantes. C.R. Acad. Sci. (Paris) **165**, 680—683 (1917).

Rathmayer, W.: Paralysis caused by the digger wasp *Philanthus*. Nature (Lond.) **196**, 1148—1151 (1962a).

Rathmayer, W.: Das Paralysierungsproblem beim Bienenwolf *Philanthus triangulum* F. Z. vergl. Physiol. **45**, 413—462 (1962b).

Rathmayer, W.: The effect of the poison of spider- and digger wasps on the prey. Mem. Inst. Butantan Simp. Int. **33**, 651—657 (1966).

Rathmayer, W., Walther, Chr.: Mode of action and specificity of *Habrobracon* venom (Hymenoptera, Braconidae) In: Animal, Plant and Microbial Toxins. A. Ohsaka, K. Hayashi, Y. Sawai eds. New York: Plenum Press 1976, Vol. **2**, pp. 299—307.

Rau, P., Rau, N.: Wasp Studies Afield, 372p., Princeton: University Press 1918.

Reinhard, E.G.: The life history and habits of the solitary wasp, *Philanthus gibbosus*. Smithsn. Inst. Ann. Rep. for 1922, 363—376 (1924).

Richards, O.W., Hamm, A.H.: The biology of British Pompilidae (Hymenoptera). Trans. Soc. Brit. Entomol. **6**, 51—114 (1939).

Rosenbrook, W., O'Connor, R.: The venom of the mud-dauber wasp. II. *Sceliphron caementarium*: protein content. Canad. J. Biochem. **42**, 1005—1010 (1964a).

Rosenbrook, W., O'Connor, R.: The venom of the mud-dauber wasp. III. *Sceliphron caementarium*: general character. Canad. J. Biochem. **42**, 1567—1575 (1964b).

Schafer, G.D.: The Ways of a Mud-dauber. Stanford Calif. 1949.

Scullen, H.A., Wold, J.L.: Biology of wasps of the tribe Cercerini, with a list of Coleoptera used as prey. Ann. entomol. Soc. Amer. **62**, 209—214 (1969).

Simon Thomas, R.T., Simon Thomas, A.M.J.: Some observations on the behavior of females of *Philanthus triangulum* (F.) (Hymenoptera, Sphecidae). Tijdschr. Entomol. **115**, 123—139 (1972).

Smith, C.E.: *Larra analis* F., a parasite of the mole cricket *Gryllotalpa hexadactyla* Perty. Proc. entomol. Soc. Wash. **37**, 65—82 (1935).

Snoddy, E.L.: Simuliidae, Ceratopogonidae and Chloropidae as prey of *Oxybelus emarginatum*. Ann. entomol. Soc. Amer. **61**, 1029—1030 (1968).

Steiner, A.L.: Contribution à l'étude biologique des Sphégides. La paralysie des proies par *Liris nigra* V.d.L. (=*Notogonia pompiliformis* Pz.). C.R. Acad. Sci. (Paris) **246**, 3526—3528 (1958a).

Steiner, A.L.: Contribution à l'étude biologique des Sphégides. L'influence des piqures de *Liris nigra* V.d.L. (=*Notogonia pompiliformis* Pz.) sur la proie. C.R. Acad. Sci. (Paris) **247**, 150—152 (1958b).

Steiner, A.L.: Étude du comportement prédateur d'un hyménoptère sphégien: *Liris nigra* V.d.L. (=*Notogonia pompiliformis* Pz.) Ann. Sci. nat., zool. Ser. 12, **4**, 1—126 (1962).

Steiner, A.L.: Interprétation neuro- et psycho-physiologique de l'état des victimes de certaines guepes paralysantes. (*Liris nigra* V.d.L.=*Notogonia pompiliformis* Pz.). C.R. Acad. Sci. (Paris) **257**, 3480—3482 (1963).

Steiner, A.L.: Digger wasp predatory behaviour (Hymenoptera, Sphecidae). II. Comparative study of closely related wasps (Larrinae: *Liris nigra*, palearctic; *L. argentata* and *L. aequalis*, nearctic) that all paralyze crickets (Orthoptera, Gryllidae). Z. Tierpsychol. **42**, 343—380 (1976).

Strandtmann, R.W.: A review of the North American species of *Philanthus*, north of Mexico. 126 p., Ohio State Univ. Press, Columbus (1946).

Theodorides, J.: Un groupe peu connu d'Insectes vulnerants pour l'Homme: les Hymenoptères Bethylides du genre *Scleroderma*. Bull. med. **44**, 769—773 (1955).

Tinbergen, N.: Über die Orientierung des Bienenwolfes (*Philanthus triangulum* F.). Z. vergl. Physiol. **16**, 305–334 (1932).

Tinbergen, N.: Über die Orientierung des Bienenwolfes. II. Die Bienenjagd. Z. vergl. Physiol. **21**, 699–717 (1935).

Vergne, M.: Sur la nidification de *Philanthus triangulum* F. Bull. Soc. entomol. France **36**, 132–136 (1931).

Visser, B.J., Spanjer, W.: Biochemical study of two paralysing insect venoms. Acta physiol. pharmacol. neerl. **15**, 107–108 (1969).

Voukassovitch, M.: Sur la biologie de *Goniozus claripennis* Forst. parasite d'*Oenophthira pilleriana* Schiff. Bul. Soc. d'Hist. Nat. Toulouse **52**, 225–246 (1924).

Walther, C., Rathmayer, W.: The effect of *Habrobracon* venom on excitatory neuromuscular transmission in insects. J. comp. Physiol. **88**, 23–38 (1974).

Walther, Chr., Reinecke, M.: On the mode of action of wasp venom on locust neuromuscular synapses. Pflügers Arch. **365**, Suppl. R. 35 (1976).

Walton, G.A.: A minute bethylid wasp of medical interest. Proc. roy. entomol. Soc. (Lond.) A, **23**, 98 (1948).

Welsh, J.H., Batty, C.S.: 5-Hydroxytryptamine content of some arthropod venoms and venom-containing parts. Toxicon **1**, 165–173 (1963).

Wheeler, W.M.: A solitary wasp (*Aphilanthops frigidus* F. Smith) that provisions its nest with queen ants. J. Anim. Behav. **3**, 374–386 (1913).

Williams, F.X.: The wasps of the genus *Solierella* in California. Proc. Calif. Acad. Sci. **26**, 355–417 (1950).

Yamada, Y.: Studies on the natural enemy of the pollen pest, *Anthrenus verbaci* L. (*Allepyris microneurus* Kieffer). (Hymenoptera: Bethylidae). Mushi **28**, 13–29 (1955).

CHAPTER 23

Venoms of Vespidae*

H. Edery[1,2], J. Ishay[2], S. Gitter[2] and H. Joshua[3]

A. Introduction

"I will send hornets before thee which shall drive out the Hivite, the Canaanite, and the Hittite before thee" (Exodus 23:28).

Ever since biblical times, many victims of Vespidae stinging are recorded every year, not only in Israel but all over the world. In most cases, local tissue injury and/or generalized systemic reactions have been reported. Fragmentary information concerning morphology, social habits of Vespidae, as well as composition and mode of action of their venoms have frequently made the provision of adequate treatment difficult. Confusion often occurs and diagnosis of Vespidae sting has been attributed to other arthropods.

Up to now, the information on Vespidae and on their venoms is scattered in specialized publications, many of which are not easily available. Therefore, the main scope of the present review is to unite the relevant data in a single work.

It is hoped that this work will provide a perspective of the areas in which adequate knowledge exists as well as of those scantily covered, thus indicating convenient directions for future research.

B. Biology of Vespidae

The family Vespidae comprises three subfamilies: the Stenogastrinae of South-East Asia; the widely distributed Polistinae; and the Vespinae, the most advanced subfamily, with distribution in the north-temperate zone and in tropical Asia (SPRADBERY, 1973). The Vespidae, together with the related Eumenidae and Masaridae, are often called Diploptera because of the ability of the adults to fold their fore-wings longitudinally when at rest. However, the Stenogastrinae and the great majority of Masaridae are in fact unable to do so, which suggests that this is most probably a secondary characteristic.

The order Hymenoptera, to which the Vespidae belong, probably originated 300 million years ago, during the late Paleozoic era which marked the end of the Carboniferous era. During the following Mesozoic era, which spanned 230 million years, the order diversified so that in the Eocene, some 60 million years

* In this review "V.v." will be used as an abbreviation for venoms of Vespidae. The literature has been surveyed up to August 1976.
[1] Israel Institute for Biological Research, Ness Ziona; [2] Department of Physiology and Pharmacology, Sackler School of Medicine, Tel-Aviv University, Tel-Aviv, and [3] Clinical Laboratory, Beilinson Hospital, Petah Tikvah, Israel.

ago, vespoid wasps related to the current social wasp fauna had evolved. The Vespidae presently comprise some 800—1000 living species.

In the layman's everyday language the word "wasp" has been loosely used to indicate all members of the order Hymenoptera, including bees, wasps, hornets, ants, and allied insects. In the strict sense, however, true wasps comprise only the families Masaridae, Euminidae, and Vespidae, while to the latter family belong only species of subsocial or social wasps.

The living species of wasps display in clearest detail the finely graded steps that had led from solitary to advanced eusocial life, with eusocial behavior being limited almost entirely to the family Vespidae.

The taxonomy of social wasps has been elucidated in numerous modern studies, of which the most comprehensive are the following: BEQUAERT (1918) on the Vespidae of Central Africa; BLÜTHGEN (1961), KEMPER and DÖHRING (1967) and GUIGLIA (1972) on the Vespidae of Europe; VAN DER VECHT (1957) on the Vespidae of Southestern Asia and New Guinea; DUCKE (1910) on the South American Polybiini; WILLINCK (1952, 1953) on the Argentine Polistinae; BEQUAERT on the Polybiini of North America and the West Indies (1933) and on the Vespidae of northern South America (1944a). The following genera of Polybiini have undergone partial revision: *Ropalidia, Parapolybia,* and *Polybioides* of the Oriental Region (VAN DER VECHT, 1962 and 1966); *Belonogaster* in Africa (DU BUYSSON, 1909); and in the New World, *Brachygastra* (Nectarina) (NAUMANN, 1968) *Synoeca* (DU BUYSSON, 1906), *Protopolybia* (BEQUAERT, 1944b), *Mischocyttarus* (RICHARDS, 1945; ZIKAN, 1949) and *Apoica* (RICHARDS and RICHARDS, 1951). Additional notes of *Polybia, Chartergus, Charterginus, Pseudochartergus, Pseudopolybia, Epipona, Tatua* and the Nearctic species of Polybiini have been supplied by BEQUAERT (1933 and 1938). The Nearctic *Vespula* (including *Dolichovespula*) have been reevaluated by MILLER (1961).

The taxonomy of the cosmopolitian genus *Polistes* has been revised by ZIMMERMANN (1930 and 1931); BERLAND (1942) and YOSHIKAWA (1962). A brief history of this group has been provided by HURD (1955), as cited by WILSON (1971).

The laboratory culturing of social wasps for the purpose of observation and experiment has received relatively little attention. Culture techniques have been developed by GAUL (1941), ISHAY (1964 and 1965), MONTAGNER (1966), ISHAY et al. (1967), ISHAY and RUTTNER (1971), and AKRE et al. (1973 and 1976). Ideally, culturing should be in a dimly lit, air-conditioned laboratory room in which the observer can sit unobtrusively in the dark and view the nests located in the artificial breeding boxes.

I. Taxonomy and Geographical Distribution

1. Stenogastrinae

The most primitive wasps in the family Vespidae are represented by some 40—60 species of the genera *Stenogaster* and *Parishnogaster,* which occur in Southeast Asia. Unlike other Vespids, the Stenogastrinae do not fold their wings longitudinally when in repose (WILLIAMS, 1919; YOSHIKAWA et al., 1969). They construct delicate nests in the shaded parts of tropical rain forests. The wasps vary in size from

12—25 mm in length, and their color ranges from black to yellow (IWATA, 1967). As for the nests, these can comprise three types: 1) an aggregate of downward-facing cylindrical or bell-like cells; 2) roughly hexagonal cells arranged in small combs with an envelope around them, and 3) one or more rows of downward-facing cells plastered to the substrate. The number of cells in these three types of nests may be up to 20, 23, and 39, respectively (WILLIAMS, 1919; IWATA, 1967; SAKAGAMI and YOSHIKAWA, 1968). The larvae do not spin silken cocoons, and at least in some species, the female seals the cell when the larva is mature (IWATA, 1967). WILLIAMS (1919) believed that the Stenogastrinae were represented by both solitary and social wasps. While there is probably no collaboration between the adults, the larvae are attended by the females and are fed on specially prepared foods, the young larvae receiving a yellowish paste which may be glandular in origin (IWATA, 1967), whereas maturing larvae are fed a masticated paste of a mixed arthropod origin.

2. Polistinae

This subfamily comprises three tribes. The tribe Ropalidiini, including the principal genus *Ropalidia* with an estimated number of species exceeding 100, is distributed in Australia, Southeast Asia, India and adjacent areas, and in Africa. The combs are either small, made up of 22 cells in a row which are either necked, enveloped, or within hollow bamboo stems (YOSHIKAWA, 1964) or large, composed of up to 200—400 cells. The nesting behavior of the different species is very diverse.

The tribe Polybiini comprises some 20 genera, the majority of which are widespread in South and Central America, with a few also in Africa Southeast Asia. The Polybiini display a wide variety of social behavior and nest architecture (SCHREMMER, 1973; JEANNE, 1975).

The genus *Belonogaster,* with some 35 species, occurs in tropical Africa extending northward to Arabia. The nest is composed of a single comb made up of some 60—450 cells, which are suspended by one or two pedicels from the substrate. Colonies are founded by single or several females (IWATA, 1966; PARDI and PICCIOLI, 1970).

Genus *Apoica* comprises nocturnal wasps which found colonies by swarming. This genus comprises five or six species and occurs from southern Mexico to Paraguay and the south of Brazil (SCHREMMER, 1972). During the day, the wasps arrange in a tight ring on the comb, with their heads towards the periphery of the comb. This behavior is most probably a defense mechanism against predators.

Genus *Brachygastra (Nectarina)* boasts large nests containing several thousand adult wasps (DU BUYSSON, 1905). Some of the species are semidomesticated by Mexican Indians, who utilize the honey produced by the wasps.

Genus *Polybia* are scattered from Mexico to Argentina. Several thousand adults and more than 18 combs may occur in a single colony. Some of the species store honey in the cells.

The tribe Polistini is composed of two genera: *Polistes* (Fig. 1) with some 150 species and *Sulcopalistes* with four socially parasitic species. The biology of the temperate species was studied by PARDI (1940, 1948, and 1951) and PARDI and CAVALCANTI (1951) in Italy, by YOSHIKAWA (1959 and 1962) in Japan, by

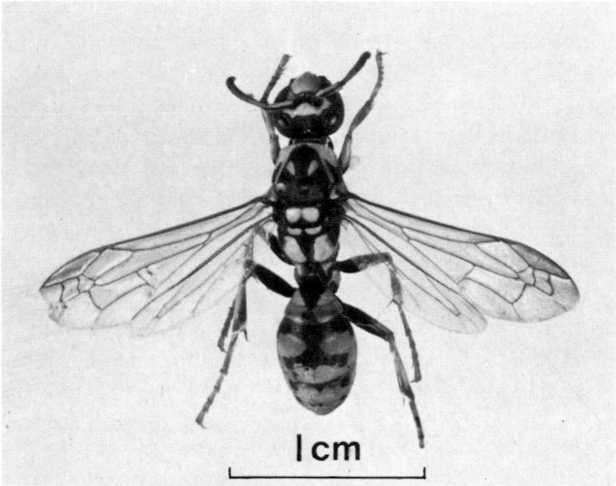

Fig. 1. *Polistes gallicus* (scale 1 cm)

DELEURANCE (1947, 1955, and 1957) and GERVET (1956, 1962, and 1964) in France, and by RAU (1928) and WEST(EBERHARD) (1967) in the United States.

The nest contains one comb whose cells are initially sustained by a single pedicel, but when the comb is enlarged, accessory pillars for support are built.

There are no envelopes aroung the combs. A new colony is founded by one or several females, and, in time, a hierarchy is established with one female becoming the queen and the other females assuming a subordinate role. Colony development lasts four to five months in temperate species and six to seven months in tropical ones.

3. Vespinae

These most socially evolved wasps are represented by three major genera: *Provespa, Vespula* (including *Paravespula* and *Dolichovespula*), and *Vespa.*

The genus *Provespa* comprises three known species: *Provespa anomala* (Saussure), *P. barthelemyi* (du Buysson) and *P. nocturna* (van der Vecht). These occur in Malaya, Sumatra, and Borneo. The nest is built above ground. The wasps are characterized by a uniform pale brown body and enlarged ocelli, characteristics also typical for several other groups of nocturnal Hymenoptera.

The genus *Vespula,* with some 33 species, is essentially Holarctic, but two of its species have expanded southwards: *Paravespula germanica* (Fig. 2), which in recent centuries has become established in South Africa, New Zealand, Tasmania, and Australia, and *P. vulgaris* (Fig. 3), which has recently become established in Australia (SPRADBERY, 1973). In the United States some of the species of the subgenus *Dolichovespula* are referred to as hornets or yellow jackets, while *D. maculata* is called the bald-faced hornet (WILSON, 1971). A list of yellow jacket literature has been compiled by AKRE et al. (1974), including extensive data on its biology, nest contents, nest associates, including parasites and other pathogens, taxonomy,

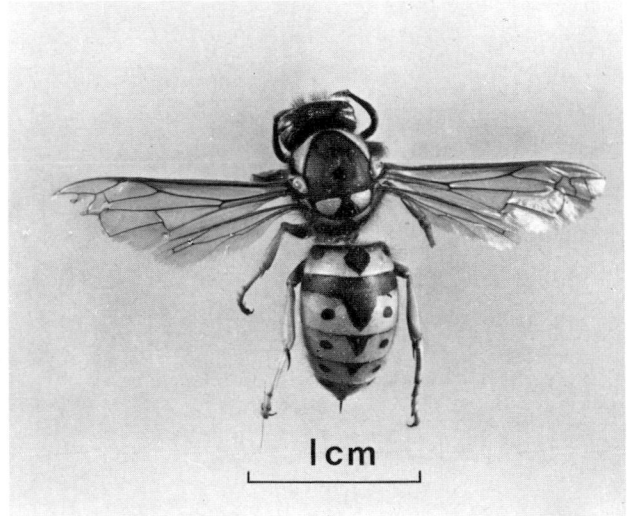

Fig. 2. *Paravespula germanica* (scale 1 cm)

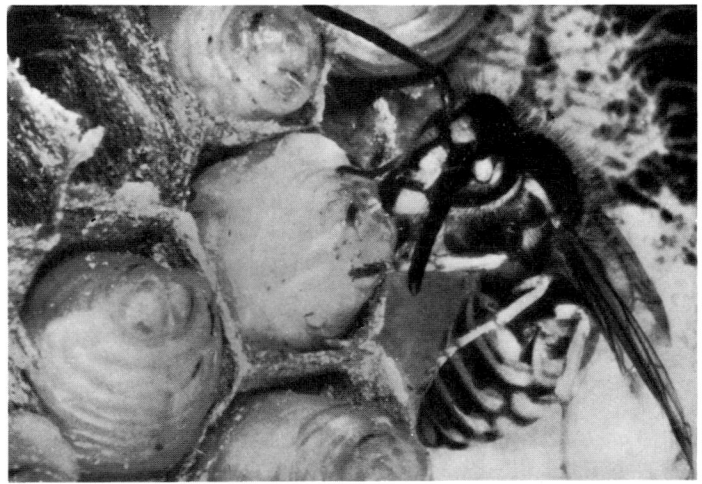

Fig. 3. *Vespa* (*Paravespula*) *vulgaris* worker feeding larvae (MASCHWITZ, 1966)

morphology, physiology, behavior economics, including damage, venoms, allergies, baits, attractants, and control. In the subgenus *Dolichovespula* the nest is aerial or arboreal, being attached to tree branches, etc. The best known species are: *D. media* (Retz) distributed in Scandinavian countries, North and East Europe, the Alpine mountains and Italy; *D. norwegica* F. in North and Central Europe, in North Asia, Japan, and Sakhalin (YAMANE, 1975); *D. saxonica* F. in North and Central Europe, Asia, and Japan; *D. pacifica* Birula in Eastern Siberia, Kamchatka, Sakhalin, Chishima, and Japan (YAMANE, 1975); and *D. sylvestris* (Scop.) in Central and Western Europe and in Central Asia. In the Nearctic the most

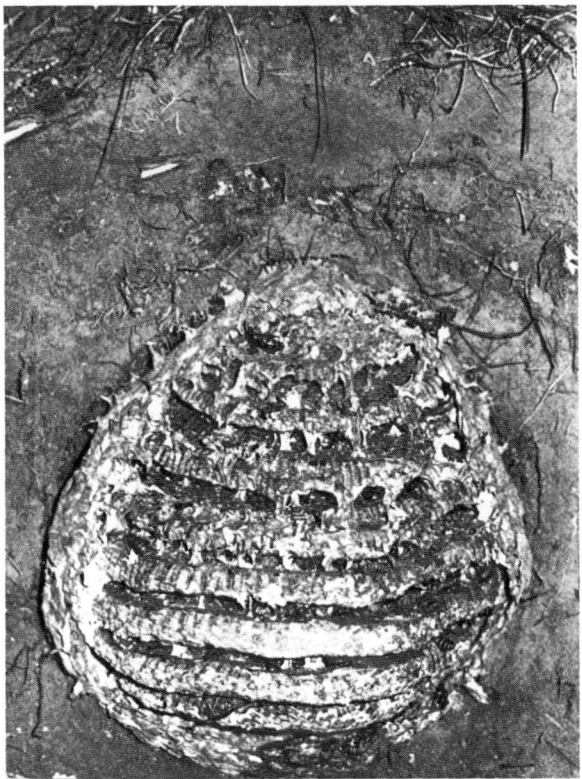

Fig. 4. Subterranean nest of *Paravespula germanica in situ* (Spradbery, 1973)

known species are *D. arenaria* F., *D. maculata* L., and *D. albida* Sladen. *D. adulterina* Buysson is a social parasite on *D. arenaria* in North America and on *D. norwegica, D. saxonica,* and *D. pacifica* in Europe, Asia, and Japan.

The other species of the genus *Vespula* build mainly subterranean nests (Fig. 4), but a few aerial nests have also been recorded (Weyrauch, 1935; Thomas, 1960). Two species groups are recognized: the *V. rufa* L.-group, with mainly small colonies and the *V. vulgaris* L.-group with large colonies. The European scholars designate the *V. vulgaris*-group species, *V. vulgaris* and *V. germanica* as *Paravespula*. Members of this group produce large colonies with several thousand adults and are human pests. The genus includes the Holarctic *Paravespula (Vespula) vulgaris* L. and *P. (V.) germanica* F., and the Nearctic *V. pennsylvanica* (Saussure) and *V. maculifrons* (du Buysson).

The *Vespula rufa* group includes the Holarctic *V. austriaca* (Panzer), the Palearctic *V. rufa* L. and the Nearctic *V. atropilosa* (Sladen), *V. intermedia* (du Buysson), *V. vidua* (Saussure), *V. acadica* (Sladen), *V. consobrina* (Saussure), *V. squamosa* (Drury) and *V. sulphurea* (Saussure) (Fig. 5). *V. austriaca* is a social parasite on *V. rufa* in Europe and North America, *V. squamosa* is evolving toward parasitism on *V. maculifrons* and is already a social parasite on *V. rufa* (MacDonald and Matthews, 1975).

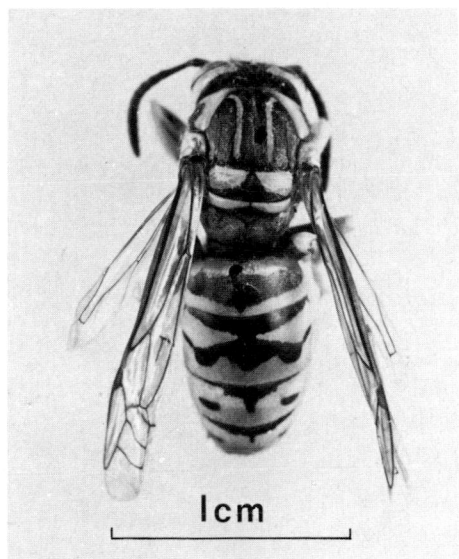

Fig. 5. *Paravespula sulphurea* (scale 1 cm)

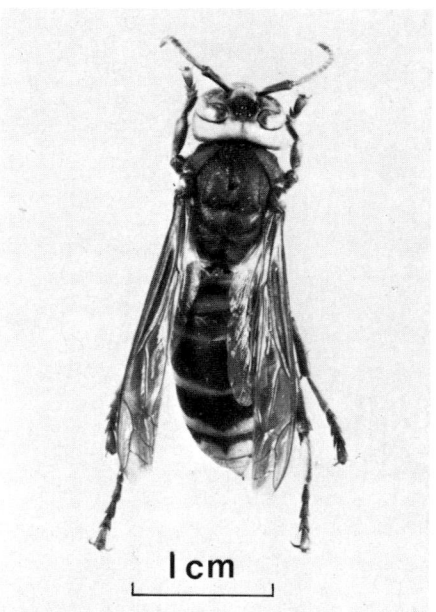

Fig. 6. *Vespa crabro* (scale 1 cm)

The genus *Vespa* has some 19 species, most of them occurring in the Indo-Australian archipelago mainly in Southeast Asia. Only two species have radiated from their origin. These are the Palearctic *Vespa crabro* L. (Fig. 6) which was accidentally introduced by man to the eastern coast of the United States, where it is called the European hornet, and the Oriental hornet (*Vespa orientalis* L.)

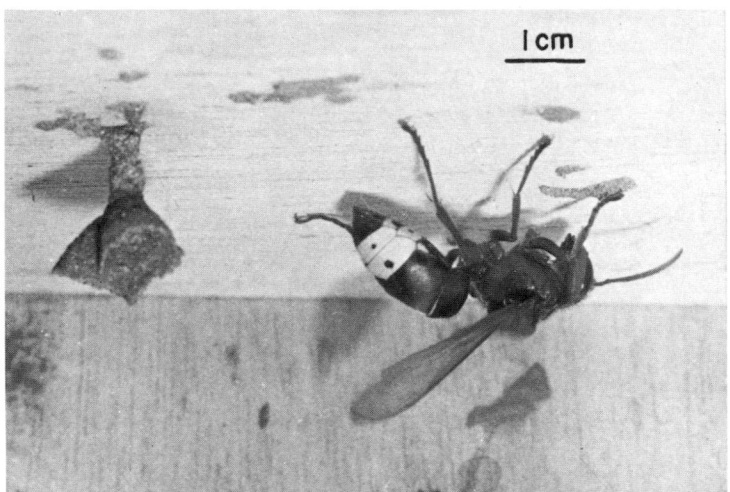

Fig. 7. *Vespa orientalis* queen near an embryonic nest

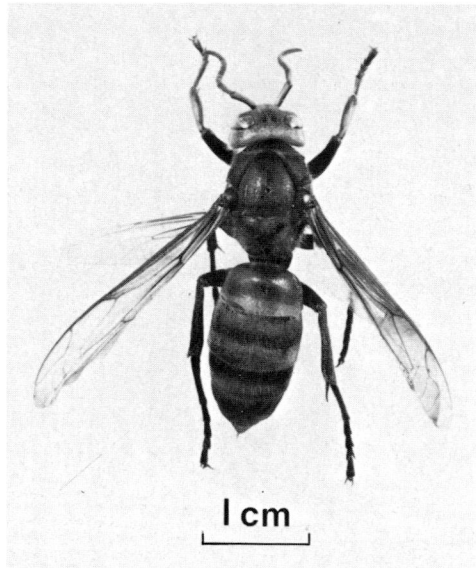

Fig. 8. *Vespa tropica* (scale 1 cm)

(Fig. 7) which extends from Southeast and Central Asia through India and Arabia to the Mediterranean basin and to North and East Africa, including Ethiopia and Malagash (BODENHEIMER, 1933). *V. orientalis* builds underground nests while *V. cra-bro* nests mostly in hollow trees.

The species *V. tropica* L. (Figs. 8 and 9) and *V. affinis* L. (Fig. 9) are widely distributed in Continental Asia as well as in the archipelago. Both these species have developed a considerable number of subspecies (VAN DER VECHT, 1957). *V. ve-lutina* (Lepeletier) is less widely distributed in Continental Asia and more so in

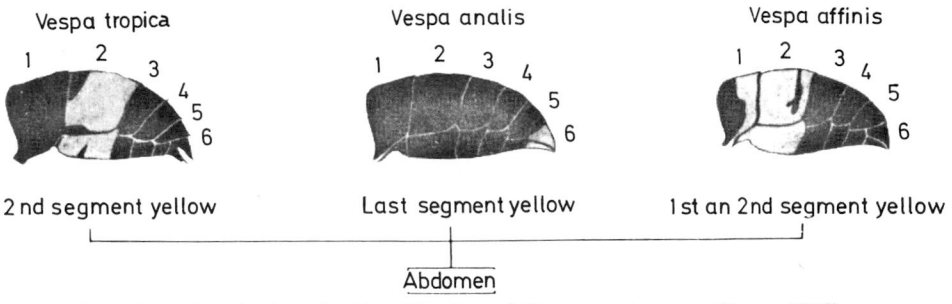

Fig. 9. Simplified pictorial key for identification of Singapore hornets (CHAN, 1972)

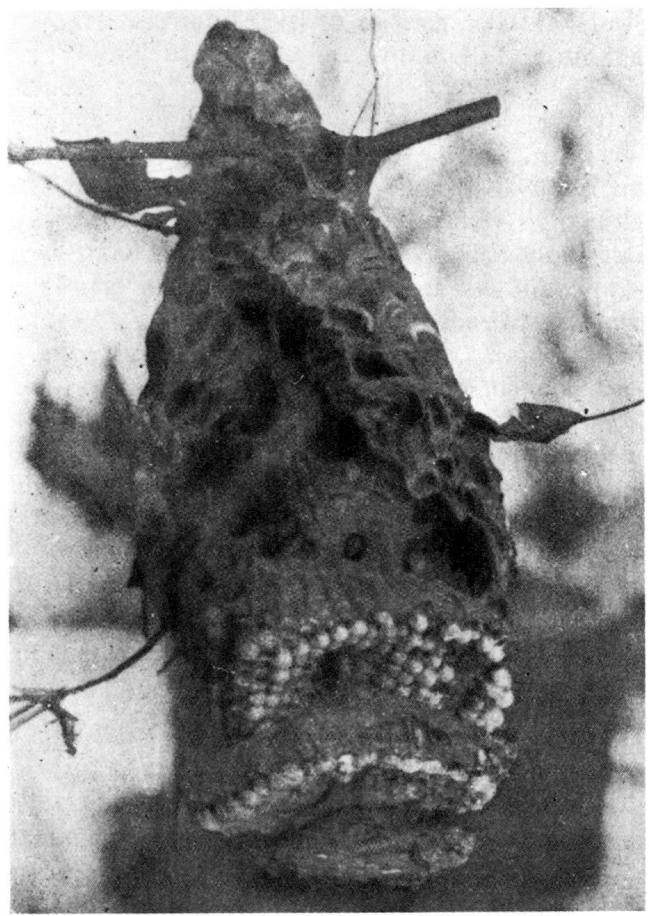

Fig. 10. A typical *V. analis* nest with the bottom part of the envelope removed to show the tiers of combs interconnected by a central stalk. Note the encapsulated pupal cells (CHAN, 1972)

the archipelago. *V. analis* F. (Figs. 9 and 10) is distributed from the Eastern Himalayas, through China, Manchuria, Singapore, and Southeastern Siberia to Japan, Formosa, Malaya, Java, and Bali.

V. basalis (Smith and *V. mocsaryna* (du Buysson) occur from the Eastern Hima-

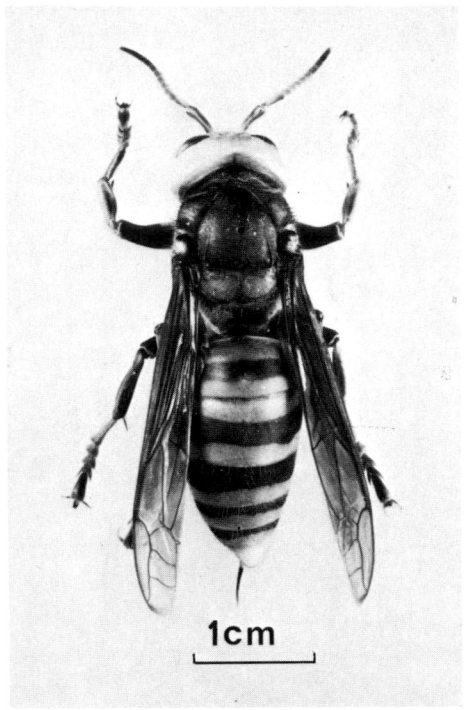

Fig. 11. *Vespa mandarinia* (scale 1 cm)

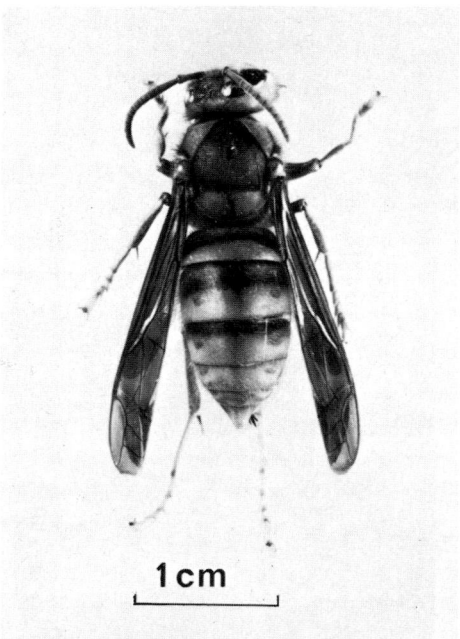

Fig. 12. *Vespa mongolica* (scale 1 cm)

layas to Sumatra. *V. luctuosa* (Saussure), *V. fervida* (Smith), *V. bellicosa* (Saussure), and *V. multimaculata* (Perez) inhabit forest areas in lowlands, the first two species occurring west of the line of Wallace on the Sunda Shelf (excluding Java), and the other two species occurring east of that line in the Philippines and Celebes. *V. mandarinia* (Smith) (Fig. 11) is distributed in India, Indochina, China, Japan, and Burma but does not invade the true humid tropics (VAN DER VECHT, 1959). This species is easily distinguished from other *Vespa* species by the gigantic size (the body weight is almost twice that of other Asiatic species), the deeply incised clypeus, and the enormously developed genae, which lend it a strange physiognomy (MATSUURA and SAKAGAMI, 1973). Fresh weight of queens is 2.0 – 3.0 g; of workers and males it is 1.0 – 1.5 g (OKADA, 1961). The relative body weight of Japanese *Vespa* species with respect to *V. crabro* are as follows: *V. crabro* 1.00, *V. mandarinia* 1.60, *V. tropica* 1.18, *V. analis* 1.15 and *V. mongolica* 0.92 (MATSUURA and SAKA-GAMI, 1973). Figure 12 shows a specimen of *V. mongolica*.

II. Social Behavior

1. Life Cycle

The life cycle of Vespinae has been elucidated by numerous investigators: JANET (1903), DUNCAN (1931), BODENHEIMER (1933), KUGLER (1938), SCHREMMER (1962), BRIAN (1965), KEMPER and DÖHRING (1967), ISHAY (1967), RICHARDS (1971), WILSON (1971), ARCHER (1972), WAFA and SHARKAWI (1972), SPRADBERY (1973), MATSUURA and SAKAGAMI (1973), and MACDONALD et al. (1974).

The early developmental stages of the *Vespa orientalis* colony has been described by DARCHEN (1964). Shortly after the first workers eclose, they assume most of the queen's duties, leaving the latter to engage mainly in egg laying. The ovarioles number in Vespinae varies from $6+6$ to $12+12$ (KUGLER et al., in press). Throughout the summer the nest is enlarged by the building of new combs. The brood, i.e., eggs, larvae, and pupae as well as the adult population, increases accordingly, the colony comprising several hundred to several thousand individuals. Social parasites on *Vespa* species: *V. dybowskii* (André) is a facultative temporary parasite on *V. crabro* L. and on *V. xanthoptera* (Cameron) (SAKAGAMI and FUKUSHIMA, 1957). Toward the end of the summer, larger cells are constructed in which males and young queens are reared. The young queens and males leave the nest and mate, the fecundated queens hibernating at the end of the season in hidden places. The population of the original nest perishes and its combs are abandoned. In New Zealand and Tasmania, *P. germanica* build enormous perennial (18 months) nests which are subterranean or attached to tree trunks and contain some 1.5 – 4 million cells (THOMAS, 1960; ANON, 1962). No wasp colonies are known to survive more than two seasons. The nest architecture of the tropic wasps has been described by JEANNE (1975), while some experiments concerning the orientation of the nest in *V. orientalis* have been reported by ISHAY (1973, 1975a, and 1976) and ISHAY and SADEH (1975).

2. The Nest Entrance

A "sentry" wasp or hornet stands at the nest entrance with its head facing outwards. The task of such sentries is to inspect and "clear" all incoming and outgoing traffic. In case of attack on the nest, the sentry alerts most of the workers inside by ejecting a drop of venom. The venom contains volatile substances, the odor of which apparently serves to warn other members of the nest. Such substances have been described by MASCHWITZ (1964), LINDAUER (1965), and SASLAVSKY et al. (1973), and are called "alarm substances."

The workers bring various building materials as well as food for the colony into the nest. As building materials the workers introduce dried woodstuff and soil particles which, when masticated and mixed with saliva, become the material from which the comb is built. Some wasp species construct combs from cellulose alone, which is obtained from paper, dry wood, etc., whereas other species mix the woody material with various amounts of available soil.

Caterpillars, mantids, bees, bugs, grasshoppers, beetles, butterflies, and moths are taken into the nest as foodstuffs (NEWPORT, 1836; ROTHNEY, 1877; HEWETT, 1889; FOREL, 1895; VIEWIG, 1896; GREEN, 1905; RIVNAY and BYTINSKI-SALZ, 1949; KUHLHORN, 1961; ISHAY et al., 1967).

3. Foraging Behavior

MATSUURA and SAKAGAMI (1973) have studied the foraging behavior of various *Vespa* species at and around Kibi, Japan. Judged by the frequency of visits to a particular site, the species ranked as follows: Visits to apiaries by *mandarinia, mongolica, crabro, analis, lewisii* (*Paravespula lewisii* which is the commonest yellow jacket in Japan), and *tropica;* visits to tree sups sources by *mandarinia, crabro, analis, tropica,* and *mongolica;* visits to houses by *tropica, crabro, mandarinia, mongolica,* and *analis.*

The foraging distance of *Vespula pennsylvanica* has been determined by employing metal labels and magnets. It was found that about 80% of the workers foraged within 1100 ft. from the nest (AKRE et al., 1975). Although the bodies of insects and other arthropods serve as the major source of protein for the larvae, the adult wasps may also "raid" butchershops and fish markets (*Vide* RAU and RAU, 1918 in North America or KEMPER and DOHRING, 1962 in Germany). Additional meat sources, apart from the carcasses of dead animals, may be the live nestlings or even adult birds (GRANT, 1959).

The attacks of hornets on beehives have been observed by numerous authors. The following is a list of such observations from various parts of the globe. *V. affinis* in Formosa: occasionally attacking beehives and removing larvae and pupae (SONON, 1927); *V. analis* in Indonesia: bee comb devastated by excited members of a hornet colony (VAN DER VECHT, 1957); *V. basalis* in Punjab: attacks on hives (SMITH, 1960); *V. crabro* in Germany and Italy: damaging bee colonies (BROCHERT, 1949 and ALBER, 1953); *V. cincta* in India and Indochina: persistently hunting at hive entrances, leading to extermination of some or most of the bee colonies (TOUMANOFF 1939; SUBBIAH and MEHADEVAN, 1957; SMITH, 1960); *V. mandarinia* in Formosa: the worst enemy of apiculture (MATSUURA, unpublished); *V. orientalis:* predatory on bees in Egypt, South Italy, Uzbekistan, Transcaucasia, Turkey, India (RIVNAY and BYTINSKY-SALZ, 1949; ADSAY, 1950; ALBER, 1953; WAFA, 1956; NOSENKO, 1963; ISHAY et al., 1967); *Vespa* sp. most probably *V. crabro* in Afghanistan: cruel enemy of the bee *Apis cerana* during all seasons (SCHNEIDER and DJALAL, 1970; KLOFT and SCHNEIDER, 1970).

The Japanese honey-bee *Apis cerana cerana* F., the largest and most easternly subspecies of the Asiatic honey-bee, when threatened by the giant hornet *V. mandarinia,* resorts to either passive retreat or active counterattack. Here is how MATSUURA and SAKAGAMI (1973) describe such an encounter: "At the arrival of a hornet, departures from the hive abruptly cease. The shimmering, a warning sound characteristic to the species (SAKAGAMI, 1960), is repeatedly emitted in the hive. Homing foragers keep a distance from the hornet and quickly enter into the hive through holes remote from the enemy. Some bees approach the hornet, directing their heads to the enemy, raising their maetasomal tips and vibrating the wings. A circle of bees is formed around the intruder and one bee pounces rapidly upon its head, while almost synchronously all the others in the circle rush upon it, so that after some 10—15 seconds the hornet is covered thickly by many bees. The bees covering the hornet keep their position for more than 20 min, meanwhile killing the hornet by stings."

The attacks of *V. mandarinia* on *Apis mellifera* bees in Japan have been observed and summarised by MATSUURA and SAKAGAMI (1973). Such attacks occur in stages as follows: (1) a hunting phase, which is basically the same as that of other hornet species, with each hornet repeating a chain of activities in the following sequence: visiting a beehive, lying in wait, catching one bee, rendering it into a ball of meat which is then carried to the nest; (2) a slaughter phase, during which the hornets kill bees whenever encountered at the hive entrance, the slaughter continuing till most of the bee population is exterminated; (3) an invasion phase during which the hornets freely enter the beehive and seizes the pupae for food, while leaving some of their mates to guard the hive entrance. The invading hornets usually destroy the honey combs but rarely utilize the honey itself. In contrast, *P. lewisii* seeks mainly the stored honey. Some of the *Vespa* species in Japan are highly predatory on *Polistes* (SAKAGAMI and FUKUSHIMA, 1957) and attack their nests mainly after emergence of the young males and queens. *V. mandarinia* attacks *Vespula* and *Vespa* species, usually in the same manner as it attacks bees. In the United States, workers of *V. pennsylvanica* and *V. atropilosa* capture prey of various sources, mainly insects of the orders Hymenoptera, Lepidoptera and Diptera. *V. pennsylvanica* workers can be a serious problem for bee-keepers in the fall (MACDONALD et al., 1974). The social wasps introduce into their nest large amounts of carbohydrates in addition to proteins. The enzymatic activity of the Oriental hornet (*Vespa orientalis*) larvae and adults have been studied extensively (IKAN et al., 1968; SONNEBORN et al., 1969; FISCHL and ISHAY, 1972; FISCHL et al., 1974; JANY et al., 1974; JANY and PFLEIDERER, 1974; ALLALOUF et al., 1972 and 1975; ISHAY, 1975b; FISCHL et al., 1975 and 1976). Reports have been published on their amino acids contents (IKAN and ISHAY, 1973), cholesterol (IKAN and ISHAY, 1965), pheromones (ISHAY et al., 1965; IKAN et al., 1969b), lipids (IKAN et al., 1969a; ISHAY et al., 1971c), catecholamines (ISHAY et al., 1974a), kinin-like substances (ISHAY, 1972), glucose level and glycemic changes in their hemolymph (ISHAY 1975c and 1975d), pteridines and purines (IKAN and ISHAY, 1967), and ubiquinones (IKAN et al., 1968b). The manganese metabolism in social Vespidae has been described by BOWEN (1950). The hemolymph composition and hemocytes have been described by Joshua et al. (1973), and the presence of insulin in the Vespinae hemolymph as well as the influence of mammalian insulin on the Vespinae glucose level have been reported by Ishay et al. (1976). Honey is obtained both by the ingestion of bees (the honey stomach of the bee) as well as by robbing honey from the beehives. Hornets and wasps also visit flowers and collect nectar from them. Meeuse (1961) noted that the flowers preferred by hornets are species of the genus *Epipactis,* of the Orchidaceae family. In Israel, hornets visit various flowers, among them the species *Ochradenus baccatus* (Resedaceae), *Zizyphus spina—christi* (Rhamnaceae) and *Urginea maritima* (Liliaceae). All of these have in common the fact that their nectar is exposed and easily accessible. Flower-visiting wasps may help to pollinate them (Schremmer, 1961). In Jamaica, coconut pollination is done by *Polistes* wasps in addition to bees (Free et al., 1975). While many flower species are visited by wasps and hornets, it is possible that they are in fact searching for insects at these foraging sites.

Carbohydrates are also collected in the form of honeydew, the sweet excretion of aphids, psyllids, and coccids (Ikan and Ishay, 1966).

4. Enemies and Parasites

The hornet (probably *V. tropica*) is attacked by a fungus *Hirsutella saussuri* (Cooke) (Garresten, 1923). During the rainy period empty cells of the wasp nest are often heavily infested with the fungi *Trichotecium* and *Fusarium* and with bacteria (Ishay, 1964).

Mason and Maxwell-Lefroy (1912) found that *V. orientalis* was preyed upon in India by four species of birds: *Merops viridis* L., *M. superciliosus* L., *Dendrocitta rufa* (Latham), and *Caprimulgus macrurus* Horsf.

In some oriental countries the immature stages of wasps are consumed by man. According to Bristowe (1932) the larvae of the hornet (probably *Vespa tropica*) are used as foodstuff in several places in Siam. The same is reported by van der Meer and Mohr (1941) from North Sumatra. Hesse (1916) lists 24 bird species predators of wasps, which among others, include the Shrike, Blackbird, Great Tit, Green Woodpecker and Magpie. Several mammals, mainly rodents, probably disrupt colonies during the incipient stage. In the British Isles (Fox-Wilson, 1946), the badger is probably the chief predator of wasp colonies. In Brazil, colonies of Polybiini wasps are attacked at night by bats (*Phylloderma stenops*), which consume the brood with apparent impunity of the adult wasp stings (Jeanne, 1970). Several species of dragon-flies (Odonata) have been found preying on *Vespula* (Hobby, 1932), and the same phenomena have been repeatedly reported on robber flies (Asilidae) (Seguy, 1927). Spiders kill wasps or trap them in their webs (Fox-Wilson, 1946) and centipeds (Chilopoda) attack founding queens (Stone, 1865). In the tropics, where the majority of social wasp species occur, predation by ants is believed to be a major force in nest evolution.

The parasitic worms (Nematoda) have been found as parasites within adult wasps. Blackith and Stevenson (1958) found up to 34.6% parasitism of *P. germanica* queens. Poinar and Ennik (1972) have infected *Vespula* workers with nematode *Neoplectana carpocapsae* which carry the bacterium *Achromobacter nematophilus,* causing septicemia in the host insect. They propose the use of the nematode in order to promote wasp control.

The beetle *Metoecus paradoxus* is frequently found in subterranean nests of *Vespula* and *Paravespula* species. The larvae are brought into the nest by wasps which collect building materials such as woodpulp. After arriving in the colony, the beetle larva enters into a wasp larva. The parasitoid larva remains within the host, feeding on its hemolymph. The life history was determined by CHAPMAN (1870) and MURRAY (1870). In Europe *M. paradoxus* was found only rarely in species other than *P. vulgaris,* where the level of parasitism in nests never exceeded 4% (POTTER, 1965). In Japan *M. paradoxus* is parasitic on *Vespula lewisii* and *M. vespae* on *V. rufa* (HATTORI and YAMANE, 1975).

5. Defensive Behavior

According to the type of nest and defensive behavior the tropical wasps can be divided into two major groups: those which construct small, uncovered nests of a single comb suspended from a petiole; *Polistes* and *Mischocyttarus* species smear the petiole with a glandular secretion that has repellent properties and those which build enclosed nests (such active defence calls for large numbers of workers as "guards" at the entrance and around the nest envelope) (JEANNE, 1975).

6. Hornet Traps

A hornet trap installed at the beehive entrance is a Japanese bee-keeper's invention (AOKI, 1950). Also, in other countries with a dense hornet population, various traps are used by apiculturists to catch and kill the hornet workers.

7. Aggressive Behavior—Stinging

The Vespinae show markedly different reactions with regard to disturbance of their nests. Wasps tend to attack intruders only close to their colony entrance. Usually, small colonies are less aggressive, even when disturbed, than more populated ones. In the latter, the defence flight of wasps is generally in response to a disturbance of the nest structure or of a solid-borne sound, i.e., a substrate vibration produced close to the nest, but not by air-borne sounds. The number of wasps responding to a stimulus is roughly proportional to the extent of the disturbance. It is the moving target which attracts most attention, thus it is safer to stand still near a nest than to run panic-stricken from a disturbed colony (SPRADBERY, 1973). The most important feature of the wasp, from the layman's point of view, is its ability to sting and to cause pain and death. GAUL (1953) determined that a defence flight lasts for 90 seconds to five minutes, the duration depending primarily on weather conditions. High temperatures tend to prolong the flight. Defending wasps will fly within a radius of about seven meters from their nest. The alarmed wasps from a disturbed colony rush out on defence flights, seeking the cause of the disturbance. Once the intruder has been located, the closest wasp starts to sting him. Most of the other wasps will try to sting the intruder as close as possible to the first sting. This happens because the venom injected into the victim contains, in addition to liquid toxic substances, volatile substances (MASCHWITZ, 1966a) which act for other wasps as an indicator of the place of the first sting. Chemical alarm systems like those occurring in social wasps are widespread in social insects (MASCHWITZ, 1964 and 1966b). The alarm pheromones are found in the venom of Vespinae species but not in Polistinae. In experiments with *V. orientalis* colonies (SASLAVSKY et al., 1973), it was possible to establish some of the structural characteristics of the alarm substances. Generally, a stronger response could be observed with adult *Vespa orientalis* workers and a weaker with the younger ones. The alarming substances are aliphatic ketones; the different location of the keto group within the molecule has a pronounced effect on the activity e.g., 2-nonanone is a very active $(+++)$ alarming substance, while 4-nonanone is not at all $(-)$; introduction of a methyl group reduces the activity, since 3-nonanone is $(+++)$, while 2-methyl-3-nonanone is $(-)$. The presence of a double bond increases the activity, 6-methyl-5-hepten-2-one $(++)$ and the saturated analog, 2-methyl-5-heptanone being $(+)$. Alarm substances are toxic to the colony members. Five stages could be observed in the behavior of individuals towards ketones: (1) a latent period lasting for 2 s to 2 min, (2) an unrest period followed by excitation, (3) loss of righting reflex and motor coordination, (4) convulsions, and (5) paralysis and death. The various members of the hornet family responded for different periods of time towards certain ketones.

8. Aggressiveness of Various Species

In general, the smaller species are less aggressive than bigger ones. Thus it is usual to be able to observe the daily activity of various species of Polistinae and also of *Vespula (Paravespula)* and *Dolichovespula* and of some *Vespa* varieties. One can watch the activity of heavily populated colonies of *V. orientalis, V. crabro, V. analis,* and *V. tropica* without difficulty. Other species, like *V. velutina* and *V. mandarinia,* are extremely aggressive and dangerous to man to the extent that there are some areas in Indonesia which cannot be cultivated until the hornet nests have been destroyed. In Laos and North Siam, people say that "to be stung by a hornet (*V. affinis*) makes one's hair go white" (BRISTOWE, 1932). In Trinidad, *Synoeca surinama* (Polistinae) is said to be the most feared of all the wasps.

C. The Venomous Apparatus

I. The Nonglandular Parts of the Sting Apparatus.
Mechanism of Stinging

Details of the mechanism of sting action have been studied in the honeybee by SNODGRASS (1956), and the essential features are applicable to most stinging Aculeate Hymenoptera. The stinging apparatus is a modified ovipositor and is absent in the male. When not used, it is kept withdrawn in the abdomen. The venom is injected in the victim's skin or cuticle through a hollow needle-like sting composed of a superior sting sheath and a pair of inferior lancets (Fig. 13). These latter

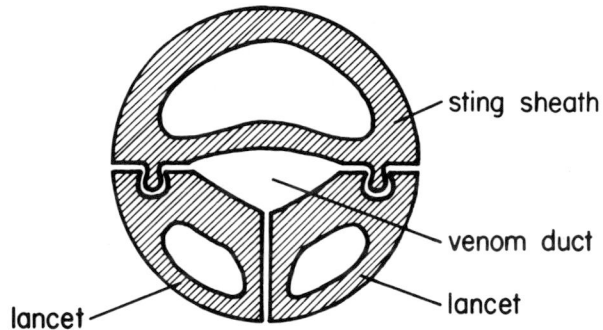

sting sheath

venom duct

lancet

lancet

Fig. 13. Schematic cross-section of Vespidae sting

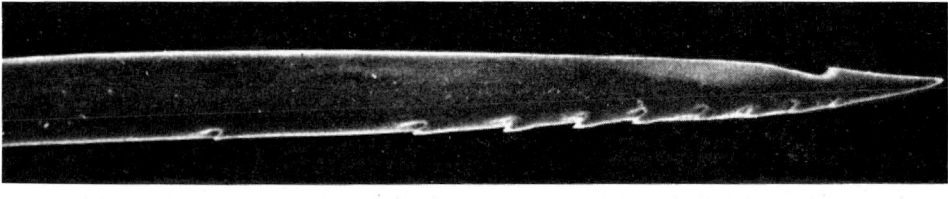

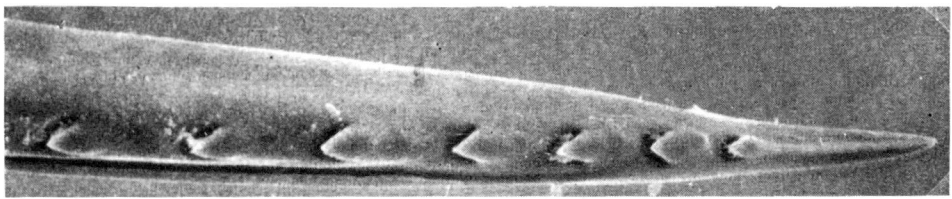

Fig. 14. Scanning electron micrograph of sting tip (lancet) showing the series of small barbs (SPRADBERY, 1973)

are long, chitinous and are *not* fused to each other. They bear at their distal end "teeth" and "barbs" (Fig. 14) and are closely held against the undersurface of the sting sheath. The latter is formed by a pair of long chitinous pieces fused into a single unit. The sting sheath is bordered ventrally on each side by a fold. These folds fit into corresponding grooves of the inferior lancets. The sting sheath, together with the pair of lancets, form the sting, whose hollow inside represents the venom duct. In this latter, the venom is transported outwards into the victim's skin. The sting is swung out by the action of the oblong and quadrate plates (Fig. 15). Both plates are actuated by contraction of muscles around them.

After the initial contact with the victim's body surface, the sting penetrates stepwise by alternating thrust movements of the lancets alongside the sting sheath (Fig. 16). During stinging, the wasps grip tightly to the victim with their legs and mandibles. In this way, they secure the penetration of the sting into the skin of vertebrates or into the cuticle of their enemy or prey. As soon as the sting has reached the appropriate depth, it remains stuck on the victim's skin with the above-mentioned "teeth" and "barbs." Wasps and hornets try to sting the enemy several times in succession. When venom injection is completed, the

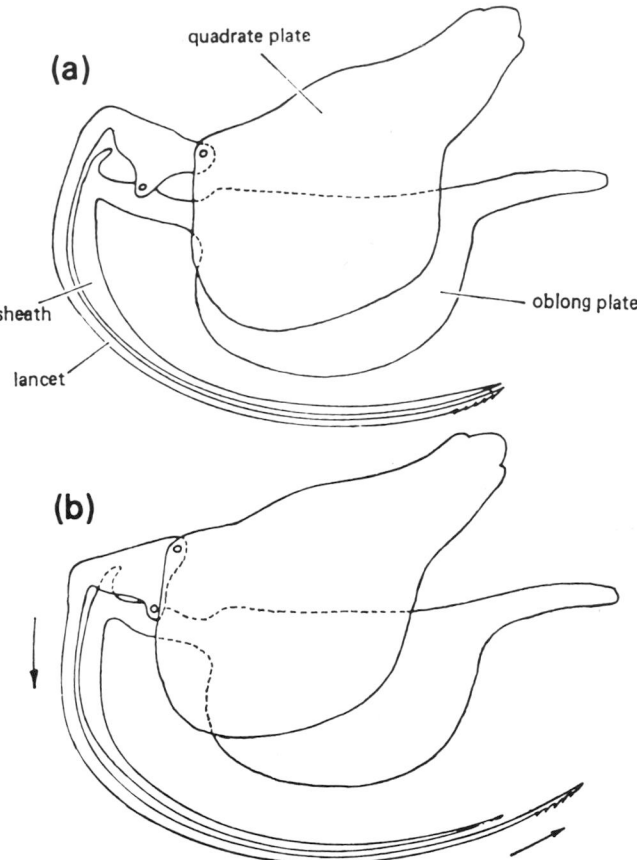

(a)

quadrate plate

sheath

lancet

oblong plate

(b)

Fig. 15a and b. Mechanics of sting action: (a) quadrate and oblong plates; (b) mechanism whereby plate swings out of the sting (SPRADBERY, 1973)

sting is withdrawn. Usually, there is no sting autotomy in Vespinae, i.e., unlike honeybees, they do not leave the sting in the victim's skin.

II. The Glandular Parts of the Sting Apparatus

As described earlier (SWAMMERDAM, 1752; LANGER, 1897; MELINOSSI, 1935), the venom gland, also called the acidic gland, is the largest in the sting apparatus. This gland is paired and is situated between the rectum and the vagina. The two venom gland tubes end in a distinct spherical reservoir, the venom sac, whose muscular wall is relatively thick and probably serves to inject the venom during the sting action. Besides the acidic venom glands, there is to be found *one* additional accessory gland called the "Dufour gland," or the alkaline gland. In *Vespa* the gland tube penetrates into the venom sac, perforates its underside, and freely ends in the sting chamber. First detailed descriptions of the venom glands in *Vespa (Paravespula) germanica* and *Vespa (Dolichovespula) media* were given by

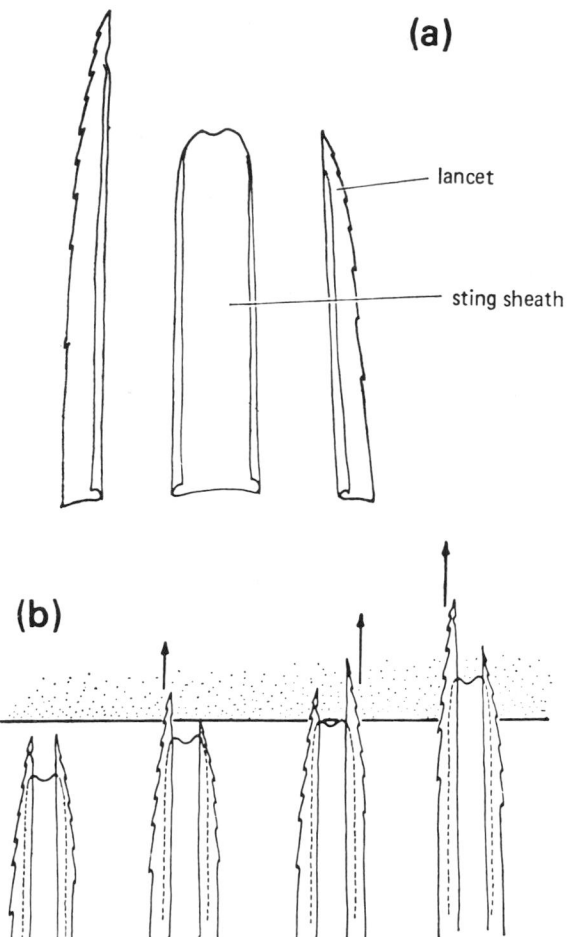

Fig. 16a and b. Vespula sting: (a) components of sting tip; (b) probable mode of penetration (SPRADBERY, 1973)

BORDAS (1894), in *V. crabro* by KOSCHEVNIKOV (1899), in *Vespa* in general by PAWLOWSKI (1927), and on the venom apparatus in various species of the order Hymenoptera by MASCHWITZ and KLOFT (1971). The venom apparatus of *V. orientalis* has been studied in detail by KANWAR and SETHI (1971), KANWAR and KANWAR (1975), and BARR-NEA et al. (1976) and is shown in Figure 17a. The average dimensions of the various components were as follows: acid glands (2), each 40—60 mm long and of 0.07—0.20 mm diameter; alkaline gland, 3.5—5.0 mm long and of 0.3—0.5 mm diameter; and the ovoid-shaped venom sac, 3.5—5.0 mm long and 2—3 mm at maximum width. The mean weight of a single dry apparatus of *V. (Paravespula) vulgaris* (JAQUES and SCHACHTER, 1954) was 0.63 mg and of *V. orientalis* 0.91 mg (ISHAY et al., in press). Protein contents (average in µg) are: acid gland, 10—20; alkaline gland, 5—15; and the venom sac, 1000—2000. The acid gland is made up of two similar tubes terminating in the venom sac.

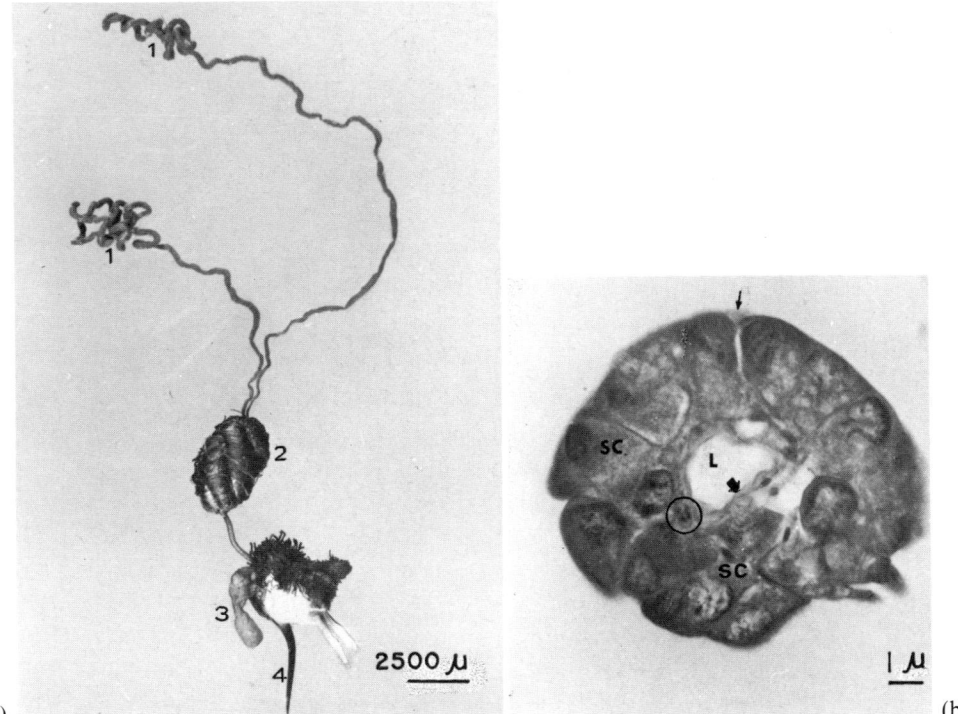

(a)   (b)

Fig. 17. (a) The venom apparatus of *Vespa orientalis*. *1* acid gland; *2*, venom sac; *3*, alkaline gland; *4*, stinger. (b) Cross-section of the acid gland, stained with luxol fast blue. *L*, lumen of the gland; *SC*, secretory cell; thick arrow, chitinous membrane; circle, squamous cell; thin arrow, basement membrane. (c) Longitudinal section of the acid gland stained with alcian blue. *L*, lumen of the gland; *CM*, chitinous membrane around the lumen; thick arrow shows net of canaliculi in intracellular space; thin arrow, opening of a canaliculus through the chitinous membrane into the lumen. (d) Cross-section of the acid gland stained with luxol fast blue. *L*, lumen of the gland; *SQ*, squamous cell; *SC*, secretory cell (Barr-Nea et al., 1976).

The distal part of the gland secretes the venom, while the proximal serves for the transport of the secretion (Melinossi, 1935). In *V. orientalis* the lumen of the tube is surrounded by a thick chitinous membrane, by some squamous cells scattered around the membrane, and two rows of secreting cells, limited externally by a basement membrane (Barr-Nea et al., 1976) (Fig. 17*b*). In the secretory part of the tube the lumen is narrow, its diameter being smaller than the width of the cell layers. The internal secreting cell layer contains large polyhedral cells with an oval nucleus generally located at the basal part of the cell. The cell cytoplasm is granular, and most of the granules are stained with alcian blue, indicating that they contain sulphated mucopolysaccharides (Lev and Spicer, 1964). The same staining is apparent in the basement membrane and throughout the chitinous one surrounding the lumen. The epithelial cells also contain lipid droplets of different sizes within their cytoplasm. Fine canaliculi connect the cells within the lumen (Fig. 17*c*) and are filled with lipid droplets. No such droplets nor mucopolysaccharides were found in the lumen. The outer secreting cell layer con-

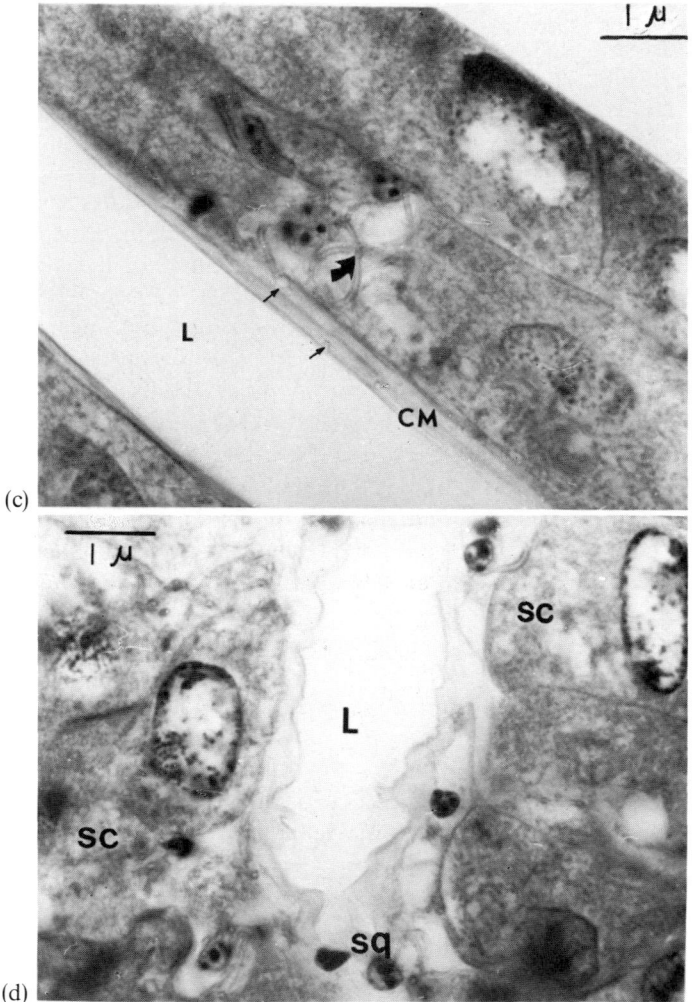

Fig. 17c and d

tains smaller cells with very few lipid droplets in the elongated cytoplasm, which is also filled with alcian blue positive granules. The squamous cells around the lumen (Fig. 17d) have practically no cytoplasm but have a nucleus containing lumps of chromatin. The fine structure of the *V. orientalis* acid gland studied by electronmicroscopy has recently been described by KANWAR and KANWAR (1975). The secretory cells, which are wedge-shaped, arrange themselves around the lumen (central duct) and drain their product through finely branched ductules or "drain pipes." Secretory cells vary in number and size, as well as in the position of the cytoplasmatic vacuoles and the location of the nucleus. This configuration suggests that secretory cycles in a particular section of the gland are asynchronous. Though secretory cells are mononuclear, the number of nucleoli per cell varies markedly. Moreover, certain features, such as irregular appearance of nuclear and nucleolar envelopes, as well as continuous shedding of electron dense emissions, strongly indicate intense protein synthetizing activity in the secretory cells. The mitochondria are small and ovoid with only few cristae and appear uniformly dispersed in a granular matrix of moderate electron density. The granular matrix contains electron-transparent vesicles of 500−800 A° diameter. These latter represent the "hyaline vacuoles" described in light-microscopy studies and are considered as the sites of water-diffusible components of the venom. Furthermore, electron-dense granules of diverse sizes were randomly found in the cytoplasm. The larger sized granules are regarded as homologous, with the "cytochemically complex secretory globules" composed of lipids, carbohydrates, and proteins described in previous studies (KANWAR and SETHI, 1971). The secretory cells are highly basophilic, their cytoplasm showing a uniformly vesiculated granular endoplasmic reticulum, though the lamellar one, as well as Golgi cisternae, is distinctively absent.

In the "transporting" part of the gland the diameter of the lumen is twice as large as in the secretory part, and the wall of the tube is made of one single cell layer. The cells themselves do not contain lipid droplets nor mucopolysaccharides; their nuclei resemble those of the squamous cells and contain lumps of chromatin. A transitory region is seen between the two parts of the gland; in this region some secretory cells, similar to those seen in the secretory part, are scattered among the nonactive cells.

The alkaline gland is made up of a single tube containing two major cell populations: an inner epithelial layer and an outer muscular layer. In most of the tube the epithelial layer is stretched, but in some places the epithelial cells proliferate inside the lumen, forming an acinar-like structure on which nets of muscles are seen (Fig. 18a). Two types of epithelial cells are present: large round cells containing some lipid droplets and flattened cells with an oval nucleus (Fig. 18b). Some of the large round cells appear to have intracellular ducts (HAMMAD, 1965). Muscle fibers, recognizable by their elongated shape, transversal striations, eosinophilic cytoplasm, and central rows of nuclei, run along the outer side of the epithelial cells and make contact with their basement membrane. Usually the muscle fibers reach the gland at a right angle and then divide into several branches, making contact with adjacent epithelial cells. The muscle fibers form consecutive nets around the epithelial cells, but the periodicity of the arrangement, if any, could not be determined. Near the junction of the alkaline gland with the stinging apparatus, the muscle fibers make a net around the gland, forming a sphincter-like structure (Fig. 18c). Toxicity tests performed both *in vivo* and *in vitro* suggest that the alkaline secretion possesses some toxic activity, since it was lethal when applied to bees, produced abnormal symptoms after i.v. injection into mice, provoked lipid accumulation within the liver cells *in vitro* (BARR-NEA et al., 1976), and exhibited phospholipase activity (ROSENBERG et al., in press).

The venom sac plays the role of a reservoir in which the secretion of the acid gland is stored. It is made essentially of a thick wall of muscle fibers arranged in four major bundles, separated by a thick membrane (Fig. 18d). The lumen is surrounded by a thick chitinous membrane. Between the lumen and the muscle layers some squamous cells are seen similar to those observed in the acid gland.

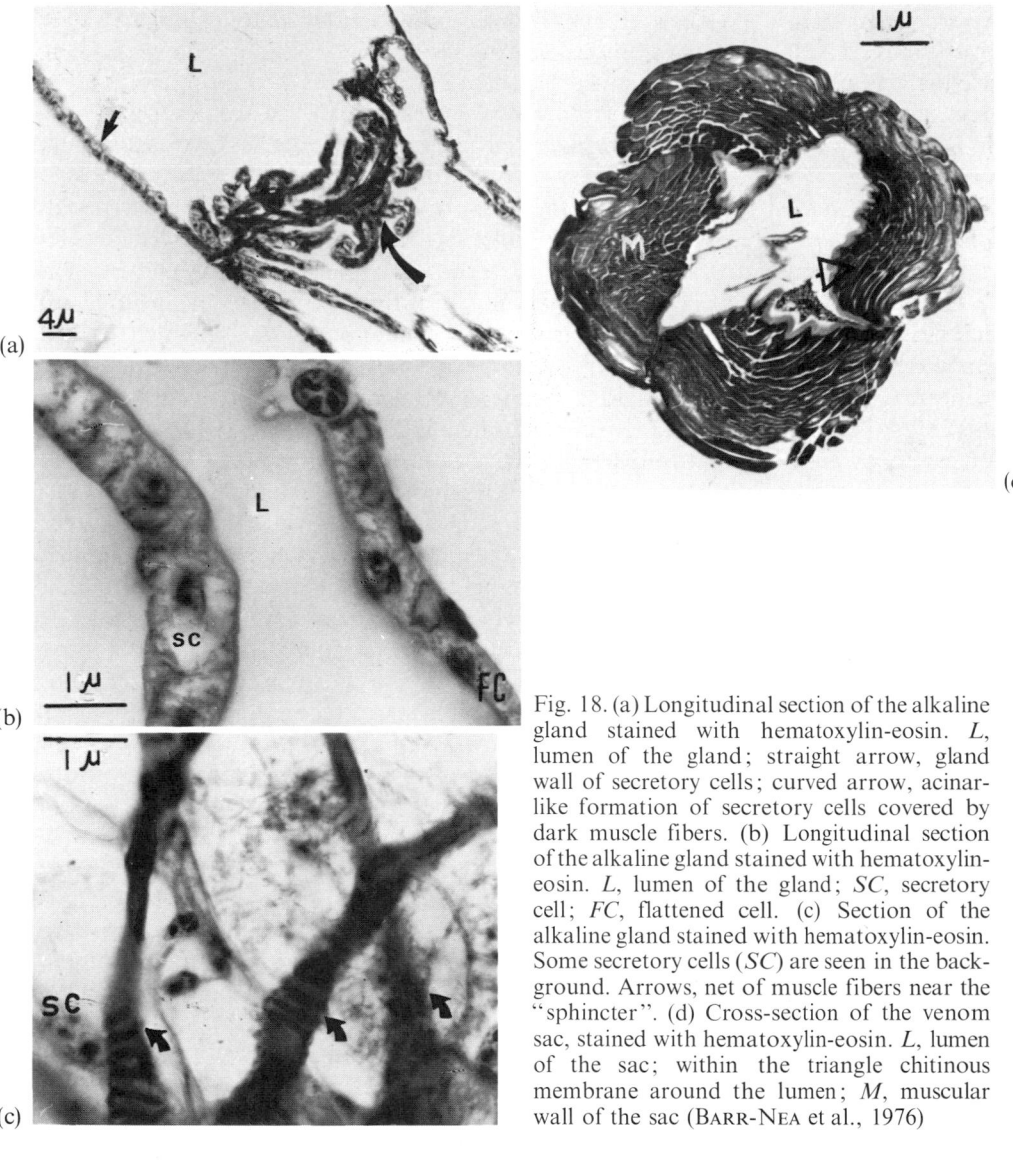

Fig. 18. (a) Longitudinal section of the alkaline gland stained with hematoxylin-eosin. *L*, lumen of the gland; straight arrow, gland wall of secretory cells; curved arrow, acinar-like formation of secretory cells covered by dark muscle fibers. (b) Longitudinal section of the alkaline gland stained with hematoxylin-eosin. *L*, lumen of the gland; *SC*, secretory cell; *FC*, flattened cell. (c) Section of the alkaline gland stained with hematoxylin-eosin. Some secretory cells (*SC*) are seen in the background. Arrows, net of muscle fibers near the "sphincter". (d) Cross-section of the venom sac, stained with hematoxylin-eosin. *L*, lumen of the sac; within the triangle chitinous membrane around the lumen; *M*, muscular wall of the sac (BARR-NEA et al., 1976)

III. Collection of the Venom

Several methods for obtaining native V.v. have been described earlier: SAID (1960) and DIRKS (1971) for *Polistes* wasps; WELSH and BATTY (1963) for various Vespinae and Polistinae wasps; JAQUES and SCHACHTER (1954) for *Vespa (Paravespula) vulgaris;* and ABRAHAMS (1955) for *V. crabro* and several other Vespinae and Polistinae wasps. General methods for obtaining native venom or venom apparatus have been proposed earlier by BENTON et al. (1963), O'CONNOR et al. (1963), BENTON and MORSE (1966), SIMON and BENTON (1969), EDERY et al. (1972), and ISHAY (1975b). The venom may be collected from living as well as from dead Vespidae.

The method of O'CONNOR et al. (1963) consists of a small hemi-cylinder of fine brass mesh about $^{1}/_{4}$ inch diameter and $^{1}/_{2}$ inch long, soldered to the end of a 2-inch length of rigid iron wire which is bent for insertion into a rubber stopper. The insect is anesthetized with carbon dioxide, placed in the cylinder, and tied in place. As the insect begins to recover it is excited by a brief high voltage shock, controlled by a key switch, until venom is secreted. With this apparatus, two or three insects can be "milked" every minute with no apparent effect on the insect. However, this method seems to be uneconomical and caused the insects to defecate, thus contaminating the venom. The method proposed by SIMON and BENTON (1969) enables mass collection of pure venom from wasps. Yields of up to 12 mg per nest were obtained, and with proper management, continuous milking from the same nest is possible. The "milking" device proposed by the above-mentioned authors is placed in the flight path near the nest entrance. Incoming wasps should strike the surface of the device, sting several times, and then retreat. Since alarm pheromones are released together with the venom droplets (MASCHWITZ, 1966b), after several stings many wasps would leave the nest and attack the device, proceeding to sting the collection sheet where the first venom droplets were deposited. The "milking" device consists of a wooden frame, over which alternately charged and grounded stainless-steel wires were stretched at 3.18 mm intervals. The circuit is closed when an insect touches any two consecutive wires. Inside this frame a wooden one is made, which is the collection area. A thin sheet of polyethylene is stretched over the inner frame, which is then pressed against the wires, thus remaining fixed. Normal stinging response could be induced by pulses of 3 volts at a frequency of 15 cycles/second. In this way, satisfactory collections were obtained from ground nests of *V. maculifrons, V. maculata,* and *V. arenaria,* but not from aerial nesting wasps like *Polistes* sp. Maximum purity of the collected venom was obtained by using two sheets of polyethylene during collection and then discarding the upper sheet. However, the collection of venom in this way has some disadvantages. After about 15 min of continuous use, the insects become too vicious for the collectors, so the device should only be used by people not sensitive to Vespidae stings. Secondly, it is not suitable for thermolabile venom, because if collection lasts for more than 5 to 10 min, the material might become partially inactivated.

EDERY et al. (1972) and ISHAY (1964, 1975b) have obtained venom from *V. orientalis* by the following technique: the hornets are traced to their nests in the field by following their diurnal flight patterns; once the nest is located, the entire colony is placed under ether anesthesia at night, when the adult population is supposed to be concentrated in the nest; the whole colony, including combs with brood and imagines, is easily collected in this way and stored either cooled or frozen; the immobilized hornet is then "milked" by hand, applying gentle pressure to the venom sac region at the distal end of the abdomen; following freezing of the hornet, its venom sac can be unsheathed by pulling the stinger at the tip of the abdomen; this maneuver exposes the sting apparatus as well as the attached spindleshaped, whitish venom sac which is then removed, placed in a test tube and kept at $-15°$ C or $-20°$ C; when enough material has been collected, it is ground, homogenized, and after centrifugation, the supernatant is used at the original concentration or dissolved in saline.

JAQUES and SCHACHTER (1954), SAID (1960), and BARR-NEA et al. (1976) have described methods for obtaining the venom apparatus comprising the acid and alkaline glands, as well as the venom sacs. The insect is immobilized in the cold, killed by crushing the head, and pinned on its back. The sting is then grasped with fine forceps, and the ventral part of the abdominal segments are cut away. The entire venom apparatus can now be seen. Care is taken to avoid rupture of the acid glands from their attachments to the venom sac. The acid glands are readily differentiated from the mass of yellowish Malpigian tubules by their large diameter and white opaque appearance. Using a stereomicroscope, it is possible to remove the venom glands uncontaminated with extraneous tissue.

IV. Quantity of Venom Collected from a Single Wasp or Hornet

ABRAHAMS (1955) obtained, by hand milking *V. crabro*, immobilized at $0°$ C $- 2°$ C, $15 - 18$ droplets totalling 0.92 mg net venom. The dry venom weight per hornet was 0.26 mg, i.e., 28% mean dry substance. The same author obtained in a similar fashion from various *Polistes* sp. $0.14 - 0.17$ mg of dry venom per insect. The whole venom glands gave 0.68 mg of dry material per wasp, i.e., four times more than the dry venom. JAQUES and SCHACHTER (1954) reported that the mean value of the soluble material in the venom apparatus of *Vespa (Paravespula) vulgaris* was $27.0 - 30.4\%$. Approximately 2 mg of pure liquid venom (300 μg protein) could be obtained by squeezing the venom sac of a single *V. orientalis* (BARR-NEA et al., 1976). Moreover, a method of quantifying the venom after repeated "milking" of the same Vespidae is described in Section VI e.

D. Chemistry of Vespidae Venoms

I. Physico-Chemical Properties

The physico-chemical properties of the Vespidae venoms have been scantily investigated. Native venom of *V. crabro* (ABRAHAMS, 1955), obtained either by mechanical stimulation of the abdomen or by spontaneous ejection, is a fine crystal clear liquid of pH $6.8 - 6.9$ (measured with indicator paper) and of bitter taste. After lyophilization, the venom becomes a hygroscopic mass of nest-like appearance, dry matter representing 28% of the total weight. The venom of *Polistes* sp. is similar to that of *V. crabro,* though it has aromatic odor (ABRAHAMS, 1955).

Freshly collected *V. orientalis* venom appears as a colorless semiviscous liquid of pH $5.5 - 6.5$ (measured with glass-electrode) with a solid contents of 27.3%, of which 76% is protein. The venom is thermolabile but loses little or none of its activity when lyophilized or stored at $-20°$ C (FISCHL et al., 1972).

II. Components of Vespidae Venoms

In fact, only in the last 25 years has comprehensive research aiming to isolate and identify substances present in V.v. been undertaken. The main components so far characterized are shown in Tables 1 and 2, which include low-molecular-weight materials, such as acetylcholine, histamine, serotonin (5-hydroxytryptamine, 5-HT), catecholamines, volatile substances (see Section II b), and kinins as well as high-molecular proteins, mainly enzymes.

Table 1. Substances identified in vespidae venoms
Quantities (mean values) are expressed as µg/mg of dry venom gland extract, or native venom (V), whereas s. refers to one single venom sac. "Id" indicates that the material was identified but not

No.	Vespidae	Low-molecular-weight substances[a]			
		Acetylcholine or acetylcholine-like material	Histamine	Dopamine	Noradrenaline
1	*Polistes exclamans annularis fuscatus pallipes* (mixed material)	Abs s.[6] V[3]	0.8[6]	Abs s.[5]	Abs s.[5]
2	*Polistes gallicus*				
3	*Polistes omissa*	Abs[5, 7]			
4	*Dolichovespula media*				
5	*Dolichovespula saxonica*			0.017[10]	0.033[10]
6	*Vespula (Dolichovespula) arenaria*			0.125 s.[11]	0.004 s.[11]
7	*Vespula (Dolichovespula) maculata*	Abs s.[5]	8 s.[5]	0.014 s.[5]	0.022 s.[5]
8	*Vespula (Paravespula) maculifrons*	Abs s.[5]	15 s.[5]	0.068 s.[5]	0.002 s.[5]
9	*Paravespula germanica*			0.038[10]	0.070[10]
10	*Vespa (Paravespula) vulgaris*		20[9]	0.284[10]	0.021[10]
11	*Vespa crabro*	37.8[1] 30−40 V[2] 50−100[3]	48[8] 10V[3]	0.160[10]	0.044[10]
12	*Vespa orientalis*	40[4]	Id[4]	0.64V[4] 0.170[4]	29V[4] 0.073[4] 0.048[10]

[a] For 5-hydroxytryptamine, see Table 2.
[b] For chemical structure as well as other kinins, see Table 3.
[1] BHOOLA et al. (1961); [2] ABRAHAMS (1955); [3] ALBL (1956); [4] EDERY et al. (1972); [5] GELLER et al. (1976); [6] PISANO (1968); [7] SAID (1960); [8] SCHACHTER (1970); [9] JAQUES and SCHACHTER (1954); [10] ISHAY et al.

1. Low-Molecular-Weight Substances

a) Acetylcholine

The presence of acetylcholine (or a very closely related cholinomimetic material) has been identified only in *V. crabro* (ABRAHAMS, 1955; ALBL, 1956; BHOOLA et al.,

quantitatively determined. "Pres" refers to presence and "Abs" to absence. Number in small type indicates reference.

				Enzymes				
Adren-aline	Kinin(s)[b]	Cholin-esterase	Histidine-decarbo-xylase	Phospho-lipase	Acid, alkaline and neutral DNA-se	Hyaluron-idase	Prote-ase	Poly- and disaccha-ridases
Abs s.[5]	Id[6]							
						Pres[16]		
						Pres[7]	Abs[7]	
						Pres[16]		
0.015[10]						Pres[16]		
Abs s.[5]	Abs[5]		Pres[5]					
Abs s.[5]	Id[5]		Pres[5]					
0.024[10]						Pres[16]	Pres[21]	
0.017[10]	Id[12]	Pres[14]		Pres[14,20]		Pres[16,17]		
0.029[10]	Id[1]			Pres[18,20]		Pres[16]		
0.24V[4] 0.047[4] 0.058[10]	Id V[4,13]	Abs V[15]		Pres[19]	Pres[22]	Pres[4,16]	Pres[4,24]	Pres[23]

(1974a); [11] OWEN (1971); [12] SCHACHTER and THAIN (1954); [13] EDERY and ISHAY (1965); [14] JAQUES (1955); [15] EDERY and KUHNBERG (1970, unpublished results); [16] ALLALOUF et al. (1972); [17] JAQUES (1956); [18] HABERMANN (1968); [19] ROSENBERG et al. (1976); [20] CONTARDI and LATZER (1928); [21] ISHAY et al. (1973); [22] SLOR et al. (1976); [23] FISCHL et al. (1974); [24] JOSHUA and ISHAY (1975).

1961) and *V. orientalis* (EDERY and ISHAY, 1965; EDERY et al., 1972). Moreover, BHOOLA et al. (1961) obtained evidence by chromatography and parallel bioassay that acetylcholine was indeed the sole choline-ester of *V. crabro* venom. The amount of acetylcholine found in *V. crabro* and *V. orientalis* venoms represent the highest source ever encountered in any biological system hitherto studied.

Table 2. 5-Hydroxytryptamine (serotonin) contents of vespidae venoms

Mean values in μg per mg of dry venom sac extract; s. refers to one venom sac, whereas s.a. to the entire stinging apparatus. Number in small type indicates reference.

No.	Vespidae	5-Hydroxytryptamine
1	*Polybia rejecta*	0.082 s.a. [6]
2	*Synoeca surinama*	2.74 s.a. [6]
3	*Polistes* *exclamans* *annularis* *fuscatus pallipes* (mixed material)	1.2 [7]
4	*Polistes fuscatus*	0.81 s.a. [6]
5	*Polistes versicolor*	1.2 s.a. [6]
6	*Polistes versicolor vulgatus*	1.94 s.a. [6]
7	*Polistes gallicus*	0.75 s.a. [6]
8	*Polistes rothneyi Iwatai*	1.2 s. [8]
9	*Vespula (Dolichovespula) maculata*	4 s. [5]
10	*Dolichovespula saxonica*	1.1 [2]
11	*Vespula (Dolichovespula) media*	0.12 s.a. [6]
12	*Vespula (Paravespula) maculifrons*	Abs s. [5 a]
13	*Paravespula germanica*	6.2 [2]
14	*Vespa (Paravespula) vulgaris*	1.3 [2], 0.03 [3]
15	*Vespa crabro*	13.6 [1], 0.77 [2]
16	*Vespa orientalis*	37 [4 b] 8 [4] 8.2 [2]
17	*Vespa mandarinia*	Id. [9 c]

[a] Serotonin has been investigated and found to be absent.
[b] Pure lyophilized venom.
[c] Serotonin has been identified but not quantitatively determined.

[1] Bhoola et al. (1961); [2] Ishay et al. (1974a); [3] Jaques and Schachter (1954); [4] Edery et al. (1972); [5] Geller et al. (1976); [6] Welsh and Batty (1963); [7] Prado et al. (1966); [8] Watanabe et al. (in press); [9] Kawai and Hori (1975).

On the other hand, the origin of acetylcholine in V.v. is not presently understood. It is not known, for instance, whether the gland possesses choline acetyltransferase activity, which is the enzyme mainly responsible for the acetylcholine synthesis in many other arthropods (Chadwick, 1963).

b) Histamine

Histamine occurs in extremely high concentrations in V.v. The amounts present in *V. crabro* and *V. vulgaris* seem to be the highest ever found in arthropod venoms. Histamine is by definition a tissular amine, and its presence as a free component of the venom still remains to be elucidated. Histamine also occurs in the feces of *V. orientalis* (BERGMANN et al., 1966) and is probably derived from the ultimate degradation of digested food. Conceivably, the venom must have been designed by nature to victimize primarily arthopods rather than humans. In these latter, V.v.'s histamine would contribute extensively to the painful reaction and local vasodilation which accompanies stinging.

c) Serotonin (5-Hydroxytryptamine, 5-HT)

Serotonin occurs widely in arthropod venoms (WELSH and BATTY, 1963). As expected, it has been found in venom sacs and in the whole stinging apparatus of a number of Vespidae (Table 2), although so far the amine has been identified in the native venom of *V. orientalis* only (EDERY et al., 1972). Furthermore, the venom glands of this latter variety as well as of *V. crabro* are the highest 5-HT containing glands among the Vespidae.

The values for some species shown in Table 2 should be considered only as acceptable approximations, as WELSH and BATTY (1963) have rightly cautioned regarding their own estimations against drawbacks which might interfere with precise 5-HT determinations. These include incomplete extractions, presence of certain interfering indoles related to 5-HT, etc. Serotonin concentration in V.v. is higher by many orders of magnitude than in the whole body of Vespidae. Moreover, its occurrence is clearly related to the evolutionary stages of the insect. It is lacking or present in barely detectable amounts only in larvae, prepupae, and pupae, whereas high concentrations are found in imagines (WELSH and BATTY, 1963; ISHAY et al., 1974a). There is a total lack of knowledge concerning the synthesis and metabolism of 5-HT in the venomous apparatus of Vespidae. Likewise, the precise role of 5-HT in the venom has not been clarified. WELSH and BATTY (1963) postulated that the amine would promote intracellular penetration of the venom by increasing cell permeability. On the other hand, it has been repeatedly postulated that 5-HT, being a potent algogen (KEELE and ARMSTRONG, 1964), would greatly contribute to the overall painful response elicited by V.v. in man. In this regard, it should be remembered that 5-HT potentiates the algogenic effect of other pain-producing substances (SICUTERI et al., 1966), including those occurring in V.v.

d) Dopamine, Noradrenaline, and Adrenaline

Catecholamines are the latest components found in V.v. (OWEN, 1971; EDERY et al., 1972; GELLER et al., 1976).

Dopamine concentration is the highest when compared with those of other catecholamines examined. On the other hand, the values for dopamine, as well as for noradrenaline and adrenaline, varied rather unevenly among the different species (Table 1). GELLER et al. (1976) reported the absence of adrenaline in the three species they examined, and their values for dopamine and noradrenaline were about one-tenth of those reported by other workers in different species. Although wide species differences might occur, it seems also likely that low values and/or variability might derive from the partial decomposition of these amines during storage of the crude material. It should be recalled that catecholamines are susceptible to spontaneous oxidation. Moreover, when determining minute amounts of catecholamines, special consideration should be given to the adequacy of the methods employed (Welsh and King, 1974).

In view of the fact that dopamine accelerates heart rate of arthropods, thus increasing hemolymph circulation, Owen (1971) suggested that catecholamines would ensure a rapid spreading of the other toxic components of the venom when Vespidae sting their prey. Furthermore, Edery et al. (1972) postulated that catecholamines of V.v. could be responsible for the immediate "blanching effect" which follows Vespidae stinging on human skin; the ensuing local vasoconstriction and concomitant reduction of local blood flow would thus prevent the rapid destruction of the other venom's algogens by the host's enzymes. An additional effect of venom catecholamines could be the sensitization of pain receptors to these algogens (Armstrong and Keele, 1964).

Catecholamines occur also in body parts and fluids of larvae, prepupae, and pupae of many Vespidae varieties (Ishay et al., 1974a). However, there does not seem to be any obvious relationship between these catecholamines concentrations and those present in the venom of the corresponding variety. Interestingly enough, noradrenaline has recently been found in the nest walls of *V. vulgaris* and *Vespula (Paravespula) germanica* (Lecomte et al., 1976). It was assumed that the amine originated in the saliva, which the adult wasp mixed with cellulose during nest building.

e) Kinins

Jaques and Schachter (1954) first showed, in extracts of *Vespa vulgaris* venom apparatus, the presence of a smooth muscle-contracting principle which could be readily differentiated from other concurring spasmogens. It was later established (Schachter and Thain, 1954) that the material was peptidic in nature, and that it could be inactivated by trypsin and chymotrypsin as well as after boiling in acid or alkali. As the pharmacological properties of the new principle closely resemble those of bradykinin, it was termed "wasp kinin" or simply "kinin." Subsequent work, which included separation by chromatography and passage through an ion-exchange resin column, showed that the venom contains three different kinins, one of which could account for 90% of the total kinin activity (Bhoola et al., 1961). From the venom of *V. crabro,* the same authors isolated a kinin, which is different from the one found in *Vespula vulgaris,* is resistent to trypsin and is degradated by chymotrypsin. They also demonstrated the different chromatographic behavior of the kinins contained in both species.

Edery and Ishay (1965) reported the presence of a kinin in *V. orientalis* fresh venom which, like that of *V. crabro,* was unaffected by trypsin and was readily inactivated by chymotrypsin. Although no purification was pursued, they concluded that the *V. orientalis* — kinin(s) differed from mammalian kinins. They based their conclusion on the fact that neither rat isolated uterus (Fig. 19) nor guinea-pig isolated ileum preparations (Fig. 20) became sensitized after application of chymotrypsin to *V. orientalis* kinin. In contradistinction, it has been shown that proteolytic enzymes specifically sensitize these preparations to bradykinin or to very closely

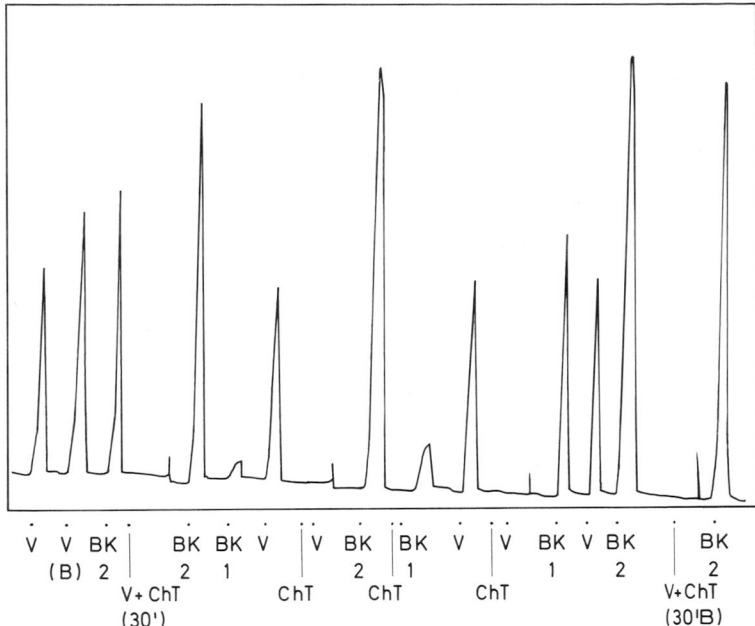

Fig. 19. Rat-isolated uterus suspended in 5 ml de Jalon solution containing 1 μg each of atropine, mepyramine, and brom-lysergic acid. Responses to kinin contained in 100 ng of *Vespa orientalis* venom: *V*, without any treatment; *V(B)*, after boiling for 5 min; *V + ChT(30′)* after incubation with 200 μg of chymotrypsin for 30 min., and *V + ChT(30′B)*, as in the latter but subsequently boiling for 5 min. Note that after the presence of *ChT* (either alone or incubated with *V*, but not boiled) the preparation became sensitized to bradykinin (*BK*, doses in ng), but not to *V. orientalis* kinin. Moreover, *ChT* did not potentiate the response to *V. orientalis* kinin but abolished it (EDERY and ISHAY, 1965)

related peptides but not to a large number of other smooth muscle-contracting substances (EDERY, 1968; EDERY and GRUNFELD, 1969).

The chemical characterization of V.v. kinins was first attempted by PRADO et al. (1966). The starting material consisted of mixed venom sacs of three *Polistes* species, namely *P. exclamans, P. annularis,* and *P. fuscatus.* Purification of kinins was accomplished by using CM-cellulose chromatography and electrophoresis, and the activity was monitored on a rat isolated uterus. A peptide was obtained, which on ultimate amino-acid analysis yielded Arg2, Pro3, Phe2, and Ser.; its sequence is shown in Table 3, peptide 1. Later on, UDENFRIEND et al. (1967) extracted, from a similar mixture of *Polistes* sacs, an octadecapeptide (Table 3, peptide 2) which was named *"Polistes* kinin". The purification of this kinin included six major steps (PISANO, 1970). Venom sacs obtained from 6000 frozen Vespidae were first homogenized in trichloracetic acid, which was subsequently removed with diethylether. The solution was then applied to a CM-sephadex column, and elution was accomplished with ammonium formate. The product was fractioned afterwards on a sephadex G-10 column and finally passed through two successive analytical CM-sephadex columns. The structure was finally established by enzymatic cleavage

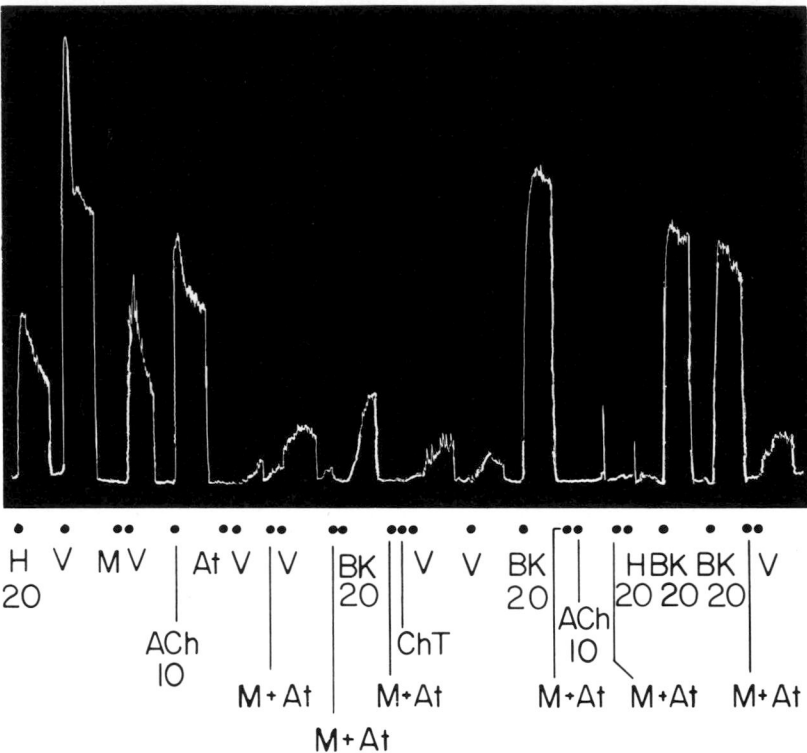

Fig. 20. *V. orientalis* venom effect on isolated guinea pig ileum. Abbreviations: Histamine (*H*), *V. orientalis* venom (*V*), acetylcholine (*ACh*), and bradykinin (*BK*). Numbers refer to µg per 5 ml bath volume (Tyrode solution). Doses of 40 µg of venom were applied the first three times, whereas 60 µg was introduced subsequently. Note that after the addition of mepyramine (M, 0.5 µg) and atropine (At, 0.5 µg), the venom caused a slow and sustained contraction. Chymotrypsin (ChT, 200 µg) did not sensitize the preparation to the venom as occurred in the case of bradykinin (EDERY et al., 1972)

and application of specific chemical reagents. STEWART (1968) first accomplished its synthesis by the solid-phase method.

Recently, WATANABE et al. (1975, 1976) succeeded in elucidating the structure of two different kinins isolated from the venom sacs and stings of 360 *Polistes rothneyi*. Their procedure included (1) homogenization of the crude material with methanol, the biological activity being determined on a rat-isolated uterus, using bradykinin as a standard, (2) double extraction with methanol, which was then evaporated under reduced pressure, (3) dissolving the dry residue in formic acid, (4) subjecting the solution to gel-permeation chromatography (SE and SG-10) sephadex columns and subsequent elution with ammonium formate; and (5), after degradation and amino acids analysis, the sequence of two peptides (Table 3, peptides 3 and 4) was established. They were termed *"Polistes* kinins—R," seemingly to incorporate the name of *Polistes* genera from which the peptides were isolated. Interestingly enough, peptide 4 (Thr-6 bradykinin) has a sequence similar to the widely occurring bradykinin, except that serine in position 6 has been

Table 3. Structure of peptide kinins isolated from Vespidae venom sacs
Number in small type indicates reference

Vespidae	Peptide Number	Structure	Amount (μg/one venom sac)
Polistes *annularis* *fuscatus* *pallipes* *exclamans*	1	Gly-Arg-Pro-Pro-Gly-Phe-Ser-Pro-Phe-Arg[a,1]	—
	2	Pyr-Thr-Asn-Lys-Lys-Lys-Leu-Arg-Gly-Arg-Pro-Pro-Gly-Phe-Ser-Pro-Phe-Arg[+,2,3]	1.5[b]
Polistes *rothneyi*	3	Ala-Arg-Arg-Pro-Pro-Gly-Phe-Thr-Pro-Phe-Arg[4,5]	0.13
	4	Arg-Pro-Pro-Gly-Phe-Thr-Pro-Phe-Arg[4,5] carbohyd carbohyd	0.70
Vespula (*Paravespula*) *maculifrons*	5	Thr-Ala-Thr-Thr-Arg-Arg-Arg-Gly-Arg-Pro-Pro-Gly-Phe-Ser-Pro-Phe-Arg[6] carbohyd carbohyd	—
	6	Thr-Thr-Arg-Arg-Arg-Gly-Arg-Pro-Pro-Gly-Phe-Ser-Pro-Phe-Arg[6]	—

[a] This kinin was isolated from mixed venom sacs of the three species.
[b] Amount refers to bradykinin equivalent (activity tested on isolated rat uterus).
(−) indicates no amount reported.

[1] PRADO et al. (1966); [2] UDENFRIEND et al. (1967); [3] PISANO (1970); [4] WATANABE et al. (1975); [5] WATANABE et al. (in press); [6] YOSHIDA et al. (1976)

replaced by threonine. Thr-6 bradykinin had been synthetized by SCHRODER and HEMPEL (1964) even before its occurrence in nature (glass activation of turtle plasma) was first reported (DUNN and PARKS, 1970).

Lately, an additional advance in the elucidation of Vespidae kinin structures has been accomplished. YOSHIDA and PISANO (1975) extracted venom sacs of 1300 *Vespula (Paravespula) maculifrons* (yellow jacket) with diluted acetic acid. The subsequent main steps were similar to those used in their previous work. Following passage through a SP-sephadex column, four active peaks were obtained, and the major one was purified by droplet countercurrent chromatography. After degradation, the sequence (Table 3, peptide 5) was determined by the dansyl—Edman procedure. Later, YOSHIDA et al. (1976) reported the structure of an additional, though shorter, peptide (Table 3, peptide 6). The newly isolated peptides have been called "*Vespula* kinins" 1 and 2, respectively and represent the first vasoactive carbohydrate-containing peptides isolated. The nature of the carbohydrates attached to threonine in position 3 has not been established with certainty, though most likely with the methods employed, hexosamines, hexoses, and pentoses could have been identified. By way of elimination, it was suggested that the carbohydrate could be N-galactosamine.

It is interesting to note that the structurally defined and active kinins of V.v., except peptide 4, possess in their sequence an amino acid chain incorporated with the N-terminal of the nonapeptide bradykinin (Arg-Pro-Pro-Gly-Phe-Ser-Pro-Phe-Arg). Contrastingly, in peptides isolated from amphibian skin (ERSPAMER and ANASTASI, 1966; ANASTASI et al., 1966; NAKAJIMA, 1968) the additional amino acid chain did not occur at the N-terminal of bradykinin but at the C-terminal. Further studies on the mechanism of kinin formation in Vespidae and in amphibians might eventually clarify the question as to whether there could be a phylogenetic relationship to explain the similarities and differences between these two kinds of kinins. One important question still to be answered concerns the formation of kinins in V.v. In mammals, structurally known kinins, such as kallidin, bradykinin, and met-lys-bradykinin, originate from cleavage by kininogenase of the precursor protein kininogen (EISEN and VOGT, 1970). It could be assumed that a similar mechanism might operate in V.v. However, such an assumption might not exactly be the case, as PRADO et al. (1966) reported the absence of kininogen and kininogenases both in venom and in protein extracts of the whole body of *Polistes*. These authors, however, did not mention the kind of kininogenases sought. This might be crucial, as Vespidae kininogenases, if at all present, might be of a different nature than the ones occurring in vertebrates. On the other hand, PRADO et al. (1966) emphasized the fact that they could isolate Gly-l-kallidin (Table 3, peptide 1) only after trypsin cleavage of a longer peptide found in large quantities in *Polistes* venom sacs. Thence, these authors conceived the hypothesis that at the first stage after stinging the large peptide would be introduced, and at the second, it could be split by enzyme(s) of the host, thus liberating the smaller Gly-l-kallidin. Undoubtedly, much work will be required, and new avenues must be explored in order to clarify the kinin origin in V.v. Conceivably, it will be necessary to develop microtechniques enabling one to follow the trail of these peptides until they reach the venom gland duct.

Presently, it is not known whether kinins contribute to the offensive action of V.v. on other arthropods. On the other hand, there is a concensus attributing a major role to kinins in eliciting the painful reaction which follows Vespidae stinging of humans. (See Sect. F, 11)

2. High-Molecular-Weight Substances: Enzymes

a) Cholinesterase

Cholinesterase activity (determined by Ellman's method, EDERY and KUHNBERG, unpublished experiments, 1970) has not been found in *V. orientalis* venom. This expected finding is consistent with the presence of a free acetylcholine-like material in this venom. Contrariwise, cholinesterase, which is present in *V. vulgaris* venom (JAQUES, 1955) may explain the lack of free acetylcholine in it. Studies of the cholinesterase-acetylcholine system extended to a larger variety of families would possibly explain whether there is any taxonomic relationship between the particular presence or absence of either material.

b) Histidine Decarboxylase

Recently, GELLER et al. (1976) found that the venom gland of *Vespula (Dolichovespula) maculata* and of *V. (Paravespula) maculifrons* possesses the capacity of synthetizing histamine through histidine-decarboxylase. The enzyme activity is about six-fold higher in fresh glands than in those stored at $-10°$ C for several weeks. The enzyme of both Vespidae species resembles the specific type found in mammalians, as it is almost totally inhibited by α-methylhistidine, a selective inhibitor of specific mammalian histidine decarboxylase. GELLER et al. (1976) postulated a double role for the venom gland enzyme: firstly, it could be responsible for the high histamine content in the venom and secondly, it could, after stinging, synthetize the amine further from the histidine of the host's tissues.

c) Phospholipases

Phospholipases have been found in the venom of *V. (Paravespula) vulgaris* (CONTARDI and LATZER, 1928), *V. crabro* (HABERMANN, 1968), and *V. orientalis* (ROSENBERG et al., 1976). In the latter, at the optimal pH of 5 the relative activities of native venom and extracts of the venom sac, acid gland, and alkaline gland were as follows: 1.0, 0.13, 0.04, and 0.03 obtained when estimated by the release of FFA from egg-yolk phospholipids. On the other hand, when activity was determined by using pure lecithine, the latter was hydrolyzed at pH 7.95 at a significantly higher rate. It is interesting to note that the alkaline gland, which has been hitherto regarded as not contributing to the enzymatic contents of V.v., has now been found to possess phospholipase and lysophospholipase activities comparable to those of the acid gland.

Many pharmacological effects induced by phospholipase A, mostly purified from snake or bee venom, have been described (HABERMANN, 1972). These effects include *in vitro* and *in vivo* hemolysis, liberation of biologically active substances (serotonin, histamine, and heparin) from rat mast cells, contraction of guinea pig-isolated ileum, lowering of blood pressure, etc. The actual amounts of phospholipase A and B present in V.v. are not known, and activity should probably vary in different batches; therefore, it is difficult to establish with certainty the share of these enzymes in the overall venom effects. Nevertheless, one can envisage at least a contributory role in the disruption of neuromuscular transmission and most likely in the general toxic effects elicited by V.v. when systemically administered (EDERY et al., 1972; ISHAY et al., 1973).

d) Acid, Alkaline, and Natural DNAses

SLOR et al. (1976) were able to demonstrate the presence of several deoxyribonucleases in the venom sac extract of *V. orientalis*. An increase in total nucleic acids in cat serum was obtained after s.c. injection of $7-8$ mg/kg of venom sac extract of *V. orientalis* or after in vitro incubation at a concentration of 2 mg/ml. After partial purification in sephadex columns, the DNAses were tested on native-stranded and U.V.-irradiated DNA and showed both endo- and exonuclease activity.

e) Hyaluronidase

JAQUES (1955) first reported the presence of hyaluronidase activity in *V. (Paravespula) vulgaris*.

The native venom, as well as venom sac extracts of *V. orientalis,* were found capable of depolymerizing hyaluronic acid (Edery et al., 1972) and to a lesser extent also chondroitin sulphate (Allalouf et al., 1972). In this respect, Oriental hornet hyaluronidase resembles the one present in mammalian testicles. Allalouf et al. (1975) reported that the optimum pH was 4.5 — 5.0, and that the enzyme was rather thermostable as, in contrast to mammalian hyaluronidase, preheating at 50° C for 3 h did not affect activity.

Concerning the role of hyaluronidase in V.v., as well as in other stinging arthropods, it has been considered responsible for ensuring the spread of venom through depolymerization of the ground substance mucopolysaccharides in and around the stinging site.

f) Protease

In contrast to hyaluronidase, proteases have not been widely searched for in V.v. Said (1960) reported that *Polistes omissa* venom did not split gelatin, fibrin, nor a variety of peptides used as substrates. On the other hand, protease activity has been detected in *V. orientalis* venom (Edery et al., 1972), though the enzyme(s) have not been fully characterized. In the venom sac extract, Joshua and Ishay (1975) found fibrinolytic activity which could be inhibited by soya bean trypsin inhibitor as well as by human serum. It might be assumed that venom protease should be capable of splitting a wide range of substrates, considering the offensive role of the venom to the victim's proteinic tissues.

g) Poly- and Disaccharidases

Fischl et al. (1972) have examined the activity of poly- and disaccharidases in various body fluids and tissues of *Vespa orientalis*. The authors were able to demonstrate the presence of trehalase, saccharase, maltase, and isomaltase in extracts of venom sac. As trehalase was by far the most active of the saccharidases, the authors postulated that Vespidae might use trehalase to predigest trehalose, which is usually the dominant carbohydrate in their prey. Lactase and cellobiase were conspicuously absent from the venom, in contrast to other body fluids and tissues.

3. Miscellaneous Substances

The presence of a number of V.v. components, such as pipecolic acid in *V. germanica* (Michl, 1957), aliesterase in *P. omissa* (Said, 1960), carbohydrates in *V. crabro* and *Polistes* sp. (Abrahams, 1955) has been reported, though the significance of the occurrence of these materials is so far unknown. For the occurrence of alarm substances, see Sect. B, 7.

E. Toxicology

In spite of the multiple stinging accidents which include a number of fatalities, very few systematic toxicological studies on Vespidae venoms have been undertaken.

The available data mostly refer to extracts of venom glands and in few cases only to the material ejected through the sting, i.e. the native venom proper. Though it seems reasonable to assume that there is a general resemblance between the biological activity, including toxicity, of venom gland extracts and the native secretion, it should be remembered that the composition, mainly proteinic contents, of gland extracts and venom might differ (DIRKS, 1971; FISCHL et al., 1972).

Moreover, the composition of V.v. and thence its toxicity may vary with the age of Vespidae and the diet which they were fed. These factors added to other batch-to-batch differences with no obvious explanation (unpublished observation) might account for variations observed while testing toxicity of V.v.

I. Systemic Toxicity of V.v.

In albino mice, after an i.v. injection of *Vespa orientalis* venom, either pure material or saline solution of sac extract (EDERY et al., 1972), the following symptoms, according to sequence were observed: dyspnea, paresis, akinesis, diarrhea, hematuria, stupor, loss of righting reflexes, and death. The component(s) responsible for the toxicity could not be determined with certainty. Nevertheless, the fact that a relatively long latent period (up to two hours) had to pass until the appearance of the symptoms would indicate that these did not derive from a direct interaction of low-molecular-weight components with particular cell receptors. Toxic effects were most likely due to generalized tissue damage elicited by proteases and phospholipases present in the venom. This view is supported by the post-mortem changes observed (see "Pathological findings"). The LD_{50} (i.v. albino mice) of pure lyophilized venom was 2.5 mg/kg, whereas that of sac extract was 70 mg/kg (ISHAY et al., 1971 b). In anesthetized dogs, i.v. administration of up to 12 mg/kg of sac extract caused profound respiratory and hemodynamic changes. Circulatory failure, shock, and death were noted after a dose of 20 mg/kg (KAPLINSKY et al., 1974).

Extract of venom sacs of *Paravespula germanica* injected i.v. into mice and chicks caused toxic symptoms similar to those by *V. orientalis*. The LD_{50} for mice resulted in 117.5 mg/kg (dry material), while chicks showed particular sensitivity, as a dose of 7 mg/kg was lethal for all the animals injected (ISHAY et al., 1973). The toxicity of the extract was probably due to its proteinic contents, because after dialysis, only the material retained inside the dialysis sac produced the same effects as the whole extract, whereas the dialysate was ineffective. The extract lost activity after boiling for 5 min, thus further indicating that the responsible material was proteinic in nature, probably enzyme(s) which became inactivated by heat.

GELLER et al. (1976) reported that seven out of 10 anesthetized rats died one hour after i.v. injection of saline extract of one venom sac of *Vespula (Dolichovespula) maculata* (hornet) or *V. (Paravespula) maculifrons* (yellow jacket). Death was preceded by a long period of bradycardia and concomitant loss of blood pressure. The former effect could be prevented by pretreating the animals with atropine, and both extracts lost their vasodepressor activity after incubation with pronase for 24 h. Furthermore, after dialysis the *V. (Paravespula) maculifrons* sac extract was inactive as far as lethality was concerned, though it still caused a fall in blood pressure after i.v. injection into rats. The toxic factor(s) present in both kinds of wasp venom sacs were not fully characterized, though the authors assumed that death resulted from a combined action of dialyzable and nondialyzable components.

JAQUES (1969) found that following the i.v. injection into guinea pigs of an extract of mixed venom from the glands of *V. vulgaris* and *Pseudovespa austriaca* (most probably *Paravespula austriaca*), death took place in all animals administered, within a few minutes. The toxic symptoms closely resembled anaphylactic or histamine shock and the estimated lethal dose was in the order of 6 mg/kg. Pretreatment of the animals with benzyl glucofuranoside (Glyvenol) by oral (100 – 1000 mg/kg) or intraperitoneal (30 – 1000 mg/kg) route conferred a dose-dependent protection against an otherwise lethal dose of the venom gland extract. Interestingly enough, the protective effect of benzyl glucofuranoside was also observed when the drug was injected a few hours before the challenge. Moreover, hydrocortisone 30 – 100 mg/kg also substantially reduced the mortality whereas two non-steroidal anti-inflammatory drugs such as aspirin and aminopyrine were practically ineffective. Benzyl glucofuranoside prevented the contraction of guinea-pig isolated ileum elicited by *V. vulgaris* venom sac extract as well as by histamine and 5-hydroxytryptamine. Thence, the protective action in the whole animal has been ascribed to antagonism of the amines present in the venom as well as to the general anti-toxic properties of benzyl glucofuranoside.

II. Toxicity of V.v. as Related to Ontogenesis

For various populations of the hornet *V. orientalis* collected from different nests in the field, the toxicity of the venom sac extract (VSE), determined by LD_{50} i.v. in albino mice, was not uniform (ISHAY et al., 1976). The toxicity levels of VSE obtained from the oriental hornet (*V. orientalis*) and the wasp *P. germanica*

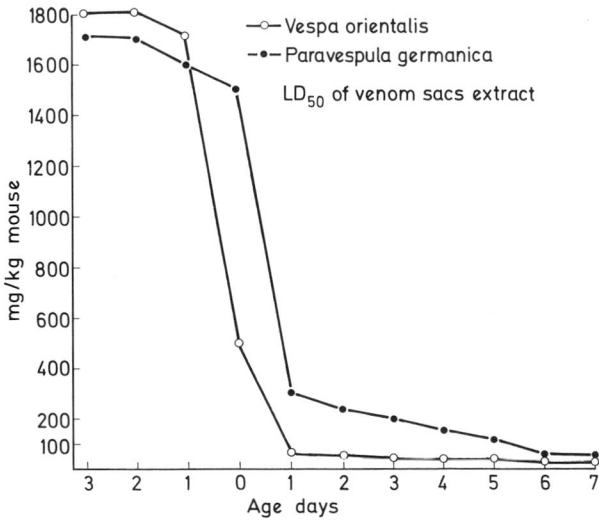

Fig. 21. Toxicity of *V. orientalis* and *Paravespula germanica* venom sacs extract related to ontogenesis. Note that the extract became toxic during and after eclosion (ISHAY et al., in press)

at different ages are presented in Figure 21. It should be noted that the hornets and wasps from which the VSE were obtained were in all cases from the same colony. As can be seen from the Figure 21, the VSE toxicity for *V. orientalis* at ages -3, -2, and -1 ($-$days before eclosion) was very low, and in fact administration of such VSE to mice was barely apparent as was injection of hemolymph from hornets or wasps of these ages. However, between age -1 and age 0, there was a significant rise in the toxicity of VSE ($p < 0.0005$), and an additional, equally significant rise between age 0 and age 1. Subsequently, there was a gradual but nonsignificant increase in toxicity up to age 7 (last age tested). Results for *P. germanica* were similar. The LD_{50} of queen VSE was invariably lower by about $30-50\%$ than that of worker VSE, but the development of the toxicity followed a similar course. The toxicity was also dependent on the diet; for instance, when hornets were fed sugar solution only, their VSE was less toxic than that of hornets also receiving protein. Toxicity tests of extracts of separated heads, thoraxes, and abdomens (minus venom sacs) dissected from adult hornets of different ages did not produce any toxic reactions ($LD_{50} > 2000$ mg/kg).

III. Pathological Findings

Macroscopic examination of mice which succumbed to a lethal dose of *V. orientalis* venom showed congestion of the lungs, with massive accumulation of fluid in the respiratory tract and congested intestines with fluid-filled lumen (EDERY et al., 1972). Light-microscopy revealed irregular vacuolization in the cytoplasm of epithelial cells in kidney proximal tubuli. In electronmicrographs of these cells, irregular pleomorphic membrane-bound dense bodies were seen. Some of these bodies showed lamellar structure, whereas others contained a compact osmophilic material. Interestingly enough, neither toxic signs nor pathological changes appeared in mice simultaneously administered with otherwise lethal doses of the venom and its antiserum (SANDBANK et al., 1973).

After injection of *V. orientalis* venom into the lower lip of a guinea pig, a mild edema developed. This was accompanied by an inflammatory exudate containing mainly polymorphonuclear leucocytes. Electronmicroscopy showed changes in the mitochondria of striated muscle, particularly at the neuromuscular junction. The cristae appeared as collapsed and agglutinating in the middle or adhering to the inner membrane of the mitochondrion. Severe damage was also observed following *in vitro* exposure of frog sartorius muscle to *V. orientalis* venom for $10-15$ min. Changes included appearance of small vacuoles randomly dispersed in the cytoplasm of muscle fibers and disappearance of myofilaments. Electronmicroscopic examination revealed enlargement of T-tubules and terminal cisterns, thus giving a disrupted appearance to the whole myofilament system (SANDBANK et al., 1971).

F. Pharmacology

A variety of pharmacological effects after administration of V.v. into experimental animals or after application to isolated biological systems have been described.

Table 4. Pharmacological effects of vespidae venoms on vertebrates
Number in small type indicates reference.

Venom[a]	Effect	Species
	Cardiovascular apparatus	
Vespula (Dolichovespula) maculata; *Vespula (Paravespula) maculifrons;* *Vespa (Paravespula) vulgaris;* *Paravespula germanica; Vespa orientalis*	Hypotension	Rat[1], rabbit[2], cat[3,16], dog[2]
Vespa crabro; Polistes sp.; *Vespa orientalis*	Hemolysis	Man[10,20], (guinea pig, cat, rabbit, rat, mouse)[20,21]
Vespa orientalis	Anticoagulation	(Man, dog)[20]
Vespa orientalis*	Hyperglycemia	Cat[12]
Vespa orientalis*	Increase in permeability of microcirculation vessels	Rat[3], rabbit[3], mouse
	Respiratory apparatus	
Vespa orientalis*	Bronchoconstriction, tachypnea, respiratory arrest	Guinea pig[3], dog[4], cat[17]
	Striated muscle	
Paravespula germanica; Vespa orientalis*	Paralysis	Cat[3], mouse[16], rat[18]
	Vision system	
Polistes sp.*; *Vespa crabro; Paravespula germanica*	Ocular irritation	Rabbit[10,13]
	Isolated organs preparations[b]	
Paravespula germanica	Uterus	Rat[16]
Polistes gallicus	Intestine (segment not specified) "C"	(Rabbit, guinea pig)[5]
Vespula (Paravespula) vulgaris; Paravespula germanica; Vespa crabro*; *Vespa orientalis**	Ileum "C"	Guinea pig[2,3,7,16]
Vespa crabro*	Intestine (segment not specified) "C"	Mouse[8]
Vespa crabro	Melanophores "C"	Carassius carassius[9]
Vespa crabro; Vespa orientalis*	Rectus abdominis "C"	Frog[7,3]
Polistes sp.*	Heart, inotropic positive and negative	Frog[10]
Vespula (Dolichovespula) arenaria	Gigant axon conduction unaffected	Squid[15]
Vespa orientalis	Spinal rootlets	Cat[3]
Vespula pennsylvanica; Vespula (Paravespula) vulgaris; Vespula (Paravespula) maculifrons; Paravespula germanica; Vespa orientalis; Vespula squamosa	Release of histamine	Cat (skin)[6,] rat (mast cells)[1,3,16,] man (white cells)[1,22,23]
	Nervous system	
Vespa orientalis	Disruption of brain-electrical activity	Cat[14,17]

Table 4 (continued)

Venom[a]	Effect	Species
	Miscellaneous	
Polistes fadwigae	Breakage of egg-cortical granules	Sea urchin [11]
Vespa orientalis	Suppression of metamorphose	Toad poles [19]

[a] Data refer to venom sac extracts though when marked with asterisk refers to native venom.
[b] "C" indicates contraction.

[1] GELLER et al. (1976); [2] SCHACHTER and THAIN (1954); [3] EDERY et al. (1972); [4] KAPLINSKY et al. (1974); [5] PAVAN (1955); [6] JAQUES and SCHACHTER (1954); [7] BHOOLA et al. (1961); [8] ALBL (1956); [9] PORA et al. (1949); [10] ABRAHAMS (1955); [11] SUGIYAMA (1953); [12] ISHAY (1975); [13] LECLERCQ et al. (1949); [14] ISHAY et al. (1974b); [15] ROSENBERG (1965); [16] ISHAY et al. (1973); [17] LASS et al. (1971); [18] ISHAY et al. (1971a); [19] BARR-NEA and ISHAY (1975); [20] JOSHUA et al. (1971); [21] JOSHUA and ISHAY (1973); [22] SOBOTKA et al. (1974); [23] KERN et al. (1976)

In most of these studies, the investigative material was not native venom, probably due to supply difficulties, but lyophilized venom gland extracts. This fact should be kept in mind when attempting to compare different V.v. activities.

The pharmacological actions of V.v. are presented in Table 4. Many of these actions could be straighforwardly deducted from the existing pharmacological knowledge of the individual components. Their contributing role has already been discussed in Section D. The main overall effects of the whole V.v. will now be considered.

I. Cardiovascular Apparatus

1. Blood Pressure

V.v. cause an immediate blood pressure fall when injected intravenously into various animal species. The minimal effective dose of dried venom sac extracts ranged from 5 to 15 µg/kg. The hypotensive effect can readily be understood if one considers the presence in the venom of histamine, acetylcholine, and kinin(s), each of which or all together could induce blood pressure fall. The extent and duration of the hypotensive response varied somewhat with the species, though in all cases the evidence strongly suggests that kinin(s) may be one of the main responsible components. The following instances seem to support this postulate. In the atropinized rabbit, after injection of *Vespa (Paravespula) vulgaris* venom, there was a long secondary hypotension which appeared when blood pressure was recovering from the initial short fall (SCHACHTER and THAIN, 1954). The cat seemed less sensitive to the same venom than the rabbit, and in both animals the hypotensive response did not occur when the venom was preheated in NaOH or incubated with either trypsin or chymotrypsin. The decrease of mean blood pressure concomitant to peripheral vasodilation observed in dogs after injection of *V. orientalis* venom could not be abolished by the prior administration of atropine, mepyramine, propranolol, or methysergide in doses which could readily block venom acetylcholine, histamine, catecholamines, and serotonin, respectively (KAPLINSKY et al., 1974). In the rat, after i.v. injection of saline extract of one single venom sac of *Vespula (Dolichovespula) maculata* or *Vespula (Paravespula) maculifrons,* there was a fatal blood pressure fall accompanied by bradycardia (GELLER et al., 1976). This latter phenomenon, as well as electrocardiographic changes, could be prevented by administration of atropine, but still hypotensive response persisted.

2. Hemolysis

Among the various pharmacological effects of vertebrate and insect venoms, those concerned with hemolysis have been the subject of numerous investigations. Most of the studies concern the hemolytic effect of bee venom (HABERMANN, 1958) as well as various snake venoms (ROY, 1945; HABERMANN and NEUMANN, 1954; GITTER et al., 1959; KLIBANSKY and DE VRIES, 1963; CONDREA et al., 1964). In all these venoms a dual hemolytic system was found, consisting of both direct and indirect hemolytic factors. The direct lytic activity was identified with basic protein(s) precipitable by heparin. The basic protein melittin present in bee venom was the most extensively studied (NEUMANN and HABERMANN, 1952; NEUMANN and HABERMANN, 1954). Melittin is a strong surface actant and a "structural" poison. It attacks the membrane integrity of washed erythrocytes and causes hemoglobin release. Indirect lytic activity is associated mostly with phospholipase A, which has no direct hydrolytic activity on the phospholipids of intact washed erythrocytes. The "indirect" hemolytic effect of phospholipase A operates through the generation of lyso-compounds from accessible phosphatides of extracorpuscular origin. Since phospholipase of lyzed cells serve also as substrate for phospholipase A, an autocatalytic character of this enzyme has also been presumed (HABERMANN, 1958). The presence of both direct and indirect factors results in a much stronger hemolytic effect, suggesting that the direct lytic factor, by changing the structure of the erythrocyte membrane, allows the simultaneous hydrolysis of its phospholipids by phospholipase A. The hemolytic effect of whole venom on washed erythrocytes reflects therefore the combined activity of both factors, although that of the direct one remains the initiating and the dominant, while the increment of hemolysis obtained upon addition of external phospholipids discriminates the indirect hemolytic activity.

The hemolytic properties of Vespidae venoms have been relatively little studied until recently, due to difficulties in obtaining sufficient amounts. ABRAHAMS (1955) studied the hemolytic activity of the native venom of *V. crabro* as well as of the picric acid precipitates of *V. vulgaris* and *Polistes* sp. venoms. Using human washed erythrocytes suspended in buffered saline, he demonstrated the presence of direct hemolytic activity in the venoms which was weakened after heating at 100° C for 15 min and almost lost if the venom was acidified with 1/10 N HCl before heating. The picric acid precipitate showed a 10 – 16 times stronger hemolytic activity than the native venom and the latter 416 times stronger than the venom sac extract.

A more detailed investigation of the *in vitro* hemolytic properties of the *V. orientalis* venom has been reported by JOSHUA et al. (1971) and JOSHUA and ISHAY (1973). Using whole venom, they obtained direct lysis of human, guinea pig, cat,

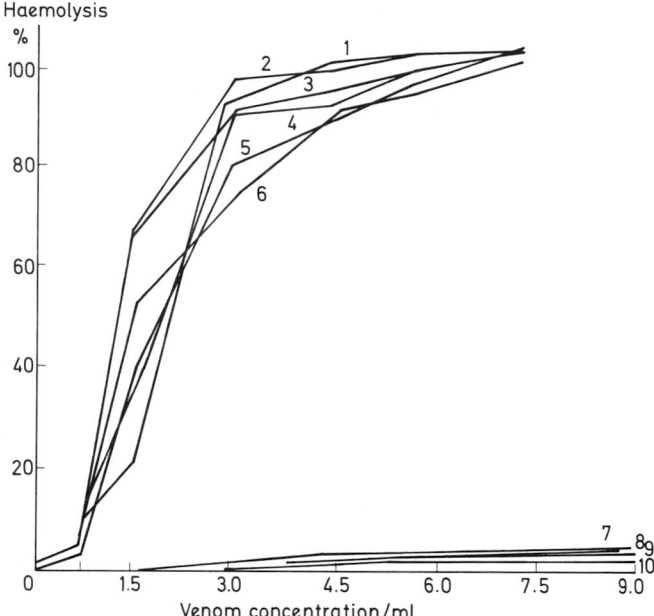

Fig. 22. Effect of *Vespa orientalis* venom concentration on the degree of hemolysis of various erythrocytes. 10% erythrocytes suspension, 120 min incubation at 37° C. Types of erythrocytes used: *1*, human; *2*, guinea pig; *3*, rat; *4*, mouse; *5*, rabbit; *6*, cat; *7*, ox; *8*, sheep; *9*, horse; *10*, camel (JOSHUA and ISHAY, 1973)

rabbit, rat, and mouse erythrocytes, whereas erythrocytes of sheep, horses, oxen, and camels resisted hemolysis (Fig. 22). The differences in species susceptibility towards wasp venom-induced hemolysis are strikingly similar to those found with some lytic snake venoms (CONDREA et al., 1964). The direct hemolysis of erythrocytes from susceptible species started at a venom concentration of 0.75 – 1.5 µg/ml and was almost completed at concentrations ranging from 3 to 6 µg/ml. Incubation of human erythrocytes with whole venom in the presence of egg yolk phospholipids resulted in a considerable increase in the hemolysis, both in terms of percent

Table 5. Lytic effect of *V. orientalis* venom on human RBC in the presence and in the absence of egg yolk phospholipids

Venom concentration (µg/ml)	Hemolysis (%)		Time of complete hemolysis (in min)	
	Without PL	With PL	Without PL	With PL
0.75	50	90	208	143
1.50	88	100	145	102
3.00	100	100	58	31
6.00	100	100	25	13

The mixtures consisted of 0.5 ml of a 5% erythrocyte suspension, 0.1 ml venom, and 0.1 ml 0.5% egg yolk phospholipids emulsion, or 0.1 ml saline, respectively. All figures represent mean values of six consecutive determinations (JOSHUA and ISHAY, 1973)

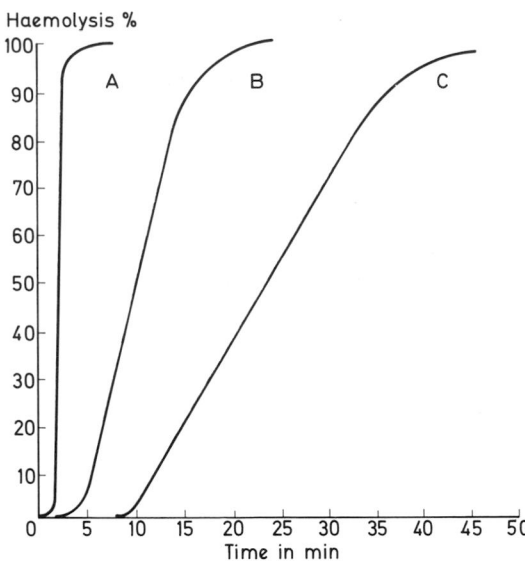

Fig. 23. Time kinetics of the hemolysis of washed human erythrocytes treated with different concentrations of whole *V. orientalis* venom. *A*, 6 µg/ml; *B*, 3.0 µg/ml; *C*, 1.5 µg/ml (Joshua and Ishay, 1973)

hemolysis for a fixed period of incubation and in terms of incubation time elapsed until a 100% hemolysis of the test system occurred (Table 5). Erythrocytes of guinea pigs, rabbits, rats, and mice behaved in a similar manner. Incubation of the hemolytic systems at 4° C yielded only a negligible degree of hemolysis (2% of the value recorded at 37° C). The degree of hemolysis was optimal at pH 7.0—7.4 and decreased at acidic pH. Time kinetics of the hemolysis caused by whole venom were studied by recording optical density fall of an erythrocyte suspension at 620 mu, measurements being carried out at 37° C. Figure 23 illustrates the curves obtained by plotting percent hemolysis versus incubation time. They are sigmoid shaped with the steepness of the slope depending on the venom concentration. A lag period preceded the initial stage of hemolysis, whose duration was inversely proportional to the venom concentration. In all the concentrations studied, the hemolysis slowed down after reaching a value of 90 to 95%. An explanation for the sigmoid-shaped curve may be that the hemolytic system consists in fact of several factors of different kinetic characteristics. Preincubation of washed erythrocytes with a sublytic concentration of whole venom (0.5 µg/ml) at 37° C resulted in potassium leakage from erythrocytes of susceptible species only (Fig. 24). Osmotic fragility of human erythrocytes after 30 min incubation with a sublytic venom concentration was markedly increased, starting at 0.7% and ending at 0.3% NaCl solutions, the osmotic hemolysis range of control erythrocyte suspension being 0.45—0.3% NaCl. A similar effect on washed erythrocytes has been shown with melittin (Habermann, 1971) and in the case of *V. orientalis* venom is due to its direct lytic factor. Prolonged dialysis of whole venom does not remove its direct lytic activity. However, heating the whole venom for 2 to 10 min in a boiling water bath at pH 6.0 or 8.0 causes the complete disappearance of the direct

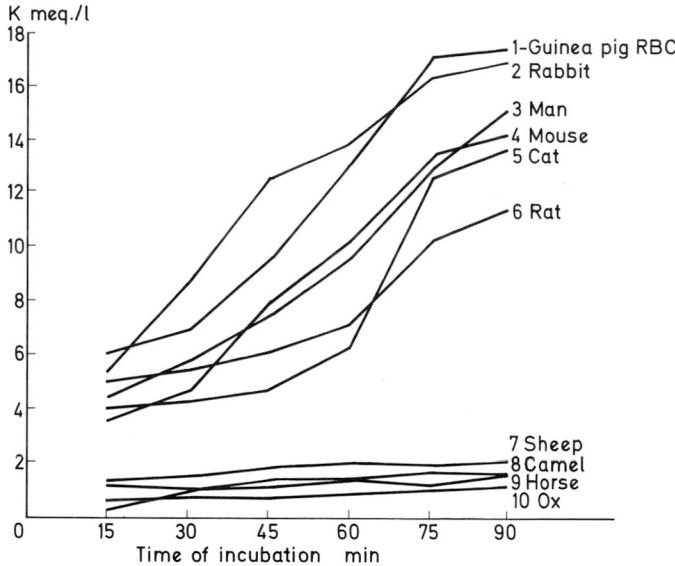

Fig. 24. Potassium leakage from erythrocytes of different species incubated with a sublytic dose (0.5 µg/ml) of *Vespa orientalis* venom (JOSHUA and ISHAY, 1973)

lytic activity of washed human RBC and of most of its indirect one. Loss of the latter could be minimized if the venom was boiled at pH 3.5. Boiling at acid pH is therefore helpful in discriminating between the direct lytic activity, which is completely lost, and the indirect one which, like phospholipase A, is preserved to a considerable extent. Addition of heparin to whole venom produces a fine precipitate, which can be separated by centrifugation for 30 min at 3.000 r.p.m. The supernatant of heparin-treated venom is completely devoid of direct lytic activity, yet it retains its ability to lyze washed erythrocytes upon addition of egg-yolk phospholipids. Dissociation of the heparin precipitate in veronal buffer containing an excess of heparin, releases a measurable direct lytic activity, mildly potentiated by the addition of egg yolk phospholipids. This effect may be due to traces of phospholipase or to complex formation of phospholipase with the direct lytic factor on the basis of ion exchange. Adsorption of the direct lytic activity of whole venom on Amberlite GC 50/200 mesh was achieved by shaking 1 ml of venom solution with 250 mg of resin powder previously equilibrated with a 0.05 M sodium citrate/citric acid buffer pH 6.0, thus confirming its basic nature. Amberlite-treated venom was also devoid of direct lytic activity, without losing the egg-yolk-prompting hemolytic activity. Heating of the heparin precipitate in boiling water completely abolishes its direct lytic activity. Whole venom direct lytic activity can be exhausted by repeated adsorption with intact erythrocytes or osmotically prepared erythrocyte stroma. The direct lytic factor seems to be firmly attached to the erythrocyte membrane; it cannot be removed by simple washing with saline and retains its hemolytic properties toward freshly added erythrocytes. Whether this is due to additional free active groups of the direct lytic factor already attached to the ghosts or to its transfer from one erythrocyte

Table 6. Neutralization of the hemolytic effect of whole venom of *V. orientalis* by rabbit anti-wasp venom immune serum[a] (JOSHUA and ISHAY, 1973)

Venom	Concentration (μg/ml)						
	384	192	96	48	24	12	6
Hemolysis	+	+	+	+	−	−	−

[a] 0.1 ml of rabbit antiwasp venom immune serum.

+ hemolysis.
− absence of hemolysis.

to another remains a matter of conjecture. Furthermore, egg-yolk phospholipids mildly potentiate the lytic effect of ghosts subjected to venom hemolysis and subsequent washing on fresh erythrocytes. Therefore, one may conclude that minute amounts of indirect lytic factor (phospholipase) may have also remained attached to the ghosts. Antiserum prepared by immunizing rabbits with whole venom and Freund adjuvant neutralises *in vitro* the lytic activity of the venom on washed human erythrocytes (Table 6). No clear cut answer can be given as to the specificity of the antibody responsible for the *in vitro* neutralization of the hemolytic activity of whole venom by the rabbit immune serum. However, since hemolysis in this system is always initiated by the direct lytic factor one may presume that antibodies against it are present in the immune serum. Most of the immunization experiments with animal venoms have mainly been concerned with the production of phospholipase antibodies (CINADER, 1957; HABERMANN, 1968), while melittin has proved to be a poor antigen. In the case of *V. orientalis* venom, however, the direct lytic factor, being nondialysable, is presumably a large molecule with better antigenic properties. FISCHL et al. (1972) separated three fractions from the native venom of *V. orientalis* using electrophoresis with cathodic migration, presumably basic proteins, nondialysable and endowed with hemolytic activity. The authors did not investigate the indirect hemolytic properties of these fractions. Electrophoresis of venom sac extracts of the oriental hornet also displayed three cathodic fractions with hemolytic activity, two of which were identical in their migration with fractions found in the pure venom. They concluded that extraction of venom from whole sacs not only introduces proteins originating in the gland tissue but also causes modification of some of the venom components either by adsorption or forming a complex with venom proteins. The fact that a basic polypeptide such as melittin can aggregate in micelles of various sizes has already been shown (FISCHER and NEUMANN, 1961). A similar phenomenon might account for the unhomogeneous separation on moving-boundaries electrophoresis and the presence of multiple chromatographic fractions with direct lytic activity in *V. orientalis* venom (JOSHUA and ISHAY, unpublished observation). The occurrence of three basic hemolytic proteins in the venom of the Oriental hornet was demonstrated also by immunoelectrophoresis against a rabbit antivenom immune serum (ISHAY et al., 1972). DIRKS (1971) also showed the presence of two low-molecular-weight basic proteins in the venom of *Polistes* sp. endowed with hemolytic properties. Variation in the hemolytic activity of Oriental hornet venom may also be due to developmental

Table 7. Direct and indirect hemolytic activity of *V. orientalis* venom sac extract obtained before, during, and following hatching (JOSHUA and ISHAY, 1976)

| Age (days) | Hemolysis (%) | | | | | |
| | Direct | | | Indirect | | |
	30′	90′	150′	30′	90′	150′
−2	—	—	—	—	—	—
−1	—	—	—	—	—	—
0	—	2	4	8	16	26
1	2	8	38	22	44	70
2	25	39	76	74	86	95
3	40	82	96	100	100	100
4	52	100	100	100	100	100

The incubation mixture consisted of 0.5% suspension of washed human RBC and 5 μg/ml (final concentration) of *V. orientalis* venom sac extract incubated at 37° C for the times indicated. — indicates absence of hemolysis.

Table 8. Hemolytic activity of *V. orientalis* venom obtained by repeated milking of four queens (A–D) during 5 consecutive days (JOSHUA and ISHAY, 1976)

Activity is expressed by (1) time in min and (2) final dilution (number in parenthesis) to obtain complete hemolysis. The system consisted of a 5% suspension of washed human RBC incubated at 37° C. In (2) incubation time was kept constant at 120 min.

| Queen | Day | | | | |
	1	2	3	4	5
A	12(1:20,000)	21(1:15,000)	32(1:10,000)	35(1:5,000)	45(1:2,000)
B	8(1:40,000)	17(1:30,000)	22(1:15,000)	30(1:10,000)	39(1:8,000)
C	12(1:20,000)	12(1:20,000)	30(1:10,000)	33(1:8,000)	37(1:5,000)
D	10(1:30,000)	21(1:15,000)	28(1:10,000)	30(1:5,000)	46(1:2,500)

and physiological factors (JOSHUA and ISHAY, 1976). Studying extracts from venom sacs obtained before, during, and following, a hornet's hatching, it was found that extracts obtained prior to hatching (days −2 and −1) were completely devoid of both direct and indirect hemolytic activity. Traces of indirect lytic activity appeared on day 0 and of direct lytic activity on day 1. Thereafter, direct and indirect activities increased on subsequent days, reaching maximal values at days 3 and 4 (Table 7). Collecting *V. orientalis* venom repeatedly from the same Vespidae for several days resulted in the gradual reduction in the amount of venom ejected as well as in the gradual decrease of its hemolytic activity (Table 8).

Briefly, these experiments were performed as follows: To evaluate the amount of native venom which could be collected by repeated "milking," the hornet's thorax was held with forceps and induced to eject its venom by stinging the surface of a cellulose acetate membrane; this maneuver was repeated daily for several consecutive days; at the end of the experiment, the membrane was immersed in a solution of 3% sulfosalycilic acid containing 0.5% brilliant green and subse-

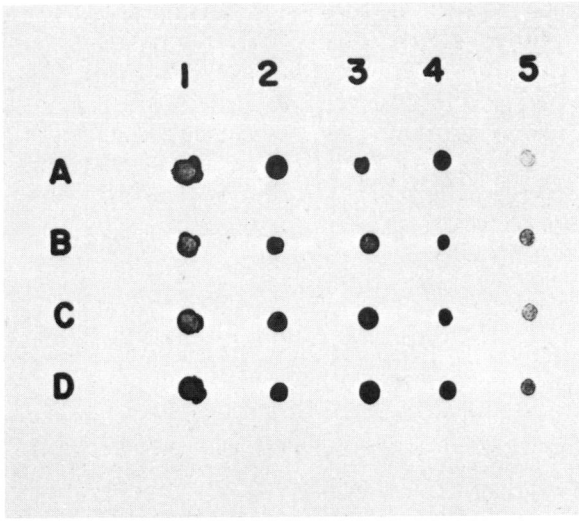

Fig. 25. Spots represent venom deposited after stinging on acetate cellulose membrane by four *V. orientalis* queens (*A–D*) during 5 consecutive days

quently decolorized with 2% acetic acid. Colored spots appeared in the areas of stinging, and the diameter as well as intensity of color was then noted. In this way a fair quantitative estimate of the venom ejected could be obtained (Fig. 25).

Adult hornets were divided into two groups, A and B. Group A was used to evaluate the amount of venom which could be obtained by repeated collection. Group B was used to titrate the hemolytic activity of the venom obtained on consecutive days. Evidence was also obtained for the synergistic participation of

Table 9. The effect of protease inhibitors on the hemolytic activity of *V. orientalis* venom (Joshua and Ishay, 1976)

Materials[a] added to hemolytic system[b]		Time (min) for 100% hemolysis	
		Direct	Indirect
1	Control	5	1
2	SBTI	33	2
3	TLCK	13	3
4	PMSF	19	3
5	N-p-TL	20	3
6	DFP	12	3

[a] 1. saline; 2. soybean trypsin inhibitor; 3. tosylamide-2-phenyl-ethyl-chloromethylketone; 4. phenyl-methyl-sulfanyl-fluoride; 5. N-p-tosyl-L-lysine; 6. diisopropyl fluorophosphate. Final concentration of the inhibitors was 5 μmol except in the case of SBTI which was 0.05%.
[b] The incubation mixture consisted of 0.5% suspension of washed human RBC and 10 μg/ml *V. orientalis* venom. Indirect lytic activity was determined by addition of 1/10 v/v of 0.5% egg-yolk phospholipid emulsion.

the venom proteases in the total hemolytic activity (JOSHUA and ISHAY, 1976), since addition of a variety of proteases inhibitors significantly reduced the degree of direct hemolysis but did not affect the indirect one (Table 9). After i.v. injection of small doses of *V. orientalis* venom into cats (ISHAY, 1975), no hemolysis occurred, though with higher doses hemoglobinemia as well as hemoglobinuria were observed in mice (JOSHUA and ISHAY, 1973). Moreover, in clinical fatal cases following multiple Vespidae stinging, hemolysis and hemoglobinuria were reported (HOH et al., 1966; TAN et al., 1966; CHUGH et al., 1976).

3. Anticoagulant Activity

A variety of animal venoms, mostly of snakes, have been shown to modify blood coagulation (HOUSSAY, 1930; ROSENFELD et al., 1968). Anticoagulant activity has been demonstrated in honey-bee venom (HABERMANN, 1968) as well as in the saliva of some blood-sucking insects (HELLMANN and HAWKINS, 1964). Recently, an extensive investigation has been reported (JOSHUA and ISHAY, 1975) concerning the *in vitro* and *in vivo* effect on blood coagulation of VSE of *V. orientalis*. The extract had no coagulating activity whatsoever on human plasma or human fibrinogen solution. On the contrary, after incubation with the VSE, prolonged recalcification and one-stage prothrombin times were recorded (Fig. 26). The addition of thrombin (10 units/ml) to plasma containing VSE did not reveal any antithrombic activity of the extract. However, incubation of tissue thromboplastin with increasing amounts of VSE or with a constant amount for varying periods of time demonstrated a clear-cut antithromboplastic activity (Fig. 27). An inhibitory activity of the extract on the formation of endogenous thromboplastin was also found. Thromboplastin inhibition was even more pronounced if isolated factors, especially serum,

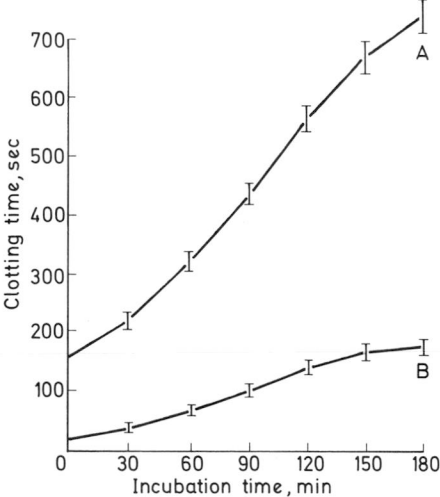

Fig. 26. The effect of various incubation times on the anticoagulant activity of a constant venom concentration (50 µg per ml) incubated with human plasma. *A*. Recalcification times (average of six determinations); *B*. Prothrombin times (average of six determinations) (JOSHUA and ISHAY, 1975)

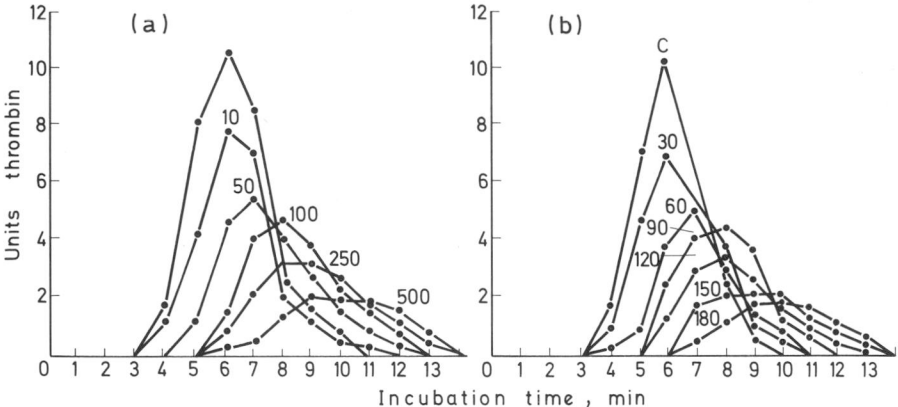

Fig. 27. Thrombin generation of human plasma in the presence of venom. *A*. plasma preincubated for 30 min with 10, 50, 100, 250, and 500 µg venom per ml; *B*. plasma preincubated with 10 µg venom per ml for 30, 60, 90, 120, 150, and 180 min.; *C*. control curves (Joshua and Ishay, 1975)

were preincubated with the extract before adding them to the reaction mixture. Thrombin generation *in vitro* was also inhibited, according to the concentration of the venom and the duration of exposure. Citrated human plasma retained its coagulability after 4 h incubation with 50 µg/ml VSE, whereas human fibrinogen solution at a concentration of 300 mg was rendered incoagulable after 90 min incubation with the same amount of venom. It took 3 hours for a thrombin-clotted fibrinogen-VSE mixture to dissolve completely, while human plasma under identical conditions exhibited a rather low fibrinolysis. Fibrinolysis of purified human fibrinogen could be abolished by the addition of either soybean trypsin inhibitor (100 µg/ml), 1/10 volume human serum, or $BaSO_4$-adsorbed plasma. The above-mentioned data indicate an anticoagulant effect of VSE manifested by inactivation of formed tissue thromboplastin as well as by inhibition of the formation of endogenous thromboplastin from its plasma precursors. Both rabbit-brain thromboplastin and a thromboplastin generation system, when mixed with VSE, promptly lose part of their thromboplastic activity. However, upon continuous incubation with VSE at 37° C, both tissue and blood thromboplastin deteriorate further, suggesting progressive degradation of their components or precursors. Of all possible thromboplastic factors, Factor X seems the most likely involved, since its inactivation would affect both thromboplastin generation and prothrombin activation (measured by the one-stage method), as indeed was observed.

Of the insect venoms, that of the honey-bee has been shown to exert antithromboplastic activity by virtue of its phospholipase A contents as well as by the presence of the basic peptide melittin (Habermann, 1968). Habermann postulated that melittin binds, by its basic groups, to the acidic ones of thromboplastin. Such a mechanism of inactivation may also possibly explain the immediate antithromboplastic effect of VSE, known to contain basic protein components (Joshua et al., 1973; Fischl et al., 1972). Furthermore, there is little doubt that a second mechanism of thromboplastic inactivation occurs. Since this effect is lost after boiling VSE at pH 4.0, it seems that phospholipase A, whose antithromboplastic properties have been shown by several authors (HECHT and SLOTTA, 1962; HABERMANN, 1968), is not the sole responsible factor. It remains therefore to be proven that this is neither due to the combined activities of phospholipase A and phospholipase B nor to the protease present in the venom. The latter enzyme most probably causes the fibrinolytic activity of the venom, since it is inhibited by soybean trypsin inhibitor or by serum known to contain an α-trypsin inhibitor but not by ε-aminocaproic acid.

The *in vivo* effect of VSE on blood coagulation was investigated by i.v. or i.p. administration of VSE (5 mg/kg) to each of two groups of six dogs anesthetized with nembutal (JOSHUA and ISHAY, 1975). Blood samples obtained from the femoral vein at different intervals were subjected to a battery of clotting tests. The i.v. injection of the extract caused a progressive prolongation of the clotting time of whole blood and of recalcified citrated plasma in all animals. This effect persisted for 90 to 120 min after envenomation, and subsequently the clotting times gradually shortened, almost equalling the initial base-line values. Recalcification times of the various plasma samples either with or without addition of protamine sulfate did not vary significantly. Throughout this period the one-stage prothrombin activity remained practically unchanged, although prothrombin consumption and thromboplastic generation were low. A definite but transient fall in the platelet count occurred after envenomation, reverting to the pre-experimental levels after $1^1/_2$ to 2 h. Plasma fibrinogen levels were not significantly reduced. All these findings point toward the inactivation of some thromboplastic factors elicited by the i.v. administered VSE. On the other hand, VSE after i.p. envenomation caused an almost unclottable state of the blood, lasting for $^1/_2$ h and followed by a marked prolongation of the clotting time, which gradually reverted to normal values after $2^1/_2$ h.

The abnormal clotting times of both whole blood and recalcified plasma reverted to normal upon addition of protamine sulfate. One may conclude, therefore, that a state of transient heparinemia induced by i.v. envenomation was most probably the result of peritoneal mast cell degranulation. Indeed *V. orientalis* venom has been shown to possess mast cell degranulating activity (EDERY et al., 1972). Plasma one-stage prothrombin activity was decreased during the period of uncoagulability. There was a transient fall of the platelet count, although milder than after i.v. administration, and plasma fibrinogen levels remained unchanged. The fact that clotting time of i.p. envenomized animals was normalized by addition of protamine sulfate suggests that the venom-induced heparinemia prevented the deterioration of thromboplastic factors observed in i.v. envenomized animals, possibly by binding the basic protein of the venom. *In vivo* anticoagulant activity associated with an antithromboplastic effect and induction of heparinemia has also been shown using *Naja flava* venom (MOHAMED and HANNA, 1973). The administration of protamine sulfate prior to envenomation reduced the heparinemia as well as the antithromboplastic activity. The thrombocytopenia following i.v. envenomation is most probably an anaphylactic manifestation. This type of thrombocytopenia is of short duration and can be antagonized by heparin administration (JOHANSSON et al., 1960). These observations are in agreement with the finding that thrombocytopenia is mild in i.p. envenomated dogs showing concomitant severe heparinemia but pronounced in i.v. envenomated dogs, which show no evidence of heparinemia.

4. Hyperglycemia

Ishay (1975) recently reported that *V. orientalis* venom could induce hyperglycemia in cats. The factor responsible was attributed to a protein or to a protein-bound substance, inasmuch as it was not removed by dialysis and was inactivated by heating the venom to 100° C.

5. Increase in Permeability of Microcirculation Vessels

The permeability-increasing effect of *V. orientalis* venom on skin microcirculation vessels was clearly evidenced after intradermal injection of 5—10 µg of venom into rats (Fig. 28) and rabbits administered with pontamine-sky blue (Edery et al., 1972). The blue spot left by the extravasated dye corresponded to areas of local increased permeability. When histamine and serotonin antagonists were injected together with the venom, a "blanching area," attributed to catecholamines, appeared. This area was interpreted as resulting from local vasoconstriction, and

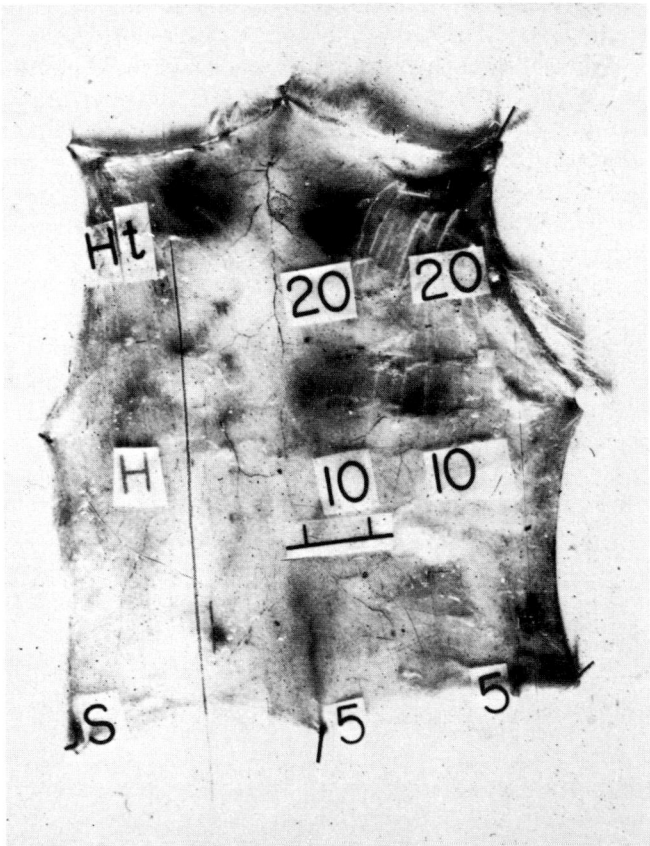

Fig. 28. Inner side of skin of a rat administered i.v. with pontamine sky blue and subsequently injected i.d. with *V. orientalis* venom (two columns on the right, numbers indicate µg); 5-hydroxytryptamine (Ht, 4 µg); histamine (H, 20 µg); and saline (S, 0.1 ml). Scale, 1 cm. Note that strength of coloring was related to the dose of venom (Edery et al., 1972)

it surrounded a smaller blue spot induced by the kinin(s). Although only the *V. orientalis* venom has been studied in some detail, it may be reasonably assumed that many other V.v. would induce increased permeability of skin's microcirculation vessels. On the other hand, it remains to be established which particular microvessels, whether capillaries, venuli, or arteriolae, would be the ones specifically affected by V.v.

6. Respiratory Apparatus

V. orientalis venom ($5-25$ µg/kg i.v.) elicited an immediate and profound bronchoconstriction in guinea pigs (EDERY et al., 1972). This effect was only partially antagonized after joint administration of atropine, mepyramine, and brom-lysergic acid which could block acetylcholine as well as biogenic amines of the venom. Conceivably, the remaining bronchoconstrictive activity was due to kinin(s). In dogs, the short-lasting tachypnea ensuing i.v. injection of *V. orientalis* venom (KAPLINSKY et al., 1974) could have been the result of primary bronchoconstriction. This latter was most probably initiated by acetylcholine present in the venom or through activation of a cholinergic mechanism, since atropinization or vagotomy suppressed the response. *V. orientalis* venom, at high doses ($150-600$ µg/kg) administered either intravenously or into a vertebral artery, caused respiratory arrest in cats (LASS et al., 1971). The effect was most likely due to disruption of the central respiratory functions, since the arrest coincided with suppression of phrenic nerve firing, though direct stimulation of the nerve elicited diaphragm contraction.

7. Striated Muscle

After injection of $200-500$ µg/kg of *V. orientalis* venom into an ipsilateral femoral artery, the directly and indirectly induced single twitches of cat leg muscles gradually diminished and eventually disappeared (Fig. 29). After administration of the highest dose, these effects were preceded by a transient muscle contracture. A protracted paralysis was also observed in mice (EDERY et al., 1972). The paralysis in cats seems to be derived from central as well as peripheral actions of the venom. The former could be due to an effect on spinal motoneurons as evidenced by

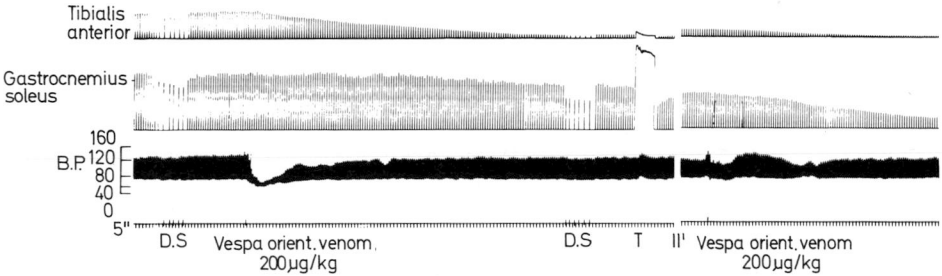

Fig. 29. Effect of *V. orientalis* venom on striated muscle and blood pressure of cat. Cat anesthetized with sodium pentobarbital. Record from top downwards: contractions of tibialis anterior: gastrocnemius-soleus; blood pressure and time (5 s). After intra-arterial injection of the venom, the amplitude of indirectly (unmarked) and directly (*D.S*) induced contractions gradually decreased, whereas ability to maintain tetanus (*T*) was preserved (EDERY et al., 1972)

suppression of semitendinous nerve potentials. The peripheral effect was manifested by neuromuscular transmission blockade and by reduction of directly induced twitches. Thence, it could be inferred that this latter phenomenon was due to muscle-fiber damage. The above-mentioned facts do not seem to support entirely the view of HABERMANN (1971). He stated that the action of hornet venom (species not stated, but most probably referring to *V. crabro*) "... on skeletal muscle is practically exclusively due to the acetylcholine present in it." Acetylcholine most probably could be held responsible for the transient contraction resulting in post-synaptic membrane depolarization, though understandably this effect could not last for long due to the hydrolytic action of cholinesterase. On the other hand, as muscular blockade elicited by the venom of *V. orientalis* was rather long lasting, it could well be possible that either venom proteases, phospholipases, or both could have injured the end-plate as well as the muscle fibers. Interestingly enough, *Paravespula germanica* venom blocked indirectly induced twitches of cat leg muscles, but unlike *V. orientalis* venom, it left the directly elicited ones unaffected (ISHAY et al., 1973).

V. mandarinia venom has been found to suppress e-p.s.p. in lobster nerve-muscle preparations (KAWAI, 1974).

8. Ocular Irritation

Topical application of various diluted V.v. on rabbit eyes caused mild conjunctival injection and increased ocular secretion. At high concentrations (1:2500) the sclera became congested, and there was also swelling of the third eyelid (ABRAHAMS, 1955). The application of saline extracts of stinging apparatus of *Polistes* sp. was about 50 times less damaging to the eye than that of the venom. It is difficult to establish which factor(s) are responsible for the effect on the eye. It does not seem to be histamine, as LECLERCQ et al. (1949) applied 10 times the amount present in *Vespula (Paravespula) germanica* venom to rabbit eyes, and, in contrast to the injury elicited by the latter, they observed no abnormalities.

9. Isolated Organ Preparations

V.v. cause contraction of a variety of isolated intestine preparations. The effective concentrations in the bathing fluid ranged from 3 to 8 µg/ml of dry venom sac extracts or native venom. The contracting effect could clearly be ascribed to the single or combined action of acetylcholine, histamine, serotonin, and kinin(s) present in the V.v. The relative contribution of these spasmogens has been readily detected by sequential application of specific blockers to appropriate isolated preparations (SCHACHTER and THAIN, 1954; EDERY et al., 1972). Figure 20 shows a typical experiment.

The frog rectus abdominis has been particularly useful in detecting acetylcholine-like activity in *V. crabro* (BHOOLA et al., 1961) and *V. orientalis* venoms (EDERY et al., 1972) as well as in ruling out its occurrence in *Polistes* sp. venom (ABRAHAMS, 1955). *Polistes* sp. venom, at a concentration of 1:10,000, increased the contraction amplitude of an isolated frog heart (ABRAHAMS, 1955). The inotropic effect lasted for several minutes and remained even after washing. Contrastingly, extracts of the stinging apparatus produce a negative inotropic effect which disappeared after washing or atropine application. The action of *V. crabro* venom on the frog heart differed essentially from that of *Polistes* sp., and it varied according to the dose (ABRAHAMS, 1955). In weak concentrations it produced an inotropic negative effect, whereas at high ones (1:500,000) it caused a diastolic standstill. Conceivably, these effects should be ascribed to the venom's acetylcholine, as it disappeared after repeated washing or after atropine application.

10. Release of Histamine

JAQUES and SCHACHTER (1954) first reported that *V. (Paravespula) vulgaris* venom occasionally released histamine when introduced into a cat's perfused skin. More consistent results have been obtained with other V.v. For instance, *V. orientalis* venom was as efficient as the potent compound 48/80 in liberating histamine from rat mast cells (EDERY et al., 1972). Likewise, 25−80% of the available histamine could be released when leucocytes obtained from a previously sensitized person were incubated with as little as 20 pg to 2 ng of *Vespula (Paravespula) maculifrons* venom sac extract (GELLER et al., 1976). The factors governing the histamine-liberating activity of V.v. cannot be established with certainty. There are some components, such as protease, phospholipase, and kinin(s), which separately or combined could be singled out, though the evidence so far available does not permit any definite conclusions. Nevertheless, when considering the particularly strong histamine-liberating activity of peptide 2 (see below), one is inclined to ascribe an important role to the kinin(s).

11. Pharmacology of Vespidae Kinins

Vespidae kinins are one of the most potent among the pharmacologically active low-molecular-weight components of V.v. Table 10 summarizes the pharmacological actions of Vespidae kinins. As a matter of fact, many of the effects elicited by V.v. were derived from their kinins. Qualitatively, some effects of Vespidae kinins, such as hypotension, contraction, or relaxation of a variety of smooth muscle-isolated preparations, increase microvessel permeability, and the distinctively important algogenesis in man overlap with those of bradykinin. Thence, in the majority of studies the Vespidae kinin activity has been examined in comparison with that of mammalian kinins. On the other hand, precise and meaningful comparisons on a molar basis have been mostly unfeasible, due to lack of pure Vespidae material. PISANO (1970) reported that *"Polistes kinin"* (Table 3, peptide 2) was 2 to 20 times more active than bradykinin in a variety of bioassays. The relative potency (considering bradykinin=1) was as follows: rat uterus, 2; rat duodenum, 2; guinea pig vascular permeability, 5; rat blood pressure by i.v. injection, 20; and pain production on human forearm (method of application not reported), 20.

Vespidae kinins, regardless of genus origin, produced a profound hypotensive response in mammalians. Contrastingly, *"Polistes* kinin" (Table 3, peptide 6) was reported to induce hypertension in chickens, though no explanation for such a conspicuous species difference has been suggested (PISANO, 1970). The effectiveness

Table 10. Pharmacological effects of Kinins derived from vespitae venoms
Number in small type indicates reference.

Kinin[a] Origin	Effect	Species
	Cardiovascular Apparatus	
Peptide 2, 5, 6; *Polistes gallicus;*		
Vespa (Paravespula) vulgaris;	Hypotension	Rat[1,2], dog[3,5],
Vespa crabro		rabbit[4], cat[6]
Peptide 2	Hypertension	Chicken[7]
Peptide 2; *Vespula (Paravespula)*	Increase in perme-	Guinea pig[1,5],
vulgaris	ability of microcir-	rabbit[5]
	culation vessels	
	Respiratory Apparatus	
Vespa orientalis	Bronchoconstriction	Guinea pig[9]
	Nervous System	
Peptide 2; *Vespa (Paravespula)*	Pain	Man[1,5]
vulgaris		
	Smooth muscle isolated	
	preparations[b]	
Peptide 2, 3, 4, 5, 6; *Vespa crabro;*		
Vespa orientalis	Uterus "C"	Cat[1,2,4,8,9,12]
Polistes gallicus	Stomach "C"	Frog[3]
Peptide 2, 5, 6; *Vespa crabro*	Duodenum "R"	Rat[4,7]
Polistes gallicus	Duodenum "C"	Dog[3]
Vespa (Paravespula) vulgaris	Jejunum "C" (contraction	Rabbit[6]
	was preceded by inhibition	
	of peristalsis)	
Peptide 2, 5, 6; *Polistes gallicus;*	Ileum "C"	Guinea pig[2,3,7,9,10]
Vespa (Paravespula) vulgaris;		
Vespa crabro, Vespa orientalis		
Peptide 2	Cecum "R"	Hen[7]
Polistes gallicus	Colon "C"	Rabbit[3]
	Miscellaneous	
Peptide 2	Release of histamine	Rat (mast cells)[11]

[a] For structure see Table 3.
[b] "C" indicates contraction and "R" relaxation.

[1] Pisano (1970); [2] Yoshida et al. (1976); [3] Erspamer and Falconieri-Erspamer (1962); [4] Bhoola et al. (1961); [5] Holdstock et al. (1957); [6] Schachter and Thain (1954); [7] Pisano (1968); [8] Watanabe et al. (1975); [9] Edery et al. (1972); [10] Schachter (1970); [11] Johnson and Erdos (1973); [12] Edery and Ishay (1965)

of "*Polistes* kinin" in inducing rat blood pressure fall varied according to the route of administration. Stewart (1968) reported that when administered via the jugular vein, it was 10 times more effective than bradykinin, whereas it was only one-sixth as active after injection into the aorta. This difference could be explained by the fact that "*Polistes* kinin," in contrast to bradykinin, does not undergo inactivation in the lung when introduced into pulmonary circulation (Ryan et al., 1970). Very recently, Yoshida et al. (1976) showed that as little as 100 ng (total dose) i.v. of "*Vespula* kinin" (Table 3, peptide 5) elicited a remarkable fall in rat blood pressure. In contrast with "*Polistes* kinin," "*Vespula* kinin" was only twice as effective as bradykinin. These authors suggested that "*Vespula* kinin" might be degraded in the rat to a similar extent as bradykinin.

All Vespidae kinins hitherto described contract isolated organ preparations of rat uterus as well as of guinea pig ileum, whereas other intestinal segments react with relaxation. Some species differences became apparent; for instance, *Polistes gallica* kinin elicited contraction of dog-isolated duodenum, while all other kinins caused relaxation in the same segment of the rat (ERSPAMER and FALCONIERI-ERSPAMER, 1962). Undoubtedly, the clarification of these species differences will become possible only when enough supply of pure synthetic kinin of the required origin is available.

As far as humans are concerned, one of the most important pharmacological actions of Vespidae kinins is the production of pain. HOLDSTOCK, MATHIAS, and SCHACHTER (1957) have shown that a purified preparation of *V. (Paravespula) vulgaris* kinin elicited a moderate sensation of pain at a concentration of 20 µg/ml when applied by the blister technique to a human subject (KEELE and ARMSTRONG, 1964). Pain sensation increased with the dose and was sometimes accompanied by itching. The way or mechanism(s) whereby Vespidae kinins interact with nervous structures subserving pain sensation are so far unknown. These aspects of research might be most rewarding in future work. It might also be possible that Vespidae kinins, in addition to their own algogenic action, could potentiate that of other pain-producers present in V.v. This distinctive possibility arises from the work of KEELE and ARMSTRONG (1964), who conducted an extensive comparative study of algogens and most descriptively said: "If we had been asked to design a reliable pain-producing mixture consisting of low-molecular-weight substances of animal origin we should very likely have concocted a brew containing histamine, 5-HT and a kinin (polypeptide) such as occurs in wasp venom. The added rapier thrust contributed by ACh in hornet venom is sheer (evil) genius." (Wasp referred to is *V. (Paravespula) vulgaris,* whereas hornet is *V. crabro*).

JOHNSON and ERDÖS (1973) examined the histamine-releasing action of a series of endogenous biologically active peptides including bradykinin and "*Polistes* kinin" (Table 3, peptide 6). The test system consisted of suspended rat mast cells, and the activity was compared with that of 48/80, the reference compound. "*Polistes* kinin" was the most potent natural substance, the ED_{50} (amount releasing 50% of the total mast cell histamine) being 3×10^{-6} M, as compared to 5×10^{-5} M for bradykinin, and 8.5×10^{-7} M for 48/80. The mast cells, when deprived of their histamine contents, appeared slightly swollen with rugged edges. These changes suggested "degranulation" similarly to that induced by 48/80. Although the mechanism of histamine liberation by kinins could not be clarified, promotion of mast-cell granules exocytosis was suggested as a possible reason. Moreover, as the potency of *Polistes* kinin was of such a magnitude (1 – 3 nmol liberated considerable amounts of histamine), the possibility was suggested that Vespidae kinins might also liberate histamine *in vivo*. If this postulate could be substantiated by evidence, a new important dimension would be added to the pharmacological activity of Vespidae kinins and particularly to their share in the overall effects of V.v.

G. Antigenicity and Immunological Aspects

Several communications in the literature deal with antigenic properties of V.v. They were first prompted with the aim to establish venom components by immunological means as well as their cross antigenicity with other body constituents of the same insect or with venoms and body constituents of related species. Later on, however, they were also stimulated by the need to study immuno-allergic reactions due to insect bites, as well as to prepare and test the neutralizing effectiveness of immune sera against various harmful venom components.

The specificity of venom sac antigens of bees, *Polistes exclamans* and *Vespula pennsylvanica,* was studied by LANGLOIS et al. (1965) and compared to those of the insect sacless body extracts. Immunization was performed in rabbits, and the antigen-antibody reactions were established by hemagglutination and inhibition of hemagglutination, agar gel diffusion, and immunoelectrophoresis. As many as seven antigens were demonstrated in the *P. exclamans* venom sac extract, compared to 12–13 components for sacless insect extracts. Common antigens were demonstrated in venom sac and sacless body extracts. At least one or possibly two antigens specific to the venom sacs of each of the species were found. Since most of the common antigens were found in the body extracts of insects, the above-mentioned authors posited the hypothesis that individuals allergic to more than one insect might have become sensitized to the insect body rather than to the venom antigens. However, as pointed out by FOUBERT and STIER (1958), clinical experience with sensitive patients indicates that the stinging insect can seldom be identified, and desensitization with material from a presumed homologous insect would not therefore be safe. These authors studied the antigenic relationships between *Apis mellifera* (honey-bee), *Polistes fuscatus aurifer* (wasp), *Dolichovespula arenaria* (yellow hornet), *Dolichovespula maculata* (black hornet), and *Vespula pennsylvanica* (yellow jacket). Whole body extracts were injected in rabbits with complete Freund adjuvant. The immune sera were tested by double gel diffusion against the various antigens. Between four and seven antigenic components were found in the various insect, of which one or two were present in all the extracts. Of all the insects investigated, the yellow jacket produced the antibody most readily reacting with heterologous antigens. Yellow jacket extract also showed the greatest tendency to cross-react with heterologous antisera. Cross sensitization was also demonstrated by anaphylactic challenge of presensitized guinea pigs. Again yellow jacket extracts were found most potent in producing sensitization to shock from heterologous antigens and also most effective in shocking animals sensitized by heterologous extracts. The authors concluded that desensitization with a combined mixture of bee, yellow jacket, and hornet antigens should be used whenever the insect causing a severe reaction cannot be identified.

Reactivity to hymenoptera antigens has also been found by *in vivo* testing of skin reactivity (PERLMAN, 1955). LOVELESS and FACKLER (1956), testing directly sensitized individuals as well as their serum on the skin of normal individuals, found that the *Vespula maculifrons* (yellow jacket), *Vespa maculata* (bald-faced hornet), *Polistes* sp. (paper wasp), honey-bee, and *Bombus* (bumble-bee) possess a common allergenic specificity, while each one of them also contains in its venom a component which is peculiar to it.

Immunologic studies in fatal anaphylactic reactions to wasp stings (McCorMICK, 1963) have demonstrated the presence of specific precipitin antibodies to antigens extracted from the insect abdomens, cross reacting with honey-bee antigens. DIRKS (1971) made an extensive immunochemical investigation of low-molecular-weight basic proteins isolated from native venom of *P. exclamans, P. annularis, P. metricus,* and *Vespula maculata.* Three to four precipitation lines were identified in each venom, using specific homologous antisera and 1−2 common components using heterologous antisera. Nonimmunological complexing also occurred with serum lipoproteins, and the possibility was raised that such complexing may be important in the etiology of hypersensitivity.

Fractionation of whole body and venom sac extracts of *P. exclamans* by DEAEcellulose chromatography (LANGLOIS et al., 1966) have shown eight to nine fractions, two of them being active in skin tests. Cross-reacting antigens were demonstrated with appropriate rabbit antisera.

Antigenicity of *V. orientalis* venom has been studied by EDERY et al. (1972), who found at least three lines of precipitation when the venom reacted with serum of immunized rabbits. ISHAY et al. (1972) studied the antigenic relationship of *Vespa orientalis* and *Paravespula germanica* venoms. Immune sera were prepared by inoculation of rabbits with native venom and complete Freund adjuvant and tested by double gel diffusion and immuno-electrophoresis. Four precipitation arcs were obtained, three of them belonging to the hemolytic fractions previously identified by electrophoretic separation (FISCHL et al., 1972). In another communication (ISHAY et al., 1971 b), the *"in vivo"* effectiveness of rabbit antiserum against *Vespa orientalis* venom was tested. The antisera used displayed three to four precipitation lines against the immunizing antigen (pure native venom), by double gel diffusion and immuno-electrophoresis. Mice envenomated with up to 2 mg venom sac extract (a dose which invariably kills the animals) were fully protected when given simultaneously 0.5 ml of rabbit immune serum. The antiserum was not effective in counteracting venom sac extracts in doses exceeding 2 mg. Since immunization was done with pure venom — while envenomation was performed with venom sac extract due to scarcity of pure venom — no answer could be given as to whether death was caused by some component for which no antibody was present in the immune serum. It should be noted that in many instances whole body insect extracts instead of native venom or venom sac extracts are currently used in immunization studies. BARR (1967), using rabbit immune serum, obtained precipitin bands with wasp, hornet (species not stated), or bee antigens, showing both specific and common components in the hornet and the bee. Positive passive cutaneous anaphylaxis was also shown with hornet, wasp, and honey-bee, but not with yellow jacket, antigens.

SHULMAN et al. (1964) used potent allergenic extracts of *Polistes exclamans, Vespula pennsylvanica,* and *Apis mellifera* for skin testing of sensitive patients, most of them reacting to more than one type of extract. Heterogenecity of the extracts was studied by zone electrophoresis and ultracentrifugation, the extracts showing varying patterns of minor fast components and major slow ones. In another investigation, SETTIPANE et al. (1971) found at least two common antigens in whole body extracts of wasps, yellow jackets, and hornets (species not stated) against immune rabbit serum, using the Ouchterlony technique. One out of 12 hymenoptera allergic patients, who was fully hyposensitized, gave a positive passive cutaneous anaphylaxis test and one out of 12 nonallergic patients recently stung showed a positive precipitin test.

SOBOTKA et al. (1974) studied histamine release together with skin testing in order to establish hypersensitivity to antigenic extracts from *Vespula pennsylvanica* (yellow jacket), yellow- and white-faced hornets, *Apis mellifera* (honey-bee), and *Bombus* (bumble-bee). The leucocytes of 13 out of 16 patients, judged clinically to have systemic reactions to stinging insects, exhibited a positive histamine release with 0.001–1.0 µg of venom. None of the 12 control patients gave positive responses with a 1000-fold greater concentration of venom. These authors emphasize the superiority of the use of Vespidae venom over whole body extracts for testing histamine release from leucocytes of sensitive patients. They conclude that the venom-induced histamine release is mediated by antibodies of the IgE class.

H. Clinical Aspects of Envenomation

I. Incidence of Sting and Dangers

In most cases, *single* Vespidae stings do not produce serious symptoms of intoxication and are more of a nuisance than a calamity. Thus, Vespidae sting may result in an experience varying from minor local pain and inflammation to generalized intoxication or allergic anaphylactic shock which may be fatal (BROCK, 1961; BEARD, 1963). Serious, nearly fatal, and fatal cases have been reported by PERLMAN (1955), KEMPER (1962), PARRISH (1963), and LECOMTE (1973). These authors analyzed many hundreds of fatalities in the United States and elsewhere. Deaths due to hymenoptera stings are probably far more numerous than those recorded in death certificates, as physicians frequently do not recognize the symptoms of the stings (FLUNO, 1961). PARRISH (1959, 1963) came to the conclusion that many coroners are not aware of anaphylactic shock as a cause of death, and many fatalities reported to be caused by "heart attacks" or "heat strokes" may actually have resulted from the sting of a venomous insect, including Vespidae. This is especially the case with regard to victims from traffic accidents whose death has been ascribed to heart attacks or to trauma and who may have suffered primarily from hymenoptera stings (MILLER, 1956). The distraction of the driver caused by the fear of the mere presence of a wasp in a moving car may be fatal. When a severe reaction to the sting occurs, the car may remain practically driverless, since the victim often loses consciousness within a few minutes.

All Vespidae venoms produce in man trauma to skin or mucosa after stinging, characterized by acute swelling and pain at the site of the sting.

It is advisable to identify the stinging insect. BARR (1974) reported that the insect had been reasonably identified in 35% and questionably in 34% of the cases; in 31% the insect remained unknown. Of the identified insects 47% were yellow jackets, 27% honey-bees, 14% wasps, 6% bumblebees, and 6% hornets. Identification of honey-bee is aided by the fact that it is the only insect that leaves its stinger at the site of the injury. Reactions of a local or systemic character may develop depending on the amount of venom injected, the specific activity of the venom components (MARSHALL, 1957; WONG, 1970), and the sensitivity of the individual. Secondary infections frequently follow Vespidae stings because of the scavenger nature of the Vespidae and the consequent greater chance of bacterial contamination (MARSHALL, 1957). Protein allergens responsible for sensitization may be found not only in the venom but also in insect feces as well as its body and wing dust (MANN and BATES, 1960). Fractions of Vespidae venom sac extracts separated by DEAE cellulose chromatography were active components in skin tests. The occurrence of common reactions to components of bee and wasp venoms is suggestive of the possibility of cross-sensitization in patients (LANGLOIS et al., 1966). Wasps and hornets contain common antigens, and, in addition, each insect contains several antigens peculiar to the individual type (FOUBERT and STIER, 1958). Cross-sensitization to various hymenoptera may occur, as severe reactions frequently appear. This phenomenon cannot be simply explained by one sting which is followed later by an additional one of the same species of Vespidae (FLUNO, 1961).

In an analysis of many hundreds of fatalities from venomous animals in the United States, PARRISH (1963) stated that hymenopteran insects, snakes, and spiders accounted for 94% of the cases. Bees appeared to kill more people in the United States than rattlesnakes, wasps being the third most deadly animal. SOMERVILLE et al. (1975) summarized 261 death cases in the Western Hemisphere and 61 cases in Western Europe produced by Hymenoptera—mostly Vespidae—stings and concluded that almost all had been caused by anaphylactic reactions except for a few cases of mechanical obstruction of the upper respiratory tract produced by intrabuccal stings. According to these authors and in agreement with many others (LOMER et al., 1958; FOUBERT and STIER, 1958; LOVELESS and FACKLER, 1956; PARRISH, 1963; JANSSEN, 1966; and BARNARD, 1967), death resulted from hypersensitivity due to insect allergy rather than the toxic effect of venom. The study of 215 death certificates of people who died from stings and bites in the United States during the five-year period 1950—1954 (PARRISH, 1959) indicated that most of the deaths from Hymenoptera stings happened within 1 h, usually within 15—30 min. Death cases from overwhelming envenomation from multiple stings were few, and most of them were the result of anaphylactic shock due to insect allergy. This is different from other insect bites: spider-bite victims died usually 18 h or more after envenomation; in snake bite victims death took place after 6—48 h. KESSLER (1975) described 240 cases of Hymenoptera stings from his experience of 20 years in Israel, all showing unusual reactions. Males were apparently more exposed than females in their outdoor activities in agriculture or as truck drivers. A familial disposition for allergic diseases was found in about 25% of the cases, one-third of which showed a positive skin test to other allergens, such as pollen, molds, or animal hair.

SOMERVILLE et al. (1975) summarize the arguments ascribing Vespidae sting accidents mainly to insect allergy, because (1) death often occurs after one single sting which at most contains an insignificant amount of venom and obviously cannot produce general toxic symptoms; (2) the affected regions of the body are widespread and the immediate spreading of the venom cannot account for such an effect; (3) death occurs rapidly in most of the fatal cases, while the symptoms of cardiovascular collapse, respiratory bronchospastic distress, and angioneurotic edema have no specific character of envenomation per se; (4) mostly adults and not children are the victims in grave stinging accidents. The latter argument is in agreement with the findings of PARRISH (1963) who underlined the different age distribution of persons dying from hymenoptera stings as compared with snake and spider victims. WONG (1970) described case histories of 45 children hospitalized in Singapore following stings from bees or hornets. In these cases there was only one instance of anaphylactic shock corroborated by reference to a previous sting in the distant past. In four cases the symptomatology was rather severe, and one of them died.

Only scant information exists concerning the actual amount of venom injected by Vespidae when stinging, most of the data being conjectural and not mentioning the species concerned. According to von SCHMIDT (1949), the amount of venom produced by the hornet is about 0.05 ml. PERLMAN (1955) cited PHISALIX (1923) and ROSS (1931) who reported that hornets may inject $0.05 - 0.3$ ml of venom, whereas SOMERVILLE et al. (1975) estimated that 1 µg may be introduced after a single stinging.

Clinical manifestations of Vespidae sting have been reported by KEMPER (1962) who rather unusually exposed himself 22 times to such stings. The intensity and type of clinical manifestations of Vespidae stings depend mainly on the following factors:

1. The species of the stinging Vespidae
2. The depth of the sting
3. The localization of the sting
4. The number of stings received simultaneously
5. The sensitivity of the victim

According to KEMPER (1962), the latter three are the most important factors, determining the seriousness of the cases as benign, serious, or life endangering. A similar classification was proposed by FLUNO (1961). Benign cases show local action of an inflammatory type, whereas serious cases are accompanied by systemic effects of a toxic or allergic character.

II. Symptomatology

1. Local Symptoms

Acute pain, local edema and erythema as well as a rise in skin temperature occur at the site of the sting. Pain may subsist for one-half to several hours and itching for days. Hemorrhage and formation of papulae at the site of the sting may occur. These are small red areas surrounded by a whitish zone and reddish flare. A wheal may be formed followed by irritation, itching, and heat. Edema of the dermis is followed by perivascular infiltration of polymorphonuclear leucocytes and lymphocytes. After several hours eosinophils, plasma-cells, and histiocytes may appear, the infiltrate being most prominent around the blood vessels. Continuous care is advisable when the localization is around the eyes, nose or throat, even in nonsensitive persons, until all symptoms of distress have disappeared (FRAZIER, 1972). Unusual swelling at the site of the sting may in some cases persist for several days and spread over adjacent joints. The swelling may interfere with normal function, such as stiffness of a finger and consequent impairment of movement (FLUNO, 1961).

Most V.v. contain relatively large amounts of 5-hydroxytryptamine. It is accepted that this substance plays an important role as a pain-producing factor together with acetylcholine, histamine, and kinins (WELSH and BATTY, 1963; KEELE and ARMSTRONG, 1963; CHAHL and KIRK, 1975). The localization of the sting may contribute to special developments. KESSLER (1975) described stings in the eyelid, producing severe, sometimes bilateral swelling and leaving the eyes practically closed but mostly without real permanent damage. In some cases stings around the eye caused atrophy of the iris, ulceration and abscess of the lens, or perforation of the eye ball, which might lead to blindness (KEMPER, 1962; FRAZIER, 1972). Eating of cakes or sandwiches into which wasps had penetrated may produce dangerous stings in the oral cavity, such as swelling of the larynx which may interrupt air passage. However, such complications are rare.

2. Generalized Symptoms

Systemic effects may be related to the toxic action of various venom components (see Section D). Cytolytic, hemolytic, neurotoxic, and hemorrhagic action may be observed, as may blood pressure lowering and peristalsis-induced activity. In addition, generalized symptoms occur, like urticaria, vertigo, and fainting. Dyspnea and bronchospasm, hemoglobinuria (CHUGH et al., 1976), paralytic and hemiplegic syndromes, as well as aphasia (KEMPER, 1962), have been described. Bilateral ptosis appeared in a patient after *Polistes* sp. stinging. The symptoms resembled the ocular form of myasthenia gravis and were reversed by i.v. injection of edrophonium chloride (BRUMLIK, 1976). Life-endangering cases are the result of:

1) Localization of the sting, as may occur in the oral cavity with ensuing swelling of the laryngo-pharynx and danger of choking.
2) Massive intoxication, as reported after multiple stinging by swarms of Vespidae (see Section B, 7).
3) Hypersensitivity and anaphylactic shock.

a) Toxic Reactions

Generalized and specific reactions may occur as a result of the toxic action of the Vespidae venom when injected in sufficient amount as a result of multiple stinging (FRAZIER, 1972). The clinical symptoms are fever, nausea, emesis, cyanosis, dyspnea, throat and chest constriction, and even asthmatic stridor. Weakness may progress, accompanied by hypotension, tachycardia, collapse, and fainting. Gastrointestinal symptoms, such as abdominal cramps and diarrhea, as well as impairment of the function of the nervous system, drowsiness, and tonic and clonic convulsions may aggravate the situation. Cardiac and respiratory arrests may occur. Case reports of this type of Vespidae sting have been summarized by JANSSEN (1966).

Severe damage to human striated muscle resulting in rhabdomyolysis has been described in cases of multiple stinging in persons who had received several hundred

Vespa affinis stings (SHILKIN, 1971; SHILKIN et al., 1972). In these cases no allergy developed, but after 24 h muscular pains, nausea, and vomiting occurred. Oliguria developed, and a critical rise in blood urea during the following days had to be treated with peritoneal dialysis. In one case complete recovery was reported, though in another the patient died from intercurrent respiratory infection. Primary nephrotoxicity, as well as a direct myolytic action of the venom, was assumed. This latter is substantiated when considering the electron-microscopic muscle changes in experimental envenomation and the effects of V.v. on cat's striated muscles (see Sections E, 3 and F, 7).

b) Allergic Reactions

BARR (1974) and KESSLER (1975) recently published reviews of many hundreds of patients who had suffered from hymenoptera sting allergy. In 77% of 249 cases studied, the former author reported a generalized reaction, while in 23% only local ones. The dissertation of HALPERIN (1936) includes references to earlier literature. COLTOIU and MATEESCU (1968) described allergy observations after Vespidae stinging in Romania. The generalized allergic reaction may elicit very severe or lethal results. The patient may fall into shock within 10–20 min of stinging, breathing being shallow and pulse and heartbeat extremely weak (FLUNO, 1961). Profuse sweating occurs, followed by edema of eyelids, glottis, larynx, and lungs as well as bronchospasm, abdominal colics, and skin and mucosa petechiae. Diarrhea and mental confusion may precede unconsciousness (KEMPER, 1962). In addition, such symptoms as stuffed nose, rashes, lymph node swelling, paresis, epigastric pain, and incontinence may be observed (BARR, 1974). Allergenic extracts from different Vespidae *(Polistes exclamans* and *Vespula pennsylvanica)* have been prepared by SHULMAN et al. (1964). Their allergenicity was determined by skin tests, and in sensitive patients a positive test may be elicited by a very dilute antigen. Most of the sensitive patients react to more than one type of insect. Very diluted antigen concentrations are recommended for diagnostic purposes (LECLERCQ, 1967; LECOMTE and LECLERCQ, 1973). Precipitin antibodies and passive cutaneous anaphylaxis were studied by SETTIPANE and HOPSON (1971) in human sera taken from subjects both sensitive and insensitive to hymenoptera, including wasps, yellow jackets, and hornets (species not quoted). The tests were negative in the nonallergic group, except for one recently stung individual.

III. Pathology

BARNARD (1973) concludes from information obtained from United States Vital Statistics Data that four main types of pathology, i.e., respiratory, vascular, anaphylactic, and neurologic, are responsible for the fatal reactions following hymenoptera sting.

Post-mortem examination shows edema of lungs and larynx, hyperemia of viscera and brain, petechial bleeding, and cyanosis of the skin, serous membranes, as well as meninges (JANSSEN, 1966). Edema is due to allergic reactions, whereas the other symptoms are due to capillary damage. The microscopic findings described by McCORMICK (1963) were those of severe congestion of all tissues and, in a case of extreme hypersensitivity, revealed enlarged lungs showing multiple bullae of various sizes. WEGELIN (1948) reports his own findings and reviews previous literature on pathology after death from a single sting. Petechial bleedings were found in pleural, epicardial, and endocardial membranes as well as in the mucosae of the respiratory and gastro-intestinal tracts. Small and large hemorrhages had been found in the renal pelvis, liver, and cerebral ventricles as well as small infarcts of lungs and adrenal cortical necrosis. In patients who had survived two to three days, extensive brain changes produced by local necrosis of vascular origin have been reported (LECOMTE and LECLERCQ, 1973).

IV Treatment

1. First Aid

The sting of the Vespidae, if left, should be removed or brushed off. Care should be taken not to squeeze the venom sac as this would empty more venom into the injury. The sting can be scooped out with the help of an adequate instrument if available, otherwise with the fingernail (FRAZIER, 1972), and the site of the sting should be cleansed. The patient should be advised to contact a physician without delay, because self-treatment may give only temporary relief. Some specialists advise the application of a proximal tourniquet (BARR, 1974). Ice packs, elevation of the limb, and topical application of antihistaminics may be of value. The latter are useful against itching but not against severe allergic reactions. STRAUSS (1949) tested the effectiveness of an antihistamine preparation applied as an ointment to the site of a sting. In all cases the intense pain sensation was relieved within a few minutes. Subcutaneous administration of $0.2-0.3$ ml of a $1^0/_{00}$ solution of adrenaline to adults or $0.1-0.2$ ml to children is recommended (BARNARD, 1970). Analgesics may be given orally, and local anesthetics may be infiltrated around the site of the sting. Steroids will reduce hives and wheezing. LECLERCQ (1973) also mentioned the therapeutic use of calcium and analeptic drugs.

2. Emergency Treatment

In case of multiple stings (more than ten at one time) hospitalization is imperative (WONG, 1970) in order to cope with the immediate dangers and with possible delayed reactions which might occur after 12 to 48 h. Parenteral infusions of antihistamines (LOMER et al., 1958; CHUGH et al., 1976) and of hydrocortisone are installed. Urinary flow, blood urea, and potassium have to be checked. Special attention has to be given to the danger of renal failure and of acute hemolysis (HOH et al., 1966; CHUGH et al., 1976), which may require blood transfusion and hemodialysis. Hemoglubinuria occurs relatively frequently (WONG, 1961; CHUGH et al., 1976). Anaphylaxis is a most difficult problem for therapeutic management. Deep subcutaneous injections of a $1^0/_{00}$ solution of adrenalin in higher doses (1 ml for adults, $0.2-0.5$ ml for children) must be given, in addition to the intravenous drip containing antihistaminics and corticosteroids. The acute danger is vascular collapse and angio-edema, as well as respiratory obstruction. Endotracheal intubation and artificial respiration may become necessary in view of the fact that death may occur very rapidly in these cases.

3. Preventive Therapy—Desensitization

FISHER and CENTER (1934) were the first to consider desensitization as a preventive treatment for people at high exposure risk. Such treatment had been given successfully to individuals previously exposed to bee stings, and it was considered that hypersensitivity to Vespidae venoms is very similar to that produced by bee venoms. In cases of anaphylactic shock, death may occur rapidly before emergency treatment can be given. Persons known to be hypersensitive to the sting of Vespidae should therefore be given the benefit of a course of hyposensitization if exposed to occupational hazards such as agricultural activities in Vespidae infected areas (FRIEDMAN and MASCIA, 1968; STOKKE, 1973). In the case of Vespidae, native venom is seldom available in sufficient quantities which would be required for hyposensitization because of collection difficulties (SHULMAN et al., 1964). LICHTENSTEIN et al. (1974) and KERN et al. (1976) recommend venom immunization as the treatment of choice for people exposed to hymenoptera sting, especially when they have shown sensitivity to repeated stings, or if there is a personal or family history with cases of anaphylaxis.

For desensitization purposes, patients are injected weekly with increasing doses, depending on the reaction to the previous one. Most studies indicate marked benefit from these desensitizing injections, and no or only slight untoward reactions have been reported (LECOMTE and LECLERCQ, 1973). Results of desensitization treatment have also been reported by SOBOTKA et al. (1974) and BARR (1971, 1972, 1974). BARR applied desensitization to all 249 patients who suffered from insect allergy. The initial dose used was the weakest one, producing a positive skin test. The skin test was carried out by the intradermal route starting with a 1×10^{-5} dilution and increasing the concentration every 10 min by a factor of 10 until a positive skin test—a wheal of at least 0.75 cm in diameter—was obtained. The highest used was 1×10^{-2} dilution.

If during hyposensitization treatment, local reactions of unusual strength occur, the subsequent doses have to be reduced until such reactions no longer appear. Furthermore, systemic reactions may also be induced by hyposensitization, and in these cases, FRAZIER (1972) recommends keeping a tourniquet and adrenaline available for immediate use. In patients who suffered life-threatening reactions, hyposensitization should be continued indefinitely. Such patients may be advised to carry a tag stating their allergy condition and instructions for first aid. Furthermore, they should carry a first aid kit containing epinephrine inhalation spray or injection, ephedrine, and antihistamine tablets. The Insect Allergy Committee of the American Academy of Allergy, in its publication on Insect Sting Allergy and based on a questionnaire study of 2606 cases (Cooperative Study, 1965), came to the conclusion that hyposensitization is of greatest value in persons sensitive to insect sting. The expectance of progressively severe reactions in about 65% of persons not hyposensitized is reduced in about 90% of the persons following hyposensitization. Protection may be maintained for years or may be lost in less than a year.

V. Prevention of Stinging

It has been pointed out by LECLERCQ (1967) that hymenoptera stings occurring during work in refineries, pastry bakeries, jam factories, etc., may legally be considered as work accidents. Dangerous exposure also exists for people working in orchards and wine plantations. Food and drinks in such surroundings should be carefully checked. Furthermore, Vespidae nests located near human quarters should be removed (KEMPER and DOHRING, 1961).

It is generally advised for people living or working near Vespidae nests to wear shoes and socks. They should avoid floral prints, bright colours, perfumes, and scented hair in order not to attract Vespidae. People who have shown severe reactions to wasp stings should not engage in wasp-control programs (FLUNO, 1961).

VI. Control of Vespidae

Vespidae nests and their surroundings may be treated with insecticides, especially during the night when the great majority of the insects are in their nests and activity is lowest. Fumigants such as carbon disulfide and gasoline are useful but highly inflammable and even explosive. Aerosolized insecticides are useful indoors. Rapid disposal of garbage around homes and in picnic areas and of fallen fruit in orchards is of importance in the prevention of Vespidae sting. This subject was analyzed in detail by WAGNER (1961) who studied feeding habits of *Vespula pennsylvanica* (yellow jacket) in parks, camps, and picnic grounds. Examination of worker wasps captured as they flew into their nests showed that they carried macerated adult flies and lepidoptera larvae to be used for feeding the larvae in the nest (see also Section B, 2). Large numbers of the wasps were found in the trash containers with high fly populations. The number of yellow jackets found per trash container formed an index of population density. Effective control was reached in Griffith Park, Los Angeles, by regular cleansing and spraying of these containers, using a 0.75% DDVP solution. When this proves unsatisfactory, the surrounding area has to be searched for nests. These nests can be destroyed effectively with a 4% aqueous DDVP sprayed into the nest entrance. WAFA et al. (1969) described the use of chlorinated hydrocarbons and of a variety of organophosphorous insecticides incorporated into honey baits for control of nests of *Vespa orientalis* in Egypt. Hornet control in Singapore is being carried out by special units (Fig. 30) equipped with hornet sting-proof suits and insecticide-proof respirators (CHAN, 1972).

"The technique employed involves throwing a ball of fire onto the nest by spraying a continuous jet of the spray mixture from a pressurized knapsack sprayer across a flame ignited at the end of an extensible aluminium pole by soaking kerosene in a ball of combustible material (Fig. 30). In this way, no time is allowed for the hornets to escape and disperse, and an average-sized hornet nest can be destroyed in about 10—15 min, the time required for the nest to be completely burnt up. When used alone, i.e., without fire, as is often necessary when dealing with nests located on buildings, the jet is directed at the hole of the nest as the hornets emerge (they invariably will) in order to prevent them from escaping, and maintained until all have died. The spray mixture consists of two insecticides in an oil base. A quick knockdown insecticide (synergized pybuthrin) is the frontline weapon. It knocks the hornets down on immediate contact. A residual insecticide (Dieldrex 15) then continues the killing action by autointoxication or by other mechanisms of poisoning. All hornets coming in contact with the spray would

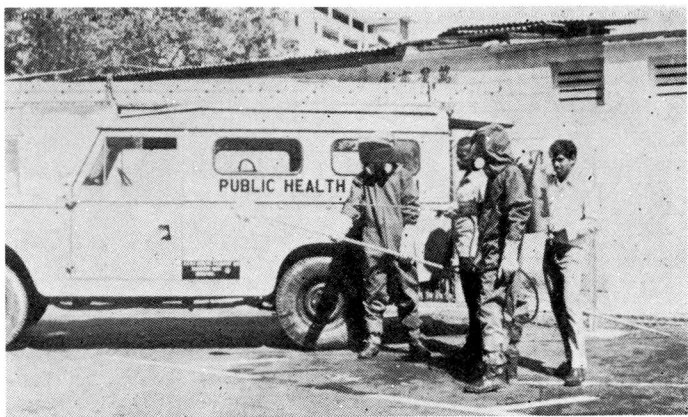

Fig. 30. Hornet control outfit, showing hornet sting-proof suits and insecticide-proof respirators. Note knapsack pressurized sprayer for throwing jet of insecticide mixture, ball of combustible material at the end of an aluminium pole, and a long ladder folded on rack at the top of land-rover (Chan, 1972)

thus eventually die even if they escaped a direct dose of the spray mixture. The oil base (antimalarial oil) acts as a carrier for the two insecticides and also as a heavy wetting agent for wetting the wings and body of the hornet so as to bring it straight down onto the floor before it could fly some distance and sting an innocent victim. The oil also serves as a fuel for the fire flame."

Davis et al. (1967) of the U.S. Department of Agriculture patented the use of 2,4-hexadienyl butyrate and related compounds as attractants for yellow jackets. Such substances selectively attract Vespidae but are without effect on most other insects (Davis et al., 1968; Davis et al., 1973; McGovern et al., 1970). In traps (see Section B, 6) containing these highly specific lures placed around orchards in fruit growing regions, hundreds of thousands of wasps were captured. Such chemical and technological developments are of importance for the prevention of Vespidae sting. The action of heptyl butyrate as an attractant was studied by MacDonald et al. (1973). It appeared that different Vespidae species do not react identically to the attractant substances, which may result in reduction of the useful and increase in the harmful species. Further investigations (Wagner and Reierson, 1969) demonstrated the importance of the choice of the insecticide which may neutralize the effect of the attractant. Construction and location of bait stations are of relevance to the efficiency of the method.

J. Concluding Remarks

After reviewing the data on V.v., the need for more thorough studies concerning their chemical composition becomes apparent. In this regard, knowledge is totally lacking with respect to a large number of species populating countries in which Vespidae stinging accidents frequently occur. The up-to-date information clearly shows that, although many V.v. contain a number of common components, their concentrations vary greatly according to species. In addition, considering the existing basic differences in V.v. composition, it would no longer be meaningful to refer—as has been done in the past—to "wasp or hornet venom" as a single homogenous entity. Though no product with therapeutic potential has hitherto been isolated from V.v., this distinct possibility may be worthwhile to explore, considering the useful materials already obtained from bee venom.

A much debated question was as to whether or not V.v., in addition to producing anaphylactic disturbances, could also cause systemic toxicity. The evidence presented in many instances of massive stinging leaves little doubt that life-endangering toxic reactions do occur after attacks by swarms of Vespidae. These cases may present serious medical problems. The identification of the responsible toxic components of V.v. will contribute to the development of rational efficient antidotes.

Acknowledgement: Our thanks are given to Mrs. G. Porath for her most efficient help in the preparation of the manuscript.

This review was partly supported by a grant from the United States-Israel Binational Science Foundation (BSF), Jerusalem, Israel, as a continuation of former agreements between the National Library of Medicine, Public Health Service, U.S. Department of Health, Education, and Welfare, Bethesda, Maryland, USA, and the *Israel Journal of Medical Sciences.*

References

Abrahams, G.: Über Gewinnung und pharmakologische Wirkungen von Hornissen- und Wespengift. Inaugural Dissertation, Medizinische Fakultät, Universität Würzburg, 1955.

Adsay, M.F.: Denizli chickens (for controlling wasps in the aviary). Aricilik dergisi **6**, 124—125 (1950).

Akre, R.D., Garnett, W.B., MacDonald, J.F., Greene, A., Landolt, P.: Behavior and colony development of *Vespula pensylvanica* and *V. atropilosa* (Hymenoptera: Vespidae). J. Kansas ent. Soc. **49**, 63—84 (1976).

Akre, R.D., Hill, W.B., MacDonald, J.F.: Artificial housing for yellow jacket colonies. J. econ. Ent. **66**, 803—805 (1973).

Akre, R.D., Hill, W.B., MacDonald, J.F., Garnett, W.B.: Foraging distances of *Vespula pensylvanica* workers. J. Kansas ent. Soc. **48**, 12—16 (1975).

Akre, R.D., MacDonald, J.F., Hill, W.B.: Yellow jacket literature (Hymenoptera: Vespidae). Melanderia **18**, 67—93 (1974).

Alber, M.A.: Il calabrone, tigre dell'aria. Apicol. ital. **20**, 188—189 (1953).

Albl, F.: Über Wirkkomponenten und Wirkungsmechanismus von Insektengiften (nach Untersuchungen am isolierten Meerscheinchen- und Mäusedünndarm). Inaugural Dissertation, Medizinische Fakultät, Universität Würzburg 1956.

Allalouf, D., Ber, A., Ishay, J.: Hyaluronidase activity of extracts of venom sacs of a number of vespinae (Hymenoptera). Comp. Biochem. Physiol. **43 B**, 119—123 (1972).

Allalouf, D., Ber, A., Ishay, J.: Properties of testicular hyaluronidase of the honey bee and Oriental hornet: comparison with insect venom and mammalian hyaluronidases. Comp. Biochem. Physiol. **50 B**, 331—337 (1975).

Anastasi, A., Erspamer, V., Bertaccini, G., Cei, J.M.: A bradykinin-like endecapeptide of the skin of phyllomedusa rohdei. In: Hypotensive Peptides, pp. 76—85 eds. E.G. Erdös, N. Back and F. Sicuteri, Berlin-Heidelberg-New York: Springer, 1966.

Anon: European wasps. Tasmania J. Agric. 341—342 (1962).

Aoki, T.: Improvement of hornet traps. Jap. biol. J. **3**, 225—257 (1950).

Archer, M.E.: Studies of the seasonal development of *Vespula vulgaris* L. (Hymenoptera: Vespidae) with special reference to queen production. J. Ent. **47**, 45—59 (1972).

Barnard, J.H.: Allergic and pathologic findings in fifty insect-sting fatalities. J. Allergy **40**, 107—114 (1967).

Barnard, J.H.: Non fatal results in third-degree anaphylaxis from Hymenoptera stings. J. Allergy **45**, 92—96 (1970).

Barnard, J.H.: Studies of 400 Hymenoptera sting deaths in the United States. J. Allergy clin. Immunol. **52**, 259—264 (1973).

Barr, S.E.: Allergy to Insect Stings. Med. Ann. D.C. **36**, 395—399 (1967).

Barr, S.E.: Allergy to Hymenoptera Stings—Review of the World Literature: 1953—1970. Ann. Allergy **29**, 49—66 (1971).

Barr, S.E.: Skin test reactivity to the stinging insects. Ann. Allergy **30**, 282—287 (1972).

Barr, S.E.: Allergy to Hymenoptera stings. J. Amer. med. Ass. **228**, 718—720 (1974).

Barr-Nea, L., Ishay, J.: Effect of the Venom sac content of the Oriental hornet (*Vespa orientalis*) on the metamorphosis of the toad tadpole (*Bufo viridis*). Experientia (Basel) **31**, 212—213 (1975).

Barr-Nea, L., Rosenberg, P., Ishay, J.: The venom apparatus of *Vespa orientalis:* Morphology and Cytology. Toxicon **14**, 65—68 (1976).

Beard, R.L.: Insect toxins and venoms. Ann. Rev. Ent. **8**, 1—18 (1963).

Benton, A.W., Morse, R.A.: Collection of the liquid fraction of bee venom. Nature (Lond.) **210**, 652—653 (1966).

Benton, A.W., Morse, R.A., Stewart, J.D.: Venom collection from honey bees. Science **142**, 228—230 (1963).

Bequaert, J.: A revision of the Vespidae of the Belgian Congo based on the collection of the American Museum congo expedition, with a list of Ethiopian Diplopterous wasps. Bull. Amer. Mus. nat. Hist. **39**, 1—384 (1918).

Bequaert, J.: The Nearctic social wasps of the subfamily Polyfunae (Hymenoptera: Vespidae). Ent. Amer. (n.s.) **13**, 87—148 (1933).

Bequaert, J.: A new *Charterginus* from Costa Rica, with notes on *Charterginus, Pseudochartergus, Chartergus, Pseudopolybia, Epipona* and *Tatua* (Hymenoptera Vespidae). Rev. Ent. Rio de Janeiro **9**, 99—117 (1938).

Bequaert, J.: The social Vespidae of the Guayanas, particularly of British Guayana. Bull. Mus. comp. Zool. Harvard **94**, 249—304 (1944a).

Bequaert, J.: A revision of *Protopolybia* Ducke, a genus of neotropical social wasps (Hymenoptera, Vespidae). Rev. Ent. Rio de Janeiro **15**, 97—134 (1944b).

Bergmann, F., Ishay, J., Kidron, M.: Pharmacologically active substances in the faeces of the Oriental wasp, *Vespa orientalis* F. Brit. J. Pharmacol. **26**, 229—236 (1966).

Berland, L.: Les *Polistes* de France (Hym. Vespidae). Ann. Soc. Ent. France **111**, 135—148 (1942).

Bhoola, K.D., Calle, J.D., Schachter, M.: Identification of acetylcholine, 5-hydroxytryptamine, histamine and a new kinin in hornet venom (*V. crabro*). J. Physiol. (Lond.) **159**, 167—182 (1961).

Blackith, R.E., Stevenson, J.H.: Autumnal populations of wasps nests. Insectes Soc. **5**, 347—352 (1958).

Blüthgen, P.: Die Faltenwespen Mitteleuropas (Hymenoptera Diploptera). Abh. Dtsch. Akad. Wiss. Berlin **2**, 1—25 (1961).

Bodenheimer, F.S.: Über die Aktivität von *Vespa orientalis* im Jahresverlauf in Palaestina. Zool. Anz. **107**, 135—140 (1933).

Bordas, L.: Sur l'appareil vénimeux des Hyménoptères C.R. Acad. Sci. (Paris), **XVI**, 385—387 (1894).

Bowen, N.T.: Manganese metabolism of social Vespidae. J. exp. Zool. **115**, 175—205 (1950).

Brian, M.V.: Social insect population. New York: Academic Press, 1965.

Bristowe, W.S.: Insects and other invertebrates for human consumption in Siam. Trans. ent. Soc. (Lond.) **80**, 387—404 (1932).

Brochert, A.: Schädlinge der Honigbiene. Leipzig: Leidloff, Loth u. Michaelis, 1949.

Brock, T.: Resumé of insect allergy. Ann. Allergy **19**, 288—291 (1961).

Brumlik, J.: Myasthenia gravis associated with wasp sting. J. Amer. med. Ass. **235**, 2120—2121 (1976).

Buysson, R. du: Monographie des Vespides du genre *Nectarina*. Ann. Soc. ent. Fr. **74**, 537—566 (1905).

Buysson, R. du: Monographie des Vespides appartenant aux genres *Appica* et *Synoeca*. Ann. Soc. ent. Fr. **75**, 333—362 (1906).

Buysson, R. du: Monographie des Vespides du genre *Belonogaster*. Ann. Soc. ent. Fr. **78**, 199—270 (1909).

Chadwick, L.E.: Actions on insects and other invertebrates. In: Cholinesterases and Anticholinesterases. Handb. exp. Pharmakol. XV, pp. 742—798, ed. G.B. Koelle, Berlin-Göttingen-Heidelberg: Springer 1963.

Chahl, L.A., Kirk, E.J.: Toxins which produce pain. Pain **1**, 3—49 (1975).

Chan, K.L.: The hornets of Singapore: their identification, biology and control. Singapore med. J. **13**, 178—187 (1972).

Chapman, T.A.: Some facts towards a life-history of *Rhipiphorus paradoxus* (=*Metoecus paradoxus*). Ann. Mag. nat. Hist. **6**, 314—326 (1870).

Chugh, K.S., Sharma, B.K., Singhal, P.S.: Acute renal failure following hornet stings. J. trop. Med. Hyg. **79**, 42—44 (1976).

Cinader, B.: Antibodies against enzymes. Ann. Rev. Microbiol. **11**, 371—390 (1957).

Coltoiu, A., Matcescu, D.: Reactii grave la intepaturi de insecte. Derm.-Vener. (Buc.) **13**, 343—348 (1968).

Condrea, E., Mammon, Z., Allalouf, S., de Vries, A.: Susceptibility of erythrocytes of various animal species to the hemolytic and phospholipid splitting action of snake venom. Biochim. Biophys. Acta **84**, 365—375 (1964).

Contardi, A., Latzer, P.: Die tierischen Gifte in der Chemie. Biochem. Z. **197**, 222—232 (1928).

Cooperative Study: Insect sting allergy: Questionnaire study of 2,606 cases. Insect Allergy Committee of the American Academy of Allergy. J. Amer. med. Ass. **193**, 115—120 (1965).

Darchen, R.: Biologie de *Vespa orientalis*. Les premières stades de development. Insectes Soc. **11**, 141—158 (1964).

Davis, H.G., McGovern, T.P., Eddy, G.W., Nelson, T.E., Bertun, K.M.R., Beroza, M., Ingangi, J.C.: New chemical attractants for Yellow Jackets (*Vespula* sp.). J. econom. Ent. **61**, 459—462 (1968).

Davis, H.G., Zwick, R.W., Rogoff, W.M., McGovern, T.P., Beroza, M.: Perimeter traps baited with synthetic lures for suppression of yellow jackets. Environ. Ent. **2**, 569—571 (1973).

Deleurance, E.P.: Le cycle evolutif du nid de *Polistes* (Hymenoptera, Vespidae). C.R. Acad. Sci. (Paris) **224**, 228—230 (1947).

Deleurance, E.P.: a. Contribution a l'étude biologique de *Polistes* (Hyménoptères, Vespides) II. Le cycle evolutif du couvain. Insectes Soc. **2**, 285—302 (1955).

Deleurance, E.P.: Contribution a l'étude des *Polistes* (Hyménoptères vespides). I. L'activité de construction. Behaviour **11**, 67—84 (1957).

Dirks, T.F.: Immunochemical analysis of vespid wasp venoms with emphasis on low-molecular weight, basic polypeptides. Diss. Abst. Int. B. **32**, 992—B (1971).

Ducke, A.: Revision des guêpes sociales polygames d'Amerique. Ann. Hist. Mus. Nation. Hungar. **8**, 449—544 (1910).

Duncan, C.D.: A contribution to the biology of North American vespine wasps. Stanford Univ. Publ. biol. Sci. **8**, 1—272 (1931).

Dunn, R.S., Parks, A.M.: A new plasma kinin in the turtle *Pseudemys scripa elegans*. Experientia (Basel) **26**, 1220 (1970).

Edery, H.: New test for biological identification of bradykinin. Nature (Lond.) **217**, 70 (1968).

Edery, H., Grunfeld, Y.: Sensitization of smooth muscle to plasma kinins: effects of enzymes and peptides on various preparations. Brit. J. Pharmacol. **35**, 51—61 (1969).

Edery, H., Ishay, J.: Pharmacologically active substances of the *vespa orientalis* venom. Proc. Israel physiol. pharmacol. Soc. **1**, 17 (1965).

Edery, H., Ishay, J., Lass, I., Gitter, S.: Pharmacological activity of oriental hornet (*Vespa orientalis*) venom. Toxicon **10**, 13—23 (1972).

Eisen, V., Vogt, W.: Plasma kininogenases and their activators. In: Bradykinin, Kallidin and Kallikrein. Handb. exp. Pharmakol. XXV, pp. 82—130, ed. E.G. Erdös. Berlin-Heidelberg-New York: Springer 1970.

Erspamer, V.: Osservazioni critiche sulle ipotesi concernenti il significato biologico della 5-idrossitriptamina (Enteramina, Serotonina). Medicina (Parma) **5**, 1—34 (1955).

Erspamer, V., Anastasi, A.: Polypeptides active on plain muscle in the amphibian skin. In: Hypotensive Peptides pp. 63—74, eds. E.G. Erdös, N. Back and F. Sicuteri. Berlin-Heidelberg-New York: Springer 1966.

Erspamer, V., Falconieri-Erspamer, G.: Pharmacological actions of eledoisin on extravascular smooth muscle. Brit. J. Pharmacol. **19**, 337—354 (1962).

Fisher, D.C., Center, C.: Hypersensitivity to bees successfully treated with whole bee extract. Allergy **5**, 519—520 (1934).

Fischer, F.G., Neumann, W.P.: Das Gift der Honigbiene. III. Mitt. zur chemischen Kenntnis der Hauptwirkstoffe (Melittin). Biochem. Z. **335**, 51—61 (1961).

Fischl, J., Ishay, J.: The glucose levels and carbohydrates autolysis in *Vespa orientalis*. Insectes Soc. **18**, 203—214 (1972).

Fischl, J., Ishay, J., Goldberg, S., Gitter, S.: Investigation of protein fractions and haemolytic properties of wasp venom. Acta pharmacol. (Kbh.) **31**, 65—70 (1972).

Fischl, J., Ishay, J., Rutenberg, A.: Poly—and disaccharidases in *Vespa orientalis* (Vespinae: Hymenoptera). Comp. Biochem. Physiol. **48B**, 299—306 (1974).

Fischl, J., Ishay, J., Talmor, N.: Monosaccharidase activity and pyruvate, lactate and carbon dioxide contents of *Vespa orientalis* hemolymph. Comp. Biochem. Physiol. **50B**, 71—74 (1975).

Fischl, J., Ishay, J., Talmor, N.: Trehalase: extraction from the midgut of larvae of the Oriental hornet and its use in microdetermination of trehalose. Insect Biochem. **6**, 53—58 (1976).

Fluno, J.A.: Wasps as enemies of man. Bull. ent. Soc. Amer. **7**, 117—119 (1961).

Forel, A.: Quelques observations biologiques sur les guêpes. Bull. Soc. Vaud. Nat. **31**, 312 (1895).

Foubert, E.L., Stier, R.A.: Antigenic relationship between honeybees, wasps, yellow hornets, black hornets and yellow jackets. J. Allergy **29**, 13—23 (1958).

Fox-Wilson, G.: Factors affecting populations of social wasps, *Vespula* species, in England. Proc. roy. ent. Soc. (Lond.) **21**, 17—27 (1946).

Frazier, C.A.: Ten points to remember in managing insect bite and sting reactions. Consultant April 1972.

Free, J.B., Raw, A., Williams, J.H.: Pollination of coconut (*Cocus nucifera* L.) in Jamaica by honeybees and wasps. Appl. Anim. Ethol. **1**, 213—223 (1975).

Friedman, E.A. Jr., Mascia, A.V.: The treatment of insect sting in children with Allpyral. Ann. Allergy **26**, 430—437 (1968).

Garresten, A.J.: Engangs aangetast door een schimmel. De Thee **4**, 91—92 (1923).

Gaul, A.T.: Experiments in housing vespine colonies, with notes on the homing and toleration instincts of certain species. Psyche, Cambridge **48**, 16—19 (1941).

Gaul, A.T.: Additions to vespine biology. XI Defence flight. Bull. Brooklyn ent. Soc. **48**, 35—37 (1953).

Geller, R.G., Yoshida, H., Beaven, M.A., Horakova, Z., Atkins, F.L., Yamabe, H., Pisano, J.J.: Pharmacologically active substances in venoms of the bald faced hornet, Vespula (*Dolichovespula) maculata*, and the yellow jacket *Vespula (Vespula) maculifrons*. Toxicon **14**, 27—33 (1976).

Gervet, J.: L'action des températures differentielles sur la monogynie fonctionelle chez les *Polistes* (Hyménoptera Vespides). Insectes Soc. **3**, 159—176 (1956).

Gervet, J.: Etude de l'effect de groupe sur la ponte dans la société polygyne de *Polistes gallicus* L. (Hyménoptères Vespides). Insectes Soc. **9**, 231—263 (1962).

Gervet, J.: Le comportement d'oophagie differentielle chez *Polistes gallicus* L. (Hymen. Vesp.). Insectes Soc. **11**, 21—40 (1964).

Gitter, S., Kochwa, S., Danon, D., de Vries, A.: Disc-sphere transformation and inhibition of rouleaux formation and sedimentation of human red blood cells induced by *Vipera xanthina palestinae* venom. Arch. int. Pharmacodyn. **118**, 350—357 (1959).

Grant, J.: Hummingbirds attacked by wasps. Canad. Fld. Nat. **73**, 174 (1959).

Green, E.E.: Rambling Notes by the Way. Spolia Zeylanica **2**, 194—197 (1905).

Guiglia, D.: Les guêpes sociales (Hymenoptera, Vespidae). Faune de l'Europe et du bassin méditerranèen. Paris: Masson et Cie, 1972.

Habermann, E.: Über die Wirkung tierischer Gifte auf Erythrozyten. Z. ges. exp. Med. **129**, 436–464 (1958).

Habermann, E.: Biochemie, Pharmakologie und Toxikologie der Inhaltsstoffe von Hymenopterengiften. Ergebn. Physiol. **60**, 220–325 (1968).

Habermann, E.: Chemistry, Pharmacology and Toxicology of Bee, Wasp and Hornet Venoms. In: Venomous Animals and their Venoms III, pp. 61–93, eds. W. Bücherl and E.E. Buckley. New York-London: Academic Press, 1971.

Habermann, E.: Bee and wasp venoms. Science **177**, 314–322 (1972).

Habermann, E., Neumann, W.: Die Hemmung der Hitzekoagulation von Eigelb durch Bienengift—ein Phospholipase-Effekt. Hoppe-Seylers Z. physiol. Chem. **297**, 179–193 (1954).

Halperin, L.: Über tödliche Wirkung der Bienen- und Wespenstiche. Inaugural Dissertation, Medizinische Fakultät, Universität Basel, 1936.

Hammad, S.M.: Morphology and history of the scent glands of *Vespa orientalis* F. and *Cataglyphis bicolor* F. Bull. Soc. ent. Egypte XLIX, 133–136 (1965).

Hattori, T., Yamane, S.: Notes on *Metoecus paradoxces* and *Metoecus vespa* parasitic on the *Vespula* species in northern Japan (Coleoptera, Rhipiphoridae; Hymenoptera, Vespidae) (I). New Entomologist **24**, 1–7 (1975).

Hecht, E., Slotta, C.H.: The chemical nature of the lipid activator of blood coagulation. Acta physiol. pharmacol. neerl. **10**, 278–279 (1962).

Hellmann, K., Hawkins, R.I.: Anticoagulant and fibrinolytic activities from *Rhodnius prolixus* Stal. Nature (Lond.) **201**, 1008–1010 (1964).

Hesse, E.: Wespenfeinde unter den Vögeln. Ornith. Monatsb. **24**, 3–4 (1916).

Hewett, H.W.: Battle between bees and wasps. J. Bombay nat. Hist. Soc. **4**, 312 (1889).

Hobby, B.M.: The prey of British Dragonflies. Trans. ent. Soc. S. Engl. **8**, 65–76 (1932).

Hoh, T.K., Soong, C.L., Cheng, C.T.: Fatal haemolysis from wasp and hornet sting. Singapore med. J. **7**, 122–126 (1966).

Holdstock, D.J., Mathias, A.P., Schachter, M.: A comparative study of kinin, kallidin and bradykinin. Brit. J. Pharmacol. **12**, 149–158 (1957).

Houssay, B.A.: Classification des actions des venins de serpents sur l'organisme animal. C.R. Soc. Biol. (Paris) **105**, 308–315 (1930).

Hurd, P.D.: The aculeate wasps. In: A century of progress in the nature sciences 1853–1953, pp. 573–575, ed. E.L. Kessel, San Francisco: California Acad. Sci., 1955.

Ikan, R., Bergmann, E.D., Ishay, J., Gitter, S.: Proteolytic enzyme activity in the various colony members of the Oriental hornet *Vespa orientalis*. Life Sci. **7**, 929–938 (1968a).

Ikan, R., Gottlieb, B., Bergmann, E.D.: Lipids of the queen of the Oriental hornet, *Vespa orientalis*. J. Insect Physiol. **15**, 1249–1257 (1969a).

Ikan, R., Gottlieb, R., Bergmann, E.D., Ishay, J.: Ubiquinones of the queens of the Oriental hornet (*Vespa orientalis*). J. Insect Physiol. **14**, 1215–1220 (1968b).

Ikan, R., Gottlieb, R., Bergmann, E.D., Ishay, J.: The pheromones of the Queen of the Oriental hornet *Vespa orientalis* L. J. Insect Physiol. **15**, 1709–1712 (1969b).

Ikan, R., Ishay, J.: The presence of cholesterol in the Oriental hornet *Vespa orientalis*. Steroids **6**, 101–103 (1965).

Ikan, R., Ishay, J.: Larval wasp secretion and honeydew of the Aphids *Chaitophorus populi* feeding on *Populus euphratica* as sources of sugars in the diet of the Oriental hornet *Vespa orientalis* L. Israel J. Zool. **15**, 64–68 (1966).

Ikan, R., Ishay, J.: Pteridines and purines of the queens of the Oriental hornet *Vespa orientalis*. J. Insect Physiol. **13**, 159–162 (1967).

Ikan, R., Ishay, J.: Free amino acids in hemolymph and venom of the Oriental hornet (*Vespa orientalis*). Comp. Biochem. Physiol. **44 B**, 949–953 (1973).

Ishay, J.: Observations sur la biologie de la Guêpe orientale *Vespa orientalis*. Insectes Soc. **11**, 193–206 (1964).

Ishay, J.: Entwicklung und Aktivität im Nest von *Vespa orientalis*. Dtsch. ent. Z. N.F. **12**, 397–419 (1965).

Ishay, J.: Observations on the behaviour of the different members of a colony of the Oriental hornet, *Vespa orientalis*. Ph. D. Thesis, Hebrew University, Jerusalem, 1967.

Ishay, J.: Kinin like substances in the saliva of larvae of wasps and hornets. J. Pharm. (Lond.) **24**, 747–748 (1972).

Ishay, J.: Thermoregulation by social wasps: Behavior and pheromones. Trans. N.Y. Acad. Sci. Ser. 2, **36**, 447—462 (1973).

Ishay, J.: Hornet Nest Architecture. Nature (Lond.) **253**, 41—42 (1975a).

Ishay, J.: Hyperglycemia produced by *Vespa orientalis* venom sac extract. Toxicon **13**, 221—226 (1975b).

Ishay, J.: Glucose levels in *Vespa orientalis:* the effect of starvation. Comp. Biochem. Physiol. **52A**, 91—96 (1975c).

Ishay, J.: Glycemic changes in social insect haemolymph (Hymenoptera). Comp. Biochem. Physiol. **52A**, 433—537 (1975d).

Ishay, J.: Comb building by *Vespa orientalis*. Anim. Behav. **24**, 72—83 (1976).

Ishay, J., Abraham, Z., Grunfeld, Y., Gitter, S.: Catecholamines in social wasps. Comp. Biochem. Physiol. **48A**, 369—373 (1974a).

Ishay, J., Bytinsky-Salz, H., Shulov, A.: Contributions to the bionomics of the Oriental hornet *Vespa orientalis*. Israel J. Ent. **2**, 45—106 (1967).

Ishay, J., Edery, H., Gitter, S., Rembold, H.: Pharmacological activity of various fractions of Oriental hornet (*Vespa orientalis*) venom. Israel J. med. Sci. **7**, 335 (1971a).

Ishay, J., Fischl, J., Gitter, S.: Investigation of wasp venom: Antigenic relationship. Acta pharmacol. (Kbh.) **31**, 71—74 (1972).

Ishay, J., Gitter, S., Fischl, J.: The production and effectivity of rabbit antiserum against *Vespa orientalis* venom. Acta allerg. (Kbh.) **26**, 286—290 (1971b).

Ishay, J., Gitter, S., Galun, R., Doron, M., Laron, Z.: The presence of insulin in and some effects of exogenous insulin on Hymenoptera tissues and body fluids. Comp. Biochem. Physiol. **54A**, 203—206 (1976).

Ishay, J., Goldberg, S., Ikan, R.: The lipids in *Vespa orientalis* larvae. Lipids **6**, 850—851 (1971c).

Ishay, J., Ikan, R., Bergmann, E.D.: The presence of pheromones in the Oriental hornet *Vespa orientalis*. J. Insect Physiol. **2**, 1307—1309 (1965).

Ishay, J., Lass, Y., Ben-Shachar, D., Gitter, S., Sandbank, U.: The effects of hornet venom sac extract on the electrical activity of the cat brain. Toxicon **12**, 159—166 (1974b).

Ishay, J., Nadler, E.Z., Gitter, S.: Pharmacological activity of *Paravespula germanica* wasp venom. Acta pharmacol. (Kbh.) **33**, 157—160 (1973).

Ishay, J., Ruttner, F.: Die Thermoregulation im Hornissennest. Z. vergl. Physiol. **72**, 423—434 (1971).

Ishay, J., Sadeh, D.: Direction finding of hornets under gravitational and centrifugal forces. Science **190**, 802—804 (1975).

Ishay, J., Shved, A., Gitter, S.: Toxicity of hornet venom as related to ontogenesis. Toxicon (in press).

Iwata, K.: Description of the nests of so called *Belonogaster griseus* var. *menelikii* (Gribodo) collected by Dr. K. Yamashita in Ethiopia, with a general consideration on the life of the genus (Hymenoptera, Vespidae). Mushi. **39**, 57—64 (1966).

Iwata, K.: Report of the fundamental research on the biological control of insect pests in Thailand. II. The report on the bionomics of subsocial wasps of Stenogastrinae (Hymenoptera, Vespidae). Nat. Life S.E. Asia. (Kira, T., and Iwata, K., eds.). **5**, pp. 259—293. Tokyo: Japan Soc. Promotion Sci., 1967.

Janet, C.: Observation sur les Guepes. Paris: Naud, 1903.

Janssen, W.: Plötzliche Todesfälle durch Insektenstiche. Morphologie, Toxikologie und forensische Bedeutung. Dtsch. Z. gerichtl. Med. **58**, 3—17 (1966).

Jany, Kl. D., Pfleiderer, G.: Purification and some physical properties of a chymotrypsin-like protease of the larva of the hornet, *Vespa orientalis*. Europ. J. Biochem. **42**, 419—428 (1974).

Jany, Kl. D., Tabatai, M.S., Pfleiderer, G.: Molecular weight determination of the chymotrypsin-like protease of the larvae of the hornet *Vespa orientalis*, by affinity of the active center. FEBS Lett. **48**, 53—55 (1974).

Jaques, R.: Vergleichende Fermentuntersuchungen an tierischen Giften (Cholinesterase, "Lecithinase", Hyaluronidase). Helv. physiol. Acta **13**, 113—120 (1955).

Jaques, R.: The hyaluronidase content of animal venoms. In: Venoms. Buckley, E.E. and Porges, N. (eds.). pp. 291—298, 1956. Washington: Amer. Ass. Advanc. Sci.

Jaques, R.: The protection afforded by a benzyl glucofuranoside and hydrocortisone against lethal wasp venom shock in guinea pigs. Pharmacology **2**, 21–25 (1969).

Jaques, R., Schachter, M.: The presence of histamine, 5-hydroxytryptamine and a potent, slow contracting substance in wasp venom. Brit. J. Pharmacol. **9**, 53–57 (1954).

Jeanne, R.L.: Note on a bat (*Phyloderma stenops*) preying upon the brood of a social wasp. J. Mammalogy **51**, 624–625 (1970).

Jeanne, R.L.: The adaptiveness of social wasp nest architecture. Quart. Rev. Biol. **50**, 267–287 (1975).

Johansson, S.A., Lundberg, A., Sjoberg, H.E.: Influence of heparin on thrombocytopenia in allergic reactions. Acta med. scand. **168**, 165–168 (1960).

Johnson, A.R., Erdös, E.G.: Release of histamine from mast cells by vasoactive peptides. Proc. Soc. exp. Biol. Med. (N.Y.) **142**, 1252–1256 (1973)

Joshua, H., Fischl, J., Henig, E., Ishay, J., Gitter, S.: Cytological, biochemical and bacteriological data on haemolymph of *Vespa orientalis*. Comp. Biochem. Physiol. **45 B**, 167–175 (1973).

Joshua, H., Ishay, J.: The haemolytic properties of the Oriental hornet venom. Acta pharmacol. (Kbh.) **33**, 42–52 (1973).

Joshua, H., Ishay, J.: The anti-coagulant properties of an extract from the venom sac of the oriental hornet. Toxicon **13**, 11–20 (1975).

Joshua, H., Ishay, J.: Factors affecting the hemolytic activity of *Vespa orientalis* venom and venom sac extracts. Proc. 5th int. Symp. Animal, Plant and Microbial Toxins, San Jose, Costa Rica, 1976 (in press).

Joshua, H., Ishay, J., Gitter, S., Edery, H.: Hemolytic activity of *Vespa orientalis* venom. Israel J. med. Sci. **7**, 703 (1971).

Kanwar, K.C., Kanwar, U.: Fine structure of the venom gland of *Vespa orientalis*. Toxicon **13**, 102–103 (1975).

Kanwar, K.C., Sethi, R.C.: Sudanophilic and PAS positive granules in venom gland of *Vespa orientalis*. Toxicon **9**, 179–182 (1971).

Kaplinsky, E., Ishay, J., Gitter, S.: Oriental hornet venom: effects on cardiovascular dynamics. Toxicon **12**, 69–73 (1974).

Kawai, N.: Actions of hornet venom on neuromuscular junctions. J. physiol. Soc. (Japan) **36**, 337 (1974).

Kawai, N., Hori, S.: Effects of hornet venom on lobster neuromuscular junctions. J. physiol. Soc. (Japan) **37**, 231 (1975).

Keele, C.A., Armstrong, D.: Substances producing pain and itch. London: Edward Arnold, 1964.

Kemper, H.: Über die Stiche der sozialen Faltenwespen und ihre Wirkung auf den Menschen. Z. angew. Zool. **49**, 351–382 (1962).

Kemper, H., Döhring, E.: Soziale Faltenwespen als Schädlinge des Obstbaues und des Obsthandels. Anz. Schädlingsk. XXXIV, 17–19 (1961).

Kemper, H., Döhring, E.: Untersuchungen über die Ernährung sozialer Faltenwespen Deutschlands, insbesondere von *P. germanica* und *P. vulgaris*. Z. angew. Zool. **49**, 227–280 (1962).

Kemper, H., Döhring, E.: Die sozialen Faltenwespen Mitteleuropas. Berlin: Paul Parey, 1967.

Kern, F., Sobotka, A.K., Valentine, M.D., Benton, A.W., Lichtenstein, L.M.: Allergy to insect sting. III. Allergenic cross-reactivity among the vespid venoms. J. Allergy clin. Immunol. **57**, 554–559 (1976).

Kessler, A.: Bee and wasp stings (Review). Harefuah **89**, 572–575 (1975).

Klibansky, Ch., de Vries, A.: Quantitative study of erythrocyte-lysolecithin interaction. Biochim. biophys. Acta **70**, 176–187 (1963).

Kloft, W., Schneider, P.: Gruppenverteidigungsverhalten bei wildlebenden Bienen (*Apis cerana* F.) in Afghanistan. Naturwissenschaften **56**, 219 (1970).

Koschevnikov, G.: Zur Kenntnis der Hautdrüsen der Apidae und Vespidae. Anat. Anz. **15**, 519–528 (1899).

Kugler, J.: Examens des nids de guêpes. MSc. Thesis, Hebrew University, Jerusalem, 1938 (in Hebrew).

Kugler, J., Orion, T., Ishay, J.: The number of ovarioles in the Vespinae (Hymenoptera). Insectes Soc. (in press).

Kuhlhorn, F.: Über das Verhalten sozialer Faltenwesepen (Hymenoptera: Vespidae) beim Stall-
    einflug, innerhalb von Viehställen und beim Fliegenfang. Z. angew. Zool. **48**, 405—422
    (1961).
Langer, J.: Über das Gift unserer Honigbiene. Naunyn-Schmiedeberg's Arch. exp. Path. Phar-
    mak. 381—419 (1897).
Langlois, C., Shulman, S., Arbesman, C.E.: The allergic response to stinging insects. J. Allergy
    36, 109—120 (1965).
Langlois, C., Shulman, S., Kozmycz, S., Arbesman, C.E.: Allergic response to stinging insects.
    VI. Fractionation of whole-body and venom sac extracts of wasp. J. Allergy **37**, 359—365
    (1966).
Lass, Y., Ishay, J., Ben-Shachar, D., Edery, H., Gitter, S.: Effects of the Oriental hornet
    (*Vespa orientalis*) venom on the nervous tissue electrical activity. Israel J. med. Sci. **7**,
    335 (1971).
Leclercq, M.: Les Problèmes concernant les piqûres d'Hyménoptères (Abeilles, Guêpes) Venins,
    Accidents, Thérapeutique. Gaz. Sanitaria (ed. française) **XVI**, 70—75 (1967).
Leclercq, M.: Les intoxications et les accidents allergiques provoqués par les insectes et acariens
    en Belgique. Rev. méd. Liège **XXVIII**, 531—537 (1973).
Leclercq, M., Fischer, P., Lecomte, J.: Nouvelle propriété des venins d'une guêpe et d'une
    abeille. Arch. int. Physiol. **LVII** 241—244 (1949).
Lecomte, J., Bourdon, V., Damas, J., Leclercq, M., Leclercq, J.: Présence de noradrenaline
    conjuguée dans les parois du nid de *Vespula germanica* Linné. C.R. Soc. Biol. (Paris)
    170, 212—215 (1976).
Lecomte, J., Leclercq, M.: Sur la mort provoquée par les piqûres d'Hyménoptères Aculéates.
    Bull. Acad. roy. Med. Belg. **128**, 615—693 (1973).
Lev, R., Spicer, S.S.: Specific staining of sulphate groups with Alcian blue at low pH. J.
    Histochem. Cytochem. **12**, 309 (1964).
Lichtenstein, L.M., Valentine, M.D., Sobotka, A.K.: A case for venom treatment in anaphylac-
    tic sensitivity to Hymenoptera sting. New Engl. J. Med. **290**, 1223—1227 (1974).
Lindauer, M.: Social behaviour and mutual communication. In: The physiology of Insects,
    pp. 123—186, ed. M. Rockstein, New York: Academic Press, 1965.
Lomer, R., Boquet, P., Izard, Y.: Sensibilité insolite et hypersensibilité aux venins des hyménop-
    tères. Presse méd. **66**, 1887—1888 (1958).
Loveless, M.H., Fackler, W.R.: Wasp venom allergy and immunity. Ann. Allergy **14**, 347—366
    (1956).
MacDonald, J.F., Akre, R.D., Hill, W.B.: Attraction of yellow jackets (*Vespula* spp.) to
    heptyl butyrate in Washington State (Hymenoptera-Vespidae). Environ. Ent. **2**, 375—379
    (1973).
MacDonald, J.F., Akre, R.D., Hill, W.B.: Comparative biology and behavior of *Vespula*
    atropilosa and *V. pennsylvanica* (Hymenoptera Vespidae). Melanderia **18**, 1—16 (1974).
MacDonald, J.F., Matthews, R.W.: *Vespula squamosa*: A Yellow-Jacket Wasp Evolving To-
    wards Parasitism. Science **190**, 1004—1005 (1975).
Mann, G.T., Bates, H.R.: The pathology of insect bites: a brief review of eleven fatal cases.
    Sth. med. J. (Bgham, Ala.) **53**, 1399—1406 (1960).
Marshall, T.K.: Wasp and bee stings. Practitioner **178**, 712—722 (1957).
Maschwitz, U.: Gefahrenalarmstoffe und Gefahrenalarmierung bei sozialen Hymenopteren.
    Z. vergl. Physiol. **47**, 596—655 (1964).
Maschwitz, U.: Das Speichelsekret der Wespenlarven und seine biologische Bedeutung. Z.
    vergl. Physiol. **53**, 228—252 (1966a).
Maschwitz, U.: Alarm substances and alarm behavior in social insects. Vitam. and Horm.
    24, 267—290 (1966b).
Maschwitz, U.W.J., Kloft, W.: Venomous insects: Morphology and function of the venom
    apparatus of insects—Bees, Wasps, Ants and Caterpillars. In: Venomous Animals and
    their Venoms III, pp. 1—60, eds. W. Bücherl and E.E. Buckley, New York-London:
    Academic Press, 1971.
Mason, C.W., Maxwell-Lefroy, H.: The food of birds in India. Mem. Dept. Agric. India,
    Ent. Ser. **3**, 1—371 (1912).
Matsuura, M., Sakagami, Sh.F.: A bionomic sketch of the giant hornet *Vespa mandarinia*,

a serious pest for Japanese apiculture. J. Fac. Sci. Hokkaido Univ. Series VI **19**, 125—162 (1973).

McCormick, W.F.: Fatal anaphylactic reactions to wasp stings. Amer. J. clin. Path. **39**, 485—491 (1963).

McGovern, T.P., Davis, H.G., Beroza, M., Ingangi, J.C., Eddy, G.W.: Esters highly attractive to *Vespula* spp. J. econ. Ent. **63**, 1534—1536 (1970).

Meer Mohr, J.C. van der: Insecten die door de Karo-Bataks gegeten morden. Trop. Nat. **30**, 41—47 (1941).

Meeuse, B.J.D.: The story of pollination. New York: Ronald Press 1961.

Melinossi, R.: Morphologia dell'apparato velenifero degli imenotteri vulneranti. Industrie Grafische V, Lischie Figli XIII, 1—43 (1935).

Michl, H.: Presence of pipecolic acid in venoms from snakes and wasps. Monatsh. Chem. **88**, 701—702 (1957).

Miller, C.D.F.: Taxonomy and distribution of Nearctic *Vespula*. Canad. Entomologist **93**, 1—52 (1961).

Miller, D.G. Jr.: Massive anaphylaxis from insect stings. In: Venoms. Buckley, E.E. and Porges, N. (eds.). Washington: Amer. Ass. Advanc. Sci., 1956.

Montagner, H.: Le mechanisme et les conséquences des comportements trophallactiques chez les guêpes du genre *Vespa*. Thèse, Faculté des Sciences de l'Université de Nancy, France, 1966.

Murray, A.: Note on *Rhipiphorus paradoxus*. Ann. Mag. nat. Hist. **6**, 204—213 (1870).

Nakayima, T.: On the third active peptide on smooth muscle in the skin of *Rana ingromaculata* Hallowell. Chem. pharm. Bull. **16**, 2088 (1968).

Naumann, M.G.: A revision of the genus *Brachygastra* (Hymenoptera: Vespidae). Kansas Univ. Bull. **47**, 929—1003 (1968).

Neumann, W., Habermann, E.: Zur papierelektrophoretischen Fraktionierung tierischer Gifte. Naturwissenschaften **39**, 286—287 (1952).

Neumann, W., Habermann, E.: Beiträge zur Charakterisierung der Wirkstoffe des Bienengiftes. Naunyn-Schmiedeberg's Arch. exp. Path. Pharmak. **222**, 367—373 (1954).

Newport, G.: On the predaceous habits of the common wasp, *Vespa vulgaris* L. Trans. ent. Soc. (Lond.) **1**, 228—229 (1836).

Nosenko, N.M.: Sershni-opasnie Khischchniki pchel. Pchelovodstvo **40**, 28—30 (1963).

O'Connor, R., Rosenbrook, W., Erickson, R.: Hymenoptera: Pure venom from bees, wasps and hornets. Science **139**, 420 (1963).

Okada, J.: Notes on the habit of giant hornet (*Vespa mandarinia*, Smith) as a noxious insect against honeybee. Bull. Fac. Agric. Tamagana Univ. **2**, 73—89 (1961).

Owen, M.D.: Insect Venoms: Identification of dopamine and noradrenaline in wasp and bee stings. Experientia (Basel) **27**, 544—545 (1971).

Pardi, L.: Richerche sui Polistini. 1. Poliginia vera ed apparente in *Polistes gallicus* L. P.V. Soc. Tosc. Sci. nat. **49**, 3—9 (1940).

Pardi, L.: Dominance order in *Polistes* wasps. Physiol. Zool. **21**, 1—13 (1948).

Pardi, L.: Richerche sui Polistini. 12. Studio della attività della divisione di lavoro in una società di *Polistes gallicus* L. dopo la comparsa delle operaie. Arch. Zool. ital. **36**, 363—431 (1951).

Pardi, L., Cavalcanti, M.: Esperienze sul meccanismo della monoginia funzionale in *Polistes gallicus* L. (Hymenoptera. Vespidae). Bull. Zool. **18**, 247—252 (1951).

Pardi, L., Piccioli, M.T.M.: Studi sulla biologia di *Belangogaster* (Hymenoptera Vespidae) 2. Differenziamento castale incipiente in *B. griseus* F. Monitore Zool. ital. N.S. Suppl. **3**, 235—265 (1970).

Parrish, H.M.: Deaths from bites and stings of venomous animals and insects in the United States. Arch. intern. Med. **104**, 198—207 (1959).

Parrish, H.M.: Analysis of 460 fatalities from venomous animals in the United States. Amer. J. med. Sci. **245**, 129—141 (1963).

Pavan, M.: Gli insetti come fonte di prodotti biologicamente attivi. Chimica e l'Industria, **XXXVII**, 714—724 (1955).

Pawlowski, E.N.: Gifttiere und ihre Giftigkeit. Jena: Fischer, 1927.

Perlman, E.: Near fatal allergic reactions to bee and wasp stings: a review and report of seven cases. J. Mt Sinai Hosp. **22**, 336—348 (1955).

Pisano, J.J.: Vasoactive peptides in venoms. Fed. Proc. **27**, 58–62 (1968).

Pisano, J.J.: Kinins of Non-Mammalian Origin. In: Bradykinin, Kallidin and Kallikrein. Handb. exp. Pharmakol. XXV, pp. 589–596. Erdös, E.G. (ed.). Berlin-Heidelberg-New York: Springer, 1970.

Poinar, G.O., Ennik, F.: The use of *Neoplectana carpocapsae* (Steinernematidae: Rhabditoidea) against adult yellow jackets (*Vespula* spp., Vespidae: Hymenoptera). J. Invertebr. Path. **19**, 331–340 (1972).

Pora, E.A., Stoicovici, F.: The effects of strophantin and of the venom of the wasp *Crabro* on the melanophores of *Carassius carassius*. Acad. Rep. Populare Romane, Bul. Stiint. **A1**, 767–775 (1949).

Potter, N.B.: Some aspects of the biology of *Vespula vulgaris* L. Ph. D. Thesis, University of Bristol, 1965.

Prado, J.L., Tamura, Z., Furano, E., Pisano, J.J., Udenfriend, S.: Characterization of kinins in wasp venom. In: Hypotensive Peptides, pp. 93–104, eds. E.G. Erdös, N. Back and F. Sicuteri. Berlin-Heidelberg-New York: Springer, 1966.

Rau, P.: The reconstruction of destroyed nest by *Polistes* wasps. Psyche **35**, 151–152 (1928).

Rau, P., Rau, N.: Wasp studies afield. Princeton: Princeton University Press, 1918.

Richards, O.W.: A revision of the genus *Mischocyttarus* de Saussure. Trans. roy. ent. Soc. (Lond.) **95**, 295–462 (1945).

Richards, O.W.: The biology of the social wasps (Hymenoptera, Vespidae). Biol. Rev. **46**, 483–528 (1971).

Richards, O.W., Richards, M.J.: Observations of the social wasps of South America (Hymenoptera, Vespidae). Trans. roy. ent. Soc. (Lond.) **102**, 1–170 (1951).

Rivnay, E., Bytinsky-Salz, H.: The Oriental hornet (*Vespa orientalis* L.) its biology in Israel. Bull. Agric. Res. Sta. Rechovot **52**, 36–42 (1949).

Rosenberg, P.: Effects of venoms on the squid giant axon. Toxicon **3**, 125–131 (1965).

Rosenberg, P., Ishay, J., Gitter, S.: Phospholipase activity of venom and venom apparatus of *Vespa orientalis*. Proc. 5th int. Symp. Animal, Plant and Microbial Toxins, San Jose, Costa Rica, 1976 (in press).

Rosenfeld, G., Nahas, L., Kelen, E.M.A.: Coagulant, Proteolytic and Hemolytic Properties of some Snake Venoms. In: Venomous Animals and Their Venoms, Vol. 1, Venomous Vertebrates, pp. 229–273, Bücherl, W., Buckley, E.E., and Deulofeu, V. (eds.). New York-London: Academic Press, 1968.

Rothney, G.A.Y.: Squirrel versus hornet (*Vespa cincta*). Ent. M. Mag. **13**, 254–255 (1877).

Roy, A.C.: Lecithin and venom hemolysis. Nature (Lond.) **155**, 171–174 (1945).

Ryan, J.W., Roblero, J., Stewart, J.M.: Inactivation of bradykinin in rat lung. In: Bradykinin and related Kinins – Cardiovascular. Biochemical and Neural actions. pp. 263–271, eds. F. Sicuteri, M. Rocha e Silva and N. Back, New York: Plenum Press 1970.

Said, E.E.: Enzymological study of the venom of *Polistes omissa* Weyr. Bull. Soc. ent. Egypte **XLIV**, 167–170 (1960).

Sakagami, Sh.F.: Preliminary report on the specific difference of behaviour and other ecological characters between European and Japanese honey bees. Acta hymenopt. **1**, 171–198 (1960).

Sakagami, Sh. F., Fukushima, K.: Some biological observations on a hornet *Vespa tropica* var *pulchra* (du Buysson), with special reference to its dependence on *Polistes* wasps. Treubia **24**, 73–82 (1957).

Sakagami, Sh. F., Yoshikawa, K.: A new ethospecies of *Stenogaster* wasps from Sarawak, with a comment on the value of ethological characters in animal taxonomy. Ann. zool. Soc. Japan **41**, 77–84 (1968).

Sandbank, U., Ishay, J., Gitter, S.: Mitochondrial changes in the guinea pig muscle after envenomation with *Vespa orientalis* Venom. Experientia (Basel) **27**, 303–304 (1971).

Sandbank, U., Ishay, J., Gitter, S.: Kidney changes in mice due to Oriental hornet (*Vespa orientalis*) Venom: Histological and Electron Microscopical Study. Acta pharmacol. (Kbh.) **32**, 442–448 (1973).

Saslavsky, H., Ishay, J., Ikan, R.: Alarm substances as toxicants in the Oriental hornet colony. Life Sci. **12**, 135–144 (1973).

Schachter, M.: Discovery of Non-Mammalian Kinins. In: Bradykinin, Kallidin and Kallikrein.

Handb. exp. Pharmakol. XXV, pp. 585–588. Erdös, E.G. (ed.). Berlin-Heidelberg-New York: Springer, 1970.

Schachter, M., Thain, E.M.: Chemical and pharmacological properties of the potent, slow contracting substance (kinin) in wasp venom. Brit. J. Pharmacol. **9**, 352–359 (1954).

Schmidt, H. von: Durch Insekten hervorgerufene Krankheiten. Stuttgart 1949, quoted by Kemper (1962).

Schneider, P., Djalal, A.S.: Vorkommen und Haltung der östlichen Honigbiene (*Apis cerana* F.) in Afghanistan. Apidologie **1**, 329–343 (1970).

Schremmer, F.: Bemerkenswerte Wechselbeziehungen zwischen Orchideenblüten und Insekten. Natur u. Volk **91**, 52–61 (1961).

Schremmer, F.: Wespen und Hornissen. Wittenberg Lutherstadt: A. Ziemsen, 1962.

Schremmer, F.: Beobachtungen zur Biologie von *Apoica pallida* (Olivier, 1791) einer neotropischen sozialen Faltenwespe (Hymenoptera, Vespidae). Insectes Soc. **19**, 343–357 (1972).

Schröder, E., Hempel, R.: Bradykinin, kallidin and their synthetic analogues. Experientia (Basel) **20**, 529–536 (1964).

Seguy, E.A.: Dipteres-Brachyceres, Asilidae etc. Faune de France **17**, Paris: P. Lechevalier, 1927.

Settipane, G.A., Hopson, C.N.: Hymenoptera allergy: precipitin and passive cutaneous anaphylaxis tests in human and rabbit sera. Acta allerg. (Kbh.) **26**, 121–130 (1971).

Shilkin, K.B.: The effect of hornet venom on human striated muscle. Proc. 2nd int. Cong. Muscle Diseases, Perth, Australia, pp. 136–139, Excerpta Medica, Amsterdam, 1971.

Shilkin, K.B., Chen, B.T.M., Khoo, O.T.: Rhabdomyolysis Caused by Hornet Venom. Brit. med. J. **1**, 156–157 (1972).

Shulman, S.: Allergic responses to insects. Ann. Rev. Ent. **12**, 323–346 (1967).

Shulman, S., Langlois, C., Arbesman, C.E.: The Allergic Response to Stinging Insects. J. Allergy **35**, 446–463 (1964).

Sicuteri, F., Franchi, P.L., Del Bianco, P.L., Fanciullacci, M.: Some physiological and pathological roles of kininogen and kinins. In: Hypotensive Peptides. Erdös, E.G., Back, N., and Sicuteri, F. (eds.). Berlin-Heidelberg-New York: Springer 1966, pp. 522–533.

Simon, R.P., Benton, A.W.: A method for mass collecting of wasp venoms. Ann. ent. Soc. Amer. **62**, 277–278 (1969).

Slor, H., Ring, B., Ishay, J.: Nucleases of the Oriental hornet (*Vespa orientalis*) venom sac extract – I. Acid, neutral and alkaline deoxyribonucleases and their pharmacological effects on cat blood *in vitro*. Toxicon (in press).

Smith, F.G.: Beekeeping in the tropics. London: Longmans, 1960.

Snodgrass, R.E.: Anatomy of the Honey Bee. London: Constable 1956.

Sobotka, A.K., Valentine, M.D., Benton, A.W., Lichtenstein, L.M.: Allergy to insect stings. J. Allergy clin. Immunology, **53**, 170–184 (1974).

Somerville, R., Till, D., Leclercq, M., Lecomte, J.: Les morts par piqûre d'hyménoptères aculeates en Angleterre et au pays de Galles. Rev. med. Liège **XXX**, 76–78 (1975).

Sonneborn, H., Pfleiderer, H., Ishay, J.: Zur Evolution der Endopeptidasen. VII: Eine Protease von Molekulargewicht 12500 aus Larven von *Vespa orientalis*, mit chymotryptischen Eigenschaften. Hoppe-Seylers Z. physiol. Chem. **350**, 389–395 (1969).

Sonon, J.: Specific names and observations of some Formosan wasps. Trans. nat. Hist. Soc. Formosa **89**, 121–138 (1927) (in Japanese).

Spradbery, J.P.: Wasps. London: Sidgwick and Jackson, 1973.

Stewart, J.M.: Synthesis and pharmacology of *Polistes* kinin, a bradykinin homolog. Fed. Proc. **27**, 534 (1968).

Stokke, D.B.: Anafylaktisk shock efter hvepsestik. Ugeskr. Laeg. **135**, 1244–1245 (1973).

Stone, S.: Scarcity of wasps. Zoologist **23**, 9757 (1865).

Strauss, W.T.: Clinical Notes, Suggestions and New Instruments, Antihistamine Therapy of Bee Stings. J. Amer. med. Ass. **140**, 603–604 (1949).

Subbiah, M.S., Mehadevan, V.: *Vespa cincta* Fabr. A predator of the hive bees and its control. Indian J. vet. Sci. **27**, 153–154 (1957).

Sugiyama, M.: Physiological analysis of the cortical response of the sea urchin egg to stimulating or non-propagating nature of the cortical changes induced by various reagents. Biol. Bull. **104**, 216–223 (1953).

Swammerdam, J.: Bibel der Natur, Leipzig, 1752.

Tan, H.K., Chew, L.S., Chao, T.C.: Fatal haemolysis from wasp and hornet sting. Singapore med. J. **7**, 122—127 (1966).

Thomas, C.R.: The European Wasp (*Vespula germanica* F.) in New Zealand. Inf. Ser. Dep. Sci. ind. Res. N.Z., **27**, 1—73 (1960).

Toumanoff, C.: Les ennemies des abeilles, Hanoi: Imprim. d'Extreme-Orient, 1939.

Udenfriend, S., Nakajima, T., Pisano, J.J.: Structure of the major kinin in wasp (*Polistes*) venom. Proc. 7th int. Cong. Biochem. VIII-4, 501 (1967).

Vecht, J. van der: The Vespinae of the Indo-Malayan and Papuan areas (Hymenoptera, Vespidae). Zool. Verh. Leiden **34**, 1—83 (1957).

Vecht, J. van der: Notes on Oriental Vespidae, including some species from China and Japan (Hymenoptera, Vespidae). Zool. Meded. R. Mus. nat. Hist. Leiden **36**, 205—232 (1959).

Vecht, J. van der: The Indo-Australian species of genus *Ropalidia* (*Icaria*) (Hymenoptera, Vespidae) (2nd. pt.). Zool. Verh. **57**, 1—72 (1962).

Vecht, J. van der: The East-Asiatic and Indo-Australian species of *Polybioides Buysson* and *Parapolybia saussure*. Zool. Verh. **82**, 1—42 (1966).

Viewig, K.: Wespen als Fliegenvertilger. Illust. Woch. Ent. **1**, 579 (1896).

Wafa, A.K.: Ecological investigations on the activity of the Oriental hornet, *Vespa orientalis*. Bull. Fac. Agric. Cairo Univ. **103**, 35—43 (1956).

Wafa, A.K., El-Borolossy, F.M., Sharkawi, S.G.: Control work of *Vespa orientalis* F. Bull. ent. Soc. Egypt, Econ. **Ser. III**, 9—16 (1969).

Wafa, A.K., Sharkawi, S.G.: Contribution to the biology of *Vespa orientalis*. Bull. Soc. Ent. Egypte LVI, 219—226 (1972).

Wagner, R.E.: Control of the yellow jacket, *Vespula pennsylvanica*, in Public Parks. J. econ. Ent. **54**, 628—630 (1961).

Wagner, R.E., Reierson, D.A.: Yellow Jacket Control by Baiting. 1. Influence of Toxicants and Attractants on Bait Acceptance. J. econ. Ent. **62**, 1192—1197 (1969).

Watanabe, M., Yasuhara, T., Nakajima, T.: New Bradykinin analogues in wasp (*Polistes rothneyi iwatai*) venom. Toxicon **13**, 131 (1975).

Watanabe, M., Yasuhara, T., Nakajima, T.: Occurrence of Thr[6]-Bradykinin and its Analogous Peptide in the Venom of *Polistes rothneyi iwatai* V. der Vecht. In: Animal, Plant and Microbial Toxins II, p. 105, ed. Y. Sawai. New York, London: Plenum 1976.

Wegelin, C.: Anatomische Befunde bei tödlichem Bienen- und Wespenstich. Schweiz. med. Wschr. **78**, 1253—1254 (1948).

Welsh, J.H., Batty, C.S.: 5-Hydroxytryptamine content of some arthropod venoms and venom containing parts. Toxicon **1**, 165—173 (1963).

Welsh, J.H., King, E.C.: Catecholamines in planarians. Comp. Biochem. Physiol. **36**, 683—688 (1970).

West (Eberhard), M.J.: Foundress association in polistine wasps: dominance hierarchies and the evolution of social behavior. Science **157**, 1584—1585 (1967).

Weyrauch, W.K.: Wie entsteht ein Wespennest. I. Teil, Beobachtungen und Versuche über Papierbereitungsinstinkt bei *Vespa, Dolichovespula* und *Macrovespula*. Z. Morph. Ökol. Tiere **30**, 401—431 (1935).

Williams, F.X.: Philippine wasp studies. II. Descriptions of new species and life history. Bull. Exper. Station, Hawaiian Sugar Planters Ass. Ent. Ser. **14**, 19—184 (1919).

Willinck, A.: Los véspidos sociales Argentinos, con exclusión del género Mischocyttarus (Hym., Vespidae). Acta Zool. Lilloana del Inst. "Miguel Lillo" Tucumán, Argentina **10**, 105—151 (1952).

Willinck, A.: Las especias Argentinas de "*Mischocyttarus*" de saussure (Hym., Vespidae). Acta Zool. Lilloana del Inst. "Miguel Lillo" Tucumán, Argentina **14**, 317—340 (1953).

Wilson, E.O.: The Insect Societies. Cambridge, Mass.: Harvard Univ. Press, 1971.

Wong, H.B.: Haemoglobinuria in Singapore. Singapore med. J. **2**, 74—78 (1961).

Wong, II.B.: Wasp and bee stings in children. J. Singapore pediat. Soc. **12**, 126—134 (1970).

Yamane, S.: Taxonomic Notes of the Subgenus *Boreovespula* Blüthgen (Hymenoptera, Vespidae) of Japan, with Notes on Specimens from Sakhalin. Kontyu, Tokyo **43**, 343—355 (1975).

Yarrow, I.H.H.: Hymenoptera (ants, bees and wasps). In: Insects and Other Arthropods of Medical Importance, pp. 409—411, ed. K.G.V. Smith, London: The Trustees of the British Museum (Natural History), 1973.

Yoshida, H., Geller, R.G., Pisano, J.J.: Vespulakinins: new carbohydrate-containing bradyki-nin derivatives. Biochemistry **15**, 61—64 (1976).

Yoshida, H., Pisano, J.J.: *Vespula* Kinin; A new carbohydrate-containing bradykinin analogue. Toxicon **13**, 113 (1975).

Yoshikawa, K.: Ecological studies of *Polistes* wasp. 5. Behaviour of *Polistes* wasps in late autumn—with reference to their mating behaviour. Akitu **8**, 50—56 (1959).

Yoshikawa, K.: Introductory studies on the life economy of polistine wasps. II. Geographical distribution and its ecological significances. J. Biol. Osaka City Univ. **13**, 19—43 (1962).

Yoshikawa, K.: Predatory hunting wasps as the natural enemies of insect pests in Thailand. In: Nat. Life S.E. Asia. (Kira, T., and Iwata, K., eds.). **3**, pp. 391—398. Tokyo: Jap. Soc. Promotion Sci. 1964.

Yoshikawa, K., Ohgushi, R., Sakagami, Sh.F.: Preliminary report on entomology of the Osaka City University 5th Scientific expedition to Southeast Asia. In: Nat. Life S.E. Asia. (Kira, T., and Iwata, K., eds.) **6**, pp. 153—182. Tokyo: Jap. Soc. Promotion Sci. 1969.

Zikan, J.F.: O gênero Mischocyttarus saussure (Hymenoptera, Vespidae) com a descrição de 82 espécies novas. Boletim Parque Nacional do Itatiáia, Rio de Janeiro **1**, 1—251 (1949).

Zimmermann, K.: Zur Systematik der palearktischen *Polistes* (Hym. Vesp.). Mitt. zool. Mus. Berlin **15**, 609—621 (1930).

Zimmermann, K.: Studien über individuelle und geographische Variabilität palearktischer *Polistes* und verwandter Vespiden. Z. Morph. Ökol. Tiere **22**, 173—230 (1931).

CHAPTER 24

Venoms of Braconidae

R.L. Beard

Introduction

Small in size, docile in behavior, some braconid wasps, as parasitoids, inactivate prey many times their size with tranquilizing drugs so potent that even minute amounts are far greater than necessary for the effect. This they do with a distinctive stinging injection apparatus (Figs. 1, 2).

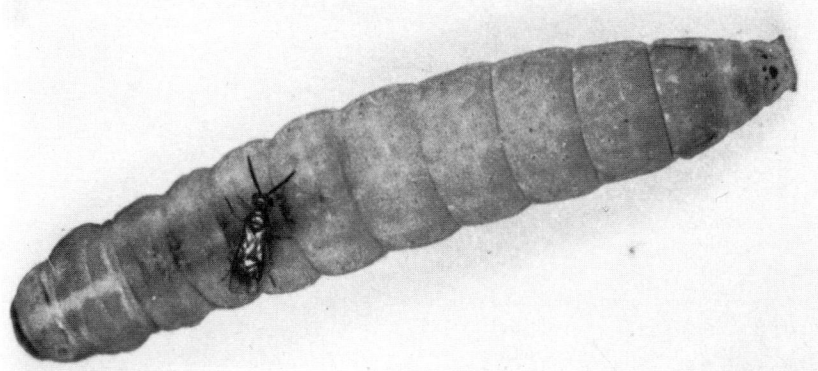

Fig. 1. *Bracon hebetor* female on larva of *Galleria mellonella*

Braconids are not alone in their use of paralyzing venoms to facilitate feeding and oviposition (Beard, 1963, 1971a; Piek and Simon Thomas, 1969). Such venoms have no simple taxonomic distribution. They occur in different families of Hymenoptera and are not a common attribute of all members of one family. This means that the evolutionary development of this system is complicated and cannot be traced until a biochemical profile of the venoms and a comparative morphology of the stinging apparatus of these taxa become revealed.

The selective advantage of the system would seem to be great inasmuch as it appears to be an easy means of acquiring a blood meal from a quiescent host and of depositing eggs that will not be dislodged by movement or molting, and that the paralyzed host will stay "fresh" for nurture of the offspring.

As compared with other solitary wasps, braconids are easy to rear, and the potency of their venom so compensates for the small size of the insect that they have attracted much investigative interest.

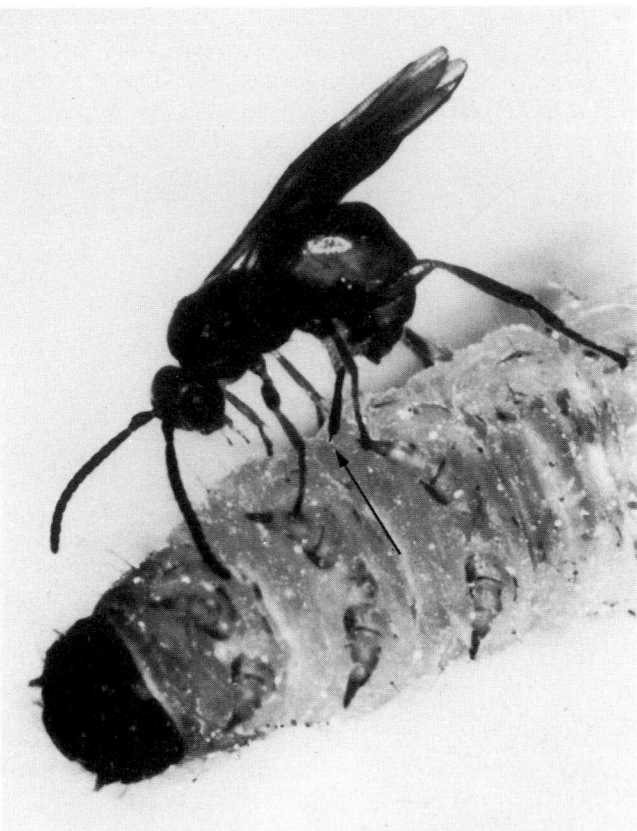

Fig. 2. *Bracon hebetor* stinging larva of *Anagasta kühniella*. Arrow points to sting. From RATH-
MAYER and WALTHER (1975)

The role of stinging in these wasps in securing food for themselves and offspring
must be viewed as offensive rather than defensive, as is the role of stinging attributed
to social Hymenoptera. In contrast to the latter, braconid wasps appear to be
incapable of stinging vertebrate animals.

A. Parasitism by Braconidae

The family Braconidae, the biology of which has been reviewed by MATTHEWS
(1974), is one of the major groups of insect parasitoids and includes many species
that exert a definite check upon the increase of numerous important plant pests.
Parasitism by Braconidae may be either internal or external, and modifications
in habit in this regard are correlated with the host stages subject to attack. In
general, internal parasitism occurs if the hosts are free-living, as illustrated by
the adult beetles attacked by the Euphorinae and others, the foliage-feeding lepidopterous larvae parasitized by Microgasterinae, Meteorinae, and others, and the

aphids, parasitized by the Aphidinae. External parasitism on the other hand predominates in hosts that live in confined quarters, such as the caterpillars in tunnels and leaf rolls attacked by the Vipioninae. Parasitoids of larvae of bark and wood-boring Coleoptera also develop in this way. Exceptions to this are the Cheloninae, Triaspinae, and Macrocentrinae which are internal parasitoids of hosts that occur in burrows or cavities in plant stems, fruits, and seeds (CLAUSEN, 1940; other relationships are discussed by CAPEK, 1965, 1971; ASKEW, 1971).

I. Stinging and Parasitism

Stinging to effect host paralysis is correlated with parasitoid life style. In general, internal parasitoids seldom even temporarily paralyze their free-living hosts. Typical of these is *Apanteles melanoscelus* Ratz., a parasitoid of the gypsy moth larva (*Porthetria dispar* (L.)). This braconid lacks the typical braconid venom apparatus and oviposits with great rapidity by inserting its ovipositor through the integument. The host only responds, presumably to the mechanical stimulus, by a momentary flexure.

It is among the external parasitoids, those that customarily attack hosts in cells, leaf rolls, burrows, or beneath a web or other covering, that the paralyzing action is to be found. This relationship is not truly based on a need of restriction for attack to occur, for host larvae removed from their habitat and exposed experimentally to parasitoids may often be stung without difficulty.

No one has demonstrated any gross effect of braconid venom experimentally (WINTERINGHAM, 1969; BEARD et al., unpubl.).

II. Paralysis of Hosts

Host paralysis resulting from braconid stinging may be temporary in some species, permanent in others.

Temporary paralysis as a physiologic event has not been studied critically, and in fact, its transitory nature makes study difficult. One example suffices to illustrate this type of parasitoid action. *Alysia manducator* Panz. parasitizes blowfly larvae such as *Sarcophaga, Lucilia,* or *Calliphora.* Attack upon a maggot is accompanied by violent writhing of the larva, apparently evoked by the actual entrance of the ovipositor (MYERS, 1927). This activity is stopped with remarkable suddenness, presumably by action of injected venom, and the maggot lies inert, usually with the head somewhat retracted. The parasitoid lays an egg, withdraws its ovipositor, and does not feed at the oviposition puncture. Paralysis lasts about half a minute, after which with little premonitory movement, the larvae begins to wriggle almost as violently as at the moment of attack. During paralysis there is no perceptible heartbeat, but normal rate of beat resumes when the postparalysis struggling begins. Repetition of attack upon the same individual may result in death, possibly (but questionably) from venom effects. This venom action differs significantly from the permanent paralyzants by its prompt action on both the bodily movement and heartbeat. A similar prompt paralysis was reported (FULTON, 1933) for Angoumois grain moths stung by *Habrocytus cerealellae.*

Other braconids causing temporary paralysis were listed by PIEK and SIMON THOMAS (1969) and include *Microbracon pini* Mues., *Cosmophorus henscheli* Ruschka, and *Apanteles glomeratus* L.

Perhaps a different type of paralysis occurs in larvae of *Dendroctonus monticolae* Hopk. parasitized by the braconid *Coeloides dendroctoni* Cushman (DELEON, 1935). This host must be in a burrow for attack to occur, and it is not certain that stinging precedes the laying of eggs externally. Nevertheless within 2 days after attack, the host larva becomes inactive, appears paralyzed, and dies a day later. This long delayed "paralysis" may actually be the result of wasp larval feeding or simply a mechanical puncture. Another example of long delayed paralysis was noted by MUNRO (1917) in *Hylobius abietus* L. stung by *Bracon hylobii* Ratz.

It is the braconid venom causing permanent paralysis which has been studied in detail, which is remarkable in several respects, and which is the principle point of discussion here. This venom (e.g. *Bracon hebetor* Say) when injected into a sensitive insect (e.g. *Galleria mellonella* L.) requires a few minutes to take effect. The following sequence of events takes place (BEARD, 1952). At the time of stinging, the larva shows some initial signs of irritation, frequently biting at the wasp or at the point of the sting. As the stung larva crawls along, its normal progress soon comes to a halt. Attempted locomotor activity continues for a fraction of a minute, but no progress is made—the insect seems to walk in one spot. As purposive movement ceases, there is a gradual loss of irritability, and the larva soon fails to respond to tactile stimulation. The mouth parts are among the last external structures to stop movement. Although the bodily muscles are flaccid, the heart and gut remain functional. Recovery can occur in some instances, but normally it does not. Death ensues because of inanition, or consumption by parasitoid larvae.

III. The Preferred Species for Study

Practically all investigations on braconid venoms causing permanent paralysis have used only three species, and these have been variously identified with three genera, with attending confusion. *Habrobracon* is the name best known and consistently used by geneticists, because *H. juglandis* Ashmead has been a favorite species for laboratory study. MARTIN (1947) encouraged the continued use of this name. Except by geneticists this species has since become more commonly referred to by its valid name, *Bracon hebetor* Say (MUESEBECK and WALKLEY, 1951), although *Microbracon* has frequently been used for the generic name. In this discussion *Bracon* will be used even though literature citations refer to the other names. The species employed have been almost limited to *B. hebetor, B. brevicornis* (Wesm.), and *B. gelechiae* (Ashm.).

Confusion exists also between *B. hebetor* and *B. brevicornis*. Taxonomic separation has largely been on the basis of number of antennal segments and of genitalia. These characters are sufficiently ambiguous as to make taxonomists cautious in determining species differences. In works reported here, *B. brevicornis* usually was obtained from India, and in some instances may be intermediate between *B. hebetor* and typical *B. brevicornis*.

B. The Venom Apparatus

I. Morphology and Histology

The poison apparatus of the braconids is sufficiently distinctive to qualify as a type contrasting with 2 others, the apid type and the vespid type (PAWLOWSKY, 1914). The braconid poison apparatus can be understood from illustrations and descriptions by BERLESE (1909) for *B. nigropedator* and *Aphidius* sp., GENIEYS (1925) for *B. brevicornis,* and BENDER (1943) for *B. hebetor.*

The apparatus, illustrated in Figure 3, consists of 8 elongated glands that surround the venom reservoir and open into the base of the reservoir which empties into the poison duct.

Each gland consists of a single layer of heavy cuboidal cells surrounding a central lumen. Nuclei are of two sizes. The larger ones are round to oval and are peripheral in the cells. Smaller nuclei are visible between the larger ones at the periphery, and many small nuclei form a layer at the lumen end of the cells. The cytoplasm appears homogeneous and finely granular, but rounded vacuoles may be present, some large ones bulging into the gland lumen. The stalk of each gland bends in a sigmoid flexure and possesses a spiral lining; it leads into a cuticular bulb at the base of the reservoir. The functional system, to be described, would seem to call for a valvular mechanism at this point, but none is evident.

The reservoir (and pump) is an ovate body lined with a distinctive cuticular spiral—a compressible helix—light brown in color. The reservoir is surrounded by a heavy muscular coat made up of longitudinal striated muscle fibers that are attached at numerous points along the spiral lining.

The poison duct runs distally from the base of the reservoir and leads to the stinging stylets. It is rather heavily sclerotized and appears rough in texture. The proximal portion of the duct is surrounded by heavily vacuolated cells that possess oval nuclei at their periphery. The vacuoles are sponge-like in appearance and occupy the larger part of each cell. These secretory cells empty individually into the poison duct by extremely fine canals. The nature of the secretion of these glandular cells is not known. BENDER (1943), apparently overlooking Dufour's gland although it was illustrated by BERLESE (1909) and GENIEYS (1925), assumed that these duct cells constituted the alkaline gland. Dufour's gland is formed of large, definite and regular cells and has no contractile fibers. It empties into the duct distal to the duct cells.

II. Mechanism of Action

The mechanism of the apparatus was described by GENIEYS (1925) and discussed by BEARD (1971 b) in terms of an automatic syringe. As the muscles of the bulblike reservoir relax, the extension of the springlike helix distends the lumen, and venom is sucked from the lumina of the secreting glands to fill the cavity. No valve mechanism can be seen to prevent backflow from the duct into the bulb unless somehow the cells of the proximal duct serve this function. As the bulb muscles contract, the cavity shortens, the spiral compresses, and venom is ejected. No valves are evident to prevent backflow into the glands, but the configuration

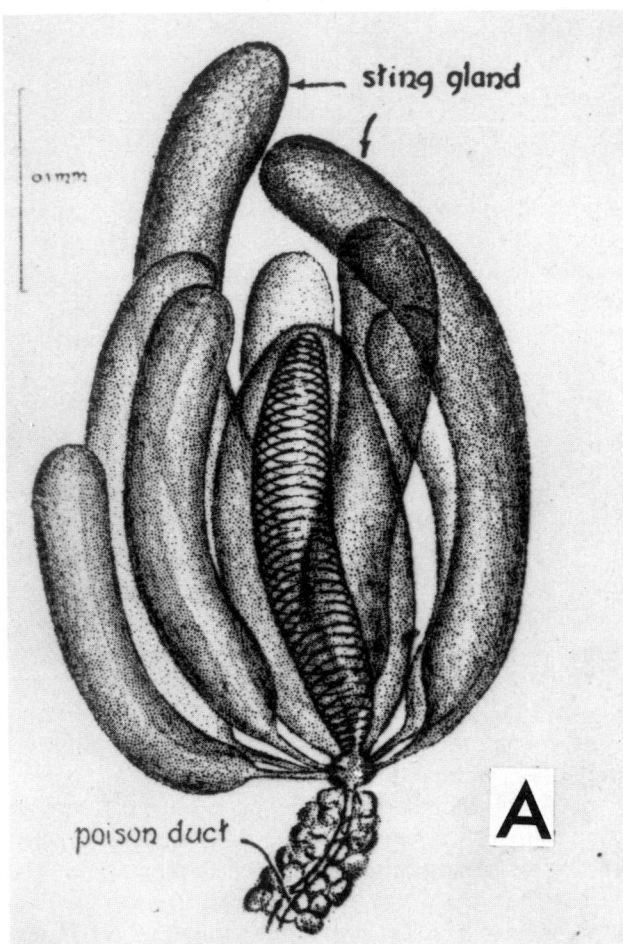

Fig. 3A and B. Details of venom apparatus. A Reservoir-pump and surrounding glands. B Sectional detail. From Bender (1943)

of the gland ducts and the base of the contractible vesicle are such as to suggest that the ducts may be wholly or partially compressed at the moment of contraction. Other secretion pressure may reduce or prevent backflow. If no backflow occurred, either from the duct on the intake stroke or into the glands on the ejection stroke, the volume of the discharge should equal the tidal volume (relaxed volume less the contracted volume of the reservoir). Otherwise, the ejected volume would equal the tidal volume diminished by the backflow volumes.

III. Volume of Ejected Venom

The helical lining of the bulb is easily measured and its extended dimensions appear to be rather uniformly about 75 μ in diameter at midlength and about 370 μ long. If this is considered to be a prolate spheroid, its volume can be

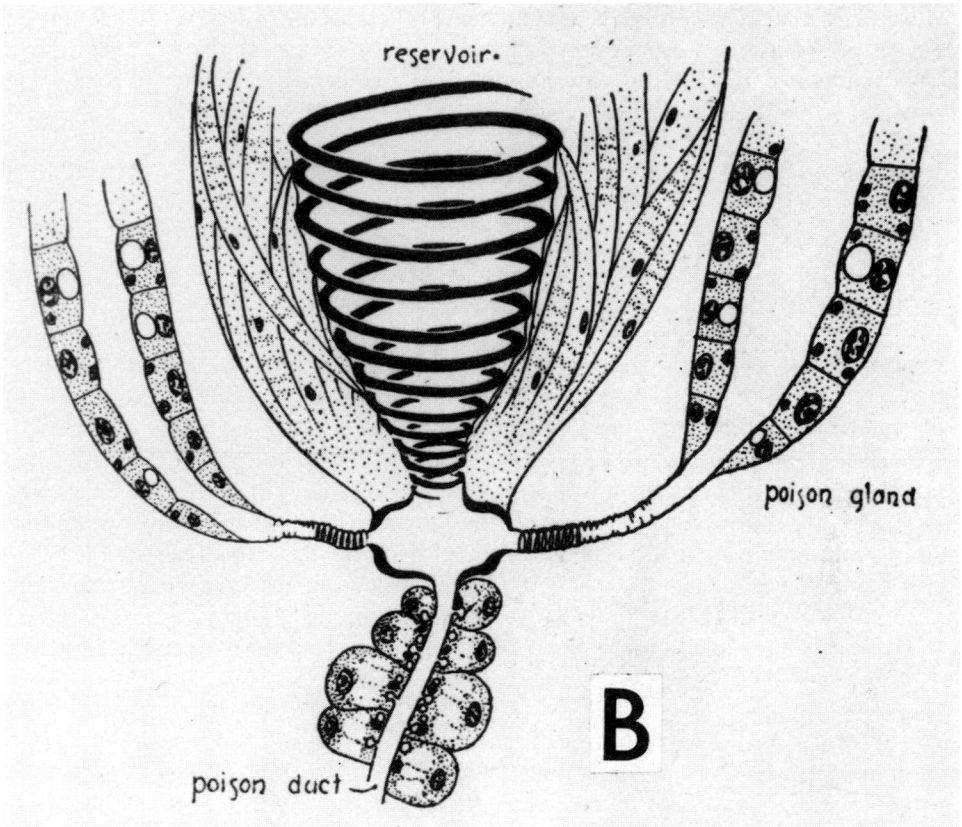

calculated to approximate 0.001 μl. The compressed volume is more difficult to assess because contraction of isolated bulbs is not readily induced. From insufficient evidence, the compressed volume is believed to be in the range of 60 percent of the total, giving a tidal volume of about 0.0004 μl if contraction is maximal. Natural stinging probably calls for maximal contraction as stinging is rapid and a sudden full stroke of the bulb as a muscular unit is likely. In isolated venom systems, partial movement can result from activity in only a portion of the contractile elements. In such cases reduced amounts of venom would be ejected, possibly in sequential droplets.

These volume relationships will be discussed further in regard to production and use of venom.

C. Methods of Obtaining Venom for Study

The ease of culturing and manipulating braconid wasps, their success in host finding, and their willingness to sting available insects mean that advantage can be taken of natural stinging in securing much information.

Experimental extraction of venom and controlled use include several techniques. Because the venom is water soluble, the whole female wasp or the abdomen alone can be macerated in water and filtered; the filtrate will contain the active paralyzing principle, contaminated with water-soluble extractives.

Hase (1924) found that restrained female wasps when mechanically stimulated would extend the stylets and discharge droplets of venom. Beard (1952) held a wasp by a suction capillary to achieve the same result. Such a method probably yields the purest venom, as contamination is minimized.

The entire venom apparatus, contaminated with portions of the gut, can be pulled from the abdomen by grasping the stylets with fine forceps.

Electric stimulation has been especially effective in inducing venom ejection in many spiders, bees, and wasps. Piek (1966) utilized this technique and developed an electric grid of stainless steel wire connected to a stimulator. From 200 to 400 wasps were exposed at one time and stimulated every 3 s for a 10 min period. The stimulus induced the wasps to eject venom, slightly contaminated with feces and other products, that could be collected upon filter paper placed below the grid. Yield of venom was comparatively low. Beard (1971 b) found electric stimulation of individual wasps to be unsatisfactory for inducing venom ejection.

Venom glands or filter paper containing venom can be extracted with water or saline solutions for use or stored under refrigeration.

Another source of venom is the circulating blood of naturally stung caterpillars.

D. Injection and Transport of Venom

To some wasps of this type has been attributed the ability to insert the sting into a ganglion of the victim, thus introducing the venom directly into the nervous system. This was inferred by Payne (1933) for braconid stinging of *Anagasta* (=*Ephestia*). This concept requires a prescience and a perception of host morphology on the part of the wasp not generally acceptable. Some observations suggested that repeated stinging by some wasps might permit some chance puncture of a ganglion.

Ganglionic stinging is not required to produce paralysis, and many experiments have demonstrated this simply and conclusively. *Bracon* can paralyze its prey by stinging at any locus (Beard, 1952). Effectiveness of the injected venom is assured by blood transport. This can be demonstrated by ligating a larva and introducing venom parenterally on one side of the ligature. Paralysis sets in only on the side of the ligature where venom was injected, regardless of the location of the ligature. Blood transport becomes confirmed if the ligature is cut and flow is restored between both body regions. The unparalyzed portion of the larva then becomes promptly paralyzed.

Artificial stinging of an insect can be achieved by introducing venom adhering to a needle or hypodermically injecting soluble extractives from venom glands, whole wasps, or even blood from paralyzed larvae.

The small amount of venom injected into a host and its high solubility account for a prompt dilution. Distribution of the venom to receptive sites must be governed by rates of mixing and transport resulting from diffusion, active circulation by

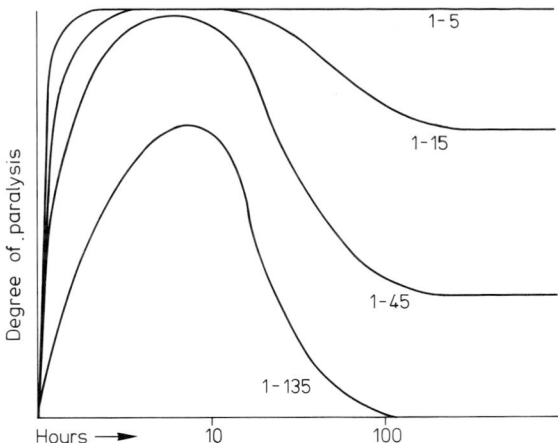

Fig. 4. Schematic relationships between venom concentration and onset of paralysis, degree of paralysis, and time of recovery. From BEARD (1952)

heart beat, and locomotion, and possibly by membrane permeability or the nature of reactive sites. These factors can explain the time required for onset of paralysis being a function of venom dose. Also physical activity can speed up and sedation retard, the onset of paralysis (PIEK and ENGELS, 1969).

Venom is not used up at reactive sites, but continues to circulate in the blood of a stung insect. Thus BEARD (1952) was able to transfer blood from one paralyzed *Galleria* larva to induce paralysis in a second larva, and thence from that, to paralyze a third larva.

Normal stinging results in reasonably prompt paralysis, but experimental diluted doses require a longer time for paralysis to occur (Fig. 4). Although some recovery from natural stinging has been reported, this is not common. Recovery from experimental injections can occur in direct relationship to the venom concentration. The factors at reaction sites that relate to recovery are not known.

This relationship of delayed onset of paralysis and early recovery with dilute venom dosages is at variance with the prompt onset and early recovery in those venoms causing only temporary paralysis. This means that the two systems are very different in one or more respects.

E. Assays of Venom Activity

No standard assay of venom activity has been developed. As different studies have used venom from diverse sources, dosages administered have been expressed variously. Sometimes quantities of venom applied are based upon body weight of the recipient (e.g. PIEK and ENGELS, 1969; DRENTH, 1974a).

Response, too, is variously recorded in terms of complete paralysis (within a given time span), incomplete paralysis with end-point defined (e.g. inability of an insect to right itself when turned on its back (DRENTH, 1974a)), or by a scoring

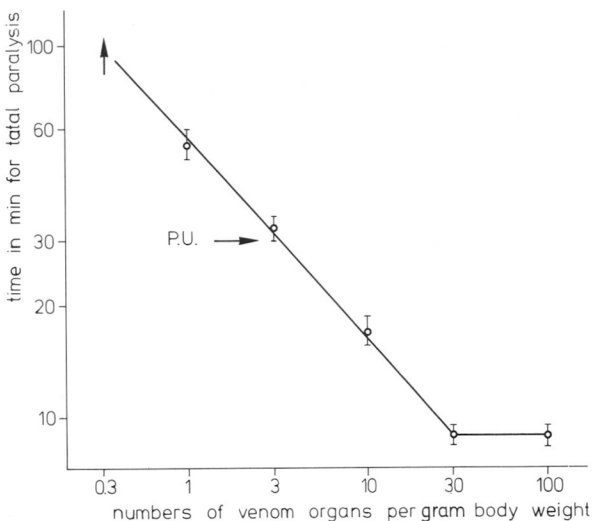

Fig. 5. Dose-effect relation of *B. hebetor* venom in larvae of *Philosamia*. *P.U.* = one *Philosamia* unit. From PIEK and ENGELS (1966)

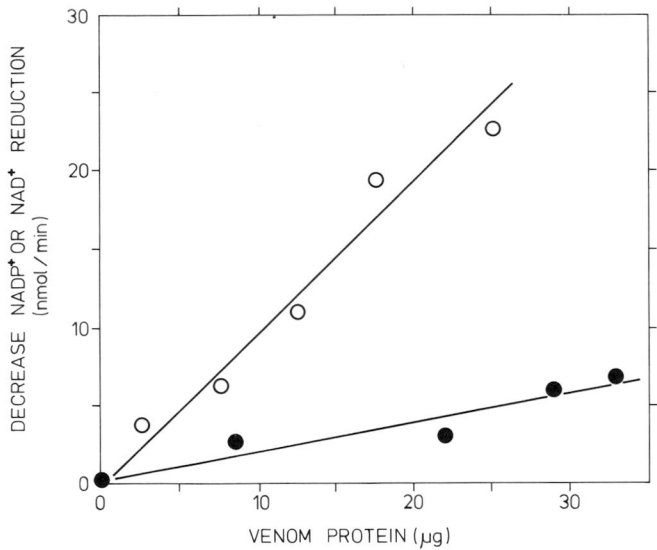

Fig. 6. Effect of *B. brevicornis* venom on oxidation-driven transhydrogenation (○) and on NAD[+] reduction by succinate (●). From BEARD et al. (1971)

system that assigns different values to different degrees of paralysis (BEARD, 1952; TAMASHIRO, 1971).

Dosage and response together may be represented in "units". BEARD (1971) used a scoring system for response, but expressed results in "*Plodia* Units" that related a sample of venom to its expected potential if fully utilized. PIEK and ENGELS (1969) used a "*Philosamia* Unit", defined as the dose, injected per g body weight, that paralyses a *Philosamia* larva of about 3 g in 30 min at 25° C. PIEK et al. (1974) referred activity to number of ED_{50} s per venom organ.

Time of response, as well as degree of response, as a function of venom dosage can serve as an assay. PIEK and ENGELS (1969) demonstrated a linear relationship between log dose of venom and log time for total paralysis in *Philosamia* larvae (Fig. 5).

On the basis that the degree of inhibition of aerobic oxidation-driven pyridine nucleotide transhydrogenation of NAD^+ reduction by succinate (observed by LEE, 1971) was proportional to the venom (*B. brevicornis*) protein concentration, and that these reactions paralleled paralytic activity, BEARD et al. (1971) suggested that such biochemical reactions could serve as a venom assay (Fig. 6).

F. Braconid Venom

I. Chemistry

BEARD (1952) concluded that braconid venom was a protein or polypeptide on the basis that it was heat labile, could be precipitated with half-saturated ammonium sulfate and adsorbed on calcium phosphate gel, was non-dialyzable, and inactivated by copper. TAMASHIRO (1971) advanced this conclusion by showing a deactivation by incubating venom with pancreatin. Although VAN DER MEER et al. (1965) questioned the proteinaceous nature of venom, it is now generally concluded that the venom is a protein or contains proteinaceous moieties (VISSER and SPANJER, 1969; PIEK et al., 1974; LEE, 1971).

LEE (1971) also found that *B. brevicornis* venom could be precipitated in presence of ammonium sulfate, in concentrations from 35 to 55 percent. She found the venom to be pH sensitive with maximal activity in the range of $6-9$.

Molecular weight determinations are not in complete agreement, possibly because of techniques of fractionation. LEE (1971) concluded on the basis of sucrose density sedimentation that *B. brevicornis* venom had a molecular weight of the order of 10^5. Gel filtration through sephadex columns types G-10 and G-25 yielded biologically active material. Although LEE (1971) found G-100 sephadex filtration unsatisfactory because of long retention time, VISSER and SPANJER (1969) succeeded with *B. hebetor* venom as did PIEK et al. (1974) with *B. gelechiae* venom to conclude that the molecular weights were 55,000 and 60,000 respectively. Discrepancies in molecular weight evaluations may have been resolved by SPANJER (personal communication) and his associates, who found two active components in *B. hebetor* venom with molecular weights of 57,000 and 42,000, both of which have the same presynaptic paralyzing effect.

Neither histamine nor 5-hydroxytryptamine has been associated with the active principle of braconid venom (D.C. CLAGETT, pers. comm.).

Some attempts to simulate, potentiate, or antagonize venom action essentially failed (BEARD, 1952).

II. Stability

DRENTH (1974b) found that venom gland extract (1 mg/ml) retained full activity after storage for 3 years either as a solution at $-20°$ C or in the dry state at either $-20°$ C or $+4°$ C. Freeze dried venom gland extracts, especially at reduced concentrations, lost activity up to 80 percent. A "trilene preparation" of venom, obtained by exposing large numbers of female wasps to trichloroethylene vapor in a glass tube provided with a glass filter and extracting with ice-cold distilled water, was less stable than venom gland extracts. Stability of trilene preparations was greatly enhanced by the addition of such proteins as crystalline bovine albumin, bovine α-globulin, bovine β-globulin, bovine fibrinogen, horse α-globulin, horse β-globulin, gelatin, casein, bovine hemoglobin, bovine γ-globulin, and others. Venom was also stabilized by hemolymph preparations of *G. mellonella* and *P. cynthia* which are susceptible to *B. hebetor* venom as well as of *Periplaneta americana, Schistocerca gregaria,* and *Locusta migratoria,* which are resistant to the venom. Among a large number of nonprotein compounds tested, a few ($ZnSO_4$, $FeSO_4$, $HgCl_2$, Ampholine (pH $7-10$), arginine, and glycerol) provided some stabilization.

Venom of *B. brevicornis* was observed to be still active in dead wasps after 6 months storage at room temperature, although much potency had been lost (Tamashiro, 1971). Refrigerated venom solutions retained some activity even after a year. Bacterial action hastened loss of potency. Beard (unpublished) found that refrigerated lyophilized venom-apparatus of both *B. hebetor* and *B. brevicornis* was active after 4 years, but potency was not assessed.

Lee (1971) observed that venom solutions left overnight at room temperature lost much activity and were completely inactivated at temperatures above $50°$ C. She observed no loss of biological activity of venom after 5 h of dialysis, but found that venom was inactivated at pH above 9 and below 5. A pH optimum of $8-9$ for stability was reported by Drenth (1974b).

III. Potency

Since the work of Hase (1924), all investigators of braconid venom have been impressed with the high potency of such small amounts of the substance.

This potency has been expressed variously. Beard (1952) reported that 1 part of venom (*B. hebetor*) in 2×10^8 parts of *G. mellonella* blood was sufficient to cause permanent paralysis, and lesser amounts caused temporary paralysis. Tamashiro (1971) found that a dosage of 30×10^{-10} ml of *B. hebetor* venom caused 100 percent paralysis (not necessarily permanent) in *G. mellonella, Angasta kühniella,* and *Plodia interpunctella. B. brevicornis* venom in a dose of 26.8×10^{-10} also caused 100 percent paralysis in these hosts, but only 70 percent in *Gnorimoschema opercullela.*

It was also concluded that the total venom produced by a braconid wasp could paralyze about 1,620,000 *Plodia* larvae if its potential could be fully utilized (Beard, 1971).

IV. Production, Storage, and Use of Venom

Only limited studies have been made on the quantities of venom produced and stored, rates of synthesis, and factors affecting these. Radio-labeling, a technique so useful in studies of this kind, has not been applied successfully. Beard (1952) fed braconid wasps ^{14}C-labeled protein hydrolysate, L-alanine, glucose, or sucrose. Not only were these wasps highly radioactive, but eggs they laid and offspring

from them were radioactive, but the venom they produced was not. Perhaps radioio-
dine would have been more successful. In the absence of such a labeling technique,
observations on extent and rate of natural stinging have been more productive.

1. Synthesis

Since female wasps and their developing larvae feed (probably) exclusively on
blood of their hosts, this must contain all the precursors that finally become
synthesized into venom. It must be the larval food that first goes into venom
synthesis, for wasps contain venom when they emerge from their coccons (TAMASH-
IRO, 1971) and sting hosts before they themselves feed. TAMASHIRO (1971) detected
venom in 4 day old pupae of both *B. brevicornis* and *B. hebetor*. He could not
confirm BEARD's observation (1960) that young pupae and male wasps sometimes
showed the presence of paralyzing substance in small amounts. BEARD found some
activity in eggs, and even less activity in *Bracon* larvae. TAMASHIRO (1971) also
found some activity in larvae. The egg substance most likely was contamination
of venom received during oviposition; the larval substance could have been a
persistence of this contamination or stuff taken up by feeding on its paralyzed
host. TAMASHIRO concluded that digestive processes in the parasitoid larva inactivate
the venom; filtrates of the meconium did not possess paralytic properties. In
any case, it can be concluded that venom synthesis begins after the midpoint
of pupal development.

BEARD (1971b) attempted to evaluate venom activity as affected by the kind
of food supplied the wasps, but he found by radiolabeling that the food sources
(*Galleria* blood, *Plodia* blood, and dextrose) could not be delimited under conditions of the experiment.

2. Storage and Volume of Venom Used

In the discussion on morphology of the venom apparatus, the "reservoir" was
viewed as a dynamic pumping system rather than a storage sac. Thus BEARD
(1971b) concluded that the volume of venom available for a single injection was
only about 0.0004 µl. Other workers have not considered the system in the same
way. PIEK and SIMON THOMAS (1969) estimated that the venom reservoir contained
0.01 µl. This calculation was based on the observation (HASE, 1924) that individual
mechanically stimulated affixed wasps could eject repeated droplets of venom,
0.0003 µl in size, at mean intervals of from 3 to 3.5 s, and that up to 36 droplets
could be elicited. BEARD (1971b) was unable to get constrained wasps to eject
venom at this regular rate, but the correspondence between his figure of 0.0004 µl
and HASE's measure of droplet size (0.0003 µl) may be significant.

TAMASHIRO (1971) also considered the volume of venom contained in the reservoir, but on a basis that overestimated the content. He assumed that the reservoir
was like a thin-walled bag of stored venom. Thus he measured the outside dimension
of the structure. He, too, calculated on the basis of a prolate spheroid, but because
of the thick muscular wall of the reservoir, his values were much higher than
those found by BEARD. TAMASHIRO also calculated the volume of the glands as
if they were thin-walled cylinders. The combined venom content of reservoir and
glands was stated to be 4.1×10^{-5} ml for *B. brevicornis* and 4.3×10^{-5} ml for *B. he-*

betor. These values were used in calculating venom content in experiments utilizing reservoir-gland extracts. Such values would be excessive for the amount naturally ejected, not only because of the method of measurement, but because of combining the venom contents. The natural ejection of venom would comprise only the tidal volume of the reservoir, whereas the intake stroke (drawing upon the supply in the glandular lumina) would replace the tidal volume.

In estimating venom content of the apparatus, structures other than the reservoir and the glands can doubtless be neglected. BEARD (1971 b) found that the other structures contained only small amounts of paralyzing substance that could be accounted for by contamination or that resident in the duct.

3. Rate of Venom Production

Rate and extent of natural stinging can serve as a measure of venom production. BEARD (1971 b) found that if excess *Plodia* larvae were supplied *B. brevicornis,* as many stings as 100 per day with a mean of 40, and as many as 1700 per lifetime with a mean of about 900 were inflicted. The rate of stinging was reasonably well sustained, but there was a slight progressive decline with age.

Somewhat similar studies (TAMASHIRO, 1971) with *B. brevicornis* stinging *Corcyra cephalonica* were conducted for 8 days. These showed a reduced amount of stinging on the first day after emergence, but thereafter the rates were essentially uniform. These rates, however, were considerably less than BEARD observed with a different host and undoubtedly a different strain of the wasp.

Although the gland-reservoir volume relationships, discussed elsewhere, clearly indicate that a life-time supply of venom is not stored from the beginning of adult life, this was given experimental support (BEARD, 1971a). Venom apparatus was assayed in wasps soon after emergence, in wasps allowed to sting at least 600 larvae, and in wasps permitted to sting only as might be necessary to obtain food from larvae already paralyzed. All 3 groups, when assayed, showed equivalent quantities of venom. Thus limited use of venom results in neither a loss of potency nor a remarkable accumulation over a period of time. Maximal stinging shows that heavy demands on the venom supply are accompanied by adequate replacement.

On the basis of volume relationships and stinging rates, BEARD (1971 b) estimated that the amount of venom present in the whole poison apparatus at any one time is almost 5 times that ejected in any one dose. This signifies a turnover of 8 times a day or some 180 times during the life of the wasp. Although this appears rapid, the actual volumes are small—approximately $0.004-0.012$ µl per day or a lifetime total of $0.1-0.3$ µl—and yet this is enough, if it could be fully utilized, to paralyze 1,620,000 *Plodia* larvae (see Section on Potency).

G. Mode of Action of Venom

I. Effect on the Heart

In contrast to maggots paralyzed temporarily by *Alysia* that show no heartbeat while paralyzed, permanent paralysis caused by braconids does not stop heart action. HASE (1924) observed an increase to twice the normal heartrate shortly after *A. kühniella* larvae had been stung by *B. hebetor,* but the frequency returned to normal after 1—2 h. BEARD (1952) noted no change from normal frequency when *G. mellonella* larvae were paralyzed by *B. hebetor.* PIEK and SIMON THOMAS (1969) noted that the heartbeat of larvae and adults of *P. cynthia* and of *Actias selene* Hbn. continued after a subcutaneous injection of *B. hebetor* venom, but a transient increase in frequency occurred. HASE (1924) also noted that temperature effects were the same on hearts of paralyzed and nonparalyzed larvae.

II. Effect on the Gut

Gut activity in paralyzed insects appears to be unimpaired, but since feeding stops, gut activity may be only physiologically normal and subject to secondary effects. BEARD (1960) electrographically recorded foregut activity in *G. mellonella* paralyzed by *B. hebetor* and found a variety of movements that could be associated with trituration of food; also the foregut was responsive to drug action that is presumed to be unaffected by paralysis. Several authors have noted that defecation by paralyzed larvae occurs (Fig. 7), but since the fecal material is excreted as a continuum, it is concluded that anal sphincter control is lost.

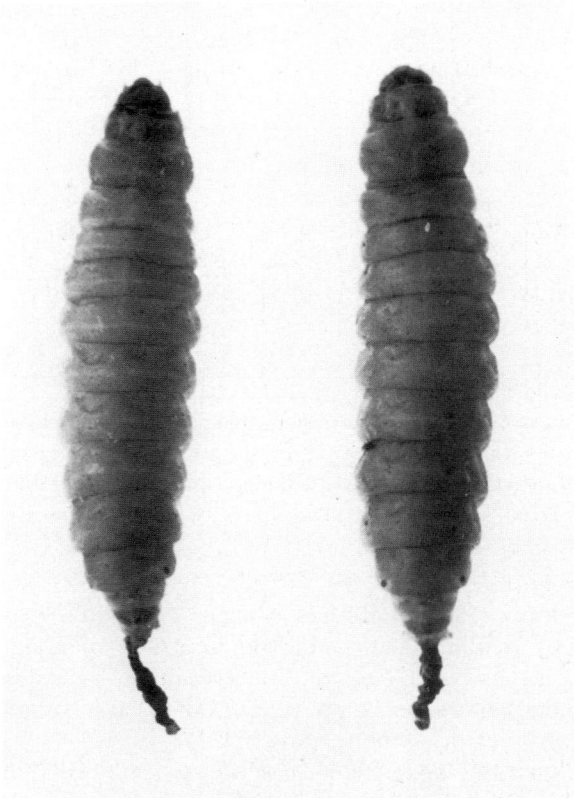

Fig. 7. Paralyzed *Galleria* larvae showing fecal discharge. From BEARD (1958)

III. Effect on Gross Respiration

Respiration in *Anagasta* larvae (PAYNE, 1937) and *Galleria* larvae (WALLER, 1965a, b; EDWARDS and SERNKA, 1969) paralyzed by braconid venom was found to be significantly less than that of unparalyzed larvae. Inhibition of oxygen uptake occurred whether larvae were paralyzed naturally or injected with venom gland extracts. WALLER (1965) found that injection of 5 μl of venom solution (1 gland/ml) reduced respiration by about 20 percent, whereas higher concentration (10 or 100 glands/ml or natural stinging) reduced the respiration by about 50 percent. Because of this concentration effect, WALLER concluded that inhibited respiration was not due only to loss of locomotor activity, but that respiratory metabolism was impaired. This conclusion was tempered by an observation that whole larval homogenates showed no inhibition of respiration.

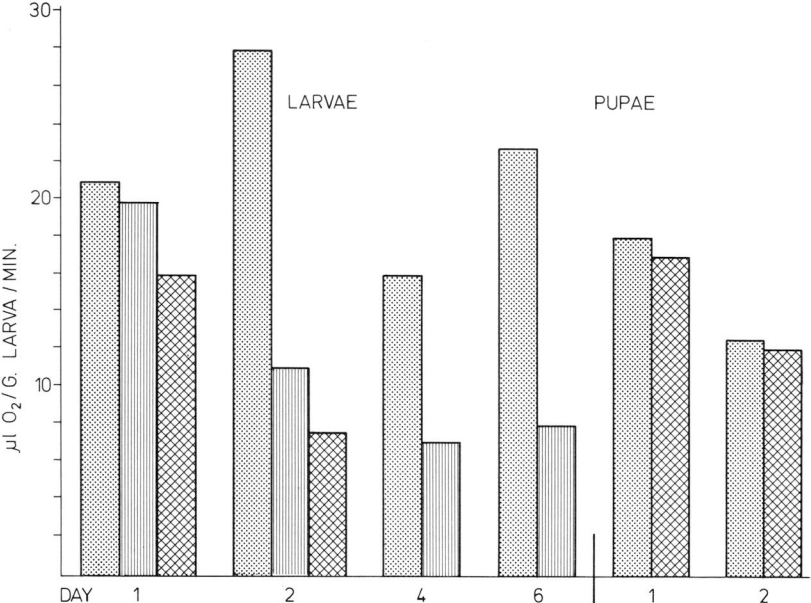

Fig. 8. Effect of *Bracon* venom on respiratory rates of *Galleria* larvae and pupae. Stippled bar = control; vertical hatching = stung larvae; cross hatching = injected larvae and pupae. From EDWARDS and SERNKA (1969)

EDWARDS and SERNKA (1969) confirmed WALLER's observed respiration inhibition in larvae, but by treating *Galleria* pupae, in which muscular activity was minimal, they found no inhibition (Fig. 8). Such results do not indicate a general metabolic effect of the venom but support the view that respiratory inhibition is related to the paralysis of the somatic musculature.

Discriminate cellular respiration could be affected and still be obscured by gross respiration. This will be discussed further below.

IV. Effect on Neuromuscular Activity

The flaccid paralysis of stung victims clearly implicates the neuromuscular system as the site affected by braconid venom, but determination of the locus and nature of the physiologic lesion has been a challenging exercise.

BEARD (1952) introduced electrophysiologic methods into the study, and as would be expected found no spontaneous action potentials in the body wall musculature. This could indicate either loss of irritability or contractility. Recording electrodes placed on interganglionic nerve connectives revealed the same kind of spontaneous action potentials in both normal and paralyzed *G. mellonella* larvae. This indicated that the central nerve cord was unaffected by venom. Likewise motor nerves from ganglia leading to the musculature generated spontaneous activity, but stimulating these nerves failed to elicit a muscular response, whereas such stimulation in unparalyzed larvae caused vigorous muscular contractions even with stimuli of low intensity. Direct stimulation of the somatic musculature of paralyzed *Anagasta* larvae caused contractions, but *Galleria* larvae were refractory to such stimulation. Chemical agents caused shortening of bodily muscles. Although these contractile experiments were somewhat equivocal, BEARD concluded that the site of venom action was the neuromuscular synapse and that the lesion was one that blocked nerve impulses that maintained muscle tone and controlled muscular movement.

Since BEARD's studies, refinements in instrumentation and techniques have confirmed the site of action, more precisely defined the lesion, and given clues as to the mechanism.

A clever experiment by PIEK (1966) confirmed that the central nerve cord was not affected by venom. He ligated a *Philosamia* larva in two places (see Fig. 9). If the ligatures were tight enough to prevent blood circulation between the three regions but not so tight as to damage the nerve cord, and if venom was injected into the middle region, only that region was paralyzed; but if the posterior region was electrically stimulated, the anterior region as well as the posterior region contracted. Furthermore, mechanical stimulation of the paralyzed middle region resulted in contraction in both the anterior and posterior regions. This confirmed, as BEARD (1952) had inferred, that sensory elements were not affected in the paralyzed region.

In a somewhat similar experiment, WALTHER and RATHMAYER (1974) using leg preparations of *Locusta migratoria,* found that stimulating paralyzed legs resulted in reflex movement in associated but unparalyzed legs; thus nervous conduction in afferent fibers was not blocked.

PIEK (1966) found that the musculature of paralyzed larvae of *Philosamia* and *Galleria* could respond, both isotonically and isometrically, to direct electrical stimulation, but only if the stimulus was sufficiently strong.

Further experiments on the flight muscles of adult moths of *Philosamia* (PIEK and ENGELS, 1969) gave additional evidence that muscle excitability was not blocked by venom action. Venom affected neither the effective membrane resistance nor response of the muscle fiber membrane to depolarizing pulses. WALTHER and RATHMAYER (1974) also found no significant effect of braconid venom on the resting membrane potential in muscle fibers of either *Anagasta* or *Locusta*.

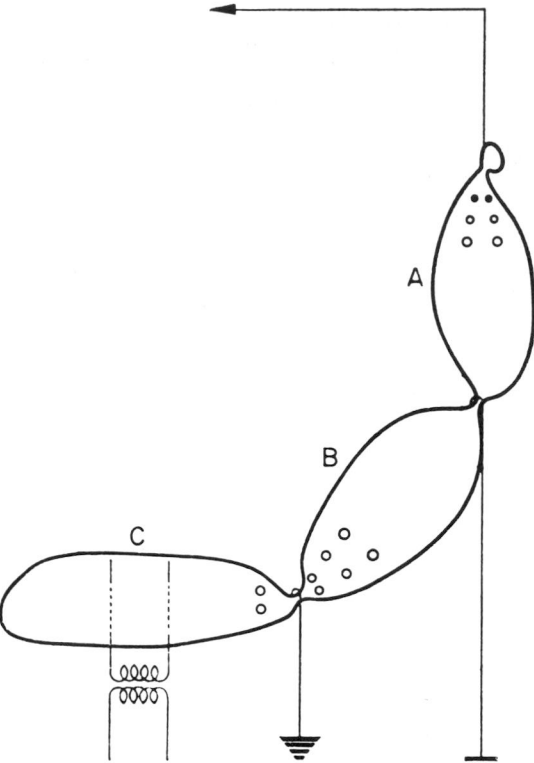

Fig. 9. Ligated larva of *Philosamia*. Contractions recorded from *A* ; Venom injected in region *B* ; Ventral nerve stimulated in *C*. From PIEK (1966)

That peripheral excitatory axons were unaffected by venom was substantiated by PIEK (1966) in *Philosamia* and WALTHER and RATHMAYER (1974) in *Anagasta* and *Locusta*. Absence of venom action on inhibitory neuromuscular transmission was found by PIEK and ENGELS (1969); PIEK and MANTEL (1970) with *Philosamia*, and WALTHER and RATHMAYER (1974) with *Anagasta* and *Locusta*.

The loss of muscle response to nervous stimulation as a result of venom activity is illustrated in Figure 10. Similar decline in excitatory postsynaptic potentials was demonstrated in *Galleria* larval muscle preparations affected by *B. gelechiae* venom (PIEK et al., 1974).

With all evidence pointing to venom action being a blocking of excitatory impulses at the neuromuscular synapse, interest has centered on what is happening there.

A postsynaptic effect has not been absolutely ruled out, but it is unlikely. WALTHER and RATHMAYER (1974) found that paralyzed and nonparalyzed hindlegs of locusts responded alike to applied preparations of glutamate, indicating no difference in postjunctional sensitivity. Thus if affected systems are glutaminergic, as is likely (RATHMAYER and WALTHER, 1975), a postsynaptic venom effect is improbable.

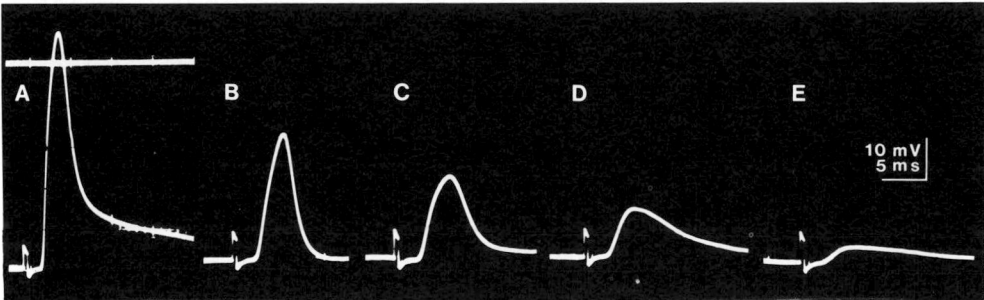

Fig. 10. Changes in postsynaptic responses of *Anagasta* muscle on application of *Bracon* venom. *A*, normal response. *B — E* decline of response 3.5, 4, 4.5, 5, and 6 min after venom application. From WALTHER and RATHMEAYER (1974)

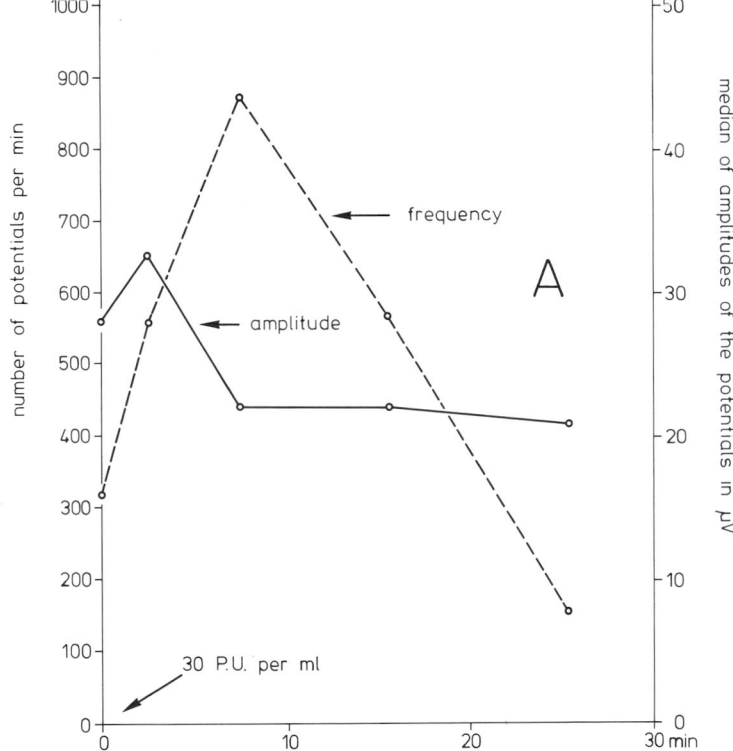

Fig. 11. Effect of *B. hebetor* venom (30 *Philosamia* units/ml) on frequency and amplitude of spontaneous miniature potentials in *Philosamia* flight muscles. From PIEK and ENGELS (1969)

A presynaptic effect of venom has been demonstrated that is sufficiently convincing that this is considered to be the locus of action (PIEK and ENGELS, 1969; PIEK and MANTEL, 1970; PIEK et al., 1974; WALTHER and RATHMAYER, 1974). The effect of *B. hebetor* venom on the spontaneous miniature potentials in flight muscle fibers of *Philosamia* was studied by PIEK and ENGELS (1969) using intracellular microelectrodes. They found that the frequency of the miniature excitatory postsynaptic potentials (mepsp's) were affected; the frequency at first increased but then decreased to zero. The amplitude was affected to a lesser degree (Fig. 11). The time course of the frequency changes could be accelerated by increasing the venom concentrations. This effect on frequency but not on amplitude of mepsp's has also been demonstrated with *B. hebetor* venom on *Anagasta* larvae and on *Locusta migratoria* (WALTHER and RATHMAYER, 1974) and with *B. gelechiae* on *Galleria* larvae (PIEK et al., 1974).

This action on mepsp's is generally considered to be an attribute of a presynaptic lesion as these potentials are probably caused by spontaneous release of small amounts of transmitter substance (AIDLEY, 1967; see discussion PIEK and ENGEL, 1969).

The action at this site could result from inhibited synthesis, hampered storage, or blocked release of the transmitter substance. These possibilities of action have been speculated upon by PIEK and ENGEL (1969), PIEK et al. (1974) RATHMAYER and WALTHER (1975) but at present conclusions favor no particular hypothesis.

Certainty that glutamate is the transmitter substance in these systems might facilitate interpretation. That braconid venom does not block either inhibitory neuromuscular transmission, where GABA is thought to be the transmitter, nor cholinergic transmission, is considered by WALTHER and RATHMAYER (1974) to favor the hypothesis that the venom acts specifically on glutaminergic synapses.

Electron micrographs of paralyzed and nonparalyzed body wall muscles do not give clues as to nature of the synaptic lesion (PIEK et al., 1974; WALTHER and RATHMAYER, 1974).

RATHMAYER and WALTHER (1975) reported no effect of braconid venom on the noninsect nerve-muscle preparations of the levator pretarsal muscle of the spider *Dugesiella hentzi,* the closer muscle in the walking legs of the crab *Eriphia spinifrons* and of the crayfish *Astacus astacus.*

Absence of paralytic action in vertebrates may be explained by the inactivity on cholinergic systems. For example, DEITMER (1973) found that application of *B. hebetor* venom even at 10 times the concentration used effectively in the locust, had no effect in the cholinergic motor endplate of the frog's sartorius muscle.

V. Biochemical Studies

ATP content in *G. mellonella* larvae was found to be unaffected by paralysis from venom of *B. hebetor* (BEARD, 1958). Likewise no difference was found between paralyzed and nonparalyzed larvae in assays for glutamic dehydrogenase or glutamic pyruvic transaminase, which are likely to be involved in glutamate synthesis (BEARD, 1971 b).

WALLER (1965) treated normal and paralyzed *Galleria* adults with Dinoseb, which stimulates respiration at the subcellular level by uncoupling the process of phosphorylation from that of oxidation. Neither the respiration of the adult moth, nor the ability of the uncoupling agent to stimulate respiration appeared to be affected by the venom.

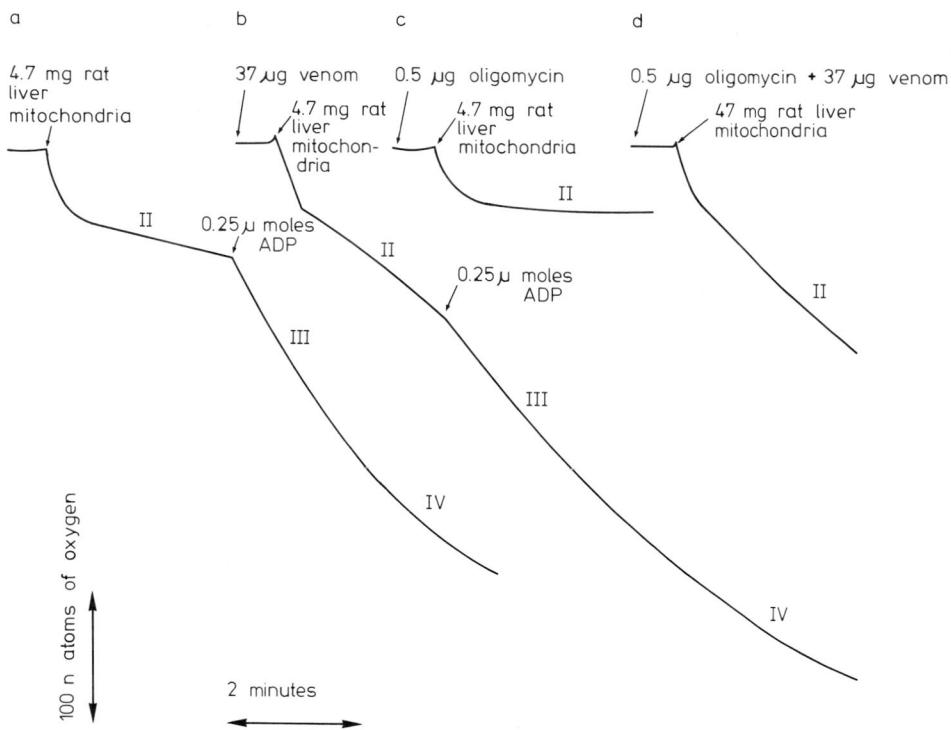

Fig. 12. Effect of *B. brevicornis* venom on respiratory control in rat liver mitochondria. For explanation see text. From LEE (1971)

The effect of venom gland (*B. brevicornis*) extracts on ATPase activity was determined (LEE, 1971) by measuring the enzyme activity as a function of inorganic phosphate released from the hydrolysis of ATP in intact rat liver mitochondria in the presence of excess added ATP. She found that 5 µg of purified venom in the medium increased phosphate release by 17 percent, and 10 µg of the venom increased phosphate release by 29 percent.

Respiratory control in intact mitochondria as affected by *B. brevicornis* venom was studied polarigraphically (LEE, 1971). The release of energy transduction suggests the uncoupling action of venom. In Figure 12, trace *a*, in the absence of venom, states *II*, *III*, and *IV* oxidation rates of the intact mitochondria were 11.2, 90.0, and 36.2 n-atom of oxygen per min, respectively. The state *III:IV* respiratory control ratio was 2.48. In the presence of 37 µg of venom protein in an identical system (trace *b*), state *II* oxidation was increased to 40 n-atom of oxygen per min, and state *III* may be regarded as 68 n-atom of oxygen per min. When the same amount of mitochondria was treated with 0.5 µg of oligomycin, state *II* oxidation was abolished (trace *c*). However, in the presence of 37 µg of venom, respiration of the oligomycin-treated mitochondria was restored, and state *II* oxidation rate became 50 n-atom of oxygen per min (trace *d*).

LEE (1971) also found venom inhibition of aerobic oxidation-driven nicotinamide pyridine nucleotide transhydrogenation, using calf liver submitochondrial particle protein. Without venom, the NADP$^+$ reduction rate was 26.6 n-moles per min per mg of particle protein. In the presence of 17.9 µg of venom protein, the rate was reduced to 7.3 n-moles per min per mg of particle protein.

LEE (1971) also found venom inhibition of aerobic oxidation-driven nicotinamide adenine dinucleotide (NAD$^+$) reduction by succinate. In the absence of venom, the activity of 0.5 mg calf heart submitochondrial particles was 262 n-moles of NADH per min per mg of particle protein. When 33 µg of venom protein was added to the system, the NADH production rate was reduced to 131.0 n-moles per min per mg of particle protein.

The electron transport activities of submitochondrial particles for succinate oxidation and ascorbate-TMPD oxidation were found to be the same with and without venom protein (LEE, 1971).

These studies led to the conclusion that the braconid venom uncoupled oxidative phosphorylation without affecting electron transport. In sucrose density gradient fractionation experiments, the inhibitory effect on the oxidation dependent transhydrogenase activity was observed in the same fractions that had the highest paralytic activity in test *G. mellonella* larvae. LEE thus speculated that the venom might interfere with the energy transduction in such a way as to account for the physiologic lesion at the neuromuscular synapse.

Considering that sulfhydryl-groups or disulphide bonds might play a role in venom action, WALTHER and RATHMAYER (1974) reported that cysteine and dithiothreitol did not inactivate braconid venom, nor was paralysis prevented by 5,5'-dithiobis-(2-nitrobenzoic acid) which oxidizes sulfhydryl-groups.

H. Host Preferences and Host Sensitivity to Venom

The relationships between different species of parasitoids and different species of insects that can be paralyzed require the following considerations: host preferences for natural parasitization; host suitability for parasite attack and development; insect sensitivity to natural or artificial envenomization.

GENIEYS (1925) lists his own and other observations on hosts of *B. brevicornis* to include:

Dioryctria (Phycis) abietella Zinck (Pyralidae)
Myelois ceratoniae Z. (Pyralidae)
Ephestia (Anagasta) kühniella Zell (Pyralidae)
Ephestia elutella Hüb. (Pyralidae)
Galleria mellonella L. (*cerella* Fabr.) (Pyralidae)
Galleria grisella Fabr. (*alvearia* Dup.) (Pyralidae)
Grapholitha rufillana Stainton (Tortricidae)
    callicana Cyn.
Hopotia corticalis
Diatraea zeacolella Fabr. (Noctuidae)
Sesamia nonagriodes (Noctuidae)
Leucania zea (Noctuidae)
Phthorimaea operculella (Tineidae)

Acrobasis obliqua
Tortrix virdana (Tortricidae)
Nothris senticella Stegr. (Gelechiidae)

A list of natural hosts of *B. hebetor* recorded in the literature as summarized by DRENTH (1974) includes:

Anagasta kühniella Zell.
Ephestia elutella Hübn.
Ephestia cautella Walk.
Plodia interpunctella Hübn.
Galleria mellonella (L.)
Paralispa (Aphomia) gularis Zell.
Vitula edmandsii Pack.
Sitotroga cerealella Ol.
Antigastra catalaunalis Dup.
Corcyra cephalonica (Staint.)
Laphygma sp.
Adisura atkinsoni Moore

These lists, which may not be complete, demonstrate that in some respects these braconid wasps are specific, but the range of natural hosts is rather broad among Lepidoptera. Experimentally GENIEYS (1925) found that *Porthetria dispar* L., *Pieris brassicae* L., and *Aporia crataegi* L. could be stung and paralyzed, were fed upon by the wasp, but could not support the parasitoid larvae. BEARD (1952) found that larvae of *Popillia japonica* Newm., *Ostrinia nubilalis* (Hübn.), and nymphs and adults of *Oncopeltus fasciatus* (Dall.) were resistant to *B. hebetor* venom; *Archips cerasivorana* (Fitch) was slightly susceptible. PIEK (1966) used *Philosamia cynthia* Hübn. as a susceptible experimental host for venom studies. DRENTH (1969) found *Musca domestica* L. (Diptera) and *Perillus bioculatus* Fabr. (Hemiptera) to be slightly susceptible.

A further study tested a broad range of insects by parenteral injections of venom gland extracts in quantities of 10, 100, or 1000 ng per 100 mg body weight (DRENTH, 1974a). The results are summarized in Table 1.

Activity of venom from *B. gelechiae* was compared with that from *B. hebetor* when administered to *G. mellonella*, *Apis mellifera*, *Musca domestica*, and *Locusta migratoria* (PIEK et al., 1974). *B. hebetor* was over 300 times as active in *G. mellonella* as *B. gelechiae* venom, but *B. gelechiae* venom was about 45 times as effective as *B. hebetor* venom in the honeybee. The two venoms were about equally effective in the other two test insects.

GENIEYS (1925) noted among the natural hosts of *B. brevicornis* differences in suitability of the host for production of parasitoids. Certainly among the studies on envenomation significant differences in sensitivity to the venom were commonly observed.

BEARD (1972) sought to relate the role of envenomation in respect to host suitability by comparing *B. brevicornis* and *B. hebetor* as to efficiencies in stinging, paralyzing action of their venoms, oviposition, larval wasp development, and yield of wasps, using as hosts larvae of *Plodia*, *Galleria*, and *Anagasta*. These hosts

Table 1. Wasp Venom Gland Extract on Insects. *Microbracon*. Groups of 10 animals of each of the species indicated below were injected with doses of 10,100, or 1000 ng of *Microbracon* venom gland extract per 100 mg body weight. After 24 hr at 20° C the number of animals paralysed was noted

Order	Species	Stage	Number or animals paralysed		
			10 ng	100 ng	1000 ng
Odonata	*Ischnura elegans*	Imago	—	—	0
Orthoptera	*Gryllus domesticus*	Imago	—	—	0
	Locusta migratoria	Imago	—	0	0
	Schistocera gregaria	Larva	—	—	0
Phasmida	*Clonopsis gallica*	Imago	—	—	0
	Dixippus morosus	Imago	0	0	0
Dictyoptera	*Blaberus giganteus*	Imago	—	0	0
	Blattella germanica	Imago	—	—	0
	Periplaneta americana	Imago	—	2	2
Hemiptera	*Rhodnius prolixus*	Imago	—	—	1
	Triatoma infestans	Imago	—	—	0
	Perillus bioculatus	Imago	0	4	10
	Naucoris cimicoides	Imago	0	0	0
	Hydrocyrius columbiae	Imago	0	0	0
	Notonecta glauca	Imago	0	0	1
Lepidoptera	*Hyponomeuta evonymella*	Larva	10	10	—
	Achroia grissella	Larva	7	10	—
	Galleria mellonella	Larva	10	10	10
	Galleria mellonella	Imago	10	10	10
	Ostrinia nubilalis	Larva	0	0	0
	Malacosoma neustria	Larva	0	9	—
	Philosamia cynthia	Larva	10	10	—
	Philosamia cynthia	Imago	10	10	—
	Actias selene	Larva	7	10	—
	Bombyx mori	Larva	—	2	10
	Pieris brassicae	Larva	10	—	—
	Pieris brassicae	Imago	10	—	—
	Vanessa urticae	Larva	10	10	—
	Vanessa urticae	Imago	10	—	—
	Vanessa atalanta	Imago	10	—	—
	Vanessa cardui	Imago	10	—	—
	Nymphalis io	Imago	10	—	—
	Tyria jacobeae	Larva	10	10	—
	Mamestra brassicae	Larva	0	4	10
Diptera	*Scopeuma stercorarium*	Imago	0	0	3
	Syrphus balteatus	Imago	—	4	10
	Lucilia caesar	Imago	—	0	0
	Phormia coerulea	Imago	0	0	0
	Musca domestica	Imago	0	1	6
Hymenoptera	*Paravespula germanica*	Imago	—	—	4
	Bombus terrestris	Imago	0	2	7
	Apis mellifera	Imago	2	9	10
Coleoptera	*Agelastica alni*	Imago	—	—	0
	Phylloperta horticola	Imago	—	—	0
	Coccinella septempunctata	Imago	—	—	0
	Tenebrio molitor	Larva	—	0	0
	Leptinotarsa decemlineata	Larva	—	—	0
	Leptinotarsa decemlineata	Imago	—	—	4

were also tested for their ability to detoxify the venoms. These three larvae are recognized hosts of both braconid species, and any one can be used for culturing either wasp. Data obtained in these experiments led to the following conclusions: *Plodia* is the best host for wasp production. *Galleria* is more sensitive to *B. brevicornis* venom than the other hosts, and is the preferred species for oviposition by both wasps. Although *Anagasta* is clearly the least sensitive to venoms of both wasps, and is inferior as a host to *B. brevicornis,* it is otherwise nearly as suitable as host to *B. hebetor. B. brevicornis* consistently differentiates hosts more sharply than does *B. hebetor.* The venoms of both wasps are lower in potency against *Anagasta,* but their relative potencies are reversed for *Plodia* and *Galleria.* These results suggest that the different attributes (one being the venom effectiveness) that result in successful parasitism are to a large degree independent of each other.

Except for one anomalous observation (*B. hebetor* venom in *Galleria*) there was no evidence that venoms circulating in the blood of these hosts were detoxified.

Somewhat similar studies were conducted by TAMASHIRO (1971) with results similar in principle but different in detail, possibly because of strain differences in the wasps used.

The very significant conclusions to be drawn from all these studies are that the braconid venoms have distinct differences in their biologic action and that natural or experimental hosts have distinct differences in sensitivity to the venoms.

J. Immune Relationships

As is now obvious, a natural immunity to braconid venom exists among many insects; such insects are neither parasitized naturally by these wasps nor are they sensitive to injected venom. The nature of this immunity is not known. It could be due to the peculiarity of the receptor system, membrane permeability, or reactive properties at the site of action, or to chemical inactivation of the injected venom.

A curious specificity of immunity was seen in *O. nubilalis* which is a natural host to *B. brevicornis,* but is refractory to venom of *B. hebetor* (BEARD, 1952; DRENTH, 1974a). BEARD (1952) showed that venom of *B. hebetor* introduced into larvae of *O. nubilalis* was circulated in the blood, had no effect, but was not antagonized. Such blood assayed by injection into *G. mellonella* larvae showed no loss of venom potency. A similar experiment by DRENTH (1974) using the resistant adult of *Locusta migratoria* further demonstrated that *B. hebetor* venom was not inactivated by hemolymph in which it circulated.

Some possible hosts to these parasitoids are not naturally attacked, but can be paralyzed by experimental injections. This "immunity" is not physiologic, but rather a behavioral characteristic of the wasps.

Most studies on acquired (induced) immunity reactions in insects have been directed toward defence mechanisms against bacteria, fungi, viruses, and protozoa as infective agents. Braconid venom as an antigenic agent that might induce an immune response has not received adequate attention. TAMASHIRO (1971) explored this by injecting an "immunizing" concentration of venom into larvae of *Corcyra cephalonica* (Stainton) to cause minor symptoms of paralysis. After allowing 2

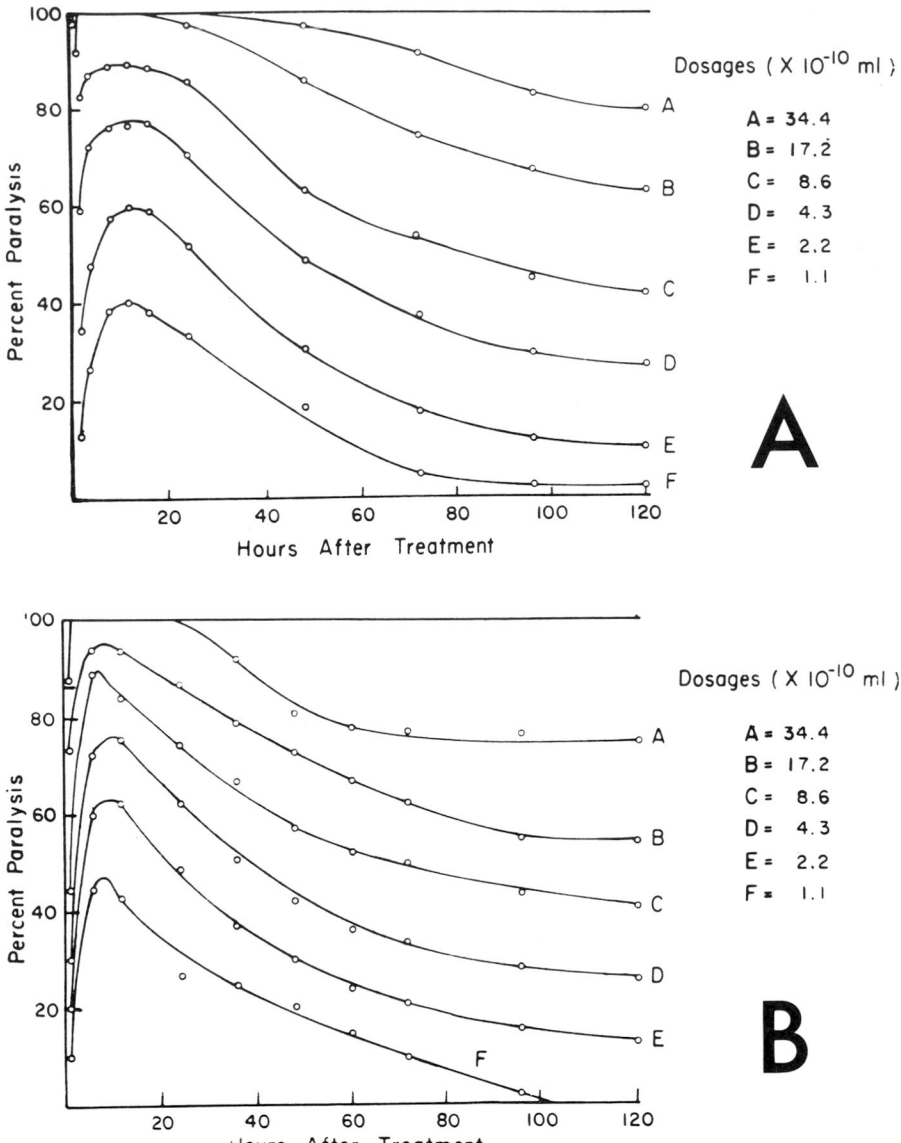

Fig. 13 A and B. Paralysis curves for *C. cephalonica*: A larvae injected with *Bracon* venom and held at room temperature; B larvae vaccinated with low dosage of venom 2 days before receiving regular dosages. From TAMASHIRO (1971)

days for recovery, the larvae were re-inoculated with a dosage series of venom, and the resulting degree of paralysis was compared with that of larvae not so "immunized." The paralysis curves for larvae so treated are shown in Figure 13. No important differences appear, and TAMASHIRO conluded that *C. cephalonica* was not detectably immunized to the effects of the braconid venom with a single "vaccination" of venom. No study was made using repeated immunizing inoculations.

References

Aidley, D.J.: The excitation of insect skeletal muscles. Adv. Insect Physiol. **4**, 1–31 (1967).

Askew, R.R.: Parasitic Insects. New York: American Elsevier, 1971.

Beard, R.L.: The toxicology of *Habrobracon* venom: a study of a natural insecticide. Conn. Agric. Exp. Stn Bull. 562 (1952).

Beard, R.L.: Secondary physiological effects of DDT in *Galleria* larvae. Entomol. Exp. Appl. **1**, 260–267 (1958).

Beard, R.L.: Electrographic recording of foregut activity in larvae of *Galleria mellonella*. Ann. Entomol. Soc. Amer. **53**, 346–351 (1960a).

Beard, R.L.: The nature of certain arthropod venoms and their effects on insect physiology. Proc. Int. Congr. Entomol., 11th, Vienna, **3**, 44–47 (1960).

Beard, R.L.: Insect toxins and venoms. Ann. Rev. Entomol. **8**, 1–18 (1963).

Beard, R.L.: Arthropod venoms as insecticides. In: Naturally Occurring Insecticides. New York: Marcel Dekker, 1971a.

Beard, R.L.: Production and use of venom by *Bracon brevicornis* (Wesm.). In: Toxins of Animal and Plant Origin. New York: Gordon and Breach, 1971b.

Beard, R.L.: Effectiveness of paralyzing venom and its relation to host discrimination by braconid wasps. Ann. Entomol. Soc. Amer. **65**, 90–93 (1972).

Beard, R.L., Clagett, D.C., Lam, W.K., Lee, Bik-Lam: *Microbracon brevicornis:* biochemical assay for active paralytic venom components. Unpublished manuscript (1971).

Bender, J.C.: Anatomy and histology of the female reproductive organs of *Habrobracon juglandis* (Ashmead) (Hymenoptera, Braconidae). Ann. Entomol. Soc. Amer. **36**, 537–545 (1943).

Berlese, A.: Gli insetti. Organi della riproduzione. Milan: Società Editrice Libraria, 1909, Vol. I Chap. 13, 891–892.

Capek, M.: The classification of Braconidae in relation to host specificity. Proc. Int. Congr. Entomol., 12th, London, 98–99 (1965).

Capek, M.: The classification of Braconidae from the viewpoint of their biology. Proc. Int. Congr. Entomol., 13th, Moscow, 1968, **1**, 120–121 (1971).

Clausen, C.P.: Entomophagous Insects. New York: McGraw-Hill, 1940.

Deitmer, J.: Die Wirkung des Giftes der Schlupfwespe *Habrobracon hebetor* Say auf die neuromuskuläre Übertragung am Sartoriusmuskel des Frosches. Diplomarbeit. Universität Bonn (1973).

Deleon, D.: The biology of *Coeloides dendroctoni* Cushman an important parasite of the mountain pine beetle (*Dendroctonus monticolae* Hopk.). Ann. Entomol. Soc. Amer. **28**, 411–424 (1935).

Drenth, D.: Some aspects of the collection and the action of the venom of *Microbracon hebetor* Say. Acta Physiol. Pharmac. Neerl. **15**, 100–101 (1969).

Drenth, D.: Susceptibility of different species of insects to an extract of the venom gland of the wasp *Microbracon hebetor* (Say). Toxicon **12**, 189–192 (1974a).

Drenth, D.: Stability of *Microbracon hebetor* (Say) venom preparations. Toxicon **12**, 541–542 (1974b).

Edwards, J.S., Sernka, T.J.: On the action of *Bracon* venom. Toxicon **6**, 303–305 (1969).

Fulton, B.B.: Notes on *Habrocytus cereallellae*, parasite of the Angoumois grain moth. Ann. Entomol. Soc. Amer. **26**, 536–553 (1933).

Genieys, P.: *Habrobracon brevicornis* Wesm. Ann. Entomol. Soc. Amer. **18**, 143–202 (1925).

Hase, A.: Die Schlupfwespen als Gifttiere. Biol. Zentr. **44**, 209–243 (1924).

Lee, Bik-Lam: An investigation on the biochemical properties of *Microbracon brevicornis* venom. Thesis. Northeastern University, Boston (1971).

Martin, A. Jr.: An Introduction to the Genetics of *Habrobracon juglandis* Ashmead. New York: Hobson Book Press, 1947.

Matthews, R.W.: Biology of Braconidae. Ann. Rev. Entomol. **19**, 15–32 (1974).

Muesebeck, C.F., Walkley, L.M.: Family Braconidae. In: Hymenoptera of America North of Mexico, Synoptic Catalog. Washington: U.S. Dep. Agric. Monograph 2, 1951.

Munro, J.W.: The structure and life history of *Bracon* sp.: a study in parasitism. Proc. Roy. Soc. Edinburgh 1915—1916, **36**, 313—333 (1917).

Myers, J.G.: Habits of *Alysia manducator*. Bull. Entomol. Res. **17**, 219—229 (1927).

Pawlowsky, E.N.: Des types principaux de glandes vénimeuses chez les Hyménoptères. C.r. Séanc. Soc. Biol. **76**, 351—354 (1914).

Payne, N.M.: The differential effect of environmental factors upon *Microbracon hebetor* Say (Hymenoptera: Braconidae) and its host *Ephestia kühniella* Zeller (Lepidoptera: Pyralidae). III Biol. Bull. **73**, 147—154 (1937).

Piek, T.: Site of action of venom of *Microbracon hebetor* Say (Braconidae, Hyménoptera). J. Insect Physiol. **12**, 561—568 (1966).

Piek, T., Engels, E.: Action of the venom of the wasp *Microbracon hebetor* Say on larvae and adults of the moth *Philosamia cynthia* Hübn. Comp. Biochem. Physiol. **28**, 603—618 (1969).

Piek, T., Mantel, P.: The effect of the venom of *Microbracon hebetor* (Say) on the hyperpolarizing potentials in a skeletal muscle of *Philosamia cynthia* Hübn. Comp. Gen. Pharmacol. **1**, 87—92 (1970).

Piek, T., Simon Thomas, R.T.: Paralyzing venoms of solitary wasps. Comp. Biochem. Physiol. **30**, 13—31 (1969).

Piek, T., Spanjer, W., Njio, K.D., Veenendaal, R.L., Mantel, P.: Paralysis caused by the venom of the wasp, *Microbracon gelechiae*. J. Insect Physiol. **20**, 2307—2319 (1974).

Rathmayer, W., Walther, C.: Electrophysiological investigations on the mode of action and specificity of *Habrobracon* venom. ms abstracted in Toxicon, **13**, 116 (1975).

Tamashiro, M.: A biological study of the venoms of two species of *Bracon*. Hawaii Agric. Exp. Stn Tech. Bull. **70**, 52 pp (1971).

Van der Meer, C., Drenth, D., Nijhof, J.K., Piek, T., Simon Thomas, R.T., Visser, B.J.: Paralyzing animal poisons. National Tech. Inform. Service Report AD 624456 (1965).

Visser, B.J., Spanjer, W.: Biochemical study of two paralyzing insect venoms. Acta Physiol. Pharmac. Neerl. **15**, 107—108 (1969).

Waller, J.B.: *Bracon* venom—a naturally occurring selective insecticide. Proc. Int. Congr. Entomol., 12th, London, 509—511 (1965a).

Waller, J.B.: The effect of the venom of *Bracon hebetor* on the respiration of the wax moth *Galleria mellonella*. J. Insect Physiol. **11**, 1595—1599 (1965b).

Walther, C., Rathmayer, W.: The effect of *Habrobracon* venom on excitatory neuromuscular transmission in insects. J. Comp. Physiol. **89**, 23—38 (1974).

Winteringham, F.P.W.: Mechanisms of selective insecticidal action. Ann. Rev. Entomol. **14**, 409—442 (1969).

CHAPTER 25

Venoms and Venom Apparatuses of the Formicidae: Myrmeciinae, Ponerinae, Dorylinae, Pseudomyrmecinae, Myrmicinae, and Formicinae

M.S. BLUM and H.R. HERMANN

A. Introduction

Ants, in the majority of subfamilies, are capable of stinging; in many cases, the reactions of human beings to such stings are severe enough to require immediate medical treatment. Because of their virtual ubiquity, ants constitute arthropods of considerable medical importance, although their role in inflicting stings is often unrecognized because of their relative inconspicuousness vis-à-vis flying hymenopterans such as bees and wasps. In all probability the venom arsenals of ants are highly varied but in addition, these insects also possess other exocrine glands which can be discharged during defensive encounters.

Poison (venom) gland constituents may be accompanied by a great variety of natural products synthesized in Dufour's gland (Figs. 7, 54, 56—58), an organ whose products are also discharged through the sting. A multitude of additional exocrine compounds, generated in the mandibular glands (Figs. 64—65), can also be evacuated prior to and during the act of stinging. Thus, ants are capable of secreting the products of at least three exocrine glands during an aggressive encounter.

With the exception of the Formicinae all the subfamilies of ants examined in this review contain species capable of stinging. The classification of these formicid subfamilies follows the scheme developed by BROWN (1954).

The subfamily classification of ants has had an interesting evolution over a period of time, beginning with contributions from EMERY, FOREL, MAYR and WHEELER and treated most recently by CLARK (1951) and BROWN (1954). At the time of BROWN's publication on internal phylogeny and subfamily classification, 9 separate subfamilies of ants were recognized: Myrmeciinae, Ponerinae, Cerapachyinae, Dorylinae, Leptanillinae, Pseudomyrmecinae, Myrmicinae, Dolichoderinae, and Formicinae. Since that time two additional subfamilies have been recognized (Aneuretinae and Sphecomyrminae) although WILSON (personal communication) recently has lumped *Aneuretus simoni* (Aneuretinae) with the dolichoderines, and *Sphecomyrma freyi* (Sphecomyrminae) is represented only by extinct members. We are thus at a point where most myrmecologists fully accept nine well-defined extant subfamilies and one extinct one.

Of the nine recognized extant subfamilies, this chapter deals with eight of them. We have omitted any discussion of the dolichoderines and their relatives, the aneuretines. Taxonomic considerations of these subfamilies are best covered by WHEELER (1950) and CREIGHTON (1950). A summary of their phylogenetic implications may be found in the paper by BROWN (1954).

Dolichoderines have been included in the following basic key to the recognized ant subfamilies.

Key to the Recognized Extant Subfamilies of the Formicidae [1]
Based on the Worker Caste

1 a   Abdominal pedicel consisting of 2 segments (petiole and postpetiole) . . 2

1 b   Abdominal pedicel consisting of only 1 segment (petiole) 5

2 a   Large eyes present, occupying approximately the anterior half of the sides of the head; long, slender mandibles present that are variously dentate on their inner margins; mandibles not squarely opposable but most often crossed over one another at full closure; restricted to the Australian Region . . . Myrmeciinae

2 b   Not as above; if eyes are large, then mandibles are not particularly long and slender 3

3 a   Frontal carinae found very close together and not covering the antennal insertions 4

3 b   Frontal carinae not close together, often being expanded laterally to more or less conceal the antennal insertions when head is viewed from above; clypeus most often prolonged back between frontal carinae . . . Myrmicinae

4 a   Eyes very large, essentially oval, occupying almost half the side of the head; ocelli most often present; mandibles not particularly elongate . . . Pseudomyrmecinae

4 b   Eyes absent or vestigial and ocellus-like; no ocelli present . . . Dorylinae

5 a   Gaster with a distinct constriction between first and second segments; if this constriction is faint, mandibles are linear and petiole bears a conical dorsal spine; sting well developed and integument well sclerotized . . . 6

5 b   Gaster without constriction between first and second segments; sting poorly developed or absent 7

6 a   Antennal scape short and stout, flattened or with a greatly reduced tip that bears a prominent lateral furrow; pygidium bearing distinct spines on its lateral and posterior boarders . . . . Cerapachyinae

6 b   Antennal scape most often long and slender; if scape is short and enlarged distally, at least the basal third is slender; pygidium not present . . . Ponerinae

7 a   Terminal gastral orifice (acidopore) circular and usually surrounded by a fringe of hairs . . . Formicinae

7 b   Terminal gastral orifice slitlike and not surrounded by a fringe of hairs . . . Dolichoderinae

---

[1] The subfamilies Leptanillinae and Aneuretinae are not included in this key since they are very rare and very little is known about their habits.

B. Venoms and Dufour's Gland Constituents

I. Myrmeciinae

1. Venom

Species in the subfamily Myrmeciinae, the bulldog ants, constitute the most primitive taxon of extant ants (BROWN, 1954). These ants are noted for their stinging propensities and analyses of the venoms of two species indicate that these proteinaceous secretions are quite similar to those produced by some species of wasps and bees (CAVILL et al., 1964; LEWIS and DE LA LANDE, 1967; WANSTALL and DE LA LANDE, 1974). Indeed, analyses of *Myrmecia* venoms represent the only detailed biochemical studies of proteinaceous ant venoms and as a consequence it is impossible to determine if these myrmeciine poison gland products are similar to the proteinaceous secretions of ants in more highly evolved subfamilies.

The venoms of *Myrmecia gulosa* (CAVILL et al., 1964) and *M. pyriformis* (LEWIS and DE LA LANDE, 1967) were obtained by dissecting out the venom gland reservoirs (plus venom gland) (Figs. 49—53, 55). In the case of *M. gulosa,* the venom was collected by rupturing the reservoir, whereas dried venom gland reservoirs were utilized for studying the venom of *M. pyriformis.* For both species, between 0.35—0.40 mg of venom were obtained from each worker, which is about 0.35 percent of the body weight.

Paper electrophoretic analyses of the venoms of both species demonstrated that these water-soluble secretions contained 6—8 constituents which possessed a wide range of pharmacologic activities (CAVILL et al., 1964; LEWIS and DE LA LANDE, 1967). Both venoms contained a biogenic amine, polypeptides, and enzymic and nonenzymic proteins. Starch gel electrophoresis demonstrated the presence of seven proteins in the venom of *M. pyriformis;* molecular weights ranged from 11,000 to greater than 23,000 (WANSTALL and DE LA LANDE, 1974).

a) Histamine

The only biogenic amine detected in the venoms of *M. pyriformis* (DE LA LANDE et al., 1963) and *M. gulosa* (CAVILL et al., 1964) is histamine. This compound accounts for about 2 percent of the dried venom of both species. Since all the biological activities described for the venom of *M. pyriformis* reside in histamine and three of the seven protein fractions, there are at least four protein constituents for which no demonstrable activity has been demonstrated (WANSTALL and DE LA LANDE, 1974).

b) Smooth Muscle Stimulant

Kininlike activity is present in the venoms of *M. pyriformis* (LEWIS and DE LA LANDE, 1967) and *M. gulosa* (CAVILL et al., 1964). The crude venom of *M. pyriformis* contracts the rat uterus and guinea pig ileum, and constricts blood vessels of the rabbit ear (LEWIS and DE LA LANDE, 1967). The minimum effective concentration of crude venom producing contraction of the rat uterus is 0.5—5.0 µg/ml. Fractionation of the venom of *M. pyriformis* by starch gel electrophoresis resulted in the isolation of a single protein (MW 11,000) which possessed, in addition to smooth muscle stimulant activity, red cell lysing and histamine-releasing activities (Wanstall and De la Lande, 1974). The smooth muscle stimulant in the venom of *M. gulosa* is identified with two protein fractions which migrate toward the cathode (Cavill et al., 1964).

c) Hyaluronidase

The venom of *M. gulosa* contains two fractions which possess about one-fifth the hyaluronidase activity of the enzyme isolated from bovine testes (Cavill et al., 1964). Five to 20 µg of the crude venom of *M. pyriformis* are required to produce detectable hydrolysis of hyaluronic acid (Lewis and De la Lande, 1967).

d) Direct Hemolytic Factor

Red blood cells are lysed by the venoms of *M. gulosa* and *M. pyriformis* (Cavill et al., 1964; Lewis and De la Lande, 1967). A single component, which migrated to the anode, was responsible for the hemolytic activity of the secretion of *M. gulosa* (Cavill et al., 1964). Fifty µg of crude *M. pyriformis* venom/ml produced marked hemolysis of human red blood cells (Lewis and De la Lande, 1967). A single component with a molecular weight of about 11,000 is responsible for the red cell lysing activity present in the venom of *M. pyriformis* (Wanstall and De la Lande, 1974).

e) Phospholipase A

The venom of *M. pyriformis* contains a phospholipase which hydrolyzes the ester bond of lecithin in the 2-position (Lewis et al., 1968). This phospholipase A may be responsible for some of the hemolytic activity of the venom through the production of lysolecithin, a known hemolysin. However, the presence of hemolytic activity in the venom in the absence of lecithin demonstrates that the poison gland secretion also contains a hemolysin other than phospholipase A (Lewis et al., 1968).

f) Histamine-Releasing Activity

Histamine is released from the intraperitoneal mast cells of the rat by the crude venom of *M. pyriformis* (Thomas and Lewis, 1965; Lewis and De la Lande, 1967). A minimum concentration of $3-7$ µg/ml of crude venom is required to cause histamine release. Although phospholipase A can contribute to some of the histamine-releasing activity of the venom by disrupting mast cells, the presence of such activity in more than one fraction of venom (Lewis and De la Lande, 1967) indicates that this enzyme cannot be solely responsible for the liberation of the biogenic amine. Two components are responsible for the histamine-releasing activity in the venom of *M. pyriformis,* a nonenzymic constituent (MW 11,000) and an enzymic component (MW > 23,000) (Wanstall and De la Lande, 1974).

2. Dufour's Gland Constituents

cis-8-Heptadecene thoroughly dominates the Dufour's gland secretion of *M. gulosa* (CAVILL and WILLIAMS, 1967). This alkene, which accounts for 62 percent of the secretion, is accompanied by *n*-tetradecane (1%), *n*-pentadecane (17%), hexadecane (1%), and heptadecane (4%). Branched hydrocarbons constitute the remaining 15 percent of the exudate. The composition of the Dufour's gland secretion of *M. tricolor* is very similar to that of *M. gulosa* (CAVILL and WILLIAMS, 1967).

II. Ponerinae

1. Venom

No detailed analyses of the venoms of ponerine species have been reported, but preliminary analyses demonstrate that proteinaceous constituents are present in the venom gland secretions. The venom of *Paraponera clavata* contains at least six proteins and that of *Neoponera villosa* is also rich in proteins (unpublished data).

2. Dufour's Gland Constituents

The Dufour's gland secretion of *Amblyopone australis* is reported to contain aliphatic hydrocarbons (CAVILL and WILLIAMS, 1967).

III. Dorylinae

1. Venom

The venom of workers of *Eciton burchelli,* obtained by rupturing the venom gland reservoir, contains proteinaceous constituents (unpublished data).

IV. Pseudomyrmecinae

1. Venom

The venom of *Pseudomyrmex pallidus,* collected in microcapillaries from the everted stings of workers, is proteinaceous (BLUM and CALLAHAN, 1963).

2. Dufour's Gland Constituents

The Dufour's gland secretion of five species contains *n*-pentadecane as a major constituent (BLUM and WHEELER, 1974). *n*-Heptadecane and heptadecene are also major constituents in some species whereas nonadecene and nonadecadiene occur as minor constituents.

V. Myrmicinae

1. Venom

Venoms of fire ant (*Solenopsis*) species were obtained by "milking" individual ants and collecting the venom in microcapillaries (BLUM et al., 1958). WILLIAMS

Table 1. Piperidine and piperideine alkaloids identified in the venoms of *Solenopsis* species

Species	Compound	Authority
S. richteri[a]	*cis-* and *trans-*2-Methyl-6-*n*-heptylpiperidine	MacCONNELL et al., 1974
S. sp.[b] and *S. richteri*[a]	*cis-* and *trans-*2-Methyl-6-*n*-nonylpiperidine	MacCONNELL et al., 1974
S. xyloni[b]	2-Methyl-6-*n*-undecyl-$\Delta^{1,2}$-piperideine	BRAND et al., 1972
S. invicta[a,b], *S. richteri*[a,b], *S. xyloni*[a,b], *S. geminata*[a,b], and *S. aurea*[a,b]	*cis-* and *trans-*2-Methyl-6-*n*-undecylpiperidine	MacCONNELL et al., 1970, 1971; BRAND et al., 1972; BLUM et al., 1973
S. invicta[b], *S. richteri*[b], *S. xyloni*[b], and *S. geminata*[b]	*cis-* and *trans-*2-Methyl-6-(*cis-*4-tridecenyl)piperidine	MacCONNELL et al., 1971; BRAND et al., 1972
S. invicta[b], *S. richteri*[b], *S. xyloni*[b], and *S. geminata*[b]	*cis-* and *trans-*2-Methyl-6-*n*-tridecylpiperidine	MacCONNEL et al., 1971; BRAND et al., 1972
S. invicta[b]	*cis-* and *trans-*2-Methyl-6-(*cis-*6-pentadecyl)piperidine	MacCONNELL et al., 1971; BRAND et al., 1972
S. invicta[b]	*cis-* and *trans-*2-Methyl-6-*n*-pentadecylpiperidine	MacCONNELL et al., 1971; BRAND et al., 1972

[a] Females.
[b] Workers.

and WILLIAMS (1965) obtained aqueous solutions of the venom of *Pogonomyrmex barbatus* by electrically stimulating the ants which were in contact with distilled water; the LD_{50} of this venom for dogs was 1.29 mg/kg.

The venom arsenals of species in myrmicine genera are remarkably diverse and constitute some of the richest sources of novel natural products in the Insecta. Proteinaceous constituents appear to be characteristic of myrmicine venoms (BLUM, 1966; WILLIAMS and WILLIAMS, 1965) but in addition, small pharmacologically active compounds may also be present in these poison gland secretions. Indeed some myrmicine venoms are highly fortified with alkaloids (MACCONNELL et al., 1970) and in at least a few cases proteinaceous compounds are present in very low concentrations relative to these alkaloids (BRAND et al., 1972). Analyses of the venoms produced by additional myrmicine genera promise to yield a wealth of surprises as regards natural products.

The venoms of fire ants (*Solenopsis* spp.) consist mostly of 2,6-dialkylpiperidines (Table 1) which possess insecticidal (BLUM et al., 1958), hemolytic (ADROUNY et al., 1959), antibacterial (JOUVANEZ et al., 1972), and necrotic (CARO et al., 1957) activities. There is considerable qualitative variation in the alkaloidal compositions of the venoms produced by *Solenopsis* species, and these alkaloidal "fingerprints" may have some value as character states. For example, the venom of *S. invicta* workers mostly contains the *trans-*isomers of five disubstituted piperidines (MAC-CONNELL et al., 1971), whereas the venoms of workers of *S. geminata* and *S. xyloni* consist essentially of the *cis-* and *trans*-isomers of a single piperidine alkaloid (BRAND et al., 1972). Furthermore, the venom gland secretions of individual workers from a single colony are subject to great quantitative variation, so that analyses of pooled samples of venom only reflect an average alkaloidal composition (BRAND et al., 1973a). Comparisons of the quantitative compositions of the venoms of individual workers from different colonies of the same species demonstrate that wide variations are common, and that high or low ratios of *cis-* and *trans*-isomers may be characteristic of particular colonies. These quantitative variations in the isomeric content of *Solenopsis* venoms are implicated even at the caste level; soldiers of *S. geminata* produce consistently higher ratios of the *cis-* and *trans*-isomers of 2-methyl-6-*n*-undecylpiperidine than their sister workers (BRAND et al., 1973a). On the other hand, numerous analyses of venom samples obtained from individual ants have demonstrated that these nitrogen heterocycles are produced with great qualitative exactitude.

Cast differences reach their ultimate expression when the compositions of the venoms of *Solenopsis* queens are compared to those of their workers. Such extraordinary quantitative and qualitative differences may characterize the venoms of the queens and their workers that they would not be recognized as originating from castes of the same species. The venom of *S. invicta* workers is dominated by five *trans*-alkaloids, and in particular two compounds with C_{15} side chains at the 6 position of their piperidine ring (Table 1) (MACCONNELL et al., 1971). On the other hand, the venom of the *S. invicta* female essentially contains both isomers of the alkaloid with a C_{11} side chain, very minor constituents in the worker venoms. Furthermore, the female venom contains a preponderance of the *cis*-alkaloid, whereas *cis*-isomers are quantitatively negligible in the venom of the workers. Indeed, in two species of *Solenopsis* BRAND et al. (1973b) found that the venoms of the females contained only the isomers of lowest molecular weight alkaloid synthesized by their workers. Even in the cases of two additional species in which the venoms of the females and workers were qualitatively similar, quantitative variations were significant.

BRAND et al. (1973b) proposed a hypothetical construct in the biochemical evolution of *Solenopsis* venoms based on: (1) thermodynamic considerations of the production of *cis-* and *trans*-isomers of the alkaloids; and (2) the compositions of the venoms of females and their workers. Considering proteinaceous venoms as the primitive state, dialkylpiperidine-rich venoms would constitute a derived condition. Since the *cis*-isomers can be biosynthesized more easily than the *trans*-isomers, on thermodynamic grounds, the former alkaloids would constitute the more primitive state. Alkaloidal evolution would proceed from species in which both females and their workers synthesize a predominance of the *cis*-isomer of the lowest molecular weight alkaloid (2-methyl-6-*n*-undecylpiperidine) as essentially their entire venom arsenal (*S. geminata, S. xyloni*-Table 1). A switch to the thermodynamically unfavorable *trans*-isomer would be followed by the addition of *trans*-isomers with longer hydrocarbon side chains (*S. richteri, S. invicta*-Table 1). This proposed biochemical evolution presupposes that the synthesis of *trans*-alkaloids is adaptively favourable to a species vis-à-vis *cis*-alkaloids, a possibility which is consistent with the much greater necrotic activity of venoms rich in *trans*-isomers (BRAND et al., 1973b).

Table 2. Dialkylpyrrolidines and pyrrolines in the venom of *Solenopsis punctaticeps* (FALES et al., 1974)

2-Ethyl-5-pentylpyrrolidine
2-Ethyl-5-pentyl-$\Delta^{1,2}$-pyrroline
2-Ethyl-5-pentyl-$\Delta^{1,5}$-pyrroline
2-Ethyl-5-heptylpyrrolidine
2-Ethyl-5-heptyl-$\Delta^{1,2}$-pyrroline
2-Ethyl-5-heptyl-$\Delta^{1,5}$-pyrroline
2-Butyl-5-pentylpyrrolidine
2-Butyl-5-pentyl-$\Delta^{1,2}$-pyrroline
2-Butyl-5-pentyl-$\Delta^{1,5}$-pyrroline
2-Butyl-5-heptylpyrrolidine

In contrast to the disubstituted piperidine produced by *Solenopsis* (*Solenopsis*) spp., the venom of *S. punctaticeps,* a South African species in another subgenus, contains only disubstituted C_4 nitrogen heterocycles (Table 2). This venom is dominated by dialkylpyrrolidines and pyrrolines (FALES et al., 1974) and contains isomeric pyrrolines in which the ring is unsaturated in either the $\Delta^{1,2}$ or $\Delta^{1,5}$-position (Table 2). Both *cis-* and *trans-*isomers of many of these alkaloids are present, but the stereochemistry of these compounds has not yet been determined. The significance of this qualitatively remarkable venom is difficult to visualize in the absence of pharmacologic investigations utilizing these compounds. The sting of *S. punctaticeps* is mild compared to those of *Solenopsis* species producing dialkyl-piperidines in their venoms (FALES et al., 1974) but it remains to be determined as to how effective these heterocycles are against the normal prey and predators or this species. However, it is now clear that some *Solenopsis* venoms can be of great qualitative diversity and investigations of the poison gland secretions of a wide range of species in this genus should be undertaken in order to establish the magnitude of this heterocyclic variation.

Substituted C_4 nitrogen heterocycles may have a wide distribution in myrmicine venoms. Methyl 4-methylpyrrole-2-carboxylate has been identified as a trail phero-mone in the venom of *Atta texana* (TUMLINSON et al., 1971), and 2-pentyl-5-butyl-pyrrolidine, a compound identified by FALES et al. (1974) in the venom of *S. puncta-ticeps,* has been detected as a poison gland product of *Monomorium pharaonis* (TALMAN et al., 1974). This dialkylpyrrolidine may be a precursor of 5-methyl-3-butyloctahydroindolizine, another compound recently identified in the venom of *Monomorium pharaonis* (RITTER et al., 1973). Another nitrogenous compound, 3-methylindole (skatole), appears to be a constituent of the venom of *Pheidole fallax* (LAW et al., 1965).

In marked contrast to the nitrogen heterocyclic theme illustrated by *Solenopsis* venoms, that of *Myrmicaria natalensis* is characterized by a terpenoid emphasis not known to be shared with species in any other myrmicine genera. This unusual poison gland secretion is dominated by *d-* and *l-*limonene (GRÜNANGER et al., 1960) but in addition, contains a diversity of other monoterpene hydrocarbons. This venom is also fortified with α-pinene, β-pinene, camphene, sabinene, myrcene, α-phellandrene, α-terpinene, and terpinolene (BRAND et al., 1974). Although several of these compounds have been identified in the frontal gland secretions of termitid soldiers, three of these monoterpenes-camphene, sabinene, and α-terpinene-had not been previously detected in animal secretions. While the poison gland products of *M. natalensis* must be regarded as constituting a novel myrmicine venom exudate, they may nevertheless be illustrative of the natural product potential of these exocrine secretions.

GRÜNANGER et al. (1960) also identified acetic, propionic, *n*-butyric, isobutyric, and isovaleric acids from whole body extracts of *M. natalensis*. These compounds are probably exocrine products which may have their origin in one of the abdominal defensive glands.

BUREN (1958) has emphasized that while the spatulate sting of *Crematogaster* spp. is not a suitable injection device, it would function ideally as an organ for topically applying venom. The venoms of many species of *Crematogaster* are emitted as a froth which accumulates on the spatulate portion of the sting where it can be easily administered to the integument of another arthropod. We have observed that the venom of *C. lineolata,* collected in microcapillaries, is very toxic when topically administered to termite workers (*Reticulitermes virginicus*). This fact is consistent with the conclusion that the venoms of *Crematogaster* spp. are adapted for integumentary application by the spatulate sting and thus may contain small molecules which exert toxic action after penetrating the cuticle. As a consequence, *Crematogaster* venoms may constitute another rich source of low molecular weight natural products possessing considerable toxicity when applied topically to invertebrates.

2. Dufour's Gland Constituents

Aliphatic hydrocarbons appear to be the only class of compounds biosynthesized in the Dufour's glands of myrmicine ants. Twenty-six hydrocarbons, in the range $C_{12}-C_{19}$, have been indentified in the secretions of species in five myrmicine genera (Table 3). The ability of some myrmicine species to synthesize isoprenoids in these exocrine tissues is illustrated by the identification of three sesquiterpenes (e.g., farnesene) as glandular products. Many of these hydrocarbons probably function as part of an alarm-defense system and it is very likely that they possess other communicative roles, as well.

Table 3. Hydrocarbons identified in the Dufour's gland secretions of myrmicine ants

Species	Compound	Authority
Pogonomyrmex rugosus and *P. barbatus*	*n*-Dodecane	REGNIER et al., 1973
Pogonomyrmex rugosus and *P. barbatus*	3-Methylundecane	REGNIER et al., 1973
Pogonomyrmex rugosus	5-Methylundecane	REGNIER et al., 1973
Pogonomyrmex rugosus	6-Methylundecane	REGNIER et al., 1973
Novomessor cockerelli, Myrmica rubra, Pogonomyrmex rugosus, and *P. barbatus*	*n*-Tridecane	VICK et al., 1969; MORGAN and WADHAMS, 1972; REGNIER et al., 1973
Pogonomyrmex rugosus and *P. barbatus*	3-Methyldodecane	REGNIER et al., 1973
Pogonomyrmex rugosus and *P. barbatus*	6-Methyldodecane	REGNIER et al., 1973
Novomessor cockerelli, Pogonomyrmex rugosus, and *P. barbatus*	*n*-Tetradecane	VICK et al., 1969; REGNIER et al., 1973

Table 3 (continued)

Species	Compound	Authority
Pogonomyrmex rugosus and *P. barbatus*	5-Methyltridecane	Regnier et al., 1973
Pogonomyrmex rugosus and *P. barbatus*	3,5-Dimethyldodecane	Regnier et al., 1973
Novomessor cockerelli, Myrmica rubra, Pogonomyrmex rugosus, and *P. barbatus*	*n*-Pentadecane	Vick et al., 1969; Morgan and Wadhams, 1972; Regnier et al., 1973
Pogonomyrmex rugosus and *P. barbatus*	6-Methyltetradecane	Regnier et al., 1973
Pogonomyrmex rugosus and *P. barbatus*	3,4-Dimethyltridecane	Regnier et al., 1973
Myrmica rubra	7-Pentadecene	Morgan and Wadhams, 1972
Aphaenogaster longiceps	α-Farnesene	Cavill et al., 1967
Novomessor cockerelli and *Myrmica rubra*	*n*-Hexadecane	Vick et al., 1969; Morgan and Wadhams, 1972
Myrmica rubra	Hexadecene	Morgan and Wadhams, 1972
Myrmica rubra	Homofarnesene	Morgan and Wadhams, 1972
Novomessor cockerelli, Myrmica rubra, Solenopsis invicta, S. richteri, and *S. geminata*	*n*-Heptadecane	Vick et al., 1969; Morgan and Wadhams, 1972; Brand et al., 1972
Myrmica rubra	*cis*-8-Heptadecene	Morgan and Wadhams, 1972
Myrmica rubra	Heptadecadiene	Morgan and Wadhams, 1972
Myrmica rubra	Bishomofarnesene	Morgan and Wadhams, 1972
Novomessor cockerelli and *Myrmica rubra*	*n*-Octadecane	Vick et al., 1969; Morgan and Wadhams, 1972
Myrmica rubra	9-Octadecene	Morgan and Wadhams, 1972
Novomessor cockerelli and *Myrmica rubra*	*n*-Nonadecane	Vick et al., 1969; Morgan and Wadhams, 1972
Myrmica rubra	9-Nonadecene	Morgan and Wadhams, 1972

VI. Formicinae

1. Venom

Formic acid appears to be a diagnostic character for all species in the subfamily Formicinae. This simple fatty acid was first isolated by Wray (1670) from workers of *Formica rufa* and since that time this compound has been identified in a wide range of formicine species. Although acidic constituents produced by a few species of ants in other subfamilies have been reported as formic acid, there is no strong evidence to indicate that this compound is indeed a constituent of the venoms of nonformicine ants.

Although formicine ants do not possess a functional sting, the utilization of venoms containing very high concentrations of formic acid provides these insects with a formidable defensive weapon. This acid is the strongest of the unsubstituted alkanoic monoacids and as a consequence, is a very powerful cytotoxin. STUMPER (1951) reported that the venoms of *Formica rufa* and *F. pratensis* contained 50 percent aqueous formic acid and OSMAN and BRANDER (1961) found that the secretion of *F. polyctena* was fortified with a 60 percent solution of this compound. Formic acid has been detected in the venoms of species in the following formicine genera: *Camponotus* (MELANDER and BRUES, 1906; STUMPER, 1922, 1952), *Formica* (MELANDER and BRUES, 1906; STUMPER, 1922, 1952; O'ROURKE, 1950; OSMAN and BRANDER, 1961), *Cataglyphis* (STUMPER, 1922, 1952), *Lasius* (STUMPER, 1952), *Plagiolepis* (STUMPER, 1952), *Polyergus* (STUMPER, 1952), *Acanthomyops* (REGNIER and WILSON, 1968), and *Anoplolepis* (SCHREUDER and BRAND, 1972).

Formic acid is the only volatile compound which has been detected in the venom gland secretions of formicine ants. However, the venoms of *Formica polyctena* and *Camponotus pennsylvanicus* also contain peptides and free amino acids (OSMAN and BRANDER, 1961; HERMANN and BLUM, 1968) whose significance as poison gland constituents is unknown. Presumably, the venoms of other formicine species are also enriched with similar nitrogenous constituents.

2. Dufour's Gland Constituents

The Dufour's gland in formicine ants must be regarded as the arthropod hydrocarbon factory par excellence. Forty six aliphatic hydrocarbons have been identified in the secretions of species in six formicine genera and these compounds cover the wide range of $C_9 - C_{23}$ (Table 4). *n*-Undecane and *n*-tridecane appear to be major alkanes produced by formicine species whereas the longer chain hydrocarbons are generally minor constituents. The alkanes are frequently accompanied by their corresponding alkenes and in several cases the dienes are also present in the Dufour's gland secretions (Table 4). Pathways for the biosynthesis of terpenes do not appear to be well developed in the tissues of the Dufour's gland and with the exception of α-farnesene (BERGSTRÖM and LÖFQVIST, 1968) and farnesyl acetate (BERGSTRÖM and LÖFQVIST, 1970), isoprenoids have not been detected in these secretions. Monomethyl-branched alkanes, generally substituted in the 3- or 5-position, appear to be characteristic of some *Formica* and *Camponotus* species (Table 4) as further testimony to the hydrocarbon diversity identified with the secretions of this exocrine gland.

A host of oxygenated compounds have been identified as concomitants of the alkane-rich secretions of the Dufour's gland. In particular, alcohols, ketones, esters, acids, and lactones have been demonstrated to be major glandular constituents, especially in the exudates of *Lasius* species (BERGSTRÖM and LÖFQVIST, 1970). Normal alcohols in the range $C_{10} - C_{16}$ are produced by *Formica* and *Lasius* species and these compounds are frequently accompanied by their acetates

Table 4. Compounds identified in the Dufour's gland secretions of formicine species

Species	Compound	Authority
Formica sanguinea, F. rufibarbis, F. nigricans, F. rufa, F. polyctena and *Camponotus ligniperda*	*n*-Nonane	BERGSTRÖM and LÖVQVIST, 1968; BERGSTRÖM and LÖFQVIST, 1973; BERGSTRÖM and LÖFQVIST, 1971
Formica sanguinea, F. fusca, F. rufibarbis, F. nigricans, F. rufa, F. polyctena, Lasius alienus, L. flavus, L. carniolicus, Camponotus ligniperda, C. herculeanus, C. americanus, C. pennsylvanicus, and *Anoplolepis custodiens*	*n*-Decane	BERGSTRÖM and LÖVQVIST, 1968; BERGSTRÖM and LÖFQVIST, 1973; BERGSTRÖM and LÖFQVIST, 1970; BERGSTRÖM and LÖFQVIST, 1971; BERGSTRÖM and LÖFQVIST, 1972; AYRE and BLUM, 1971; SCHREUDER and BRAND, 1972
Formica nigricans and *Anoplolepis custodiens*	3-Methylnonane	BERGSTRÖM and LÖFQVIST, 1973; SCHREUDER and BRAND, 1972
Anoplolepis custodiens	Decene	SCHREUDER and BRAND, 1972
Formica rufa, F. sanguinea, F. rufibarbis, F. neogagates, F. subsericea, F. schaufussi, F. exsectoides, F. rubicunda, F. pergandei, F. subintegra, F. nigricans, F. polyctena, Lasius umbratus, L. fuliginosus, L. alienus, L. niger, L. flavus, L. carniolicus, L. sitkaensis, L. neoniger, L. nearcticus, L. speculiventris, Acanthomyops claviger, A. latipes, A. subglaber, Camponotus americanus, C. pennsylvanicus, C. herculeanus, C. ligniperda, C. noveboracensis, C. intrepidus, Anoplolepis custodiens, and *Polyergus rufescens*	*n*-Undecane	BERGSTRÖM and LÖFQVIST, 1968; BERGSTRÖM and LÖFQVIST, 1973; WILSON and REGNIER, 1971; BERGSTRÖM and LÖFQVIST, 1970; REGNIER and WILSON, 1969; QUILICO et al., 1957a; BERNARDI et al., 1967; REGNIER and WILSON, 1968; BERGSTRÖM and LÖFQVIST, 1971; BERGSTRÖM and LÖFQVIST, 1973; AYRE and BLUM, 1971; BROPHY et al., 1973; SCHREUDER and BRAND, 1972
Formica nigricans, F. rufa, F. polyctena, Camponotus ligniperda, C. herculeanus, and *Anoplolepis custodiens*	9-Undecene	BERGSTRÖM and LÖFQVIST, 1973; BERGSTRÖM and LÖFQVIST, 1971; BERGSTRÖM and LÖFQVIST, 1972; SCHREUDER and BRAND, 1972
Formica fusca, F. rufibarbis, F. nigricans, F. rufa, F. polyctena, Lasius alienus, Camponotus ligniperda, C. herculeanus, C. intrepidus, and *Anoplolepis custodiens*	*n*-Dodecane	BERGSTRÖM and LÖFQVIST, 1968; BERGSTRÖM and LÖFQVIST, 1973; BERGSTRÖM and LÖFQVIST, 1970; BERGSTRÖM and LÖFQVIST, 1971; BERGSTRÖM and LÖFQVIST, 1972; SCHREUDER and BRAND, 1972
Formica nigricans, F. rufa, F. polyctena, Camponotus ligniperda, C. herculeanus, C. intrepidus, and *Anoplolepis custodiens*	1-Dodecene	BERGSTRÖM and LÖFQVIST, 1973; BERGSTRÖM and LÖFQVIST, 1971; BERGSTRÖM and LÖFQVIST, 1972; BROPHY et al., 1973; SCHREUDER and BRAND, 1972
Formica fusca, F. nigricans, F. rufa, F. polyctena, Lasius carniolicus, Camponotus ligniperda, C. herculeanus, and *C. intrepidus*	3-Methylundecane	BERGSTRÖM and LÖFQVIST, 1968; BERGSTRÖM and LÖFQVIST, 1973; BERGSTRÖM and LÖFQVIST, 1970; BERGSTRÖM and LÖFQVIST, 1971, BERGSTRÖM and LÖFQVIST, 1972; BROPHY et al., 1973
Formica nigricans and *F. polyctena*	Dodecadiene	BERGSTRÖM and LÖFQVIST, 1973
Formica nigricans, F. polyctena, and *F. rufa*	5-Methylundecane	BERGSTRÖM and LÖFQVIST, 1973; BROPHY et al., 1973

Table 4 (continued)

Species	Compound	Authority
Formica sanguinea, F. fusca, F. rufibarbis, F. subintegra, F. subsericea, F. nigricans, F. rufa, F. polyctena, Lasius fuliginosus, L. alienus, L. niger, L. flavus, L. carniolicus, Acanthomyops claviger, Camponotus ligniperda, C. americanus, C. pennsylvanicus, C. herculeanus, C. intrepidus, and *Anoplolepis custodiens*	*n*-Tridecane	BERGSTRÖM and LÖFQVIST, 1968; BERGSTRÖM and LÖFQVIST, 1973; BERNARDI et al., 1967; BERGSTRÖM and LÖFQVIST, 1970; REGNIER and WILSON, 1969; BERGSTRÖM and LÖFQVIST, 1971; BERGSTRÖM and LÖFQVIST, 1972; AYRE and BLUM, 1971; BROPHY et al., 1973; SCHREUDER and BRAND, 1972
Formica fusca, Lasius flavus, Camponotus ligniperda, C. herculeanus, C. americanus, C. pennsylvanicus, C. intrepidus, and *Anoplolepis custodiens*	9-Tridecene	BERGSTRÖM and LÖFQVIST, 1968; BERGSTRÖM and LÖFQVIST, 1970; BERGSTRÖM and LÖFQVIST, 1971; BERGSTRÖM and LÖFQVIST, 1972; AYRE and BLUM, 1971; BROPHY et al., 1973; SCHREUDER and BRAND, 1972
Camponotus intrepidus	3-Methyldodecane	BROPHY et al., 1973
Formica nigricans	4-Methyldodecane	BERGSTRÖM and LÖFQVIST, 1973
Camponotus intrepidus	5-Methyldodecane	BROPHY et al., 1973
Camponotus ligniperda	Tridecadiene	BERGSTRÖM and LÖFQVIST, 1971
Formica nigricans, F. rufa, F. polyctena, Camponotus ligniperda, C. herculeanus, C. intrepidus, and *Anoplolepis custodiens*	*n*-Tetradecane	BERGSTRÖM and LÖFQVIST, 1973; BERGSTRÖM and LÖFQVIST, 1971; BERGSTRÖM and LÖFQVIST, 1972; BROPHY et al., 1973; SCHREUDER and BRAND, 1972
Formica nigricans, F. rufa, F. polyctena, Camponotus ligniperda, C. herculeanus, and *C. intrepidus*	3-Methyltridecane	BERGSTRÖM and LÖFQVIST, 1973; BERGSTRÖM and LÖFQVIST, 1971; BERGSTRÖM and LÖFQVIST, 1972; BROPHY et al., 1973
Formica nigricans, F. rufa, F. polyctena, Camponotus ligniperda, C. herculeanus, and *C. intrepidus*	5-Methyltridecane	BERGSTRÖM and LÖFQVIST, 1973; BERGSTRÖM and LÖFQVIST, 1972; BERGSTRÖM and LÖFQVIST, 1971; BROPHY et al., 1973
Formica nigricans, F. rufa, F. polyctena, Camponotus ligniperda, and *Anoplolepis custodiens*	Tetradecene	BERGSTRÖM and LÖFQVIST, 1973; BERGSTRÖM and LÖFQVIST, 1972; SCHREUDER and BRAND, 1972
Formica fusca, F. rufibarbis, F. nigricans, F. rufa, F. polyctena, Lasius fuliginosus, L. alienus, Camponotus ligniperda, C. herculeanus, C. americanus, C. pennsylvanicus, C. intrepidus, and *Anoplolepis custodiens*	*n*-Pentadecane	BERGSTRÖM and LÖFQVIST, 1968; BERGSTRÖM and LÖFQVIST, 1973; BERNARDI et al., 1967; BERGSTRÖM and LÖFQVIST, 1970; BERGSTRÖM and LÖFQVIST, 1971; BERGSTRÖM and LÖFQVIST, 1972; AYRE and BLUM, 1971; BROPHY et al., 1973; SCHREUDER and BRAND, 1972
Formica rufibarbis, F. nigricans, F. rufa, F. polyctena, Camponotus ligniperda, C. herculeanus, C. americanus, C. intrepidus, and *Anoplolepis custodiens*	7-Pentadecene	BERGSTRÖM and LÖFQVIST, 1968; BERGSTRÖM and LÖFQVIST, 1972; AYRE and BLUM, 1971; BROPHY et al., 1973; SCHREUDER and BRAND, 1972

Table 4 (continued)

Species	Compound	Authority
Formica nigricans and *F. polyctena*	Pentadecadiene	BERGSTRÖM and LÖFQVIST, 1973
Formica sanguinea, F. fusca, Camponotus ligniperda, C. herculeanus, and *Polyergus rufescens*	α-Farnesene	BERGSTRÖM and LÖFQVIST, 1968; BERGSTRÖM and LÖFQVIST, 1971; BERGSTRÖM and LÖFQVIST, 1972
Formica nigricans, F. rufa, F. polyctena, Camponotus ligniperda, C. herculeanus, and *Anoplolepis custodiens*	n-Hexadecane	BERGSTRÖM and LÖFQVIST, 1973; BERGSTRÖM and LÖFQVIST, 1971; BERGSTRÖM and LÖFQVIST, 1972; SCHREUDER and BRAND, 1972
Formica nigricans and *Anoplolepis custodiens*	Hexadecene	BERGSTRÖM and LÖFQVIST, 1973; SCHREUDER and BRAND, 1972
Camponotus intrepidus	3-Methylpentadecane	BROPHY et al., 1973
Formica nigricans and *Camponotus intrepidus*	5-Methylpentadecane	BERGSTRÖM and LÖFQVIST, 1973; BROPHY et al., 1973
Formica fusca, F. rufibarbis, F. nigricans, F. rufa, F. polyctena, Lasius niger, L. alienus, Camponotus ligniperda, C. herculeanus, C. intrepidus, Anoplolepis custodiens, and *Polyergus rufescens*	*n*-Heptadecane	BERGSTRÖM and LÖFQVIST, 1968; BERGSTRÖM and LÖFQVIST, 1973; BERGSTRÖM and LÖFQVIST, 1970; BERGSTRÖM and LÖFQVIST, 1971; BERGSTRÖM and LÖFQVIST, 1972; BROPHY et al., 1973; SCHREUDER and BRAND, 1972
Formica nigricans, F. rufibarbis, F. rufa, F. polyctena, Lasius niger, L. alienus, Camponotus ligniperda, C. herculeanus, and *Anoplolepis custodiens*	*cis*-8-Heptadecene	BERGSTRÖM and LÖFQVIST, 1968; BERGSTRÖM and LÖFQVIST, 1973; BERGSTRÖM and LÖFQVIST, 1970; BERGSTRÖM and LÖFQVIST, 1971; BERGSTRÖM and LÖFQVIST, 1972; SCHREUDER and BRAND, 1972
Formica nigricans, F. rufa, F. polyctena, Camponotus ligniperda, and *C. herculeanus*	Heptadecadiene	BERGSTRÖM and LÖFQVIST, 1973; BERGSTRÖM and LÖFQVIST, 1971; BERGSTRÖM and LÖFQVIST, 1972
Camponotus intrepidus	3-Methylheptadecane	BROPHY et al., 1973
Camponotus intrepidus	5-Methylheptadecane	BROPHY et al., 1973
Formica nigricans, F. rufa, F. polyctena, Camponotus ligniperda, C. ligniperda, and *Anoplolepis custodiens*	*n*-Octadecane	BERGSTRÖM and LÖFQVIST, 1973; BERGSTRÖM and LÖFQVIST, 1971; BERGSTRÖM and LÖFQVIST, 1972; SCHREUDER and BRAND, 1972
Formica nigricans, F. rufa, F. polyctena, and *Anoplolepis custodiens*	9-Octadecene	BERGSTRÖM and LÖFQVIST, 1973; SCHREUDER and BRAND, 1972
Formica rufibarbis, F. rufa, F. polyctena, F. nigricans, Lasius niger, Camponotus ligniperda, C. herculeanus, and *Anoplolepis custodiens*	*n*-Nonadecane	BERGSTRÖM and LÖFQVIST, 1968; BERGSTRÖM and LÖFQVIST, 1973; BERGSTRÖM and LÖFQVIST, 1970; BERGSTRÖM and LÖFQVIST, 1971; BERGSTRÖM and LÖFQVIST, 1972; SCHREUDER and BRAND, 1972
Formica nigricans, F. rufa, F. polyctena, Lasius alienus, Camponotus ligniperda, and *Anoplolepis custodiens*	9-Nonadecene	BERGSTRÖM and LÖFQVIST, 1973; BERGSTRÖM and LÖFQVIST, 1970; BERGSTRÖM and LÖFQVIST, 1971; SCHREUDER and BRAND, 1972

Table 4 (continued)

Species	Compound	Authority
Formica nigricans, F. rufa, and *F. polyctena*	Nonadecadiene	BERGSTRÖM and LÖFQVIST, 1973
Formica nigricans, F. rufa, F. polyctena, and *Anoplolepis custodiens*	*n*-Eicosane	BERGSTRÖM and LÖFQVIST, 1973; SCHREUDER and BRAND, 1972
Formica rufa and *Anoplolepis custodiens*	Eicosene	BERGSTRÖM and LÖFQVIST, 1973; SCHREUDER and BRAND, 1972
Formica nigricans, F. rufa, Lasius alienus, and *Anoplolepis custodiens*	*n*-Heneicosane	BERGSTRÖM and LÖFQVIST, 1973; BERGSTRÖM and LÖFQVIST, 1970; SCHREUDER and BRAND, 1972
Formica nigricans, F. rufa, F. polyctena, and *Anoplolepis custodiens*	Heneicosene	BERGSTRÖM and LÖFQVIST, 1973; SCHREUDER and BRAND, 1972
Formica nigricans and *F. rufa*	*n*-Docosane	BERGSTRÖM and LÖFQVIST, 1973
Camponotus ligniperda	*n*-Tricosane	BERGSTRÖM and LÖFQVIST, 1971
Formica nigricans, F. rufa, and *F. polyctena*	Tricosene	BERGSTRÖM and LÖFQVIST, 1973
Formica sanguinea	1-Decanol	BERGSTRÖM and LÖFQVIST, 1968
Formica sanguinea and *Lasius niger*	1-Undecanol	BERGSTRÖM and LÖFQVIST, 1968; BERGSTRÖM and LÖFQVIST, 1970
Formica sanguinea and *Lasius niger*	1-Dodecanol	BERGSTRÖM and LÖFQVIST, 1968; BERGSTRÖM and LÖFQVIST, 1970
Camponotus ligniperda	1-Tridecanol	BERGSTRÖM and LÖFQVIST, 1971
Camponotus ligniperda and *C. herculeanus*	1-Pentadecanol	BERGSTRÖM and LÖFQVIST, 1971; BERGSTRÖM and LÖFQVIST, 1972
Camponotus ligniperda, C. herculeanus, and *Lasius niger*	1-Hexadecanol	BERGSTRÖM and LÖFQVIST, 1971; BERGSTRÖM and LÖFQVIST, 1972; BERGSTRÖM and LÖFQVIST, 1970
Formica nigricans, F. polyctena, and *Camponotus ligniperda*	Hexadecenol	BERGSTRÖM and LÖFQVIST, 1973; BERGSTRÖM and LÖFQVIST, 1971
Formica nigricans, F. rufa, and *F. polyctena*	all-*trans*-Geranyl geraniol	BERGSTRÖM and LÖFQVIST, 1973
Formica rufibarbis, F. neogagates, F. rubicunda, F. subsericea, Lasius umbratus, L. speculiventris, L. alienus, L. neoniger, L. carniolicus, Acanthomyops claviger, A. latipes, A. subglaber, Camponotus ligniperda, and *C. herculeanus*	2-Tridecanone	BERGSTRÖM and LÖFQVIST, 1968; WILSON and REGNIER, 1971; QUILICO et al., 1957a; BLUM et al., 1968a; BERGSTRÖM and LÖFQVIST, 1970; REGNIER and WILSON, 1969; REGNIER and WILSON, 1968; BERGSTRÖM and LÖFQVIST, 1971; BERGSTRÖM and LÖFQVIST, 1972
Lasius carniolicus	3-Tetradecanone	BERGSTRÖM and LÖFQVIST, 1970
Lasius carniolicus, L. fuliginosus, L. alienus, L. umbratus, L. nearcticus, L. speculiventris, Acanthomyops claviger, A. latipes, A. subglaber, and *Camponotus ligniperda*	2-Pentadecanone	BERGSTRÖM and LÖFQVIST, 1970; BERNARDI et al., 1967; REGNIER and WILSON, 1969; WILSON and REGNIER, 1971; REGNIER and WILSON, 1968; BERGSTRÖM and LÖFQVIST, 1971
Lasius carniolicus	3-Hexadecanone	BERGSTRÖM and LÖFQVIST, 1970

Table 4 (continued)

Species	Compound	Authority
Lasius alienus and *L. fuliginosus*	2-Heptadecanone	Bergström and Löfqvist, 1970; Bernardi et al., 1967
Lasius alienus	2-Nonadecanone	Bergström and Löfqvist, 1970
Lasius flavus	4-Hydroxyoctadec-9-enoic acid	Bergström and Löfqvist, 1970
Formica sanguinea (females)	*n*-Nonyl acetate	Bergström and Löfqvist, 1968
Formica sanguinea, F. rufibarbis, F. pergandei, F. subintegra, Lasius niger, and *Camponotus ligniperda*	*n*-Decyl acetate	Bergström and Löfqvist, 1968; Wilson and Regnier, 1971; Bergström and Löfqvist, 1970; Bergström and Löfqvist, 1971
Formica sanguinea, F. rufibarbis, Lasius niger, and *Camponotus ligniperda*	*n*-Undecyl acetate	Bergström and Löfqvist, 1968; Bergström and Löfqvist, 1970; Bergström and Löfqvist, 1972
Formica sanguinea, F. rufibarbis, F. pergandei, F. subintegra, and *Lasius niger*	*n*-Dodecyl acetate	Bergström and Löfqvist, 1968; Wilson and Regnier, 1971; Bergström and Löfqvist, 1970
Camponotus ligniperda	*n*-Tridecyl acetate	Bergström and Löfqvist, 1972
Formica pergandei, F. subintegra, F. nigricans, F. rufa, F. polyctena, Lasius niger, Camponotus ligniperda, and *C. herculeanus*	*n*-Tetradecyl acetate	Wilson and Regnier, 1971; Bergström and Löfqvist, 1973; Bergström and Löfqvist, 1970; Bergström and Löfqvist, 1971; Bergström and Löfqvist, 1972
Formica nigricans, F. rufa, F. polyctena, Camponotus ligniperda, and *C. herculeanus*	Tetradecenyl acetate	Bergström and Löfqvist, 1973; Bergström and Löfqvist, 1971; Bergström and Löfqvist, 1972
Lasius alienus	Methyl *n*-hexadecanoate	Bergström and Löfqvist, 1970
Camponotus ligniperda and *C. herculeanus*	*n*-Pentadecyl acetate	Bergström and Löfqvist, 1971; Bergström and Löfqvist, 1972
Lasius niger, Camponotus ligniperda, and *C. herculeanus*	Farnesyl acetate	Bergström and Löfqvist, 1970; Bergström and Löfqvist, 1971; Bergström and Löfqvist, 1972
Formica nigricans, F. rufa, F. polyctena, Lasius niger, L. alienus, Camponotus ligniperda, and *C. herculeanus*	*n*-Hexadecyl acetate	Bergström and Löfqvist, 1973; Bergström and Löfqvist, 1970; Bergström and Löfqvist, 1971; Bergström and Löfqvist, 1972
Formica nigricans, F. rufa, F. polyctena, Camponotus ligniperda, and *C. herculeanus*	Hexadecenyl acetate	Bergström and Löfqvist, 1973; Bergström and Löfqvist, 1971; Bergström and Löfqvist, 1972
Formica nigricans, F. rufa, F. polyctena, Lasius niger, and *Camponotus ligniperda*	*n*-Octadecyl acetate	Bergström and Löfqvist, 1973; Bergström and Löfqvist, 1970; Bergström and Löfqvist, 1971
Formica nigricans, F. rufa, and *F. polyctena*	Geranylgeranyl acetate	Bergström and Löfqvist, 1973
Lasius flavus	4-Hydroxyhexadec-9-enolide	Bergström and Löfqvist, 1970
Lasius flavus	4-Hydroxyoctadec-9-enolide	Bergström and Löfqvist, 1970

which may constitute major glandular products (BERGSTRÖM and LÖFQVIST, 1968, 1970). $C_{13}-C_{19}$ methyl ketones are commonly produced by formicine species and 2-tridecanone is often a major glandular constituent (Table 4). The identification of two ethyl ketones- 3-tetradecanone and 3-hexadecanone—in the secretion of *Lasius carniolicus* (BERGSTRÖM and LÖFQVIST, 1970) clearly demonstrates the ability of the formicine Dufour's gland to biosynthesize 3-alkanones as well as 2-alkanones. *Lasius flavus* is distinguished by its ability to synthesize two γ-hydroxy lactones and one of their corresponding acids (BERGSTRÖM and LÖFQVIST, 1970).

The Dufour's gland secretions of formicine ants constitute the most qualitatively complex exocrine secretions that have been characterized from arthropods. The identification of about 40 of the 50 compounds detected in the secretion of *Camponotus ligniperda* (BERGSTRÖM and LÖFQVIST, 1971) is indicative of the chemical diversity associated with this exocrine organ and should provide a spur for the detailed analyses of the Dufour's gland secretions of additional formicine species.

C. Morphology of the Hymenopterous Venom Apparatus

The formicid venom apparatus is well known primarily as a defensive system. It was derived first from an ovipositor, such as we find in the Thysanura, Orthoptera, Thysanoptera, Hemiptera, and Homoptera (Figs. 1, 1—4) (MICHENER, 1944; SCUDDER, 1961a, 1961b; SMITH, 1969; SNODGRASS, 1935, 1956).

In the early Hymenoptera (Symphyta) it retained its function solely as a system of oviposition (CHRYSTAL, 1928; COOPER, 1953; MALYSHEV, 1968; SMITH, 1970) (Fig. 5). In the Terebrantia (Parasitica) it took on a new role, one of an offensive nature (COPLAND and KING, 1971; RATCLIFFE and KING, 1967). The glandular secretions that once were employed in adhering eggs to a substrate (CHRYSTAL, 1928) now became chemicals with a paralytic function (PIEK and THOMAS, 1969; CLAUSEN, 1940; EVANS, 1966); the sclerites (1) formed a needlelike structure through which the paralytic chemicals flowed, and (2) retained their function as an ovipositor.

Through time, the gonapophyses represented by the ovipositor lost their association with the reproductive system (ROBERTSON, 1968) and became chiefly a mechanism of defense (most aculeates). An examination of most ant species reveals that this is the phyletic stage in which they reside (HERMANN, 1978a).

D. General Formicid Venom Apparatus

Information on the anatomy, function, and evolution of the formicid venom apparatus has been treated by BEYER (1891), BLUM and CALLAHAN (1963), BORDAS (1895), CALLAHAN et al. (1959), CAVILL et al. (1964), FOERSTER (1912), FOREL (1878, 1887), HERMANN (1968a, 1968b, 1969a, 1969b, 1978a), HERMANN and BLUM (1966, 1967a, 1967b, 1968), JANET (1898), MASCHWITZ and KLOFT (1971), PAVAN and RONCHETTI (1955), ROBERTSON (1968) and WHELDEN (1957, 1958a, 1958b, 1960, 1963).

The formicid venom apparatus in its entirety would include the seventh abdominal segment (Fig. 6) since some of the muscles that function in moving the apparatus

Abbreviations Used in Figures

AA	Anal arc	Ln	Lancet
AE	Anterior extension of sting base	LS	Lancet shaft
A-L E	Anterolateral extensions	Mes	Mesal side
AP	Anal pad	OP	Oblong plate
Bb	Barbs of lancets	PC	Venom canal
Cap	Capsule	PGS	Proximal gonostylar segment
CC	Cuboidal cells	PP	Pivot point
CG	Convoluted gland	PS	Venom sac
CU	Cuticle	QP	Quadrate plate
DA	Dorsal apodeme	Ra 1	First ramus
DE	Duct exit	Ra 2	Second ramus
DG	Dufour's gland	Res	Reservoir
DGS	Distal gonostylar segment	S VII	Seventh sternite
DT	Distal tip	SB	Sting bulb
DT	Duct	SE	Squamous epithelium
FA	Fulcral arm	SP	Spiracular plate
FG	Filamentous glands	Sph	Sphincter muscle
Flx Pt	Point of flexion	SS	Sting shaft
Fu	Furcula	St	Sting
Gon	Gonangulum	T VII	Seventh tergite
Go	Gonostyli	T 8	Eighth tergite
1 Gop	First gonapophysis (=first gonacoxite)	T 9	Ninth tergite
		T 10	Tenth tergite
2 Gop	Second gonapophysis (=second gonacoxite)	TP	Triangular plate
		TS	Tracheal sac
GR	Gland reservoir	VA	Valve
1 Gs	First gonostyle	VA	Ventral apodeme
2 Gs	Second gonostyle	1 Vlf	First valvifer
1 Gx	First gonacoxite (=first valvifer)	2 Vlf	Second valvifer
2 Gx	Second gonacoxite (=second valvifer)	1 Vlv	First valvula
		2 Vlv	Second valvula
In	Intima	VII	Seventh abdominal segment

have their origin on the seventh segment (Table 8 and Fig. 41). Also, a considerable amount of abdominal manipulation results from the contraction of other abdominal muscles throughout most of the gastral segments, thus affording indirect manipulative control of the sting.

The venom apparatus proper is composed of several specialized sclerites and two glands (Fig. 7). The sclerites have undergone a process of internalization (Remane, 1952) so that their position is inside the gaster. Other glands, such as Koshewnikow's gland, Bordas' gland, and the sting sheath gland, have been found associated with sclerites of the hymenopterous venom apparatus (Ghent and Gary, 1962; Maschwitz and Kloft, 1971; Oeser, 1961; Snodgrass, 1935, 1956; Wilson, 1965) but their presence in ants has not been firmly established (Hermann, 1978a; Robertson, 1968). Also, they apparently do not produce venom components and therefore are not included in our discussion here. The venom and Dufour's glands are responsible for the production of venom and other substances while the sclerites are responsible for dispersing these substances.

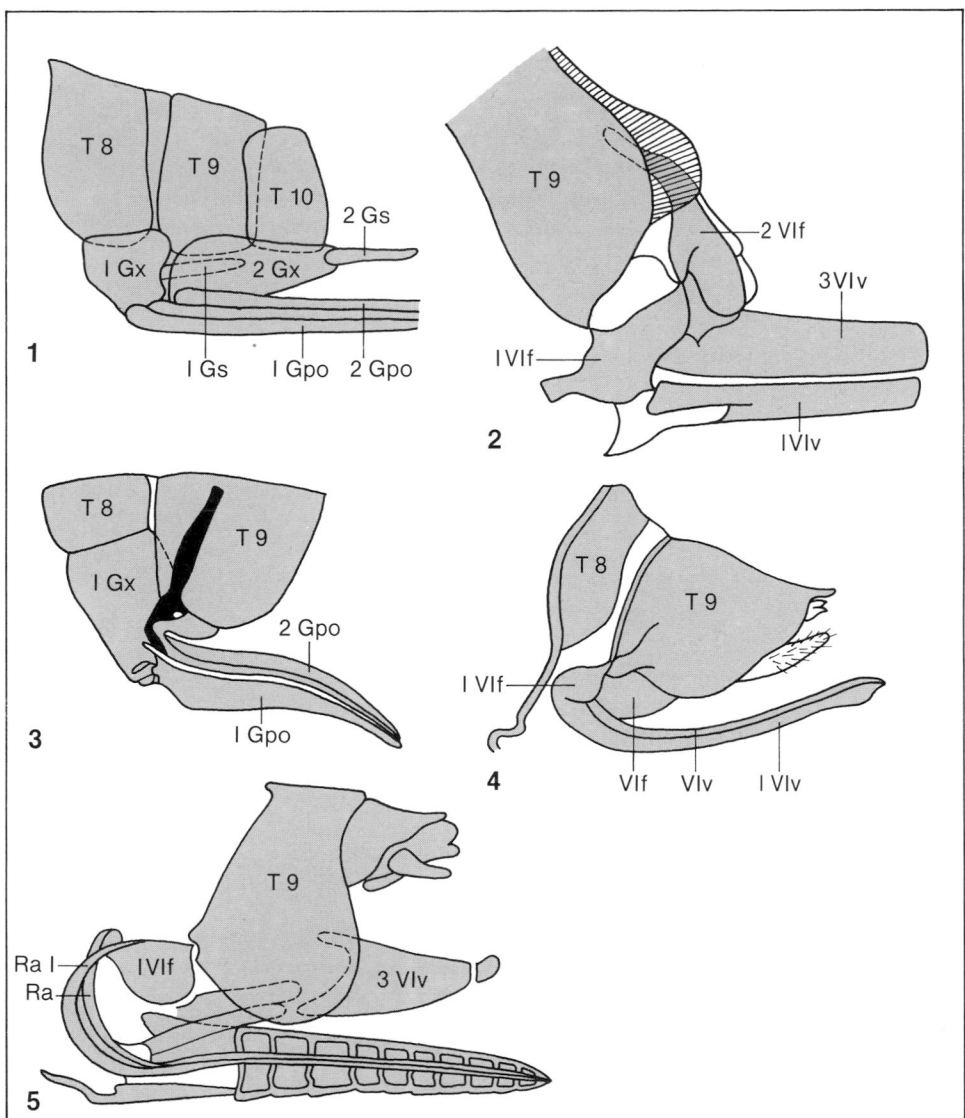

Figs. 1—5. Sclerites of the genital segments. Fig. 1. *Petrobius maritimus* (Thysanura) (after SCUDDER, 1961a). Fig. 2. *Gryllus assimilis* (Orthoptera) (after SNODGRASS, 1935). Fig. 3. *Thrips validus* (Thysanoptera), showing gonangulum (black) (after SCUDDER, 1961a). Fig. 4. *Magicicada septendicim* (Homoptera) (after SNODGRASS, 1935). Fig. 5. Symphyta (composite) (Hymenoptera) (after SMITH, 1970)

E. Venom Apparatus Sclerites and their Musculature
General Formicid Structure

Like other members of the Hymenoptera, sclerites that make up the formicid venom apparatus have originated from tergites and sternites of the 8th through

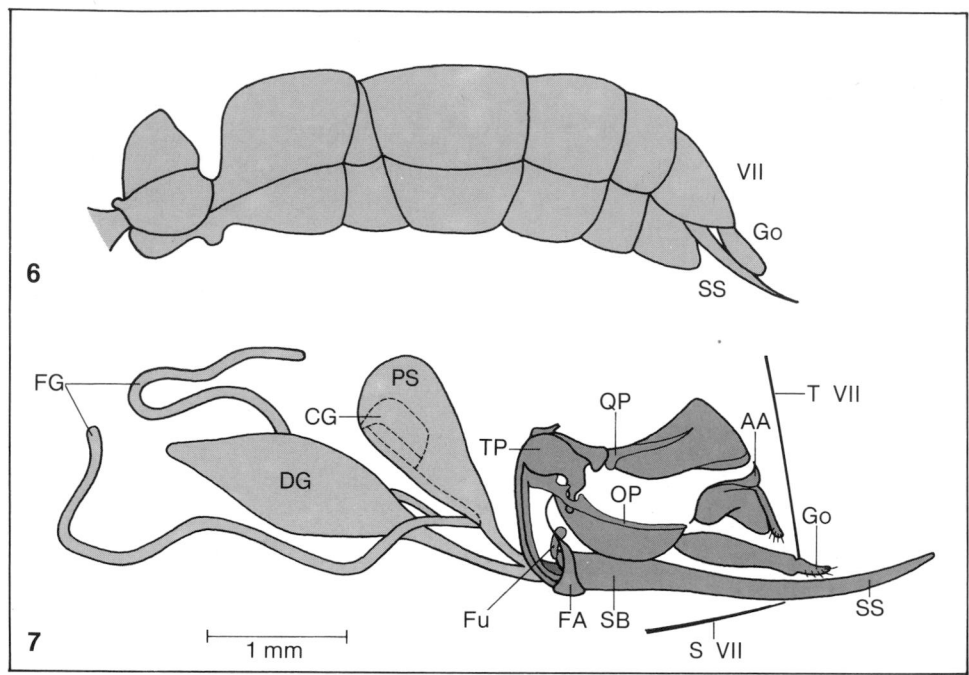

Figs. 6 and 7. Abdomen of a ponerine, showing exsertile condition of the sting. Fig. 7. Lateral view of the venom apparatus of *Paraponera clavata* (Ponerinae). (After Hermann and Blum, 1966)

10th abdominal segments and the gonapophyses extending from the 8th and 9th segments (Figs. 1—5) (Betts, 1923; Beyer, 1891; Davis, 1955; Derwitz, 1878; D'Rozario, 1942; Flemming, 1957; Gustafson, 1950; Gupta, 1950; Kahlenberg, 1895; Kraepelin, 1873; Lacaze-Duthiers, 1850; Matsuda, 1957; Michener, 1944; Morison, 1927; Oeser, 1961; Ouljanin, 1872; Rietschel, 1937; Scudder, 1957a, 1957b, 1959, 1961a, 1961b; Snodgrass, 1931, 1933b, 1935; Trojan, 1935; Walker, 1919; and Zander, 1899, 1911). In their most primitive form they may resemble the original tergal and sternal plates to some degree (Scudder, 1961a, 1961b) (Figs. 1—5). In the ants these sclerites for the most part have been extensively modified toward partial or complete reduction (Foerster, 1912; Hermann, 1978a, 1977; Hermann and Blum, 1968).

In the Formicidae, large paired spiracular plates (8th hemitergites) are well represented (SP, Fig. 8). They have originated from the 8th tergum and largely cover most of the remaining venom sclerites (Hermann, 1978a). In more primitive Hymenoptera (*Ammophila, Polistes, Vespa*), the spiracular plates are fused or partially separated while in the Formicidae they represent two distinct sclerites joined only by a posterodorsal bar (Rietschel, 1937; Zander, 1899). There is a close association between the spiracular plate and the smaller quadrate plate, a more integral part of the venom apparatus. Muscles from the abdominal tergum insert on the spiracular plate and upon moving it, indirectly affect the movement of the entire venom apparatus (Callahan et al., 1959; Hermann, 1978a).

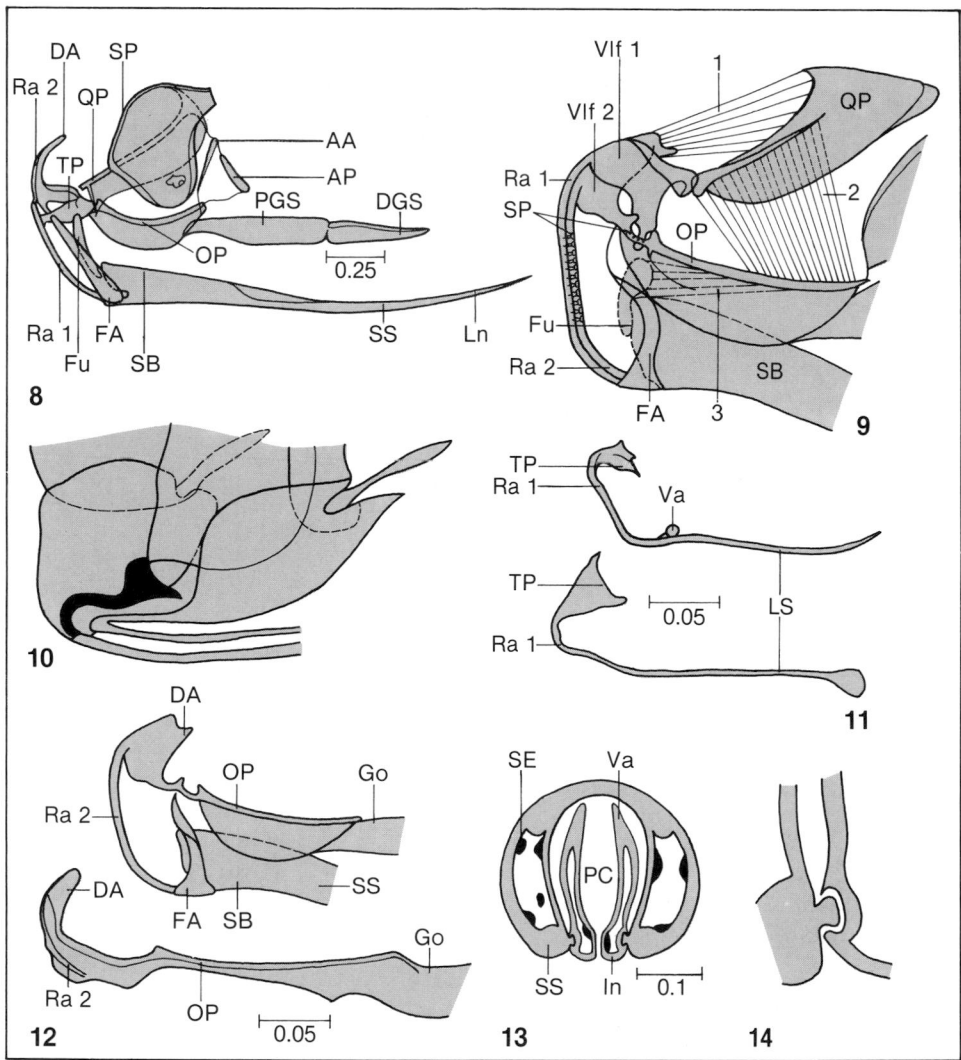

Figs. 8—14. Sclerites of the formicid venom apparatus. Fig. 8. *Leptogenys elongata* (after Hermann, 1969a). Fig. 9. *Paraponera clavata* (after Hermann and Blum, 1966). Fig. 10. *Lepisma
saccharina* (Thysanura), showing gonangulum (dark structure) (after Scudder, 1961a). Fig. 11.
Lancets of *Pogonomyrmex badius* (Myrmicinae) (upper) and *Camponotus pennsylvanicus* (Formicinae) showing valve on one and not on the other (after Hermann and Blum, 1968). Fig. 12.
Sting and associated sclerites of *Pogonomyrmex badius* (upper) and *Camponotus pennsylvanicus*,
showing reduced state of the latter. Fig. 13. Transverse section of sting of *Paraponera clavata*,
through lancet valves. Fig. 14. Enlarged view of tongue and groove articulation between sting
and lancet

The two quadrate plates (outer plates, epipygium écaille anale) have originated
from the 9th tergum (QP, Fig. 8). They have separated mesally except for a light
mesoposterior connection and are thus called 9th hemitergites. There is a strong
connection between the proximal condyle of the quadrate plate and the dorsal
condyle of the triangular plate (TP). This connection represents the pivot point

for movement of the paired quadrate plates (QP) and paired oblong plates (OP). The two muscles originating on the quadrate plate are antagonistic (14, 15, Fig. 43). One serves to indirectly extend the lancets (14) while the other causes a retraction of the same (15) (CALLAHAN et al., 1959; HERMANN and BLUM, 1966). Contraction of this latter muscle also results in a levation of the genostyli.

The paired triangular plates (first valvifers, piece triangulaire, fulcral plates), representing the eighth sternites (TP, Fig. 8), have strong but moveable dorsal connection with the oblong plates. According to SCUDDER (1961b), the triangular plate is correctly called the gonangulum (Gng, Fig. 10), a sclerite that may have arisen from the second gonocoxa; if it did arise from this sclerite, it actually belongs to the ninth abdominal segment.

The triangular plates extend anteriad to the thin first rami (Ra 1, Fig. 8) which in turn pass through the sting as the paired lancets (1st valvulae, stylets, anterior gonapophyses, stechborsten) (Fig. 11). Although the connection between triangular plate and first ramus has been reported by some authors as flexible (LACAZE-DU-THIERS, 1850; SOLLMAN, 1863; LEUENBERGER, 1954), it appears to be a rigid connection in the Formicidae and apparently in most other members of the Hymenoptera (HERMANN, 1978a; MASCHWITZ and KLOFT, 1971).

The basal region of each lancet shaft (1st valvula) of most ant species bears a valvular lobe (Va, Fig. 11). However, such a lobe is missing in some species that have a reduced venom apparatus (HERMANN, 1969a, 1978a; HERMANN et al., 1970).

Each distal lancet tip is usually barbed (Fig. 18) to some degree. Barb size varies considerably among formicid species from completely lacking (e.g., in the Attini and Dorylinae) (HERMANN and BLUM, 1967b; HERMANN et al., 1970) to highly developed (e.g., in *Pogonomyrmex* spp.), where barb size often causes sting autotomy (HERMANN, 1971; HERMANN and BLUM, 1967a). Sensilla campaniformia also have been found on the lancets (RATHMAYER, 1962; JANET, 1898).

The paired oblong plates (second valvifers, inner plates, lamina interna, écaille laterale) (OP, Fig. 8) represent the lateral parts of the 9th sternum (MICHENER, 1944). They are elongate sclerites that connect anteriorly with the second rami (Ra 2) (and indirectly to the sting) and posteriorly to the gonostyli (3rd valvulae) (Go, Fig. 8). Two sets of important muscles originating on the oblong plate indirectly cause a depression (muscle 25) and rotation (muscle 23) of the sting (HERMANN, 1968a; HERMANN and BLUM, 1967b) (Figs. 12, 43, 45—48). At the point of articulation between the ventral apodeme of the triangular plate and the oblong plate there is a distinct sensory bristle field on the latter sclerite (OESER, 1961). The bristles of ants are setaceous (trichoid sensilla) in appearance (HERMANN and BLUM, 1967a) and apparently are mechanoreceptors.

The slender paired second rami (Ra 2) extending from the oblong plates connect distally with the venter of the sting (Fig. 12). At this connection point a pair of fulcral arms (FA, Fig. 8), representing remnants of the eighth sternum, are connected to the base of the sting bulb. The basal region of these fulcral arms represents a pivot point (PP) for the depression and levation of the sting (HERMANN 1968a; HERMANN and BLUM, 1967b).

The sting itself is made up of the fused second valvulae (Vlv 2, Fig. 2) dorsally and laterally and the lancets ventrally; the lancets move alternately back and forth, pushing out venom with each movement.

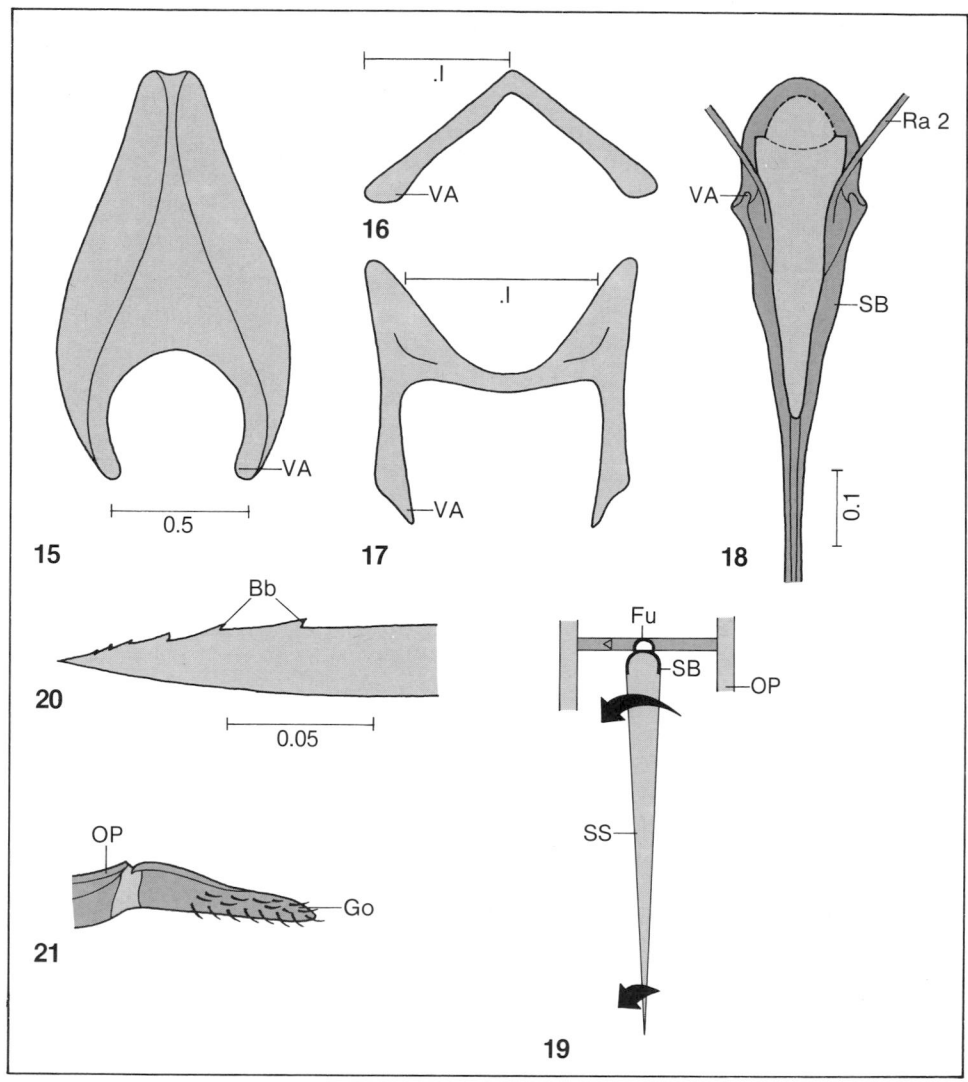

Figs. 15–21. Formicid venom sclerites. Fig. 15. Ponerine furcula. Fig. 16. Same, *Pogonomyrmex* sp. (after HERMANN and BLUM, 1967a). Fig. 17. Same, *Atta* sp. (after HERMANN et al., 1970). Fig. 18. Ventral view of *Eciton hamatum* sting, showing how furcula probably formed from anterior tip of sting (outlined by dotted line). Fig. 19. Resultant rotation of sting upon concentration of muscles inserting on furcula. Fig. 20. Distal tip of lancet, showing barbs. Fig. 21. Gonostylus with abundant trichoid sensilla

A small sclerite, the furcula (detached notum) (Fu, Fig. 15), is responsible for most of the manipulative control of the sting (HERMANN, 1977). As pointed out by SMITH (1970), a considerable amount of abdominal manipulation, and indirectly sting manipulation, is due to intersegmental muscle contraction. Contrary to the reports of TROJAN (1935) and FLEMMING (1957), the furcula has arisen from the anterior end of the sting bulb (Sternite 9) (HERMANN, 1977; ZANDER,

Table 5. Muscles of the Seventh Abdominal Segment that Affect the Movement of the Venom Apparatus. (As reviewed by DALY, 1953; HERMANN, 1975a; RIETSCHEL, 1937; and SNODGRASS, 1933b) (Fig. 11 A)

No.	Muscle	Point of origin	Point of insertion	Function
1.	First lateral tergo-sternal muscle	Lateral part of tergum seven	Lateral apodeme of sternum seven	Dorsoventral compression of abdomen with slight posterior movement of sternum seven
2.	Second lateral tergosternal muscle	Lateral part of tergum seven, just dorsad of muscle	Lateral margin of sternum seven	Dorsoventral compression of abdomen with slight anterior movement of sternum seven
3.	Third lateral tergo-sternal muscle	Lateral margin of tergum seven	External margin of tergum seven	Slight lateral compression of abdomen
4.	First lateral internal dorsal muscle	Posterior to ante-costa of tergum seven and mesad of second lateral internal dorsal muscle	Just anterior to second lateral internal dorsal muscle on dorsal anterior margin of tergum eight	Intersegmental muscle-abdominal contraction, especially in dorso-mesal region, also some abdominal rotation
5.	Second lateral internal dorsal muscle	Anterior and posterior to ante-costa of tergum seven	Dorsal anterior margin of tergum eight	Intersegmental muscle-abdominal contraction, especially in dorso-mesal region. Also some abdominal rotation
6.	Third lateral internal dorsal muscle	Lateral part of tergum seven ventral to second lateral internal dorsal	Anterior ventral margins of tergum eight	Intersegmental muscle-abdominal contraction, especially in lateral region
7.	Lateroexterodorsal muscle	Posterolateral margin of tergum seven	Anteroventral or anterolateral margin of tergum eight	Posterior movement of spiracular plate and entire venom apparatus, especially in ventral region, affording some rotation of the spiracular plate
8.	First lateral inter-segmental sterno-tergal muscle	Mesal surface of lateral apodeme of sternum seven	Ventral margin of tergum eight	Anterior movement of spiracular plate and entire venom apparatus, causing some rotation of the spiracular plate
9.	Second lateral inter-segmental sterno-tergal muscle	Anterolateral part of sternum seven	Posteroventral margin of tergum eight	Anterior movement of spiracular plate and entire venom apparatus, causing some rotation of the spiracular plate

1899) (Fig. 19) and only in certain ants has it fused again with the sting (HERMANN, 1968c; HERMANN and BLUM, 1967b). Movement of the furcula comes about through muscles from the oblong plates (Figs. 20, 46). SMITH (1970) recognized the insertion of a single pair of muscles, the posterior gonocoxapophyseal muscles, on the dorsal furcular apodeme, while an antagonistic pair, the anterior gonocoxapophyseal muscles, insert on the anterior border of the second valvulae. In aculeates, however, there are two distinct pairs of muscles inserting on the dorsal and lateral furcular apodemes, one being responsible for sting depression and the other being responsible for sting rotation (HERMANN, 1977). When the furcula moves it in turn moves the sting base (HERMANN, 1968a; HERMANN and BLUM, 1967b) (Fig. 4, D). Due to the points of rotation by the fulcral arms, any slight movement of the sting base in turn causes extensive movement of the sting tip (HERMANN, 1975b).

The gonostyli (3rd) valvulae, posterior lateral gonapophyses) (Go, Fig. 8) are sensory in nature, apparently being functional in mechanoreception, as well as acting as a sting sheath. They are generally covered with numerous trichoid sensilla (HERMANN and MULLEN, 1974) (Fig. 21). The gonostyli in ants are elevated above and away from the sting by muscles that have their origin on the quadrate plates (Fig. 9).

Table 6. Muscle of the Formicid Venom Apparatus. (As reviewed by DALY, 1953; HERMANN, 1975a; RIETSCHEL, 1937; and SNODGRASS, 1933b)

No.		Point of origin	Point of insertion	Function
10.	First muscle of terga eight and nine[a]	Lateral, dorsal, anterolateral or anterodorsal region of tergum eight	Anterodorsal, externoposterio-dorsal or dorsal region of tergum nine	Lateral and possibly some ventral movement of the quadrate plates (ninth hemitergites).
11.	Second muscle of terga eight and nine[a]	Lateral, dorsolateral or anterolateral region of tergum eight	Externoventral or externolateral region of tergum nine	Lateral and possibly some ventral and posterior movement of quadrate plates (ninth hemitergites).
12.	Third muscle of terga eight and nine[a]	Ventroposterior or ventroanterior region of tergum eight	Externolateral or externoventral region of tergum nine	Lateral and possibly some ventral and posterior movement of quadrate plate (ninth hemitergites).
13.	Tergovalvifer muscle	Posteroventral or posterodorsal region of tergum eight	Posterodorsal region of the first valvifer	Posterior movement of triangular plate. Lancet retraction.
14.	Anterior tergo-valvifer[b]	Anterodorsal region of tergum nine	Anterodorsal apodeme of second valvifer	Lancet protraction— Works through anterior pressure of the triangular plate.
15.	First posterior tergovalvifer muscle[b]	Anteromesoventral part of tergum nine	Posterodorsal region of second valvifer	Lancet retractor— Works indirectly on triangular plate.

Table 6 (continued)

No.		Point of origin	Point of insertion	Function
16.	Second posterior tergovalvifer muscle	Posteromesodorsal region of tergum nine	Posterodorsal region of second valvifer	Levator of gonostyli
17.	First muscle of proctiger	Anterodorsomesal region of tergum nine	Lateral part of proctiger	Retraction of proctiger
18.	Second muscle of proctiger (may not appear in ants)	Posterodorsal region of tergum nine	Lateral part of proctiger	Retraction of proctiger
19.	Third muscle of proctiger (may not appear in ants)	Posterodorsal region of tergum nine	Mesal plate of proctiger	Retraction and lateral movement of proctiger
20.	Fourth muscle of proctiger (may not appear in ants)	Posterodorsal region of tergum nine	Anus	Protraction and some lateral movement of proctiger
21.	Muscles of second ramus	Lateral margin of second ramus	Base of sting bulb (fused second valvulae)	Sting levator
22.	Flexor of venom canal	Anterior part of second valvifer	Lateral part of duct from venom sac	Found in formicine ants; is homologous with the sting rotator inserting on the furcula; directs venom flow toward the acidopore
23.	First muscle of the furcula (sting rotator)	Anteromesal part of second valvifer	Laterodistal part of furcula	Homologous with transverse muscle of second valvula above—rotates sting
24.	Pivoting muscle of sting base	Anteromesal part of second valvifer	Anterolateral part of sting base	Pivots sting laterally; homologous with flexor of venom canal and sting rotator above. Found in the Dorylinae and some Ponerinae.
25.	Second muscle of furcula (first sting depressor)	Posteromesal part of second valvifer	Laterobasal part of furcula	Sting depression
26.	Second sting depressor	Posteromesal part of second valvifer	Anterolateral region of sting base	Sting depression—homologous with the first sting depressor above—found in dorylines and some ponerines

[a] There are some differences in the points of origin and insertion of these muscles in different members of the Hymenoptera and hence some difference in the movement of the plates upon which they insert.

[b] These muscles are also discussed in the text.

The aforementioned special muscles of the formicid venom apparatus and other muscles that function in manipulating the venom apparatus or its glands are summarized in Tables 5 and 6.

I. Myrmeciinae and Ponerinae

Of the six subfamilies that will be discussed in this chapter (Ponerinae, Dorylinae, Pseudomyrmecinae, Myrmicinae, and Formicinae), the Myrmeciinae and Ponerinae are beyond a doubt the most primitive groups (BROWN, 1954; CAVILL et al., 1964; EISNER and BROWN, 1958; HERMANN, 1969a, 1978a; ROBERTSON, 1968; WILSON, 1958, 1963; WILSON et al., 1967a, 1967b). The venom apparatus of myrmeciine ants has been discussed in detail by CAVILL et al. (1964) and ROBERTSON (1968). The sclerites and glands look remarkably like those in the Ponerinae. All of the sclerites are strong and there is a well defined furcula. Since investigations of these two subfamilies have revealed that they are similar anatomically, a discussion of the ponerine apparatus will serve as an explanation of the same structure in the Myrmeciinae.

In general, ponerines are independent foragers. They feed their young insect parts directly, they partially provision their nests and they readily employ their stings both in prey capture and in the defense of themselves and their colonies. Their venom apparatus is strongly developed and wasplike in general appearance (Figs. 7–9, 22–23).

Most contributions to our knowledge of the ponerine venom apparatus have been by CAVILL et al. (1964), FOERSTER (1912), HERMANN (1968c, 1969a, 1969b), HERMANN and BLUM (1966), ROBERTSON (1968), STUMPER (1960), and WHELDEN (1957, 1958a, 1958b, 1960).

The ponerine venom apparatus is strongly constructed and highly sclerotized (Fig. 22). The sting tip usually is exsertile and slightly curved upward (HERMANN, 1968c, 1969a, 1969b). In some cases the sting is extremely curved (*Onychomyrmex hedleyi*) (HERMANN, 1969a) (Fig. 23).

The basal region of the sting may be truncate or extended anteriorly to some degree (Fig. 24). All ponerine species but one have been found to possess a furcula (HERMANN, 1968c) articulating with the anterior sting base (Fu, Fig. 24).

The furcula, except in *Simopelta oculata* (HERMANN, 1968c) (Fig. 25), is very well developed and strongly attached to the anterior sting tip (HERMANN, 1977). It generally is X- or Y-shaped in the ponerines (Figs. 15, 46), the dorsal apodeme serving as a point of insertion for strong sting rotating muscles that originate on the oblong plate (HERMANN and BLUM, 1967b) (Figs. 24, 46). This furcula is important in sting manipulation (HERMANN, 1968a, 1969a, 1977) and is understandably well developed in those ant species that utilize their stings for gathering food and for defense.

The lancets are barbed (Fig. 18) and possess valves that control the flow of venom through the sting shaft (Va, Fig. 11). Their alternating movement is primarily for venom flow control and not particularly for cutting a wound, as was previously thought.

One ponerine species, *Simopelta oculata* (Fig. 25), stands out as a unique member of that subfamily based both on behavioral and anatomic evidence (GOT-

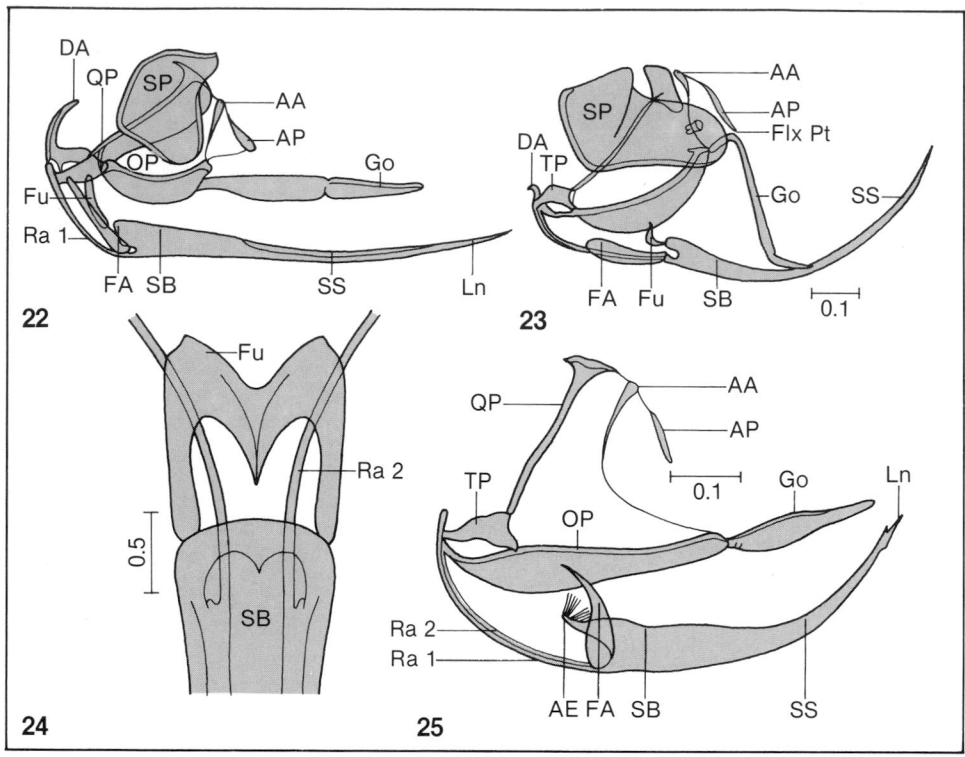

Figs. 22—25. Ponerine venom apparatuses. Fig. 22. *Leptogenys elongata* (after Hermann, 1969a). Fig. 23. *Onychomyrmex hedleyi,* showing strongly recurved sting shaft (after Hermann, 1969b). Fig. 24. Dorsal view of sting base and furcula of *Neoponera villosa* (after Hermann, 1969b). Fig. 25. *Simopelta oculata,* showing dorylinelike sting base and gonostylus (after Hermann, 1968c)

Wald and Brown, 1966; Hermann, 1968c). The venom apparatus of this species is distinctly dorylinelike in appearance, supporting the contention that dorylines and ponerines are either closely related or convergently resemble each other (Brown, 1954; Brown and Nutting, 1950). The anterior end of the sting extends cephalad as it does characteristically in most New World members of the Dorylinae (Figs. 26—30). The gonostyli also are similar to those found in doryline species (Go, Fig. 25).

II. Dorylinae

Doryline ants represent a unique group because of their well known group raiding behavior (Rettenmeyer, 1963). Behaviorally and anatomically they are linked to the Ponerinae and Cerapachyinae and possibly to the Leptanillinae (Brown, 1954; Hermann, 1969a).

Although there are obviously a number of anatomic differences between the ponerines and dorylines (Brown, 1954), the chief differences in the venom appa-

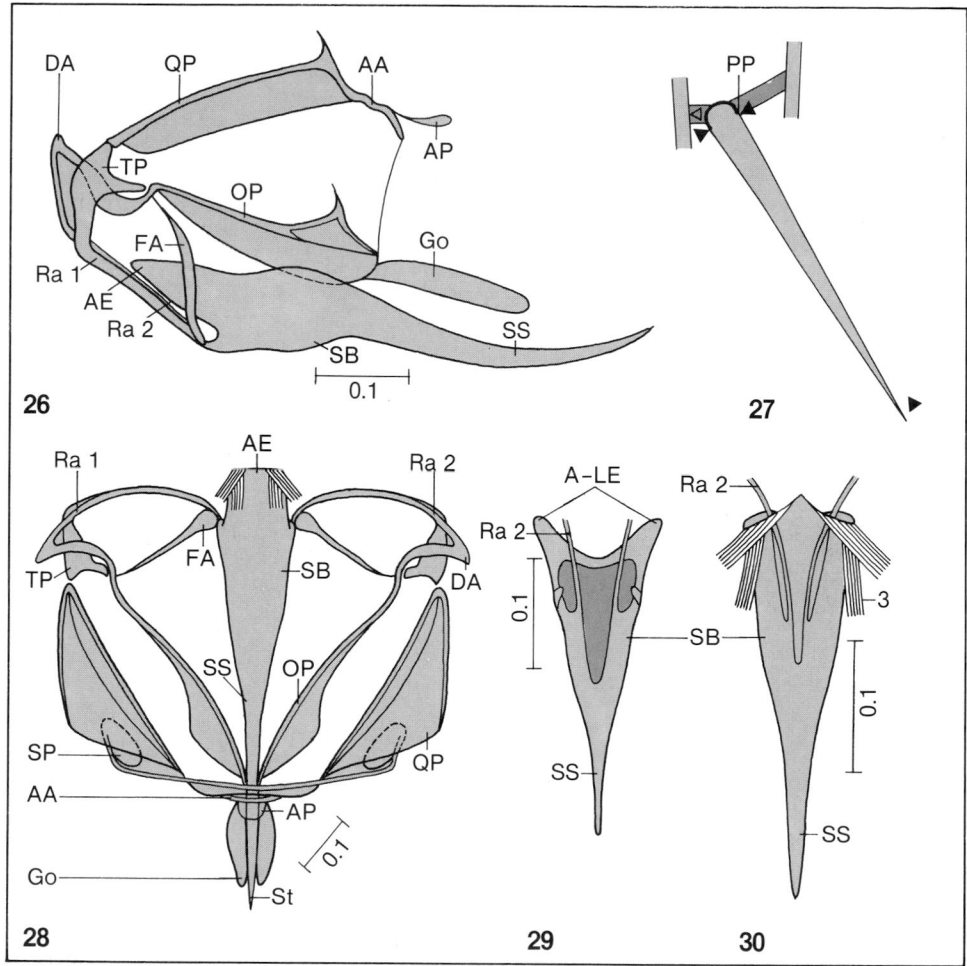

Figs. 26–30. Doryline and cerapachyine venom apparatuses. Fig. 26. *Eciton vagans* (Dory-linae). Fig. 27. Diagrammatic representation of a doryline sting, showing sting pivoting upon contraction of muscle 24 (Fig. 48). Fig. 28. *Cheliomyrmex morosus* (Dorylinae). Fig. 29. *Dorylus* (*Anomma*) *molestus* (Dorylinae). Fig. 30. *Syscia typhla* (Cerapachyinae). (After HERMANN, 1969b)

ratus involve the general appearance of the gonostyli (Go, Fig. 26) and the change in the importance of the sting in prey capture and defense. Along with these anatomic changes there also has been considerable behavioral change.

The gonostyli of doryline ants are generally simple in appearance and chiefly membranous in structure (HERMANN and BLUM, 1967b; WHELDEN, 1963). They do not have the bilobed appearance of ponerine gonostyli (HERMANN and BLUM, 1966) (Go, Fig. 22). They nevertheless have retained their function as mechanore-ceptors and possess numerous trichoid sensilla on their lateral and distal surfaces.

Fusion has occurred between the furcula and anterior sting base in the Dorylinae (HERMANN and BLUM, 1967b) (Fig. 26). This has resulted in a loss of manipulative control of the sting (HERMANN, 1977) (Fig. 27). A similar phyletic development has occurred in the Cerapachyinae and in *Simopelta oculata* (Ponerinae) (HERMANN, 1969a) (Fig. 24). Such a change indicates the lack of importance of the venom apparatus in these ant species in capturing prey. Emphasis changes from a single individual encountering its prey and having to subdue it (in the Ponerinae) to the mass capture and dismembering of prey (in the Dorylinae) during group raids (RETTENMEYER, 1963). Stings became less significant and mandibles became more significant, hence the phyletic acquisition of larger mandibles especially in the Old World dorylines.

III. Pseudomyrmecinae

Pseudomyrmecine ants have a relatively primitive venom apparatus (Fig. 31). Many of the sclerites are ponerinelike (BLUM and CALLAHAN, 1963; HERMANN, 1978a).

Most of the sclerites are slender and well developed. The gonostyli (Go) are distinctly bilobed and thus ponerinelike in appearance. The furcula is Y-shaped (Fig. 32), facilitating manipulative control of the sting. The lancets are barbed.

It is in this group that phyletic development toward sting autotomy (HERMANN, 1971; MASCHWITZ and KLOFT, 1971) first appears in the Formicidae. Lancet-barb size in some cases is sufficient to keep a worker ant attached to its victim for an increased period of time, thus allowing the ant to inject additional venom. Sting autotomy develops to a greater degree in the Myrmicinae.

IV. Myrmicinae

This large group of ant species is extremely diverse in its anatomy and behavior. The venom apparatus varies considerably (Fig. 33).

The sting base of both queen and worker Attini is spatulate, an anatomic condition perfectly correlated with attine behavior and use of the sting sclerites (Fig. 34). These sclerites function in the deposition of trail pheromones and in no way are they employed as a defensive mechanism. A spatulate sting tip has been found in species of *Crematogaster* (Fig. 38) (HERMANN, unpublished data) (Fig. 28), while a spatulate sting base is characteristic of the Old World Dorylinae (HERMANN, 1969a).

Some myrmicine species have a well-developed sting which is not very different from the sting of ponerine or pseudomyrmecine ant species (Fig. 35).

The furcula is usually small, weakly structured, and most often U- or V-shaped (Fig. 36). Such a furcula indicates a venom apparatus that is normally insignificant in defense. Reduction in the furcula results in a reduction in the manipulative control of the sting (HERMANN, 1968a, 1978b; HERMANN and BLUM, 1967b).

Other species have developed a sting autotomous apparatus, in which the lancet barbs are extremely well developed (Fig. 37). Sting autotomy has been recognized as a natural phenomenon in certain social Hymenoptera (HERMANN, 1971; HERMANN and HAMILTON, 1978; MASCHWITZ, 1964; MASCHWITZ and KLOFT, 1971; RIETSCHEL, 1937). Prior to these investigations, DARWIN (1859) correctly attributed sting autotomy to lancet-barb size but incorrectly assumed that such a phenomenon was due to an accidental development of the barbs. The phenomenon of sting

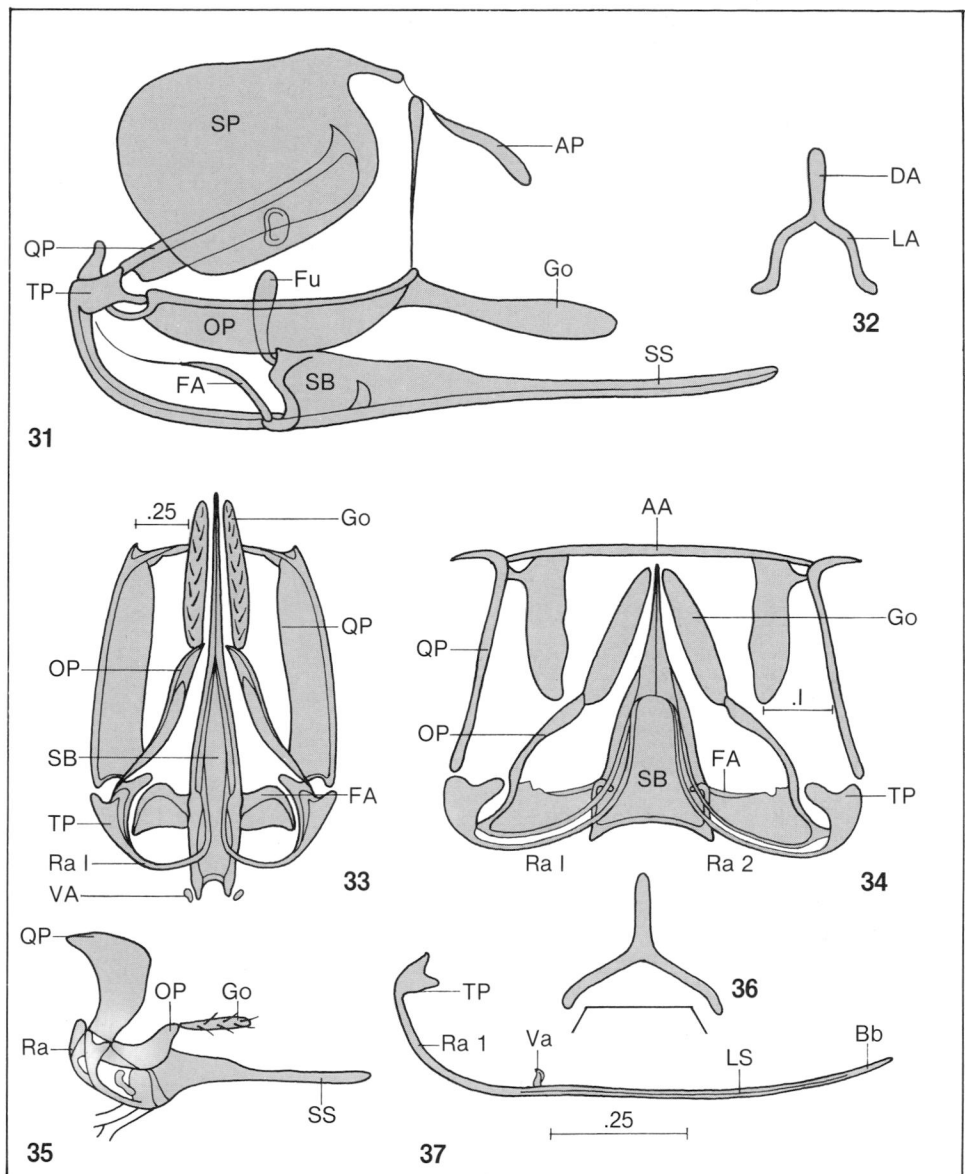

Figs. 31 – 37. Venom sclerites of pseudomyrmecine and myrmicine ants. Fig. 31. *Pseudomyrmex spinicola* (Pseudomyrmecinae). Fig. 32. Same, furcula. Fig. 33. *Pogonomyrmex badius* (Myrmicinae) (after HERMANN and BLUM, 1967a). Fig. 34. *Atta texana* (Myrmicinae) (after HERMANN et al., 1970). Fig. 35. *Solenopsis invicta* (Myrmicinae) (after CALLAHAN et al., 1959). Fig. 36. Myrmicine furcula. Fig. 37. Myrmicine lancet with large distal barbs

autotomy was later understood to represent a natural selective phyletic development of lancet-barbs that is extremely important to some of the social Hymenoptera.

Other myrmicine species have lost the function of the gonapophyses and its associated sclerites as a mechanism of defense and now use them in producing and dispersing pheromones (Fig. 34).

The sclerotized portion of the attine apparatus consists of the entire complement of sclerites found in even the most primitive ant species (Hermann et al., 1970). However, certain of the sclerites have become reduced to some degree, but not to the extent of being lost.

V. Formicinae

Formicine ant species undoubtedly have undergone the most anatomic changes in the venom apparatus in all of the Formicidae (Fig. 39). Reduction is the rule (Forbes, 1938; Hermann and Blum, 1968).

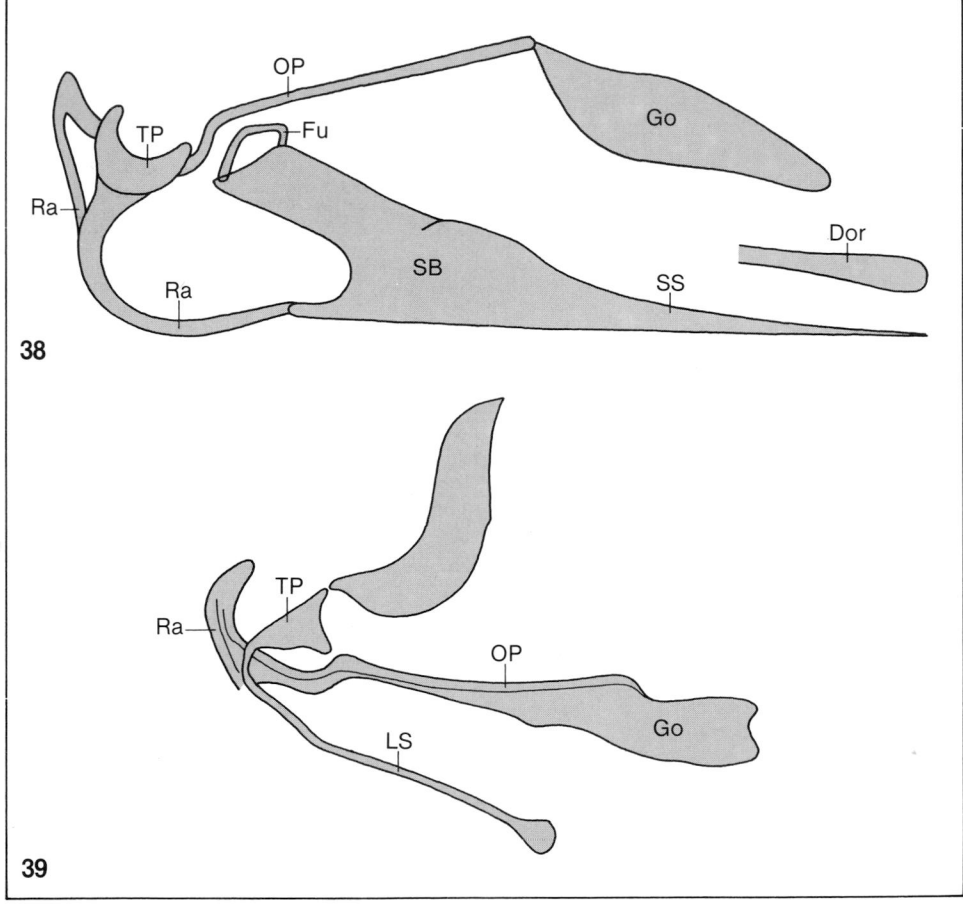

Figs. 38 and 39. Venom apparatuses of two nonstinging ant species. Fig. 38. *Crematogaster* sp., showing spatulate sting tip (small drawing is dorsal view). Fig. 39. *Camponotus pennsylvanicus,* showing reduced rami and valvulae. (After Hermann and Blum, 1968)

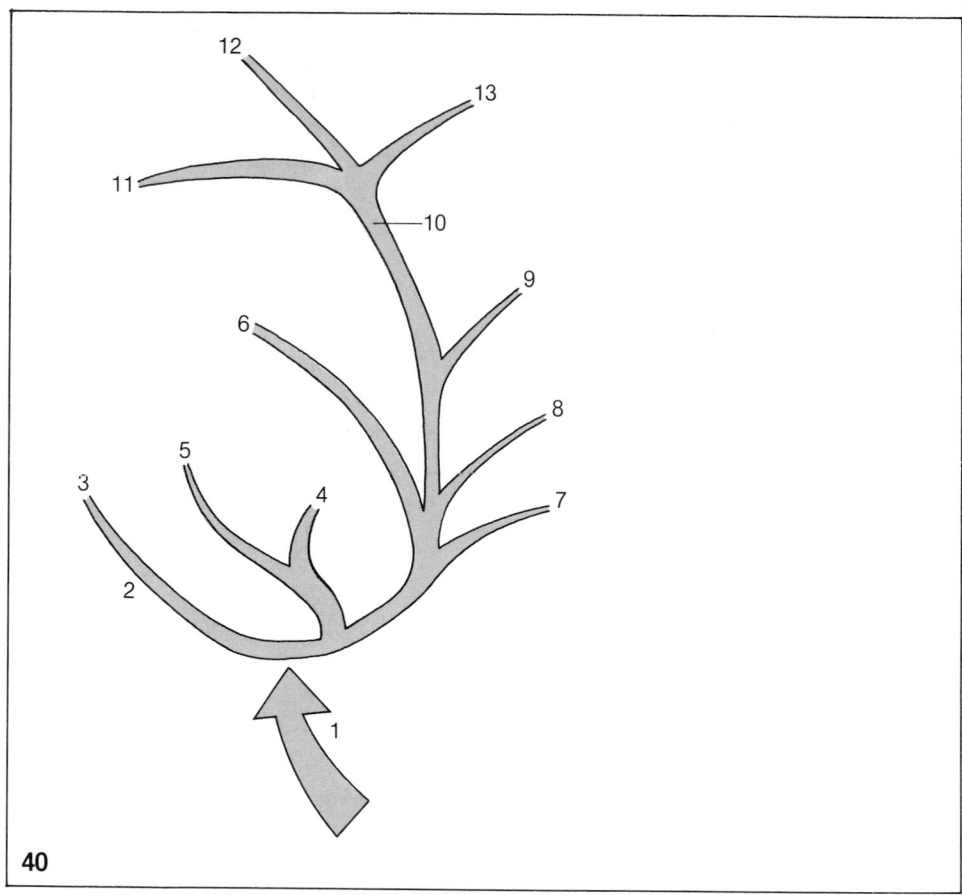

Fig. 40. Phyletic trends in the formicid venom apparatus. A pre-ant ancestor with a familial or semifamilial way of life (*1*) gave rise to the euformicids. Sphecomyrminae and the Formicinae broke off from the main line early. *Sphecomyrma* (*2*) retained its venom apparatus while formicine ants (*3*) lost most of the important venom sclerites. In another direction, the Ponerinae retained their very strong venom apparatus (*4*), while *Simopelta* and possibly other ponerines (*5*) underwent some reduction in the venom apparatus. Dolichoderines (*6*) separated from the main line before the acquisition of a second petiole. The dorylines left the main line as two separate branches, one right after the other. The first to leave were the Old World dorylines (*7*), followed by the New World species (*8*). Pseudomyrmecines, with two well-defined petiolar nodes but still with many primitive characters, left next (*9*) before the myrmicines. The myrmicines (*10*) diverged in many directions; many retained the sting sclerites as a defensive weapon (*11*), while the venom apparatus of others became weak in appearance so that either the sting base (*12*) (*Atta* spp.) or the sting tip (*13*) (*Crematogaster* spp.) became spatulate. This diagram indicates only phyletic trends. It does not reflect on the relationships between subfamilies

Both first and second valvifers (triangular and oblong plates) (TP and OP) are well represented in the Formicinae. Their respective rami and valvulae are reduced. The first ramus (Ra 1, Fig. 39) is thin and leads to a lancet shaft (Sft) with a spatulate distal end. The second ramus (Ra 2) is represented only in its proximal region; the distal portion and normally associated second valvulae (sting) are not present. The acidopore represents a short channel through which venom flows; the old sting rotating muscle of the furcula (22, Fig. 45) now controls the direction of venom flow (Hermann, 1978b) while the venom reservoir is constricted both by abdominal pressure and circular muscles primarily around the basal region of the sac (Hermann et al., 1975).

Formicine ants have a dual defensive mechanism of biting and introducing acid into the wound or, merely the spraying of acid and other substances at its attacker (Hung and Brown, 1964). Although some of the sclerites are markedly reduced, the glands and reservoir associated with the apparatus are well developed (Hermann et al., 1975).

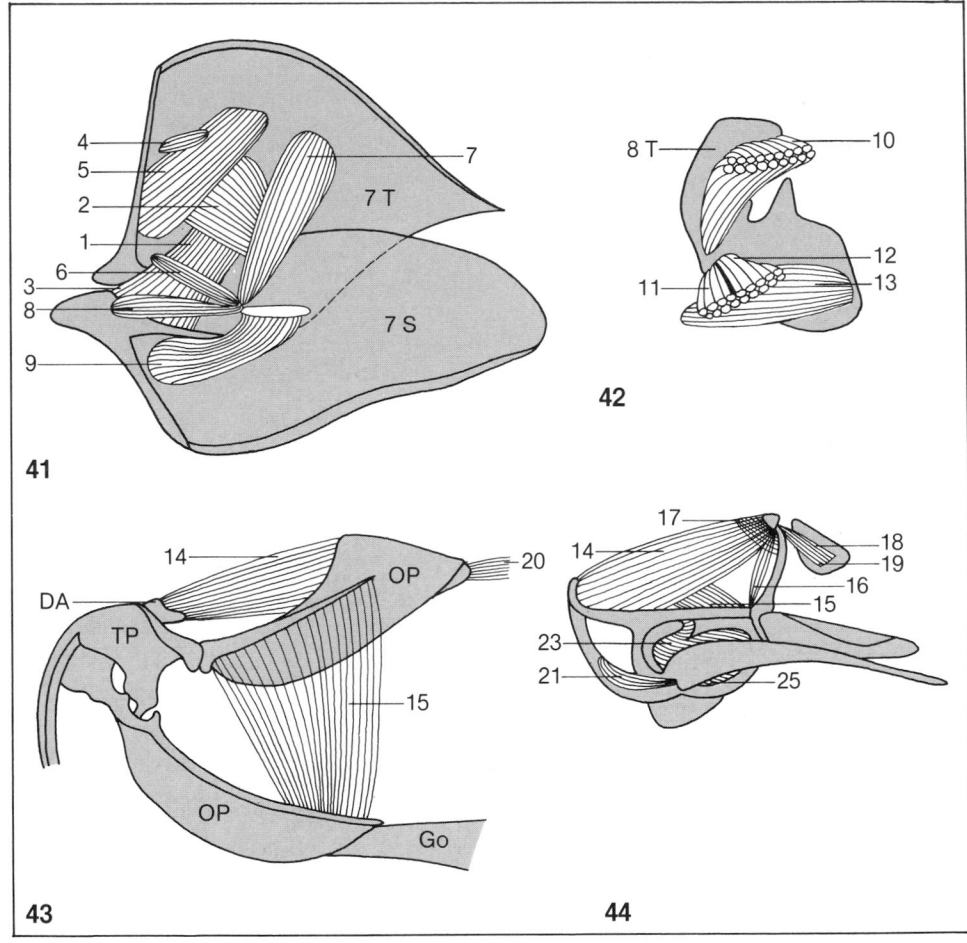

Figs. 41—44. Muscles of the formicid venom apparatus (Redrawn from Daly, 1953; Hermann, 1978a; Rietschel, 1937; and Snodgrass, 1933b). Fig. 41. Muscles of the seventh abdominal segment (right side) which indirectly affect movement of the venom apparatus (see Table 8). Fig. 42. Muscles 10—13 (right side) of venom apparatus (Table 9). Fig. 43. Antagonistic muscles 14 and 15, responsible for protracting and retracting the lancets (Table 9). Fig. 44. Muscles 14—21, 22 and 25 (Table 9)

F. Abdominal Muscles that Indirectly Affect the Movement of the Venom Apparatus

Other than the direct muscles of the venom apparatus, a number of abdominal muscles affect the manipulative control of the venom sclerites (DALY, 1953; HERMANN, 1978a; RIETSCHEL, 1937; SNODGRASS, 1933a, 1933b). Of these muscles, contraction of the tergosternal and intersegmental muscles of all of the pregenital abdominal segments results in abdominal manipulation and thus indirectly assists venom apparatus manipulation.

Muscles of the seventh segment and sting have never been completely homologized with the pregenital musculature. Some attempts at homology have been made by DALY (1953) on *Bombus, Formica, Melipona, Paraponera,* and *Vespula,* by RIETSCHEL (1937) on *Bombus, Prosopis,* and *Vespa,* by SNODGRASS (1933a, 1933b) on *Apis* and by TROJAN (1935).

Muscles of the seventh and eighth abdominal segments are especially influential on the venom apparatus and are outlined in Table 8 and figured in Figs. 41—44. They cause movement of the plates of the seventh abdominal segment and spiracular plate. The latter structure is the only plate of the venom apparatus that is directly controlled by pregenital segment seven.

G. Muscles of the Venom Apparatus

Muscles of the venom apparatus itself (Figs. 45—48) are those that originate or insert on any of the genital plates or their gonapophyses. These muscles and their function have been discussed by a number of investigators (DALY, 1953; CALLAHAN et al., 1959; HERMANN, 1968a, 1978a; HERMANN and BLUM, 1966, 1967b, 1968; RIETSCHEL, 1937; SNODGRASS, 1933a). Their points of origin and insertion and their function are described in Table 9. If any of these muscles have been discussed in the text they will be noted with a double asterisk.

This list by no means represents every muscle found associated with the hymenopterous venom apparatus. Others have been reported by SNODGRASS (1933b) but they may represent a summary of muscles by SNODGRASS that may have been erroneously reported by other authors. Also, additional muscles have been reported in other hymenopterans (HAUPT, 1952; MORISON, 1927) that apparently are not found in the ants. This list includes most of the muscles reported from the Formicidae (HERMANN, 1978a). The remaining muscles, those affecting movement of venom or Dufour's gland contents, have been reported on by HERMANN (1978a). There are reservoir constrictors, dilators, and occlusors of the venom canal within or adnate to the sting base.

H. Evolution of the Venom Sclerites

From the wasplike structures found in the venom apparatus of ponerine ants (Fig. 8), many phyletic changes have occurred in the Formicidae, resulting in a characteristic apparatus for each ant subfamily.

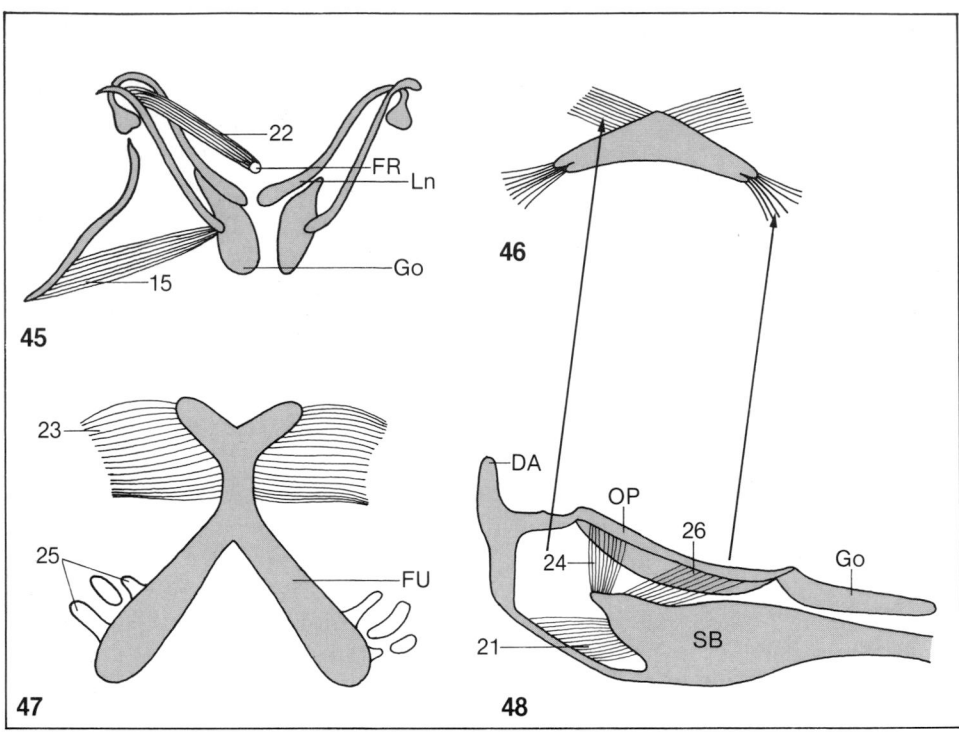

Figs. 45—48. Muscles of the formicid venom apparatus (Redrawn from DALY, 1953; HERMANN, 1978a; RIETSCHEL, 1937; and SNODGRASS, 1933b) (Table 9). Fig. 45. Formicine apparatus (Dorsal view) with muscles 15 and 22 and reduced venom sclerites. Fig. 46. Ponerine furcula, showing sting rotator (23) and sting depressor (25). Fig. 47. Doryline sclerites-sting tip in dorsal transverse section. Fig. 48. Lateral view of second valvifer (*OP*) and second and third valvulae (*SB* and *Go*) with pivoting muscle (24) and depressor (26)

In summary (Fig. 40), the basic wasplike venom apparatus, similar to the one we find in the Ponerinae and Myrmeciinae, led to a number of derived conditions. An explanation of these changes merely demonstrates what happened phyletically to the venom apparatus sclerites. It does not attempt to draw phyletic connections between the ant subfamilies. In one direction (3) (Formicinae), probably resulting from an early departure of one ant group, there was an extensive loss of many of the sting sclerites (FOERSTER, 1912; HERMANN, 1978a; HERMANN and BLUM, 1968). At the same time, there was a retention of large body size and a single petiole. In other directions (4, 5, 7, 8) (Ponerinae, Dorylinae, Cerapachyinae, Leptanillinae) behavioral changes occurred convergently toward group raiding (WILSON, 1958). Two specific and important anatomic changes occurred simultaneously in the Dorylinae: (1) the mandibles became larger and more important both in prey capture and colony defense and (2) the furcula fused with the anterior sting base, giving the venom apparatus less manipulative control. This latter change resulted in a less important role for the venom apparatus in prey capture and colony defense.

Other ant groups changed in other ways. A reduction in body size but retention of the venom sclerites occurred in the Dolichoderinae (JANET, 1898) (6), although some of the sclerites have been reduced in size (HERMANN, 1978a). Changes in this subfamily also occurred in the filamentous glands (HERMANN, 1978a; JANET, 1898).

In yet another direction the furcula and other sclerites were retained with little change. This led to a new branch (9), the Pseudomyrmecinae. Very little change occurred anatomically and relatively small colonies were still the rule. One modification leading to increased colony defense efficiency was the acquisition of enlarged lancet-barbs (HERMANN, 1971). This enables the defending ants to inject more venom into their victims than if they stung and left quickly. Along with these changes there was also some reduction in body size and a slender body developed.

Most of the remaining ant species retained the venom sclerites, although considerable modification occurred. This led to the Myrmicinae (10), a large and diverse group both anatomically and behaviorly. Changes occurring in the venom apparatus followed many directions, such as the spatulate sting of *Crematogaster* species (13) in which frothing is its defensive mechanism; the broadly spatulate sting base of attines (12), which have acquired large mandibles to use in colony defense; and the sting of *Pogonomyrmex* species (HERMANN and BLUM, 1967a) (11) that has weak manipulative powers but demonstrates sting autotomy because of enlarged lancet-barbs (HERMANN, 1971; HERMANN and HAMILTON, 1978; MASCHWITZ, 1964; MASCHWITZ and KLOFT, 1971; RIETSCHEL, 1937).

I. Glands Associated with the Venom Apparatus

The formicid venom producing and storage organ is a complex system of ducts through which venom precursors pass, are transformed into venom, and are stored (BLUM and HERMANN, 1969; HERMANN et al., 1975).

The venom components (Fig. 49) consist of a venom reservoir (*Res*) (venom storage area), a convoluted gland (*CG*) and filamentous glands (*FG*) (HERMANN et al., 1975). Venom formed and stored by these components flows through a venom canal (VC) prior to passing through a sting or comparable structure. The general arrangement of the venom components varies in the Formicinae while the gross change in appearance of the filamentous glands occurs chiefly in the Dolichoderinae.

I. Myrmeciinae, Ponerinae, Dorylinae and Pseudomyrmecinae

The venom sac in myrmeciine, ponerine (Fig. 50), doryline, (Fig. 51) and pseudomyrmecine (Fig. 52) ant species characteristically has a convoluted gland inside, near its apex (CAVILL et al., 1964; HERMANN, 1968c, 1969a, 1969b; HERMANN and BLUM, 1966; ROBERTSON, 1968). The convoluted gland is connected to a relatively long duct that exits from the base of the reservoir. A single duct (CD) extends from the reservoir base and eventually branches into two elongate filaments

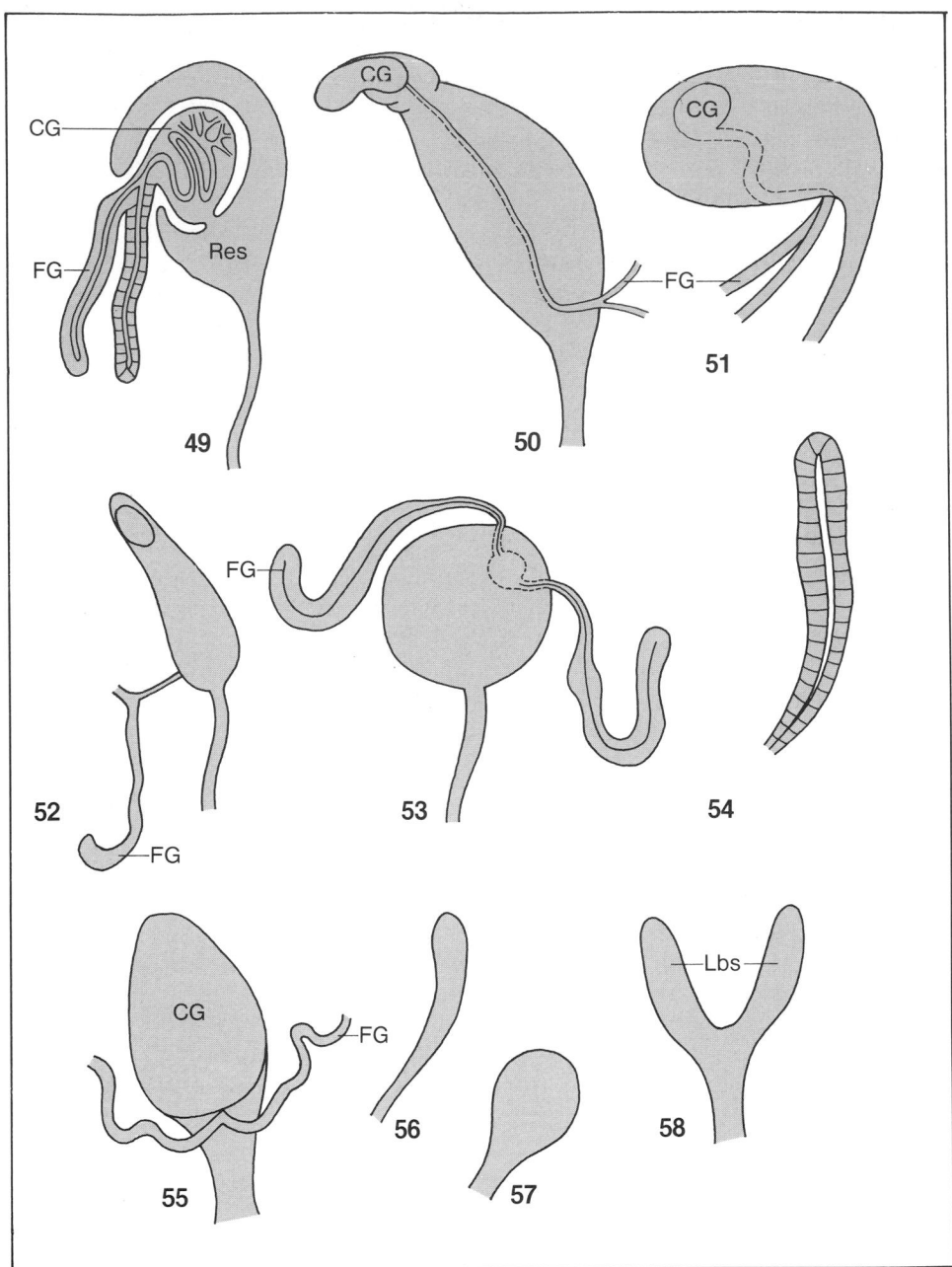

Figs. 49 — 58. Glandular regions of the formicid venom apparatus. Fig. 49. Diagrammatic representation of venom components showing connections between reservoir, convoluted and filamentous glands (after HERMANN et al., 1971). Fig. 50. Ponerine venom components, showing common duct from filamentous glands attached to base of reservoir. Fig. 51. Same, doryline. Fig. 52. Same, pseudomyrmecine. Fig. 53. Same, myrmicine, but filaments leave reservoir near reservoir apex. Fig. 54. Dufour's gland. Its appearance is much the same in all of the Formicidae except some Formicinae. Fig. 55. Formicine venom components, showing convoluted gland on outside of reservoir. Fig. 56. Dufour's gland in *Lasius sitkaensis* (Formicinae). Fig. 57. Same, *Acanthomyops claviger* (Formicinae). Fig. 58. Same, *Camponotus* and *Formica* (Formicinae)

(*FG*). A relationship between the various glandular parts, as has been described for the Ponerinae with the common filament extending from the reservoir base, is considered the most primitive condition found in ants and all of the other sacs are derived from it. This type of arrangement also is found in the Myrmeciinae, Cerapachyinae, and Leptanillinae (HERMANN, 1978a).

Dufour's gland remains much the same in these subfamilies as it is in most wasps. It is an elongate sac lined with simple cuboidal or columnar cells (Fig. 54). It is always found entering the sting bulb beneath the duct from the venom sac (Fig. 7).

II. Myrmicinae

Myrmicine ant species characteristically have a round or oval venom reservoir with the filaments branching directly from the reservoir's apical surface (Fig. 53). Often there is considerable difference between the proximal and distal filamentous diameters.

As a whole, the venom components of myrmicine ants are much the same in appearance, regardless of the variation in sting sclerites.

Generally, Dufour's gland in myrmicine ant species is not different from the gland in ponerines, dorylines, and pseudomyrmecines. It is an elongate sac lined with a simple columnar or cuboidal epithelium (Fig. 54).

III. Formicinae

The greatest departure from the general arrangement of venom components occurs in the subfamily Formicinae (HERMANN and BLUM, 1968; HERMANN et al., 1975). The venom reservoir (Fig. 55) is large as is the duct through which venom flows during its release through the acidopore. The convoluted gland (*CG*) is positioned on the sac's dorsum, a condition unique to the Hymenoptera. The filaments (*FG*) extend to fatty tissue from the base of the convoluted gland.

With the main glandular mass positioned outside the venom reservoir in all formicine species it is difficult to understand just how the difference came about. Like most anatomic and behavioral characteristics of this group, there is a wide anatomic hiatus between it and any of the other ant groups.

Functionally, the synthesizing portion of the venom components in formicine ants falls into two categories, a filamentous gland (*FG*) and a convoluted gland (*CG*). HERMANN et al. (1975) clearly showed that the filaments contained distinct gland cells and stated that significant chemical changes appeared to occur in these structures. Cells of the convoluted gland appeared glandular to a lesser degree, although the convoluted gland cortex definitely appeared glandular in function.

Dufour's gland in most formicine ants is unique. In *Lasius* species (Fig. 56) it has retained the typical elongate appearance of the same gland in most other ant species. In *Acanthomyops* (Fig. 57), Dufour's gland is globate in appearance. In species of *Camponotus* and *Formica* (Fig. 58) Dufour's gland is bilobed, a condition found only rarely in other members of the Hymenoptera.

J. Gland Phylogeny

Glands associated with the venom apparatus have had an interesting phylogeny (Fig. 63). Assuming they arose from paired reproductive accessory glands, their original function was one of producing proteinaceous compounds that either coated the eggs of facilitated the adhering of the eggs to a substrate. At this stage the glands were paired and similar in appearance. Through time this function changed in the Terebrantia (=Parasitica) so that the chemicals produced caused a paralyzing effect on their host. At this stage the gonopods remained functional as an ovipositor but the glands no longer looked alike. One developed into a complex venom gland while the other (Dufour's gland) remained relatively simple in structure.

Slight chemical changes but significant behavioral and anatomic changes occurred during the phyletic development of lower aculeates, insects that employed their gonopods in stinging a host. It was between the Parasitica and the rise of the lower Aculeata that the gonopods lost their association with the reproductive system, thus becoming a sting. These lower aculeates also readily employed their sting in defense.

Most ant species use their stings to subdue their prey. However, other changes occurred in the venom apparatus. The glands changed their function to produce various types of pheromones and an assortment of defensive compounds.

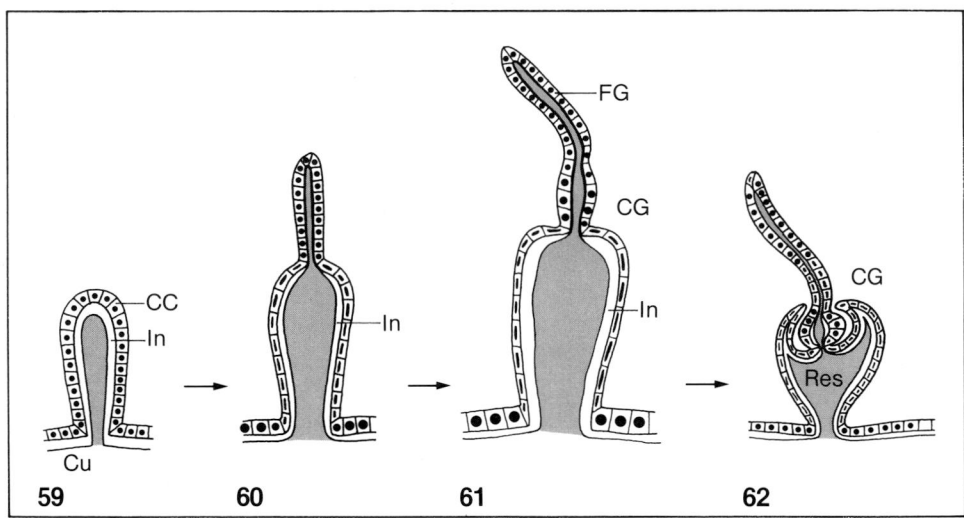

Figs. 59–62. Apparent stages of development of the reproductive accessory glands from a simple invagination to the highly complex venom gland found in ant species. Fig. 59. A simple sac with cells similar to the hypodermis or perhaps more glandular in appearance (similar to Dufour's gland in most ant species). Fig. 60. Cell differentiation, in which an apical filamentous gland develops (similar to the venom gland in *Apis* spp.). Fig. 61. Further cell differentiation to form a new glandular mass at the base of the filament adnate to the reservoir. There has been an increase in the thickness of the intima (somewhat simpler than the formicine venom components). Fig. 62. The basal gland may convolute and sink into the venom reservoir, leaving only the filamentous gland showing (in many ways similar to the myrmicine venom components)

In summary, we can elaborate on the original tentative description of venom glands by PAWLOWSKY (1927). He listed: (1) a braconid type in which there are numerous filamentous glands ending on the reservoir, and circular muscles but no elements of a filamentous gland; (2) a vespid type in which there are two filamentous glands that come together on the very muscular wall of the reservoir; and (3) an apid type in which there is an unpaired filamentous gland that is connected directly to the large reservoir. These different gland types were not correctly described by PAWLOWSKY (1927), and a more up-to-date description was presented by HERMANN (1978a).

Most venom glands of hymenopterous insects appear to have arisen from one basic pattern. The initial gland arose as an invagination from the chitinous ectoderm (Fig. 59), resulting in a saclike structure with an internal intima (*In*). This is very like Dufour's gland, although much of the obvious intima has been lost in that gland. Further development toward what we know of as a venom gland came about with cell differentiation within the gland (Fig. 60). With further enlargement of the basal region of the chamber the cells in that area lost their function in producing substances to pass through the ovipositor (Fig. 61), but the intima (*In*) thickened to protect these new cells from the compounds that were produced in the apical region.

Continued differentiation produced an envelopment of the basal glandular region (Fig. 62); the gland elongated and became convoluted. From this basic plan, in which there are three well defined areas, all of the present venom glands arose (Fig. 63). Some of the basic changes that occurred were: (1) branching and later numerical reduction of the filamentous glands (parasitic Hymenoptera); (2) exsertion of the convoluted gland (Formicinae); (3) bilateral enlargement and shortening of the filamentous glands (Dolichoderinae); (4) enlargement in the transverse gland muscles (Vespidae); (5) change in position of association of the filamentous glands and the venom reservoir (Ponerinae, Myrmeciinae, Dorylinae, Cerapachyinae, Leptanillinae, and Pseudomyrmecinae); (6) reduction of musculature around the reservoir (Attini and others).

With these changes in mind we revise PAWLOWSKY's original grouping to the following: (1) the *symphyte type*, in which the venom sac is large and there are numerous branches of the filamentous glands (ROBERTSON, 1968); (2) *the terebrant (parasitic) type*, in which the venom sac is elongate and there are numerous filamentous gland branches (RATCLIFFE and KING, 1967; ROBERTSON, 1968); and (3) the *basic aculeate type*, in which there is an elongate duct leading to the sting from a well-defined reservoir and the filamentous glands extend from the reservoir base (Scolioidea). All other venom sacs, including the sac present in ants, arose from a sac like the one described in (3) as follows: (4) the *exserted convoluted gland or formicine type*, in which the convoluted gland is outside the venom reservoir (Formicinae); (5) the *dolichoderine type*, in which the filamentous glands are globate (Dolichoderinae); (6) the *myrmicine type*, in which the filamentous glands enter the reservoir near the latter structure's apex; (7) the *vespid type*, in which the muscle supply around the reservoir is extensive (Vespidae); (8) the *apid type*, in which there appears to be no internal convoluted gland and the single filamentous gland extends from the reservoir apex.

In reviewing these various types of sacs we must realize that there is overlap

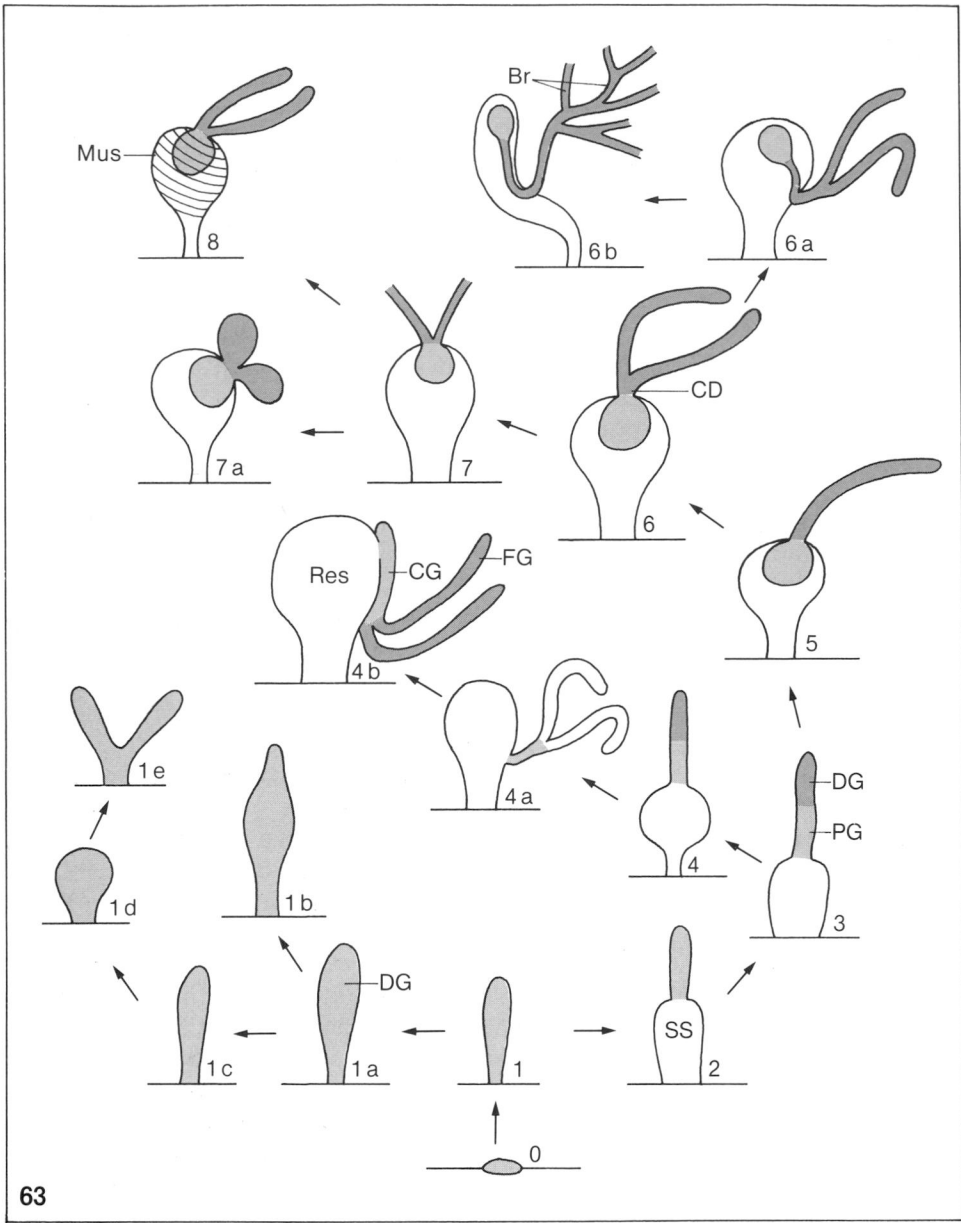

Fig. 63. Gland phylogeny. Venom and Dufour's gland started as a pocket of modified hypodermal cells (*0*) and later developed into a simple saclike structure (*1*). Very little change occurred in the development of Dufour's gland (*1a*) throughout most of the Formicidae other than enlargement (*1b*). However, in the Formicinae the gland retained its simple form in *Lasius* (*1c*), became globate in *Acanthomyops* (*1d*) and bilobed in *Camponotus* and *Formica*. The venom components changed in other ways. A new area developed, a secondary sac (SS), so that the new sac functioned as a reservoir while the original structure produced compounds (*2*). Differentiation between the proximal (*PG*) and distal glandular (*DG*) regions (*3*) and the constriction of the reservoir base (*4*) led to a structure similar to that in the honey

between the groups. For instance, the *terebrant* type of sac is not found in all of the Parasitica; the venom sac and associated components of some members of this group (Ichneumonoidea) are of the *aculeate type*.

In the Formicidae the sacs are usually distinct within the groups outlined. There is considerable anatomic diversity in the subfamily Myrmicinae, along with an equal amount of behavioral diversity.

K. Envenomization

Venoms kill between 35,000 and 50,000 people a year (RUSSELL, 1967) and an estimated additional 10 million people are victims of envenomization annually (HUNT and HERMANN, 1973). Of the venomous animals in the world, the order Hymenoptera apparently heads the list as the most important group (ANONYMOUS, 1965; BARNARD, 1967; BEARD, 1971; BOWEN, 1951; PARRISH, 1963).

According to STUMPER (1960), of the 3500 species of ants known to have a well-developed venom apparatus, the sting of only a small percentage (about 3%) produces a noticeably painful sensation in man. For an unknown reason STUMPER excluded the myrmicines, which are, nevertheless, capable of producing an irritating feeling at the site of the sting (HERMANN and BLUM, 1966).

Probably one of the most painful stings is delivered by the large *Paraponera clavata* (Ponerinae) of the New World (HERMANN and BLUM, 1966). BEQUAERT (1926) described this species as fierce, vicious, and extremely aggressive. SPRUCE (1908) reported on the affects of several stings that he received about the feet and legs. He had no alleviation of pain for about three hours. The pain returned on two occasions during the night, causing an hour of acute suffering after each return.

WEBER (1937) received a sting from a worker of this species on the patella. Paralyzing symptoms were produced, and finally a large, persistent blister developed. He also stated that there is lymphatic involvement and fever. On another occasion, when he was stung by a queen of this species (WEBER, 1939), the sting seemed considerably less painful than the stings he received by workers in 1937.

The most painful stings delivered by myrmicines are delivered by members of the genus *Pogonomyrmex*. Within minutes after the sting is administered large edematous structures appear around the point of the sting (HERMANN and BLUM, 1967a). WEBER (1959) noted that the sting of *P. occidentalis* produced edematous and erythematous areas, throbbing sensations with intense pain, and usually profuse sweating in the areas around the sting.

---

bee (*4*). In the Formicinae the distal gland branched (*4a*) to form paired filamentous glands (*FG*) and the proximal gland elongated to form the convoluted gland (*CG*) (*4b*). In another direction the proximal convoluted gland became enveloped by the reservoir (*5*). Further changes led to branching of the filamentous gland with a short common duct (*CD*) (Myrmicinae) (*6,6b*), a change in the point in which the filamentous glands leave the reservoir (Myrmeciinae, Ponerinae, Dorylinae, Pseudomyrmecinae) (*6a*), a loss of the common duct (*7*), formation of globate filamentous glands (Dolichoderinae) and the elaboration of extensive circular muscle (*Mus*) around the reservoir (Vespidae) (*8*). This phyletic representation does not indicate relationships between subfamilies. It merely represents phyletic stages through which the glands passed

McCook (1879) noted a sharp, severe pain upon being stung by *P. barbatus*. Before the effects terminated he experienced chilling sensations, a steady heavy pain that continued for about three hours and a light numbness in the area of the sting.

Based on the findings of Hermann and Blum (1967a), there is a dampness to the stung area within 6 min after a sting. Tenderness of the lymph nodes occurred within 12 min after a sting. The dampness faded within $6^1/_2$ hr after a sting and an itching commenced at the sting locus.

Williams and Williams (1964, 1965) stated that children in the Southwest frequently suffer from nausea and vomiting following sting encounters with two or more of these ants. They established an LD_{50} of 1.9 mg/kg for male Swiss Webster mice and attributed the toxicity to a protein or polypeptide.

Experiments with the genus *Pogonomyrmex* (Hermann and Blum, 1967a) have shown that all species in this genus demonstrate sting autotomy (Hermann, 1971). Sting autotomy (self amputation of the sting) is important to the welfare of their social organization.

The public and investigators have devoted most of their attention to members of the genus *Solenopsis* (Lockey, 1974), primarily *S. invicta*. Typical symptoms accompanying a sting in an allergic victim are swelling, generalized urticaria, pruritus, nausea, wheezing, and shortness of breath. This is followed by the formation of a pustule within 24 hr of the sting.

Histologically, edema appears in the upper corium within a few minutes after the sting occurs. Epidermal edema, dermal vessel dilation, and slight lymphocytic, histiocytic and plasma cell infiltration follows. Some necrosis occurs within 30 min. At 24 hr the characteristic pustule contains many necrotic polymorphonuclear and lymphocytic cells.

Lockey (1974) summarized the work done on reactions to ant stings (Table 3) and concluded that further information is needed on additional documented case reports, identification of the species of ant responsible for the reaction, the natural history of ant hypersensitivity (Barr, 1972; Spence, 1963; Vansclow, 1969), identification of the antigen or antigens responsible for the hypersensitivity state, and whether cross reactivity exists among the more commonly recognized Hymenoptera.

Hunt and Hermann (1973) investigated what they considered the three basic venom reactions in mammalian tissues, exemplified in the reactions mentioned here for *Paraponera clavata*, *Pogonomyrmex* spp. and *Solenopsis* spp.

The reaction produced by *Paraponera* is in many ways comparable to the reaction produced by *Polistes annularis* (Vespidae) (Hunt and Hermann, 1973).

These three ant species produce quite distinct sting reactions; however, hematologic data showed marked similarities in the fluctuation of both white cell counts and white cell differentials following massive envenomization.

L. Mandibular Gland Constituents

I. Ponerinae

Although the mandibular gland chemistry of relatively few ponerine species has been analyzed, it is nevertheless possible to conclude that the genera in this primitive subfamily produce an extraordinary variety of natural products. The results of

Table 7. Compounds identified in the mandibular gland secretions of ponerine species

Species	Compound	Authority
Paltothyreus tarsatus	Dimethyldisulfide	CASNATI et al., 1967; CREWE and FLETCHER, 1974
Paltothyreus tarsatus	Dimethyltrisulfide	CASNATI et al., 1967; CREWE and FLETCHER, 1974
Odontomachus hastatus	2,5-Dimethyl-3-isopentylpyrazine	WHEELER and BLUM, 1973
Odontomachus brunneus	2,6-Dimethyl-3-*n*-pentyl-, *n*-butyl-, *n*-propyl-, and ethylpyrazine	WHEELER and BLUM, 1973
Neoponera villosa	4-Methyl-3-heptanone	DUFFIELD and BLUM, 1973
Neoponera villosa	4-Methyl-3-heptanol	DUFFIELD and BLUM, 1973
Gnamptogenys pleurodon	Methyl 6-methylsalicylate	DUFFIELD and BLUM, 1974

these investigations are presented in Table 7 and refer to analyses of workers only.

At this juncture, no common chemical denominators characterize the natural products identified in the mandibular glands of ponerine species (Table 7). Completely unrelated compounds are synthesized by species in each of the four genera examined, and all of these diverse natural products appear to function in both defensive and communicative contexts. The two alkyl sulfides produced by *P. tarsatus* (CASNATI et al., 1967) are excellent defensive compounds and function as releasers of digging behavior as well (CREWE and FLETCHER, 1974). These sulfides are only known as animal natural products because of their production by workers of this ponerine species.

Nitrogen-containing natural products are not commonly encountered in the nonpoison gland secretions of arthropods and the pyrazines produced by *Odontomachus* species are particularly distinctive because both 2, 5- and 2, 6-dialkylpyrazines are synthesized (WHEELER and BLUM, 1973). These compounds function both as defensive substances and alarm pheromones. Similarly, 4-methyl-3-heptanone and its corresponding carbinol possess the same duality in functions for workers of *Neoponera villosa* (DUFFIELD and BLUM, 1973) as do the pyrazines produced by workers of *Odontomachus*. 4-Methyl-3-heptanone is a relatively characteristic compound of myrmicine species and its occurrence in the mandibular gland secretion of *N. villosa* workers demonstrates that ponerine species possess the capacity to synthesize and utilize the same natural products for defensive and communicative roles as do species in more highly evolved taxa. On the other hand methyl 6-methyl-salicylate, the main compound in the alarm-defense system of *Gnamptogenys pleurodon* (DUFFIELD and BLUM, 1974), is utilized as a sex pheromone by males of formicine species in the genus *Camponotus* (BRAND et al., 1973c).

Analyses of the mandibular gland products of additional ponerine genera will undoubtedly enlarge the natural products repertory of the species in this subfamily.

II. Dorylinae

4-Methyl-3-heptanone is present in the mandibular gland secretions of males of *Neivamyrmex harrisii, N. melsheimeri,* and *Labidus coecus* (BLUM et al., 1974b).

Workers of *N. nigrescens* also produce this compound in their mandibular glands, in addition to 3-methylindole (skatole) (BLUM and WATKINS, 1969). The ethyl ketone functions as an alarm pheromone and defensive compound whereas skatole is presumably utilized solely as a deterrent substance.

III. Pseudomyrmecinae

Workers of *Pseudomyrmex gracilis* produce 4-methyl-3-heptanone in their mandibular glands and in workers of two other species this alkanone is accompanied by 3-methyl-2-heptanone (BLUM and WHEELER, 1974). In another group of species the mandibular gland secretion is dominated by methyl ketones in admixture with an ethyl ketone. 2-Heptanone is a major constituent in the secretions of three *Pseudomyrmex* species but in addition, the exudate contains 3-methyl-2-heptanone, 5-methyl-2-heptanone, 2-octanone, and 2-nonanone. These remarkable ketonic blends are also fortified with 6-methyl-3-octanone. These secretions are particularly distinctive of pseudomyrmecine species, especially since only 2-heptanone and 6-methyl-3-octanone have been previously identified in ants. These ketones function as defensive compounds in addition to being powerful releasers of alarm behavior.

IV. Myrmicinae

The mandibular glands of myrmicine ants constitute a veritable storehouse of ethyl ketones which are often accompanied by their corresponding carbinols. Seven 3-ketones have been identified in these glandular secretions and four of these carbonyl compounds occur along with their alcoholic counterparts (Table 8). Ethyl ketones would thus appear to be a hallmark of myrmicine ants, particularly among species in the genus *Manica* in which five of these compounds have been identified (FALES et al., 1972 – Table 8). The biosyntheses of the 3-ketones and 3-carbinols would appear to be related, but the absence of detectable quantities of alcohols in the mandibular gland secretions of *Manica* species (FALES et al., 1972) indicates that, in at least some cases, ketonic biogenesis may not involve an alcoholic precursor or vice versa.

Methyl ketones, which are characteristic anal gland products of dolichoderine ants, have a limited distribution in the Myrmicinae (Table 6). 2-Heptanone appears to be an invariant concomitant of 4-methyl-3-heptanone in *Atta* species (MOSER et al., 1968; BLUM et al., 1968a) but is not characteristic of genera in the tribe Attini which includes *Atta* (CREWE and BLUM, 1972). The recent identification of 2-heptanol as a mandibular gland product of *A. texana* (RILEY et al., 1974b) demonstrates that as in the case of the ethyl ketones, methyl ketones may be accompanied by their corresponding alcohols.

The methyl-branched 3-alkanones may be biosynthesized with an extraordinary sterospecific exactitude. RILEY et al. (1974a) have demonstrated that workers of *A. texana* produce exclusively the S-(+)-isomer of 4-methyl-3-heptanone and are far more sensitive to this enantiomer than they are to the unnatural (−)-isomer. 4-Methyl-3-heptanone is a powerful releaser of alarm behavior for *Atta* species which, by possessing chemoreceptor sites that selectively accomodate the spatial disposition of the natural S-(+)-isomer, exhibit maximal sensitivity to this phero-

Table 8. Mandibular gland constituents identified in myrmicine ants

Species	Compound	Authority
Crematogaster africana, C. sp., C. buchneri, C. depressa, C. jullieni, and C. luciae	*trans*-2-Hexenal	BEVAN et al., 1961; BLUM et al., 1969a; CREWE et al., 1972
Veromessor pergandei	Benzaldehyde	BLUM et al., 1969b
Mycocepurus goeldii	*o*-Aminoacetophenone	BLUM et al., 1974a
Atta sexdens	Neral	BUTENANDT et al., 1959; BLUM et al., 1968a
Atta sexdens	Geranial	BUTENANDT et al., 1959; BLUM et al., 1968a
Crematogaster africana and *C. buchneri*	*trans*-2-Hexenol	CREWE et al., 1972
Atta texana	2-Heptanol	RILEY et al., 1974b
Atta texana	3-Heptanol	RILEY et al., 1974b
Myrmica brevinodis, M. punctiventris, M. fracticornis, M. americana, M. ruginodis, M. rubra, M. sabuleti, M. scabrinodis, Crematogaster navajoa, C. peringueyi, C. castanea, C. cerasi, C. ashmeadi, C. atkinsoni, C. monticola, C. liengmei, C. clara, C. jehovae, C. minutissima, C. striatulata, C. gambiensis, C. gabonensis, C. stadelmanni, C. depressa, C. africana, C. jullieni, C. buchneri, C. clariventris, C. luciae, C. scutellaris, Trachymyrmex septentrionalis, T. seminole, Acromyrmex octospinosus, Cyphomyrmex rimosus, Atta texana, and A. cephalotes	3-Octanol	CREWE and BLUM, 1970a; CREWE and BLUM, 1970b; CREWE et al., 1970; CREWE et al., 1972; SCHLUNNEGGER and LEUTHOLD, 1972; RILEY et al., 1974b
Pogonomyrmex badius, P. barbatus, P. californicus, P. desertorum, P. occidentalis, P. rugosus, Trachymyrmex septentrionalis, Atta texana, and *A. cephalotes*	4-Methyl-3-heptanol	McGURK et al., 1966; CREWE and BLUM, 1972; RILEY et al., 1974b
Myrmica brevinodis, M. rubra, M. punctiventris, M. fracticornis, M. americana, M. ruginodis, M. sabuleti, M. scabrinodis, Crematogaster navajoa, C. cerasi, C. ashmeadi, C. atkinsoni, C. jehovae, C. minutissima, C. striatulata, C. gambiensis, C. gabonensis, C. stadelmanni, C. depressa, C. africana, C. jullieni, C. buchneri, C. clariventris, C. luciae, C. peringueyi, C. castanea, C. monticola, and *C. liengmei*	6-Methyl-3-octanol	CREWE and BLUM, 1970b; CREWE et al., 1970; CREWE et al., 1972
Atta laevigata and *A. capiguara*	Citronellol	BLUM et al., 1968a
Atta sexdens	Geraniol	BLUM et al., 1968a

Table 8 (continued)

Species	Compound	Authority
Atta texana, A. robusta, A. capiguara, A. laevigata, A. columbica, A. cephalotes, and *Crematogaster jehovae*	2-Heptanone	Moser et al., 1968; Blum et al., 1968a; Riley et al., 1974b; Crewe et al., 1972
Manica mutica and *M. hunteri*	4-Methyl-3-hexanone	Fales et al., 1972
Myrmica brevinodis, M. punctiventris, M. fracticornis, M. americana, M. ruginodis, M. rubra, M. sabuleti, M. scabrinodis, Crematogaster navajoa, C. peringueyi, C. castanea, C. cerasi, C. ashmeadi, C. atkinsoni, C. monticola, C. liengmei, C. clara, C. jehovae, C. minutissima, C. striatulata, C. gambiensis, C. gabonensis, C. stadelmanni, C. depressa, C. africana, C. jullieni, C. buchneri, C. clariventris, C. luciae, C. scutellaris, Manica mutica, M. hunteri, Trachymyrmex septentrionalis, T. seminole, Acromyrmex octospinosus, Atta texana, and *A. cephalotes*	3-Octanone	Crewe and Blum, 1970a; Crewe and Blum, 1970b; Crewe et al., 1969; Crewe et al., 1972; Schlunnegger and Leuthold, 1972; Fales et al., 1972; Crewe and Blum, 1972; Riley et al., 1974b
Pogonomyrmex badius, P. barbatus, P. californicus, P. desertorum, P. occidentalis, P. rugosus, Atta texana, A. robusta, A. capiguara, A. laevigata, A. sexdens, A. bisphaerica, A. columbica, A. cephalotes, Trachymyrmex seminole, Manica mutica, and *M. hunteri*	4-Methyl-3-heptanone	McGurk et al., 1966; Moser et al., 1968; Blum et al., 1968a; Riley et al., 1974b; Crewe and Blum, 1972; Fales et al., 1972
Myrmica brevinodis, M. punctiventris, M. fracticornis, M. americana, M. ruginodis, M. rubra, M. sabuleti, M. scabrinodis, Crematogaster navajoa, C. peringueyi, C. castanea, C. cerasi, C. ashmeadi, C. atkinsoni, C. monticola, C. liengmei, C. clara, C. jehovae, C. minutissima, C. striatulata, C. gambiensis, C. gabonensis, C. stadelmanni, C. depressa, C. africana, C. jullieni, C. buchneri, C. clariventris, and *C. luciae*	3-Nonanone	Crewe and Blum, 1970b; Crewe et al., 1970; Crewe et al., 1972
Myrmica brevinodis, M. punctiventris, M. fracticornis, M. americana, M. ruginodis, M. rubra, M. sabuleti, M. scabrinodis, Crematogaster navajoa, C. peringueyi, C. castanea, C. cerasi, C. ashmeadi, C. atkinsoni, C. monticola, C. liengmei, C. clara, C. jehovae, C. minutissima, C. striatulata, C. gambiensis, C. gabonensis, C. stadelmanni, C. depressa, C. africana, C. jullieni, C. buchneri, C. clariventris, and *C. luciae*	6-Methyl-3-octanone	Crewe and Blum, 1970b; Crewe et al., 1970; Crewe et al., 1972
Manica mutica and *M. hunteri*	3-Decanone	Fales et al., 1972
Manica mutica and *M. hunteri*	4,6-Dimethyl-4-octen-3-one	Fales et al., 1972

mone. Similarly, workers of *A. cephalotes* produce only S-(+)-4-methyl-3-hepta-none and are considerably more responsive to this enantiomer than they are to the (−)-enantiomer (RILEY et al., 1974b). Recently, BENTHUYSEN and BLUM (1974) reported that the workers of *Pogonomyrmex barbatus*, which also utilize 4-methyl-3-heptanone as an alarm releaser, were considerably more sensitive to the S-(+)-isomer than to the R-(−)-enantiomer of this ethyl ketone. It remains to be deter-mined if 4-methyl-3-hexanone and 6-methyl-3-octanone, two other methyl-branched ketones produced by myrmicine species (Table 6), are similarly biosynthesized with such stereospecific exactitude.

Some of the 3-alkanols present in myrmicine mandibular gland secretions do not appear to be synthesized as sterospecifically as 4-methyl-3-heptanone. RILEY et al. (1974b) showed that both *A. texana* and *A. cephalotes* produced a pair of diastereomers of 4-methyl-3-heptanol in a 1:1 ratio. If this alcohol is a precursor of 4-methyl-3-heptanone in *Atta* species, it is likely that only one of the diastereo-mers is oxidized to the ketone.

Although monoterpenes do not appear to be particularly characteristic products of myrmicine mandibular glands, the presence of citral (BUTENANDT et al., 1959), geraniol, and citronellol (BLUM et al., 1968a) in *Atta* secretions demonstrates that isoprenoids are produced by some species. Similarly, aromatic natural products have not been frequently encountered in these glandular exudates but the occurrence of benzyldehyde in the secretion of *Veromessor pergandei* (BLUM et al., 1969b) and *o*-aminoacetophenone in that of *Mycocepurus goeldii* (BLUM et al., 1974a) demonstrates that aromatics are sometimes produced in the mandibular gland tissues.

V. Formicinae

The mandibular gland secretions of formicine ants are dominated by terpenoid constituents, especially those of species in the genus *Lasius* (BERGSTRÖM and LÖFQVIST, 1970). Thirteen isoprenoids have been identified in these glandular exu-dates and these compounds include mono-, sesqui-, and diterpenes (Table 9). Oxy-

Table 9. Compounds identified in the mandibular gland secretions of formicine ants

Species	Compound	Authority
Acanthomyops claviger, Lasius alienus, and *L. carniolicus*	2,6-Dimethyl-5-heptenal	REGNIER and WILSON, 1968; REGNIER and WILSON, 1969; BERGSTRÖM and LÖFQVIST, 1970
Acanthomyops claviger, A. latipes, A. sub-glaber, Lasius umbratus, L. alienus, L. carniolicus, L. flavus, L. speculiventris, and *L. spathepus*	Citronellal	CHADA et al., 1962; REGNIER and WILSON, 1968; WILSON and REGNIER, 1971; BLUM et al., 1968b; REGNIER and WILSON, 1969; KISTNER and BLUM, 1971
Acanthomyops claviger, A. subglaber, and *A. latipes*	Neral	CHADHA et al., 1962; WILSON and REGNIER, 1971

Table 9 (continued)

Species	Compound	Authority
Acanthomyops claviger, A. subglaber, and *A. latipes*	Geranial	Chadha et al., 1962; Wilson and Regnier, 1971
Lasius fuliginosus	Farnesal	Bernardi et al., 1967
Lasius alienus and *L. flavus*	2,3-Dihydrofarnesal	Bergström and Löfqvist, 1970
Lasius niger	1-Octanol	Bergström and Löfqvist, 1970
Lasius niger	1-Nonanol	Bergström and Löfqvist, 1970
Lasius carniolicus	Geranylgeranial	Bergström and Lövqvist, 1970
Lasius carniolicus	Geranylcitronellal	Bergström and Lövqvist, 1970
Acanthomyops claviger (males and workers), *Lasius neoniger* (males), and *L. alienus*	2,6-Dimethyl-5-heptenol-1	Law et al., 1965; Regnier and Wilson, 1968; Regnier and Wilson, 1969
Acanthomyops claviger (males), *Lasius neoniger* (males), *L. umbratus, L. alienus,* and *L. speculiventris*	Citronellol	Law et al., 1965; Blum et al., 1968b; Regnier and Wilson, 1969; Wilson and Regnier, 1971
Lasius carniolicus and *L. fuliginosus*	6-Methyl-5-hepten-2-one	Bergström and Lövqvist, 1970; Bernardi et al., 1967
Camponotus nearcticus (males)	2,4-Dimethyl-2-hexenoic acid	Brand et al., 1973c
Camponotus ligniperda (males), *C. herculeanus* (males), *C. pennsylvanicus* (males), and *C. noveboracensis* (males)	10-Methyldodecanoic acid	Brand et al., 1973d
Lasius fuliginosus	Perillene	Bernardi et al., 1967
Lasius fuliginosus	Dendrolasin	Quilico et al., 1957b
Camponotus nearcticus (males), *C. rasilis* (males), and *C. ligniperda* (males)	Methyl anthranilate	Brand et al., 1973c; Brand et al., 1973d
Camponotus nearcticus (males), *C. pennsylvanicus* (males), *C. subbarbatus* (males), *C. noveboracensis* (males), *C. ligniperda* (males), and *C. herculeanus* (males)	Methyl 6-methylsalicylate	Brand et al., 1973c; Brand et al., 1973d
Camponotus ligniperda (males), *C. herculeanus* (males), *C. pennsylvanicus* (males), and *C. noveboracensis* (males)	Mellein (3,4-dihydro-8-hydroxy-3-methyl isocoumarin)	Brand et al., 1973d
Camponotus spp.	Massoilactone (δ-Dec-2-enoic acid lactone)	Cavill et al., 1968

genated monoterpenes such as citronellal and the isomers of citral appear to be particularly characteristic of the secretions of *Lasius* and *Acanthomyops* species (Bergström and Löfqvist, 1970; Wilson and Regnier, 1971) and these compounds function admirably as both defensive and communicative substances (Ghent, 1961).

The presence of perillene—a monoterpene furan—in the secretion of *Lasius fuliginosus* (BERNARDI et al., 1967) further emphasizes the biosynthetic versatility of the mandibular glands of formicine ants. Perillene is accompanied by dendrolasin — a sesquiterpene furan—as the major constituent in the secretion of *L. fuliginosus.* On the other hand, the mandibular gland exudate of *Lasius carniolicus* is dominated by geranycitronellal, and another diterpene, geranylgeranial, represents a minor concomitant (BERGSTRÖM and LÖFQVIST, 1970—Table 9).

Massoilactone and mellein, two lactones isolated from *Camponotus* species (CAVILL et al., 1968; BRAND et al., 1973 d), in common with many of the other formicine mandibular gland products, have been previously isolated from plant sources. However, unlike massoilactone, mellein is known to be a sex-specific compound, along with the acids and aromatic esters identified in the glandular exudates of *Camponotus* species (BRAND et al., 1973 c, 1973 d). These compounds, which have only been detected in the mandibular gland secretions of males, function to regulate the swarming activity of the females (HÖLLDOBLER and MASCHWITZ, 1965) but in addition, they undoubtedly play a role as defensive substances for the males themselves. Novel sex-specific compounds may be widespread in the Formicinae, and investigations of these glandular exudates in species in other genera should yield results of considerable comparative value.

M. Morphology of the Mandibular Glands

Mandibular glands probably occur in all of the Formicidae and most of the Insecta, although they have been investigated in very few insects. They have been reported in *Mantis religiosa* (SUSLOV, 1912) and in a number of ant species (BLUM et al., 1968 b).

They appear to be large in some of the ants (Formicinae) but small in others (Ponerinae). Anatomically there is very little variation in the glands throughout the Formicidae (Fig. 64). They consist of a reservoir and a flattened glandular mass that is found on the surface of the reservoir. CHADHA et al. (1962) apparently lost the glandular region in dissection. The exit ducts apparently are always connected to the mesal side of the mandibles and open near the anterior edge of the preoral cavity (BLUM et al., 1968 b).

The mechanism behind the release of mandibular gland secretion is at present a controversial subject (HERMANN et al., 1971) (Fig. 65). SIMPSON (1960) believed that depressing the floor of the hypopharynx caused the mouth of the gland to open and release the secretion. KRATKY (1931) suggested that the duct opens automatically when the mandible is abducted.

Longitudinal mandibular grooves have been suspected as channels through which mandibular secretions flow (BUREN et al., 1970). SNODGRASS (1956) also stated that mandibular gland secretion apparently flows down the mandibular groove, although SIMPSON (1960) pointed out that the groove does not extend to the gland orifice. In considering that the mandibular grooves always appear to be on the opposite side of the mandible from the orifice of the mandibular gland, it seems unlikely that the two are related (HERMANN et al., 1971).

Mandibular gland secretions sometimes produce a definite stinglike reaction.

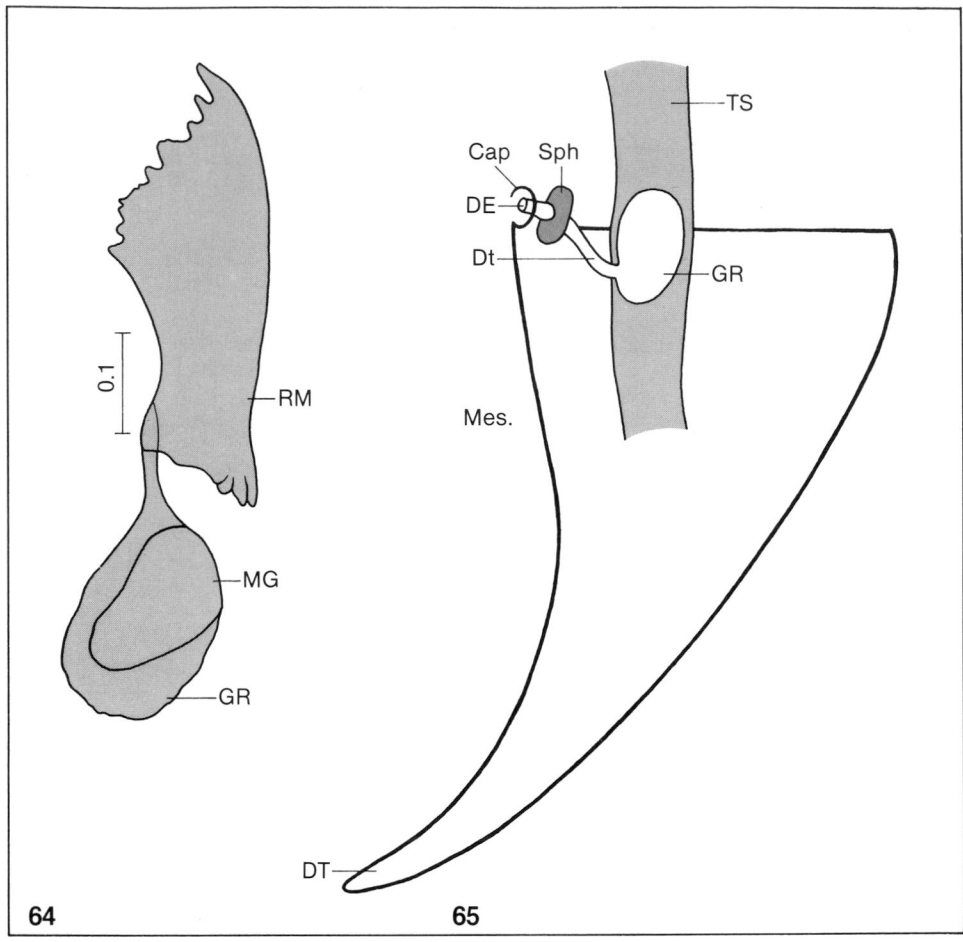

Figs. 64 and 65. Mandibular glands. Fig. 64. *Lasius umbratus* (Formicinae) (after Blum et al., 1968b). Fig. 65. Diagrammatic, showing circular muscle (Sph) around duct on mesal side of mandible (after Hermann et al., 1971)

A spreading of the mandibles during biting may assist the release of mandibular gland secretion. Mandible spreading also is commonly seen in some ant genera in attempts to defend their colonies (e.g., *Iridomyrmex*).

GHENT (1961) found that *Acanthomyops claviger,* in the defense of its colonies, first bites and discharges mandibular gland secretion and then sprays formic acid through the acidopore into the wound (HERMANN, 1978a; HERMANN and BLUM, 1968; HUNG and BROWN, 1964). He found that both the abrasion and the mandibular gland secretion enhance the penetration of insect cuticle for formic acid.

WHEELER (1928) and DELEURANCE (1946) record that certain wasps (*Eumenes*) macerate their prey in conjunction with stinging. Other wasps (*Pemphredon* and *Xylocelia*) are thought to be able to induce paralysis in their prey by macerating the thorax with their mandibles without stinging (JANVIER, 1955; POWELL, 1964).

Ants of the genus *Camponotus* are known to discharge quantities of mandibular fluid during the act of biting (CREIGHTON, 1952; CREIGHTON and SNELLING, 1966).

Other ants of various genera (*Crematogaster, Veromessor, Liometopum,* and *Azteca*) are able to produce irritatingly painful bites, seemingly out of proportion to their size, without stinging. Of these four genera, *Crematogaster* and *Veromessor* are in the subfamily Myrmicinae and possess stings but do not use them for stinging purposes (BUREN, 1958; CREIGHTON, 1953), while functional stings are absent in *Azteca* and *Liometopum,* in the subfamily Dolichoderinae.

We suspect that biting as an aggressive or defensive measure must be widespread in the aculeate Hymenoptera and that it may often involve concomitant discharge of mandibular gland fluid. We also have noticed a slight stinging sensation from the bites of some *Neivamyrmex* species (subfamily Dorylinae) and feel certain that future investigations will reveal that defensive reactions through the use of mandibles and mandibular gland secretions are widespread among the Formicidae.

N. Metapleural Gland Products

I. Myrmicinae

The metapleural glands of myrmicine ants have proven to be the source of an unusual mixture of natural products. Phenylacetic acid has been identified as the major glandular product of *Atta sexdens* (SCHILDKNECHT and KOOB, 1970), *Messor barbarus,* and *Myrmica rubra* (SCHILDKNECHT and KOOB, 1971). In addition, the well known plant auxin, indole-3-acetic acid, is present as a trace constituent in the glandular exudates of *A. sexdens* (SCHILDKNECHT and KOOB, 1970), *M. barbarus,* and an *Acromyrmex* species (SCHILDKNECHT and KOOB, 1971). The secretions of *A. sexdens, M. barbarus, Acromyrmex* sp., and *Myrmica rubra* are also fortified with β-hydroxydecanoic acid (SCHILDKNECHT and KOOB, 1971), a compound which has been designated as myrmicacin. β-Hydroxyoctanoic acid and β-hydroxyhexanoic acid are minor concomitants of myrmicacin in the exudate of *A. sexdens.*

These acids are regarded by SCHILDKNECHT and KOOB (1971) as critical growth regulators in the fungus gardens of *A. sexdens.* β-Hydroxydecanoic acid is viewed as a selective fungicide whereas phenylacetic acid is considered to be a bactericide (MASCHWITZ et al., 1970) and indole-3-acetic acid a mycelial growth stimulant. On the other hand, although these acids could be readily detected in the fungus gardens of *A. sexdens,* they were present in concentrations which were effective as fungal growth stimulants but not as antibiotics (SCHILDKNECHT et al., 1973). Thus, the precise role of these acidic compounds in the ant-fungus relationship must still be regarded as *terra incognita.* MASCHWITZ (1974) has reported that the metapleural gland secretions of ant species in six of seven subfamilies contain acidic constituents, and it is thus likely that aliphatic and aromatic acids are not limited in their distribution to myrmicine ants. In one species, *Crematogaster difformis,* the glandular exudate is sticky and odorous, functioning both to immobilize arthropod predators and to release alarm behavior in the ant workers. Therefore, this exocrine discharge constitutes part of the alarm-defense system of *C. difformis* (MASCHWITZ, 1974) and presumably is used in conjunction with other secretions which also function in this capacity.

O. Morphology of the Metapleural Glands

Metapleural glands apparently are present in most members of the Formicidae with only a few exceptions (BROWN, 1968). These glands are evident externally by the presence of a bulla, which covers an atrium, and a slitlike or porelike meatus that passes to the outside from the atrium. The atrium has a cribriform wall into which the ducts of single gland cells enter. These structures are situated at the posterolateral corners of the alitrunk.

Anatomic studies on the metapleural glands have been reported chiefly by JANET (1898), MASCHWITZ (1974), TULLOCH (1936), and TULLOCH et al. (1962). Additional research on these glands was reviewed by MASCHWITZ (1974). The glands were unknown functionally as late as 1968 when BROWN proposed a theory that they produced repellent substances. Since that report MASCHWITZ (1974) and SCHILDKNECHT et al. (1973) have indicated that they have a multifunction nature.

Other theories on metapleural gland function involve theories of nest odor and grooming compounds (BROWN, 1968). Based on the work of GÖSSWALD (1953) and a brief summary by BROWN (1968), there are four anatomic classes of metapleural glands: (1) the glands of doryline males; (2) the glands of male myrmicine ants and a few nonmyrmicine genera; (3) the glands of certain slave makers of the genus *Polyergus;* and (4) the glands of queens of social parasites.

P. Natural Products of the Formicidae—An Overview

Although investigations of the comparative exocrinology of the Formicidae are still in their early exploratory stages, it is already obvious that ants possess the ability to biosynthesize a dazzling variety of natural products. Many of the compounds identified in the exocrine secretions of these arthropods have not been detected in any other animal taxa or for that matter in plants either. In particular, the venoms of ants have proven to be a particularly rich source of small pharmacologically active compounds which appear to be limited in their distribution to the poison gland secretions of species in a few myrmicine genera. The dialkylpiperidines (MACCONNELL et al., 1971), dialkylpyrrolidines (FALES et al., 1974), and indolizine (RITTER et al., 1973) identified in the venoms of *Solenopsis* and *Monomorium* species typify the nitrogen heterocyclic themes that are characteristic of the poison gland tissues of some myrmicine genera. This emphasis on the biosynthesis of small nitrogenous compounds may be a by-product of the proteinaceous themes that are characteristic of the venoms of primitive myrmicine genera (BLUM, 1966). However, until the venoms of species in other subfamilies are examined for the presence of small nitrogen heterocycles, it is impossible to ascertain whether the synthesis of these compounds is the exclusive domain of myrmicine ants.

LEWIS and DE LA LANDE (1967) and LEWIS et al. (1968) have concluded that the venom of the myrmeciine *Myrmecia pyriformis* is very similar to that of the honeybee (*Apis mellifera*) and they have suggested that the venom of this ant more closely resembles honeybee venom than those of other stinging ants. More recently, WANSTALL and DE LA LANDE (1974) characterized a protein in the venom of *M. pyriformis* which possessed smooth muscle stimulant, red cell lysing, and histamine-releasing activites, as does melittin, the major peptide in bee venom. Furthermore, since the *M. pyriformis* compound behaves like melittin when fractionated by gel filtration, WANSALL and DE LA LANDE (1974) suggest that the two compounds may be closely related. However, although the compounds present in the venoms of the bulldog ant *M. pyriformis* and the honeybee possess several comparable activities, it would be premature to conclude that they are homologous proteins. In view of the fact that not one of the protein-rich venoms produced by stinging ants in the subfamilies Ponerinae, Dorylinae, Pseudomyrmecinae, and Myrmicinae has been biochemically or pharmacologically analyzed in any detail, it is impossible at this time to compare the venoms of *Myrmecia* species to those of other stinging ants. Hemolysins may be widespread in the venoms of stinging ants, and we have found that the venoms of *Paraponera clavata* (Ponerinae), *Myrmica americana,* and three *Pogonomyrmex* species (Myrmicinae) possess easily demonstrable hemolytic activity (unpublished observations). Furthermore, the venoms of many ponerine (WEBER, 1939) and myrmicine (MCCOOK, 1879; WILLIAMS and WILLIAMS, 1965) ants are potently algogenic and thus may be fortified with high concentrations of histamine-releasing substances or histamine, as is the venom of *M. pyriformis* (THOMAS and LEWIS, 1965; LEWIS and DE LA LANDE, 1967). Since the proteinaceous venoms of nonmyrmeciine ants constitute virtual *terra incognita,* there appear to be no substantive grounds for examining the comparative exocrinology of these secretions at this time.

In general, it appears that proteinaceous venoms are characteristic of species in the subfamilies Myrmeciinae, Ponerinae, Dorylinae, Pseudomyrmecinae, and Myrmicinae (CAVILL et al., 1964; BLUM, 1966). Indeed even the alkaloidrich venoms of *Solenopsis* species contain proteinaceous constituents (BRAND et al., 1972), and we are unaware of any known examples of venoms derived from stinging ants which lack macromolecular compounds. Nothing is known about the chemistry of the venom gland secretions of species in the subfamily Dolichoderinae. At this juncture it would seem that the only generalization that can be made about any venoms is that formic acid is an ubiquitous venom gland product of species in the subfamily Formicinae. This acid is produced as a very concentrated aqueous solution and an elucidation of the biosynthesic pathway for this compound in formicine species should yield results of great comparative interest. CASTELLANI et al. (1969) reported that labeled formic acid was isolated from workers of *Formica lugubris* which had ingested D, L-serine 3-C_{14}. They further reported that formylglycine was the precuror of formic acid. This latter finding is of considerable interest since formylglycine has not been usually implicated in the biogenesis of formic acid in either plants or animals. Additional investigations on the biosynthetic origin of formic acid in formicine ants should further illuminate the metabolic pathways of one carbon units in arthropods.

The Dufour's gland secretions of nonformicine ants appear to consist exclusively of aliphatic hydrocarbons, generally in the range of $C_{14}-C_{19}$. Although C_{12} and C_{13} alkanes have been identified in a few myrmicine secretions (REGNIER et al., 1973), C_{15} and C_{17} hydrocarbons appear to predominate in myrmeciine (CAVILL and WILLIAMS, 1967), pseudomyrmecine (BLUM and WHEELER, 1974) and myrmicine (MORGAN and WADHAMS, 1972) glandular exudates. Since the Dufour's gland secretion of *Anoplolepis custodiens* also contains only alkanes and alkenes (SCHREUDER and Brand, 1972), it is obvious that hydrocarbon exclusivity can characterize the exudates of some formicine species as well. However, in general, the products discharged from the Dufour's glands of formicine ants contain, in addition to a wealth of aliphatic hydrocarbons, a multitude of oxygenated compounds as well (Bergström and Löfqvist, 1968, 1973).

Hydrocarbon diversity is a hallmark of the formicine Dufour's gland tissue. These formicine secretions often contain both shorter-chain (C_9-C_{10}) (Bergström and Löfqvist, 1968, 1971) and longer-chain alkanes ($C_{20}-C_{23}$) than have been detected in the exudates of nonformicine species. The formicine discharges further contrast with those of species in other subfamilies by the presence of *n*-undecane and *n*-tridecane as major defensive constituents. However, it is the presence of primary alcohols, often accompanied by their esters, as well as a series of methyl ketones ($C_{13}-C_{19}$), which distinguish the defensive arsenals of the formicine Dufour's gland from those of species in the other subfamilies. These oxygenated compounds are probably derived from the rich hydrocarbon store produced in the tissue of the Dufour's gland. From a biosynthetic standpoint this development would reflect in the Dufour's tissues of formicine ants the presence of more highly evolved metabolic pathways than are characteristic of the glands of species in other subfamilies. This exocrine diversity of the Formicinae may represent an adaptation for discharging a defensive exudate which is considerably more potent than the hydrocarbon-exclusive secretions utilized by ants in subfamilies which possess penetrating stings. Thus, it is likely that selection for more effective defensive compounds has accompanied the loss of a functional sting in formicine ants. Furthermore, the acquisition of larger numbers of oxygenated compounds may have occurred in the more highly evolved formicine species, a hypothesis which could be examined by analyzing the Dufour's gland secretions of formicine species which reflect the major phylogenetic development in this subfamily.

The variety of compounds already identified in the mandibular gland secretions of ants indicates that these tissues will continue to be an outstanding source of arthropod natural products. Investigations of the mandibular gland products of four ponerine genera have yielded four different classes of compounds, a strong indication that the members of this primitive subfamily have independently evolved a diversity of metabolic pathways for producing these exocrine compounds. It seems almost certain that as additional ponerine genera are analyzed, the mandibular gland chemistry of this subfamily will be considerably enlarged. 4-Methyl-3-heptanone, one of the compounds synthesized by *Neoponera villosa* (Duffield and Blum, 1973), currently possesses the widest subfamily distribution of any compound identified in ants. This ketone has also been identified in doryline (Blum et al., 1974b), pseudomyrmecine (Blum and Wheeler, 1974) and myrmicine (McGurk et al., 1966) species, and species in all taxa utilize it for both defensive and communicative functions. Ultimately, ponerine genera may be demonstrated to produce many of the same natural products that are biosynthesized by species in more advanced subfamilies.

Although species in only about a dozen genera in the large subfamily Myrmicinae have been chemically analyzed, it would appear that the biosynthesis of ethyl ketones has been strongly emphasized by the members of this taxon. Seven 3-ketones have been identified in species in myrmicine genera and five of these compounds are produced by species in the genus *Manica* (FALES et al., 1972). Since *Manica* is regarded as a primitive myrmicine genus, ethyl ketone diversity may have been a characteristic of the less highly evolved genera in this subfamily. Although 3-alkanones appear to be a hallmark of certain myrmicine tribes, surprising natural product deviations from this ketonic theme may be uncovered if chemical analyses are undertaken on a wide range of tribal genera. CREWE and BLUM (1972) presented a phylogenetic treatment of several genera in the tribe Attini which was based on the presence of two ethyl ketones and their corresponding carbinols. However, the recent identification of *o*-aminoacetophenone as a mandibular gland product of the attine *Mycocepurus goeldii* (BLUM et al., 1974a) demonstrates that generalizations about the natural products synthesized by closely related genera may be susceptible to easy demolition.

If 2-alkanones are characteristic of myrmicine species, then terpenes must be regarded as a trademark of the formicine mandibular glands. The large variety of isoprenoids identified in the secretions of the relatively few formicine genera that have been analyzed is indicative of the terpenoid emphasis identified with these exocrine tissues. Monoterpene aldehydes appear to be biosynthesized by the conventional isoprenoid pathway (HAPP and MEINWALD, 1965) and it is very probable that the host of C_{10} and C_{15} isoprenoids identified in formicine mandibular gland exudates are similarly produced. These compounds are very effective defensive compounds, especially when utilized in conjunction with formic acid (GHENT, 1961) and analyses of additional formicine genera promise to expand the list of terpenes produced in the mandibular glands of formicine ants. On the other hand, the occurrence of a host of novel nonterpenoid constituents in the exudates of *Camponotus* species (BRAND et al., 1973c, 1973d; CAVILL et al., 1968) indicates that these formicine glands will continue to yield a wealth of natural products belonging to a diversity of chemical classes.

Q. The Formicid Venom Apparatus — Phyletic Implications

I. Relationship to Wasps

Examination of the formicid venom apparatus gives us some anatomic clues to an understanding of the relationships between the Formicidae and between the Formicidae and the hymenopterans that presumably gave rise to the ants. There are only two presently outstanding theories concerning the rise of ants (HERMANN, 1978a): (1) the Tiphioid theory, outlined repeatedly by BROWN (1954), EISNER and BROWN (1958), and WILSON et al. (1967a, 1967b); and the (2) Bethylid theory, presented in detail by MALYSHEV (1968).

MALYSHEV listed 4 primary phases of phyletic development from the stem from which he felt ants arose: (1) a *Predatory Semi-Familial Phase;* (2) an *Ectoparasitic Semi-Familial Phase;* (3) a *Familial Ectoparasitic (Hemiformicoid) Phase;* and (4) a *Primary Ant (Proformicoid) Phase.* This last phase led to the *Secondary Ant (Formicoid) Phase,* represented by modern ants.

Althoug MALYSHEV (1968) no doubt put a lot of time and thought into his organization of pre-ant hymenopterans, it is our feeling that MALYSHEV described *the trend of some hymenopterous groups toward sociality,* a phenomenon which has occurred or has partially occurred on many occasions.

Malyshev neglected one main point characteristic of the most primitive extant ant species: the primitive Myrmeciinae and Ponerinae are large ants, whereas the bethylid from which ants presumably arose is very small. Malyshev's thoughts were not fruitless, however. His research brought to light the fact that "*a wide gulf separates the Formicidae from the truly solitary wasps such as the Mutillidae, Tiphiidae, Scoliidae and Myzine, in whose behavior and mode of life not a trace remains of any possibility of their change to familial or even a semi-familial life.*"

For a better understanding of why Malyshev's statement is so important we must first examine part of Sudd's list of characteristics of the earliest ants (1967): (1) early ants nested in the soil or in moist rotting wood or humus; (2) early ants hunted insect prey or collected dead insects. At the same time they took nectar and possibly honeydew (Hermann, 1975) as the extant thipiid *Myrmosia* does (Krombein, 1939); (3) early ants mated in the air; the flight is still a behavioral necessity even in many ants that make no use of flight for dispersion; (4) the colonies of early ants were founded by solitary queens.

Probably one of the earliest and most primitive extant ant groups is the Amblyoponini. The form of the petiole appears to be one of the most important characters used by Wilson et al. (1967a, 1967b) to link the Formicidae with the Tiphiidae. In this case the petiolar region is considered an important tool to indicate a close relationship; yet, relating the Myrmicinae and Pseudomyrmecinae through the presence of a petiole and postpetiole seems to be of little importance (Brown, 1954).

To further our understanding of these relationships, the following characteristics of the Tiphiidae may be of help: (1) prey is left *in situ* or they nest in a preexisting cavity that may or may not be modified. *Methocha* may encounter prey outside of its burrow and drag it back inside; (2) they are predators on beetle larvae in the soil or rotten wood; most attack white grubs (Scarabaeidae), but the Methochinae attack the larvae of tiger beetles; (3) females of many Tiphiidae that attack larvae living in the ground or in wood are wingless; (4) some of the apterous females are smaller and very different in appearance from the males; in some cases the male carries the female about during a prolonged mating flight (e.g., *Dimorphathynnus haemorrhoidalis*).

From this list, it is obvious that the tiphiids are far from social insects. The wide gulf becomes more obvious when we examine the list of possible preadaptations for sociality presented by Evans and Eberhard (1970). With their major steps toward sociality, plus additional, more detailed substeps (Hermann, 1978a), they pointed out the complexity in the rise of sociality. They also pointed out that the tiphiids demonstrate only the first two steps toward a social existence.

Looking for wasps that are apterous is not necessarily a prerequisite for a formicid ancestor. Ant queens are winged and only the workers ar secondarily apterous. Ponerine queens usually are winged and much the same size as the workers; ergatoid, apterous, or gynaecoid females are found in some forms, characters that undoubtedly are secondary and evolving in the Formicidae and convergently with any other group of the Hymenoptera in which they occur. Doryline females are secondarily apterous and physogastric. Cerapachyine females often are apterous and dichthadiiform. Leptanilline females apparently are like doryline females. All of the other ant subfamilies, presumably derived groups, have winged females.

We can clearly see that the lack of wings is a derived condition, a condition that convergently has appeared in some scolioid families, including some members of the Formicidae. Using the apterous condition of scolioids as an indicator of ant ancestry may possibly lead to invalid assumptions.

When we look at the tiphiid venom apparatus we see first that the sclerites are wasplike; secondly, and probably of more importance we see an apparatus that is not particularly antlike. Here again it appears that there is a wide anatomic gap between the Tiphiidae and the Formicidae.

It is therefore apparent that regardless of whatever superficial or convergent characters the Tiphiidae have in common with the Formicidae, MALYSHEV's statement that a wide gulf separates these two groups is a fact that must be regarded as important in our understanding of familial interrelationships. That the ants are closely related to any of the other Aculeata is purely theoretical.

II. Formicinae

An examination of the venom apparatus within the subfamilies of the Formicidae also gives us some clues as to their relationship with each other. The phyletic studies reported to date (BROWN, 1954; EISNER and BROWN, 1958; ROBERTSON, 1968; WILSON et al., 1967a, 1967b) have been vague about where to place the Formicinae; yet, most investigators speak of the formicines as advanced.

As pointed out here, there are considerable anatomic and behavioral differences between this subfamily and other ant subfamilies. Based on venom apparatus anatomy, the Formicinae are extremely different and often unique in the structures that they possess (HERMANN, 1978a; HERMANN et al., 1975; HERMANN and BLUM, 1968). The lightly sclerotized venom apparatus is highly reduced and the sclerites have been modified beyond simple reduction to suit their tremendously modified mode of action. Dufour's gland and the venom components are unique among the Formicidae. The acidopore (HUNG and BROWN, 1964) has taken the place of the sting and through the function of muscles attached to the enlarged venom canal there is some directional control during the release of venom and associated compounds.

Such a wide anatomic and behavioral hiatus between the formicines and other ants strongly indicates that the formicines are a group separated from the other ants by a significant phyletic gap. It appears that other members or subfamilies did not lead to the Formicinae at all, but that the Formicinae stands alone as a subfamily; they obviously have a common origin with the other ants but they split off from the main formicid line early in ant phylogeny.

III. Pseudomyrmecinae

Although the pseudomyrmecines superficially resemble the myrmicines there appears to be some sort of gap between the two groups. Based on the anatomy of the venom apparatus the pseudomyrmecines are primitive. They have venom sclerites and venom gland components like those found in the Ponerinae. The close similarity with the myrmicines in lancet development leading to sting autotomy (Hermann, 1971; Hermann and Hamilton, 1978) is due to convergence just as it is in other hymenopterous insects.

IV. Myrmicinae

Myrmicine ants are widely divergent in their anatomic and behavioral characteristics. The venom apparatus, in most cases, indicates trends towards reduction often to the point of losing the function of the sclerites in the role of stinging. This loss is accompanied by behavioral changes and usually anatomic changes that enable the ants to continue defending their colonies while employing their defunct venom apparatus for other behavioral functions.

V. Ponerinae, Dorylinae, Cerapachyinae

Probably some of the most important interrelationships among ant subfamilies that have been brought out by investigations of the venom apparatus are those between the Ponerinae, Dorylinae, and Cerapachyinae (Hermann, 1969a). Although the Cerapachyinae have been thought of as linking the Ponerinae with the Dorylinae (Emery, 1901; Wheeler, 1920), their venom apparatuses indicate that they are dorylinelike.

The relationship between the Ponerinae and Dorylinae indicates that the two groups may have had a common ancestor, the Dorylinae being a derived group both behaviorally and anatomically (Hermann, 1969a; Hermann, 1978a). The presence of a legionary ponerine (Gotwald, 1970; Hermann, 1968c), also anatomically similar to the dorylines, probably indicates convergent evolution.

VI. Old and New World Dorylinae

Studies of the doryline venom apparatus strongly indicate a well-recognized distinction between the Old World and New World dorylines, although they also have indicated some similarities. In brief the Old World and New World dorylines are related and apparently monophyletic but they have been separated for a considerable period of time.

Acknowledgement: The research reported upon in this chapter was partially supported by NSF Grant 38482.

References

Adrouny, G.A., Derbes, V.J., Jung, R.C.: Isolation of a hemolytic component of fire ant venom. Science **130**, 449 (1959).
Anonymous: Insect sting allergy, Questionaire study of 2606 cases. J.A.M.A. **193**, 115 (1965).
Ayre, G.L., Blum, M.S.: Attraction and alarm of ants (*Camponotus* spp.-Hymenoptera: Formicidae) by pheromones. Physiol. Zool. **44**, 77—83 (1971).

Barnard, J.H.: Allergic and pathologic findings in fifty insect sting fatalities. J. Allergy **40**, 107 (1967).

Barr, S.E.: Skin test reactivity to the stinging insects. Ann. Allergy **30**, 282 (1972).

Beard, R.L.: Arthropod venoms as insecticides. In: *Naturally Occurring Insecticides.* Jacobson, M., Crosby, D.G. (eds.). New York: Marcel Dekker, 1971.

Benthuysen, J.L., Blum, M.S.: Quantitative sensitivity of the ant *Pogonomyrmex barbatus* to the enantiomers of its alarm pheromone. J. Georgia Ent. Soc. **9**, 235—238 (1974).

Bequaert, J.C.: Medical report of the Hamilton Rice Seventh Expedition to the Amazon, in conjuction with the Department of Tropical Medicine of Harvard University, 1924—25. Cambridge, Mass.: Harvard Univ. Press, 1926, pp. 250—253.

Bergström, G., Löfqvist, J.: Odour similarities between the slave-keeping ants *Formica sanguinea* and *Polyergus rufescens* and their slaves *Formica fusca* and *Formica rufibarbis.* J. Insect Physiol. **14**, 995—1011 (1968).

Bergström, G., Löfqvist, J.: Chemical basis for odour communication in four species of *Lasius* ants. J. Insect Physiol. **16**, 2353—2375 (1970).

Bergström, G., Löfqvist, J.: *Camponotus ligniperda* Latr.-a model for the composite volatile secretions of Dufour's gland in formicine ants. In: *Chemical Releasers in Insects* (Tahori, A.S., ed.) New York: Gordon and Breach, 1971, Vol. III, pp. 195—223.

Bergström, G., Löfqvist, J.: Similarities between the Dufour's gland secretions of the ants *Camponotus ligniperda* (Latr.) and *Camponotus herculeanus* (L.). Ent. Scand. **3**, 225—238 (1972).

Bergström, G., Löfqvist, J.: Chemical congruence of the complex odoriferous secretions from Dufour's gland in three species of ants of the genus *Formica.* J. Insect Physiol. **19**, 887—907 (1973).

Bernardi, R., Cardani, C., Ghiringhella, D., Selva, A., Baggini, A., Pavan, M.: On the components of secretion of mandibular glands of the ant *Lasius* (*Dendrolasius*) *fuliginosus.* Tetrahedron Lett. **40**, 3893—3896 (1967).

Betts, A.D.: Pratical Bee Anatomy. Benson, England: The Apis Club, 1923, 88 pp.

Bevan, C.W.L., Birch, A.J., Caswell, H.: An insect repellent from black cocktail ants. J. Chem. Soc. **1961**, 488 (1961).

Beyer, O.W.: Der Giftapparat von *Formica rufa,* ein reduziertes Organ. Jena'sche Zeitschrift für Naturwissenschaft **25**, 26—112 (1891).

Blum, M.S.: The source and specificity of trail pheromones in *Termitopone, Monomorium* and *Huberia,* and their relation to those of some other ants. Proc. Roy. Ent. Soc. London Ser. A **41**, 155—160 (1966).

Blum, M.S., Brand, J.M., Amante, E.: Unpublished data (1974a).

Blum, M.S., Brand, J.M., Duffield, R.M., Snelling, R.R.: Chemistry of the venom of *Solenopsis aurea* (Hymenoptera: Formicidae). Ann. Ent. Soc. Amer. **66**, 702 (1973).

Blum, M.S., Brand, J.M., Watkins, J.F.: Unpublished data (1974b).

Blum, M.S., Callahan, P.S.: The venom and poison glands of *Pseudomyrmex pallidus* (F. Smith). Psyche **70**, 69—74 (1963).

Blum, M.S., Crewe, R.M., Sudd, J.H., Garrison, A.W.: 2-Hexenal: Isolation and function in a *Crematogaster (Atopogyne)* sp. J. Georgia Ent. Soc. **4**, 145—148 (1969a).

Blum, M.S., Hermann, H.R.: The hymenopterous poison gland: Probable functions of the main glandibular elements. J. Georgia Ent. Soc. **4**, 23—28 (1969).

Blum, M.S., Padovani, R., Amante, E.: Alkanones and terpenes in the mandibular glands of *Atta* species. Comp. Biochem. Physiol. **26**, 291—299 (1968a).

Blum, M.S., Padovani, F., Curley, A., Hawk, R.E.: Benzaldehyde: Defensive secretion of a harvester ant. Comp. Biochem, Physiol. **29**, 461—465 (1969b).

Blum, M.S., Padovani, F., Hermann, H.R., Kannowski, P.B.: Chemical releasers of social behavior. XI. Terpenes in the mandibular glands of *Lasius umbratus* (Hymenoptera: Formicidae: Formicinae). Ann. Ent. Soc. Amer. **61**, 1354—1359 (1968b).

Blum, M.S., Walker, J.R., Callahan, P.S., Novak, A.F.: Chemical, insecticidal and antibiotic properties of fire ant venom. Science **128**, 306—307 (1958).

Blum, M.S., Watkins, J.F.: In: Attractant-repellent secretions in blind snakes (*Leptotyphlops dulcis*) and army ants (*Neivamyrmex nigrescens*) (Watkins, J.F., Gehlbach, F.R., Kroll, J.C.). Ecology **50**, 1098—1102 (1969).

Blum, M.S., Wheeler, J.W.: Unpublished data (1974).

Bordas, M.L.: Appareil glandulaire des Hymenopteres. Ann. Sci. Nat. Zool. Paleon. **19**, 1—363 (1895).

Bowen, R.B.: Insects and allergic problems. South Med. J. **44**, 836 (1951).

Brand, J.M., Blum, M.S., Barlin, M.R.: Fire ant venoms: Intraspecific and interspecific variation among castes and individuals. Toxicon **11**, 325—331 (1973a).

Brand, J.M., Blum, M.S., Fales, H.M., MacConnell, J.G.: Fire ant venoms: comparative analyses of alkaloidal components. Toxicon **10**, 259—271 (1972).

Brand, J.M., Blum, M.S., Lloyd, H.A., Fletcher, D.J.C.: Monoterpene hydrocarbons in the poison gland secretion of the ant *Myrmicaria natalensis* (Hymenoptera: Formicidae). Ann. Ent. Soc. Amer. **67**, 525—526 (1974).

Brand, J.M., Blum, M.S., Ross, H.H.: Biochemical evolution in fire ant venoms. Insect Biochem. **3**, 45—51 (1967b).

Brand, J.M., Duffield, R.M., MacConnell, J.G., Blum, M.S. Fales, H.M.: Caste-specific compounds in male carpenter ants. Science **179**, 388—389 (1973c).

Brand, J.M., Fales, H.M., Sokoloski, E.A., MacConnell, J.G., Blum, M.S., Duffield, R.M.: Identification of mellein in the mandibular gland secretion of carpenter ants. Life Sci. **13**, 201—211 (1973d).

Brophy, J.J., Cavill, G.W.K., Shannon, J.S.: Venom and Dufour's gland secretions in an Australian species of *Camponotus*. J. Insect Physiol. **19**, 791—798 (1973).

Brown, W.L., Jr.: Remarks on the internal phylogeny and subfamily classification of the family Formicidae. Insectes Soc. **1**, 21—31 (1954).

Brown, W.L., Jr.: An hypothesis concerning the function of the metapleural glands in ants. Amer. Natur. **102**, 188—191 (1968).

Brown, W.L., Jr., Nutting, W.L.: Wing venation and the phylogeny of the Formicidae (Hymenoptera). Trans. Amer. Ent. Soc. **75**, 113—132 (1950).

Buren, W.F.: A review of the species of Crematogaster, *sensu stricto*, in North America (Hymenoptera: Formicidae). Part I. J.N.Y. Ent. Soc. **66**, 118—134 (1958).

Buren, W.F., Hermann, H.R., Blum, M.S.: The widespread occurence of mandibular grooves in aculeate Hymenoptera. J. Georgia Ent. Soc. **5**, 185—196 (1970).

Butenandt, A., Linzen, B., Lindauer, M.: Über einen Duftstoff aus der Mandibeldrüse der Blattschneiderameise *Atta sexdens rubropilosa* Forel. Arch. Anat. Microscop. Morph. Exptl. **48**, 13—19 (1959).

Callahan, P.S., Blum, M.S., Walker, J.R.: Morphology and histology of the poison glands and sting of the imported fire ant (*Solenopsis saevisima* v. *richteri* Forel). Ann. Ent. Soc. Amer. **52**, 573—590 (1959).

Caro, M.R., Derbes, V.J., Jung, R.: Skin responses to the sting of the imported fire ant (*Solenopsis saevissima*). A.M.A. Arch. Dermatol. **75**, 475—488 (1957).

Casnati, G., Ricca, A., Pavan, M.: Sulla secrezione difensiva delle glandole mandibolari *Paltothyreus tarsatus* (Fabr.). Chimica Ind. (Milano) **49**, 57—61 (1967).

Castellani, A.A., Gabba, A., Laterza, L., Pavan, M.: Sulla biogenesi dell'acido formico in *Formica lugubris* Zett. Memorie Soc. Ent. Ital. **48**, 147—152 (1969).

Cavill, G.W.K., Clark, D.V., Whitfield, F.B.: Insect venoms, attractants, and repellents. XI. Massoilactone from two species of formicine ants, and some observations on constituents of the bark oil of *Cryptocarya massoia*. Aust. J. Chem. **21**, 2819—2823 (1968).

Cavill, G.W.K., Robertson, P.L., Whitfield, F.B.: Venom and venom apparatus of the bull ant, *Myrmecia gulosa* (Fabr.). Science **146**, 79—80 (1964).

Cavill, G.W.K., Williams, P.J.: Constituents of Dufour's gland in *Myrmecia gulosa*. J. Insect Physiol. **13**, 1097—1103 (1967).

Cavill, G.W.K., Williams, P.J., Whitfield, F.B.: α-Farnesene, Dufour's gland secretion in the ant *Aphaenogaster longiceps* (F. Sm.). Tetrahedron Lett. **23**, 2201—2205 (1967).

Chadha, M.S., Eisner, T., Monro, A., Meinwald, J.: Defense mechanisms of arthropods. VII. Citronellal and citral in the mandibular gland secretions of the ant *Acanthomyops claviger* (Roger). J. Insect Physiol. **8**, 175—179 (1962).

Chrystal, R.N.: The *Sirex* wood-wasps and their importance in forestry. Bull. Ent. Res. **19**, 219—247 (1928).

Clark, J.: The Formicidae of Australia. Subfamily Myrmeciinae. Melbourne, Australia: Commonwealth Sci. Ind. Res. Org., 1951, Vol. I.

Clausen, C.P.: Entomophagous Insects. New York: McGraw Hill, 1940.

Cooper, K.W.: Egg gigantism, oviposition, and genital anatomy: Their bearing on the biology and phylogenetic position of *Orussus* (Hymenoptera: Siricoidea). Proc Rochester Acad. Sci. **10**, 39—68 (1953).

Copland, M.J.W., King, P.E.: The structure of the female reproductive system in the Chalcididae (Hym.). Ent. Monthly. **107**, 230—239 (1971).

Creighton, W.S.: The ants of North America. Bull. Mus. Comp. Zool. **104**, 1—585 (1950).

Creighton, W.S.: Studies on Arizona ants. 1. The habits of *Camponotus ulcerosus* Wheeler and its identity with *C. bruesi* Wheeler, Psyche **58**, 47—64 (1952).

Creighton, W.S.: New data on the habits of the ants of the genus *Veromessor*. Amer. Mus. Novitates. **1612**, 1—18 (1953).

Creighton, W.S., Snelling, R.R.: The rediscovery of *Camponotus* (*Myrmaphaenus*) *yogi*. (Wheeler) (Hymenoptera: Formicidae). Psyche **73**, 187—195 (1966).

Crewe, R.M., Blum, M.S.: Identification of the alarm pheromones of the ant *Myrmica brevinodis*. J. Insect Physiol. **16**, 141—146 (1970a).

Crewe, R.M., Blum, M.S.: Alarm pheromones in the genus *Myrmica* (Hymenoptera: Formicidae). Their composition and species specificity. Z. Vergl. Physiol. **70**, 363—373 (1970b).

Crewe, R.M., Blum, M.S.: Alarm pheromones of the Attini: Their phylogenetic significance. J. Insect Physiol. **18**, 31—42 (1972).

Crewe, R.M., Blum, M.S., Collingwood, C.A.: Comparative analysis of alarm pheromones in the ant genus *Crematogaster*. Comp. Biochem. Physiol. **43b**, 703—716 (1972).

Crewe, R.M., Brand, J.M., Fletcher, D.J.C.: Identification of an alarm pheromone in the ant *Crematogaster peringueyi*. Ann. Ent. Soc. Amer. **62**, 1212 (1969).

Crewe, R.M., Brand, J.M., Fletcher, D.J.C., Eggers, S.H.: The mandibular gland chemistry of some South African species of *Crematogaster* (Hymenoptera: Formicidae). J. Georgia Ent. Soc. **5**, 42—47 (1970).

Crewe, R.M., Fletcher, D.J.C.: Ponerine ant secretions: The mandibular gland secretion of *Paltothyreus tarsatus* Fabr. J. Ent. Soc. South Africa **37**, 291—298 (1974).

Daly, H.V.: A comparative survey of the sting of aculeate Hymenoptera. Thesis, Univ. Kansas, USA, 67 pp. (1953).

Darwin, C.: On the origin of species by means of natural selection. London: Murray, 1859.

Davis, N.T.: Morphology of the female organs of reproduction in the Miridae (Hemiptera). Ann. Ent. Soc. Amer. **48**, 132—150 (1955).

Deleurance, E.P.: Les *Eumenes* de la région nicoise. Essai de monographic biologique. Bull. Soc. Zool. France. **70**, 85—100 (1946).

Derwitz, H.: Über Bau und Entwicklung des Stachels der Ameisen. Zeitschr. f. wiss. Zool. **28**, 527—556 (1878).

D'Rozario, A.M.: On the development and homologies of the genitalia and their ducts in Hymenoptera. Trans. R. Ent. Soc. Lond. **92**, 362—415 (1942).

Duffield, R.M., Blum, M.S.: 4-Methyl-3-heptanone: Indentification and function in *Neoponera villosa* (Hymenoptera: Formicidae). Ann. Ent. Soc. Amer. **66**, 1357 (1973).

Duffield, R.M., Blum, M.S.: Unpublished data (1974).

Eisner, T., Brown, W.L., Jr.: The evolution and social significance of the ant proventriculus. Proc. 10th Int. Congr. Ent. (Montreal, 1956) **2**, 503—508 (1958).

Emery, C.: Notes sur les sous-familles des Dorylines et Ponérines. (Famille des Formicides). Ann. Soc. Belg. **45**, 32—54 (1901).

Evans, H.E.: The comparative ethology and evolution of the sand wasps. Comstock Publ. Assoc. Cambridge, Mass. **I-XVI.** 526 pp. (1966).

Evans, H.E., Eberhard, M.J.W.: The Wasps. Ann. Arbor: Univ. Michigan Press, 1970.

Fales, H.M., Blum, M.S., Crewe, R.M., Brand, J.M.: Alarm pheromones in the genus *Manica* derived from the mandibular gland. J. Insect Physiol. **18**, 1077—1088 (1972).

Fales, H.M., Pedder, D., Blum, M.S., Crewe, R.M., MacConnell, J.G.: Unpublished data (1974).

Flemming, H.: Die Muskulatur und Innervierung des Wehrstachelapparates von Aculeaten. Z. Morphol. Oekol. Tiere **46**, 321–341 (1957).

Foerster, R.: Vergleichendanatomische Untersuchungen über den Stechapparat der Ameisen. Zool. Jahrb. (Sect. 2) Abt. Anat. Ontog. Tiere. **34**, 347–380 (1912).

Forbes, J.: Anatomy and histology of the worker *Camponotus herculeanus pennsylvanicus* De Geer (Formicidae, Hymenoptera). Ann. Ent. Soc. Amer. **31**, 181–195 (1938).

Forel, A.: Der Giftapparat und die Analdrüsen der Ameisen. Z. Wiss. Zool. **3**, 28–68 (1878).

Forel, A.: Der Giftapparat und die Analdrüsen der Ameisen. Z. Wiss. Zool. **30**, 28–66 (1887).

Ghent, R.L.: Adaptive refinements in the chemical defense mechanisms of certain Formicinae. Doctoral Thesis, Cornell University, Ithaca, New York (1961).

Ghent, R.L., Gary, N.E.: A chemical alarm releaser in honey bee stings (*Apis mellifera* L.). Psyche **69**, 1–6 (1962).

Gösswald, K.: Histologische Untersuchungen an der arbeiterlosen Ameise *Teleutomyrmex schneideri* Kutter (Hym. Formicidae). Mitteilungen Schweiz. Ent. Ges. **26**, 81–126 (1953).

Gotwald, W.H., Jr.: Mouthpart morphology of the ant *Aneuretus simoni*. Ann. Ent. Soc. Amer. **63**, 950–952 (1970).

Gotwald, W.H., Jr., Brown, W.L., Jr.: The ant genus *Simopelta* (Hymenoptera: Formicidae). Psyche **73**, 261–277 (1966).

Grünanger, P.A., Quilico, A., Pavan, M.: Sul secreto del formicide *Myrmicaria natalensis* Fred. Accad. Nazion. Lincei **28**, 293–300 (1960).

Gupta, P.D.: On the structure, development and homology of the female reproductive organs in Orthopteroid insects. Indian J. Ent. **10**, 75–123 (1950).

Gustafson, J.F.: The origin and evolution of the genitalia of the Insecta. Microent. **15**, 35–67 (1950).

Happ, G.M., Meinwald, J.: Biosynthesis of arthropod secretions. I. Monoterpene synthesis in an ant (*Acanthomyops claviger*). J. Amer. Chem. Soc. **87**, 2507–2508 (1965).

Haupt, H.: Alte und neue *Pepsis*-arten (Sphecoidea) Pompilidae, olim Psammocharidae auct. mit einem Anhang: Der Stachelapparat der spinnenfangenden Raubwespen. Nova Acta Leopoldina, N.S. **15**, **109**, 309–414 (1952).

Hermann, H.R.: The hymenopterous poison apparatus. IV. *Dasymutilla occidentalis* (Hymenoptera: Mutillidae). J. Georgia Ent. Soc. **3**, 1–10 (1968a).

Hermann, H.R.: The hymenopterous poison apparatus. V. *Aneuretus simoni*. Ann. Ent. Soc. Amer. **61**, 1315–1317 (1968b).

Hermann, H.R.: The hymenopterous poison apparatus. VII. *Simopelta oculata* (Hymenoptera: Formicidae: Ponerinae). J. Georgia Ent. Soc. **3**, 163–166 (1968c).

Hermann, H.R.: The hymenopterous poison apparatus: Evolutionary trends in three closely related subfamilies of ants (Hymenoptera: Formicidae). J. Georgia Ent. Soc. **4**, 123–141 (1969a).

Hermann, H.R.: The hymenopterous poison apparatus. VIII. *Leptogenys (Lobopelta) elongata* (Hymenoptera: Formicidae). J. Georgia Ent. Soc. **42**, 239–243 (1969b).

Hermann, H.R.: Sting autonomy, a defensive mechanism in certain social Hymenoptera. Insectes Soc. **18**, 111–120 (1971).

Hermann, H.R.: Crepuscular and nocturnal activities of *Paraponera clavata* (Hymenoptera: Formicidae: Ponerinae). Ent. News **86**, 94–98 (1975).

Hermann, H.R.: The hymenopterous venom apparatus-Morphology and evolution. Ann. Ent. Soc. Amer. (in press) (1978a).

Hermann, H.R.: The furcula, a major component in the formicid venom apparatus. Inter. J. Insect Morph. and Embryol. (in press) (1977).

Hermann, H.R.: Muscles of the sting base in hymenopterous insects. Inter. J. Insect Morph. and Embryol. (in press) (1978b).

Hermann, H.R., Baer, R., Barlin, M.: Histology and function of the venom gland system in formicine ants. Psyche **82**, 67–73 (1975).

Hermann, H.R., Blum, M.S.: The morphology and histology of the hymenopterous poison apparatus. I. *Paraponera clavata* (Formicidae). Ann. Ent. Soc. Amer. **59**, 397–409 (1966).

Hermann, H.R., Blum, M.S.: The morphology and histology of the hymenopterous poison apparatus. II. *Pogonomyrmex badius* (Formicidae). Ann. Ent. Soc. Amer. **60**, 661—665 (1967a).

Hermann, H.R., Blum, M.S.: The morphology and histology of the hymenopterous poison apparatus. III. *Eciton hamatum* (Formicidae). Ann. Ent. Soc. Amer. **60**, 1282—1291 (1967b).

Hermann, H.R., Blum, M.S.: The hymenopterous poison apparatus. VI. *Camponotus pennsylvanicus* (Hymenoptera: Formicidae). Psyche **75**, 216—227 (1968).

Hermann, H.R., Hamilton, W.D.: Sting anatomy and autotomy in tropical polistine wasps (In preparation) (1975).

Hermann, H.R., Hunt, A.N., Buren, W.F.: Mandibular gland and mandibular groove in *Polistes annularis* (L.) and *Vespula maculata* (L.) (Hymenoptera: Vespidae). Int. J. Insect Morph. Embryol. **1**, 43—49 (1971).

Hermann, H.R., Moser, J.C., Hunt, A.N.: The hymenopterous poison apparatus. XI. Morphological and behavioral changes in *Atta texana* (Hymenoptera: Formicidae). Ann. Ent. Soc. Amer. **63**, 1552—1558 (1970).

Hermann, H.R., Mullen, M.A.: The hymenopterous poison apparatus. XI. *Xylocopa virginica* (Hymenoptera: Xylocopidae). J. Georgia Ent. Soc. **9**, 246—252 (1974).

Hölldobler, B., Maschwitz, V.: Der Hochzeitsschwarm der Roßameise *Componotus herculeanus* (Hym. Formicidae). Z. Vergl. Physiol. **50**, 551—568 (1965).

Hung, A.C.F., Brown, W.L.: Structure of gastric apex as a subfamily character of the Formicinae (Hymenoptera: Formicidae). J.N.Y. Ent. Soc. **74**, 198—200 (1964).

Hunt, A.N., Hermann, H.R.: Insect envenomization: Some hematological reactions in guinea pigs to three hymenopterous venoms. J. Georgia Ent. Soc. **8**, 249—264 (1973).

Janet, C.: Études sur les fourmis, les guêpes et les abeilles. Note 18. Aiguillon de la *Myrmica rubra*. Appareil de fermeture de la glande à venin. Georges Carré et C. Naud, éditeurs, Paris **11**, 393—449 (1898).

Janvier, H.: Paralysie des pucerons par constriction thoracique. C.R. Acad. Sci. **241**, 608—609 (1955).

Jouvanez, D.P., Blum, M.S., MacConnell, J.G.: Antibacterial activity of venom alkaloids from the imported fire ant, *Solenopsis invicta* Buren. Antimicrob. Ag. Chemotherap. **2**, 291—293 (1972).

Kahlenberg, H.: Thesis, Univ. Erlangen, Germany (1895).

Kistner, D.H., Blum, M.S.: Alarm pheromone of *Lasius (Dendrolasius) spathepus* (Hymenoptera: Formicidae) and its possible mimicry by two species of *Pella* (Coleoptera: Staphylinidae). Ann. Ent. Soc. Amer. **64**, 589—594 (1971).

Kraepelin, C.: Untersuchungen über den Bau, Mechanismus und die Entwicklungsgeschichte des Stachels der bienenartigen Tiere. Zeitschr. f. wiss. Zool. **23**, 289—330 (1873).

Kratky, E.: Morphologie und Physiologie der Drüsen in Kopf und Thorax der Honigbiene. Z. wiss. Zool. **139**, 120—200 (1931).

Krombein, K.V.: Habits of Tiphiidae. Trans. Ent. Soc. Amer. **65**, 415—466 (1939).

Lacaze-Duthiers, H.: Recherches sur l'armure génitale des Insectes. Ann. Sci. Nat. **14**, 17—52 (1850).

Lande, I.S., de la, Thomas, D.W., Tyler, M.J.: Pharmacological analysis of the venom of the "Bull dog" ant. In: Recent Advances in the Pharmacology of Toxins, Proc. 2nd Int. Pharm. Meeting, Prague. Oxford: Pergamon Press, 1963, Vol. IX, p. 71.

Law, J.H., Wilson, E.O., McCloskey, J.A.: Biochemical polymorphism in ants. Science **149**, 544—545 (1965).

Leuenberger, F.: Die Biene. Aarau: Sauerländer, 1954.

Lewis, J.C., Lande, I.S. de la: Pharmacological and enzymic constituents of the venom of an Australian "Bull Dog" ant *Myrmecia pyriformis*. Toxicon **4**, 225—234 (1967).

Lewis, J.C., Day, A.J., Lande, I.S., de la: Phospholipase A in the venom of *Myrmecia pyriformis* (an Australian bull dog ant). Toxicon **6**, 109—112 (1968).

Lockey, R.F.: Systemic reactions to stinging ants. J. Allergy Clin. Immunol. **54**, 132—146 (1974).

MacConnell, J.G., Blum, M.S., Fales, H.M.: Alkaloid from fire ant venom: Identification and synthesis. Science **168**, 840—841 (1970).

MacConnell, J.G., Blum, M.S., Fales, H.M.: The chemistry of the fire ant venom. Tetrahedron **26**, 1129—1139 (1971).

MacConnell, J.G., Williams, R.N., Brand, J.M., Blum, M.S.: New alkaloids in the venoms of fire ants. Ann. Ent. Soc. Amer. **67**, 134—135 (1974).

Malyshev, S.I.: Genesis of the Hymenoptera. London: Methuen, 1968.

Maschwitz, U.: Gefahrenalarmstoffe und Gefahrenalarmierung bei sozialen Hymenopteren. Z. vergl. Physiol. **47**, 596—655 (1964).

Maschwitz, U.: Vergleichende Untersuchungen zur Funktion der Ameisenmetathorakaldrüse. Oecologia **16**, 303—310 (1974).

Maschwitz, U., Koob, K., Schildknecht, H.: Ein Beitrag zur Funktion der Metathorakaldrüse der Ameisen. J. Insect Physiol. **16**, 387—404 (1970).

Maschwitz, U.W.J., Kloft, W.: Morphology and function of the venom apparatus of insects—Bees, wasps, ants, and caterpillars. In: Venomous Animals and Their Venoms. Bücherl, W., Buckley, E.E. (eds.). Chap. 44, **3**, 1—60 (1971). Academic Press, N.Y.

Matsuda, R.: Comparative morphology of the abdomen of a machilid and a rhaphidiid. Trans. Amer. Ent. Soc. **83**, 39—63 (1957).

McCook, H.C.: The Natural History of the Agricultural Ant of Texas. Philadelphia: Lippincott, 1879.

McGurk, D.J., Frost, J., Eisenbraun, E.J., Vick, K., Drew, W.A., Young, J.: Volatile compounds in ants: identification of 4-methyl-3-heptanone from *Pogonomyrmex* ants. J. Insect Physiol. **12**, 1435—1441 (1966).

Melander, A.L., Brues, C.T.: The chemical nature of some insects' secretions. Bull. Wis. Nat. Hist. Soc. N.S. **4**, 22—36 (1906).

Michener, C.D.: A comparative study of the appendages of the eighth and ninth abdominal segments of insects. Ann. Ent. Soc. Amer. **37**, 336—351 (1944).

Michener, C.D.: Hymenoptera. In: Taxonomist's Glossary of Genitalia in Insects. Tuxen, S.L. (ed.). Copenhagen: 1951, pp. 131—140.

Morgan, E.D., Wadhams, L.J.: Chemical constituents of Dufour's gland in the ant, *Myrmica rubra*. J. Insect Physiol. **18**, 1125—1135 (1972).

Morison, G.D.: The muscles of the adult honey-bee (*Apis mellifera* L.). Quart. J. Micr. Sci. **71**, 395—463 (1927).

Moser, J.C., Brownlee, R.G., Silverstein, R.M.: The alarm pheromones of *Atta texana*. J. Insect Physiol. **14**, 529—535 (1968).

Oeser, R.: Vergleichend-morphologische Untersuchungen über den Ovipositor der Hymenopteren. Mitt. Zool. Mus. Berlin **37**, 1—119 (1961).

O'Rourke, F.J.: Formic acid production among the Formicidae. Ann. Ent Soc. Amer. **43**, 437—443 (1950).

Osman, M.F.H., Brander, J.: Weitere Beiträge zur Kenntnis der chemischen Zusammensetzung des Giftes von Ameisen aus der Gattung *Formica*. Z. Naturforsch. **16b**, 749—753 (1961).

Ouljanin, H.: Entwicklung des Stachels der Arbeitsbiene. Z. Wiss. Zool. **22**, 289 (1872).

Parrish, H.M.: Analysis of 460 fatalities from venomous animals in the United States. Amer. J. Med. Sci. **245**, 129 (1963).

Pavan, M., Ronchetti, G.: Studi sulla morfologia esterna e anatomia interna dell' operaia di *Iridomyrmex humilis* Mayr e ricerche chimiche e biologiche sulla iridomercina. Atti Soc. Ital. Sci. Nat. Milan. **94**, 379—477 (1955).

Pawlowsky, E.N.: Gifttiere und ihre Giftigkeit. Jena: Fischer, 1927.

Piek, T., Thomas, R.T.S.: Paralysing venoms of solitary wasps. Comp. Biochem. Physiol. **30**, 13—31 (1969).

Powell, J.A.: Biology and behavior of nearctic wasps of the genus *Xylocelia* with special reference to *X. occidentalis* (Fox) Wasmann. J. Kansas Entomol. Soc. **37**, 240—258 (1964).

Quilico, A., Piozzi, F., Pavan, M.: Ricerche chimiche sui Formicidae. Sostanze prodotte dal *Lasius* (*Chthonolasius*) *umbratus* Nyl. Rend. Ist. Lomb. Sc. Lett., Cl. Sc. **91**, 271—279 (1957a).

Quilico, A., Piozzi, F., Pavan, M.: The structure of dendrolasin. Tetrahedron **1**, 177—185 (1957b).

Ratcliffe, N.A., King, P.E.: The venom system of *Nasonia vitripennis* (Walker) (Hymenoptera: Pteromolidae). Proc. R. Ent. Soc. London (A) **42**, 49—61 (1967).

Rathmayer, W.: Das Paralysierungsproblem beim Bienenwolf *Philanthus triangulum* F. (Hym. Spec.) Z. Vergleich. Physiol. **45**, 413—462 (1962).

Regnier, F.E., Nieh, M., Hölldobler, B.: The volatile Dufour's gland components of the harvester ants *Pogonomyrmex rugosus* and *P. barbatus*. J. Insect Physiol. **19**, 981—992 (1973).

Regnier, F.E., Wilson, E.O.: The alarm-defensive system of the ant *Acanthomyops claviger*. J. Insect Physiol. **14**, 955—970 (1968).

Regnier, F.E., Wilson, E.O.: The alarm-defensive system of the ant *Lasius alienus*. J. Insect Physiol. **15**, 893—898 (1969).

Remane, A.: Die Grundlagen des natürlichen Systems der vergleichenden Anatomie und der Phylogenetik. Leipzig: Geest and Portig, 1952.

Rettenmeyer, C.W.: Behavioral studies of army ants. Kansas Univ. Sci. Bull. **44**, 281—465 (1963).

Rietschel, P.: Bau und Funktion des Wehrstachels der staatenbildenden Bienen und Wespen. Zeitschr. Morph. Ökol. Tiere **33**, 313—357 (1937).

Riley, R.G., Silverstein, R.M., Moser, J.C.: Biological responses of *Atta texana* to its alarm pheromone and the enantiomer of the pheromone. Science **183**, 760—762 (1974a).

Riley, R.G., Silverstein, R.M., Moser, J.C.: Isolation, identification, synthesis, and biological activity of the volatile compounds from the heads of *Atta* ants. J. Insect Physiol. **20**, 1629—1637 (1974b).

Ritter, F.J., Rotgans, I.E.M., Talman, E., Verwiel, P.E.J., Stein, F.: 5-Methyl-3-butyloctahydroindolizine, a novel type of pheromone attractive to Pharaoh's ants. Experientia **29**, 530—531 (1973).

Robertson, P.L.: A morphological and functional study of the venom apparatus in representatives of some major groups of Hymenoptera. Aust. J. Zool. **16**, 133—166 (1968).

Russell, F.E.: Pharmacology of animal venoms. Clin. Pharmacol. Ther. **8**, 849—873 (1967).

Schildknecht, H., Koob, K.: Pflanzliche Bioregulatoren als Inhaltsstoffe der Metathorakaldrüsen der Knotenameisen. Angew. Chem. **82**, 181 (1970).

Schildknecht, H., Koob, K.: Myrmicacin, das erste Insekten-Herbicid. Angew. Chem. **83**, 110 (1971).

Schildknecht, H., Reed, P.B., Reed, F.D., Koob, K.: Auxin activity in the symbiosis of leaf-cutting ants and their fungus. Insect Biochem. **3**, 439—442 (1973).

Schlunnegger, U.P., Leuthold, R.H.: Rapid identification of volatile compounds in insects with direct gas chromatography/mass spectrometry procedure: 3 octanone and 3-octanol in *Crematogaster scutellaris* and *C. ashmeadi*. Insect Biochem. **2**, 150—152 (1972).

Schreuder, G.D., Brand, J.M.: The chemistry of Dufour's gland and the poison gland secretions of *Anoplolepis custodiens* (Hymenoptera, Formicidae). J. Georgia Ent. Soc. **7**, 188—195 (1972).

Scudder, G.G.E.: Reinterpretation of some basal structure in the insect ovipositor. Nature. Lond. **180**, 340—341 (1957a).

Scudder, G.G.E.: The systematic position of *Dicranocephalus* Hahn, 1826 and its allies (Hemiptera-Heteroptera). Proc. R. Ent. Soc. Lond. (A) **32**, 147—158 (1957b).

Scudder, G.G.E.: The female genitalia of the Heteroptera: Morphology and bearing on classification. Trans. R. Ent. Soc. Lond. **111**, 405—467 (1959).

Scudder, G.G.E.: The comparative morphology of the insect ovipositor. Trans. R. Ent. Soc. Lond. **113**, 25—40 (1961a).

Scudder, G.G.E.: The functional morphology and interpretation of the insect ovipositor. Can. Ent. **93**, 267—272 (1961b).

Scudder, G.G.E.: Further problems in the interpretation and homology of the insect ovipositor. Can. Ent. **96**, 405—417 (1964).

Simpson, J.: The functions of the salivary glands of *Apis mellifera*. J. Insect Physiol. **4**, 107—121 (1960).

Smith, E.L.: Evolutionary morphology of the external insect genitalia. I. Origins and relationships, to other appendages. Ann. Ent. Soc. Amer. **62**, 1051—1079 (1969).

Smith, E.L.: Evolutionary morphology of the external insect genitalia. 2. Hymenoptera. Ann. Ent. Soc. Amer. **63**, 1—27 (1970).

Snodgrass, R.E.: Morphology of the insect abdomen. Part I. General structure of the abdomen and its appendages. Smithsonian Misc. Coll. **85**, 1—128 (1931).

Snodgrass, R.E.: How the bee stings. The Bee World **14**, 3—6 (1933a).

Snodgrass, R.E.: Morphology of the insect abdomen. Part II. The genital ducts and the ovipositor. Smithsonian Misc. Coll. **89**, 1—148 (1933 b).

Snodgrass, R.E.: Principles of Insect Morphology. New York: McGraw-Hill, 1935.

Snodgrass, R.E.: Anatomy of the honey bee. Ithaca, N.Y.: Cornell Univ. Press, 1956.

Sollman, A.: Der Bienenstachel. Zeitschr. Wiss. Zool. **13**, 528—540 (1863).

Spence, J.E.: A comparison of the allergic and immunological effects of the hemolytic component of fire ant venom. Tulane Univ. La. Med. School Prize Essay 7, 212 (1962, 1963).

Spruce, R.: Notes of a botanist on the Amazon and Andes. II. London 366 pp (1908).

Stumper, R.: Nouvelles observations sur le venin des fourmis. C.R. Acad. Sci. **174**, 413—415 (1922).

Stumper, R.: Sur la sécrétion d'acide formique par les fourmis. C.R. Acad. Sci. **233**, 1144—1146 (1951).

Stumper, R.: Données quantitatives sur la sécrétion d'acide formique par les fourmis. C.R. Acad. Sci. **234**, 149—152 (1952).

Stumper, R.: Die Giftsekretion der Ameisen. Naturwissenschaften **47**, 457—463 (1960).

Sudd, J.H.: An Introduction to the Behavior of Ants. New York: St. Martin's Press, 1967.

Suslov, S.: Über die Kopfdrüsen einiger niederen Orthopteren. Zool. Jahrb. Anat. **34**, 96—120 (1912).

Talman, E., Ritter, F.J., Verwiel, P.E.J.: Structure elucidation of pheromones produced by the Pharoah's ant. *Monomorium pharaonis* L. In: Proc. Int. Symp. on Mass Spectrometry in Biochem. and Med. Milan, 1973 (Frigerio, A., Castagnoli, N., eds.) New York: Raven, 1974, pp. 197—217.

Thomas, D.W., Lewis, J.C.: Histamine release by the ant. Aust. J. Exp. Biol. Med. Sci. **43**, 275—276 (1965).

Trojan, E.: Zur Frage der Oligomerie weiblicher Akuleaten. Z. Morphol. Oekol. Tiere **30**, 597—628 (1935).

Tulloch, G.S.: The metasternal glands of the ant, *Myrmica rubra,* with special reference to the Golgi bodies and the intracellular canaliculi. Ann. Ent. Soc. Amer. **29**, 81—84 (1936).

Tulloch, G.S., Shapiro, J.F., Hershenov, B.: The ultrastructure of the metasternal glands of ants. Brooklyn Ent. Soc. Bull. **77**, 91—101 (1962).

Tumlinson, J.H., Silverstein, R.M., Moser, J.C., Brownlee, R.G., Ruth, J.M.: Identification of the trail pheromone of a leaf-cutting ant, *Atta texana.* Nature **234**, 348—349 (1971).

Vansclow, N.R.: Hypersensitivity to Hymenoptera insects. J. Arkansas Med. Soc. **63**, 723—725 (1969).

Vick, K., Drew, W.A., McGurk, D.J., Eisenbraun, E.J., Waller, G.R.: Identification of hydrocarbons from *Novomessor cockerelli.* Ann. Ent. Soc. Amer. **62**, 723—725 (1969).

Walker, E.M.: The terminal abdominal structures of Orthopteroid insects: A phylogenetic study. Ann. Ent. Soc. Amer. **12**, 267—326 (1919).

Wanstall, J.C., Lande, I.S. de la: Fractionation of bulldog ant venom. Toxicon **12**, 649—655 (1974).

Weber, N.A.: The sting of an ant. Amer. J. Trop. Med. **17**, 765—768 (1937).

Weber, N.A.: The sting of the ant, *Paraponera clavata.* Science **89**, 127—128 (1939).

Weber, N.A.: The stings of the harvesting ant *Pogonomyrmex occidentalis* (Cresson), with a note on populations (Hymenoptera). Ent. News **70**, 85—90 (1959).

Wheeler, G.C.: Ant larvae of the subfamily Cerapachyinae. Psyche **57**, 102—113 (1950).

Wheeler, J.W., Blum, M.S.: Alkylpyrazine alarm pheromones in ponerine ants. Science **182**, 501—503 (1973).

Wheeler, W.M.: The Social Insects; Their Origin and Evolution. New York: Harcourt Brace, 1920.

Wheeler, W.M.: Social Life among the Insects. New York: Harcourt, Brace, 1928.

Whelden, R.M.: Additional notes on *Rhytidoponera convexa* Mayr (Hymenoptera, Formicidae). Ann. Ent. Soc. Amer. **51**, 80—85 (1957).

Whelden, R.M.: Additional notes on *Rhytidoponera convexa* Mayr (Hymenoptera, Formicidae). Ann. Ent. Soc. Amer. **51**, 80—84 (1958 a).

Whelden, R.M.: Notes on the anatomy of the Formicidae. I. *Stigmatomma pallipes* (Haldemann). J. New York Ent. Soc. **65**, 1—21 (1958 b).

Whelden, R.M.: The anatomy of *Rhytidoponera metallica* F. Smith (Hymenoptera: Formicidae). Ann. Ent. Soc. Amer. **53**, 793—808 (1960).

Whelden, R.M.: The anatomy of the adult queen and workers of the army ants *Eciton burchelli* Westwood and *Eciton hamatum* Fabricius. J.N.Y. Ent. Soc. **71**, 158—178 (1963).

Williams, M.W., Williams, C.S.: Collection and toxicity studies of ant venom. Proc. Soc. Exp. Biol. and Med. **116**, 161—163 (1964).

Williams, M.W., Williams, C.S.: Toxicity of ant venom. Further studies of the venom from *Pogonomyrmex barbatus*. Proc. Soc. Exp. Biol. Med. **119**, 344—346 (1965).

Wilson, E.O.: The beginnings of nomadic and group-predatory behavior in the ponerine ants. Evolution **12**, 24—31 (1958).

Wilson, E.O.: The social biology of ants. Ann. Rev. Ent. **8**, 345—368 (1963).

Wilson, E.O.: Chemical communication in the social insects. Science **149**, 1064—1071 (1965).

Wilson, E.O., Carpenter, F.M., Brown, W.L., Jr.: The first Mesozoic ants. Science **157**, 1038—1040 (1967a).

Wilson, E.O., Carpenter, F.M., Brown, W.L., jr.: The Mesozoic ants, with the description of a new subfamily. Psyche **74**, 1—19 (1967b).

Wilson, E.O., Regnier, R.E.: Evolution of the alarm-defense system in the formicine ants. Amer. Nat. **105**, 279—289 (1971).

Wray, J.: Some uncommon observations and experiments made with an acid juyce to be found in ants. Phil. Trans. Roy. Soc. London **1670**, 2063—2069 (1970).

Zander, E.: Beiträge zur Morphologie des Stacheapparates der Hymenopteren. Z. Wiss. Zool. **66**, 289—333 (1899).

Zander, E.: Handbuch der Bienenkunde III. Der Bau der Biene. Stuttgart: Ulmer, 1911.

CHAPTER 26

Venoms and Venom Apparatuses of the Formicidae: Dolichoderinae and Aneuretinae

S. BLUM and H.R. HERMANN, JR.

A. Introduction and Taxonomy

In many areas of the world, ants in the subfamily Dolichoderinae constitute one of the dominant groups of invertebrates. This is especially true of the American and certain regions of the Old World tropics where many species of dolichoderine ants form populous colonies. The aggressive and fast-moving workers can represent a formidable force when unleashed against either invertebrate or vertebrate intruders. Although these formicids lack a penetrating sting, they have an extraordinary defensive capability derived from one of the most variegated exocrine arsenals produced by any group of invertebrates. A multitude of unique defensive compounds are biosynthesized in the anal glands, structures which have arisen *de novo* in the Dolichoderinae and function as both social organs and defensive glands. Among the Formicidae, the anal glands may constitute the chemical arsenal par excellence and are probably, to a great extent, responsible for the success of the dolichoderines in exploiting a multitude of habitats despite intense competition from other groups of ants.

Species in some dolichoderine genera are particularly pugnacious, and can deliver a painful bite to mammals such as man. This is particularly true of certain arboreal species in the genera *Azteca* and *Liometopum* (unpublished data) and must reflect venomous constituents in the cephalic secretions of their workers. Thus, apparently in addition to the anal glands, the cephalic glands of species in some genera are a source of potent defensive compounds. Obviously, too, the lack of a functional sting has not been a severe defensive liability for some dolichoderine species.

In addition to the Dolichoderinae, the subfamily Aneuretinae is included in this review. Since the Aneuretinae, represented by a single Ceylonese species, *Aneuretus simoni,* are closely related to the Dolichoderinae, these two taxa form a logical formicid unit for discussion.

The taxonomy and phylogeny of the Dolichoderinae and Aneuretinae are discussed by WHEELER (1922), CREIGHTON (1950), BROWN (1954), and WILSON et al. (1956). These two subfamilies can be readily separated from the other formicid subfamilies by employing the following dichotomous key (modified from CREIGHTON, 1950).

Key to the Subfamilies Dolichoderinae and Aneuretinae

Myrmeciinae, Ponerinae, and *Cerapachyinae.*
1. Gaster with a distinct constriction between the first and second segments . .
   Gaster without any constriction between the first and second segments 2
   Myrmicinae, Leptanillanae, Dorylinae, and *Pseudomyrmecinae*
2. Abdominal pedicel consisting of two segments . . . .
   Abdominal pedicel consisting of one segment 3
3. Cloacal orifice distinctly circular and usually surrounded by a fringe
   of hairs . . . . *Formicinae*
   Cloacal orifice slit-like, the hairs, when present, not forming an
   encircling fringe 4
4. Sting well developed and exsertile . . . .   Aneuretinae
   Sting not well developed or exsertile . . . .   Dolichoderinae

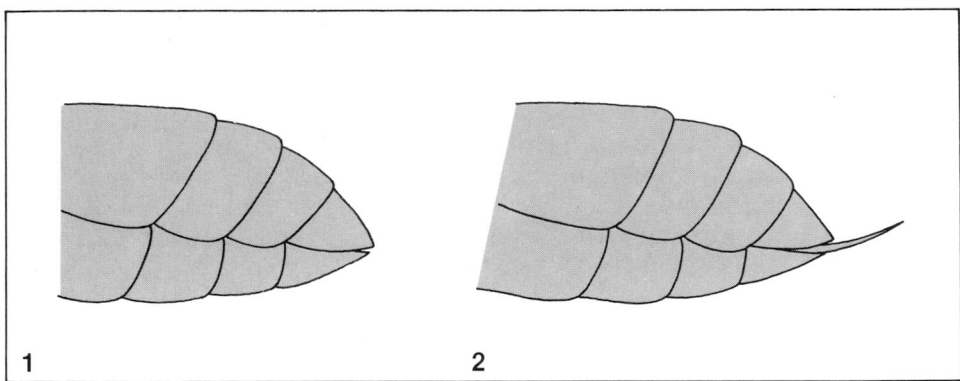

Figs. 1 and 2. Insertile sting, not evident or only slightly evident upon gross examination (Fig. 1). Exsertile sting, strongly evident upon gross examination (Fig. 2)

The biology of the Dolichoderinae and Aneuretinae is discussed by Wheeler (1910), Sudd (1967) and Wilson (1971).

B. Dolichoderine Natural Products and Anatomy of the Venom Apparatus

I. Mandibular Gland Constituents

Cavill and Houghton (1974a) identified a series of pyrazines from total extracts of the Argentine ant, *Iridomyrmex humilis*. Subsequently, these weakly basic compounds were demonstrated to be produced in the heads of worker ants (Cavill and Houghton, 1974b). These pyrazine derivatives are probably derived from the mandibular glands (Fig. 3).

The trisubstituted pyrazines identified in *I. humilis* are presented in Table 1. (*E*)-2,5-Dimethyl-3-styrylpyrazine is the major pyrazine present, comprising 200 p.p.m. of the body weight of a worker ant. On the other hand, 2,5-dimethyl-3-

Table 1. Compounds identified in the mandibular gland secretion of *Iridomyrmex humilis*

Compound	Species	Authority
2,5–Dimethyl–3–propylpyrazine	*Iridomyrmex humilis*	CAVILL and HOUGHTON, 1974a, b
2,5–Dimethyl–3–isopentylpyrazine	*Iridomyrmex humilis*	CAVILL and HOUGHTON, 1974 a, b
(*E*)–2,5–Dimethyl–3–styrylpyrazine	*Iridomyrmex humilis*	CAVILL and HOUGHTON, 1974a, b

n-propylpyrazine is a trace constituent which is present at approximately 5 p.p.m. 2,5-Dimethyl-3-isopentylpyrazine (Table 1) comprises about 70 p.p.m. of the worker body weight and is accompanied by a trace constituent (ca. 5%) which appears to be 2,5-dimethyl-3-isopentyldihydropyrazine (CAVILL and HOUGHTON, 1974a).

CAVILL and HOUGHTON (1974a) reported that (*Z*)-2,5-dimethyl-3-styrylpyrazine was the major styrylpyrazine present when extracts of whole ant workers were analyzed. However, these investigators established that the (*E*)-isomer is rapidly photoisomerized to the (*Z*) form, a finding of major significance in view of the fact that analyses of ant extracts are normally carried out under laboratory conditions in sunlight. When analyses were undertaken in the dark, the (*E*)-isomer of 2,5-dimethyl-3-styrylpyrazine (Table 1) constituted 80% of the styrylpyrazine mixture and if the extract was exposed to light for one hour, it consisted of the pure (*Z*)-isomer. Thus, (*E*)-2,5-dimethyl-3-styrylpyrazine is considered to be the predominant, if not the only, 3-styryl-isomer present in the ant (CAVILL and HOUGHTON, 1974a).

It has been suggested that both 2,5-dimethyl-3-isopentylpyrazine and (*E*)-2,5-dimethyl-3-styrylpyrazine could arise from alanine via 2,5-dimethylpyrazine (CAVILL and HOUGHTON, 1974a). The isoprenoid or styryl moiety would be introduced into the symmetrical pyrazine intermediate.

No pyrazine derivatives were detected in extracts of the endemic Australian dolichoderine, *Iridomyrmex detectus* (CAVILL and HOUGHTON, 1974a).

II. Poison Gland Constituents

None of the compounds synthesized in the dolichoderine poison gland have been chemically characterized. Indeed, in view of the lack of any known function for the poison gland products, it is difficult to visualize what role these compounds play in dolichoderine biology.

III. Anatomy of the Venom Apparatus Components in the Dolichoderinae

In spite of our lack of chemical knowledge about dolichoderine venom components, the venom reservoir, filamentous and convoluted glands are well developed (Figs. 4—6). Indeed, the filamentous glands (*FG*) in this subfamily are unlike those in any of the other formicid subfamilies. They are globose in appearance and attach to the reservoir near the latter structure's apex. If we would say anything about the appearance of these glands we would have to hypothesize that they probably have enlarged to increase the production of whatever chemicals they produce. The reservoir (*RES*) is round to oval and most often filled with liquid. We suspect that these glands and their associated structures must have an important function in the biology of these ants.

The convoluted gland (*CG*) is inside the reservoir. Except for the globate appearance of the filamentous glands, the general structure of the venom apparatus components is myrmicine-like. The venom apparatus components of the Dolichoderinae in no way resemble those of the Ponerinae.

The venom apparatus components of all dolichoderine species appears to be similar to those illustrated by PAVAN and RONCHETTI (1955) for *Iridomyrmex humilis*

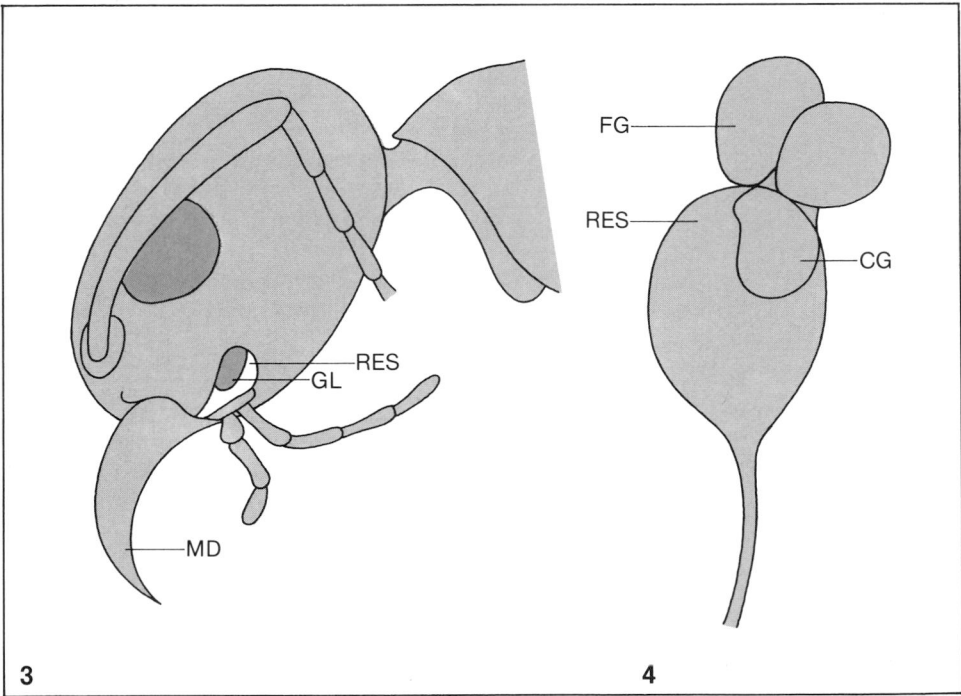

Figs. 3 and 4. Two pheromone-producing glands in *Iridomyrmex* spp. Fig. 3. Mandibular gland. Fig. 4. Venom reservoir and associated glandular regions. *CG* Convoluted gland, *FG* Filamentous gland, *GL* Gland, *MD* Mandible, *RES* Reservoir

except in the connection between the venom duct, Dufour's gland, and the sting base. PAVAN and RONCHETTI pictured Dufour's gland entering the sting bulb dorsad of the venom duct. Further investigation (HERMANN and BLUM, unpublished data), however, demonstrated that Dufour's gland in all members of the Aculeata enters the sting bulb ventrad of the venom duct.

Glandular components in the Aneuretinae have not been examined and therefore no comments can be made on comparisons of these structures with those of the Dolichoderinae and Ponerinae.

IV. Anatomy of Venom Sclerites

The venom sclerites of both the Dolichoderinae and Aneuretinae (Figs. 4—8) are present in their entirety, except for the furcula (HERMANN, 1968, 1978). The furcula has fused to the anterior string base so that the muscles originating on the oblong plate articulate to the sting base (HERMANN, 1977).

This feature alone indicates a close relationship between the Dolichoderinae and Aneuretinae. Although the ponerine *Simopelta oculata* demonstrates a similar condition at the sting base (GOTWALD and BROWN, 1966; HERMANN, 1968a), the authors feel that this character is convergent between the Ponerinae and Aneuretinae (GOTWALD, 1970; HERMANN, 1968b). Other characters support a relationship

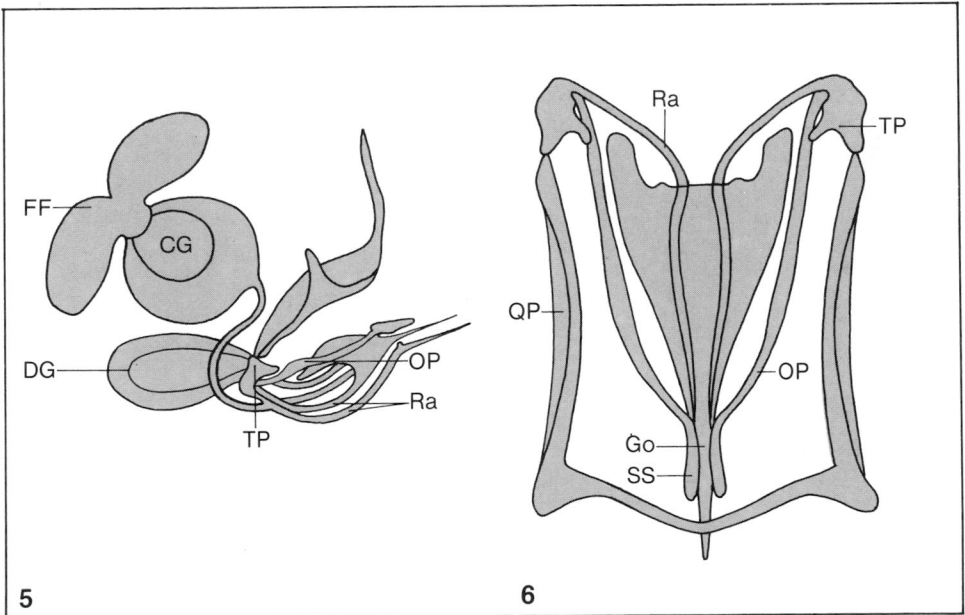

Figs. 5 and 6. Venom sclerites of *Iridomyrmex pruinosus* (Fig. 5) and *Dolichoderus analis* (Fig. 6). *Go* Gonostylus, *OP* Oblong plate, *QP* Quadrate plate, *Ra* Rami, *SS* Sting shaft, *TP* Triangular plate

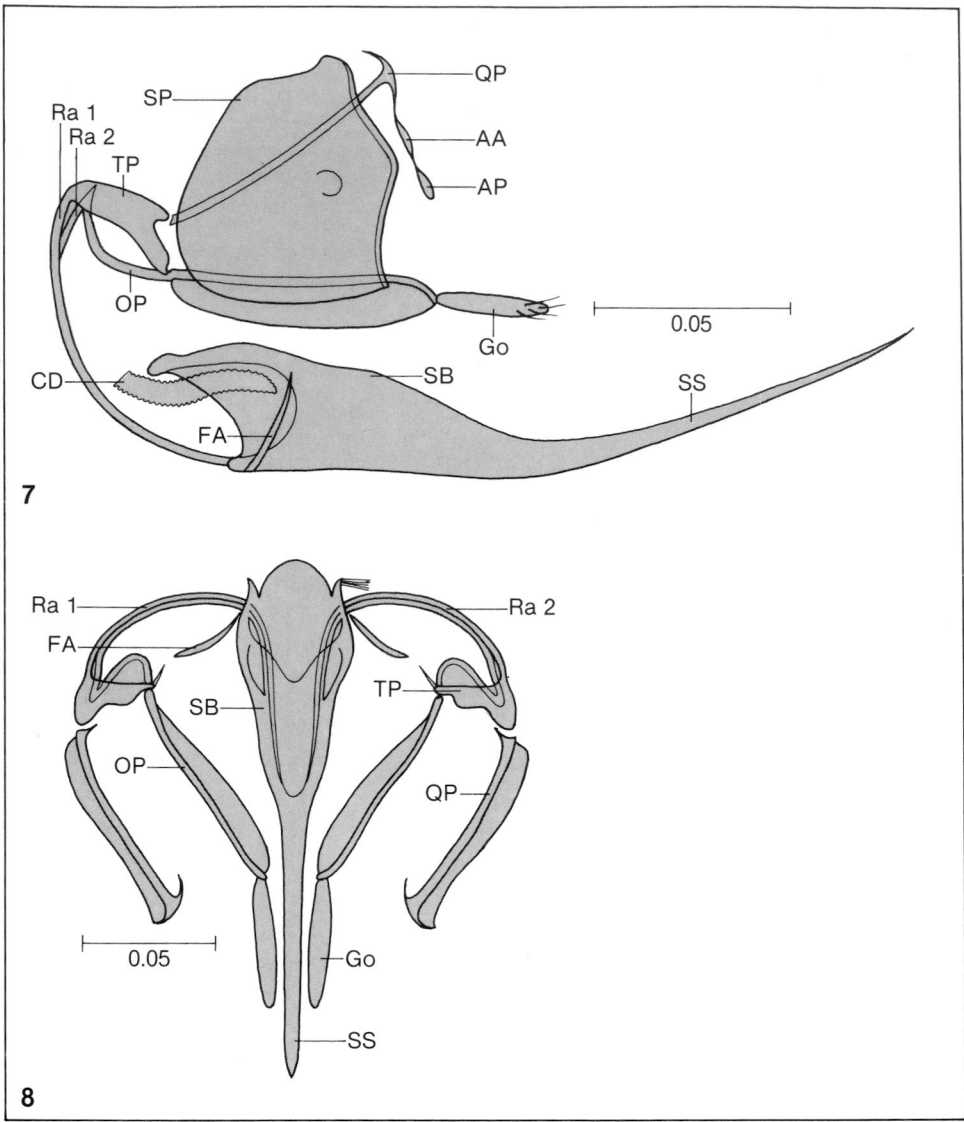

Figs. 7 and 8. Lateral Fig. 7 and dorsal Fig. 8 views of venom sclerites of *Aneuretus simoni* (after Hermann 1968). *AA* Anal arc, *AP* Anal pad, *CD* Common duct of venom reservoir, *FA* Fulcral arm, *Go* Gonostyli, *OP* Oblong plate, *QP* Quadrate plate, *Ra* Rami, *SB* Sting bulb, *SP* Spiracular plate, *SS* Sting shaft, *TP* Triangular plate

between the Aneuretinae and Dolichoderinae and very little support has been obtained for a close relationship between the Aneuretinae and Ponerinae.

The sting base in the Dolichoderinae flares out broadly in dorsal view. This is characteristic of ants that have lost their ability to sting. *Aneuretus* has a relatively narrow sting base. There is little phyletic significance in this character. Broadening of the sting base occurs in Symphyta and appears in some species of the Dorylinae and Myrmicinae of the family Formicidae. Also the distal half of the sting is membranous in the Dolichoderinae and unable to penetrate any type of tissue. In this character the Aneuretinae and Dolichoderinae differ. The sting shaft of *Aneuretus simoni* is strong and apparently employed as a sting (HERMANN, 1968b). Such a difference may be used to separate the two subfamilies, since it indicates a different biology for each group. However, we feel that the degree of sclerotization of the sting is not as important as some of the other characters that closely link the two subfamilies.

Venom sclerites nevertheless are well formed and easy to identify. The lancets possess a valve, characteristically present in all stinging ants that move venom down the sting shaft and out of the sting tip. However, the distal lancet tip, like the sting tip, is membranous and there are no lancet barbs.

The gonostyli are small and simple in structure. Gonostyli like these are much the same in both subfamilies. Ponerine gonostyli are distinctly composed of two lobes (HERMANN, 1975).

V. Dufour's Gland Constituents

Recently, CAVILL and HOUGHTON (1973, 1974b) have analyzed the compounds in the Dufour's gland of *Iridomyrmex humilis* and BLUM and WHEELER (1975) have examined the secretions of species in the genera *Monacis* and *Azteca*. Twenty-seven hydrocarbons have been identified in the glandular exudate of *I. humilis* and six hydrocarbons have been detected in the secretions of *Azteca* and *Monacis* species (Table 2).

CAVILL and HOUGHTON (1974b) exclude hydrocarbons with a chain length greater than C_{19} as Dufour's gland constituents because $C_{20}-C_{27}$ alkanes are normal constituents of the epicuticular waxes of insects. However, BERGSTRÖM and LÖFQVIST (1971) have detected tricosane (C_{23}) in the Dufour's gland secretion of workers of *Camponotus ligniperda* and MOORE (1968) has identified heptacosane (C_{27}) in the frontal gland secretion of termite soldiers of *Coptotermes lacteus*. Therefore, there are no substantive grounds for excluding long-chain alkanes as possible exocrine products, especially since both the epicuticle and Dufour's gland are derived from ectodermal cells and thus share the potential for synthesizing similar compounds. CAVILL and HOUGHTON (1974b) also indicate that several of the hydrocarbons identified from *I. humilis* workers may be derived from the head.

Hydrocarbons in the range $C_{13}-C_{27}$ are produced in the Dufour's glands of dolichoderine species in three genera (Table 2). The alkenes produced by *I. humilis* are all unsaturated toward the center of the hydrocarbon chain ($\Delta_7-\Delta_9$), and only one diene, nonadecadiene, has been identified as a Dufour's gland product. In *I. humilis* heptadecane is the major alkane, whereas (Z)-9-nonadecene is the dominant alkene (CAVILL and HOUGHTON, 1973, 1974b). In general, *n*-pentadecane is the major hydrocarbon in *Azteca* species, whereas in *Monacis bispinosa* *n*-heptadecane and heptadecene are also major constituents (BLUM and WHEELER, 1975).

The Dufour's gland secretion of *I. humilis* is rich in 3- and 5-branched alkanes (Table 2). Two 4-methylalkanes—4-methylhexadecane and 4-methylheptadecane—have also been demonstrated to be constituents of the Dufour's gland secretion of *I. humilis* (CAVILL and HOUGHTON, 1973, 1974b).

Table 2. Compounds identified in the Dufour's gland secretion of dolichoderine ants

Compound	Species	Authority
n—Tridecane	*Monacis bispinosa*	blum and wheeler, 1975
n—Tetradecane	*Iridomyrmex humilis*	cavill and houghton, 1973; 1974 b
3—Methyltridecane	*Iridomyrmex humilis*	cavill and houghton, 1973; 1974 b
n—Pentadecane	*Iridomyrmex humilis, Monacis bispinosa, Azteca parzensis, A. chartifex,* and *A.* spp.	cavill and houghton, 1973; 1974 b; blum and wheeler, 1975
7—Pentadecene	*Iridomyrmex humilis*	cavill and houghton, 1973; 1974 b
n—Hexadecane	*Iridomyrmex humilis*	cavill and houghton, 1973; 1974 b
3—Methylpentadecane	*Iridomyrmex humilis*	cavill and houghton, 1973; 1974 b
5—Methylpentadecane	*Iridomyrmex humilis*	cavill and houghton, 1973; 1974 b
n—Heptadecane	*Iridomyrmex humilis, Azteca nr. constrictor, A.* sp. and *Monacis bispinosa*	cavill and houghton, 1973; 1974 b; blum and wheeler, 1975
7—Heptadecene	*Iridomyrmex humilis*	cavill and houghton, 1973; 1974 b
(Z)—8—Heptadecene	*Iridomyrmex humilis*	cavill and houghton, 1973; 1974 b
4—Methylhexadecane	*Iridomyrmex humilis*	cavill and houghton, 1973; 1974 b
n—Octadecane	*Iridomyrmex humilis*	cavill and houghton, 1973; 1974 b
3—Methylheptadecane	*Iridomyrmex humilis*	cavill and houghton, 1973; 1974 b

Compound	Species	Authority
4–Methylheptadecane	*Iridomyrmex humilis*	CAVILL and HOUGHTON, 1974 b
5–Methylheptadecane	*Iridomyrmex humilis*	CAVILL and HOUGHTON, 1973; 1974 b
9–Octadecene	*Iridomyrmex humilis*	CAVILL and HOUGHTON, 1973; 1974 b
n–Nonadecane	*Iridomyrmex humilis*	CAVILL and HOUGHTON, 1973; 1974 b
(*Z*)–9–Nonadecene	*Iridomyrmex humilis*	CAVILL and HOUGHTON, 1973; 1974 b
Nonadecadiene $C_{19}H_{36}$	*Azteca* nr. *instabilis* and *A.* spp.	BLUM and WHEELER, 1975
n–Eicosane	*Iridomyrmex humilis*	CAVILL and HOUGHTON, 1973; 1974 b
3–Methylnonadecane	*Iridomyrmex humilis*	CAVILL and HOUGHTON, 1973; 1974 b
n–Heneicosane	*Iridomyrmex humilis*	CAVILL and HOUGHTON, 1973; 1974 b
n–Docosane	*Iridomyrmex humilis*	CAVILL and HOUGHTON, 1973; 1974 b
n–Tricosane	*Iridomyrmex humilis*	CAVILL and HOUGHTON, 1973; 1974 b
n–Tetracosane	*Iridomyrmex humilis*	CAVILL and HOUGHTON, 1973; 1974 b
n–Pentacosane	*Iridomyrmex humilis*	CAVILL and HOUGHTON, 1973; 1974 b
n–Hexacosane	*Iridomyrmex humilis*	CAVILL and HOUGHTON, 1973; 1974 b
n–Heptacosane	*Iridomyrmex humilis*	CAVILL and HOUGHTON, 1973; 1974 b

VI. Anatomy of Dufour's Gland

Dufour's gland (*DG*, Figs. 4—6) in the Dolichoderinae appears to be much like the same gland in all other subfamilies of the Formicidae except the Formicinae. It is an elongate sac that enters the sting base ventrad of the venom canal.

C. Anal Gland Constituents

The chemical hallmarks of the dolichoderine anal glands (Figs. 9—11) are the cyclopentanoid monoterpenes. PAVAN (1949) isolated iridomyrmecin (Table 3) from *Iridomyrmex humilis* and reported that this compound possessed insecticidal activity against a wide variety of species (PAVAN, 1952). Subsequently, FUSCO et al. (1955a, b) elucidated the structure of iridomyrmecin which, in common with the other dolichoderine cyclopentanoid monoterpenes, contains the 1,2-dimethyl-3-isopropylcyclopentane nucleus. CAVILL et al. (1956a) identified a second lactone, isoiridomyrmecin (Table 3), as an anal gland product of the Australian dolichoderine *Iridomyrmex*

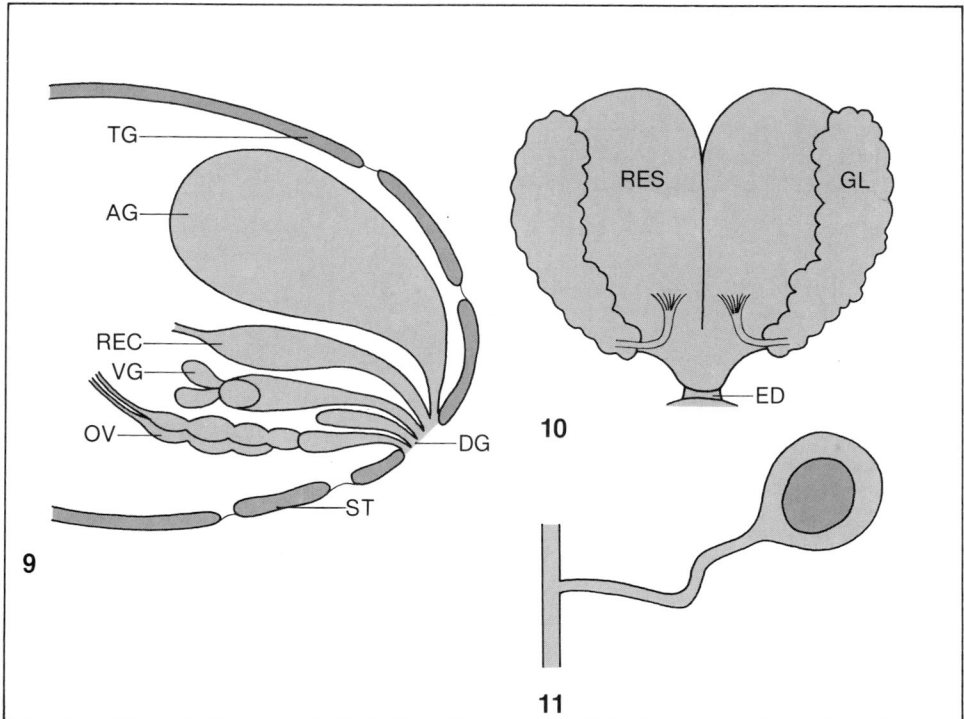

Figs. 9—11. Gaster and pheromone-producing glands of dolichoderine ants. Fig. 9. Schematic lateral view of glands and other structures exiting from distal tip of gaster (gland of Pavan not illustrated). Fig. 10. Dorsal view of anal glands and their reservoir. Fig. 11. Single anal gland cell and its collecting duct. *AG* Anal gland, *DG* Dufour's gland, *ED* Exit duct from anal gland reservoir, *GL* Gland, *OV* Ovary, *REC* Rectum, *RES* Reservoir, *ST* Sternum, *TG* Tergum

nitidus, and more recently isodihydronepetalactone (Table 3) has been shown to be an additional glandular constituent of this species (CAVILL and CLARK, 1967). Iridomyrmecin and isoiridomyrmecin are often referred to as iridolactones, and these ant-derived compounds are structurally related to nepetalactone, a major constituent of the catnip plant, *Nepeta cataria* (BATES et al., 1958).

In addition to the iridolactones, two dialdehydes, iridodial and dolichodial (Table 3), have been identified as anal gland products of species in a wide range of dolichoderine genera (CAVILL et al., 1956b; TRAVE and PAVAN, 1956; CAVILL and HINTERBERGER, 1961; McGURK et al., 1968). The dialdehydes, together with the iridolactones, are referred to as iridoids. Iridodial has been converted into iridomyrmecin, a significant finding in view of the proposed biosynthesis of the iridolactones via iridodial (CLARK et al., 1959; CAVILL and HINTERBERGER, 1960a). More recently, McGURK et al. (1968) have identified both iridodial and iridolactones in the anal gland secretions of two dolichoderine species and have demonstrated that the lactones possess the stereochemistry of the predominant iridodial isomer.

Iridomyrmecin (*IV* — Fig. 12) can be readily epimerized to isoiridomyrmecin (*V* — Fig. 12) (FUSCO et al., 1955a; CAVILL and LOCKSLEY, 1957) which is identical to the naturally occurring iridolactone isolated from *I. nitidus*. Both of these iridolactones yield nepetalinic acids (*II* and *III* — Fig. 12) on oxidation with potassium permanganate (FUSCO et al., 1955b; CAVILL and LOCKSLEY, 1957), further establishing the relationship of the iridolactones to nepetalactone (*I* — Fig. 12) and the nepetalinic acids. The isolation of nepetalinic acids *II* and *III* from the oxidation of iridomyrmecin (*IV*) and isoiridomyrmecin (*V*), respectively (Fig. 12), establishes that the epimerization of *IV* into *V* involves the C_4 center in the iridolactones, that is, the C_8 center in the nepetalinic acids. Based on the conversion of iridomyrmecin and isoiridomyrmecin into *cis*- and *trans*-nepetalinic acids (Fig. 12), the *cis*-fusion of the δ-lactone ring and the *trans*-relationship of the methyl group attached to the cyclopentane nucleus are proven (CAVILL and CLARK, 1971). Employing X-ray crystallography, McCONNELL et al. (1962) have established that each of the iridolactones possesses a boat conformation of the lactone ring with the methyl group at C_4 in the equatorial position. Thus, iridomyrmecin has the *endo* (*VI* — Fig. 12) and isoiridomyrmecin the *exo* boat (*VII* — Fig. 12) conformation.

CAVILL and HINTERBERGER (1960b) and CAVILL and HOUGHTON (1974b) have isolated cyclopentanoid monoterpene acids from *Dolichoderus anthoclinea dentata* and *Iridomyrmex. humilis,* respectively. Extracts of *I. humilis* workers contained two oxo-acids in which either aldehyde group of dolichodial was oxidized. The corresponding dicarboxylic acid was also present as well as a dicarboxylic acid corresponding to oxidized iridodial. *D. anthoclinea dentata* workers contained only the oxo-acids. These acids have been demonstrated to be oxidation artifacts arising during the work up of the extracts (CAVILL and HOUGHTON, 1974b).

The anal glands have proven to be a rich source of ketones of both terpenoid and nonterpenoid origin (Table 3). Initially the identification of 6-methyl-5-hepten-2-one (CAVILL et al., 1956a; TRAVE and PAVAN, 1956), 2-methyl-4-heptanone (TRAVE and PAVAN, 1956), and 4-methyl-2-hexanone (CAVILL and HINTERBERGER, 1960a, b) indicated that the ketonic products of the anal glands were of exclusive terpenoid origin. However, the identification of 2-heptanone as an anal gland

Table 3. Compounds identified in the anal gland secretions of dolichoderine ants

Compound	Species	Authority
Benzaldehyde	*Azteca* sp.	BLUM and WHEELER, 1975

Iridodial	*Iridomyrmex detectus, I. conifer, I. pruinosus, Tapinoma nigerrimum, T. sessile, Dolichoderus scabridus, Conomyrma pyramicus, Azteca* nr. *instabilis, A.* nr. *velox, A. chartifex, A. parzensis, A.* spp., and *Monacis bispinosa*	CAVILL *et al.,* 1956 a, b; CAVILL and HINTERBERGER 1960 a, b; CAVILL and FORD, 1960; TRAVE and PAVAN, 1956; McGURK *et al.,* 1968; BLUM and WHEELER, 1975

Dolichodial	*Dolichoderus clarki, D. dentata, D. scabridus, Iridomyrmex detectus, I. rufoniger,* and *I. humilis*	CAVILL and HINTERBERGER, 1960 a, b; CAVILL and HINTERBERGER, 1961; CAVILL and HOUGHTON, 1974 b

Iridomyrmecin	*Iridomyrmex humilis* and *I. pruinosus*	FUSCO *et al.,* 1955 a, b; McGURK *et al.,* 1968

Isoiridomyrmecin	*Iridomyrmex nitidus, Dolichoderus scabridus,* and *Tapinoma sessile*	CAVILL *et al.,* 1956 a, b; CAVILL and HINTERBERGER, 1960 a, b; McGURK *et al.,* 1968

Isodihydronepetalactone	*Iridomyrmex nitidus*	CAVILL and CLARK, 1967

2–Heptanol	*Azteca* sp.	BLUM and WHEELER, 1975

6–Methyl–5–hepten–2–ol	*Iridomyrmex* nr. *pruinosus*	CREWE and BLUM, 1971

2–Pentanone	*Azteca* sp. and *Monacis bispinosa*	BLUM and WHEELER, 1975

Compound	Species	Authority
2–Methylcyclopentanone	*Azteca* nr. *instabilis, A.* nr. *nigriventris,* and *A.* nr. *velox*	WHEELER *et al.,* 1975
2–Heptanone	*Iridomyrmex pruinosus, Conomyrma pyramicus, Azteca chartifex, A. parzensis, A.* nr. *constrictor, A.* spp., and *Monacis bispinosa*	BLUM *et al.,* 1963; BLUM and WARTER, 1966; McGURK et al., 1968; WHEELER *et al.,* 1975; BLUM and WHEELER, 1975
4–Methyl–2–hexanone	*Dolichoderus clarki*	CAVILL and HINTERBERGER, 1960 a, b
6 Methyl–5–hepten–2–one	*Iridomyrmex detectus, I. conifer, I. rufoniger, I.* nr. *pruinosus, I. nitidiceps, Liometopum microcephalum, Conomyrma pyramicus, Tapinoma nigerrimum, Dolichoderus scabridus, Azteca chartifex, A. parzensis, A.* sp., and *Monacis bispinosa*	CAVILL *et al.,* 1956 a, b; CREWE and BLUM, 1971; TRAVE and PAVAN, 1956; McGURK *et al.,* 1968; CAVILL and HINTERBERGER, 1960 a, b; WHEELER *et al.,* 1975; BLUM and WHEELER, 1975
2–Methyl–4–heptanone	*Tapinoma nigerrimum* and *T. sessile*	TRAVE and PAVAN, 1956; BLUM and WHEELER, 1975
cis–1–Acetyl–2–methyl cyclopentane	*Azteca* nr. *velox* and *A.* nr. *nigriventris*	WHEELER *et al.,* 1975
2–Acetyl–3–methyl cyclopentene	*Azteca* nr. *nigriventris* and *A.* nr. *instabilis*	WHEELER *et al.,* 1975
Acetic acid CH_3COOH	*Liometopum microcephalum*	CASNATI *et al.,* 1964
n–Butyric acid	*Liometopum microcephalum*	CASNATI *et al.,* 1964
Isovaleric acid	*Liometopum microcephalum* and *Iridomyrmex nitidiceps*	CASNATI *et al.,* 1964; CAVILL and CLARK, 1971

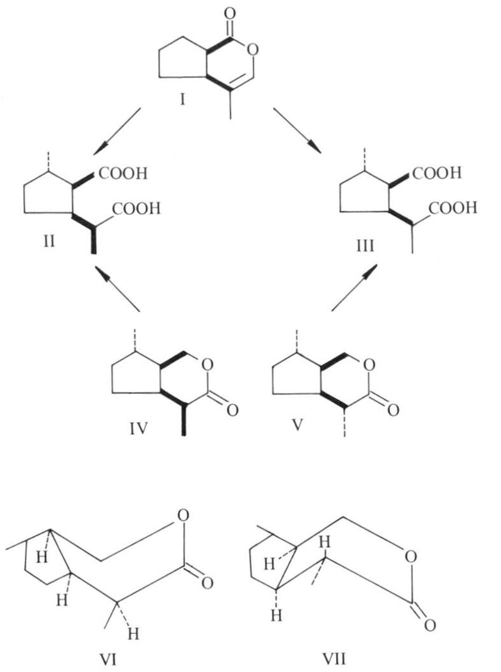

Fig. 12. Configuration and conformations of iridolactones based on their relationship with nepetalactone and nepetalinic acid

product of species in several dolichoderine genera (Blum et al., 1963; Blum and Warter, 1966; Blum and Wheeler, 1975) and the recent identification of 2-pentanone (Table 3) in an *Azteca* species and *Monacis bispinosa* (Blum and Wheeler, 1975), demonstrate that nonterpenoid methyl ketones have a wide distribution in the anal gland secretions of dolichoderine ants. The novel cyclopentyl ketones (Table 3) fortifying the glandular secretions of *Azteca* species (Wheeler et al., 1975) further enlarge the list of nonterpenoid ketones produced by dolichoderines in their anal glands.

Benzaldehyde has been identified as a major anal gland constituent in a single *Azteca* species (Table 3), but the significance of this atypical dolichoderine natural product is not known. The presence of two alcohols, 2-heptanol and 6-methyl-5-hepten-2-ol (Table 3), as concomitants of the corresponding ketones, indicates that these carbinols may be involved in the biogenesis of the carbonyl compounds. The occurrence of three simple fatty acids in the anal gland secretions of a *Liometopum* and *Iridomyrmex* species (Casnati et al., 1964; Cavill and Clark, 1971) undoubtedly increases the deterrent potency of the glandular exudates and further demonstrates the capacity of these exocrine structures to biosynthesize very short-chain compounds.

I. Anatomy of the Anal Glands in the Dolichoderinae

Dolichoderinae anal glands (=repugnatorial glands) (Figs. 9, 10) are little understood anatomically, the only detailed accounts of them being the reports by Forel

(1878) and PAVAN and RONCHETTI (1955). These glands exit from the posterior opening in the gaster just dorsad of the anus (Fig. 9).

The true anal glands are bilobed (Fig. 10) and composed of numerous single gland cells (Fig. 11) that empty their contents into a main collecting duct. Anal gland products pass through the main collecting duct to a large bilobed reservoir for storage. Dispersal of the substances stored in the reservoir occurs through a large common orifice (Fig. 10). Forcing of its contents through the orifice is facilitated by a muscle sheath around the reservoir.

II. Biological Activities of Dolichoderine Anal Gland Products

PAVAN has undertaken extensive investigations on the physiological properties of iridomyrmecin, the lactone first isolated from *I. humilis* (PAVAN, 1949). The insecticidal and acaricidal properties of this compound were evaluated by comparing its contact toxicity to those of DDT and γ-BHC (PAVAN, 1952). Iridomyrmecin-sensitive insects exhibited a symptomatology similar to that observed in DDT-poisoned insects; initial irritation was eventually followed by a lack of coordination and ultimate paralysis.

At a concentration of 1 $\mu g/cm^2$ iridomyrmecin was reported to be as effective as γ-BHC against a wide range of insect species and two species of mites. Iridomyrmecin was considerably more toxic to the louse *Linognathus setosus* than either DDT or γ-BHC. Tests utilizing insects from seven different orders demonstrated that iridomyrmecin was generally superior to DDT as a contact insecticide (PAVAN, 1952).

KERR (1961) topically treated individual houseflies with iridomyrmecin and isoiridomyrmecin and reported that the lactones exhibited no toxicity at a dosage of 670 μg. However, the iridolactones caused a 50% knockdown within $20-30$ min. It thus appears that iridomyrmecin acts primarily as a knockdown agent which may promote the toxic effects of other anal gland products as well. In this regard it may be significant that dolichodial has been recently identified as an additional anal gland product of *I. humilis* (CAVILL and HOUGHTON, 1974b).

Iridomyrmecin is active in inhibiting the development of certain species of plants. In the *Allium cepa* test it interferes with mitotic activity, particularly at the interphase stage (PAVAN, 1958). The lactone also slows development of the legume *Lupinus albus* (PAVAN and BAGGINI, 1955) and antagonizes the tumor-inducing effects of both γ-BHC and colchicine (PAVAN and VALCURONE, 1955). Iridomyrmecin is also reported to possess antibacterial activity against both gram-negative and gram-positive species (PAVAN, 1950).

The oral toxicity of iridomyrmecin for the white mouse is 1.5 g/kg (PAVAN, 1952). When incubated with chick embryo heart fibroblasts, the lactone caused about an 80% inhibition of development at a concentration of 1 p.p.m. (PAVAN, 1959).

Unlike iridomyrmecin, iridodial rapidly polymerizes and it is likely that this dialdehyde may function as a fixative for the more volatile carbonyl compounds in the anal gland secretion (PAVAN, 1959). The variety of ketones produced in the anal glands of dolichoderine species are probably excellent deterrent substances in themselves, and several of these carbonyl compounds are found in the defensive secretions of solitary arthropods. WHEELER et al. (1975) have demonstrated that the cyclopentyl ketones present in the anal gland exudates of *Azteca* species effectively repel workers of the fire ant *Solenopsis invicta.*

D. Dolichoderine Natural Products — An Overview

A meaningful analysis of the natural products chemistry of the Dolichoderinae is essentially equivalent to an examination of the exocrine products generated in the capacious anal glands of these formicids. Dolichoderine mandibular gland products are presently limited to the three trisubstituted pyrazines identified from workers of *I. humilis* (CAVILL and HOUGHTON, 1974a, b) but it appears that this class of compounds has a widespread distribution in the Formicidae. WHEELER and BLUM (1973) have identified pyrazines in several species of *Odontomachus* in the subfamily Ponerinae, and MOORE (1974) has detected pyrazines in a species of *Calomyrmex* in the subfamily Formicinae. The Dufour's gland products of *I. humilis* (CAVILL and HOUGHTON, 1973, 1974b), *Azteca* spp., and *Monacis bispinosa* (BLUM and WHEELER, 1975) are fairly typical of those of ants in all the other subfamilies and as such, possess little diagnostic value. *I. humilis* workers share alkanes and alkenes with myrmeciines (CAVILL and WILLIAMS, 1967), myrmicines (MORGAN and WADHAMS, 1972; REGNIER et al., 1973), and formicines (BERGSTRÖM and LÖFQVIST, 1972, 1973; BROPHY et al., 1973). The 3- and 5-methylalkanes which fortify the Dufour's gland secretion of workers of *I. humilis* (CAVILL and HOUGHTON, 1973, 1974b) are thematic of the 3- and 5-monomethyl-branched alkanes present in the secretions of myrmicines (REGNIER et al., 1973) and formicines (BERGSTRÖM and LÖFQVIST, 1972, 1973; BROPHY et al., 1973). Thus, constituents of the dolichoderine Dufour's glands appear to be rather typical of the natural product chemistry of the Formicidae.

Among the subfamilies of ants, the Dolichoderinae appear to have a monopoly on the biosynthesis of cyclopentanoid monoterpenes. Whereas these compounds appear to be especially typical anal gland products of the Dolichoderinae, they have not been encountered in species in any other subfamily of ants. Their ubiquitous occurrence in the anal gland secretions of dolichoderine species appears to indicate that the metabolic pathways for the synthesis of these compounds were present in ancestral dolichoderines and thus constitute a biosynthetic trademark of these formicids. Although the biogenesis of cyclopentanoid monoterpenes appears to be limited among ants to this subfamily, some insect species in unrelated taxa have also developed the capacity to produce these compounds. The phasmid, *Anisomorpha buprestoides,* secretes anisomorphal, structurally identical to iridodial (MEINWALD et al., 1962), and the cerambycid *Aromia moschata* as well as four staphylinids — *Staphylinus olens, Thyreocephalus lorquini, Eulissus orthodoxus,* and *Creophilus erythrocephalus* — produce this compound as a major constituent of their metasternal or pygidial gland secretions (VIDARI et al., 1973; ABOU-DONIA et al., 1971; BELLAS et al., 1974).

In terms of biochemical systematics, the restriction of the cyclopentanoid monoterpenes to the Dolichoderinae indicates that this taxon is not closely related to any of the other formicid subfamilies. BROWN (1954) places the Dolichoderinae in the "Myrmecioid Complex" along with the Myrmeciinae, Formicinae, and

Pseudomyrmecinae. The dolichoderines are considered to have developed from aneuretine stock, while the formicines are believed to have descended directly either from a myrmeciine ancestor or, like the Dolichoderinae, from an aneuretine ancestor. However, on biochemical grounds, the Dolichoderinae and Formicinae do not appear to be closely related. Formicines emphasize the biosynthesis of oxygenated *acyclic* monoterpenes, whereas the dolichoderine terpenoid pathways stress the biogenesis of *cyclic* monoterpenes as well as distinctive acyclic terpenoids. Three oxygenated acyclic monoterpenes—6-methyl-5-hepten-2-one, 2-methyl-4-heptanone, and 4-methyl-2-hexanone—have been identified as dolichoderine anal gland products and only 6-methyl-5-hepten-2-one has a widespread subfamily distribution. Indeed, 4-methyl-2-hexanone has only been detected in *Dolichoderus clarki* (CAVILL and HINTERBERGER, 1960a, b) and 2-methyl-4-heptanone appears to be limited to the anal gland secretions of *Tapinoma* species (TRAVE and PAVAN, 1956). Aside from being detected as a trace mandibular gland constituent in workers of *Lasius carniolicus* (BERGSTRÖM and LÖFQVIST, 1970) and *L. fuliginosus* (BERNARDI et al., 1967), 6-methyl-5-hepten-2-one has not been encountered in any nondolichoderine ant species.

An examination of the frequency of occurrence of dolichoderine anal gland compounds in other ant subfamilies reinforces the conclusion that this subfamily is not closely related to any of the formicid subfamilies in terms of natural products. Seventy percent of these compounds are restricted to dolichoderine species, while only six of these natural products have been detected as exocrine products of species in two other ant subfamilies. 6-Methyl-5-hepten-2-one, which is the only dolichoderine anal gland compound identified in formicines, *Lasius carniolicus* (BERGSTRÖM and LÖFQVIST, 1970) and *L. fuliginosus* (BERNARDI et al., 1967), appears to be a very atypical exocrine product of *Lasius* species, and has not been detected in ten other species in this genus.

On the other hand, 25% of the dolichoderine anal gland constituents have been encountered as natural products of species in the Myrmicinae. Acetic and isovaleric acids have been identified in the myrmicine *Myrmicaria natalensis* (GRÜNANGER et al., 1960) and the dolichoderine *Liometopum microcephalum* (CASNATI et al., 1964). Benzaldehyde is a major exocrine product of the myrmicine *Veromessor pergandei* (BLUM et al., 1969) and is a major constituent in the anal gland secretion of an *Azteca* species (BLUM and WHEELER, 1975). 6-Methyl-5-hepten-2-ol, which accompanies the corresponding ketone in the anal gland secretion of an *Iridomyrmex* species (CREWE and BLUM, 1971), has been recently identified in the mandibular gland secretion of *Atta texana* (RILEY et al., 1974), a species in a highly evolved myrmicine genus. 2-Heptanone, which is a major glandular constituent of some dolichoderine species in the genera *Iridomyrmex* (BLUM et al., 1963), *Conomyrma* (BLUM and WARTER, 1966; McGURK et al., 1968), *Azteca* (WHEELER et al., 1975), and *Monacis* (BLUM and WHEELER, 1975), is a typical mandibular gland product of *Atta* species (MOSER et al., 1968; BLUM et al., 1968) and has been detected in a *Crematogaster* species (CREWE et al., 1972). Thus, from an exocrinological standpoint, the Dolichoderinae currently have far more in common with the Myrmicinae than any other formicid subfamily.

CLARK et al. (1959) and CAVILL and HINTERBERGER (1960a) have proposed a pathway for the biosynthesis of the cyclopentanoid monoterpenes from acyclic

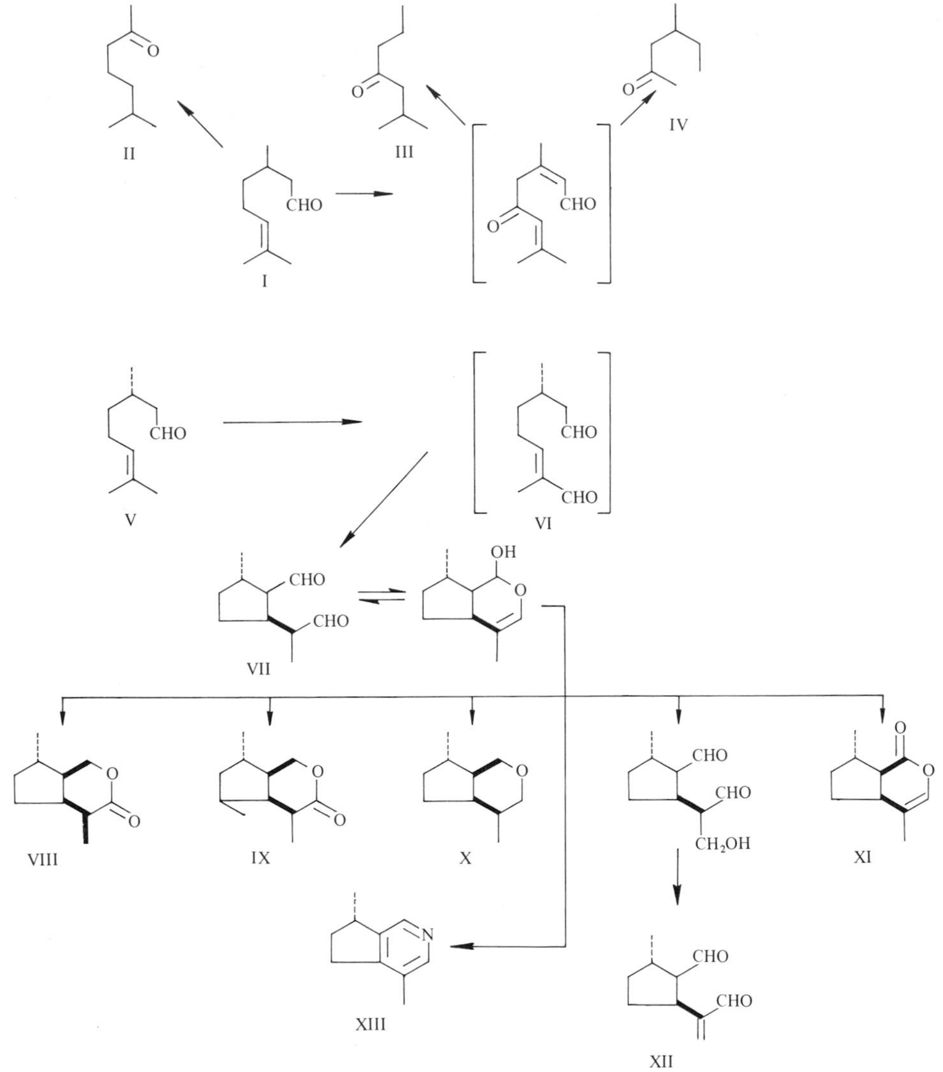

Fig. 13. Proposed biogenetic scheme for the cyclopentanoid monoterpenes. (From Cavill and Hinterberger, 1960a and Cavill and Clark, 1971)

terpene precursors (Fig. 13). Citral (*I* — Fig. 13) is considered to be the basic precursor of the ant extractives. The volatile ketones (*II, III, IV* — Fig. 13) would be produced after citral had undergone oxidation and reduction processes, coupled with the reverse aldol reaction. L-Citronella (*V* — Fig. 13) would be produced by stereospecific reduction of citral followed by a terminal oxidation of the isopropylidene group of citronellal, yielding 2,6-dimethyloct-2-en-1,8-dial (*VI* — Fig. 13). Iridodial (*VII* — Fig. 13) would then be produced from the dial by the equivalent of a Michael condensation. Iridodial would be converted into a iridomyrmecin (*VIII* — Fig. 13), isoiridomyrmecin (*IX* — Fig. 13), and isodihydronepetalactone (*X* — Fig. 13) by the equivalent of a Cannizaro reaction. Dolichodial (*XII* — Fig. 13) would be produced from iridodial by β-hydroxylation followed by the elimination of water. Iridodial could also serve as the precursor of the well known plant products nepetalactone (*XI* — Fig. 13) and actinidine (*XIII* — Fig. 13). Nepetalactone would result from an oxidation of the lactone form of iridodial (Fig. 13) whereas the alkaloid actinidine would result from the action of ammonia or its equivalent on the dial.

The laboratory conversion of L-citronellal to iridodial (CLARK et al., 1959) and the synthesis of both isoiridomyrmecin and actinidine from iridodial (CAVILL and FORD, 1960) are consistent with the proposed biosynthetic pathway for the cyclopentanoid monoterpenes. However, the key precursors in this biogenetic scheme, citral and citronellal (*I, IV* — Fig. 13), have never been detected in dolichoderine species, although these monoterpenes have been identified in both myrmicine (BUTENANDT et al., 1959) and formicine (CHADHA et al., 1962) species. Thus, although this proposed metabolic pathway is very attractive on biosynthetic grounds, the apparent absence of the key oxygenated monoterpene precursors from dolichoderine anal gland secretions raises the possibility that the cyclopentanoid monoterpenes may be derived from unknown acyclic precursors. On the other hand, BELLAS et al. (1974) identified citronellal, geranial, iridodial, and actinidine in the pygidial gland secretions of staphylinid beetles, a finding which is completely consistent with the biosynthetic scheme proposed by CLARK et al. (1959) and CAVILL and HINTERBERGER (1960a).

McGURK et al. (1968) have demonstrated that dolichoderines do not biosynthesize iridodial with absolute stereospecificity. There are four possible isomers of iridodial because of epimerization at the carbon γ to each carbonyl group and all four isomers have been detected as anal gland products of three dolichoderine species. Workers of *Iridomyrmex pruinosus, Conomyrma pyramicus,* and *Tapinoma sessile* synthesize α, β, γ, and δ iridodial but in each species a different isomer predominates (McGURK et al., 1968). *T. sessile* workers emphasize the α-isomer whereas the β-isomer predominates in *C. pyramicus* and the δ-isomer in *I. pruinosus.* Significantly, iridodial is accompanied by iridomyrmecin in *I. pruinosus* and isoiridomyrmecin in *T. sessile,* and the iridolactones possess the stereochemistry of the major iridodial isomer biosynthesized by each species. This finding is in accord with the biosynthetic route first proposed by CLARK et al. (1959).

Although the biogenetic pathways for the cyclopentanoid monoterpenes have been the subject of considerable speculation, the biosynthetic routes for the nonterpenes constitute *terra incognita,* notwithstanding their emphasis by species in some dolichoderine genera. 2-Heptanone, which is a major anal gland product of some dolichoderine species in four of the seven genera examined (Table 3), obviously represents a product derived from a well-developed metabolic pathway. An additional methyl ketone, 2-pentanone (Table 3), has been recently identified as an anal gland constituent of *Monacis bispinosa* and an *Azteca* species (BLUM and WHEELER, 1975) and WHEELER et al. (1975) have recently characterized cyclopentyl ketones from a variety of *Azteca* species. Therefore it is evident that dolichoderines produce a wide variety of nonterpenoid ketones in their anal glands, and it is no exaggeration to state that their biosyntheses constitute a remarkably fertile area for natural products research. Since different species (WHEELER et al., 1975; McGURK et al., 1968) produce both nonterpenoid and terpenoid compounds in their anal glands, it seems evident that pathways for both classes of compounds can be well developed in these exocrine structures.

If dolichoderine natural products are to possess any value as additional character states, it will be necessary to analyze these compounds in different populations of a species over a wide area. Obviously, the value of these compounds as chemotaxonomic indicators must be predicated on a firm taxonomic base, which, unfortunately, is lacking for most dolichoderine genera. Therefore, the qualitative variation in natural products observed in different colonies of a single "species" must be cautiously interpreted without fairly recent and comprehensive revisionary studies of the genus under consideration. For example, McGURK et al. (1968) identified 6-methyl-5-hepten-2-one in two different subspecies of *Conomyrma pyramicus* and 2-heptanone in another subspecies. However, two of these forms had already been separated as species based on sympatry (WILSON, 1957) and the third form is probably a valid species (BLUM, 1969) as well.

Similar sympatry observed with two colonies of *Iridomyrmex rufoniger,* which produce different anal gland constituents (CAVILL and HINTERBERGER, 1960a, b), may also indicate that the ants in each nest belong to different taxa. Dolichodial was identified in ants in one colony whereas 6-methyl-5-hepten-2-one and iridodial were detected in workers from another colony only about 16 meters from the first. CAVILL and HINTERBERGER (1960a, b) also reported that different colonies of *Dolichoderus scabridus* yielded a) isoiridomyrmecin or, b) dolichodial or, c) iridodial and 6-methyl-5-hepten-2-one. However, the presence of different anal gland constituents in colonies of black-legged and red-legged ants may not be insignificant from a classificatory standpoint and it would seem highly desirable to exercise considerable caution in regarding these forms as taxonomically identical. Indeed, CREWE and BLUM (1971) identified 6-methyl-5-hepten-2-one in a population of *Iridomyrmex pruinosus,* a species which had been previously demonstrated to produce 2-heptanone in the anal glands (BLUM et al., 1963). The methyl-heptenone-producing species was subsequently determined to be a cryptic species of *Iridomyrmex,* closely related to *I. pruinosus* (CREWE and BLUM, 1971). Thus, natural product inconsistencies among different population elements of a "species" may often be easily explicable after careful taxonomic analyses.

The Dolichoderinae will undoubtedly continue to yield a wealth of new natural products as additional genera are subjected to detailed chemical analysis. Our knowledge of the chemistry of dolichoderine exocrine glands is predicated on analyses of relatively few species in only seven genera (Table 3) and new chemical surprises have emerged as each new genus has been subjected to careful analytical scrutiny. Ultimately, the success of the Dolichoderinae may become more comprehensible as a function of the biosynthetic versatility of their anal glands, exocrine organs par excellence.

E. Phyletic Implications Based on Venom Sclerites and Associated Glands

There is a paucity of information on the anatomy of the exocrine glands and venom apparatus in the Dolichoderinae. Consequently, the phyletic standing of this group and the Aneuretinae is not well understood.

Based on the venom components it appears obvious that the Dolichoderinae is unlike all other ant subfamilies (with the possible exception of the Aneuretinae). The filamentous glands are large and globate in appearance. That they extend from the apex of the venom reservoir indicates a similarity with the Myrmicinae. The glands and reservoir do not resemble the same structures in the Ponerinae in any way. Since only preserved specimens of *Aneuretus simoni* were available for dissection (HERMANN, 1968 b), details of the venom components were not observed. Examination of the venom reservoir and associated filamentous glands will probably give us some insight into the little understood relationships of this subfamily.

Two characters, broadened sting base and membranous sting tip, indicate that the Dolichoderinae and Aneuretinae have different biologies, although we are not sure that these characters are very important phyletically. A broad sting base occurs in some members of the Dorylinae and Myrmicinae, two widely separated groups of the Formicidae. Likewise, a membranous sting tip is found in some myrmicines (e.g., *Myrmicaria* spp.).

Fusion of the sting base with the furcula is commonly found in both the Aneuretinae and Dolichoderinae. Such a fusion between these sclerites has occured in a number of cases in the Formicidae and may indicate convergence between these two subfamilies.

The simple appearance of the gonostyli may link the Dolichoderinae with the Aneuretinae. However, in most of the Formicidae loss of the proximal and distal gonostylar lobes has been the case in ant groups that have undergone considerable change in the venom sclerites. There is nevertheless a significant difference between the gonostyli of aneuretines and dolichoderines on the one hand and ponerines on the other.

We have not decided whether the dolichoderines and aneuretines are close enough to lump into a single group, although Wilson (pers. comm.) has lumped them. With a different sting, and consequenty a different biology, we feel that they may represent two separate groups. However, many external characters indicate a close relationship between the two. We see no reason to speculate on the relationship between the Aneuretinae and Ponerinae as has been done by GOTWALD (1970), HERMANN (1968 b) and WILSON et al. (1956), since very few characters are shared by these two subfamilies. Those characters that are primitive (long anterior petiolar peduncle and low, rounded node) are not characteristically ponerine characters. GOTWALD (1970) showed that the stipes of *Aneuretus* is like that found in some ponerine species but in other mouthpart characters *Aneuretus* is similar to the dolichoderines.

References

Abou-Donia, S.A., Fish, L.J., Pattenden, G.: Iridodial from the odoriferous glands of *Staphylinus olens* (Coleoptera: Staphylinidae). Tetrahedron Lett. **43**, 4037—4038 (1971).

Bates, R.B., Eisenbraun, E.J., McElvain, S.M.: The configurations of the nepetalactones and related compounds. J. Amer. Chem. Soc. **80**, 3420—3424 (1958).

Bellas, T.E., Brown, W.V., Moore, B.P.: The alkaloid actinidine and plausible precursors in defensive secretions of rove beetles. J. Insect Physiol. **20**, 277—280 (1974).

Bergström, G., Löfqvist, J.: Chemical basis for odour communication in four species of *Lasius* ants. J. Insect. Physiol. **16**, 2353–2375 (1970).

Bergström, G., Löfqvist, J.: *Camponotus ligniperda* Latr.—a model for the composite volatile secretions of Dufour's gland in formicine ants. In: Chemical Releasers in Insects. Tahori, A.S. (ed.). New York: Gordon and Breach, 1971, Vol. III, 195–223.

Bergström, G., Löfqvist, J.: Similarities between the Dufour's gland secretions of the ants *Camponotus ligniperda* (Latr.) and *Camponotus herculeanus* (L.). Ent. Scand. **3**, 225–238 (1972).

Bergström, G., Löfqvist, J.: Chemical congruence of the complex, odoriferous secretions from Dufour's gland in three species of ants of the genus *Formica*. J. Insect Physiol. **19**, 887–907 (1973).

Bernardi, R., Cardani, C., Ghiringhella, D., Selva, A., Baggini, A., Pavan, M.: On the components of the secretion of mandibular glands of the ant *Lasius* (*Dendrolasius*) *fuliginosus*. Tetrahedron Lett. **40**, 3893–3896 (1967).

Blum, M.S.: Alarm pheromones. Ann. Rev. Ent. **14**, 57–80 (1969).

Blum, M.S., Padovani, F., Amante, E.: Alkanones and terpenes in the mandibular glands of *Atta* species. Comp. Biochem. Physiol. **26**, 291–299 (1968).

Blum, M.S., Padovani, F., Curley, A., Hawk, R.E.: Benzaldehyde: Defensive secretion of a harvester ant. Comp. Biochem. Physiol. **29**, 461–465 (1969).

Blum, M.S., Warter, S.L.: Chemical releasers of social behavior — VII. The isolation of 2-heptanone from *Conomyrma pyramica* (Hymenoptera: Formicidae: Dolichoderinae) and its *modus operandi* as a releaser of alarm and digging behavior. Ann. Ent. Soc. Amer. **59**, 774–779 (1966).

Blum, M.S., Warter, S.L., Monroe, R.S., Chidester, J.C.: Chemical releasers of social behaviour. I. Methyl-*n*-amyl ketone in *Iridomyrmex pruinosus*. J. Insect Physiol. **9**, 881–885 (1963).

Blum, M.S., Wheeler, J.W.: Unpublished data (1975).

Brophy, J.J., Cavill, G.W.K., Shannon, J.S.: Venom and Dufour's gland secretions in an Australian species of *Camponotus*. J. Insect Physiol. **19**, 791–798 (1973).

Brown, W.L., Jr.: Remarks on the internal phylogeny and subfamily classification of the family Formicidae. Insectes Soc. **1**, 21–31 (1954).

Butenandt, A., Linzen, B., Lindauer, M.: Über einen Duftstoff aus der Mandibeldrüse der Blattschneiderameise *Atta sexdens rubropilosa*. Archs. Anat. Microscop. Morph. Exptl. **48**, 13–19 (1959).

Casnati, G., Pavan, M., Ricca, A.: Ricerche sul secreto delle glandole anali di *Liometopum microcephalum* Panz. Boll. Soc. Ent. Ital. **94**, 147–152 (1964).

Cavill, G.W.K., Clark, D.V.: Insect venoms, attractants, and repellents. — VII. Isodihydronepetalactone. J. Insect Physiol. **13**, 131–135 (1967).

Cavill, G.W.K., Clark, D.V.: Ant secretions and cantharidin. In: Naturally Occurring Insecticides. Jacobson, M., Crosby, D.G. (eds.). New York: Marcel Dekker, 1971, 271–304.

Cavill, G.W.K., Ford, D.L.: The chemistry of ants. — III. Structure and reactions of iridodial. Aust. J. Chem. **13**, 296–310 (1960).

Cavill, G.W.K., Ford, D.L., Locksley, H.D.: Iridodial and iridolactone Chem. Ind. **1956**, 465 (1956a).

Cavill, G.W.K., Ford, D.L., Locksley, H.D.: The chemistry of ants — I. Terpenoid constituents of some Australian *Iridomyrmex* species. Aust. J. Chem. **9**, 288–293 (1956b).

Cavill, G.W.K., Hinterberger, H.: Dolichoderine ant extractives. Proc. XIth Int. Kongr. Ent., Vienna, 1960. **3**, 53–59 (1960a).

Cavill, G.W.K., Hinterberger, H.: The chemistry of ants. IV. Terpenoid constituents of some *Dolichoderus* and *Iridomyrmex* species. Aust. J. Chem. **13**, 514–519 (1960b).

Cavill, G.W.K., Hinterberger, H.: The chemistry of ants. V. Structure and reactions of dolichodial. Aust. J. Chem. **14**, 143–149 (1961).

Cavill, G.W.K., Houghton, E.: Hydrocarbon constituents of the Argentine ant, *Iridomyrmex humilis*. Aust. J. Chem. **26**, 1131–1135 (1973).

Cavill, G.W.K., Houghton, E.: Some pyrazine derivatives from the Argentine ant, *Iridomyrmex humilis*. Aust. J. Chem. **27**, 879–889 (1974a).

Cavill, G.W.K., Houghton, E.: Volatile constituents of the Argentine ant, *Iridomyrmex humilis*. J. Insect Physiol. **20**, 2049–2059 (1974b).

Cavill, G.W.K., Locksley, H.D.: The chemistry of ants. II. Structure and configuration of iridolactone (isoiridomyrmecin). Aust. J. Chem. **10**, 352–358 (1957).

Cavill, G.W.K., Williams, P.J.: Constituents of Dufour's gland in *Myrmecia gulosa*. J. Insect Physiol. **13**, 1097–1103 (1967).

Chadha, M.S., Eisner, T., Monro, A., Meinwald, J.: Citronellal and citral in the mandibular gland secretions of the ant *Acanthomyops claviger* (Roger). J. Insect Physiol. **8**, 175–179 (1962).

Clark, K.J., Fray, G.I., Jaeger, R.H., Robinson, R.: Synthesis of D- and L-isoiridomyrmecin and related compounds. Tetrahedron **6**, 217–224 (1959).

Creighton, W.S.: The ants of North America. Bull. Mus. Comp. Zool. **104**, 1–585 (1950).

Crewe, R.M., Blum, M.S.: 6-Methyl-5-hepten-2-one: Chemotaxonomic significance in an *Iridomyrmex* sp. (Hymenoptera: Formicidae). Ann. Ent. Soc. Amer. **64**, 1007–1010 (1971).

Crewe, R.M., Blum, M.S., Collingwood, C.A.: Comparative analysis of alarm pheromones in the ant genus *Crematogaster*. Comp. Biochem. Physiol. **43B**, 703–716 (1972).

Forel, A.: Der Giftapparat und die Analdrüsen der Ameisen. Zeitschr. Wiss. Zool. **30**, Suppl., 28–66 (1878).

Fusco, R., Trave, R., Vercellone, A.: La struttura dell'iridomirmecina. Chim. Ind. (Milano) **37**, 958–959 (1955a).

Fusco, R., Trave, R., Vercellone, A.: Ricerche sulla iridomirmecina, l'insetticida naturale secreto dalla *Iridomyrmex humilis* Mayr. Chim. Ind. (Milano) **37**, 251–259 (1955b).

Gotwald, W.H., jr., Brown, W.L., jr.: The ant genus *Simopelta* (Hymenoptera: Formicidae). Psyche **73**, 261–277 (1966).

Gotwald, W.H., jr.: Mouthpart morphology of the ant *Aneuretus simoni*. Ann. Ent. Soc. Amer. **63**, 950–952 (1970).

Grünanger, P., Quilico, A., Pavan, M.: Sul secreto odoroso del formicide *Myrmicaria natalensis* Fred. Accad. Nazion. Lincei **28**, 293–300 (1960).

Hermann, H.R.: The hymenopterous poison apparatus. VII. *Simopelta oculata* (Hymenoptera: Formicidae: Ponerinae). J. Georgia Ent. Soc. **3**, 163–166 (1968a).

Hermann, H.R.: The hymenopterous poison apparatus. V. *Aneuretus simoni*. Ann. Ent. Soc. Amer. **61**, 1315–1317 (1968b).

Hermann, H.R.: The furcula, a major component of the hymenopterous venom apparatus. Inter. J. Ins. Morph. Embryol. (in press) (1977).

Hermann, H.R.: The hymenopterous venom apparatus. XV. Dolichoderinae (Hymenoptera: Formicidae). Ann. Ent. Soc. Amer. (in press) (1978)

Hermann, H.R.: The ant-like venom apparatus of *Typhoctes peculiaris*, a primitive mutillid wasp. Ann. Ent. Soc. Amer. (in press) (1978)

Kerr, R.W.: In Cavill, G.W.K., Ford, D.L., Hinterberger, H., Solomon, D.H.: Bisnoriridodial, bisnoriridolactone, and related compounds. Aust. J. Chem. **14**, 276–283 (1961).

McConnell, J.F., Mathieson, A. Mcl., Schoenborn, B.P.: Conformation of iridomyrmecin and isoiridomyrmecin. Tetrahedron Lett. **10**, 445–448 (1962).

McGurk, D.J., Frost, J., Waller, G.R., Eisenbraun, E.J., Vick, K., Drew, W.A., Young, J.: Iridodial isomer variation in dolicherine ants. J. Insect Physiol. **14**, 841–845 (1968).

Meinwald, J., Chadha, M.S., Hurst, J.J., Eisner, T.: Defense mechanisms of arthropods–IX. Anisomorphal, the secretion of a phasmid insect. Tetrahedron Lett. **1**, 29–33 (1962).

Moore, B.P.: Studies on the chemical composition and function of the cephalic gland secretion in Australian termites. J. Insect Physiol. **14**, 33–39 (1968).

Moore, B.P.: In Cavill, G.W.K., Houghton, E.: Some pyrazine derivatives from the Argentine ant, *Iridomyrmex humilis*. Aust. J. Chem. **27**, 879–889 (1974a).

Morgan, E.D., Wadhams, L.J.: Chemical constituents of Dufour's gland in the ant, *Myrmica rubra*. J. Insect Physiol. **18**, 1125–1135 (1972).

Moser, J., Brownlee, R.G., Silverstein, R.M.: The alarm pheromones of *Atta texana*. J. Insect Physiol. **14**, 529–535 (1968).

Pavan, M.: Ricerche sugli antibiotici di origine animale. Nota riassuntiva. Ricerca Sci. **19**, 1101–1107 (1949).

Pavan, M.: Summary on original research on antibiotic substances of insects. VIIIth Int. Congr. Ent., Stockholm. 1948, 866–869 (1950).

Pavan, M.: Iridomyrmecin as insecticide. IX Congr. Int. Ent., Amsterdam, 1951. **1**, 321–327 (1952).

Pavan, M.: Significato chimico e biologico di alcuni veleni di Insetti. Tipografia Artigianelli, Pavia **1**, 1—75 (1958).

Pavan, M.: Biochemical aspects of insect poisons. Trans. 4th Int. Congr. Biochem., Vienna, 1958. **12**, 15—36 (1959).

Pavan, M., Baggini, A.: Ricerche sull'attivitá fitoinibitrice della iridomyrmecina su *Lupinus albus*. Boll. Zoll. **22**, 393—404 (1955).

Pavan, M., Ronchetti, G.: Studi sulla morfologia esterna e anatomia interna dell'operaia di *Iridomyrmex humilis* Mayr e ricerche chimiche e biologiche sulla iridomirmecina. Atti Soc. Ital. Sci. Nat. Museo Civico Storia Nat. Milano **94**, 379—477 (1955).

Pavan, M., Valcurone, M.L.: Ricerche sull'antagonismo della iridomyrmecina verso l'attivitá oncogena della colchicina e del gammaesano su *Lupinus albus*. Boll. Zool. **22**, 405—419 (1955).

Regnier, F.E., Nieh, M., Hölldobler, B.: The volatile Dufour's gland components of the ants *Pogonomyrmex rugosus* and *P. barbatus*. J. Insect Physiol. **19**, 981—992 (1973).

Riley, R.G., Silverstein, R.M., Moser, J.C.: Isolation, identification, synthesis, and biological activity of the volatile compounds from the heads of *Atta* ants. J. Insect Physiol. **20**, 1629—1637 (1974).

Sudd, J.H.: An Introduction to the Behavior of Ants. London: Arnold, Ltd., 1967.

Trave, R., Pavan, M.: Veleni degli insetti. Principi estratti dalla formica *Tapinoma nigerrimum* Nyl. Chim. Ind. (Milano) **38**, 1015—1019 (1956).

Vidari, G., De Bernardi, M., Pavan, M., Ragozzino, L.: Rose oxide and iridodial from *Aromia moschata* L. (Coleoptera: Cerambycidae). Tetrahedron Lett. **41**, 4065—4068 (1973).

Wheeler, W.M.: Ants: Their Structure, Development and Behavior. New York: Columbia Univ. Press, 1910.

Wheeler, W.M.: Ants of the American Museum Congo Expedition. A contribution to the myrmecology of Africa. VII. Key to the genera and subgenera of ants. Bull. Amer. Mus. Nat. History **45**, 631—710 (1922).

Wheeler, J.W., Blum, M.S.: Alkylpyrazine alarm pheromones in ponerine ants. Science **182**, 501—502 (1973).

Wheeler, J.W., Evans, S.L., Blum, M.S., Torgerson, R.L.: Cyclopentyl ketones: Identification and function in *Azteca* ants. Science **187**, 254—255 (1975).

Wilson, E.O.: Sympatry of the ants *Conomyrma bicolor* (Wheeler) and *C. pyramica* (Roger). Psyche **64**, 76 (1957).

Wilson, E.O.: The Insect Societies. Harvard Univ. Press. Cambirdge, Mass.: The Belknap Press, 1971.

Wilson, E.O., Eisner, T., Wheeler, G.C., Wheeler, J.: *Aneuretus simoni* Emery, a major link in ant evolution. Bull. Mus. Comp. Zool. **115**, 81—99 (1956).

Author Index

Page Numbers in *italics* refer to the bibliography

Subject Index

Handbuch der experimentellen Pharmakologie/ Handbook of Experimental Pharmacology

Heffter-Heubner,
New Series

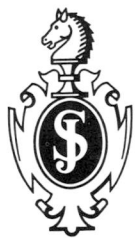

Springer-Verlag
Berlin
Heidelberg
New York

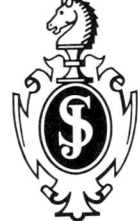

Springer-Verlag
Berlin
Heidelberg
New York

AFRICA AND THE MIDDLE EAST

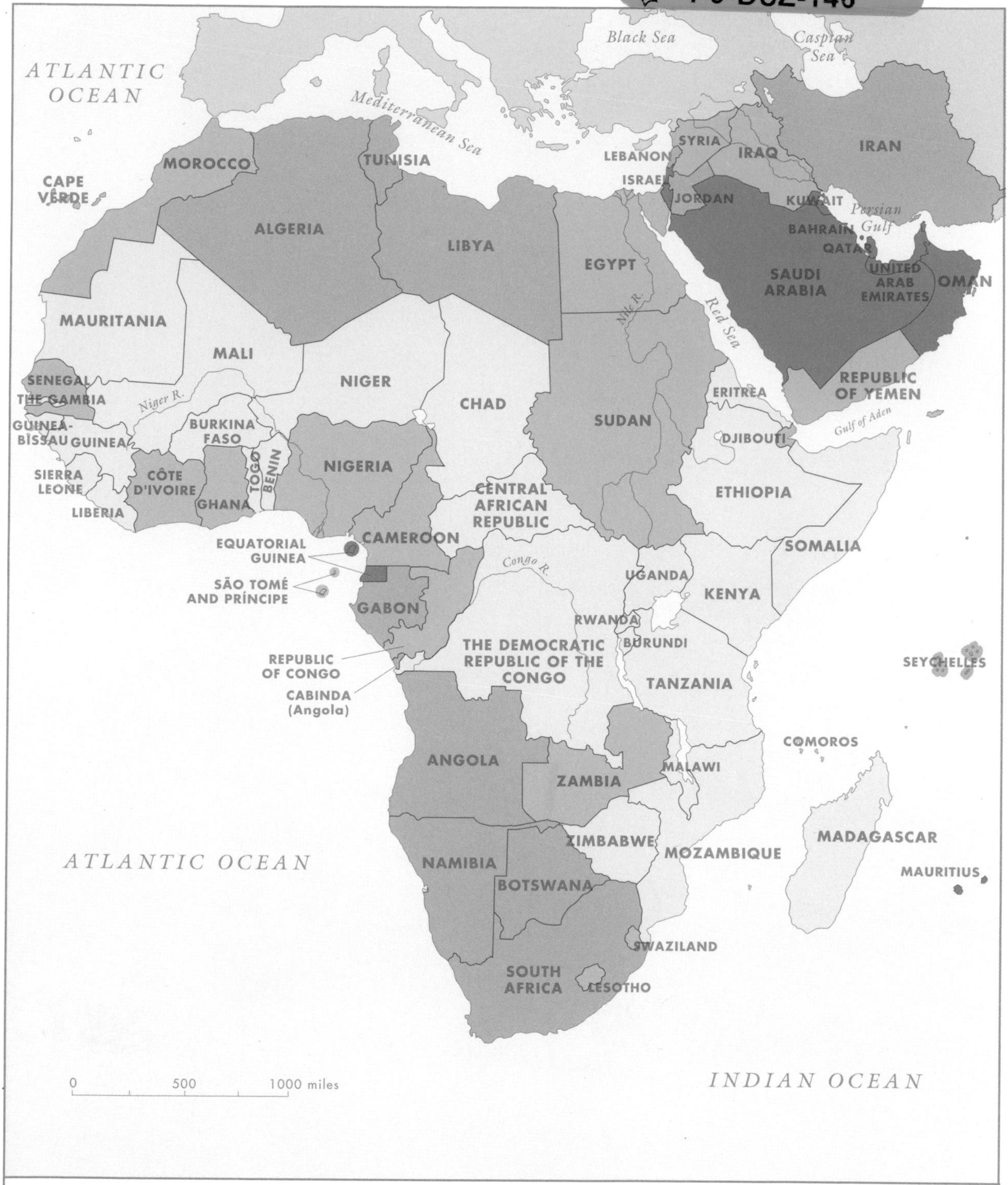

Income status, 2011

Low income   Lower-middle income   Upper-middle income   High income

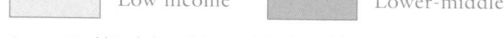

Source: World Bank, http://data.worldbank.org/about/country-classifications
/country-and-lending-groups

ECONOMICS OF DEVELOPMENT

SEVENTH EDITION

ECONOMICS OF DEVELOPMENT

SEVENTH EDITION

Dwight H. Perkins
Harvard University

Steven Radelet
U.S. Agency for International Development

David L. Lindauer
Wellesley College

Steven A. Block
Tufts University

W. W. Norton & Company
New York • London

W. W. Norton & Company has been independent since its founding in 1923, when William Warder Norton and Mary D. Herter Norton first published lectures delivered at the People's Institute, the adult education division of New York City's Cooper Union. The firm soon expanded its program beyond the Institute, publishing books by celebrated academics from America and abroad. By midcentury, the two major pillars of Norton's publishing program—trade books and college texts—were firmly established. In the 1950s, the Norton family transferred control of the company to its employees, and today—with a staff of four hundred and a comparable number of trade, college, and professional titles published each year— W. W. Norton & Company stands as the largest and oldest publishing house owned wholly by its employees.

Editor: Jack Repcheck
Assistant Editor: Hannah Bachman
Manuscript Editor: Candace Levy
Project Editor: Rachel Mayer
Electronic Media Editor: Nicole Sawa
Marketing Manager, Economics: Sasha Levitt
Production Manager: Sean Mintus
Permissions Manager: Megan Jackson
Permissions Clearing: Bethany Salminen
Text Design: JoAnn Simony
Art Director: Rubina Yeh
Composition: Jouve North America—Brattleboro, VT
Manufacturing: Quad Graphics—Taunton, MA

Library of Congress Cataloging-in-Publication Data
Economics of development / Dwight H . Perkins . . . [et al.].—7th ed.
        p. cm.
    Rev. ed. of: Economics of development / Dwight H. Perkins, Steven Radelet, David L. Lindauer.
6th ed. c2006.
    Includes bibliographical references and index.
    ISBN 978-0-393-93435-9 (hardcover)—ISBN 0-393-93435-7   1. Developing countries—Economic
policy.   2. Economic development.   I. Perkins, Dwight H. (Dwight Heald), 1934-   II. Perkins,
Dwight H. (Dwight Heald), 1934- Economics of development.
    HC59.7.E314 2013
    338.9—dc23
                                                                                        2012029688

W. W. Norton & Company, Inc., 500 Fifth Avenue, New York, NY 10110-0017
                            wwnorton.com

W. W. Norton & Company Ltd., Castle House, 75/76 Wells Street, London W1T 3QT

1 2 3 4 5 6 7 8 9 0

Brief Contents

Contents

PART ONE
Development and Growth

1 Patterns of Development   3

2 Measuring Economic Growth and Development   23

3 Economic Growth: Concepts and Patterns   55

PART TWO
Distribution and Human Resources

PART THREE
Macroeconomic Policies for Development

13 Foreign Debt and Financial Crises 455

14 Foreign Aid 499

15 Managing Short-Run Crises in an Open Economy 545

PART FOUR
Agriculture, Trade, and Sustainability

19 Trade Policy 709

20 Sustainable Development 757

Index 803

Preface

In 1983, when the first edition of this textbook was published, 50 percent of the world's population lived in nations the World Bank classified as low income. By 2010 the number had dropped to 12 percent. Much of that change is the result of rapid economic growth in China and India. Today, both are middle-income economies. But economic growth and development has not been limited to these two Asian giants. "Africa Rising" was the cover story of a 2011 issue of *The Economist*, reflecting more than a decade of rapid growth in a region *The Economist* 10 years earlier referred to as "The Hopeless Continent." Throughout Africa, East and South Asia, Latin America, and elsewhere, dramatic improvements have been taking place in the education, health, and living standards of billions of people.

The study of the economics of development has had to keep pace with these historic changes. We have tried to keep pace as well. In this as in previous editions, we have incorporated new ideas and new data and provide fresh insights from the experiences of the nations that make up the developing world. While there is much that is new in this seventh edition, the distinguishing features of this text remain the same:

- It is based primarily on the real-world experiences of developing countries. It explores broad trends and patterns and uses numerous real-country examples and cases to illustrate major points, many of which are drawn from the authors' own experiences.
- It draws heavily on the empirical work of economists who believe that attention to the data not only reveals what the development process entails but permits us to test our beliefs about how that process works.
- It relies on the theoretical tools of neoclassical economics to investigate and analyze these real-world experiences in the belief that these tools contribute substantially to our understanding of economic development.
- It highlights the diversity of development experience and recognizes that the lessons of theory and history can be applied only within certain institutional and national contexts.

As in previous editions, the seventh edition of *Economics of Development* is intended to be both accessible and comprehensive. The discussion is *accessible* to those students, whether undergraduates or those pursuing advanced degrees in international relations, public policy, and related fields, who have only an elementary background in economics. At the same time, the text provides a *comprehensive* introduction to all students, including those with significant training in economics, who are taking their first course in development economics.

Major Changes for the Seventh Edition

The seventh edition of *Economics of Development* continues and extends the major revisions of the book initiated in previous editions. The substantial changes reflect the contributions of three new coauthors—Steven Radelet in the fifth edition, David Lindauer in the sixth, and Steven Block in the seventh—working alongside original coauthor Dwight Perkins. The seventh edition features fundamental revisions of many chapters. The revised chapters take full advantage of research on development economics over the past decade. In addition, there are more and better tables, charts, and other exhibits chronicling the lessons and remaining controversies of the development field. The chapter summaries that follow highlight the major changes in the seventh edition. Asterisks indicate chapters that are essentially or entirely new for this edition.

Chapter 1 (Patterns of Development) has been condensed. It begins with the three vignettes—on Malaysia, Ethiopia, and Ukraine—that were introduced in the previous edition and updated for this one. The chapter includes a new table on the classification of world economies and populations according to income status. Also added is a section on how the study of development economics differs from the study of economics as applied to developed nations.

Chapter 2 (Measuring Economic Growth and Development) reflects important updates by various agencies and authors, including the 2005 International Comparison Program (ICP) estimates of purchasing power parity; Angus Maddison's latest and last estimates of world economic growth; and the United Nations Development Programme's (UNDP) 2010 revision of the human development index (HDI). The analysis of economic growth and happiness has been fully revised and expanded, reversing some of the conclusions first reported in the sixth edition. A new box has been added on the determinants of long-run economic growth suggested by Jared Diamond's *Guns, Germs, and Steel*. There is also a new box on the use of logarithms, essential to understanding the HDI and other development measures.

Chapter 3 (Economic Growth: Concepts and Patterns) has been reorganized and updated to include the latest data and country examples. This edition features a new box on the calculation of growth rates, future values, and doubling times. Previous material on the characteristics of production functions and on growth convergence has been moved to Chapter 4. The previous discussion of structural change has been entirely rewritten and relocated to Chapter 16, where it supports the discussion of economic dualism.

Chapter 4 (Theories of Economic Growth) has also been streamlined and consolidated. This edition integrates into its presentation of growth theory the discussions of production functions and growth convergence previously found in Chapter 3. The previous discussion of dual-sector growth models has been eliminated from the discussion of growth theory and relocated to Chapter 16, where its primary purpose is to illustrate sectoral interactions as a foundation for discussing the role of agriculture in development. Chapter 4 also provides newly updated data and illustrative figures.

*Chapter 5 (States and Markets) raises the central question, What makes economic development happen? For this edition, senior author, Dwight Perkins, takes a fresh look, tracing the evolution of thinking about development from Adam Smith, through notions of The Big Push advanced in the 1940s by economist Paul Rosenstein-Rodan, to more recent debates over Structural Adjustment and the Washington Consensus.

Chapter 6 (Inequality and Poverty) updates the analysis of poverty by examining the revision of the global poverty line from $1 per day to $1.25 per day. Combined with recent measures of purchasing power parity (PPP), the latest estimates on levels of both inequality and poverty are presented. A new section, "Living in Poverty," has been added that includes insights from the work by economists Abhijit Banerjee, Esther Duflo, and others on the economic lives of the poor. The use of conditional cash transfers also receives more attention.

Chapter 7 (Population) incorporates the United Nations 2010 Revision to its world population projections. The chapter now includes more discussion of the demographic dividend and a new section on population issues for the twenty-first century.

Chapter 8 (Education) benefits from recent revisions to the Barro-Lee data set on school attainment and from recent results of the Organisation for Economic Co-Operation and Development's (OECD) Programme for International Student Assessment (PISA). Fuller use is made of econometric approaches, including natural experiments and randomized controlled trials (RCTs) in determining rates of return to schooling and the effectiveness of alternative interventions to improve learning outcomes. A new box on combating teacher absence has been added.

Chapter 9 (Health) now includes an extended discussion of the relationship between income and health. The Preston curve, showing the relationship between life expectancy and per capita income is presented and the debate over causality more fully developed. A box has been added on creating markets for vaccines for diseases that primarily affect populations in low-income settings.

*Chapter 10 (Investment and Savings) draws on material from two chapters in the sixth edition. The chapter assumes students have had some background in the principles of macroeconomics and focuses on topics central to developing nations. These include barriers to both public and private investment and alternative sources of savings to finance productive investments. Special attention is given to foreign direct investment and its role in promoting economic growth.

Chapter 11 (Fiscal Policy) continues to focus on the key components of government expenditures and revenues. Data have been updated and a box added on the challenges of fiscal decentralization in Brazil and China.

Chapter 12 (Financial Development and Inflation) reorders some of the material on monetary policy and price stability, providing a more intuitive flow to the material. The discussion of microcredit has been expanded and includes a new box based on an RCT in India.

Chapter 13 (Foreign Debt and Financial Crises) is updated to provide the most recent data on foreign debt and provides current examples of financial crises (including the 2010–11 Euro Zone crisis, though the focus remains on developing countries).

Chapter 14 (Foreign Aid) has been updated to reflect recent trends in official development assistance, which, in part, are the results of events in Afghanistan, Iraq, and Pakistan. New boxes have been added on the commitment to development index and on Chinese foreign aid.

Chapter 15 (Managing Short-Run Crises in an Open Economy), formerly Chapter 21, now concludes the section on macroeconomic policies for developing countries. Presentation of the Australian model of short-run macroeconomic management has been clarified and illustrated with updated examples. New boxes cover real versus nominal exchange rates and the Greek debt crisis of 2010–11 (with an application of the Australian model). This chapter also features a new appendix for this edition, providing a review of national income and balance of payments accounting.

*Chapter 16 (Agriculture and Development) is the first of two entirely new chapters on agriculture. This chapter places agriculture in its broad developmental context, emphasizing the potential contributions of agriculture to both growth and poverty alleviation. Specific topics include structural transformation, dual-sector growth models, agriculture and growth, and agriculture as a pathway out of poverty.

*Chapter 17 (Agricultural Development: Technology, Policies and Institutions) builds on the broad discussion of agriculture and development in the previous chapter, concentrating on policies and institutions to promote agricultural development. Specific topics introduced in this chapter include a typology of agricultural systems common in developing countries, a broad framework for analyzing constraints to agricultural production growth, the role of technical change and the green revolution, the role of institutions and land reform in agricultural development, and a review of the global food price crisis of 2005–08.

*Chapter 18 (Trade and Development) presents an overview of trends and patterns in world trade. It reviews the theory of comparative advantage, discussing both the benefits of trade and its distributional consequences. Special attention is paid to trade in primary products, including export pessimism and the terms of trade, Dutch disease and the real exchange rate, and the resource curse and responses to it.

*Chapter 19 (Trade Policy) builds on the broad discussion of trade and development in the previous chapter. It reviews import substitution as a trade strategy and the consequences of trade protection. This is followed by discussion of export orientation, including experience with export processing zones. Evidence is presented on trade, growth, and poverty alleviation. The chapter concludes with an examination of key issues on the global trade agenda, such as the impact of China and India on global trade competition, sweatshops and labor standards, the Doha Round of trade negotiations, and temporary labor migration as a strategy to alleviate world poverty.

*Chapter 20 (Sustainable Development) is essentially a new treatment of the subject, retaining from the previous edition only the discussion of market and policy failures. New topics addressed in this edition are the environmental Kuznets curve hypothesis, an expanded and more analytical treatment of the concept and measurement of sustainable development, institutional perspectives on externalities (drawing on the work of Elinor Ostrom), payments for environmental services as a response to externalities, a substantially expanded treatment of poverty-environment linkages, and a new section on the economics of climate change. New boxes in this edition cover the Malthusian effect of population growth on adjusted net savings in Ghana, taxation of water pollution in Colombia, and, policy failures and deforestation in Indonesia.

About the Authors

Of the four original authors of *Economics of Development* only Dwight Perkins remains as an active contributor to this edition. Michael Roemer's death in 1996 took from the development field one of its most thoughtful and productive writers and practitioners. Mike, in many ways, was the single most important contributor to the earlier editions, and his legacy endures in this edition. Malcolm Gillis, an expert in issues of public finance and economic development, played the central role in getting this book started in the early 1980s. He later went on to a distinguished career as president of Rice University, from which he retired. Donald Snodgrass was responsible for Part Three, "Human Resources," for the first five editions. Both Malcolm Gillis's and Donald Snodgrass's strong contributions are evident in the current edition as well. The new authors are privileged to be part of a text that, thanks to the scholarship of the original authors, helped to define the field of development economics.

Dwight H. Perkins is the H. H. Burbank Professor of Political Economy Emeritus at Harvard University and former director of the Harvard Institute for International Development. Professor Perkins is a leading scholar on the economies of East and Southeast Asia. Professor Perkins's legacy is contained not only in the many chapters he has contributed to *Economics of Development* and in his many scholarly books and articles but also in the thousands of students he has taught over his distinguished academic career (including all of his current coauthors!).

Steven Radelet joined *Economics of Development* for its fifth edition. At the time he was a fellow at Harvard's Institute for International Development and taught in both Harvard's economics department and the Kennedy School of Government. He subsequently was deputy assistant secretary of the U.S. Treasury for Africa, the Middle East, and South Asia; a Senior Fellow at the Center for Global Development; and Senior Advisor on Development for Secretary of State Hillary Clinton. He is an expert on foreign aid, developing country debt and financial crises, and economic growth and has extensive experience in West Africa and Southeast Asia. He currently serves as Chief Economist for the U.S. Agency for International Development (USAID). In that capacity he was unable to contribute to this edition but his prior work on the textbook significantly informs this edition as well.

David L. Lindauer is the Stanford Calderwood Professor of Economics at Wellesley College, where he has taught since 1981. He has frequently served as a consultant to the World Bank and was a faculty associate of the Harvard Institute for International Development. Professor Lindauer's area of expertise is in labor economics. His research and policy advising has included work on industrial relations, labor costs and export potential, minimum wages, poverty and unemployment, public sector pay and employment, and racial affirmative action. He has worked on labor market issues in East and Southeast Asia, Sub-Saharan Africa, and elsewhere. Professor Lindauer, an award-winning teacher of economics, brings his considerable experience teaching undergraduates to this edition.

Steven A. Block is Professor of International Economics and head of the International Development Program at the Fletcher School of Law and Diplomacy, Tufts University. He joins *Economics of Development* beginning with this edition and has been teaching development economics at the Fletcher School since 1995. Professor Block also holds a faculty appointment at the Friedman School of Nutrition Science and Policy at Tufts University, and has been a visiting scholar at the Harvard University Center for International Development and at Harvard's Weatherhead Center for International Affairs. He has published numerous scholarly articles in the areas of agricultural development and political economy, and worked extensively on policy advisory teams across Sub-Saharan Africa and in Southeast Asia.

Acknowledgments

Any textbook that makes it to a seventh edition accumulates many debts to colleagues who read chapters, provided feedback, or contributed in some way to the success and longevity of the work. We owe many thanks to many people. In these acknowledgments, we wish to thank those individuals who contributed to this edition.

Dwight H. Perkins is grateful to the hundreds of colleagues and students from around the developing world and at Harvard and other universities in the United States and elsewhere who, over the past five decades, have taught him what he knows about development economics and to his wife, Julie, who has joined him on many of his trips to developing countries.

David L. Lindauer thanks his research assistants, Yue Guan and Teju Vela-yudhan. They did a tremendous job creating the charts and figures in many of the chapters. Dana Lindauer, Pasinee Panitnantanakul, and Anisha Vachani provided additional assistance. Thanks are owed David Johnson and Joseph Stern for help in drafting several of the text Boxes. He also received excellent comments from Akila Weerapana (Wellesley College), Jere Behrman (Pennsylvania), Lant Pritchett (Harvard), Martin Ravallion (World Bank), and Paul Glewwe (Minnesota). He greatly appreciates the sabbatical leave provided by Wellesley College that provided the time needed to produce this edition and wishes to thank his family for all their support.

Steven A. Block thanks his research assistant, Bapu Vaitla, for his impeccable support and useful suggestions. He is particularly grateful to Peter Timmer (emeritus, Harvard University) and Jeffrey Vincent (Duke University) for their critical reading and constructive suggestions for Chapters 16, 17, and 20 of this edition. In addition, he is grateful to his family—Avi; Ruthie; and wife, Maria—for their love and patience.

All three of us wish to thank everyone at W. W. Norton and Company for their continued support. We are especially grateful for the continued guidance and efforts of our editor, Jack Repcheck.

D.H.P. *Cambridge*
S.R. *Washington, D.C.*
D.L.L. *Wellesley*
S.A.B. *Tufts*

International Development Resources on the Internet

International Organizations

1. The World Bank (*www.worldbank.org*) hosts specific sites dedicated to country information (*www.worldbank.org/html/extdr/regions.htm*), data on a range of development indicators (*www.worldbank.org/data*), specific development themes (*www.worldbank.org/html/extdr/thematic.htm*), poverty reduction (*www.worldbank.org/poverty*), and governance and anticorruption (*www.worldbank.org/wbi/governance*).
2. The International Monetary Fund (*www.imf.org*) hosts individual country information (*www.imf.org/external/country/index.htm*) and an index of over 100 economic, commodity, and development organizations (*www.imf.org/np/sec/decdo/contents.htm*).
3. African Development Bank (*www.afdb.org*), Asian Development Bank (*www.adb.org*), and Inter-American Development Bank (*www.iadb.org*).
4. The United Nations development organizations, including the United Nations Development Programme (*www.undp.org*), the Food and Agriculture Organization (*www.fao.org*), the World Health Organization (*www.who.org*), the United Nations Children's Fund (*www.unicef.org*), the Joint United Nations Programme on HIV/AIDS (*www.unaids.org*), and the United Nations Millennium Project with information on the Millennium Development Goals (*www.unmillenniumproject.org*).

Independent Research Organizations

5. The Center for Global Development (*www.cgdev.org*).
6. The Center for International Development at Harvard University (*www.hks.harvard.edu/centers/cid*).
7. The Earth Institute at Columbia University (*www.earthinstitute.columbia.edu*).
8. The Overseas Development Institute (*www.odi.org.uk*).
9. The World Institute for Development Economics Research (*www.wider.unu.edu*).
10. The World Resources Institute (*www.wri.org*).

Information Gateways

11. The Development Gateway (*www.developmentgateway.org*).
12. Institute of Development Studies (*www.ids.ac.uk*).
13. The International Development Research Centre (*www.idrc.ca*).
14. Netaid.org (*www.netaid.org*).
15. Oneworld.net (*www.oneworldgroup.org*).
16. International Economics Network, Development Resources (*www .internationaleconomics.net/development.html*)

Data Sources

In addition to the other sites listed, the following offer useful data.

17. The Center for International Comparisons (Penn World Tables, *www.pwt.econ .upenn.edu*).
18. The Development Assistance Committee of the Organization for Economic Cooperation and Development (*www.oecd.org/dac*).
19. The Living Standards Measurement Study of Household Surveys (*www .worldbank.org/LSMS*).
20. The Roubini Global Economics Monitor (*www.rgemonitor.com*).
21. The World Factbook (*www.cia.gov/cia/publications/factbook*).

Foundations

22. The Bill and Melinda Gates Foundation (*www.gatesfoundation.org*).
23. The Ford Foundation (*www.fordfound.org*).
24. The Open Society Institute (*www.soros.org*).
25. The Rockefeller Foundation (*www.rockfound.org*).
26. The William and Flora Hewlett Foundation (*www.hewlett.org*).

PART ONE

Development and Growth

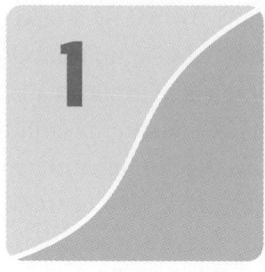

Patterns of Development

MALAYSIA

During the early 1980s, when she was 17 years old, Rachmina Abdullah did something no girl from her village had ever done before. She left her home in a beautiful but poor part of the state of Kedah in Malaysia, where people grew rice in the valleys and tapped rubber trees in the nearby hills, and went to work in an electronics plant in Penang, 75 miles away. Rachmina's family was poor even by the modest standards of her village, and her parents welcomed the opportunity for their daughter to earn her own keep and possibly even send money back to help them feed and clothe the family, deal with recurrent emergencies, and raise their five younger children. With these benefits in mind, they set aside their reservations about their unmarried daughter's unheard-of plan to go off by herself to work in the city.

---

[1] The three narratives that follow are fictional. The vignette on Malaysia is loosely based on Fatimah Daud, *Minah Karan: The Truth about Malaysian Factory Girls* (Kuala Lumpur: Berita Publishing, 1985), and Kamal Salih and Mei Ling Young, "Changing Conditions of Labour in the Semiconductor Industry in Malaysia," *Labour and Society* 14 (1989), 59–80. The narratives on Ethiopia and Ukraine are based on discussions with experts who have lived and worked in these nations. The named individuals are constructs rather than actual people. Data used in all three vignettes are from *World Development Indicators Online*.

Rachmina got a job assembling integrated circuits in a factory owned by a Japanese company. Every day, she patiently soldered hundreds of tiny wires onto minute silicon chips. It was tedious, repetitive work that had to be performed at high speed and with flawless accuracy. From a long day of hard work with few breaks, Rachmina could earn the equivalent of a few dollars. Because their wages were low, Rachmina and her colleagues welcomed opportunities to work overtime. Often they put in two or three extra hours a day, for up to seven days a week. They particularly liked working Sundays and holidays, when double wages were paid. Rachmina shared a small house in a squatter area with seven other factory workers. By living simply and inexpensively, most of the young women managed to send money back home each month and generally enjoyed the unfamiliar freedom of living apart from their families and villages.

Five years later, Rachmina, who had accumulated some savings, decided it was time to return to her village, where she soon married a local man and settled down. She later had two children—fewer than her friends who had stayed in the village and married earlier. Her savings helped provide for her family, and she was able to enroll her children in the local school.

Rachmina's chance to work in an electronics factory came about because, starting in the 1970s, American and Japanese electronics manufacturers were moving into export processing zones (EPZs) established by the Malaysian government. The national unemployment rate was high, and the government was particularly anxious to find more urban, nonagricultural jobs for the indigenous Malay population. In the mid-1970s, demand for electronic devices was growing by leaps and bounds, and international firms were looking for overseas locations where they could carry out parts of their operations at lower cost. The first beneficiaries of this migration were the newly industrializing nations of East Asia: Hong Kong, Singapore, South Korea, and Taiwan. Malaysia, with its good infrastructure, English-speaking workforce and stable political environment, also attracted foreign investors. Although the wages were lower than those paid in Japan and the United States, they were much higher than most Malays could earn through farm work, and people lined up for the opportunity to secure these prized jobs.

Malaysia, which previously had been known mainly for the export of rubber, tin, and palm oil, became one of the world's largest exporters of electronic components and other labor-intensive manufactured goods. Partly because of these exports, Malaysia emerged as one of the fastest growing economies in the world and a leading development success story. The income of the average Malay more than *quadrupled* in real terms between 1970 and 2010, infant mortality fell from 41 to 6 infants per thousand, and life expectancy rose from 61 to 75 years. Adult literacy jumped from 58 to 92 percent and the ratio of girls to boys enrolled in school increased from 83 to 103 percent. (In other words, if Rachmina had grandchildren, today her granddaughters would be slightly *more likely* to attend school than would her grandsons.)

The Malaysian economy changed as well. Agriculture accounted for about one third of national output in 1970; today it accounts for less than 10 percent. Households in Kedah still grow rice, and young women still work in electronics assembly in Penang as they did in the 1970s. (If you own a Dell laptop, it very well may have been assembled in Penang.) But Penang must now look to the future. Low wage competition from Vietnam and elsewhere in Southeast Asia is attracting the electronic assembly plants that once came to Malaysia. Penang is hoping to develop a more knowledge-based economy, which might include biotechnology, business-process outsourcing, and medical tourism.[2] Rachmina's grandchildren in all likelihood will live in a Malaysia far different from the one she knew.

ETHIOPIA

On another continent and at about the same time that Rachmina was on her way to begin working in Penang, Getachew was born in Ethiopia. Getachew's family and many of his relatives lived in a rural area outside of Dese, a drought-affected area in Amhara region and a day's bus ride from the capital city of Addis Ababa. The family lived in a thatched hut and had few possessions. They owned cooking utensils, some blankets and clothing, a radio, and a bicycle. Getachew's sisters spent two hours a day fetching water from a small stream outside their village. The village did not have a paved road or electricity. In addition to growing tef, a cereal crop similar to millet, the family grew vegetables and relied on its own production for most of its consumption needs. The family was especially proud of their livestock. Getachew's father raised and traded oxen, which earned the family most of their meager cash income.

Getachew was the fifth of eight children, one of whom died at birth and another before her third birthday. Getachew received five years of schooling, but the years were not in succession. In some years, he needed to tend the family's crops and livestock with his father and brothers. In other years, the family did not have enough money to pay for uniforms and other school fees and could afford to send only one or two of their children to school. Priority was given to Getachew's older brothers. By the time he was 16, Getachew was able to read and write, although not well.

Getachew and his family have known hard times. His mother died shortly after the birth of her last child. This was due, in part, to her weakened state as a result of the drought and famine in 1984, compounded by multiple births and lack of emergency postpartum care. Despite worldwide attention to Ethiopia's plight that year, relief came too late to help them. The area has been affected by drought and shortages of food since then, but none as severe. Political transition in 1991 brought a lot of uncertainty, even to the countryside. The village school remained closed that year, as the teacher returned to live in the capital. Prices for most commodities went up at the same time that Getachew's father earned little for his oxen. In 1998, war broke out between Ethiopia and neighboring Eritrea. Getachew was staying with his brother in Addis at the time and escaped the draft, but several of his friends were conscripted to serve. One lost a

---

[2]Homi Kharas, Albert Zeufack, and Hamdan Majeed, *Cities, People & the Economy: A Study on Positioning Penang*, Khazanah Nasional Berhad and the World Bank (Kuala Lumpur, 2010).

leg during the war and returned home but was no longer much help tending livestock. Another contracted HIV/AIDS and, without treatment, died soon after.

Getachew's second oldest brother is a truck driver and occasionally provides the family with goods and cash. Getachew went with his brother to Addis Ababa and lived there for a time, finding only occasional casual day labor. Life was hard in the city, in some ways harder than in the countryside. Back home everyone lived similarly. In Addis, many people had money to spend while Getachew did not. When his father fell ill from tuberculosis, Getachew went back to help out on the farm. He would like to get married but land has become increasingly scarce in his village, and it is unclear when he will be able to support a family of his own.

Getachew's life has been much like his father's and parallels that of most Ethiopians and many Africans. Per capita incomes in 2004 were at about the same levels as in 1981. In the intervening years, incomes at times increased and at other times declined, but overall, economic stagnation characterized the nation. Since 2004, however, economic growth has been faster and more consistent, averaging 6.6 percent per year. This is much faster than at any time over the past three decades. Despite the global recession of 2008–09, Ethiopia's economy continues to grow rapidly, although it is hard to know if this will be sustained.

Looking at other indicators of living standards, infant mortality rates fell from an estimated 136 per thousand in 1970 to 67 per thousand in 2009, reflecting the potential for health outcomes to improve even when income does not. Life expectancy, at 56 years, is 13 years more than in 1970 but still well below the levels in Malaysia and other more affluent economies. Adult literacy is less than one out of three, but this will improve in the future. Four out of every five of Ethiopia's children of school age are now enrolled in primary school—double the level of a decade ago. The economy is changing too, albeit slowly. In 1970, 61 percent of national output was derived from agriculture; today this figure is 51 percent. Growing crops and tending livestock remain the main economic activities for Getachew and three quarters of all Ethiopians.

With more than 80 million people, Ethiopia is one of the most populous poor nations in the world. But it is also one of Africa's emerging economies. Exports of primary products (including coffee), remittances from Ethiopians working abroad, and foreign direct investment are all fueling the nation's recent growth. Underlying these trends are better economic policies and management; the spread of new technologies, including cell phones; and increasing economic relations with China, India, and the Middle East.

UKRAINE

Unlike Getachew or Rachmina, Viktor and Yulia are relatively well educated. Both were born in L'viv in western Ukraine, about 300 miles from the capital, Kyiv. They graduated from secondary school in 1980 and went on to study for several more years at the local polytechnic institute, which is where they met. Viktor studied engineering, and Yulia architectural drawing. After finishing their studies, they married, and Viktor began work at a local glass factory. Yulia was hired by a municipal agency. As was common during the Soviet era, the couple moved into the one-bedroom apartment where Yulia's parents lived. Viktor and Yulia owned a refrigerator and other kitchen appliances, a television, furniture, some musical instruments, many books, and a telephone. They went on vacations, often going to a state-subsidized "sanatorium" in the Carpathian Mountains in Ukraine's southwest. Their daughter, Tetiana, was born in 1986, and Yulia was able to take a paid maternity leave.

Viktor's and Yulia's lifestyle in the 1980s was certainly modest by American or western European standards. They enjoyed few luxuries but most of their everyday needs were met. Often this required standing in long lines at government stores for staples such as bread, cooking oil, milk, and sugar. They also had their own garden plot where they grew flowers, fruit, and vegetables. Occasionally they purchased Polish goods in the gray market (technically illegal but not enforced). Healthcare and daycare were publicly provided.

Like many other ethnic Ukrainians in L'viv, Viktor, Yulia, and Yulia's parents longed for national independence. They spoke and maintained their native language even though the official language of the Soviet Union was Russian. Beyond their nationalist leanings, they thought their lives would be better in a less-centralized economy but were unaware of the severe consequences the breakup of the Soviet Union would entail.

Ukraine became independent in December 1991, with 90 percent of voters in support of a referendum on independence. Street celebrations and emotional speeches about freedom marked the event. But independence also had negative consequences. Trade with Russia collapsed and, with it, so did orders at the glass factory where Viktor was employed. Viktor was paid less and less often. A common refrain heard throughout the former Soviet Union was "they pretend to pay us and we pretend to work." Ukraine relied on energy supplies from Russia, but without foreign exchange to pay for them, Russian fuel exports dwindled, and many Ukrainians had to endure cold winters without much heat in their homes or offices. Mismanagement of the domestic economy led to hyperinflation in 1993–94, with prices rising almost 5,000 percent. The hyperinflation destroyed the purchasing power of pensioners, like Yulia's aging parents, and others living on fixed incomes. The healthcare system fell apart. Medicine, at times, had to be obtained on the black market, and one could never be sure of its efficacy. Life became harsher, with more anxiety, stress, and uncertainty about the future. Life expectancy for Ukrainian men was 66 years in 1989 but fell to 62 years by 1995. In 2009, it was still lower than two decades earlier, at 64 years.

Ukrainians had hoped that after independence foreign investment would flow into their country. It did not. Foreigners looked at Ukraine's situation and found existing technology backward, products of poor quality, and corruption rife. Instead of foreign purchase of factories, company officials often stripped factories of whatever assets they had and kept the proceeds themselves. Per capita income in 1998 was only 40 percent of its pretransition peak in 1989. All of this was happening in a society in which adult literacy was universal and where the nation's boys *and* girls were all well educated.

Viktor was one of many Ukrainian men who had a difficult time with the transition. He could not adjust to changing circumstances and never found a new job. He spent a lot of time at home, doing some carpentry and other odd jobs now and then. His health was poor as a result of smoking too much and, Yulia believes, the environmental hazards of the glass factory. Many of Viktor's friends from the factory have similar health problems; a few have died prematurely. Yulia is holding the family together. She has reinvented herself. She still is employed at the municipal agency, although her wages are not always paid. She spends much of her time at work drawing plans for some of the newly rich Ukrainians who are building summer villas and renovating apartments. She prefers not to discuss where the money to pay for these villas, and for her services, is coming from.

Ukraine's economy rebounded during the 2000s, and Viktor and Yulia were starting to feel more optimistic about the prospects for their daughter. By 2008 income per capita had risen to three quarters of its level in 1989. But the global recession hit Ukraine hard, in part because of a sharp decrease in demand for steel, one of the nation's major exports. A weak domestic banking sector also proved vulnerable to the world financial crisis. The economy shrank by 15 percent in 2009. (By way of comparison, during the Great Recession the U.S. economy contracted by only 2.5 percent.) Although the economy improved again in 2010, the nation is plagued by political turmoil and poor governance. Problems of corruption, cronyism, and unresponsive public institutions remain unresolved.

DEVELOPMENT AND GLOBALIZATION

These three development vignettes, about Malaysia, Ethiopia, and Ukraine, are meant to capture the range of experiences of individual nations over the past three to four decades. Some nations, including Malaysia, have experienced historically unprecedented rates of economic growth, which have dramatically changed the lives of their populations. In other parts of the world, including Ethiopia and much of sub-Saharan Africa, economic growth, at least until fairly recently, has been minimal, and standards of living have changed far less from one generation to the next. A third group of nations experienced a fundamental transition from one economic system to another. In many nations, including Ukraine, this resulted in an abrupt and steep decline in living standards. Recovery occurred in some but not all areas during the 2000s; the global financial crisis in 2008–09 hit some nations harder than others. Understanding the causes and consequences of these different patterns of economic development is the central goal of this textbook.

Economic growth, stagnation, and transition have had a profound impact on the lives of Rachmina, Getachew, and Viktor and Yulia, respectively, and on the more than 5.6 billion people of the developing countries these individuals are meant to personify. As different as the outcomes have been across nations, all countries have been affected by dramatic changes both within their borders and outside of them.

- Political systems have undergone profound changes, especially since the end of the cold war. Many low-income countries have adopted more democratic political systems since the early 1990s. The relationship between these political changes and the process of economic development and poverty reduction remains a matter of considerable debate.
- Substantial demographic shifts have led to a fall in population growth rates in many countries, with a decline in the number of dependent children and a corresponding growth in the share of workers in the population. Looking forward, many low-income countries will soon see large segments of the population reaching retirement age, with important implications for savings, tax revenues, pension systems, and social programs.
- The spread of endemic disease, including the HIV/AIDS pandemic, threatens development progress in many countries. In more than half a dozen African countries, more than a quarter of the adult population is HIV-positive. HIV/AIDS, malaria, tuberculosis, and other diseases bring a heavy human toll and substantial economic costs.
- Global trade has grown rapidly in line with sharply falling transportation and communication costs, giving rise to far more sophisticated global production networks. Instead of products being made start to finish in one location, firms in one country specialize in one part of the production process, while firms in another country play a different role. There has been a dramatic shift away from producing goods for the local market under government protection toward greater integration with global markets.[3]
- Capital moves much more quickly across borders than it did several decades ago. More sophisticated financial instruments and a greater emphasis on private capital have opened opportunities for low-income countries to access foreign capital for local investment. In some countries rapid financial liberalization resulted in deep financial crises when local financial institutions were weak and foreign capital was quickly withdrawn. On the other hand, the financial crisis of 2008–09 that originated in the United States and other advanced economies had far less of an impact on many developing economies than was expected.

---

[3]Malaysia has been most obviously helped by this process, and, at least in the short run, Ukraine has been hurt. Even rural Ethiopians who engage in subsistence agriculture are not insulated from global economic events. The Asian financial crisis of the late 1990s provides an example. The crisis resulted in a sharp decline in global demand for shoes, handbags, and other goods made from leather. This in turn lowered the demand and price for animal hides, a traditional Ethiopian export, and reduced the cash income of rural Ethiopians who might have had no idea why the prices they received for their animal skins had fallen.

- Information and ideas spread much faster around the globe than in earlier times. Cell phones, the Internet, and other communications technology have created new opportunities for low-income countries. Farmers can get pricing information that previously was unavailable, and family members can send money without the need of traditional banks. The new technology has created jobs that provide services via satellite and through the Internet, such as accounting, data entry, and telephone help lines.

Many forces are at work behind these changes. One of the most important is the process of **globalization**. *Globalization* is a term used by different people to mean many different things. Columbia University economist Jagdish Bhagwati defines *economic globalization* as the integration of national economies into the international economy through trade in goods and services, direct foreign investment, short-term capital flows, international movements of people, and flows of technology. Globalization has important noneconomic aspects as well, including integration of cultures, communications, and politics. It is not a new phenomenon: The early voyages of Ferdinand Magellan, Christopher Columbus, Zheng He, Marco Polo, and others opened an early epoch of globalization, and the late nineteenth and early twentieth centuries saw increased global integration until the process abruptly ended with the onset of World War I. But the current era has included more parts of the world and affected far more people than earlier episodes.

These broad global trends and the individual stories of Rachmina, Getachew, Viktor and Yulia raise many issues central to the process of economic development addressed in this book. How do governments promote investment, industrialization, and exports? How do countries educate their citizens and protect their health, enabling them to become productive workers? Who benefits from foreign investment and integration with global trading networks, and who loses? How does the shift from agriculture to manufacturing affect the lives of the majority of people in developing countries who still are rural and poor? How will climate change affect the lives of those who already face extreme poverty? This book explores the economics of these and other issues in an attempt to understand why some countries develop rapidly, whereas others seem not to develop at all. Remember that within each nation are people like Rachmina, Getachew, Viktor and Yulia, whose lives are deeply affected by the progress their nations make along the path toward economic development.

RICH AND POOR COUNTRIES

The countries with which this book is concerned have been labeled with many different terms. A term in vogue during the 1980s, especially in international forums, was the **third world**. Perhaps the best way to define it is by elimination. Take away the industrialized economies of western Europe, North America, and the Pacific (the first world, although it was rarely called that) and the industrialized, formerly centrally planned economies of eastern Europe (the second world), and the remaining countries constitute the third world. This terminology is used much less frequently today. The geographic configuration of the third world has led to a parallel distinction of **North** (first and second worlds) versus **South**, which still has some currency.

The more popular classifications used today implicitly put all countries on a continuum based on their degree of development. Therefore, we speak of the distinctions between developed and underdeveloped countries, more and less developed ones, or—to recognize continuing change—**developed countries** and **developing countries**. The degree of optimism implicit in the words *developing countries* and the handy acronym **LDCs** (less-developed countries), make these widely used terms, although they suffer from the problem that *developed* implies the process is fully complete for wealthier countries. The United Nations employs a classification scheme that refers to the poorest nations as the **least-developed countries**. Some Asian, eastern European, and Latin American economies, whose industrial output is growing rapidly, are sometimes referred to as **emerging economies**. Richer countries are frequently called **industrialized countries**, in recognition of the close association between development and industrialization. The highest-income countries are sometimes called postindustrial countries or service-based economies because services (finance, research and development, medical services, etc.), not manufacturing, account for the largest and most rapidly growing share of their economies.

The rich–poor dichotomy, based simply on income levels, has been refined by the World Bank[4] to yield a four-part classification:

- **Low-income economies**, with average incomes less than $1,005 per capita in 2010, converted into dollars at the current exchange rate.
- **Lower-middle-income economies**, with incomes between $1,006 and $3,975.
- **Upper-middle-income economies**, with incomes between $3,976 and $12,275.
- **High-income economies**, with incomes over $12,275.

The World Bank's classification system dates back to the 1970s. The Bank wanted poorer countries to receive better lending terms. To do so required some way to distinguish economic capacity for repaying loans. Gross national product

---

[4]The World Bank, formally the International Bank for Reconstruction and Development (IBRD), borrows funds on private capital markets in developed countries and lends to developing countries; through its affiliate the International Development Association (IDA), it receives contributions from the governments of developed countries and lends to low-income countries at very low interest rates with long repayment periods. The Bank, as it often is called, is perhaps the world's most important and influential development agency. Its role is explored in more detail in the discussion of foreign aid in Chapter 14.

(GNP) per capita, also referred to as GNI (gross national income) per capita, was adopted as such a measure. The actual cutoffs used to distinguish between low-, middle-, and high-income economies were based on natural gaps among countries. The threshold income levels are updated annually to account for international price inflation.[5]

Table 1–1 divides the world according to the Bank's classification scheme. It may surprise you that the largest number of countries, 70, falls into the high-income category. This is because in addition to the well-known rich nations such as France, Japan, and the United States, there are a large number of small rich nations, including Aruba, Brunei, Isle of Man, Liechtenstein, and Qatar. Despite the number, the high-income economies represent only 16 percent of the world's population. The middle-income economies represent 72 percent. China and India alone account for almost half of the population of the middle-income economies. The 35 low-income economies, the poorest nations in the world, represent 12 percent of humanity. These economies can be found mostly in sub-Saharan Africa. Haiti is the only nation in the Western Hemisphere that is still a low-income country. Other low-income nations are located throughout Asia, with Bangladesh being the most populous of these. As a group, the low-income nations in 2010 averaged just over $1,200 GNI per capita, measured in terms of **purchasing power parity (PPP)**. PPP is a way of accounting for the difference in prices between nations and gives a more accurate comparison of incomes among countries. (PPP is discussed at greater length in Chapter 2.) Average GNI per capita in low-income nations in 2010 was a mere 3.4 percent of the average GNI per capita of high-income nations, $37,183. We will have more to say about global income inequality in Chapter 6.

Table 1–1 provides a snapshot of the world in 2010. It tells us that one out of every two people in the world live in low- or lower-middle-income countries where the average standard of living is well below that in the upper-middle-income and high-income economies. But it does not tell us much about how things have changed over time. In 1983, when this textbook was first published, 16 percent of the world's population lived in high-income countries, the same percentage as today. But 50 percent of the world's population in 1983 lived in low-income countries, compared to only 12 percent today. This is a dramatic change, the result of rapid economic growth in China, India, and many other previously very poor nations.[6]

---

[5]The inflation rate used today is an average of inflation in the Euro Zone, Japan, the United Kingdom, and the United States.

[6]According to World Bank estimates, India graduated from low-income to lower-middle-income status in 2009. China became a lower-middle-income economy in the late 1990s and graduated into the upper-middle-income group in 2010. Because of systematic undervaluation of its currency, China actually graduated from one income category to the next earlier than reported by the World Bank. When China officially became an upper-middle-income economy in 2010, the average GNI per capita of both the lower and the upper-middle-income groups fell. Do you see why?

TABLE 1-1 Classification of World Economies, 2010

COUNTRY CLASSIFICATION	GNI PER CAPITA* (US$)	COUNTRIES† (NO.)	POPULATION IN MILLIONS (% OF WORLD TOTAL)	AVERAGE GNI PER CAPITA‡ (US$, PPP)	REGIONAL EXAMPLES§
Low-income	≤ $1,005	35	817 (12%)	$1,247	Ethiopia, Bangladesh, Cambodia, Haiti, Tajikistan
Lower-middle-income	$1,006–3,975	57	2,466 (36%)	$3,701	Senegal, Sri Lanka, Philippines, Ecuador, Jordan, Ukraine
Upper-middle-income	$3,976–12,275	54	2,449 (36%)	$9,904	Gabon, Malaysia, Brazil, Iran, Romania
High-income	>$12,275	70	1,123 (16%)	$37,183	Australia, France, Japan, Norway, Saudi Arabia, Taiwan, United States
World**	$9,097	216	6,855 (100%)	$11,058	

*Gross national income (GNI) per capita expressed in terms of current market exchange rates.
†Countries with populations of 30,000 or more people are included.
‡Average GNI per capita by income group in terms of current purchasing power parity (PPP).
§For the low- and middle-income groups, the examples are listed by World Bank geographical regions in the following order: Sub-Saharan Africa, South Asia, East Asia and Pacific, Latin America and the Caribbean, Middle East and North Africa, and Europe and Central Asia.
**World GNI per capita values are based on the population weighted average of all 216 countries.

Source: World Bank, "World Development Indicators," http://databank.worldbank.org.

GROWTH AND DEVELOPMENT

While the labels used to distinguish one set of countries from another can vary, one must be more careful with the terms used to describe the development process itself. The terms **economic growth** and **economic development** are sometimes used interchangeably, but they are fundamentally different. *Economic growth* refers to a rise in national or per capita income. If the production of goods and services in a country rises, by whatever means, and along with it average income increases, the country has achieved economic growth. Economic growth explains why the percentage of the world's population living in low-income countries, defined in terms of GNI per capita, has fallen so rapidly over the past three decades. *Economic development* implies more—particularly, improvements in health, education, and other aspects of human welfare. Countries that increase their income but do not also raise life expectancy, increase schooling, and expand individual opportunities are missing out on some important aspects of development. The extent to which economic growth supports these broader criteria for development is related to **income distribution** within countries. The average income figures cited earlier tell us nothing about how widely (or narrowly) the benefits of growth are shared within countries. If all of the increased income is concentrated in the hands of a few or spent on monuments or a military apparatus, there has been very little development in the sense that we mean.

Development is also usually accompanied by significant shifts in the structure of the economy, as more and more people typically shift away from rural agricultural production to urban-based and higher-paying employment, usually in manufacturing or services. Economic growth without structural change is often an indicator of the new income being concentrated in the hands of a few people. Situations of growth without development are the exceptions rather than the rule, but they do happen. Take the case of Equatorial Guinea, a small nation of fewer than 700,000 people on the west coast of Africa. The discovery and development of vast oil deposits off the nation's coast raised its GNI per capita income from an estimated US$330 in 1990 to US$12,420 in 2009. During the 2000s, Equatorial Guinea was the fastest-growing economy in the world, averaging growth rates of 25 percent per year, far greater than China, India, or any other successful economy. With growth rates of this magnitude, Equatorial Guinea moved from being a low- to a high-income economy in about a decade.

Does this also mean that Equatorial Guinea became a developed economy? By 2009, Equatorial Guinea had a per capita income comparable to Hungary's, but this is where the similarity between the two nations ends. Life expectancy in Equatorial Guinea stands at 50 years. In Hungary it is 74 years. About 90 percent of school-aged Hungarian children are enrolled in primary school; for Equatorial Guinea it is closer to 50 percent. Despite Equatorial Guinea's sudden high level of per capita income there has been little transformation in the low levels of education and poor health care of most Equatorial Guineans. Nor has there been much change in their economic activity. Rapid economic growth has not brought economic development to most of the population of Equatorial Guinea. But again, this case is the exception rather than the rule. In most cases, increases in per capita incomes and economic development have moved together.

Modern economic growth, the term used by Nobel laureate Simon Kuznets, refers to the current economic epoch as contrasted with, say, the epoch of merchant capitalism or the epoch of feudalism. The epoch of modern economic growth still is evolving, so all its features are not yet clear, but the key element has been the application of science to problems of economic production, which in turn has led to industrialization, urbanization, and even explosive growth in population. Finally, it should always be kept in mind that, although economic development and modern economic growth involve much more than a rise in per capita income or product, no sustained development can occur without economic growth.

DIVERSITY IN DEVELOPMENT ACHIEVEMENTS

A large number of less-developed countries have experienced growth in income over the past four decades and many have enjoyed substantial growth. The most rapidly growing economies have been in Asia and include China, India, Indonesia, Korea, Malaysia, and Thailand. But several non-Asian countries also are among the fast growers, such as Botswana, Chile, Estonia, and Mauritius. Since 1970, Botswana, a landlocked country in southern Africa, has been one of the fastest-growing economies in the world and one that has used its increased income to improve the lives of its citizens. Botswana's experience challenges the stereotype that all African countries have been stuck with little growth and development. At the same time, several Asian countries have grown slowly or not at all, including Myanmar (Burma), North Korea, and Papua New Guinea.

There are many examples of countries that have had an income growth exceeding 2 percent a year over the past four decades. At 2 percent annual growth, average income doubles in 35 years; at 4 percent, it doubles in 18 years. In most of these countries, manufacturing grew more rapidly than the gross domestic product and thus moved these economies through the inevitable structural change that reduces the share of income produced and labor employed in agriculture. Many other countries experienced slower (albeit positive) growth and development, with incomes growing 1 or 2 percent per year. In still others, incomes stagnated or declined. Most of the countries in this latter group are in Africa, although income also fell elsewhere, including in many of the transition economies of eastern Europe and Central Asia.

Perhaps the most remarkable changes in low-income countries in recent decades have been the virtually universal improvement in health conditions and the availability of schooling. From 1970 to 2009, the infant mortality rate in today's low-income nations fell dramatically from 147 to 76 per thousand births. This means that within this group of nations an additional 71 children out of every 1,000 lived to see their first birthday. For today's middle-income nations, which in 1970 included many countries that were still low-income, the results are similarly dramatic. Primary school enrollment became nearly universal in middle-income economies and rose substantially in most of the low-income countries. With few exceptions, more than three-quarters of eligible children attend primary school in poor countries. Despite this good news, more than 1 billion people in the developing world continue to live in extreme poverty.

The study of economic development is not mainly a review of what has and has not been accomplished in the past. It is a field concerned most of all with the future, particularly the future of the least-advantaged people in the world. To comprehend the future, one must first try to understand how we got to the point where we are now. But the future will not be just a replay or a projection of trends of the past, as new forces that will shape that future also are at work. Some of these forces can be seen clearly today, whereas others are only dimly perceived, if they are seen at all.

Any list of changes that will make the future of economic development different from the past should probably start with the information revolution. Greatly enhanced communication around the world as represented by the Internet has sped up the flow of ideas across oceans and borders to an unprecedented degree. Lower transport costs, together with better information, contribute to global production networks and the expansion of global trade and investment. The rapid flow of information is also having an impact on politics by making it harder for authoritarian regimes to control what their people are allowed to know. Partly for this reason, democratic regimes are becoming more the norm than the exception in developing countries, and there is reason to expect this trend to continue.

Not all the foreseeable trends of the future are positive. Despite the benefits of advanced technology and the information revolution, some groups in society, notably the better educated, may capture most of the gains while other large groups are left behind. The experience with HIV/AIDS must keep us vigilant for whatever the next new infectious disease might be. Natural disaster—droughts, earthquakes, hurricanes, and tsunamis—hit rich and poor nations alike, but the effects are usually far more severe the poorer the country. Environmental degradation is much more serious today than it was a century ago, when Europe and North America were in the early stages of economic growth. Global warming, as a result, is a problem likely to play an important role in our future. The one positive change in the environmental sphere is that people around the world are becoming aware of the danger at a much faster pace than in the past, though international cooperation in limiting climate change remains a challenge.

We probably are not even aware of many of the forces that will shape the future economic development of nations. No one at the end of the nineteenth century had heard of nuclear energy, DNA, or integrated circuits. No one in the 1970s had heard of cell phones, laptop computers, or antiretroviral (ARV) drugs used to treat HIV/AIDS. Given the pace of change in the current world of the new millennium, similar and possibly greater discoveries will profoundly influence how economies develop. That said, we cannot rely on future discoveries to solve the problems of economic development and poverty among nations. We must try to understand how the nations of the world got to where they are today so that we can do a better job of raising living standards for all in the future.

APPROACHES TO DEVELOPMENT

This book is not for readers looking for a simple explanation of why some countries are still poor or how poverty can be overcome. Library shelves are full of studies explaining how development will occur if only a country will increase the amount it saves and invests or intensify its efforts to export, among other prescriptions.

For two decades in the mid-twentieth century, industrialization through import substitution—the replacement of imports with home-produced goods—was considered by many to be the shortest path to development. In the 1970s, labor-intensive techniques, income redistribution, and provision of basic human needs to the poor gained popularity as keys to development. More recently, economists have counseled governments to avoid high protective barriers and to depend substantially on markets to set prices and allocate resources. A different theme for some analysts is that development will be possible only with a massive shift of resources, in the form of foreign aid and investment, from the richest countries to the poorest. Others call for debt forgiveness for poor nations that have found it difficult to repay earlier loans.

No single factor is responsible for poverty, and no single policy or strategy can set in motion the complex process of economic development. Each of the various explanations and solutions to the development problem makes sense if placed in the proper context and makes no sense at all outside that set of circumstances. Import substitution has carried some countries toward economic development, but export promotion has helped others when import substitution bogged down. Prices badly distorted from their free-market values can stifle initiative and hence growth, but removing those distortions leads to development only when other conditions are met as well. Finally, where leaders backed by interests hostile to development rule countries, those leaders and their constituents must be removed from power before growth can occur. Fortunately, the majority of developing countries have governments that want to promote development.

This book is not neutral toward all issues of development. Where controversy exists we shall point it out. Indeed, the authors of this book differ among themselves over some questions of development policy. But we share a common point of view on certain basic points.

This text extensively uses the theoretical tools of mainstream economics in the belief that these tools contribute substantially to our understanding of development problems and their solution. The text does not rely solely or even primarily on theory, however. For five decades and more, development economists and economic historians have been building up an empirical record against which these theories can be tested, and this book draws heavily on many of these empirical studies. We try to give real-country examples for the major points made in this book. In part, these examples come from the individual country and cross-country comparative studies of others, but they also are drawn extensively from our own personal experiences working on development issues around the world. The several authors who contributed to this textbook, both the current and past editions, have been fortunate enough to study and work over long periods of time in Bolivia, Chile, China, the Gambia, Ghana, Indonesia, Kenya, Korea, Malaysia, Nepal, Peru, Samoa, Sri Lanka, Tanzania, Vietnam, and Zambia. At one time or another, at least one nation from this group has exemplified virtually all the approaches to development now extant.

THE STUDY OF DEVELOPMENT ECONOMICS

If you are like most students taking a course in development economics this will not be your first course in economics. Most likely, you have taken courses in principles of microeconomics and macroeconomics. Some of you may have also studied intermediate economic theory, statistics, econometrics, and other economic subfields. Your study of these subjects will prove extremely useful in your examination of development economics. In your introductory microeconomics class you learned the importance of incentives and how markets tend to clear when quantity demanded equals quantity supplied. In macroeconomics you learned how expanding the money supply can lead to inflation. These insights are as applicable to poor nations as they are to rich ones. But there also are important differences between your earlier study of economics and the study of development. Context matters.

If you took your micro principles courses in a college or university in the United States or other high-income country, the examples you were given and the problems you studied reflected those of a rich nation. Rent control is a common example included in principles textbooks to explain price ceilings and how they can have unintended effects, including housing shortages and black market prices. In a developing country, price ceilings will have the same impact but are unlikely to be used to control apartment prices. A better example might be how governments have attempted to use price ceilings to *lower* urban food prices for urban consumers (usually at the expense of farmers, who are often much poorer than urban consumers). Rich nations are more prone to employ price floors to *raise* food prices and support farm incomes.

When discussing taxes, authors of principles textbooks in the United States will focus on how marginal tax rates can affect the supply of labor—the higher the tax, the less likely workers will want to work. In poor nations, the presence of such taxes is most likely to encourage growth in the informal sector in which people are employed, although those workers evade paying taxes on their earnings. This happens in rich nations too but is a much less common response. In low-income nations, the lack of secure property rights to land helps explain squatter settlements and urban slums. This is not much of a problem in rich nations and is less likely to be discussed.

In learning macroeconomics, you may have studied how an expansion in the money supply may cause a nation's exchange rate to depreciate. You were less likely to have learned how a country can fix its exchange rate intentionally to undervalue its currency. Such practices are far more common in developing nations (including China) than in developed ones. You might have read about the importance of the independence of the Federal Reserve System in the United States, which helps insulate decisions about monetary policy from domestic politics. But in developing nations, the lack of independence of central banks is far more likely.

The study of macroeconomics in high-income economies tends to focus on economic stabilization—that is, on how monetary and fiscal policy can be used to keep unemployment down and inflation low. Economic growth is less of a focus, in part because of the success high-income economies have had in growing their economies. To the extent you studied economic growth, much of the focus was on technological change as a determinant of growth. In the development setting, economic growth and structural change are central issues in the field. Growth rates depend not only on the technological frontier but also on the ability to mobilize savings and engage in productive investment. These issues will capture much of our attention in the chapters that follow.

A final difference between the study of economics in a developed versus a developing nation context is the role of **institutions**. Economic theory tends to take institutions (the rules of the game that govern the functioning of markets, banking systems, enforcement of property rights, and so on) as a given. But development is concerned with how one creates and strengthens institutions that facilitate development in the first place. How, for example, does a country acquire a government interested in and capable of promoting economic growth? Can efficiently functioning markets be created in countries that currently lack them, or should the state take over the functions normally left to the market elsewhere? Is a fully developed financial system a precondition for growth, or can a country do without at least some parts of such a system? Is land reform necessary for development and, if so, what kind of land reform? What legal systems are needed to support market-based growth? These institutional issues and many others like them are at the heart of the development process and will reappear in different guises throughout this book.

The economics you have studied before is an important foundation for the study of development economics. Be prepared to build on it.

ORGANIZATION

This book is divided into four parts. Part 1 examines the main factors, both those suggested by economic theory and those supported by empirical investigations, that contribute to differing rates of economic growth. This discussion involves the deliberate choices by governments, including the debate over how economic development should be guided or managed.

Part 2 goes beyond issues of economic growth and focuses directly on inequality and poverty. Because economic development first and foremost is a process involving people, who are both the prime movers of development and its beneficiaries, Part 2 deals with how human resources are transformed in the process of economic development and how that transformation contributes to the development process itself. Individual chapters are devoted to population, education, and health.

The other major physical input in the growth process is capital. Part 3 is concerned with how capital is mobilized and allocated for development purposes. From where, for example, do savings come and how are they transformed into investment? How does government mobilize the resources to finance development? What kind of financial system is consistent with rapid capital accumulation? Will inflation enhance or hinder the process, and what roles will foreign aid and investment play?

Especially in the early stages of development, countries depend heavily on agriculture and on the export of food, fuel, and raw materials. Part 4 discusses strategies to enhance the productivity of such primary industries as a first, and often a continuing, task in stimulating economic development. Part 4 also explores trade in primary products, in manufactured goods and increasingly in services, too. In a more globalized world economy, trade plays a larger role in low- and middle-income nations than ever before. Part 4 concludes with the all-important question of environmental sustainability and the challenges developing nations confront in the face of climate change.

SUMMARY

- The last 40 years have seen a wide diversity of development experiences around the world. Some countries, including some very large ones like China, India, and Indonesia, have experienced rapid growth and development. Others, particularly many African countries and some in eastern Europe, have experienced stagnation or even a decline in incomes. Understanding the differences in these experiences and the lessons for the future is the core purpose of this book.

- Many different terms are used to differentiate poor from rich countries, but this text mainly uses the terms *developing* and *low-* and *middle-income economies* to refer to those nations with incomes substantially lower than the *developed* and *high-income* nations.

- Only 12 percent of the world's population today lives in low-income economies, nations with a GNI per capita falling below US$1,005 (in 2010). Twenty-five years ago, *half* of the world's population lived in low-income nations. Economic growth in China, India, and many other previously poor nations accounts for this historic change. Of course, many very poor people still live in these economies, but their numbers have fallen significantly.

- *Economic growth* refers to an increase in per capita incomes, whereas *economic development* involves, in addition, improvements in health and education and major structural changes, such as industrialization and urbanization. Some countries may have economic growth, usually because of the discovery of great mineral wealth, but not development because they retain many of the structural features of a traditional society.

- No single factor is responsible for poverty, and no single policy or strategy can set in motion the complex process of economic development. We can learn much from the past experience of other nations, especially those that have achieved rapid growth and experienced economic development in recent decades.

- We must also be aware that new forces, from new diseases to new technologies, will influence the path and opportunities facing today's developing nations. Changes in the global climate, including the planet's physical climate as well as its economic and political climate, will also impact the course nations follow.
- The economics of development bears a lot in common with the economics you may have studied in other courses. But it is also different. Context matters. A focus on long-term economic growth and structural change in the economy and on the role of institutions commands the attention of development economists.

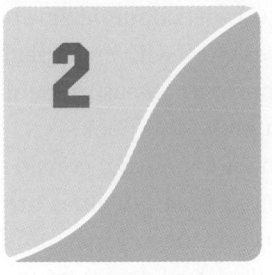

2

Measuring Economic Growth and Development

A native American saying recommends, "One should not go hunting a bear unless one knows what a bear looks like." This is sound advice for bear hunters; it also has meaning for our inquiry. Understanding how to achieve economic development requires some agreement on what we want to achieve.

The previous chapter drew a distinction between economic growth and economic development. Economic growth refers to a rise in real national income per capita— that is, a rise in the inflation-adjusted, per person, value of goods and services produced by an economy. This is a relatively objective measure of economic capacity. It is widely recognized and can be computed with varying degrees of accuracy for most economies. There is far less of a consensus on how to define economic development. Most people would include in their definition increases in the material well-being of individuals as well as improvements in basic health and education. Others might add changes in the structure of production (away from agriculture toward manufacturing and services), improvement in the environment, greater economic equality, or an increase in political freedom. Economic development is a normative concept, one not readily captured by any single measure or index.

To understand the magnitude of the global challenge of development, it is essential to be able to track what has happened to an economy over time and make comparisons between countries. If we want to understand why some nations experienced more rapid growth and development than others, we need measures of economic performance that are relatively accurate and comparable. Poor countries are environments in which information is scarce and data can be of questionable quality, so we have to assure ourselves that our indicators, though imperfect, are sufficiently robust to help us understand the outcomes we observe. The study of economic development requires us to combine our insights on how economies work with an appeal to the evidence to check if our insights are consistent with experience. Measurement is central to this process and will be an issue we return to throughout this book.

To get started, this chapter introduces measures of national income and considers the problem of making cross-country comparisons when national incomes are expressed in different currencies. Equipped with a means of making comparisons of national income levels, we examine the record both over time and across countries. These data highlight the enormous differences in economic growth that have characterized different regions of the world over the past 500 years as well as over the more recent past. Much of the rest of this book is devoted to understanding what has caused these differences.

Economic growth may be central to achieving economic development, but there is much more to economic development than growth alone. Not only the level of per capita income but how that income is produced, spent, and distributed within and between countries determines development outcomes. There is much debate about how to define and measure economic development. We introduce two widely cited indicators of economic development, the human development index and the millennium development goals, and consider their strengths and weaknesses. The information presented in this chapter may not make you a better bear hunter but it will inform the rest of your study of development economics.

MEASURING ECONOMIC GROWTH

At the core of studies of economic growth are changes in national income. Two basic measures of national income are commonly employed. **Gross national product (GNP)** is the sum of the value of finished goods and services produced by a society during a given year. GNP excludes intermediate goods (goods used up in the production of other goods, such as the steel used in an automobile or the chips that go into a computer). GNP counts output produced by citizens of the country, including the value of goods and services produced by citizens who live outside its borders. GNP is one of the most common terms used in national income accounting. The World Bank and other multilateral institutions often refer to this same concept as gross national income (GNI). **Gross domestic product (GDP)** is similar to GNP, except that it counts all output produced within the borders of a country, including output produced by resident foreigners, but excludes the value of production by citizens living abroad. GNP or GDP divided by total population provides a measure of **per capita income**. Economic growth refers to changes in per capita income over time.

The distinction between GNP and GDP can be illustrated using examples from two very different economies, Angola and Bangladesh. More than three-quarters of

Angola's national income is derived from oil. Multinational companies drill for most of the oil and repatriate their profits. These profits count as part of Angola's GDP but not its GNP. In 2009, Angola's GDP was 12 percent higher than its GNP. By contrast, Bangladesh has few natural resources and little foreign investment. Large numbers of Bangladeshis work abroad, especially in the Persian Gulf: men often as construction workers and Bangladeshi women as domestics. The value of the output produced by these Bangladeshi workers counts as part of Bangladesh's GNP (since these workers are Bangladeshi nationals) but not as part of its GDP (because the work is performed outside of the country). In 2009, Bangladesh's GNP was 9 percent higher than its GDP. In most countries the differences between GNP and GDP are much smaller. In part because it is easier to track economic activity within a nation's borders, GDP has become the more widely used measure of national income by the International Monetary Fund (IMF), UN Development Programme, World Bank, and other multilateral agencies as well as by researchers engaged in analyzing cross-country data and trends. We follow this convention and refer primarily to GDP and GDP per capita as measures of national income from here on. Unless otherwise indicated, when discussing trends over time, we refer to **real GDP** and real GDP per capita—that is, per capita gross domestic product adjusted for domestic price inflation.[1]

The contribution of a sector or component of GDP, such as manufacturing or agriculture, is measured by the value added by that sector. **Value added** refers to the incremental gain to the price of a product at a particular stage of production. Therefore, the value added of the cotton textile industry is the value of the textiles when they leave the factory minus the value of raw cotton and other materials used in their production. At the same time, the value added is equal to the payments made to the factors of production in the textile industry: wages paid to labor plus profits, interest, depreciation of capital, and rent for buildings and land. Because the total value added at all stages of production equals total output, GDP is a measure of both total *income* and total *output*.

MEASURING GDP: WHAT IS LEFT OUT?

One way to calculate GDP is to add up the value of all the goods and services produced within a country and then sold on the market. The focus on goods and services sold in the market creates a measurement problem because many valuable contributions to society are excluded. When a farm household pays someone else to dig an irrigation ditch or repair a roof, such economic activity is included in GDP because these activities are purchased "in the market." However, when unpaid members of

---

[1]Real GDP is computed by deflating nominal GDP (GDP measured in current prices) by a price index. National statistical offices often calculate a variety of price indices, including the consumer price index (CPI), the GDP deflator, and others. What these indices share in common is an attempt to isolate any general increase (or decrease) in the price level for all goods.

the household perform these same tasks, they tend not to enter GDP. The scale of this problem tends to be larger in low-income countries and is evident in a poor nation like Cambodia, where about one-third of the labor force is classified as unpaid family workers, most of whom are engaged on family farms, producing food and other goods and services for their own consumption.

In most developing countries, a large number of activities do not enter the market. Much of what is produced by the agricultural sector is consumed by the farm household and never exchanged in the marketplace. To not include this production would seriously underestimate a nation's GDP. The usual practice is to include estimates from sample surveys of farm output consumed by the producer, which are then valued at the prices of marketed farm produce. This is done, for example, in Moldova and even includes the output of household garden plots. In India, estimates are made for the construction of traditional homes made out of mud, straw, and other local materials. Even illegal activity may be included, as in Afghanistan where estimates of poppy production, a banned crop, are part of the nation's GDP. Despite these adjustments, not all household production is accounted for. As economies grow, more output is transacted in the marketplace and gets included in GDP. The resulting estimates of GDP may overestimate the growth in economic activity because some of what is now captured is merely a transfer of production from within the household to the market.

An additional measurement problem for GDP arises from the need to compare apples with oranges in calculating the value of national output. A typical economy might produce thousands of different goods and services. Adding up the total value of goods and services that are traded in markets requires using their market prices. But accurate price information may not be available or may not be representative of market prices at the national level. Government agencies in poor countries may lack the means to conduct thorough market surveys of prices or may rely too heavily on information from major urban centers (where prices may be easier to track but are unrepresentative of markets around the country).

Another criticism of GDP is that it may be a measure of the goods and services produced by an economy, but does not account for the "bads" society produces. If a steel mill pollutes a river or the air, the value of the steel produced is included in GDP but the cost of pollution is not deducted. Should crime, congestion, and other social bads be deducted from estimates of GDP? *Gross* domestic product also does not account for the depreciation of goods (for example, when machinery or trucks wear out) or depletion of natural resources (when forests are cut, fisheries depleted, or mines exhausted). Proposals for making adjustments to GDP to account for these factors have been raised, but none has been widely adopted yet.[2] Although there are

---

[2] In 2008, President Nicolas Sarkozy of France established the international Commission on the Measurement of Economic Performance and Social Progress that included discussion of GDP as a useful measure. The commission, chaired by Joseph Stiglitz, a Nobel laureate in economics, raised many concerns about GDP as a measure of economic production and as a measure of the quality of life and of sustainability. More information is available at www.stiglitz-sen-fitoussi.fr/documents/rapport_anglais.pdf.

obvious flaws in GDP as a measure of national income, there are also many benefits. Having a widely agreed on approach to measuring national income facilitates comparisons of nations' economic activity both over time and relative to other countries. Both types of comparisons are essential to understanding the process of economic development.

EXCHANGE-RATE CONVERSION PROBLEMS

Another measurement issue we need to consider is how to compare *levels* of GDP per capita across countries. The problem arises because each nation measures national income in its own currency: dinar in Tunisia, guarani in Paraguay, leu in Moldova, and so on. Economic growth rates can be computed in a nation's own currency, but if we want to understand better what is required to transform a nation from low to high income, it is useful to compare nations at different income levels. To do so requires converting GDP per capita into a common currency. The shortcut to accomplishing this goal is to use the market exchange rate between one currency, usually U.S. dollars, and each national currency. For example, to convert India's GDP per capita (2009) of about 57,000 rupees into U.S. dollars, use the appropriate exchange rate between the two currencies (about 49 rupees per US$1 in 2009), which in this case yields an estimate of about US$1,160.

A common reaction to this low figure by anyone who has lived in or visited India (or for that matter any developing nation) is that one U.S. dollar goes much further in India than it does in the United States. A basic woman's haircut in a less-affluent part of Mumbai, for example, might cost 200 rupees (US$4 at the official exchange rate), whereas a basic haircut in Boston might run US$40. If one can buy more for $1 in India than one can in the United States—in this example, 10 haircuts in Mumbai for the price of 1 in Boston—then India's true level of per capita income must be higher than the one given by converting currency using the official exchange rate.

There is considerable merit to this argument. One problem with converting per capita income levels from one currency to another is that exchange rates, particularly those of developing countries, can be distorted. Trade restrictions or direct government intervention in setting the exchange rate make it possible for an official exchange rate to be substantially different from a rate determined by a competitive market for foreign exchange.

But even the widespread existence of competitively determined market exchange rates would not eliminate the problem. The huge price difference in haircuts between Boston and Mumbai is not the result of trade restrictions or a managed Indian exchange rate. Instead, a significant part of national income is made up of what are called **nontraded goods and services**—that is, goods that do not and often cannot enter into international trade. Haircuts are one example. Internal transportation, whether by bus, taxi, or train, cannot be traded, although many transport inputs, such automobiles and rail cars, can be imported. Wholesale and retail trade and elementary school education also are nontraded services. Land, homes, and office buildings are other obvious examples of goods that are not exchanged across national borders. Generally speaking, whereas the prices of traded goods tend to be similar across countries (because, in the absence of tariffs and other trade barriers, international trade could exploit any price differences), the prices of nontraded goods can differ widely from one country to the next. This is because the markets for nontraded goods are spatially separated and the underlying supply and demand curves can intersect in different places, yielding different prices.

Exchange rates are determined largely by the flow of traded goods and international capital and generally do not reflect the relative prices of nontraded goods. As a result, GDP converted to U.S. dollars by market exchange rates gives misleading comparisons of income levels if the ratio of prices of nontraded goods to prices of traded goods is different in the countries being compared. The way around this problem is to pick a set of prices for all goods and service prevailing in one country and to use that set of prices to value the goods and services of all countries being compared. In effect, one is calculating a purchasing power parity (PPP) exchange rate. Thus a cement block, a computer chip, or a haircut is assigned the same value whether it is produced in New Delhi or New York.

The essence of the procedure can be illustrated by the numerical exercise presented in Table 2–1. The two economies in the table are called the United States and India for illustrative purposes, and each economy produces one traded commodity (steel) and one nontraded service (retail sales). Each economy produces a different amount of each good. GDP, expressed in local currencies, is equal to the total value of production of steel plus retail sales. A ton of rolled steel sells for about $1,000 in the United States and Rs 50,000 in India. The value of the services of retail sales personnel is estimated in the most commonly used way, which is to assume the value of the service is equal to the wages of the worker providing the service. (For the United States we assume earnings of $10 per hour, working 40 hours per week for 50 weeks, for annual earnings of $20,000. In India, we assume annual earnings of Rs 60,000.) Wages are likely to differ widely across countries and to be determined almost exclusively by domestic labor supply and labor demand conditions. This is because workers cannot easily migrate from one country to another to take advantage of any differences in wages (partly because of immigration rules and partly because the cost of moving to a new country can be high, both financially and psychically). From the data in Table 2–1 we determine that GDP in the United States equals $240 billion and in India, Rs 1,490 billion.

One way of comparing the GDP levels in the two economies is to convert them into a single currency, say, the U.S. dollar. In this simple world of two goods and two nations, the exchange rate is determined solely by trade in steel. If steel is freely traded between the two countries, then the exchange rate settles where the price per ton of steel in the two countries is equal—that is, at the point at which the U.S. price of $1,000 per ton equals India's price of Rs 50,000 per ton or

TABLE 2-1 **Market Exchange Rate Versus Purchasing Power Parity Methods of Converting GDP**

	UNITED STATES			INDIA		
	QUANTITY	PRICE (US$)	VALUE OF OUTPUT (BILLION US$)	QUANTITY	PRICE (RUPEES)	VALUE OF OUTPUT (BILLION RUPEES)
Steel (million tons)	200	1,000 per ton	200	25	50,000 per ton	1,250
Retail sales personnel (millions)	2	20,000 per person per year	40	4	60,000 per person per year	240
Total GDP (local currency, billions)			240			1,490

Market exchange rate based on steel prices = Rs 50,000/$1,000 or Rs 50 = US$1.

1. India's gross domestic product (GDP) in U.S. dollars calculated by using the official exchange rate: Rs 1,490 billion/Rs 50 = US$29.8 billion.

2. India's GDP in U.S. dollars calculated by using U.S. prices for each individual product or service and applying that price to India's quantities (that is, using purchasing power parity [PPP]):
   Steel: 25 million tons $\times$ $1,000/ton = $25 billion
   Retail sales personnel: 4 million people $\times$ $20,000/person = $80 billion
   GDP: $25 billion + $80 billion = $105 billion

3. Ratio of PPP calculation of India's GDP to official exchange rate calculation: $105 billion/$29.8 billion = 3.5

where US$1 = Rs 50.[3] Using this market-determined exchange rate, India's GDP of Rs 1,490 billion equals US$29.8 billion, or about 12 percent of U.S. GDP in this hypothetical example.

The problem with this comparison is that, although Rs 50 and US$1 purchase the same amount of steel in both countries, they purchase different amounts of the nontraded good. To compare the GDP levels of the two nations taking into account this difference in the purchasing power of the respective currencies, we cannot rely on market exchange rates. An alternative approach is to use a common set of prices applied to the output of both countries. We can calculate Indian GDP in U.S. dollars by applying U.S. prices for each product or service to India's quantities. (We could also compute U.S. GDP in terms of India's prices but the convention is to express PPP estimates in terms of U.S. dollars.) This PPP calculation results in India's steel production valued at US$25 billion and retail sales valued at US$80 billion, for an estimated India GDP of US$105 billion. In this example, the PPP calculation of

[3]At any other exchange rate, there would be profitable opportunities to buy more steel from one of the two countries, causing changes in the market for foreign exchange until the two steel prices were equivalent and the exchange rate settled at US$1 = Rs 50. This is sometimes referred to as *the law of one price,* reflecting how opportunities for arbitrage in traded goods lead to price convergence in these goods.

India's GDP is more than three times as large as the calculation that relied on market exchange rates. In terms of PPP, India's GDP is over 40 percent of the U.S. GDP.

Table 2–1 presents a hypothetical PPP conversion for two countries using two goods. The task becomes significantly more complicated in a world of tens of thousands of goods and more than 200 nations. The **International Comparison Program (ICP)**, which began in 1968 under the auspices of the United Nations and is now overseen by the World Bank, tackles this difficult task by deriving a set of **international prices** in a common currency. Detailed price data on a basket of hundreds of specific goods have been collected periodically for an ever-increasing number of nations. International prices are then derived by aggregating the price data from the individual countries and are used to determine the value of national output at these standardized international prices. The most recent round of international price comparisons released by the ICP was based on 2005 data and represented a significant quality improvement over the previous round of price data from 1993. Key elements of this improvement were coverage of a larger number of countries (146 countries in 2005 as compared to only 118 in 1993) and more careful comparison of specific goods and services across countries. (The next update of the ICP will be based on 2011 data, to be released in 2013.) Estimates of national income in terms of PPP are reported in the publications of the IMF, UN Development Programme (UNDP), World Bank, and other multilateral agencies. Researchers have made extensive use of these data.[4]

The ratio of GDP per capita based on international prices relative to GDP using official exchange rates ranged in 2009 from about 0.7 in Norway to 3.3 in the Gambia (Table 2–2). For high-income countries, like Germany, Japan, and the United Kingdom, the ratio is close to 1.0. This means market exchange rate conversion is a close approximation of what is obtained when converting German, Japanese, or UK GDP into international price dollars using the PPP method. This is to be expected because at similar levels of income the prices of nontraded goods tend to be similar as well. For low- and middle-income economies the ratio is greater than 1, consistent with the finding that the degree to which the official exchange rate conversion method understates GNP is related, generally, to the average income of the country. For China the ratio is 1.8, for Bolivia 2.5, for Vietnam and Ethiopia 2.7, and for India 2.8.

With differences of this magnitude, comparisons of per capita income levels using market exchange rate conversions can be misleading. Market exchange rates suggest that per capita incomes in the United States were about 40 times those in India in 2009. PPP calculations narrow the multiple to about 14 times—still a huge gap but maybe a more reasonable indicator of relative income levels. Another way of appreciating the difference between making comparisons of GDP using market exchange rates versus PPP is to think about world GDP as a whole. When world GDP

---

[4]If you read *The Economist* you may be familiar with another measure of PPP, the Big Mac index, which was introduced, lightheartedly, in 1986 and has been reported on annually ever since. The common basket of goods is a cheese hamburger with lettuce, onions, and pickles on a sesame bun. For a discussion of the Big Mac index as a measure of PPP, see M. Pakko and P. Pollard, "Burger Survey Provides Taste for International Economics," Federal Reserve Bank of St. Louis, *The Regional Economist* (January 2004), 12–13.

TABLE 2-2 Comparing GDP per Capita Using Market Exchange Rates and PPP in 2009 (US$)

COUNTRY	GDP AT MARKET EXCHANGE RATES	GDP AT PPP	RATIO OF PPP CALCULATION TO MARKET EXCHANGE RATE CALCULATION
Norway	79,089	56,214	0.7
Japan	39,738	32,417	0.8
Germany	40,670	36,378	0.9
United Kingdom	35,165	35,155	1.0
United States*	45,989	45,989	1.0
Hungary	12,868	20,312	1.6
Lebanon	8,175	13,070	1.6
China	3,744	6,828	1.8
Botswana	6,064	13,384	2.2
Bolivia	1,751	4,419	2.5
Vietnam	1,113	2,953	2.7
Ethiopia	344	934	2.7
India	1,192	3,296	2.8
The Gambia	430	1,415	3.3

*Gross domestic product (GDP) per capita in the United States is unchanged when measured in terms of purchasing power parity (PPP). This must be the case because the United States is used as the reference country by the International Comparison Program (ICP). As with any index number, the price index at the heart of the ICP must be compared relative to some base, and by convention, U.S. prices were selected.

Source: World Bank, "World Development Indicators," http://databank.worldbank.org.

is calculated by converting each nation's GDP into a common currency using market exchange rates, the low- and middle-income economies account for 29 percent of world output. When the calculation is based on PPP, the low- and middle-income economies account for 44 percent of world output.

PPP allows for more valid comparisons of real income levels across economies. But PPP has its limits too. Trade and capital flows are transacted at market exchange rates and should be converted at those rates. The ICP provides a consistent set of PPP estimates of national income, but these are only estimates and critics have pointed out flaws in data collection and methodology.[5] PPP conversions cannot correct for

[5]Angus Deaton provides a useful introduction to the ICP in "Reshaping the World: The 2005 Round of the International Comparison Program," in Prasada Rao and Fred Vogel, eds., *Measuring the Size of the World Economy: The Framework, Methodology, and Results from the International Comparison Program* (Washington, DC, World Bank, in press). Problems associated with constructing PPP estimates are discussed in Angus Deaton and Alan Heston, "Understanding PPPs and PPP-Based National Accounts," *American Economic Journal: Macroeconomics* 2, no. 4 (2010), 36–45.

underlying problems in the measurement of GDP in a nation's own currency. Variations in the quality of goods cloud cross-country comparisons. In addition, the specific price index constructed by the International Comparison Project gives more weight to the goods consumed in rich nations and tends to bias upward the GDP of poorer nations that consume a different basket of goods. This index number problem occurs whenever one studies the aggregate performance of an economy over time or compares the performance of different economies. But, despite these problems, much can be learned from the data at hand, and PPP estimates of GDP per capita are central to the study of economic growth and development.

ECONOMIC GROWTH AROUND THE WORLD: A BRIEF OVERVIEW

We now turn from exploring the measurement of GDP to examining the actual performance of countries around the world in terms of the rate of growth of GDP per capita.[6] We begin by looking at the findings of economic historian Angus Maddison, who estimated income levels and corresponding rates of economic growth for the world economy as far back as the year 1 B.C.E. Such an exercise requires a lot of conjecture, especially the further back in time one goes. To perform the analysis, Maddison compiled estimates of population, GDP, and a price index for determining PPP.[7]

According to Maddison's calculations, average world income in 1000 was virtually the same as it had been 1,000 years earlier. In other words, growth in per capita income between 1 B.C.E. and 1000 was effectively zero. The next 820 years (from 1000 to 1820) were barely any better, with world income per capita growing, on average, by just 0.05 percent per year. (Note: This is not a growth rate of 5 percent; it is a growth rate of 0.05 percent.) During those 820 years, world GDP grew by only slightly more than the growth in world population. After eight centuries, world per capita income had increased by only 50 percent. To place this in some perspective, China today is one of the world's fastest-growing economies. With more than 1 billion people (about four times the entire world's population in 1000), economic growth in China averaged about 9.5 percent over the past decade, raising Chinese per capita incomes by 50 percent, not in 820 years but in just under 5 years!

---

[6]In this section we derive the growth rate of real GDP per capita in PPP using the formula for annual compound growth, $Y_t = Y_0(1 + r)^t$, where Y refers to real GDP per capita in PPP; t, the number of years under consideration; r, the rate of growth of real GDP per capita; and Y_0 refers to real GDP per capita in the base year and Y_t in the final year. Alternative ways of estimating growth rates are discussed in Box 3–2.

[7]Angus Maddison died in 2010. His work is being maintained by his colleagues. The data reported here are from Maddison's original web page titled "Statistics on World Population, GDP and Per Capita GDP, 1–2008 AD." Links are available at www.ggdc.net/MADDISON/oriindex.htm, accessed February 2012.

Maddison's estimates indicate considerable uniformity in per capita incomes throughout the first millennium. The little bit of economic growth that did take place over the next 800 years was centered in western Europe and in what Maddison calls the western "offshoots" (Australia, Canada, New Zealand, and the United States). By 1820, these regions already had a decided advantage over the rest of the world. For example, whereas China and India may have been slightly ahead of the western European countries in 1000, average per capita incomes in western Europe and in their offshoots were already double those of China and India by 1820. Box 2–1 offers one explanation for some of the early and divergent trends and their consequences for the world we live in today.

Maddison's research suggests that rapid economic growth as we know it really began around 1820. He estimates that over the subsequent 190 years, the average growth in world income increased to 1.3 percent per year. Note that the difference between annual growth of 0.05 percent and 1.3 percent is huge. With the world economy growing at 0.05 percent per year, it would take more than 1,400 years for average income to double. With annual growth of 1.3 percent, average income doubles in just 55 years. The world had changed from no growth at all during the first millennium, to slow growth for most of the second millennium, to a situation in which, in the past two centuries, average real income began to double in less than every three generations.

Maddison's estimates of average income levels for the world's major regions since 1820 are shown in Figure 2–1.[8] Several features of these data are notable. First, economic growth rates clearly accelerated around the world since the early 1800s and especially after 1880. Second, and perhaps most striking, the richest countries recorded the fastest growth rates and the poorest countries recorded the slowest growth rates, at least until 1950. Per capita income in the Western offshoots grew by about 1.6 percent per year between 1820 and 1950, while in Asia it grew by only 0.16 percent. As a result, the ratio of the average incomes in the richest regions to those in the poorest regions grew from about 2:1 in 1820 to about 13:1 in 1950.

Between 1950 and 2008, the patterns of economic growth changed, at least in several regions. The gap between the Western offshoots and western Europe, which had been widening through 1950, narrowed significantly. The poorest region in 1950 (Asia) recorded the fastest subsequent growth rate (3.6 percent), thereby beginning to close the income gap with the richer regions of the world. By contrast, Latin America's growth stagnated during the 1980s and 1990s, and eastern Europe's collapsed after the fall of the Berlin Wall in 1989. Both regions resumed economic growth during the 2000s.

[8]Note that the *y*-axis in Figure 2–1 expresses GDP per capita in PPP using Geary-Khamis (GK) dollars, another PPP index. Figure 2–1 also expresses per capita income in logarithms. We will have more to say about the use of log scales later in this chapter. For now, it will be useful to know that when using a log scale, the slopes of the lines for each region are estimates of the growth rate of GDP per capita.

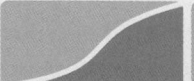

BOX 2-1 JARED DIAMOND: GUNS, GERMS, AND STEEL

Most of this textbook is devoted to understanding why over the past 50 years some countries have experienced rapid economic growth and development while others have not. Jared Diamond, a physiologist, geographer, and Pulitzer Prize–winning author, poses a related but different question. The world as we know it is the result of the historical dominance of Eurasians, especially people of Europe and East Asia. Why, Diamond asks, did history turn out this way? Why did things not work in reverse with Native Americans, Africans, and Aboriginal Australians conquering Europeans? We know that Hernán Cortés, the conquistador, overthrew the Aztec Empire and began Spanish colonization of the Americas. But Diamond wants to understand why the opposite did not happen. Why didn't Emperor Montezuma cross the Atlantic and conquer Europe? World history would have turned out differently had he done so.

For Diamond, much of the history of the last two centuries is the result of what happened in the previous 10,000 years. It was the advantages Europe and Asia had over other continents by 1500 that determined much of what followed. Diamond is interested in the early divergence of regional incomes. He identifies the "proximate causes" of Eurasian dominance over other regions: guns, germs, and steel. Eurasians had guns and steel for swords, which gave them their military advantage; they carried diseases, such as measles and smallpox, which decimated other populations; and they had political structures that could finance seaworthy ships and organize expeditions that led to the conquest of other lands.

But these are only proximate causes. Diamond digs deeper asking why Eurasians had these advantages more than 500 years ago. Diamond's explanation is geography. Eurasia has a land mass that has an east–west axis whereas Africa and the Americas have a north–south orientation. An east–west axis permitted the more rapid spread of both domesticated animals (cattle, chickens, horses) and edible grains, which in turn permitted more rapid development of settled farming communities. In time, these communities became productive enough to support craftsmen and others who developed the technologies that led to the guns, ships, and steel necessary for foreign adventures and conquest. If a continent has a north–south axis, plant and animal varieties cannot spread as rapidly because they need to adapt to different climates as they move from one area to the next, thus significantly limiting the opportunity for economic growth.

Domesticated agriculture also lies behind the germs that decimated indigenous populations in the Americas and elsewhere. Many infectious diseases result from microbes crossing over from animal populations to humans. Eurasians acquired these diseases and built up their immunity to them as a consequence of developing settled agriculture early. As more densely populated communities came in close contact with their farm animals, diseases spread as did immunity to them. Eurasia also happened to have more animal species suitable for domestication than other continents. As Diamond writes, "Just think what the course of world history might have been if Africa's rhinos and hippos had lent themselves to domestication! If that had been possible, African cavalry mounted on rhinos and hippos would have made mincemeat of European cavalry mounted on horses."

Sources: Jared Diamond, *Guns, Germs and Steel: The Fates of Human Societies* (New York, W. W. Norton, 1998). A summary is contained in a 1997 talk by Jared Diamond, "Why Did Human History Unfold Differently on Different Continents for the Last 13,000 Years?" April 22, 1997, transcript available at http://edge.org/conversation/why-did-human-history-unfold-differently-on-different-continents-for-the-last-13000-years, accessed February 2012.

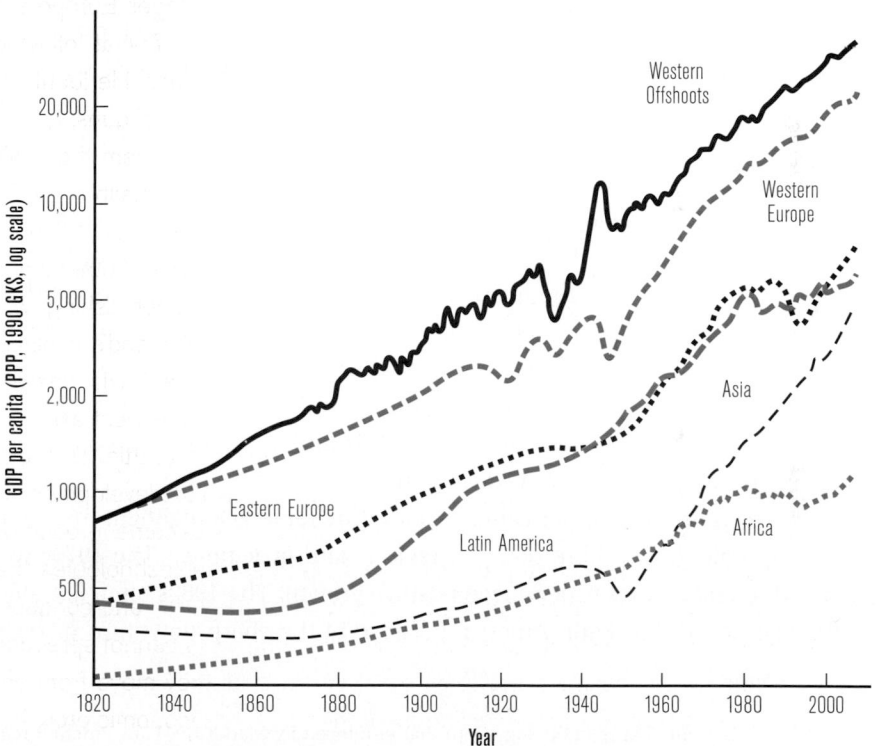

FIGURE 2-1 Levels of GDP per Capita by Region: 1820–2008

Notes: Western offshoots include Australia, Canada, New Zealand, and the United States. GDP, gross domestic product; GK$, Geary-Khamis dollars; PPP, purchasing power parity.
Source: Angus Maddison, "Statistics on World Population, GDP, and Per Capita GDP, 1–2008 AD," www.ggdc.net/MADDISON/Historical_Statistics/vertical-file_02-2010.xls.

In Africa, as elsewhere, average growth rates accelerated after 1820 and did so again after 1950, in the period associated with the end of the colonial era. But as in Latin America, economic growth in Africa faded after 1980, continued to stagnate in the 1990s, and rebounded only recently. As a result, the income gap between the world's richest regions (the Western offshoots) and the poorest in 2000 (Africa) reached 19:1. According to Maddison's work, this is the largest gap in income between rich and poor regions the world has ever known.[9] Because of resurgence in economic growth in Africa during the 2000s, this gap has narrowed but still remains huge by historical standards.

Maddison's broad sweep of world economic history indicates how differential rates of economic growth, especially over the past two centuries, have produced the divergence in income levels that characterizes the world's economy today.

ECONOMIC GROWTH, 1970–2010

Table 2–3 takes a closer look at the pattern of growth rates over the past four decades. The selection of decades as the unit of observation is somewhat arbitrary. The 1970s often are associated with two oil price shocks and other significant changes in commodity prices; the 1980s, with the first wave of international debt crises; the 1990s, with the major transition toward market economies, especially in eastern Europe and the republics of the former Soviet Union; and the 2000s, with the global consequences of the attacks of September 11, 2001, and of the financial crisis of 2008–09. The regional divisions in Table 2–3 differ from those in Maddison and conform to conventions used by the World Bank, a major source of data on economic development. Most of the regional definitions are self-explanatory; however, all high-income economies are combined in one category regardless of geographic location. Therefore, East Asia does not include Japan, Korea, Singapore, Taiwan, and a few small and affluent island economies. Similarly, Europe and Central Asia refers primarily to eastern Europe and Central Asia and excludes all (mostly western) European economies classified as high-income.

The growth rates in GDP per capita reported in Table 2–3 highlight major differences in economic growth both between regions and over time.[10] The 1970s were a decade in which *all* regions experienced positive growth. The 1980s often are referred to as "the lost decade" in Latin America because of the sharp downturn in regional

---

[9]Using a somewhat different methodology from that employed by Maddison, Lant Pritchett reached similar conclusions in "Divergence, Big Time," *Journal of Economic Perspectives* 11, no. 3 (1997), 3–17.

[10]The growth rates in Table 2–3 are based on constant US$. Although large differences in the *level* of GDP per capita are observed depending on whether PPP or market exchange rates are used, this is not the case when comparing *growth rates* of national income. The growth rates reported in the table are the differences between World Bank estimates of GDP growth and population growth by region and by decade.

TABLE 2-3 Rate of GDP per Capita Growth (Percent/Year)

	1970s	1980s	1990s	2000s
East Asia and Pacific	5.0	6.4	6.1	8.6
Europe and Central Asia	4.4	1.5	−2.9	5.7
Latin America and Caribbean	3.0	−0.3	1.7	2.5
Middle East and North Africa	3.0	−1.1	0.8	2.9
South Asia	1.2	3.5	3.8	5.7
Sub-Saharan Africa	1.1	−1.2	−0.2	2.6
High income	2.4	2.5	1.8	1.3

Sources: World Bank, *World Development Report 1995* (New York: Oxford University Press, 1995). World Bank, *World Development Report 2000/2001* (New York: Oxford University Press, 2001). World Bank, *World Development Report 2011* (Washington, DC: World Bank, 2011).

growth, from +3.0 percent in the 1970s to –0.3 percent in the following 10 years. Negative growth and falling per capita income also were features of the Middle East and North Africa region and sub-Saharan Africa in the 1980s. Growth in sub-Saharan Africa also remained negative, but by a smaller amount, throughout the 1990s. The economies of Europe and Central Asia collapsed in the 1990s after the transition from a planned to a market-based economic system. But the region rebounded during the 2000s, in some cases because of large improvements in commodity prices, especially oil, and in other cases because of the integration of these countries with the global economy. The poor performance of some regions during the 1980s and 1990s stands in sharp contrast to the accelerating growth rates—and the associated improvements in living standards—in both East and South Asia. The term *economic miracle* has been used to describe the historically unprecedented rates of growth achieved by some nations in these two regions.

The growth rates in Table 2–3 also reveal that the 2000s were the best decade since the 1970s for the low- and middle-income nations as a group. The political and economic events that rocked the high-income economies, especially the United States and the European Union, did not have the same impact elsewhere. Such resiliency on the part of low- and middle-income nations was not expected based on the experience of the 1980s and 1990s. Sub-Saharan Africa's improved growth performance is especially noteworthy. Some of it is due to much higher commodity prices. Emerging economies in the region are also benefiting from improved economic policies and management, more democratic and accountable governments, new technologies, and a new generation of development-oriented African leaders and entrepreneurs.[11]

[11]Steven Radelet, *Emerging Africa: How 17 Countries Are Leading the Way* (Washington, DC, Center for Global Development, 2010).

There are a few more points to take away from the growth rates presented in Table 2–3. First, remember that even small differences in growth rates imply huge differences in the potential for economic development. In the 1970s, economic growth in South Asia was 1.2 per year. At this rate, GDP per capita in the region expanded by a mere 12.5 percent in a decade. In the 1980s, South Asia achieved a growth rate a few percentage points higher, 3.5 percent, and ended the decade with a 41 percent increase in GDP per capita. In the 2000s, growth rates again grew by a few more percentage points, reaching 5.7 percent. That decade ended with per capita incomes 75 percent higher than they began. Second, the regional averages in Table 2–3 are weighted averages, where the weights are the population size of each nation in the region. Such averages are heavily influenced by the experience of the most populous country in the region, especially China in East Asia and India in South Asia, and disguise the wide range in individual country performance. For example, in East Asia, the Philippines' annual growth rate from 1979 to 2009 was only 0.7 percent, a fraction of its region's performance; Botswana grew at 4.4 percent per annum over these three decades, far exceeding not only the sub-Saharan Africa average but the performance of most nations worldwide.

The successful growth performance in Asia and a few countries in other regions relative to the high-income economies illustrates an observation by economic historian Alexander Gerschenkron. When Gerschenkron refers to "**the advantages of backwardness**," he is not suggesting that it is good to be poor. Instead, he means that being relatively poorer might allow low-income countries to grow more quickly. For the first nations to experience modern economic growth, in western Europe and its offshoots, growth rates were constrained by the rate of technological progress. That same constraint operates today. Growth rates in the high-income economies reported in Table 2–3 range from 1.3 to 2.5 percent, far lower than the growth rates of the successful regions in the developing world. Poor countries can borrow and adapt existing technology and have the potential to grow faster and to catch up to the more advanced economies. Over the past three decades, this is what enabled growth rates in Asia to exceed the average growth rate of the high-income nations. For development economists, the challenge is to understand why some countries have been able to realize the advantages of backwardness whereas others have fallen further behind.

WHAT DO WE MEAN BY *ECONOMIC DEVELOPMENT*?

As indicated in Chapter 1, economic growth is a necessary but not sufficient condition for improving the living standards of large numbers of people in countries with low levels of GDP per capita. It is necessary because, if there is no growth, individuals can become better off only through transfers of income and assets from others. In a poor country, even if a small segment of the population is very rich, the potential for this kind of redistribution is severely limited. Economic growth, by contrast, has the potential for all people to become much better off without anyone becoming worse off. Economic growth has led to widespread improvements in living standards in Botswana, Chile, Estonia, Korea, and many other countries.

Economic growth, however, is not a sufficient condition for improving mass living standards for several reasons. First, governments promote economic growth not just to improve the welfare of their citizens but also, and sometimes primarily, to augment the power and glory of the state and its rulers. Governments in developing nations may use national income to expand their militaries or construct elaborate capital city complexes in deserts and jungles. Political leaders may be corrupt and expropriate income for personal gain, whether for conspicuous consumption at home or the accumulation of wealth in overseas bank accounts and property. When gains from growth are channeled in such ways, they often provide little benefit to the country's citizens. Second, resources may be heavily invested in further growth, with significant consumption gains deferred to a later date. In extreme cases, such as the Soviet collectivization drive of the 1930s, consumption can decline dramatically over long periods. When the Soviet Union fell in 1991, its consumers were still waiting for the era of mass consumption to arrive. Normally, the power to suppress consumption to this extent in the name of economic growth is available only to totalitarian governments. Third, income and consumption may increase, but those who already are relatively well off may get all or most of the benefits. The rich get richer, the old saw says, and the poor get poorer. (In another version, the poor get children.) This is what poor people often think is happening. Sometimes, they are right.

If economic growth does not guarantee improvement in living standards, then GDP per capita may not be a meaningful measure of economic development. In addition to problems associated with how income is spent and distributed, any definition of economic development must include more than income levels. Income, after all, is only a means to an end, not an end itself. More than 2,000 years ago, Aristotle wrote, "The life of money-making is one undertaken under compulsion and wealth is evidently not the good we are seeking, for it is merely useful for the sake of something else."

If economic growth and economic development are not the same thing, how should we define economic development? Amartya Sen, economist, philosopher, and Nobel laureate, argues that the goal of development is to expand the *capabilities* of people to live the lives they choose to lead. Income is one factor in determining such capabilities and outcomes, but it is not the only one. To be capable of leading a life of one's own choice requires what Sen calls "elementary functionings," such as escaping high morbidity and mortality, being adequately nourished, and having at least a basic education. Also required are more complex functionings, such as achieving self-respect and being able to take part in the life of the community. Income is but one of the many factors that enhance such individual capabilities.

In his 1998 Nobel address, Sen identified four broad factors, beyond mere poverty, that affect how well income can be converted into "the capability to live a minimally acceptable life":

- *Personal heterogeneities*: including age, proneness to illness, and extent of disabilities.
- *Environmental diversities*: shelter, clothing, and fuel, for example, required by climatic conditions.
- *Variations in social climate*: such as the impact of crime, civil unrest, and violence.
- *Differences in relative deprivation*: for example, the extent to which being impoverished reduces one's capability to take part in the life of the greater community.

According to Sen, economic development requires alleviating the sources of "capability deprivation" that prevent people from having the freedom to live the lives they desire.

Sen's seminal contributions played a key role in the formulation of the human development approach to economic development. This approach is also associated with the UNDP and the work of Pakistani economist Mahbub ul Haq. Part of the motivation of Haq and Sen was a concern over the focus by other development economists on economic growth. Like Aristotle, they wanted to explore how "money-making" was "useful for the sake of something else." They wanted to see the focus shift from the production of commodities to a focus on human lives, including the enhancement of individual capabilities and the enlargement of people's choices.

MEASURING ECONOMIC DEVELOPMENT

The UNDP published its first human development report in 1990 with "the single goal of putting people back at the center of the development process." Although the terminology is different, human development and economic development are the same idea. The distinction is intended to expand the perception of development as encompassing more than increases in per capita income (Box 2–2).

The UNDP attempted to quantify what it saw as the essential determinants of human development: to live a long and healthy life, acquire knowledge, and have access to the resources needed for a decent standard of living. For each of these elements, a specific measure was constructed and aggregated into an index, the **Human Development Index (HDI)**. Every year since 1990, the UNDP has calculated the value of the HDI for as many of the world's nations as the data permit and assessed the relative progress of nations in improving human development. Because the HDI combines outcomes with different units of measurement—years of life expectancy, years of schooling, and dollars of income—each outcome must be converted into an index number to permit aggregation into a composite measure. In response to criticisms of

BOX 2-2 HUMAN DEVELOPMENT DEFINED

Human development is a process of enlarging people's choices. In principle, these choices can be infinite and change over time. But at all levels of development, the three essential ones are for people to lead a long and healthy life, to acquire knowledge, and to have access to resources needed for a decent standard of living. If these essential choices are not available, many other opportunities remain inaccessible.

But human development does not end there. Additional choices, highly valued by many people, range from political, economic, and social freedom to opportunities for being creative and productive, and enjoying personal self-respect and guaranteed human rights.

Human development has two sides: the formation of human capabilities—such as improved health, knowledge, and skills—and the use people make of their acquired capabilities—for leisure, productive purposes, or being active in cultural, social, and political affairs. If the scales of human development do not finely balance the two sides, considerable human frustration may result.

According to this concept of human development, income is clearly only one option that people would like to have, albeit an important one. But it is not the sum total of their lives. Development must, therefore, be more than just the expansion of income and wealth. Its focus must be people.

Source: United Nations Development Programme, *Human Development Report 1990* (Oxford: Oxford University Press, 1990), p. 10.

the index, the HDI has evolved over time, including different variables and changing how the index is computed. In the *Human Development Report 2010*, the 20th anniversary of the HDI, significant changes were made to the variables used, the construction of the indices for each dimension, and the method of aggregation.

As a proxy for living a long and healthy life, the HDI employs a nation's life expectancy at birth and compares progress on this measure relative to other nations. The goalposts for assessing life expectancy are a minimum value of 20 years and a maximum of 83.2. Twenty years represents the minimum life expectancy that permits a society to sustain itself. Anything less than 20 years would be below the prime reproductive age range and a society would eventually die out. Historical evidence bears this out. The maximum value of 83.2 years is what Japan achieved in 2010, the highest level recorded in any nation over the 20 years the HDI has been calculated. A country's score on this dimension is a measure of its populations' life expectancy compared to the maximum and minimum scores. For example, in 2010, El Salvador had life expectancy at birth of 72 years. El Salvador's HDI life expectancy index is calculated as (72 – 20) ÷ (83.2 – 20) = 0.82; in other words, El Salvador has attained 82 percent of the potential range in life expectancy.

As a proxy for acquiring knowledge, the HDI includes two variables. One is the mean years of schooling achieved by the adult population, those 25 years and older. The second variable is expected years of schooling for children of school-going ages. It is based on enrollment data. The goalposts of the adult schooling variable are 0 and 13.2, the observed maximum from the United States. For expected years of schooling, the goalposts are 0 and 20.6, the maximum referring to Australia. El Salvador's mean years of schooling among adults is 7.7 years (58 percent of the way in between the two goalposts); for expected years of schooling it is 12.1 years (59 percent). These values are then aggregated to form one composite index for education.

Access to resources is measured by transforming GNI per capita (PPP in US$).[12] The goalposts are $163 and $108,211; the minimum is the value attained in Zimbabwe in 2008, and the maximum is from the United Arab Emirates in 1980. The relative standing of a nation's GNI per capita is determined by taking the logarithms of all dollar values. The transformation into logarithms decreases the significance of income gains as income increases. This reflects the conclusions made by all the human development reports that there are diminishing returns to income as a means of securing a *decent* standard of living (or, alternatively, that the marginal utility of an extra dollar of income falls as income rises). El Salvador, with an estimated 2010 GNI per capita of $6,498, falls 57 percent between the logarithm-adjusted income goalposts (Box 2–3).

All three dimensions of the HDI are expressed in terms of a percentage, solving the problem of different units of measurement. The next challenge is how to aggregate the three dimensions. Up until 2010, this was done by giving the index of each dimension an equal weight of one third and computing the *arithmetic mean* of the three. In 2010, the three dimensions still have equal weight but now a *geometric mean* of the three percentages is computed.[13] The UNDP explains the reason for this change. Using an arithmetic mean implied "perfect substitutability" among the three components of HDI. If a nation lost, say, 10 percent on its schooling measure this could be compensated by a 10 percent improvement in income and the HDI would remain unchanged. The geometric mean does not have this property. Low achievement in one dimension is no longer linearly compensated by high achievement in another dimension. The level of each index matters, creating a situation of imperfect substitutability across

[12]Before 2010, the HDI was based on GDP values. The change to GNI was made to include remittances and foreign assistance income and to exclude income generated within a country but repatriated abroad. All three can be significant, especially for low-income countries. This recalls our earlier discussion of the differences between GDP and GNP/GNI.

[13]The calculation requires taking the cube root of the product of the three indices on life expectancy, schooling, and income.

BOX 2-3 WHY USE LOGARITHMS?

Logarithms have been used several times in this chapter and will be referred to throughout this text. It is worth reviewing some of their properties. It is easiest to understand logarithms if you remember that the answer to any question involving a logarithm is an exponent. If we want to know the logarithm of 100 in base 10, the answer would be 2, because 10 raised to the second power is 100. In mathematical notation,

$$log_{10}\,(100) = 2 \text{ because } 10^2 = 100$$

The base of the logarithm merely determines what number will be raised to a given power to arrive at the value whose logarithm we are seeking. If our base were 2 instead of 10, then the logarithm of 16 would be 4, because 2 raised to the fourth power is 16:

$$log_2\,(16) = 4 \text{ because } 2^4 = 16$$

The HDI uses the logarithm of income per capita rather than the level of income per capita in determining the importance of incomes in a country's human development. To see the implications, we build off our example. Assume that two nations have incomes of 10 and 100, respectively. Using these values implies a 10-fold importance to the higher income because 100 is 10 times as large as 10. What if we use logarithms instead? If we use base 10 logarithms, we can easily see how the relative importance of the higher income is reduced. As we already determined, the logarithm of 100 in base 10 is 2. What is the logarithm of 10 in base 10? It is 1, because 10 raised to the first power is 10. Using logarithms in this case reduced the relative importance of the higher income from a factor of 10 to a factor of only 2.

This reduced *relative importance* becomes more pronounced as the spread between incomes grows. If the two incomes were 10 and 1,000, using base 10 logarithms reduces the relative importance of the higher income from a factor of 100 to a factor of only 3! Logarithms are consistent with the UNDP's position that income exhibits diminishing returns in achieving human development.

Economists, including the authors of the HDI, often use the mathematical constant *e* as the base for their logarithms; these are called natural logarithms. Base *e* is closely related to the concept of continuous compounding and is a useful tool when examining economic variables that grow over time. Box 3–2 discusses this further.

One more property of logarithms is worth noting. If we track a variable in logs rather than in levels, differences in the log values imply equal *percentage* changes. For example, using logarithms in base 2,

$$log_2 (2) = 1 \text{ as } 2^1 = 2$$

$$log_2 (4) = 2 \text{ as } 2^2 = 4$$

$$log_2 (8) = 3 \text{ as } 2^3 = 8$$

$$log_2 (16) = 4 \text{ as } 2^4 = 16$$

As we move from the log values 1 to 2 to 3 to 4, the absolute change of the underlying value increases by 2 then 4 then 8, but the percentage change always remains the same at 100 percent.

This property of logarithms can be observed by considering the logarithmic scales used in Figures 2–1 and 2–2. In Figure 2–2, notice that the distance between $500 and $1,000 on the horizontal axis is the same as the distance between $20,000 and $40,000. We know that the absolute change is different along those two intervals (clearly $500 is smaller than $20,000), but both intervals represent a doubling (a 100 percent increase) of the variable. GNI per capita expressed in logarithms must behave this way.

the HDI's three dimensions. The UNDP argues that a geometric mean better reflects intrinsic differences across the indices than did the arithmetic mean.

Once the geometric mean is applied, El Salvador had a 2010 HDI of 0.659, placing it in the medium human development range, ranked 90th out of the 169 nations for which an HDI was computed. El Salvador's HDI improved from an estimated value of 0.456 in 1980, to 0.562 in 1995, to its most recent value of 0.659 in 2010. These trends suggest significant progress in El Salvador's human development over the past 30 years.

WHAT CAN WE LEARN FROM THE HUMAN DEVELOPMENT INDEX?

The basic concept behind human development is one with which many people would agree. But when we move from concept to measurement, problems arise. Many criticisms have been leveled against the HDI since it was first introduced. Some are concerned with limiting the index to only three dimensions of human development. In response, the human development reports now compute additional indices focusing on human poverty and gender-related development. An inequality-adjusted HDI was added in 2010.

Some commentators criticize the HDI for assuming diminishing returns only to income but not to either life expectancy or schooling. If the marginal utility of income declines with the more income one has, can the same be said for an extra year of life or schooling? Specific criticisms also have been raised about the introduction of a geometric mean to aggregate the three dimensions. Geometric means are sensitive to low values; in the extreme, if one index equaled zero then the HDI would equal zero too. The same principle applies if one index is close to zero. As economist William Easterly put it, "The new HDI has a 'you're only as strong as your weakest link' property, and in practice the weakest link turns out to be very low income."[14] This is due to both the construction of the HDI and to the greater convergence across nations in life expectancy and schooling than in income. The implication for nations with the lowest HDI, including Zimbabwe, the Democratic Republic of the Congo, and Niger seems to be focus on economic growth rather than health or education. This seems the opposite of the message behind the entire human development approach. It may be the right message for these nations but it is also an unintended artifact of how the HDI is now constructed.[15]

Beyond these criticisms lies the central question of how much of an improvement the HDI is over national income per capita as an index of economic or human development. Figure 2–2 presents a comparison of HDI values and levels of GNI per capita. The scatter diagram of values for individual countries indicates, as might be predicted, that rising incomes raise the HDI. This is expected because incomes are a component of the HDI, and health and schooling also rise with incomes. According to the trend line, income alone explains 90 percent of the variation in the HDI. But the scatter diagram also indicates variance around this trend. Angola and Georgia have similar levels of per capita GNI (around US$4,900, PPP) but Angola has much lower life expectancy than does Georgia (48 versus 72 years). There is also an almost eight-year gap in schooling between the two nations. Despite identical per capita incomes, there is low human development in Angola, with an HDI of 0.403, and high human development in Georgia, with an HDI of 0.698. If one compares Mozambique and Togo the story is similar. Both have per capita incomes of close to $850, but life expectancy and schooling are much higher in Togo, raising its HDI value. In terms of HDI values, Angola and Mozambique lay well below the trend line in Figure 2–2, Georgia and Togo lay well above it.

We can conclude that alternative measures of economic development are significantly but not perfectly correlated with levels of income. This suggests that with economic growth, increasing levels of income can predict a lot about economic development. But the data also suggest that improved health and education depend on factors other than income. We elaborate on this point in the discussion of income and health in Chapter 9.

From an advocacy perspective, the HDI has been useful in calling attention to development issues. It is widely reported in the media and gets the attention of

[14]William Easterly, "The First Law of Development Stats: Whatever Our Bizarre Methodology, We Make Africa Look Worse," *AIDWATCH* (blog), December 2, 2010. http://aidwatchers.com/2010/12/the-first-law-of-development-stats-whatever-our-bizarre-methodology-we-make-africa-look-worse/.

[15]Allen Kelley, "The Human Development Index: 'Handle with Care,'" *Population and Development Review* 17, no. 2 (June 1991), 315–24 provides an early critique of the original HDI. Concerns about the 2010 version are discussed in Martin Ravallion, "Troubling Tradeoffs in the Human Development Index," Policy Research Working Paper 5484, World Bank, November 2010.

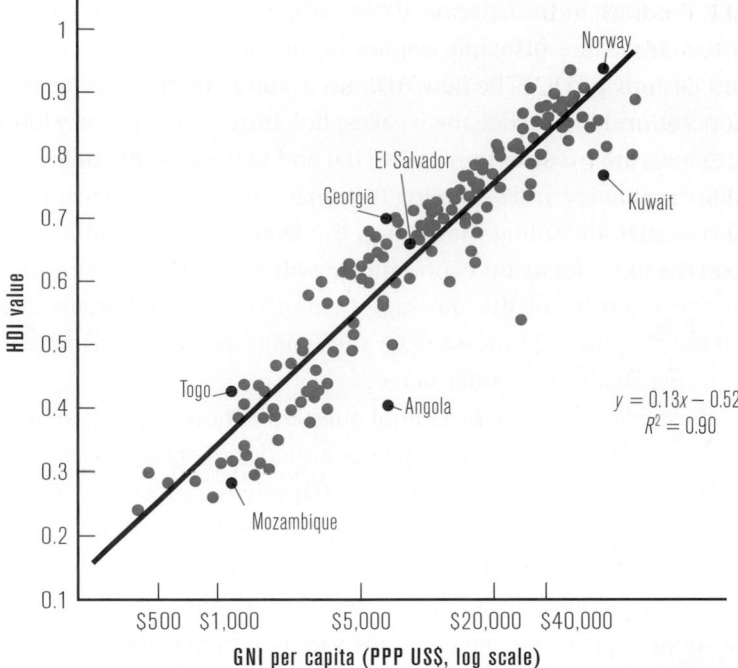

FIGURE 2-2 HDI Versus GNI per Capita by Country (2010)

Source: UN Development Programme, *Human Development Report 2010* (New York: UN Development Programme, 2010), http://hdr.undp.org/en/media/HDR_2010_EN_Contents_reprint.pdf.

political leaders. But the construction of the HDI is far from transparent and the aggregation of different dimensions of human development may not be better than a dashboard of several indicators. How much additional insight the HDI offers as a means of *measuring* economic development remains open to debate.

MILLENNIUM DEVELOPMENT GOALS

Defining economic development is inherently difficult. As with any normative concept, people have different opinions as to what should be included in the definition and on what weight to give to different goals. But even without a commonly agreed-on definition, policy makers need specific targets. One such set of targets is known as the **millennium development goals (MDGs)**.

In September 2000, 189 nations adopted the "United Nations Millennium Declaration," a broad-reaching document that states a commitment "to making the right to development a reality for everyone and to freeing the entire human race from want."[16] The declaration specifies a set of eight goals consistent with this commitment:

---

[16]UN General Assembly, "United Nations Millennium Declaration," section III, paragraph 11, September 18, 2000.

- Goal 1. Eradicate extreme poverty and hunger.
- Goal 2. Achieve universal primary education.
- Goal 3. Promote gender equality and empower women.
- Goal 4. Reduce child mortality.
- Goal 5. Improve maternal health.
- Goal 6. Combat HIV/AIDS, malaria, and other diseases.
- Goal 7. Ensure environmental sustainability.
- Goal 8. Develop a global partnership for development.

To more fully define these goals, a panel of experts developed a comprehensive set of targets and indicators for each of the MDGs. The eight MDGs contain 21 targets, which correspond to 60 indicators (Box 2-4). This combination of multiple goals, targets, and indicators is an articulation of what most of the world's governments believe should be achieved to make "development a reality for everyone." The

BOX 2-4 TARGETS OF THE MILLENNIUM DEVELOPMENT GOALS

Target 1A. Halve, between 1990 and 2015, the proportion of people whose income is less than one dollar a day.

Target 1B. Achieve full and productive employment and decent work for all, including women and young people.

Target 1C. Halve, between 1990 and 2015, the proportion of people who suffer from hunger.

Target 2A. Ensure that, by 2015, children everywhere, boys and girls alike, will be able to complete a full course of primary schooling.

Target 3A. Eliminate gender disparity in primary and secondary education, preferably by 2005, and to all levels of education no later than 2025.

Target 4A. Reduce by two-thirds, between 1990 and 2015, the under-five mortality rate.

Target 5A. Reduce by three-quarters, between 1990 and 2015, the maternal mortality ratio.

Target 5B. Achieve, by 2015, universal access to reproductive health.

Target 6A. Have halted by 2015 and begun to reverse the spread of HIV/AIDS.

Target 6B. Achieve, by 2010, universal access to treatment for HIV/AIDS for all those who need it.

Target 6C. Have halted by 2015 and begun to reverse the incidence of malaria and other major diseases.

Target 7A.   Integrate the principles of sustainable development into country policies and programs and reverse the loss of environmental resources.

Target 7B.   Reduce biodiversity loss, achieving, by 2010, a significant reduction in the rate of loss.

Target 7C.   Halve, by 2015, the proportion of people without sustainable access to safe drinking water and basic sanitation.

Target 7D.   By 2020, to have achieved a significant improvement in the lives of at least 100 million slum dwellers.

Target 8A.   Develop further an open, rule-based, predictable, nondiscriminatory trading and financial system.

Target 8B.   Address the special needs of the least developed countries.

Target 8C.   Address the special needs of landlocked countries and small island developing states.

Target 8D.   Deal comprehensively with the debt problems of developing countries through national and international measures in order to make debt sustainable in the long run.

Target 8E.   In cooperation with pharmaceutical companies, provide access to affordable essential drugs in developing countries.

Target 8F.   In cooperation with the private sector, make available the benefits of new technologies, especially information and communications.

Source: United Nations Statistics Division, "Official List of MDG Indicators," January 2008, available at http://unstats.un.org/unsd/mdg/Host.aspx?Content=Indicators/OfficialList.htm, accessed February 2012.

millennium declaration even suggests ways in which this development agenda might be financed. For example, Target 8B, which focuses on the least developed countries, makes recommendations for debt relief and for more official development assistance from the rich nations. But none of these recommendations is binding.

The MDGs were drawn up in 2000 and their due dates are soon approaching. It is possible to assess progress thus far. Poverty reduction at the global level, for which the poverty indicator is living on less than US$1.25 (PPP) per day, is on track to meet or exceed the global target by 2015 (although the target will not be met in every country or region). Access to clean drinking water is proceeding well and should exceed the original target. More disappointing are trends in under-five mortality. In 1990, the developing regions experienced child mortality in the neighborhood of 100 deaths per 1,000 children. This fell to 66 per 1,000 by 2009. To reach the target of a two-thirds reduction in child mortality by 2015 will take, according to the United Nations, "substantial and accelerated action," especially in Sub-Saharan Africa and South Asia where child mortality rates remain high. Target 6B, universal treatment for HIV/AIDS, has met with some success. But because only 35 to 40 percent of those who

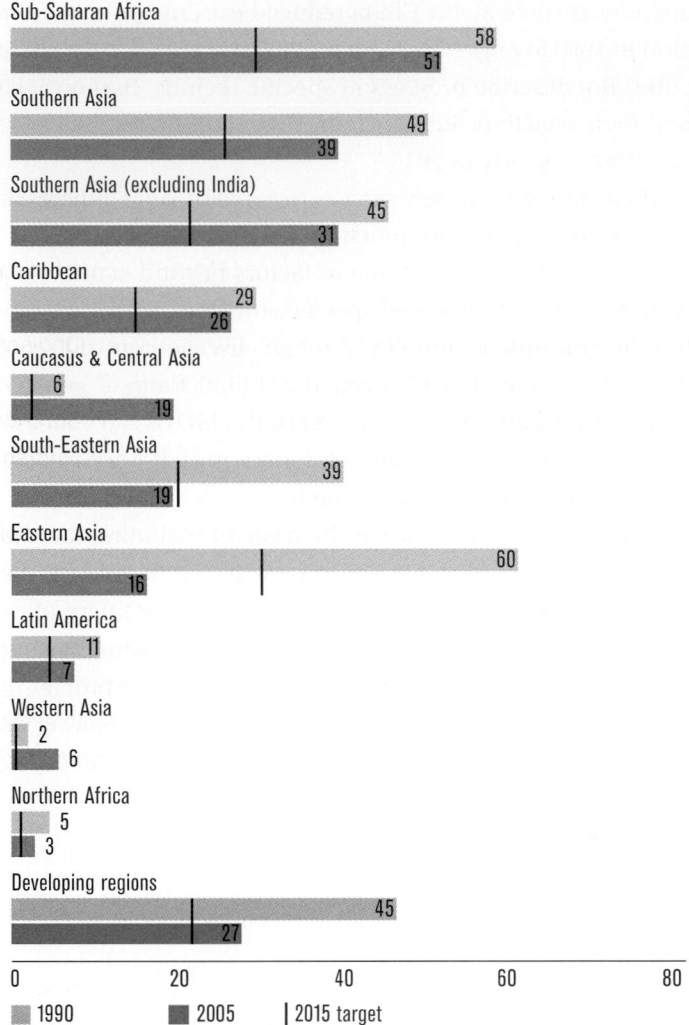

FIGURE 2-3 Proportion of People Living on Less Than $1.25 a Day, 1990 and 2005 (Percentage)

Source: Figure from the *Millennium Development Goals Report*, 2011. The World Bank. Reprinted by permission of United Nations Publications.

needed antiretroviral treatment received it in 2009, universal coverage will not be achieved by the target date. Universal treatment by 2010 was an ambitious and probably unrealistic goal.

Evaluating progress toward achieving the MDGs requires caution, especially regarding the level of aggregation across countries. Relative success and failure at meeting the MDGs varies not only among specific targets but also by region. Some of the explanation for differential performance is based on disparities in the rate of economic growth between countries. Success at cutting global poverty in half owes a lot to China's performance alone. China reduced extreme poverty from 60 percent of its population in 1990 to only 16 percent by 2005. Yet Figure 2–3 illustrates that this global result does not describe progress in specific regions. Based on data for 2005, the most recent data available, Sub-Saharan Africa and South Asia appear far from being on track to halve poverty by 2015.

Rapid economic growth is widely seen as responsible for China's success at poverty alleviation and, by implication, much of global achievements. But *some* of the difficulty in achieving other MDGs is due to factors beyond economic growth. Better use and distribution of income and specific strategies aimed at some of the targets (such as reducing infant mortality through disease control), combined with economic growth, are essential to achieving the United Nations' goal of "freeing the entire human race from want." By setting targets, the MDGs have focused the attention of governments in poor nations and of donors in rich ones to achieve specific outcomes that promote economic development.

The MDGs have been challenged on the basis of including too much and setting targets that may be either too high or too low based on historical experience.[17] The MDGs also fail to address the fundamental economic problem of trade-offs and priorities. If one cannot fulfill all 21 targets simultaneously, which takes precedence: maternal mortality or access to safe drinking water, reducing hunger or promoting environmental sustainability? This is less of a problem for defining development: Economic development involves all these goals. But it is a practical problem for those charged with realizing such an ambitious development agenda.[18]

IS ECONOMIC GROWTH DESIRABLE?

After discussing the MDGs, which convey the absolute and relative deprivation of so many people around the world, and recognizing the positive correlation between economic growth and human development, it may seem odd to end this chapter by asking, Is economic growth desirable? The answer would seem to be an obvious and emphatic yes! But there are other perspectives. Some decry the spread of materialism, the Westernization of world cultures, and the destruction of traditional societies that seem to accompany economic growth. Others are troubled by environmental degradation, whether species loss or global warming, that has accompanied rising per capita incomes. Still others in the high-income world may wonder if we should be so quick to encourage people to follow the path we have taken: seemingly insatiable

---

[17]Michael Clemens, Charles Kenny, and Todd Moss, "The Trouble with the MDGs: Confronting Expectations of Aid and Development Success," *World Development* 35, no. 5 (2007), 735–51; and William Easterly, "How the Millennium Development Goals Are Unfair to Africa," *World Development* 37, no. 1 (2009), 26–35.

[18]A strategy for achieving the MDGs is laid out in a report by the UN Millennium Project, *Investing in Development: A Practical Plan to Achieve the UN Millennium Development Goals* (New York: United Nations Development Programme, 2005).

consumerism, the withering of extended and nuclear families, high levels of stress, and all the other ills associated with modern life.

Richard Easterlin, an economic historian, once observed that, although per capita incomes in the United States had risen dramatically over the preceding half century, people did not seem to be any happier. He based this conclusion, which came to be known as the **Easterlin paradox**, on survey data taken over time in which people were asked how happy they were with their lives. Easterlin found similar results when looking across a small number of high-income nations. The Easterlin paradox and, more generally, the analysis of subjective well-being, often referred to as the study of happiness, have received a great deal of attention over the past decade by economists and other social scientists. This research has been enabled by newly conducted surveys of happiness and life satisfaction covering countries at all income levels. The motivation behind this research has included many of the concerns raised throughout this chapter about whether GDP or GNI per capita is a useful measure of economic well-being.

How can happiness be measured? One set of surveys asks individuals, "Taking all things together, would you say you are: very happy, quite happy, not very happy, or not at all happy?" Responses are coded from 1 to 4, with 4 signifying "very happy." Easterlin's work was based on questions like this. Another set of surveys directed at life satisfaction asks a related but different question:

> Please imagine a ladder with steps numbered from 0 at the bottom to 10 at the top. Suppose we say that the top of the ladder represents the best possible life for you, and the bottom of the ladder represents the worst possible life for you. On which step of the ladder would you say you personally feel you stand at this time, assuming that the higher the step the better you feel about your life, and the lower the step the worse you feel about it? Which step comes closest to the way you feel?

Surveys that ask both of these questions find that responses are well but not perfectly correlated. Happiness and life satisfaction are not identical.

Based on data from the life satisfaction question, which include a relatively large sample of countries, the plots in Figure 2–4a show the life satisfaction score against GDP per capita (US$, PPP). In Panel b, GDP per capita (US$, PPP) is entered in log values. Both graphs tend to reject the Easterlin paradox. Life satisfaction rises with per capita income. One reason Easterlin did not observe this relationship is the small sample of rich nations he had to work with. The graph using log values suggests that, in relative terms, life satisfaction increases with percentage changes in per capita incomes across the entire range of observed incomes. Although economic growth and happiness are correlated, within income categories (low, middle, and high) there appears to be much less of a trend than between them. Among any given income category the Easterlin paradox may hold.[19]

[19]Angus Deaton, "Income, Health, and Well-Being around the World: Evidence from the Gallup World Poll," *Journal of Economic Perspectives* 22, no. 2 (Spring 2008), 53-72; Betsey Stevenson and Justin Wolfers, "Economic Growth and Subjective Well-Being: Reassessing the Easterlin Paradox," *Brookings Papers on Economic Activity* 39, no. 1 (Spring 2008), 1–102.

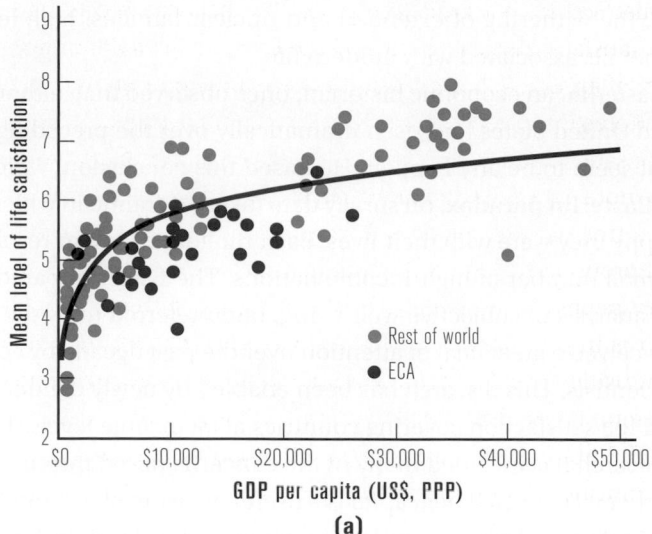

(a)

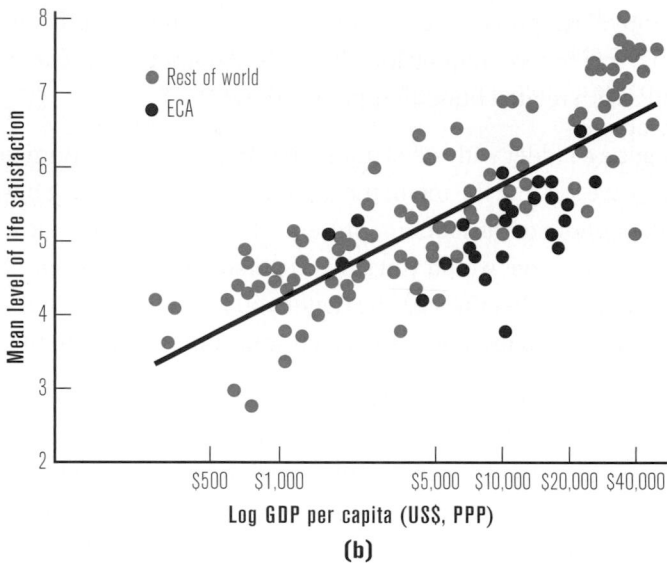

(b)

FIGURE 2-4 **Life Satisfaction as a Measure of Well-Being (2008)**

Life satisfaction measures the mean level of life satisfaction of a random group of people who were asked the following question: "Please imagine a ladder with steps numbered from zero at the bottom to ten at the top. Suppose we say that the top of the ladder represents the best possible life for you, and the bottom of the ladder represents the worst possible life for you. On which step of the ladder would you say you personally feel you stand at this time, assuming that the higher the step the better you feel about your life, and the lower the step the worse you feel about it? Which step comes closest to the way you feel?"

Source: Gallup World Poll.

There is also variance around the trend line because more than income levels determine life satisfaction. Costa Rica and the United States both have mean levels of life satisfaction of around 7.2, but Costa Rica has only one-quarter the income of the United States; Korea is more than three times richer than Thailand, but both share similar levels of life satisfaction (around 6.1). For reasons other than income, Costa Ricans and Thais are more satisfied than are Americans and Koreans. One group of nations stands out in terms of lower life satisfaction than expected based on income alone. Countries in Europe and Central Asia almost always lie below the trend line. After accounting for income level, mean life satisfaction is systematically lower for these nations than it is in other regions. Much of this can be explained by the wrenching effects of the transition from planned to market economies. People who benefited from the former system, including those who had decent jobs or relied on pensions, were made worse off. Public goods deteriorated, inequality rose, and growth rates turned negative. All contributed to declining measures of average life satisfaction. There is some evidence that with the resumption of growth in many of these economies during the 2000s, levels of happiness are rising and falling more in line with other regions.[20]

Recent research suggests that happiness and income levels are correlated, implying that economic growth improves happiness. But even in those situations in which the relationship is less certain, a case for economic growth still can be made. More than half a century ago, W. Arthur Lewis, one of the pioneers of the field of development economics and a Nobel laureate, provided one. Lewis was writing before there was survey evidence on happiness and at a time when the distinction between the terms *economic growth* and economic development were not as nuanced as they are today. The concluding chapter of his 1955 book, *The Theory of Economic Growth,* is titled, "Is Economic Growth Desirable?" Lewis's answer: "The case for economic growth is that it gives man greater control over his environment, and thereby increases his freedom."[21]

SUMMARY

- Understanding the process of economic development requires methods of measuring economic performance across countries and over time. Gross domestic product (GDP) per capita is a measure of the aggregate value of national output and, despite a number of limitations, is the most common standard for measuring economic growth.
- For cross-country comparisons, GDP per capita is best measured in terms of purchasing power parity (PPP). PPP estimates are superior to

---

[20]Sergei Guriev and Ekaterina Zhuravskaya, "(Un)Happiness in Transition," *Journal of Economic Perspectives* 23, no. 2 (Spring 2009), 143–68.

[21]W. Arthur Lewis, *The Theory of Economic Growth* (Homewood, IL: Richard D. Irwin, 1955), p. 420–21.

comparisons based solely on market exchange rates. Market exchange rates tend to underestimate the GDP levels of poorer nations. This is because market exchange rates are based on traded goods and capital flows and fail to account for the much lower prices of nontraded goods in poor nations. The PPP estimates obtained from the UN International Comparison Program correct this problem by expressing every nation's GDP per capita in terms of a common set of international prices.

- Angus Maddison provides a broad overview of economic growth over the past 2,000 years. For most of this period and in most regions, growth in output was just about sufficient to match growth in population, resulting in more or less stagnant per capita incomes. According to Maddison, modern economic growth began only around 1820, with the escalation of growth rates in western Europe and its offshoots. These regions had achieved higher per capita income levels by 1500 but accelerated these differences, especially, over the last 190 years. Rapid growth rates began to characterize other regions, especially in Asia, only in the decades after 1950. As a result of these divergent patterns of economic growth, there is much greater disparity in world incomes today than in the past.

- Unlike economic growth, which is a relatively objective measure of economic capacity, economic development is a normative concept. Various scholars and organizations offer specific indicators or goals for achieving development. Prominent among these is the human development index (HDI), a composite measure reflecting the goals of leading a long life, acquiring knowledge, and achieving material well-being. The millennium development goals (MDGs) rely on a multiplicity of goals and targets for advancing human well-being within the decade.

- Analysis of the HDI and the MDGs reveals the centrality of economic growth to achieving both. HDI ranks are well correlated with per capita income levels, and differential performance in achieving specific MDGs often is tied to differential growth performance. But economic growth is not a panacea. Achieving economic development also involves questions of distribution and strategies to reach specific development targets.

- Citizens of rich nations can engage in a debate over whether further economic growth will advance their well-being, but this is not a meaningful debate for poor nations. Even if rising per capita incomes are not perfectly correlated with perceptions of happiness, economic growth and development are essential for poor nations as a means of increasing choices and advancing human capabilities and freedoms.

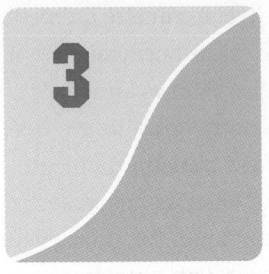

Economic Growth: Concepts and Patterns

Why are some countries rich and others poor? Why do some economies grow quickly with their citizens enjoying rapid increases in their average incomes, while others grow slowly or not at all? How did some East Asian countries advance from poverty to relative prosperity in just 30 years, while many African countries remain mired in deep poverty, with few signs of sustained growth and development? These are some of the most important questions in the study of economics and indeed touch on some of the deepest problems facing human society.

As we saw in the last chapter, rapid economic growth and wide divergences of economic performance across countries are fairly recent phenomena in world history. Up until about 500 years ago—a relatively short period of time in human history—most people lived in conditions that we now would consider abject poverty. Housing was poor, food supplies were highly variable and dependent on the weather, nutrition was inadequate, disease was common, healthcare was rudimentary, and life spans rarely exceeded 40 years. Even as recently as 125 years ago, the vast majority of people living in the world's most modern cities, including New York, London, and Paris, lived in extremely difficult conditions on very meager incomes. One decade into the twenty-first century, however, income levels around the world generally are both much higher and far more diverse. A significant minority of the world's population has recorded relatively rapid and sustained income growth during the last several decades and now enjoys much longer and healthier lives, higher levels of education, and much-improved standards of living. Other countries have achieved important but more modest gains and now are middle-income countries.

The majority of the world's population, however, continues to live in poverty, in most cases better off than their ancestors but living at levels of income and welfare far below those of the world's richest countries.

Economic growth and economic development are not synonymous, as we discovered in Chapter 2. Yet economic growth is at the heart of the development process, and sustained development and poverty reduction cannot occur in the absence of economic growth. This chapter and the next explore in some detail the puzzles of economic growth and divergent levels of income across countries. Our objectives are to better understand the processes by which economies grow and develop and the characteristics that distinguish rapidly growing economies from those with slower growth. This chapter explores the basic empirical data on economic growth, the concepts underlying the leading ideas of what causes growth, and some of the patterns of changing economic structure that typically accompany growth. Chapter 4 expands the analysis by introducing some formal models of economic growth. Later chapters explore other dimensions of development introduced earlier, including the distribution of income, poverty, and improvements in health and education.

DIVERGENT PATTERNS OF ECONOMIC GROWTH SINCE 1960

As we begin to explore differences in growth rates, consider Thailand and Zambia. In 1960, the annual income of the average Zambian was almost twice as high as that of the average Thai, around $1,800 in Zambia and $960 in Thailand in constant 2005 purchasing power parity (PPP) dollars. Since that time, Thailand achieved very rapid economic growth of around 4.3 percent per person per year, so that the average income in Thailand is now around $7,800. In 2009, the income of the average Thai was over *eight times* higher in real terms than that of his or her grandparents 50 years ago. As a result, Thais can consume much more (and much higher-quality) food, housing, clothing, healthcare, education, and consumer goods. Thais are better off in other ways as well: life expectancy increased from 54 to 69 years, infant mortality dropped from 103 to 12 per thousand (meaning that an additional 91 children per thousand infants lived beyond their first birthday), and the percentage of adults that were literate grew from 80 (in 1970) to 94 percent. In Zambia, by contrast, average income actually fell slightly to $1,765, about 2 percent lower than in 1960. Life expectancy remained at around 45 years, pulled down to a large extent because of the dramatic spread of the HIV/AIDS pandemic in the 1990s. Infant mortality rates improved (from 126 to 86 per thousand), as did literacy rates (from 48 to 71 percent), but overall Zambians are arguably worse off than their parents and grandparents.

The different growth records of Thailand and Zambia are mirrored by the experiences of many other developing countries, as shown in Table 3–1. Madagascar joins

TABLE 3-1 Economic Growth across Countries, 1960–2009

COUNTRY	GDP PER CAPITA (2005 PPP) 1960	GDP PER CAPITA (2005 PPP) 2009	RATIO OF 2009 TO 1960 GDP/ CAPITA	AVERAGE ANNUAL GROWTH RATE (%)	INCOME AS A SHARE OF U.S. INCOME* 1960	INCOME AS A SHARE OF U.S. INCOME* 2009
Negative growth						
Madagascar	842	753	0.89	−0.23	0.07	0.02
Zambia	1,803	1,765	0.98	−0.04	0.14	0.04
Slow growth						
Senegal	1,421	1,492	1.05	0.01	0.11	0.04
Kenya	1,020	1,206	1.18	0.34	0.08	0.03
Rwanda	860	1,031	1.2	0.37	0.07	0.03
Nigeria	1,528	2,034	1.33	0.58	0.12	0.05
Venezuela	6,663	9,115	1.37	0.64	0.52	0.22
Chad	819	1,277	1.56	0.91	0.06	0.03
Jamaica	5,609	8,795	1.57	0.92	0.44	0.21
El Salvador	3,397	6,338	1.87	1.28	0.26	0.15
Argentina	6,244	11,961	1.92	1.33	0.49	0.29
Peru	3,759	7,280	1.94	1.36	0.29	0.18
South Africa	3,850	7,589	1.97	1.4	0.3	0.18
Ghana	603	1,239	2.05	1.48	0.05	0.03
Philippines	1,314	2,838	2.16	1.58	0.1	0.07
Moderate growth						
Turkey	3,243	9,909	3.06	2.31	0.25	0.24
Papua New Guinea	887	2,746	3.1	2.34	0.07	0.07
Brazil	2,581	8,160	3.16	2.38	0.2	0.2
Chile	3,780	11,999	3.17	2.39	0.29	0.29
Pakistan	728	2,353	3.23	2.43	0.06	0.06
Lesotho	401	1,311	3.27	2.45	0.03	0.03
Dominican Republic	2,355	9,911	4.21	3.06	0.18	0.24
Mauritius	2,208	9,484	4.29	3.01	0.17	0.23
Rapid growth						
India	711	3,239	4.55	3.14	0.06	0.08
Egypt	1,036	4,956	4.78	3.24	0.08	0.12
Sri Lanka	765	4,035	5.27	3.45	0.06	0.1
Indonesia	693	4,075	5.88	3.69	0.05	0.1
Malaysia	1,470	11,296	7.68	4.25	0.11	0.27
Thailand	961	7,794	8.11	4.36	0.07	0.19
Singapore	4,300	47,373	11.02	5.02	0.33	1.15
South Korea	1,782	25,034	14.05	5.54	0.14	0.61
Botswana	578	8,872	15.35	5.73	0.05	0.22
China	403	7,634	18.94	6.18	0.03	0.19
Industrialized countries						
United Kingdom	12,841	33,383	2.6	1.97	1	0.81
United States	15,438	41,099	2.66	2.02	1.2	1
Canada	12,988	36,209	2.79	2.11	1.01	0.88
France	10,101	30,822	3.05	2.31	0.79	0.75
Japan	5,850	30,008	5.13	3.4	0.46	0.73

*Growth rates are trend-growth calculated by ordinary least squares regressions and do not necessarily match endpoint-to-endpoint growth rates. Growth rates are listed in order of magnitude, but the ordering of magnitudes in the third and fourth columns sometimes differ.

PPP, purchasing power parity; GDP, gross domestic product.

Source: Penn World Tables 7.0, http://pwt.econ.upenn.edu/php_site/pwt_index.php, accessed May 2011.

Zambia in the unfortunate experience of shrinking incomes. Because incomes were very low to begin with in many of these countries, negative growth has been a major tragedy. A second group of countries attained positive growth but at relatively slow rates. Average incomes in these countries increased but not by as much as in many other countries around the world. In Venezuela, for example, per capita growth averaged about 0.6 percent per year since 1960, enough for incomes to increase by around 37 percent, but less than what many Venezuelans may have hoped for.

A third group of countries has been more successful and has achieved moderate growth, shown in the table as per capita growth between 2 and 3 percent per year. By world historical standards (calculated by Angus Maddison and shown in Figure 2–1), these growth rates are relatively high and allow for solid increases in average income. For example, Egypt recorded a growth of 3.2 percent a year, enough for average income to double every 22 years and nearly quintuple between 1960 and 2009, a significant achievement. India, home to over 1 billion people, saw similar growth.

A fourth group of countries has done even better, recording rapid growth of more than 3 percent per capita per year. A few have achieved extraordinary growth exceeding 5 percent, including Singapore, South Korea, Botswana, and China. These are some of the fastest growth rates ever recorded over a 50-year period in the history of the world, and they have led to enormous changes. In South Korea, income expanded by a mind-boggling factor of 14, while in Botswana (Box 3–1), average income is *more than 15 times* what it was 50 years ago. (Unfortunately, Botswana's great success is now threatened by the HIV/AIDS pandemic, as we discuss later in the book.) China, where growth has averaged 6 percent per year (with almost all of it coming after 1980, meaning the growth rate since then has been much faster), has undergone perhaps the most remarkable transformation of all: For one-fifth of the world's population, including a huge number of people living in or near poverty, average incomes have increased by a factor of nearly 19 between 1960 and 2009. China's rapid growth is one of the most important events of the last century, and its continued growth will have profound implications for this century, as well.

There are some clear regional differences in growth rates, as the data in Table 3–1 suggest and as we saw in Table 2–3. Most of the rapidly growing countries are in East Asia, while most of the slowly growing countries are in Africa. But beware of taking these general statements too far because there are important exceptions. In East Asia, Myanmar (Burma) and Laos both recorded slow growth, and the Philippines' performance has been modest at best. In Africa, Botswana and Mauritius are among the fastest-growing countries in the world, and tiny Lesotho and Swaziland have also achieved steady growth.

Remember, apparently small differences in growth rates can make a huge difference over time. The difference between 1 percent growth and 2 percent growth is huge: It is not a 1 percent difference but a 100 percent difference. With growth of 1 percent per year, average income increases by about 65 percent over 50 years, and

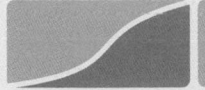

BOX 3-1   BOTSWANA'S REMARKABLE ECONOMIC DEVELOPMENT[a]

Whereas most of sub-Saharan Africa has achieved little or no economic growth in per capita income on average over the past 50 years, Botswana stands out as a clear exception. Indeed, during the 20-year period between 1970 and 1990, Botswana was the fastest-growing economy in the world, with growth averaging an astonishing 7.9 percent per year, easily outpacing the more widely noted rapid growth in Singapore (6.3 percent), Korea (6.9 percent), and other countries around the world. Table 3–1 shows that over the longer period from 1960 to 2009, Botswana's growth rate was second only to China's. Over the 50-year period, average real income increased by a factor of more than 15 in just over two generations. A wide array of other development indicators improved dramatically as well. Life expectancy increased from 46 to 61 years in 1987 (before plunging again because of the HIV/AIDS pandemic), infant mortality fell from 118 to 43 per thousand by 2009, and literacy rates jumped from 46 percent (in 1970) to 83 percent by 2008.

Botswana did not seem to have strong prospects when it achieved independence from Great Britain in 1965. At that point, there were only 12 kilometers of paved roads in the entire country. Only 22 Batswana had graduated from university, and only 100 had graduated from secondary school. The country is landlocked, and more than 80 percent of the country is in the Kalahari Desert, leaving only a small amount of arable land. Yet, despite the long odds, Botswana prospered. What was behind this remarkable transformation?

Diamonds are part of the story, because Botswana sits atop some of the world's richest diamond deposits, and mining now accounts for about 40 percent of the country's output. But the answer is not that simple: Many other developing countries have rich natural resources, and in many cases, these have created more problems than benefits (see Chapter 17). More broadly, most observers point to Botswana's strong policies and institutions as key determinants of its development success.

Botswana clearly managed its resources much more prudently than other countries. Most of the receipts were invested productively: Botswana has built an impressive infrastructure, with paved roads connecting much of the country,

[a]This account draws heavily from Daron Acemoglu, Simon Johnson, and James Robinson, "An African Success Story," in Dani Rodrik, ed., *In Search of Prosperity: Analytic Narratives on Economic Growth* (Princeton, NJ: Princeton University Press, 2003); and Clark Leith, "Why Botswana Prospered," paper presented at the 34th Annual Meeting of the Canadian Economics Association, University of British Columbia, Vancouver, Canada, June 2000, available at www.ssc.uwo.ca/economics/faculty/Leith/Botswana.pdf, accessed February 2012.

a reasonably reliable electricity generation and distribution system, a substantial stock of housing, and many schools and clinics. Some of the diamond receipts were saved as reserves to help manage macroeconomic fluctuations. Corruption has been much less of a problem than in other countries. Overall macroeconomic policies were strong; inflation was relatively low, for the most part; and supporting fiscal, monetary, and exchange-rate policies were in place. Trade policies were relatively open, with the external tariff set through Botswana's membership in the Southern Africa Customs Union. The public sector has remained small, with a civil service based on merit rather than patronage and relatively few state-owned companies. Property rights and other legal protections have been generally well respected. Strong economic management, in turn, may have been due partly to the fact that Botswana is a democracy, and one of the few countries in Africa that has been so since independence.

However, not everything in Botswana is positive. Income inequality is high and has not declined over time. Unemployment remains high, particularly for migrants coming from rural to urban areas. Although democratic traditions are solid, with fair elections and a vibrant free press, one party has dominated politics since independence. The biggest concern, however, is HIV/AIDS. According to the World Health Organization, Botswana has the second-highest prevalence of HIV in the world; around 24 percent of the adult population is HIV-positive. The scourge of HIV/AIDS threatens to turn back much of the progress Botswana has realized in recent decades. With all that Botswana has achieved, its greatest challenges may lie ahead in fighting the disease and ensuring continued growth and development.

incomes double in about 70 years. With 2 percent growth, average income increases by 270 percent over 50 years, and it takes only 35 years for income to double. (Box 3–2 demonstrates the methods behind these calculations.)

FACTOR ACCUMULATION, PRODUCTIVITY, AND ECONOMIC GROWTH

Economists have been trying to understand the determinants of economic growth and the characteristics that distinguish fast-growing from slower-growing countries at least since Adam Smith wrote *An Inquiry into the Nature and Causes of the Wealth of Nations,* published in 1776. More than 200 years later, our knowledge about the growth process has expanded but is far from complete. A broad range of factors could

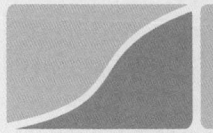

BOX 3-2 CALCULATING FUTURE VALUES, GROWTH RATES, AND DOUBLING TIMES

The illustrative growth calculations presented in the text are based on simple, yet quite useful mathematical techniques. Let us take a look at how to perform the calculations required to answer three basic questions.

QUESTION 1

If a country's current level of income per capita is X_0 and that country's income per capita grows for t years at rate r, what will its income per capita be at the end of that period (X_t)?

To answer this question, we will use the basic formula for compound growth over discrete periods (such as years),

$$X_t = X_0 \times (1 + r)^t$$

For example, we see from Table 3–1 that Senegal's income per capita in 2009 was $1,492, and its historical growth rate was 1.05 percent per year (which we will round down to 1 percent per year to simplify this calculation). Suppose we want to project Senegal's per capita income 10 years into the future (in 2019), assuming that its income continues to grow at 1 percent per year. Plugging in $1,492 for X_0, 0.01 for r, and 10 for t:

$$\$1,492 \times 1.01^{10} = \$1,648$$

The key here is to recognize that this future value is not simply 1 percent times 10 years (or 10 percent) greater than the initial value. Compound growth calculations take into account that after one year of 1 percent growth (starting at $1,492), Senegal's income is $1,507; the second year's growth of 1 percent thus starts from this new base. That is, for the first year, we'd calculate $1,492 × 1.01 = $1,507; for the second year we'd calculate ($1,492 × 1.01) × 1.01, or $1,492 × 1.01^2 = $1,522, and so on.

QUESTION 2

If, instead, we know a country's initial level of per capita income (X_0) and its level of per capita income t years hence (X_t), what was its annually compounded average rate of growth?

To solve for the growth rate we begin with the basic compound growth formula from Question 1. With a bit of algebraic manipulation, we can solve that equation for r, resulting in the following formula:

$$\left(\frac{X_t}{X_0}\right)^{\frac{1}{t}} - 1 = r$$

If we knew that Senegal's per capita income in 2009 was $1,492 and that it would be $1,648 10 years later, we could calculate its average compound growth rate as:

$$\left(\frac{\$1,648}{\$1,492}\right)^{\frac{1}{10}} - 1 = 0.01 \text{ or } 1 \text{ percent}$$

Calculating growth rates using these endpoint data is potentially misleading if either the start or end year observation is unusually high or low relative to the underlying trend (that is, if there was a shock of some sort in either the start or end year, making it unrepresentative of the trend). It is possible to avoid this problem by using regression analysis to estimate the growth rate. This approach uses all of the observations in a given time series, rather than relying entirely on the first and last observations.

To estimate average growth rates by least-squares regression, we begin by transforming the basic formula for discrete periods of compound growth into a linear function by taking the natural logarithm of both sides of the formula:

$$\ln X_t = \ln X_0 + \ln(1 + r) \times t$$

We can estimate this equation as the least-squares regression $\ln X_t = a + bt$, where $a = \ln X_0$, $b = \ln(1 + r)$, and t is time. That is, we regress the natural log of the series against a linear time trend. To recover the direct estimate of the compound growth rate t, we calculate $r = e^b - 1$.

QUESTION 3

If income (or, for that matter, population) were to grow at rate r, how long would it take to double?

To calculate doubling times (commonly used for illustrative purposes), we resort to the rule of 70. The rule of 70 is based on a slightly different concept of compounding from the one used for the other questions. In the previous examples, we compounded once each year. The rule of 70 is based on continuous compounding, in which the base is increased at each instant. The basic equation for continuous compounding uses the exponential function (e),

$$X_t = X_0 \times e^{rt}$$

In general, continuous compounding using this formula is more appropriate when calculating growth rates for populations, which growth continuously. (When the available data for a series consist of annual observations, such as is common for countries' gross domestic product [GDP], then it may be more appropriate to apply annual compounding for those discrete periods, as described earlier.) We can use this formula to calculate the time it takes for income (or population) to double by setting $X_t = 2$ and $X_0 = 1$,

$$2 = 1 \times e^{rt}$$

If we transform this equation by taking natural logarithms of both sides, we have

$$\ln 2 = \ln 1 + (r \times t)$$

Conveniently, $\ln 1 = 0$ so that term drops out. This calculation is called the *Rule of 70* because $\ln 2 \approx 0.70$. So if we know r, we can solve for the doubling time:

$$\text{doubling time } (t) = \frac{0.70}{r}$$

If Senegal's economy grows at 1 percent per year, its level doubles every $(0.70/0.01) = 70$ years. If, instead, Senegal's economy grows at 2 percent per year, it would double in size every $(0.70/0.02) = 35$ years.

plausibly be important to growth, including the amount and type of investment, education and healthcare systems, natural resources and geographical endowments, the quality of government institutions, and the choice of public policy. All these play some role, as we see later in the chapter, but some are more central to the process of growth than others.

At the core of most theories of economic growth is a relationship between the basic factors of production—capital and labor—and total economic production. Some countries also are endowed with specific natural resources assets, such as petroleum deposits, gold, rubber, land, rich agricultural soil, forests, lakes, and oceans. These assets are often included as parts of a broad definition of the capital stock, but sometimes are treated separately. For simplicity, we focus our analysis on capital and labor. Depending on the products being produced, different combinations of these inputs are required. Growing rice requires significant amounts of labor (at least around planting and harvesting time), but not much machinery other than a plow. Garment production also requires lots of unskilled labor, but needs many sewing machines as well as decent infrastructure to get goods to overseas markets. A steel or chemical factory requires substantial amounts of machinery and other capital, including a reliable source of energy, and (relatively) less labor.

A country's total output—and thus its total income—is determined by how much capital and labor it has available and how productively it uses those assets. In turn, *increasing* the amount of production—that is, economic growth—depends on increasing the amount of capital and labor available and increasing the productivity of those assets. In other words, economic growth depends on two basic processes:

- **Factor accumulation**, defined as increasing the size of the capital stock or the labor force. Producing more goods and services requires more machines, factories, buildings, roads, ports, electricity generators, computers, and tools along with more and better educated workers to put this capital equipment to work.
- **Productivity growth**, defined as increasing the amount of output produced by each machine or worker. Productivity can be increased in two broad ways. The first is to improve the **efficiency** with which current factors are being used. A small furniture maker might initially have each worker make a chair from start to finish. By reorganizing the workers so each specializes in one task (for example, cutting, assembling, finishing), total production might be increased. The second is **technological change**, through which new ideas, new machines, or new ways of organizing production can increase growth. Countries that can either invent new technologies or quickly adopt technologies invented elsewhere (a more relevant path for most developing countries) can achieve more rapid economic growth than other countries. Productivity growth often entails shifting resources from producing one good to another. The process of economic growth in low-income countries almost always corresponds to major structural shifts in the composition of output, generally from agriculture to industry, as we discuss in Chapter 15.

Understanding that factor accumulation and productivity gains are at the heart of the growth process is important but takes us only so far. To gain a deeper understanding of growth, we must understand what drives factor accumulation and productivity growth themselves. We begin with saving and investment.

SAVING, INVESTMENT, AND CAPITAL ACCUMULATION

Perhaps the most influential model of economic growth was developed by MIT economist Robert Solow in 1956.[1] At the heart of the **Solow growth model** (which we explore in depth in Chapter 4) and many other influential growth models is the process of capital accumulation. As mentioned previously, classical and neoclassical growth models typically give much less attention to the process of expanding the

---

[1]Robert Solow, "A Contribution to the Theory of Economic Growth," *Quarterly Journal of Economics* 70 (February 1956), 65–94, and "Technical Change and the Aggregate Production Function," *Review of Economics and Statistics* 39 (August 1957), 312–20.

labor force (because labor is not seen as a binding constraint on growth), which usually is assumed to grow in line with the population. The key ideas in these kinds of models are relatively straightforward:

- *New investment increases the capital stock.* Investment in new factories or machines directly increases the capital stock, which facilitates greater production. For the capital stock to grow, the value of new investment must be greater than the amount of depreciation of existing capital. Factories and machines deteriorate over time, and a certain amount of new investment is needed simply to keep pace and maintain the current size of the capital stock. Investment greater than the amount of depreciation directly adds to the capital stock. Investment must be greater than depreciation and the growth of the labor force for there to be an increase in capital per worker.

- *Investment is financed by saving.* We know from standard national accounts identities that investment equals saving.[2] Thus the models postulate that the key to increasing investment (and the capital stock) is to increase saving.

- *Saving comes from current income.* Households save whatever income they do not consume. Corporations save in the form of retained earnings after distribution of dividends to stockholders. Governments either add to saving to the extent that they receive tax payments in excess of government current (noninvestment) spending (that is, a budget surplus, excluding investment spending) or detract from saving if they spend more than tax receipts (a budget deficit, excluding investment spending). We discuss these concepts in more depth in Chapters 10 and 11. Gross domestic saving, which combines all three sources of saving, provides the resources to finance investment.[3]

A key decision facing households, corporations, and governments is how much income to consume and how much to save. Individuals do not care about the level of capital or even the level of output, but they do care about the amount of goods and services they consume. However, there is a clear trade-off: The more that is consumed now, the less that is available for saving and therefore for investment, growth, and increased future consumption. On the one hand, people prefer to consume sooner rather than later. Given a choice between better housing now or in five years, everyone would choose now. On the other hand, people also recognize that consuming all income now is shortsighted. At a minimum, enough needs to be saved to compensate for depreciation of existing assets: to fix the roof on the house when it leaks, repair

---

[2]On the production side of the national accounts (for a closed economy with no trade), everything that is produced (total output, usually designated as Y) must be used for either consumption (C) or investment (I). On the income side, total income (also designated as Y because the value of total output must equal total income) is either used to purchase consumption goods (C) or saved (S). Putting these two identities together (because Y and C appear in both), saving must be equal to investment.

[3]In an open economy with trade and international capital flows, foreign saving (for example, borrowing from an overseas bank) can add to the total pool of available saving.

the motorbike, or replace a worn-out hoe. Additional saving can provide the basis for even higher income in the future. Deferring current consumption can lead to greater consumption later. For example, a farmer who wants to buy a water buffalo may have to reduce his or her consumption for several years to save enough to eventually make the purchase. The farmer's reward comes later, when (ideally) the water buffalo increases farm production and income by far more than the amount saved, allowing for even larger consumption in the future.

As the last sentence hints, although generating saving and investment is necessary for growth, it is not sufficient. The investments actually have to pay off with higher income in the future, and not all investments do so. The farmer who buys the water buffalo will not earn the reward if the field is too rocky to plow or the land does not have enough nutrients to support the crop. If the government forces down the price of the crop (for example, to try to keep food prices low for urban consumers), the farmer's income will fall and the investment will be much less profitable. If property rights are not secure, the farmer could lose the water buffalo or the land. Changes in world market prices (well out of the farmer's control) could also affect income. These issues highlight a key point: *Sustaining economic growth requires both generating new investment and ensuring that the investment is productive.* This idea is a recurrent theme in the next two chapters and throughout this book.

SOURCES OF GROWTH ANALYSIS

So far, we have identified factor accumulation and productivity gains as the two core determinants of growth. But how important are each of these in explaining growth? Robert Solow pioneered early efforts to quantify the contribution of each of the proximate causes of increased output—capital accumulation, labor accumulation, and productivity gains—to economic growth. This approach is more of an accounting framework based on actual data than an economic model. It seeks to answer the following question: What proportions of recorded economic growth can we attribute to growth in the capital stock, growth of the labor force, and changes in overall productivity?[4]

One way to explore how factor accumulation and productivity growth affect output and economic growth is by examining a **production function**, which characterizes how inputs (capital and labor) are combined to produce various levels of output. Figure 3–1 shows an example of a common production function. The horizontal axis shows one measure of factor inputs (the amount of capital per worker),

---

[4]Solow, "Technical Change and the Aggregate Production Function." A year before Solow's paper, Moses Abramovitz found similar estimates of the contribution of productivity gains to U.S. growth between 1870 and 1953 using a less formal methodology. See his "Resource and Output Trends in the United States since 1870," *American Economic Review* 46, no. 2 (May 1956), 5–23.

and the vertical axis shows the amount of output per worker (in this example, pairs of running shoes). Combining capital and labor into the single "capital per worker" term is a convenient way to simplify the analysis, but it also reflects the dominant role that capital has played in thinking on economic growth over the years. In most models, insufficient capital is seen as the binding constraint on growth. Labor is usually assumed to be in plentiful supply, based on the observation of unemployed or underemployed workers. Thus, in this formulation, increasing the amount of capital available for each worker is seen as key to growth.

Factor accumulation is shown in Figure 3–1a as a movement to the right along the *x*-axis. As the economy accumulates more capital for each of its workers, output expands, shown by the upward slope of the production function. Note that this particular production function begins to flatten out as capital per worker expands, a characteristic that we explore more fully later. In this case, as the value of capital

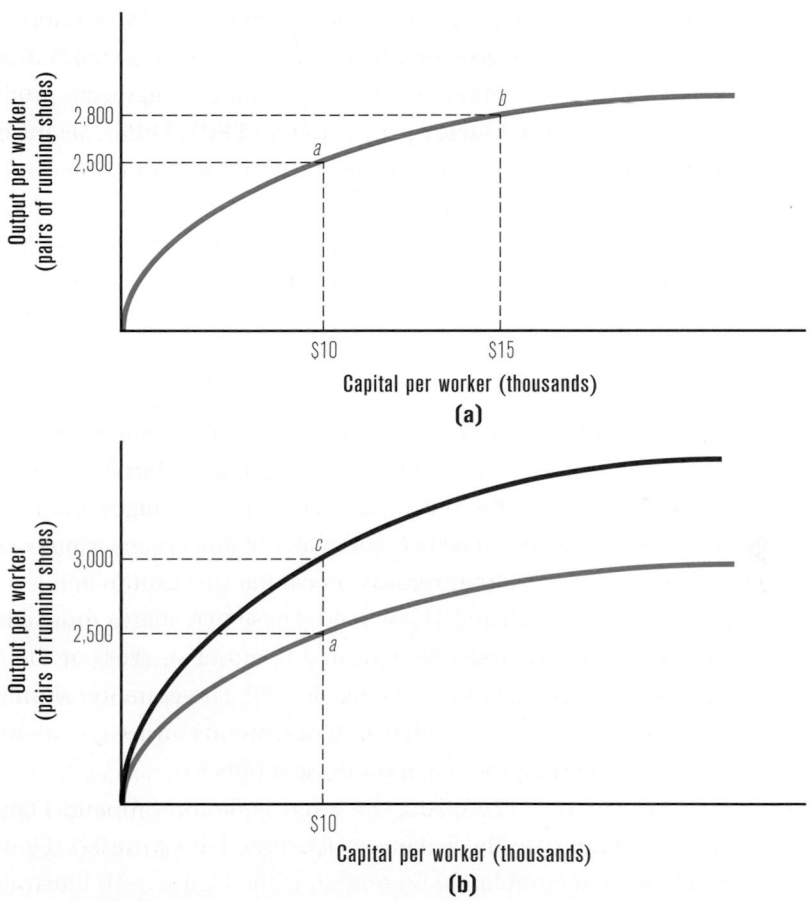

FIGURE 3-1 **Basic Sources of Economic Growth**

(a) Factor accumulation. As capital per worker expands, output per worker increases.
(b) Productivity gains. As the factors of production are used more efficiently or the economy acquires new technology, the same level of capital per worker can produce more output.

per worker increases from \$10,000 to \$15,000, output per worker grows from 2,500 to 2,800 pairs of shoes. The movement from point *a* to point *b* on the production function is the process of economic growth. Of course, growth of this magnitude (12 percent) does not happen instantaneously. It might take two years or so, in which case the annual rate of growth would be a brisk 5.8 percent.

Figure 3-1b shows the relationship between productivity change and economic growth. As factors of production are used more efficiently or as new technology is adopted, the production function shifts upward. With this productivity gain, any amount of capital per worker produces more output than it did before. The production function shifts upward so that \$10,000 worth of capital per worker can now produce 3,000 pairs of running shoes, whereas it originally produced 2,500 pairs. This expansion of output of 20 percent might take four years, in which case the annual rate of growth would be 4.7 percent. In this case, the movement along the path from point *a* to point *c* depicts the process of economic growth through productivity gains.

Solow's procedure for measuring these relationships usually is referred to as **growth accounting** or **sources of growth analysis**. He starts with a standard production function relating the contribution of labor and capital to aggregate production, then adds a term to capture **total factor productivity (TFP)**. TFP is meant to measure the contribution to production of efficiency, technology, and other influences on productivity. This production function is then converted into a form that makes it possible to measure the contribution of changes in each term—expansion of the labor force, additions to the capital stock, and growth in TFP—to overall growth. The resulting equation is

$$g_Y = (W_K \times g_K) + (W_L \times g_L) + a \qquad [3\text{-}1]$$

where g_Y stands for the growth of total income, or gross domestic product (GDP); g_K and g_L are the growth rates of the capital stock (K) and the labor force (L), respectively; and W_L and W_K represent the shares in total income of wages and returns on capital, respectively. For example, if 60 percent of all income comes from wages and the remaining 40 percent comes from returns on capital (for example, interest payments and rent), then $W_L = 0.60$ and $W_K = 0.40$. These two shares must add up to 100 percent because all income must be allocated to either workers or the owners of capital. The final term, a, is the rate of change in TFP. The equation should make intuitive sense: It shows us how the growth in output depends on the growth in inputs (K and L) and the growth in the productivity of those inputs (a).

It is important to see the relationship between equation 3-1 and Figure 3-1. Equation 3-1 simply summarizes the two effects illustrated in Figure 3-1. Figure 3-1a shows the effect of factor accumulation on output, while Figure 3-1b illustrates productivity growth as a vertical shift of the production function (for example, getting more output per unit of input). Equation 3-1 combines these two dimensions of growth in a way that allows us to distinguish between them. The first two terms on the right-hand side of the equation, $(W_K \times g_K) + (W_L \times g_L)$, describe movements along the production function (that is, using more inputs to increase output). TFP growth (indicated by a in equation 3–1) measures the upward shift in the production function in Figure 3–1b.

The basic procedure is to substitute actual data for all the variables in equation 3-1 except a, which cannot be measured directly, then calculate a as the residual. This is the famous **Solow residual**. In this way, the contribution of each of these variables to growth can be measured and identified. A straightforward numerical example illustrates the way in which this equation is used. From the statistical records of a developing country, we find the following values for the variables in the equation:

g_Y = 0.05 (GDP growth rate of 5 percent a year).

g_K = 0.07 (capital stock growth of 7 percent a year).

g_L = 0.02 (labor force growth of 2 percent a year).

W_L = 0.6 (the share of labor in national income is 60 percent).

W_K = 0.4 (the share of capital is 40 percent).

By substituting these figures into equation 3–1, we get

$$0.05 = (0.4 \times 0.07) + (0.6 \times 0.02) + a$$

Solving for a, we find that a = 0.01, meaning that TFP growth is 1 percent per year. These figures tell us the degree to which capital accumulation, labor accumulation, and TFP growth each contribute to the overall rate of output growth of 5 percent. TFP growth of 1 percent counts for one fifth (20 percent) of total growth. The growth in the capital stock accounts for slightly more than half (56 percent) the total growth: $(0.4 \times 0.07)/0.05$. Finally, growth in the labor force accounts for the remaining 24 percent of total growth: $(0.02 \times 0.6)/0.05$. In this particular example, capital accumulation is the main driver of growth, with labor accumulation and TFP growth each contributing similar amounts.

This type of accounting analysis has been used widely in many countries to examine the sources of growth, with particular attention paid to calculating TFP growth. Before examining some of these results, however, it is important to recognize the limits of this kind of study, arising from the fact that we can estimate productivity growth only as the residual output growth unexplained by having used more inputs. There are at least two kinds of problems:

- First, a represents a combination of influences that this analysis cannot entirely disentangle. Should improvements in a be attributed to efficiency gains stemming from improved trade policies, reduced corruption, or streamlined bureaucratic procedures? Or are they due to the introduction of faster computers, new seed varieties for agricultural crops, or other technologies? The limited growth accounting framework cannot definitively answer these questions without adding many more variables for which data do not exist (although that has not stopped analysts from assigning their own favorite explanation to the results).

- Second, *a* invariably is measured inaccurately because it is the residual in the equation. All economic data are measured with some inevitable errors, including all the data used in equation 3–1. As a result, in addition to TFP, *a* captures the net effect of all the errors and omissions in the other data.

What is labeled TFP actually, in practice, is a combination of errors in the data, omission of other factors that should be included in the growth equation, and efficiency gains and changes in technology. As a result, there is a danger in trying to read too much into these data when analysts interpret them as strictly efficiency gains or the effects of new technology. Rather than truly being TFP growth, *a* simply is the part of measured growth that cannot be explained by data on the traditional factors of production. For this reason, economist Moses Abramovitz famously referred to the residual *a* as a "measure of our ignorance" about the growth process.[5]

Sources of growth analyses have been carried out for many countries. Solow's initial study on the United States attributed a surprisingly large share of growth to the residual and a correspondingly small share to changes in the capital stock: 88 percent to TFP growth and only 12 percent to increases in capital per worker. Subsequent work by Abramovitz, Edward Denison, Zvi Griliches, Dale Jorgenson, and others attempted to measure, in a more precise way, the contribution of various inputs to the growth process. They divided labor into different skill categories, based on the amounts of formal education workers had received. A worker having a high school education and earning $50,000 a year is treated as the equivalent of two people having only primary school education and earning $25,000 a year each. Similar procedures are used to measure the increase in productivity that occurs when workers shift from low-productivity occupations in rural areas to higher-productivity occupations in urban areas. Other methods are used to measure improvements in the quality of capital and increasing economies of scale.

Many of these more detailed analyses of the U.S. economy found results similar to Solow's initial work: The bulk of the growth process could be attributed to the residual, with relatively small amounts apportioned to various categories of labor, capital, and other inputs. Over the years, many more studies have been completed for the industrialized countries. Increases in the capital stock frequently account for less than half the increase in output, particularly in rapidly growing countries. These results came as a bit of a surprise for most economists because most basic models put capital formation at the heart of the growth process.

Similar studies have now been carried out for a wide range of developing countries. Data problems and price distortions tend to be more severe for developing countries than for the industrialized countries, making the results even harder to interpret. Few developing countries, for example, have reliable measures for differences in the quality of alternative capital input and labor skill categories.

---

[5]Abramovitz, "Resource and Output Trends in the United States since 1870."

Generally speaking, sources of growth analyses in developing countries attribute a larger role to capital formation than in the industrialized country studies. This is consistent with the idea that developing countries have lower levels of capital per worker than the industrialized countries and can catch up (or converge incomes) through the investment process. Much of the capital equipment imported by developing countries (counted as investment) embodies advances in technology. Therefore, the mobilization of capital remains a major concern of policy makers in developing countries.

Economists Barry Bosworth and Susan Collins explored the relative contributions of physical capital, human capital (in the form of education), and TFP to economic growth in a large number of countries around the world between 1970 and 2000. Some of their results are shown in Table 3–2.[6] As with other studies, they found a fairly consistent pattern that capital accumulation was the main contributor to growth for developing countries, whereas for industrialized countries, the main contributions were more evenly split between capital accumulation and TFP growth. In East Asia, capital accumulation accounted for about two-thirds of total growth, with TFP growth accounting for a smaller share. In comparing TFP growth across countries, the rapidly growing East Asian economies generally (but not always) recorded faster TFP growth than did developing countries from other regions of the world. TFP growth in East Asia was generally faster than that of the industrialized countries during the 1970s and 1980s and about the same during the 1990s.

Average TFP growth was negative in all three decades in Africa, during the 1980s in Latin America, during the 1970s in South Asia, and during the 1970s and 1990s in the Middle East! What does this mean? Inputs actually became less productive over time. This might be the result of capital and labor lying idle, as often happens during wars, political unrest, or recessions. During Latin America's deep recession, induced by the debt crisis of the 1980s, growth was negative while new investment was essentially zero, implying less productive use of existing capital. Negative TFP growth also might reflect the accumulation of increasingly unproductive assets, like presidential palaces or so-called white elephant projects. For example, Ethiopia built one of the largest tanneries in the world, but it usually operates at a fraction of its capacity, and Nigeria's Ajaokuta Steel factory cost nearly $5 billion in construction costs over 25 years and has yet to produce any steel.

In a more recent study, Bosworth and Collins provide a detailed comparative analysis of the sources of growth in the world's two most populous countries—India and China.[7] Since 1980, GDP per capita has more than doubled in India and increased more than sevenfold in China. While China's growth has been driven by its

[6]Susan M. Collins and Barry Bosworth, "The Empirics of Growth: An Update," *Brookings Papers on Economic Activity* 2 (2003), 113–79.

[7]Barry Bosworth and Susan M. Collins, "Accounting for Growth: Comparing India and China," *Journal of Economic Perspectives*, 22, no. 1 (Winter 2008), 45–66.

TABLE 3-2 Sources of Growth in East Asia and Other Regions, 1960–2000
(Average Annual Growth Rate, Percent)

| | CONTRIBUTION BY COMPONENT | | |
	GROWTH OF OUTPUT PER WORKER	PHYSICAL CAPITAL PER WORKER	EDUCATION PER WORKER	TOTAL FACTOR PRODUCTIVITY
Brazil				
1970s	4.86	2.02	0.12	2.72
1980s	−1.63	0.16	0.68	−2.47
1990s	0.71	0.07	0.38	0.25
Ecuador				
1970s	5.96	1.05	0.89	4.03
1980s	−1.42	−0.28	0.16	−1.30
1990s	−1.40	−0.46	0.31	−1.24
Egypt				
1970s	4.39	2.33	0.54	1.52
1980s	2.91	1.98	0.89	0.03
1990s	1.46	−0.12	0.64	0.94
Ethiopia				
1970s	0.55	0.22	0.13	0.20
1980s	−1.74	1.11	0.27	−3.12
1990s	1.84	0.81	0.29	0.74
Ghana				
1970s	−2.01	−0.24	0.24	−2.00
1980s	−1.14	−1.23	0.15	−0.07
1990s	1.62	0.80	0.16	0.65
India				
1970s	0.70	0.61	0.36	−0.27
1980s	3.91	1.06	0.36	2.48
1990s	3.13	1.35	0.49	1.29
Singapore				
1970s	4.41	3.53	0.11	0.78
1980s	3.79	2.01	0.39	1.38
1990s	5.08	1.96	0.91	2.22
Taiwan				
1970s	5.93	3.69	1.11	1.14
1980s	5.36	2.19	0.24	2.94
1990s	4.84	2.66	0.41	1.77
United States				
1970s	0.83	0.11	0.71	0.01
1980s	1.82	0.55	0.12	1.15
1990s	1.84	0.74	0.11	0.98
Africa				
1970s	1.03	1.28	0.08	−0.32
1980s	−1.06	−0.07	0.42	−1.41
1990s	−0.16	−0.09	0.40	−0.48
East Asia				
1970s	4.27	2.74	0.67	0.86
1980s	4.36	2.45	0.66	1.25
1990s	3.36	2.35	0.50	0.52

Industrial countries				
1970s	1.75	0.95	0.52	0.28
1980s	1.82	0.69	0.24	0.90
1990s	1.52	0.75	0.22	0.54
Latin America				
1970s	2.69	1.25	0.34	1.10
1980s	−1.77	0.04	0.47	−2.28
1990s	0.91	0.16	0.34	0.41
Middle East				
1970s	1.92	2.08	0.45	−0.61
1980s	1.15	0.55	0.53	0.07
1990s	0.84	0.34	0.52	−0.01
South Asia				
1970s	0.68	0.56	0.34	−0.23
1980s	3.67	1.02	0.40	2.25
1990s	2.78	1.19	0.42	1.17

Source: Susan M. Collins and Barry Bosworth, "The Empirics of Growth: An Update," *Brookings Papers on Economic Activity* 2 (2003), 113–79.

industrial sector, India's less traditional growth pattern has been driven by its service sector. Comparing these two economies in the aggregate for the years 1978–2004, Bosworth and Collins estimate that TFP growth accounted for just under half of the growth in output per worker in both countries. Yet, the absolute rate of TFP growth in China over that period was 3.6 percent per year compared with 1.6 percent per year in India. The contribution of TFP to growth in output per worker in India and China, they find, differs sharply from the broader pattern in East Asia (excluding China), where average TFP growth was slower (0.9 percent per year) and accounted for less than 25 percent of growth in output per worker.

The aggregate figures for the contribution of TFP to output growth in Sub-Saharan Africa presented in Table 3–2 are bleak. Yet, a more recent and more detailed analysis of that region by economist Steven Radelet demonstrates that for the 17 countries of the region that succeeded in stabilizing their economic and political circumstances by the mid-1990s, average TFP growth rates soared from negative and unstable rates to positive TFP growth since 1995 on the order of 1.5 percent per year.[8] In summary, sources of growth analyses suggest that capital accumulation is the main source of growth for developing countries, consistent with the Solow growth model. TFP can play an important part in the growth process in the appropriate

[8]Steven Radelet, *Emerging Africa: How 17 Countries Are Leading the Way*. Washington, DC: Center for Global Development, 2010. Radelet's 17 emerging African countries are Botswana, Burkina Faso, Cape Verde, Ethiopia, Ghana, Lesotho, Mali, Mauritius, Mozambique, Namibia, Rwanda, São Tomé and Príncipe, Seychelles, South Africa, Tanzania, Uganda, and Zambia.

policy and structural context. In rapidly growing economies, both factor accumulation and TFP growth appear to play an important role. TFP growth tends to become more important as income rises and is a major contributor to growth in the high-income industrialized countries.

CHARACTERISTICS OF RAPIDLY GROWING COUNTRIES

We identified the key proximate causes of economic growth: factor accumulation (accumulating additional productive assets) and productivity growth. Productivity growth, in turn, comes either from efficiency gains or new technology. Sustaining economic growth requires both generating new investment and ensuring that the new investment is productive. These basic points, however, raise a new set of questions. What are the more fundamental characteristics that explain a country's ability to attract investment and accumulate capital, increase efficiency, and obtain new technologies? More broadly, what are the deep characteristics that distinguish more rapidly growing economies from slowly growing ones?

A large body of research over the last few decades tried to answer this question by searching for broad characteristics common to rapidly growing economies. Until relatively recently, it was difficult for researchers to systematically examine these issues due to severe data limitations. Many researchers examined trends in individual countries, but it was difficult to draw general conclusions from these case studies. A few pioneering efforts, such as Irma Adelman and Cynthia Taft Morris's *Society, Politics, and Economic Development—A Quantitative Approach*,[9] paved the way for today's cross-country empirical growth research. In recent years, this type of research has grown very rapidly, in line with the emergence of many new and large data sets on income in PPP terms, education levels, health characteristics, quality of governance, and a host of related items.[10]

Most of the recent studies are modeled on research conducted by economist Robert Barro in the early 1990s. These studies try to explain the variance in growth rates across countries. With country growth rates as the dependent variable, this approach examines several variables that might affect growth through one of the channels identified earlier (controlling for the initial level of income in each country). These variables include levels of education and health, policy choices, resource endowments, geographic characteristics (latitude, whether the country is landlocked, etc.), and political systems.

---

[9]Irma Adelman and Cynthia Taft Morris, *Society, Politics, and Economic Development—A Quantitative Approach* (Baltimore, MD: Johns Hopkins University Press, 1967).

[10]The vast literature on cross-country growth empirics began with Robert Barro, "Economic Growth in a Cross Section of Countries," *Quarterly Journal of Economics* 106, no. 2 (May 1991), 407–43. For the most comprehensive recent survey of this type of research, see S. Durlauf, P. Johnson, and J. Temple, "Growth Econometrics," in P. Aghion and S. Durlauf eds., *Handbook of Economic Growth* (Amsterdam: North Holland, 2005).

This type of research has been controversial, and there is far from a consensus on the exact group of variables that affects growth.[11] For one thing, although this research starts with the Solow model, for many of the variables tested, there is no well-developed theoretical link between the variable and either economic growth or the proximate causes of growth (factor accumulation or productivity growth). The existing theories on economic growth simply are not explicit enough about exactly what variables determine the shape of the production function, the rate of investment, the profitability of investment, efficiency, and the rate of change in technology. Some characteristics may appear statistically important in one research study that includes a certain group of variables but unimportant in another study with a different group of variables.[12]

A second issue has to do with interpretation of the statistical results. For example, most economists would agree that high saving rates are associated with rapid economic growth. But which causes which? Higher saving can lead to more rapid growth, as suggested by the Solow model, while faster economic growth might provide more disposable income and a higher saving rate (we discuss this issue more in Chapter 10). It is a major statistical challenge to precisely estimate the magnitude of these two effects.

Despite these issues, such empirical growth research has helped analysts better understand some of the broad characteristics associated with rapid growth, albeit very imperfectly. The broad thrust of the conclusions from research across countries is consistent with many studies of individual countries. Although the debate is far from over about which variables influence long-run growth, how they do so, and the magnitude of the effect, this research has helped provide broad clues about why some economies grow faster than others. The most rapidly growing developing countries tend to share six broad characteristics.[13]

1. MACROECONOMIC AND POLITICAL STABILITY

Stability is good for growth. Economic and political instability undermine investment and growth and are especially hard on the poor, who are least able to protect themselves against volatility. Consider the Democratic Republic of the Congo (formerly Zaire), which suffered through inflation rates averaging an astonishing 2,800 percent

[11]For critiques of the cross-country approach, see Durlauf et al., "Growth Econometrics;" and David Lindauer and Lant Pritchett, "What's the Big Idea? The Third Generation of Policies for Economic Growth," *Economia* 3, no. 1 (Fall 2002).

[12]A seminal study on the robustness of explanatory variables across different specifications is Ross Levine and David Renelt, "A Sensitivity Analysis of Cross-Country Growth Regressions," *American Economic Review* 82, no. 4 (September 1992), 942–63.

[13]Economist Xavier Sala-i-Martin has examined a wide range of studies and identified a list of variables that are most consistently and robustly found to be closely associated with economic growth. See Xavier X. Sala-i-Martin, "I Just Ran Two Million Regressions," *American Economic Review* 87, no. 2 (May 1997), 178–83. The specific list of key areas used here is similar to that suggested by Lawrence Summers and Vinod Thomas in "Recent Lessons of Development," *World Bank Research Observer* 8, no. 2 (July 1993), 241–54.

per year between 1990 and 2002 and civil and cross-border wars involving troops from at least five other countries. It is not surprising that its growth and development performance was about the worst in the world: "growth" of −7.2 percent per year (meaning that average incomes fell by 60 percent over 12 years), life expectancy fell from 52 to 45 years, and infant mortality rose from 128 to 139 per thousand.

Relatively low budget deficits over time (with corresponding high rates of government saving), prudent monetary policy (which keeps inflation in check), appropriate exchange rates, suitable financial markets (depending on the stage of development), and judicious foreign borrowing at sustainable levels are the key elements to macroeconomic stability. Stability reduces risk for investors, whether they are multinational conglomerates or coffee farmers considering planting more trees. A high rate of inflation, for example, makes prices and profits much less predictable, undermining growth.[14] Volatile short-term capital flows can lead to wide swings in the exchange rate, affecting prices throughout the economy and undermining investment. In extreme situations, volatile capital flows can lead to full-blown financial crises, as we explore more deeply in Chapter 13.

Political stability is, of course, also good for growth and development. Civil and cross-border wars, military coups, and other incidences of political instability undermine investment and growth. Once again, the poor are the most vulnerable and least able to protect themselves from the consequences of political unrest. In the late 1990s, nearly one-third of the 42 countries in sub-Saharan Africa were embroiled in cross-border or civil wars, which took a huge toll on human lives, infrastructure, institutions, and economic activity and commerce. Figure 3–2 shows sharp declines in income, averaging 28 percent, after civil war in seven developing countries. By contrast, most of the relatively successful developing countries during the last several decades were politically stable for long periods of time. Although some of the successful countries experienced periods of instability, for the most part they were short-lived. Economist Paul Collier and others have pointed out the insidious negative cycle of civil war in low-income countries: poverty increases the risk of conflict, and conflict undermines growth and entrenches poverty.[15] Of course, the absence of war is no guarantee of economic growth. Cuba, Jamaica, and Kenya were politically stable for decades but still experienced low growth.

---

[14]The negative association between inflation and growth has been demonstrated in numerous studies, prominent among them Robert Barro, "Inflation and Growth," *Review* [Federal Reserve Bank of St. Louis] 78, no. 3, 153–69 (May–June 1996).

[15]See Paul Collier, "On the Economic Consequences of Civil War," *Oxford Economic Papers* 51 (1999), 168–83; and Paul Collier, V. L. Elliot, Håvard Hegre, Anke Hoeffler, Marta Reynal-Querol, and Nicholas Sambanis, *Breaking the Conflict Trap: Civil War and Development Policy* (Washington, DC: World Bank and Oxford University Press, 2003). Collier summarizes this and related work in *The Bottom Billion: Why the Poorest Countries are Failing and What Can Be Done About It,* (Oxford: Oxford University Press, 2007).

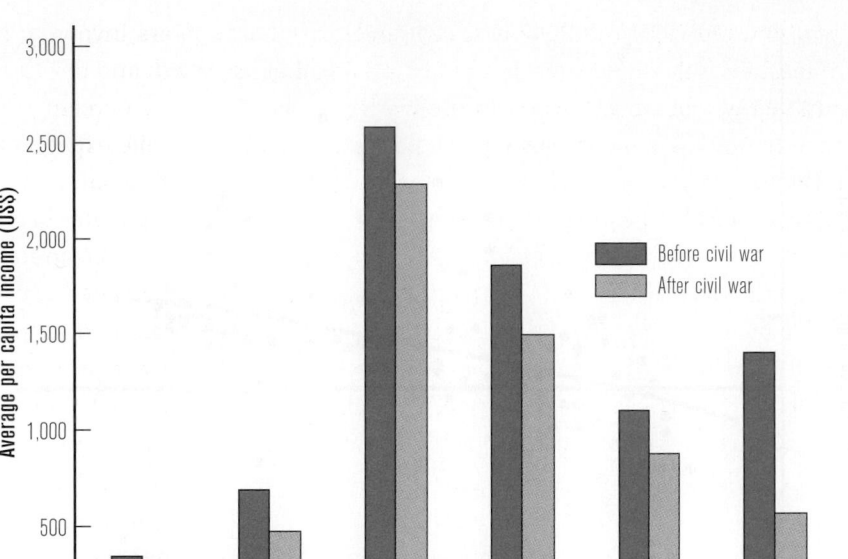

FIGURE 3-2 **GDP per Capita before and after a Civil War**

In these six countries, average income was 28 percent lower after the civil war than before.

Sources: Civil war data from Paul Collier, V. L. Elliot, Håvard Hegre, Anke Hoeffler, Marta Reynal-Querol, and Nicholas Sambanis, *Breaking the Conflict Trap: Civil War and Development Policy* (Washington, DC: World Bank and Oxford University Press, 2003). Gross domestic product per capita data from *World Development Indicators 2004*, (Washington, DC: World Bank), http://data.worldbank.org/data-catalog/world-development -indicators.

2. INVESTMENT IN HEALTH AND EDUCATION

Countries with *longer life expectancy* (and therefore better health) tend to grow faster, after accounting for other factors affecting growth, as shown in Figure 3–3.[16] A longer life expectancy indicates general improvements in the health of a population, which in turn means a healthier and more productive labor force. Thus, one way that life expectancy affects growth is by influencing productivity. In addition, a higher life expectancy might also boost saving and capital accumulation because businesses may be more likely to invest where workers are healthier and more productive. Moreover, people are more likely to invest in education to deepen their skills if they expect to live longer and reap greater benefits. Accessible basic healthcare facilities, clean water and sanitation, disease control programs, and strong reproductive and

---

[16]See, for example, World Health Organization, *Macroeconomics and Health: Investing in Health for Economic Development, Report of the Commission on Macroeconomics and Health* (Geneva: World Health Organization, 2001). For a brief nontechnical summary, see David E. Bloom, David Canning, and Dean Jamison, "Health, Wealth, and Welfare," *Finance and Development* 41, no. 1 (March 2004), 10–15.

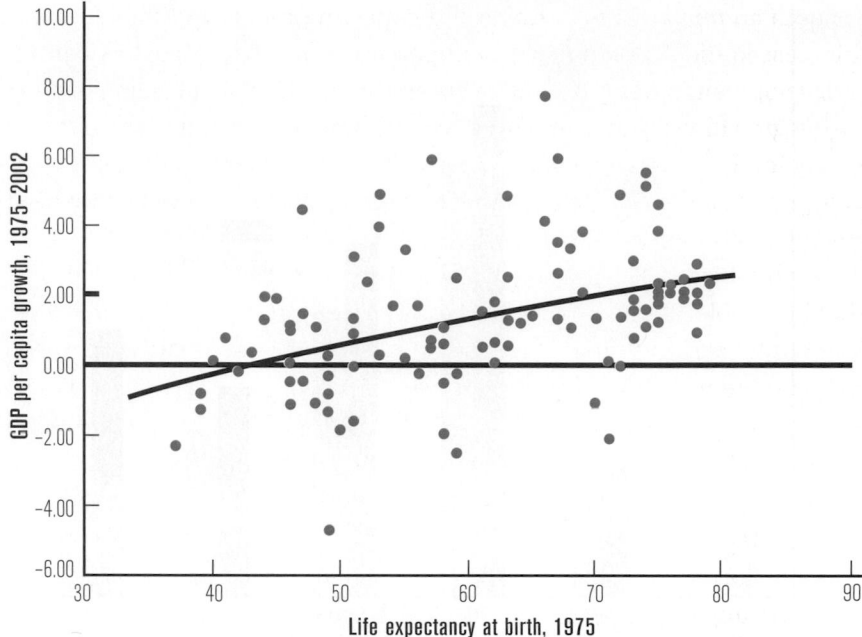

FIGURE 3-3 Growth and Life Expectancy

maternal and child health programs help countries lengthen life expectancy and improve worker productivity.

Malaysia's efforts to reduce malaria and improve health are a good example. When settlers first began to arrive in what is now Kuala Lumpur in the 1850s in search of tin, nearly half died of malaria. A century later, things had improved, but malaria and other diseases were still a problem, and life expectancy in 1960 was just 54 years. Growth during the 1960s was still a respectable 3.4 percent per year. An active government malaria control program began to make significant inroads, and by 1975, the number of malaria cases had been cut by two-thirds relative to 1960. Partly as a result, life expectancy increased to 64 years. Improved health (along with several other factors) contributed to a surge in growth, which accelerated to about 5 percent per year between 1976 and 1996, slowing only in the wake of the 1998 East Asian financial crisis. The incidence of malaria has continued to decline, falling to just above 7,000 confirmed cases in 2009.[17]

Note that the relationship between life expectancy and growth works both ways: Better health helps spur faster growth, and faster growth (and higher income) helps improve life expectancy, as we discuss in more detail in Chapter 9. That is, better

[17]The data on the incidence of malaria come from the World Health Organization, World Malaria Report 2011," available at www.who.int/malaria/world_malaria_report_2011/en, accessed February 2012. The country profile for Malaysia is available at www.who.int/entity/malaria/publications/country-profiles/profile_mys_en.pdf, accessed February 2012.

health is both an *input* to and *outcome* of the growth process. In Chapter 2, we discussed increased life expectancy as an important development goal as part of the human development index (HDI). Here we emphasize the role of good health as an input to the growth process. These two positions are not contradictory—far from it. Rather, they imply a positive reinforcing cycle in which better health supports faster economic growth, and the higher income from growth facilitates even better health.

Similarly, both *increased levels and improved quality of education* should translate into a more highly skilled workforce and increased productivity. A skilled workforce should be able to work more quickly with fewer errors, use existing machinery more effectively, and invent or adapt new technologies more easily. As with better health, a more highly educated workforce may also help attract new investment, thereby contributing to capital accumulation as well. Also, like better health, education has a pro-cyclical relationship with growth, in which better education helps support growth and growth generates the resources to finance stronger educational systems. Education of girls has a particularly strong effect on growth, both the direct impact on their skills and the indirect impact in the next generation on their children's health and education. The impact of education on growth can take a long time because investments in primary school education today may not show up as improved worker productivity for many years. The quality of service delivery is just as important as quantity. It is not enough to build schools and increase enrollment rates; teachers have to show up, be motivated, and have adequate basic supplies (such as textbooks) to do their job.[18]

As discussed in Chapter 8, most micro-level studies in individual developing countries show very high rates of return to education, especially girl's education. However, in macro-level cross-country studies, the statistical strength of the relationship often is relatively modest. This may be due to difficulties in accurately measuring the quantity and quality of education across a large number of countries in a consistent way. It also suggests that a better-educated workforce is no guarantee of more rapid economic growth. Human capital, just like physical capital, can be squandered in an environment that is not otherwise supportive of economic growth.

3. EFFECTIVE GOVERNANCE AND INSTITUTIONS

The role of governance and institutions in economic growth in development began to receive serious attention only beginning in the early 1990s (Box 3–3). This work was heavily influenced by the research and writing of Nobel Prize–winning economist Douglass C. North of Washington University.[19] Since that time, many studies have found a positive relationship between economic growth and the strength of the rule

---

[18]These issues are explored more deeply in Chapter 8 and in the World Bank's world development report, *Making Service Work for Poor People* (Washington, DC: World Bank and Oxford University Press, 2004).

[19]See, for example, Douglass C. North, *Institutions, Institutional Change, and Economic Performance* (New York: Cambridge University Press, 1990).

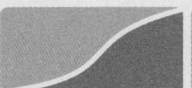

BOX 3-3 INSTITUTIONS, GOVERNANCE, AND GROWTH[a]

The role of institutions and governance in supporting and sustaining economic growth began to receive strong attention in the 1990s, following the path-breaking work by Nobel Prize–winning economist Douglass C. North.[b] In its broadest definition, institutions include a society's formal rules (for example, constitutions, laws, and regulations), informal constraints (such as conventions, norms, traditions, and self-enforced codes of conduct), and the organizations that operate within these rules and constraints.[c] There are many different kinds of institutions that influence growth and development. Dani Rodrik and Arvind Subramanian suggest four broad types of economic institutions, to which we add a fifth for political institutions:

- *Market-creating institutions* protect property rights, ensure that contracts are enforced, minimize corruption, and generally support the rule of law. Without these institutions in place, markets are likely not to exist or to perform poorly; by contrast, strengthening them can help boost investment and entrepreneurship. Examples include an independent judiciary, an effective police force, and enforceable contracts.
- *Market-regulating institutions* deal with market failures, such as imperfect information and economies of scale. These institutions limit monopoly power and help provide the basis for building and managing public goods, such as roads and fisheries. Examples include regulatory agencies in telecommunications, transportation, water and forestry resources, and financial services.
- *Market-stabilizing institutions* ensure low inflation, minimize macroeconomic volatility, ensure fiscal stability, and avert financial crises. Central banks, exchange rate systems, ministries of finance, and fiscal and budgetary rules are all market-stabilizing institutions.
- *Market-legitimizing institutions* provide social protection and insurance, focus on redistribution, and manage conflict. These institutions help

[a]This text draws heavily on the discussion of institutions found in *Finance and Development* 40, no. 2 (June 2003), particularly Dani Rodrik and Arvind Subramanian, "The Primacy of Institutions (and What This Does and Does Not Mean)"; and Jeffrey D. Sachs, "Institutions Matter, but Not for Everything."

[b]Douglass C. North, *Institutions, Institutional Change, and Economic Performance* (New York: Cambridge University Press, 1990).

[c]North distinguishes between the formal rules and informal constraints (which he includes in his definition of institutions) and organizations (which he excludes). He refers to institutions as the "rules of the game" and organizations as "the players." In common usage, however, many people use the term *institutions* to cover both the rules and the organizations.

protect individuals and corporations from shocks or disasters or from adverse market outcomes. Examples include pension systems, unemployment insurance schemes, welfare programs, and other social funds.
- *Political institutions* determine how society is governed and the extent of political participation. In many countries, there is a strong focus on the key institutions that support democracy, including a free press, elections, competitive political parties, and participatory politics.

A large body of evidence now shows a robust relationship between stronger institutions, rapid economic growth, and improved development outcomes. The evidence is based partly on major advancements in the ability to better measure governance and institutions, such as the data compiled by Dani Kaufmann and Aart Kraay at the World Bank Institute.[d] Strong institutions are central to managing financial systems, building public education and health systems, ensuring efficient trade and commerce, and governing legal systems. Much of neoclassical economic theory on well-functioning markets is based on the assumption that fundamental institutions are in place (such as contract enforcement, perfect information, and the rule of law). But in many low-income countries, these key institutions are weak or nonexistent.

Understanding the importance of institutions for growth brings us only so far, however. Economic analysis tells us very little about the specific forms of institutions that are best suited for a particular environment (for instance, common law versus civil law). There is significant debate about which institutions are most important for low-income countries, their specific form, and the relative importance of institutions versus other factors. Although some analysts claim that institutions dominate all other factors in the growth process, the bulk of the evidence suggests that other factors play an important role, such as policies, geography, and resource endowments. Much of the research indicates that institutions themselves are heavily influenced by geography, history, resource endowments, and the extent of integration with the global economy.

Perhaps even more important, theory and research do not tell us much about how institutions change and how a country with weak institutions can best strengthen them. Institutions change only slowly, but fortunately they do change. Deepening our understanding of how institutions affect growth and development, the appropriate form for institutions in different circumstances and how institutions change over time are major challenges for economists and development specialists in the future.

[d]Available at http://info.worldbank.org/governance/wgi/index.asp.

of law, the extent of corruption, property rights, the quality of government bureau-cracies, and other measures of governance and institutional quality.[20]

Stronger governance and institutions help improve the environment for invest-ment by reducing risk and increasing profitability. Investors are more likely to make long-term investments where they feel property rights are secure and their factory, machines, or land will not be confiscated. Strong legal systems can help settle commercial disputes in a predictable, rational manner. Low levels of corrup-tion help reduce the costs of investment, reduce risks, and increase productivity, as managers focus their attention on production rather than influencing politicians and government officials. Strong government economic institutions, such as the central bank, ministry of finance, ports authority, and ministry of trade can help establish effective government policies that influence both factor accumulation and productivity.

The most effective governments established institutions that helped facilitate (rather than hinder) strong economic management, effective social programs, and a robust private sector. Governance in the most rapidly growing countries varied widely from very effective (Singapore and Botswana) to more mixed (Indonesia and Thailand) but generally was better than in slower-growing countries.

4. FAVORABLE ENVIRONMENT FOR PRIVATE ENTERPRISE

Sustained economic growth requires millions of private individuals to make deci-sions every day regarding saving, investment, education, and job opportunities. Small-scale farmers, business owners, factory workers, and market stall vendors all strive daily to increase their incomes, and the regulatory and policy environment has a significant effect on their success or failure. For many countries, *agricultural policies* are central to the growth process. Where governments have pushed farm-gate prices low to keep food prices cheap or forced farmers to sell their products to government-owned marketing boards, agricultural production (and farmer income) has suffered. The most dramatic example of reducing restrictions of farmers is China's moves to decollectivize agricultural production in the early 1980s and to allow farmers to sell their produce on markets. China's agricultural output soared in the decade that fol-lowed. Farmers need reasonable access to fertilizers, seeds, and pesticides, and the construction of rural roads has had a dramatic impact on rural incomes in many countries, such as Indonesia. Absolute free markets are not necessarily the solution—some countries have subsidized fertilizer or other inputs to encourage their use,

[20]See, for example, Stephen Knack and Philip Keefer, "Institutions and Economic Performance: Cross Country Tests Using Alternative Institutional Measures," *Economics and Politics* 7, no. 3 (1995), 207–27; Daniel Kaufmann, Aart Kraay, and Pablo Zoido-Lobatón, "Governance Matters," World Bank Policy Research Paper No. 2196, October 1999; World Bank, Washington, DC; and Daron Acemoglu, Simon Johnson, and James Robinson, "The Colonial Origins of Comparative Development: An Empirical Investigation," *American Economic Review* 91, no. 5 (December 2001), 1369–401.

whereas others have used buffer stocks to counter large swings in prices—but policies that consistently push against markets (rather than helping strengthen markets) almost always fail in the long run.

The climate for small-scale businesses and manufacturing is also important for long-term growth. While some regulation is crucial for well-functioning markets, most governments in developing countries impose unnecessarily high costs on businesses through licensing, permits, and other restrictions. Hernando de Soto's *The Mystery of Capital* demonstrated the damaging effects of heavy business regulation and weak property rights.[21] When the regulatory burden to start a business is high, fewer entrepreneurs bother to start businesses, and when they do, they tend to operate on a smaller scale and in the informal sector. Moreover, government investments in infrastructure, at the core of capital formation, are central. No matter how favorable the policy environment, businesses cannot operate if the electricity shuts off every day, the water is brown, and the phones do not work.

5. TRADE, OPENNESS, AND GROWTH

Most economists agree that international trade plays an important role in economic growth. In discussing this role, however, it is important to distinguish between the volume of trade and trade policy. Economists Jeffrey Frankel and David Romer surmounted significant statistical challenges to demonstrate that trade (as a proportion of GDP) causes growth.[22] They find that a 1 percentage point increase in the ratio of trade to a country's GDP increases income per capita by at least 0.5 percent. Trade, they conclude, plays this role by encouraging countries to accumulate both physical and human capital and by increasing productivity. This finding is consistent with earlier studies that hypothesized trade could contribute to growth by facilitating transfers of both capital and technology and by creating incentives for competitiveness. Yet the conclusion that trade as a share of GDP contributes to growth says nothing directly about the relationship between trade *policy* and growth.

Casual observation suggests that outward orientation (a set of policies designed to encourage exports) contributes to growth. For instance, it's widely accepted that outward-oriented trade policies contributed to the rapid growth of many economies in East Asia, whereas inward-oriented trade policies (that had the effect of discouraging exports) contributed to slow growth in much of Latin America and sub-Saharan Africa. Yet, economists continue to debate the evidence in support of such

---

[21]Hernando de Soto, *The Mystery of Capital: Why Capitalism Triumphs in the West and Fails Everywhere Else* (New York: Basic Books, 2000). The World Bank and International Finance Corporation maintain an extensive program to monitor the costs of doing business in 183 economies. Data and publications from the Doing Business project are available at www.doingbusiness.org, accessed February 2012.

[22]Jeffrey Frankel and David Romer, "Does Trade Cause Growth?" *American Economic Review* 89, no. 3 (June 1999), 379–99.

conclusions. Part of the controversy lies in constructing measurable indicators of trade policy orientation. For instance, economist David Dollar constructed an indicator of outward orientation based on real exchange rate distortion and volatility.[23] He found that, for the period 1976–85, the developing countries that were most open to trade had an average annual growth rate of 2.9 percent per capita, whereas the most closed portion of his sample countries experienced negative growth of −1.3 percent.

In a highly influential study, economists Jeffrey Sachs and Andrew Warner constructed a composite indicator of openness to trade in which countries were deemed either open or closed based on several trade policy indicators.[24] They found openness to have a substantial influence on growth, concluding that open countries (between 1970 and 1989) grew at least 2 percentage points faster on average than did closed countries. Applying the Sachs-Warner indicator to a longer time period, economists Romain Wacziarg and Karen Horn Welch found that open economies over the period 1950–1998 had an average growth rate of income per capita of 2.7 percent as compared with an average growth of of 1.18 percent in closed economies, a margin of nearly 1.5 percentage points.[25] In a prominent response to these studies, however, economists Francísco Rodriguez and Dani Rodrik question the validity, interpretation, and robustness of these policy indicators, concluding that the evidence linking pro-trade policies to growth remains inconclusive.[26] We address these issues in depth in Chapters 17 and 18.

6. FAVORABLE GEOGRAPHY

A striking fact is that there are no rich economies located between the Tropic of Cancer and the Tropic of Capricorn other than Singapore and a few small, oil-rich countries. Figure 3–4 shows that the poorest countries in the world are almost all in the tropics, while the richest countries tend to be in more temperate zones. Even within the temperate zones, the regions closer to the tropics tend to be less well off: Northern Europe is richer than southern Europe, the northern part of the United States is wealthier than the southern parts, and southern Brazil is better off than the north part of the country. In Latin America and Africa, the wealthiest countries are located in the temperate south: Chile, Argentina, and South Africa.

---

[23]David Dollar, "Outward-Oriented Developing Economies Really Do Grow More Rapidly: Evidence from 95 LDCs, 1976–1985," *Economic Development and Cultural Change*, 40, no. 3 (April 1992), 523–44.

[24]Jeffrey Sachs and Andrew Warner, "Economic Reform and the Process of Global Integration," *Brookings Papers on Economic Activity* 26 (1995), 1–118.

[25]Romain Wacziarg and Karen Horn Welch, "Trade Liberalization and Growth: New Evidence," *World Bank Economic Review* 22, no. 2 (June 2008), 187–231.

[26]Francísco Rodriguez and Dani Rodrik, "Trade Policy and Economic Growth: A Skeptic's Guide to the Cross-National Evidence" (pp. 261–338), in Ben S. Bernanke and Kenneth Rogoff, eds., *NBER Macroeconomics Annual 2000* (Cambridge, MIT Press: National Bureau of Economic Research, 2001).

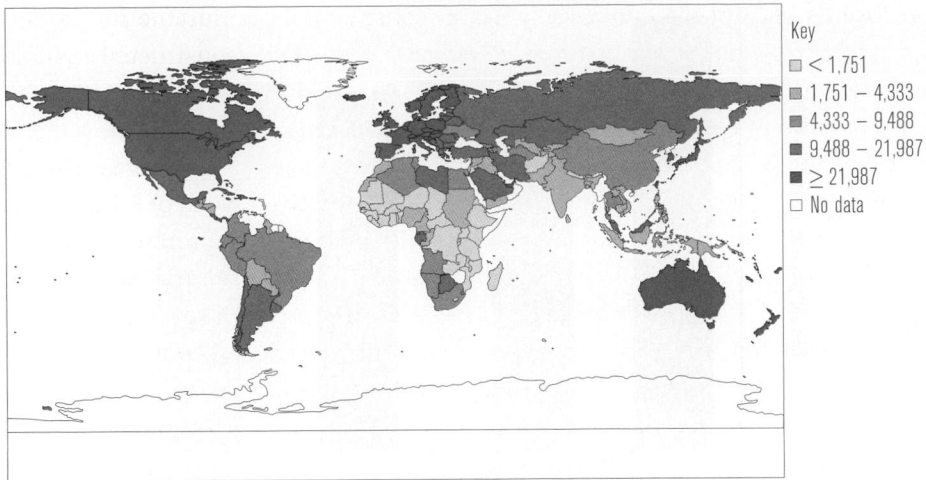

Key
- ☐ < 1,751
- ☐ 1,751 − 4,333
- ☐ 4,333 − 9,488
- ■ 9,488 − 21,987
- ■ ≥ 21,987
- ☐ No data

FIGURE 3-4 **Income Levels and Geography**

Data are gross domestic product per capita in 2009 (constant 2005 international dollars, PPP).

Source: World Bank, "World Bank Indicators," http://databank.worldbank.org.

Several studies have shown a strong relationship between location in the tropics, other geographical characteristics, and growth.[27] Figure 3–5 shows that the average growth rate per capita between 1975 and 2009 for countries located in the tropics was significantly lower than for countries outside the tropics. Tropical countries have to deal with a greater burden from virulent diseases, erratic climate, and at least in some areas, very poor-quality soil for agriculture. Most of the world's most virulent diseases are centered in the tropics, including malaria and HIV/AIDS. These diseases seriously undermine worker productivity and add to healthcare costs. Similarly, although erratic climate can occur anywhere around the world, floods, droughts, and violent storms tend to be more concentrated in the tropics. Hurricanes and typhoons, of course, are by definition tropical phenomena. Hotter climates make a long, hard day of outdoor work much more difficult, reducing labor productivity (one way Singapore has compensated for being in the tropics is by air-conditioning the vast majority of buildings in the country, a step that is much easier for a small city-state like Singapore than for most other countries). And while some tropical regions have very fertile soils (as in the rich lands in Java, one of the main islands of Indonesia), most of the great Sahara desert is in the tropics, as are the arid lands of northern Brazil. These characteristics work to reduce both factor productivity and

[27]Studies that explore the impact of geographical factors on levels of income and growth rates include Robert Hall and Charles Jones, "Why Do Some Countries Produce So Much More Output per Worker Than Others?" *Quarterly Journal of Economics* 114 (February 1999), 83–116; and John Gallup and Jeffrey Sachs, "Geography and Economic Development" (127–78), in Boris Pleskovic and Joseph Stiglitz, eds., *World Bank Annual Conference on Development Economics 1998* (Washington, DC: World Bank, 1998).

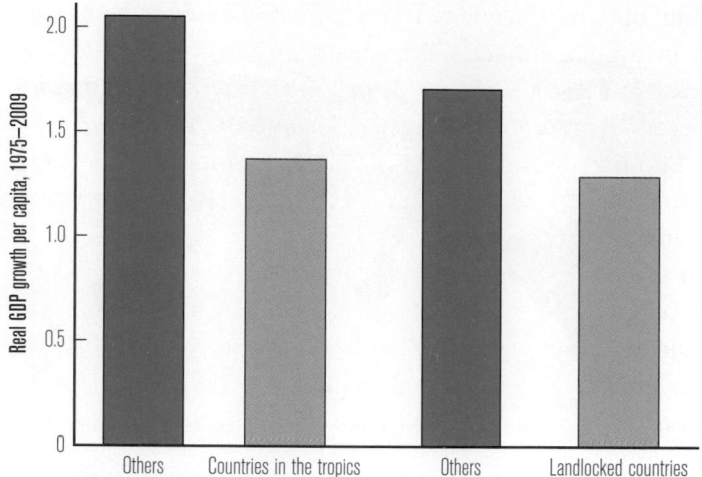

FIGURE 3-5 **Geography and Growth**

GDP, gross domestic product.

Source: Penn World Tables 7.0, http://pwt.econ.upenn.edu/php_site/pwt_index.php, accessed May 2011.

the incentives for investment and factor accumulation. Location in the tropics does not necessarily preclude growth and development because some of the burdens can be alleviated at least partially through policies and institutional development, but it clearly creates difficulties and obstacles that make growth and development more difficult.

Another geographical feature that can affect growth is isolation from major markets, such as for landlocked countries and for small island nations (for example, located in the Pacific Ocean). These isolated countries face higher transport costs and fewer economic opportunities than do coastal economies and countries located nearer to major markets. Landlocked African countries face overland shipping costs that can be three times higher than their coastal neighbors'. Higher transport costs make imports more expensive, which both reduces income left for consumption and raises production costs. They also make it more expensive to export products to other countries, reducing profits.

Not all landlocked countries have had poor economic performance. Switzerland and Austria are in some ways the exceptions that prove the rule. Although they are landlocked, they are far from being isolated, as they are located in the heart of Europe. Perhaps the clearest exception is Botswana, which has deftly managed its vast diamond mines to generate sustained growth for the last four decades. Figure 3–5 shows that economic growth in landlocked countries has averaged 1.29 percent since 1975 (excluding Bhutan and Botswana, this figure falls to 0.99 percent), while in coastal economies, growth averaged 1.71 percent, about one-third higher (and nearly twice as high excluding Botswana). Being landlocked does not mean growth is impossible, but it does limit options and add to production costs. Geographical isolation can be overcome by investments that reduce overland transport costs (for example, better roads or trucks) or by producing goods that rely more on air rather than sea transport. Landlocked Uganda, for example, grows flowers near its international airport for export to Europe. Advancements in satellite communications open up new possibilities for isolated countries, such as data entry or accounting services provided for firms located in other countries.

Note that some countries face multiple geographical obstacles that significantly limit their development options. Perhaps the most challenging are the landlocked countries in the midst of the Sahara desert; Burkina Faso, Chad, Ethiopia, Mali, Niger, and Sudan are among the very poorest countries in the world. These countries have far fewer options and face much more difficult challenges than the average developing country.

These six broad areas are not a complete list of the characteristics that influence factor accumulation, productivity, and economic growth, but they are among the most prominent attributes identified by research and experience. It is important to recognize that this list is not absolute: There is significant variation across countries, and these characteristics are neither a guarantee of success nor a set of rigid requirements for growth. Some countries have done relatively well in many of these areas and still have not experienced rapid economic growth. At the same time, while almost all of the fastest-growing countries score well in most of these areas, some do not. Our understanding of the precise pathways through which each of these factors influence growth is far from complete. However, the evidence does show that these characteristics are among the most important factors supporting factor accumulation, productivity, and growth.

SUMMARY

- Countries have varied widely in their experiences of economic growth since 1960. While some economies, such as Madagascar and Zambia shrank slightly in per capita terms, others such as Botswana and China increased their per capita incomes by factors of 15 to 19 between 1960 and 2009.
- Theories of economic growth have identified several key dimensions of the growth process. Factor accumulation—the expansion of a country's capital stock along with the growth of its labor force—is critical. These are the principal inputs for production of national output.
- In the long run, factor accumulation alone cannot sustain rapid growth in per capita income. Long-run growth depends on being able to produce more output per unit of input. This is the definition of productivity growth. Productivity growth is ultimately a reflection of technical change (which

we can think of as the invention of better recipes for producing national output).

- Productivity growth is measured as a residual. It is the increase in output that is not explained by increased use of inputs. Any errors in the measurement of either inputs or output spill over into our estimate of productivity growth. The goal of sources of growth analysis is to decompose a change in output into the portion explained by the changing use of each input and the unexplained portion that we designate as productivity growth.

- Sources of growth analyses indicate that capital accumulation tends to contribute substantially to growth in low-income countries, while increases in the size and quality of the labor force and productivity growth also make important contributions. Productivity growth tends to account for a larger share of growth in high-income countries.

- Some of the key country characteristics most closely associated with rapid growth include economic and political stability, investments in health and education, strong governance and institutions, a favorable environment for private enterprise (including agricultural, regulatory policies), and more-favorable geography. Participation in international trade is also strongly associated with economic growth. Our understanding of precisely how these and other factors affect the growth process is far from complete.

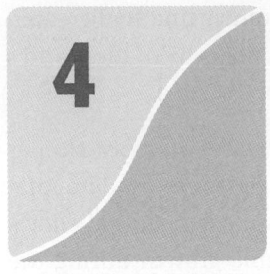

4

Theories of Economic Growth

Economists have long puzzled over the question of economic growth. What is it that makes some countries rich while others remain poor? Formal studies of this question date back at least to the eighteenth-century writings of Scottish social philosopher Adam Smith. The search for answers continues to dominate economic thinking. In a lecture presented in 1985, Nobel Prize–winning economist Robert Lucas noted the then-rapid economic growth of Indonesia and Egypt and slow growth of India, famously asking,

> Is there some action a government of India could take that would lead the Indian economy to grow like Indonesia's or Egypt's? If so, what exactly? If not, what is it about the "nature of India" that makes it so? The consequences for human welfare involved in questions like these are simply staggering: Once one starts to think about them it is hard to think of anything else.[1]

More than a quarter century later, economists Dani Rodrik, Arvind Subramanian, and Francesco Trebbi noted,

> Average income levels in the world's richest and poorest nations differ by a factor of more than 100. Sierra Leone, the poorest economy for which we have national income statistics, has a per-capita GDP of $490, compared to Luxembourg's $50,061. What accounts for these differences, and what (if anything) can we do

---

[1]Robert E. Lucas, "On the Mechanics of Economic Development," *Journal of Monetary Economics* 22, no. 1 (July 1988), 3–42.

to reduce them? It is hard to think of any question in economics that is of greater intellectual significance, or of greater relevance to the vast majority of the world's population.[2]

Two observations emerge from the juxtaposition of these strikingly similar quotations: (1) Long-run economic growth may be the single most fundamental determinant of human welfare around the world, and (2) despite substantial efforts and significant progress toward solving the puzzle of economic growth during the 27 years that separate these comments, we remain far from a complete and policy-relevant understanding of the deep determinants of growth.

This chapter explores key contributions to the theory of economic growth. We began to explore these issues in the last chapter by examining some of the basic processes and patterns that characterize economic growth in low-income countries. We emphasized that growth depends on two processes: the *accumulation of assets* (such as capital, labor, and land), and *making those assets more productive*. Saving and investment are central, but investments must be productive for growth to proceed. Our approach was largely empirical, as we examined much of the data on growth and some of the key findings from research on the determinants of growth across countries. We saw that government policy, institutions, political and economic stability, geography, natural resource endowments, and levels of health and education all play some role in influencing economic growth. We emphasized that growth is not the same as development, but it remains absolutely central to the development process.

This chapter develops these ideas more formally by introducing the underlying theory and the most important basic models of economic growth that influence development thinking today. These models provide consistent frameworks for understanding the growth process and provide a theoretical foundation for the empirical approach we took in the last chapter. Here, we identify specific mathematical relationships between the quantity of capital and labor, their productivity, and the resulting aggregate output. It is important that these models also explore the process of accumulating *additional* capital and labor and *increasing* their productivity, which shifts the model from determining the *level* of output to the *rate of change* of output, which of course is the rate of economic growth.

As we begin to examine the models, it is useful to consider the words of Robert Solow, the father of modern growth theory, who once wrote: "All theory depends on assumptions that are not quite true. That is what makes it theory. The art of successful theorizing is to make the inevitable simplifying assumptions in such a way that

---

[2]Dani Rodrik, Arvind Subramanian, and Francesco Trebbi, "Institutions Rule: The Primacy of Institutions over Geography and Integration in Economic Development," *Journal of Economic Growth*, 9, no. 2 (2004), 131–65.

the final results are not very sensitive."[3] The best models are simple, yet still manage to communicate powerful insights into how the real world operates. In this spirit, the models presented here make assumptions that clearly are not true but allow us to simplify the framework and make it easier to grasp key concepts and insights. For example, we begin by assuming that our prototype economy has one type of homogeneous worker and one type of capital good that combine to produce one standard product. No economy in the world has characteristics even closely resembling these assumptions, but making these assumptions allows us to cut through many details and get to the core concepts of the theory of economic growth.

THE BASIC GROWTH MODEL

The most fundamental models of economic output and economic growth are based on a small number of equations that relate saving, investment, and population growth to the size of the workforce and capital stock and, in turn, to aggregate production of a single good. These models initially focus on the *levels* of investment, labor, productivity, and output. It then becomes straightforward to examine the *changes* in these variables. Our ultimate focus is to explore the key determinants of the *change in output*—that is, on the rate of economic growth. The version of the basic model that we examine here has five equations: an aggregate production function, an equation determining the level of saving, the saving-investment identity, a statement relating new investment to changes in the capital stock, and an expression for the growth rate of the labor force.[4] We examine each of these in turn.

Standard growth models have at their core a production function. At the individual firm or microeconomic level, a production function relates the number of employees and machines to the size of the firm's output. For example, the production function for a textile factory would reveal how much more output the factory could produce if it hired (say) 50 additional workers and purchased five more looms. Production functions often are derived from engineering specifications that relate given amounts of physical input to the amount of physical output that can be produced with that input. At the national or economywide level, production functions describe the relationship of the size of a country's total labor force and the value of its capital stock with the level of that country's gross domestic product (GDP; its total output). These economywide relationships are called **aggregate production functions**.

---

[3]Robert Solow, "A Contribution to the Theory of Economic Growth," *Quarterly Journal of Economics* 70 (February 1956), 65–94.

[4]This five-equation presentation is based on teaching notes compiled by World Bank economist Shantayanan Devarajan, to whom we are indebted.

Our first equation is an aggregate production function. If Y represents total output (and therefore total income), K is the capital stock, and L is the labor supply, at the most general level, the aggregate production function can be expressed as

$$Y = F(K, L) \qquad [4\text{-}1]$$

This expression indicates that output is a function (denoted by F) of the capital stock and the labor supply. As the capital stock and labor supply grow, output expands. Economic growth occurs by increasing either the capital stock (through new investment in factories, machinery, equipment, roads, and other infrastructure), the size of the labor force, or both. The exact form of the function F (stating precisely *how much* output expands in response to changes in K and L) is what distinguishes many different models of growth, as we will see later in the chapter. The other four equations of the model describe how these increases in K and L come about.

Equations 4–2 through 4–4 are closely linked and together describe how the capital stock (K) changes over time. These three equations first calculate total saving, then relate saving to new investment, and finally describe how new investment changes the size of the capital stock. To calculate saving, we take the most straightforward approach and assume that saving is a fixed share of income:

$$S = sY \qquad [4\text{-}2]$$

In this equation, S represents the total value of saving, and s represents the average saving rate. For example, if the average saving rate is 20 percent and total income is $10 billion, then the value of saving in any year is $2 billion. We assume that the saving rate s is a constant, which for most countries is between 10 and 40 percent (typically averaging between 20 and 25 percent), although for some countries it can be higher or lower. China's savings rate in 2008 (along with those of several large oil exporters) exceeded 50 percent, while several countries (including Mozambique, Guinea, the Seychelles, and Georgia) reported savings rates less than 5 percent of GDP. Actual saving behavior is more complex than this simple model suggests (as we discuss in Chapter 10), but this formulation is sufficient for us to explore the basic relationships between saving, investment, and growth.

The next equation relates total saving (S) to investment (I). In our model, with only one good, there is no international trade (because everyone makes the same product, there is no reason to trade). In a closed economy (one without trade or foreign borrowing), saving must be equal to investment. All output of goods and services produced by the economy must be used for either current consumption or investment, while all income earned by households must be either consumed or saved. Because output is equal to income, it follows that saving must equal investment. This relationship is expressed as

$$S = I \qquad [4\text{-}3]$$

We are now in a position to show how the capital stock changes over time. Two main forces determine changes in the capital stock: new investment (which adds to the capital stock) and depreciation (which slowly erodes the value of the existing capital stock over time). Using the Greek letter delta (Δ) to represent the change in the value of a variable, we express the change in the *capital* stock as ΔK, which is determined as follows:

$$\Delta K = I - (dK) \qquad [4\text{-}4]$$

In this expression d is the rate of depreciation. The first term (I) indicates that the capital stock *increases* each year by the amount of new investment. The second term $-(d \times K)$ shows that the capital stock *decreases* every year because of the depreciation of existing capital. We assume here that the depreciation rate is a constant, usually in the range of 2 to 10 percent.

To see how this works, let us continue our earlier example, in which total income is $10 billion and saving (and therefore investment) is $2 billion. Say that the value of the existing capital stock is $30 billion and the annual rate of depreciation is 3 percent. In this example, the capital stock increases by $2 billion because of new investment but also decreases by $0.9 billion (3 percent $\times$ $30 billion) because of depreciation. Equation 4–4 puts together these two effects, calculating the change in the capital stock as $\Delta K = I - (d \times K) = $2\,\text{billion} - (0.03 \times $30\,\text{billion}) = $1.1\,\text{billion}$. Thus the capital stock increases from $30 billion to $31.1 billion. This new value of the capital stock then is inserted into the production function in equation 4–1, allowing for the calculation of a new level of output, Y.

The fifth and final equation of the model focuses on the supply of labor. To keep things simple, we assume that the labor force grows exactly as fast as the total population. Over long periods of time, this assumption is fairly accurate. If n is equal to the growth rate of both the population and the labor force, then the change in the labor force (ΔL) is represented by

$$\Delta L = nL \qquad [4\text{-}5]$$

If the labor force consists of 1 million people and the population (and labor force) is growing by 2 percent, the labor force increases annually by 20,000 (1 million $\times$ 0.02) workers. The labor force now consists of 1.02 million people, a figure that can be inserted into the production function for L to calculate the new level of output. (If we divide both sides of equation 4–5 by L, we can see directly the rate of growth of the labor force, $\Delta L / L = n$.)

These five equations represent the complete model.[5] Collectively, they can be used to examine how changes in population, saving, and investment initially affect

---

[5]Note that because the model has five equations and five variables (Y, K, L, I, and S) it always can be solved. In addition, there are three fixed parameters (d, s, and n), the values of which are assumed to be fixed exogenously, or outside the system.

the capital stock and labor supply and ultimately determine economic output. New saving generates additional investment, which adds to the capital stock and allows for increased output. New workers add further to the economy's capacity to increase production.

One way these five equations can be simplified slightly is to combine equations 4–2, 4–3, and 4–4. The aggregate level of saving (in equation 4–2) determines the level of investment in equation 4–3, which (together with depreciation) determines changes in the capital stock in equation 4–4. Combining these three equations gives us

$$\Delta K = sY - dK \qquad [4\text{-}6]$$

This equation states that the change in the capital stock (ΔK) is equal to saving (sY) minus depreciation (dK). This expression allows us to calculate the change in the capital stock and enter the new value directly into the aggregate production function in equation 4–1.

THE HARROD-DOMAR GROWTH MODEL

As we have stressed, the aggregate production function (shown earlier as equation 4–1) is at the heart of every model of economic growth. This function can take many different forms, depending on what we believe is the true relationship between the factors of production (K and L) and aggregate output. This relationship depends on (among other things) the mix of economic activities (for example, agriculture, heavy industry, light labor-intensive manufacturing, high-technology processes, services), the level of technology, and other factors. Indeed, much of the theoretical debate in the academic literature on economic growth is about how to best represent the aggregate production process.

THE FIXED-COEFFICIENT PRODUCTION FUNCTION

One special type of a simple production function is shown in Figure 4–1. Output in this figure is represented by **isoquants**, which are combinations of the inputs (labor and capital in this case) that produce equal amounts of output. For example, on the first (innermost) isoquant, it takes capital (plant and equipment) of $10 million and 100 workers to produce 100,000 keyboards per year (point a). Alternatively, on the second isoquant, $20 million of capital and 200 workers can produce 200,000 keyboards (point b). Only two isoquants are shown in this diagram, but a nearly infinite number of isoquants are possible, each for a different level of output.

The L-shape of the isoquants is characteristic of a particular type of production function known as **fixed-coefficient production functions**. These production

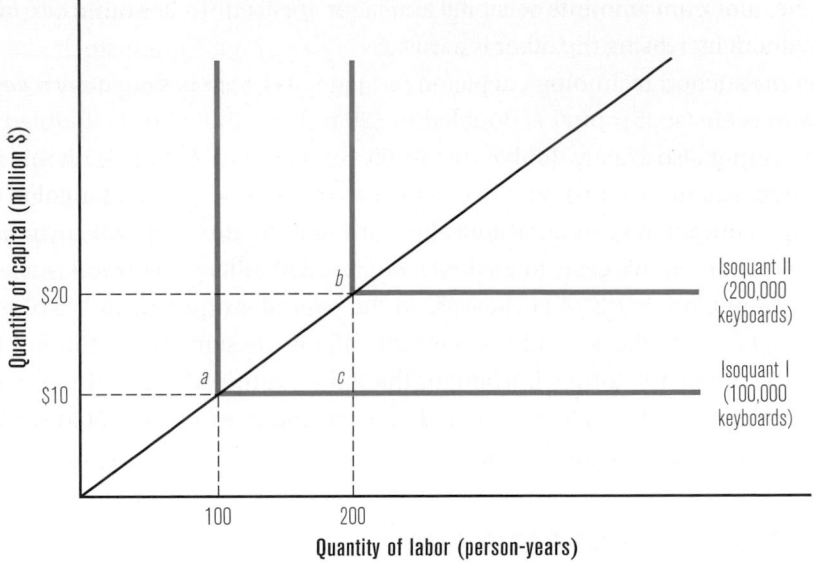

FIGURE 4-1 **Isoquants for a Fixed-Coefficient Production Technology**

With constant returns to scale, the isoquants will be L-shaped and the production function will be the straight line through their minimum-combination points.

functions are based on the assumption that capital and labor need to be used in a fixed proportion to each other to produce different levels of output. In Figure 4–1, for the first isoquant, the **capital–labor ratio** is 10 million:100, or 100,000:1. In other words, $100,000 in capital must be matched with one worker to produce the given output. For the second isoquant, the ratio is the same: $20 million:200, or 100,000:1. This constant capital–labor ratio is represented in Figure 4–1 by the slope of the ray from the origin through the vertices (*a* and *b*) of the isoquants. These vertices represent the least cost and hence most efficient mix of capital and labor to produce a given quantity of output. In the case of fixed coefficients, this mix is the same for every quantity of output.

With this kind of production function, if more workers are added *without* investing in more capital, output does *not* rise. Look again at the first isoquant, starting at the elbow (with 100 workers and $10 million in capital). If the firm adds more workers (say, increasing to 200 workers) without adding new machines, it moves horizontally to the right along the first isoquant to point *c*. But at this point, or at any other point on this isoquant, the firm still produces just 100,000 keyboards. In this kind of production function, new workers need more machines to increase output. Adding new workers without machines results in idle workers, with no increase in output. Similarly, more machinery without additional workers results in underused machines. On each isoquant, the most efficient production point is at the elbow, where the minimum amounts of capital and labor are used. To use any more of either factor without increasing the other is a waste.

The production technology depicted in Figure 4–1 also is drawn with **constant returns to scale**, so if capital is doubled to $20 million and labor is doubled to 200 workers, output also exactly doubles to 200,000 keyboards per year.[6] With this further assumption, two more ratios remain constant at any level of output: capital to output and labor to output. If keyboards are valued at $50 each, then 100,000 keyboards are worth $5 million. In this case, in the first isoquant, $10 million in capital is needed to produce $5 million worth of keyboards, so the **capital–output ratio** is $10 million: $5 million, or 2:1. In the second isoquant the ratio is the same ($20 million:$10 million, or 2:1). Similarly, for each isoquant the **labor–output ratio** is also a constant, in this case equal to 1:50,000, meaning that each worker produces $50,000 worth of keyboards, or 1,000 keyboards each.

THE CAPITAL–OUTPUT RATIO AND THE HARROD-DOMAR FRAMEWORK

The fixed-coefficient, constant-returns-to-scale production function is the centerpiece of a well-known early model of economic growth that was developed independently during the 1940s by economists Roy Harrod of England and Evsey Domar of MIT, primarily to explain the relationship between growth and unemployment in advanced capitalist societies.[7] It ultimately focuses attention on the role of capital accumulation in the growth process. The **Harrod-Domar model** has been used extensively (perhaps even overused) in developing countries to examine the relationship between growth and capital requirements. The model is based on the real-world observation that some labor is unemployed and proceeds on the basis that capital is the binding constraint on production and growth. In the model, the production function has a very precise form, in which output is assumed to be a *linear* function of capital (and only capital). As usual, the model begins by specifying the level of output, which we later modify to explore changes in output, or economic growth. The production function is specified as follows:

$$Y = 1/v \times K \quad or \quad Y = K/v \qquad [4\text{--}7]$$

where v is a constant. In this equation, the capital stock is multiplied by the fixed number $1/v$ to calculate aggregate production. If $v = 3$ and a firm has $30 million in capital, its annual output would be $10 million. It is difficult to imagine a simpler

---

[6]In a constant-returns-to-scale production function, if we multiply both capital and labor by any number, w, output multiplies by the same number. In other words, the production function has the following property: $wY = F(wK, wL)$.

[7]Roy F. Harrod, "An Essay in Dynamic Theory," *Economic Journal* (1939), 14–33; Evsey Domar, "Capital Expansion, Rate of Growth, and Employment," *Econometrica* (1946), 137–47; and Domar, "Expansion and Employment," *American Economic Review* 37 (1947), 34–55.

production function. The constant v turns out to be the capital–output ratio because, by rearranging the terms in equation 4–7, we find

$$v = K/Y \qquad [4\text{-}8]$$

The capital–output ratio is a very important parameter in this model, so it is worth dwelling for a moment on its meaning. This ratio essentially is a measure of the productivity of capital or investment. In the earlier example in Figure 4–1, it took $10 million in investment in a new plant and new equipment to produce $5 million worth of keyboards, implying a capital-output ratio of 2:1 (or just 2). A larger v implies that more capital is needed to produce the same amount of output. So, if v were 4 instead, then $20 million in investment would be needed to produce $5 million worth of keyboards.

The capital–output ratio provides an indication of the capital intensity of the production process. In the basic growth model, this ratio varies across countries for two reasons: either the countries use different technologies to produce the same goods or they produce a different mix of goods. Where farmers produce maize using tractors, the capital–output ratio will be much higher than in countries where farmers rely on a large number of workers using hoes and other hand tools. In countries that produce a larger share of **capital-intensive products** (that is, those that require relatively more machinery, such as automobiles, petrochemicals, and steel), v is higher than in countries producing more **labor-intensive products** (such as textiles, basic agriculture, and foot wear). In practice, as economists move from the v of the model to actually measuring it in the real world, the observed capital–output ratio can also vary for a third reason: differences in efficiency. A larger measured v can indicate less-efficient production when capital is not being used as productively as possible. A factory with lots of idle machinery and poorly organized production processes has a higher capital–output ratio than a more-efficiently managed factory.

Economists often calculate the **incremental capital–output ratio (ICOR)** to determine the impact on output of additional (or incremental) capital. The ICOR measures the productivity of additional capital, whereas the (average) capital–output ratio refers to the relationship between a country's total stock of capital and its total national product. In the Harrod-Domar model, because the capital–output ratio is assumed to remain constant, the average capital–output ratio is equal to the incremental capital–output ratio, so the ICOR $= v$.

So far, we have been discussing total output, not growth in output. The production function in equation 4–7 easily can be converted to relate *changes* in output to *changes* in the capital stock:

$$\Delta Y = \Delta K/v \qquad [4\text{-}9]$$

The growth rate of output, g, is simply the increment in output divided by the total amount of output, $\Delta Y/Y$. If we divide both sides of equation 4-9 by Y, then

$$g = \Delta Y/Y = \Delta K/Yv \qquad [4\text{-}10]$$

Finally, from equation 4–6, we know that the change in the capital stock ΔK is equal to saving minus the depreciation of capital ($\Delta K = sY - dK$). Substituting the right-hand side of equation 4–6 into the term for ΔK in equation 4–10 and simplifying[8] leads to the basic Harrod-Domar relationship for an economy:

$$g = (s/v) - d \qquad [4\text{-}11]$$

Underlying this equation is the view that capital created by investment is the main determinant of growth in output and that saving makes investment possible.[9] It rivets attention on two keys to the growth process: saving (s) and the productivity of capital (v). The message from this model is clear: Save more and make productive investments, and your economy will grow.

Economic analysts can use this framework either to predict growth or to calculate the amount of saving required to achieve a target growth rate. The first step is to try to estimate the incremental capital–output ratio (v) and depreciation rate (d). With a given saving rate, predicting the growth rate is straightforward. If the saving (or investment) rate is 24 percent, the ICOR is 3, and the depreciation rate is 5 percent, then the economy can be expected to grow by 3 percent (because $0.24/3 - 0.05 = 0.03$).

How does this model work in practice? Consider Indonesia, which from 2002 to 2007 had an investment rate of about 30 percent and recorded a GDP growth just under 5.5 percent per year. Assuming a depreciation rate of 5 percent, the implied ICOR was approximately $v = 2.86$.[10] Would these figures have helped the Indonesian government predict the 2007–08 growth rate? In 2008, the investment rate was 29 percent, so the Harrod-Domar model would have predicted growth of 5.1 percent ($g = 0.29/2.86 - 0.05$). The actual growth rate in 2007–08 was 6.0 percent, within sight of the prediction but not highly accurate.

STRENGTHS AND WEAKNESSES OF THE HARROD-DOMAR FRAMEWORK

The basic strength of the Harrod-Domar model is its simplicity. The data requirements are small, and the equation is easy to use and to estimate. And, as we saw with the example of Indonesia, the model can be somewhat accurate from one year to the next. Generally speaking, in the absence of severe economic shocks (such as a drought, a financial crisis, or large changes in export or import prices), the model can do a reasonable job of estimating expected growth rates in most countries over very short periods of time (a few years). Another strength is its focus on the key role of saving. As discussed

---

[8]Substituting equation 4–6 into 4–10 leads to $g = (sY - dK)/Y \times 1/v$, which can be simplified to $g = (s - d \times K/Y) \times 1/v$. Since $K/Y = v$, we have $g = (s - dv) \times 1/v$, which leads to $g = s/v - d$.

[9]For an important early contribution to the discussion of the importance of capital accumulation to the growth process, see Joan Robinson, *The Accumulation of Capital* (London: Macmillan, 1956).

[10]Because $g = s/v - d$, then $v = s/(g + d)$. For Indonesia between 2002 and 2007, $v = 0.30/(0.055 + 0.05) = 2.86$.

in Chapter 3, individual decisions about how much income to save and consume are central to the growth process. People prefer to consume sooner rather than later, but the more that is consumed, the less that can be saved to finance investment. The Harrod-Domar model makes it clear that saving is crucial for income to grow over time.

The model, however, has some major weaknesses. One follows directly from the strong focus on saving. Although saving is necessary for growth, the simple form of the model implies that it is also sufficient, which it is not. As pointed out in Chapter 3, the investments financed by saving actually have to pay off with higher income in the future, and not all investments do so. Poor investment decisions, changing government policies, volatile world prices, or simply bad luck can alter the impact of new investment on output and growth. Sustained growth depends both on generating new investment and ensuring that investments are productive over time. In this vein, the allocation of resources across different sectors and firms can be an important determinant of output and growth. Because (for simplicity) the Harrod-Domar assumes only one sector, it leaves out these important allocation issues.

Perhaps the most important limitations in the model stem from the rigid assumptions of fixed capital-to-labor, capital-to-output, and labor-to-output ratios, which imply very little flexibility in the economy over time. To keep these ratios constant, capital, labor, and output must all grow at exactly the same rate, which is highly unlikely to happen in real economies. To see why these growth rates must all be the same, consider the growth rate of capital. If the capital stock grew any faster or slower than output at rate g, the capital–output ratio would change. Thus the capital stock must grow at g to keep the capital–output ratio constant over time. With respect to labor, in our original five-equation model, we stipulated (in equation 4–5) that the labor force would grow at exactly the same pace as the population at rate n. Therefore, the only way that the capital stock and the labor force can grow at the same rate is if n happens to be equal to g. This happens only when $n = g = s/v - d$, and there is no particular reason to believe the population will grow at that rate.

In this model, the economy remains in equilibrium with full employment of the labor force and the capital stock *only* under the very special circumstances that labor, capital, and output all *grow* at the rate g. On the one hand, if n is larger than g, the labor force grows faster than the capital stock. In essence, the saving rate is not high enough to support investment in new machinery sufficient to employ all new workers. A growing number of workers do not have jobs and unemployment rises indefinitely. On the other hand, if g (or $s/v - d$) is larger than n, the capital stock grows faster than the workforce. There are not enough workers for all the available machines, and capital becomes idle. The actual growth rate of the economy no longer is g, as the model stipulates, but slows to n, with output constrained by the number of available workers.

So, unless $s/v - d$ (or g) is exactly equal to n, either labor or capital is not fully employed and the economy is not in a stable equilibrium. This characteristic of the Harrod-Domar model has come to be known as the *knife-edge* problem. As long as

$g = n$, the economy remains in equilibrium, but as soon as either the capital stock or the labor force grows faster than the other, the economy falls off the edge with continuously growing unemployment of either capital or labor.

The rigid assumptions of fixed capital–output, labor–output, and capital–labor ratios may be reasonably accurate for short periods of time or in very special circumstances but almost always are inaccurate over time as an economy evolves and develops. Each of these varies among countries and, for a single country, over time. Consider the incremental capital–output ratio. The productivity of capital can change in response to policy changes, which in turn affects v. Moreover, the capital intensity of the production process can and usually does change over time. A poor country with a low saving rate and surplus labor (unemployed and underemployed workers) can achieve higher growth rates by utilizing as much labor as possible and thus relatively less capital. For example, a country relying heavily on labor-intensive agricultural production will record a low v. As economies grow and per capita income rises, the labor surplus diminishes and economies shift gradually toward more capital-intensive production. As a result, the ICOR shifts upward. Thus a higher v may not necessarily imply inefficiency or slower growth. ICORs can also shift through market mechanisms, as prices of labor and capital change in response to changes in supplies. As growth takes place, saving tends to become relatively more abundant and hence the price of capital falls while employment and wages rise. Therefore, all producers increasingly economize on labor and use more capital and the ICOR tends to rise.

Consider again the example of Indonesia. The ICOR changed from approximately 2.4 during the 1980s, to 4.1 during the 1990s, to 3.6 during 2000–09, reflecting a trend toward more capital-intensive production processes. To continue to use the 1980s ICOR in 2009 would have been very misleading and betrayed a significant misunderstanding of the growth process. The structure of the economy had changed substantially during that time period and, with it, the ICOR. Thailand provides a similar example, as described in Box 4–1.

As a result of these rigidities, the Harrod-Domar framework tends to become increasingly inaccurate over longer periods of time as the actual ICOR changes and, with it, the capital–labor ratio. In a world with fixed-coefficient production functions, little room is left for a factory manager to increase output by hiring one more worker without buying a machine to go with the worker or to purchase more machines for the current workforce to use. The fixed-proportion production function does not allow for any substitution between capital and labor in the production process. In the real world, of course, at least some substitution between labor and capital is possible in most production processes. As we see in the next section, adding this feature to the model allows for a much richer exploration of the growth process.

A final weakness of the Harrod-Domar model is the absence of any role for productivity growth—the ability to produce increasing quantities of output per unit of input. In Figure 4–1, increased factor productivity can be represented by an inward shift of each isoquant toward the origin, implying that less labor and capital would

BOX 4-1 ECONOMIC GROWTH IN THAILAND

In the 1960s, Thailand's agrarian economy depended heavily on rice, maize, rubber, and other agricultural products. About three-quarters of the Thai population derived its income from agricultural activities. Gross domestic product (GDP) per capita in 1960 (measured in 2005 international dollars) was around $1,200—less than one-tenth the average income in the United States. Life expectancy was 53 years and the infant mortality rate was 103 per 1,000 births. Few observers expected Thailand to develop rapidly.

However, since the mid-1960s, the Thai economy has grown rapidly (if not always steadily), benefiting from relatively sound economic management and a favorable external environment. The government regularly achieved surpluses on the current account of its budget and used these funds (plus modest inflows of foreign assistance) to finance investments in rural roads, irrigation, power, telecommunications, and other basic infrastructure. At least until the mid-1990s, the government's fiscal, monetary, and exchange rate policies kept the macroeconomy relatively stable with fairly low inflation, despite the turbulent period of world oil price shocks in the 1970s and 1980s. Beginning in the 1970s, the government began to remove trade restrictions and promote the production of labor-intensive manufactured exports. These products found a ready market in the booming Japanese economy of the 1980s and provided a growing number of jobs for Thai workers.

Thailand's ability to make investments and deepen its capital stock depended on its capacity to save. The country's saving rate averaged about 20 percent in the 1960s, already high for developing countries, and increased steadily over time to an average of 35 percent in the 1990s, falling to about 32 percent during the 2000s. These high saving rates, combined with relatively prudent economic policies, supported very rapid economic growth and development.

Thailand's development experience has been far from completely smooth, however. In mid-1997, a major financial crisis erupted. Huge short-term offshore borrowing combined with a fixed exchange rate and weak financial institutions led to a collapse of a real estate bubble, rapid capital flight, a substantial depreciation of the Thai baht, and a deep recession (see Chapter 13). In some ways, Thailand had become the victim of its own success, with its rapid growth attracting significant numbers of investors looking to gain quick profits, who rapidly fled once the bubble began to collapse. After two years of negative growth (with GDP falling 10 percent in 1998), the economy began to recover and growth rebounded to 3.9 percent between 1999 and 2007.

Over the longer period between 1960 and 2007, per capita growth averaged 4.5 percent, so that the average income in Thailand is now more than eight times higher than it was in 1960. By 2009, life expectancy grew to 69 years, infant mortality fell to 12 per thousand, and adult literacy reached 93 percent. During this period, the structure of the economy changed significantly. By 2009, manufacturing accounted for 34 percent of GDP, up from just 14 percent in 1965, while the share of agricultural production dropped commensurately. The composition of exports shifted away from rice, maize, and other agricultural commodities toward labor-intensive manufactured products, which now account for a large majority of all exports. As the Harrod-Domar model predicts, Thailand's high saving rate and resulting capital accumulation was accompanied by a dramatic increase in output (and income) per capita. Contrary to the Harrod-Domar model, however, the ICOR did not remain constant. As the stock of capital grew and the economy shifted toward more capital-intensive production techniques, the ICOR increased from 2.6 in the 1970s to nearly 5 by the early 2000s. The rising ICOR indicated that, as the Thai economy expanded and the level of capital per worker increased, an ever-larger increment of new capital was required to bring about a given increase in total output.

be needed to produce the same amount of output. The simplest way to capture this in the Harrod-Domar framework is to introduce a smaller ICOR, but of course, this would contradict the idea of a constant ICOR.

Despite these weaknesses, the Harrod-Domar model is still used to a surprisingly wide extent. Economist William Easterly documented how the World Bank and other institutions use the model to calculate "financing gaps" between the amount of available saving and the amount of investment supposedly needed to achieve a target growth rate.[11] He shows how simplistic and sometimes careless use of the model can lead to weak analysis and faulty conclusions. In essence, analysts enamored by the simplicity of the model tend to overlook its shortcomings when applying it to the real world.

The Harrod-Domar model provides some useful insights but does not take us very far. The fixed-coefficient assumption provides the model with very little flexibility and does not capture the ability of real world firms to change the mix of inputs in the production process. The model can be reasonably accurate from one year to the next (in the absence of shocks), and it rightly focuses attention on the importance

---

[11]See William Easterly, "Aid for Investment," *The Elusive Quest for Growth* (Cambridge: MIT Press, 2001), chap. 2; and Easterly, "The Ghost of the Financing Gap: Testing the Growth Model of the International Financial Institutions," *Journal of Development Economics* 60, no. 2 (December 1999), 423–38.

of saving. But it is quite inaccurate for most countries over longer periods of time and implies that saving is sufficient for growth, although it is not. Indeed, in the late 1950s, Domar expressed strong doubts about his own model, pointing out that it was originally designed to explore employment issues in advanced economies rather than growth per se and was too rigid to be useful for explaining long-term growth.[12] Instead, he endorsed the new growth model of Robert Solow, to which we now turn our attention.

THE SOLOW (NEOCLASSICAL) GROWTH MODEL

THE NEOCLASSICAL PRODUCTION FUNCTION

In 1956, MIT-economist Robert Solow introduced a new model of economic growth that was a big step forward from the Harrod-Domar framework.[13] Solow recognized the problems that arose from the rigid production function in the Harrod-Domar model. Solow's answer was to drop the fixed-coefficients production function and replace it with a **neoclassical production function** that allows for more flexibility and substitution between the factors of production. In the Solow model, the capital–output and capital–labor ratios no longer are fixed but vary, depending on the relative endowments of capital and labor in the economy and the production process. Like the Harrod-Domar model, the Solow model was developed to analyze industrialized economies, but it has been used extensively to explore economic growth in all countries around the world, including developing countries. The Solow model has been enormously influential and remains at the core of most theories of economic growth in developing countries.

The isoquants that underlie the neoclassical production function are shown in Figure 4–2. Note that the isoquants are curved rather than L-shaped as in the fixed-coefficient model. In this figure, at point *a*, $10 million of capital and 100 workers combine to produce 100,000 keyboards, which would be valued at $5 million (because, as stated earlier, keyboards are priced at $50 each). Starting from this point, output could be expanded in any of three ways. If the firm's managers decided to expand at constant factor proportions and move to point *b* on isoquant II to produce 200,000 keyboards, the situation would be identical to the fixed propor-

---

[12]Evsey Domar, *Essays in the Theory of Economic Growth* (Oxford: Oxford University Press, 1957).

[13]The two classic references of Solow's work are his "A Contribution to the Theory of Economic Growth" and "Technical Change and the Aggregate Production Function," *Review of Economics and Statistics* 39 (August 1957), 312–20. For an excellent and very thorough undergraduate exposition of the Solow and other models of economic growth, see Charles I. Jones, *Introduction to Economic Growth* (New York: W. W. Norton and Company, 2001). In 1987, Solow was awarded the Nobel Prize in economics, primarily for his work on growth theory.

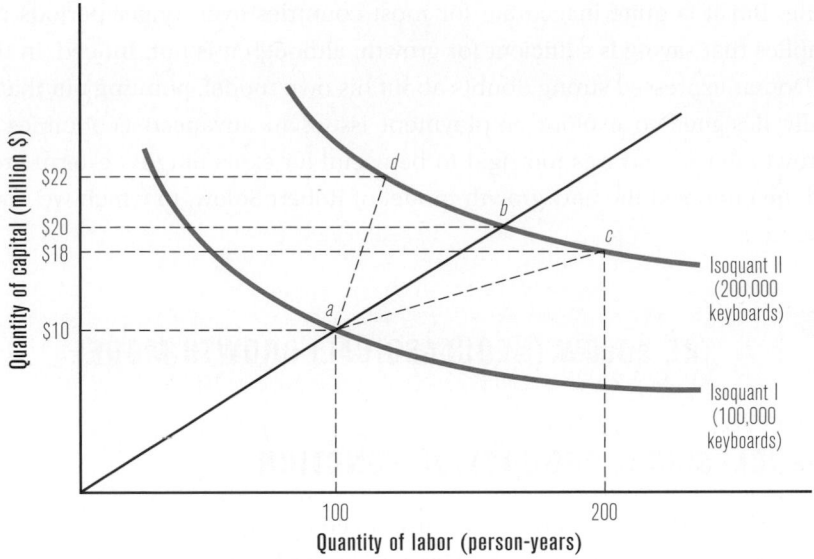

FIGURE 4-2 Isoquants for a Neoclassical Production Technology

Instead of requiring fixed factor proportions, as in Figure 4–1, output can be achieved with varying combinations of labor and capital. This is called a *neoclassical* production function. Note that the isoquants are curved rather than L-shaped.

tions case of Figure 4–1. The capital–output ratio at both points *a* and *b* would be 2:1, as it was before ($10 million of capital produces $5 million of keyboards at point *a*, and $20 million of capital produces $10 million of keyboards at point *b*). Note that the Solow model retains from the Harrod-Domar model the assumption of constant returns to scale, so that a doubling of labor and capital leads to a doubling of output. But by dropping the fixed-coefficients assumption, production of 200,000 keyboards could be achieved by using different combinations of capital and labor. For example, the firm could use more labor and less capital (a more labor-intensive method), such as at point *c* on isoquant II. In that case, the capital–output ratio falls to 1.8:1 ($18 million in capital to produce $10 million in keyboards).

Alternatively, the firm could choose a more capital-intensive method, such as at point *d* on isoquant II, where the capital–output ratio would rise to 2.2:1 ($22 million in capital to produce $10 million in keyboards). The kinds of tools that policy makers use to try to decrease or increase the capital–output ratio are discussed in depth in several chapters later in this text.

THE BASIC EQUATIONS OF THE SOLOW MODEL

The Solow model is understood most easily by expressing all the key variables in per-worker terms (for example, output per worker and capital per worker). To do so, we divide both sides of the production function in equation 4–1 by L, so that it takes the form

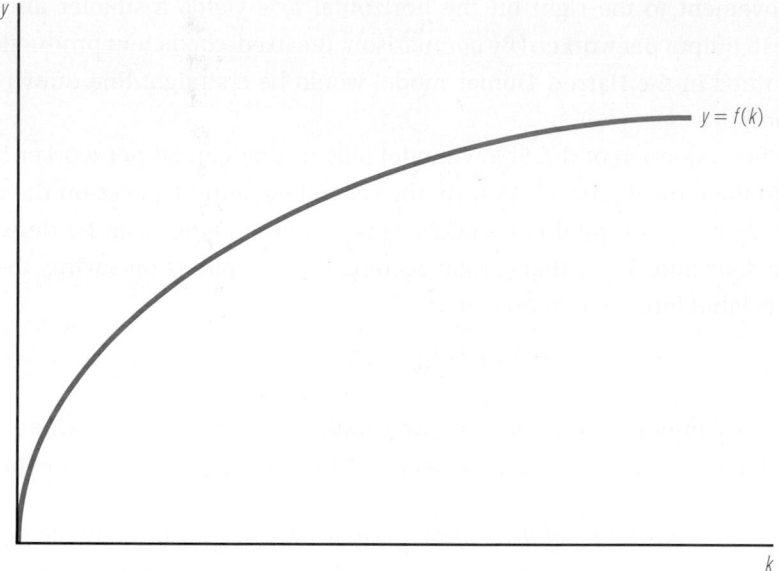

FIGURE 4-3 The Production Function in the Solow Growth Model

The neoclassical production function in the Solow model displays diminishing returns to capital so that each additional increment in capital per worker (k) is associated with smaller increases in output per worker (y).

$$Y/L = F(K/L, 1) \qquad\qquad [4\text{--}12]$$

The equation shows that output per worker is a function of capital per worker.[14] If we use lower-case letters to represent quantities in per-worker terms, then y is output per worker (that is, $y = Y/L$) and k is capital per worker ($k = K/L$). This gives us the first equation of the Solow model, in which the production function can be written simply as

$$y = f(k) \qquad\qquad [4\text{--}13]$$

Solow's model assumes a production function with the familiar property of **diminishing returns to capital**. With a fixed labor supply, giving workers an initial amount of machinery to work with results in large gains in output. But as these workers are given more and more machinery, the addition to output from each new machine gets smaller and smaller. An aggregate production function with this property is shown in Figure 4–3. The horizontal axis represents capital per worker (k), and the vertical axis shows output per worker (y). The slope of the curve declines as the capital stock increases, reflecting the assumption of the diminishing marginal product of capital.

---

[14]We can divide both sides by L because the Solow model (like the Harrod-Domar model) assumes the production function exhibits constant returns to scale and has the property that $wY = F(wK, wL)$. To express the Solow model in per-worker terms, we let $w = 1/L$.

Each movement to the right on the horizontal axis yields a smaller and smaller increase in output per worker. (By comparison, the fixed-coefficient production function assumed in the Harrod-Domar model would be a straight line drawn through the origin.)

The first equation of the Solow model tells us that capital per worker is fundamental to the growth process. In turn, the second equation focuses on the determinants of changes in capital per worker. This second equation can be derived from equation 4–6[15] and shows that capital accumulation depends on saving, the growth rate of the labor force, and depreciation:

$$\Delta k = sy - (n + d)k \qquad\qquad [4\text{–}14]$$

This is a very important equation, so we should understand exactly what it means. It states that the change in capital per worker (Δk) is determined by three things:

- *The Δk is positively related to saving per worker.* Because s is the saving rate and y is income (or output) per worker, the term sy is equal to saving per worker. As saving per worker increases, so does investment per worker, and the capital stock per worker (k) grows.
- *The Δk is negatively related to population growth.* This is shown by the term $-nk$. Each year, because of growth in the population and labor force, there are nL new workers. If there were no new investment, the increase in the labor force would mean that capital *per worker* (k) falls. Equation 4–14 states that capital per worker falls by exactly nk.
- *Depreciation erodes the capital stock.* Each year, the amount of capital per worker falls by the amount $-dk$ simply because of depreciation.

Therefore, saving (and investment) adds to capital per worker, whereas labor force growth and depreciation reduce capital per worker. When saving per capita, sy,

---

[15]To derive equation 4–14, we begin by dividing both sides of equation 4–6 by K so that
$$\Delta K/K = sY/K - d$$
We then focus on the capital per worker ratio, $k = K/L$. The growth rate of k is equal to the growth rate of K minus the growth rate of L:
$$\Delta k/k = \Delta K/K - \Delta L/L$$
With a little rearranging of terms, this equation can be written as $\Delta K/K = \Delta k/k + \Delta L/L$. We earlier assumed that both the population and the labor force were growing at rate n, so $\Delta L/L = n$. By substitution we obtain
$$\Delta K/K = \Delta k/k + n$$
Note that in both the first equation of this footnote and the equation just given, the left-hand side is equal to $\Delta K/K$. This implies that the right-hand sides of these two equations are equal to each other, as follows:
$$\Delta k/k + n = sY/K - d$$
By subtracting n from both sides and multiplying through by k, we find that
$$\Delta k = sy - nk - dk \quad \text{or} \quad \Delta k = sy - (n + d)k$$

is larger than the amount of new capital needed to compensate for labor force growth and depreciation, $(n + d)k$, then Δk is a positive number. This implies that capital per worker k increases.

The process through which the economy increases the amount of capital per worker, k, is called **capital deepening**. Economies in which workers have access to more machines, computers, trucks, and other equipment have a deeper capital base than economies with less machinery, and these economies are able to produce more output per worker.

In some economies, however, the amount of saving is just enough to provide the same amount of capital to new workers and compensate for depreciation. An increase in the capital stock that just keeps pace with the expanding labor force and depreciation is called **capital widening** (referring to a widening of both the total amount of capital and the size of the workforce). Capital widening occurs when sy is exactly equal to $(n + d)k$, implying no change in k. Using this terminology, equation 4–14 can be restated as saying that *capital deepening (Δk) is equal to saving per worker (sy) minus the amount needed for capital widening $[(n + d)k]$.*

A country with a high saving rate can easily deepen its capital base and rapidly expand the amount of capital per worker, thus providing the basis for growth in output. In Singapore, for example, where the saving rate has averaged more than 40 percent since the early 1980s, it is not difficult to provide capital to the growing labor force and make up for depreciation and still have plenty left over to supply existing workers with additional capital. By contrast, Kenya, with a saving rate of about 15 percent, has much less saving to spare for capital deepening after providing machines to new workers and making up for depreciation. As a result, capital per worker does not grow as quickly, and neither does output (or income) per worker. Partly because of this large difference in saving rates, output per person in Singapore grew by an average of 4.9 percent per year between 1960 and 2009, while Kenya's growth averaged about 0.34 percent.

We can summarize the two basic equations of the Solow model as follows. The first $[y = f(k)]$ simply states that output per worker (or income per capita) depends on the amount of capital per worker. The second equation, $\Delta k = sy - (n + d)k$, says that change in capital per worker depends on saving, the population growth rate, and depreciation. Thus, as in the Harrod-Domar model, saving plays a central role in the Solow model. However, the relationship between saving and growth is not linear because of diminishing returns to capital in the production function. In addition, the Solow model introduces a role for the population growth rate and allows for substitution between capital and labor in the growth process.

Now that we are equipped with the basic model, we can proceed to analyze the effects of changes in the saving rate, population growth, and depreciation on economic output and economic growth. This is accomplished most easily by examining the model in graphical form.

THE SOLOW DIAGRAM

The diagram of the Solow model consists of three curves, shown in Figure 4–4. The first is the production function $y = f(k)$, given by equation 4–13. The second is a saving function, which is derived directly from the production function. The new curve shows saving per capita, sy, calculated by multiplying both sides of equation 4–13 by the saving rate, so that $sy = s \times f(k)$. Because saving is assumed to be a fixed fraction of income (with s between 0 and 1), the saving function has the same shape as the production function but is shifted downward by the factor s. The third curve is the line $(n + d)k$, which is a straight line through the origin with the slope $(n + d)$. This line represents the amount of new capital needed as a result of growth in the labor force and depreciation just to keep capital per worker (k) constant. Note that the second and third curves are representations of the two right-hand terms of equation 4–14.

The second and third curves intersect at point A, where $k = k_0$. (Note that, on the production function above the sy curve, $k = k_0$ corresponds to a point directly above A where $y = y_0$ on the vertical axis.) At point A, sy is exactly equal to $(n + d)k$, so capital per worker does not change and k remains constant. At other points along the horizontal axis, the *vertical difference* between the sy curve and the $(n + d)k$ line determines the *change* in capital per worker. To the left of point A (say, where $k = k_1$

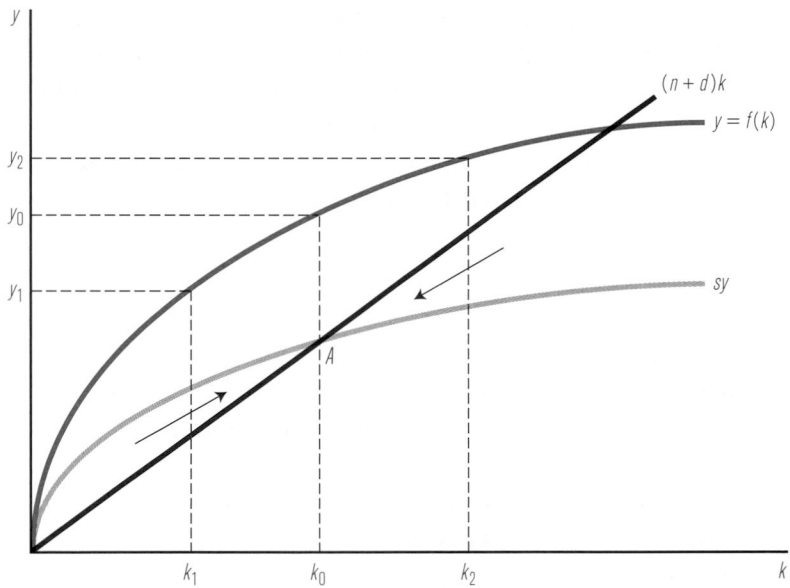

FIGURE 4-4 The Basic Solow Growth Model Diagram

In the basic Solow diagram, point A is the only place where the amount of new saving, sy, is exactly equal to the amount of new capital needed to compensate for growth in the workforce and depreciation $(n + d)k$. Point A is the steady state level of capital per worker and output per worker.

and on the production function $y = y_1$), the amount of saving in the economy per person (sy) is larger than the amount of saving needed to compensate for new workers and depreciation $[(n + d)k]$. As a result, the amount of capital per person (k) grows (capital deepening) and the economy shifts to the right along the horizontal axis. The economy continues to shift to the right as long as the sy curve is *above* the $(n + d)k$ curve, until eventually the economy reaches an equilibrium at point A. In terms of the production function, the shift to the right implies an increase in output per worker, y (or income per capita), from y_1 to y_0. To the right of point A (say, where $k = k_2$ and $y = y_2$), saving per capita is smaller than the amount needed for new workers and depreciation, so capital per worker falls and the economy shifts to the left along the horizontal axis. Once again, this shift continues until the economy reaches point A. The shift to the left corresponds to a decline in output per worker from y_2 to y_0.

Point A is the only place where the amount of new saving, sy, is exactly equal to the amount of new capital needed for growth in the workforce and depreciation. Therefore, at this point, the amount of capital per worker, k, remains constant. Saving per worker (on the vertical axis of the saving function) also remains constant, as does output per worker (or income per capita) on the production function, with $y = y_0$. As a result, point A is called the **steady state** of the Solow model. Output per capita at the steady state (y_0) is alternatively referred to as the **steady state**, **long run**, or **potential level of output per worker**.

It is very important to note, however, that all the values that remain constant are expressed as *per worker*. Although output per worker is constant, *total* output continues to grow at rate n, the same rate the population and workforce grow. In other words, *at the steady state GDP (Y) grows at the rate n, but GDP per capita (y) is constant (average income remains unchanged)*. Similarly, although capital per worker and saving per worker are constant at point A, total capital and total saving grow.

CHANGES IN THE SAVING RATE AND POPULATION GROWTH RATE IN THE SOLOW MODEL

Both the Solow and Harrod–Domar models put saving (and investment) at the core of the growth process. In the Harrod-Domar model, an increase in the saving rate translates directly (and linearly) into an increase in aggregate output. What is the impact of a higher saving rate in the Solow model?

As shown in Figure 4–5, increasing the saving rate from s to s' shifts the saving function sy up to $s'y$, without shifting either the production function or the capital widening line $(n + d)k$. The increase in the saving rate means that saving per worker (and investment per worker) now is greater than $(n + d)k$, so k gradually increases. The economy shifts to a new long-run equilibrium at point B. In the process, capital per worker increases from k_0 to k_3 and output per worker increases from y_0 to y_3. The aggregate economy initially grows at a rate faster than its steady-state growth

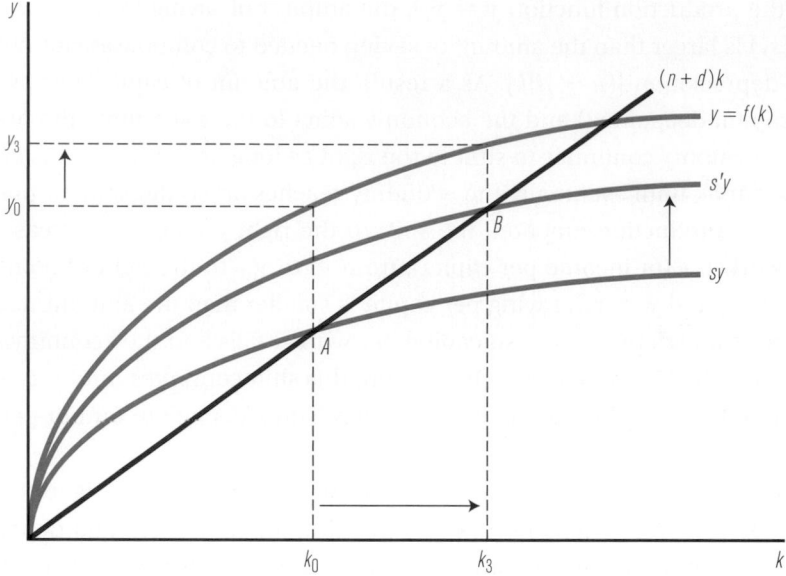

FIGURE 4-5 An Increase in the Saving Rate in the Solow Model

An increase in the saving rate from s to s' results in an upward shift in the capital deepening curve, so that capital per worker increases from k_0 to k_3.

rate of n until it reaches point B, where the long-run growth rate reverts to n. Thus, the higher saving rate leads to more investment, a permanently higher stock of capital per worker, and a permanently higher level of income (or output) per worker. In other words, the Solow model predicts that economies that save more have higher standards of living than those that save less. (The increase in per capita income, however, is smaller than for a similar increase in s in the Harrod-Domar model because the Solow model has diminishing returns in production.) Higher saving also leads to a *temporary* increase in the economic growth rate as the steady state shifts from A to B. However, the increase in the saving rate does *not* result in a permanent increase in the long-run rate of output growth, which remains at n.

The Solow diagram also can be used to evaluate the impact of a change in the population (or labor force) growth rate. An increase in the population growth rate from n to n' rotates the capital widening line to the left from $(n + d)k$ to $(n' + d)k$, as shown in Figure 4–6. The production and saving functions do not change. Because there are more workers, savings per worker (sy) becomes smaller and no longer is large enough to keep capital per worker constant. Therefore, k begins to decline, and the economy moves to a new steady state, C. More workers also means that capital per worker declines from k_0 to k_4 and saving per worker falls from sy_0 to sy_4. Output per worker (or income per capita) also declines, from y_0 to y_4. Thus, an increase in the population growth rate leads to lower average income in the Solow model. Note, however, that the new steady-state growth rate of the entire economy has increased

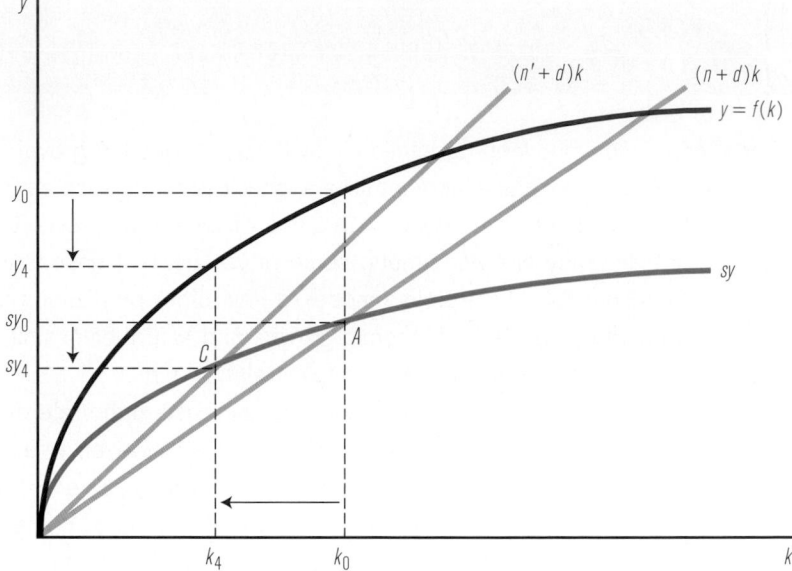

FIGURE 4-6 **Changes in the Population Growth Rate in the Solow Model**

An increase in the rate of population growth from n to n' causes the capital widening curve to rotate to the left. Equilibrium capital per worker drops from k_0 to k_4.

from n to n' at point C. In other words, with a higher population growth rate, Y needs to grow faster to keep y constant.[16] By contrast, a *reduction* in the population growth rate rotates the $(n + d)k$ line to the right and leads to a process of capital deepening, with an increase in both k and in the steady-state level of income per worker, y. However, the relationship between population growth and economic growth is not quite so simple, as described in Box 4–2.

The Solow growth model (as described to this point) suggests that growth rates differ across countries for two main reasons:

- Two countries with the same current level of income may experience different growth rates *if one has a higher steady-state level of income than the other*. To the extent that two countries with the same current level of income have different aggregate production functions, saving rates, population growth rates, or rates of change in productivity (described later), their steady-state income levels will differ and so will their growth rates during the transition to their respective steady states.
- Two countries with the same long-run steady-state level of income may have different growth rates *if they are in different points in the transition to*

---

[16]A similar exercise can be used to determine the impact of an increase in the depreciation rate, d. Such an increase results in a reduction in k and y to a lower steady-state income per capita. The subtle difference between an increase in n and an increase in d is that the latter case does not lead to a change in the long-run growth rate of Y, which remains equal to n.

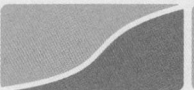

BOX 4-2 POPULATION GROWTH AND ECONOMIC GROWTH

The inverse correlation between population growth and economic growth suggested by the Solow model has a lot of intuitive appeal. Countries such as Belize, Burkina Faso, Liberia, Niger, and Yemen have some of the world's fastest rates of population growth. They are also among some of the poorest nations in the world. But closer inspection of the Solow model reveals other predictions about how population growth may affect economic growth, and a further examination of empirical trends suggests a much more complex relationship.

Figure 4–6 illustrates that, in the Solow model, an increase in the rate of population growth lowers the steady-state level of income, y. However, y refers to output per *worker*, whereas the more common measure of aggregate economic welfare is output per person, y^*. These two measures of output, of course, are related to one another, as follows:

$$y^* = y \times (N/Pop)$$

where N equals the number of workers, and Pop is the total population. Differences in the level of output per capita, therefore, depend on both the amount of output per worker and the ratio of workers to total population. Growth in per capita output, similarly, depends on growth in output per worker and the growth in the worker-to-population ratio.

The Solow model suggests that more rapid population growth reduces capital deepening and hence reduces growth in output per worker. But the effect of population growth on the ratio of workers to total population is more complex. It depends on the age structure of the population. Because of rapid population growth, most developing countries have a young age structure, with a larger share of younger people than is the case in developed nations that have growing populations of more elderly people. As a result of previously higher population growth rates, many developing nations today are experiencing an increase in their ratio of workers to total population. This positive effect of a changing age structure on per capita incomes, sometimes referred to as a *demographic gift*, can play a positive and large role in determining economic growth rates.

The impact of population growth on economic growth goes beyond its effects on capital widening and a nation's age structure. In the Solow model, saving and technological change are considered exogenous. But population growth can affect these parameters as well. The net effect of population growth on economic growth is therefore an empirical matter. Econometric investigations of the impact of population growth on economic growth generally show no systematic relationship (see Chapter 7). Population growth influences many aspects of economic growth and development, not only those described by the Solow model.

the steady state. For example, consider two countries that are identical in every way except that one has a higher saving rate than the other and, so, initially has a higher steady-state level of income. At the steady states, the country with the higher saving rate has a higher level of output per worker, but both are growing at the rate *n*. If the country with the lower saving rate suddenly increases its saving to match the other country, its growth rate will be higher than the other country until it catches up at the new steady state. Thus, even though everything is identical in the two countries, their growth rates may differ during the transition to the steady state, which may take many years.

TECHNOLOGICAL CHANGE IN THE SOLOW MODEL

The Solow model, as described to this point, is a powerful tool for analyzing the interrelationships between saving, investment, population growth, output, and economic growth. However, the unsettling conclusion of the basic model is that, once the economy reaches its long-run potential level of income, economic growth simply matches population growth, with no chance for sustained increases in average income. How can the model explain the historical fact reported in Chapter 2 that many of the world's countries have seen steady growth in average incomes since 1820? Solow's answer was technological change.[17] According to this idea, a key reason why France, Germany, the United Kingdom, the United States, and other high-income countries have been able to sustain growth in per capita income over very long periods of time is that technological progress has allowed output per worker to continue to grow.

Technological progress is a key driver, but not the only driver, of productivity growth. Historically, most technological innovation has originated in today's developed countries, where technological progress has played a central role in explaining productivity growth. Technological progress is also important for today's developing countries; yet, most such progress in developing countries is adopted and adapted from developed countries. In developing countries, the productivity-enhancing effects of technological innovation have played a smaller role in driving productivity growth than in developed countries. In the former, productivity growth has also resulted from improvements in physical infrastructure, increased education of the labor force, and improvements in regulatory environments and incentives. Absent these (and related) factors, technology adoption in developing countries tends to be more limited and less effective in enhancing factor productivity. With these important caveats, we proceed to introduce productivity growth into the Solow model using technological progress as a shorthand.

---

[17]See Solow, "Technical Change and the Aggregate Production Function." For an early discussion about the relationship between capital accumulation and technological progress, see Joan Robinson, *Essays in the Theory of Economic Growth* (London: Macmillan, 1962).

To incorporate an economy's ability to produce more output with the same amount of capital and labor, we slightly modify the original production function and introduce a variable, T, to represent technological progress, as follows:

$$Y = F(K, T \times L) \tag{4-15}$$

In this specification, technology is introduced in such a way that it directly enhances the input of labor, as shown by the specification in which L is multiplied by T. This type of technological change is referred to as *labor augmenting*.[18] As technology improves (T rises), the efficiency and productivity of labor increases because the same amount of labor can now produce more output. Increases in T can result from improvements in technology in the scientific sense (new inventions and processes) or in terms of **human capital**, such as improvements in the health, education, or skills of the workforce.[19]

The combined term $T \times L$ is sometimes referred to as the amount of **effective units of labor**. The expression $T \times L$ measures both the amount of labor and its efficiency in the production process. An increase in either T or L increases the amount of effective labor and therefore increases aggregate production. For example, an insurance sales office can increase its effective workforce by either adding new workers or giving each worker a faster computer or better cell phone. An increase in T differs from an increase in L, however, because the rise in aggregate income from new technology does not need to be shared with additional workers. Therefore, *technological change and productivity growth more broadly allow output (and income) per worker to increase.*

The usual assumption is that technology improves at a constant rate, which we denote by the Greek letter theta (θ), so that $\Delta T/T = \theta$. If technology grows at 1 percent per year, then each worker becomes 1 percent more productive each year. With the workforce growing at n, growth in the effective supply of labor is equal to $n + \theta$. If the workforce (and population) grows by 2 percent per year and technology grows by 1 percent per year, the effective supply of labor increases by 3 percent per year.

To show technological change in the Solow diagram, we need to modify our notation. Whereas earlier we expressed y and k in terms of output and capital *per worker*, we now need to express these variables in terms of output and capital *per effective worker*. The change is straightforward. Instead of dividing Y and K by L as

---

[18]Two other possibilities are *capital-augmenting technological change* $[Y = F(T \times K, L)]$, which enhances capital inputs, and *Hicks-neutral technological change* $[Y = F(T \times K, T \times L)]$, which enhances both capital and labor input. For our purposes, the specific way in which technology is introduced does not affect the basic conclusions of the model.

[19]Keep in mind, however, that, while these two broad categories of improvements in technology have similar general effects in this aggregate model, their true effects are somewhat different in the real world. Technological change in the mechanical sense or from the spread of a new idea can be shared widely across the workforce and considered a public good. Improvements in human capital, by contrast, are specific to individual workers and are not necessarily widely shared. However, both have the effect of augmenting the supply of labor and increasing total output.

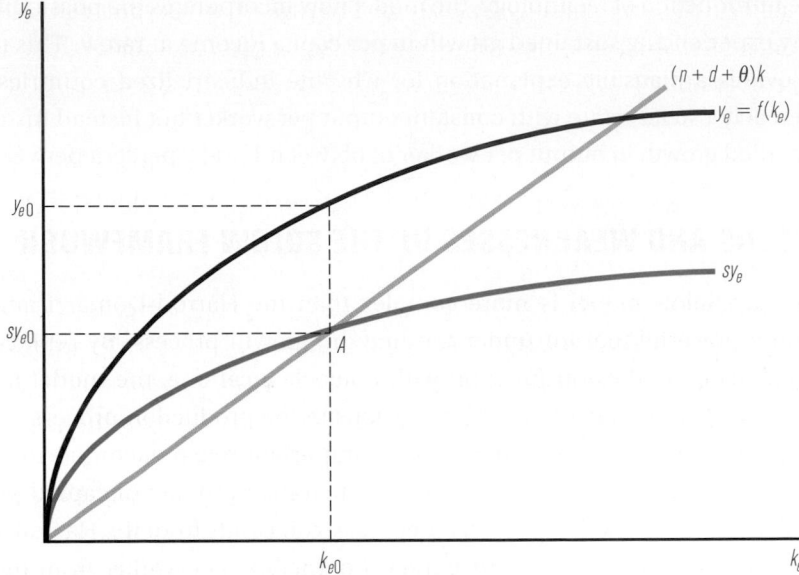

FIGURE 4-7 **The Solow Model with Technical Change**

In the Solow model with technical change, the equilibrium level of effective capital per worker (K_{e0}) is determined by point A, the intersection of the effective capital widening curve $(n + d + \theta)$ and the effective saving curve (sy_e).

previously (to obtain y and k), we now divide each by $(T \times L)$. Thus **output per effective worker** (y_e) is defined as $y_e = Y/(T \times L)$. Similarly, **capital per effective worker** (k_e) is defined as $k_e = K/(T \times L)$.[20]

With these changes, the production function can be written as $y_e = f(k_e)$ and saving per effective worker expressed as sy_e. With effective labor now growing at the rate $n + \theta$, the capital accumulation equation (4–14) changes to

$$\Delta k_e = sy_e - (n + d + \theta)k_e \qquad [4\text{–}16]$$

The new term $(n + d + \theta)k_e$ is larger than the original $(n + d)k$, indicating that more capital is needed to keep capital *per effective worker* constant.

These changes are shown in Figure 4–7, which looks very similar to the basic Solow diagram, with only a slight change in notation. There still is one steady-state point, at which saving per effective worker is just equal to the amount of new capital needed to compensate for changes in the size of the workforce, depreciation, and technological change in order to keep capital per effective worker constant.

One change, however, is very important. At the steady state, output per *effective* worker is constant, rather than output per worker. *Total output now grows at the rate $n + \theta$, so that output per actual worker (or income per person) increases at rate θ.*

---

[20]Note that this is consistent with the earlier notation. If there is no technological change (our earlier assumption), so that $T = 1$ (and remains unchanged), then $y_e = y$ and $k_e = k$.

With the introduction of technology, the model now incorporates the possibility of an economy experiencing sustained growth in per capita income at rate θ. This mechanism provides a plausible explanation for why the industrialized countries never seem to reach a steady state with constant output per worker but instead historically have recorded growth in output per worker of between 1 and 2 percent per year.

STRENGTHS AND WEAKNESSES OF THE SOLOW FRAMEWORK

Although the Solow model is more complex than the Harrod-Domar framework, it is a more powerful tool for understanding the growth process. By replacing the fixed coefficients production function with a neoclassical one, the model provides more reasonable flexibility of factor proportions in the production process. Like the Harrod-Domar framework, it emphasizes the important role of factor accumulation and saving, but its assumption of diminishing marginal product of capital provides more realism and accuracy over time. It departs significantly from the Harrod-Domar framework in distinguishing the current level of income per worker from the long-run steady-state level and focuses attention on the transition path to that steady state. The model provides powerful insights into the relationship between saving, investment, population growth, and technological change on the steady-state level of output per worker. The Solow model does a much better job, albeit far from perfect, of describing real world outcomes than the Harrod-Domar model.

A particularly important contribution of the model is the simple yet powerful insights it provides into the role of technological change and productivity growth in the growth process. For policy makers, key questions then become how to best acquire new technologies and how to magnify their potential contributions to productivity growth through complementary investments and policies. For most low-income countries, while some domestic innovation is possible, for many industries it is probably most cost-effective for entrepreneurs to acquire the bulk of their new technologies from other countries (one of the benefits of "globalization") and adapt them to local circumstances. The willingness of entrepreneurs to make such investments, however, may depend on a number of factors that government can influence. Investments in education (for example, improvements in the *quality* of the labor force) may enable firms in developing countries to make better use of imported technologies. Investments in physical infrastructure might motivate technology adoption by better connecting firms to markets. Improved public institutions to protect property rights and extend the rule of law may also provide powerful incentives for firms to invest in improving their own productivity. However, the model's focus on the role of factor accumulation and productivity (including technology) as the proximate determinants of the steady state raises a new set of questions that the model does not answer.

The model's most troubling limitation is that Solow specified productivity growth as exogenous (that is, determined independently of all the variables and parameters specified in the model). He did not spell out exactly how it takes place or how the growth process itself might affect it. In this sense, productivity growth has been called "manna from heaven" in the Solow model. This is an appropriate abstraction for the purpose of explaining the theoretical role of technological change. In practice, policy makers in developing countries need to know the sources of this manna.

What are the more fundamental determinants of factor accumulation and productivity that affect the steady state and the rate of economic growth? The empirical evidence in Chapter 3 suggests that the most rapidly growing developing countries share certain common characteristics: greater economic and political stability, relatively better health and education, stronger governance and institutions, more export oriented trade policies, and more favorable geography. Box 4-3 provides an estimate of the quantitative importance of these factors in East Asia's rapid growth relative to other countries. In the language of the Solow model, these characteristics operate through factor accumulation and productivity to help determine the precise shape of the production function and the steady-state level of output per worker. Changing any of these factors—say, encouraging more open trade—changes the steady-state level of output per worker and therefore the current rate of economic growth as the economy adjusts to the new steady state. Thus, the model helps us focus attention on these more fundamental influences on the steady state and the growth rate, but it does not provide a full understanding of the precise pathways through which these factors influence output and growth.

Certain characteristics of the neoclassical production function embedded in the Solow model also lead to one of the model's broadest and most problematic empirical predictions—that initially poorer countries will grow more rapidly than initially wealthier countries and eventually catch up. To understand this theoretical prediction, we begin by reviewing the neoclassical production function introduced in Chapter 3.

DIMINISHING RETURNS AND THE PRODUCTION FUNCTION

For output and income to continue to grow over time, a country must continue to attract investment and achieve productivity gains. But as the capital stock grows, the magnitude of the impact of new investment on growth may change. Most growth models are based on the assumption that the return on investment declines as the capital stock grows. We illustrate this aspect of the aggregate neoclassical production in Figure 4-8. The shape of this production function reflects the important but common assumption of diminishing returns to capital or, more precisely, a **diminishing marginal product of capital (MPK)**. This property is indicated by the gradual

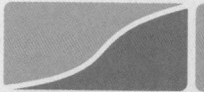

BOX 4-3 EXPLAINING DIFFERENCES IN GROWTH RATES

Many recent studies have shown that the initial levels of income, openness to trade, healthy populations, effective governance, favorable geography, and high saving rates all contribute to rapid economic growth. But which are most important? One study sought to explain differences in growth during the period 1965–90 among three groups of countries: 10 East and Southeast Asian countries (in which per capita growth averaged 4.6 percent), 17 sub-Saharan African countries (in which growth averaged 0.6 percent), and 21 Latin American countries (in which growth averaged 0.7 percent).[a]

Policy variables explained much of the differences in growth rates. The East and Southeast Asian countries recorded higher government saving rates, were more open to trade, and had higher-quality government institutions. Together, the differences in these policies accounted for 1.7 percentage points of the 4.0 percentage point difference between the East and Southeast Asian and sub-Saharan African growth rates, and 1.8 percentage points of the difference between East and Southeast Asia and Latin America. Openness to trade stood out as the single most important policy choice affecting these growth rates.

Initial levels of income also were important, as the Solow model predicts. Because the Latin American countries had higher average income (and therefore greater output per worker) than the East Asian countries in 1965, the Solow model would predict somewhat slower growth in Latin America. Sure enough, this study estimates that Latin America's higher initial income slowed its growth rate by 1.2 percentage points relative to East and Southeast Asia, after controlling for other factors. By contrast, the sub-Saharan African countries had lower average initial income, indicating that (all else being equal) these countries could have grown 1.0 percentage point faster than the East and Southeast Asian countries, rather than the actual outcome of 4.0 percentage points slower. This suggests that the other factors had to account for a full 5.0 percentage point difference in growth rates between East and Southeast Asia and sub-Saharan Africa.

Initial levels of health, as indicated by life expectancy at birth, were a major factor contributing to sub-Saharan Africa's slow growth. Life expectancy at birth averaged 41 years in sub-Saharan Africa in 1965, compared to 55 years in East

---

[a]Steven Radelet, Jeffrey Sachs, and Jong-Wha Lee, "The Determinants and Prospects for Economic Growth in Asia," *International Economic Journal* 15, no. 3 (Fall 2001), 1–30. These results are summarized in the Asian Development Bank's study *Emerging Asia: Changes and Challenges* (Manila: Asian Development Bank, 1997), 79–82.

and Southeast Asia. The study estimates that this reduced sub-Saharan Africa's growth rate by 1.3 percentage points relative to East and Southeast Asia. By contrast, because average life expectancy in Latin America in 1965 was almost the same as in East and Southeast Asia, health explains little of the difference in growth between these regions.

Favorable geography helped East and Southeast Asia grow faster. The combination of fewer landlocked countries, longer average coastline, fewer countries located in the deep tropics, and less dependence on natural resource exports all favored Asia. Taken together, these factors accounted for 1.0 percentage point of East and Southeast Asia's rapid growth compared to sub-Saharan Africa, and 0.6 percentage points relative to Latin America. Differences in initial levels of education and the changing demographic structure of the population accounted for the remaining differences in growth rates across these regions.

Of course, this simple accounting framework does not fully explain the complex relationships that underlie economic growth. Each of the variables in the study captures a range of other factors that affect growth rates. For example, differences in government saving rates probably reflect differences in fiscal policy, inflation rates, political stability, and many other factors. Because of lack of sufficient data, the analysis omits several factors (such as environmental degradation) that may be important. And it certainly does not begin to explain why different policy choices were made in different countries. As a result, studies like these should be seen as a first step to understanding growth, rather than as a precise explanation for the many complex differences across countries.

---

flattening (or declining slope) of the curve as capital per worker grows. It is important, however, to bear in mind the distinction between diminishing returns to individual factors of production holding constant the use of all other factors and the **returns to scale** of the entire production function. The production functions illustrated in Figure 4–8 exhibit diminishing returns to capital per worker but (by assumption) still have constant returns to scale. This latter characteristic means that if producers doubled all inputs (rather than just one input) then total output would also double.

Looking at the production function in Figure 4–8, we can see that at low levels of capital per worker (such as point *a*), new investment leads to relatively large increases in output per worker. But at higher levels of capital per worker (such as point *b*), the same amount of new investment leads to a smaller increment in output. Each addition of a unit of capital per worker (moving to the right along the *x*-axis) yields smaller and smaller increases in output per worker. More generally, giving the same number of workers more and more machinery yields smaller and smaller additions to output.

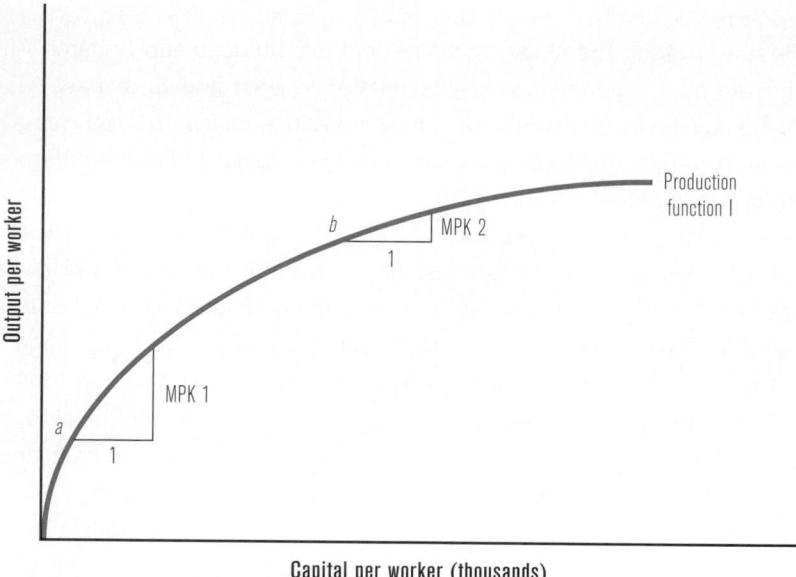

FIGURE 4-8 **Diminishing Marginal Product of Capital**

Along production function I, an addition of 1 unit of capital per worker at point *a* yields a much larger increase in output per worker than the same investment at point *b*. The incremental output produced by adding an additional unit of capital is called the marginal product of capital (MPK).

The assumption of a diminishing marginal product of capital has many implications, but three are particularly important for developing countries. Consider countries located toward the left on the *x*-axis of Figure 4–8, such as at point *a*. These countries have both relatively small amounts of capital per worker and low levels of output per worker. *The latter means, by definition, that these countries are relatively poor.* By contrast, countries toward the right have both higher levels of capital per worker and more output per worker, the latter implying that they are relatively rich. In general, low-income countries tend to have much less capital per worker than do richer countries. Therefore, if all else is equal between the two countries—a crucial qualifier—new investment in a poor country will tend to have a much larger impact on output than the same investment in a rich country. The three key implications are as follows:

- If all else is equal, poor countries have the *potential* to grow more rapidly than do rich countries. In Figure 4–8, a country located at point *a* has the potential to grow more rapidly than does a country at point *b* because the same investment will lead to a larger increase in output.
- As countries become richer (and capital stocks become larger), growth rates tend to slow. In other words, as a country moves along the production

function from point *a* to point *b* over a long period of time, its growth rate tends to decline.

- Because poor countries have the *potential* to grow faster than do rich countries, they can catch up and close the gap in relative income. To the extent this happens, income levels between rich and poor countries would converge over time.

These are very powerful implications. It is important to recognize that they rest on the assumption that all else is equal between the two countries, in particular that countries have the same rates of savings, population growth, and depreciation, and hence the same steady-state level of capital and income per capita. As this interpretation of the Solow model is not conditional on countries differing from one another in these key parameters, it is known as **unconditional convergence**. For all else to be equal, both countries also have to be operating along the same production function, have access to the same technology. If they are not, the predictions for rich and poor countries do not necessarily hold. For instance, a given poor country might actually be operating along different, and perhaps much flatter, production function than the one shown in Figure 4-8 if it does not have access to the same technology as reflected in the production function in Figure 4-8. In that case, each new investment (at a given level of the capital stock) would produce less output on the margin than that same additional investment would produce on the steeper production function. In that case, the poor country might not be expected to grow faster than the rich country and may never catch up. The phrase *ceteris paribus* (all else being equal), which is much used and often overlooked in economics, is of great importance in the convergence debate.

THE CONVERGENCE DEBATE

If it were true that poorer countries could grow fast while richer countries experience slower growth, poorer countries (at least those in which all else is equal) could begin to catch up and see their income levels begin to converge with the rich countries. Has this actually happened?

The short answer is that it has for some countries but not for most. Consider the example of Japan. In the 1960s, Japan's income per capita was only about 35 percent of average U.S. income, and it had a much smaller capital stock, giving it the potential for very rapid growth. (We use the United States as the benchmark for convergence because it has among the highest per capita incomes in the world and is usually considered the global technological leader.) Indeed, Japan's GDP growth rate exceeded 9 percent during the 1960s. By the time Japan had reached 70 percent of U.S. per capita income in the late 1970s, its GDP growth rate had slowed to about 4 percent. As its income continued to grow, its growth rate fell further, and growth was very slow after Japan reached about 85 percent of U.S. income in the early 1990s. Japan's experience illustrates the preceding three points very well: (1) When it was relatively poor, it could grow fast; (2) as its income increased, its growth rate declined; and (3) as a result, its income converged significantly toward U.S. income. People who boldly predicted in the 1960s and 1970s that Japan could grow at 7 to 9 percent per year indefinitely—and many people did—ignored the impact of diminishing returns of capital on long-term growth rates.

Japan is not the only country whose income has converged with the world leaders since 1960. Look again at the group of rapidly growing countries shown in Table 3–1. All these countries were relatively poor in 1960, and all grew by an average of between 3 and 6 percent per capita for nearly 50 years. Rich countries cannot grow that fast over a period of many years (in the absence of a continuous infusion of new technology), but poor countries can because they start with low levels of capital.

However, being poor and having low levels of capital per worker by no means guarantees rapid growth. As the upper sections of Table 3–1 show, many low-income countries recorded low growth. Not only did these countries not catch up but they fell further behind and their incomes diverged even more from the world leaders. The point is that low-income countries have the potential for rapid growth, *if* they can attract new investment and *if* that new investment actually pays off with a large increment in output.

Looking beyond the experience of a few individual countries, is there a general tendency for poor countries to grow faster and catch up with the richer countries? Broadly across all countries, the short answer is no. Figure 4–9 shows the initial level of per capita income in 1960 and subsequent rates of growth from 1960 to 2009 for

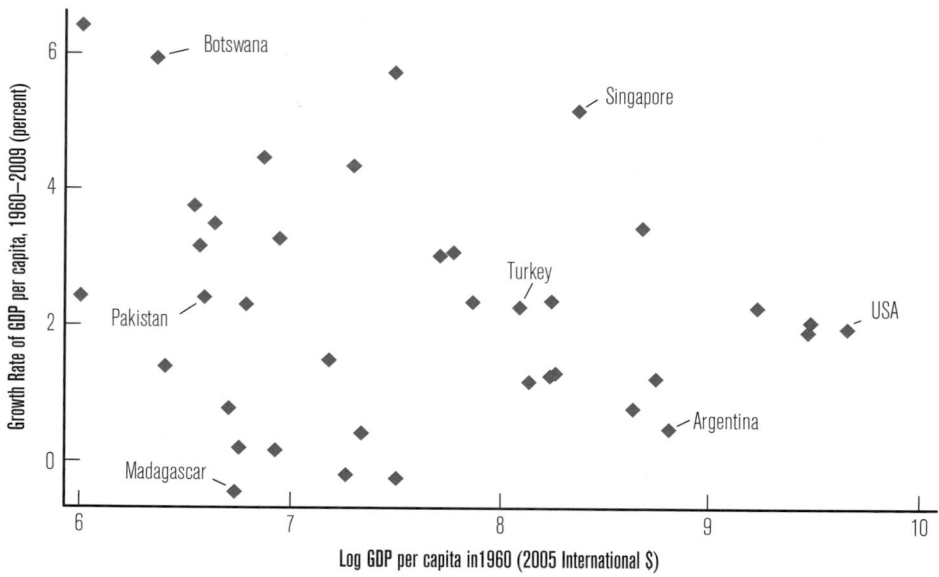

FIGURE 4-9 **Gross Domestic Product (GDP) Growth, Unconditional**

See Table 3–1 for data.

Source: Penn World Tables 7, http://pwt.econ.upenn.edu/php_site/pwt_index.php, accessed June 2011.

the 38 countries listed in Table 3–1. If it were true that poor countries were growing faster than rich countries, the graph would show a clear downward slope from left to right. Poor countries would record a high rate of growth (and appear in the upper left part of the figure) and rich countries would display a slower growth rate (and be in the bottom right). But there is no clear pattern evident in the figure. For example, income per capita in 1960 was approximately the same in Botswana, Pakistan, and Madagascar; yet while Botswana subsequently grew at nearly 6 percent per year, Pakistan's subsequent growth was only 2.3 percent per year and Madagascar's income per capita actually declined. Similarly, Pakistan, Turkey, and the United States all grew at roughly the same rate from 1960 to 2009, yet they began the period with quite different levels of income. The only part that seems accurate is that almost all the rich countries display relatively slow growth rates, as expected. Such results have been documented in many studies using larger samples and more sophisticated statistical techniques. The empirical fact is clear: There has been no *general* tendency for poor countries to catch up to the world leaders. If anything, the opposite has been true. As we saw in Figure 2–1, for the last two centuries, the gap between the richest and the poorest regions of the world has grown, implying a divergence of incomes for these countries.

However, the simple graph in Figure 4–9 does not really do justice to the predictions of convergence, which are based on the critical assumption that all else is equal across countries. This assumption clearly is not true for all countries in the world. Instead, if convergence were to occur, we should expect to find it among countries that share some broad key characteristics, such as a similar underlying production function and similar rates of saving, population growth, depreciation, and technology growth. Some of the poor countries in Figure 4–9, for example, have low saving rates or very little growth in technology compared with other countries and, therefore, have much less potential for rapid growth. To see if the convergence predictions of the Solow model hold under these stricter conditions, we have to dig a little deeper.

Figure 4–9 demonstrates the lack of unconditional convergence, *unconditional* in the sense that it imposes the assumption that all countries share the same key parameters (depreciation, savings, and population growth rates in particular). Digging deeper into the Solow model's predictions, however, we consider the implications for convergence of allowing each country to take on its own individual combination of these key parameters. This allows each country to have its own individual steady-state level of capital and income per capita. Once we allow that, the question is whether initially poorer countries grow faster as they approach their own steady state. Figure 4–10 applies statistical techniques to relax the previous assumption that all countries have the same rates of population growth. Looking at the data from the same countries as in Figure 4–9, but conditional on the countries' population growth rates, we begin to see the predicted negative association between initial income levels and subsequent growth rates. This is known as **conditional convergence**.

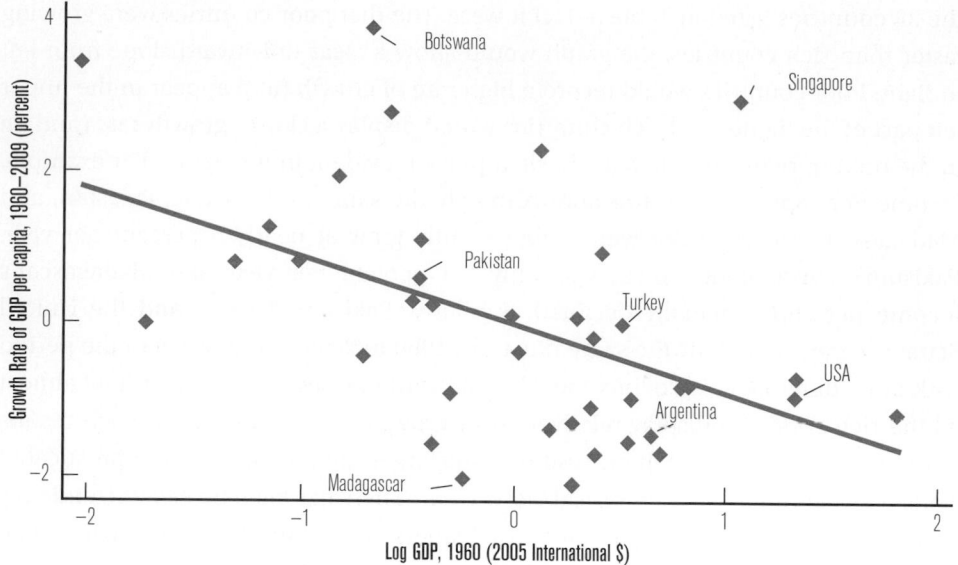

FIGURE 4-10 **Gross Domestic Product (GDP) Growth, Conditional on Population Growth**

See Table 3-1 for data.

Sources: Penn World Tables 7, http://pwt.econ.upenn.edu/php_site/pwt_index.php, accessed June 2011; World Bank, "World Development Indicators," http://databank.worldbank.org.

Another approach is to pick a group of countries from all income levels that are similar in their policy choices, geographic characteristics, or some other variable. Economists Jeffrey Sachs and Andrew Warner, for example, examined the evidence for convergence among all countries that had been consistently open to world trade since 1965.[21] Open economies, as discussed in Chapter 3, are similar in that they have similar (global) markets for their products, purchase their inputs on world markets, and can acquire new technology relatively quickly from other open economies through imports of new machinery and their connections to global production networks. What if we include countries' openness to trade among the conditioning variables? Figure 4–11 conditions GDP growth on countries' rates of savings and population growth in addition to the proportion of time between 1960 and 2009 that they were open to trade. Clearly, these additional conditioning variables sharpen the inverse correlation between initial income and subsequent growth as indicated by the tighter fit around the trend line.[22] Initially wealthier countries may still grow faster in absolute terms than initially poorer countries if the former are converging toward

---

[21]Jeffrey D. Sachs and Andrew Warner, "Economic Reform and the Process of Global Integration," *Brookings Papers on Economic Activity*, 26, no. 1 (1995), 1–118.

[22]Tracing the countries highlighted in Figure 4–9 through Figures 4–10 and 4–11, we note that, despite the additional conditioning variables, Botswana and Singapore consistently grew faster than predicted for their initial incomes (indicated by their positions above the trend lines), whereas Madagascar and Argentina consistently grew more slowly than predicted.

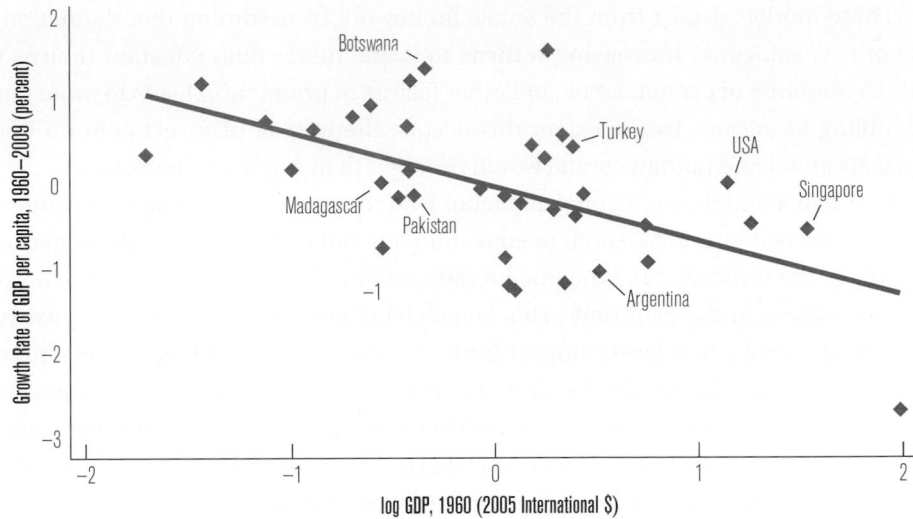

FIGURE 4-11 Gross Domestic Product (GDP) Growth, Conditional on Openness, Savings, and Population Growth

See Table 3-1 for data.

Sources: Penn World Tables 7, http://pwt.econ.upenn.edu/php_site/pwt_index.php, accessed June 2011; World Bank, "World Development Indicators," http://databank.worldbank.org.

much higher steady-state levels of capital per capita. That is why we do not observe unconditional convergence across rich and poor countries' levels of income. On the other hand, if each country is allowed to have its own steady-state level, we do see faster growth among initially poorer countries, as predicted by the Solow model and its implication of conditional convergence.

BEYOND SOLOW: NEW APPROACHES TO GROWTH

A new generation of models takes off where Solow left off, by moving beyond the assumptions of an exogenously fixed saving rate, growth rate of the labor supply, workforce skill level, and pace of technological change. In reality, the values of these parameters are not just given but are determined partially by government policies, economic structure, and the pace of growth itself. Economists have begun to develop more-sophisticated models in which one or more of these variables is determined within the model (that is, these variables become endogenous to the model).[23]

[23]The seminal contributions to the new growth theory are Paul Romer, "Increasing Returns and Long-Run Growth," *Journal of Political Economy* 94 (October 1986), 1002–37; Robert Lucas, "On the Mechanics of Economic Development," *Journal of Monetary Economics* 22 (January 1988), 3–42; and Paul Romer, "Endogenous Technological Change," *Journal of Political Economy* 98 (October 1990), S71–S102.

These models depart from the Solow framework by assuming that the national economy is subject to **increasing returns to scale**, rather than constant returns to scale. A doubling of capital, labor, and other factors of production leads to *more* than a doubling of output. To the extent this occurs, the impact of investment on both physical capital and human capital would be larger than suggested by Solow.

How can a doubling of capital and labor lead to more than a doubling of output? Consider investments in research or education that not only have a positive effect on the firm or the individual making the investment but also have a positive "spillover" effect on others in the economy. This beneficial effect on others, called a **positive externality**, results in a larger impact from the investment on the entire economy. The benefits from Henry Ford's development of the production line system, for example, were certainly large for the Ford Motor Company, but they were even larger for the economy as a whole because knowledge of this new technique soon spilled over to other firms that could benefit from Ford's new approach.

Similarly, investments in research and development (R&D) lead to new knowledge that accrues not only to those that make the investment but to others who eventually gain access to the knowledge. The gain from education is determined not just by how much a scientist's or manager's productivity is raised by investment in his or her own education. If many scientists and managers invest in their own education, there then will be many educated people who will learn from each other, increasing the benefits from education. An isolated scientist working alone is not as productive as one who can interact with dozens of well-educated colleagues. This interaction constitutes the externality. In the context of the "sources of growth" analysis introduced in Chapter 3, such externalities suggest that the measured contribution of physical and human capital to growth may be larger than that captured by the Solow framework. Among other implications, this outcome could account for a significant portion of the residual in the Solow accounting framework, meaning that actual TFP growth is smaller than many studies have suggested.

Another important implication is that economies with increasing returns to scale do not necessarily reach a steady-state level of income as in the Solow framework. When the externalities from new investment are large, diminishing returns to capital do not necessarily set in, so growth rates do not slow, and the economy does not necessarily reach a steady state. An increase in the saving rate can lead to a *permanent* increase in the rate of economic growth. These models can explain continued per capita growth in many countries without relying on exogenous technological change. Moreover, they do not necessarily lead to the conclusion that poor countries will grow faster than rich countries because growth does not necessarily slow as incomes rise, so there is no expectation of convergence of incomes. Initial disparities in income can remain, or even enlarge, if richer countries make investments that encompass larger externalities.

Because growth can perpetuate in these models without relying on an assumption of exogenous technological change, they often are referred to as **endogenous**

growth models. They are potentially important for explaining continued growth in industrialized countries that never reach a steady state, especially those engaged in R&D of new ideas on the cutting edge of technology.

For developing countries, the new models reinforce some of the main messages of the Solow and Harrod-Domar models. Like their forerunners, these models show the importance of factor accumulation and increases in productivity in the growth process. The potential benefits from both of these sources of growth are even greater in endogenous growth models because of potential positive externalities. The core messages of saving, investing in health and education, using the factors of production as productively and efficiently as possible, and seeking out appropriate new technologies are consistent across all these models.

The applicability of endogenous growth models to developing countries is questionable, however, because many low-income countries can achieve rapid growth by adapting the technologies developed in countries with more advanced research capacities rather than making the investments in R&D themselves. For many low-income countries, the Solow model's assumptions of exogenous technological change and constant returns to scale in the aggregate production function may be more appropriate. Productivity growth in such countries may also depend as much on appropriate complementary investments and policies as on technological change itself.

SUMMARY

- Formal growth models provide a more precise mechanism to explore the contributions to economic growth of both factor accumulation and productivity gains. These models allow us to understand better the implications of changes in saving rates, population growth rates, technological change, and other related factors on output and growth.
- The Harrod-Domar model assumes a fixed-coefficients production function, which helps simplify the model but introduces strict rigidity in the mix of capital and labor needed for any level of output. In this model, growth is directly related to saving in inverse proportion to the incremental capital–output ratio.
- The Harrod-Domar model usefully emphasizes the role of saving, but at the same time overemphasizes its importance by implying that saving (and investment) is sufficient for sustained growth, which it is not. Also, the model does not directly address changes in productivity. In addition, the model's assumption of a fixed ICOR leads to increasing inaccuracy over time as the structure of production evolves and the marginal product of capital changes.

- The Solow model improves on some of the weaknesses in the Harrod-Domar framework and has become the most influential growth model in economics. The model allows for more flexibility in the mix of capital and labor in the production process and introduces the powerful concept of diminishing marginal product of capital. It allows for exploration of the impact on growth of changes in the saving rate, the population growth rate, and technological change. The model helps provide a deeper understanding of a much wider range of growth experiences than the Harrod-Domar model. Nevertheless, the model does not provide a full explanation for growth. It does not provide insights into the more fundamental causes of factor accumulation and productivity growth and, as a one-sector model, does not address the issue of resource allocation across sectors.

- The Solow model has several powerful implications, including (1) poor countries have the *potential* to grow relatively rapidly; (2) growth rates tend to slow as incomes rise; (3) across countries that share important common characteristics, the incomes of poor countries potentially can converge with those of the rich countries; and (4) acquiring new technology is central to both accelerating and sustaining economic growth.

- Some poor countries have achieved rapid growth and seen their incomes converge with those of richer countries, but many have not and have seen their incomes fall further behind. There is no evidence of unconditional convergence across countries, but there is strong evidence of *conditional* convergence, in which countries sharing certain characteristics are able to achieve rapid growth and begin to catch up with the richer countries. We find evidence of conditional convergence in the inverse relationship between initial income and subsequent growth rates, when we account for countries differing in key parameters and hence in their steady-state levels.

- In the 1990s, new theories of economic growth gained popularity. These theories sought to fill in key gaps in the neoclassical model. In particular, these models sought to explain the rate of technological progress, which Solow had identified as the determinant of long-term growth in per capita income but that remained exogenous in his model. These new growth theories are thus known as endogenous growth models.

5

States and Markets

Who is it that makes economic development happen? Is it all done by individuals pursuing their various goals, relying on the market to coordinate and make sense of their diverse actions? Or does the government play a central role in achieving sustained increases in per capita income and output? The debate over the proper role for government in achieving economic progress has been going on for more than two centuries. In the *Wealth of Nations* (1776) Adam Smith argued against conventional wisdom of the time, which assumed it was government that led the development process. For example, the king and queen of Spain supported Columbus's exploration of the Americas, and a royal monopoly gave the British East India Company its dominant role in development of trade with India and beyond. Smith proposed instead that economic progress was achieved by individuals who worked through the market to specialize in the production of one particular product (his example was the manufacture of pins) and then exchanged that product on the market for what else they, as producers, needed.

In England at least, Smith's view dominated development thinking for much of the country's growth in the 1800s, as the leaders of the nation promoted free trade and a minimal role for government in the economy. Elsewhere, the state often played a major role in the development of new industries. As one moved eastward from England to France, Germany, and finally Russia, the government played a steadily increasing role in nineteenth-century economic development.[1]

---

[1] This is the basic thesis of Alexander Gerschenkron in *Economic Backwardness in Historical Perspective* (Cambridge: Belknap Press of Harvard University Press, 1962).

After David Ricardo and later Karl Marx, however, the attention of most economists shifted to trying to understand how markets worked, and economic growth was more or less taken for granted, at least in Europe and North America.[2] This focus changed dramatically after the end of World War II, which had devastated much of Europe and Japan. The challenge was how to achieve economic recovery before wartime devastation brought to power new totalitarian regimes and further warfare. In what we now know as the developing countries of the world, former colonies were rapidly becoming independent states. These countries wanted programs that would facilitate their rise out of poverty and make it possible for them to catch up with the already industrialized nations. The United States, the one industrialized country not devastated by war, stood ready to help.

The first decades after the end of World War II witnessed a major effort to achieve modern economic growth throughout the world. There were some successes, mainly the rapid recovery of western Europe, but also many failures, and that set off a debate that continues to this day over just what countries need to do to achieve sustained economic development. At the center of this debate is the question of the proper role for government in development. In the remainder of this chapter we trace the evolution of ideas since the end of World War II about the proper role of the state in economic development. For the most part thinking about the role of the state has been a learning process because successes and failures have helped develop a more sophisticated understanding of the role of government and government-created institutions in the development process. In addition, old ideas that did not initially work well have crept back into the debate. And despite all of the development thinking since the 1950s, there are still a great many poor countries and poor people in the world. In the remainder of this chapter we describe and analyze how thinking about the role of the state has evolved through these debates. In the chapters that follow we return again and again in much greater detail to the role of government as part of the solution to the full panoply of specific development questions.

DEVELOPMENT THINKING AFTER WORLD WAR II

There were several key influences on development thinking after the end of World War II. For economists, the main ideas about growth dated back a century or more. Adam Smith had stressed markets and technological progress as the key, but David Ricardo writing three decades later stressed the importance of saving and investment and of the accumulation of capital. Karl Marx published *Das Kapital* in 1867 and also took the accumulation of capital as the central driving force of growth. Furthermore, the Harrod-Domar model (see Chapter 4) put investment and capital at the center of

[2]The notable exception in the first half of the twentieth century was Joseph Schumpeter.

growth. One influential book published in 1960 argued that the key to growth was to raise the rate of investment and capital formation to a level above 15 percent of gross domestic product (GDP), although there were numerous voices at the time that said the process was more complicated than that.[3]

If capital is at the center of the growth story, it would seem to follow that one key to growth would be to raise the rate of saving so that one could increase the rate of investment. But in poor countries, it was argued, there was a vicious circle of poverty that had to be broken first. Poor countries were too poor to save much and so did not have the resources to invest and so could not grow. The obvious solution was for rich countries to contribute some of their saving to poor countries to break this cycle. In the 1960s the idea was refined further with the development of Hollis Chenery's two-gap model.[4] There was not just a saving gap but also a foreign exchange gap, and the latter was the major constraint on development in most countries. Emphasis on the foreign exchange gap reinforced the view that the key to economic development was for rich countries to provide aid (in the form of dollars or another convertible currency) to fill both the savings and foreign exchange gaps.

This view of development was greatly reinforced at the time by the experience of the Marshall Plan in rescuing the economies (and the democracies) of western Europe and Japan. The Marshall Plan supplied $25 billion to rebuild western Europe, with immediate and dramatic results.[5] Europe recovered rapidly, with GDPs growing so quickly that these countries caught up to the level of income that they would have achieved if they had not been engulfed by war. Much the same experience occurred in Japan. In 1945 virtually all of the cities of Japan lay in ruins, and malnutrition was common throughout the country. But by the 1950s the nation was well launched on two decades of unprecedented 10 percent a year GDP growth. Large injections of capital, mostly from the United States, had done the trick, or so it seemed.

What was missing from the analysis of these success stories was the role of the supporting institutions required for economic development. Western Europe had fully developed legal systems designed for a modern industrial economy; had education systems capable of providing required training; and despite the enormous loss of life, had large numbers of people who knew how to organize a company (and a government) and who understood modern technology. Much of the physical infrastructure was gone, but many of the key institutions were embodied in people, and all that was needed was a little help to get started. When the same emphasis on foreign aid, capital, and foreign exchange was applied a decade later to developing countries,

---

[3]Walter W. Rostow, *The Stages of Economic Growth: A Non-Communist Manifesto* (Cambridge: Cambridge University Press, 1960).

[4]Hollis Chenery and Alan Strout, "Foreign Assistance and Economic Development," *American Economic Review*, 56, no. 4 (1966).

[5]Technically the Marshall Plan itself supplied only half of the $25 billion; the other half was contributed by the United States in the years between the end of World War II and the formal beginning of the plan in April 1948. The total amount of aid converted into today's dollars would be over US$200 billion.

many of the critical institutions were missing. *Developing* poor and underdeveloped nations proved to be a very different process from *reconstructing* already developed economies destroyed by war.

Most developing countries did not start with the Smith view that well-functioning markets were the key to successful development. To begin with, markets in developing countries were associated with capitalism, and capitalism in the minds of many was associated with colonialism and being kept poor by colonial powers. Many leaders in developing countries were looking for an alternative path, and they had plenty of support from people and events elsewhere.

In the industrialized West there was the obvious fact that markets had not functioned all that well before the war. The Great Depression of the 1930s was a market failure on an unprecedented scale. But economists and others had long been aware that all economies suffer market failures, albeit on a smaller scale (Box 5–1). The question was not whether these market failures existed but how prevalent they were and thus what (if anything) the government should do about them. Among the Fabian socialists in Britain whose ideas were reflected in the Labour Party then in power in Britain, market failures were common and called for active intervention by government in many areas of economic activity. The British Labour government of the time also supported outright government takeover of certain major businesses. The relevance of this to developing countries is that many were former British colonies whose leaders had been educated in Britain at universities where Fabian socialist views were common and widely discussed. It is interesting to note that this was true of Jawaharlal Nehru and other leaders of the Indian Congress Party, which ruled India for several decades after the country achieved independence from Britain in 1948.

Some of the most prominent theories of development economists in this early period also argued that the situation facing developing countries required broad government intervention. The **big push** idea of economist Paul Rosenstein-Rodan argued that it was difficult for one modern industry to start up in a developing country (his example was shoes) because there would not be enough people with the money to buy the products of one shoe factory.[6] Instead one needed to develop a wide range of industries all at the same time so that the workers in each factory would have the income needed to buy the products of the other factories. The only way to achieve this broad-based development of a wide range of industries was to have a government plan that could guide individual producers and guarantee that the demand would be there when they went into production. Economist Albert Hirschman countered this argument with the view that countries instead could start by emphasizing industries with strong **linkages** so the creation of one industry, machinery for example, would create demand for steel and steel would create

---

[6]Paul Rosenstein-Rodan, "Problems of Industrialization of Eastern and South-Eastern Europe," *Economic Journal* 53, nos. 210–11 (1943), 202–11.

BOX 5-1 MARKET FAILURE

The term *market failure* refers to situations in which markets fail to achieve efficient outcomes. *Efficiency* in this context has a precise definition, based on the concept of **Pareto efficiency**. A Pareto efficient market outcome is one in which no one can be made better off without making someone else worse off. (Note that this definition, conceived by nineteenth-century Italian economist Vilfredo Pareto, says nothing about equity.) Market failures can occur for various reasons, including the presence of externalities and the existence of monopolies, public goods, and information asymmetries. The common theme across these categories of market failure is the divergence in equilibrium between **marginal social costs** and **marginal social benefits**. Market equilibrium occurs when private actors equate their marginal costs with their marginal benefits. Under conditions of perfect competition, with no externalities and no public goods, the marginal costs and benefits faced by private actors equal the marginal social costs and benefits faced by society. Yet, imagine a situation in which a factory sits along a riverbank upstream from a fishery. That factory chooses a profit-maximizing quantity of output by equating its private marginal costs and benefits and thus releases the related quantity of effluent into the river. If the cost of the pollution is reflected in the loss of revenue to the fishery, that cost is borne by society but does not enter into the private cost–benefit calculations of the factory owner. It is an externality and leads to a divergence between marginal private costs and marginal social costs. This constitutes a market failure in which the factory overproduces both its output and pollution. On a larger scale, the overproduction of greenhouse gasses, widely seen as a cause of global warming, has been called, "the biggest market failure the world has ever seen."[a] (We return to this theme extensively in Chapter 19.)

A similar divergence between private and social marginal costs and benefits occurs in the presence of monopolies. Profit-maximizing monopolists restrict output below the level that would occur under perfect competition. In doing so, the monopolist is equating private marginal costs and benefits (the basic condition for profit maximization). Yet, reducing the quantity of product available in the monopolized market results in an equilibrium in which the marginal social benefits of an additional unit of output exceed the marginal social costs of producing that last unit, another instance of market failure. Society would be better off with additional output in this market.

The market failure associated with public goods arises from the incentive for individuals to act as free riders. Public goods have the characteristic that no

[a]N. Stern, *Stern Review on the Economics of Climate Change* (London: HM Treasury, 2006).

one can be excluded from consuming them (for example, national defense). The resulting distinction between public and private goods is that to consume the latter, each individual must reveal his or her true willingness to pay for that good, but with the former, because no one can be excluded, the incentive is for individuals to conceal their true willingness to pay for consumption. Markets thus fail by undersupplying public goods (here, too, implying a divergence between private and social marginal costs and benefits).

Information asymmetries are situations in which one party to a transaction has more information than the other party. Such situations commonly arise in insurance markets, where the insured knows more about his or her own risk profile and behavior than does the insurer. Thus, high-risk individuals will tend to drive up the price of insurance for low-risk individuals and drive them out of the market (the adverse selection problem). Similarly, having insurance might lead some to engage in riskier behavior than otherwise, thus driving up the price of insurance for those who continue to behave more cautiously (the "moral hazard" problem). In both cases, the information asymmetry creates an externality, leading to market failure.

Faced with these (and other) potential sources of market failure, the challenge for government policy makers lies in deciding if, when, and how to intervene. Potential policy interventions to correct market failures are varied and complex. They might include taxing polluters (to internalize the cost of externalities), breaking or regulating monopolies, and directly providing public goods. In practice, diagnosing market failures is rarely a straightforward task, and public intervention brings with it the risk of making the situation worse than it would have been without the intervention. Such instances are known as **government failure**. The tension between the risks of market failure and government failure lies at the heart of the debates described in this chapter.

demand for iron ore and coal (what Hirschman called **backward linkages**).[7] The big push theory implicitly assumed that solving the demand problem by exporting a new product was not a realistic option, an assumption that was not unreasonable given that Rosenstein-Rodan was writing during and shortly after World War II. Some analysts still use the term *big push*, but mostly when arguing for making a large effort, such as an unprecedented increase in foreign aid to get over one or another major

[7]Albert O. Hirschman, *The Strategy of Economic Development* (New Haven, CT: Yale University Press, 1958).

obstacle to growth. More recent uses of the big push terminology are discussed at greater length in Chapter 14.

Of comparable or greater influence than these intellectual debates was the perceived success of the model of growth pioneered by the Soviet Union.[8] This model had three basic components:

1. The proponents of the model, like Marx, emphasized the role of capital and high rates of investment achieved by limiting consumption by farmers and others.
2. The model gave priority to the development of heavy industry that would provide physical capital products, such as machinery, that were assumed not to be available unless produced domestically.[9]
3. Management of the economy rejected the use of market forces except in areas peripheral to most economic activity.

The allocation of goods was to be done by large government bureaucracies guided by a central plan drawn up in Moscow. The appeal of the Soviet approach was based on the widely held perception that it had transformed a poor and backward country into an industrial powerhouse that defeated the strongest military power in the world, Nazi Germany. Three decades later this economic model would appear to be far less formidable within the Soviet Union itself as well as elsewhere, but in the 1950s many developing countries were inspired by it. Ghana under Kwame Nkrumah, for example, the first African nation to achieve independence from its colonial ruler, focused on heavy industry during its initial growth phase. India went even further in attempting to adapt major parts of the Soviet economic model, and China, after the 1949 revolution, adopted the Soviet system in its entirety.

Finally, the attitude toward the prospects of achieving growth through reliance on foreign trade had limited appeal in most developing countries. The belief among many was that dependence on foreign trade would force these countries to be forever the source of raw material from their mines and agriculture and never industrialized countries in their own right. More important, the one region of the developing world that had begun industrial development before World War II (South America, in particular Brazil, Argentina, Columbia, and Chile) had done so by developing industry behind high protective barriers, called *import substituting industrialization* (discussed at greater length in Chapter 18). There was no belief at the time that growth could be achieved to a large degree by the export of manufactures, and there was a solid reason for this belief. During World War I and II, there were few international markets for South American manufactures because submarine war, among other

---

[8]Strictly speaking, the Soviet model of economic growth was patterned in part on the German wartime economic model used during World War I (1914–18).

[9]Strictly speaking, the Soviet model assumed that the economy was basically closed to foreign trade; hence exporting consumer goods or natural resources to purchase capital goods from abroad was not an option or was, at best, a very limited option.

things, prevented most normal trading relationships. In between the two wars was the Great Depression, when industrialized countries vied with each other to raise tariff barriers to protect their own domestic industry. The very high Smoot-Hawley Tariff, enacted in 1930, was the American contribution to this trade war.

By the 1950s and 1960s this emphasis on import substituting industrialization was further reinforced in South America. Industries developed behind high trade barriers were an important part of those economies and gave them substantial political influence to keep the trade barriers in place. In addition, economists such as Raul Prebisch, based at the Economic Commission for Latin America (ECLA) in Santiago, Chile, and Hans Singer, based at the United Nations Industrial Development Organization (UNIDO) provided an intellectual rationale for import substituting industrialization. The low income and price elasticities of demand for developing countries' exports of raw materials and the inability of such nations to compete against the economic head start of the industrialized nations meant that all or most of the benefits of foreign trade went to the already industrialized nations, or so Prebisch and Singer argued.

The result of these various influences is that most developing countries in the 1950s and 1960s believed that a high level of government planning and government intervention in the economy was desirable and even absolutely necessary if economic growth were to be achieved. All over the world, countries introduced one government intervention after another. Sometimes these interventions were based on strategy articulated in a national plan; at other times they had a much narrower focus, including the personal interests of the government officials introducing the measures. All of this was occurring, however, while the governments of the industrialized nations were in the process of dismantling most of their trade barriers under the auspices of the General Agreement on Tariffs and Trade (GATT), formed in 1949 and now superseded by the World Trade Organization (WTO). Economists from industrialized countries who had lived through the trade wars of the 1930s and a much wider group of political leaders felt that these trade disagreements had contributed directly to global warfare and were determined to move the industrialized world back to the open trading system that had existed before World War I. Some of these same economists argued vigorously against the protectionist trends in the developing world, but not many policy makers in developing countries were listening.

The main approach of economists working with developing countries in the 1950s and 1960s was not to try to reduce the role of government in the economy but to try to make government intervention more rational and geared to achieving well thought out development objectives. One such measure was to help countries set up planning commissions that would draw up economic development plans and provide sound economic advice to development officials in general. The Harvard Development Advisory Service (later the Harvard Institute for International Development), heavily funded by the Ford Foundation, for example, provided technical support mostly in the form of economic analysis and training to planning commissions in Iran, Pakistan, Indonesia, Malaysia, Ghana, and other countries in the 1960s and early 1970s.[10]

By the early 1970s, therefore, a high level of intervention and a high level of government investment in the economy of developing countries was the norm, although there were exceptions. The role of industrialized countries was to provide aid mainly to governments either through bilateral or multilateral aid programs (for example, the World Bank) and to provide technical assistance to help design and manage aid projects and help more generally with government economic policy making. In countries within the sphere of influence of the Soviet Union, the full Soviet model, where the government controlled and administered most economic activity outside of agriculture, was the norm.

FUNDAMENTAL CHANGES IN THE 1970s AND 1980s

By the 1970s a reaction against the approaches of the earlier decades was building, particularly among economists and other policy makers in the bilateral and multilateral aid agencies and in the governments of the industrialized world. There was a growing disillusionment with the results of the considerable amounts of aid given out over the previous two decades. In Africa, most governments that had gained independence in the 1960s were experiencing little or no growth, and total factor productivity in the continent as a whole was negative. In Latin America import substituting industrialization had run into the limits caused by the small size of most of the domestic markets and growth had slowed in much of the region. By the 1980s (and in China by the late 1970s), interest in the Soviet model had waned because most of the countries with a Soviet-type economic system began to stagnate and in certain cases to build up unsustainable levels of international debt.

The analysis of what had gone wrong, however, had several different strains to it, and analysts and policy makers often did not agree about which one was the major source of weak performance. One strain of criticism of the policies of the 1950s and 1960s argued that too much attention had been paid to the growth rate of GDP and not enough to how the benefits of growth were distributed.

Too many of the benefits of growth, it was argued, were going to a narrow group of wealthy business people and their government and politician supporters. The share of the population trapped in poverty was not declining rapidly enough even in areas where GDP growth was relatively robust, and it was not declining at all in

---

[10]Edward S. Mason, *The Harvard institute for International Development and Its Antecedents* (Cambridge: Distributed by Harvard University Press, 1986).

much of the developing world.[11] Inequality also had a regional component. In many countries growth appeared to be concentrated in one part of the country, often near the capital city, while other regions stagnated. The breakup of West Pakistan and East Pakistan with the latter becoming Bangladesh in 1971, for example, was in part caused by the belief that all or most of the benefits of foreign aid and development were flowing to West Pakistan.

Economists had recognized for decades that an efficient economic system did not necessarily mean the system was equitable or that the fruits of the system were fairly distributed. Efficiency in economic theory was typically defined as a system that could not make anyone better off without making someone else worse off, a concept called **Pareto optimality**. Markets were efficient in this sense (or at least perfectly competitive markets were efficient), but that could be consistent with an economy with a concentration of income and wealth in the hands of the few. If markets could not necessarily solve the problem of inequality, it seemed to many economists that it was up to the government to correct this failure. They argued that government was best suited to address basic needs and target aid to the poor. Private charities and other nongovernmental organizations (NGOs) could play a role in these efforts, but they lacked the resources possessed by governments.

Counter to this argument for even more government intervention in the economy was a growing awareness based on research and experience that many government interventions did not work out as intended or planned. Many simply created obstacles to economic growth. Trade restrictions in Indonesia, for example, forced importers to obtain 70 different stamps of approval before a good could be brought into the country. This approach may have protected a few domestic industries, but it made it difficult for most businesses to get needed inputs in a timely manner, something that was essential if they were to compete in the international marketplace. Other interventions such as those of Kwame Nkrumah in Ghana were based on a flawed development strategy unsuited to the conditions then prevailing in the country (Box 5-2). Many governments had no economic rationale at all for their interventions or justified their actions as solving some particular market failure when the real motivation lay elsewhere. Often policies that had the stated goal of helping the poor were really designed to provide jobs or illicit income for well-off government officials. Other interventions, whether well intended or not, provided government officials with discretionary authority to issue permits, providing the opportunity for illegal payments.

For the increasing number of economists and policy makers who held these views, the clear implication was that governments of developing countries needed to

---

[11]One study at the time that had an important influence on thinking about redistribution, particularly in the World Bank, was the book by Hollis Chenery, Richard Jolly, Montek S. Ahluwalia, C. L. Bell, and John H. Duloy, *Redistribution with Growth: Policies to Improve Income Distribution in Developing Countries in the Context of Economic Growth* (World Bank, 1974).

BOX 5-2 GHANA AFTER INDEPENDENCE

On March 6, 1957, with great celebration, Ghana became the first sub-Saharan African country to gain its independence. Optimism was in the air: Ghana was the world's largest cocoa producer, it had the highest per capita income in sub-Saharan Africa (except South Africa), and its foreign exchange reserves were equivalent to over three years of imports. Ghana's prospects looked bright.

But it was not to be. President Kwame Nkrumah, who was brilliant in leading Ghana to independence, proved to be much less effective as an economic and political leader. In a push for rapid industrialization, Nkrumah introduced extensive state intervention in the economy, with many controlled prices, restrictions on trade and investment, and state-owned enterprises. Based on its cocoa earnings, Ghana borrowed heavily to establish a wide range of industries designed to substitute for imports and for processing many of Ghana's raw materials. But cocoa prices collapsed in the mid-1960s, and the state's heavy hand led to widespread corruption, poor investment decisions, distorted prices, and growing instability. In 1966, a group of army officers overthrew Nkrumah in what was only the first of a series of coups and countercoups over the following 17 years. The economy fluctuated wildly, with growth plunging to −6 percent in 1966, then climbing to 7 percent in 1970 as cocoa prices recovered, only to collapse again to −5 percent 2 years later and to a disastrous −14 percent in 1975. By 1983, the economy had collapsed. Cocoa production was only half as large as it once had been, inflation exceeded 120 percent, growth had been below −6 percent for 3 years in a row, and per capita income was about one-third lower than it had been 26 years before at independence.

In 1983, President Jerry Rawlings (who had taken power himself in a coup 2 years earlier as Flight Lieutenant Rawlings), with few options at his disposal, turned to the International Monetary Fund (IMF) and World Bank for financial assistance and, in return, accepted their strict conditions for changes in economic policy. Rawlings introduced Ghana's Economic Recovery Program, which in many ways was a prototype for reform programs introduced by many other developing countries under the auspices of the IMF and World Bank in the 1980s and early 1990s. The reforms were widespread: Ghana devalued its currency, freed interest rates from restrictions, and substantially reduced its budget deficit. It removed or modified a range of price controls (including raising the price paid to cocoa farmers), reduced tariffs on many imported products, and otherwise took steps to liberalize the trade regime. It partially or fully privatized dozens of enterprises over several years, including transport, the marketing of cocoa, banking, and other areas. The IMF and World Bank heralded Ghana's progress in reforms and predicted that these changes would lay the foundation for greater macro-economic stability, sustained economic growth, and a reduction in poverty.

The results were a clear improvement although not as dramatic as many at the time had hoped. The economy stabilized: Inflation fell (although it still remained above 20 percent), the trade deficit shrank, and foreign exchange reserves grew. Growth became far less volatile, and per capita GDP grew at 1.6 percent through the mid-1990s and at a higher rate of just over 2.9 percent from 1996 through 2010. Growth after 2004 was further boosted by the international community forgiving nearly $6 billion of Ghana's debt, although Ghana then borrowed another $750 million in 2007. The discovery, also in 2007, of major off-shore oil reserves promised further support for Ghana's economy. The first oil began to flow in 2010 and the per capita GDP growth rate in 2011 jumped to over 8 percent. Whether this oil windfall will lead to sustained higher growth or will be mismanaged with negative consequences for growth remains to be seen. The evidence as to whether this will be the case as of 2011 is mixed.

step back from meddling in the economy and better design whichever existing policies seemed to be working. The shortcomings of import substituting industrialization have been particularly well documented.[12] Even Nobel laureate Gunnar Myrdal, an early advocate of import substituting protection as a means of mobilizing under-employed labor, eventually recognized that intervention often leads to corruption, which in turn inhibits development.[13] By the 1970s and early 1980s the World Bank also began to push harder on these issues.

While these debates over the role of government were proceeding, two major developments occurred that were to have a profound impact on how the role of government in development was perceived. The first development was the rise in oil prices engineered by the Organization of the Petroleum Exporting Countries (OPEC) in 1973 and 1979. These price increases led to large amounts of money flowing into the treasuries of oil-exporting countries, expanding the role of government investment in those countries, often by a very large amount. Of equal if not greater importance over the

---

[12]One of the early influential articles questioning import substitution industrialization was John Sheahan, "Import Substitution and Economic Policy: A Second Review," Research Memorandum No. 50 (Williamstown: Williams College, Center for Development Economics, 1972). See also his study of import substitution in Latin America, John Sheahan, *Patterns of Development in Latin America: Poverty, Repression and Economic Strategy* (Princeton: Princeton University Press, 1987).

[13]In his *Asian Drama: An Inquiry into the Poverty of Nations,* 3 vols. (New York: Twentieth Century Fund, 1968), Gunnar Myrdal introduced the concept of the *soft state,* which was ineffective in carrying out its development goals and was typically riddled with corruption arising from these ineffective efforts.

longer run, however, was that several of the largest exporters acquired large reserves of foreign exchange that they reinvested with the cooperation of the international banks.

The enormous amount of money involved led to low interest rates on loans world-wide, and governments of developing countries were encouraged to borrow large sums to fund their development programs. Particularly in Latin America, debts to the major private international banks began to accumulate. By the mid-1980s, the situation had changed dramatically. Alarmed by rising inflation, due in part to the OPEC oil shocks, the U.S. Federal Reserve sharply contracted the U.S. money supply, causing interest rates to rise precipitously. This had two highly detrimental effects on developing nations that had borrowed abroad. First, many loans were written with variable interest rates; second, they were denominated in dollars, not local currency. When the U.S. dollar rapidly appreciated as markets responded to the policies of U.S. monetary authorities, heavily indebted nations had trouble servicing their debts as their interest payments rose and the value of their currencies against the U.S. dollar fell. The ensuing debt burden on Latin American countries forced several major countries to consider defaulting on their debts. The full nature of the debt problem in this period is discussed at length in Chapter 13; here we note that the buildup of debt first made it possible for developing country governments to finance a wide array of development projects, and then created a payment crisis that brought many of these projects to a premature end in what in Latin America has often been called the lost decade of the 1980s. The impact of this lost decade went far beyond the immediate debt problems. It called into question the whole subject of the appropriate role for government in development.

The other profound event of the 1970s really began in the 1960s, but its impact on development thinking was felt only a decade later, and its lessons are still being debated today. This event was the rise of the Four East Asian Tigers: South Korea, Taiwan, Hong Kong, and Singapore. By the late 1970s these economies had been growing at rates comparable to those of Japan for over a decade and were increasingly seen as economic success stories. The basis for their growth was a direct challenge to the view that the path to successful development rested on an emphasis on import substituting industrialization. All four built their rapid economic growth on the export of labor-intensive manufactures. There was a period of import substitution, but the four quickly moved to a reliance on exports, manufactured exports in particular. The model for the economies of South Korea and Taiwan was Japan, which had pioneered a similar strategy during the first phases of its development and again after World War II. Hong Kong and Singapore had long been trading entrepôts and possessed all of the infrastructure and institutions that trading economies required. What was added in the latter two economies was a manufacturing sector oriented toward export markets. In Hong Kong's case, it was manufacturers in Shanghai who moved their base of operation to Hong Kong after the Communist revolution in China in 1949. All Four East Asian Tigers exported first and foremost to the United States whose market, unlike in the 1930s, was wide open to foreign imports. These nations demonstrated that a development strategy based on the export of manufactures was not only possible but superior to the import substituting strategies then prevailing in much of the developing world.

More controversial is the influence of the Four East Asian Tigers on the role of government in their economic development strategy. The facts themselves are not really in dispute. The governments of South Korea and Taiwan were actively involved in export promotion and in industrial development more generally. They devalued their currencies, subsidized exports in various ways, and promoted education and research in technology in support of industry. Government support, including temporary protection against imports, was predicated on performance, and performance by Korean and Taiwanese firms was measured by their ability to export. By any standard these governments were interventionist, but they had a clear strategy behind their intervention, which was not allowed to be diverted toward the private interests of government officials. Corruption existed in the two economies, but it had little influence on industrial and export policies. It is also the case, however, that state-led economic development became less and less viable as these economies became more sophisticated and complex. By the first decade of the twenty-first century, both South Korea and Taiwan had eliminated much of the intervention that characterized their first decades of rapid growth (Box 5-3).

The experience with the role of government in development in Hong Kong and to a large degree Singapore as well could not be more different. Hong Kong was as close to a pure laissez faire market economy as any in the world. The government of Hong Kong maintained a completely open free trade economy. In the few areas in which it did intervene, such as land policy, the government imposed policies unrelated to the main development strategy. The role of government was to maintain a stable macroeconomic environment, support education and health, and maintain security. Singapore's government was similar in most respects, but there the government did play a role in supporting particular industries and several of the key corporations (Singapore Airlines, for example) were government owned. For the most part, however, Singapore's industrial policy focused on creating a favorable climate for foreign direct investment (see Chapter 10).

Some studies have tried to press these rather different experiences of the Four East Asian Tigers into a story consistent across all the groups.[14] More common has been the selective choice of one experience over another to support a particular preconceived view of the role of government intervention (Hong Kong for those who support laissez faire markets;[15] South Korea's heavy and chemical industry drive of

---

[14]World Bank, *The East Asian Miracle: Economic Growth and Public Policy* (New York: Oxford University Press, 1993), ably describes many of the reasons for the success of the four economies but less successfully tries to fit the experiences of the four into a single development model that relied mostly on market forces for its success. This reasonably portrays the policies of Hong Kong and Singapore but not those of South Korea and Taiwan.

[15]See for example Milton Friedman, "The Real Lesson of Hong Kong," *National Review,* December 31, 1997.

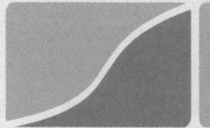

BOX 5-3 THE DECLINING EFFECTIVENESS OF GOVERNMENT INTERVENTION IN THE MARKET: KOREA, 1960s-2010

South Korea in the 1960s and 1970s pursued an industrial policy that involved heavy intervention by the government to promote exports in general and specific industries in particular. The government provided bank loans to favored industries at below-market rates, gave these industries special access to government-controlled foreign exchange and imports, and helped build the infrastructure they required. The president of the country even met monthly with the heads of the major industries to review and help solve their problems, many of them related to intervention by government in their efforts to expand. The government saw itself as correcting for market failures, even though many of these market failures were the creation of earlier and continuing government controls that were part of its import substituting policies.

These industrial policies appear to have worked reasonably well, although the heavy industry and chemical industry drive of the 1970s remains controversial to this day. President Park Chung Hee, who led this effort, kept politics and corruption out of most of these industrial policy decisions. Because he ran an authoritarian regime supported mainly by a modern army, he felt no need to use industrial policies to pay off his political supporters. By the early 1980s, however, many Korean economists and others felt that this activist government industrial policy was causing too many economic distortions and the country should move toward a more market-oriented system. This change proved to be difficult because of promises made to private companies that had carried out the government's wishes in the past. Such companies felt that they had an implicit guarantee that they would be helped out if, by doing the government's bidding, they got into trouble. In the 1980s, they did get into trouble, and the government spent much of its time in that decade providing them with subsidies and other means of support.

By the 1990s, Korea had a democratic government led, from 1992 to 1997, by President Kim Young Sam, who had little interest in an activist industrial policy. Like his predecessors, however, he saw how these policies could be used to raise large sums of money to support his political campaigns. Increasingly the principal criterion for getting government support for a particular firm or industry depended on whether that firm contributed to the political campaigns. Such contributions existed in the 1960s and 1970s as well, but they were not allowed to influence major industrial policy decisions. By contrast, in the 1990s, industrial policy interventions were driven more by politics than by a concern for building efficient, competitive industries. Industrial policy in the earlier period had produced such firms as POSCO, one of the largest and most efficient steel companies in the world, a firm that remained profitable right through the Asian financial crisis of 1997–98. The industrial policy in the 1990s produced such firms as the Hanbo Steel company, whose bankruptcy contributed in a significant way to Korea's involvement in the Asian financial crisis.

Finally, in the 1998–2008 period, the Korean government under two new presidents, Kim Dae Jung and then Roh Moo Hyun, began to make a major effort to get themselves out of the business of supporting particular industries and firms. The objective was to create a level playing field for all, but to do so without triggering another financial crisis caused by the collapse of the older firms that had relied so much on government support. Moving away from extensive government intervention and relying entirely on market forces, however, is not as simple as simply telling the government to stop intervening. In many cases, the government felt it had to introduce new interventions to undo the damage of previous ones. This same conflict of goals continued during the government of President Lee Myung-Bak who took office in 2009.

the 1970s for those who believe in extensive government intervention). As the experience of these four economies became better understood, however, two conclusions became increasingly clear. One was that developing countries could grow at very rapid rates with the right policies. The other was that growth could be based on exports, at least on exports of manufactures. Exports based on natural resources (discussed in Chapter 17) were another matter, but none of the four tigers had significant exports of natural resources.

The influence of the experience of the Four East Asian Tigers was particularly strong regionally, notably in China after 1978 and Vietnam after 1986, but it also changed the thinking of many economists and policy makers in South America and elsewhere in the developing world.

STRUCTURAL ADJUSTMENT, THE WASHINGTON CONSENSUS, AND THE END OF THE SOVIET MODEL

The response of the multilateral and bilateral aid agencies, particularly the World Bank, was to use their aid programs to support changes in the approach to development in countries whose economic performance was weak. By the late 1980s the list of countries struggling but largely failing to achieve rapid economic development included most of those in Africa, Latin America, and South Asia. The term used by the World Bank for many of the changes it proposed was *structural adjustment,* a broad term that includes reforms aimed at changing the structure of the economy to be more market based, more efficient, more open to international trade, and more focused on the production of tradable commodities. The result was a wide range of reform proposals, initially somewhat ad hoc, that were often made conditional if a country wanted to receive assistance from the World Bank or other aid agencies.

A major objective of structural adjustment reforms was to reduce or remove distortions generated by government intervention. In the majority of developing countries, the list of distorted prices was long and included high and uneven tariffs, cheap interest rates on loans (which discourage saving and lead to poor loan decisions), high minimum wages that help some workers but hurt others, subsidized fuel or food, and limits on prices paid to farmers to control food prices. For every government-determined price, there are winners who receive more for their output or pay less for their inputs, and losers who experience the opposite. Price distortions most often occur when the beneficiaries of a price change are few and concentrated, and the losers are many and dispersed. A tariff raises profits for the well-connected factory owner. But even though millions of people might be paying a higher price for the tariff-protected goods, they are scattered unevenly across the country and unlikely to organize to protest the increase. Because the tariff is built into retail prices, consumers may not even be aware that government intervention caused the higher prices. The owners of the company, however, know and are happy to share their increased profits with those who helped them, thus creating political barriers to reform.

Sometimes, correcting a distortion may lead to lower prices, as in removing a tariff, but it can also lead to higher consumer prices, as in the removal of food or fuel subsidies. These subsidies are often paid for out of the budget and can be major contributors to budget deficits and inflation, or they can come from scarce tax revenues that might be better spent on schools, roads, or health clinics. However, removing such subsidies can create enormous political pressure because consumers immediately see the costs but not always the benefits. Removal of a food or fuel subsidy frequently triggers rioting that can topple governments.

Thus there is often stiff resistance to structural adjustment reforms designed to correct price distortions, either because they hurt powerful and well-connected people or because they affect many consumers. In central and eastern Europe and in Russia and China, most state enterprises saw themselves as beneficiaries of state price controls because it meant that they received key inputs at artificially low prices. To get around the resistance of large state enterprises, China created a dual price system in the 1980s by which steel going to a large enterprise in accordance with the annual plan was charged a low state-set price and all other steel was sold on the market at much higher market-determined prices. This dual system overcame much of the political resistance to price reform, but it also created opportunities for corruption by those who could use their influence to buy at the low state price and quickly resell at the high market price, corruption that contributed to the discontent that fueled the demonstrations on Tiananmen Square in 1989. Many of the other social-ist and former socialist countries, from Russia to Vietnam, therefore, opted for elimi-nating state-set prices altogether and using one market-determined price for most goods and services. By the latter half of the 1990s, China had largely eliminated the two-price system in favor of a unified market-price system. The gradual elimination of the dual price system resulted in part from deliberate decisions by the Chinese government to reduce the quantity of goods sold at low state-set prices. For the most part, however, the state-set prices disappeared because producers increasingly were unwilling to sell their goods at below market prices, and they found numerous ways to circumvent government instructions requiring them to do so.

There were many other elements to most structural adjustment programs, and over time what started as an ad hoc country-by-country approach gradually evolved into a comprehensive view of what successful development involved. In later years this came to be known as the Washington Consensus, but a comprehensive view of what was wrong began to appear well before that term was coined. In 1981, for example, the World Bank published an influential report, *Accelerated Development in Sub-Saharan Africa: An Agenda for Action*, better known as the Berg Report after its principal author, economist Eliot Berg. It presented a wide range of policy changes that would be needed if Africa were to reach its potential growth. The report focused heavily on agriculture because that is where most people lived and worked. The Berg Report called for an end to overvalued exchange rates then common in Africa, and an elimination of trade restrictions that favored inefficient industries over effi-cient farms. The expanding role of the state in managing the economy, particularly the role of state marketing boards as substitutes for private marketing mechanisms, came in for criticism. These marketing boards, such as the Ghana Cocoa Board, often extracted high taxes from farmers by setting output prices far below the true export price for the commodity. There also were recommendations for better debt and aid management and more emphasis on improving human resources through education and health measures. Similar reports followed in subsequent years but through the 1980s African development remained sluggish.

It was a seminal essay by economist John Williamson, however, that laid out clearly the view of what the international and bilateral aid agencies thought was the core set of problems that countries needed to face if they were to accelerate their development. This growing strong agreement among the International Monetary Fund (IMF), the World Bank, the U.S. government, and other key international actors focused on the steps that were necessary for Latin American countries to reform their economies, but the implications went beyond Latin America. Williamson was the first to label this broadly agreed reform agenda *the Washington Consensus*.[16] Williamson's

---

[16]The original article is John Williamson, "What Washington Means by Policy Reform" in Williamson, ed., *Latin American Readjustment: How Much Has Happened* (Washington, DC: Institute for International Economics, 1989).

purpose was to identify "the lowest common denominator" of policy advice prevailing at the time. In so doing, he highlighted how these policies differed from the conventional wisdom that had prevailed 20 years before. The 10 components of Williamson's Washington Consensus are as follows.

- *Fiscal discipline.* Balanced government budgets are essential to avoid inflation, balance of payments deficits, and capital flight. Government budget deficits of more than 1 or 2 percent of GDP are considered to be excessive and evidence of policy failure.
- *Reordering public expenditure priorities.* Expenditures on subsidies of various kinds (gasoline, food, and many other products) and politically sensitive areas, including the military, should be cut back and instead should be concentrated on education, health, key infrastructure, and maintaining essential public administration (but cutting back on bloated bureaucracies).
- *Tax reform.* To alleviate budget deficits, improve incentives, and achieve equity, reforms call for modest marginal tax rates and a broadening of the tax base.
- *Liberalization of interest rates.* Market forces should determine interest rates and the allocation of credit. Interest rates need to be positive in real terms— that is, the nominal interest rate should be higher than the rate of inflation.
- *Competitive exchange rates.* The exchange rate also should be determined by market forces and at a level that maintains a balance-of-payments equilibrium and, in particular, facilitates the expansion of exports.
- *Trade liberalization.* Elimination of quantitative restrictions (import quotas and import licensing) and a move toward uniform and low tariffs on imported goods. Such measures, in part, would encourage domestic firms to sell to foreign markets rather than focus on protected domestic ones.
- *Liberalization of foreign direct investment.* Restrictions on foreign direct investment should be removed so as to facilitate the inflow of needed capital, skills, and know-how.
- *Privatization.* Public enterprises should be privatized, to both relieve pressures on the government budget (from subsidies to loss-making public enterprises) and promote greater efficiency. This reflected the prevailing view that private firms generally are more efficient than those in the public sector.
- *Deregulation.* The primary vehicle for promoting competition within the domestic economy is to greatly reduce or eliminate government regulation, especially those that limit the entry and exit of firms. However, regulations that ensure safety, environmental protection, and the supervision of the banking sector remain justified.
- *Secure property rights.* Private property rights matter and steps should be taken to strengthen these rights, including providing them at reasonable cost to the small-scale, informal sector.

The common thread of all of these recommendations was that growth was being inhibited by major distortions in the market, distortions for the most part introduced by inappropriate government policies. Removing these distortions was seen as the key to accelerating growth. Government failure, more so than market failure, was viewed as the primary impediment to economic growth and development.

Williamson's original essay was written at the end of what was referred to above as the *lost decade* for economic growth and development in Latin America. The paper was meant both as a *description* of the policy reforms recommended to Latin American economies and a *prescription* for reforms needed in the region. This package of reforms, or close variants of it, which advocated prudent macroeconomic policies, greater outward orientation, and increased reliance on free markets, was also applied outside of Latin America. After the fall of the Berlin Wall in 1989, a large group of transition economies emerged, and they were encouraged to pursue similar policies. Sub-Saharan Africa, which had been stuck in its own growth crisis, also was urged to follow this same approach. When financial crises reemerged, first in Mexico in 1994, then in East Asia in 1997, followed soon thereafter by crises in Russia, Brazil, Turkey, and Argentina, elements of the Washington Consensus were applied to these situations, even though the underlying reasons for financial crises (see Chapters 12 and 13) were often different from a failure to achieve sustained economic growth.

The 1980s and 1990s witnessed a significant shift toward the reform agenda captured by the Washington Consensus. The pendulum swung away from state planning toward the market. Fiscal discipline became more widespread, with budgets moving in the direction of greater balance; hyperinflation, which especially had plagued Latin America, became less common; exchange rates worldwide became less overvalued, with black market premiums tending to fall if not disappear entirely; financial repression (by which nominal interest rates are held below the rate of price inflation, with governments allocating scarce credit to favored firms) fell out of favor; produce marketing boards were disbanded and other forms of direct price control dismantled; trade barriers were reduced; and privatization of state-owned enterprises proceeded on all continents.[17]

SOVIET COMMAND MODEL TO MARKET ECONOMIES: THE GREAT TRANSITION

As the Latin American economies were beginning to pull out of the debt crisis of the 1980s and were moving in the direction of the Washington Consensus, one of the

---

[17]In Latin America, fiscal discipline reduced the average budget deficit from 5 percent of GDP to about 2 percent—and lowered public external debt from about 50 percent of GDP to less than 20 percent. Trade liberalization brought average tariffs down from more than 40 percent to nearly 10 percent. . . . Banks, power plants, telecommunication systems, and even roads and water and health services were sold off to the private sector. More than 800 public enterprises were privatized between 1988 and 1997. Nancy Birdsall and Augusto de la Torre, *Washington Contentious: Economic Policies for Social Equity in Latin America* (Washington, DC: Carnegie Endowment for International Peace, 2001).

major events of the late twentieth century was occurring in Eastern Europe. Under the leadership of Mikhail Gorbachev of the Soviet Union, the countries in Eastern Europe were freed up to go their own way. In rapid succession beginning in 1989, the wall separating East Germany from West Germany was torn down and throughout the countries of Eastern Europe, the ruling authoritarian communist parties were replaced by multiparty parliamentary systems. Soon thereafter, the Soviet Union itself collapsed and was broken up into 15 separate and independent countries.

For the countries of central and eastern Europe that had been independent before World War II and in the newly independent three Baltic states, the economic goal of the new governments was clear—they wanted to become as much like western Europe as possible, and that included the rapid replacement of Soviet-style central planning and administrative allocation of most industrial products with a market economy. In Russia there was more division of opinion, but there too under President Boris Yeltsin the country set out to transform itself into a market economy as well as a more democratic polity.

The question in all of these transition economies was how to carry out this transformation. Should the transition be carried out across the board in one dramatic leap, as many foreign and domestic economists were advising? Or should the process be gradual? What exactly did the transition to a market economy involve? Some of these economies had allowed the market to exist alongside the command economy, notably in agriculture and in the distribution of many consumer products, but now the challenge was how to introduce market forces into the economy as a whole. Introducing a market system into an economy governed primarily through nonmarket mechanisms is not the same as removing distortions in an existing market system, but that difference was not well understood at the time. In a distorted market system, the institutions needed for a market system to function are often in place but are being distorted by government interference—for example, in the setting of prices. In a command economy in which most goods are distributed through government bureaucracies and not through markets, many of the institutions needed for a well-functioning market system do not exist.

There are five key elements required for a market to function well:

1. *There must be a reasonable degree of macroeconomic stability.* High inflation, large balance of payments deficits, and large-scale unemployment are generally not consistent with a well-functioning market economy.
2. *Most goods and services must be distributed through the market.* This seems obvious, but remember that the Soviet-type economy mostly distributed goods and services using administrative means implemented by large government bureaucracies. Even in Western economies during wartime, it is typical for a large part of distribution to be handled by government officials rather than by the market. Commanders in the field do not buy their weapons on the market—the weapons are allocated to them by a government bureaucracy, such as a defense ministry. For goods to be distributed on the market, a

market must exist. In the case of simple markets (for example, a farmer selling an egg to a consumer), markets can spring up overnight. More complicated markets, however, require institutions that often do not exist. Stock markets and futures markets, for example, operate in accordance with an elaborate set of rules that define what kinds of activities are allowed and what kinds are not allowed. Even the sale of automobiles typically requires a distribution network of dealers who not only sell the car but also service it. Because automobiles are expensive relative to the income of the typical consumer, there must also be a mechanism set up to help finance the purchase of the auto.

3. If the goods are going to go to their most efficient uses, *prices must be freed up to reflect the relative scarcities in the economy.* Prices are the signals that guide producers on what to produce and consumers on what best to consume. The wrong prices send the goods to the wrong (less efficient) uses.

4. *There must be competition in the markets.* Monopoly power distorts prices and hence distorts the signals sent by prices to producers and consumers. A mechanism thus needs to be in place that prevents producers from colluding with each other to establish monopoly control of particular markets.

5. Getting prices right in part through competition, however, is only half of the battle. If goods and services are to be directed to their most efficient uses, producers must respond to these prices in the appropriate way—they must behave in accordance with the rules of the market, which in their most basic form say that *producers should attempt to maximize profits.* Furthermore they need to maximize profits by increasing their sales or cutting their costs, not by getting larger subsidies through their connections with government.

The standard advice of economists involved in the Eastern European and Russian transitions was similar in many key respects to the program of the Washington Consensus, and it dealt with many key aspects of what a well-functioning market requires but not all. These economic advisers typically recommended that governments should eliminate high levels of inflation and restructure the international debts that had built up because of long periods with balance of payments deficits. Assuming that as background, or going ahead even if the macro situation was not under control, the remaining steps were to have all or most goods and services sold on a market and prices freed up to find their appropriate level. The final step was to privatize as much of the economy as possible so that producers would thus focus on the maximization of profit. All of these steps were to be taken as quickly as possible, preferably all at once in a year or two.

Not all of the countries involved in this transition process followed this advice closely, but many did. The result in almost all cases was a catastrophic drop in GDP and a rise in unemployment. The transition economies fell into an economic depression that lasted for years. What went wrong? Were the recommendations about how to make the transition from a state managed economy to a market economy wrong or did the transition uncover problems in several of these economies that had been hidden from view? The answer involves some of both.

The Soviet Union and several Eastern European countries had industries whose products were no longer as much in demand as in the past. The end of the cold war, for example, meant that the demand for military products fell off sharply in both Eastern Europe and the former states of the Soviet Union. Many other products had enjoyed captive markets through the trading system developed by the Soviet Bloc. The quality of many of those goods was too low to compete with similar products from Western Europe and other market economies, and it would take considerable time and learning to upgrade them to a competitive level. Many enterprises simply could not accomplish the necessary upgrading, and they lost their markets as consumers in the former Soviet Bloc switched to higher quality goods that were available from elsewhere if one had the necessary foreign exchange to pay for them.

But the model of how to make the transition to a market economy was itself seriously flawed in two ways. One was the view that everything had to be done together and rapidly more or less at the same time, the so-called big bang or shock therapy approach to reform. It was easy enough quickly to free up the prices of many products. It was also plausible to try to get inflation under control quickly. Bringing down inflation gradually from say 1,000 percent the first year to 500 percent the next, 200 percent the next, and so on seldom makes sense. The anti-inflationary effort is much more likely to be credible and sustaining if the money supply is brought down sharply to a level compatible with price stability in a matter of weeks or months.

What does not make sense is the view that one can change the behavior of the management of a large industrial sector over night simply by privatizing the industries involved. Most of the enterprises in the Soviet Union and Eastern Europe were run by managers who had learned to manage in the context of the Soviet command economy. They knew little about markets or how one organized a company to meet market demand. The concept of marketing as something that could be taught in business schools was unknown to most of these people. They produced what the plan told them to produce, and another bureaucracy delivered the end product to its user. Privatization could be a first step toward changing the behavior of these managers, but there were many other steps required to obtain the necessary knowledge and skills, and those took time.[18]

It is also the case that markets that did not exist in the past do not necessarily spring up quickly. This is particularly true for financial markets such as stock markets for which elaborate rules to guide and control transactions on the stock exchange need to be devised and enforcement mechanisms need to be introduced. But it also applies to less complex markets. In the early stages of the reforms in eastern Europe, the rush

---

[18]Privatization of state-owned enterprises was done for political and economic reasons. Privatization was seen by many reformers as a way of breaking the power of the existing political system in which senior government and party officials were closely allied with state enterprise managers.

to change sometimes led to the abolition of the existing state-run purchasing and distribution system (for grain in one case) before an alternative system was in place.

In terms of the five criteria needed for a functioning market economy, the reforms advocated by those reflecting an approach similar to that of the Washington Consensus were on target with respect to items 1 (control of macro imbalances), 3 (freeing up prices), and 4 (promoting market competition), but were less than adequate with respect to 2 (creating the institutions needed for well functioning markets) and fell far short of what was required with respect to item 5 (changing the incentives and hence the behavior of plant managers in an appropriate way).

While Latin America was recovering from its lost decade, and the countries of eastern Europe and the former Soviet Union were undergoing their radical transformation, at the other end of the Eurasian continent a similar and equally radical economic transition was already under way, only this one by any reasonable measure was a success. China began its reform effort in late 1978 with decisions to open up its economy to foreign trade and foreign direct investment and to return the management of agricultural production back to the household where before it had been managed by production teams of 20 to 30 households working together collectively. China did not begin these reforms with a complete well thought out theory or view about how reform should proceed. What China's leaders did know was that the previous system had worked badly and they wanted a system that would make China wealthy and powerful in as short a time as possible. The reforms in agriculture were followed in 1984 by replacing allocation of products by the administration with allocation through markets at market prices. That led to a boom in what was called township and village industries. By the 1990s the legal and incentive environment for foreign investors had improved to a point where foreign companies were investing more than $50 billion a year in China—a figure that would more than double by 2010. GDP growth continued at over 9 percent per year for three decades, and China was well on its way to transforming a poor rural economy into a middle-income urban and industrial economy.

China, therefore, demonstrated that a sustained high growth rate was possible if one opened up the economy to the outside world, promoted the export of manufactures, and introduced competitive market forces into most transactions. For simpler markets and production, China made some of these changes rapidly, but when large enterprises had to be transformed from creatures of central planning into internationally competitive market-oriented firms, change was very gradual. Further, China still lacks, for example, many of the institutions needed for a Western-style market economy and a legal system capable of settling major economic disputes without political interference. The more complex the institutions required, the longer it takes to introduce them and make them function properly.

Beginning in 1986 and accelerating after 1989, Vietnam followed a reform path similar to that of China. This demonstrated, among other things, that the success of China's step-by-step approach was not a fluke.

The other major country that introduced broad-based reforms designed to increase the role of market forces and free up technical and entrepreneurial energy was India. India, as pointed out earlier, had been heavily influenced by both the Soviet economic model and the British Fabian socialists' views on the importance of active regulation of the economy. The result for decades had been a slow rate of growth of GDP that raised per capita incomes by a little under 2 percent per year between 1952 and 1980 a rate similar to that of China in the same period. Modest reforms reducing regulation and freeing up markets led to some acceleration in per capita growth in the 1980s to a bit over 3 percent a year; then major reforms beginning in and after 1991 led to East Asian–style growth rates of nearly 5 percent per capita through 2010. (Total GDP grew at nearly 8 percent per year over the reform period.) Unlike China where the most rapid growth was in industry, in India the highest growth sector was in services. The reason is that industry still retained a high degree of regulation and India's political leaders had not yet made a full commitment to opening their economy. Hence, Indian manufactured exports remained far below those of the Four East Asian Tigers and particularly China, but India did achieve significant success in exporting services. India's lower level of dependence on exports, it should be noted, also reduced the impact of the 2008–10 world recession on India.

China and India thus present important examples of large economies that grew with a mixed model of state involvement, both adopting selective dimensions but neither adopting all of the Washington Consensus. Together India and China account for 37 percent of the world's population, in contrast to 16 percent for all of the high-income countries of Europe, North America, and Japan combined. Arguably their rise out of extreme poverty into middle-income status is the most significant event of the past half century.

WAS THE WASHINGTON CONSENSUS A SUCCESS OR A FAILURE?

During the first decade of the twenty-first century there has been a growing backlash against the forces of globalization, which in effect is also a backlash against many elements of the Washington Consensus. Demonstrations, often violent, have disrupted some international meetings set up to further the liberalization of international trade, for example in Seattle in 1999 and Cancun in 2003. The global recession of 2008–10 also led many economists to question the effort of the past decades to reduce sharply the amount of government regulation in the economy. All of the high-income countries introduced new regulatory measures for their financial markets, and many developing countries have pulled back from efforts to further liberalize their systems. Was the earlier effort to reduce the government regulatory role in the economy wrong? Was it wrong for all countries or for only the few that took the process too far?

The issue for developing countries as of 2010 was whether the Washington Consensus approach to development was wrong or whether it furthered their economic goals, even if it did not offer a complete solution. To begin with we note that many developing countries across the globe did make an effort to implement many of the recommended policies contained in the Washington Consensus. In Latin America in particular most countries succeeded in ending decade after decade of high rates of inflation. Exchange rates for the most part were no longer overvalued and import barriers were greatly reduced. Fiscal discipline was much improved, although this was not universal. Argentina, for example, tried to ensure stability by pegging its currency to the dollar from 1991 to 2002 in what amounted to a currency board arrangement (that is, allowing full convertibility between the peso and the dollar at a fixed rate of exchange), but the central government could not control the spending of local governments, and maintaining the currency peg became impossible.

The data in Table 5–1 compare Latin America's ability to control inflation and its rate of per capita GDP growth starting with the lost decade of the 1980s through to 2008 and the beginning of the global financial crisis and inflation. The data are for the region as a whole (including the Caribbean nations) and for several of its largest and most important countries. The rate of inflation is chosen not only because it is an important indicator in its own right of the quality of government economic management but because high rates of inflation are closely associated with government budgets that are out of control and with a wide variety of other undesirable interventions, many of which are designed to ameliorate the effects of inflation.

The data in Table 5–1 make clear what was meant by the lost decade of the 1980s. Per capita GDP growth in the region as a whole and in most of the major countries was low or negative. In per capita terms the region as a whole suffered a decline in income. The 1980s were also a period of hyperinflation, the kind of inflation in which prices change almost daily (see Chapter 12). During the 1990s, particularly during the later years, Latin America began to get control of inflation, and by the first decade of the next century the rate of annual price increase was in the single digits throughout the region.

TABLE 5-1 **Economic Growth and Inflation in Latin America**

REGION/COUNTRY	PER CAPITA GDP GROWTH (%)			INFLATION RATES (%)		
	1980–90	1991–2000	2001–08	1980–90	1991–2000	2001–08
Latin America and Caribbean	−0.4	1.6	2.3	14.6	17.5	6.1
Brazil	0.1	1.0	2.3	396.4	308.9	8.1
Mexico	0.3	1.8	1.3	60.7	16.3	7.8
Colombia	1.5	0.7	3.0	24.7	22.5	6.7
Argentina	−2.4	2.2	3.2	490.7	10.3	12.7
Venezuela	−2.4	0.0	2.7	22.1	40.1	25.0
Chile	2.5	4.8	3.1	20.9	8.5	5.7

GPD, gross domestic product.

Source: World Bank, "World Development Indicators," http://databank.worldbank.org.

Did control of inflation together with all of the other reforms introduced in the 1990s and after improve the overall performance of the economy? For the most part economic stagnation came to an end in the region as growth resumed, but the growth rates achieved were modest, particularly compared with what was happening in East and Southeast Asia and in India. The most plausible explanation for this performance was that the reforms designed to improve the functioning of markets in Latin America were necessary if higher growth was to be achieved, but were not by themselves sufficient to achieve the very high catch-up growth rates experienced in Asia in recent years. There is more to achieving a high rate of GDP growth than simply getting the prices right by removing market distortions caused by inappropriate government interventions. There is a need for new technologies appropriate to the conditions in specific countries. It is also essential to have high-quality human resources, people who are well educated and healthy. Investors also require a stable political environment. These other elements in the development equation will come up again and again in the chapters that follow. Here we simply note that the level and nature of government intervention in Latin American in the 1980s and before was excessive, and the efforts to reduce and redirect the nature of government intervention in the 1990s and during the first decade of the twenty-first century appear to have had a positive impact but not as large an impact as many of the advocates of the Washington Consensus reform program had hoped for.

It is also the case that market-oriented reforms in Latin America did little to improve the highly unequal distribution of income that characterizes many of the countries in the region. This in turn is part of the reason for the reaction in the first decade of the twenty-first century that brought many leftist governments to power. Some of these governments, notably Brazil, retained market oriented reforms while making a greater effort to improve social welfare initiatives. Others, notably Venezuela, reverted to earlier approaches that used high oil prices to increase subsidies to political supporters, an approach that has generally proved to be unsustainable once oil prices fall.

Any attempt to assess the impact of market reforms on development in Africa is even more complex than for Latin America. Many countries in sub-Saharan Africa during the turn of the century did make a major effort to remove distortions in markets caused by inappropriate government intervention. Overvalued exchange rates were devalued, and the role of government marketing organizations was reduced. Trade restrictions were also cut back in much of the region. But sub-Saharan Africa is made up of 47 countries, some of which have made a major effort to reform, while others are mired in civil war or rampant corruption. To understand the impact of market-oriented reforms, therefore, one needs to separate out the countries that have made a major reform effort from those that have not. A recent study by Steven Radelet has done precisely that, dividing the countries in sub-Saharan Africa into three groups: emerging nations that have made major reforms and have enjoyed sustained increases in per capita income, oil-exporting countries whose income has

TABLE 5-2 Emerging African Countries and Growth in Average Incomes, 1996–2008

EMERGING COUNTRIES	ANNUAL PER CAPITA INCOME GROWTH (%)	CUMULATIVE INCREASE IN AVERAGE REAL INCOME (%)
Botswana	4.1	68
Burkina Faso	2.8	43
Cape Verde	4.0	67
Ethiopia	4.1	65
Ghana	2.6	40
Lesotho	2.3	33
Mali	2.5	37
Mauritius	3.7	61
Mozambique	5.3	96
Namibia	2.4	36
Rwanda	3.7	60
São Tomé and Principe	5.0	40
Seychelles	2.5	37
South Africa	2.0	29
Tanzania	3.0	46
Uganda	3.8	61
Zambia	1.8[*]	25
Average	3.2	50

[*]We include Zambia even through its 13-year growth rate is slightly lower than 2 percent because its annual average growth rate for the 10-year period was 2.3 percent.

Source: Steven Radelet, *Emerging Africa: How 17 Countries Are Leading the Way* (Washington, DC: Center for Global Development, 2010).

tended to fluctuate with the ups and downs of petroleum prices, and the others that have not made much of a reform effort and/or are mired in civil war. He identifies 17 emerging African countries that have carried out substantial reforms and have achieved sustained per capita growth since 1996 (Table 5–2).

These reforming or emerging African economies have lowered tariff rates, eliminated overvalued exchange rates, and in a variety of other ways improved the climate for private businesses more than in the countries in Africa that did not perform as well (Table 5–3). Among the countries that had generally not done as well were the oil exporters that took in large amounts of foreign exchange from oil revenues; African governments typically could not manage the funds efficiently or without large-scale corruption. The poorest performers included countries wracked by civil war (notably the Congo) or those that were badly managed by an oligarchy willing to do almost anything to hold on to power (for example, Zimbabwe).

As in the case of Latin America, market-oriented reforms in parts of Africa did not eliminate all of the barriers to high growth in the region. The growth rates achieved by the emerging African countries were far below the per capita GDP growth rates achieved in Asia. But the growth rates in the 17 emerging African countries were also

TABLE 5-3 Average Rank in Doing Business of Sub-Sahara African (SSA) Countries out of 181 Countries Worldwide, 2009

INDICATOR*	EMERGING SSA	OTHER SSA	LOW INCOME (WORLDWIDE)
Total ease of doing business	108	158	141
Starting a business	97	146	118
Dealing with construction permits	109	121	124
Employing workers	100	132	114
Registering property	113	129	118
Getting credit	100	135	123
Protecting investors	87	131	115
Paying taxes	85	128	120
Trading across borders	128	139	141
Enforcing contracts	92	134	113
Closing a business	108	140	135

*The lower the ranking, the greater the ease of doing business.

Source: Steven Radelet, *Emerging Africa: How 17 Countries Are Leading the Way* (Washington, DC: Center for Global Development, 2010).

far above what those countries had achieved in the past before 1996 and were also significantly above what other sub-Saharan African countries were achieving after 1996.

What then can one conclude about the appropriate mix of market influences and the role of government intervention? Was the Washington Consensus approach and its variant dealing with reform of former Soviet-type economies the right answer? Or was that approach far off the mark? Economists and others continue to actively debate this question. Discussions of a post–Washington Consensus have tended to moderate the original's exclusive focus on market liberalization, highlighting instead the role of good governance and strong institutions as pillars of development.[19]

The first conclusion that can be derived from an overview of the actual experience of developing countries is that there was considerable variation in the degree to which these countries, including the most reform minded among them, applied the policies recommended by the Washington Consensus. China and Vietnam, for example, did not carry out privatization of most of their state-owned enterprises. Other countries retained restrictions on imports, and the Four East Asian Tigers model that inspired many reform efforts actually retained tight restrictions on imports during the first three decades of rapid growth. While few if any of the countries that attempted to implement market-oriented reforms carried out all of them, virtually all of the more successful countries, whether in Asia, Latin America, or sub-Saharan Africa, did make significant moves in the direction of reduced government intervention and greater

[19]A good review of these debates as seen by one analyst is Derek Heady, "Appraising a post-Washington Paradigm: What Professor Rodrik Means by Policy Reform," *Review of International Political Economy* 16, no. 4 (2009), 698–728.

reliance on market forces. No country, however, had to move all the way to a perfect market economy to achieve positive results.

When it comes to the question of what is the appropriate level and nature of government intervention in the economy of a developing country, there is no one-size-fits-all formula. The governments of some countries such as South Korea and Taiwan have actively promoted particular industries using a variety of subsidies and other interventions and have done so successfully, at least in the early stages of their accelerated growth period. Governments elsewhere, Indonesia in the 1990s, for example, pursued government-led industrial policies that put increasing emphasis on large state-supported import substituting industrial projects with disastrous results. Yet, Indonesia before the 1990s had done well as a result of policies that had steadily reduced the regulation of trade and industry and had created an environment conducive to the export of labor-intensive products. Governments in most developing countries have played a dominant role in the provision of infrastructure (roads, railroads, electric power, and so on), and some have carried out these large capital investments with comparative efficiency, while in others the process has been riddled with corruption and waste.

The point here is that some governments in developing countries are capable of carrying out a relatively efficient interventionist industrial and infrastructure development policy, but other countries lack this ability. The terms sometimes used to describe these two kinds of governments are **hard governments**, which can intervene actively in a way that promotes growth, and **soft governments**, which are not able to do so. Hard governments can carry out Korean-style interventionist policies with success; soft governments can also achieve successful development but must rely as much as possible on market forces to guide the effort. Being hard or soft is not something that is a permanent condition for the government of a particular country. Governments can move from being unable to set priorities and stick to them when implementing a development program to being able to do so and vice versa. What makes some governments hard and others soft at a point in time takes one back to the underlying conditions prevailing in particular countries—the nature of their colonial experience, their culture and politics, their natural resources, and much else. These topics go far beyond what can be covered in this book. Hard or soft, however, as economies become more advanced and sophisticated intervention becomes more and more difficult, market forces need to play a larger and larger role. Government intervention should be carefully targeted toward areas in which market guidance alone is clearly insufficient (the financial sector, environmental controls, and amelioration of extreme poverty are three important areas).

A second conclusion is that market-oriented reforms do not require that everything be done at once and as quickly as possible. Reform can be achieved step by step over a substantial period of time—the big bang or shock therapy approach was not necessary, and in most cases was probably not feasible or even desirable. Finally, making greater use of market forces and reducing the role of government intervention in the economy is not a magic bullet that solves all of the problems of development. A highly interventionist approach by which government actions are driven as much by politics and rent seeking or corruption can slow or even stop growth, but reliance on market forces by itself does not guarantee high economic growth rates. A large degree of reliance on market forces is generally helpful to development, but there is much more to the development process, as the chapters that follow make clear.

SUMMARY

- The respective roles of states and markets in shaping economic development have been a central focus of debate since the time of Adam Smith. This debate took on new urgency in the period after World War II, when today's developing countries began to emerge from colonial rule.
- Early postwar development thinking focused on the accumulation of capital as the key to economic growth. This idea was formalized in early growth models, such as Harrod-Domar; yet, the intellectual origins of the focus on capital accumulation arose from such divergent sources as David Ricardo and Karl Marx.
- The experience of rebuilding western Europe after the war bolstered the capital-oriented view of development, but early analysts failed to note the important role played by supporting institutions that had long existed on the Continent.
- The experience of the Great Depression and massive market failure before World War II contributed to widespread skepticism among economists and policy makers in both emerging industrialized countries and developing countries about the ability of markets to guide development. The perceived early success of the Soviet growth model that rejected reliance on market forces in favor of an economy run almost entirely by large state bureaucracies also influenced developing country thinking, particularly in China and India.
- Market skepticism extended to international trade as well, leading many countries to turn inward and erect trade barriers to protect their domestic economies from what appeared to be unreliable international market forces. This import substituting approach to development was particularly prevalent in South America, where early industrialization had begun in the first half of the twentieth century, when two world wars and the Great Depression made export-oriented industrial growth virtually impossible; but industry began to stagnate as small domestic markets became saturated.

- By the late 1970s, poor economic performance in many developing countries following government-led models of development and import substitution, together with the rising debt burden of many Latin American countries, led to a broad questioning of that approach and a reexamination of the potential benefits of markets and trade for development. At the same time, economists and policy makers were becoming more aware of alternative and successful growth models being pursued in East Asia. These models stressed the export of manufactures as central to growth and limited import substituting protection to the first few years when a new industry was learning how to compete. The role of government in these successful countries, however, varied considerably from the highly interventionist model of South Korea, Taiwan, and Japan to the almost laissez faire model of Hong Kong.

- By the 1980s and early 1990s, the perceived development failures in the developing world outside of East Asia had led the major international development agencies and the U.S. government, among others, to be advocates of a development model that came to be known as the Washington Consensus. This model called for developing countries to practice fiscal discipline and rely for the most part on market forces to guide the economy. Foreign assistance and debt relief was often made conditional on a country implementing the components of this consensus.

- The Washington Consensus was first promoted in sub-Saharan Africa, even before the term was coined, but it was later central to international efforts to help Latin America recover from the lost decade caused by the debt crisis of the 1980s. This same set of policy prescriptions was then advocated for and to some degree implemented by the states of Eastern Europe and the former Soviet Union as they rejected the Soviet-style command economy in favor of market forces. The economic performance of the countries that adopted many or even most of the policies called for by the Washington Consensus, however, was often disappointing.

- While much of the international aid effort was focused on implementing the goals of the Washington Consensus, China, beginning in 1978, was implementing a model that had some of the components of that consensus but lacked many others. China moved step by step toward a model that relied increasingly on markets but with a high degree of state intervention and continued state ownership of many of the larger enterprises. By 2011, that model had produced decades of high, near double-digit growth.

- India and Vietnam by the 1990s were also moving away from the extreme levels of government intervention in the economy that characterized their earlier development strategies, but like China they implemented only some of the components of the Washington Consensus. Like China, they began to grow very rapidly throughout the 1990s and the first decade of the twenty-first century.

- Was the Washington Consensus a failure? There is no question that it oversimplified what was required to achieve sustained economic development. Not all of the elements in the consensus were necessary in all developing countries, and certain key elements, notably the quality of governance, were largely absent from the consensus. Nevertheless, when one looks at the performance of nations in Africa and Latin America, it is the countries that implemented much of what was called for by the consensus that have performed better than those that did not do so.

PART TWO

Distribution
and Human Resources

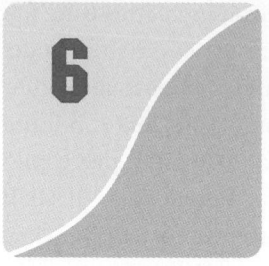

Inequality and Poverty

Bangladesh is one of the world's most heavily populated low-income nations. In 2010, per capita income among Bangladesh's 164 million people was $1,486 (US$, PPP). On a daily basis, this amounts to a bit more than $4 per person per day, which would permit a meager standard of living at best. But $4 per day refers only to the average, the income level that would prevail if all of GDP was available for consumption and then was divided equally among the entire population, which, of course, it is not. What income level is earned by those who fall below the average? How much do the poorest Bangladeshis depend on for their survival? Evidence from the World Bank suggests that 50 percent of Bangladeshis survive on $1.25 a day or less, the standard international definition for absolute poverty.[1]

The most recent estimates for global poverty are for 2005, although projections have been made for more recent years. In 2005, 1.4 billion people, or more than one out of every five people, were estimated to live below the $1.25 a day poverty line; 2.6 billion people, about half the population of the developing world in 2005, survived on less than $2 a day. For most readers of this book, who are enrolled in a college or

---

[1]The World Bank's international poverty line originally referred to $1 a day, in 1985 US$ (PPP). It has been revised several times. The most recent estimates identify two poverty lines: $1.25 a day in 2005 US$ (PPP) is the mean of the national poverty lines for 15 of the world's poorest countries and is considered a measure of extreme poverty; $2.00 a day is the mean national poverty line among all developing countries. The selection of these poverty lines is discussed in more detail later in the chapter. Global poverty estimates refer to 2005 and are from S. Chen and M. Ravallion, "The Developing World Is Poorer Than We Thought, but No Less Successful in the Fight Against Poverty," *Quarterly Journal of Economics* 125, no. 4 (2010). Estimates for Bangladesh and other countries referred to in this chapter are from World Bank, "World Development Indicators," http://databank.worldbank.org unless otherwise indicated.

university, the idea of living on $1 to $2 a day is close to inconceivable. But these are the circumstances facing tens of millions of Bangladeshis and billions of people worldwide.

The major explanation for the degree of absolute poverty in Bangladesh and other low income nations is the low level of total production per capita. But this is not the only factor. Mexico is an upper-middle-income nation with a 2010 GDP per capita income of US$15,224 (PPP), more than 10 times the level in Bangladesh. If GDP were distributed equally in Mexico, each Mexican would have about $42 per day. But income is not equally shared in Mexico, or in Bangladesh, or for that matter, in any other country. The richest 20 percent of Mexicans receive over 50 percent of total household income, almost *15 times* as much as the poorest 20 percent who receive only 3.5 percent of total income. The distribution of income in Mexico results in over 3.5 million Mexicans (about 3.4 percent of the population in 2008) living below the $1.25 a day poverty line and 8.1 percent living below $2 a day.

Raising people out of poverty requires economic growth. Increases in GDP per capita typically benefit those below the poverty line as well as those who live near or considerably above it. Without sustained economic growth, the most Bangladesh could achieve is the low level of income that $4 a day permits. But the distribution of national income plays a vital role, too. Inequality affects the amount of poverty generated by a given level of income. It may affect growth just as growth may affect levels of inequality, and inequality *itself* is something people care about, independent of its effects on poverty and growth.

If both economic growth and distribution affect poverty levels, what does this suggest about policy? Toward the end of this chapter, we consider potential elements of a pro-poor development strategy. These elements include encouraging more rapid economic growth, improving opportunities for the poor via investments in basic education and healthcare, and designing social safety nets and other programs for especially vulnerable groups.

MEASURING INEQUALITY

Economists often are interested in the distribution of *income* among households within a nation. But these are not the only dimensions of inequality we might want to investigate. Instead of income, development economists often look at the distribution of household *consumption*, usually measured by household expenditures, whether in-kind or in money terms. In poor countries income can be hard to measure, especially for subsistence farm households who consume rather than market most of what they produce. Consumption also may be a more reliable indicator of welfare than is income, in part because consumption tends not to fluctuate as much as income from one period to the next.

One might also be interested in the distribution of *wealth,* which always is more unequal than the distribution of either income or consumption. Distributions of assets, whether of land or education, are useful in understanding the opportunities individuals have to be productive and generate household income. The distribution of income depends on ownership of factors of production (including the value of the labor services that one "owns") and the role each factor plays in the production process. Ownership of land and capital often is highly concentrated, so anything that enhances the relative returns to these factors makes the distribution of income more unequal. Conversely, relatively higher wages for unskilled labor, the most widely distributed factor of production in developing nations, tend to lead to a more equal distribution.

In addition to deciding whether to look at the distribution of income, consumption, or wealth *within* one nation, one might want to look at how each is distributed *among* nations. We assess the level of global inequality at the end of the chapter. One can also look within the household at patterns of intrahousehold inequality, which are critical for understanding gender issues and the welfare of children.

No matter what dimension of distribution one is interested in, one needs a set of analytical tools for describing and understanding distributional outcomes. The simplest way of depicting any distribution is to display its **frequency distribution**, which tells us how many (or what percent of) families or individuals receive different amounts of income. Figure 6–1a presents the frequency distribution of household consumption per capita for Bangladesh. This distribution is based on a survey of about 7,000 Bangladeshi families, selected to represent the over 24 million households in Bangladesh. Surveyed households responded to detailed questionnaires about their sources of income and consumption of a wide variety of goods. Researchers used this information to derive an estimate of each household's per capita consumption.

Figure 6–1a tells us the percentage of individuals with different levels of annual consumption starting from the lowest reported level and rising in increments of 650 taka, the Bangladeshi currency. Almost 1 million people, less than 1 percent of Bangladesh's population, reported the lowest annual consumption expenditures in the survey, under 3,250 taka per year (less than $270, PPP); 8.4 percent (the highest bar in the figure) had per capita consumption of between 5,850 and 6,500 taka (around $500, PPP); and less than 0.5 percent had the top amounts reported in Figure 6–1a, over 22,750 taka (almost $1,900, PPP). There are households with even higher consumption in Bangladesh, but Figure 6–1a reports the distribution for only 95 percent of individuals ranked by per capita consumption. Had the top 5 percent been included in the figure, the tail of the distribution would continue to extend much farther to the right of the diagram.[2]

---

[2]Household income and expenditures surveys, like the one for Bangladesh, often fail to capture two groups of households. Both the poorest and richest families are likely to be underrepresented. The poorest families, including those who are homeless and live in places such as railway stations or river gullies, tend not to be adequately enumerated. Similarly, the most affluent, few in number, are unlikely to be part of the statistical sample. There also is a tendency for more affluent households not to respond to such surveys or to underreport their incomes. Thus even in the best of surveys, the degree of inequality may be underestimated.

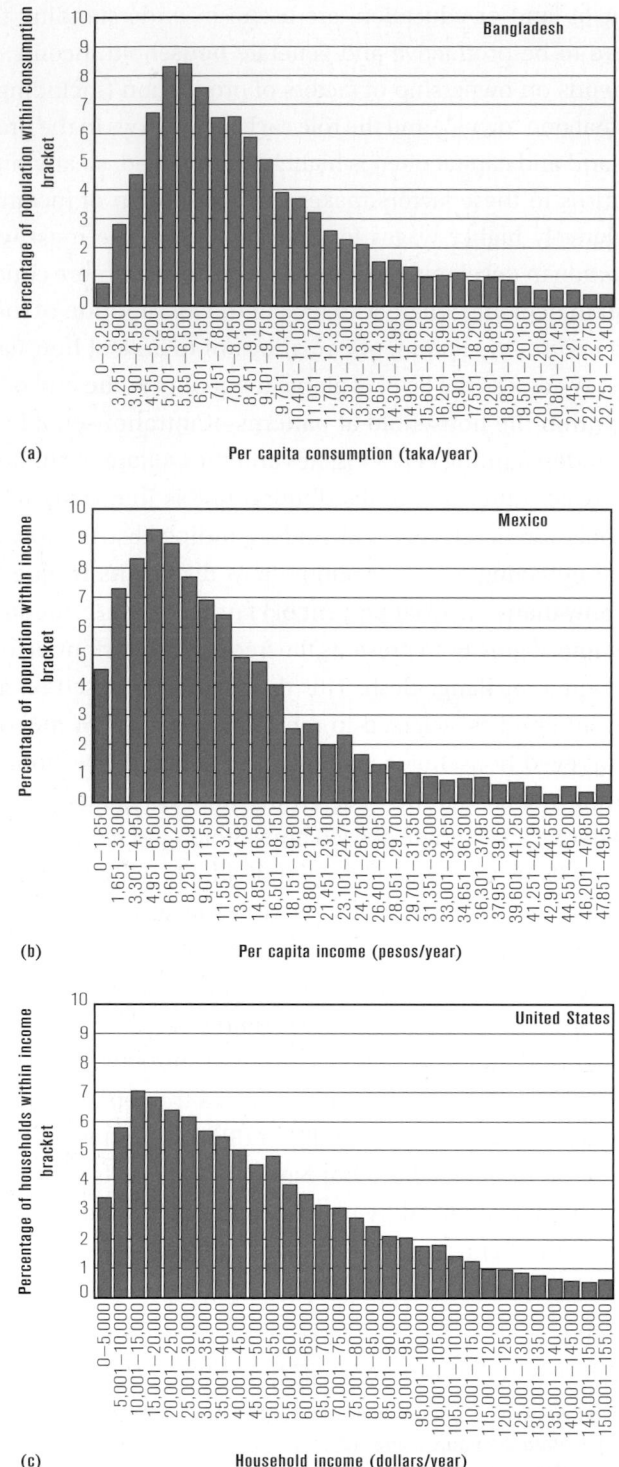

(a)

(b)

(c)

FIGURE 6-1 **The Distribution of Income: Bangladesh, Mexico, and the United States, 2000s**

Sources: Collaboration with Claudio E. Montenegro, World Bank; *U.S. Current Population Survey* (March 2004).

Take a look at the shape of the frequency distribution for Bangladesh in Figure 6-1a. The distribution is not rectangular, with every level of consumption represented by the same percentage of individuals, nor was it expected to be. The height of the bars, each bar representing a different consumption level, initially rises and then grows progressively shorter. If distributions were very equal, there would be a small number of very tall bars in the middle of the diagram, indicating that just about everyone had nearly the same level of consumption. The distribution also is not a normal distribution, the so-called bell curve, with which you may be familiar from courses in statistics. If consumption or income were distributed normally, there would be an equal number of households on either side of the mean and symmetric tails to the distribution suggesting equal percentages of the population at both low and high consumption and incomes. IQs are distributed normally, but consumption and income are not. The distribution instead is described as lognormal, meaning that if you took the logarithms of household consumption or incomes and redrew the frequency distribution it would approximate the more familiar bell curve.

The lognormal distribution captures what you already know about incomes. In virtually all societies there are a relatively small number of rich households (captured in the long, flat tail to the right) and a much larger number of lower-income families who make up "the hump" of the distribution, which is located at the lower end of the income range. This particular shape of the distribution of income is not unique to Bangladesh. Similar distributional outcomes characterize low-, middle-, and high-income economies. Figure 6–1b–c illustrate this point. These income distributions are based on micro-level household surveys for Mexico and the United States. Note that all three nations exhibit similar lognormal distributions, each with its own long, flat tail to the right.

Bangladesh, Mexico, and the United States all have similarly shaped frequency distributions, but they are not identical. This means that the degree of inequality in the three nations varies. To get a sense of the differences we need to rearrange the data contained in the frequency distributions; these distributions have complex shapes and are difficult to compare across nations or within nations over time. Calculating the **size distribution** provides an easier way of identifying the degree of inequality present in the underlying distribution.

Size distributions tell us the share of total consumption or income received by different groups of households, ranked according to their consumption or income level. One can rank households or individuals by deciles or even percentiles, but the convention is to report on quintiles, ranking households from the poorest 20 percent, to the next 20 percent, all the way to the richest 20 percent of households. In the case of Bangladesh, each quintile represents about 30 million people. Summing all individual consumption expenditures in each quintile and dividing by the country's total consumption yields each quintile's share.

Table 6–1 contains World Bank estimates of the size distribution of consumption for Bangladesh and household income for Mexico and the United States. This way of

TABLE 6-1   **Size Distributions of Consumption or Income within Quintiles in Bangladesh, Mexico, and the United States, 2000s**

| | SHARE OF TOTAL CONSUMPTION OR INCOME | | |
QUINTILE	BANGLADESH	MEXICO	UNITED STATES
Bottom 20%	9.0	3.5	3.4
Second 20%	12.5	8.2	8.7
Third 20%	16.0	13.3	14.8
Fourth 20%	21.5	21.2	23.4
Top 20%	41.0	53.7	49.8

Sources: Collaboration with Claudio E. Montenegro, World Bank; *U.S. Current Population Survey* (March 2004).

presenting the data makes it clear that, of the three nations, Bangladesh has the relatively most equal distribution because the quintile shares are closer to one another than is the case for either Mexico or the United States. (If the distribution were completely equal, each quintile would receive 20 percent of the total.) In Bangladesh, the top 20 percent receive 41 percent of total consumption, about 4.5 times the amount received by the poorest 20 percent. In Mexico and the United States, the ratio is much larger, roughly 15:1.[3] Some of these differences are due to what precisely is being measured—consumption or income and whether on a per capita or household basis—but much of the difference is due to the underlying distribution within each nation.

The size distribution provides a means for introducing some other techniques commonly used to measure inequality, including some that reduce the entire distribution to a single number. Data from the size distribution can be used to draw a **Lorenz curve** (Figure 6–2), named after Max Lorenz, a statistician. Income recipients are arrayed from lowest to highest income along the horizontal axis. The curve itself shows the share of total income received by any cumulative percentage of recipients. Its shape indicates the degree of inequality in the income distribution. By definition, the curve must touch the 45-degree line at both the lower-left corner (0 percent of recipients must receive 0 percent of income) and the upper-right corner (100 percent of recipients must receive 100 percent of income). If everyone had the same income, the Lorenz curve would lie along the 45-degree line (perfect equality). If only one household received income and all other households had none, the curve

[3]Unlike most low- and middle-income nations, the United States has a comprehensive system of taxation of household incomes and government transfer payments (such as Social Security). The data reported here are for money incomes before taxes and after cash transfer payments. Noncash transfers, such as food stamps and Medicare, are not accounted for. Once taxes and all government transfer payments are included, the distribution becomes somewhat more equal. The ratio of the shares of the top 20 to the bottom 20 falls to closer to 10:1 than the 15:1 reported in Table 6–1.

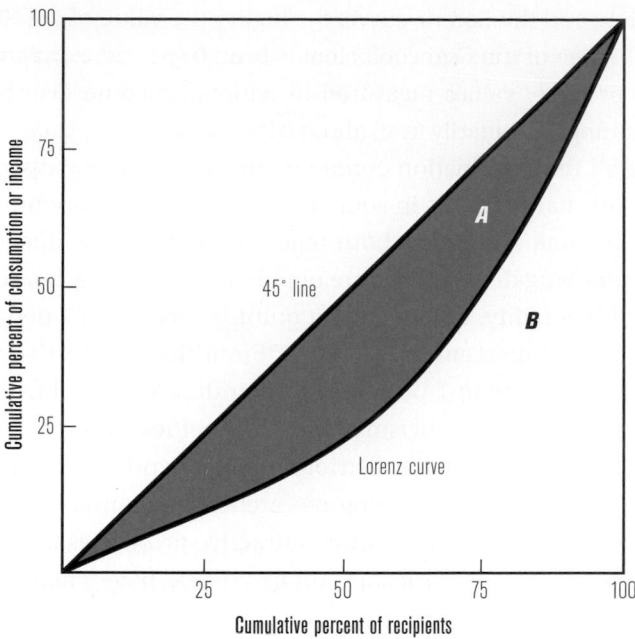

FIGURE 6-2 **Lorenz Curve**

would trace the bottom and right-hand borders of the diagram (perfect inequality). In all actual cases the Lorenz curve lies somewhere in between. The farther the Lorenz curve bends away from the 45-degree line of perfect equality (the larger the shaded area, *A*) the greater the inequality. When comparing Lorenz curves, either for the same country at different points of time or for different countries, it is possible for the separate curves to intersect. When this happens it is ambiguous if inequality has increased or decreased over time (or if one country has more inequality than the other).[4]

Single numbers can also be used to describe the distribution of income. One commonly used statistic is the ratio of the income share of the top 20 percent of households to the share received by the bottom 20 or 40 percent. The most frequently used statistic, the **Gini coefficient** (named after statistician Corrado Gini,), can be derived from the Lorenz curve. This ratio is understood most easily as the value of area *A* divided by area *A* + *B* in Figure 6-2.[5] The larger the share of the area between

[4]To see the reason for this ambiguity, draw two Lorenz curves and label the point of intersection *X*. Below point *X*, there is relatively more equality along the Lorenz curve closer to the 45-degree line; but above point *X*, there is relatively more equality along the other Lorenz curve. Because both Lorenz curves have sections of greater equality, there is no way to decide, overall, if one represents a more equal distribution than the other.

[5]The Gini coefficient can be calculated using a relatively complex formula based on the absolute income differences across all observations in a population, which are then normalized by both the size and mean income of the population.

the 45-degree line and the Lorenz curve, the higher the value of the Gini coefficient. The theoretical range of the Gini coefficient is from 0 (perfect equality) to 1 (perfect inequality). In practice, values measured in national income distributions have a much narrower range, ordinarily from about 0.25 to 0.65.

Collapsing all the information contained in the frequency distribution into a single number inevitably results in some loss of information about the underlying distribution. Argentina and Kenya both report similar Gini coefficients of around 0.48, but the underlying distributions are not identical. Both nations have considerable amounts of inequality, but the lowest quintile received 4.7 percent of income in Kenya, and only 3.6 percent in Argentina. From the perspective of the poor in these countries, a more than 1 percentage point difference in income shares is a significant amount. Another criticism of the Gini coefficient is that it is more sensitive to changes in some parts of the distribution than in others. Despite these shortcomings of the Gini, the desire among researchers to summarize inequality in a single number combined with some other attractive properties of the Gini, including its geometric interpretation using Lorenz curves, have encouraged its widespread use.[6]

PATTERNS OF INEQUALITY

Simon Kuznets, one of the early Nobel Prize winners in economics and a pioneer of empirical work on the processes of economic growth and development, was one of the first economists to investigate patterns of inequality. In his presidential address to the 1954 meeting of the American Economic Association, Kuznets reported on historical data on income shares for England, Germany, and the United States. He then introduced a few data points for the developing world: Ceylon (now Sri Lanka), India, and Puerto Rico. The data were so limited that Kuznets did not include them in a table or figure; he simply listed them in the text.[7] Some 50 years later, researchers are far less constrained. Data on inequality are available for most nations of the world, although for most countries they are updated only once or twice a decade. The quality and comparability of these data also are sometimes a concern: The World Bank, one of the primary compilers of such information, offers more than the usual caveats about data comparability across countries and over time.

Figure 6–3 presents one set of estimates of Gini coefficients of the distribution of household consumption or income for countries by region. What is immediately

[6]There are other single-number measures of inequality in addition to the Gini coefficient and top 20 to bottom 20 or 40 ratios. Discussion of the alternatives and the desirable properties of measures of inequality can be found in Gary Fields, *Distribution and Development: A New Look at the Developing World* (Cambridge: MIT Press, 2001).

[7]Simon Kuznets, "Economic Growth and Income Inequality," *American Economic Review* 45, no. 1 (1955).

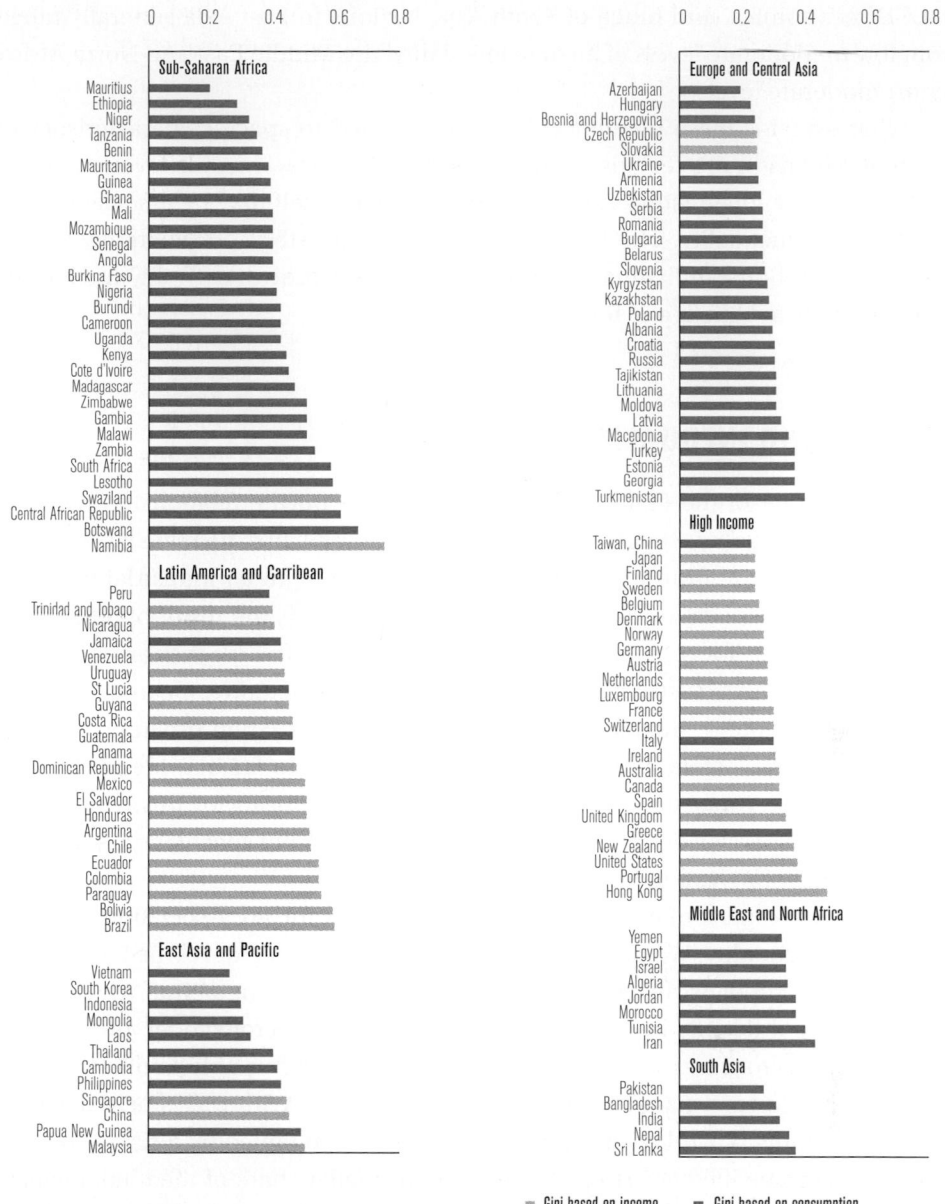

FIGURE 6-3 Gini Coeffiecients by Country and Region

Sources: Figure 2.9 from The International Bank for Reconstruction and Development. The World Bank: *World Development Report*, 2006. Reprinted with permission.

apparent is the variance in inequality both within and across regions. There is evidence of a tendency toward higher inequality, with the Gini coefficient generally above 0.40 and in some cases approaching 0.65, in Latin America and parts of Africa (especially southern Africa). Low inequality is characteristic of the transition economies of eastern Europe and central Asia, many of the high-income economies of the Organisation for Economic Co-Operation and Development

(OECD) economies, and much of South Asia. Nations in East Asia generally range from low to moderate levels of income inequality; the Middle East and North Africa report moderate levels.

What explains these differences? Are they related to specific characteristics of different regions or are regions a proxy for something else—income level, perhaps? One idea with a long history is that economic growth itself may be associated with the degree of inequality. The basic intuition is that growth is an inherently unbalanced process. Some individuals capture the benefits of growth early on, and it takes time for others to benefit and for returns to equalize.

GROWTH AND INEQUALITY

Kuznets was one of the first economists to speculate on the relationship between growth and inequality, suggesting that inequality might first increase as a nation makes the transition from a mostly agricultural economy to an industrial one. The underlying mechanism for this rise in income inequality is the result of differences in the returns to factors of production between agriculture (where they are lower and less dispersed) and industry. When everyone works in agriculture, income is distributed relatively equally, but as industrialization and urbanization progress, inequality rises. As more factors make the transition from farm to factory, inequality may then start to fall. Kuznets readily acknowledged that the basis for this relationship was "perhaps 5 percent empirical information and 95 percent speculation, some of it possibly tainted by wishful thinking."

Other economists offered alternative explanations for an association between growth and inequality. W. Arthur Lewis, a Nobel Prize winner, developed a theoretical model that predicts rising inequality followed by a "turning point," which eventually leads to a decline in inequality. Employing a two-sector model, the modern or industrial sector faces "unlimited supplies" of labor as it is able to draw workers with low or even zero marginal product from agriculture. With wages held down by the elastic supply of workers, industrial growth is accompanied by a rising share of profits. As average incomes rise, labor receives a smaller share of the total, increasing inequality. The turning point is reached when all the surplus labor has been absorbed and the supply of labor becomes more inelastic. Wages and labor's share of income then start to rise and inequality falls.[8]

In Lewis's **surplus labor model**, inequality is not just a necessary effect of economic growth; it is a cause of growth. A distribution of income that favors high-income groups contributes to growth because profit earners save to obtain funds

---

[8]W. Arthur Lewis, "Economic Development with Unlimited Supplies of Labor," *Manchester School* 22 (1954). The Lewis model is more fully developed in Chapter 16.

for expanding their enterprises. The more income they receive, the more they invest. Their saving and investment increase the economy's productive capacity and thus bring about output growth. Not only does inequality contribute to growth according to Lewis, but attempts to redistribute income prematurely run the risk that economic growth will be slowed. These were powerful conclusions. Could they be maintained in light of the empirical evidence on economic growth and inequality?

The ideas of Kuznets, Lewis, and others about growth and inequality held considerable sway among development economists for several decades. During the 1960s, a period of strong growth in many regions, some economists wondered why growth was not yielding more rapid reductions in poverty. One idea was that the relationship that came to be known as Kuznets inverted-U, or the **Kuznets curve**, might be at work. Twenty years after Kuznets's original paper, researchers were armed with more data on inequality and reexamined the relationship using primarily cross-section analyses of countries, including many developing countries. A key assumption in this approach was that nations at different levels of per capita income could approximate what individual nations might experience over time as they achieved economic growth. Studies using this approach supported the existence of the Kuznets curve.[9] The tendency for inequality to rise and then fall with rising levels of per capita income was maintained as a stylized fact about development until the late 1980s. Subsequent research has overturned this perspective.

Better and more abundant data on income inequality, especially time-series data on individual countries, coupled with more rigorous econometric methods, permitted researchers to identify patterns over time within individual nations. In India, a low-income nation with generally low-income inequality, there is evidence of some decline in inequality from 1950 until the mid-1960s, but at least into the 1990s there was no distinct trend in either direction.[10] Figure 6–4 illustrates the trend in the Gini coefficient since 1980 for Chile and Taiwan. Chile, one of Latin America's most successful economies, has been a middle-income nation throughout this period; Taiwan has gone from middle- to high-income status. Chile's Gini coefficient fluctuates minimally from year to year but exhibits no particular pattern over time, except perhaps for a recent slight downward trend. What is most apparent in Chile's case is the persistence of a relatively high level of inequality. Taiwan also exhibits little fluctuation over time. The most notable feature of Taiwan's

[9]Montek S. Ahluwalia, "Inequality, Poverty and Development," *Journal of Development Economics* 3 (1976).

[10]Michael Bruno, Martin Ravallion, and Lyn Squire, "Equity and Growth in Developing Countries: Old and New Perspectives on the Policy Issues," in Vito Tanzi and Ke-young Chu, eds., *Income Distribution and High-Quality Growth* (Cambridge: MIT Press, 1998).

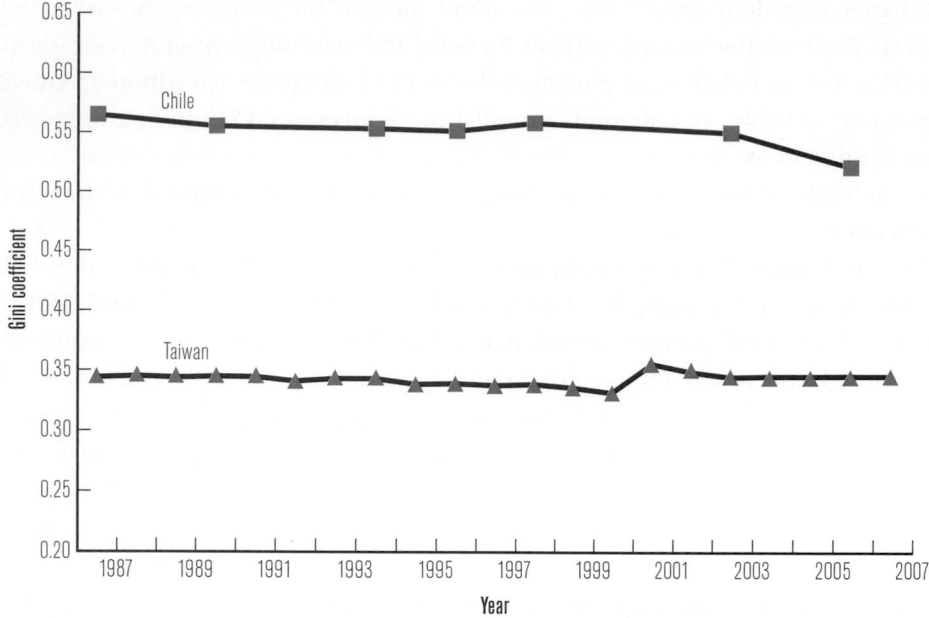

FIGURE 6-4 **Trends in Inequality: Gini Coefficients in Chile and Taiwan**

Sources: Data for Chile: World Bank, "World Development Indicators," http://databank.worldbank.org. Data for Taiwan: Statistical Bureau of the Republic of China (Taiwan), Report on the Survey of Family Income and Expenditure, "Percentage Share of Disposable Income by Percentile Groups of Income Recipients and Measures of Income Distribution," 2007, link available at http://eng.stat.gov.tw/ct.asp?xItem=3417&CtNode=1596, accessed June 2009.

experience is the persistence of a very low level of inequality.[11] There is no evidence of any inverted-U for India, Chile, or Taiwan.

One should not generalize from a few cases, so it is important to look at the experience of a larger number of nations. Researchers who have done so find little evidence of a general tendency for income inequality to first rise and then fall with economic growth. It is as common for Gini coefficients to rise as per capita income grows as it is for them to fall.[12] The persistence of a given level of inequality within nations may be the strongest trend. Support for the Kuznets curve in earlier cross-section analysis was driven by the higher inequality of a subset of middle-income nations. Better econometric tests reveal that the inverted-U was driven not by

[11]Taiwan's record of rapid economic growth with low income inequality is somewhat unique. Some transition economies have similarly low or even lower levels of income inequality but none has yet achieved Taiwan's per capita income level. Among rapidly growing economies, China has achieved similar growth rates, although not yet for as many years, but China has done so with significantly higher inequality. The same is true for Malaysia, Thailand, and Singapore. Korea's record on growth and inequality comes closest to Taiwan's.

[12]Klaus Deininger and Lyn Squire, "New Ways of Looking at Old Issues: Inequality and Growth," *Journal of Development Economics* 57 (1998); Martin Ravallion and Shaohua Chen, "What Can New Survey Data Tell Us about Recent Changes in Distribution and Poverty?" *World Bank Economic Review* 11, no. 2 (1997).

economic growth but by the coincidence of Latin America's high levels of inequality and middle-income ranking. Investigation of the Kuznets curve offers a cautionary tale for empirical work on developing nations. Patterns observed across nations may not always provide reliable insight into what ultimately are dynamic processes that occur within nations.[13]

Rejection of the Kuznets curve as an overall tendency does not imply that economic growth has no impact on inequality, nor does it deny that something like the Kuznets curve might occur in some countries. The lack of one general pattern simply confirms the complexity of the process that determines inequality. Research on the Kuznets curve identifies the large role played by country- or region-specific circumstances, which appear far more important in determining distributional outcomes than the level of per capita income. This is an encouraging finding. That all nations do not follow a similar distributional path suggests that there may be greater scope for government policy to influence the distributional outcomes that accompany economic growth.

WHAT ELSE MIGHT CAUSE INEQUALITY?

If inequality is not systematically associated with the level of income, what else accounts for the observed differences across countries and regions shown in Figure 6–3? There is little doubt that history and politics have played an important role. An obvious example is South Africa, which has one of the world's highest levels of income inequality. For decades, the apartheid government excluded blacks and other nonwhite South Africans from owning prime agricultural land, getting a decent education, and living in major urban areas. The legacy of these policies remains today, reflected in South Africa's highly unequal distribution of income. According to the World Bank's country brief on South Africa, the Gini coefficient in 2008 was 0.67—one of the highest in the world.

History and politics also played key roles in other parts of the world. At the end of World War II, the United States administered a land reform in South Korea as part of the dissolution of 50 years of Japanese colonial rule. These reforms redistributed land from Japanese to Korean households, providing millions of Korean families with a key asset from which they could earn a living, resulting in a relatively equal distribution of rural incomes. Low levels of inequality in eastern Europe and central Asia are, in part, the product of years of legislated wages and state ownership of the means of production. Citizens of these countries had limited opportunity to accumulate

---

[13]Even the experience of the United States now rejects Kuznets's original hypothesis. Income inequality in the United States fell over the four decades after the great Depression. But, after 1975, during a period of continued growth in the U.S. economy, household incomes became increasingly *unequal,* the opposite of the predictions of the Kuznets curve. Economists believe technological change, immigration, increased international trade, and a slowdown in the growth of school attainment are some of the factors that explain this post-1975 shift.

any productive assets other than an education. It is not surprising that, with the turn toward the market, inequality is now rising in many of these countries; in some of them this is happening alongside renewed economic growth.

Some of the high levels of inequality in Latin America may be traced to patterns of land ownership dating back centuries. Not only was the colonial legacy part of this process but the demands of specific crops, including the advantages of plantation-style agriculture, were also a factor. In East Asia, rice cultivation was better suited to family farming and established a basis for higher income equality in this region. Conversely, mineral wealth, whether in diamonds or oil, tends to produce higher inequality. Factor endowments shaped distributional outcomes in the past and continue to do so today.

Resource endowments and the "persistence of the past" play significant roles in shaping a nation's distribution of income, but policy choices made today also affect these outcomes. Government policy influences the accumulation of assets, including education. Policy decisions affect the diffusion of technology and access to markets, which condition productivity growth and the returns to factors of production. Taxes and government spending, including expenditures on social safety nets, directly influence how income is divided. The level of inequality in any nation is the result of complex interactions among history, politics, resource endowments, market forces, and government policies.

WHY INEQUALITY MATTERS

If economic development requires a reduction in the amount of poverty, then the simplest explanation for why income inequality matters is that the degree of inequality plus the level of income determines the extent of poverty. Even without a discussion of how to define poverty (which we will get to shortly), some examples of the relationship between economic growth, income inequality, and poverty should be clear. If an economy grows and inequality remains unchanged, the income of the poor has grown in line with everyone else's. The poorest quintiles have more income, which potentially helps raise some households out of poverty. If per capita income remains unchanged and inequality rises, the poorest quintiles have less income and some households probably have fallen into poverty. These propositions merely express the basic mathematics governing the relationship among poverty, growth, and inequality.

But inequality and growth are not determined independently of one another. There may not be one systematic tendency for how inequality changes as nations grow, but inequality often changes with rising per capita incomes. Similarly, inequality may affect the rate of growth an economy achieves. Do nations with more inequality tend to experience slower growth, thus doubly hurting the well-being of the poor?

Finally, income inequality also matters in its own right. Societies have preferences concerning inequality and may (or may not) wish for their governments to intervene to achieve distributional outcomes.[14]

Just as there has been a long debate over the impact of growth on inequality, there is ongoing debate over how inequality affects economic growth. As discussed previously in this chapter, some early theories of economic development concluded that inequality might raise growth rates. By concentrating income in fewer hands, there might be more savings available to finance investments critical for capital accumulation. But this simple view of distribution and growth fails to capture other channels in which income inequality can be a drag on economic growth. Contemporary discussion of the relationship between inequality and growth explores these channels.

When inequality is high, worthwhile investments may not be undertaken. Poor people may have promising investment opportunities. Buying a farm animal or improving irrigation, investing in a piece of equipment or building a store, or sending a child to school all may yield a good economic return. But the individuals or families may not undertake these investments because they cannot afford them. Credit market imperfections and the inability of the poor to offer lenders collateral lowers the amount of productive investment they engage in and leads to less economic growth. If the economy had a more equal income distribution, more of these productive investments could be financed and pursued.

Another channel that links inequality and growth is the political process. There are numerous "political economy" connections between distribution and growth. Some argue that, when inequality is high, the rich use their wealth to secure outcomes favorable to their interests, influencing everything from government spending (disproportionate amounts spent on public universities, which the children of the rich attend, as compared to primary schools) to trade policy (using tariffs and other forms of trade protection to maintain domestic monopolies). These policies can lead to inefficient outcomes that lower growth rates. Others argue the opposite political response occurs. When inequality is high, populist movements may arise that focus more on redistribution and less on growth, leading, for example, to higher taxes and less investment. High inequality also tends to be associated with more violence, both personal and political, which in turn can reallocate expenditures to less productive activities (more police and private security services) and discourage greater investment.

Given the multitude of connections between inequality and growth, the net effect is an empirical matter. Studies that attempt to sort out the relationship tend to rely on the cross-country growth regressions introduced in Chapter 3. Early studies found statistical support that high initial inequality, especially of landholdings, was

---

[14]Evidence that people prefer fairness is presented in World Bank, "Equity and Well-Being," *2006 World Development Report: Equity and Development* (Washington, DC: World Bank, 2005.)

associated with slower subsequent growth. But later studies, using larger data sets and different econometric techniques, either found no such effect or even an opposing one.[15] The inconclusive nature of these results is not surprising, given both the complexity and potential circularity of the relationship. Inequality affects growth and growth affects inequality, complicating statistical identification. It also is unlikely that one systematic pattern describes the relationship between inequality and growth for all countries at all times. This does not imply that, in a specific-country context, inequality and growth are unrelated. High inequality may be a constraint on growth, but easing this constraint is always a daunting challenge for policy makers.

MEASURING POVERTY

People sometimes refer to inequality and poverty as if they were the same thing. They are not. Inequality is an important determinant of poverty, but the two concepts are distinct. To see why, consider the following. Assume your lot in life was to fall in the bottom quintile of the income distribution. If you could pick the nation you would live in, would it be one where the bottom 20 percent received 3.4, 3.5, or 9.0 percent of household income? If your answer is the nation where the poorest receive 9.0 percent, you are confusing inequality with poverty. You also probably are forgetting the results presented in Table 6–1. Recall from that table that the share of household income of the poorest quintile in Bangladesh was 9.0 percent; in Mexico, 3.5 percent; and in the United States, only 3.4 percent!

In the United States the bottom 20 percent refers to over 60 million people. Some of these people are destitute but the overwhelming majority is not. Almost all live in a permanent dwelling with electricity, a gas or electric stove, clean water, and indoor plumbing. Most have access to medical care (even if it means an emergency room at a local hospital) and, during childhood, receive a full regimen of vaccinations against many infectious diseases. The likelihood of contracting malaria or dying of a diarrheal disease is remote, although both were common in the United States in its earlier history. For those with children, the probability of an infant dying before its first birthday is low, and that child is likely to receive at least 12 years of education. Those in the bottom quintile in the United States are likely to own a television and a landline or cellular phone and perhaps a car, and have some access to a computer at a public library if not in their own homes.

---

[15]Two frequently cited papers that reach opposite conclusions relating inequality and growth are Alberto Alesina and Dani Rodrik, "Distributive Politics and Economic Growth," *Quarterly Journal of Economics* 109, no. 2 (1994); and Kristin Forbes, "A Reassessment of the Relationship between Inequality and Growth," *American Economic Review* 90, no. 4 (2000).

The poorest 20 percent are poor relative to most other Americans and may find this demoralizing, but they have a substantially higher material standard of living than the poor in either Bangladesh or Mexico. No one in the bottom quintile in Bangladesh (or in most any quintile) is likely to receive the health or education benefits or the material goods consumed by America's poorest individuals. The 30 million individuals who make up the bottom quintile in Bangladesh are likely to live in the most rudimentary of dwellings, those that can be washed away in a bad storm. Food is often scarce and clean water unavailable. Living with intestinal parasites is a regular occurrence; infectious diseases take a regular toll on young and old and infant deaths are a common event. School enrollment rates are rising, but the educational attainment of poor Bangladeshis, especially females, is well below that of their American counterparts. Consumer goods consist of a few articles of clothing, some cooking utensils and little else. Most of those in the bottom 20 percent have never placed a phone call or clicked on a mouse.

The bottom quintile in the United States receives only 3.4 percent of household income, whereas the bottom quintile in Bangladesh consumes 9.0 percent of total consumption expenditures in Bangladesh. But America's bottom 20 percent commands a much larger amount of *total* income and, therefore, enjoys a higher standard of living even if its relative share is so much less. The Gini coefficient is thus a measure of relative equity; it describes the outcomes for one group relative to other groups but provides no information about absolute standards of living.

POVERTY LINES

Just as a set of analytical tools is needed for describing and understanding distributional outcomes, a similar set of tools is needed to define and measure poverty. We focus mostly on a consumption or income definition of **absolute poverty**, but it is important to recognize that poverty is multidimensional and encompasses deprivations not readily captured by income measures alone. This should be a familiar idea because it parallels the debate over how to define economic development. Both the human development index (HDI) and the millennium development goals (MDGs), discussed in Chapter 2, go well beyond GDP per capita as a measure of well-being and similar approaches are used in defining poverty.

Poverty lines, defined as having a certain amount of taka or pesos or dollars to spend per day, can capture the degree of material deprivation but may not reflect securing basic health and education. A family may have sufficient funds to purchase a minimal basket of food, but if they have no ready access to safe drinking water, food purchases are no guarantee of meeting nutritional needs because waterborne microbes may result in gastrointestinal illness and reduce the absorption of key nutrients. In this critical sense, access to safe drinking water joins money income as a determinant of absolute poverty. The availability of public services, including basic health and education, can also have an impact on poverty status today and the transmission of poverty across generations, independent of current consumption levels. Another dimension of poverty is vulnerability to adverse shocks. Expenditures in one period may raise a family above the poverty line, but in a subsequent period, natural disasters, economywide downturns, or even the ill health or death of a family's breadwinner can push the family below the poverty line. Families often move in and out of poverty and reducing vulnerability is intrinsic to improving well-being.

Poverty is multidimensional, and it is possible to quantify many of its dimensions.[16] A great deal of attention is paid to quantifying income or consumption poverty. Development economists often use a definition of absolute poverty by which a specific monetary value is defined as a dividing line between the poor and nonpoor. Most nations define their own poverty lines, usually basing the amount on the per capita cost of some minimal consumption basket of food and a few other necessities (Box 6–1). Food dominates these consumption bundles because it may account for two-thirds to three-quarters of poor people's total expenditures. In many low-income nations, poverty lines are based on a standard of obtaining 2000 or more calories per day. While these caloric requirements seem "scientific," the actual poverty line remains a social construct. The food purchased to achieve these calories depends on what individuals actually choose to buy. Expenditures even lower than the poverty line might achieve required calories but hardly anyone would actually purchase such a consumption basket.

Often governments specify more than one poverty line. Because of regional price differences, distinct poverty lines may be applied for urban versus rural areas or, as is the case in Bangladesh, for different regions of the country. Once a poverty line (or lines) is established and expressed in a nation's own currency, that level of consumption or income has to be adjusted on an annual basis to account for changes in the price of the underlying bundle of goods. The goal is to maintain a constant poverty line over time, holding constant the ability to purchase the core consumption basket of food and other necessities.[17] This permits policy makers and researchers to chart the progress a country or region is making in lifting people out of absolute poverty.

[16]Multidimensional indices of poverty have been developed by scholars at the Oxford Poverty & Human Development Initiative (www.ophi.org.uk). With their assistance, the multidimensional poverty index (MPI) was introduced by the UN Development Programme (UNDP) in its 2010 human development report and serves as an alternative to measuring income poverty. The MPI defines someone as poor if he or she experiences deprivation in a number of areas, including education (for example, "if no household member has completed five years of schooling"), health (for example, "if any household member is malnourished"), and standard of living (for example, "if the household has no electricity" or "if the household has a dirt, sand, or dung floor").

[17]Poverty lines also can be expressed in relative terms. In the European Union, poverty is sometimes defined as living below 60 percent of median income. With this definition, the poverty line does not represent the ability to purchase a fixed bundle of goods but changes as median incomes change. Using this approach, absolute poverty declines only if incomes become more equally distributed, not if there is a general increase in per capita incomes.

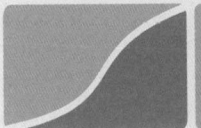

Instead of one official poverty line, Bangladesh has many. Separate poverty lines exist for each of 14 regions to reflect varying costs. Regional lines are further divided into upper and lower levels to capture different intensities of poverty. All poverty lines are based on securing a minimum daily caloric intake of 2,112 calories. The representative bundle of food to obtain these calories was specified in the early 1990s and is made up of 11 items: rice, wheat, pulses, milk, oil, meat, freshwater fish, potatoes, other vegetables, sugar, and fruit. The cost of this bundle is adjusted using a domestic price index. The lower poverty line in each region represents the level of poverty at which a person does not have the resources to meet both food and nonfood requirements and must sacrifice some minimum daily caloric requirement to afford essential nonfood needs. The upper poverty line represents a level of poverty at which a person is able to meet minimum daily food requirements and afford some nonfood expenditures.

Mexico has three official poverty lines that capture a range of conditions of poverty. Within these lines, there is differentiation between rural and urban populations. The lowest poverty line is estimated by calculating the cost of a representative bundle of food, taking into account the differing nutritional requirements of rural versus urban dwellers in terms of daily calories and grams of protein. Falling below this poverty line indicates that a person cannot meet even these minimal daily nutrition requirements. Falling below the second poverty line means the person does not have the resources to meet both daily nutritional requirements and minimum health and educational expenses. The third line indicates that resources are insufficient to pay for all necessary costs of living, including food, education, health, clothing and footwear, housing, and public transportation expenses.

The United States also specifies multiple poverty lines that vary, not by location, but according to household size and age of household members. U.S. poverty lines, like those in Bangladesh and Mexico, start with the cost of a basket of food items. Designed to meet a person's nutritional needs at minimum cost, the bundle of food items used is still based on a 1955 survey of household food consumption. It is made up of servings of milk, cheese, and ice cream; meat, poultry and fish; eggs; dry beans, peas, and nuts; flour, cereal, and baked goods; citrus fruit and tomatoes; dark-green and deep-yellow vegetables; potatoes; other vegetables and fruits; fats and oils; and sugars and sweets. The cost of the bundle of food was multiplied by three to arrive at the poverty threshold because the 1955 survey found that the average family of three or more people spent approximately one-third of its disposable income on food. Since adopting these poverty lines in 1965, the dollar value is adjusted annually to account for price inflation. Neither the bundle of food items nor the portion of income a family spends on food has been adjusted in almost 60 years despite changes in diets and evidence that even poor Americans spend less than one-third of their after-tax income on food.

Sources: Fernando Cortés, Daniel Hernández, Enrique Hernández Laos, Miguel Székely, and Hadid Vera Llamas, "Evolución y características de la pobreza en México en la última década del siglo XX," Economia Mexicana NUEVA EPOCA, vol. XII (2003), available at www .economiamexicana.cide.edu/num_anteriores/XII-2/Fernando_Cortes.pdf. Eloise Cofer, Evelyn Grossman, and Faith Clark, "Family Food Plans and Food Costs: For Nutritionists and Other Leaders Who Develop or Use Food Plans," Home Economics Research Report 20 (Washington, DC: U.S. Government Printing Office, November 1962), available at http://aspe.hhs.gov/poverty/ familyfoodplan.pdf, accessed July 2005; Constance Citro and Robert T. Michael, *Measuring Poverty: A New Approach* (Washington, DC: National Academy Press, 1995); World Bank, "Poverty in Bangladesh: Building on Progress," Report 24299-BD (Washington, DC: World Bank, December 2002).

Most nations have their own poverty lines, and these could be used to make international comparisons. One could combine the number who are deemed poor in Bangladesh (daily per person regional poverty lines of between roughly 19 and 32 taka, or US\$1.70 and \$2.80, PPP) with the number said to be poor in Mexico (poverty lines of 30 to 45 pesos, or US\$4.60 to \$6.60, PPP) and in the United States (daily per person poverty line of around \$15).[18] This would offer a measure of poverty as perceived by each nation. But the resulting differences in poverty rates across nations would themselves be functions of the poverty lines the nations choose. An alternative and more widely adopted approach is to establish a single global poverty line. By applying one common poverty line, often the \$1.25-a-day or \$2-a-day measure, it may be possible to obtain a more consistent picture of the degree of absolute poverty across countries and regions and of how the number of poor is changing over time.

Before investigating the origins of the \$1.25-a-day line and regional trends in poverty, it is worth examining the use of poverty lines in a bit more detail and defining some alternative measures of poverty that can be based on such lines. Figure 6–5 reproduces the frequency distribution of consumption per capita in Bangladesh with

[18]The United States defines poverty depending on the size and composition of a household. Households with children or elderly members are assumed to have different food requirements, leading to different poverty lines. Households with more members are assumed to achieve economies of scale in consumption and this, too, affects their poverty lines. In 2009, daily per capita requirements ranged from \$30 for a household with one nonelderly member to \$12 for a household of eight with six children. The \$15 refers to the average poverty line for households with four members. The reported values for Bangladesh and Mexico refer to their upper poverty lines, as discussed in Box 6–1, for the years 2000 and 2002, respectively.

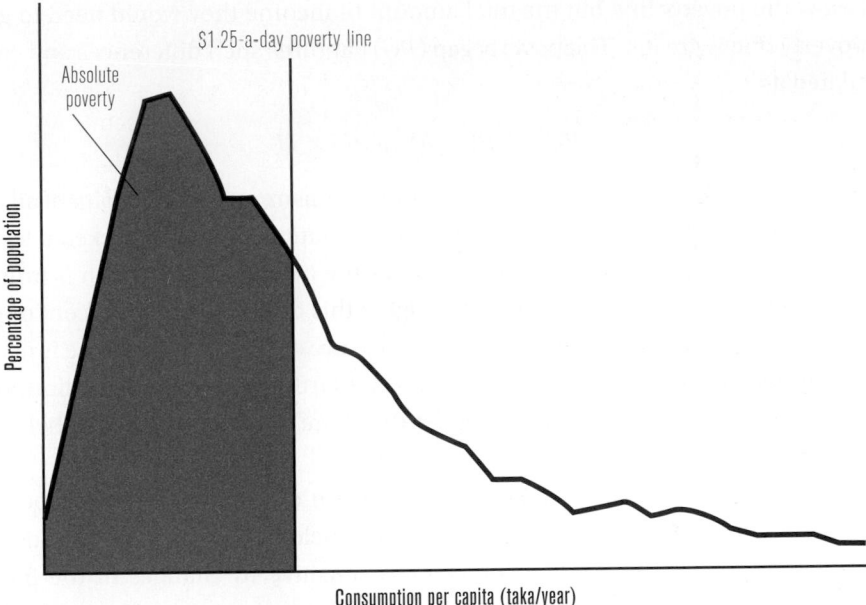

FIGURE 6-5   Absolute Poverty in Bangladesh

Source: Collaboration with Claudio E. Montenegro, World Bank.

the addition of the $1.25-a-day poverty line. Individuals with consumption below the poverty line, some 50 percent of all Bangladeshis, are considered absolutely poor. It should be evident that there is something arbitrary about this distinction between the poor and the nonpoor. Is someone just above the poverty line, with a few taka more of consumption expenditures, living that much differently from someone just below the poverty line? This arbitrary character of poverty lines is inevitable. But poverty lines still are useful in providing a sense of the extent of absolute poverty, a means for assessing the success of policies designed to alleviate poverty, and a mechanism for calling attention to and mobilizing support for reducing human deprivation. Strategies that succeed in reducing the numbers below the poverty line usually spill over and also help the "near poor," those just to the right of the poverty line in the frequency distribution.

Once a poverty line is selected, the extent of absolute poverty can be identified in a number of ways. The simplest is to report the number of people below the poverty line. Equally straightforward is the **head-count index**, the ratio of the number below the poverty line to total population. A third measure, the **poverty gap**, describes the severity of poverty. The severity of poverty refers to both how many people fall below the poverty line and how far they are from that line. Look again at Figure 6–5. Imagine if the frequency distribution below the $1.25-a-day poverty line was somewhat higher closer to the origin and somewhat lower closer to the poverty line. This would mean that poverty was more severe. The same number of individuals might fall below the poverty line but the total amount of income they would need to get to the poverty line is greater. The poverty gap (*PG*) captures such differences and can be calculated as

$$PG = [(PL - MC)/PL] \times H$$

where *PL* stands for the poverty line, *MC* is mean consumption per capita of all individuals below the poverty line, and *H* is the head-count index. The bracketed term in the equation indicates in relative terms how far the average poor person is from the poverty line; the head-count index then weights this amount by the percent of poor people in the population. The poverty gap, a measure of how much income is needed to get the poor to the poverty line, increases the farther mean consumption of the poor is from the poverty line and the higher the share of the population is below the poverty line.

The head-count index, tells us what proportion of the population is poor, and the poverty gap tells us proportionately how far below the poverty line the mean income of the poor falls. Neither indicator is sensitive to changes in the income distribution among the poor, and by relying on the mean income gap, *PG* places equal weight on an individual just below the poverty line and on another individual who might be quite far below the line. These shortcomings are addressed simply by squaring *PG*. This third indicator, known (it's not surprising) as the poverty gap squared, places greater weight on incomes that fall farther below the poverty line and thus more fully captures the severity of poverty. These three indicators together provide a much richer picture of the various dimensions of poverty than any one of them alone.

WHY $1.25 A DAY?

The first widely used global poverty line was a $1 a day and had its origins in the late 1980s. To determine the extent of absolute poverty in the world, the World Bank's 1990 World Development Report (WDR) examined a set of 34 country-specific poverty lines from both developing and developed nations. As expected, these poverty lines generally rose with income level. Focusing only on the low-income nations in this group, the country-specific poverty lines tended to fall within a range of $275 to $370, measured in terms of 1985 PPP dollars per person per year. The upper bound of this range, just over $1 a day, was adopted as a global poverty threshold.

To chart changes in poverty over time, it is necessary to increase the poverty line in local currencies in response to changes in domestic prices. Ideally, this would be done using a price index based on the goods the poor tend to consume. In practice, a nation's consumer price index is used. To assess what happened to regional and global poverty since 1985, researchers have done more than just adjust the original $1-a-day poverty line by domestic price inflation. The most recent estimate defines *extreme poverty* as living below $1.25, measured in terms of 2005 PPP dollars.

To compute this latest global poverty line, researchers were aided by an expanded compilation of poverty lines, now including 74 developing countries, as well as new estimates of purchasing power parity, which, for the first time, included price surveys for China. The new compilation of poverty lines was especially important because the composition of low-income nations changed between 1985 and 2005. The original $1-a-day poverty line reflected national poverty lines, including those of Bangladesh, Egypt, India, Indonesia, Kenya, Morocco, and Tanzania. Economies in sub-Saharan Africa were underrepresented. Rather than relying on an inflation-adjusted value of the poverty line defined by this earlier group of countries, researchers at the World Bank repeated the original exercise and determined a new poverty line based on 15 of today's poorest countries.[19] The new group includes 13 sub-Saharan countries, Nepal, and Tajikistan. The average of the national poverty lines of this group is $1.25 a day, which is thought to be more representative of how the poorest nations define absolute poverty. The median poverty line of all developing economies in the sample was $2.00 a day, which is often used as a measure of poverty in middle-income economies, especially in Latin America and eastern Europe.

New estimates of purchasing power parity were equally important in establishing the $1.25-a-day poverty line and in assessing the extent of poverty. If two people have the same purchasing power, they should be considered poor or not poor independent of where they live. But if they live in different countries they use different currencies and face different prices. As discussed in Chapter 2, we cannot rely on comparisons made using market exchange rates as a way to ensure that these two people living in different countries will be evaluated similarly. This is because of the importance of nontraded goods in consumption. To capture PPP, economists rely on detailed price surveys in individual countries. Prices in shops and stalls of specific items, including everything from 500-gram packages of durum spaghetti to low-heeled ladies' shoes, are collected. These surveys are conducted under the auspices of the United Nations International Comparison Program (ICP) and offer estimates of PPP.

The most recent poverty estimates rely on ICP surveys from 2005, which have several important advantages over previous rounds. One problem in comparing prices in different countries is accounting for the quality of goods. Nontraded goods may be cheaper in poor countries than in rich countries, but some of this difference may be due to inferior quality, leading to an underestimation of PPP in poor countries. The 2005 ICP made corrections for this problem. It also expanded country coverage; China participated for the first time. Given the size of China's population and its success in reducing poverty, accurate measures of its PPP were critical for improved estimates of global poverty. Finally, the most recent estimates of global poverty were aided by improved coverage of the household surveys needed to make poverty estimates. Over 1.2 million households were part of 1 of 675 surveys taken

[19]S. Chen, M. Ravallion, and P. Sangraula, "Dollar a Day Revisited," *World Bank Economic Review* 23, no. 2 (2009).

in 115 countries and covering over 90 percent of the population of low- and middle-income nations. Based on these new sources of information, it was possible not only to estimate poverty in 2005 but also to reestimate values back to 1981.

Figure 6–6 presents the most recent poverty estimates by World Bank economists Shaohua Chen and Martin Ravallion. The headline news from these new estimates was that "the developing world is poorer than we thought, but no less successful in the fight against poverty." The key reason for finding more poverty was that the latest PPP estimates indicated that the cost of living in developing countries, including China and India, was higher than previously thought. Consumption expenditures therefore purchased less, causing poverty levels to rise, not only for 2005 but also in the revised poverty counts going back to 1981. As far as the world's poor was concerned, nothing had changed. The difficulty of their circumstances remained the same. It was only the official count of the number of poor that had gotten worse.

Employing the $1.25-a-day poverty line, the good news is that the number of people living in absolute poverty fell by almost 520 million people, from 1.90 in 1981 to 1.38 billion in 2005. This represents an incredible achievement in reducing human deprivation. The bad news is that 1.38 billion people in poverty still accounts for more than one out of every five people living in developing nations. A closer look at regional patterns also reveals how isolated and uneven the fall in poverty has been. Almost the entire decline occurred in East Asia, and within East Asia most of the

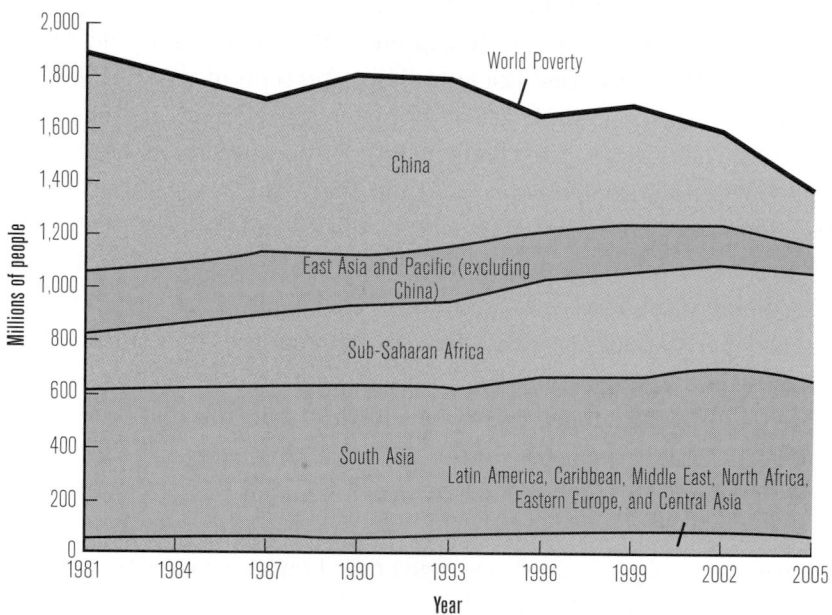

FIGURE 6-6 **Number of People Living Below $1.25 a Day**

Source: S. Chen and M. Ravallion, "The Developing World Is Poorer Than We Thought, but No Less Successful in the Fight Against Poverty," *Quarterly Journal of Economics* 125, no. 4 (2010).

decline is due to China's success. Over 600 million fewer Chinese people lived below $1.25 a day in 2005 than did in 1981. Many observers trace the start of China's success to the economic reforms of the late 1970s, which decollectivized agriculture and encouraged farm households to produce and market more of their output, pulling them out of poverty.

Poverty reduction was dramatic throughout all of East Asia, with large declines in Indonesia, Malaysia, South Korea, Taiwan, and Thailand. But in absolute terms, given the size of China's population, China's success dominates the global decline. By comparison, South Asia, dominated by India, saw an increase of almost 50 million in the number of poor. In sub-Saharan Africa, the trend was worse. As the population of this region grew, so did absolute poverty, from 214 million in 1981 to 391 million in 2005.[20] Trends in other regions add little to the aggregate picture for two reasons: Their population size is relatively small and, as mostly middle-income nations, the share of their populations living at only $1.25 a day was and remains low.

Trends in absolute numbers are one way to mark the progress made against absolute poverty. But it is not the only way. The head-count index presents poverty relative to population size and reinforces both the good and bad news on poverty (Table 6–2). In 1981, China's head-count index was 84 percent; by 2005, it was down to only 16 percent. In South Asia, the incidence of poverty also declined significantly, from just over 59 percent to 40 percent. Sub-Saharan Africa showed a modest decrease, from 54 to 51 percent. Latin America also had limited success at decreasing its poverty rate; the head-count index fell from 11.5 to 8.4 percent. Given their generally middle-income status, $1.25 a day is not the most meaningful poverty line for eastern Europe and central Asia (ECA) or for the Middle East and North Africa (MENA). Both regions have had poverty rates in the single digits for the past 25 years, although ECA experienced an increase in poverty since 1981 while MENA saw a decline. For the developing world as a whole, there has been a significant decline in the percentage of people who experience the grinding poverty of living below $1.25 a day. Approximately 52 percent of the developing world fell below the $1.25-a-day poverty line in 1981; 24 years later, this ratio stood at 25. Can similar progress be made over the next 20 years?

Before trying to answer that question, it is worth considering the severity of poverty as measured by the poverty gap (Table 6–2). In 1981, absolute poverty was severe in the most populous regions of the developing world. In East and South Asia, as well as in sub-Saharan Africa, the poverty gap ranged from 20 to 36 percent. But, by 2005, the poverty gap had fallen to 10 percent or less everywhere but in sub-Saharan Africa,

---

[20]S. Chen and M. Ravallion, "How Have the World's Poorest Fared Since the Early 1980s?" *World Bank Research Observer* 19, no. 2 (2004). The authors point out that the earlier their estimates, the less confident they are in the results because of the paucity of household surveys from the early 1980s. This is especially true in Africa. The trend toward increasing absolute poverty in sub-Saharan Africa is not in doubt, but the magnitude of this increase may not be precise.

TABLE 6-2 Absolute Poverty* by Region, 1981–2005

REGION	NUMBER OF POOR (MILLIONS)			HEAD-COUNT INDEX (PERCENT)			POVERTY GAP (PERCENT)		
	1981	1990	2005	1981	1990	2005	1981	1990	2005
East Asia	1,071.5	873.3	316.2	77.7	54.7	16.8	35.5	18.2	4.0
(China only)	(835.1)	(683.2)	(207.7)	(84)	(60.2)	(15.9)	(39.3)	(20.7)	(4.0)
South Asia	548.3	579.2	595.6	59.4	51.7	40.3	19.6	15.2	10.3
Sub-Saharan Africa	213.7	299.1	390.6	53.7	57.9	51.2	22.9	26.6	21.1
Latin America and Caribbean	42.0	42.9	46.1	11.5	9.8	8.4	4.0	3.6	3.2
Middle East and North Africa	13.7	9.7	11.0	7.9	4.3	3.6	1.6	0.9	0.8
Eastern Europe and Central Asia	7.1	9.1	17.3	1.7	2.0	3.7	0.4	0.6	1.1
Total†	1,896.2	1,813.4	1,376.7	51.8	41.6	25.2	21.3	14.2	7.6
(Total excluding China)	(1,061.1)	(1,130.2)	(1,169.0)	(39.8)	(35.0)	(28.2)	(n.a.)‡	(n.a.)	(n.a.)

*Absolute poverty refers to a poverty line of $1.25 a day (PPP, 2005).
†Total refers to low- and middle-income nations only.
‡n.a., not available.

Source: S. Chen and M. Ravallion, "The Developing World Is Poorer Than We Thought, but No Less Successful in the Fight Against Poverty," *Quarterly Journal of Economics* 125, no. 4 (2010).

where it remained at over 20 percent. Almost 1.4 billion people still lived on less than $1.25 a day in 2005, but most of them had gotten a good deal closer to this bare minimum of consumption.

China's success at lowering its poverty gap from 39 to 4 percent is an unprecedented achievement in human history. It also holds some promise for what is possible and, therefore, what nations in sub-Saharan Africa might achieve in the next few decades. Much of sub-Saharan Africa began the twenty-first century with a poverty gap well below China's level 25 years earlier. However, the challenge facing Africa is greater. In 1981, China had a more equal distribution of income than is typical of most African nations. Therefore, African growth rates have to be even faster than China's or policies of redistribution greater for absolute poverty to fall as rapidly. It is hard to envision such outcomes. China benefited from a fundamental transformation in its economy, which brought tremendous economic progress. It is hard to identify anything in Africa comparable to China's transition out of socialism and toward the market that has the potential to produce sustained growth rates in output approaching double digits. Reducing absolute poverty in sub-Saharan Africa remains a huge challenge to both African nations and the global community.

DISSENTING OPINIONS ON THE EXTENT OF ABSOLUTE POVERTY

With something as complex as estimating the amount of absolute poverty in the world, it should come as no surprise that not everyone agrees with the numbers. Some criticize the estimates as too low; others claim they are too high.

The somewhat arbitrary nature of any poverty line already has been identified. Is someone living on just less than $1.25 a day poor, whereas someone consuming just over $1.25 a day not poor? Princeton economist Angus Deaton has a different concern. He devoted his 2010 presidential address to the American Economic Association to the latest round of poverty estimates and argued that the $1.25-a-day poverty line is *too high*! The latest poverty estimates raise the number of poor in 2005 by close to half a billion people compared to using the previous method and applying it to 2005. This is a huge increase for a measure of *absolute* poverty, which is intended to stay constant in real terms over time.

Deaton traces the problem to how the poverty line was constructed. He is not persuaded that the 15 countries used to establish the new poverty line were the right ones. He notes that the small nation of Guinea-Bissau, with a population of about 1.5 million people, was included in the construction of the new poverty line, but India, with a population exceeding 1 billion people, was excluded. India has a national poverty line below $1.25 a day but is now judged as having many more poor people because of a standard determined by the poverty conditions prevailing in Guinea-Bissau (where the poverty line is above $1.25 a day) and other smaller economies. Deaton favors using a weighted average of national poverty lines from a much larger group of developing nations so that the weights reflect the number of poor people living in each nation. These and other recommended adjustments result in a global poverty line of less than $1 a day and a world poverty count in 2005 of well under 1 billion.[21]

Some commentators disagree with Deaton and see $1.25 a day as *too low* a threshold for defining absolute poverty at a global level. This cutoff has been described as "destitution" and may be too low to serve as an effective benchmark for poverty alleviation. Others are critical of what they consider the particularly arbitrary nature of any international poverty line. They argue that the use of one global poverty line bears too little relationship to national poverty lines and therefore defines poverty in way that may have little relevance to the actual bundles of goods poor people need to purchase to attain their basic needs.[22] This latter argument has special merit for middle-income nations whose poverty lines tend to be above $1.25 a day. Still others contend that even $2 a day is too low a threshold for a *global* poverty line (Box 6–2).

[21]A. Deaton, "Price Indexes, Inequality, and the Measurement of World Poverty," *American Economic Review* 100, no. 1 (2010).

[22]See *In Focus: Dollar a Day: How Much Does It Say?* International Poverty Centre, UN Development Programme, September 2004. www.ipc-undp.org/pub/IPCPovertyInFocus4.pdf.

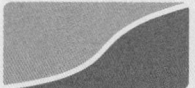

BOX 6-2 WHO IS *NOT* POOR?

Economist Lant Pritchett argues against $1.25 a day and even $2 a day as legitimate measures of *global* poverty. He suggests instead a poverty line no less than $15 a day (2000, PPP), close to the lower bound of the prevailing poverty lines in high-income nations. Pritchett argues as follows:

> Because poverty is a social construct each country should be free to set its own definitions of poverty and its own poverty line. . . . But for setting a common, international standard for income poverty—for what constitutes "unacceptable" deprivation in the human condition or inadequate income in a globalized world—it seems grossly unfair that a person is "poor" if born in one country and yet is "not poor" with a level of real income *ten times* lower if born in another. That is, while India might set a poverty line that is attuned to its capabilities and circumstances and the USA another, for international comparisons choosing the lower line implies that what is "unacceptable" deprivation for a US resident is acceptable for another human being simply because of their residence.

Pritchett goes on to demonstrate that the World Bank's poverty lines are grossly inconsistent with achieving minimally acceptable levels of such indicators of physical well-being as infant mortality and stunting, the latter referring to the fraction of children whose height for age is less than two standard deviations below medical norms.

Pritchett recommends defining $1.25 a day as "destitution," $2 a day as "extreme poverty," and $15 a day as *global* poverty. He concludes, "This simple shift in definitions allows continuity and comparability with previous measures of poverty while embracing a new bold vision of what the dream of a world free of poverty really means."

Sources: Lant Pritchett, "Who Is *Not* Poor? Proposing a Higher International Standard for Poverty," CGD Working Paper 33 (Washington, DC: Center for Global Development, November 2003); Lant Pritchett, "Who Is *Not* Poor? Dreaming of a World Truly Free of Poverty," *World Bank Research Observer* 21, no. 1 (2006).

POVERTY TODAY

In 2005, 2.6 billion people, 47 percent of the population of all low- and middle-income economies, fell below the $2-a-day poverty line. Regional head-count indices reached as high as 73 percent in South Asia and sub-Saharan Africa. China stood at 36 percent, and Latin America at 17 percent. When comparing world regions at $2 a day, poverty remained most severe in sub-Saharan Africa (it has the highest poverty gap), but there were still more than three times the number of poor in all of Asia than in sub-Saharan Africa (Figure 6–7). What has happened since 2005?

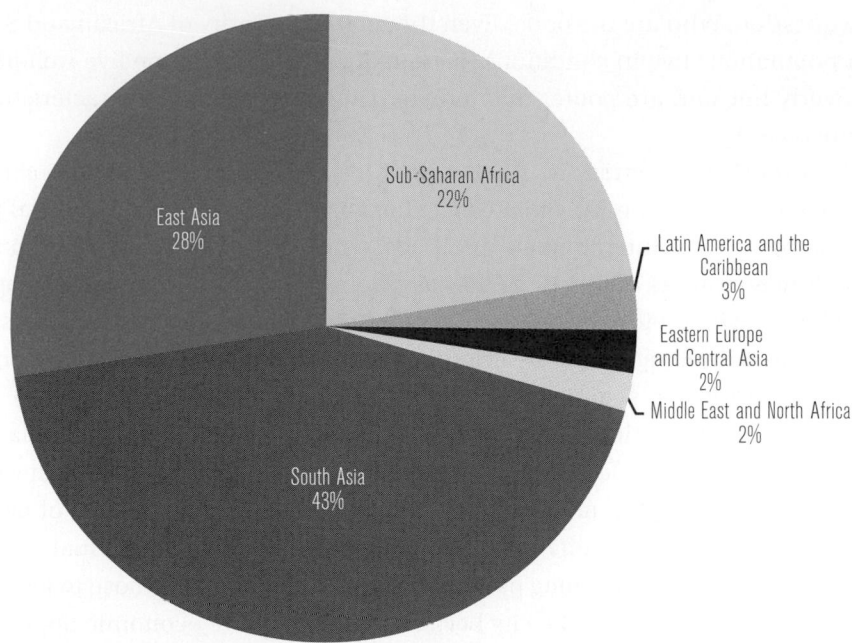

FIGURE 6-7 **Regional Distribution of People Living below the $2-a-Day Poverty Line, 2005**

Source: S. Chen and M. Ravallion, "The Developing World Is Poorer Than We Thought, but No Less Successful in the Fight Against Poverty," *Quarterly Journal of Economics* 125, no. 4 (2010).

The simple answer is that we do not really know. The data required for making estimates of global poverty are considerable and the exercise is not undertaken frequently. Following the financial crisis of 2008, which began in the United States and quickly spread to other nations, there was considerable fear that developing nations would be hit hard. Many were but certainly not all; China and India continued to grow rapidly. The World Bank estimated that 64 million people in developing nations were pushed into "extreme poverty" (under $1.25 a day) because of the crisis. But the years leading up to the crisis were years of strong growth in many regions of the world, and 2010 saw a faster rebound for developing regions than many expected. Far more people are thought to have escaped poverty between 2005 and 2010 than the number pushed back into poverty because of the global financial crisis. Because economic growth tends to be good for the poor, a point we return to below, there is every reason to believe that the number of absolutely poor people as well as the percentage that are poor will be much lower in the second decade of the twenty-first century than in the first.

WHO ARE THE POOR?

If the World Bank's estimates for 2005 are correct and nearly three out of every four Africans and South Asians lived below the $2-a-day poverty line, it might be easier to identify the nonpoor than the poor. This is a somewhat cynical response to the question, Who are the poor? Even though the majority of African and South Asian populations live in conditions that qualify as poverty, some live well below the poverty line and are poorer than others. There are defining characteristics of extreme poverty.

The twenty-first century is the first time in human history that the majority of the world's population lives in areas defined as urban. Nevertheless, rural poverty, in terms of absolute numbers and rates, tends to be higher than urban poverty. This may come as a surprise to the casual observer who contrasts the image of rural villages, with their open spaces and often picturesque arrangements of straw huts and basic dwellings, with the urban squalor and densely settled and seeming disorganization in the shantytowns and favelas[23] common to large cities in low- and middle-income nations. What the casual observer fails to see are the lack of opportunities in rural areas. There are fewer ways to earn income, less education and healthcare, and often more vulnerability to the weather and forces of nature. Within rural areas, poverty often is most common among landless casual laborers or, in sub-Saharan Africa, among pastoralists. Individuals often choose to leave the countryside for the slums of the city because there are more economic opportunities in urban areas.

In addition to the rural–urban divide, poverty rates vary by regions within countries. Two examples are northeast Brazil and the Indian state of Uttar Pradesh, which for decades have been pockets of deep and persistent poverty compared to the rest of their respective countries. The persistence of regional poverty reflects both the limits of spreading development from one region to another and the constraints individuals may face in escaping poverty by migrating from one region to another. Poverty also has a racial and ethnic face. Scheduled castes in India, certain ethnic minorities in eastern Europe including Roma, and indigenous groups in the Andean region all experience poverty rates in excess of others in their societies.

Looking at poverty from the perspective of gender requires consideration of intra-household distribution, the sharing of resources within family units. Most studies of gender roles and opportunities in developing and developed nations conclude that women are disadvantaged relative to men along many dimensions.[24] Women have less access to property rights, including ownership of land, and often are denied inheritance. Girls have tended to receive less primary and secondary education than boys, although in many countries and regions this is no longer the case. Labor markets tend to discriminate against women, paying them less than men for the same work. Combining the work done at home with that done for income,

---

[23]The origin of the word *favela* is the Morro de Favela hillside in Rio de Janeiro, Brazil, where freed slaves established a community of squatters in the late nineteenth century. Over time the term has been adopted to describe any urban slum, especially in Latin America.

[24]This discussion draws from World Bank, *Engendering Development* (Washington, DC: Oxford University Press, 2001).

women tend to work many more hours per week. Domestic violence against women is all too common. Sex-selective abortion favors the birth of boys over girls in many parts of the world.

Given all these disadvantages, the feminization of poverty seems straightforward. But it is not. Measures of individual consumption are based on household data, and it is difficult to disentangle who consumes what within the family. Some goods, including housing, are jointly consumed. Given the lack of data on individual consumption by gender, some studies compare poverty rates between households headed by men and women. The results are inconclusive. Some categories of women-headed households do quite poorly. For example, widows without male heirs in India and elderly women on pensions in eastern Europe have particularly high poverty rates. But other women-headed households, including unmarried women working in urban areas and married women with husbands working abroad and sending remittances, may experience lower-than-average poverty rates. Studies of nutrition that assess the degree to which the needs of females versus males are met find some evidence of the relative deprivation of females but the results vary widely across regions of the world and even within countries. Despite the lack of evidence on the feminization of poverty, it is hard to imagine that reducing gender inequality would not also help reduce poverty in general.

LIVING IN POVERTY

You now know how economists define poverty, how many poor people there are, and a bit about the characteristics of the poor. What do we know about the lives of the poor? You might think living below $1.25 a day implies living on the edge of subsistence and leading a monotonous life with few choices. But this is not the case. The poor are a heterogeneous group who do not devote all their resources to food, who engage in a variety of economic activities, and who pursue strategies to reduce the risks associated with their vulnerable economic situations.

Social scientists, especially anthropologists, have been studying the poor for a long time.[25] This work has been complemented more recently with the collection of household-level surveys that include the poorest families. Many of these surveys have been part of the World Bank's Living Standards Measurement Study (LSMS) surveys, the first of which were undertaken in Côte-d'Ivoire and Peru in 1985. The LSMS and other similar surveys have been used to obtain counts of the poor and to understand the circumstances and behavior of poor households. MIT economists

[25]In 1953, Sol Tax, an anthropologist, published *Penny Capitalism* (Washington, DC: Smithsonian) based on his observation of the lives of a poor indigenous community in Guatemala. Tax observed that members of the community were efficient in their use of time and other resources despite their poverty.

Abhijit Banerjee and Esther Duflo employ 13 of these surveys from around the developing world to create a profile of the economic lives of the poor.[26]

Banerjee and Duflo find that, on average, poor households do not put every penny into purchasing more calories. Food represents about half to three-quarters of total consumption expenditures. For those living under $1.25 a day, the elasticity of spending on calories relative to total food expenditures is about 0.5,[27] suggesting that the poor care about what they eat as well as how much they eat; how food tastes matters even when one is poor. The poor, like the rest of us, spend money on nonessential items, including alcohol, tobacco, festivals (funerals, weddings, and religious holidays), radios, and televisions. The health of the poor is far more compromised than that of the nonpoor. In a number of surveys that ask about health, Banerjee and Duflo find that a family member often is reported to have been bedridden for a day or more during the past month. In the Udaipur district in India, 43 percent of households reported that members did not have enough to eat throughout the year, and 55 percent of adults were anemic.

In their productive activities, the poor tend to diversify their labor time, pursuing multiple opportunities rather than specializing. Among rural households, almost all farm their own land, but this is not their only or even their primary source of income. Poor men often work as daily laborers; poor women might sew, gather fuel, or run small eateries (for example, selling dosas in the morning in India). In one survey of rural West Bengal in India, the median family had three working members engaged in *seven* different occupations. Household members in poor families may engage in temporary migration to obtain work, usually for not more than a month or two. Permanent migration of the poor out of West Bengal is rare, and most migration for work is not far from where the poor live. Reliance on multiple occupations and a willingness to temporarily migrate to find work are strategies that reduce risk. If one activity is no longer available or remunerative, another can be pursued. Such a strategy has its costs. By not specializing and investing in specific skills, it is hard to achieve economies of scale and to gain the productivity required for higher income.

While the poor are often entrepreneurial and lead diverse lives, it would be a mistake to romanticize their situation. Living under $1.25 is a constant struggle filled with uncertainty and vulnerability. Among the poor we can identify a group of "ultra-poor," who find themselves barely surviving. A study by the International Food Policy Research Institute (IFPRI) found that in 2004, 162 million people were ultra-poor,

---

[26]A. Banerjee and E. Duflo, "The Economic Lives of the Poor," *Journal of Economic Perspectives* 21, no. 1 (2007). Also see their book *Poor Economics: A Radical Rethinking of the Way to Fight Global Poverty* (New York: Public Affairs, 2011).

[27]Calories are obtained from different types of food. Coarse grains, like rice and wheat, are inexpensive to buy and offer an individual relatively cheap calories. Meat is expensive making the calories obtained from meat consumption more costly ones. By investigating the foods poor households consume to obtain their calories, it is possible to estimate the elasticity of spending on calories relative to total food expenditures.

living on *less than* 50 cents a day.[28] In another series of studies, researchers asked the poor to describe poverty. Some of their responses follow:[29]

> Don't ask me what poverty is because you have met it outside my house. Look at the house and count the number of holes. Look at my utensils and the clothes that I am wearing. Look at everything. . . . What you see is poverty.—A man in Kenya

> Poverty is hunger, loneliness, nowhere to go when the day is over, deprivation, discrimination, abuse, and illiteracy.—A mother in Guyana

> Poverty is pain; it feels like a disease. It attacks a person not only materially but also morally. It eats away one's dignity and drives one into total despair.—A woman in Moldova

When asked to describe poverty and its causes, poor people reveal poverty to be more than just a lack of money. Not only do the poor suffer from material deprivation but poverty exacts an often severe psychological toll. There are many causes of poverty. The poor lack assets, especially land, and are aware that illiteracy often constrains their opportunities. Illness is dreaded because it can drive a family into destitution. The poor are vulnerable to environmental risks as well, whether droughts or floods or the degradation of their land. The poor often feel exploited by markets, in which private traders charge exorbitant prices for necessities or levy usurious rates for credit, and by governments, who do not provide essential services to the essentially voiceless poor unable to affect change.

STRATEGIES TO REDUCE POVERTY

The World Bank's *1990 World Development Report* not only provided an estimate of the amount of world poverty but also outlined a strategy for alleviating it. The strategy had two main elements: (1) promote market-oriented economic growth and (2) direct basic health and education services to the poor. Market-oriented growth included many of the familiar recommendations of the Washington Consensus discussed in Chapter 5: macroeconomic stability, greater economic openness to trade and investment, increased public investment in infrastructure, improved credit markets, and the

---

[28]Estimates of the number of ultra-poor are from Akhter U. Ahmed, Ruth Vargas Hill, Lisa C. Smith, Doris M. Weismann, and Tim Frankenberger, "The World's Most Deprived," 2020 Discussion Paper 43, International Food Policy Research Institute, Washington, DC, 2007. This study was undertaken before the latest round of the ICP. With the new PPP estimates, the number of ultra-poor would be higher. At over 160 million, the ultra-poor collectively represent a population similar to that of Pakistan's, the world's sixth most populous nation.

[29]The quotations are from United Nations Development Programme, *Human Development Report 1997* (New York: Oxford University Press, 1997), and D. Narayan, *Voices of the Poor: Can Anyone Hear Us?* (Washington, DC: World Bank, 2000).

like. Combined, these policies would lead to labor-demanding growth, which would benefit the poor because the primary asset the poor rely on is their labor. The second element of the strategy called for investing in people. Directing government health and education services to the poor would increase their productivity and thereby contribute to poverty reduction. A third but less emphasized part of the strategy was to develop social safety nets to assist individuals unable to take advantage of market opportunities. This group includes the sick and the old but also all those who suffer from systemic shocks, such as natural disasters and macroeconomic crises.

Most strategies for reducing poverty call for increasing the rate of overall economic growth, because the poor are expected to benefit from economic growth along with the rest of the population. To quote a popular metaphor for development economists, "A rising tide lifts all boats." But there are dissenting voices. In 1996, the United Nations Development Progamme (UNDP) wrote in its flagship publication, *The Human Development Report*, "Policy-makers are often mesmerized by the quantity of growth. They need to be more concerned with its structure and quality." The report goes on to specify problems with economic growth: "*jobless*—where the overall economy grows but does not expand opportunities for employment," "*ruthless*—where the fruits of economic growth mostly benefit the rich, leaving millions of people struggling in ever-deepening poverty," "*voiceless*—where growth in the economy has not been accompanied by an extension of democracy or empowerment," *rootless*—which causes people's cultural identity to wither," and "*futureless*—where the present generation squanders resources needed by future generations."[30]

The UNDP report raises many concerns. One of them is to question whether (or at least how often) economic growth is good for the poor or whether the benefits are more likely to be concentrated on the rich. The basic mathematics of growth, distribution, and poverty suggests that, generally, growth should be good for the poor. Earlier in this chapter, we saw that inequality does not systematically increase with economic growth. This implies that in most cases growth should benefit the poor just as it benefits others in a society. As long as GDP grows faster than the population, average incomes within each quintile usually also increase. Numerous studies support this conclusion.

GROWTH IS GOOD FOR THE POOR

Figure 6–8 reproduces the data from one of the studies supporting the notion that growth is good for the poor.[31] This figure compares the growth in income of the poor, here defined as the bottom 20 percent of the income distribution, with overall eco-

[30]United Nations Development Programme, *Human Development Report* (New York: Oxford University Press, 1996), p. 3–4.

[31]David Dollar and Aart Kraay, "Growth Is Good for the Poor," *Journal of Economic Growth* 7, no. 3 (2002). Earlier studies that reached similar conclusions are Michael Roemer and Mary Kay Gugerty, "Does Economic Growth Reduce Poverty?" CAER Discussion Paper No. 5, Harvard Institute for International Development, Cambridge, 1997; and John Gallup, Steve Radelet, and Andrew Warner, "Economic Growth and the Income of the Poor," CAER Discussion Paper No. 36, Harvard Institute for International Development, Cambridge, 1999.

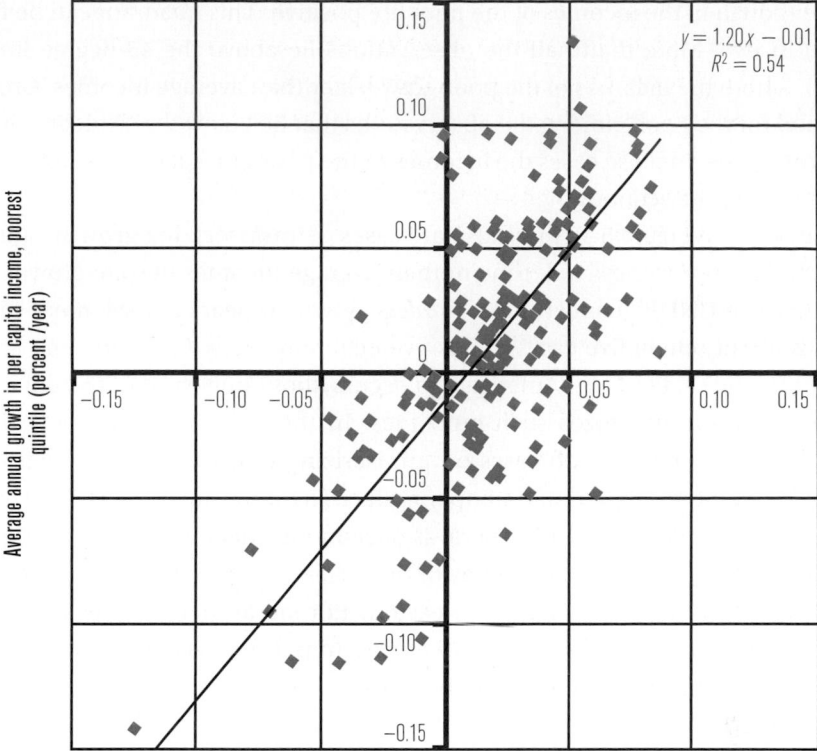

FIGURE 6-8   Is Growth Good for the Poor?

Source: David Dollar and Aart Kraay. "Growth Is Good for the Poor," *Journal of Economic Growth* 7 (September 2002). Dataset available at http://econ.worldbank.org/WBSITE/EXTERNAL/EXTDEC/0,,contentMDK :22802584~pagePK:64165401~piPK:64165026~theSitePK:469372,00.html.

nomic growth (growth in GDP per capita). Each observation refers to a growth spell of five or more years in a given country. In many cases, there is more than one observation per country. This occurs when information on the distribution of income is available for multiple years. Growth spells have a median length of six years. These spells occur between the years 1956 to 1999, with most taking place in the 1980s and 1990s. Not all countries are represented in the data set, but there is good coverage by region and for the world population as a whole.[32]

The trend shown in Figure 6–8 is consistent with the view that growth is generally good for the poor. The fitted regression line has a *positive* slope of 1.2, indicating that, *on average*, the incomes of the poor grow at a slightly higher rate than does GDP per capita. The slope of 1.2 means that if GDP per capita grows, say, at 5 percent, the regression predicts that the incomes of the poor will grow by 6 percent. Most observations lie in the quadrant in which both the growth in per capita income

[32]Departing from the original study, the Organisation for Economic Co-Operation and Development (OECD) economies are excluded from the figure, as are a few statistical outliers.

and the growth in the incomes of the poor are positive. This quadrant can be further divided in two. More than half the observations lie above the 45-degree line (not shown), where the incomes of the poor grow faster than average incomes. Growth is still "good for the poor" among the observations that lie below the 45-degree line but above the x-axis. In these cases the incomes of the poor grow at a rate somewhat less than the rest of the economy.

Returning to Figure 6–8, there also are cases of **immiserizing growth**, situations in which the poor witness a decline in their average incomes despite growth in the economy. The UNDP's concern over *ruthless* growth appears to have merit in some cases. In about one in five cases of positive economic growth, the income levels of the poor decrease. For Latin America this occurs about one-third of the time. Rapid growth, however, minimizes such outcomes. In these data, when growth is over 5 percent, there are only two cases of immiserizing growth.[33] Rapid growth seems especially good for the poor and nonpoor alike. The opposite also is true. The poor are particularly vulnerable during periods of economic decline. This is shown in the lower-left-hand quadrant, where many of the observations lie well below the regression line (a substantial number from eastern Europe and central Asia during the late 1980s and early 1990s). Although there are important exceptions, the empirical record suggests that economic growth benefits the poor more often than it leaves the poor behind.

SOMETIMES GROWTH MAY NOT BE ENOUGH

The centrality of economic growth in achieving economic development is a major theme of this textbook, as is the role of markets in achieving more rapid economic growth. But, in some situations, more than economic growth and market forces may be needed to reduce absolute poverty. First, there are the cases just identified, in which the well-being of the bottom quintile falls despite increases in GDP per capita. These are cases in which the increase in income inequality that accompanied economic growth was so large as to reverse any potential gains for the poor from rising GDP per capita. Second are cases in which, despite economic growth, too few of the poor cross the poverty line because their initial share of income is so low. This situation is not depicted by the data in Figure 6–8 because the vertical axis measures changes in the mean income of the bottom 20 percent, not changes in the head-count index or poverty gap. This makes a difference. Imagine an economy in which average incomes are low and inequality is high. If the bottom 20 percent receives only 2 to 3 percent of the total income, as they do in many countries in Latin America and southern Africa, the well-being of the poor makes little progress even if their

---

[33]The two cases are Puerto Rico (1963–69) and Singapore (1978–83).

incomes grow at the same rate as the nation's average income. If high levels of inequality further reduce the prospects for more rapid economic growth, the situation of the poor is that much worse.

A third situation is where distributional changes reduce the amount of poverty alleviation generated by economic growth. Latin America during the 1990s experienced only modest economic growth accompanied by rising income inequality. Even the modest growth that was achieved, assuming no change in inequality, would have reduced the numbers living under $2 a day by 90 million people.[34] But, because inequality increased during the 1990s, the number of people living in poverty fell by only 45 million. Poverty in Latin America would have fallen further had there been both faster growth and less inequality.

The data in Figure 6–8 report on rates of growth. But how does growth affect the *absolute amount* of income individuals in different quintiles actually receive? Even when the growth in income of the poor exceeds that of the rich, higher income quintiles usually still receive a much larger increase in absolute income. This is because a small percentage of a large number always represents much more additional income than a larger percentage of a small number. Consider the cases of Bangladesh and Mexico presented at the beginning of this chapter. If economic growth is distributionally neutral (GDP per capita rises but inequality remains the same), then for each increase of 100 taka or 100 pesos going to someone in the bottom 20 percent, someone in the top 20 percent, on average, receives roughly 450 more taka in Bangladesh and 1,500 more pesos in Mexico. In other words, even when growth is good for the poor and the number below the poverty line falls,[35] the absolute income gap between rich and poor continues to widen.

PRO-POOR GROWTH

With increasing attention paid to global poverty, captured by the MDG of cutting poverty in half by 2015, development experts frequently refer to the need for development strategies that adopt a poverty focus (Box 6–3). Sometimes this is referred to as **pro-poor growth**. This is not a well-defined term. Pro-poor growth is sometimes described as the situation in which income growth among the poor is faster than average income growth. The problem with this definition is that it favors circumstances in which the incomes of the poor grow, for example, at 3 percent while the GDP per capita grows at 2 percent over situations in which the incomes of the poor

---

[34]"Is Growth Enough?" *Latin American Economic Policies* 14 (2001).

[35]The elasticity of the poverty rate with respect to growth in GDP per capita is reported by Ravallion to be around –2 but with lots of variation. With a 95 percent confidence interval, a 2 percent rate of growth in average household income generates a 1 to 7 percent decline in the poverty rate. Martin Ravallion, "Poverty and Growth" in David Clark, ed., *The Elgar Companion to Development Studies* (Cheltenham, UK: Elgar Publishing, 2006).

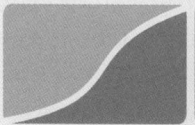

BOX 6-3 WHY SHOULD DEVELOPMENT STRATEGIES HAVE A POVERTY FOCUS?

In an interview appearing in *Finance and Development*, a journal of the International Monetary Fund, Harvard University economist Dani Rodrik makes a compelling case for reform strategies to adopt a poverty focus.

First, in considering social welfare, most people, and democratically elected governments in particular, would give more weight to the well-being of the poor than to that of the rich. The economy's growth rate is not a sufficient statistic for making welfare evaluations because it ignores not only the level of income but also its distribution. A policy that increases the income of the poor by one rupee can be worthwhile at the margin, even if it costs the rest of society more than a rupee. From this perspective, it may be entirely rational and proper for a government considering two competing growth strategies to choose the one that has a greater potential payoff for the poor, even if its impact on overall growth is less assured.

Second, even if the welfare of the poor does not receive extra weight, interventions aimed at helping the poor may still be the most effective way to raise average incomes. Poverty is naturally associated with market imperfections and incompleteness. The poor remain poor because they cannot borrow against future earnings to invest in education, skills, new crops, and entrepreneurial activities. They are cut off from economic activity because they are deprived of many collective goods (such as property rights, public safety, and infrastructure) and lack information about market opportunities. It is a standard tenet of economic theory that raising real average incomes requires interventions designed to close gaps between private and social costs. There will be a preponderance of such opportunities where there is a preponderance of poverty.

Third, focusing on poverty is also warranted from the perspective of a broader, capabilities-oriented approach to development. An exclusive focus on consumption or income levels constitutes too narrow an approach to development. As Nobel Laureate Amartya Sen has emphasized, the overarching goal of development is to maximize people's ability to lead the kind of life they value. The poor face the greatest hurdles in this area and are therefore the most deserving of urgent policy attention.

Source: Excerpt from Dani Rodrik, "Growth Versus Poverty Reduction: A Hollow Debate," *Finance and Development* 37, no. 4 (December 2000). Reprinted by permission of the International Monetary Fund.

grow at 4 percent while the GDP per capita grows at 6 percent, even though more rapid poverty reduction would occur in the latter case. This is not a hypothetical distinction; China's experience reflects the second scenario. An alternative and more general definition of pro-poor growth is economic growth that includes any growth in the incomes of the poor.

While not well-defined, at least the intentions of pro-poor growth are clear. What can governments do to achieve economic growth that rapidly improves the well-being of the poor? Answers lie in better understanding the complex interactions among growth, inequality, and poverty. Pro-poor growth does not represent a choice between being pro-growth and being pro-poor. The strategy calls for combining more rapid growth with increased opportunities for the poor to participate in that growth. Policies that both accelerate growth and address inequality may be needed to achieve these goals.

Those who question whether growth is good for the poor may also be skeptical about the ability of markets to help poor people. Competition may be seen as exploiting poor people, by paying them too little for their labor or by charging too much for the inputs they purchase or the goods they buy. Policies associated with the Washington Consensus are often viewed critically as protecting the interests of rich countries or rich citizens in poor nations at the expense of the masses of poor people in low- and middle-income countries. But are these criticisms valid? Can market-friendly strategies serve the interests of the poor?

Consider China's experience. Before 1980, China's farm system was dominated by collectives and communes. Market forces played little role in the allocation of farm inputs or in returns to agricultural work. Market reforms under the household responsibility system changed everything. It transferred control (but not ownership) over farmland to individual farmers. After meeting output quotas to the state, farmers were free to keep or sell additional output on relatively open markets. The unleashing of personal incentives resulted in a massive supply response and lifted hundreds of millions of Chinese peasants out of poverty. This outcome was supported by a relatively equal distribution of land, which occurred after the breakup of the communes. Low inequality in access to farmland was essential for the pro-poor growth that followed.[36]

Macroeconomic stability and economic openness are major elements of the Washington Consensus. What impact do these policies have on the poor? Maintaining fiscal discipline and reducing price inflation are key features of macroeconomic stability. Such stability usually entails reducing budget deficits, achieved by cutting government expenditures. This in turn often brings forth protests that the poor are hurt by reduced government spending on basic services. There can be considerable truth to such concerns, but it is not the whole picture. Government spending frequently fails to reach the poor, as programs, including those on health and education, often are targeted at higher income quintiles.

Maintaining unsustainable budget deficits also leads to price inflation, which tends to hurt the poor much more than the rich. Higher income individuals have ways to avoid the negative consequences of rapid price inflation. They can send

---

[36]Martin Ravallion, "A Comparative Perspective on Poverty Reduction in Brazil, China and India," *World Bank Research Observer* 26, no. 1 (2011).

their savings abroad or hold their wealth in land or real estate, which often are a hedge against inflation. But the poor lack these options. What minimal savings they have can disappear under persistent price inflation, the costs of even their minimal borrowing escalate, and any type of fixed income, like a pension, for example, soon becomes relatively worthless. Price inflation usually leads to the depreciation of the currency, which raises the price of imported goods, including fuel and other essential commodities. When fuel prices go up, transportation costs increase, affecting many items the poor depend on. Price inflation also acts like a brake on investment and economic growth, and slower economic growth is not in the interests of the poor. Overall, macroeconomic stability tends to be good for both economic growth and the poor.

Trade liberalization and greater economic openness entail reducing trade barriers, encouraging foreign direct investment and freeing up exchange rates. Anti-globalization advocates see such measures as hurting the poor, who cannot protect themselves from the vagaries of world capital markets or the onslaught of cheap exports. Once again, there is merit to this position in some circumstances. The Asian financial crisis of the late 1990s hurt both the rich and the poor in many economies. Cheap crops, the result (in part) of farm subsidies in the European Union and the United States, hurt farmers in some economies. Cotton growers in West Africa are often cited as an example.

But there is another side to increased economic openness. If nations export goods in which they have a comparative advantage, many low-income nations specialize in goods that rely on unskilled labor. This leads to an increase in the employment of such workers and, over time, to an increase in their wages. Because poverty is likely to be common among the least skilled, trade increases labor demand and reduces poverty. Greater openness, including the exchange of technology and the capital accumulation that results from foreign direct investment, can improve productivity and raise overall economic growth. In addition, trade may also reduce the prices the poor must pay for goods and services, further improving their welfare.

The textbook case for trade is compelling, and the success in poverty reduction throughout East Asia often identifies trade, especially exports of labor-intensive manufactured products, as an engine of growth. But there is more to economic openness than increasing exports, and a full account of the impact of globalization on poverty does not yield one simple conclusion. Trade reform can help some of the poor while hurting others. In Mexico, the North American Free Trade Agreement (NAFTA) brought more liberalized trade, which hurt farmers who previously were protected by tariffs on corn at the same time that it helped those who found employment in the growing export sector. (See Chapters 18 and 19 for a fuller account of the impact of trade on growth, development, and poverty.) Trade reforms illustrate an important principle: Market forces create new opportunities that benefit some and hurt others. Helping the poor get the most out of new opportunities is a challenge facing all economies.

IMPROVING OPPORTUNITIES FOR THE POOR

Improving the operation of markets helps the poor only if they can take advantage of these opportunities. This is why expanding basic education and health services is often a main element of strategies to reduce poverty. Education tends to make people more productive. It permits them to access new information and helps them take advantage of new opportunities, from new seed varieties that increase farm yields to new jobs that require the ability to read and write and new medicines that increase child survival or improve adult health. Education is not, however, a panacea. In a bad economic environment, education can yield a low return (see Chapter 8). But without an education, many of the poor may get trapped in intergenerational cycles of poverty. Similar arguments can be made for the importance of basic health (see Chapter 9). The debilitating effects of a host of diseases, including malaria and HIV/AIDS, prevent those who are infected from engaging in work and seizing new opportunities. No matter how well markets work, if someone is too sick to take advantage of such opportunities, poverty persists.

Investing in education and health—that is, in the human capital of the poor—is part of an agenda for improving the opportunities of the poor. Other reforms also warrant consideration. Most of the poor live in rural areas and either directly or indirectly depend on agriculture as a source of income. Studies of India find that growth in the rural economy alleviates both rural and urban poverty, whereas urban growth primarily reduces only urban poverty.[37] Supporting the rural economy is not something governments in low- and middle-income nations always do. More attention needs to be paid to rural infrastructure, including better roads and telecommunications, so that poor farmers can more easily market their crops and obtain information about prices. Tube wells for safe drinking water, improved irrigation, agriculture extension services, research and development on crop varieties, and expanded access to credit are other interventions that can contribute to the improved performance of the rural economy and a decline in rural poverty (see Chapters 16 and 17 for further discussion of agricultural development and its impact on the poor.)

Spending more on the poor, whether on their education or healthcare, on the infrastructure on which they depend, or in the rural economy where most of the poor live, means spending less on other groups in society. Reforming the allocation of government expenditures can be both pro-poor and pro-growth. But it is bound to encounter resistance as interest groups act to maintain government expenditures they have come to expect. Even more controversial are proposals to redistribute assets, most often land, to the poor.

Explanations for the economic growth and success at poverty alleviation among East Asian countries, including China, Korea, and Taiwan, often point to the role

---

[37]Martin Ravallion and Gaurav Datt, "Why Has Economic Growth Been More Pro-Poor in Some States of India than Others?" *Journal of Development Economics* 68 (2002).

played by earlier policies of land redistribution. These were fairly radical interventions that included the expropriation of land by the state with minimal or no compensation to owners. Land reforms in East Asia occurred during times of extreme political upheaval, whether social revolution in China or the end of foreign occupation in Korea. Despite the ultimate success of these economies and the role redistribution of agricultural land played in these nations' subsequent economic development, land reforms and other types of asset redistribution receive less support today. They often are seen as politically difficult, if not unfeasible, by both national governments and multilateral institutions like the International Monetary Fund and World Bank. Land reforms also have gone badly in many countries. Zimbabwe's land reform is but one element of the destructive actions taken by the government of Robert Mugabe that turned Zimbabwe from a net food exporter into a nation dependent on food aid. Zimbabwe's experience is an extreme example; it demonstrates that solely redistributing assets offers little promise of alleviating poverty. A much broader set of complementary policies is needed to permit the poor to take advantage of any increase in their assets. But even when such policies are in place, asset redistribution is often politically too difficult to play much of a role in a pro-poor growth strategy.

INCOME TRANSFERS AND SAFETY NETS

Every nation has individuals who are poor because they lack economic opportunity or are beyond the reach of the market. The latter include those who are too old, too young, or too sick to work and are without family networks to care for them. There are also situations in which systemic shocks, whether due to natural catastrophes or economic crises, require government action because the marketplace cannot resolve them.

Situations of chronic poverty tend to call for income transfers. These may take the form of cash grants or food pricing/distribution programs. The challenge facing all such programs is making them cost effective and having them reach the target population and not "leak" to higher-income groups. Food price subsidies, for example, aid the poor but also subsidize the purchases of the nonpoor. The net result can be an unsustainable fiscal burden on the budget.

Conditional cash transfers (CCTs) increasingly are employed in all regions to address both current and future poverty. These programs provide cash payments to eligible households and in return families must satisfy program goals, usually enrolling children in school and requiring them to attend at least 80 to 85 percent of school days. Some CCTs also require families to visit health clinics for periodic checkups, vaccinations of young children, prenatal care for expecting mothers, and other services. Cash payments address current poverty. By encouraging school enrollment and better healthcare, the programs simultaneously increase the human capital of children with the goal of reducing the transmission of poverty from one generation to the next.

Two of the most well known programs are Bolsa Familia Program (family allowance) in Brazil and Oportunidades (opportunities) in Mexico (originally called PROGRESA: Programa de Educación, Salud y Alimentación). Oportunidades uses geographic targeting based on census data to identify the poorest rural areas and urban blocks. It then uses household surveys on income and assets ("Do you have a dirt or cement floor?" "Do you own a hot-water heater?") in the identified areas to direct benefits to eligible households. This approach reduces the leakage of program benefits to the nonpoor. Transfers are made to the female head of a household (usually the mother, but sometimes a grandmother), consistent with evidence that women are more likely than men to spend financial resources on their children and to improve the well-being of their families. Banks rather than government agencies handle the transfer of funds to individual recipients, reducing the number of intermediaries involved and cutting down on corruption. A high percentage of the program's budget goes directly to beneficiaries who spend the money on local businesses, often small in scale and located within the poor Mexican communities where recipients live. From its inception, Oportunidades set up systems for data collection and rigorous program evaluation so that the impact of CCTs could be determined and verified.[38]

Bolsa Familia offers eligible households about $13 a month per child, helping to lift many families above Brazil's poverty line. The program has been especially effective in rural areas but somewhat less so in urban ones, where costs are higher and the $13 does not go as far. Problems of drug addiction, violence, child labor, and family breakdown also compound the causes of income poverty in urban areas. Bolsa Familia today covers families representing almost 50 million Brazilians, about one quarter of the population, but the aggregate cost is small, about 0.5 percent of Brazil's GDP and 2.5 percent of total government expenditures. This modest amount is seen as having played a role in reducing poverty *and* inequality in Brazil.

Social safety nets are similar to income transfers but, in their design, recognize that household poverty often is transitory rather than chronic. Panel data that trace individuals or households over time find that there are fewer families who are always poor than there are families who are poor some of the time. This outcome is true in low- and middle-income economies as well as in high-income settings. The transitory nature of poverty does not minimize the hardship families endure nor does it imply that those living on amounts just over a nation's poverty line are satisfying their material needs. But it does recommend designing policies that help individuals and households when income and consumption shortfalls occur, not in a permanent fashion. Public employment schemes are one example.

---

[38]Because of the linkage with schooling, we discuss CCTs again in Chapter 8; see especially Box 8–3. A comprehensive review of CCTs is provided by Ariel Fiszbein and Norbert Schady, *Conditional Cash Transfers: Reducing Present and Future Poverty* (Washington, DC: World Bank, 2009).

The Employment Guarantee Scheme (EGS) in the Indian state of Maharashtra and the Trabajar program in Argentina were designed to ensure poor people a source of income and reduce the variability of their incomes. The EGS guarantees employment within a few weeks of the individual's request and provides a job relatively close to a person's home. These jobs involve public works, such as road construction and repair, irrigation systems, and prevention of soil erosion. To solve the targeting problem, wages in public employment schemes must be kept low relative to market alternatives. By offering the prevailing market wage for unskilled rural labor, EGS encourages self-targeting, which increases the likelihood that those who choose to participate are individuals the program is intended to benefit. This maintains the cost-effectiveness of the scheme by minimizing the number of nonpoor people seeking these jobs. There also is a ceiling on the number of days per year such employment will be available.

To encourage self-targeting, Trabajar in Argentina offered a monthly wage set at 75 percent of the average monthly earnings of workers in the bottom 10 percent of households living in and around Buenos Aires. Evaluation of these public employment schemes finds that they were well used and well targeted. ESG provides about 100 million person-days of employment, varying both by season and by year. Participation falls during the busy season in agriculture, confirming that poor families use the program to counter the variability in monthly incomes. The majority of participants in the ESG and Trabajar programs were from the lowest income deciles. Participants realized significant increases in their incomes, lifting many above poverty.[39] The experience with ESG is one of the reasons why India launched a similar nationwide initiative, the Mahatma Gandhi National Rural Employment Guarantee Act, which promises up to 100 days of unskilled manual labor on rural public works projects per family per year. Pay is equal to the official minimum wage rate for agricultural labor.

GLOBAL INEQUALITY AND THE END OF POVERTY

Our discussion of inequality and poverty reduction has so far focused on nations. We looked carefully at levels and trends in inequality within nations and pro-poor policies that governments might pursue. Most policy making occurs at a national level, so this focus is warranted. But there also is a global dimension to issues of inequality and poverty. The gap between rich and poor across countries tends to be greater than it is within most nations. Should anything be done to change this outcome? Is

---

[39]World Bank, "Principles of Successful Workfare Programs," *World Development Report 2000/2001: Attacking Poverty* (Washington, DC: World Bank, 2001), Box 8.9.

reducing world poverty a global goal? Is there a role for actions that go beyond the nation-state? There is considerable debate over the answers to these questions.

A simple way of portraying global inequality is to divide the world into the high- versus low- and middle-income economies. In 2010, the high-income nations accounted for 16 percent of world population and consumed 55 percent of world output. The low- and middle-income nations represented the rest: 84 percent of world population and 45 percent of world output. This level of global inequality is comparable to that in Brazil and South Africa, two of the world's most unequal nations. This degree of global inequality is not a recent outcome. About 30 years ago the results were similar: in 1980 the high-income nations represented 18 percent of world population and consumed 62 percent of world output.[40] This simple division of the world provides a fairly reliable snapshot of global inequality, but it ignores important differences between countries within each of these groups. In addition, not everyone in a high-income economy is rich, nor is everyone in a low-income nation poor. To resolve these problems, three measures often are used in debates over whether the world is becoming a more equal or unequal place.

One approach is to define **international inequality** by comparing average incomes across countries. For some questions, it is appropriate to rely on this method. For example, the convergence debate, discussed in Chapter 4, asks whether there is a tendency for the income levels across nations to converge over time. Comparing mean incomes is warranted here. This approach treats each of the world's nations equally, whether the Caribbean nation of Dominica, with a population of about 75,000, or China with more than 1.3 billion people. But for a discussion of human welfare, treating each nation the same without regard to its population seems less warranted. An alternative index of international inequality is to weight each nation's mean income by its population. A population-weighted measure of international inequality is better suited for some questions but still leaves a key issue unresolved. By multiplying the average level of income by population, no account is taken of the domestic distribution of income; everyone in China or Dominica is assumed to have the same income as everyone else in the nation. To avoid this problem, one needs a measure of global inequality that compares the income or consumption of each individual regardless of where that person lives. Such a measure describes inequality among all individuals, not just among all nations. It is not surprising that the level of inequality and its trend varies according to which of these definitions is employed.

Figure 6–9 compares two estimates of international inequality, one weighted and the other unweighted by population, from 1961 to 2008. Gini coefficients are

---

[40]The share of world output refers to gross national income (GNI) measured in terms of PPP. If GNI is measured at market exchange rates, the high-income nations' share of GNI was closer to 80 percent in 1980 and 70 percent in 2010.

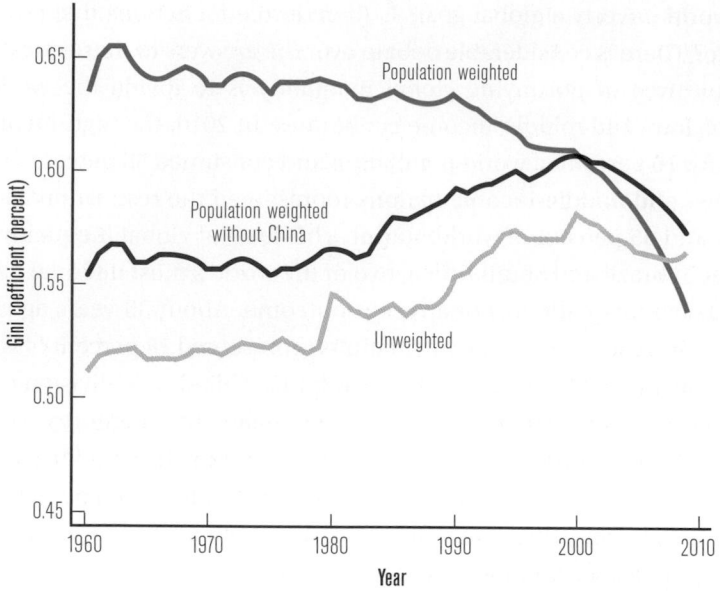

FIGURE 6-9 **Trends in International Inequality, 1961–2008**

Source: Figure 1 from The International Bank for Reconstruction and Development. The World Bank: *Policy Research Working Paper 5061* by Branko Milanovic, 2009. Reprinted with permission.

estimated annually for each of these series.[41] The unweighted trend (counting each country the same) shows little systematic change until the early 1980s, after which there is an almost continuous rise in inequality until 2000, when it begins to decline. The weighted series (giving larger countries more influence) shows something different. First, it suggests a higher level of inequality until the very end of the series. Second, the time trend never systematically rises and starts to decrease earlier and more rapidly, beginning around 1990.

The differences in trends between the two series are easy to explain. The rise in the unweighted measure of international inequality between 1980 and 2000 reflects the regional growth trends we first encountered in Chapter 2. The 1980s were a "lost decade" for Latin America, with debt crises followed by economic stagnation and decline. In the 1990s, the transition experience in eastern Europe and central Asia was accompanied by steep declines in income. These reversals of fortune contrast with positive growth in the high-income economies and parts of Asia and account for rising international inequality. Decreasing international inequality in the 2000s is evidence of faster growth in most low- and middle-income economies.

[41]Much of this discussion of trends in global inequality draws from Branko Milanovic, *Worlds Apart: Measuring International and Global Inequality* (Princeton, NJ: Princeton University Press, 2005); and Branko Milanovic, "Global Inequality Recalculated: The Effect of New 2005 PPP Estimates on Global Inequality," Policy Research Working Paper 5061 World Bank, Washington, DC, September 2009.

The population-weighted measure of international inequality shows a different trend. For four decades, the measure declined, picking up speed after 1990. Given the construction of this measure, what happened in heavily populated nations drives the outcome. China's experience explains much of the observed trend. This is evident when one compares the population-weighted trend in Figure 6–9 that includes China versus the one that excludes it. China's post-1978 economic transformation quickly moved the nation from low- to middle-income status. This closed some of the gap between China and the high-income nations, especially the heavily populated United States, but increased the income gap between China and the remaining low-income nations. On net, the Chinese population's move toward the middle of the world distribution of income resulted in a significant decline in the population-weighted Gini ratio. Rapid growth since 2000 in India, another heavily populated nation, accounts for the decrease in the population-weighted trend in international inequality excluding China. Rapid income growth in China and India helps explain why by 2008 the population-weighted measure finally falls below the unweighted measure.

Population-weighted international inequality assigns all citizens within a nation the same level of per capita income or consumption—that is, it assumes "perfect income equality" within every nation. This is a poor assumption for measuring inequality for the world's population. Correcting this problem requires more than data on GDP per capita and population size. Household-level data are needed to assign a more precise estimate of income levels to every person in the world and to compute what might be called global inequality. There is considerable variance in the level of global inequality predicted by various studies and no consensus on trends in recent decades. But what all these studies show is that global inequality is significantly higher than population-weighted international inequality. Estimates of global Gini coefficients range from about 0.60 to 0.80.[42] China, India, and the United States, the three most populous nations in the world, contribute significantly to this level of inequality. In recent decades, all three have had economic growth accompanied by rising domestic Gini coefficients.

Measured this way, global inequality at the beginning of the twenty-first century exceeds the level of inequality of almost any nation in the world. It should come as no surprise that the world is a very unequal place, but the *degree* of inequality is striking. Your response to the evidence on the degree of global inequality may be, "Something should be done about this!" If it is, it is important to be clear on the nature of the problems created by global inequality that you wish to resolve.

Consider the following: Global inequality would be lower if, all else equal, economic growth in high-income economies were slower. Some may be in favor of slower economic growth in the United States and elsewhere, but their reasons

---

[42]Reviews of alternative studies can be found in Branko Milanovic, *Worlds Apart: Measuring International and Global Inequality* (Princeton, NJ: Princeton University Press, 2005), 119–27; and in World Bank, *World Development Report 2006: Equity and Development* (Washington, DC: World Bank, 2006), chap. 9.

may have little to do with global inequality or with the well-being of people in poor nations. You may reject the relentless consumerism of the United States. Americans buy ever-larger houses, fill them with a seemingly endless supply of goods, and drive bigger vehicles on increasingly congested roads. There is much in the life-styles and consumption habits of high-income economies to criticize. But slower economic growth in rich nations, even if it led to lower global inequality, might have an adverse impact on low- and middle-income nations. If rich nations grew more slowly, their demand for goods from other nations would fall, affecting these nations' growth rates. Global inequality brought about by slower growth in high-income economies could prove a detriment to progress in reducing global poverty. There is no reason to believe that if the United States grew more slowly, Africa or some other poor region would grow more quickly. In all likelihood, the opposite would be true.

There are many ways in which global inequality could be lower today. What if income inequality in China had not risen over the past 20 years? Remember that China has had an exceptionally high growth rate for more than two decades and has been able to lift over 400 million of its citizens above the $1.25-a-day poverty line. China's economic miracle also contributed to reducing global inequality, but the effect would have been even greater if income inequality within China had not risen. Could China have grown rapidly, dramatically reduced poverty, *and* kept its level of inequality from rising? We really do not know because we cannot observe the coun-terfactual. But there is some chance that lower inequality within China might have required slower economic growth.

Calls for reducing global inequality may be misplaced unless proper consider-ation is taken of how greater equality might be achieved. Even before considering how to achieve greater global equality, the question of why to do so remains. We have encountered some of these arguments before on a national level and some are also applicable on a global level. First, on the grounds of economic efficiency, the con-centration of world incomes may lower productivity growth. Market failures limit poor people from borrowing to finance worthwhile projects, and some redistribution of income could increase the return on total global investments. Second, it may be in the self-interest of higher-income households, wherever they may live, to support redistribution. Health risks, for example, cross borders faster than in the past. The rapid transmission of HIV/AIDS across continents is one example. A redistribution of world resources might mitigate the health risks facing both the poor and the rich. Another reason why it may be in the interest of high-income households to favor greater global equality is that, in an information age, people around the world are aware of the gap between rich and poor. This knowledge and frustration over feeling left out may play a destabilizing role in international affairs, affecting the interests of the rich as well as the poor. Third, a more equitable distribution may be the right goal to strive for on moral grounds. Philosophers since Plato have been writing about this subject. Especially given the size of the income gap between those on the top versus those on the bottom, global inequality should be seen as an opportunity to address the absolute poverty that has been a central focus of this chapter.

If those in higher income quintiles are averse to high levels of inequality and willing to move toward a world of less poverty and greater equality of incomes and opportunities, what might they do? Columbia University economist Jeffrey Sachs offers both a diagnosis and a blueprint. In his book *The End of Poverty*, he writes,

> The greatest tragedy of our time is that about one sixth of humanity is not even on the development ladder. A large number of the extreme poor are caught in a poverty trap, unable on their own to escape from extreme material deprivation. They are trapped by disease, physical isolation, climate stress, environmental degradation, and by extreme poverty itself. Even though life-saving solutions exist to increase their chances for survival—whether in the form of new farming techniques, or essential medicines, or bed nets that can limit the transmission of malaria—these families and their governments simply lack the financial means to make these critical investments. The world's poor know about the development ladder: they are tantalized by images of affluence from halfway around the world. But they are not able to get a first foothold on the ladder, and so cannot even begin the climb out of poverty.[43]

Sachs proposes a global compact to end absolute poverty by 2025. As with any compact there are at least two parties: poor countries and rich ones. Poor countries are to be held accountable for their efforts to reduce poverty. Corrupt regimes and those that pursue war rather than development cannot be part of this compact. Sachs makes it clear, however, that even among low- and middle-income nations that sign onto the compact, their actions alone may not be enough to end poverty. Conditions in parts of Africa are so dire that many of the poor, lacking the basics of food, clean water, medicines, and healthcare facilities, are, in Sachs's words, "too poor to stay alive."

Given the degree of absolute poverty in the world, there is a need for rich nations to do more to alleviate poverty. Some of Sachs's suggestions meet with wide support among development economists: the need for rich countries to keep their markets open to exports from poor nations and the need for rich nations to invest in global public goods, such as basic science on combating tropical diseases and improving agricultural yields. Other elements of his global compact are more controversial: the need for better environmental stewardship by the rich nations to minimize the impact of climate change on poor nations, the need for debt forgiveness of the accumulated international debts of poor nations owed to multilateral institutions like the IMF and World Bank, and the need for a significant increase in the foreign aid from rich nations to poor ones. We explore these ideas in later chapters. Despite

---

[43]Jeffrey Sachs, *The End of Poverty: Economic Possibilities for Our Time* (New York: Penguin Press, 2005), p. 19–20.

disagreement about elements of this global compact to end poverty, it is hard to argue against one of its central ideas: Rich nations have a critical role to play in reducing global poverty.

SUMMARY

- The number of people in poverty in a given country depends on both the level of per capita income or consumption and its distribution. Distributional outcomes are described using size distributions, which report inequality in terms of shares going to each population quintile ranked from poorest to richest; the Lorenz curve, which offers a geometric portrait of inequality; and the Gini coefficient, which provides a single summary statistic.

- Income and consumption inequality exhibits significant regional variation. Latin America and sub-Saharan Africa have relatively high levels of inequality; eastern Europe and central Asia, South Asia, and the high-income economies generally have low levels; and inequality in East Asia generally falls in the medium range. These regional patterns seem to have less to do with the *level* of per capita income than with underlying historical and political determinants as well as factor endowments.

- According to World Bank studies, in 2005 nearly 1.4 billion people, representing 25 percent of the developing world's population, lived below the international poverty line of $1.25 a day, sometimes referred to as *absolute poverty* or *extreme poverty*. The number of people living in absolute poverty declined by 520 million between 1981 and 2005. Most of this decline happened in East Asia, especially in China. With generally strong economic growth in many low- and middle-income economies since 2005, absolute poverty probably has declined since then.

- Because world population grew significantly from 1981 to 2005, success at poverty reduction can also be measured in relative terms. Estimates of the head-count index suggest that the incidence of poverty fell significantly in East and South Asia. In sub-Saharan Africa, the level remained at over 50 percent. Most of the world's poor still live in East and South Asia, although both the poverty rate (head-count index) and the severity of poverty (poverty gap) are highest in sub-Saharan Africa.

- Poverty tends to be greater in rural than in urban areas. Racial and ethnic minorities often face higher poverty rates. Women are discriminated against throughout the world. They earn lower wages on average, often are denied inheritance or the right to own land, and traditionally have received less education than men. However, because household resources tend to be shared as a result of intra-household distribution decisions, there is less evidence that income poverty rates for women are higher than for men.

- Empirical studies confirm that economic growth tends to be good for the poor. Across countries, the incomes of the bottom 20 percent grew at the same rate as GDP per capita. This is an average tendency, and in some cases and in some time periods, the average income of the poorest quintile *fell* despite increases in GDP per capita.

- *Pro-poor growth* refers to a development strategy that combines more rapid economic growth with increased opportunities for the poor to participate in the economy. Many economists believe that market-friendly policies, including maintaining fiscal discipline, reducing price inflation, and increasing economic openness, serve the interests of the poor. But these interventions alone are not enough; some of the poor will benefit and others will be hurt.

- Growth strategies designed to include the poor may have the greatest potential to promote pro-poor growth. Because poverty tends to be disproportionately rural, growth strategies that include agricultural development may be particularly important to pursue.

- Governments must also invest in the education and health of the poor and in the infrastructure on which the poor rely. Conditional cash transfer programs, such as Bolsa Familia in Brazil and Oportunidades in Mexico, have proven cost-effective in reducing current poverty and making investments in children that should reduce future poverty. Social safety nets, such as guaranteed employment schemes, are designed for those temporarily unable to take advantage of the opportunities markets provide.

- Just as we can measure inequality within nations, it is possible to estimate the degree of global inequality. The most comprehensive measure of global inequality compares the income (or consumption) of each individual regardless of where that person lives. Estimates of this measure report Gini coefficients of global inequality of 0.60 to 0.80, values higher than for almost any single nation. Given both the level of absolute poverty in the world and the degree of global income inequality, it is important to consider the steps rich nations can take to help poor nations.

7

Population

n 1973, marking the completion of his first term as president of the World Bank, Robert McNamara wrote *One Hundred Countries, Two Billion People,* which brings together his basic views on economic development. There is no ambiguity about McNamara's beliefs. He writes, "The greatest single obstacle to the economic and social advancement of the majority of the peoples in the underdeveloped world is rampant population growth."[1]

Before coming to the World Bank, McNamara was a professor at the Harvard Business School, president of the Ford Motor Company, and secretary of defense in the Kennedy and Johnson administrations. A man of incredible intellectual reach, McNamara understood much about the role of capital accumulation and technological change and their contributions to economic growth. But he maintained the view that rapid population growth was a threat that would have "catastrophic consequences" unless dealt with. "The underdeveloped world needs investment capital for a whole gamut of productive projects, but nothing would be more unwise than to allow these projects to fail because they are finally overwhelmed by a tidal wave of population."[2]

The "Two Billion People" in the title of McNamara's book refers to the early 1960s when the world's population was close to 3 billion, with 2 billion, or about two-thirds of the total, living in the developing nations. Since then the world has grown,

[1]Robert McNamara, *One Hundred Countries, Two Billion People* (New York: Praeger, 1973), p. 31.
[2]MacNamara, *One Hundred Countries,* p. 31.

reaching 7 billion in 2011. Over 5.8 billion of these people reside in low- and middle-income economies.

Despite this massive increase in numbers of people, the views of James Wolfensohn, World Bank president from 1995 to 2005, could not be more different from those of his predecessor. Wolfensohn's speeches and publications reveal only limited reference to population growth. Most often these references indicate how population growth exacerbates another problem, whether improving access to clean water or making a dent in the numbers suffering from absolute poverty. The same is true for Wolfensohn's successor, Robert Zoellick. After his first 100 days in office, Zoellick delivered a speech identifying six strategic themes to meet global challenges. Reducing population was not one of them; in fact, "population growth" is not mentioned even once.[3]

Was McNamara unnecessarily alarmist? Or did Wolfensohn and Zoellick make irreversible mistakes by not focusing on rising population numbers? Was the United Nations similarly wrong in not including reductions in population growth as one of the original millennium development goals (MDGs; introduced in Chapter 2)? We begin to address these questions by reviewing the world's population history and exploring the demographic transition that has characterized today's high-income nations and increasingly the low- and middle-income nations as well. We also consider population projections for the future before turning our attention to the complex relationship between population growth and economic development. This relationship is viewed both at an aggregate level and at the level of individual families making decisions about how many children to have. We conclude by reviewing the options nations face in pursuing policies to limit the size of their populations.

A BRIEF HISTORY OF WORLD POPULATION

Anthropologists debate when our first ancestors appeared. For our purposes, we do not have to go that far back in time. We might begin at the end of the last Ice Age, about 13,000 years ago, when humans on all continents were still living as hunter–gatherers, or 12,000 years ago with the first signs of agricultural settlements, or 7,000 years ago with the first indications of urbanization. For most of the thousands of years since then, population growth has been close to zero, with annual births roughly offsetting annual deaths. Opportunities for human survival slowly improved, and by 1 C.E. the world's population is estimated at about 230 million.[4] To gain some perspective on this number, today Indonesia by itself has a population that size.

---

[3]Robert Zoellick, "An Inclusive & Sustainable Globalization," speech to the National Press Club, Washington, DC, October 10, 2007.

[4]Angus Maddison, *The World Economy: Historical Statistics* (Paris: Development Centre of the Organisation for Economic Co-operation and Development, 2003).

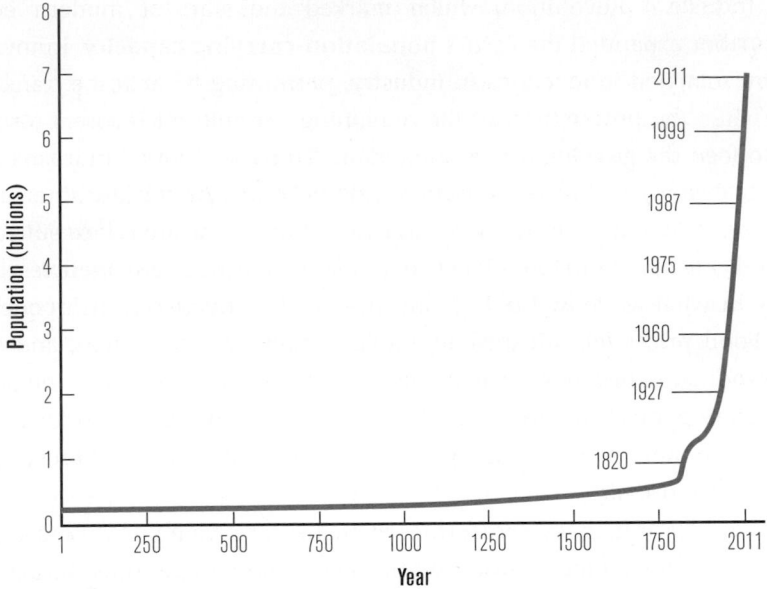

FIGURE 7-1   World Population Growth through History: Years Needed to Add 1 Billion More People

Source: Angus Maddison, "Statistics on World Population, GDP, and Per Capita GDP, 1–2008 AD," www.ggdc
.net/MADDISON/Historical_Statistics/vertical-file_02-2010.xls.

Figure 7-1 charts world population from 1 C.E. through 2011. The figure makes it abundantly clear that population growth is a recent and unprecedented event in human history. From the beginning of human settlements, it took more than 10,000 years for the world's population to reach 1 billion in 1820. But the next billion were added in only about 110 years and, for the last four decades, the world added 1 billion people every 12 to 15 years. No wonder McNamara was so worried.

We have a broad understanding of how world population went from a period of relatively small and stable population numbers to the 7 billion (and still growing) that inhabit the planet today. The introduction of settled agriculture revolutionized the earth's capacity to sustain human life. During the years leading up to the Industrial Revolution of the late eighteenth and early nineteenth centuries, the food supply grew and became more reliable. The death rate fell, life expectancy increased, and population growth gradually accelerated. This growth, however, was set back at intervals by famines, plagues, and wars, any of which could wipe out as much as half of the population in a given area. As late as the fourteenth century, the black death (bubonic plague) killed one-third of the population of Europe. Despite these catastrophic events, by 1800, the world's population had grown to almost 1 billion, implying an annual growth rate of a mere 0.08 percent between 1 C.E. and 1800.

The Industrial Revolution, which marked the start of modern economic growth, further expanded the earth's **population-carrying capacity**. Innovations in agriculture matched innovations in industry, permitting labor to be transferred to industry while the productivity of the remaining agricultural laborers rose quickly enough to feed the growing urban population. Transcontinental railroads and fast, reliable ocean shipping further boosted world food output in the late nineteenth century, making it possible to grow more basic foodstuffs in the areas best suited for this activity and get supplies to food-deficit areas in record time in emergencies. Famines, especially in what are now the high-income nations, decreased in frequency and severity. Food prices fell. Meanwhile, modern medicine, sanitation, and pharmaceutical production began to develop. All these factors helped reduce the death rate and accelerate population growth. By 1945, the population of the world was slightly less than 2.5 billion, meaning that global population grew by 0.6 percent per year between 1800 and 1945.

After World War II, there were further dramatic improvements in food supply and disease control. Techniques introduced in the developed countries during the preceding era spread throughout the globe. The result was a veritable revolution in falling death rates and rising life expectancy in both the developed and the developing world. Plummeting death rates in many areas raised population growth rates to levels the world had never known before. Reference to a worldwide **population explosion**, unthinkable for most of human history, became commonplace in the 1960s and 1970s as the world's population grew to 3 and then 4 billion. World population passed 5 billion in 1987, 6 billion in 1999, and 7 billion early this decade; almost all this growth has occurred in the developing countries. Between 1945 and 2009, the growth in world population averaged a historically unprecedented rate of 1.6 percent per annum, twenty times faster than the estimated 0.08 percent between 1 C.E. and 1800.

THE DEMOGRAPHIC TRANSITION

The relationship between annual births and deaths determines population growth. Figure 7–2 depicts the basic stages in the **demographic transition** in a now-developed nation, Finland. Finland's experience is typical of what most high-income countries have experienced over the past several centuries. The top line in Panel a refers to the **crude birth rate**, the number of live births per year per 1,000 people. The lower line refers to the **crude death rate**, the number of deaths per year also per 1,000 people. The difference between these two rates, the excess of births over deaths, is the rate of **natural increase** in the population, which often is expressed as a percentage. For the world as a whole, the natural increase in the population equals the population growth rate; for an individual country, population growth is the difference between the rate of natural increase and net migration.

For hundreds of years before the eighteenth century, Finland was in the first stage of the classic demographic transition. High birth rates were matched by high death rates and the natural increase in population was close to zero. In some years,

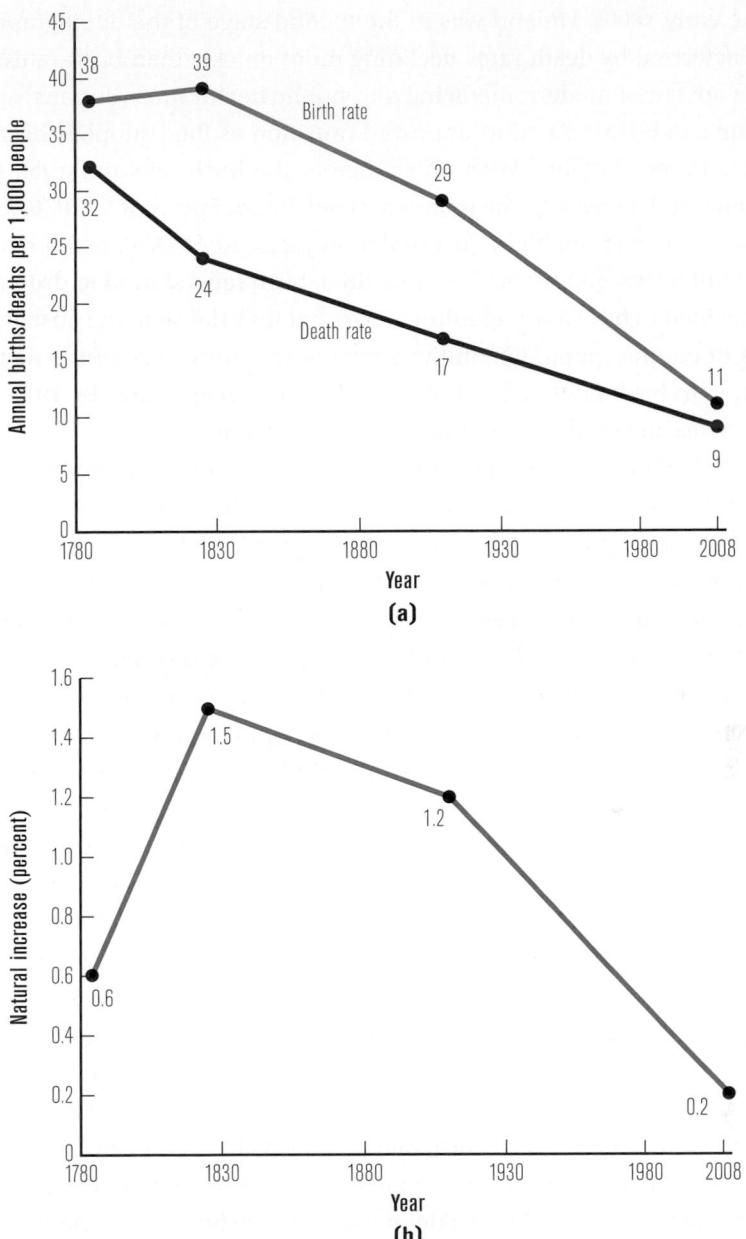

FIGURE 7-2 Demographic Transition for Finland (1785–2008)

Source: Arthur Haupt, Thomas Kane, and Carl Haub, *PRB's Population Handbook* 6th edition (Washington, DC: Population Reference Bureau, 2011).

births exceeded deaths; in other years, the opposite occurred. By 1785, before the start of industrialization and the first year for which data are available, Finland still had high birth and death rates, but the gap between the two resulted in a 0.6 percent rate of natural increase. If this rate had been maintained, it would have taken 117 years for Finland's population to double.

By the early 1800s, Finland was in the second stage of the demographic transition, characterized by death rates declining more quickly than birth rates. This was before the advent of modern medicine and public health interventions; so much of this decline can be attributed to improved nutrition as food supplies became more abundant and less variable. With no change in the birth rate and a fall in deaths, the rate of natural increase in the population reached 1.5 percent by 1830. At this rate, the population would double in just under 50 years. After 1830, death rates continued to fall but not as quickly. At the same time, birth rates started to drop as Finnish families decided to have fewer children. Note that they did so in the absence of modern forms of contraception. Finland was now in the third stage of the demographic transition, with birth rates falling more quickly than death rates. By 1915, Finland's natural increase in population had slowed to 1.2 percent.

By 2008, Finland reached the fourth stage of its demographic transition in which its population growth had fallen close to zero, this time with low birth and death rates. The nation had gone from relatively high birth and death rates producing a low rate of population growth before 1785, through a period of more rapid natural increase in the nineteenth and early twentieth centuries, back down to a very low rate of population growth characterized by both low birth and death rates. Today, Finland has a population of 5 million, growing at 0.2 percent per annum. Abstracting from changes due to migration, at this rate Finland's population would require 350 years to double in size. But Finland's population probably will never double again. As has happened elsewhere in Europe, birth rates may fall even further and the crude death rate will rise as the population ages. In coming decades, Finland may even experience negative population growth, just as Germany and Italy already are.

Based on the few observations available, Finland's rate of natural increase never exceeded 1.5 percent. Compare this to the experience of the developing countries where, as a group, the rate of natural increase reached 2.5 percent during the 1960s. Even today, Pakistan's population is growing by 2.1 percent, Jordan's by 3.2 percent, and Madagascar's by 2.9 percent. Why draw so much attention to a 1- or 1.5-percentage point difference in population growth rates? Because doubling time drops from around 50 years at a growth rate of 1.5 percent to only 28 years at 2.5 percent to 22 years at 3.2 percent. Seemingly small differences in growth rates provide societies with even less time to achieve a demographic transition before population levels increase by substantial amounts.

Clearly, there are major differences between the historical experience of today's industrialized nations and the contemporary demographic transition of the developing nations. Figure 7–3 portrays the movement of crude birth and death rate for the less-developed nations as a group from 1950 to 2005. Panel b charts the corresponding rate of natural increase over the same years. By 1950, the rate of natural increase in the developing nations was 2.1 percent, far larger than the rate ever experienced by today's industrialized countries. The higher rate was the result of somewhat higher birth rates than historically had been the case in today's high-income nations due,

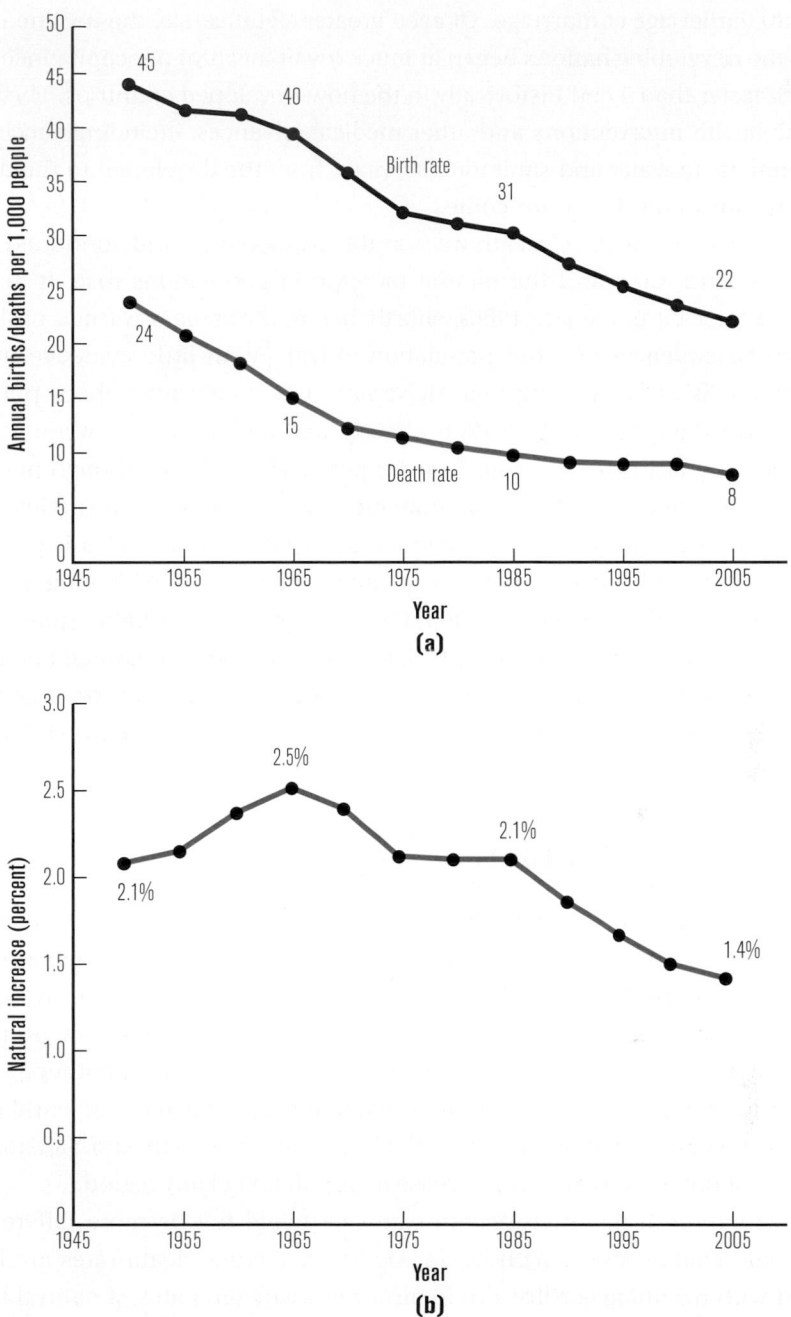

FIGURE 7-3 Demographic Transition for Less-Developed Regions (1950–2008)

Source: Population Division of the Department of Economic and Social Affairs of the United Nations Secretariat, *World Population Prospects: The 2002 Revision* and *World Population Prospects: The 2008 Revision.*

in part, to earlier age at marriage. Of even greater significance, the decline in death rates in the developing nations began at much lower levels of per capita income and fell much faster than it had historically in the now-developed countries. The transfer of public health interventions and other medical advances, including vaccines and improvements in water and sanitation services, from the developed to the developing world contributed to this outcome.

Between 1950 and 1970, death rates in the developing world continued to drop faster than birth rates, and the natural increase in populations rose. It peaked at around 2.5 percent in the late 1960s, shortly before McNamara warned of the catastrophic consequences of rapid population growth. With little evidence of falling birth rates, it is not surprising that McNamara was so alarmist about population trends. But a demographic transition already was under way. Between 1950 and 2005, the crude birth rate fell from 45 to 22 per 1,000, and even though death rates also fell, from 24 to 8 per 1,000,[5] the natural increase of the developing nations slowed to 1.4 percent, still high by historical standards but with an unmistakable trend. In all regions of the world and in almost every nation, women started having fewer children and **total fertility rates (TFRs)** fell (Box 7–1). These trends help explain why the World Bank and other multilateral organizations appear less concerned about population growth today. The world population is still growing and will continue to do so for several more generations, but the *rate of growth* has slowed and population *explosion* no longer seems an appropriate metaphor.

THE DEMOGRAPHIC SITUATION TODAY

In 2009, world population exceeded 6.7 billion. Only 16 percent resided in the high-income countries, 84 percent lived in the low- and middle-income nations (Table 7–1). Almost 3 out of every 10 inhabitants of the planet lived in East Asia. China alone accounted for just under 20 percent of world population. South Asia, dominated by India's more than 1 billion inhabitants, represented another 23 percent of the world's people. Sub-Saharan Africa accounted for 12 percent of world population, but this share is expected to rise in the future. At 2.4 percent, sub-Saharan Africa had the most rapid rate of natural increase in population of any region.

The situation in the high-income countries could not be more different from that in sub-Saharan Africa. With aging populations, crude death rates are likely to rise, and with declining fertility, crude birth rates will fall. Rates of natural increase already have slowed to 0.4 percent. Almost all *population growth* in the high-income countries is attributable to immigration, with openness to immigrants at a higher

---

[5]Careful inspection of Figures 7–2 and 7–3 reveals that the death rate in 2008 in Finland, at 9 per 1,000 people, is almost identical to the death rate in 2005 in the less-developed regions. This does not mean that life expectancy and the overall survival chances in the two places are the same. If one compares age-specific mortality rates, survival probabilities in Finland exceed those of the developing countries for every age group, especially for infants. But, in the aggregate, because Finland has a much older population than the developing world, the crude death rates, coincidentally, average to almost the same number.

BOX 7-1 TOTAL FERTILITY RATES

Another way to assess population trends is to examine fertility behavior. One of the most common measures of fertility is the total fertility rate (TFR). TFR sometimes is thought of as a measure of the average number of children a woman will bear, but this is not entirely correct. TFR is a *synthetic* measure. It sums the age-specific fertility rates of women in a given year, where age-specific fertility rates refer to the average number of children born to women of a specific age (usually, 15–19, 20–24, . . . , 40–44). In other words, TFR is the number of children the average woman would have in her lifetime if age-specific fertility rates remained constant. But these rates change over time as younger women delay having their children and as women have fewer children over all. TFR is a reliable indicator of the number of children women *currently* are having, and trends in TFR reveal a great deal about the world's demographic transition.

The figure below charts TFRs over the past 40 years for the World Bank's seven geographical regions. In 1967 in Africa, Asia, and Latin America, TFR was 5.5 children or more. Only the high-income economies and the nations of Europe and central Asia had reached low TFRs of fewer than 3 children. Over the next four decades, and at varying speeds, fertility rates fell in every region. In East and

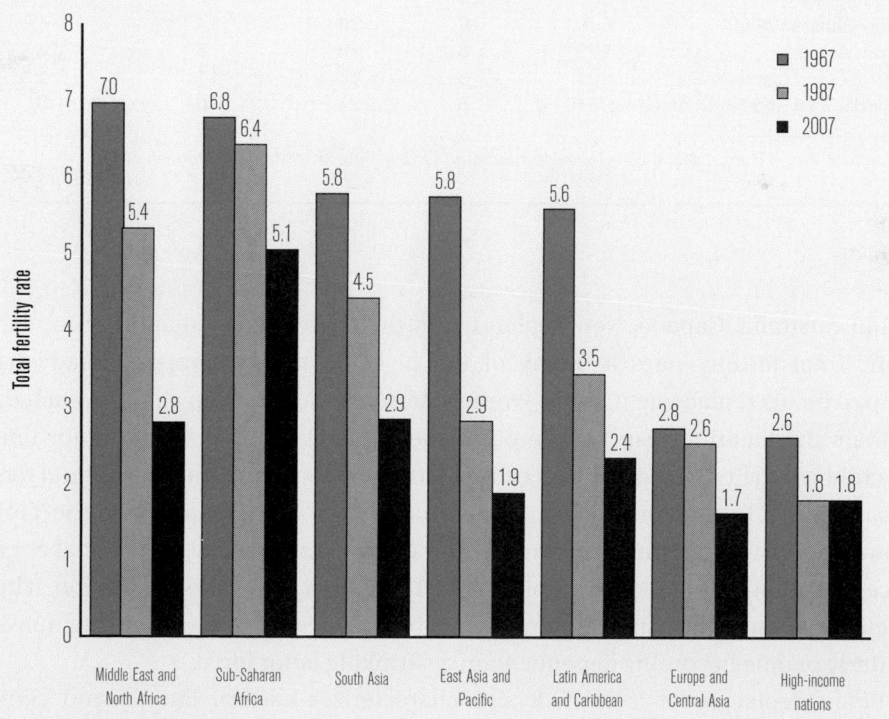

South Asia and in Latin America and the Middle East, TFR fell by half or more. Sub-Saharan Africa's demographic transition took longer to begin, but even in this poorest part of the world, TFR, now at 5.1 children per woman, has fallen by more than one child since 1987. Most demographers expect the decline in Africa's TFR to follow that of other regions and the rate to continue to fall.

TABLE 7-1 Levels and Trends in the World Population, 2009

| | TOTAL POPULATION | | POPULATION GROWTH | | |
	NUMBER (MILLIONS)	PERCENT OF TOTAL	BIRTH RATE (PER 1,000)	DEATH RATE (PER 1,000)	NATURAL INCREASE (PERCENT)
World	6,775	100	20	8	1.2
Income category					
Low income	846	13	34	11	2.3
Middle income	4,813	71	19	8	1.1
High income	1,117	16	12	8	0.4
Region					
East Asia	1,944	29	14	7	0.7
South Asia	1,568	23	24	7	1.7
Sub-Saharan Africa	840	12	38	14	2.4
Latin America	572	8	18	6	1.2
Europe and Central Asia	404	6	15	11	0.4
Middle East and North Africa	331	5	24	6	1.8

Source: World Bank, "World Development Indicators Online," http://databank.worldbank.org.

level in Australia, Canada, New Zealand, and the United States than in Europe and Japan. Total fertility rates in many of the high-income economies already have dropped below replacement levels. Women must have at least two children each during their childbearing years for the population to replace itself. Allowing for infant and child mortality, demographers estimate that the replacement level of total fertility is around 2.1. In countries such as Germany, Italy, and Japan, where the TFR is below the replacement level and immigration rates also are low, policy makers are concerned about a population implosion rather than a population explosion. These societies can anticipate smaller populations overall as well as an increasing number of elderly people becoming dependent on a shrinking labor force.

Below replacement level, TFR also characterizes eastern Europe and central Asia, where the rate of natural increase is only 0.4 percent. East Asia's TFR has dipped below replacement levels (1.9 in 2007). By contrast, neither Africa, Latin America, nor the Middle East has progressed as far along its demographic transitions, implying faster growth in population and an increasing share of the world's total.

THE DEMOGRAPHIC FUTURE

When extrapolated into the future, even modest population growth rates generate projected total populations that seem unthinkable. Continued growth at the world's 2010 rate of natural increase, 1.2 percent, would bring population to 11 billion by 2050 and 26 billion by 2100. This type of projection, beloved by some popular writers, is frightening to many. It is hard to imagine life in a world with three to four times as many people as there are today. How will this expanded population live? How will the globe's finite supplies of space and natural resources be affected?

While a significant increase in world population can be expected during your lifetime, it is unlikely to double. Linear extrapolations of current trends are badly misleading because after accelerating for more than two centuries, world population growth has been slowing down for the past four decades. This trend is likely to continue, but no one can be certain how quickly the transition to lower fertility levels will be or whether there will be any reversals in recent trends.

Every few years the United Nations produces forecasts of future population growth.[6] These projections offer a variety of scenarios based on a similar set of assumptions about declining mortality but using different assumptions about the amount and speed of fertility declines. Figure 7–4 combines estimates of the world population from 1820 to 2000 with the United Nations' low-, medium-, and high-population projections for the twenty-first century. The high scenario assumes the world TFR does not reach replacement levels, world population reaches 10.8 billion people by 2050, and continues to expand to over 15 billion by 2100. The medium scenario has the world reaching slightly less than replacement levels by 2050. Under the medium variant, world population rises to over 9 billion by 2050. Population growth then continues to slow throughout the century, leveling off at around 10 billion in 2100. The low scenario assumes a future TFR well below replacement levels. Under these assumptions world population hits a maximum of 8.1 billion shortly before 2050 and declines to 6 billion by the end of the century. The United Nations offers the three variants as alternative projections without assigning probabilities to which outcomes are more likely.

What all three scenarios share in common is the projection that world population will continue to grow over the next 50 years, in other words, over the adult lifetime of a university student today. The scenarios differ in the size of the projected

---

[6]In addition to the United Nations, the International Institute for Applied Systems Analysis in Austria, the U.S. Census Bureau, and the World Bank produce independent population projections. A useful introduction to how such projections are made appears in Brian O'Neill and Deborah Balk, "World Population Futures," *Population Bulletin* (Population Reference Bureau) 56, no. 3 (September 2001).

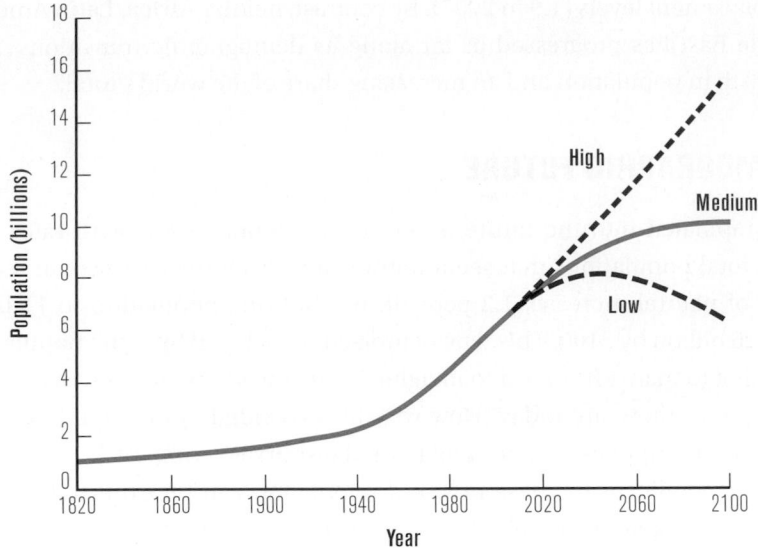

FIGURE 7-4 **World Population Historical Trends and Projections**

UN population projections for 2000–2100. The scenarios presented here represent different future levels of fertility.

Source: Angus Maddison, "Statistics on World Population, GDP, and Per Capita GDP, 1–2008 AD," www.ggdc .net/MADDISON/Historical_Statistics/vertical-file_02-2010.xls. U.N. Department of Economic and Social Affairs, Population Division, Population Estimates and Projection Section, *World Population Prospects, The 2010 Revision*, October 20, 2011, available at http://esa.un.org/unpd/wpp/index.htm; accessed February 2012.

growth within a broad range: from 1 to almost 4 billion. There are three basic reasons for this projected continued increase. The first two explain why the TFR may remain above replacement levels: (1) a desire for large families and (2) a failure to achieve the desired number of children (so-called unwanted children). The third reason is **population momentum**, a demographic concept requiring some explanation.

Populations that have been growing rapidly, as they have been especially in the developing world, have large numbers of people in, or about to enter, the most fertile age brackets. Even if all the world's couples today were to start having just enough children to replace themselves, the total population would continue to grow for many more decades before eventually leveling off. This is because today's children, who outnumber their parents, will become tomorrow's parents. Stated differently, past fertility decisions echo far into the future (Box 7-2). Population momentum alone could add several billion more people to the world's population in the twenty-first century.[7]

Another way of appreciating the demographic future is to focus on specific countries, especially those projected to be the world's most populous. Table 7-2 lists the

---

[7]John Bongaarts estimated that half of the projected increase in the world's population during the twenty-first century could be attributed to population momentum alone. John Bongaarts, "Population Policy Options in the Developing World," *Science* 263, no. 5148 (February 11, 1994).

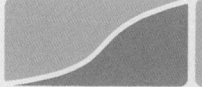

BOX 7-2 POPULATION MOMENTUM

The impact of population momentum on future population levels can be illustrated by the following example of two families. The first generation of each family consists of one man and one woman. Each woman has four children over her reproductive life. This second generation includes four females and four males.

PERIOD ONE
Fertility above Replacement Level; Total Population, 12

First generation:

Second generation:

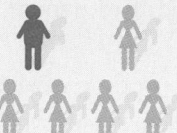 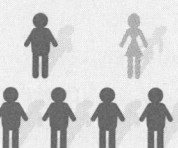

PERIOD TWO
Fertility at Replacement Level; Total Population, 16

First generation dies:

Second generation marries:

Third generation is born:

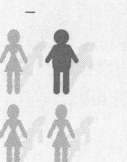 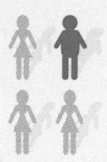 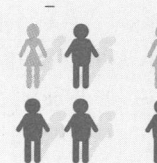 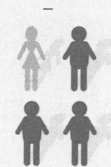

PERIOD THREE
Fertility at Replacement Level; Total Population, 16

Second generation dies:

Third generation marries:

Fourth generation is born:

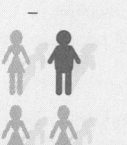 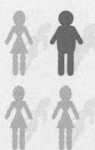 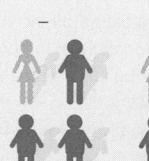 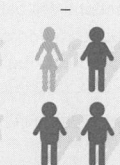

In period two, the first generation dies and everyone in the second generation marries. Each woman in the four resulting couples has two children, producing a third generation of four males and four females. Even though the second generation reaches replacement levels of fertility, population momentum causes a 33 percent increase in total population, from 12 to 16, between period one and period two.

The process is repeated in period three. The second generation dies; the third generation marries and produces a fourth generation. If the third generation remains at replacement levels of fertility, the total population stabilizes. The size of the steady-state population in the final period is the result not only of the fertility decisions of the second and third generations, but of those of the first generation as well.

Population momentum also can work in reverse. If subsequent generations have lower than replacement fertility, the decline in total population could be rapid, reflecting the fertility decisions of both current and previous generations.

TABLE 7-2 Projections: The World's 10 Most Populous Nations in 2050*

COUNTRY	2050 POPULATION (MILLIONS)	RANK	2010 POPULATION (MILLIONS)	RANK	POPULATION INCREASE MILLIONS	PERCENT
India	1,748	1	1,189	2	559	47
China	1,437	2	1,338	1	99	7
United States	423	3	310	3	113	36
Pakistan	335	4	185	6	150	81
Nigeria	326	5	158	8	168	106
Indonesia	309	6	235	4	74	31
Bangladesh	222	7	164	7	58	35
Brazil	215	8	193	5	22	11
Ethiopia	174	9	85	13	89	105
Congo	166	10	68	19	98	144
Total (share of world's population)	5,355 (0.56)		3,925 (0.57)		1,430 (0.55)[†]	

*Projections are based on the "United Nations" medium variant.
[†]The absolute increase in the population of the 10 most populous nations in 2050 divided by the change in total world population between 2010 and 2050.

Source: Population Reference Bureau, *2010 World Population Data Sheet,* www.prb.org/ pdf10/10wpds_eng.pdf.

10 most populous nations in 2050 according to the United Nations' medium-variant projections. The table also lists the population of those countries in 2010. These 10 nations are projected to account for 5.4 billion people in 2050, over half of the projected world population at that time.

China, India, and the United States will continue to be the three most populated nations, although India will replace China in the top spot. Increases in China's population, which already is well below TFR replacement levels, will be due exclusively to population momentum; in the United States, immigration will be the primary factor for increasing numbers; and in India, both population momentum and fertility above replacement levels will contribute to a projected increase of over 550 million *more* inhabitants than the 1.1 billion who live in India today.

Just as striking are the expected population gains elsewhere in South Asia. Pakistan is projected to increase its population by 81 percent and Bangladesh by 35 percent. In sub-Saharan Africa, the Democratic Republic of the Congo, Ethiopia, and Nigeria all are projected to experience even greater percentage increases in their populations. Projections for the Congo and Ethiopia are so large as to catapult them into the top-10 category in 2050, replacing Japan and Russia, which were among the top 10 in 2010.

It must be remembered that all these estimates of population trends are only projections, which become less and less reliable the further out in time one goes, and much could happen to change these outcomes. The impact on future population size of infectious diseases, some unknown today, is difficult to predict. Civil strife and migration will play a role as well. But what these projections make clear is that we should expect significant increases in world population, almost exclusively in today's low- and middle-income nations, over the next 50 years. Given the current difficulties many of these nations face today, the challenge of achieving economic development for ever-larger numbers of people seems daunting.

THE CAUSES OF POPULATION GROWTH

Discussions of the world's population future often turn acrimonious. Questions of whether and whose populations are to be limited and by what means are sensitive. Before we can confront such issues intelligently, we must consider what is known about both the causes and the effects of rapid population growth. We must concern ourselves with the two-way relationship between the growth of population and economic development—that is, with how population growth affects economic development and how economic development affects population growth. We deal with the latter relationship first.

THOMAS MALTHUS, POPULATION PESSIMIST

The most famous and influential demographic theorist of all time was **Thomas Malthus** (1766–1834). Malthus believed that "the passion between the sexes" would cause population to expand as long and far as food supplies permitted. People generally would not limit procreation below the biological maximum. Should wages somehow rise above the subsistence level, workers would marry younger and have more children, more of whom would survive. But this situation could be only temporary. In time, the rise in population would create an increase in labor supply, which would press against fixed land resources. Eventually, through diminishing returns, food prices would rise and real wages would fall back to the subsistence level. If this process went too far, famines and rising deaths would result. Malthus did not think that the growth of the food supply could stay ahead of population growth in the long run. In a famous example, he argued that food supplies grow according to an arithmetic (additive) progression, whereas population follows an explosive geometric (multiplicative) progression.

In the grim Malthusian world, population growth is limited primarily by factors working through the death rate, what he called *positive checks*. In this deceptively mild phrase, Malthus included all the disasters that exterminate people in large numbers: epidemics, famines, and wars. These phenomena, he believed, generally constitute the operative limitation on population. Only in later editions of his famous *Essay on the Principle of Population* did he concede the possibility of a second, less drastic, category of limiting factors: "preventive checks" that work through the birth rate. Here, Malthus had in mind primarily measures of "restraint," such as a later age of marriage. Unlike latter-day Malthusians, he did not advocate birth control, which as a minister he considered immoral. Although he grudgingly admitted that humanity might voluntarily control its own numerical growth, Malthus invested little hope in the possibility.

The gloominess of the Malthusian theory is understandable when one considers that its author lived during the early years of the Industrial Revolution. In all prior history, population had tended to expand in response to economic gains. With unprecedented economic growth under way in the world he knew, what could Malthus expect except an acceleration of natural increase as death rates fell? That indeed was happening during his lifetime.

Malthus did not live to witness the next stage in the European demographic transition. The early decline in death rates was followed, with a lag, by a fall in fertility; beginning in the middle of the nineteenth century, wages began to increase dramatically in contrast to Malthus's prediction. Why did all this happen? Wages rose, despite accelerating population growth, because capital accumulation and technical change offset any tendency for the marginal product of labor to decline. Death rates fell through a combination of higher incomes (better nutrition and living conditions) and better preventive and curative health measures. The fall in the birth rate is harder to understand. There are both biological and economic reasons to expect, as Malthus did, that fertility would rise, not fall, as income went up. Healthier, better-fed women have a greater biological capacity to conceive, carry a child full term, and give birth to a healthy infant. Also, people might marry earlier when times are good, and better-off families have the financial capacity to support more children. Why, then, do increases in income seem to lead to declines in fertility? An answer to this question must be sought in post-Malthusian demographic theory.

WHY BIRTH RATES DECLINE

Two kinds of demographic change affect the crude birth rate. The first is change in the population shares of different age groups. A rise in the share of people of reproductive age (roughly 15 to 45) increases the birth rate, as we saw earlier in the discussion of population momentum. Conversely, if the proportion of older people in the population goes up, as is happening in many industrial countries today, the birth rate drops. The second factor is fertility, the rate at which women have children.

Why, then, do people have as many children as they do? Is it because they are moved by Malthus's "passion between the sexes" and do not know how to prevent the resulting births? Or is it because they are tradition bound and custom ridden? Or is it rational in some economic and social settings to have large families? All three positions have some merit. The case for the first one, implicitly, is what those who recommend providing birth control as a response to rapid population growth probably have in mind. A Latin American doctor at an international conference put it bluntly. "People don't really want children," he said. "They want sex and don't know how to avoid the births that result." This viewpoint captures the element of spontaneity inevitably present in the reproductive process. Yet the evidence suggests that all societies consciously control human fertility. Rarely does the number of children that the average woman has over her childbearing years even approach her biological capacity to bear children. One exceptional case is that of the Hutterites, a communal sect that left Russia and settled in Canada and the northern Great Plains in the late 1800s. The group's religious beliefs and lifestyle encouraged maximum fertility. Hutterite women, on average, bore over 10 children, a fertility rate no contemporary low- or middle-income nation comes close to approaching. All societies practice some method of controlling their numbers whether by aborting pregnancies, disposing of unwanted infants, or inhibiting conception. (Recall our earlier discussion of fertility decline in nineteenth-century Finland.)

As for the second proposition, it has been said that many children are the social norm in traditional societies, that society looks askance at couples who have no or few children, that a man who lacks wealth at least can have children, and that a woman's principal socially recognized function in a traditional society is to bear and rear children. Such norms and attitudes are important, but they probably are not the decisive factors in human fertility. Fertility is determined by a complex combination of forces. Social scientists in recent years have given increasing credence to elements of individual rationality in the process. Simply stated, they believe that most families in traditional societies have many children because it is in their interest to do so.

This brings us to the third explanation. Although some might regard it as a cold, inhumane way of looking at the matter, it is nevertheless true that children impose certain costs on their parents and confer certain benefits. In some low-income settings, especially in rural areas, children may supplement family earnings by working. On family farms and in other household enterprises, there usually is something that even a young child can do to increase production. In many poor societies, children work outside the home. In the longer run, children also provide a form of social security, which is important in societies that lack institutional programs to assist the elderly. In some cultures, it is considered especially important to have a son who survives to adulthood; if infant and child mortality is high, this can motivate couples to keep having children until two or three sons have been born, just to be safe. In addition to these economic benefits, which are probably more important in a low-income society than a more-affluent one, children also can yield psychic benefits (and costs!), as all parents know.

The economic costs of children can be divided into explicit and implicit costs. Children entail cash outlays for food, clothing, shelter, and often for education. Implicit costs arise when childcare by a member of the family, usually the mother, involves a loss of earning time. Some of the costs felt by parents parallel the costs of population growth experienced at the national level. For example, more children in a family may mean smaller inheritances of agricultural land, an example of a natural resource constraint operating at the family level. Similarly, it may be harder to send all the children in a larger family to school; this reflects the pressures on social investment felt when population growth is rapid.

Viewing childbearing as an economic decision has several important implications:

1. Fertility should be higher when children earn income or contribute to household enterprises than when they do not.
2. Reducing infant deaths should lower fertility because fewer births are needed to produce a given desired number of surviving children.
3. The introduction of an institutionalized social security system should lower fertility by reducing the need for parents to depend on their children for support in their old age.
4. Fertility should fall when there is an increase in opportunities for women to work in jobs that are relatively incompatible with childbearing, essentially work outside the home.
5. Fertility should be higher when income is higher because the explicit costs are more easily borne.

The first four predictions have received substantial support from empirical studies. The fifth, however, conflicts with observation. Fertility usually is negatively related to income. The negative relationship shows up both in time-series data (that is, fertility usually declines over time as income rises) and in cross-section data (fertility generally is higher in poor countries than in rich ones; also, in most societies, middle- and upper-income families have fewer children than poor families).

Several theorists have wrestled with the seeming anomaly that household demand for children falls as income rises; in other words, children are "inferior goods." Economist Gary Becker of the University of Chicago, a pioneer of *the new household economics*, analyzes children as a kind of consumer durable that yields benefits over time.[8] Couples maximize a joint (expected) utility function in which the "goods" they can "buy" are (1) number of living children, (2) child quality (a vector of characteristics including education and health), and (3) conventional goods and services. The constraints faced by parents in Becker's model are (1) their time and (2) the cost of purchased goods and services.

Becker explains the fall in fertility as income rises over time by saying that the cost of children tends to rise, especially because the opportunity cost of the parents' time, particularly the mother's, goes up. The familiar income and substitution effects that result from any price change are at work here. As a woman's market wage rises, her income also rises, leading to an increase in her demand for any normal good, presumably including the demand for more children. But as a woman's wage rises, the opportunity cost of her time also goes up, so the price of raising children rises. As a result, her demand for any activity that is intensive in the use of her time decreases, including child rearing. If the substitution effect is greater than the income effect, couples may decide to have fewer offspring. Becker also argues that given the rising cost of child *quantity*, many parents opt to invest in child *quality* and spend more time and money on a smaller number of children. Wanting "higher-quality" children as income rises also reverts the demand for children back to the demand for a "normal good."

Much of Becker's work on the family was directed at understanding declining fertility levels in the United States and other high-income economies. But the application of the new household economics to the circumstances of developing nations also offers keen insights. Replacing Malthus's assumption that people are driven solely by their passions, fertility now is seen as the outcome of a rational process. This does not mean that every child born, in rich and poor nations alike, is the result of a conscious cost–benefit calculation. Economics rarely can explain individual outcomes; its power is in explaining average tendencies. What the new household economics suggests is that rich and poor people alike weigh the consequences of their actions, and to understand behavior, we may gain more insights by assuming people act in what they perceive as their own best interests. Having large numbers of children then may be seen not as an irrational act but as the result of the difficult choices poor people face. For poor families, having many children may make economic sense.

---

[8]Gary Becker, *A Treatise on the Family* (Cambridge, MA: Harvard University Press, 1981).

The new household economics provides insights into the fertility decisions of families in the developing world and, in so doing, raises an apparent contradiction. If individual decisions about fertility are rational and in the perceived best interest of the family, why did McNamara, and many others, identify population growth as "the greatest single obstacle" to economic development? How could rational decisions at the household level result in so dire a society wide outcome?

POPULATION GROWTH AND ECONOMIC DEVELOPMENT

Even if population growth is not the greatest obstacle, has population growth been a major impediment to achieving economic development and is it still one today? To a casual observer who has spent time in Cairo or Calcutta, Manila or Mexico City, or in hundreds of other cities or villages in the developing world, the answer might seem obvious. Looking at the masses of poor people in these places, it would be hard not to conclude that the situation could be measurably improved if only there were fewer people. (A casual observer might draw the same conclusion in New York or Tokyo.)

But more than casual observation is needed to understand the complex relationship between population growth and economic development, especially if one is going to consider policy interventions to reduce population growth. First, we must be clear on the question we are asking. We cannot ask whether people who have been born would have been better off having never been born. This is a question economics cannot possibly answer. Our question can only be whether per capita income, life expectancy, educational attainment, or any other indicator of economic development would be higher if a nation's population had grown more slowly. Given the centrality of economic growth to the development process, much of our attention is on the relationship between population growth and economic growth.

Simon Kuznets, a Nobel Prize winner in economics and a pioneer in the use of data to examine trends in economic growth, reported on a lack of correlation between population growth and per capita output growth for 40 less-developed nations between the early 1950s and 1964.[9] Similar studies have been conducted since Kuznets's work, many of which also report a low correlation between the two growth rates over various time periods.[10] Starting in the 1980s, it was more common

[9]For the 40 less-developed countries in Kuznets's sample, the rank correlation between rates of population growth and growth in per capita GDP was 0.111. From Simon Kuznets, "Population and Economic Growth," *Proceedings of the American Philosophical Society* 3 (June 1967), as reported in United Nations, *The Determinants and Consequences of Population Trends,* Department of Social Affairs, Population Division, Population Studies No. 17 (New York: United Nations, 1973).

[10]Discussion of these studies can be found in Allen Kelley and Robert Schmidt, "Economic and Demographic Change: A Synthesis of Models, Findings and Perspectives," in Nancy Birdsall, Allen Kelley, and Steven Sinding, eds., *Population Matters: Demographic Change, Economic Growth, and Poverty in the Developing World* (Oxford: Oxford University Press, 2001).

to find a negative correlation between them. In growth regressions, which include many possible determinants of economic growth, the significance of population growth varies depending on what other variables are included.

The lack of one pattern relating population growth to economic growth should not be misinterpreted. It does not mean that population has no systematic effect on economic growth; it simply means that the relationship is complex. We need to ask, How does population growth affect the determinants of economic growth? What direction of causality is there between population growth and economic growth? And how important are the individual components of population growth—fertility, mortality, and migration—to gross domestic product (GDP) growth (and vice-versa)?

We begin by challenging a *naïve view* of how population growth and economic growth are related. The growth rate in GDP per capita equals the growth rate of GDP minus the growth rate in population.[11] The naïve view then holds that, for any given rate of GDP growth, per capita growth would be faster the slower the growth in population. This conclusion is true, but its implicit assumption is false. Growth in output is not independent of growth in the population. The simplest reason is that children born today are the labor force of the future, and labor, along with land and capital, is one of the main factors of production for any economy. Stated differently, population growth affects both the level of GDP and how many people must share in that GDP. Once one recognizes these connections, the critical question becomes how population growth affects the core determinants of economic growth: the accumulation of factors of production and the productivity of those factors.

POPULATION AND ACCUMULATION

A pioneering model of population's effect on material welfare was written in 1958 by demographer Ansley Coale and economist Edgar Hoover.[12] Their work falls squarely into the camp of **population pessimists**, or anti-natalists, those who perceive population growth as harmful to economic development. Coale and Hoover argue that a reduction in the birth rate could raise per capita income in three important ways. First, lower fertility levels would slow future labor force growth. The amount of investment then needed to provide a constant amount of capital per worker for a growing number of workers (*capital widening*) would go down and permit more investment to be used to increase capital per worker (*capital deepening*).[13] Second, with lower

---

[11]The growth rate of any fraction, A/B, is equal to the growth of the numerator, A, minus the growth of the denominator, B. This is because the growth rate of any variable, X, can be found by taking the derivative of the log of the variable with respect to time: $d(\ln X)/dt = (dX/dt)/X = g(X)$, where g is the rate of growth. If $X = (A/B)$, then $\ln(A/B) = \ln A - \ln B$, and $d[\ln(A/B)]/dt = d(\ln A)/dt - d(\ln B)/dt$, or $g(A/B) = g(A) - g(B)$. In the case of GDP per capita, $g(\text{GDP}/\text{population}) = g(\text{GDP}) - g(\text{population})$.

[12]Ainsley Coale and Edgar Hoover, *Population Growth and Economic Development in Low-Income Countries: A Case Study of India's Prospects* (Princeton, NJ: Princeton University Press, 1958).

[13]The implications of capital widening and capital deepening for economic growth are developed more fully in the discussion of the Solow growth model in Chapter 4.

fertility and fewer children, public funds could be diverted away from education and health expenditures and toward physical capital, which Coale and Hoover assumed would be a more productive use of government spending. Third, slower population growth would lower the **dependency ratio**, the ratio of the non-working-age population (usually 0 to 14 years and 65 and over) to the working age population (Box 7–3). A lower dependency ratio, in turn, would reduce consumption and increase saving at any given level of income, permitting a higher rate of asset accumulation. Taken together, these three benefits from slower population growth could raise income levels at both the household and aggregate levels.

Coale and Hoover's conclusions, generally, have not always been supported by later research.[14] For a given amount of investment, a larger labor force results in less capital per worker, but the quantitative significance of this effect on output often appears small. Coale and Hoover's concern about the diversion of resources toward education also has not held up to later research. Demographic factors do not exert much of an independent effect on the share of GDP allocated to education and other social welfare programs. In addition, education and health increasingly are seen, not as consumption expenditures, but as investments in human capital that may have returns equal to or higher than the returns on investments in physical capital.

The third relationship highlighted by Coale and Hoover, among population growth, dependency ratios, and saving, has attracted a great deal of analysis. Some studies find little correlation. This may be because business and government savings are relatively independent of demographic change. Even household saving may be fairly insensitive to changes in population growth if most saving comes from wealthy families. Such households' saving behavior would be affected by neither their own fertility decisions nor those of the poor. On the other hand, there is cross-country evidence that, as the share rises of the population 15 years of age and younger, the aggregate saving rate falls.

This last insight is part of a more recent analysis often referred to as the **demographic dividend** or **bonus**. The dividend refers to the opportunity created when a nation with rapid population growth experiences a fall in fertility. As fertility falls, population growth falls too, but for a period of time the working age population (15- to 65-year-olds) grows *more rapidly* than the youth population (0 to 14). This is because the growth of the working age population depends on earlier and higher birth rates. The age pyramids in Box 7–3 experience a bulge in the number of young adults and a shrinking of the number of children. Not only are there now more potential workers per child, but more women join the labor force as fewer years are spent on childbearing. With relatively more workers, the productive potential of the economy expands. During this phase of the demographic transition, the society still has a relatively small older age cohort so the problem of the dependency of the elderly is not yet a concern. It will eventually become one, as it has in an increasing number of developed and developing nations today, making the demographic dividend a temporary opportunity.

---

[14]Nancy Birdsall, "Economic Analysis of Rapid Population Growth," *World Bank Research Observer* 4, no. 1 (January 1989).

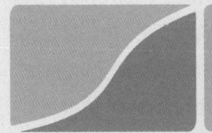

BOX 7-3 POPULATION GROWTH, AGE STRUCTURE, AND DEPENDENCY RATIOS

In 2009, Nigeria had a population of 153 million people compared to Russia with 142 million. Although similar in population size, the two nations are at very different points in their demographic transitions. Nigeria has a total fertility rate

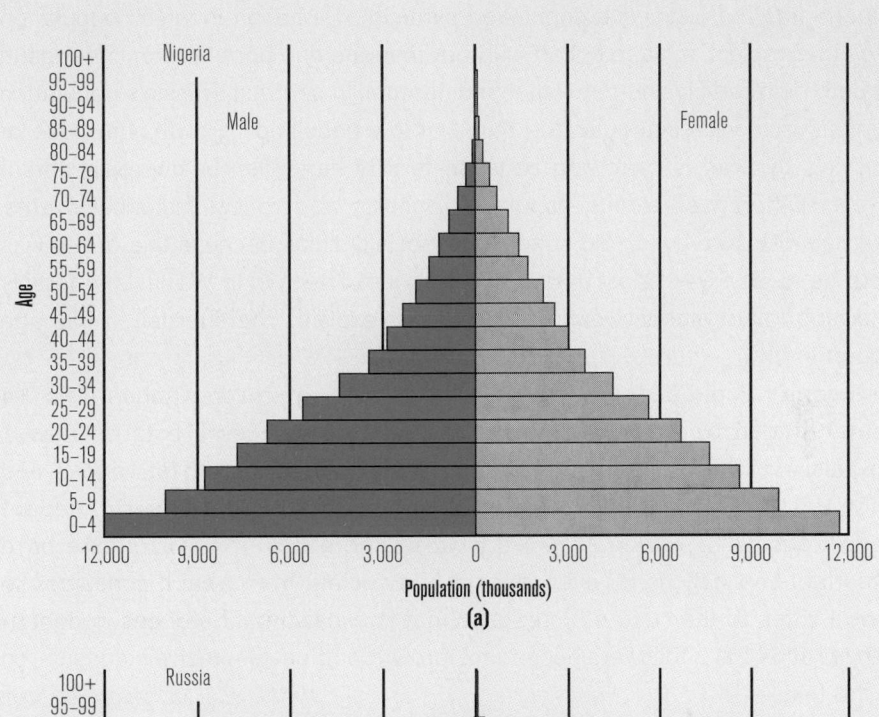

(a)

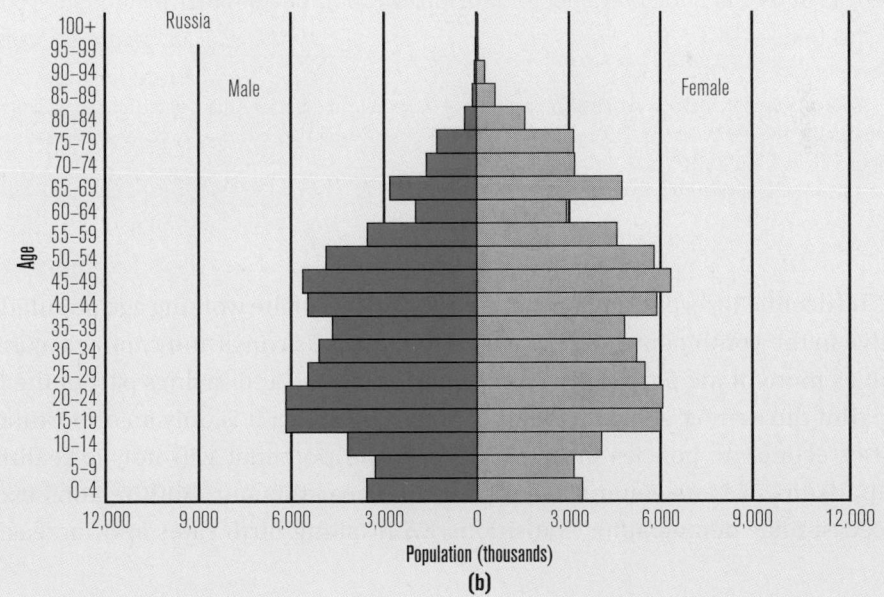

(b)

of 5.7; Russia's is 1.5. Nigeria's population growth rate this past decade was +2.1 percent per year; Russia's was −0.35 percent. Only recently has Nigeria reached the stage of the demographic transition where birth rates have started to fall. Russia passed through this phase decades ago.

Differences in crude birth and death rates, in addition to their impact on population growth, have a large effect on a nation's age structure. Population pyramids (on previous page) illustrate these effects. Each bar of the pyramid refers to the number of males and females, respectively, in a given age cohort. Nigeria has the distinctive population pyramid of a nation in which population growth is rapid. Each age cohort is larger than the one born before it, the result of both high fertility and population momentum. In contrast, Russia's population pyramid is more rectangular, the result of low population growth. The base of Russia's pyramid is narrowing because fertility has fallen below replacement levels. (Differences among population cohorts also reflect historical events. Russia's 60- to 64-year-old cohort is especially small because this group was born between 1944 and 1948, during and just after World War II. Low fertility and high infant mortality during those years explains the shortfall in this age cohort today.)

Nigeria's youth dependency ratio, the number of children (ages 0 to 14 years) divided by the number of people of working ages (15 to 64 years), obviously will be higher than Russia's. The ratio equals 0.87 for Nigeria and only 0.21 for Russia. But Russia has a higher elderly (older than 64) dependency ratio of 0.14 than Nigeria's (0.03). Differences in age structure have important implications for every aspect of a society, from what it consumes to how it votes to the culture it creates. What implications differences in dependency ratios have for overall economic growth and development is considered in the text.

Source: Population Division of the Department of Economic and Social Affairs of the United Nations Secretariat, *World Population Prospects: The 2008 Revision*, available at www.un.org/esa/population /publications/wpp2008/wpp2008_highlights.pdf.

The decline in fertility not only increases the size of the working age population relative to the youth population. It may also increase savings and capital accumulation as more of the population is now in the working and savings part of the life cycle. But the demographic dividend is not a sure thing; it is only an opportunity. If other economic policies are not in place, the potential will not be realized. Comparisons of Latin America with East Asia bear this out. Both regions experienced similar demographic transitions, with falling birth rates and increasing working age cohorts. But the similarity ends there. East Asia boomed; Latin America did not.

Some researchers argue that East Asia's demographic transition contributed substantially to the region's rapid economic growth. Using cross-country growth regressions, they attribute one-third or more of the region's growth to the rapid increase in its working age population after the decline in fertility. Others think the effect on growth was far smaller, finding little empirical evidence at the household level to support the life-cycle hypothesis of saving central to the demographic dividend.[15] The relationship between population growth and saving remains unresolved.

POPULATION AND PRODUCTIVITY

In addition to its potential effects on the accumulation process, population growth also can influence the other important determinant of economic growth, the productivity of assets. Concern over these impacts dates back to Thomas Malthus. Malthus saw population growth leading to an inevitable decline in agricultural productivity and having devastating consequences for humanity. What Malthus did not envisage is the revolution in agricultural technology that would raise, not lower, the productivity of land. Malthus never would have believed that, in a world of 7 billion people, individuals, on average, would eat better than they did in his day, when world population was closer to 1 billion. Economic historian Robert Fogel cites evidence that, in the late eighteenth century, about the time Malthus wrote his famous essay, the average daily caloric consumption in France was 1,753 and in England in the neighborhood of 2,100. Contrary to Malthus's predictions, in the developing world today the average is much higher, exceeding 2,600 calories.[16]

[15]The significance of the demographic dividend is presented in David Bloom and Jeffrey Williamson, "Demographic Transitions and Economic Miracles in Emerging Asia," *World Bank Economic Review* 12, no. 3 (1998); David Bloom, David Canning, and Jaypee Sevilla, *The Demographic Dividend: A New Perspective on the Economic Consequences of Population Change* (Santa Monica: Rand, 2003). A dissenting view is presented in Angus Deaton and Christina Paxson, "Growth, Demographic Structure and National Saving in Taiwan," *Population and Development Review* 26 (2000; Suppl.), 141–73.

[16]There is a group of countries that in recent years have consumed fewer than 1,750 calories per day, the level in France in the late eighteenth century. In 1999–2001, this group included Afghanistan, Burundi, the Congo, Eritrea, Somalia, and Tajikistan. Although all but Tajikistan had extraordinarily high TFRs of 6.0 or more at the time, what also distinguishes this group is that they were all failed states. It is likely that their malnutrition was caused less by overpopulation than by the disruption of agriculture due to massive political instability. Historical data on caloric intake are from Robert Fogel, "The Relevance of Malthus for the Study of Mortality Today: Long-Run Influences on Health, Mortality, Labor Force Participation, and Population Growth" (231–84), in Kerstin Lindahl-Kiessling and Hans Landberg, eds., *Population, Economic Development, and the Environment* (Oxford: Oxford University Press, 1994). More recent data are from United Nations Food and Agriculture Organization, *The State of Food Insecurity in the World* (Rome: FAO, 2003).

Despite these improvements, neo-Malthusian ideas still are popular. Concern over an imbalance between population and food supplies continues to be voiced, as is concern over how population pressures will affect the availability of fresh water and energy, the spread of infectious diseases, the degree of biodiversity and climate change, and the overall sustainability of the environment. Neo-Malthusians, like their intellectual predecessor, believe that there are limits to the carrying capacity of the planet and that science and technology cannot resolve fundamental problems of diminishing returns.[17]

Malthus's thinking placed him squarely in the camp of population pessimists. But some later economists, **population optimists**, would view population growth as having the potential to increase factor productivity. Several reasons for such a relationship have been proposed. First, a larger population, the result of more rapid population growth, can yield economies of scale in production and consumption. Roads are a good example. The return on an investment in a rural road is higher, up to a point, the more people there are to use the road. Other forms of infrastructure as well as public services in health and education exhibit similar scale effects. Second, there is some evidence that population pressures can induce technological change. Increasing population density in previously underpopulated regions can encourage more labor-intensive farming systems, increasing the return to land and, perhaps, to other inputs. Third, economist Julian Simon, perhaps the greatest population optimist of all, argued that a larger population contains more entrepreneurs and other creators, who can make major contributions to solving the problems of humanity. Simon called human ingenuity the "ultimate resource" that can overcome any depletion of other resources.[18]

Just as is true for the population pessimists, empirical support for the positions of the population optimists is spotty. Scale effects exist but often are realized at population densities that already have been achieved; a possible exception is some sparsely settled regions of Africa. Diseconomies of scale also exist and city sizes in parts of the world may be approaching those levels. Finally, there is no simple one-for-one correspondence between population pressures and technological change. Population is only one of many factors that affect the nature and quality of the institutional environment that conditions the introduction of new technologies and methods of pro-

---

[17]The neo-Malthusian perspective is presented in Lester Brown, Gary Gardner, and Brian Halweil, *Beyond Malthus: Nineteen Dimensions of the Population Challenge* (New York: Norton, 1999). The opposing view, that the planet is not overreaching its carrying capacity, is presented in Bjorn Lomborg, *The Skeptical Environmentalist: Measuring the Real State of the World* (Cambridge: Cambridge University Press, 2001).

[18]The seminal work on population pressures inducing changes in agricultural production is Ester Boserup, *The Conditions of Agricultural Growth* (Chicago: Aldine, 1965.) On human ingenuity, see Julian Simon, *The Ultimate Resource* (Princeton, NJ: Princeton University Press, 1981).

duction. Green revolution technologies, which can dramatically increase agricultural output for specific crops, such as rice and wheat, have been adopted in some densely populated areas but not in others. This suggests that population pressures alone have not been the deciding factor.

POPULATION AND MARKET FAILURES

In addition to the population pessimists and the population optimists who present such conflicting views, there is a third school of thought on population and development: the **population revisionists** (referred to by some as population neutralists). The revisionists situate themselves between the two extreme camps, arguing that there is no one size that fits all on population matters. Because of the varied influences of population growth on economic and social variables, growing populations may or may not be detrimental to economic development, depending on time, place, and circumstances.

The revisionists also bring together micro models of fertility behavior with macro assessments of the consequences of population growth. This merging of micro and macro is critical. According to the prevailing microeconomic model of fertility, individuals have control over their fertility decisions and behave rationally. In other words, couples, on average, make decisions on the number of children they want in their own best interest. If this insight is correct, how is it possible that actually tens of millions of rational individual decisions concerning the number of children to have could result in detrimental outcomes for nations or even for the planet as whole? The revisionist answer is a familiar one to economists: **market failures**, situations in which the costs or benefits of reproductive behavior by individuals (households) are not fully borne by them.

Revisionists agree with some neo-Malthusians that rapid population growth may hasten depletion of natural resources or harm the environment. But unlike the neo-Malthusians, revisionists argue the fundamental problem is not too many people, but the lack of well-defined property rights. As in the classic "Tragedy of the Commons," population growth can destroy a common resource—for example, common grazing lands or a fishery—because no one family takes into consideration the impact of its use on others. A larger family might help that family gain greater benefits from the common resource (at least in the short run) but, at the same time, help speed its destruction, to the detriment of all.[19] A similar argument can be made about many government services, whether in education, health, sanitation, or transport. Each family may be acting rationally, but if the population grows too quickly, government services may not expand quickly enough. The resulting congestion of government services may produce lower quality of life for all. The root cause of the problem is not

[19]Garret Hardin, "The Tragedy of the Commons," *Science* 162, no. 1 (1968), 243–48.

population growth but the inability of government to finance the increased demand for publicly provided goods and services. In both these examples, population growth may exacerbate an existing market failure.

Revisionists also call attention to a failure in the market for contraception. If there are poor, incomplete, or imperfect markets either for information on contraception or for the contraceptives themselves, women have more children than they want and population growth is higher. One study reports that in Haiti 40 percent of women 15 to 49 years old preferred to avoid a pregnancy but were not using contraception.[20] To the extent that this was the result of a lack of information about or access to birth control, there is a market failure for contraceptives. In such circumstances, fertility levels do not fully reflect individual preferences and are too high. The ultimate source of the market failure is less apparent. Is it due to lack of information, government restrictions on the sale of birth control devices, or something else? The price of birth control is far less than the price of raising a child. Free markets deliver Coca-Cola worldwide, why not contraceptives?[21]

In addition to drawing attention to market failures, population revisionists focus on the impact of fertility decisions on dimensions of human welfare other than growth in per capita income, such as income distribution. At a household level, high fertility may benefit parents, in terms of earnings from child labor and old age support. But these same advantages for parents may work to the disadvantage of children if they result in fewer resources available per child for human capital investments. Higher-birth-order children may be at a particular disadvantage. Looking across households, because higher fertility is inversely correlated with household income level, more rapid population growth may increase income inequality and worsen poverty outcomes.

Population revisionists have contributed to the otherwise polarized debate on population between the pessimists and optimists. The revisionists emphasize that rapid population growth is unlikely to be the primary impediment to economic development, focusing instead on how population growth can exacerbate the failings in other markets or particular government policies. Even these negative effects are likely to be mitigated over the long run as households adjust to changing circumstances. Despite their more nuanced approach, the population revisionists seem unable to identify the specific circumstances and country settings in which market failures are large and policies to limit births are warranted. Their perspectives, however, help frame the debate over appropriate population policies.

---

[20]Sara Maki, "Unmet Need for Family Planning Persists in Developing Countries" Population Reference Bureau (October 2007), www.prb.org/Articles/2007/UnmetNeed.aspx accessed March 2012.

[21]Adapted from William Easterly, *The Elusive Quest for Growth* (Cambridge: MIT Press, 2001), p. 89–90.

POPULATION POLICY

While economic analysis cannot provide a definitive answer as to where, or even whether, intervention is warranted to slow population growth, most governments in developing nations and most donors favor slower population growth. In pursuit of this objective, governments implement a variety of population policies. Economic reasoning can help evaluate the relative merits of specific policies when the stated goal is to lower population growth rates.

The growth of a population can be reduced either by lowering the birth rate or raising the death rate. In practice, the only acceptable policy solution is reducing the birth rate. No one would advocate increasing the death rate as a way to slow population growth, but nations and donors do not always follow a strictly anti-mortality approach. The initially slow donor response to the HIV/AIDS crisis in sub-Saharan Africa is a case in point.

If slowing the rate of population growth is the goal, then reducing the birth rate is the solution. This can be achieved by reducing the share of the population of reproductive age or the fertility rate. Raising the average age of women at childbearing slows down population momentum and, in time, leads to a reduction in the share of the population of reproductive age. Providing women with more education and better employment opportunities can achieve these results. These interventions will also reduce fertility levels. And reduction in fertility, whether by direct or indirect means, is the primary target of population policies.

Two controversies surround population policies aimed at reducing fertility. One is the debate over the significance of family planning efforts versus broad-based socioeconomic development. The other is the debate over the use of relatively authoritarian tactics, including elements of China's 1979 one child campaign, to achieve population goals. Before getting to either of these controversies, we can identify some noncontroversial elements of population policy.

Educating girls is one of the least controversial and most effective means of achieving a long-term decline in fertility. As predicted by the new household economics, women with more education have a higher opportunity cost of time and choose to have fewer children. This result has been born out empirically by numerous studies. (Figure 7–5 provides evidence from four nations.) Because educating girls is valuable in its own right, all schools of thought on population agree to support improvements in girls' education. Any subsequent impact on fertility is as much a consequence as a motivation for such policies. The same can be said for interventions that reduce infant and child mortality. Such interventions, usually involving prenatal care, better birthing practices, and health initiatives directed at the young, can significantly improve survival chances. These interventions need not be motivated by a desire to lower fertility, even though they have this effect.

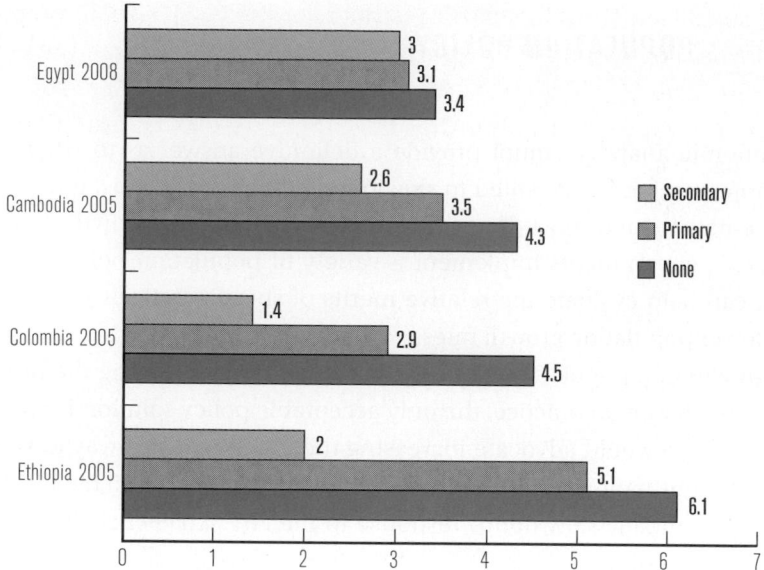

FIGURE 7-5 Total Fertility Rates by Mother's Education

Source: Demographic and Health Surveys, available at www.measuredhs.com.

All policies that promote economic development and lead to more education, better health, higher per capita incomes, and less poverty are associated with declining fertility, even if this is not their primary purpose. At the first United Nations World Population Conference, held in Bucharest in 1974, a popular slogan was, "Take care of the people and the population will take care of itself." Some development specialists go so far as to conclude that economic development is the best contraceptive. But others disagree and argue that more direct interventions to control fertility outcomes are needed.

FAMILY PLANNING

Family planning refers to a range of reproductive health information and services. It includes information on contraception and provision of contraceptives of various types, often highly subsidized or delivered at no cost to the user. Without government family planning services, couples could purchase contraceptives available at market prices or could control their fertility using traditional methods (abstinence, rhythm method, withdrawal). More modern forms of contraception (condoms; hormone therapies including birth control pills, patches, and injections; IUDs; male and female sterilization), however, are more reliable and associated with a greater probability of achieving desired fertility. One of the most important contributions of family planning services, whether provided publicly or through the market, is to help families reach their desired fertility levels. As levels of desired fertility fall, modern forms of contraception provide the means for achieving these goals.

Some population specialists also draw attention to the significant proportion of births in the developing world that are unwanted. Information on unwanted births is obtained from household survey data in which women report the number of births they have had as well as the number of children they would like to have. Using data from the 1970s and 1980s, demographer John Bongaarts estimated that approximately one out of every four children born in the developing world (excluding China) was unwanted.[22] Estimates for the past decade suggest much smaller numbers; for a sample of developing nations representing about two-thirds of the developing world excluding China, the total "not wanted" was only 8 percent, with another 9 percent "wanted later."[23] Reducing the number of unwanted births is another way of reducing population growth.

Whether family planning programs are effective at reducing unwanted births is a matter of some debate. This may sound surprising: Isn't the lack of contraception the reason women have births they do not want? Some further explanation is needed. When women reduce their desired level of fertility, contraception plays an important role in achieving these lower levels. Desired levels of fertility and contraceptive prevalence are well correlated, with causality most likely running from the former to the latter. When women desire small families, contraceptive prevalence is high. However, contraceptive use is less well correlated with reported differences between actual and desired fertility—that is, with the number of unwanted births. Using data from the 1970s and 1980s, development economist Lant Pritchett found that after controlling for desired fertility there was little correlation between contraceptive prevalence and excess births.[24] Women may have more births than they want but the availability of contraception may not explain why.

Family planning programs may influence individual preferences about how many children to have. This dimension of family planning efforts involves providing information, counseling, and various forms of "persuasion" concerning the number and spacing of children. Public campaigns to discourage high fertility are employed by many countries. In the 1980s, the slogan of India's national family planning program was *"Hum Do, Hamaray Do,"* which when translated means "Us Two, Our Two," or for two parents, two kids—a model family. The slogan was displayed widely on the sides of buses, billboards, and in TV advertisements and came with a logo, a silhouette of two parents holding the hands of two children, a boy in shorts and a pigtailed girl in skirts. The slogan on India's Ministry of Health and Family Welfare website recently flashed, "Control Population! Have fun with one!" In Indonesia, the *"Dua cukup"* program recommended "two is enough"; in the Philippines, public ads showed two happy children and advised, "If you love them, plan for them;" and in Zimbabwe, a family planning poster suggested,

---

[22]Bongaarts, "Population Policy Options," p. 771–76.

[23]Population Reference Bureau, *Family Planning Worldwide: 2008 Data Sheet,* www.prb.org/Publications/Datasheets/2008/familyplanningworldwide.aspx.

[24]Lant Pritchett, "Desired Fertility and the Impact of Population Policies," *Population and Development Review* 20, no. 1 (March 1994), 1–55.

"A small family brings a better life." These campaigns can affect social norms and the desire to have many children.

Family planning information also can be more personalized. One widely studied program of this type began in the late 1970s in the Matlab region of Bangladesh. It included fortnightly visits to each married woman in half the villages in the region. The visit was from a project employee, who discussed family planning needs and provided contraceptives. As a result of these visits, fertility rates fell dramatically by 1.6 births relative to the half of villages in the region that did not receive such visits. One evaluation of the program in Matlab considered its long-term consequences. After roughly 20 years, families who lived in the program villages not only had fewer children with greater spacing between them but were healthier and more prosperous than residents of similar villages that had not been served.[25] An important lesson of the Matlab experiment is that family planning can be effective at reducing fertility and providing other benefits, but it can entail substantial costs. Fortnightly field visits, free contraceptives, and administrative expenses per woman amounted to 10 percent of per capita income, sums that could not be sustained at a national level.[26]

Family planning programs need not be as expensive as in the Matlab program to be effective, but the general point remains. If the goal is to reduce fertility levels, is it better to devote scarce resources to expand family planning programs, or might it be more effective to devote these same resources to general improvements in socioeconomic status, which, in turn, could result in an equal or greater decline in fertility? In their evaluations of Indonesia's rapid decline in fertility rates, economists Paul Gertler and John Molyneaux determined that heavy subsidization of contraceptives, representing about half of the family planning program's expenditures, had a marginal impact on reducing fertility. Expansion of the distribution network into rural areas had a more significant effect. But most of the increased use of contraceptives was induced through economic development and the improved education and opportunities facing Indonesian women.[27]

Family planning may not play a large independent role in reducing fertility but this does not suggest that governments should abandon these programs or limit the availability of contraceptives. Modern forms of contraception enable families to better control their fertility. In this sense, family planning and development are complements, not substitutes. Family planning services also help people lead healthier and more satisfying lives. By being better able to time pregnancies, women can better space their children. Children born three to five years apart have higher rates of survival than children born within two years of one another. Avoiding unintended pregnancies can also reduce the need for abortions. In many low- and middle-income

---

[25]James Gribble and Maj-Lis Voss, "Family Planning and Economic Well-Being: New Evidence from Bangladesh," *Policy Brief* (Population Reference Bureau, May 2008).

[26]Pritchett, "Desired Fertility and the Impact of Population Policies," p. 37.

[27]Paul Gertler and John Molyneaux, "How Economic Development and Family Planning Programs Combined to Reduce Indonesian Fertility," *Demography* 31, no. 1 (February 1994), 33–63; John Molyneaux and Paul Gertler, "The Impact of Targeted Family Planning Programs in Indonesia," *Population and Development Review* 26 (2000; Suppl.), 61–85.

nations, abortions are illegal and take place under unsafe circumstances, contributing to maternal mortality. Increased use of contraceptives can help reduce the amount of premature deaths of both women and children in poor nations.

The 1994 Cairo International Conference on Population and Development endorsed the idea that family planning be replaced by a broader program of reproductive health. The World Health Organization defines the goals of this new approach as follows:

> Reproductive health implies that people are able to have a responsible, satisfying, and safe sex life and that they have the capability to reproduce and the freedom to decide if, when, and how often they do so. Implicit in this last condition are the right of men and women to have access to safe, affordable, and acceptable methods of fertility regulation of their choice, and the right of access to appropriate health care services that will enable women to go safely through pregnancy and childbirth and provide couples with the best chance of having a healthy infant.[28]

In the same spirit, the United Nations in 2007 added achieving universal access to reproductive health as a target to the MDG to Improve Maternal Health.[29]

AUTHORITARIAN APPROACHES

Some countries, concerned over the growth of their populations, have resorted to relatively authoritarian approaches to reduce their birth rates. In India, during the 1970s, the government added male sterilization to its list of promoted family planning methods. It did so because the government felt unable to control population growth by conventional means. Incentives were offered to men who agreed to be sterilized, and quotas were assigned to officials charged with carrying out the program. Problems arose when force allegedly was used against low-status individuals by officials anxious to fill their quotas. The sterilization campaign provoked an adverse political reaction because the methods of population control were regarded as excessively zealous and callous in their disregard of individual rights. Indira Gandhi's surprising defeat in India's 1977 general election was attributed in part to the population policy of her emergency government.

China's experience has been different. Chinese leaders have expressed concern about the size of the nation's population since the census of 1953 revealed a population of almost 600 million. Modest attempts to influence fertility outcomes followed, but not until 1971 was a more aggressive stance adopted. In that year the "planned births" campaign was initiated and established three reproductive norms, *wan, xi, shao* ("later, longer, fewer"): later marriage, longer spacing between births,

---

[28]Cited in World Bank, *Population and Development* (Washington, DC: World Bank, 1994), p. 81.

[29]Specific goals and strategies for improving reproductive health are presented in, World Bank, "The World Bank's Reproductive Health Action Plan, 2010–2015" (April 2010), http://siteresources.worldbank .org/INTPRH/Resources/376374-1261312056980/RHActionPlanFinalMay112010.pdf.

and fewer children. To implement these norms, birth targets were set for administrative units at all levels throughout China. The responsibility for achieving these targets was placed in the hands of officials heading units ranging from provinces of 2 to 90 million people down to production brigades of 250 to 800. The national government held information and motivation campaigns to persuade people to have fewer children, but it was left to local officials to fill out many details of the program and finance much of its cost. In China's villages, where much of the population lived, IUD insertions, abortions, and, later, sterilizations were offered. A wider range of contraceptives was provided in the cities. National spokespeople maintained that participation in the program was voluntary, but local officials with targets to fulfill often applied pressure. At the production brigade level, birth planning became intensely personal, as couples were required to seek approval to have a child in a particular year. (The application might be accepted or they might be asked to wait a year or two.)

The *wan xi shao* campaign began by discouraging couples from having more than two children; by the end of the 1970s, couples were encouraged to have only one. During the 1970s, total fertility rates in China plummeted from around six children per woman to less than three, a rate of fertility decline without precedent in world history. But, despite lowered fertility, population projections continued to cause concern, and in 1979, the **one child campaign** was promulgated. Couples, initially, were required to apply for official approval before conceiving the one allowed child. Those who complied could receive income supplements, extra maternity leave, and preferential treatment when applying for public housing. Couples bearing more than one child might be fined or lose access to education or other privileges. Early in the campaign, the government employed harsh methods to enforce its population goals. A system of incentives and penalties, plus other forms of social pressure, moved women to undergo sterilization after two births. China's one child approach has gone through various phases since its inception, with periods of stricter and looser interpretations. Since the late 1980s, rural couples in most provinces were allowed to have two children if their first was a daughter. Chinese couples still are obliged strictly to limit the number of children they have but elements of the earlier coercion to force such outcomes have waned.[30]

Several lessons can be learned from China's experience. First, the dramatic decline in fertility that took place in China is the result of more than the government's population policies. At the same time that these programs were implemented, economic reforms ushered in a period of rapid economic growth and urbanization, which decreased desired fertility. Even without the one child campaign, Chinese fer-

---

[30]For a survey of demographic trends and policies in the People's Republic of China, see Nancy Riley, "China's Population: New Trends and Challenges," Population Reference Bureau *Population Bulletin* 59, no. 2 (June 2004). The human face of China's policy is captured in the multimedia presentation by American Public Media, *Marketplace*, "China's One Child Policy" (June 2010), available at http://marketplace .publicradio.org/projects/project_display.php?proj_identifier=2010/06/21/china-one-child-policy; accessed February 2012.

tility levels would have fallen but probably not as far. Today, many Chinese couples would likely choose on their own to have only one child or even none. Second, the sharp fall in births may have longer-term adverse consequences. China will face a rapidly aging population in the decades ahead, which may stress both private and public systems of old-age support. China also faces a growing imbalance between the number of males and females (Box 7–4). This is the result of a traditional preference

---

BOX 7–4 MISSING GIRLS, MISSING WOMEN

Most parents believe that the chances of having a daughter or a son are fifty–fifty. But this is not true. For most human populations, the expected ratio of boys to girls at birth is closer to 105:100. Scientists are not entirely sure why this is the case, but believe it compensates for biological weaknesses in males resulting in higher mortality rates for boy versus girl infants. Because more than biology determines survival, social scientists draw attention to sex ratios, at birth and throughout the life cycle, when they deviate from what is expected in a gender-neutral environment.

The chart on the next page compares the sex ratio of children 0 to 4 years old in various regions. Europe and North America have ratios close to 105:100. The lower ratios in some regions may be due to a tendency for populations of African descent to record male to female ratios at birth closer to 102:100 or to the higher rates of male infant and child mortality. The most striking result is the pattern in East Asia, where in 2005 there were close to 121 boys for every 100 girls. This is neither a recent outcome nor is it biologically driven. The shortage of girls 0 to 4 years old is the result of long-standing son preference in the region. In previous periods, the shortage of young females was the result of deliberate female infanticide and neglect. Today, sex-selective abortion is another mechanism causing male children to outnumber female children, one facilitated by the increasing availability of ultrasound and other prenatal screening devices.

Sex-selective abortions, abandonment of female infants, and differential neglect of girls, especially in medical care, are all means of realizing son preference. They have been common in many parts of East Asia but none more so than in China. Although son preference has a long history in China, the one-child campaign and the overall move to low fertility rates among Chinese households have contributed to these outcomes. In 1982, at the beginning of the one-child policy, the sex ratio of first births was 107; second births, 105; and all subsequent births, 110. The change by 2000 was dramatic. The sex ratio of first births in China was still 107, but for second births it rose to 152 and for any subsequent

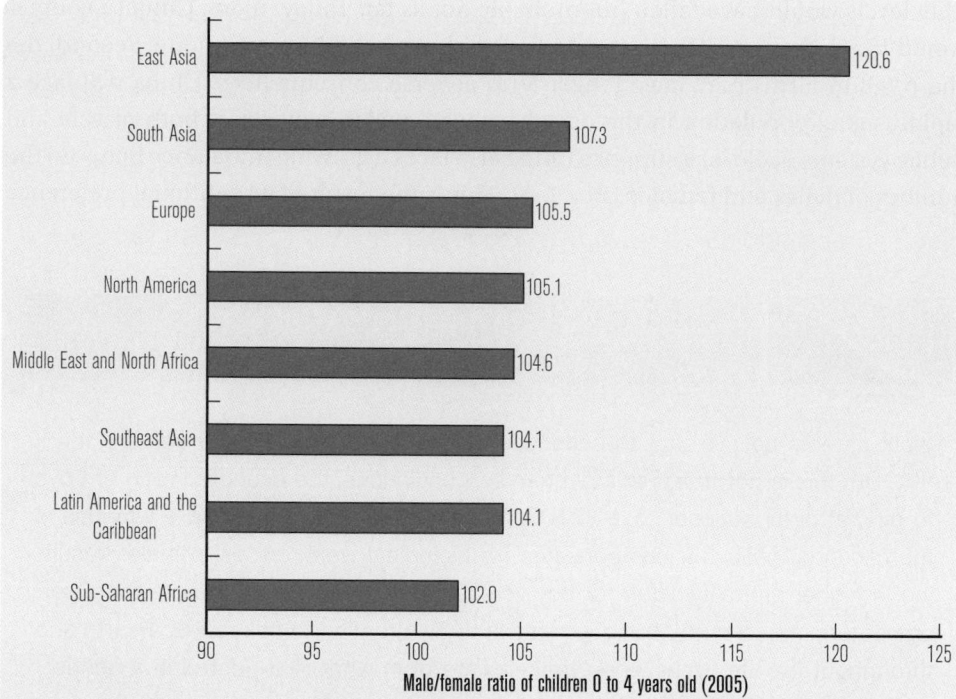

Source: Population Division of the Department of Economic and Social Affairs of the United Nations Secretariat, *World Population Prospects: The 2008 Revision,* available at www.un.org/esa /population/publications/wpp2008/wpp2008_highlights.pdf.

births it was almost 160. Second and higher-order births represented only one-third of all births in 2000, but sex selection for these births resulted in the high and grossly imbalanced sex ratio for all Chinese births.

China is not alone in this extreme form of discrimination against females, which has been referred to as *gendercide.* Amartya Sen examined the issue of differential mortality of males versus females and found that survival chances vary across countries and over the life cycle. In India, the differential used to show up less at birth and more during childhood and the late teen years. Today, sex-selective abortions are on the rise in India. Sen and other researchers concluded in 1990 that more than *100 million women were missing* worldwide, 80 million from China and India combined, as a result of sex-selective abortions and the relative neglect of girls and women. Today the numbers may well be higher.

Sources: Nancy E. Riley, "China's Population: New Trends and Challenges," Population Reference Bureau, *Population Bulletin* 59, no. 2 (June 2004); Amartya Sen, "More Than 100 Million Women Are Missing," *New York Review of Books* (December 20, 1990); Stephan Klasen and Claudia Wink, "'Missing Women': Revisiting the Debate," *Feminist Economics* 9, nos. 2–3 (November 2003). The cover story of the March 6, 2010, issue of *The Economist* was on gendercide.

for sons combined with policies that limited the number of children a couple could have. This most severe form of discrimination against females has human rights implications and may result in a host of social problems for future generations of Chinese women and men.

Finally, nations that today are worried about the growth in their populations are unlikely to be able to follow the Chinese approach. Few states can exercise as much social control as Chinese governments have in the recent past. India's experience in the 1970s suggests that a democracy is unlikely to accept the authoritarian approaches employed in China. But, even if a nation could do so, should they? Amartya Sen argues that, if freedom is valued at all, depriving people of the freedom to regulate their own fertility, one of life's most personal decisions, must represent a significant social loss.[31] Such a loss can be justified only if the social cost of not intervening is high. As this chapter has shown, it is hard to make the case that individuals systematically make poor decisions when it comes to childbearing or that the negative externalities of these decisions are large. If this is true, what justification is there for coercion to regulate fertility? Noncoercive approaches, including broad-based socioeconomic improvements, can achieve similar ends and should be pursued instead.

POPULATION ISSUES FOR THE TWENTY-FIRST CENTURY

In retrospect, the fears of Robert McNamara and many others about a population explosion no longer seem warranted. Population growth has slowed dramatically, and the expectation is no longer that world population will increase indefinitely. By mid-century, the world's population is expected to peak, admittedly with billions more people then when McNamara first expressed his fears.

But the drop in population growth rates does not mean that demographic concerns are a thing of the past. The world economy, if the United Nation's medium term projection comes to pass, still must accommodate another 2 billion more people over the next 40 years, almost all of whom will be born in today's developing nations. A second major demographic development will be the change in the age distribution of the world's population. There will be fewer children and many more elderly; not only are the developed nations aging but so are many of the developing ones. According to United Nations' projections, those 65 and older made up 6.7 percent of Asia's population in 2010; in 2050 they will make up 17.3 percent. In China alone, in part due to the one child policy, the percentage of seniors is projected to rise from

---

[31]Amartya Sen, "Population: Delusion and Reality," *The New York Review of Books* 41, no. 15 (September 22, 1994).

8.2 to 23.3 percent of the population. In Latin America the change will be similar to that in Asia. Only in sub-Saharan Africa, where fertility rates remain high, will the share of the elderly remain in single digits.

How will the needs of the elderly be met? As households grow smaller in size, traditional systems of family support are likely to breakdown. Financing old-age pensions, a huge problem now in developed nations, will increasingly confront emerging economies. Chile's pension system is often cited as a model for dealing with old age security. It no longer relies on a traditional pay-as-you-go (PAYGO) system similar to Social Security in the United States, where workers pay taxes each year that finance the pensions of those who already are retired. Starting in 1981, Chile developed a national system of mandatory personal retirement accounts, similar to 401K plans in the United States. This system of prefunded retirement savings relieves some of the burden of publicly financed old-age support. But it is not a complete solution, as many Chilean workers are self-employed or work in the informal sector and do not participate. About half of Chilean women were not covered because they did not work outside of their homes. Low-income workers may not earn enough for their accounts to lift them above poverty after their working years. Recent reforms, which include more public funding of old-age security, address some of these limitations but continue to build on the personal retirement account system.[32]

A changing age structure will challenge some economies; others will continue to face high fertility and the burdens (and opportunities) of a young population. This will be the case for many nations in sub-Saharan Africa. If this region follows what has happened elsewhere, economic growth and development will reduce the demand for children and accelerate a demographic transition to lower birth and death rates, and a slower rate of population growth.

SUMMARY

- The twentieth century will be remembered for populating the planet. In 1900, the world population stood at about 1.5 billion. By 2000, there were over 6 billion people; 5 billion living in developing nations. In no prior century did the world population increase by even 1 billion. World population growth has slowed since the 1960s, and current projections do not envision that the twenty-first century will see increases as large as those of the last century.
- The driving force behind the population increases of the last 100 years is the demographic transition, especially in the developing world. Improvements

[32]Estelle James, Alejandra Cox Edwards, and Augusto Iglesias, "Chile's New Pension Reforms," Policy Report No. 326, National Center for Policy Analysis, Dallas, TX, March 2010.

in nutrition, medical knowledge, and public health led to a rapid decline in death rates. Birth rates took longer to fall, and in the interim, the rate of natural increase in the populations of low- and middle-income nations soared to unprecedented levels. Today, most regions of the world are experiencing a decline in fertility and are approaching replacement levels. Sub-Saharan Africa is the one exception, where total fertility remains high, but even in this region, some decline is evident.

- There is considerable debate over the consequences of population growth on economic development. This is because of the multitude of ways population growth affects the determinants of growth; population growth, for example, may inhibit capital deepening, but it also may encourage institutional and technological innovations that increase factor productivity.

- In trying to understand the impact of population growth on economic development it is important to reconcile micro behavior with macro outcomes. If individual couples are making rational choices over the number of children they have, then at a macro level, why might a problem arise? The answer is market failures—for example, if the social costs of raising children exceed the private costs. In practice, it has proven difficult to identify the precise circumstances in which this happens and how large the resulting costs are.

- The debate over whether population growth is an obstacle to economic development is reflected in the choice of population policies governments pursue. If household behavior is rational and market failures are small, then development may be the best contraceptive. With better education, especially for girls; better employment opportunities, especially for women; and improved healthcare, especially for the young; couples desire fewer children. Family planning programs also may influence social norms about family size and assist individuals in attaining desired fertility levels in a safe and reliable manner.

- Some governments, especially in China, decided that the macro consequences of population growth are so negative that authoritarian steps must be taken to limit fertility. Such approaches have proven effective at reducing fertility levels and rates of population growth. But their development benefits are less obvious. Coercive population policies entail high social costs and loss of individual freedom. It is difficult to justify these actions with such limited evidence that reduced fertility contributes to faster economic growth and development.

- Despite the slowing of world population growth, the twenty-first century will face demographic challenges of its own, including a rising share of the elderly. With fewer workers per nonworking senior, nations will need to craft fiscally sustainable systems of old age support.

8

Education

Belief in the importance of education for economic development is not a new idea. The Chinese philosopher Guan Zhong, writing in the seventh century B.C.E., advised, "If you plan for a year, plant a seed. If for ten years, plant a tree. If for a hundred years, teach the people. When you sow a seed once, you will reap a single harvest. When you teach the people, you will reap a hundred harvests."

Contemporary scholars voice similar perspectives. Nobel laureate Theodore Schultz, in his 1960 presidential address to the American Economic Association, highlighted the importance of investing in people. Schultz referred to the acquisition of skills and knowledge as investments in human capital. Economists consider resources spent on physical capital as an investment that yields a future return rather than as consumption. Schultz argued that expenditures on people should be viewed in a similar way. He believed that most of the "impressive rise" in the earnings of workers in the industrialized countries was due to the growth in human capital, and a limiting factor in the advance of poor countries was insufficient investment in people.[1]

Among the major categories of human capital investments, Schultz included formal education at the elementary, secondary, and higher levels; health services; on-the-job training; and private and government sponsored training programs. In this chapter, we focus on formal education, specifically on schooling, and its implications for economic growth and development. In the next chapter, we consider health. On-the-job training includes everything from a parent teaching a child to

[1]Theodore W. Schultz, "Investment in Human Capital," *American Economic Review* 51, 1 (March 1961), 1–17.

farm to an apprentice learning a craft from a master tradesman to a multinational corporation offering courses to newly hired or experienced workers. All these forms of on-the-job training are important sources of human capital investment, but they ordinarily take place with limited amounts of policy intervention and public spending, especially when compared to education and healthcare. Schooling also provides *general* human capital, which is a prerequisite to the *specific* human capital more often associated with different forms of training. For these reasons, we restrict our attention in this chapter to schooling.

Over the past 40 years, there has been tremendous growth in schooling in all regions of the world. It is estimated that in 1960, 55 percent of the population age 15 and over in the developing world had never attended school. By 2010, this percentage had fallen to only 17 percent. It will fall even further in the decades ahead. In many countries expansion in schooling has contributed significantly to the human capital of the labor force and subsequent economic growth and development. But in other settings, schooling has not yet delivered what Guan Zhong and Theodore Schultz predicted in terms of growth and development. It is not that the Chinese philosopher and the American Nobel laureate were wrong. Instead, education, like so many other prescriptions for economic development, is not a panacea. It is not the sole determinant of economic success. If economic conditions do not encourage productive economic activity, the demand for educated workers will be weak, and even those with schooling may struggle to generate income for themselves and their families.

After considering recent trends in schooling and learning, this chapter examines the evidence on schooling as an investment. Schooling generally displays attractive rates of return, but even when this is the case, spending on schooling often delivers less than it might. Countries often underinvest in schooling overall, misallocate resources across the different levels of schooling, and inefficiently use resources within schools themselves. In some cases, the problem is insufficient or misallocated resources; in others, it is a lack of accountability among teachers, principals, and others responsible for the education of the young. The seventh-century Chinese philosopher Guan Zhong may have been right in his overall view of education but he did not spell out the details: How does one induce parents to send and keep their children in school; how does one combat rampant absenteeism among teachers; and, even more fundamental, how does one increase the amount of learning students achieve by attending school?

TRENDS AND PATTERNS

If you are reading this book for a course in development economics, you are among a privileged group in the world who has the opportunity to attend university. You may not feel part of an especially select group as you make your way through the crowded hallways of your college or university, but you are part of one. Worldwide, gross enrollment rates in any type of tertiary education (schooling beyond high school) amount to about one out of every four members of your age group. In the high-income countries, the rate exceeded 67 percent in 2008; in the middle-income nations, it reached 25 percent; and in the low-income countries, it was only 7.5 percent. Just as striking is a comparison with the generations that came before you. In the United States today, about one out of every three adults over the age of 25 received schooling beyond the secondary level. In France, the ratio is closer to one in five. In the developing nations it is often much lower: around 6 percent for both China and India; 7 percent in Brazil; and between 2 and 3 percent in Ghana and Kenya.[2] The experience of your age cohort, as compared to the schooling experience of earlier generations, tells us a lot about the stocks and flows of education in the world today. **Stocks** refer to the amount of schooling embodied in a population; **flows**, to the net change in those stocks as the result of school enrollment patterns.

STOCKS AND FLOWS

The scarcity of education in the developing nations is evident in the data on the levels of schooling completed among today's adult population (Figure 8–1). In the United States, an advanced economy, only 3 percent of adults did not complete six

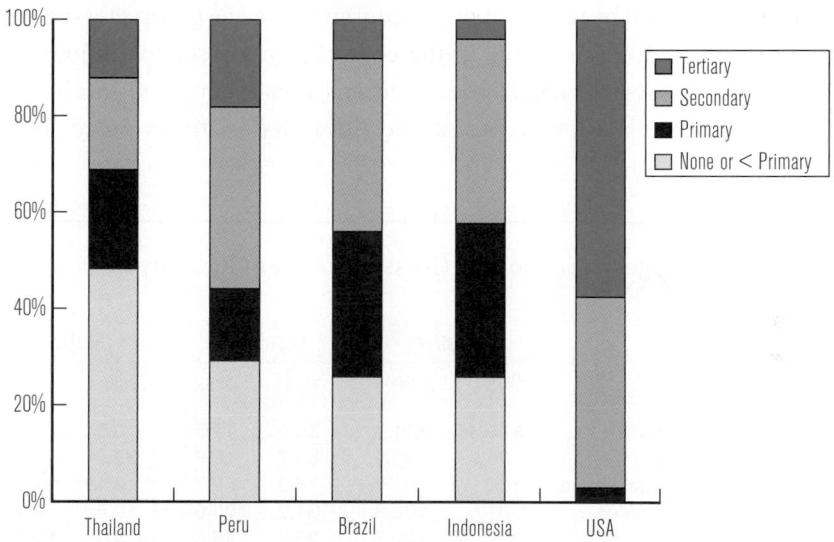

FIGURE 8-1 Educational Attainment of the Adult Population (ages 25 to 64)

Sources: Data for Thailand, Peru, Brazil, and Indonesia are from United Nations Educational, Scientific and Cultural Organization (UNESCO). Data for the United States are available from the U.S. Census Bureau.

[2]Estimates from the Barro-Lee Educational Attainment Dataset (2010), available at www.barrolee.com, accessed February 2012.

years of schooling (that is, did not complete primary school). The situation in low- and middle-income nations could not be more different. In Brazil about one out of every four adults did not attend or complete primary school; in Thailand almost one out of every two adults. Household data from the two Indian states of Uttar Pradesh and Bihar tell a similar story. By the late 1990s these two states had a combined population of 250 million people and were among the poorest states in India and hence among the poorest people in the world. Over two-thirds of their adult population did not complete primary school, most of them having never attended school.

Minimal levels of education characterize today's labor force in many low- and middle-income countries, but the situation is changing. Throughout the world, parents and governments, as well as bilateral donors and international agencies, are advocating that current and future generations receive more schooling. This trend is evident in a comparison of school enrollment rates by region over the past three decades (Table 8–1). At the primary school level, **gross enrollment rates** either have been high for decades (East Asia, Europe and central Asia, Latin America) or have expanded rapidly (Middle East and North Africa, South Asia and sub-Saharan Africa). Consistent with the millennium development goal (MDG) on achieving universal primary education, regional trends indicate real progress in increasing the amount of schooling children receive. But there is more progress to be made; in 2008, close to 70 million children were not in school.

Gross enrollment rates refer to the total number of children enrolled in a given school category divided by the number of children of the age group that officially corresponds to that level of schooling. In the case of primary school, the relevant age group usually is 6 to 11 years old. If older children (or younger ones) enroll in primary school, the gross enrollment ratio can exceed 100, as it does in several regions. Gross

TABLE 8-1 Changes in Schooling, Gross Enrollment Rates by Region, 1975–2005

REGION*	PRIMARY		SECONDARY		TERTIARY	
	1975	2005	1975	2005	1980	2005
East Asia and the Pacific	112.8	111.4	36.5	72.5	2.5	20.1
Europe and central Asia	96.9	96.9	84.7	87.9	32.9	54.7
Latin America and the Caribbean	109.1	117.7	38.3	89.7	13.1	29.6
Middle East and North Africa	81.5	106.3	31.2	75.6	10.5	26.1
South Asia	76.7	109.7	26.5	49.5	4.5	10.4
Sub-Saharan Africa	58.8	92.0	11.3	31.8	1.2	5.3
High-income economies	98.4	99.8	78.6	97.7	34.3	62.3

*Data for each region are aggregated from country-level data. Countries in the region were not included if data were unavailable.

Source: United Nations Educational, Scientific and Cultural Organization (UNESCO), Institute of Statistics, available at http://stats.uis.unesco.org/unesco/tableviewer/document.aspx?ReportId=143.

enrollment ratios that exceed 100 often are a mixed blessing. The good news is that they indicate lots of children are enrolled in school; the bad news is that they usually imply that many children are repeating grades. If repetition rates are high, as they often are in poor countries, gross enrollment rates can be high even though a substantial number of children never attend school.[3]

Alternative measures of school attendance take account of this problem. **Net enrollment rates** refer to enrollments of only those of the relevant age group. **Grade survival rates** estimate how many children actually complete a certain grade level. Estimates of these measures confirm the substantial progress nations have made in expanding primary education but also highlight that universal *completion* of primary school remains a challenge. In 2008, net enrollment ratios in low- and middle-income countries were 81 and 88 percent, respectively; in sub-Saharan Africa they were 75 percent. Estimates of grade survival rates suggest that 1 out of 5 children in some of the poorest nations did not complete five years of schooling; in some middle-income nations, more than 1 in 10 failed to do so. These failures are most pronounced among the poorest children, those with families in the bottom quintile of the income distribution. Because of these tendencies, the MDG of achieving universal primary education for all children by 2015 is unlikely to be met.

Achieving universal primary education remains an important goal. Another challenge is to expand secondary and tertiary enrollments. Huge enrollment gains in secondary education have been realized in virtually all regions (Table 8–1). Latin America's gains are the greatest, with gross secondary school enrollment expanding from approximately 38 to 90 percent between 1975 and 2005. The poorest regions, sub-Saharan Africa and South Asia, still lag the other regions, but much progress has been made in 30 years. It is not surprising that both the absolute level and expansion of tertiary enrollments remain low in almost all developing regions relative to the high income group. Even the current star performers in terms of economic growth, East and South Asia, do not stand out in terms of the level of tertiary enrollment rates achieved to date. Faced with limited resources, governments must decide whether to allocate additional resources to achieving universal primary education or to expanding opportunities at either the secondary or tertiary levels. We return to this controversial issue later in the chapter.

Trends in school enrollment rates across regions, combined with the age structure of today's developing world, tell us how human capital endowments will change in the decades ahead. Subsequent generations will be more numerous and have

---

[3]Paul Glewwe and Michael Kremer offer the following hypothetical example, "In a school system with 6 years of primary education, a 100 percent gross enrollment rate is consistent with 75 percent of children taking 8 years to complete primary school (because each child repeats two grades) and 25 percent of children never attending school." From "Schools, Teachers, and Education Outcomes in Developing Countries," in E. Hanushek and F. Welch, eds., *Handbook on the Economics of Education* (Boston: Elsevier, 2006).

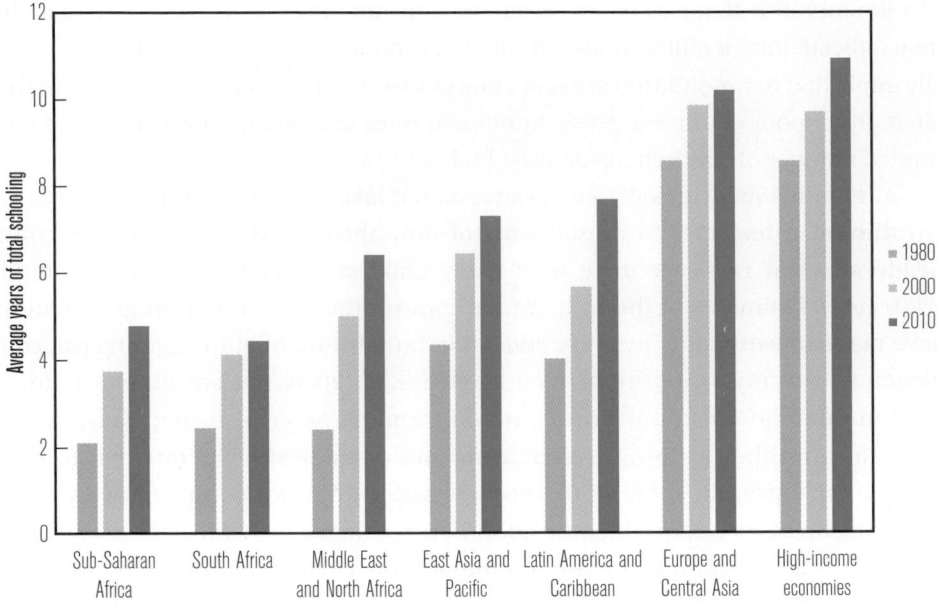

FIGURE 8-2 **Education Attainment, Adult Population 25 and over**

Source: Robert Barro and Jong-Wha Lee, "A New Data Set of Educational Attainment in the World, 1950–2010." NBER Working Paper No. 15902, (Cambridge, MA: NBER, April 2010). Data available at www.barrolee.com/data/dataexp.htm.

more schooling than their parents. This trend already is evident. Figure 8–2 provides estimates of the increase in the average years of schooling completed by adults 25 and over for all regions between 1980 and 2010.[4] As expected, average years of schooling have gone up everywhere. What is striking about these numbers is the extent of this increase. The educational attainment of the potential workforce in East Asia has gone from a predicted mean of 4.4 years to 7.4 years of schooling; in South Asia from 2.5 to 4.5 years, and in the Middle East and North Africa from 2.5 years to 6.5 years. The average level of educational attainment may still seem low, especially relative to the high-income economies (11 years in 2010), but remember these estimates are population means. In the developing nations, people in their 50s and 60s with no or little schooling are averaged together with people in their 20s and 30s whose educational attainment exceeds the mean. The trend is unmistakable; younger workers are entering the labor force with more years of schooling and are enriching the

---

[4]Calculating average years of schooling for a nation would seem a straightforward task. It is not, in part, because census and survey data in many developing nations are not conducted on a regular basis. Economists estimate educational attainment using a perpetual inventory method, which combines available census and survey data reflecting the stock of human capital with information on enrollment and repetition rates, which reflects the flow of schooling. Economists Robert Barro and Jong-Wha Lee provide the most-often-cited estimates and projections of educational attainment. Their most recent estimates are reported in Robert Barro and Jong-Wha Lee, "A New Data Set of Educational Attainment in the World, 1950–2010," NBER Working Paper No. 15902, (Cambridge, MA: NBER, April 2010).

human capital of the developing countries. It is fair to say that since 1980 there has been a global revolution in the provision of schooling.

BOYS VERSUS GIRLS

Progress has been achieved not only in the number of years of schooling received but also in the distribution of who receives this schooling. There has been considerable progress in spreading the opportunity to attend school to girls as well as boys, although girls' education still lags. Favoring the education of boys over girls is a long-standing and pervasive practice throughout much of the world, but this practice is changing. The MDGs called for eliminating gender disparity in primary and secondary education by 2005 and at all levels by 2015.

Estimates of average years of schooling for men and women over the age of 15 reveal a gender gap that has declined significantly over time. For all developing nations, the mean number of years of schooling for men in 1960 was only 3.1 years and for women even less, 2.0 years. Taking the ratio of the two, women completed only 62 percent the schooling of men. By 1980, this gap had narrowed a bit with the gender ratio at 74 percent. Much more progress has been made since 1980. For the developing world as a whole in 2010, women were estimated to have completed an average of 6.5 years of schooling as compared to 7.6 years for adult men, meaning a gender ratio of 86 percent.

Regional patterns show considerable variation (Table 8-2) around these trends. All regions have narrowed the gender gap in schooling, with Europe and central Asia and Latin America having almost achieved gender parity. South Asia, by comparison, has a long way to go. Estimates for 1980 show that adult women had received virtually

TABLE 8-2 **Estimates of School Attainment for Adults 25 and over by Gender and Region, 1980 and 2010**

	1980			2010		
REGION	WOMEN (YEARS)	MEN (YEARS)	RATIO (%)	WOMEN (YEARS)	MEN (YEARS)	RATIO (%)
East Asia and Pacific	3.0	4.7	65	6.8	8.0	85
Europe and central Asia	6.9	8.2	84	10.2	10.4	98
Latin America and the Caribbean	3.9	4.3	89	7.7	7.9	97
Middle East and North Africa	1.4	3.2	43	5.5	7.5	74
South Asia	0.9	2.8	33	3.4	5.6	60
Sub-Saharan Africa	1.5	2.9	53	4.0	5.7	70
High-income economies	8.1	8.9	91	10.9	11.2	97

Source: Robert Barro and Jong-Wha Lee, "A New Data Set of Educational Attainment in the World, 1950–2010." NBER Working Paper No. 15902, (Cambridge, MA: NBER, April 2010). Data available at www.barrolee.com/data/dataexp.htm.

no schooling (0.9 years), only one third of what adult men received (2.8 years). By 2010, outcomes had improved. Women averaged 3.4 years of schooling, now about 60 percent of what men completed. South Asia's gender gap is expected to continue to narrow. Today in South Asia, gross primary school enrollment rates for boys and girls both exceed 100 percent, with the rate for girls equal to 95 percent those of boys; the secondary school enrollment rate is 56 percent for boys and 48 percent for girls. When these young people move on to replace their parents and grandparents in the labor force, the region's stock of human capital will be larger and its distribution between men and women relatively more equal.

SCHOOLING VERSUS EDUCATION

Years of schooling and the gender distribution of that schooling are two ways of charting the accumulation of human capital. But schooling is only a means to an end; the real goal is education—that is, the skills individuals acquire from time spent studying and learning. Students can sit through many years of schooling and learn very little. Measuring learning outcomes is notoriously difficult within one nation let alone across many. But there have been attempts to apply basic tests of core competencies in reading and mathematics across nations. The results are sobering because of both the gap between rich and poor nations and the implications for the quality of schooling available in many low- and middle-income nations.

One source of cross-country information on learning outcomes is the Programme for International Student Assessment (PISA). Initially, PISA administered examinations only among Organisation for Economic Co-Operation and Development (OECD) members—that is, mostly high-income economies. But interest in their work led to an expansion of testing to some non-OECD and mostly middle-income settings. PISA's goal is to assess how well 15-year-olds, approaching the end of their compulsory schooling years, are prepared "to meet the challenges of today's societies." Representative samples of 15-year-olds attending school are selected from participating nations, with the total number of students tested ranging from 4,500 to 10,000 per country. Average scores on the 2009 reading test for a subset of the more than 60 participating nations are presented in Figure 8–3. Korea had the highest mean score, with Korean students performing better than many nations with considerably higher incomes. Finland was 2nd; the United States ranked 16th (tied with Poland).

The middle-income nations in the table have scores that are almost always lower than the high-income nations. This is not surprising. We expect these scores to be income elastic. At higher incomes, economies have more to spend on schooling and we believe there is some association between school expenditures and student learning. At higher incomes, children may be healthier and more able to learn. They also are more likely to have parents who attended school, another predictor of student performance. Of course, income is not all that matters. Korea and Poland's superior performance relative to much richer nations cannot be due to income.

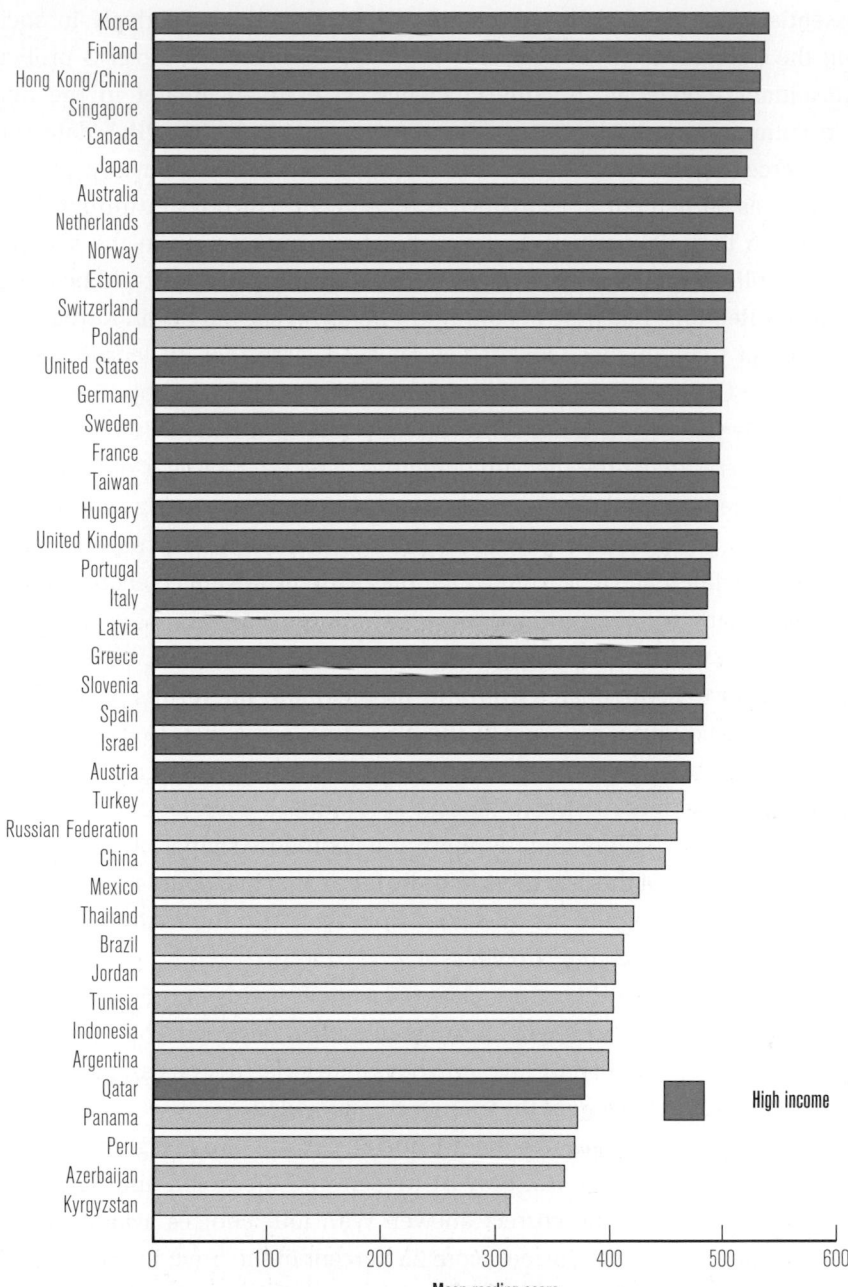

FIGURE 8-3 **Learning Outcomes: Reading Achievement of 15-Year-Olds, 2009**

Source: Organisation for Economic Co-Operation and Development (OECD), *PISA: 2009 Results: Executive Summary*, available at www.pisa.oecd.org/dataoecd/34/60/46619703.pdf, accessed February 2012.

What is alarming about the findings is not that middle-income nations have lower scores, that was expected, but how much lower these scores are relative to high-income economies. On the reading achievement test, 19 percent of all OECD students failed to achieve proficiency Level 2: a level low enough that students "lack the essential skills needed to participate effectively and productively in society."[5] Raising the percentage of 15-year-olds in OECD countries to Level 2 proficiency is a formidable challenge. But the challenge is so much greater in the middle-income nations. Among the 26 middle-income nations in the PISA data set, the median percentage of 15-year-old boys who did not achieve Level 2 proficiency in reading was 50 percent; for girls it was 33 percent. For boys in Indonesia it was 65 percent; in Peru, 70 percent. In the only low-income nation in the sample, the Kyrgyz Republic, it was 88 percent. Clearly, the education a 15-year-old boy received in the Kyrgyz Republic had little in common with a 15-year-old boy in Korea.

Results on mathematical skills show an even larger gap in learning between students in OECD countries and those outside of the OECD group. Because most middle-income nations have not achieved universal secondary school enrollments, PISA results *overestimate* the measured abilities of all their 15-year-olds. Those who are not in school are unlikely to know as much as those attending school; and the PISA exam was given to only those in school! If PISA surveyed more low-income economies, the difference in learning outcomes with the advanced economies would likely be even starker.

It is possible that the disparity in results is due to cultural bias, because any test is likely to suffer to some degree from this problem, but the results on student performance across countries reported by the PISA study are similar to those from other evaluations. One study from Bangladesh found that 58 percent of a sample of rural children age 11 and older failed to identify seven out of eight letters; a similar percentage had difficulty identifying numbers and geometric shapes. A 2007 nationally representative survey of third-graders in India found that half could not read a simple first-grade paragraph. One of the questions from the Third International Mathematics and Science Study asks the following:

Three-fifths of the students in a class are girls. If 5 girls and 5 boys are added, which statement is true? (a) There are more girls than boys; (b) There are the same number of girls as boys; (c) There are more boys than girls; (d) You cannot tell whether there are more girls or boys from the information provided.

Approximatley 82 percent of Japanese and 62 percent of U.S. eighth-graders provided the correct answer (a). But only 31 percent of Colombian and South African eighth-graders identified the correct answer. With four choices available, random guessing would result in the correct score 25 percent of the time; the schoolchildren in Colombia and South Africa performed only marginally better.[6]

---

[5]OECD, *PISA at a Glance* (Paris: OECD, 2010), p. 12.

[6]The Bangladesh results are from Vincent Greaney, Shahidur Khandker, and Mahmudul Alam, *Bangladesh: Assessing Basic Learning Skills* (Dhaka: University Press, 1999) as reported by Glewwe and Kremer, *Handbook on the Economics of Education*. The Trends in International Mathematics and Science Study results are cited in Lant Pritchett, "Access to Education," in Bjorn Lomborg, ed., *Global Crises, Global Solutions* (London: Cambridge University Press, 2004).

That learning outcomes in developing nations, on average, are below the levels prevailing in developed nations is not a surprising finding. Rich nations have many advantages over poorer ones. Given the rapid expansion in school enrollments over the past few decades, many developing nations had no choice but to focus on expanding quantity, not on improving quality. There simply could not have been, for example, enough experienced teachers and principals to handle the primary and secondary schooling needs resulting from the increase in school enrollments. Anyone with firsthand experience of schools in poor countries, especially in rural areas, is familiar with the problems: too many unqualified teachers, endemic absenteeism among students *and* teachers, and too few books and other teaching materials. In such environments, it is no wonder that learning outcomes are so poor.

EDUCATION AS AN INVESTMENT

Despite problems of low quality, the demand for education remains high in most countries. Parents want their children to have better lives and often see getting an education as a way to achieve them. In terms of material well-being, what parents perceive is borne out by the data. On average, people with more schooling earn more than people with less schooling. Few economic outcomes are as robust as the relationship between earnings and schooling. Primary school graduates tend to earn more than those with no schooling, secondary school graduates earn more than their counterparts who completed only primary school, and those with tertiary education tend to earn the most. Of course, these are average tendencies. A professor with many years of schooling may earn less than a plumber who went to school for fewer years, but on average, the relationship holds. It holds for both men and women, it holds in fast growing economies and stagnant ones, and it holds across income levels and regions.

Figure 8–4 illustrates the relationship between schooling and earnings for one country, Nicaragua. Using household data, Figure 8–4 charts **age-earnings profiles** for men and women separately, by level of education attained. Workers at all schooling levels tend to see their earnings rise quickly in their early years, reach a plateau, and sometimes fall off in later years. The more educated the worker, the higher the age-earnings profile tends to be. In Nicaragua, the earnings premiums for more educated men are unambiguous. As level of schooling rises, each age-earnings profile lies above the one that preceded it. For Nicaraguan women, the trends are not as definitive due, in part, to the relatively small number of observations on working women in this data set. A larger sample would most likely produce the same non-overlapping earnings profiles that characterize Nicaraguan men. Comparison of the earnings of Nicaraguan men and women reveals one other relationship. At every education level women tend to earn less than their male

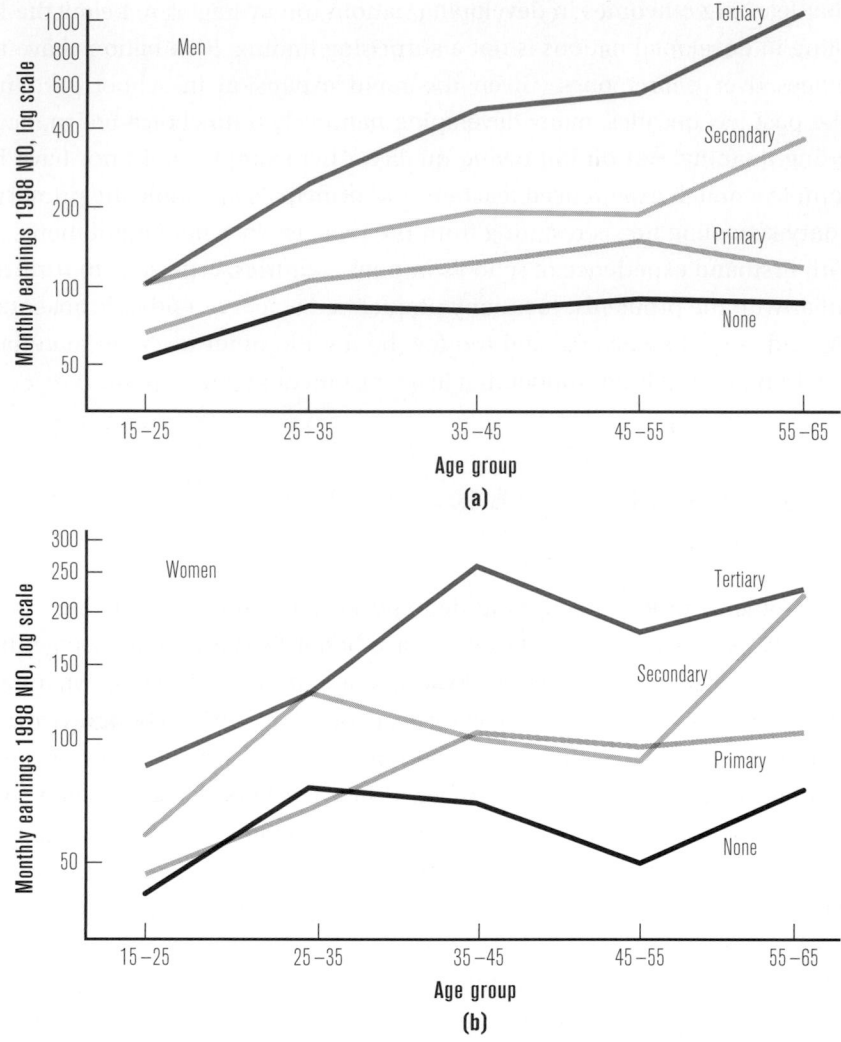

FIGURE 8-4 Earnings by Age, Education, and Gender, Nicaragua, 1998

Source: World Bank, Nicaragua Living Standards Measurement Study Survey, Encuesta Nacional de Hogares sobre Medición de Niveles de Vida (ENMV), 1998, available via www.worldbank.org/lsms/country/ni98/ni98docs.html#English.

counterparts, a worldwide result almost as common as the tendency for earnings to rise with education levels.

If Figure 8-4 were reproduced for any country the results would be similar: People with more years of schooling tend to earn more than people with fewer years. This suggests thinking about education as an investment. Economists define investment as the flow of resources into the production of new capital. In the case of schooling, resources by both governments and households are spent in the expectation that schooling produces human capital. The expectation is also that these investments will yield a positive return. By attending school, an individual hopes to acquire human capital, which makes that individual more productive and, therefore, better compensated. This relationship holds whether the individual becomes a farmer or trader, laborer or artisan, professional or government official.

There are several benefits to thinking of education as an investment. Schooling competes with many other activities on which governments and households spend their scarce resources. How does a government decide how much to devote to schooling? Should more resources be spent on schools as opposed to health clinics, tube wells for clean water, or rural roads? Even within the education sector, how should a government allocate its spending: Is achieving universal primary education a better use of resources than expanding colleges and universities? Governments must make these decisions and thinking about education as an investment can help. Households make similar decisions. When education is viewed as an investment it becomes easier to understand why some families send their children to work and not to school, while other families do everything in their power to make sure a child receives an education.

THE RATE OF RETURN TO SCHOOLING

Figure 8–5 illustrates the factors that determine the **private return** on schooling. The figure presents two stylized streams of future earnings, one if the individuals complete only primary school and the other if they complete a secondary education. All individuals are assumed to complete primary school at age 11. If they

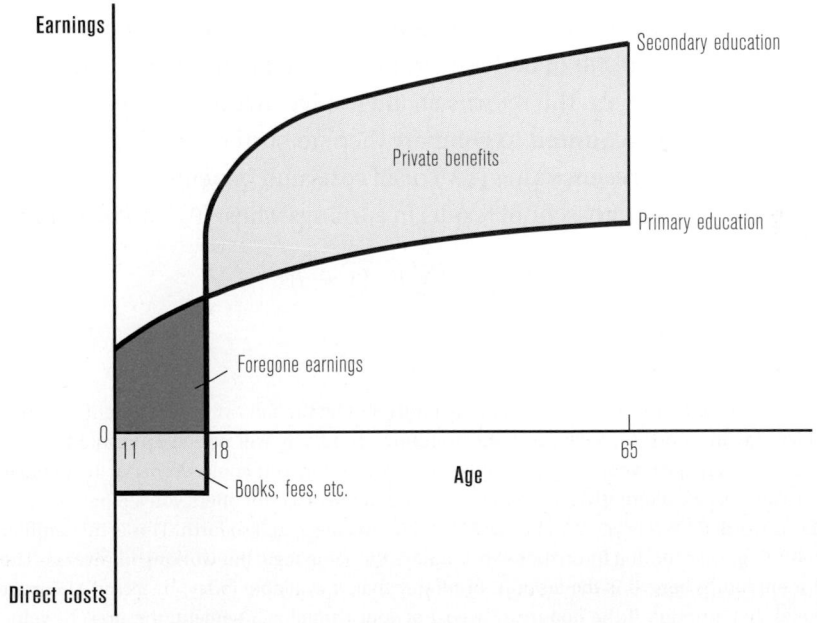

FIGURE 8-5 **Determinants of the Private Returns to Schooling**

do not continue with their education, they begin to work and follow the earnings profile marked as primary education. Alternatively, individuals might complete secondary education and remain in school until age 18. For ease of exposition, we assume that individuals do not work while in school and, therefore, have zero earnings while in school. Once secondary school is completed, these individuals follow the higher of the two earnings profiles. The private pecuniary benefits of a secondary education, as we saw in Figure 8–4, are the earnings the individual expects to receive beyond what they would have earned with only a primary school education.

But costs also are associated with the decision to remain in school. These costs include any foregone earnings, sacrificed because an individual is in school and not working. These costs may seem low for a young person considering attending primary or secondary school. But for the majority of households in the developing nations, the opportunity costs of sending a child to school are real. In rural households, for example, children work in the fields, take care of animals, or watch siblings, permitting others, including adults, to be engaged in farming or other productive activities. In addition to foregone earnings, households face direct costs in sending a child to school. These costs may include school or uniform fees, payments for books and other materials, transportation costs, or other "unofficial" fees to ensure a child gets the attention of a teacher. Although the sums may seem small, to a poor family they may be overwhelming.

To think of education as an investment, we need a systematic way to compare the costs and benefits of schooling depicted in Figure 8–5. Economists argue that one cannot simply add up the costs and compare them to the benefits because money received in the future is worth less than money that can be spent today. Such positive time preference is the result of both uncertainty about the future and the opportunity cost of resources—namely, the returns an alternative investment might yield. Future benefits need to be **discounted** to compare them to current costs. One way of doing so is to compute the **present value (PV)** of all costs and benefits.[7]

Completing secondary school results in earnings whose PV can be computed as

$$PV_B = \sum_{t=1}^{n} B_t/(1 + i)^t \qquad\qquad [8\text{–}1]$$

---

[7]The need to discount future benefits can be motivated by the following example. If you are asked to trade $100 today in return for $100 one year from now, you likely will not accept the offer. Beyond any uncertainty you may have about being paid back in 12 months, you could do better by depositing your $100 in a relatively safe alternative, like a bank account. If that account offers you a 5 percent return, your $100 today is worth $105 one year from now, $110.25 in two years, and so forth. This is the familiar process of compounding. Discounting future benefits employs the same logic but working in reverse. The present value of some future benefit is the amount of money that, if available today, by virtue of compounding, would equal that amount. If the opportunity cost of your capital is 5 percent, the present value of $105 received one year from now equals [$105 ÷ (1 + 0.05)] = $100; similarly, the present value of $110.25 received in two years also is $100 since [$110.25 ÷ (1 + 0.05)²] = $100.

where PV_B equals the sum of the present value of all future private benefits (the earnings differential received with more schooling) over an individual's n years of working; B_t equals the benefits in year t; and i is the interest rate (the household's opportunity cost of capital), which discounts future benefits. A similar calculation can be made for the private costs of schooling (or for any other investment option):

$$PV_C = \sum_{t=1}^{n} C_t/(1 + i)^t \qquad\qquad [8\text{-}2]$$

where PV_C now refers to the sum of the present value of all anticipated private costs and C_t equals the costs, including foregone earnings while attending school plus any direct costs paid by the household, incurred in each of the t years.

There are several ways one can then determine whether a particular investment is worthwhile. In the analysis of education, a common way is to estimate an internal rate of return for the investment. The **internal rate of return** is a derived interest rate, r, which equates PV_B to PV_C. In other words, the level of r such that

$$\sum_{t-1}^{n} (B_t - C_t)/(1 + r)^t = 0 \qquad\qquad [8\text{-}3]$$

Even though the dollar value of the private benefits of an education is likely to far exceed the dollar value of the private costs, a value for r can be found because future benefits, occurring many years from now, are much more heavily discounted than are costs incurred more immediately. Once the private rate of return to schooling is estimated, it can be compared to the rates of return available to other household investments. This helps rank the economic benefits of education as compared to alternative uses of household resources.

Schooling represents not only a private investment; it also is a social one. We, therefore, can define a **social return** to schooling. Figure 8–6 presents a schematic representation. On the cost side, schooling entails more than the foregone earnings of the individual and the payments of households. Primary school is "free" in most parts of the world, yet someone pays for teachers, the construction of schools, and the like. When evaluating education as an investment from society's perspective, these costs must be taken into consideration. The social return includes all the costs entailed in the provision of schooling. On the benefit side, schooling benefits the individual through higher earnings but schooling may also produce a positive **externality**: benefits that accrue to members of society above and beyond the benefits to the individual who receives the education. Potential positive externalities from school include health spillovers (the children of educated mothers tend to be healthier, which benefits children in other families because it reduces the transmission rate of certain diseases), reductions in crime, and more-informed political participation and decisions. More schooling, especially higher education, may also lead to technological progress that is not fully captured by private returns. To calculate a social rate of return to education use equation 8–3, but all the benefits of schooling, not just private earnings, and all the costs, private and public, should be included.

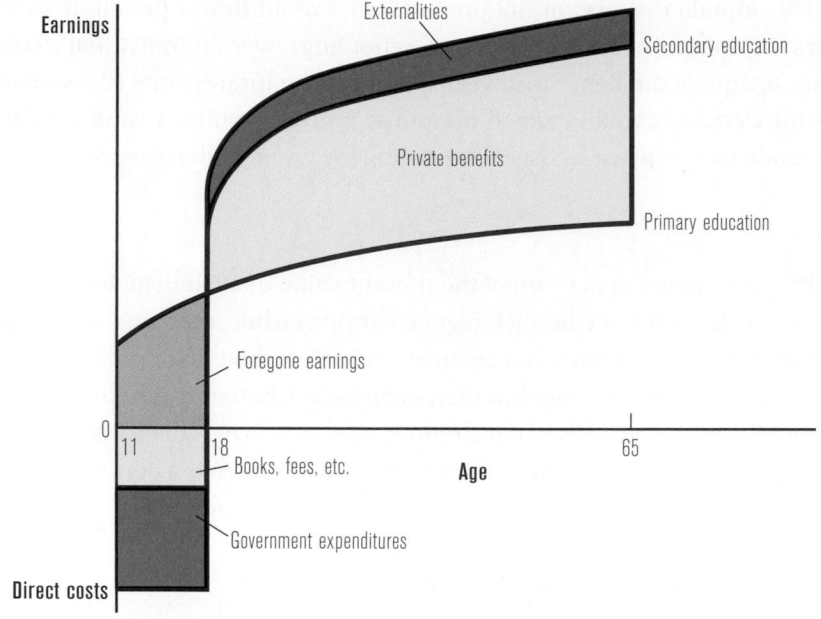

FIGURE 8-6 Determinants of the Social Returns to Schooling

Note: For ease of exposition, the figure is drawn without any positive externalities arising from primary education.

ESTIMATED RATES OF RETURN

Moving from the conceptual to the empirical, a large number of rate-of-return estimates for schooling are available for both developed and developing nations. To interpret these estimates it is important to be familiar with many of their implicit assumptions. First, there is no way of knowing what anyone's future earnings will be. Economists use the current earnings of individuals at various ages as an estimate of the expected age-earnings profile of someone with a particular level of education. Substituting such cross-sectional findings (comparing wages for different ages at one point in time) for what may happen over time to the wages of individuals as they grow older is a common empirical technique in economics; however, especially in a rapidly changing economy, estimates based on cross-sectional findings may not be a good proxy for events that will occur in the future.

Second, estimates of the return on education require some measure of individual earnings. In low-income nations and in many middle-income nations, the vast majority of workers do not work for wages. They are self-employed, often subsistence farmers or unpaid family workers engaged in petty trading or other informal sector activity. Such workers do not report the kind of earnings data included in standard rate of return on schooling estimations. By relying only on those who receive earnings, most rate-of-return estimates are based on a fraction of a nation's labor force.

Third, problems of **identification** confront most empirical studies. Returns to schooling are no exception. If individuals who have more years of schooling earn more than those with fewer, how do we know schooling caused the higher earnings? Perhaps people who are innately more talented both earn more and receive more schooling. Is the increase in earnings a result of their schooling or their innate abilities? If we do not control for innate ability—something that is not easy to measure—and for many other variables that might influence future earnings, how can we be certain that our estimates of the rate of return to schooling are correct?

FIRST-GENERATION ESTIMATES

Economists have developed different techniques for estimating rates of return to education, and it is instructive to see how methodological advances have replaced earlier approaches and dealt with problems of identification. Some of the first studies have been compiled in meta-analyses by World Bank economists George Psacharo-poulos and Harry Patrinos. Table 8–3 is from their work and includes calculations of internal rates-of-return for over 75 nations. Some of these studies refer to outcomes as far back as the late 1950s, whereas others refer to the 1990s.[8] Rates of return esti-mated for individual countries are averaged together and presented as a mean value for different income categories and regions. These are simple cross-country averages and are not weighted by population size. They are *real* not nominal rates of return because they are based on cross-sectional estimates that measure earnings in the same current dollars.

A number of patterns can be observed in these data. Returns on all levels of schooling and in all income categories are almost always in double digits. Returns

TABLE 8-3 **Returns to Schooling by Level and Country Income Group**

INCOME CATEGORY	PRIVATE RATE OF RETURN			"SOCIAL" RATE OF RETURN*		
	PRIMARY	SECONDARY	TERTIARY	PRIMARY	SECONDARY	TERTIARY
Low	25.8	19.9	26.0	21.3	15.7	11.2
Middle	27.4	18.0	19.3	18.8	12.9	11.3
High	25.6	12.2	12.4	13.4	10.3	9.5

*The estimates of social rates of return account for only government expenditures on schooling and do not include estimates of any positive externalities resulting from schooling.

Source: G. Psacharopoulus and H. Patrinos, "Returns to Investment in Education: A Further Update," *Education Economics* 12, no. 2 (August 2004).

[8]George Psacharopoulos and Harry Patrinos, "Returns to Investment in Education: A Further Update," *Education Economics* 12, no. 2 (August 2004).

to schooling also tend to be greater for developing versus developed economies. This may seem surprising given the much higher wages and salaries workers earn in high-income nations. But, remember, rates of return measure something different from the level of earnings. Take the case of graduates of tertiary education. Given the relative scarcity of students with a tertiary education in poorer nations, the pay premium to having such an education may be greater than the relative pay gap between university and high school graduates in richer nations. It is the relative scarcity of labor skills, a combination of the strength of labor demand and the extent of labor supply, that contributes to the attractiveness of schooling as an investment. In poorer nations, educated workers are relatively scarce, often making schooling (at the primary, secondary, and tertiary levels) an investment with a higher rate of return than in advanced economies, where educated workers are far more abundant.

Looking across levels of schooling, returns are highest for primary schooling. This is probably because the opportunity cost of attending school in terms of foregone earnings is lowest when attending primary school and rises thereafter. Returns to secondary school are below or close to those of a tertiary education. This may be due to much larger pay differentials between tertiary and secondary school graduates versus between secondary and primary school graduates. Or it may reflect opportunities tertiary school students have to earn some income while studying (so there is less cost from foregone earnings), including receipt of government stipends for attending a school, a common practice in many developing nations, especially during the time period of the studies represented in the table.

Estimated "social" returns in Table 8–3 are lower than private ones at every level of schooling. Theoretically this need not be the case (see Figure 8–6). If positive externalities are sufficiently large, social returns could exceed the private rate of return even if social costs are greater than private costs. However, no direct means are available for estimating the positive externalities of schooling; the average "social" rates of return to schooling reported in Table 8–3 account for only social costs, using private not social benefits; hence our use of quotation marks around the word *social.* By incorporating the full cost of schooling but not any positive externalities, "social" returns for a given level of schooling must be less than the corresponding private return. Note also that the relative gap between private and "social" returns is especially large for tertiary schooling in low- and middle-income nations. This reflects the relatively high per pupil cost and high degree of state subsidy for tertiary education, often including free tuition. Even though the "social" returns are below private returns, the rates are sufficiently high to make schooling an attractive public investment compared to many alternatives, including investments in physical capital.

Another approach to estimating the rate of return to education is to estimate wage equations by which regressions are run to determine the impact on earnings of schooling adjusting for age and other demographic characteristics. The coefficient on schooling can be interpreted as an estimate of the private return to an additional year of schooling (Box 8–1). The return is based on all years of schooling rather than distinguishing between primary, secondary, and tertiary. Psacharopoulos and Patrinos report on these estimates as well and find the range for low- and middle-income nations by region is 7 to 12 percent per additional year of schooling. The attractiveness of such returns can be illustrated by comparing them to estimates of the return on other investment opportunities. For example, U.S. government securities, one of the world's safest investments, have yielded an average real (inflation-adjusted) return of about 1 percent per year over the last 50 years; an index of the U.S. stock market, a riskier investment, over the same period yields an annual real return of 2 to 3 percent. Of course, most families do not choose between investing in U.S. stocks or government securities versus sending a child to primary school; a comparison of these rates of return is intended only to put into perspective the relative magnitudes and to highlight the attractiveness of human capital as an investment.

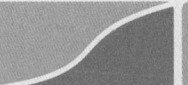

BOX 8–1 ESTIMATING RATES OF RETURN FROM WAGE EQUATIONS

Conceptually, the notion of rates of return to schooling is relatively straightforward. Estimating such returns is more complex. One of the most common approaches is to estimate the impact on earnings of schooling, age, and other demographic characteristics. Data on these variables can be obtained from either household or firm surveys and used to estimate a human capital earnings function or wage equation like the following:

$$\ln E_i = \alpha + \beta_1 S_i + \beta_2 \exp_i + \beta_3 \exp_i^2 + \varepsilon_i$$

where E_i refers to the earnings or wages of each individual; S_i, the years of schooling completed; and $\exp_i$ and $\exp_i^2$, the years of work experience of the individual and its square, often approximated by the individual's age and its square. The reason for including the squared term is to capture the expected nonlinearity in age-earnings profiles because earnings tend to rise at a decreasing rate over a worker's lifetime. The regression equation also includes an error term, ε_i.

In this specification of the wage equation, the coefficient on schooling (β_1), where $\beta_1 = (\partial E/E)/\partial S$, provides an estimate of the average percent increase in earnings received by workers per additional year of schooling. It is an estimate of how wages in an economy vary by education for the year in which the data are obtained.

The term β_1 is also interpreted as the average annual private rate of return to one additional year of schooling, regardless of the level of schooling already attained. This interpretation requires a number of assumptions, including the same assumption used in the internal rate-of-return calculation: that earnings differentials by education *in a cross-section* are a good approximation of what will happen to pay differentials *over time* as workers age. Another assumption (one not required by the internal rate-of-return approach) requires that foregone earnings represent the only private cost of schooling. In some instances these are reasonable assumptions, in others not.

Estimates of wage equations tend to find a higher return to schooling for women than men.[9] This does not mean that women earn more than men; we already noted that for a given level of education men, on average, always earn more than women. Once again, the higher return indicates that the *relative benefit*, in terms of earnings, of an extra year of schooling is higher for women than men. There is further evidence to believe that the social return to educating women may exceed that of men because of the positive health and fertility externalities that are generated. This is because educating women reduces child mortality more than educating men does; educating women reduces fertility and, in so doing, reduces maternal mortality; and educating women is more effective than educating men in reducing the spread of HIV/AIDS. A 1992 study concluded that providing 1,000 girls in India with an extra year of primary school would avert 2 maternal deaths, 43 infant deaths, and 300 births. The cost of providing this education was about 60 percent of the estimated discounted social benefit, suggesting a huge social rate of return on sending girls to school.[10] This is powerful evidence in support of the MDG of reducing gender disparities in schooling.

SECOND-GENERATION ESTIMATES

The estimates of internal rates of return to education presented in Table 8–3 are subject to some debate. We already pointed out the limitations of using cross-section results to approximate a time series event, especially in environments in which labor market outcomes are changing rapidly. Another concern is the quality of studies included in the Psacharopoulos and Patrinos compilations. One critical review of rate-of-return estimates for Africa found many of the original studies were based on

[9]In the survey by Psacharopoulos and Patrinos, the average return to a year of schooling for women was 9.8 percent for women and 8.7 for men. In a different study, Peter Orazem and Elizabeth King use harmonized household data sets from 48 developing countries to estimate wage equations separately for women and men. The average return for women was 9.7 percent, for men 6.7 percent. Even more telling than the average, out of 71 cases the return was higher for women 59 times and for men only 5 times. "Schooling in Developing Countries: The Roles of Supply, Demand and Government Policy," in T. Paul Schultz and John Strauss, eds., *Handbook of Development Economics*, vol. 4 (Amsterdam: Elsevier, 2008).

[10]Lawrence Summers, "Investing in All the People: Educating Women in Developing Countries," EDI Seminar Paper No. 45 (Washington, DC: World Bank, 1994).

guesstimates of prevailing wages by consultants rather than on data from surveys. Another problem was limiting observations to those workers earning wages—that is, to those employed in the formal sector.[11] This is especially tricky when many formal sector jobs are in the public sector where wage setting may not reflect productivity criteria as is more likely in the private sector. Private rates of return to primary education for Africa in the Psacharopoulos and Patrinos sample range from 7.9 percent in Tanzania in 1991 to 99 percent in Botswana and Liberia in 1983. This large a range in estimates strains the creditability of the reported findings. Better data and more careful analysis might result in smaller estimates of the average returns to schooling, especially for low-income nations.

Another criticism of studies that form the basis of the results reported in Table 8–3 is the failure to account for all the school costs facing families. In Honduras, for example, the private return to primary school is estimated at 21 percent, if it is assumed that there are no direct costs to the family of attending school and if the child is considered to have foregone earnings only during the last two years of primary school, at ages 11 and 12. If the actual direct costs for uniforms, school supplies, transportation, and other parental contributions are included, the private returns drop to 16 percent; if foregone earnings are added for age 10, the returns drop to below 15 percent.[12] These criticisms challenge the magnitude of some of the reported rates of return to schooling but generally do not reverse the conclusion that schooling has a sufficiently high rate of return to make it a good investment for both the individual and society.

An additional criticism concerns the identification problems mentioned earlier that plague many of the studies that contributed to the first-generation estimates contained in Table 8–3 and to many of the estimates derived from the wage equations discussed in Box 8–1. One solution to these identification problems is to identify a **natural experiment** in which a set of circumstances permits the researcher to better isolate the effect of an intervention on one group (the treatment group) versus another (the control group). In a seminal paper, MIT economist Esther Duflo identifies a natural experiment in Indonesia that permits estimation of the return on schooling. Following the oil boom of 1973, the Indonesian government undertook a massive construction program, resulting in over 60,000 new primary schools. It stands as one of the world's fastest school-building programs ever undertaken. The natural experiment involves the subsequent educational attainment and adult wages of those who were 12 to 17 years old in 1974 and finished school just before the program began and were therefore not impacted by it versus those who were 2 to 6 years old in 1974 and immediately benefited from the new schools. Because the location of the new schools was not random, there is another dimension to the natural experiment involving the region where the

[11]Paul Bennell, "Rates of Return to Education: Does the Conventional Pattern Prevail in sub-Saharan Africa?" *World Development* 24, no. 1 (January 1996).

[12]Patrick McEwan, "Private Costs and the Rate-of-Return to Education," *Applied Economic Letters* 6 (1999).

child lived. Using state-of-the-art econometrics, Duflo is able to identify the expansion in the supply of schools as responsible for an increase in the number of years of schooling received by the treatment group and the impact of this increase on their earnings some 20 years later relative to the control group. She estimates a return on schooling ranging from 6.8 to 10.6 percent, results consistent with many earlier estimates.[13]

Results of other studies that grapple with identification problems reach somewhat different conclusions. In a recent review article, University of Pennsylvania economist Jere Behrman draws attention to problems stemming from omitted variables, including measures of innate cognitive skills, early-life nutrition and school quality. Studies that attempt to account for these determinants find that in addition to years of schooling, the quality of the school and the ability of the student have a significant effect on future earnings. When these variables are included in the regressions, the estimated return on *years* of schooling declines, sometimes by a significant amount.[14] Better data and improved econometric techniques are generating refined estimates of the return not only to years spent in school but also to other dimensions of schools and attributes of students. While differences in magnitudes remain, these newer estimates continue to support the notion that education is a worthwhile investment.

PUZZLES

Beyond disagreements about how high the rate of return to schooling is for different levels of schooling and for different countries and regions, several puzzles emerge about the relationship between these returns and both microeconomic and macroeconomic outcomes. One of the microeconomic puzzles concerns schooling and learning. The key issue is why does education have an economic return? The usual answer is that education provides the individual with cognitive skills, skills learned as distinct from innate ability, which makes him or her more productive in the marketplace. Higher productivity, in turn, is associated with higher compensation, a result that holds if one is discussing farm labor or professionals (Box 8–2). If schools produce cognitive skills, then we expect to observe a positive correlation between years of schooling and earnings and a positive rate of return on attending school. The puzzle involves results reported earlier in the chapter that reveal schooling in many developing countries often produces little in the way of learning. If true, why in these settings is there a continued association between schooling and earnings and significant rates of return to education? One possibility is that schools may have been better in the past, accounting for the higher earnings of older workers today. If school quality is more of a recent problem, it is less likely to show up in the cross-section studies

---

[13]Esther Duflo, "Schooling and Labor Market Consequences of School Construction in Indonesia: Evidence from an Unusual Policy Experiment," *American Economic Review* 91, 4 (September 2001).

[14]Jere Behrman, "Investment in Education: Inputs and Incentives," in Dani Rodrik and Mark Rosenzweig, eds., *Handbook of Development Economics*, vol. 5 (Amsterdam: Elsevier, 2010).

relating schooling to earnings that combine younger and older workers. And if school quality is a more contemporary problem, as younger workers age they may not realize as much of a return on their education as did today's older workers.

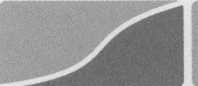

BOX 8-2 RETURNS TO SCHOOLING AND INCOME OPPORTUNITIES

In a series of studies, Andrew Foster and Mark Rosenzweig, economists at Brown and Yale Universities, respectively, examine the interaction between returns to schooling and technological change in agriculture. Their core argument is that schooling has a return primarily when new income-generating opportunities arise. In one study of worker productivity, data were assembled on workers engaged primarily in harvesting in Bukidnon, the Philippines. Controlling for a worker's physical ability, proxied by gender and height, there was no impact of the worker's education on the wage received. In this situation, workers performed a routine task and little was gained from additional schooling.

A different outcome was observed in India. In a study of over 4,000 rural households between the years 1968 and 1981, the authors assessed the impact schooling had on farm profitability. The time period studied covered the introduction of the green revolution to India, when imported high-yield variety (HYV) seeds were introduced that could dramatically increase farm output (usually because it permitted double and even triple cropping during a calendar year). HYV seeds are particularly sensitive to the use of complementary inputs, including irrigation and fertilizer, and it was especially important for farmers to be able to learn how to use these seeds because the required farming techniques were different from traditional methods.

In areas where conditions were suitable for the introduction of the HYV, farmers with primary schooling had higher profits than those without schooling, holding all other inputs constant. Investments in education had a high return to these farmers because of increased returns to learning and new information. In other areas of the country, including the Indian state of Kerala, where farmers had above average years of schooling, conditions were not suitable for the new seeds. These farmers got little return because there were no new opportunities that required education.

Rosenzweig concludes that "schooling returns are high when the returns to learning are also high." This can be because of a new technology, like the green revolution or new opportunities created by changes in market or political regimes. Not only do those with more schooling reap a return in these situations but they also tend to invest more heavily in the schooling of their children. School enrollment rates increased more rapidly in those Indian communities that benefited from the technological change than in those that did not.

Sources: Andrew Foster and Mark Rosenzweig, "Technical Change and Human-Capital Returns and Investments: Evidence from the Green Revolution," *American Economic Review* 86, no. 4 (September 1996); Mark Rosenzweig, "Why Are There Returns to Schooling?" *American Economic Review* 85, no. 2 (May 1995).

One of the macroeconomic puzzles results from trying to reconcile another set of empirical observations. Earlier in this chapter, we reported on trends in schooling by region. The evidence is clear. There has been rapid growth in schooling throughout the world over the past decades, resulting in some convergence in years of schooling per worker across countries. Given the rates of return to education reported by Psacharopoulos and Patrinos and others, such an expansion of schooling should have produced more rapid aggregate economic growth in many regions and some convergence in incomes. This is expected because schooling has grown much more rapidly in developing than developed nations and the returns to schooling are higher in low- and middle-income nations than in high-income settings. But this is not what the aggregate data show. Instead, there has been considerable divergence in per capita incomes at the same time there has been some convergence in schooling.

Schooling, of course, is not the only determinant of aggregate growth, and other factors may be more important in determining growth rates of gross domestic product (GDP) per capita. But there remains something disconcerting about the micro evidence on the accumulation of schooling and on the attractive rates of return to these investments and the subsequent lack of evidence that increased schooling results in significantly higher economic growth rates. Exploration of this puzzle led one researcher to ask, "Where has all the education gone?" and then to speculate that, in environments not conducive to growth, those with more education may engage in rent seeking and other unproductive activities that are privately remunerative but "socially dysfunctional."[15] This may be part of the explanation, but a fuller reconciliation of micro and macro evidence on schooling outcomes remains a challenge for future research.

---

[15]Excellent discussion of the macroeconomic puzzles involving schooling and economic growth can be found in Lant Pritchett, "Where Has All the Education Gone?" *World Bank Economic Review* 15, no. 3 (2001) and "Does Learning to Add Up Add Up? The Returns to Schooling in Aggregate Data," *Handbook on the Economics of Education* (Boston: Elsevier, 2006). A less-technical review of some of these points can be found in William Easterly, "Educated for What?" in *The Elusive Quest for Growth* (Cambridge, MA: MIT Press, 2001).

MAKING SCHOOLING MORE PRODUCTIVE

Despite debate and puzzles over the rate of return to schooling, no one would conclude that parents or governments in developing nations should invest less in schooling. Schooling has benefits that go well beyond narrow economic returns. It often is considered a merit good, a good that a society determines all members should have access to regardless of ability or willingness to pay. There is also evidence that schooling improves health, with educated mothers having fewer and healthier children. The challenge facing policy makers and all those concerned with promoting economic development is to understand how to make schooling a better investment: better for students and their families who devote so much of their time to education, and better for governments and donors who finance much of the direct costs.

Rates of return on schooling depend on what happens both in schools and in the labor market after students graduate. Much of this textbook is devoted to the latter, to understanding how to increase the rate of economic growth in an economy and with it an increase in the demand for labor. We will not go over these elements again here. But it is worth noting that low returns to education often have a lot to do with failures to increase the demand for labor. High unemployment among school leavers, including graduates of universities, often reflects failures in promoting economic growth rather than failures in schools. This has been true in transition economies but also is apparent in countries such as Argentina and Egypt, which have not made good use of the human capital they accumulated. High dropout rates, as well as low and even declining school enrollment rates (the latter occurred throughout sub-Saharan Africa during the 1990s), may have as much to do with low returns in the labor market as with a family's resource constraints or problems with the schools themselves. Students and their families may decide that the benefits of schooling do not justify the costs. And in many instances they may be right. The provision of schooling is no guarantee that getting an education will yield a high return. Problems with labor demand highlight that schooling is not a panacea; it is not *the one solution* to problems of poverty and economic backwardness.

But problems on the demand side do not imply that the supply of education is without flaws. The remainder of this chapter focuses on the supply of education in an attempt to understand how investments in schooling can be made more productive. In many countries schooling is not doing as much as it can to promote development. Some of the reasons for this are that there is underinvestment in schooling overall, that governments misallocate resources across different levels of schooling, and that there are systematic inefficiencies in the use of resources within schools.[16]

---

[16]Two early reviews of resource use and schooling are World Bank, *Financing Education in Developing Countries* (Washington, DC: World Bank, 1986) and *Priorities and Strategies for Education* (Washington, DC: World Bank, 1995). Recent surveys of improving school outcomes in developing nations are Glewwe and Kremer, "Schools, Teachers, and Education Outcomes" and Pritchett, "Access to Education."

UNDERINVESTMENT

Despite attractive economic returns and other benefits to schooling, many developing countries spend too little on educating their children. Determining the right amount that should be spent is no simple matter. First, estimates of rates of return are imprecise at best; second, spending more money on schooling is no guarantee that the money will be well spent and produce better education outcomes. But money does matter, and cross-country data reveal considerable variance in public spending on schooling (comparable data on private spending are not available). In Figure 8–7, among low- and lower-middle-income nations, the range in public expenditures on education as a share of GDP is from about 1.5 to over 12 percent. We cannot be sure that the average spending share within these income groups is the "right" amount, especially because we do not know the corresponding amount of private spending. But nations such as Cambodia, Chad, and Zambia, where public spending on schooling is under 2 percent of GDP (well below the 3.6 percent median of the low-income group) stand as candidates for increasing the amount their governments spend on education. Similarly, Angola, Georgia, and Peru devote well below the lower-middle-income median of 4.3 percent of GDP to schooling and may be seriously underinvesting in education. To the extent that any of these and other countries also have a high dependency burden of young people, they especially need to devote a larger share of GDP to schooling because those expenditures must be spread among a large number of students.

There are many explanations for why nations may underinvest in schooling. One is as a response to fiscal crises. Education and the social sectors in general, as opposed to the military or debt service, often are victims of budget cuts. Economic downturns and negative growth rates have impacts on education spending and can result in an entire cohort of children getting less schooling than would have been the case in a more stable economy. Protecting schooling and the other social sectors is a major challenge nations face whenever government revenues start to fall.

MISALLOCATION

Misallocation of resources between different levels of schooling refers to government decisions on how much to spend on primary, secondary, and tertiary levels. The estimates of rates of return to schooling in Table 8–3 indicate that the social returns are highest for primary school followed by secondary then tertiary schooling. Given the construction of these estimates, the results are not surprising. The direct costs of tertiary schooling (everything from junior colleges through doctoral programs) per student, including expenditures on computers, laboratories, libraries, professors, and the like, are much higher than the per student costs of either primary or secondary education. Because the government often pays for all or most of these costs, social returns to higher education are going to be significantly less than are private returns.

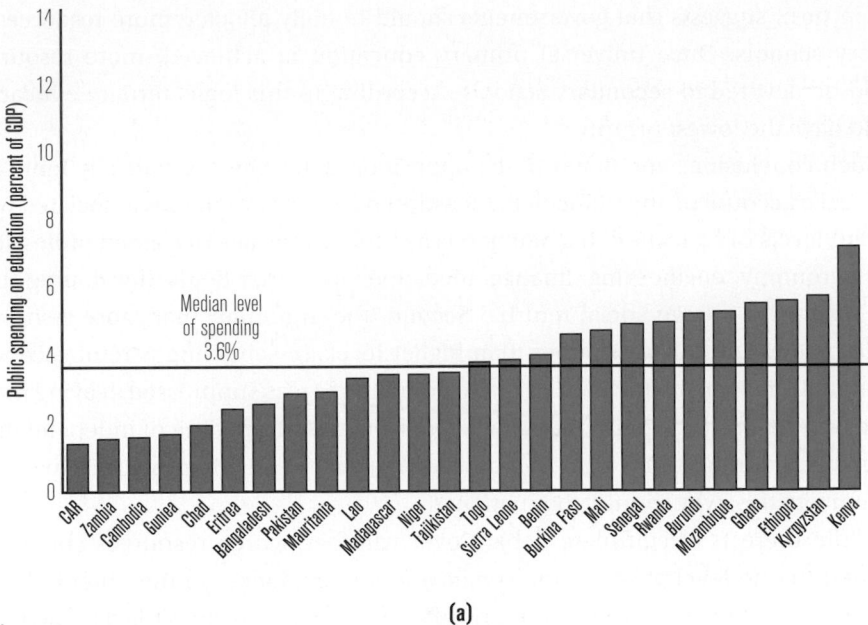

(a)

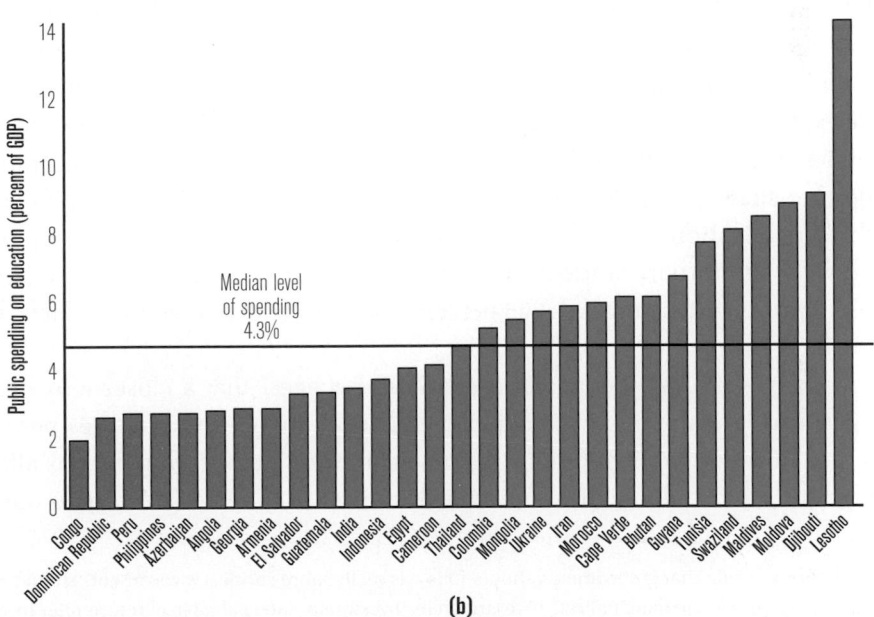

(b)

FIGURE 8-7   Public Spending on Education, 2005–07

(a) Lower-income economies. (b) Lower-middle-income economies.

GDP, gross domestic product.

Source: World Bank, "World Development Indicators Online," http://databank.worldbank.org.

This, in turn, suggests that governments should initially allocate more resources to primary schools. Once universal primary education is achieved, more resources should be devoted to secondary schools. According to this logic, tertiary education should have the lowest priority.[17]

Such conclusions encounter much opposition. First, the estimates in Table 8–3 do not take account of any (difficult to measure) positive externalities associated with different levels of education. If a nation has a chronic shortage of trained professionals in agronomy, engineering, finance, medicine, and other fields, developing such skills may yield a large social return.[18] Second, the argument that more resources should be devoted to lower rather than higher levels of schooling is reminiscent of the colonial era, when education of native populations was suppressed, leaving many nations with a minuscule number of educated citizens at the time of independence. Rich nations did not wait to achieve universal primary education before expanding their universities; why should poor nations?

While there is a legitimate debate over whether scarce resources should be allocated to one level of schooling versus another, evidence on the potential misallocation of public resources among different levels of schooling is suggested by comparing enrollment rates and expenditure patterns on tertiary education. Among sub-Saharan African countries for which the relevant data are available, the gross enrollment rate for tertiary education is 5.3 percent, while the median share of total government education expenditures devoted to the tertiary sector is 16 percent. In Latin America, tertiary enrollment rates are almost six times bigger, but the expenditure share is the same as in sub-Saharan Africa. In the high-income economies, the gross enrollment rate is over 60 percent, but the median public expenditure share is only 24 percent. United Nations Educational, Scientific, and Cultural Organization (UNESCO) computes a related and telling statistic: public expenditures per tertiary student as a percentage of gross national income (GNI) per capita. In 2007 this ratio was 206 percent in Senegal, 39 percent in Mexico, and 30 percent in France.

Gaps between enrollments and expenditures suggest that a closer look needs to be given to how the money is being spent. Much higher expenditures per student enrolled in tertiary institutions in some countries stem from generous allowances given to those enrolled in university; in essence, paying students to obtain

---

[17]The theoretical rule that governments should follow is really more subtle. Governments should allocate resources to equate the marginal rate of return on its investment. Internal rates of return refer to average returns (the average for all graduates of primary, secondary, or tertiary schooling) not the marginal return, which refers to the economic rate of return for the last student educated. When a particular level of schooling gets close to universal enrollment and completion, it is likely that the marginal social return will be below the average return, perhaps well below it.

[18]Arguments in favor of for devoting more resources to higher education in developing nations is presented in World Bank, *Higher Education in Developing Countries: Perils and Promise* (Washington, DC: World Bank, 2000).

an education that is likely to yield them considerably higher earnings in the future. Noneducational expenditures in the form of student allowances and scholarships as well as subsidized housing, healthcare, loans, and so on, accounted for 50 percent of public expenditures on tertiary education among Francophone African countries, 20 percent in Latin America, and only 14 percent in OECD countries. Such allowances are often given in addition to free tuition.[19] With growing numbers of tertiary school students, such expenditures add further stress to tight education budgets. Given the tendency for those of higher socioeconomic status to have the opportunity to attend tertiary school, allowances and free tuition are also regressive uses of public money. A review of enrollment in public and private tertiary schools in Latin America found that 75 percent of the students in Colombia were from the top two quintiles of the income distribution; in Mexico, it was 83 percent, and in Brazil, 92 percent.[20] Many of these families have resources that could be devoted to higher education. When the state finances so much of the education of their sons and daughters, the outcome is a regressive one.

One approach to correcting the misallocation of resources across schooling levels is to have university students pay for some of their education. This can be justified because higher education is likely to have a high private rate of return, even if the student pays (including by taking out loans) for some of his or her education. The use of tuition reduces public contributions and permits some shifting of state spending from tertiary to primary and secondary schooling. The economic logic of charging students, especially those with the ability to pay, for some of the cost of their tertiary schooling may be clear, but instituting such fees may be far from straightforward. In Mexico, the constitution calls for free public education at all levels. Confronted with rising numbers of university students and the rising costs of providing that education, the National Autonomous University of Mexico (UNAM) in 1999 decided to raise student fees from the level last set in 1948. By 1999, these fees, adjusted for price inflation, amounted to only 2 cents ($US) per year. The administration of UNAM proposed new fees of about $150 for those with the economic means to cover these costs. Such fees would have offset less than 10 percent of the government's expenditures on the university. In response to the proposal, many of the school's 270,000 students went on strike and the school remained closed for almost a full year. In the end, the school modified its proposal, making the $150 fee voluntary, and the university's president resigned. Despite the economic logic behind the user fees on the grounds of both economic efficiency and social equity, the politics surrounding the proposal made it unworkable.

---

[19]World Bank, *Constructing Knowledge Societies: New Challenges for Tertiary Education* (Washington, DC: World Bank, 2002), pp. 51–52.

[20]World Bank, *Constructing Knowledge Societies,* p. 195.

IMPROVING SCHOOLS

In addition to spending more on schooling overall and reallocating some expenditures between levels, the use of resources *within* schools needs to be improved. Parents complain about schools in almost every community in the world, from suburban Boston to rural India. Some of these complaints are the same, "My child is not getting enough attention" or "My child is not learning enough." But some are quite different, "Why are teachers absent so much of the time?" or "Why are there no books for students to read?" In some instances the solutions to these problems require more financial resources; in others, they require spending available resources better; and in still others, the problems are less about resources than about holding teachers and principals more accountable for their actions.

Inefficient use of resources and lack of accountability within schools are not new issues. But recent research has given new insight into these long-standing concerns. Especially important have been the use of **randomized controlled trials (RCTs)**, also referred to as randomized evaluations. Research organizations like the Abdul Latif Jameel Poverty Action Lab (J-PAL) at MIT are pioneering the use of experiments in the field to learn more about what works in schooling, health, microcredit, and other areas. Unlike the natural experiments discussed earlier, RCTs are *actual* experiments that researchers design to determine if a particular intervention shows promise. Similar to natural experiments and to studies in medicine, one group receives a treatment and outcomes are compared to a control group that does not receive a treatment. Experimental design focuses on making sure the treatment and control groups, whether individuals, households, or entire villages, are the same in order to isolate the impact of the treatment on later outcomes.

A well-designed RCT can help resolve problems of causality that confront other types of analysis. In a conventional cross-section regression analysis of reading and mathematic achievement in Ghanaian middle schools, one of the most statistically significant variables in raising student test scores was repairing leaking roofs. Maybe this was because by repairing the leaks, school remained open and students attended school more often, which led to greater learning. Or maybe the underlying relationship was that more motivated teachers, principals, and parents were more likely to keep the building in good order. If the latter explains the statistical finding, then a nationwide initiative to repair leaky school roofs would not yield the hoped-for improvement in children's learning.[21] An RCT that experimented, for example, with building maintenance might resolve this question. Insights obtained from RCTs and other types of research offer suggestions on how to improve the participation and retention of students as well as how to enhance student learning.

---

[21]Glewwe and Kremer, "Schools, Teachers, and Education Outcomes."

REDUCING THE COSTS OF GOING TO SCHOOL

Earlier we noted that the MDG of achieving universal primary education by 2015 is not likely to be met. Data on grade survival rates suggest that 20 percent of children in low-income nations do not complete even four years of schooling. One reason why children may not be in school is because there is no conveniently located school to attend. This certainly can be a problem in remote regions, and many children continue to travel long distances to get to school. However, research findings suggest lack of attendance is much more often a problem of household demand than of school supply.[22]

On the demand side, households may not send their children to school, including primary school, because poor families cannot afford the fees required for school attendance. These can be user charges to attend school or fees to pay for textbooks or mandatory school uniforms. A school uniform in Kenya costs $6, a nontrivial amount in a nation where one fifth of the population lives below the $1.25-a-day poverty line. Starting in the late 1990s, governments in several East African nations (including Kenya, Tanzania, Uganda, and Zambia) eliminated all user fees for primary schools; in some cases, school uniforms were no longer compulsory. Governments subsequently reported substantial increases in enrollment.

It is not surprising that eliminating school fees would lead to an increase in enrollment, but it comes at a cost. Many families previously had paid the fees and sent their children to school. By eliminating fees, the government lost much-needed revenue to pay for teachers and other school needs. Financing schooling now requires new revenues or reallocating funds from some other use. The critical economic question is whether reducing school fees represents an efficient use of resources. Michael Kremer, a development economist at Harvard University and a leading proponent of the use of RCTs and other experimental approaches, evaluated one program in Kenya where 7 out of 14 poorly performing schools were randomly selected. The treatment schools provided free uniforms and textbooks to their students, paid for by a Dutch NGO, and also received improved classrooms. Dropout rates fell considerably, and many students from nearby schools transferred into the treatment group, raising class size by 50 percent. Kremer and his co-authors concluded that the financial benefit of free uniforms was a significant factor in improving school attendance. (By keeping girls in school longer, free uniforms were also associated with a more than 10 percent reduction in teen childbearing.) The researchers concluded that, because parents accepted larger class sizes in return for these benefits, the government could have reallocated education spending, trading off larger classes for lower fees, and thereby increasing school completion rates.[23]

Another approach to increasing enrollments and school retention is to design means-tested and targeted programs in which families are paid to send their children

[22]Pritchett, "Access to Education."
[23]Glewwe and Kremer, "Schools, Teachers, and Education Outcomes."

to school. Several countries have adopted this approach, referred to as **conditional cash transfers (CCTs)**. Bolsa Familia (family allowance) in Brazil and Oportunidades in Mexico provide modest stipends to millions of poor families as long as their children remain in school. Both have been associated with gains in enrollment and retention (Box 8–3). So has a program in Cambodia financed by the Japan Fund for Poverty Reduction. The 45 neediest girls in each of 93 participating schools were awarded a $45 scholarship, a large sum in this low-income nation, as long as the student enrolled in school, maintained a passing grade, and had a good record of attendance. Evaluation of the program reports large increases in desired outcome measures. The Food for Schooling program in Bangladesh provides a free monthly ration of wheat or other grains to eligible families, where eligibility is means tested. To qualify, households must own less than half an acre of land and the household head must be a woman, a day laborer, or work in a very low-wage activity. The family can consume the grain or sell it and use the cash for other expenses. To maintain eligibility, children must attend 85 percent of classes each month. The program has been successful in increasing primary school enrollment, promoting school attendance, and reducing dropout rates, especially among girls.

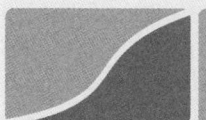

BOX 8–3 MEXICO'S PROGRAMA DE EDUCACIÓN, SALUD Y ALIMENTACIÓN (PROGRESA)/OPORTUNIDADES

When Ernesto Zedillo became Mexico's president in 1995, a fifth of the population could not afford the minimum daily nutritional requirements, 10 million Mexicans lacked access to basic health services, more than 1.5 million children were out of school, and student absenteeism and school desertions were three times higher in poor and remote areas than in the rest of the country. His administration decided that a new approach to poverty alleviation was needed. The Education, Health, and Nutrition Programs of Mexico, called PROGRESA, introduced a set of *conditional cash transfers* to poor families—the families would receive cash if their children were enrolled in school and if family members visited health clinics for checkups and nutritional and hygiene information.

The program was intended to remedy several shortcomings of earlier programs. First, it would counter the bias in poor families toward consumption by bolstering investment in human capital. Second, it would recognize the interdependencies among education, health, and nutrition. Third, it would link cash transfers to household behavior, aiming at changing attitudes. Fourth, to reduce political interference, the program's goals, rules, requirements, and evaluation methods would be widely publicized.

Children over the age of seven were eligible for education transfers. Benefits increased by grade (because the opportunity costs of being in school increase with age) and were higher for girls in middle school, to encourage their enrollment. To retain the benefits, children needed to maintain an 85 percent attendance record and could not repeat a grade more than once. Transfers went to mothers, who were thought to be more responsible for caring for children. In 1999, the average monthly transfer was around $24 per family, nearly 20 percent of mean household consumption before the program, with benefits available for up to three years.

By the end of 2002, the program had about 21 million beneficiaries, roughly a fifth of the Mexican population. Almost 60 percent of program transfers went to households in the poorest 20 percent of the national income distribution and more than 80 percent went to the poorest 40 percent.

School enrollment of participating households rose, especially in middle school and more so for girls than boys. Much of the increase came from increases in the transition from primary to middle school. The program worked principally by keeping children in school, not by encouraging those who had dropped out to return. Grade repetition decreased among participating families even for children in grades one and two who were not eligible for program benefits. Perhaps, this was because household income was higher or because older siblings were now spending more time in school. The impact of the program on learning is less clear. Teachers reported improvements, attributing them to better attendance, student interest, and nutrition. But a study conducted one year after the program started found no difference in test scores. Follow-up studies on longer-term effects are planned.

In 2001 and under a new Mexican president, PROGRESA was renamed, *Oportunidades*. The success of the program is reflected not only in schooling and health outcome measures but in its ability to survive changes in political leadership. It also has become a model for similar programs throughout Latin America and the rest of the world.

Source: Adapted from World Bank, "Spotlight on PROGRESA," 2004 World Development Report, "Making Services Work for Poor People" (Washington, DC: World Bank and Oxford University Press, 2004), 30–31. (World Bank, 2009).

CCTs like the ones just described all have multiple aims and can be seen as part of a package to alleviate poverty. If such transfers of cash or grain were going to be made on poverty grounds alone, then making them conditional on sending children to school makes the education component highly cost-effective. If they are intended primarily as interventions to expand enrollment and school retention, cost-effectiveness depends, in part, on how carefully the targeting is done. If eligibility is too broad, recipients will include families that already were sending their children to school and the cash or food expenditures will yield no marginal improvements in schooling for these households. Despite such concerns over cost-effectiveness, the success of CCTs such as Bolsa Familia and Oportunidades in raising school enrollments has resulted in their adoption in dozens of nations.

INEFFICIENT USE OF RESOURCES

Improving the efficient use of resources within schools also involves making decisions about spending. Should scarce resources be allocated to buildings or teachers, to teachers or school supplies (blackboards, desks, textbooks, etc.), or to any of a number of other alternatives? The problems that schools in poor nations face can be overwhelming. There usually are shortages of everything. There are too few textbooks and sometimes there are none. Roofs leak, and many students are crammed around simple desks if there are desks at all. Teachers often are untrained and children often too sick to learn effectively. Deciding on how to allocate resources in such environments is not easy.

In the 1980s, some of the debate over resource allocation within schools concerned building schools versus expenditures on recurrent costs to run schools. These recurrent costs included teacher and administrative salaries as well as nonwage expenditures on school supplies and equipment. Donors, who often financed much of the spending on schools, especially in low-income nations, had a preference for constructing new school buildings. The donors could point to the tangible product of their aid, something constituents back home might want to see. Donors also expected a partnership with those governments who received aid and assumed that governments would cover the recurrent costs. The result of these arrangements often was the construction of schools, often at higher standards than necessary and sometimes requiring imported building materials, met by an underfunding of recurrent costs. Schools without teachers or classrooms without chalk or writing paper often resulted.

By the 1990s, the approach had changed. Concern over the quantity and availability of schools diminished, and increasing attention was paid to improving the quality of schools. Resources were redirected toward recurrent expenditures, especially nonwage items. But this approach also proved wanting; improvements in learning outcomes remained elusive.

One cost-effective intervention for increasing school attendance (in addition to lowering fees) is not an educational input; it is biannual dosages of albendazole or praziquantel, two medications used to reduce intestinal worms such as hookworms or schistosomes. Such intestinal worms affect a quarter of the world's population and are especially common among children. Severe infections can cause anemia, protein-energy malnutrition and other health problems. On the basis of an RCT, students in some schools in rural Kenya, where worm infestation was particularly severe, received treatments and others did not. Researchers found that school absenteeism decreased by 25 percent in treatment versus control schools. Some children who previously were weak or listless were able to attend school because of the drugs; in other cases, deworming improved concentration and may have made attending more worthwhile. Beyond their effect on school attendance, these drugs also improved health outcomes.

Deworming proved highly cost-effective because the treatment cost is low, about $0.50 per child per year. Deworming increased school attendance by an average of 0.15 year per pupil or $3.50 per an additional full year of school participation. By comparison, school uniforms cost $6 per child. Because provision of school uniforms increased school attendance at a somewhat lower rate than deworming, the school uniform program was less cost-effective at $99 per additional year of school participation. Even though deworming was associated with improved school attendance and was cost-effective in doing so, there was no discernible improvement in learning as measured by student test scores at the time of treatment.[24]

New findings from the original deworming RCT reveal its long-term benefits. A follow-up study conducted in 2007–09 located a large percentage of the original Kenyan school children, some 6 to 11 years after the experiment began. By then their median age was 22 years. Comparing those who attended schools where the treatment was provided with those where it was not reveals significant differences. Deworming is associated with more subsequent years enrolled in school, better self-reported adult health, more hours spent working, higher earnings among those employed in wage-paying jobs, and improvements in adult food consumption.[25] Consistent with a growing literature, these investments in the childhood years had significant pay-offs when these children reach adulthood because of improved childhood health and schooling.

More traditional school input issues involve reducing class size, increasing the availability of textbooks and other instructional materials, and improving teacher training. Appropriate class size is a matter of debate in school systems throughout the world, in rich and poor nations alike. The basic argument is straightforward. In smaller classes, teachers can provide more attention, even individualized work, for each student. Running a 25-pupil class of 7-year-olds (let alone 13-year-olds) is daunting enough, but what must it be like to teach a class two, three, or more times as large?

---

[24]Edward Miguel and Michael Kremer, "Worms: Identifying Impacts on Education and Health in the Presence of Treatment Externalities," *Econometrica* 72, no. 1 (2004).

[25]Michael Kremer, Sarah Baird, Joan Hamory Hicks, and Edward Miguel, "Worms at Work: Long-Run Impacts of Child Health Gains" (May 2011), www.economics.harvard.edu/faculty/kremer/files/KLPS-Labor_2011-05-13-Circulate-B-No-IRR.pdf.

Eric Hanushek, a senior fellow at the Hoover Institution and a leading expert on the economics of education in the United States, surveyed almost 100 studies on the determinants of student test scores in developing countries. Of the 30 studies that looked at class size, 8 found a statistically significant positive effect (the fewer students per teacher, the better students performed); 8 found a statistically significant negative effect (the fewer students per teacher, the *worse* students performed); and 14 found no significant effect at all.[26] We need to be careful interpreting these findings. They do not suggest that class size never matters; the results say only that there is no evidence of a robust and significant correlation (let alone causation) between class size and student performance.[27] In some instances, reducing class sizes is warranted; in others, the extra expenditure on teachers and additional classrooms yields no return. Without being able even to identify a simple correlation between reduced class size and student achievement, it is that much harder to move to the question of cost-effectiveness or economic efficiency of allocating scarce resources so that outcomes per dollar are equalized across alternative inputs.

The failure to easily identify strategies to improve student outcomes is not restricted to studies of student–teacher ratios. Studies of teacher training or textbook use yield a similar range of outcomes. According to the survey by economists Paul Glewwe and Michael Kremer, the introduction of textbooks in Jamaican primary schools improved reading scores, while in the Philippines the impact of textbooks was "unstable," including positive *and negative* effects on the mathematics and reading scores of first graders. An RCT in rural Kenya found no evidence that provision of textbooks improved scores for the average student. However, Kenyan students who were above average before textbooks were provided realized improvements. This may be because textbooks provided by the government were in English, often the second or even third language of many local children, and only the most able students had sufficient English language skills to benefit from the textbooks they received. What the textbook studies suggest is that the central problem may not be an absence of learning materials but systemic problems in the education system. Textbooks that help only the best students highlight problems with a centralized national

[26]Eric Hanushek, "Interpreting Recent Research on Schooling in Developing Countries," *World Bank Research Observer* 10, no. 2 (1995). In an earlier study, Hanushek reached the same conclusion about the impact of class size on student performance in the United States ("The Economics of Schooling: Production and Efficiency in Public Schools," *Journal of Economic Literature* 24 [1986]).

[27]One of the difficulties of identifying the impact of class size on student learning is the problem of *endogeneity*. Class size may not be determined independently of other determinants of student performance. For example, if school administrators decide to keep class sizes small for students who are disruptive or have difficulty learning in the hope that teachers can manage such classes better if they have fewer students, then class size will be inversely correlated with student performance but not a cause of low performance. Similarly, if better-educated and higher-income communities effectively lobby for more teachers and smaller classes, class size will be positively correlated with better student performance even though better performance may mostly be due to having students with better-educated parents enrolled in smaller classes. Once again the causal effect of class size on performance would be hard to identify.

curriculum oriented to educating the children of the politically influential elite and failing to recognize the heterogeneity among students.

Most schools in developing nations can do better, and RCTs are providing useful insights, including the benefits of some technology-assisted approaches and linking teacher pay to student test scores.[28] One single intervention, however, will not work all the time. Local conditions make a difference, such as the accountability of teachers, principals, and other school officials.

IT IS ABOUT MORE THAN THE MONEY

If there has been a trend in thinking about education and development, it has gone from concern primarily over increasing the quantity of schooling, achieved by building more schools, hiring more teachers, and most recently, reducing the cost of attending to improving the quality of schools by improving the amounts and mix of inputs within schools themselves. Both these approaches have had some measure of success, with the huge increases in enrollments (discussed earlier) and success in learning outcomes, at least in some settings, due to different or better use of school inputs. But widespread and persistently low student achievement has resulted in a call not only for more money but also for reform of school systems. School reform and more resources need not be substitutes. Both may be required to realize better outcomes, but more money without school reforms will be insufficient to achieve these ends. Calls for school reforms echo those for institutional reforms in other areas of government. Improvements in governance are needed not only to improve the climate for private enterprises and encourage investment in physical capital but to improve investment in human capital.

One critical area of school reforms is to better motivate teachers, many of whom fail to show up for work and to engage in teaching when they do. With weak incentives, teacher motivation often is low. The need for improved accountability among teachers is starkly demonstrated by a nationwide study of teacher absence in India.[29] Researchers made three unannounced visits to 3,700 Indian primary schools. The presence or absence of teachers assigned to each school was determined by *direct physical verification*—that is, by a member of the research project looking for the teacher in the school building and not by checking logbooks or other records. On average, one in four primary school teachers was absent on the day of a visit. And only 45 percent (less than half) of primary school teachers were actively engaged in teaching their students at the time of the visit. Some percentage of these absences

---

[28]The use of RCTs has increased dramatically in recent years. J-PAL records many of the latest findings on its website at www.povertyactionlab.org/. Also, see Michael Kremer and Alaka Holla, "Improving Education in the Developing World: What Have We Learned from Randomized Evaluations?" *Annual Review of Economics* 1 (September 2009).

[29]Michael Kremer et al., "Teacher Absence in India: A Snapshot," *Journal of the European Economic Association* 3, nos. 2–3 (April–May 2005).

and involvement in nonteaching matters was due to excused absences for health or other reasons or performing required administrative or other duties. But even after correcting for these factors the degree of absence remains high.

The authors of the India study looked at the correlates of teacher absence and did not find that relatively higher pay or more education among teachers reduces absences. Stronger ties to the local community do not seem to play much of a role either. Schools with better infrastructure (for example, with electricity or staff toilets), more frequent inspections, and closer proximity to roads have somewhat lowered absenteeism, but the overwhelming conclusion is that getting more teachers to do their jobs is a significant challenge. The research includes similar investigations in other countries. While India's teacher absence rate is on the high end (Uganda is higher at 27 percent), rates of 14 percent in Peru, 15 percent in Papua New Guinea, and 19 percent in Indonesia are not encouraging. Discussions of appropriate curriculums, better teaching methods, or more school resources almost seem secondary if so many teachers are not minimally engaged in the daily routines of educating their pupils. In explaining why teacher absence is so high, Michael Kremer and his co-authors note that teachers face little risk of being fired. They found that only one head teacher (school principal) in nearly 3,000 primary schools in India had ever dismissed a teacher for repeated absences. (An innovative solution to reducing teacher absence in some schools in India is discussed in Box 8–4.) The absence of repercussions is one explanation for high absence rates but the problem of accountability runs far deeper.

BOX 8–4 COMBATING *TEACHER* ABSENCE

When a student misses a class his or her learning suffers; when the teacher is absent the whole class suffers. Or does it? In an attempt to reduce teacher absence and assess its impact, Esther Duflo and colleagues collaborated with an Indian nongovernment organization (NGO), Seva Mandir, on an innovative policy experiment.

Seva Mandir runs single-teacher primary schools in tribal villages in a sparsely populated and remote rural area. Tens of millions of Indian children attend schools like these. Their goal is to teach basic skills to prepare students for the regular government-run school system. Teachers are employed by the NGO on flexible contracts and are not civil servants, as are most Indian schoolteachers. This made it easier to implement a program that provided monetary incentives to reduce teacher absences. Because of their remote location, it is difficult to monitor such schools. Teacher absence was at the alarming rate of 44 percent. This was despite Seva Mandir's threat to dismiss teachers with too many absences, although that threat rarely was carried out.

Seva Mandir selected 120 of its schools to participate in a randomized control trial (RCT). These one-room schools usually have about 20 students and run a six-hour school day. The teacher is drawn from the local community and has about 10 years of education. There is only one teacher per school, and when the teacher is absent the school is closed. Half of the schools, the treatment group, were given a camera with a tamper-proof date and time function. Each day, teachers were instructed to have a child in the school take a picture of the teacher and the other children at the beginning and end of the school day. A *valid school day* was defined as one in which at least five hours elapsed between the two pictures and when at least eight students were present in each picture. Teacher pay was a function of the number of valid days they worked based on the photographs submitted. The nontreatment group was paid their regular monthly salary. They continued to be told that they could be dismissed for poor performance, including too many unexcused absences. There was one unannounced visit to control schools each month. Average salaries ended up almost identical in the two groups.

Over an 18-month period, the absence rate in the treatment schools fell by half, to 22 percent. The use of cameras to monitor teacher presence completely eliminated extremely delinquent behavior—absences of over 50 percent. It also increased the number of teachers with perfect or very high attendance from under 1 percent in the control group to 36 percent in the treatment group.

Did students learn more? The incentives built into the program encouraged teachers only to be present. It did not reward spending more time teaching or improving student performance, the true goal of the intervention. Based on observations during the unannounced visits, teachers in treatment and control groups were equally likely to be engaged in teaching. Because the treatment group was present far more often, more teaching was taking place, equivalent to almost 3 days per month. After one year, this resulted in a 0.17 standard deviation increase in children's test scores in basic Hindi and math skills, and a significantly higher matriculation rate of children in the treatment group to government schools. These benefits were highly cost-effective. Outside of salaries, which were the same in the two groups, all other costs, including cameras, film, and administrative expenses, amounted to roughly $6 per child or to $3.58 per 0.10 increase in the standard deviation in test scores.

Seva Mandir continued to monitor attendance with cameras long after the RCT ended and improved attendance has been maintained. The effects appear to be long lasting. The success of this monitoring system, however, may not be applicable to government schools in India, in part, because of resistance from teacher unions. But the potential of incentive schemes that reward teacher performance remains.

Source: Esther Duo, Rema Hanna, and Stephen P. Ryan, "Incentives Work: Getting Teachers to Come to School," *American Economic Review* (forthcoming).

Teacher absence or, for that matter, the absence of health workers or any number of other government workers is not the only example of the breakdown in accountability that compromises the delivery of public services in low- and middle-income-nations.[30] In another often-cited study, researchers followed the money allocated by Uganda's national government for local primary schools.[31] Despite the government authorizing 20 percent of public expenditures to education, most of it to primary education, a program to finance nonwage expenditures rarely resulted in money reaching the schools it was intended for. Over the period 1991–95, an average of only 13 percent of such grants actually reached the schools; almost three-quarters of the 250 primary schools surveyed in the study received less than 5 percent of what had been authorized. Local officials and politicians captured much of the money along the way.

The identification of the massive leakage of funds in Uganda led to a number of institutional improvements. The central government responded by launching an information campaign, where the amounts of centrally disbursed grants were reported in newspapers. Primary schools were also required to post notices of grants actually received. Local parent teacher associations (PTAs), which are very powerful in the Ugandan school system, thus were made aware of grants due their schools and could monitor outcomes. By reducing information asymmetries, it was possible to hold local officials more accountable. The information campaign, coupled with more attention from central government officials (including stiff penalties against offenders), increased the receipt of funds by schools from 20 percent in 1995 to 80 percent in 2001.[32]

The Ugandan example ultimately relied on local or community control as a means of increasing accountability, this time of local officials who received funds

[30]The problem of improving service delivery by the public sector is the focus of the *2004 World Development Report, Making Services Work for Poor People* (Washington, DC: World Bank and Oxford University Press, 2004). Specific chapters are devoted to basic education, health and nutrition, and drinking water, sanitation, and electricity.

[31]Ritva Reinikka and Jakob Svensson, "Local Capture: Evidence from a Central Government Transfer Program in Uganda," *Quarterly Journal of Economics* 119, no. 2 (May 2004).

[32]Ritva Reinikka and Jakob Svensson, "The Power of Information: Evidence from a Newspaper Campaign to Reduce Capture," Policy Research Paper 3239 (Washington, DC, World Bank, March 2004). See also Paul Hubbard, "Putting the Power of Transparency in Context: Information's Role in Reducing Corruption in Uganda's Education Sector," Working Paper Number 136 (Washington, DC, Center for Global Development, December 2007), which argues that the improved flow of resources to intended beneficiaries was the product of many reforms in government practice, including but not solely the result of more transparent information.

from the central government. Expanding local control, often through decentralization of authority over schools, is one of several reform strategies to hold all providers—officials who control funds as well teachers and principals—more accountable. The Educo program (Educación con Participación de la Comunidad) in El Salvador provides another example of this approach.

A prolonged civil war in the 1980s left the Salvadorian school system in a woeful state. One-third of the country's primary schools were closed, and in many regions, traditional government schools, and their teachers, were viewed with distrust by local people who may have been fighting against the government. During the war, some communities had recruited local teachers and established community schools in place of government-run ones. Seizing on this model, the government decided to incorporate community schools into the national system and encourage new ones to open. These *popular* schools enter into one-year renewable agreements with the ministry of education. The local schools are run by parent groups, which receive grants from the government, hire teachers on renewable contracts, and determine the salaries and other terms of these contracts. Turnover rates arc high; teachers who are frequently absent or perform poorly are dismissed. Parents visit schools more often and are more involved than in traditional schools. The results of these arrangements are encouraging. Educo reached far into the countryside. Rural primary school enrollments grew rapidly with most new students enrolled in the *popular* schools. Student performance in Educo and traditional schools was comparable. This was an impressive outcome because Educo students tended to come from poorer and less-educated families than students who attended the traditional government schools.[33]

The relative success of Educo does not mean that all school systems should adopt a similar model or that greater parental involvement and control always improves school outcomes. Results from some RCTs in Kenya and India suggest otherwise.[34] But all these cases speak to the need for nations to experiment with alternative modes of service delivery. School reforms are part of a larger agenda of institutional reforms that many nations, whether low, middle, or high income, are pursuing to improve schooling, health, and other outcomes. Evidence from such reforms indicates that one size does *not* fit all and continued experimentation and evaluation is needed to identify what works in different settings. School systems need to enroll and retain more students and improve learning outcomes at all levels of education. Teachers must be adequately trained and motivated. Schools need clear objectives, adequate financing, and some autonomy on how to operate and achieve stated goals. They also must be held accountable to the taxpayers (at home and abroad) who finance school systems and, most important, to the students and their parents who count on schools to provide an education.

[33]World Bank, *2004 World Development Report,* pp. 131–32.
[34]Kremer and Holla, "Improving Education in the Developing World."

SUMMARY

- By historical standards, the last three decades have witnessed a revolutionary change in the number of men and *women* who have attended school and received a basic education. By 2010, 80 percent of the developing world's adults had attended school as children. These investments in human capital have profound implications for improving the well-being of much of humanity in the twenty-first century.

- Despite these achievements, much remains to be done. More than four out of every five children in the world live in low- and middle-income nations, and far too many of them have never attended school or failed to complete even four years of primary school. And those who attend school often learn far too little, with their education lagging well behind what comparably aged children master in high-income nations.

- Attending school remains a worthwhile private and social investment. In every nation, if you have more years of schooling, on average, you earn more than those with less schooling. Estimated rates of return, which take account of both the benefits and costs of schooling, indicate that schooling at all levels yields attractive returns when compared to other investments.

- But schooling is not a panacea. Many nations have expanded enrollments and sent their young people through years of schooling and still have not grown. In a bad economic environment, schooling, like other investments, can be wasted. Increasing the demand for all workers, educated and not educated, raises the private and social return on education and remains a key challenge to achieve economic development.

- Much also needs to be done to make schools more productive. Some developing nations underinvest in education overall; many misallocate resources by spending too much on the tertiary sector at the expense of primary and secondary levels; and most could improve the use of resources within schools themselves, including reducing the frequency of absent *teachers.*

- Decreasing user fees and other costs, offering households cash transfers conditional on school attendance, and improving child health and nutrition have all proven effective in getting the children of poor families to enroll in and more regularly attend school.

- Prescriptions for how to improve learning outcomes have proven harder to identify, although use of randomized controlled trials are offering many new insights. Changing the mix of school inputs has shown limited promise; making teachers, administrators, and government officials accountable for school outcomes may be the most important factor of all.

Health

Grab a pencil, here comes a pop quiz. Denmark, a high-income nation, had a population of 5.4 million people. With a death rate of 10 per 1,000, about 54,000 Danes died that year. Here is your first question: What was the median age of those who died? In other words, pick the age at which half of those who died were older and half were younger than that age. Now turn to Sierra Leone, one of the poorest nations in the world, which has a population about the same size as Denmark's. But Sierra Leone's death rate was much higher, estimated at 24 per 1,000, resulting in roughly 130,000 deaths. Here is your second question: What was the median age of those who died in Sierra Leone? Write down your predictions; we will provide the answers in a moment.

The difference in the age distribution of deaths between a very poor nation like Sierra Leone and a wealthy developed country like Denmark is that most deaths occur before age 5 in Sierra Leone, whereas most deaths occur among the elderly in Denmark. This is graphically illustrated by the age pyramids in Figure 9–1. We examined age pyramids in Chapter 7, contrasting those of rapidly versus slowly growing populations (Box 7–3). The age pyramids of Figure 9–1 look entirely different. They refer only to those who died in a given year. In Sierra Leone, more deaths occur in the first 4 years of life than in all other age brackets combined; in Denmark, child deaths rarely occur. Here are the answers to the quiz: The median age of death in Denmark is 77; in Sierra Leone, it is under 4. The striking difference between these numbers tells us a lot about life and death in the richest and poorest nations of the world.

One of the best indicators of a county's overall health status is the **under-five mortality rate**. This measure is the probability (expressed as per 1,000 live births)

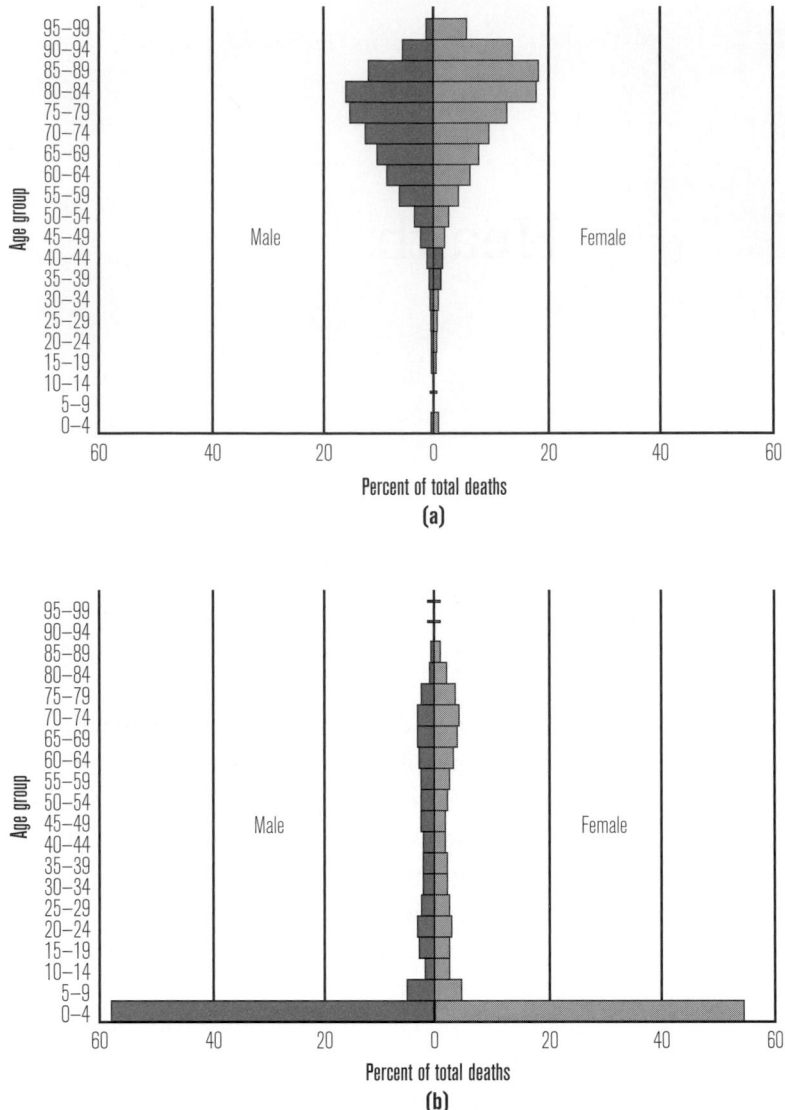

FIGURE 9-1 Distribution of Age at Death, 2005

(a) Denmark. (b) Sierra Leone. Values are projections.

Source: World Bank, *Health Financing Revisited*, processed (Washington, DC: World Bank, 2005).

that a child born in a specific year dies before reaching five years of age, if subjected to current age-specific mortality rates. In Sierra Leone, there were 194 deaths of children under-five per 1,000 live births compared to only 4 in Denmark (Table 9–1). About a quarter of all under-five mortality occurs in the first month of life in Sierra Leone. Early childhood is an especially risky period for Sierra Leone's children.

There are many explanations for the massive disparity in the chances that a child born in Sierra Leone versus one born in Denmark will survive and for the lower health status these numbers suggest for the rest of the population. At birth, less

TABLE 9-1   Selected Health-Related Measures for Sierra Leone and Denmark, Mid-2000s

	SIERRA LEONE	DENMARK
Mortality statistics		
Life expectancy at birth (years)		
Both sexes	40	79
Males	39	76
Females	42	81
Mortality rates (per 1,000)		
Neonatal (first 28 days)	56	3
Under 5 years	269	4
Adult (15–60 years) men	556	111
Adult (15–60 years) women	460	65
Healthy life expectancy at birth (HALE, years)		
Males	27	69
Females	30	71
Morbidity statistics		
Children under 5 years, stunted for age (%)	38	–
Children under 5 years, underweight for age (%)	25	–
Environmental risk factors		
Access to improved water sources, urban (%)	83	100
Access to improved water sources, rural (%)	32	100
Access to improved sanitation, urban (%)	20	100
Access to improved sanitation, rural (%)	5	100
Health services coverage		
Immunization coverage among 1-year-olds (%)		
Measles	67	89
Diphtheria, tetanus, pertussis, three doses	64	75
Births attended by skilled health personnel (%)	43	–
Health system statistics		
Number of physicians per 10,000	< 1	36
Number of nurses and midwives per 10,000	5	101
Hospital beds per 10,000	4	38
Per capita total expenditures on health (US$, PPP)	41	3,349

HALE, health-adjusted life expectancy; PPP, purchasing power parity.

Source: World Health Organization, Statistical Information System, *World Health Statistics 2009*, available at www.who.int/whosis/en, accessed February 2012.

than half of all mothers in Sierra Leone are tended to by a skilled health worker; in Denmark, such services are available to all mothers. In Sierra Leone, malnutrition is common, especially among children. One out of every three children under age five is stunted and one out of five is underweight. **Stunting** refers to the percentage of children under five years that have a height to age ratio more than two standard deviations below the **World Health Organization (WHO)** global reference median. Being **underweight** refers to the percentage of children under five years that have a weight to age ratio more than two standard deviations below the WHO global reference median. Both outcomes are rare in Denmark.

Sierra Leone and Denmark also differ significantly in terms of health services received and resources available to the health system. The majority of rural inhabitants in Sierra Leone have no access to clean water or improved sanitation, and many in the urban areas lack those services as well. Everyone in Denmark has access to safe drinking water and modern sanitation. Almost all 1-year-olds (89 percent) are immunized in Denmark for measles and receive three doses of the diphtheria, tetanus, and pertussis (DTP) or whooping cough vaccine, designated DTP3. About 60 percent of 1-year-olds in Sierra Leone are immunized for measles and for DTP3; thus 40 percent are not immunized and at risk of infection. A person who gets sick in Denmark has many more resources to turn to for medical care. Denmark has almost 50 times as many nurses and midwives per 10,000 persons as Sierra Leone (98 versus 2). There are 32 trained physicians per 10,000 people in Denmark; in Sierra Leone, there is less than 1. Denmark also spends almost 100 times as much per person per year on healthcare ($3,513 versus $32 in purchasing power parity [PPP]). Poor access to health services from childhood through adulthood increases adult mortality. In Sierra Leone, adult men (ages 15–60) are four times more likely to die than in Denmark; adult women are five times more likely.

The data for Denmark and Sierra Leone reflect the experience of their geographical regions, Europe and Africa. Africa has the highest rate of under-five mortality with 142 deaths per 1,000 compared to 14 per 1,000 for Europe, the region with the lowest rate[1] (Table 9-2). The eastern Mediterranean region, which includes 21 nations in North Africa and the Middle East, has the next highest regional under-five mortality rate at 78; and Southeast Asia, encompassing 11 nations (including Bangladesh, India, and Indonesia), is the third highest at 63. Poor health outcomes are correlated with low incomes, which in turn are associated with low levels of education and environmental risk factors, such as lack of access to safe drinking water and the absence of improved sanitation, especially in rural areas. Absence of medical personnel and low levels of health spending are other characteristics of high mortality among both children and adults. As we shall see, low incomes explain much, but certainly not all, of the disparity in health outcomes across countries and regions.

WHAT IS HEALTH?

The WHO defines *health* as a state of complete mental, physical, and social well-being and not merely the absence of disease.[2] However, such a complex construct would be difficult to measure and would likely vary between cultures and over time.

---

[1] WHO is the primary United Nations agency responsible for global health issues. WHO data rely on a regional breakdown that is different from the one used by the World Bank and frequently referred to throughout this textbook.

[2] Preamble to the Constitution of the World Health Organization as adopted by the International Health Conference, New York, June 19–22, 1946. The definition has not been amended since 1948.

TABLE 9-2 Selected Health-Related Measures for World Health Organization Regions, 2009

	AFRICA	AMERICAS	SOUTHEAST ASIA	EUROPE	EASTERN MEDITERRA- NEAN	WESTERN PACIFIC
Mortality statistics						
Life expectancy at birth, males (years)	51	73	63	70	63	72
Life expectancy at birth, females (years)	54	78	66	78	66	77
Mortality rates (per 1,000)						
Neonatal (first 28 days)	40	11	35	10	38	17
Under 5 years	145	19	65	15	82	22
Adult (15–60 years) men	429	163	252	221	229	144
Adult (15–60 years) women	374	91	187	94	175	85
Healthy life expectancy at birth, males (HALE years)	45	65	56	64	55	65
Healthy life expectancy at birth, females (HALE years)	46	69	57	70	57	69
Morbidity statistics						
Prevalence of HIV among adults aged > 15 (per 100,000)	4,735	448	295	336	202	89
Environmental risk factors						
Access to improved water sources, urban (%)	82	98	94	100	93	98
Access to improved water sources, rural (%)	46	81	84	92	75	82
Access to improved sanitation, urban (%)	46	92	58	97	85	79
Access to improved sanitation, rural (%)	26	68	27	85	43	61
Health services coverage						
Immunization coverage among 1-year-olds (%)						
Measles	74	93	73	94	84	92
Diphtheria, tetanus, pertussis, three doses	74	93	69	96	87	92
Births attended by skilled health personnel (%)	46	92	48	96	59	92
Health system statistics						
Number of physicians per 10,000	2	19	5	32	10	14
Number of nurses and midwives per 10,000	11	49	12	79	15	20
Hospital beds per 10,000	10	24	9	63	14	33
Per capita total expenditures on health (US$, PPP)	111	2,788	85	1,719	259	461

HALE, health-adjusted life expectancy; PPP, purchasing power parity.

Source: *World Health Statistics 2009* (Geneva: World Health Organization, 2009).

The measures most often used to express health are those that describe the absence of health: mortality and morbidity statistics. **Mortality** measures deaths in a population; **morbidity** measures rates of disease and illness.

Because death is an unambiguous event indicating a complete failure of health, mortality statistics offer a summary of a population's health status and reveal much about a population's standard of living and healthcare. Most countries record and publish death rates with various levels of coverage and accuracy. In a very poor country, such as Sierra Leone, less than 25 percent of deaths were covered by the country's own vital registration system. In such cases, mortality rates are estimated from sample surveys or other existing data.

Perhaps the most common summary statistic used to provide a snapshot of a country's health status is life expectancy, which is derived from data on mortality. Because death rates are affected by factors such as age, sex, and race, life expectancy is often calculated for specific demographic subgroups. The life expectancy for a male born in 2008 in Sierra Leone was 48 years and 50 years for a female. A Danish baby boy born in 2008 had a life expectancy of 77 and a girl had a life expectancy of 81. To put these numbers in some historical perspective, life expectancy in Sierra Leone today is about what it was in the United States in 1900.

One might think that in a country where life expectancy is 49 (or 79) years, most people die by that age. That is clearly not the case, as Figure 9–1 demonstrates. Many people have shorter lives whereas others live well past the average life expectancy. Confusion arises because life expectancy is an average with variance around the mean; it is a "synthetic" statistic. It is based on the probability of surviving from one year to the next assuming that today's age-specific death rates remain unchanged into the future. But this is unlikely. Rising incomes and advances in medicine suggest that age-specific death rates are likely to fall in coming decades, expanding lifetimes beyond the predictions of current life expectancy estimates. However, new diseases, like HIV/AIDS, can cause the opposite, leading to shorter lifetimes and declining life expectancy.

Box 9–1 describes in detail how life expectancy is computed using data from Malaysia. Even though life expectancy in Malaysia was 69 years, people in the 70–75 age group had a life expectancy of 10 more years, a sort of "bonus" for surviving. In countries with high infant mortality, like Sierra Leone, life expectancy for children who survive the early years can be higher than at birth. For example, life expectancy at birth for Sierra Leone was 49 years in 2008. For the 5- to 9-year-old age group, life expectancy was 55 additional years for a total of 60 years for a 5-year-old—a full 11 years more than a newborn.[3] A 5-year-old child in Sierra Leone today will probably live even longer than 60 years. Now that years of civil war finally have ended, it is hoped that economic growth and development can begin. If this happens, age-specific death rates should start to fall, and Sierra Leone's children should tend to live beyond current estimates of life expectancy.

---

[3]WHO Global Health Observatory Repository, available at http://apps.who.int/ghodata; *World Health Statistics 2010,* World Health Organization, Geneva, 2010.

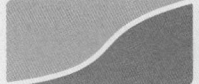

BOX 9-1 LIFE EXPECTANCY

Life expectancy is an estimate of the average number of additional years a person could expect to live if the age-specific death rates for a given year prevail for the rest of the person's life. Life expectancy is a hypothetical measure because it is based on current death rates, and actual death rates change (they usually fall) over the course of an individual's lifetime.

Life tables are used to calculate life expectancy; with life expectancy at birth the most commonly cited life expectancy measure. The table in this box contains selected portions of a life table for men in Malaysia in 1995. Age-specific death rates are applied to a hypothetical population of 100,000 people born in the same year. Column 1 shows the proportion of each age group dying in each age interval. These data are based on the observed mortality experience of the Malaysian population.

Column 2 shows the number of people alive at the beginning of each age interval, starting with 100,000 at birth. Each age group contains the population that survived from the immediately preceding group. Column 3 shows the number who would die within each age interval (Column 1 × Column 2 = Column 3). Column 4 shows the total number of person-years that would be lived within each age interval, including estimates of those who remain alive for only part of the interval. Column 5 shows the total number of years of life to be shared by the population in the age interval in all subsequent intervals. This measure takes into account the frequency of deaths that will occur in this and subsequent intervals. As age increases and the population shrinks, the total person-years that the survivors have to live necessarily diminish.

Abridged Life Table for Males in Malaysia, 1995

AGE	1 PROPORTION DYING IN THE AGE INTERVAL	2 NUMBER LIVING AT THE BEGINNING OF THE AGE INTERVAL	3 NUMBER DYING DURING THE AGE INTERVAL	4 PERSONS-YEARS LIVED IN THE AGE INTERVAL	5 IN THIS AND SUBSEQUENT INTERVALS	6 YEARS OF LIFE REMAINING (LIFE EXPECTANCY)
<1	0.01190	100,000	1,190	98,901	6,938,406	69.38
1–5	0.00341	98,810	337	394,437	6,839,505	69.22
5–10	0.00237	98,473	233	491,782	6,445,067	65.45
10–15	0.00270	98,240	265	490,536	5,953,285	60.60
–	–	–	–	–	–	–
65–70	0.16050	70,833	11,368	325,743	928,004	13.10
70–75	0.25762	59,464	15,319	259,024	602,260	10.13
75–80	0.34357	44,145	15,167	182,808	343,237	7.78
80+	1.00000	28,978	28,978	160,428	160,428	5.54

Source: Department of Statistics, Malaysia, 1997.

Life expectancy is shown in Column 6. The total person-years lived in a given interval plus subsequent intervals, when divided by the number of persons living at the beginning of that interval, equals life expectancy — the average number of years remaining for a person at a given age interval (Column 5 ÷ Column 2 = Column 6). For example, dividing the number of person-years associated with Malaysian men who survive to age 70 (602,260) by the number of these men (59,464) shows they have an additional life expectancy of 10.1 years. With age, life expectancy actually rises, a kind of "bonus" for surviving. The 59,464 Malaysian men who survive to age 70 can expect to live more than 10 additional years, well past their life expectancy at birth of 69 years.

Source: Adapted from, Arthur Haupt and Thomas T. Kane, *Population Handbook*, 5th ed. (Washington, DC: Population Reference Bureau, 2004), p. 29–30.

Cause-specific death rates provide information on why people die and can be a useful policy tool. Morbidity statistics provide information on how people live, whether they live in full health or experience disabilities that may limit their participation in work or family life. Researchers have developed several innovative approaches to measuring health status that address the limitations of morbidity and mortality statistics by combining the information from both into a single unit. The WHO uses a single measure of death and disability that recognizes that years lived with a disability are not the same as healthy years. **Health-adjusted life expectancy (HALE)** reduces life expectancy by years spent with disabilities, and disabilities are weighted according to their level of severity and duration. The balance remaining is the expected number of years of healthy life.[4]

Using the HALE measure, healthy life expectancy in Sierra Leone for males is cut by 14 years from 48 to 34 and for females it is reduced from 50 to 37. This is the lowest healthy life expectancy of all 192 WHO member countries. In Denmark, disabilities reduce healthy life expectancy from 77 to 70 for males; females live 73 healthy years compared to an average life expectancy of 81. The percentage of life lost to disability tends to be higher in poorer countries because some limitations strike children and young adults, such as injury, blindness, paralysis, and the debilitating effects of several tropical diseases such as malaria. People in the healthiest regions (Europe) lose about 11 percent of their lives to disability, versus 15 percent in the least healthy region (Africa; Table 9–2).

[4]*World Health Report 2002: Reducing Risks, Promoting Healthy Life* (Geneva: World Health Organization, 2002), statistical annex.

TRANSITIONS IN GLOBAL HEALTH

The past two centuries have seen a remarkable improvement in health and life expectancy. Until 1800, life expectancy at birth averaged around 30 years, but it could be lower. In France between 1740 and 1790, life expectancy of males fluctuated between 24 and 28 years. In England between the 1500s and the 1870s, life expectancy ranged from 28 to 42 with an average of only 35 years.[5] Many people died in infancy or early childhood while a few lived on to old age. Life expectancy has steadily increased since the late nineteenth century, making dramatic gains in the twentieth century. From 1960 to 2008, life expectancy around the world increased from 50 to 69 years (Table 9–3). Among the low- and middle-income countries, the increase is especially dramatic. Life expectancy was only 44 years in 1960; in 2008, it was 67 years, more than a 50 percent increase. By comparison, the increase in the high-income countries over this time period was 11 years, from 69 to 80. This smaller increase is because the high-income countries had achieved significant gains in life expectancy earlier in their history.

All regions of the world experienced gains in life expectancy since 1960, whether or not they also experienced economic growth. In East Asia, where economic growth has been rapid (and China dominates the regional average), life expectancy has risen from only 39 years in 1960 to 72 years in 2008. In 2008, per capita income in East Asia was only 15 percent that of high-income countries, but its life expectancy was already 90 percent the level achieved by high-income nations. Despite its slow growth between 1960 and 1990, South Asia added more than five years of increased life expectancy per decade. Latin America, even with its lost decades, by 2008, had achieved the world's second-highest regional life expectancy, at 73 years.

TABLE 9-3 Increased Life Expectancy, 1960–2007

REGION	LIFE EXPECTANCY, YEARS			CHANGE IN YEARS PER DECADE	
	1960	1990	2007	1960–1990	1990–2007
Low and middle income	44	63	67	6.3	2.4
East Asia and Pacific	39	67	72	9.3	2.9
Europe and Central Asia	n.a.	69	70	n.a.	0.6
Latin America and Caribbean	56	68	73	4.0	2.9
Middle East and North Africa	47	64	70	5.7	3.5
South Asia	43	59	64	5.3	2.9
Sub-Saharan Africa	41	50	51	3.0	0.6
High Income	69	76	79	2.3	1.8
World	50	65	69	5.0	2.4

Source: World Bank, "World Development Indicators," http://databank.worldbank.org.

[5]James C. Rile, *Rising Life Expectancy: A Global History* (Cambridge: Cambridge University Press, 2001).

But not all the news is this positive. Sub-Saharan Africa experienced an increase in life expectancy between 1960 and the early 1990s, but many African nations have recorded declines since then, as young adults and children died prematurely due to HIV/AIDS. Tragically, life expectancy in parts of southern Africa has been reduced by a decade or more. Life expectancy declined in some other countries as well. In Russia, life expectancy fell sharply in the 1990s. Between 1990 and 1994, life expectancy for Russian men fell from 64 years to 58 years and for Russian women from 74 to 71 years.[6] Increases in cardiovascular disease (heart disease and stroke) and injuries accounted for two-thirds of the decline in life expectancy. Causes for this decline include high rates of tobacco and alcohol consumption, poor nutrition, depression, and a deteriorating health system. The underlying causes of these determinants of increased morbidity and mortality have been traced to both the cumulative effects of often poor living standards under communist rule of the Soviet Union and to the upheaval and stresses associated with Russia's transition. It took two decades, but today life expectancy in Russia is back to the levels of 1990, the start of its economic transition.

The examples from Africa and Russia demonstrate that declines in health and life expectancy can take place rapidly. But these outcomes remain exceptions to the general trend of improving health and increasing life expectancy. The gaps in health outcomes between the richest and the poorest regions of the world have become markedly smaller since 1960. The difference in life expectancy between low- and middle-income compared to high-income nations was 25 years in 1960 but fell to only 13 years by 1990—the level it is also at today. Despite a lack of income convergence across nations (see Chapter 4), there is strong evidence of a convergence in life expectancy.[7]

THE EPIDEMIOLOGIC TRANSITION

Dramatic improvements in life expectancy and reductions in infant and child mortality during the past century resulted in equally dramatic demographic and socioeconomic changes. These changes led to the lower fertility rates and slower rates of population growth discussed in Chapter 7. Worldwide, youth dependency declined while elderly dependency rose. In 1970, 40 percent of the populations of all low- and middle-income nations were children 14 years and under. In 2009, the percentage had fallen to 29 percent. The elderly, those 65 and older, were only 4 percent of the population of developing nations in 1970 and today are still only 6 percent; they are 15 percent of the population in high-income countries. In coming decades, demographic change will

[6]Francis Notzon et al., "Causes of Declining Life Expectancy in Russia," *JAMA* 279, no. 10 (1998), 793–800.

[7]In the second half of the twentieth century, world life expectancy (computed as life expectancy by country weighted by each country's population) rose by about 18 years, while the weighted standard deviation *fell* from 13 to 7 years. See Charles Kenny, "Why Are We Worried About Income? Nearly Everything That Matters Is Converging," *World Development* 33, no. 1 (January 2005). See also Gary S. Becker, Tomas J. Philipson, and Rodrigo R. Soares, "The Quantity and Quality of Life and the Evolution of World Inequality," *American Economic Review* 95, no. 1 (2005), 277–91.

accelerate as the consequences of the developing world's transition from high to low population growth rates combine with falling child mortality and rising life expectancy.

As societies age and health improves, the pattern of disease and causes of death also shift in a generally predictable pattern. This shift in disease pattern is referred to as the **epidemiologic transition**. One early characterization of the epidemiologic transition identified three main stages: the age of pestilence and famine, the age of receding pandemics, and the age of degenerative and human-made diseases.[8] The age of pestilence and famine, which covered most of human history, was a time of frequent epidemics and famines. Chronic malnutrition existed, as did severe maternal and child health problems. Health outcomes were affected by environmental problems such as unsafe water, inadequate sanitation, and poor housing. During the age of receding pandemics, death rates fell as infectious disease and famines declined. As people lived longer, they began to experience heart disease and cancer in greater numbers. In the age of degenerative and human-made diseases, mortality rates are low and chronic degenerative diseases, such as heart disease, diabetes, and hypertension; lifestyle diseases, the result of smoking and excessive use of alcohol, for example; and environmental diseases, such as those caused by pollution, take the place of infectious diseases as the primary causes of death. Changes have been made to this initial theory, but it remains a useful framework.

Some researchers add other stages of epidemiologic transition, such as emerging and reemerging infectious disease.[9] Old infectious diseases may cause increased morbidity and mortality due to resistance to antimicrobial therapies, as is the case for drug-resistant tuberculosis, and new pathogens continue to emerge. HIV/AIDS is the best known of these new infections, although other new infectious diseases have emerged over the past 30 years, including the Ebola virus, severe acute respiratory syndrome (SARS), and recent strains of avian and H1N1 swine flu.

The twentieth century has seen a major shift in causes of death and disability from infectious diseases to noncommunicable disease. However, not all countries made this transition fully. Many of the poorest countries and poor subpopulations in middle-income countries still suffer from high rates of infectious diseases, maternal and perinatal conditions, and nutritional deficiencies that ceased to be problems in high-income nations. Table 9–4 demonstrates the extent of these disparities for 2004, the most recent update assembled by WHO. Globally, 60 percent of mortality is due to noncommunicable conditions such as cardiovascular disease and cancer, 30 percent of mortality is due to communicable conditions, and 10 percent is due to injuries. High-income countries have reduced mortality from communicable disease to only 7 percent, with 87 percent due to noncommunicable conditions. In stark

[8]A. R. Omran, "The Epidemiologic Transition: A Theory of the Epidemiology of Population Change," *Millbank Memorial Fund Quarterly* 49, no. 4 (1971), 509–37.

[9]Ronald Barrett, Christopher W. Kuzawa, Thomas McDade, and George J. Armelagos, "Emerging and Re-Emerging Infectious Diseases: The Third Epidemiologic Transition," *Annual Review of Anthropology* 27 (1998), 247–71.

TABLE 9-4 **Mortality by Cause, 2002**

CAUSE OF DEATH*	WORLD	AFRICA	AMERICAS	SOUTHEAST ASIA	EUROPE	EASTERN MEDITERRANEAN	WESTERN PACIFIC
I. Communicable diseases, maternal and perinatal conditions, and nutritional deficiencies (%)	32.1	71.9	14.7	39.3	5.9	41.7	14.2
II. Non-communicable conditions (%)	58.8	21.1	76.3	50.6	85.8	48.9	75.5
III. Injuries (%)	9.1	7.0	9.1	10.0	8.3	9.4	10.3

*Total mortality.

Source: *World Health Report 2004: Changing History* (Geneva, World Health Organization 2004), annex table 2.

contrast, 68 percent of mortality in sub-Saharan Africa remains due to communicable diseases and only 25 percent to noncommunicable conditions. The situation in India (characteristic of all of South Asia) and Latin America lies in between sub-Saharan Africa and the high-income countries. The differences in causes of death are also seen in Table 9-5. In high-income countries, such as Denmark, all but one of the 10 leading causes of death are from noncommunicable disease. In sub-Saharan Africa, the top four leading causes of mortality are infectious conditions.

China, a country that experienced rapid economic growth, also experienced a substantial epidemiologic transition. The distribution of the causes of death in China is rapidly approaching those of the high-income nations (Table 9-4). Heart diseases, cancers, and strokes are now the leading causes of death, accounting for approximately two-thirds of total deaths among adults 40 years and older. As recently as the early 1960s, famines in China accounted for tens of millions of deaths. China no longer faces the threat of famine but must instead contend with the more modern health risks of smoking; obesity; and the various causes of cancers, heart disease, and other noncommunicable conditions.

THE DETERMINANTS OF IMPROVED HEALTH

Improved health and increases in life expectancy are due to several factors. Major advances in agriculture and food distribution in Europe led to the disappearance of famine and starvation, a concern up to the nineteenth century in some parts of

TABLE 9-5 Leading Causes of Mortality, 2002

RANK	CAUSE*	PERCENT OF TOTAL
World		
1	(II) Ischemic heart disease	12.6
2	(II) Cerebrovascular disease	9.7
3	(I) Lower respiratory infections	6.8
4	(I) HIV/AIDS	4.9
5	(II) Chronic obstructive pulmonary disease	4.8
6	(I) Diarrheal diseases	3.2
7	(I) Tuberculosis	2.7
8	(I) Malaria	2.2
9	(II) Trachea/bronchus/lung cancers	2.2
10	(III) Road traffic accidents	2.1
Total for 10 causes		51.2
Africa		
1	(I) HIV/AIDS	19.6
2	(I) Malaria	10.7
3	(I) Lower respiratory infections	10.4
4	(I) Diarrheal diseases	6.6
5	(I) Childhood diseases	4.9
6	(II) Cerebrovascular disease	3.4
7	(I) Tuberculosis	3.3
8	(II) Ischemic heart disease	3.1
9	(III) Road traffic accidents	1.8
10	(III) Violence	1.3
Total for 10 causes		65.1
Europe		
1	(II) Ischemic heart disease	24.8
2	(II) Cerebrovascular disease	15.1
3	(II) Trachea/bronchus/lung cancers	3.8
4	(II) Lower respiratory infections	2.9
5	(II) Chronic obstructive pulmonary disease	2.7
6	(II) Colon/rectum cancer	2.4
7	(II) Hypertensive heart disease	1.9
8	(II) Cirrhosis of the liver	1.8
9	(III) Self-inflicted	1.7
10	(II) Stomach cancer	1.6
Total for 10 causes		58.7

*(I), communicable diseases; (II), noncommunicable diseases; (III), injuries.

Source: *World Health Report 2004: Changing History* (Geneva, World Health Organization 2004), annex table 2.

the region. Famines were common and devastating in East and South Asia through-out much of the twentieth century. With few exceptions, North Korea being one, famine no longer appears as a threat in most of Asia. The same cannot be said for sub-Saharan Africa, where famines still occur regularly. Even without famine, malnu-trition continues to plague billions of people in Africa and elsewhere and contributes to lower life expectancy. Malnutrition makes individuals more susceptible to infec-tions and less able to fight them off.

Rising incomes generally allow for better nutrition and housing and improved survival rates. Throughout the twentieth century, life expectancy has been strongly associated with per capita income. Life expectancy rises rapidly with income, especially at low levels of income. Increased income allows people, particularly the poor, to buy more food, better housing, and more health care. However, since 1900, on an almost decade by decade basis, life expectancy has shifted upward, so that more health is realized for a given income. This upward shift indicates that health depends on more than income.[10]

Public health measures such as clean water, sanitation, and food regulation contributed to the decline in child mortality in the late nineteenth century and continue to do so today. In the late nineteenth century, Robert Koch showed that the bacterium *Mycobacterium tuberculosis* causes tuberculosis and people began to understand germs. Many other pioneers of science and medicine, such as Louis Pasteur and Joseph Lister, made equally important discoveries. Simple precautions such as preparing food and disposing of waste hygienically, eliminating flies and rodents, and quarantining the sick had far-reaching benefits. The discovery that cholera and typhoid were transmitted through impure water dates to the 1850s, but access to safe drinking water is still far from universal. Medical technology became important to controlling infectious diseases in the 1930s, when antibacterial drugs and new vaccines were introduced. All these developments coupled with the rise of public health institutions that provide for improved sanitation, distribute vaccines, control disease vectors such as mosquitoes, and offer surveillance of disease outbreaks protect societies against the major infectious causes of death.

The critical role of science and institutions as determinants of health, independent of income, is reflected in the historical record. In 1900, life expectancy in the United States was 47 years and per capita income US$5,500 (2005). Compare this to the situation in low- and middle-income countries in 2009. Life expectancy was substantially higher at 67 years, even though per capita income, at about US$5,000 (2005, PPP) was about 10 percent lower. The explanation is straightforward. Penicillin and other antibiotics were unknown in 1900. Urban living conditions were overcrowded, and few vaccines were available. Infectious diseases took their toll on the U.S. population just as they do in many low-income nations today.

Finally, education plays an important role in improving health. This was not always the case. Child mortality differed little by education or income in the United States in the last decade of the nineteenth century, but these factors made a big difference by the early twentieth century. The implication is that affluence and education did not matter much until the underlying scientific knowledge was present. Better-educated individuals acquire and use new information more quickly. This helps explain the large differences in child mortality by mother's education observed in developing countries.[11]

---

[10]World Bank, "Health in Developing Countries: Successes and Challenges," in *World Development Report 1993: Investing in Health* (Oxford: Oxford University Press, 1993), pp. 17–36.

[11]World Bank, "Health in Developing Countries."

HEALTH, INCOME, AND GROWTH

As indicated before, in both rich and poor countries, there is a strong positive relationship between better health and economic growth. In Chapter 3, we saw that countries with higher life expectancy have faster economic growth. Figure 9–2 takes a different perspective, showing the relationship between under-five mortality and the *level* of income. Mortality rates are highest in the poorest countries, and they drop off sharply in conjunction with higher incomes. In countries with per capita income below US$2,000 (PPP), on average, 129 out of every 1,000 children do not live to their 5th birthday. Whereas in rich nations people reaching their 100th birthday is no longer that unusual, in poor nations 1 out of every 8 children still does not live to see his or her 5th birthday. For incomes between $4,000 and $6,000, the child mortality rate is much lower, falling to just 44 per 1,000. For countries with incomes above $10,000, only 12 out of 1,000 die early in life.

Because key measures of health are strongly related to both income levels and growth rates, it should be no surprise that they are also strongly related to poverty. Figure 9–3 makes the link with poverty, showing that countries with higher life expectancies have much lower rates of poverty. In countries with life expectancy below 45 years,

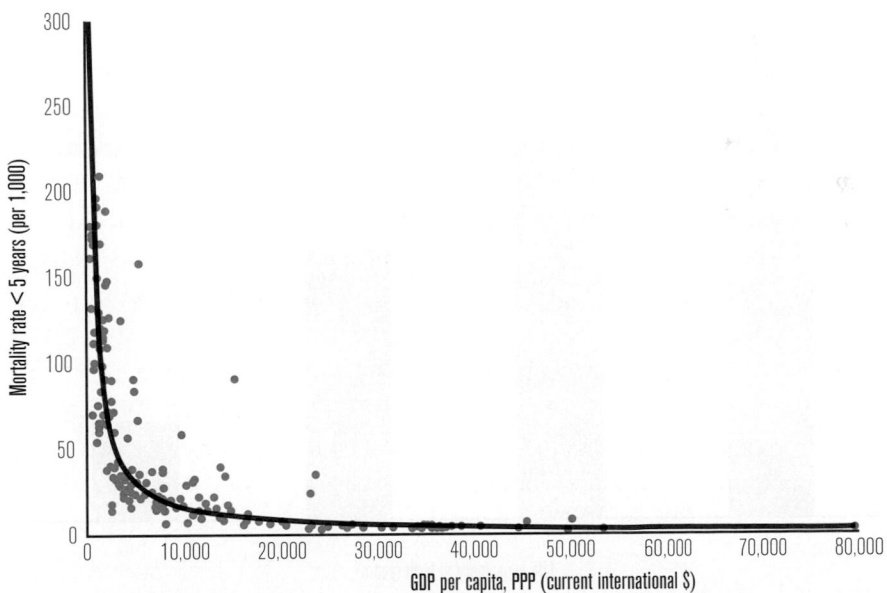

FIGURE 9-2 Child Mortality and Income, 2007

Based on data for 2007 from 168 countries of all income levels around the world.

GDP, gross domestic product; PPP, purchasing power parity.

Source: World Bank, "World Development Indicators," http://databank.worldbank.org.

81 percent of the population lives below the $2-a-day poverty line; in countries with life expectancy greater than 70 years, only 17 percent live below the poverty line.

The strength of these relationships is not in doubt. The question is this, What is causing what? Higher income and reductions in poverty could lead to better health. But the causality could run in the opposite direction; improved health could lead to faster economic growth, higher incomes, and less poverty. In fact, both channels probably are at work. Better health and higher incomes work together in a mutually reinforcing and virtuous cycle, in which improvements in health support faster economic growth leading to higher incomes, and higher incomes facilitate even better health. Unfortunately, the cycle can also work in reverse, as declines in income can weaken health (as in Russia and other transition economies), and the onset of new diseases, such as HIV/AIDS, can lead to a fall in income.

INCOME AND HEALTH

As incomes increase, individuals, households, and societies at large are able to increase spending on a range of goods and services that directly or indirectly improve health. Individuals and households can buy more and better food, so there is a strong causal link from higher income to improved nutrition to better health.[12] Research

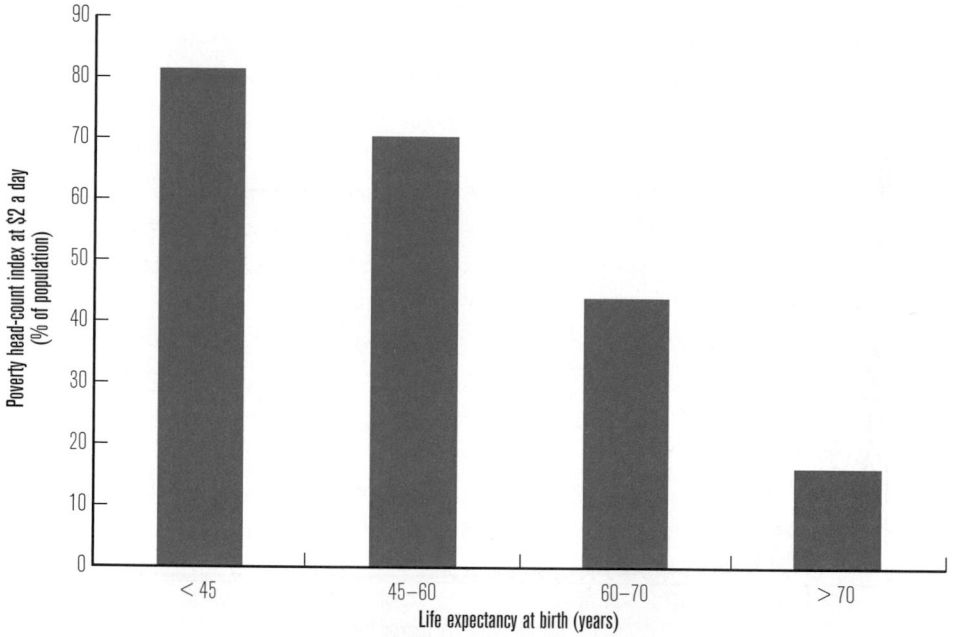

FIGURE 9-3 **Poverty and Life Expectancy, 2000–2007 (Average)**
Source: World Bank, "World Development Indicators," http://databank.worldbank.org.

[12]John Strauss and Duncan Thomas, "Health, Nutrition and Economic Development," *Journal of Economic Literature* 36 (June 1998).

shows that, as incomes rise, child height (an indicator of long-term nutrition) tends to increase in many low-income countries. With higher incomes, poor households can more easily afford clean water and basic sanitation facilities, either as an outhouse or through indoor plumbing, which can help control disease. Also, as incomes rise, poor households can afford better shelter, which in turn should keep them healthier. They are also more likely to be able and willing to seek medical care when it is needed, either because they can afford the transportation costs to the clinic or pay for medicines or other out-of-pocket expenses. For individuals living on subsistence incomes, paying for even the most basic medicines and healthcare can sometimes be a struggle. As incomes rise, such expenditures become more routine.

For society as a whole, as incomes rise, there is greater ability to build public health clinics and hospitals, train more doctors and nurses, and pay for public health services such as immunization campaigns or insect-spraying programs. Poor countries cannot afford to build the same kinds of public and private health systems that richer countries can, and they may not be able to afford to pay their doctors and nurses the kinds of salaries needed to keep them home rather than taking positions in richer countries. Interruptions in the supply of electricity can reduce the efficacy of medications—for example, many vaccines need to be kept refrigerated before inoculation, and when the electricity grid fails, the stock of vaccines is damaged. It is not uncommon in developing countries to find hospitals and clinics without medicines or clean water. Often, because operating budgets are so small and patients cannot afford to pay much, the patient's family must supply basic food and care to a family member in the hospital. As a society's income rises, it is much better able to pay for a reasonable healthcare system. Both sub-Saharan Africa and Latin America devote about 7 percent of GDP to health, including both private and public expenditures. In sub-Saharan Africa with 2009 GDP per capita of US$2,138 (PPP), spending 7 percent of national income on health translates to about $150 per person per year. In Latin America, where per capita incomes average a much higher US$10,555 (PPP), a similar 7 percent allocation to health expenditures provides $740 per person per year, which can buy far more hospital beds and medicine.

Economists Lant Pritchett and Lawrence Summers provide one estimate of the potential impact of rising incomes on health. They find that the long-run income elasticity of under-five mortality is between −0.2 and −0.4, meaning that each 10 percent increase in income is associated with a 2 to 4 percent decline in child mortality rates. According to this result, if income growth in low- and middle-income nations during the 1980s had been 1 percent higher, as many as half a million child deaths would have been averted in 1990 alone.[13] Pritchett and Summers' article is titled, "Wealthier Is Healthier," suggesting that improvements in income, holding other factors constant, lead to lower child mortality and increased life expectancy. The relationship between income levels and life expectancy is captured in Figure 9–4,

---

[13]Lant Pritchett and Lawrence H. Summers, "Wealthier Is Healthier," *Journal of Human Resources* 31, no. 4 (1996), 841–68.

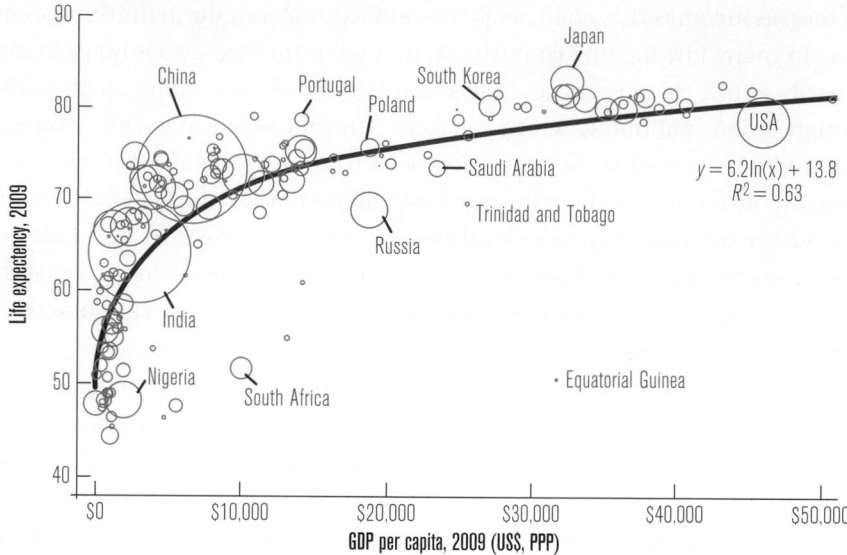

sometimes referred to as the **Preston curve**, after the work of demographer Samuel Preston. In this "bubble" graph, in which each bubble is proportional to the population of the country represented, life expectancy climbs rapidly at lower levels of per capita income and then levels off at higher incomes.

But as we have observed before, correlation does not imply causation. Income is not the only barrier to the use of even life-saving treatments and the significance of rising incomes in explaining health trends is, perhaps surprisingly, a matter of some debate. Preston makes this point in his 1975 article, arguing that most of the gains in life expectancy result from upward shifts in curves like the one depicted in Figure 9–4 rather than from movements along them.[14] A similar conclusion is reached by economists David Cutler, Angus Deaton, and Adrianna Lleras-Muney, who write,

> We tend to downplay the role of income. Over the broad sweep of history,
> improvements in health and income are both the consequence of new ideas
> and new technology, and one might or might not cause the other. Between
> rich and poor countries, health comes from institutional ability and political
> willingness to implement known technologies, neither of which is an automatic
> consequence of rising incomes.[15]

[14]Samuel Preston, "The Changing Relation between Mortality and Level of Economic Development," *Population Studies* 29, no. 2 (1975).

[15]David Cutler, Angus Deaton, and Adrianna Lleras-Muney, "The Determinants of Mortality," *Journal of Economic Perspectives* 20, no. 3 (2006), 116.

They cite historical improvements in life expectancy in countries across Europe in the nineteenth century, which happened at more or less the same time despite quite different rates of economic growth. They note that in the twentieth century both China and India made substantial gains in reducing child and infant mortality *before* the reforms that resulted in rapid economic growth. And once reforms were in place, further progress in infant mortality slowed down. Neither the historical record nor the cross-country evidence suggests "that economic growth will improve health without deliberate public action."

The creation and dissemination of medical knowledge and public health practices was central to the historical rise in life expectancy in the now-developed nations (Box 9–2). The diffusion of this knowledge to poor nations today remains a key determinant of health outcomes in developing countries. It is also a determinant somewhat independent of the per capita income levels of the poorer nations. This is another example of economic historian Alexander Gerschenkron's hypothesis about the advantages of backwardness. Poor countries can learn from the scientific knowledge, most of it generated in the developed nations, about disease transmission and interventions to promote health and extend people's lives.

While these cross-country associations between income levels and various measures of health indicate broad trends, the decisions of individual households are important as well. This is a theme of the widely acclaimed book *Poor Economics*, by Abhijit Banerjee and Esther Duflo. The MIT economists provide many examples of poor households making decisions that run counter to the health of their children and families that cannot be explained by low incomes alone. Take the case of oral rehydration therapy (ORT), a simple mixture of water, salts, and sugar that is an effective treatment for common, and often fatal, diarrheal diseases in children. It is extremely inexpensive, at under 50 cents per treatment, especially when viewed relative to its life-saving benefits. Poverty alone is an unlikely explanation for the failure to use ORT. Instead, in western India, mothers may not believe that ORT works and prefer that health workers give their children an antibiotic. Despite being prescribed oral rehydration salts for their children, these mothers may simply not use them. Banerjee and Duflo also discuss insecticide-treated bed nets that have proven effective at reducing exposure to mosquitoes that transmit malaria. They also are inexpensive—at less than $10 for a net that provides protection for up to five years. But even when bed nets (or childhood immunizations) are provided for free, the take-up rates are far from universal. More than low incomes must be involved.

Banerjee and Duflo conclude, "The poor seem to be trapped by the same kinds of problems that afflict the rest of us—lack of information, weak beliefs, and procrastination among them." People living in developed nations do not have to worry about chlorinating their water because it comes that way automatically. Poor households

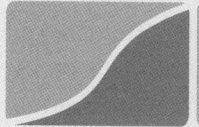

BOX 9-2 "HOW BENEFICENT IS THE MARKET? A LOOK AT THE MODERN HISTORY OF MORTALITY"

Richard Easterlin, a distinguished economic historian and demographer, investigated the reasons behind the decline in mortality rates that began in Europe in the nineteenth century. While rising levels of income improved nutrition and generally contributed to increased resistance to disease, economic growth in this period also increased exposure to disease as industrialization gave rise to urbanization and the concentration of people in closer quarters.

In explaining the great improvement in life expectancy that occurred in parts of Europe in the nineteenth century, Easterlin identifies the centrality of scientific discoveries and the role of public health initiatives. Easterlin also reflects on the role of markets versus the state in achieving these outcomes:

> Only with the growth, first, of epidemiological and, then, bacterial knowledge did effective techniques emerge for controlling infectious disease. These techniques focused primarily on the prevention of the spread of disease—first via controlling the mode of transmission, and subsequently via immunization. It is these methods of prevention that have been chiefly responsible for the great improvement in life expectancy. In the last half century the advance of knowledge has added methods of curing disease to the arsenal available to fight infectious disease, particularly with the development of antibiotics, but the great bulk of the reduction in infectious disease has been accomplished largely by preventive methods.
>
> The control of infectious disease involves serious issues of market failure—information failures, externalities, public goods, principal-agent problems, and so forth. The market cannot be counted on for such things as the provision of pure water and milk, the proper disposal of sewage, control of pests such as mosquitoes and rats, the supply of uncontaminated food and other manufactured products, immunization of children and adults against major infectious diseases, and the dissemination of new knowledge regarding personal hygiene, infant and child care, food handling and preparation, care of the sick, and the like. There is also a serious market failure problem with regard to the distribution of anti-microbials because of externalities associated with the development of disease-resistant bacteria.
>
> The title of this article posed the question, how beneficent is the market? The ubiquity of market failure in the control of major infectious disease supplies the answer: if improvement of life expectancy is one's concern, the market cannot do the job . . . [T]he assumption that the market, in solving the problem of economic growth, will solve that of human development is belied by the lessons of experience. Rather than a story of the success of free market institutions, the history of mortality is testimony to the critical need for collective action.

need to take active steps each day to ensure their water is safe, a far more difficult process even without the tough constraints the poor face. We trust the advice of our health professionals based on experience; given the low quality of medical care in many poor nations such trust is understandably absent. To overcome some of these constraints Banerjee and Duflo recommend *nudges*, whether providing small monetary incentives for childhood vaccines (2 pounds of dal per vaccination and a set of stainless-steel plates for completing the course) or just making it easier to do the right thing (a "one turn" chlorine dispenser next to a village well that makes chlorinating water as easy as possible).[16] Understanding the behavior of households and individuals is critical to improving health outcomes.

HEALTH AND PRODUCTIVITY

There is increasingly strong evidence of the causality also running in the opposite direction, in which improved health leads to faster economic growth, higher incomes, and reduced poverty. Several studies have shown that higher life expectancy in an early period (say, 1960) leads to faster subsequent economic growth (say, from 1960 to 2000). The relationship is usually found to have diminishing returns, meaning that an extra year of life expectancy at birth has a big effect on growth when life expectancy is 45 years but a smaller effect when life expectancy reaches 70 years. A typical estimate suggests that, after controlling for other factors that influence growth, each 10 percent improvement in life expectancy at birth translates into an increase of 0.3 to 0.4 percentage points per year in economic growth.

Better health affects both fundamental causes of economic growth: productivity gains and increased investment. Healthier people tend to be more economically productive because they are more energetic and mentally alert. A healthier worker is able to harvest more crops, build more furniture, assemble more computers, or make more service calls than a worker who is ill or lethargic. A study of sugarcane workers in Tanzania showed that workers with schistosomiasis, a disease caused by a parasitic worm that causes fever, aches, and fatigue, were able to cut much less cane and therefore earn much less in wages (because they were paid by the amount they cut) than workers in the same estate that did not have the disease.[17] Healthier workers not only are more productive while they work but also lose fewer workdays because of illness. The types of work available to many low-income, low-skilled workers put a premium on physical health because they typically rely more on strength and endurance than higher-skilled desk jobs. Moreover, aside from their own health, if a worker's

[16]Abhijit Banerjee and Esther Duflo, *Poor Economics: A Radical Rethinking of the Way to Fight Global Poverty* (New York: Public Affairs, 2011), chap. 3.

[17]A. Fenwick and B. M. Figenschou, "The Effect of *Schistosoma mansoni* on the Productivity of Cane Workers in a Sugar Estate in Tanzania," *Bulletin of the World Health Organization* 47, no. 5 (September 1972), 567–72.

family is healthier, the worker loses fewer workdays in caring for family members that are ill. A dramatic example of the latter point involves HIV/AIDS. Firms in southern Africa, where HIV prevalence rates are the highest in the world, lose workdays due not only to the illnesses of employees but also in time lost to attending the high number of funerals of coworkers and family members.

A family member's health can also have an impact on children's education, which in turn has implications for future income. Families that cope with long-term illnesses, such as HIV/AIDS or tuberculosis of an adult, may rely on children to work the fields, find other ways to bring in income, or care for the sick family member, thus preventing the child from attending school and investing in his or her own human capital. The child's health also directly affects his or her schooling. Poor health can reduce cognitive ability in students and undermines schooling through absenteeism and shorter attention spans. As noted earlier, experimental evidence from Kenya finds that students in schools that received a simple treatment for hookworms had higher school enrollment rates and, in cases of wage employment, higher earnings as young adults. When child mortality declines, parents tend to have fewer children, allowing them to invest more in each child's health and education, as discussed in Chapter 7.

Childhood health can affect labor productivity years later when children grow older and join the workforce. The early effects of health on physical strength and cognitive ability can have lasting impacts. Nobel laureate Robert Fogel found a strong relationship among nutrition, body size, and labor productivity.[18] Research on Brazil inspired by Fogel's earlier work identifies a relationship between a worker's height and wages. Taller workers, who, after controlling for other factors, are likely to have had better nutrition during childhood, earn much higher wages, reflecting higher levels of productivity. The relationship in Brazil is strong: A 1 percent increase in height is associated with a nearly 8 percent increase in wages. When workers are healthier and more productive, firms are willing to pay them higher wages.

HEALTH AND INVESTMENT

Beyond its impact on labor productivity, improved health can influence the other key channel for achieving economic growth, increased saving and investment.

As people expect to live longer, they have greater incentives to make long-term investments in their farm or other business and their human capital. By contrast, people with poor health have to divert more of their income into medical expenses, reducing their capacity to save. Poor people facing catastrophic illness sometimes must sell some of their assets, such as livestock or farm tools, thus depleting their capital stock, to pay for medicines or simply to feed their family if they no longer can

---

[18]See, for example, Robert Fogel, "New Findings on Secular Nutrition and Mortality: Some Implications for Population Theory," in M. R. Rosensweig and O. Stark, eds., *Handbook of Population and Family Economics*, vol. 1a (Amsterdam: Elsevier Science, 1997) pp. 433–81.

work. Health can also affect public saving and investment. Governments fighting endemic diseases must allocate more of their spending to these purposes, reducing the amount available for building roads or other capital investment.

In South Africa, the high prevalence of HIV/AIDS is viewed as both a public health challenge and as a macroeconomic problem that reduces economic growth. The disease reduced the size of the workforce and its productivity at the same time as it has decreased the ability of households, firms, and the government to invest in the future. Households face lost labor income and increased expenditures on health; firms confront increased expenditures on health benefits and insurance, higher absenteeism and job turnover, and greater training costs due to premature deaths; and government finds that health expenditures crowd out other high-priority expenditures. Some studies suggest that HIV/AIDS may have cost South Africa a full percentage point of annual economic growth—a huge amount for an economy averaging GDP per capita growth of only 1.5 percent.[19]

Reduction or elimination of diseases can help substantially increase the amount of usable productive assets, including land. The classic example of disease impeding a critical investment is the construction of the Panama Canal in the late nineteenth century (Box 9–3). Contemporary examples include large tracts of land rendered uninhabitable by endemic disease. The dramatic reduction of river blindness in west Africa allowed increased farming in the fertile lands near riverbanks that previously were breeding grounds for the disease (see Box 14–4 for a discussion of the fight against river blindness in the context of foreign aid programs). Schistosomiasis makes it unsafe for people to enter lakes and streams in sections of Africa, and trypanosomiasis (sleeping sickness) restricts the range of the livestock industry. The reduction of malaria allowed farmers to work new lands in Malaysia, Sri Lanka, and the Terrai area of northern India. Singapore's economic prosperity was made possible partly because rampant malaria was brought under control on the island. Similarly, disease can undermine foreign investment, as investors shun environments where HIV/AIDS, malaria, tuberculosis, and other diseases are more prevalent.

THREE CRITICAL DISEASES

Dramatic changes are taking place in global health. The reduction of infectious disease allows the survival of many individuals to old age. Reductions in fertility rates contribute to a change in population structure so that the elderly represent a larger portion of

---

[19]Jeffrey D. Lewis, "Assessing the Demographic and Economic Impact of HIV/AIDS," in Kyle Kauffman and David Lindauer, eds., *AIDS and South Africa: The Social Expression of a Pandemic* (Hampshire, UK: Palgrave Macmillan, 2004).

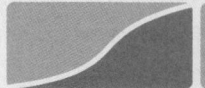

BOX 9-3 MALARIA, YELLOW FEVER, AND THE PANAMA CANAL

On February 1, 1881, capitalized by over 100,000 mostly small investors, the French Compagnie Universelle du Canal Interocéanique began work on a canal that would cross the Isthmus of Panama and unite the Atlantic and Pacific Oceans. Ferdinand de Lesseps, builder of the Suez Canal, led the project. In the first months, the digging progressed slowly but steadily. Then, the rains began, and the crew soon discovered what they were up against: mile upon mile of impassable jungle, day upon day of torrential rain, insects, snakes, swamps, heat, and endemic disease—smallpox, malaria, and yellow fever.

In 1881, the company recorded about 60 deaths from disease. In 1882, the number doubled, and the following year, 420 died. The most common killers were malaria and yellow fever. Because the company often fired sick men to reduce medical costs, the numbers probably reflect low estimates. By the time the company halted the project and went out of business in December 1888, about $300 million had been spent, and 20,000 men had died.

In 1904 President Theodore Roosevelt instigated a treaty with Panama that gave the United States the right to build the canal and create the 10-mile-wide Canal Zone, which amounted to sovereign American territory surrounding the waterway. The U.S. Army dispatched surgeon Colonel William Gorgas to Panama to tackle malaria and yellow fever. Gorgas was fresh from Havana where he had helped eradicate yellow fever, following discoveries by his colleague Major Walter Reed and others that the disease was carried by a mosquito. The fight against yellow fever also substantially reduced malaria, building on discoveries by British bacteriologist Ronald Ross that the parasite that causes malaria was transmitted by the *Anopheles* mosquito.

The efforts to control the two diseases were successful. Yellow fever was totally eradicated. Deaths due to malaria in employees dropped from 11.6 per 1,000 in November 1906 to 1.2 per 1,000 in December 1909. But the impact spread well beyond the canal workers. Deaths from malaria in the Panamanian population fell from 16.2 per 1,000 in July 1906 to 2.6 per 1,000 in December 1909. The canal was completed in 1914, one of the greatest construction miracles of the early twentieth century. The project powerfully demonstrated that malaria and yellow fever could be controlled over a wide geographical area, paving the way for investment and increased economic activity.

Sources: Adapted from the Public Broadcasting Service's film series *The American Experience: The Story of Theodore Roosevelt,* "TR's Legacy—The Panama Canal," www.pbs.org/wgbh/amex/tr/panama.html; and Centers for Disease Control and Prevention, *Malaria: The Panama Canal,* www.cdc.gov/malaria/history/panama_canal.htm.

the population, imposing new demands on healthcare systems. The process of industrialization, urbanization, and modernization creates its own set of health problems. Pollution damages the environment and affects health. Increased tobacco use adds to the burden of diseases such as lung cancer and heart disease. Alcohol abuse, injuries, and stress create their own set of health problems. A shift in diet from vegetables and cereals to highly processed foodstuffs coupled with a decline in activity levels leads to rising obesity in both rich and poor nations and contributes to chronic illnesses.

While the burden of noncommunicable disease grows, the unfinished agenda of infectious diseases remains. There is a great disparity in what has been achieved in healthcare between the developed and developing nations and even between groups within nations. The rest of this chapter focuses on a handful of diseases that are preventable, treatable, or curable, yet pose significant problems in developing countries. This is followed by examples of how countries and the international community have addressed some of these and other diseases. A disease-based approach offers a snapshot of some of the health issues facing developing countries and some of the ways these challenges have been met.

Three of the developing world's most prominent and deadly infectious diseases are HIV/AIDS, malaria, and tuberculosis (Box 9-4). They were the first, fourth, and sixth leading causes of death in sub-Saharan Africa (Table 9-5). These three diseases have spread steadily in recent decades and together kill nearly 4.5 million people every year. Relative to high-income countries, the burden of these diseases (in terms of deaths per capita) was 23 times greater in developing countries, resulting in tremendous economic loss and social disintegration. One of the many tragedies of each of these diseases is that they are preventable and, with adequate resources and institutions, can be treated effectively.

HIV/AIDS

Although HIV/AIDS[20] has affected humans since at least the 1930s, it was virtually unknown until it was first recognized in 1981. Since then, the pandemic[21] has spread inexorably around the globe, exacting a terrible toll on the health and welfare of the world's poorest communities. More than 33 million people were living with HIV/AIDS in 2009, about 1 of every 200 people in the world, and almost 2 million people died that year of AIDS-related causes. HIV/AIDS is the leading cause of death among adults aged 15 to 59 worldwide and has killed an estimated 25 million people.

[20]This section draws on information from UNAIDS, 2010 *Report on the Global AIDS Epidemic* (Geneva: UNAIDS, 2010); Global Fund, *2004 Disease Report* (Geneva: Global Fund to Fight AIDS, Tuberculosis, and Malaria, 2004); and information from WHO (www.who.int) and the U.S. Centers for Disease Control and Prevention (CDC; www.cdc.gov).

[21]HIV/AIDS is usually referred to as a pandemic rather than an epidemic. Both terms often refer to the spread of an infectious disease. *Epidemics* refer to an illness that shows up in a larger number of cases than is normally expected. *Pandemics* refer to an even higher number of cases spread over a larger geographic area.

BOX 9-4 HIV/AIDS, MALARIA, AND TUBERCULOSIS: SOME BASICS

HIV stands for human immunodeficiency virus. Once infected with HIV, a person will always carry the virus. The disease primarily is a sexually transmitted disease, but it can also be transmitted through needles or contaminated blood. Over time, HIV infects and kills white blood cells called CD4 lymphocytes (or T cells), leaving the body unable to fight off infections and cancers. **AIDS** stands for acquired immune deficiency syndrome and is caused by HIV. A person with AIDS has an immune system so weakened by HIV that he or she usually becomes sick from one of several opportunistic infections or cancers, such as pneumonia, Kaposi sarcoma (KS), diarrhea, or tuberculosis. AIDS usually takes several years to develop from the time a person acquires HIV, usually between 2 and 10 years. AIDS can be treated but not cured. With successful antiretroviral (ARV) therapy, which requires medication for life, the body can remain healthy and fight off most viruses and bacteria, and people living with HIV can resume a relatively normal life.

Malaria is a serious and sometimes fatal disease caused by a plasmodium parasite transmitted by the female *Anopheles* mosquito. The mosquito transmits malaria by taking blood from an infected individual and passing it to another. Malaria can also be transmitted by blood transfusion and contaminated needles and syringes. Patients with malaria typically are very sick with high fevers, shaking chills, and flulike illness. Four species of plasmodium infect humans, but the most dangerous is *Plasmodium falciparum,* which causes the most severe disease and deaths and is most prevalent in sub-Saharan Africa and some parts of Southeast Asia. Although malaria can be a fatal disease, illness and death from malaria are largely preventable.

Tuberculosis (TB) is a bacterium that infects the lungs and is spread through the air when someone with active TB coughs, sneezes, talks, or otherwise releases microscopic droplets containing *Mycobacterium tuberculosis,* which then enter the respiratory system of another person. Because proximity and poor ventilation speed transmission, TB is a particular problem in densely populated or enclosed settings, such as urban slums or prisons. Each person with active TB infects an average of 10 to 15 people each year. Only about 10 percent of people infected with the bacterium develop active TB and the accompanying symptoms: fever, weight loss, chronic cough, chest pain, bloody sputum, loss of appetite, and night sweats. A third of those with active TB die within a few weeks or months if they are not treated. The remainder struggle with recurrent infections or the disease goes into remission, but it reemerges from time to time to cause pain, fever, and possibly death. The HIV epidemic fueled the resurgence of TB. HIV weakens the immune system, and people who are infected with HIV are particularly vulnerable to TB. Antibiotics to treat and cure TB patients have been available for over 50 years. Successful treatment requires strict patient compliance. Antibiotics must be taken regularly for six months or more. Failure to do so has contributed to the spread of multidrug-resistant TB, which is much harder to cure.

Sources: "HIV InSite," University of California at San Francisco; WHO; Centers for Disease Control and Prevention; and the Global Fund to Fight AIDS, Tuberculosis, and Malaria.

Sub-Saharan Africa bears the largest burden, with two-thirds the world's infection, even though it is home to only one-tenth the world's population. Across sub-Saharan Africa nearly 1 in 20 adults carries the virus, but huge variations exist across the region. Some west African countries, such as Senegal, have maintained adult prevalence rates of less than 1 percent for more than a decade. In these low-prevalence countries, the disease is confined primarily within groups that practice high-risk behavior, such as sex workers and their clients. In southern Africa, HIV/AIDS has taken hold within the general population. In Swaziland, prevalence rates among pregnant women are a mind-boggling 42 percent. In three countries in southern Africa, more than one-fifth of all adults are HIV positive: Botswana, Lesotho, and Swaziland. Nearly 1.3 million people died of HIV/AIDS-related causes in 2009 in sub-Saharan Africa, more than two-thirds the global total.

The good news is that HIV epidemics in the region are either stable or declining. Among the five countries in sub-Saharan African with the largest HIV epidemics, four (Ethiopia, South Africa, Zambia, and Zimbabwe) reduced new HIV infections by more than a quarter between 2001 and 2009. Prevalence rates are falling in several African countries, including Kenya, Uganda, and Zimbabwe, representing an important achievement in turning the tide on the pandemic. However, even these trends convey a mixed message. Some claim that declines in prevalence rates in Uganda can be attributed at least partially to behavioral changes linked to the government's ABC program: promoting abstinence, being faithful to one partner, and using condoms. But studies demonstrated that, in some regions of the country, falling prevalence rates are less the result of behavioral change than of high mortality. Because of AIDS-related deaths, there were simply fewer HIV-positive adults in 2003 than there were a decade earlier.[22]

The pandemic is less severe in other regions but still a major threat that continues to spread. Adult prevalence rates stabilized around 1 percent in the Caribbean, where there is wide variation between and within countries. In 2009 adult HIV prevalence

[22]In the Rakai region in Uganda, researchers attribute approximately 5 percentage points of the 6.2 percent decline in HIV prevalence between 1994 and 2003 to increased mortality. UNAIDS, *AIDS Epidemic Update* (Geneva, UNAIDS, 2005), p. 26.

was 0.1 percent in Cuba but 3.1 percent in the Bahamas. In Asia, Thailand has implemented a successful campaign to limit the spread of the disease, and the rate of new infections fell more than 25 percent between 2001 and 2009 in India and Nepal; in other countries, however, the number of infected people is growing. With 2.4 million people living with HIV, India has the third largest number of infected people in the world behind South Africa and Nigeria. The epidemic is evolving in China, where unsafe blood transfusion and drug abuse traditionally accounted for the majority of HIV cases. Of the 740,000 HIV-positive people in China in 2009, 59 percent were infected through sexual transmission. The epidemic is worsening in eastern Europe and central Asia (the number of people living with HIV in this region has almost tripled since 2000), fueled by a surge in infections among people who inject drugs.

Women are increasingly vulnerable to HIV, and globally, girls and women account for more than half of those living with HIV. In Africa, the picture is especially grim for young women; those aged 15 to 24 are as much as eight times more likely than men to be HIV-positive. Socioeconomic factors contribute significantly to women's vulnerability to HIV infection. Most are infected by partners who practice high-risk behavior. Compounding this problem is that as many as 9 out of 10 HIV-positive people in sub-Saharan Africa do not know that they are infected. Social disempowerment and lack of access to HIV education or services further contribute to the soaring pandemic among women. In 24 sub-Saharan countries, two-thirds or more of young women aged 15 to 24 years lacked comprehensive knowledge of HIV transmission.[23] Children are also vulnerable. More than 2.5 million children are HIV-positive, and there were more than 0.25 million AIDS-related deaths among children in 2009. The vast majority of infected children acquire HIV through transmission from their mother during pregnancy, labor and delivery, or breast-feeding. Antiretroviral (ARVs) drugs, such as nevirapine, significantly reduce mother to child transmission but still are not always available in sub-Saharan Africa.

The HIV/AIDS pandemic has had a crippling effect on many countries that were making significant progress in health. Whereas most countries in sub-Saharan Africa had achieved steady increases in life expectancy in the 1960s, 1970s, and early 1980s, in several countries this progress stopped in the late 1980s and has since reversed. Figure 9–5 shows changes in life expectancy for six of the most severely infected countries. Tragically, life expectancy dropped from an average of 61 years in 1992 to just 47 years in 2007. But as Figure 9–5 suggests, some countries (Botswana, Namibia, Zimbabwe) seem to have reached a turning point, with life expectancy rising once again.

The effects on communities and families are devastating as parents, children, and community leaders become sick and die. Unlike most diseases, HIV/AIDS attacks primarily young adults and the economically active segment of the population. Other diseases tend to incapacitate the very young, the old, or those already weakened by other

---

[23]UNAIDS and World Health Organization, "HIV Infection Rates Decreasing in Several Countries but Global Number of People Living with HIV Continues to Rise," press release, November 21, 2005, available at www.who.int/hiv/epiupdate2005/en/index.html.

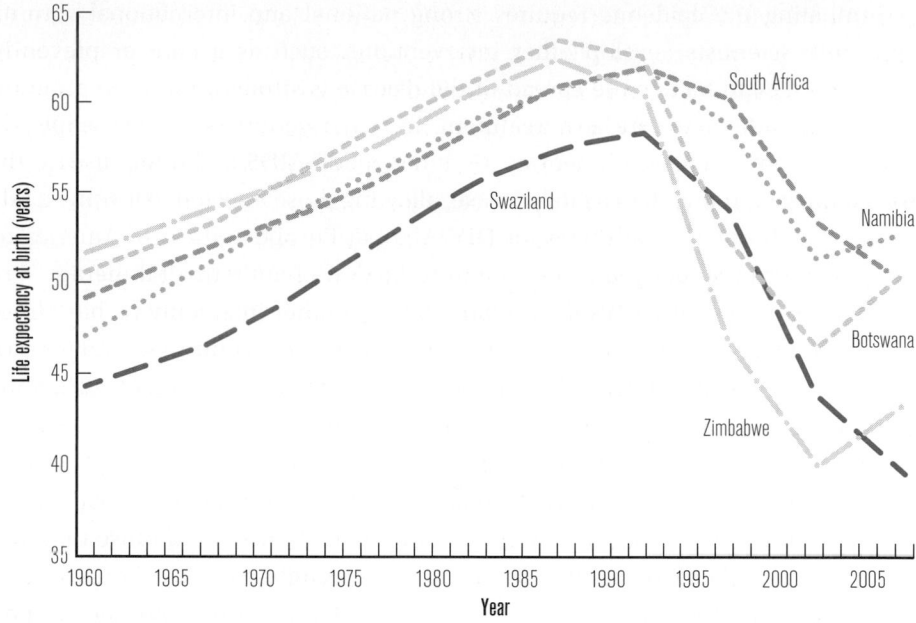

FIGURE 9-5 **Life Expectancy at Birth in Selected Most HIV-Affected Countries**
Source: World Bank, "World Development Indicators," http://databank.worldbank.org.

conditions. HIV/AIDS is different. In Africa, HIV disproportionately destroys the lives of society's most productive members. Households face catastrophe as income earners fall ill and eventually succumb to the disease. The long duration of AIDS illness makes it particularly costly. In addition to these losses, others in the family must stop work to care for those that are ill. Small farms and gardens go untended, and children may be taken out of school to tend to sick family members or to go to work to earn extra income. Families become further impoverished as they face increasing medical costs and have less income to pay for food, clothing, or other expenses. In some cases, funeral costs may be higher than healthcare costs and add to a family's burden. Studies in Tanzania and Thailand estimate that the cost of medical care and funerals can be greater than the household's annual income, triggering borrowing, asset sales, or other coping strategies that can have long-term financial welfare implications.[24] Many of the effects of HIV/AIDS are intergenerational: Worldwide there are now 16.6 million AIDS orphans who have had one or both parents die from the disease.

[24]Steven Russell, "The Economic Burden of Illness for Households: A Review of Cost of Illness and Coping Strategy Studies Focusing on Malaria, Tuberculosis and HIV/AIDS." Disease Control Priorities Project (DCPP) Working Paper 15, August 2003, available at http://www.dcp2.org/file/30/wp15.pdf. Funeral costs have become a significant expense to both households and firms. They have become so common that firms are beginning to limit the number of days that employees can take for funeral leave each month. This is an issue, in part, because family members often are buried in their traditional villages, requiring days of travel for mourners.

Combating the epidemic requires strong national and international commitment. Until scientists develop other interventions, such as a cure or preventive vaccine, the key to halting the spread of the disease is strong prevention programs coupled with adequate care and treatment. In richer countries, where people can afford treatment, the development of ARVs has made AIDS a chronic disease that can be managed, rather than a fatal disease, allowing those infected to resume a relatively normal lifestyle. Death rates for HIV/AIDS in Europe and North America fell by 80 percent in the four years after the introduction of antiretroviral therapy. Prophylactic treatment with ARVs in combination with other interventions has almost entirely eliminated HIV infection in infants in industrialized countries.[25] But for most people in the poorest countries, ARVs remain out of reach. At the end of 2009, about one in three Africans who needed treatment had access to these drugs. Beginning in 2003, access to ARVs in developing countries began to improve, and in a few countries, treatment coverage is now widespread. In Botswana, Cambodia, Croatia, Cuba, Guyana, Namibia, Romania, and Rwanda, more than 80 percent of those that need ARVs are now receiving them, but these are exceptions rather than the norm.

Delivering antiretroviral therapy on a global level requires not only good science and health policy but also political and economic initiatives. The most cost-effective way to provide the massive quantities of drugs required at hugely discounted prices is to encourage the manufacture of generic versions of these antiretroviral agents. Issues of trade-related intellectual property rights and patents must be considered here. One challenge is to encourage such manufacture while providing incentives for major pharmaceutical companies to develop newer medicines as patients develop resistance to the current stock.[26]

The international community was slow to respond to the growing crisis during the 1990s, but that has begun to change. In 1996, only about US$300 million was available to fight the disease globally. By 2009, an estimated US$15.9 billion was available, a figure that includes not just donor funds but the steadily increasing funding that comes from country governments and out-of-pocket spending by directly affected individuals and families. Yet this amount is still $10 billion short of what the Joint United Nations Programme on HIV/AIDS (UNAIDS) has estimated was required in 2010. Due to fiscal constraints in response to the global financial crisis, 2009 was the first time that international assistance did not increase from the previous year. Finding the needed funds will be a continuing challenge, and even when they are found, they will have significant opportunity costs because funding is diverted from other key challenges to fight HIV/AIDS.

[25]World Health Organization, *World Health Report 2004: Changing History* (Geneva: World Health Organization, 2004).

[26]Diane V. Havlir and Scott M. Hammer, "Patents Versus Patients? Antiretroviral Therapy in India," *New England Journal of Medicine* 353, no. 8 (August 25, 2005), 749–51.

MALARIA

Malaria[27] is estimated to claim the lives of 2,000 children every day and is a major contributor to illness in the developing world. WHO estimates that approximately half of the world's population is at risk of malaria in over 106 countries, primarily poor countries located in the tropics. Malaria contributes to almost 800,000 deaths and 225 million cases of severe illness each year. Africa, again, bears the heaviest burden, with about 78 percent of the cases of clinical malaria and 91 percent of the world's malaria deaths. Almost one-fifth of the deaths in children under five in Africa are caused by malaria. Malaria also continues to be a problem in Southeast Asia, India, Latin America, and some parts of Oceania.

Most diseases in developing countries have a disproportionate impact on the poor, but this is especially the case with malaria. Poor families are more likely to live in slum areas or in the countryside where malaria is common, less likely to be able to afford simple prevention steps (like insecticide-treated bed nets), and less likely to receive treatment once fever strikes. In the 1990s, more than half of malaria deaths occurred in the poorest 20 percent of the world's population, a higher percentage than for any other disease of major public health importance. This percentage is

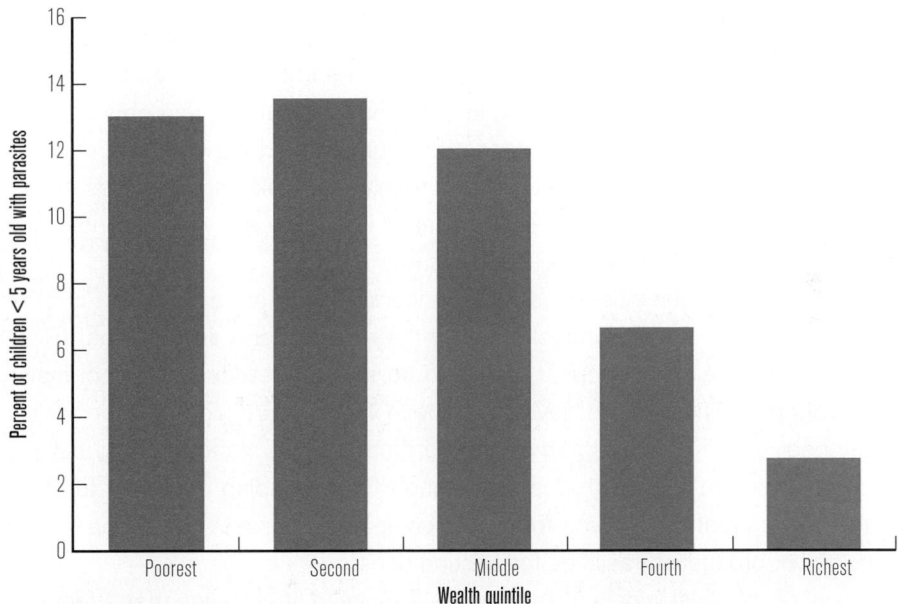

FIGURE 9-6 **Parasite Prevalence Is Higher in Poor Children**

Source: Government of the Republic of Zambia Ministry of Health, *Zambia National Malaria Indicator Survey 2008*, available at www.nmcc.org.zm/files/ZambiaMIS2008Final.pdf, accessed February 2012.

[27]This section draws on information from UNICEF and WHO, *2010 World Malaria Report*, (Geneva: World Health Organization, 2010); the Global Fund, 2004 *Disease Report*; and Tina Rosenberg, "What the World Needs Now Is DDT," *New York Times* (April 11, 2004).

probably higher today. Figure 9–6 shows that in Zambia 13 percent of children from the poorest quintiles had malaria, whereas less than 3 percent of children from the richest quintile were infected.

Many countries have begun to make progress in reducing malaria. Prevention strategies include the use of insecticide-treated bed nets for those at highest risk of malaria, intermittent preventive drug treatment of pregnant women, and spraying with insecticides and other forms of vector control. For those who become sick with malaria, the disease can be controlled with early treatment. As of yet, there is no vaccine against the disease, although research is under way to find one. Unfortunately, because this is a disease of the poor, commercial opportunities are limited for selling a vaccine and recouping expensive research and development costs, and research on this vaccine has been underfunded. Box 9–5 describes one idea aimed at overcoming this market failure.

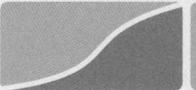

BOX 9-5   MAKING MARKETS FOR VACCINES

Vaccines save 3 million lives a year, prevent long-term disability and illness in millions more, and are one of the most cost-effective ways of enhancing health and reducing poverty in developing countries. Yet, there are no vaccines for some of today's biggest killers, such as malaria, HIV, and tuberculosis; and new vaccines developed for hepatitis B, pneumococcus, rotavirus, and cervical cancer, which kill millions of people a year, are not affordable in developing countries. If vaccines are so cost-effective and save so many lives, why are vaccines not being developed and used for these killer diseases?

In some cases, the science is highly uncertain, such as for HIV. But in other cases, private firms that conduct much of the research and development (R&D) for vaccines have no financial incentive to do so for diseases that affect mainly poor countries. The costs of developing these vaccines are high, and incomes in many poor countries are too low to afford them. Private markets fail to develop vaccines because a price that is low enough for developing countries to afford is too low to create incentives for private companies to invest in developing new vaccines or production facilities for existing ones.

Many of the most widely used vaccines are aimed at diseases that affect children in both rich and poor countries, such as diphtheria, tetanus, pertussis, and polio. Because these vaccines are used around the world, the market is large enough to cover a pharmaceutical company's costs for both R&D and production. In some cases, vaccines could be sold at a higher price in richer countries, to recover R&D costs, and a lower price in poorer countries. But some of the highest-priority diseases for developing countries lack the high priority for rich countries. AIDS, diarrheal diseases, malaria, and other diseases, which are some of the biggest killers in developing countries, are not nearly as high on the list for rich countries, so the total potential market for vaccines for these diseases is much more limited. The pharmaceutical industry tends to respond to where the financial pay-off is the greatest, serving the health needs of the richer countries while neglecting diseases concentrated in low-income countries.

The costs of development and the risks of failure for vaccines are high. Vaccine development can take 7 to 20 years for basic research, clinical testing, regulatory approval, production, and distribution, and even the most promising vaccine candidates can fail at any stage. Estimates of the total costs of developing a new vaccine vary but range from several hundred million dollars to $1.5 billion. It is not realistic to hope that private companies will spend the money necessary to develop urgently needed vaccines then just give them away or sell them at a low price to poor countries.

One way to overcome this market failure is for donors to provide an advance market commitment (AMC) to provide private firms the financial returns they need to develop new vaccines while keeping the cost low for consumers in low-income countries. Sponsors and donors, such as governments, international agencies, and foundations, make binding commitments to pay for a desired vaccine if and when it is developed. Developing countries could buy the vaccine at a low and affordable price, and sponsors would commit to providing the balance up to a guaranteed price, thus guaranteeing market returns for the vaccine developer that are comparable to other products. Once a specified number of vaccines was purchased at the guaranteed price (enough to cover R&D costs), the supplier would be committed to selling further treatments at a lower, affordable price without the sponsor's top-up. This step would ensure that developing countries could afford to continue purchasing the vaccine once payments under the commitment had been made.

A commitment creating a market comparable to the sales revenue of an average new medicine would cost about $3 billion. As an example, sponsors could make a legally binding commitment to purchase 200 million treatments of a malaria vaccine for $15 each. Poorer nations would decide to buy the vaccine at a low price (say, $1 per treatment) and the sponsors would provide the additional $14. After the first 200 million treatments, the company would be committed to sell additional treatments at $1, enough to cover ongoing production costs. These purchases, along with sales to the military, travelers, and some middle-income countries that can afford a higher price, would create the $3 billion market.

This approach complements rather than substitutes for other approaches for developing vaccines, such as support for public research facilities and universities.

R&D in public health often involves government-funded research into the "public good" of knowledge about diseases, which can then be appropriated by the private sector for commercial development. AMC provides clear incentives for private firms to invest in the development of critical vaccines. It also respects intellectual property rights for vaccines and removes pressures on firms to sell new products at a loss. For donors, there would be no cost unless a vaccine is actually developed, minimizing their risks. AMC would use public funds to make markets work more effectively to solve some of the developing countries' most pressing health problems.

In 2009 the first AMC was launched by the Global Alliance for Vaccines and Immunisations (now GAVI Alliance), a public–private partnership including major donors, pharmaceutical companies, and foundations. This pilot AMC is designed to accelerate access to existing vaccines against pneumococcal diseases. Such diseases include pneumonia, which is estimated to kill 1.6 million people per year, most of them children and about 90 percent occurring in developing nations. A pneumococcal vaccine has existed since 2000 and is part of regular immunization programs in developed countries. But the existing pneumococcal vaccine sells at over $70 per dose, far too expensive for widespread adoption in low-income countries. Funding from GAVI Alliance will permit the long-term price of the vaccine to fall to $3.50 and prevent an estimated 7 million childhood deaths by 2030.

Sources: The idea for the AMC was developed by a working group hosted by the Center for Global Development and is based on an earlier idea by Harvard University economist Michael Kremer. See Owen Barder, Michael Kremer, and Ruth Levine, *Making Markets for Vaccines: Ideas to Action* (Washington, DC: Center for Global Development, 2005). Much of the text in this box is drawn from this report. Also see Michael Kremer and Rachel Glennerster, *Strong Medicine: Creating Incentives for Pharmaceutical Research on Neglected Diseases* (Princeton, NJ: Princeton University Press, 2004).

Malaria can have substantial economic costs on top of its public health impact. Research by economists John Gallup and Jeffrey Sachs concluded that the presence of a high malaria burden reduces economic growth by 1.3 percent per year.[28] Although that figure probably incorporates the impact of other diseases that occur in tandem with malaria (such as HIV/AIDS), there is little doubt that malaria creates a heavy burden in countries with high prevalence rates. Malaria programs can be very cost-effective. One study, based on data from sub-Saharan Africa, estimated that the net benefits of a complete package of malaria interventions were about 18 times higher than the costs.[29]

[28]John Gallup and Jeffrey Sachs, "The Economic Burden of Malaria," *American Journal of Tropical Medicine and Hygiene Special Supplement* (June 2001).
[29]Global Fund, 2001 *Disease Report*, p. 37.

But even cost-effective programs can prove controversial. The insecticide of choice for combating malaria is dichlorodiphenyl-trichloroethane (DDT), but donors rarely pay for its use. The irony is that DDT was once used extensively and successfully in the United States, southern Europe, and many developing countries as a means of malaria control and eradication. But overuse of DDT in the United States, especially to control agricultural pests, was linked to environmental damage affecting wildlife. Author and social activist Rachel Carson brought attention to the problem in her seminal book *Silent Spring*, published in 1962. (The title refers to the impact of DDT on bird populations.) DDT use eventually was banned in the United States and other countries, but remains a highly effective and inexpensive (its patent expired long ago) means of eradicating the mosquito that transmits malaria. When sprayed on the interior walls of dwellings (the preferred mode for preventing the spread of malaria), DDT has minimal environmental consequences and has not been found harmful to humans. But given its pariah status in the West and the fear of maintaining a double-standard (selling an insecticide to poor countries that is banned in rich ones), DDT has not played a significant role in saving lives in Africa and other malaria-endemic regions for many years.

The level of international attention to and spending on malaria control in poor regions has been dismal. Funds by the major external financers of malaria control (the Global Fund, the World Bank, and the U.S. President's Malaria Initiative) stagnated at US$1.8 billion in 2010. Estimates by the WHO find that effective malaria control requires more than US$5 billion annually.

TUBERCULOSIS

Until 20 years ago, tuberculosis (TB)[30] was uncommon in the industrialized world and many assumed that the disease had been largely conquered. But, in recent years, TB has reemerged as a virulent killer. More than 2 billion people, one-third of the world's population, are infected with the TB bacterium. Most people who are infected carry the bacterium in their body without symptoms, but each year 9.4 million people develop active TB and exhibit fever and other symptoms. TB causes or contributes to 1.7 million deaths each year, with 90 percent of the deaths occurring in developing countries. About a quarter of those who die also are infected with HIV, which weakens the immune system and makes people more vulnerable to developing active TB.

As with other diseases, the poor are particularly vulnerable to TB. Studies in India have shown that the prevalence of TB is two to four times higher among groups with low income and no schooling. The poor are more likely to live in overcrowded conditions where the airborne bacterium can spread easily. Poor nutrition and

---

[30]This section draws on information from WHO, *Global Tuberculosis Control 2010* (Geneva: World Health Organization, 2010).

inadequate sanitation also add to the risk. And as with other diseases, once the poor are infected, they are less likely to be diagnosed and treated. The economic costs of TB can be significant, stemming from lost work for the patient and caregivers, extra nutritional needs, treatment costs, transportation to and from clinics, and withdrawal of children from schools. In the developing world, an adult with TB can lose an average of three to four months of work.[31] Every year in India alone, more than 300,000 children leave school because of their *parent's* TB. By some estimates, TB depletes the incomes of the world's poorest communities by up to $12 billion every year, and lost productivity can cost an economy on the order of 4 to 7 percent of GDP.[32]

The internationally recommended strategy to control TB is directly observed treatment, short course (DOTS), which combines a regular TB drug dosage with clinical observation visits. Full treatment takes many months, but unfortunately some patients stop taking their medicines during that period because they start to feel better or the drug supply is unreliable. This may lead to the emergence of drug-resistant TB. A particularly dangerous form of drug-resistant TB is multidrug-resistant TB (MDR-TB). Rates of MDR-TB are high in some countries, including Russia, and threaten TB-control efforts. From a public health perspective, poorly supervised or incomplete treatment of TB is worse than no treatment at all. When people fail to complete the treatment regime, they may remain infectious and develop a resistance to treatment. People they infect have the same drug-resistant strain. While drug-resistant TB generally is treatable, it requires extensive chemotherapy (up to two years of treatment), which is often prohibitively expensive (often more than 100 times more expensive than treatment of drug-susceptible TB) and more toxic to patients. Direct observation of treatment helps TB patients adhere to treatment. According to WHO, the DOTS strategy produces cure rates of up to 95 percent, even in the poorest countries. A six-month supply of drugs for treatment under the DOTS strategy costs as little as $10 per patient. The World Bank has identified the DOTS strategy as one of the most cost-effective of all health interventions.[33]

For DOTS to be effective, there must be access to TB sputum microscopy for TB detection; standardized short-course treatment of six to eight months, including direct observation of treatment; an uninterrupted supply of high-quality drugs; a reporting system to monitor patient outcome and program performance; and a political commitment to sustained TB control. Since its inception in 1995, more than 41 million TB patients have been treated under DOTS and 184 countries have adopted the DOTS strategy. However, 1.8 million people fail to get access to TB treatment each year.

---

[31]World Health Organization, *Treatment of Tuberculosis: Guidelines for National Programmes*, 3rd ed. (Geneva: World Health Organization, 2003).

[32]Global Fund, 2004 *Disease Report*, p. 26.

[33]World Health Organization, "Tuberculosis," Fact Sheet No. 104 (Geneva: World Health Organization, 2005).

WHAT WORKS? SOME SUCCESSES IN GLOBAL HEALTH

Despite many challenges to health in the developing world, there are also many successes. The examples that follow recount specific actions by the health sector that saved millions of lives and improved millions more. These cases are excerpted from *Millions Saved: Proven Successes in Global Health*, by Ruth Levine and the What Works Working Group.[34] (The What Works Working Group is a group of 15 development specialists convened by the Center for Global Development.) *Millions Saved* describes 17 successful public health interventions in the developing world. The programs highlighted were implemented on national, regional, or global scales, addressed problems of substantial public health significance, demonstrated a clear and measurable impact on a population's health, lasted at least five consecutive years, and were cost-effective.

The cases presented in *Millions Saved* demonstrate what the health sector can do, even in the poorest countries. Innovative interventions that involve the community can reach the most remote regions. These cases also demonstrate that governments in poor countries can get the job done, including being the chief sources of funds for the interventions. In almost all the cases, the public sector, so often maligned for its corruption and inefficiency, was responsible for delivering care to the affected populations. The interventions included technological developments as well as basic changes in behavior that had a great impact on health. In the control of guinea worm in Africa, for example, families learned to filter their water conscientiously; and in the fight against deaths from dehydration due to diarrheal disease in Bangladesh, mothers learned how to mix a simple salt and sugar solution and taught the technique to their daughters. Interventions can also benefit from international coalitions or partnerships. Such cooperative ventures can break through bureaucracies, provide funding, bring technical capabilities, and generate the political will to sustain an effort in the face of competing priorities. It is also possible to determine whether improvements in health outcomes are due to specific interventions; in most cases, because special efforts were made to collect data that look at outcomes. Finally, these cases illustrate that success comes in all shapes: disease-specific programs, initiatives that improve access and quality, traditional public health interventions, and legal and regulatory reforms all can work, individually or in combination.

---

[34]Ruth Levine and the What Works Working Group with Molly Kinder, *Millions Saved: Proven Successes in Global Health* (Washington, DC: Center for Global Development, 2004). We summarize 5 of the 17 cases presented. Interested students should consult *Millions Saved* for more complete coverage of these five cases and to learn about the other cases.

PREVENTING HIV/AIDS IN THAILAND

Well-documented stories of large-scale success in HIV prevention are few, although many small programs have been shown to be effective. But in Thailand, a large-scale program was successful in changing behaviors associated with increased risk of HIV among sex workers and those who use their services. Thai authorities initially recognized the severity of the situation in 1988, when the first wave of HIV infections spread among injecting-drug users. Between 1989 and 1990, they found that brothel-based sex workers infected with HIV tripled from 3.1 percent to 9.3 percent, and a year later it reached 15 percent. Over the same period, the proportion of male conscripts who were HIV positive when tested on entry to the army rose from 0.5 percent to 3 percent, a sixfold increase in only two years.

Although prostitution is illegal in Thailand, and there was fear that the government's intervention could imply that it tolerated or even condoned it, officials agreed that the higher priority was preventing HIV from spreading further. To do this the government launched the "100 percent condom program," in which all sex workers in brothels were required to use condoms with clients. There was one straightforward rule: no condom, no sex. By creating a monopoly environment, clients, most of whom preferred unprotected sex, could not go elsewhere to find it. Health officials provided free boxes of condoms and local police held meetings with brothel owners and sex workers. Men seeking treatment for sexually transmitted diseases were asked to name the brothel they had used, and health officials would then visit the establishment to provide more information. In principle, the police could shut down any brothel that failed to adopt the policy. Such sanctions were used a few times early on but authorities generally preferred to work with the brothels rather than alienate them.

The campaign was successful: Nationwide condom use in brothels increased from 14 percent in 1989 to more than 90 percent in 1992. The rate of new HIV infections fell fivefold between 1991 and 1993–95. The program may have prevented 200,000 HIV infections during the 1990s. While the program was successful among sex workers, the program did little to encourage men and women, especially among teens and young adults, to use condoms in casual but noncommercial sex. A substantial risk remains that HIV will spread through unprotected sex in Thailand. In addition, HIV continues to spread among injecting-drug users, where the rate is as high as 39 percent. The cost of treating AIDS with antiretroviral drugs, as well as the cost of treating opportunistic infections, is a major challenge facing the Thai government and its citizens. The expense of the government's ARV program, in part, was responsible for a two-thirds decline between 1997 and 2004 in the budget for HIV prevention.

CONTROLLING TUBERCULOSIS IN CHINA

In 1991, China revitalized its TB program and launched the 10-year Infectious and Endemic Disease Control Project to curb its TB epidemic in 13 of its 31 mainland provinces. The program adopted the DOTS strategy. Trained health workers watched patients at local TB dispensaries every other day for six months as they swallowed their antibiotic treatment. Information on each treatment was sent to the county TB dispensary, and treatment outcomes were sent quarterly to the National Tuberculosis Project Office.

China achieved a 95 percent cure rate for new cases within two years of adopting DOTS, and a cure rate of 90 percent for those who had previously undergone unsuccessful treatment. The number of people with TB declined by over 37 percent between 1990 and 2000, and an estimated 30,000 TB deaths were prevented each year. The program cost $130 million in total. The World Bank and WHO estimate that successful treatment was achieved at less than $100 per person. One life year was saved for an estimated $15 to $20.

Despite China's success in curing TB, the program achieved lower-than-hoped-for rates of case detection. China is not alone in this shortcoming and had an experience similar to other high-burden countries. One of the main contributing factors to the low case detection rate was inadequate referral of suspected TB cases from hospitals to the TB dispensaries. Because hospitals can charge for TB diagnosis and treatment, they have little economic incentive to direct patients to the dispensaries. As a result, despite regulations requiring referrals to dispensaries, most TB patients are diagnosed in hospitals, where treatment is often abandoned prematurely.

TB remains a deadly threat in China. Hundreds of millions of people are infected and 10 percent of these are predicted to develop active TB. The government of China faces the challenge of maintaining high cure rates in the provinces covered by the project while scaling up the DOTS program to the remaining half of the population. In response to the 2004 SARS epidemic, the government established a web-based reporting system throughout the country, making it mandatory to report 37 infectious diseases, including TB, within 24 hours. From 2004 to 2007 the proportion of TB cases referred from hospitals to dispensaries increased from 59 percent to 78 percent, and in 2009 China had one of the highest case detection rates for high burden countries.

ERADICATING SMALLPOX

Smallpox, which had affected 10 to 15 million people globally in 1966 and resulted in 1.5 to 2 million deaths, has been completely eradicated. The last recorded case of smallpox occurred in Somalia in 1977. Its eradication has been heralded as one of the greatest achievements of public health in world history. In addition to the direct impact on smallpox, the campaign brought important benefits to other health issues, such as improvements in routine immunization. During the smallpox eradication campaign it was discovered that more than one vaccine could be given at a time, an idea now taken for granted. In 1970, the Expanded Program on Immunization was proposed, which sought to add several vaccines to routine smallpox inoculation. By 1990, 80 percent of the children throughout the developing world were receiving vaccines against six childhood killers, compared to only 5 percent when the program started.

The cost of smallpox eradication can be compared to its benefits, captured by the costs of the disease that have been averted. In developing countries, the costs averted include expenditures for caring for patients as well as lost economic productivity due to illness. In 1976, it was estimated that the cost of caring for someone with smallpox in India was about $3 per patient, which translated to an annual cost of $12 million for the country due to the widespread nature of the disease. Although $3 per patient may seem small, bear in mind that, in many developing countries, public health spending in total is typically only $7 to $8 per person. In addition to the costs of care, by one estimate, India lost about $700 million each year due to diminished economic performance. Assuming 1.5 million deaths due to smallpox worldwide in 1967, smallpox cost developing countries at least $1 billion each year at the start of the eradication campaign.

In the industrialized countries, eradication allowed governments to save the cost of vaccination programs that had been in place to prevent the reintroduction of the disease. In the United States, the bill for 5.6 million primary vaccinations and 8.6 million revaccinations in 1968 alone was $92.8 million, or about $6.50 per vaccination. With other indirect costs of the vaccination program, expenditures in all developed countries were around $350 million per year. Therefore, combining developing and industrialized countries, the estimated global costs, both direct and indirect, of smallpox in the late 1960s was more than $1.35 billion per year. This figure represents the economic benefits of eradication.

The ultimate expenditures of the intensified eradication program were around $23 million per year from 1967 to 1979, financed with $98 million from international contributions and $200 million from the endemic countries. Thus the benefits of eradication far outweighed the costs. It has since been calculated that the largest donor, the United States, saved, in terms of costs averted, the total of all its contributions every 26 days, making smallpox prevention through vaccination one of the most cost-beneficial health interventions of our time.

ELIMINATING POLIO IN LATIN AMERICA

The world's largest public health campaign, the Global Polio Eradication Initiative, follows in the footsteps of smallpox eradication. In 1988, 125 countries were endemic for polio with an estimated 350,000 cases. By 2006, the number of cases had dropped to below 1,400 and only 6 countries and territories remained polio endemic: Afghanistan, Egypt, India, Niger, Nigeria, and the Palestinian Territories. However, poliovirus continues to spread to previously polio-free regions. In late 2004 and 2005, 10 previously polio-free countries were reinfected. Worldwide success is due to the coordinated efforts of regional and international polio eradication campaigns that have immunized hundreds of millions of children. The regional polio campaign in the Americas eliminated polio in just six years.

Polio, short for poliomyelitis, is caused by the intestinal poliovirus. Its most feared effect, paralysis, develops in less than 1 percent of all victims, when the virus affects the central nervous system. The most serious form of the disease causes paralysis that leaves a person unable to swallow or breath. Respiratory support is needed to keep patients alive and mortality runs as high as 40 percent.

In the 1930s and 1940, after a series of polio outbreaks, the American public called for a vaccine. The mobilization effort was led by the disease's most famous victim, U.S. President Franklin D. Roosevelt. In 1938, President Roosevelt created the National Foundation for Infantile Paralysis, later renamed the March of Dimes, to raise funds "a dime at a time" to support the quest for a vaccine. In 1952, the campaign paid off with Dr. Jonas Salk's discovery of an inactivated polio vaccine (IPV). Between 1955 and 1961, more than 300 million doses were administered in the United States, resulting in a 90 percent drop in the incidence of polio. In 1961, a second scientific breakthrough resulted in a new form of the vaccine. Dr. Albert Sabin's oral polio vaccine (OPV) had several advantages over the previous vaccine. The vaccine prevented paralysis, as did the IPV, but OPV went further by helping to halt person-to-person transmission. At approximately $0.05 per dose, OPV was cheaper than its predecessor, and because it is an oral vaccine that requires no needles, it is easier to administer on a wide scale by volunteers.

Successful vaccination programs in Latin America eventually led the Pan American Health Organization in 1985 to launch a program to eradicate polio from the Americas. The immunization strategy of the campaign centered around three primary components: achieving and maintaining high immunization coverage, prompt identification of new cases, and aggressive control of outbreaks. In countries where polio was endemic, national vaccine days (NVDs) were held twice a year, one to two months apart, reaching nearly all children younger than five. The NVDs were designed to vaccinate as many children as possible. While aggressive vaccination strategies helped slow polio's transmission in most of the region, the disease still lingered.

Operation Mop-Up was launched in 1989 to aggressively tackle the virus in its final bastions. The initiative targeted the communities where polio cases had been reported, where coverage was low, or where overcrowding, poor sanitation, weak healthcare infrastructure or heavy migration pervaded. In these communities, house-to-house vaccination campaigns were held to finally wipe out the disease. The last reported case in Latin America was in Peru in 1991. Polio was declared eradicated from the Americas a few years later when no further cases emerged.

Administration of an oral polio vaccine proved both inexpensive and cost-effective. The cost of immunizing a child with three doses of the polio vaccine (along with diphtheria, tetanus, and pertussis vaccine) is just $21. Even without taking into consideration such benefits as increased productivity, strengthened capacity to fight other diseases, and reduced pain and suffering, the polio eradication campaign was

economically justified based on the savings of medical costs for treatment and reha-
bilitation alone. The first five years of the polio campaign cost $120 million: $74 from
national sources and $46 million from international donors. Taking into consider-
ation the savings from treatment avoided, donor contributions paid for themselves
in 15 years. Today, war and politics, not money, are the primary barriers to the total
eradication of polio.

PREVENTING DEATHS FROM DIARRHEAL DISEASE

Diarrheal disease is one of the leading causes of death among children, causing
nearly 20 percent of all child deaths. Worldwide, dehydration from diarrhea kills
between 1.4 and 2.5 million babies each year, mostly in developing countries where
children suffer an average of three episodes a year. Nearly 20 out of 1,000 children die
of diarrheal disease before the age of two. This is a great public health failure because
such deaths easily can be prevented at very low cost. Nevertheless, there has been
some progress. Many countries, including Egypt, as documented later, have succeeded in disseminating knowledge about a life-saving treatment that resulted in
dramatic declines in mortality associated with diarrhea and a large improvement in
infant and child survival.

Diarrhea is an intestinal disorder characterized by abnormally frequent and
watery stools. It is caused by a number of agents, including bacteria, protozoa, and
viruses. Unclean water, dirty hands during eating, and spoiled food are the primary
sources of transmission. The most effective modes of prevention include improved
water supply and sanitation, improved hygiene, and immunization against measles (which can cause diarrhea). Dehydration is the most serious effect of diarrhea. When fluid loss reaches 10 percent of body weight, dehydration becomes
fatal. In cases that are not fatal, dehydration can leave a child susceptible to future
infections.

Avoiding death from dehydration requires the swift restoration of lost fluids and
electrolytes. Until the development of oral rehydration therapy in the 1960s, the only
effective treatment was through intravenous (IV) infusions in a hospital or clinic.
IV therapy is not a treatment of choice in the developing world because of its high
cost, the hardship of traveling to clinics, and shortage of both trained personnel and
supplies. Many people turn to drugs, including antibiotics, which can stop diarrhea.
However, the majority of these drugs have no proven health benefit and some can
cause dangerous side effects.

Oral rehydration therapy has been called the most important medical discovery
of the twentieth century. Developed in the 1960s in Bangladesh and India, it consists
of a simple solution of water, salt, and sugar that is as effective in halting dehydration as intravenous therapy. It is immensely cheaper at just a few cents per dose,
safer and easier to administer, and more practical for mass treatment. The effectiveness of ORT was proven during cholera outbreaks in refugee camps on the border of

India and Bangladesh in the 1970s. In 1971, the war for independence in what is now Bangladesh created 10 million refugees. The unsanitary conditions in overcrowded refugee camps resulted in outbreaks of cholera with fatality rates approaching 30 percent. Resources were not available for mass treatment with IV fluids. Oral treatment was proposed as an alternative. The results were extraordinary. Cholera fatalities in the camp using ORT dropped to less than 4 percent, compared to 20 to 30 percent in camps treated with intravenous therapy.

Egypt was one of the pioneers of national-level administration of oral rehydration therapy. In 1977, 1 in 20 children died of diarrhea before his or her first birthday. That year packets of oral rehydration salts were introduced at public clinics and for sale at pharmacies, but few mothers were aware of the treatment and even fewer used it. In 1982, only 10 to 20 percent of diarrhea cases used the packets of oral rehydration salts. Physicians also did not recommend them.

In 1980, the government launched the Strengthening of Rural Health Delivery Project to test how mothers and physicians could be persuaded to use ORT. Initially, in 29 rural villages, nurses taught mothers in their homes how to use ORT and physicians were educated about the therapy. ORT use rose dramatically, and as a result, child mortality was 38 percent lower than in control villages, and diarrhea-associated mortality during the peak season was 45 percent lower. Based on the success of these community trials, in 1981 Egypt began a massive program to promote ORT use among the country's 41 million residents. Financial and technical support came from the U.S. Agency for International Development (USAID) and the public health organization John Snow, Inc. The program involved the entire Ministry of Health, other branches of government, WHO, and UNICEF. The program worked through the existing health infrastructure in order to strengthen the capacity of the health services to deliver care.[35]

The program used several innovative approaches to increase the use of ORT. Packets were redesigned in smaller quantities and the project logo became the most recognized product label in Egypt. Production and distribution channels were developed. Health workers, nurses, and physicians were trained. A mass media campaign was launched in 1984 that took advantage of the 90 percent of households that had televisions. The campaign was very successful. By 1986, nearly 99 percent of mothers were aware of ORT. Infant mortality dropped by 36 percent and child (under-five) mortality by 43 percent between 1982 and 1987. Mortality due to diarrhea dropped 82 percent among infants and 62 percent among children during this same period. The program achieved success with an extremely cost-effective intervention. The average cost per child treated with ORT was less than $6, and the cost per death averted was between $100 and $200.

[35]M. el-Rafie et al., "The Effect of Diarrheal Disease Control on Infant and Childhood Mortality in Egypt: Report from the National Control of Diarrheal Diseases Project," *The Lancet* 335, no. 8690 (March 17, 1990).

ORT continues to be the most cost-effective means of treating dehydration, and its use has been adapted to the unique challenges found in different countries. In Bangladesh, where 90 percent of the over 100 million residents lives in rural areas with poor transportation in a country 10 times the size of Egypt, distribution of ORT packets was not feasible. In 1980, a program to promote ORT in rural Bangladesh began by training workers to go door to door and teach mothers about dehydration and ORT. Mothers were also taught how to make a homemade solution by mixing a three-finger pinch of salt, a fistful of sugar, and a liter of water. (Today, packaged oral rehydration salts are available in most of the country.) Between 1980 and 1990, 13 million mothers were taught to make oral rehydration mixtures. An evaluation of more than 7,000 households found that between 25 and 52 percent of cases of severe diarrhea used the mixture. Today, the usage rate of ORT in Bangladesh is 80 percent, and ORT is part of Bangladeshi culture. An increase in the use of ORT across the globe has slashed diarrhea mortality rates in children by at least half. ORT saves the lives of an estimated 1 million children each year.

LESSONS LEARNED

There is no simple prescription for success that comes out of comparing the cases presented in *Millions Saved*. Nor can one easily place blame for the dismal failures that let HIV/AIDS ravage southern Africa or prolong malaria's devastating toll on so many. Poverty is one of the explanations for the failures but it is not sufficient. Even poor nations have had success in combating diseases. The health sector is one with pervasive market failures: There are all the common problems of negative externalities, principal-agent problems, information failures, and public goods. An inability to resolve these issues reflects equally pervasive government failures at the local, national, and international levels.

Successful health initiatives are characterized by strong leadership. Former World Bank president Robert McNamara was personally committed to controlling river blindness in West Africa, the Thai government had charismatic leaders with the vision to launch a program to prevent the spread of HIV/AIDS, and Egyptian officials stood firmly behind plans to expand ORT from community trials to a national program. In contrast, South African presidents Nelson Mandela and Thabo Mbeki generally ignored HIV/AIDS as an issue until the disease had already turned into a pandemic and national tragedy. Malaria, after having been resolved in the developed nations, has been neglected elsewhere.

In addition to strong leadership and program champions, one needs a combination of a technological solution and an affordable delivery system. Affordability can require concessions from patent holders, as has happened with generic ARVs mass produced by pharmaceutical companies in Brazil and India. Public–private partnerships also have worked, in which drugs are provided at cost and distribution is handled by government authorities. Donors, whether public or private, can play important roles. The Global Fund to Fight AIDS, Tuberculosis and Malaria; USAID; the World Bank; and others have provided critical finance as has the private Bill & Melinda Gates Foundation. Local commitment is equally essential. Delivering improved health requires the actions of millions of individuals, whether those trained as doctors, nurses, or engineers or relatively unskilled workers and volunteers who watch patients take their medications as part of DOTS programs or help administer oral vaccines in remote villages.

HEALTH CHALLENGES

The challenge for the twenty-first century is to continue the battle against communicable disease while developing strategies to combat emerging epidemics of noncommunicable conditions. The developing world continues to face the illnesses of poverty. Over 8 million children and 300,000 mothers die each year, even though most of these deaths can be avoided through cost-effective vaccine programs, rehydration therapy for diarrheal diseases, improved nutrition status, and better birthing practices. Many people believe that infectious diseases in low- and middle-income countries should be a high priority because the technical means exist to control them and they disproportionately affect the young. The Millennium Development Goals (MDGs) placed maternal and child health as a high priority and an integral part of poverty reduction. Over the past decade, the MDGs have moved maternal and child health from a primarily technical concern to one that is increasingly seen as a "moral and political imperative."[36]

The battle against infectious disease will be ongoing this century. New diseases will emerge and, in a more globalized world, move quickly across borders. Drug resistance will make disease eradication much harder, as the discovery of new drugs races against the ability of microbes to adapt and mutate into even more virulent strains. But infectious diseases are not the only challenge the low- and middle-income nations face. The *2002 World Health Report: Reducing Risks, Promoting Healthy Life* highlighted other factors that have adverse effects on health. The report identified 10 major global risk factors in terms of the burden of disease. Listed in order of their expected health risks, they are underweight children; unsafe sex; high blood pressure; tobacco consumption; alcohol consumption; unsafe water, sanitation, and hygiene; iron deficiency; indoor smoke from solid fuels; high cholesterol; and obesity and physical inactivity. These 10 risk factors already account for more than one-third of deaths worldwide.

[36]*World Health Report 2005: Make Every Mother and Child Count* (Geneva: World Health Organization, 2005), p. 3.

Underweight children are strongly related to poverty as are unsafe water, inadequate sanitation, and indoor air pollution. Unsafe sex is the main factor in the spread of HIV/AIDS, with a major impact in the poor countries of Africa and Asia. Some of these risk factors, such as high blood pressure and high cholesterol, tobacco and excessive alcohol consumption, obesity and physical inactivity, are more commonly associated with wealthy societies. However, with epidemiologic transitions, poor and middle-income countries increasingly face these risks as well. For improvements in health and life expectancy to continue, it will be necessary to address this *double burden* of disease in the decades ahead.

SUMMARY

- Life expectancy is among the most common measures for assessing health outcomes. In 2008, the high-income nations had life expectancy at birth of 80 years; in Latin America, 73 years; in South Asia, 64 years; and in sub-Saharan Africa, only 52 years. Most of the differences can be explained by the much higher rates of mortality during the first 5 years of life in poorer regions.

- Since the 1960s, the gap in life expectancy between nations, unlike the gap in per capita incomes, has fallen rapidly. Many low- and middle-income nations have made substantial and historically unprecedented progress in increasing life expectancy. This stands as one of the great successes of human development in the past half century although there are exceptions, including several nations in sub-Saharan Africa.

- In many developing nations, where life expectancy has risen and fertility fallen, the age structure of the population has changed and so has the pattern of disease. This has resulted in an epidemiologic transition. Heart disease, a noncommunicable disease, is now the leading cause of death worldwide. Diseases common in high-income nations, including heart disease and cancers, are becoming more prevalent in low- and middle-income nations. But infectious diseases, which take a relatively small toll in high-income nations, remain a major threat to children and adults in developing countries.

- Improving health and rising levels of per capita income are well correlated. But significant improvements in health can occur even at low incomes. Preventative measures long practiced in developed countries are vital. They include access to clean water and proper sanitation, control of insects and other disease vectors, and widespread vaccination programs. In addition to these public health measures, education, especially of females, is correlated with better health outcomes.

- Better health helps children remain at school and makes workers more productive in their fields and at their jobs. Better health increases the opportunity nations and individuals face to save and invest in their futures. Higher incomes, in turn, permit governments and families to devote more resources, whether for water, sanitation, vaccines, drugs, or health workers, to improving health.

- Infectious disease continues to plague poor nations. HIV/AIDS, malaria, and tuberculosis are three of the best known. Together they kill 4.5 million people a year, accounting for about 8 percent of all deaths worldwide. Other infectious diseases kill millions more, especially children, and debilitate those who are sick but do not die. Many of these infectious diseases, including HIV/AIDS, malaria, and tuberculosis, are preventable and with adequate resources and institutions can be treated effectively. That this is not happening is both an economic failure and a human tragedy.

- The spread of HIV/AIDS, the failure to attack malaria, and the reemergence of TB, including new drug-resistant strains, provide evidence of what has gone wrong in addressing world health. But there are also abundant examples of health successes, ranging from the eradication of smallpox to the near eradication of polio to the diffusion of oral rehydration therapies as a means of saving children from diarrheal diseases.

- The challenge of the twenty-first century will be for low- and middle-income countries to win the battle against both old and new infectious diseases, while addressing the increasing prevalence of chronic noncommunicable diseases long associated with higher incomes.

PART THREE

Macroeconomic Policies for Development

10

Investment and Savings

I n Chapter 4 we learned that economic growth occurs because of increases in a country's capital stock and in its employed labor force together with increases in the productivity of those two factors of production. In this section of the book we go in depth into the mechanisms that lead to increases in the capital stock and to the increases in productivity that are embodied in capital. Capital increases because individuals and companies decide to invest their funds in the purchase of machinery, buildings, and other capital equipment. If they invest wisely, their production and profits increase. If they invest poorly the capital stock and profits may not increase at all. A farmer in Kenya will plant coffee trees and expect to reap a return when the coffee beans are ripe several years in the future. A large corporation in China will invest in furnaces and rolling mills to produce finished steel products.

To invest, however, the farmer or corporation must first obtain the funds and other resources that make their investments possible. The Kenyan farmer must have money to buy coffee seedlings and to hire labor to help in the preparation of the land. The Chinese steel corporation must find the funds to pay workers to build the furnaces and rolling mills and to purchase the best steel-rolling technology from abroad or from another corporation in China. The funds required may come from savings from the farmer's own income, may be borrowed from members of his or her extended family, or may be a loan from a microcredit institution. The large corporation may sell ownership shares in the company, use its own retained earnings, or borrow from a major bank. All of these sources of funds require that some person or business first save at least part of their income. If all income is consumed for food by the farmer or spent on an expensive limousine for the steel plant manager, there will be nothing left over to invest. Both the farmer and the steel corporation, however, can borrow from someone else who has saved and use the money to invest, paying it back at some future time.

In this chapter, we start first with the fundamentals of what constitutes good investments—what leads to investments that promote growth either of the individual farmer, the large corporation, or the country as a whole? The principles of good investments from a country's point of view apply equally to investments made by individuals, by private companies, or by governments. However, differences in ownership, in who is making the investment decisions, have a powerful influence on whether the investor applies the principles of good investment correctly. Government officials do not have the same objectives as private companies, and large corporations can pursue goals quite different from a small farmer or proprietor of a five person factory. Foreign investors may have different incentives and goals from domestic investors. As already noted, no one can invest either well or poorly unless someone or some company or government agency first saves. We will briefly explore why households, corporations, and governments save. Of particular interest is that some of the saving done for many developing countries is done by foreigners, not just by citizens of the country itself.

In some cases investors save and invest their own money, but more commonly those who invest are different from those who save. The gap between the savers and investors is filled by a wide variety of financial institutions ranging from banks and the stock market to the government itself. This separation of investors and savers makes possible much higher rates of investment than would otherwise be the case, but it also depends on institutions and government policies that can behave in ways that lead to economic crises, as occurred throughout much of the world in 2008–09. There is, of course, much more to the role of the government in managing the economy than just what it can accomplish through a central bank. Government is both an investor itself and a spender of funds in a wide variety of areas, ranging from income transfers to the poor to paying the salaries of civil servants and the military, that have little to do with investment. In Chapter 11 we explore how the government raises the revenue it needs to make these expenditures and how it uses these resources to help cope with economic crises as they occur.

Chapter 12 deals with the role of the financial sector first in its role as the intermediary that mobilizes savings from individuals and then allocates savings to investors. Efficient management of the financial sector, however, can be undermined by inflation and thus control of inflation is a critical component of any effective growth strategy. The chapter reviews how developing countries have tried to control inflation and avoid financial crises and how their success or failure in these efforts has fostered or undermined the development of the intermediation role of the sector. Chapter 13 explores in greater depth the central role of developing country debt in triggering many financial crises. Developing country debt that leads to crises also involves foreign savings, both private and government, that is then lent to developing countries by international banks and other financial institutions including multilateral agencies, such as the International Monetary Fund (IMF) and World Bank. Chapter 14 focuses on the role of foreign aid to developing countries (a major form of foreign savings made by aid-giving governments that is transferred to developing countries).

USING INVESTMENT PRODUCTIVELY: COST–BENEFIT ANALYSIS

In many low-income countries, there appear to be abundant opportunities for increased investment that could have significant economic and social benefits, but these investments do not happen. Roads are absent or of poor quality, electricity and telecommunications facilities are in short supply and unreliable, and there seem to be many workers with few factories to employ them. Sometimes, this is because investment funds are not always available, but it is also because the investments that do take place are not always particularly productive. But this in itself is a puzzle: The Solow growth model discussed in Chapter 4 suggests that, in low-income countries where capital is scarce, new investment has the *potential* to be highly productive but that potential is not always realized. Questions about the quantity and productivity of investment become more complicated when foreigners make the investments. Although foreign capital appears to be a ready source of additional investment funds, foreign investment does not always have a good reputation, and in some cases, even where it is productive, it is not always welcomed.

How does one judge whether an investment is likely to be productive or not? One of the most powerful tools for answering this question is **cost–benefit analysis**, which is also referred to as **project appraisal**. This tool is applicable to both private and public investment and to investment made by foreign firms as well. Public or government investors, however, should use the tool somewhat differently from private investors because their objectives are different.

PRESENT VALUE

The investor's calculation normally involves four steps. First, the firm will forecast the **net cash flow** of an investment, measuring the difference between the cash revenues from the sale of the product and the cash outlays on investment, material inputs, salaries and wages, purchased services, and other items.

Second, investors have to adjust their valuation of costs and benefits, depending on whether they happen soon or far into the future. Investors recognize that cash received in the future is less valuable than cash received immediately because in the interim they could earn interest (or profits) on these funds by investing them in bonds or savings accounts (or in additional, revenue-earning production facilities). Any firm or individual asked to choose between $1,000 today or $1,000 next year would take the money now and place it in a savings account earning, say, 2 percent a year. Then, after one year, the interest payment would boost the savings account balance to $1,020. Equivalently, the prospect of $1,000 a year from now should be evaluated as equivalent today to only $1,000/1.02 = $980. This process of reducing the value of future flows is called **discounting**. Because the interest rate provides a first approximation of the rate at which future cash flows must be discounted, it is usually called the **discount rate**. Discounting takes place over several years, so the discount rate must be compounded over time. In the second year another 2 percent would be earned on the balance of $1,020, and increase it to $1,040.40. The payment of $1,000 two years from now then would be discounted to yield a present value of only $1,000/1.040 = $961. A general expression for the present value, P, is

$$P = F/(1 + i)^t \qquad\qquad [10\text{--}1]$$

where F is the value in the future, i is the discount rate, and t is time, usually represented by the number of years. As the interest rate or the number of years increases, the present value of the future cash flow decreases. Note that because project appraisals are most conveniently done at **constant prices**, netting out inflation, the discount rate is a **real rate of interest**, net of inflation.

Investment projects usually have negative cash flows in the early years, when there are large expenditures, then generate positive cash flows in later years, as the new facilities begin to earn revenues. Tree crops such as palm oil and rubber take several years before they become productive and must be cut down and replanted when production falls off because of aging. Such a **time profile** of net cash flow is depicted in Figure 10–1; it is the most common of several possible profiles. To summarize the value of this net cash flow in a single number, each year's net cash flow is divided by the respective discount factor, and the resulting present values are added to give the **net present value (NPV)**:

$$NPV = \sum (B_t - C_t)/(1 + i)^t \qquad\qquad [10\text{--}2]$$

where B_t and C_t are the benefits (revenue) and costs in each year t, and i is the discount rate. For a firm, the correct discount rate is the average cost at which additional funds may be obtained from all sources (that is, the firm's cost of capital).

If the NPV of a project happens to equal 0, the project will yield a net cash flow just large enough to cover all the projects costs. In that case, when NPV = 0, the discount rate has a special name, the internal rate of return (IRR), a term we introduced in the discussion of education as an investment in Chapter 8. If the net present value is positive, then the project can cover all its financial costs with some profit left over for the firm. If negative, the project cannot cover its financial costs and should not be undertaken. The higher the net present value, the better the project's financial

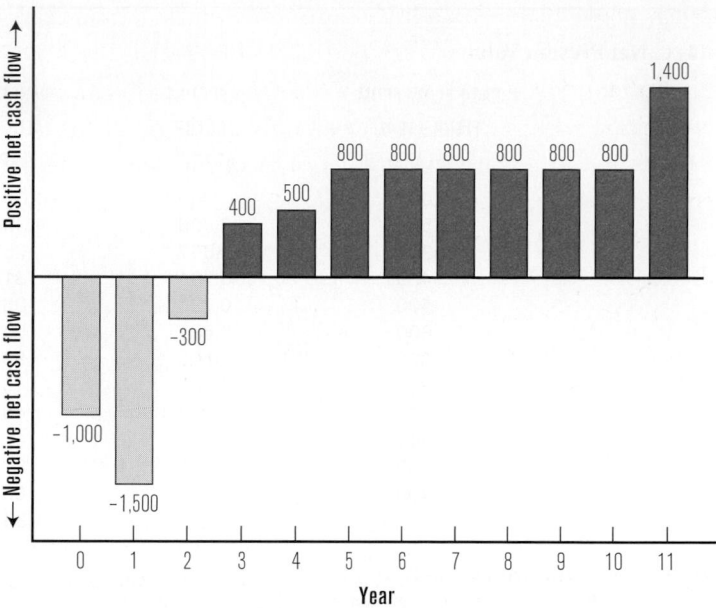

FIGURE 10-1 **Time Profile for Investment: Net Cash Flow**

The cash flow of a project can be represented by a bar diagram. Cash outflows are shown by bars below the horizontal axis; inflows, by bars above the axis. Year 0 and 1 show investment in construction and equipment, hence the negative cash flows. Year 2 is the startup period, years 3 and 4 show gradually increasing output and cash inflows, and years 5 through 10 show steady output and cash inflows. The project is assumed to end in year 11, when the salvage value of equipment swells the cash inflow.

profile. If the cash flow of Figure 10–1 is discounted at a rate of 8 percent,[1] the net present value is a positive $1,358 (Table 10–1). This calculation indicates that the investment will earn enough to repay the total costs ($2,500 over years 0 and 1) with a (discounted) surplus of $1,358.

Third, investors must consider the risks to both the costs and the benefits of their investments. Simple NPV analysis such as that in Table 10–1 can be misleading because it generates a single summary number for the answer, giving a false sense of precision. In reality, investors cannot be sure in advance of all the costs or the cash flows their investment might generate. Fuel prices might skyrocket or electricity supplies might be cut off, forcing the investor either to buy a new generator or to curtail production. The prices for their products might be either much higher or much lower than the original projections. Political instability might increase costs and disrupt

---

[1]The return on investment in developing countries can be much higher and much lower than 8 percent, depending on circumstances. We have used 8 percent in our example because it is a common rate of return for such investments.

TABLE 10-1 **Net Present Value**

YEAR	CASH FLOW FROM FIGURE 10-1 (DOLLARS)	DISCOUNT FACTOR AT 8%*	PRESENT VALUE† (DOLLARS)
0	−1,000	1	−1,000
1	−1,500	0.926	−1,389
2	−300	0.857	−257
3	400	0.794	318
4	500	0.735	368
5	800	0.681	544
6	800	0.63	504
7	800	0.583	467
8	800	0.54	432
9	800	0.5	400
10	800	0.463	371
11	1,400	0.429	600
Net Present Value‡			1,358

*Calculated as $1/(1 + i)^t$ from equation 10–2.
†Calculated as the cash flow times the discount factor.
‡Sum of the present value of each year.

the firm's ability to purchase supplies or sell its products. Therefore, prudent investors calculate a range of NPVs for their investment based on best case and worse case scenarios, testing the sensitivity of the outcome to changes in specific costs or benefits. An investor may decide not to make an investment even if it generates a positive NPV under baseline calculations if the risks around actually achieving that outcome are too great.

Fourth, investors must compare across projects. Just because a project generates a positive NPV does not mean it is the best possible use of investment funds, especially if the firm has a set of alternative projects to consider and a budget that can accommodate several but not all of them. Under these circumstances, investors should select the set of projects that will yield the highest total net present value for the entire investment budget.

Up to this point the methodology is the same for both private and public investors. The next steps calculate the costs and benefits from an economywide perspective. Private investors are typically only interested in whether a project provides an adequate rate of return or profit to themselves. Governments, in contrast, should be concerned with whether a project contributes to the growth of the economy as a whole or to social welfare more broadly. This concern of governments applies both to public investment undertaken by the government itself and to the impact of private investments. Governments are often called on to support private investments in various ways, and their decisions in this regard need to be based on the economy-wide impact of the project, not just on whether the private investors will make a profit or not.

OPPORTUNITY COSTS

Every investment uses goods and services that could otherwise be used for other purposes. In evaluating the investment from an economywide perspective, these goods and services should be valued in terms of the net benefits they would have provided if used in some alternative project—that is, they have **opportunity costs**. An investment in a dam requires saving that otherwise could be invested in a rural road or in elementary schools. Cotton used in a textile factory otherwise could have been exported and sold abroad. The labor used to build a road might have otherwise been used to sink water wells or grow millet. For a private firm, the cost is the market value that it pays for wages, goods, and services. For society at large, the cost is the value of the resources in terms of their next best use. Public sector investments, in particular, should be evaluated using opportunity costs rather than market costs where the two differ.

The opportunity cost to society might differ from the market wage rate if the government pays wages higher than the market clearing value. If 10 farm workers take jobs building a new highway, their opportunity cost is the value of the lost agricultural output due to their leaving the farm, net of the nonlabor recurrent costs of producing that output. This reduction in net output is the value of the **marginal revenue product** and, in this situation, is equal to the opportunity cost of labor.[2] Similarly, if the highway project means that savings will be drawn away from other projects that on average would have earned a return of 5 percent, then the opportunity cost of capital is 5 percent, and this should be used as the discount rate in evaluating the project, even if the government borrows money at 2 percent.

In some countries, the market price of foreign exchange might differ from the opportunity cost, especially in countries where governments manipulate or control the exchange rate. Cotton used in a textile mill otherwise might have been exported; if so, its opportunity cost would be the foreign currency it would have earned as an export. If the cloth produced by the mill would have been imported in the absence of the project, its opportunity cost (a benefit in this case) would be the foreign exchange that otherwise would have been spent on cloth imports.

SHADOW PRICES

The opportunity costs of goods and services for the economy as a whole are called **shadow prices** or **economic opportunity costs**. The first approximation of a shadow price (for land, labor, capital, and foreign exchange) is the price paid by private participants in the market. Interference in the market distorts market prices from their economic opportunity cost: taxes and subsidies of all kinds, monopoly power, minimum wages, interest rate controls, tariffs and import quotas, price controls, and

[2]The value of the marginal product of a factor of production can be calculated as the price of a commodity multiplied by the additional physical output that results when one unit of the factor is added to the production process with all other factors held constant (e.g., that factor's marginal product).

so forth. When a private firm undertakes investment analysis, it conducts a **commercial project appraisal** based on market prices and focusing on profitability. When governments consider public investments, they want to measure the full economic impact of the investment on the country. To do so, they must use shadow prices when market prices do not fully reflect true scarcity values. This kind of evaluation is called **economic project appraisal**. To estimate shadow prices, market prices must be adjusted to reflect full opportunity costs.

Estimating shadow prices is not easy and requires intimate knowledge of the workings of an economy, both its macroeconomic relationships and the microeconomic behavior of its factor markets. But such adjustment can be important. In many countries, the shadow foreign exchange rate is higher than the official rate in terms of local currency per dollar. In most cases, this reflects the impact of import duties and quotas or intervention by central banks in establishing or modifying the exchange rate. As a consequence, any export project that earns more foreign exchange than it uses or any import-substituting project that saves more than it uses gets a boost from the shadow exchange rate. Although the salaries and wages of skilled employees usually require no adjustment from market to shadow prices, frequently the opportunity cost of unskilled workers is lower than the wage in formal urban labor markets. Therefore, any project using unskilled labor, especially if it is located in a rural area, gets a boost because the shadow wage reduces costs without changing benefits.

Discount rates might also be adjusted from market interest rates to shadow discount rates if a government treats capital as a very scarce factor of production or if it has a strong preference for projects that realize their benefits relatively quickly. This approach would tend to discourage any public investment project with high initial investment costs, long gestation periods, and low net cash flows. A higher shadow discount rate would favor projects that generate their net benefits early because these can be reinvested in other productive projects for continued growth and projects that use relatively abundant factors of production, especially labor, instead of scarce ones, like capital.

An illustration of the power of shadow pricing is contained in Table 10–2, which depicts two projects with identical cash flows. One project (the textile mill) earns more foreign exchange but uses more labor. Because the shadow wage rate is below the market rate, the economic NPV of both projects is raised, but the more labor-intensive textile project benefits more (shown in Part 2 of the table). When the shadow exchange rate is applied, the NPV of the textile mill is raised considerably, and that of the telecommunications system becomes negative (Part 3).

WELFARE WEIGHTS

Under some circumstances, governments want to incorporate broader social goals into the evaluation of public sector projects, such as the impact on income distribution, poverty alleviation, or environmental degradation. To do so, governments can use welfare weights to further adjust shadow prices in a project analysis. This process

TABLE 10-2 Effects of Shadow Pricing on Cost–Benefit Analysis

PROJECT	INVESTMENT (FIRST YEAR)	NET ANNUAL CASH FLOW (NEXT 5 YEARS)	NET PRESENT VALUE (10%)
1. Take two projects with identical cash flows. Project A earns more net foreign exchange and uses more labor than project B:			
A. Textile mill, of which	−1,000	+300	+137
Net foreign exchanged earned	−500	+400	
Wages paid	−350	−100	
B. Telecommunications system, of which	−1,000	+300	+137
Net foreign exchange earned	−800	0	
Wages paid	−100	−50	
2. The shadow wage is 75% of market wage, so all wage costs are reduced by 25%. This results in the following net cash flows:			
A. Textile mill	−913	+325	+319
B. Telecommunications system	−975	+313	+212
3. The shadow exchange rate is 20% above official rate, so the net foreign exchange flow is raised by 20%. This results in the following net cash flows:			
A. Textile mill	−1,100	+380	+340
B. Telecommunication system	−1,160	+300	−23

might place a higher value on net additional income to certain target groups, such as the very poor. Then projects generating more income for these groups have higher NPVs than otherwise and tend to be selected more frequently. Similarly, it might adjust benefits to capture environmental goals or further reduce the shadow wage rate if it was particularly interested in creating new jobs. When welfare weights are introduced or shadow prices are further adjusted to reflect social goals, the process is called **social project appraisal**.

The method is potentially powerful but has its dangers. Welfare weights are arbitrary, subject to policy makers' or politicians' judgment. This, in itself, is not bad, but these weights can so overwhelm economically based shadow prices that project selection comes down to a choice based almost entirely on arbitrary weights. This gives a false sense of precision and sometimes can be misused. In most cases, it is best to do the calculations without these weights and then look separately at the welfare implications of the project.

BARRIERS TO PRODUCTIVE PUBLIC AND PRIVATE INVESTMENT

In Chapter 3 we explored at a macro level many of the variables that influence the rate of growth of gross domestic product (GDP) in a country. Many of these same variables have an influence on the productivity of investment, both public and private.

Political instability can lower the rate of return and increase the risk, particularly to private investors but to government investors as well. Macroeconomic instability can distort investment decisions away from investments that promote long-term growth and toward investments that protect the investor from inflation. Excessive investment in high-income housing and office buildings often characterized the high inflation period that characterized some South American countries in the 1950s through the 1980s. Investment by governments and the private sector in education and health increase the quality of the labor force and that in turn raises the rate of return on investment in projects other than the investments in education and health themselves. More open economies provide opportunities for high return investments not only for exporters but also for any investment that needs to use imported inputs. In closed economies imported inputs are often very expensive if they are available at all.

Our focus here, however, is on what in the macroeconomic analysis in Chapter 3 is referred to as effective governance and institutions. There are a wide range of elements that are included under the rubric of good governance and effective institutions. We focus here at the micro level on two: the extent and nature of government intervention in the economy and on corruption. The two are closely related. As we have indicated in many chapters in this book, government regulation is often necessary to correct for market failures that could do damage to the environment, to health, or to growth. In all countries, however, government intervention can create opportunities for private investors and public officials alike to seek what economists call rents. **Rent-seeking** behavior refers to activities by private and public officials to extract value from a project without providing any compensation in return or contributing any increased productivity to the project. An example would be for an investor in a cement plant to negotiate with the government to provide high tariffs on imported cement so that the investor could raise the domestic price on cement, thus earning a higher level of profit. The cement producer in this case has done nothing to raise the quality of the cement or to increase the efficiency with which the cement is produced. The increase in profits is due solely to this investor's ability to persuade the government to raise the cement tariff and hence the domestic cement price. Purchasers of the cement then must pay more money to the producer without getting any increased value for themselves. Not only can rent-seeking behavior lead to poor policy choices, but the rent-seeking behavior itself entails the diversion of potentially substantial resources from productive uses.

The relevance of these concepts to this chapter is that excessive or inappropriate kinds of regulation together with high levels of corruption are a major reason public investment projects in low- and middle-income countries often have a low rate of economywide return. They can also explain why many private investors also face a low rate of return on their investments despite trying to provide a badly needed product or service that under more normal circumstances would provide the investor with a substantial profit. The World Bank has compiled quantitative indicators of how government interventions affect the ease of doing business in individual countries. Transparency International, a nongovernmental organization (NGO), also has carried out and collected surveys of perceptions of the level of corruption in most of these same countries. We take up each of these two efforts in turn.

BARRIERS TO DOING BUSINESS

Starting and running a business is often described as an individual coming up with a good idea (a new or better product, an old product in a new location, or a new way to produce a good), building a factory, hiring workers to produce the good, and creating a marketing office to sell it to customers. In most countries that individual must first get a license to open that business and in many countries it takes a large number of such licenses. In Malaysia, for example, in the early years of the twenty-first century, it took 70 licenses or permits to open a new hotel. The business must then hire labor, and typically there are many regulations governing the hiring of labor. Many of these regulations make good sense in the right context. Employers in many countries, including the United States, are not allowed to discriminate in hiring based on gender, race, or religion. More problematic are the rules in countries that make it extremely difficult to dismiss employees even if their performance is subpar or an economic downturn limits the work that is available. This new business, early on and throughout its existence, must enter into numerous contracts with suppliers, with clients, and with its own employees. The question then becomes who if anyone will enforce these contracts. In a high-income country it is typically the legal system and the judiciary that is responsible for deciding whether a contract should be enforced or not, and these decisions are made according to rules typically written into law by the legislature. In many low- and middle-income countries, however, the judiciary is poorly trained, has little power, and is often corrupt. Enforcement of contracts tends to depend more on the power and influence of the company seeking (or trying to avoid) enforcement.

The World Bank has measured the degree to which these many government interventions affect the ability to open a new business or carry on an existing one. They report on a number of government interventions that are widely believed to affect the ease of doing business in a country. For each of these indicators, they measure the time it took to get the necessary permits, the number of permits or procedures required, the cost of getting these permits, and a variety of other indicators in areas such as the employment of labor or obtaining credit. The full list of categories is as follows: Starting a Business, Dealing with Construction Permits, Employing Workers, Registering Property, Getting Credit, Protecting Investors, Paying Taxes, Trading across Borders, Enforcing Contracts, and Closing a Business.[3] Table 10-3 presents data for a number of economies on their overall ranking as a place where it is easy or difficult to do business.

[3]World Bank, *Doing Business 2010: Reforming through Difficult Times* (Washington, DC: World Bank, 2010).

TABLE 10-3 **The Business Environment**

COUNTRY	DOING BUSINESS RANK, 2011	CORRUPTION PERCEPTION RANK, 2011
Singapore	**1**	**5**
United States	**4**	**24**
Georgia	16	64
Thailand	17	80
Japan	**20**	**14**
Mauritius	23	46
Latvia	21	61
South Africa	35	64
Taiwan	**25**	**32**
Chile	39	22
Spain	**44**	**31**
Turkey	71	61
Jamaica	88	86
Pakistan	*105*	*134*
China	91	75
Vietnam	98	112
Kenya	109	154
Egypt	110	112
Greece	**100**	**80**
Bangladesh	*122*	*120*
Russia	120	143
Nigeria	133	143
Brazil	126	73
India	132	95
Iran	144	120
Philippines	136	129
Haiti	*174*	*175*
Afghanistan	*160*	*180*
Bolivia	153	118
Venezuela	177	172
Chad	*183*	*168*
Central African Republic	*182*	*154*

Bold, high-income economies; italics, low-income economies.

Sources: The World Bank, *Doing Business 2011*,4 (Washington, DC: The World Bank) available at www.doingbusiness.org/Rankings. Transparency International, *Corruption Perception Index 2011* (Berlin: Transparency International) available at www.transparency.org/policy_research/surveys_indices/cpi/2011.

Virtually all the high-income countries are ranked among the top 30 (out of 183) in the overall ease of doing business, with Singapore occupying the top spot. Six middle-income nations also made it into the top 30 in 2010: Georgia, Thailand, Mauritius, Malaysia, Lithuania, and Latvia. We find some poor performers among the high-income nations: Taiwan, Spain, Italy, Brunei, and Greece. Most middle-income countries rank in the top half of this index but there are notable exceptions, such as Russia, Brazil, India, and Iran. The bottom 20 countries are 17 sub-Saharan African countries, some of them plagued by war (Chad, Congo), plus Timor-Leste, Laos, and Venezuela.

Most of these countries are among the poorest in the world, although Venezuela is a major oil exporter. The Central African Republic ranked as the most difficult nation in the world with which to do business in 2010, according to this index.

The reasons for the differences in these rankings between the highly and lowly ranked can be best understood by looking at the specific categories measured. In Singapore, only 3 procedures were required to start a business, and it took only 3 days to complete those procedures, there were no restrictions on firing unwanted employees (rated 0 out of 100, with 0 indicating no difficulty), and the fired employee was entitled to only 4 weeks of severance pay. Registering property involved 3 procedures and took a mere 5 days. In Kenya, a country ranked close to the middle on ease of doing business, 12 procedures were required to start a business and it took 34 days to complete them; the difficulty of firing workers was rated 30 out of 100 and 47 *weeks* of severance pay was required. In addition, there were 8 procedures to register property, which took 64 days to complete. In the bottom quarter was Bolivia, where the 15 procedures involved in starting a business took 50 days; the difficulty of firing an employee was rated 100 out of 100, meaning you could not fire an employee so severance pay was not relevant. Registering property in Bolivia involved 8 procedures that took 2 months to complete. For these and other countries, the money cost of completing all the necessary procedures was a relatively low share of per capita income in high-ranked countries and a much larger share of per capita income in low ranked countries.

Time is also money for an investor, thus the more procedures that exist and the longer they take, the less likely the investor will go ahead with the investment. The result is that in countries with an unfriendly business climate, investments are lower, the costs of doing business are higher, and the rate of return on investments is lower. All of this translates at the macro level into a lower rate of growth.

Excessive regulation that creates any number of obstacles to doing business is not just a matter of lost time or the direct legal costs of the procedures. Large numbers of procedures involving licenses and permits also create broad opportunities for rent seeking and outright **corruption**. The difference between corruption and rent seeking is that corruption involves rent seeking that is illegal, whereas many forms of rent seeking are perfectly legal even though they damage the productivity of the economy. Large numbers of regulatory procedures are not the only cause of widespread corruption. Construction, especially public construction, often involves large elements of rent seeking and corruption. Road construction and the building of government offices involve costs that are difficult to measure for someone not involved directly in the business, making it easier for a construction contract to include hidden costs needed to bribe politicians to provide the necessary project funding and to pay off those in charge of granting construction permits.

Data on perceptions of corruption in countries around the world estimated by Transparency International, a non-profit organization based in Berlin but with a global network, are presented in Table 10–3. Even a casual comparison of the two columns in the table reveals the rough correlation between the ease of doing business and the perception of corruption. Countries with friendly business procedures typically have low levels of corruption, and the reverse is equally true.

Complete elimination of corruption from public construction and from government business relations is virtually impossible. Even the wealthiest countries regularly discover that an official has taken a bribe to issue a permit and a politician has received illegal payments so that a vote to fund a public investment project would go forward. It is often assumed that the solution to the problem of corruption is to increase the number of police investigating corruption and raising the penalties for being caught. Certainly law enforcement has a role in curbing corruption, but law enforcement alone cannot accomplish much if the opportunities for corruption are pervasive (or if law enforcement is itself corrupt). In China, the death penalty has frequently been applied to cases of corruption, but there is little evidence that corruption has declined as a result.

Key elements in the fight against corruption are similar to what it takes to improve the climate for doing business. The number of regulations should be kept to the minimum necessary to control fundamental violations of public health, the environment, or other important social goals. The officials administering those regulations should have as little discretion as possible on whether to grant a permit. The more discretion they have, the more opportunity they have to delay and obfuscate the procedures until they receive illegal payments to do what they should be doing without payment. The process should be fully transparent with clear deadlines for the officials making the decisions. Putting the whole process online where all applicants can go to find out the status of their application has proved to be a powerful tool in countries where computer literacy is the norm. For public construction contracts the key is to have competitive bidding with controls to ensure that the companies bidding do not collude with each other or with the official contract awarding agency. If all of these steps are taken, the amount of corruption that remains will be less, and the anticorruption law enforcement agencies will not be overwhelmed and will be able to root out much of the corruption that remains. That, in essence, is the Singapore story, and Singapore is ranked 3 on Transparency International's 2009 Corruption Perception Index. Central African Republic is ranked 158.

Overcoming corruption becomes almost impossible if the corruption starts not at lower levels of government, such as in the customs office where those issuing import permits work, but instead at the highest levels of government, including those closest to the president or prime minister of the country. The motive for high-level corruption is partly personal greed, as the family of Ferdinand Marcos in the Philippines demonstrated, but it is also a result of the difficulties most countries have in finding legal and transparent ways of funding the political organization needed to win elections or hold on to power in more authoritarian situations. Raising money for a political organization is easy if the politician can offer favored access to government decisions in exchange. Two presidents of the Republic of Korea and the son of another were convicted of receiving hundreds of millions of dollars in this way. More than a few low-income countries have a serious problem in this regard, and even the American political process has yet to find a way to fund elections in a way in which buying political influence is minimal.

FOREIGN DIRECT INVESTMENT

The vast majority of investment in developing countries is undertaken by local citizens, either through small individual projects, larger investments by local firms, or by the government. But in some countries, an increasingly larger share of investment is made by foreign individuals or firms. Since 1990, **foreign direct investment (FDI)** has been the largest of all international capital flows to middle-income developing countries, larger than either cross-border bank lending or foreign aid (in low-income countries, FDI is smaller). FDI is defined as a long-term investment in which a non-resident entity exerts significant management control (usually at least 10 percent of voting stock) over an enterprise in the host country. A second type of cross-border investment is **portfolio equity**, in which an investor takes a smaller stake in an enterprise, either through a direct purchase or through a stock exchange. Portfolio equity flows to developing countries, starting from a low base, grew rapidly in the early 1990s, but then fell sharply following the financial crises of 1997 and 1998. A similar pattern occurred in the last decade. Portfolio equity increased 10-fold between 2000 and 2007, only to turn *negative* in 2008 as investors withdrew their investments. With the end of the most recent financial crisis such flows have resumed, and by the end of 2009 were approaching 2007 levels. Even at their peak, however, portfolio flows were still only one-quarter the size of FDI and about half the size of long-term international commercial bank loans.

In the 1960s and 1970s, many developing countries were suspicious of FDI and often took steps to actively discourage it. At the time, because of the colonial history in many countries and the sometimes offensive behavior of certain foreign investors in taking advantage of weak political and legal systems to gain monopoly rights, make huge profits, and influence domestic politics, this suspicion often was well founded. Starting in the mid-1980s, however, these attitudes began to change, and developing countries increasingly sought to attract FDI as a means of financing investment, creating jobs, and importing technology and ideas. FDI to developing countries grew rapidly from $22 billion in 1990 to $148 billion in 2000 to almost $600 billion in 2008 (more than half of all foreign capital flows). The sharp increase was due partly to worldwide advances in technology in communications and transportation (and the accompanying reduction in costs) and was closely related to the rapid expansion in world trade during the period. It was also the result of much greater enthusiasm on the part of developing countries in trying to attract FDI. The financial crisis reduced these flows by 2009, but they still were more than double the level of 2000.[4]

FDI continues to generate extensive controversy on a range of issues, including repatriation of profits, loss of control over domestic natural resources to foreign-owned entities, the extent of the transfer of technology, the impact on tax revenues, and the content of incentive packages. For some, foreign ownership of domestic companies should always be discouraged, even if it brings economic benefits. For others, FDI is a critical avenue to integrate the domestic economy with global markets that brings with it new technology and skills. The evidence on the relationship between FDI and development suggests that it is hard to make broad generalizations, and the impact depends critically on the purpose and type of the investment as well as policies and institutions in the recipient country. FDI in firms producing manufactured products sold on competitive global markets is more likely to be positively related to economic growth and other development outcomes, whereas FDI in firms producing primary products or manufactures or services for protected domestic markets tends to have more mixed outcomes.

FDI PATTERNS AND PRODUCTS

The majority of direct foreign investment in developing countries is undertaken by **multinational corporations (MNCs).** A multinational corporation is a firm that controls assets of enterprises located in countries other than its home country in which foreign operations are central to its profitability. Multinational enterprises are quite diverse, coming in all sizes, from all regions of the world, and are engaged in a wide variety of activities. The majority of MNCs are from industrialized countries, but a growing number are based in developing countries. Six developing countries had companies in *Fortune* magazine's list of the world's largest 500 firms in 2010, including China (46 entries), India (8), and Brazil (7). Not all of these firms operate outside of their own nations, but most of them do. Many MNCs are private corporations, but not all: *Fortune*'s top 500 includes a number of giant, state-owned companies producing petroleum, such as China National Petroleum (ranked 10 in the world) and Mexico's PEMEX (64).[5] But multinationals are not always large; small companies, especially in East and Southeast Asia, have been investing overseas for many years, particularly producing labor-intensive manufactured products such as textiles, shoes, toys, and electronics.

It is no surprise that the vast majority of FDI comes from rich-country investors. Globally, most multinational investment is also directed toward other wealthy countries, but the share aimed at developing countries has been rising. In the late 1980s, less than one-fourth of global FDI flows were directed toward developing countries.

[4]World Bank, *Global Development Finance, 2011,* 36 (Washington, DC: World Bank, 2010).
[5]Walmart Stores, Inc. is the largest corporation in the world.

The developing country share of global FDI flows increased rapidly during the early 1990s, peaking at 40 percent in 1994 and averaging 31 percent over that decade. By 2000, the developing country share had fallen below 20 percent; yet, that share grew throughout the first decade of the 21st century, reaching 46 percent by 2010.[6] Then, in the wake of the financial crisis of 2008–09, total FDI flows fell steeply, but the amounts going to low- and middle-income economies stayed relatively stable. However, FDI (as well as portfolio equity) is highly concentrated in a few developing countries. By 2010, half of all FDI in developing countries went to just 10 countries. China (including Hong Kong), received one-quarter of the total at the same time as China was becoming a major investor in Africa and elsewhere. Russia is another large recipient of FDI, followed by Brazil and India. By contrast, the UN's category of least-developed nations, making up much of sub-Saharan Africa, received just 5 percent of the total.[7]

FDI is aimed at a very wide range of activities that are sometimes difficult to classify, but three broad categories stand out:

- Natural resource-based activities, such as petroleum, minerals, and agricultural production. Firms engaged in these activities tend to be quite large and the investments capital intensive. These investments are usually negotiated directly with the host government, and the government is often a partner in the investment.
- Manufacturing and services aimed at the domestic market in the host country, including consumer goods (such as processed food or apparel); capital-intensive products such as steel or chemicals; and a range of services such as transportation, communication, finance, electricity, business services, and retail trade. In many cases, these activities are protected at least partially against competition from imports through tariffs or other restrictions.
- Labor-intensive manufacturing aimed for export on world markets, including apparel, electronics, food processing, footwear, textiles, and toys. Firms in these activities tend to be efficient and competitive, but they also can move quickly from one country to another in response to changes in production costs or macroeconomic or political instability.

BENEFITS AND DRAWBACKS OF FDI

Viewed most narrowly, FDI is a **source of capital** that adds to total investment. FDI is relatively small compared to domestic investment, but its share has grown rapidly in the last three decades. It accounted for between 2.2 and 3.6 percent of GDP in all

---

[6]United National Conference on Trade and Development (UNCTAD) on-line data, UNCTADSTAT http://unctadstat.unctad.org/ReportFolders/reportFolders.aspx, accessed March 23, 2012.

[7]United Nations Conference on Trade and Development, *World Investment Report 2010*, annex table A-1.

developing countries throughout the first decade of the twenty-first century compared to close to 1 percent in the early 1990s and less than 1 percent in the 1980s. In terms of investment, FDI amounted to about 12 percent of gross capital formation during the past decade,[8] but its importance varies widely. In some countries, FDI can be equivalent to well over 10 percent of GDP in some years, especially in countries with oil or other natural resources (for example, Kazakhstan). In other countries, FDI is less than 1 percent. By the end of 2010, Vietnam was averaging foreign direct investments equal to 9 percent of its GDP; Bangladesh attracted barely 1 percent.

Foreign capital in general tends to be more volatile than domestic capital, but FDI is usually more stable than other forms of private foreign capital. One key reason is that FDI is often attracted by either resource endowments or long-term fundamental economic strengths, factors that generally do not change as quickly as interest rates and exchange rates, which are stronger determinants of short-term bank loans and portfolio capital. Moreover, because FDI is characterized by significant management control in large, fixed-production facilities such as factories and mines, investors are less likely (and less able) to flee during economic downturns. During the 1997–98 Asian financial crises, FDI fell somewhat but much less than bank loans and portfolio capital, which dropped sharply. FDI in emerging market countries fell between 2008 and 2009.

Along with providing new capital, recipient countries hope that FDI will add to the demand for labor and **generate employment**. It is not surprising that because FDI is a relatively small source of investment in most developing countries, its contribution to employment also tends to be small, accounting for less than 5 percent of total employment in most developing countries. However, the impact on employment varies greatly depending on the activity. FDI focused on resource-based capital-intensive industries, such as mining or petroleum, creates relatively few jobs, whereas investments in labor-intensive manufacturing create more jobs. The impact of FDI on wages and working conditions is controversial, with some people charging that MNCs pay low wages and impose harsh working conditions. While conditions vary, and this may be true in some instances, on the whole, evidence suggests that MNCs pay higher average wages and have better average working conditions than do domestic firms.[9]

Another benefit of at least some kinds of FDI, especially FDI in manufactured exports, is that it can help increase **specialization** in production. When firms in developing countries are part of a global production process, they can focus on the particular activity in which they have a comparative advantage and produce most efficiently. Although domestically financed investment can also engage in very specialized production, FDI has the advantage of stronger links to other parts of a global supply chain. Firms in the automobile business need not make the entire car (and

---

[8]Calculated from World Bank, "World Development Indicators," http://databank.worldbank.org.

[9]Edward Graham, *Fighting the Wrong Enemy: Antiglobal Activists and Multinational Enterprises* (Washington, DC: Institute for International Economics, 2000), chap. 4.

if they did, they might not be able to compete on world markets). Instead, they can specialize in assembly, production of basic components (such as door parts or wiring), manufacturing of more sophisticated parts (for example, engines or transmissions), design, or other aspects of the production process. In today's production environment, it is difficult to classify an automobile as American, German, Japanese, or Korean because the parts are made all over the world. Moreover, the particular activity that makes sense in an economy can change over time as resource endowments, skills, and economic policies change. When Intel made its first investments in the electronics industry in Malaysia in the early 1970s, it focused on low-skill activities such as simple assembly. Over the years, as the Malaysian workforce gained new skills and more Malaysians became experienced managers, activity shifted toward production of basic parts (such as keyboards), then to more-advanced components (such as microprocessors), and later to testing and research. More recently, electronics production in the Philippines has followed a similar progression.

FDI can also bring with it **access to world markets**. Developing countries capable of producing at competitive costs often find it difficult to penetrate foreign markets. Many multinationals, particularly in natural resources, chemicals, and other heavy industries, are vertically integrated, oligopolistic firms, for which many transactions take place within the firm. Multinationals develop preferential access to customers by fashioning and adhering to long-term contracts in standardized products, such as petroleum, or by acquiring a reputation for delivering a specialized product of satisfactory quality on a reliable schedule, as in electronics and engineering. On their own, firms from a developing country often require years to overcome such marketing advantages, and an affiliation with an MNC can help accelerate the process.

Among the most important potential benefits from foreign investment is the **transfer of technology, skills, and ideas**. Because much of the world's research and development activity takes place within North America, Europe, and East Asia, firms from these areas are a potentially rich source of innovative products, machinery, manufacturing processes, marketing methods, quality control, and managerial approaches. MNCs potentially can bring these new ideas and technologies with them, helping reduce costs and increase productivity in the host country. FDI is most valuable when these kinds of benefits spread beyond the local affiliate of the MNC itself and help other local firms and enterprises, generating positive externalities called **spillovers**. For example, local firms competing against the MNC may observe and adopt the technology brought from abroad to try to improve their own productivity. A domestic furniture maker might learn about new machinery, a special technique to finish wood products, or a different way to organize production that could lower its costs and increase its competitiveness. Competition from the MNC can push rival firms to reduce their costs through more-efficient use of all inputs and by introducing new technologies and techniques, generating an indirect benefit to all firms that buy from the MNC and its competitors.

While this kind of "horizontal" spillover to competitors can be important, MNCs clearly have the incentive to limit technology transfer to their rivals. They have stronger incentives to encourage "vertical" spillovers to firms operating up and down the supply chain that either sell to or buy from the MNC. MNCs want their local suppliers to produce at the lowest possible cost, so it is in their interest to work with suppliers to increase the suppliers' productivity by introducing new methods to improve quality and reliability and reduce costs. These changes provide indirect benefits to other firms that buy from these suppliers.[10]

One important way these kinds of spillovers can occur is through the **training of workers and managers**. Most developing countries do not have many well-trained managers with experience in organizing and operating large industrial projects, such as those undertaken by multinational firms. MNCs have the incentive to train local managers and workers (both their own employees and their supplier's) and, in some circumstances, will send employees abroad to the parent company for training in production methods or management techniques. It is not uncommon for local managers to spend six months or more working in the parent company and then return to senior positions in the local affiliate. The immediate impact is to help increase productivity and profitability of the MNC. However, over time, these managers and workers may move to other firms or even start their own companies, bringing this new knowledge with them. When textile companies began to move from Korea and Taiwan to Indonesia in the 1980s, initially most senior managers were expatriates. Over time, more Indonesians were trained to fill those positions, and eventually some started their own companies, competing against the MNCs. When Mauritius first began to produce textiles and footwear in the early 1980s, virtually 100 percent of the export firms were foreign owned, but within 15 years, foreign firms controlled just 50 percent of total equity capital.[11]

However, just as FDI can create positive spillovers, it can create negative ones. MNCs might create air or water pollution or cause other environmental damage, generating a negative externality for the host country. (Of course, local investors also cause environmental damage, in some cases even worse damage.) While some MNCs have been guilty of causing extreme environmental damage, others bring with them cleaner and more efficient production techniques that help reduce environmental damage.

FDI in protected or inefficient activities can lead to net economic losses rather than gains by misallocating capital, labor, and other resources. If a government encourages an MNC to invest in a petrochemicals company that can be profitable

---

[10]See Howard Pack and Kamal Saggi, "Vertical Technology Transfer via International Outsourcing," *Journal of Development Economics* 65, no. 2 (2001), 389–415; Garrick Blalock and Paul Gertler, "Foreign Direct Investment and Externalities: The Case for Public Intervention," in Theodore Moran, Edward Graham, and Magnus Blomstrom, eds., *Does Foreign Direct Investment Promote Development?* (Washington, DC: Institute for International Economics and Center for Global Development, 2004).

[11]See Blalock and Gertler, "Foreign Direct Investment and Externalities."

only with government subsidies or regulations that limit competition (like high import tariffs on competing products), the costs to the country are likely to be higher than the benefits. Firms operating under protection tend to use more outdated technologies and are less likely to be able to compete eventually on world markets. The firm might boast large profits and appear to be thriving, but the costs to taxpayers and to downstream customers forced to pay higher prices might be even larger.

Perhaps the biggest concern about FDI is the loss of local control over business. MNCs can drive out local businesses, and even where this might be economically efficient it can be politically very unpopular. A large efficient MNC can drive out small local business that operate at higher costs, particularly in countries with high trade barriers and other regulations where local firms may be relatively weak. Also, MNCs are more likely to repatriate their profits abroad, although some reinvest locally (and many local businesses also send their profits abroad). Concerns are most acute for the largest MNCs, whose size and control over resources often match and sometimes outstrip that of the recipient country governments. Investment by a multinational corporation raises the specter of interference by, and dependence on, foreign economic powers beyond the control of the host country. In some cases valid social preferences over the control and distribution of income might outweigh economic efficiency arguments.

FDI AND GROWTH

Ultimately, broad statements about whether FDI is beneficial or harmful are difficult to make and can be misleading. Because FDI is so varied, much depends on the specific activity, the actions taken by the MNC and the government, and the reaction by local suppliers, competitors, and customers. Debate continues as to the existence and magnitude of spillovers, both positive and negative. Research examining the relationships between FDI and growth has reached mixed conclusions. Some research has found a positive relationship, particularly when the workforce in the recipient country has achieved a minimum level of education, whereas other studies have found no relationship or even a negative one.[12]

Clearer patterns begin to emerge when researchers take into account the purpose and context of the FDI. Foreign investment that produces for the domestic

[12]The research on FDI, spillovers, and growth is extensive. For an example of a study finding a positive relationship in the presence of a minimum level of education in the recipient country, see E. Borensztein, J. DeGregorio, and Jong-Wha Lee, "How Does Foreign Investment Affect Growth?" *Journal of International Economics* 45, no. 1 (1998), 115–72. For an influential study finding negative spillovers in Venezuela, see Brian Aitken and Ann E. Harrison, "Do Domestic Firms Benefit from Direct Foreign Investment? Evidence from Venezuela," *American Economic Review* 89, no. 3 (June 1999), 605–18. For a recent survey, see Robert Lipsey and Fredrik Sjöholm, "The Impact of Inward FDI on Host Countries: Why Such Different Answers?" in Theodore Moran, Edward Graham, and Magnus Blomstrom, eds., *Does Foreign Direct Investment Promote Development?* (Washington, DC: Institute for International Economics and Center for Global Development, 2004).

market and relies heavily on subsidies or protection from competition is much less likely to be beneficial and may even generate economic losses for the host country. FDI in natural resource-based industries depends heavily on the impact of the industries themselves. As described in Chapter 18, while primary product exports have at times helped spur development in some countries (such as diamonds in Botswana and petroleum in Indonesia and Malaysia), in other countries, natural resource abundance has been as much as curse as a blessing, such as oil in Nigeria and Venezuela, copper in Zambia, and diamonds in the Democratic Republic of the Congo and Sierra Leone.

FDI aimed at firms producing manufactured exports and operating in competitive global markets most often is found to have a positive relationship with growth and development. This type of activity tends to be economically efficient and conducive to importation of new technologies, training new workers and managers, and positive spillovers to suppliers and even competitors. Georgetown University economist Theodore Moran finds significant differences in operating characteristics between subsidiaries that are integrated into the international sourcing networks of their parent multinationals and those that serve protected domestic markets. Where parent firms use local affiliates as a part of a strategy to remain competitive in international markets, they maintain those affiliates at the cutting edge of technology, management, and quality control. But Moran finds that FDI in protected industries can hinder an economy, as these firms typically use older technologies and operate under restrictions that raise costs, hinder exports, and reduce productivity gains.[13]

POLICIES TOWARD FOREIGN DIRECT INVESTMENT

Developing countries interested in attracting FDI and ensuring maximum benefit generally use some combination of three broad strategies:

- Improve the general environment for all kinds of investment (foreign or domestic) by strengthening infrastructure, reducing red tape, and improving the quality of labor.
- Introduce specific policies and incentives to attract FDI, such as export processing zones, worker training, import protection, or tax holidays.
- Impose requirements on MNCs (such as limits on equity holdings or repatriation of profits) in an attempt to capture more benefits locally.

IMPROVE THE GENERAL INVESTMENT ENVIRONMENT The least-controversial approach, and one that can bring benefits beyond those associated with FDI, is to take steps to improve the general environment for investment and business operations. As

---

[13]Theodore Moran, "How Does FDI Affect Host Country Development? Using Industry Case Studies to Make Reliable Generalizations," in Theodore Moran, Edward Graham, and Magnus Blomstrom, eds., *Does Foreign Direct Investment Promote Development?* (Washington, DC: Institute for International Economics and Center for Global Development, 2004).

discussed earlier, businesses in poor countries usually face much larger regulatory burdens and higher costs than those in rich countries. To try to improve the general investment environment, governments can improve road and ports infrastructure, invest in utilities to make them more reliable and less expensive, reduce trade tariffs, strengthen the judicial process and the rule of law, and reduce unnecessary regulations and red tape that add to the cost of doing business. These steps should help attract new investment, both domestic and foreign, and help make existing investments more productive and profitable.

INTRODUCE POLICIES AIMED SPECIFICALLY AT ATTRACTING FDI The question of whether governments should take specific measures to encourage FDI even more than domestic investment turns on views on the existence and size of spillovers: If FDI brings with it positive spillovers that generate benefits to firms other than the MNC, then policies and incentives aimed specifically at attracting FDI may be appropriate. Where there are few if any positive spillovers and possibly negative ones, the argument for government action and special treatment is much weaker.

Three kinds of specific policies are common. First, host governments can provide effective and timely **information** to potential investors that markets might not provide on their own. Investors might not come to a particular country if they simply do not know much about it. Many governments in developing countries have established investment promotion agencies to market their countries and provide information on business costs, port facilities, natural resources, levels of education, climate, and other factors that might make their country attractive to investors. In some countries, this kind of promotion can help, but in others it seems to make little difference.

Second, governments can undertake specific expenditures aimed at making their country more attractive for FDI. Many governments have established industrial parks or **export-processing zones (EPZs)** to increase investment and manufactured exports. The basic idea is that building infrastructure and improving the investment climate for an entire economy are likely to take a long time, so as an interim measure, the government could establish an enclave located near port facilities in which infrastructure is of high quality, utilities are reliable and of relatively low cost, and there are fewer regulations and less red tape. Typically, countries welcome both domestic and foreign investment in EPZs, but FDI tends to account for a greater share of the investment. Most of the countries that have been highly successful in producing manufactured exports have established EPZs or similar facilities, including EPZs in Malaysia, Korea, Mauritius, the Dominican Republic, and Indonesia; special economic zones in China; and maquiladoras in Mexico and similar stand-alone facilities in Tunisia and other countries. But EPZs and related facilities are not always successful and have failed when they have been poorly located, badly managed, or in other ways added to rather than reduced the producer's costs (see Chapter 19).

Third and more controversial, governments can provide specific incentives to MNCs to increase their profitability, including protection from import competition, subsidies, or tax breaks. Governments provide **protection** by introducing tariffs and quotas to reduce imports of competing goods or provide outright monopoly control over local markets. These steps are most relevant for FDI aimed at producing for the domestic market, rather than for exports. Because import protection and monopoly control create higher domestic prices and profits, in effect local consumers pay higher prices as a transfer to the multinationals' foreign stockholders. Because evidence suggests that FDI aimed for protected domestic markets brings with it the least benefits (and sometimes net economic losses), it is often difficult to justify this kind of intervention.

Perhaps the most controversial of all steps taken to encourage FDI is income tax incentives. While these incentives can take a wide variety of forms, the most common is income **tax holidays**, which exempt firms from paying taxes on corporate income, usually for three to six years. Most countries otherwise would tax profits at rates anywhere from 20 percent to as high as 50 percent. For tax holidays to help the multinationals, they must be creditable against income taxes due to their home country governments. Otherwise, if home countries tax firms on worldwide income, as all industrial countries except France do, then the MNC would pay less tax to the developing country but more to its home country. In effect, taxes foregone by the developing country would simply be transferred to tax revenues of the multinational's home country. Most industrial countries now permit their firms to take credit for tax holidays granted abroad through tax treaties negotiated between host- and home-country governments.

There is substantial debate about the circumstances, if any, under which tax holidays are justified. Most studies conclude that, for many kinds of FDI, income tax holidays have only marginal effects on multinational investment decisions and reward the multinationals for doing what they would have done in any case. This is especially true for firms attracted by natural resources or those intending to produce in protected domestic markets of the host countries. Under these circumstances, MNCs are attracted by specific characteristics of the host country, such as the presence of gold or petroleum deposits or a large domestic consumer market. These MNCs may have few other serious location options, so tax treatment may not be a critical factor in their investment decision. Moreover, tax holidays cannot turn an unprofitable investment into a profitable one: Taxes become relevant only once a firm is earning profits.

Evidence suggests that export-oriented, labor-intensive, "footloose" industries may be more sensitive to tax holidays and other incentives because they have a much wider set of location options. Firms producing electronics products, shoes, textiles, clothing, games, and toys can choose among dozens of countries that offer the basics of political and economic stability, relatively low transport costs, and a pool of unskilled and semiskilled workers. Under these circumstances, tax holidays may be an important factor for the MNC in choosing its location. Because research suggests that these kinds of investments are more likely to provide positive spillovers to the host country, limited tax holidays may be justified. These steps always are controversial, however, because local firms and other MNCs quickly demand similar tax treatment, and it may be difficult for governments to resist this pressure.

REQUIREMENTS AND RESTRICTIONS ON FDI Many governments impose restrictions and requirements on MNCs in an attempt to capture as much as possible of the expected benefits from foreign direct investment, including performance requirements, local ownership requirements, labor requirements, and restrictions on profit repatriation. It is possible that these policies can increase the benefits to the host country; however, under most circumstances, they discourage FDI.

Many host countries have made it mandatory for foreign investors to sell a specified share of equity, usually at least 51 percent, to local partners to form **joint ventures**. Through local ownership requirements, host governments hope to ensure the transfer of technology and managerial skills, limit the repatriation of profits, and maintain local control. However, parent multinationals often are more reluctant to allow diffusion of technology to joint ventures than to wholly owned subsidiaries. Moreover, many local joint-venture partnerships are pro forma arrangements involving local elites close to the centers of political power with little knowledge or expertise in business that simply receive occasional payment from the MNC as a figurehead partner. This is not always the case, however. In some cases, skilled local partners eventually can take greater control and possibly buy out the MNC.

Many countries impose **domestic content requirements** on MNCs, requiring them to purchase a certain share of their inputs locally (as opposed to through imports), often with the share increasing over time. The idea is to encourage local suppliers and ensure stronger links between the MNC and local firms. Ideally, MNCs would choose to purchase locally in any case, but when they are forced to do so it usually indicates that the local suppliers are not producing at low enough prices and high enough quality to compete with imports. These requirements add directly to the costs of the MNC and can discourage investment. Domestic content requirements today, however, typically violate the rules of the World Trade Organization (WTO) and thus cannot be used by developing countries subject to those rules. Similar production requirements can be aimed at labor or technology transfer. Policies that make foreign firms use local personnel are aimed not only at job creation but also at increasing absorptive capacity for the transfer of technology from multinationals. Developing countries have tried to promote technology transfer by imposing standards requiring multinational firms to import only the most-advanced capital equipment rather than used machinery. Other common restrictions include ceilings on repatriation of profits to the parent corporation and stiff taxes on profit remittances. As with domestic content requirements, if not carefully designed, these restrictions can deter investment and may do little in the long run to help transfer benefits to local entities.

Overall, the accumulated evidence indicates that some types of FDI bring large benefits and others bring small or even negative benefits. This suggests that the best general policy is to get the basics right to make the investment climate more attractive for both domestic and foreign investment: reliable transportation, power, and communications facilities; freedom from unnecessary or onerous government regulations; capable institutions; adherence to the rule of law; macroeconomic and political stability; and labor markets in which wages are matched by productivity.

SAVINGS

As pointed out at the beginning of this chapter investment is not possible without first some person, company, or government saving part of their income. The saver can then invest the funds saved directly or deposit them in an intermediary (a bank or other financial institution) that specializes in identifying promising investments and lending it the money needed to make those investments a reality.

In the early years after the end of World War II it was commonly assumed that a lack of savings was at the heart of why so many of the countries in the world were poor. Because people in those countries were so poor, it was argued, they had to use all of their income to maintain a subsistence level of income and had nothing left over to save and invest. This problem was seen as the most fundamental of the various vicious circles of poverty that plagued low-income countries. To break the circle and get these countries on the path out of poverty, an outside source of savings (and hence investment) had to be found. The answer for many was to increase foreign aid provided by high-income countries to those mired in this rut. Arguments for foreign aid of this sort are still heard today but the rationale for most analysts has moved away from this view. (Foreign aid and the rationale for it are the subject of Chapter 14.)

Foreign aid is a form of **foreign savings** that is transferred to low-income countries and either invested or consumed. Other forms of foreign savings include FDI (discussed earlier in this chapter); portfolio equity by foreigners in developing country stock markets; and loans to developing countries by private (usually high-income-country) financial institutions, high-income governments, and international financial institutions (such as the World Bank, the IMF, and the regional international development banks).

Domestic sources of savings, however, are far larger in most developing countries than all of the sources of foreign savings combined. **Domestic savings** is made up of household, domestic corporation, and government savings. Domestic savings tend on average to be higher in high- and middle-income countries than in low-income countries but there is enormous variation within each group, and the savings rate among low-and middle-income countries has risen from two or three decades ago. China had a savings rate in 2005–09 of roughly 50 percent of GDP, an extraordinarily high rate. India, a country with lower income than China's, had a savings rate of over 30 percent in the same period, also a high amount. But some nations save very little; Nepal saved about 10 percent of its GDP, whereas Ghana and Guatemala had domestic savings rates of 5 percent or less. High-income countries such as the United States and the United Kingdom had savings rates below 15 percent of GDP. Savings and investment data for a selection of countries are presented in Table 10-4.

How does a low-income country with a low savings rate increase that rate to contribute to a higher rate of growth in income? Can government policy have a major influence on a country's savings rate? Since the nineteenth century it has been assumed that higher incomes would raise the savings rate. In all countries the highest income earners in the population typically save far more than the lowest income earners. It would seem to follow that if a country's income increased, the average rate of savings of the country as a whole would rise along with income. But when economists set out to measure the change in savings rate over time, they quickly discovered

TABLE 10-4 Domestic Capital Formation (Investment) and Savings

	GROSS CAPITAL FORMATION (% OF GDP)		GROSS DOMESTIC SAVINGS (% OF GDP)	
	1975–1979	2005–2009	1975–1979	2005–2009
Economy				
Low income	14	23	7	10
Middle income	26	28	25	30
High income	24	20	24	20
Region				
East Asia and Pacific	30	38	30	44
Europe and Central Asia	n.a.	23	n.a.	24
Latin America and Caribbean	25	21	23	23
Middle East and North Africa	30	26[*]	24	32[*]
Sub-Saharan Africa	25	21	23	16
South Asia	18	33	16	28
Country				
Brazil	24	18	21	19
China	32	44	32	51
Egypt	31	20	16	16
Ghana	9	22	9	5
Guatemala	20	18	16	3
India	20	36	19	32
Indonesia	24	27	29	30
Mexico	24	25	23	23
Nepal	16	29	12	10
Russian Federation	n.a.	22	n.a.	32
South Africa	27	20	31	18
United Kingdom	20	17	20	14
United States	20	18	20	13

[*]Data from 2005–2007 only.
GDP, gross domestic product.

Source: World Bank, "World Development Indicators," http://databank.worldbank.org.

that as average per capita income rose, the national average domestic savings rate did not change much if at all.[14] It turns out that we do not really even know whether it is a rise in savings that leads to a rise in investment that in turn leads to higher growth or whether the causation goes in reverse. Is it instead the rise in the rate of growth brought about by various reforms in government policy that leads to a higher rate of domestic savings? In the economies of South Korea and Taiwan, for example, reforms in economic policy in the early 1960s jump-started growth at a time when the savings rate, particularly the savings rate in South Korea, was very low. Rapid growth during the 1960s and into the 1970s then led to a rising rate of domestic savings and domestic investment that sustained the high growth sparked by the earlier reforms.

Although there is much not known about what determines a country's overall rate of domestic savings, we do know something about what drives household savings, typically the most important part of the overall level of domestic savings. We also can say something about government savings but much less about savings by domestic corporations. We will look at each of these sources of domestic savings in turn. The chapter ends with a return to the issue of foreign savings and what drives whether a country is a net lender (that transfers savings abroad) or a net borrower (which receives other countries' savings, as in the case of FDI).

HOUSEHOLD SAVING AND CONSUMPTION

Individuals and households save for two main reasons. First, they want to generate higher future income by saving and investing some of their current income. Second, they want to save some current income to protect themselves from the risk of unexpected falls in income in the future, often from a serious illness on the part of the major income earner; the loss of employment for some other reason; a drought that undermines next year's food crop; the loss of productive assets from fire, flood, theft, or disease (that kills crops or livestock); or other loss of income. This precautionary motive can be particularly important for poor people living on subsistence levels, for whom a sudden loss of income can be catastrophic, or where insurance markets are not well developed and individuals, families, and businesses must self-insure against the risks of a sudden loss of income or assets. In most low-income countries insurance markets are weak, especially in poor rural areas.

Given these motivations, a key decision is how much to save and how much to consume. The more a person saves, the more he or she can invest to increase future income and the more he or she can safeguard against future shocks. But saving comes at a cost: The only way to save is to reduce current consumption. Households

---

[14]This discovery led to the works of Milton Friedman on the permanent income hypothesis and James Duesenberry on the relative income hypothesis, which, in different ways, attempted to explain this paradox.

will sacrifice current consumption to save only if they believe either that the ensuing investment will increase their income and consumption in the future or they will need to draw on that saving to finance basic consumption in the event of a severe income shock. A wide variety of factors might influence saving: the current level of income, anticipated future levels of income, the number of dependents that must be supported, the opportunities for productive investment, and the quality of the financial institutions through which some saving might be channeled.

The **life-cycle model** of household savings captures an important element of why some household savings in developing countries is high whereas with other kinds of households it is low. The life-cycle model, associated most closely with Nobel Prize–winning economist Franco Modigliani, is specific about how saving and consumption would be expected to vary systematically during a person's lifetime.[15] In this model, young adults tend to have lower saving rates because they have lower incomes (and expect higher incomes in the future) and are raising children. Indeed, many people would be expected actually to dissave (go into debt) during this stage of life. Saving rates tend to rise and peak toward the middle and end of a person's working years, when incomes are higher and there are fewer consumption-related expenses for children. During this stage of life, people accumulate the bulk of their saving to be used during retirement. Once workers retire, their income falls and they again dissave by drawing down on their previous saving. Thus saving rates tend to be low or even negative during the younger years, high during middle age, and negative again after retirement.

The life-cycle hypothesis suggests that the demographic structure of a society may have a strong effect on overall saving rates. As discussed in Chapter 7, all societies tend to pass through a demographic transition with three basic stages: (1) high birth and death rates, with low population growth, (2) falling death rates with continued high birth rates and consequently high population growth rates, and (3) falling birth rates with continued low death rates and lower population growth. As countries pass through these stages, the share of the population too young to work, of working age, or retired tends to change dramatically, and saving rates may change with them. A society in stage 2 of the demographic transition is likely to have a relatively large number of surviving children because of falling death rates and continued high birth rates. Children, of course, earn very little or no income, so their consumption effectively is negative saving. At this stage of the demographic transition, each worker in the society has more young dependents to care for, so saving rates are expected to be relatively low. Later on, as a country enters stage 3 of the transition, the number of

[15]See Franco Modigliani and Richard Brumberg, "Utility Analysis and the Consumption Function: An Interpretation of Cross-Section Data," in K. Kurihara, ed., *Post Keynesian Economics* (New Brunswick, NJ: Rutgers University Press, 1954); Alberto Aldo and Franco Modigliani, "The Life-Cycle Hypothesis of Saving: Aggregate Implications and Tests," *American Economic Review* 53, no. 1, (March 1963), 55–84. For a classic early work on the subject, see Ansley J. Coale and Edgar M. Hoover, *Population Growth and Economic Development in Low-Income Countries* (Princeton, NJ: Princeton University Press, 1958).

children tends to fall and the large number of children from the previous generation enters the workforce. As a result, society as a whole tends to have a far larger share of workers and fewer dependents. Because each worker has fewer children to care for, saving rates are expected to rise. Later still, these workers retire and saving rates tend to decline. This hypothesis is consistent with an income-saving relationship in which saving rates are high for middle-income countries and lower for high-income countries. Higher-income countries tend to have longer life expectancies and more people living in retirement, which would suggest lower average saving rates for these countries.

Figure 10–2 shows the relationship in 100 low- and middle-income economies between saving rates and the *dependency ratio*, which compares the size of the dependent population (children and retirees, the population aged 0 to 15 years and those over 60) to the working-age population. The figure shows a tendency for saving rates to be lower in countries with a larger number of dependents relative to the workforce. Note that there is significant variation around the line. Gabon and Tajikistan, for example, both have similar levels of dependency, but Gabon had a gross domestic savings rate of almost 50 percent while Tajikistan had one of *negative* 21 percent. Clearly, more than the dependency burden determines the rate of national savings. Some studies that controlled for more variables found little connection between dependency ratios and saving rates, while others detected a relationship.[16] The relationship seems to be more robust with respect to the young-age dependency ratio (the ratio of the population between 0 and 15 years of age to the working-age population). The evidence is weaker with respect to the old-age dependency ratio, which compares the size of the population aged over 60 to the working-age population, suggesting that this cohort may not reduce its saving as much as the life-cycle theory suggests.

The life-cycle hypothesis may capture a reason for the high savings rates in East Asia. When the East Asian economies such as South Korea and Taiwan began to grow rapidly, their societies also went through a rapid demographic transition as birth rates came down soon after the decline in death rates, leading to a population largely concentrated in the working ages of 15 to 65 and a declining young population. As time passed, those of working age gradually retired and with increasing life expec-

---

[16]Studies that find no relationship between demographic structure and saving include Angus Deaton, *Understanding Consumption* (Oxford: Clarendon Press, 1992); M. Gersovitz, "Savings and Development," in Hollis Chenery and T. N. Srinivasan, eds., *Handbook of Development Economics*, vol. 1 (Amsterdam: North-Holland, 1988). Studies that reach the opposite conclusion include Sebastian Edwards, "Why Are Saving Rates So Different across Countries? An International Comparative Analysis," NBER Working Paper 5097 (Cambridge, MA: NBER, 1996); Paul R. Masson et al., "International Evidence on the Determinants of Private Saving" *The World Bank Economic Review* 12, no. 3 (September 1998), 483–501; Norman Loayza, Klaus Schmidt-Hebbel, and Luis Serven, "What Drives Private Saving across the World?" *Review of Economics and Statistics* 82, no. 2 (May 2000), 165–81; Steven Radelet, Jeffrey Sachs, and Jong-Wha Lee, "Economic Growth in Asia" (Cambridge, MA: Harvard Institute for International Development, May 1997).

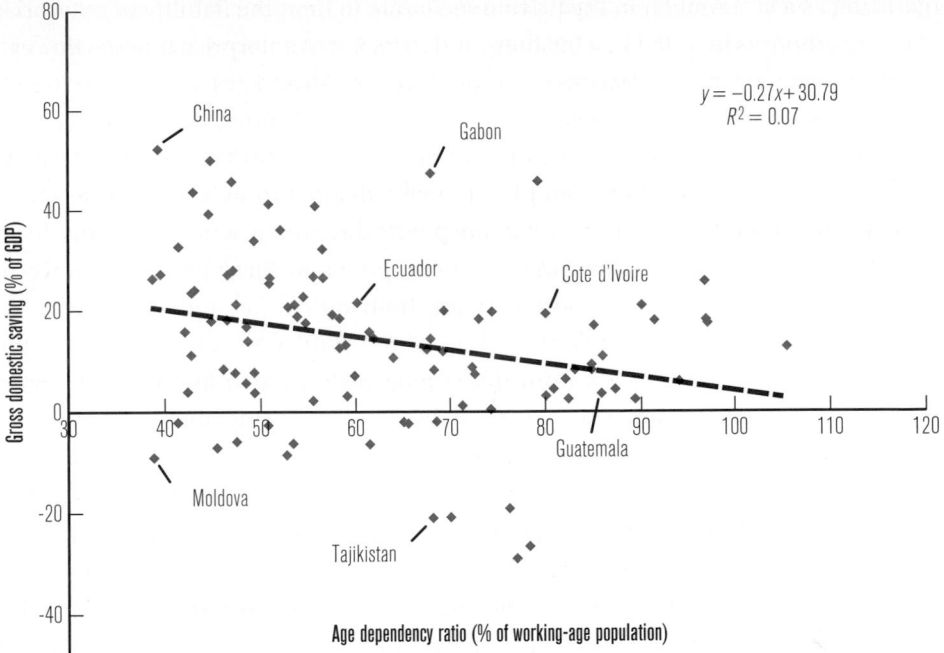

FIGURE 10-2 Gross Domestic Saving and the Age Dependency Ratio, 2009

GDP, gross domestic product.

Source: World Bank, "World Development Indicators," http://databank.worldbank.org.

tancy, elderly dependents made up a rapidly rising share of the population, but this did not occur until after these economies had experienced three or more decades of high savings, high investment, and rapid economic growth. China's one child policy has produced a similar phenomenon. The one child policy was instituted in the first part of the 1970s and had taken full effect by the time the economic reform began in 1978 that jump-started economic growth. Rapid growth thus benefited from and was sustained to an important degree by the dwindling share of dependent young people, which in turn made high rates of household savings possible. A rising share of elderly dependents in China is only now beginning to occur and will not have a major impact on the overall dependency ratio for another decade.

CORPORATE SAVING

Corporate saving is relatively small in most developing countries primarily because the corporate sector generally is small. For a variety of reasons, there are fewer pressures and incentives in developing countries for doing business in the corporate form (as opposed to operating as an unincorporated business). The principal reasons for organizing as a corporation in the private sector are to limit the liability of enterprise owners to amounts invested in a business and to facilitate enterprise finance through the issue of equity shares (stocks). Although these advantages are substantial in higher-income countries with well-developed commercial codes, civil court systems, and capital markets, they are smaller in most developing countries, where the collection of commercial claims (for example, company debts) through the courts is relatively difficult and where capital markets are poorly developed, when they exist at all.

As usual, however, there are important exceptions to these generalizations. In some developing countries, corporations are both numerous and quite large. As noted earlier, *Fortune* magazine's annual list of the 500 largest corporations in the world (in 2010) includes MNCs from developing nations such as China's Sinopec Corporation, Shanghai Automotive Industry Corporation, and the Industrial and Commercial Bank of China. The giant firms in India included Tata Steel and in Brazil the financial conglomerate Banco Bradesco. But less than 15 percent of the *Fortune* list was from low- and middle-income nations and two-thirds of them were located in China. The vast majority of developing countries had none. There are, of course, many good-size corporations that do not make it into the *Fortune* 500 largest list. Thus in most developing countries, even when corporations of say a billion dollars in sales are accounted for, such corporations do not account for a large share of private-sector business activity and do not provide a high proportion of domestic saving.

In all but a few of the highest-income developing countries, the great bulk of private sector farming and commercial and manufacturing activity is conducted by unincorporated, typically family-owned enterprises. Some of these businesses fall into the category of medium-scale establishments (from 20 to 99 workers). The great majority are small-scale operations with fewer than 20 employees. The noncorporate sector, including most small family farms and urban informal sector enterprises, manages to generate more than half of all domestic saving in most developing countries, and this sector is the only consistent source of surplus in the sense that the sector's saving exceeds its investment. For those closely held, largely family-owned and -managed firms, enterprise profits become an important part not only of corporate saving but also of gross household income. The available evidence indicates, and economic theory suggests, that household saving accounts for the overwhelming share of private saving in developing countries and the chief source of household saving is probably household income from unincorporated enterprises.

GOVERNMENT SAVING

Unlike private saving, there are no well-developed theories for government saving and consumption behavior. Government saving arises when tax revenues exceed public consumption expenditures (that is, government spending excluding public investment expenditures).[17] Government saving in most countries tends to be smaller than private saving (although not always), typically averaging between 3 and 10 percent of GDP in most developing countries. In countries where governments run large budget deficits, government saving is negative. Government saving also tends to be much smaller in low-income countries than in middle- and upper-income countries. One reason is that poorer countries generally do not generate as much tax revenue as richer countries.

Even though government saving usually is smaller than private saving, historically it has been given strong emphasis in development policy. This is partly because private saving is often seen as inherently constrained by such factors as low per capita income and high private consumption propensities among wealthy families with the greatest capacity for saving. But it is also because government saving can be controlled more directly by policy makers, and public sector investment financed by that saving (roads, bridges, ports) plays an important role in supporting economic growth.

Government saving can be changed by either increasing revenues or reducing consumption expenditures. Historically, most effort has focused on increasing tax revenues, either by strengthening tax structures and collection systems or by altering tax rates. In this line of thinking, tax ratios in many developing countries are too low, and policy changes aimed at increasing tax revenues help increase domestic saving (and ultimately the rate of economic growth). But there are several steps in between, and the extent to which this occurs depends on three key questions:

1. To what extent can governments increase the tax ratio, if they want to do so?
2. Will an increase in the tax ratio lead to an increase government saving?
3. Will an increase in government saving increase total domestic saving?

On the first question, it is not easy to judge the appropriate level of taxation in developing countries. If taxes are too low, governments cannot provide essential services, such as basic education, public health, a well-functioning judicial system, basic security, and public infrastructure. Tax rates that are too high (or fall too heavily on some groups) can undermine private entrepreneurs and reduce the incentives for new investment and economic growth. As a general matter, developing countries generally do not (and cannot be expected to) have tax ratios as high as is common in wealthier countries (except for developing countries with significant natural-resource endowments, which are easier to tax). Moreover, it is not easy to increase tax collection in developing countries, if for no other reason than their much lower per capita income allows a much smaller margin for taxation after subsistence needs are met. Figure 10–3 shows that in the 1990s, whereas typical tax ratios for low-income countries averaged around 15 percent, the ratio of government revenue to GDP in the industrialized countries averaged over 30 percent.

---

[17]In some countries saving by government-owned enterprises contributes to government saving, but it generally plays a minor role, so our discussion of government saving is confined to budgetary saving.

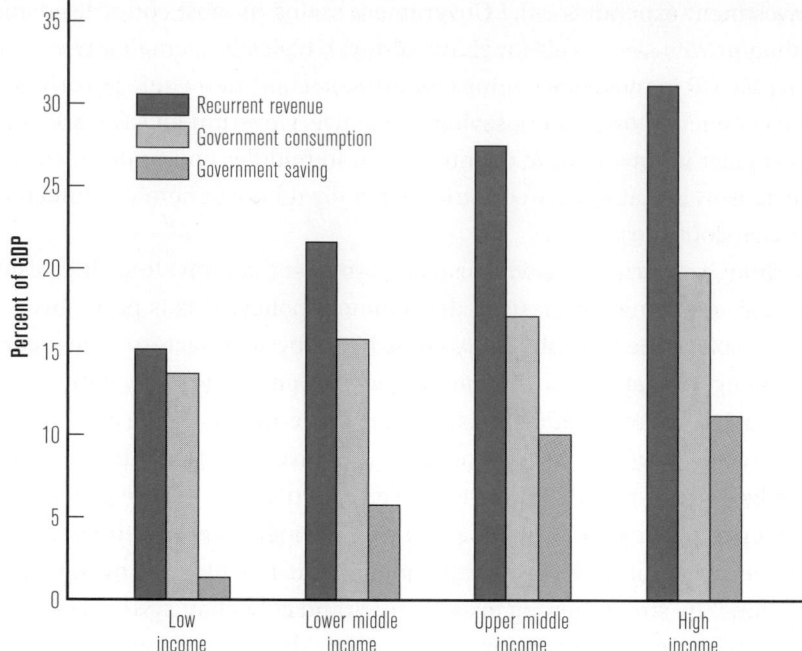

FIGURE 10-3 Government Revenue, Consumption, and Saving, 1990–2002

Tax revenues as a share of income tend to be much smaller in low-income countries than in high-income countries. Government consumption also grows with income but not nearly as much. Therefore, government saving generally is much smaller in low-income countries than in high-income countries.

GDP, gross domestic product.

Turning to the second question, a higher tax ratio does not necessarily lead to a higher government saving rate. It depends on what the government does with the revenue. To the extent that it spends the revenue on consumption (that is, increased government employment or higher salaries), government saving does not increase; to the extent it uses the revenue to reduce a budget deficit or for investment, government saving increases. More specifically, the impact of increased tax revenue on the government saving rate depends on the government's propensity to save (as opposed to consume) an additional peso or rupiah of tax revenue. In many countries, the government's marginal propensity to save out of taxes has been sufficiently small that higher taxes often have had relatively little effect on government saving and in some cases none at all.

It is worth emphasizing that increasing government consumption (rather than saving) may or may not be bad policy. Some consumption expenditures may be a waste, such as fancy cars, luxurious government offices, or a rapid buildup of military purchases. But other consumption expenditures may be vitally important, such as purchasing vaccines; making salary adjustments to keep and attract qualified civil servants; maintaining roads, schools, health facilities, and communication networks; and strengthening the judicial system or financial institutions.

Government consumption tends to rise less sharply with income than does revenue, as shown in Figure 10-3. There is much less difference in government consumption ratios between low-income countries (14 percent) and high-income countries (19 percent) than there is in tax ratios. This difference leads to a substantial divergence in average government saving rates. The poorest countries tend to have very low (and sometimes negative) government saving rates; government saving rates tend to rise with income as tax ratios increase.

On the third question, perhaps counter intuitively, an increase in government saving does not automatically increase domestic saving. How can this be when government saving plus private saving equals domestic saving? It depends on how private saving responds to the increase in government saving. If the government raises taxes, government saving might increase, but private individuals might respond by lowering their saving to pay the higher taxes, thereby dampening the impact on aggregate domestic saving. Thus the effect on saving of raising taxes depends on both the government's and the private sector's propensity to save out of the marginal dollar of income. As a general statement, increased tax revenue increases the domestic saving rate only if the government's propensity to save is greater than the private sector's propensity to save.

Debates about the private sector's reaction to increased government saving date back at least as far as the early part of the nineteenth century to the writings of the great British economist David Ricardo. Ricardo postulated—and largely rejected—the idea that, under certain circumstances, a change in taxes will have absolutely no effect on total domestic saving. Ricardo's theory has come to be known as **Ricardian equivalence**: Any increase in public saving is offset by an equivalent decline in private saving, with total domestic saving remaining unchanged. The basic idea is that when private actors receive a tax cut and see that government spending does not change, they anticipate a commensurate tax increase in the future and prepare for it by increasing their current saving. Thus, if the government reduces taxes, government saving may fall, but households and firms increase private saving in anticipation of a future tax increase. The fall in government saving is offset exactly by a rise in private saving, and the tax cut has no impact on total saving. Similarly, a tax increase may lead to higher government saving, but private saving is expected to decline by the same amount with no change in total saving. Ricardo's original idea was rejuvenated and formalized by economist Robert Barro in 1979.[18]

Ultimately, of course, this is an empirical issue that comes down to measuring the extent to which private agents alter their saving behavior in response to changes in government tax and expenditure policies. The abundance of evidence suggests partial, but only partial, truth to Ricardo's hypothesis. Many studies have shown that an increase in government saving tends to be associated with a decline in private saving, but by less

---

[18]Robert Barro, "Are Government Bonds Net Wealth?" *Journal of Political Economy* 82, no. 6 (November–December 1974), 1095–117.

than the strict one-to-one relationship postulated by Ricardo. Most studies have found an offset of between 0.40 and 0.65, meaning that a 1 percentage point of GDP increase in the government saving rate is associated with a 0.40- to 0.65-percentage-point decline in the private saving rate. This would imply a net increase in the total domestic saving rate of between 0.35 and 0.60 percentage points.[19]

The salutory impact of higher government saving may go beyond the effect on domestic saving. Because higher government saving is derived largely from smaller budget deficits, it reduces the government's borrowing requirements. Government deficits in developing countries typically are financed through domestic money creation (that is, borrowing from the central bank, which prints money to fund the deficit) or by borrowing in either local or overseas markets. Larger budget deficits can lead to higher rates of inflation (from money creation), larger government debts, or both. Lower budget deficits (or higher public saving) tend to have the opposite outcomes: lower inflation and indebtedness. Thus higher public saving is likely to enhance general macroeconomic stability.

FOREIGN SAVING

Historically, many countries have augmented domestic saving with foreign saving to help finance investment and growth. The United States relied heavily on foreign saving, particularly during the antebellum period from 1835 to 1860 and again in the late nineteenth century to finance, among other things, the expansion of the railway system. Likewise, Russia used foreign saving to help propel its development in the three decades before World War I and the Communist revolution. However, not all countries have followed this pattern: Japan became a wealthy nation even though it actively discouraged inflows of foreign saving and investment throughout its history. Therefore, foreign saving can help development but is not necessarily essential for it.

In decades past, some developing countries actively tried to shut out private capital flows; today almost all developing countries actively try to encourage them. But controversy surrounds foreign aid, foreign investment, short-term private capital flows, and the debt that has accrued from foreign borrowing. The remainder of this chapter provides a brief overview of some basic concepts and data on foreign saving. Foreign saving in the form of FDI was discussed earlier in this chapter; foreign savings transferred through loans to developing countries and the resulting accumulation of foreign debt is the subject of Chapter 13, and more in-depth analyses of foreign aid as a source of savings is the subject of Chapter 14. The appendix to Chapter 15 provides related background on balance-of-payments accounting.

[19]See, for example, Edwards, "Why Are Saving Rates So Different across Countries?;" Masson et al., "International Evidence on the Determinants of Private Saving"; Loayza et al., "What Drives Private Saving across the World?"; Radelet et al., "Economic Growth in Asia."

The relationships between investment, domestic saving, foreign saving, and the trade balance can best be seen from standard national accounts identities, which tell us that total investment (I) must equal total saving (S), which in turn consists of domestic saving (S_d) and foreign saving (S_f). To see this, recall from the income side of the national accounts that

$$Y = C + I + G + X - M \qquad\qquad [10\text{-}3]$$

where G is government consumption, X is exports of goods and services, and M is imports of goods and services. On the expenditure side, all income must be consumed, saved, or given to the government as taxes:

$$Y = C + S_p + T \qquad\qquad [10\text{-}4]$$

Note that the saving term (S_p) in this identity refers to private saving. Because both equations equal Y, the right-hand sides must be equal:

$$C + I + G + X - M = C + S_p + T \qquad\qquad [10\text{-}5]$$

Subtracting C from both sides and rearranging the terms yields

$$I = (T - G) + S_p + (M - X) \qquad\qquad [10\text{-}6]$$

The first term on the right-hand side ($T - G$) is government saving, and the second term (S_p) is private saving. The third term ($M - X$) is both the current account deficit of the balance of payments and foreign saving. When a country's imports (M) exceed its exports (X), the difference must be financed by inflows of capital from abroad (foreign aid, bank loans, equity flows, etc.), which is foreign saving. The right-hand side of the equation is the sum of domestic and foreign saving, yielding

$$I = S_d + S_f \qquad\qquad [10\text{-}7]$$

or the more traditional

$$I - S_d = M - X \qquad\qquad [10\text{-}8]$$

Thus, as the difference between investment and domestic saving grows (or shrinks), the trade deficit grows (or shrinks) commensurately. The two balances must move together in tandem. One can think of this in many ways. As investment increases (without an increase in domestic saving), imports tend to increase and exports decrease to provide the materials needed for the investment project. A firm building a new factory requires steel, concrete, lumber, and machinery, which can come from either new imports or purchasing the goods domestically, leaving less for export. Alternatively, an export boom without a commensurate increase in imports generates profits that can contribute to domestic saving, closing the gap between investment and domestic saving.

Foreign saving includes both a public sector component (called *official foreign saving*) and a private component. Most **official foreign saving** is foreign aid provided on **concessional terms** as either *grants* (outright gifts) or *soft loans*, meaning that they bear lower interest rates and longer repayment periods than would be available in private international capital markets. Industrialized-country governments and international agencies also provide some financing as loans on commercial terms (*hard loans*), particularly to middle-income countries.

Private foreign saving consists of four elements. *Foreign direct investment* (discussed at length earlier in this chapter) is made by nonresidents, typically but not always by multinational corporations, in enterprises located in host countries. Direct investment implies that funds go directly to an enterprise (as opposed to indirectly through a stock market), with the foreigner gaining full or partial control of the enterprise. *Portfolio equity* is the purchase by foreigners of host country bonds or stocks, without managerial control. Portfolio equity was a very important form of financing in the nineteenth and early twentieth centuries, but fell into disuse after World War II. It was revived in the 1990s, however, as rich-country investors showed interest in emerging stock and bond markets, especially in Asia and increasingly in Latin America. *Commercial bank lending* to developing country governments and enterprises supplanted portfolio investment in importance for a time but waned beginning in the 1980s when debt crises afflicted many developing countries. It expanded quickly in the early 1990s, then dropped sharply toward the end of the decade, as several developing countries experienced major financial crises. In some cases it had not fully recovered when the global financial crisis hit in the latter half of 2008. Finally, exporting firms from the industrialized countries, their commercial banks, and official banks (such as the U.S. Export-Import Bank) offer *export credits* (or credit guarantees) to firms in developing countries that import from the industrialized countries. These credits help the exporters promote sales by permitting delayed payment, often at commercial interest rates.

Capital flows to developing countries changed dramatically in several important ways between 1990 and 2008, as shown in Table 10–5. First, private capital flows grew extremely rapidly until 1996, growing from $82 billion to $281 billion in 1996. All the major categories of private finance expanded rapidly: long-term loans, short-term loans, portfolio equity, and foreign direct investment. But this trend changed abruptly in 1997 after the financial crises that struck Thailand, Indonesia, Korea, Russia, and several other countries. Private capital flows fell sharply for several years and then grew rapidly between 2000 and 2008 (and declined again in 2009 after the financial crisis that originated in the United States).

Second, and in sharp contrast to private flows, official development flows fell during the 1990s. In particular, net official lending dropped significantly and turned negative, meaning that developing countries were repaying old loans more than they were receiving new loans from donor governments. Whereas official development finance and private finance differed by a factor of two in 1990, private flows were 35 times larger in 2008. While these two patterns hold for developing countries as a whole, the patterns differ between low-income and middle-income countries. In particular, the large increase in private capital flows was concentrated in middle-

TABLE 10-5   Financial Flows from and to Developing Countries, 1990–2008
(billions, US$)

	1990	1996	2000	2008
Inflows	81.6	281.3	172.3	727.3
Official development finance				
Official loans (net)	26.4	3.8	−5.8	20.4
Private finance	55.2	281.3	178.1	706.9
Long-term debt flows (net)	16.6	82.5	7.4	124.2
Short-term debt flows (net)	13.2	37.4	−7.9	−16.3
Portfolio investment	3.4	32.9	12.4	15.7
FDI into developing countries	22.1	128.6	166.2	583.0
Outflows	53.5	200.5	226.6	1,105.0
Accumulation of reserves	32.4	90.4	46.8	447.3
FDI from developing countries	5.0	10.0	16.5	164.0
Other items/errors and omissions	16.1	100.1	163.3	493.7
Memo item: aggregate current account balance of developing countries	−28.1	−83.6	43.6	377.9

FDI, foreign direct investment.

Source: World Bank, *Global Development Finance 2005* (Washington, DC: World Bank, 2005)
http://go.worldbank.org/581EDYH6R0; IMF, *International Financial Statistic* (Washington, DC: IMF);
Annual Yearbook and World Bank, *Global Development Finance 2009* (Washington, DC: World Bank,
2009) http://go.worldbank.org/581EDYH6R0.

income countries. Private capital flows to low-income countries were small in 1990, and while they were larger after the year 2000, the increase accounted for a relatively small share of the increase in total private capital flows. Official flows to low-income countries were only slightly larger in 2008 than they were in 1990, particularly if the figures are adjusted for inflation; in middle-income countries, the picture is similar.

Third, whereas capital inflows to developing countries in aggregate grew rapidly, capital outflows grew even more rapidly. The aggregate current account deficit of developing countries (shown at the bottom of Table 10–5) moved from a deficit position to a surplus position in 2000. In other words, aggregate exports of all goods and services exceeded imports of goods and services, so developing countries as a whole were exporting capital to the richer countries. Correspondingly, total net capital flows (or net foreign saving, summing together all inflows and outflows) shifted from positive to negative. The main channel through which this occurred was a small number of developing countries running large balance of payments surpluses and accumulating foreign exchange reserves, especially China. In 2007 and 2008, China accumulated foreign exchange reserves at a rate of over $400 billion per year. Typically balance of payments surplus countries (along with other central banks in developing countries) hold their foreign exchange reserves in one of two ways: (1) as deposits in banks in the United States, Europe, or Japan, which is a form of saving available to finance new loans in those countries, or (2) by purchasing government securities, such as U.S. Treasury bills. China's central bank (the People's Bank of China) became one of the largest purchasers of U.S. Treasury bills. In effect, the balance of payments surpluses generated by these countries are providing the saving necessary to finance the U.S. budget deficit. Historically and under normal circumstances, capital tends to flow from rich countries (which tend to have larger capital stocks) to low-income countries (where capital is scarce), but since 2000 that pattern has been reversed. However, this pattern is heavily concentrated in a small number of developing countries that are exporting a large amount of capital by accumulating reserves. The majority of low-income countries continue to be net importers of capital from rich countries.

SUMMARY

- Both public investment and private investment are central to economic growth and development. Public investment generally focuses on roads, ports, telecommunications facilities, schools, and health facilities. Private investment tends to be larger than public investment and provides the dynamism for the vast majority of new jobs, new technologies, and growth in economic output.
- Cost–benefit analysis provides a rigorous technique for evaluating both public and private investments and calculating the net present value over time of each investment. This technique can be used for commercial evaluation (to calculate private-sector financial benefits), economic evaluation (to measure the economic costs and benefits to society as a whole), or social evaluation (incorporating the impact of investments on important social goals).
- The key factors that influence investment at the macro level are similar to the variables discussed in Chapter 3 that promote economic growth. At the micro level the quality of the business environment is the main influence on the level and productivity of the investment. Governments that intervene excessively, thus delaying and raising the cost of business investment decisions, lead to rent seeking and corruption that further reduce the quantity and quality of investment.
- Foreign direct investment can generate important benefits, but not all FDI is alike. FDI focused on firms producing exports on competitive global markets appears to be most beneficial, creating jobs and bringing new technologies and ideas from abroad, among other spillovers. FDI for natural resources or for firms operating in protected domestic markets generally has had more mixed benefits and sometimes has been costly to recipient countries. Policies specifically aimed at attracting FDI, such as tax

holidays, are more controversial than those aimed at improving the general investment environment.

- Investment requires that there first be savings. Savings can be either by domestic individuals and organizations (corporations, governments) or by foreigners who then allow their savings to be transferred abroad through foreign aid, foreign direct investment, portfolio equity, or commercial lending.

- Domestic savings tend on average to be higher in high- and middle-income countries than in low-income countries, but there is enormous variation within each group.

- A determinant of the level of savings is the demographic makeup of a country. A country in the early stages of a demographic transition with a low death rate and a high birth rate will have a high rate of growth in the number and share of children not yet old enough to work, which may lower the savings rate. Countries further along in the demographic transition have lower birth rates and hence a higher share of the population is of working age (and not of retirement age), which can lead to higher rates of saving.

- Government saving makes an important contribution to total saving in many developing countries, although it is usually much smaller than private saving. An increase in government saving generally increases total domestic saving but typically by less than one for one, as it can be partially offset by a decline in private saving.

- Foreign saving is relatively small compared to domestic saving, but is often more controversial. The composition of foreign capital flows has changed markedly since the early 1990s. The amount of official finance flowing to low-income countries dropped sharply. By contrast, private finance grew even more quickly, at least until severe financial crises affected several countries in the late 1990s, but recovery and growth to even higher levels than in the past occurred through 2008. The increase in private capital flows has been concentrated in middle-income countries, with much less flowing to low-income countries. In a change from the normal pattern, in recent years some developing countries, particularly China, have been providing financing to rich countries.

11

Fiscal Policy

Beginning in late 2007, what had been a booming market for housing in the United States evolved instead into a depressed market with house prices falling and many homeowners forced into foreclosure. Financial instruments created by packaging large numbers of mortgages that were rated as safe investments suddenly dropped sharply in value, triggering losses not only for individuals but for major financial institutions such as Bear Stearns, Lehman Brothers, and the American International Group (AIG). The failure of these financial institutions in turn threatened the viability not only of other financial institutions but of the entire U.S. economy. The potential failure of many American financial institutions and the related sharp decline in economic activity in the United States in turn led to similar threats to financial institutions in the rest of the world, notably in Europe, and initiated a global recession that was the most severe recession worldwide since the Great Depression of the 1930s. Developing countries had not caused the global recession. Many had gone through a similar financial crisis in 1997–98, which had led to a major recession in several large developing economies, particularly in Asia. That crisis in turn led many of those economies to reform their financial systems in ways that protected them from the kind of financial meltdown being experienced in the high-income European countries and the United States. Developing countries, however, did feel the impact of the global recession as they saw their exports to the United States and Europe fall.

The magnitude of the recession in the United States and globally was so large that the normal mechanisms used to reverse the downturn, mainly monetary policies that lowered interest rates and increased the money supply, were not sufficient to end the decline. Instead, first the United States, together with several major European economies, had to revert to large expenditures through the government budget to reverse the sharply falling demand for goods and services in the economy. Soon thereafter a number of developing economies also introduced their own stimulus packages in an effort to reverse falling export demand that threatened to drive their economies into recession only a decade after their last crisis. The largest of these developing country stimulus packages was China's. China initiated a program of nearly US$600 billion to be spent mainly on infrastructure, such as a national high-speed highway system, eight new north–south and east–west high-speed rail lines, and new and modernized ports and airports. The stimulus package kept Chinese gross domestic product (GDP) growth from falling despite a large drop in the demand for Chinese exports in 2009. The average rate of GDP growth in China, thanks to a large degree to these government expenditures, was 9.8 percent a year in 2009 and 2010.

When a government raises its expenditures or cuts taxes on individuals and corporations so that they can raise their expenditures, these actions are referred to as **fiscal policy**. When government efforts instead rely on the central bank to adjust the money supply and interest rates to raise or lower individual and corporate expenditures, this is referred to as the exercise of **monetary policy**.

In this chapter we focus on fiscal policy and begin by noting that the main purpose of fiscal policy is not to deal with economic crises, whether crises of inadequate demand leading to recessions as in 2009–10 or of excess demand leading to inflation. The first function of fiscal policy is to manage government expenditures used to fund whatever activities government policy makers and the people they represent think the government should support. The next closely related function of fiscal policy is to find a way of financing those government expenditures, either through the collection of taxes, issuance of government bonds, or in more desperate cases by printing money.

This chapter starts with a discussion of what expenditures are typically undertaken by governments and follows with an analysis of the kinds of taxes commonly used to pay for those expenditures. With this as background, we then return to the question of what happens when something goes wrong either in the public or the private sphere of the economy. What is it that a government can do to repair what has gone wrong?

In many respects these issues are similar in high-, middle-, and low-income economies, but there are significant differences. Developing countries often have to rely more on fiscal policy to curb inflation or recover from a recession because many of the instruments of monetary policy are not as effective or do not even exist. Underdeveloped markets in developing countries are also often a major reason why they rely on government to take responsibility for investments and other expenditures that in a more advanced economy would be handled by the private sector.

The limitations of markets in developing countries would seem to suggest that government expenditures would be a higher share of GDP than in high income countries. But, as the data in Table 11–1 indicate, the opposite is the case. Governments in

TABLE 11-1 Central Government Expenditure as a Share of GDP, 2009

COUNTRY	PERCENT OF GDP
Low-income economies	
Bangladesh	11.3
Cambodia	11.0
Ghana	17.9
Lower-middle-income economies	
Indonesia	15.8
El Salvador	21.6
Morocco	27.9
Upper-middle-income economies	
Colombia	19.4
Thailand	19.7
Mauritius	20.9
High-income economies	
South Korea	21.9
Denmark	42.5
United Kingdom	46.4

Source: World Bank, "World Development Indicators," http://databank.worldbank.org.

developing countries on average spend a smaller share of GDP than do high-income countries. A major reason is that high-income countries typically spend a larger share of GDP on social welfare measures (old-age pensions, poverty reduction, healthcare for all) largely because the people of these countries demand such expenditures for reasons of fairness and feel that at their relatively high incomes they can afford to do so. Developing country governments are more apt to focus on measures to increase investment for overall growth. There is, however, considerable variation in the share of government expenditures in GDP among countries at both ends of the income spectrum.

GOVERNMENT EXPENDITURES

At the most general level all countries rely on government for certain activities because of public goods and market failures discussed in Chapter 5. For private goods, such as rice, saris, or TV sets, the signals provided by unfettered competitive market mechanisms guide producers to satisfy consumer demand efficiently. For pure public goods, the market fails entirely. There are few examples of pure public goods; national defense and basic scientific research generally are cited as illustrations. The term *public good* refers to a good or service that exhibits two traits: **nonrival consumption** and **nonexcludability**.

In *nonrival consumption,* one person's use of a good does not reduce the benefits available to others. That being the case, no one has any incentive to offer to pay for the good: If it is available to one, it is available to all. *Nonexcludability* means that it is either impossible or prohibitively expensive to exclude anyone from the benefits once the good is available. In either case, the private market cannot provide the good: Market failure is total. For most public goods, the characteristics of nonrival consumption and nonexcludability are present but less pronounced, and the market can function only in an inefficient way. Examples include vaccination against contagious diseases, police protection, and mosquito abatement. Therefore, it is evident that the appropriate role of the public sector, to a significant degree, is a technical issue.

In practice in all countries, government expenditures designed to offset market failures of this sort account for only a portion of government expenditures even in the most laissez faire, small government–oriented societies. In democratic societies the people through their elected representatives generally want government to do more, such as provide pensions for the elderly and healthcare for the sick regardless of income. In authoritarian societies, the leadership often does much the same because failure to do so can threaten the leaderships' ability to govern.

CATEGORIES OF GOVERNMENT EXPENDITURES

The principal distinction between types of government expenditure is between **capital** or **public investment** expenditures also called **development expenditures**, on the one hand, and **recurrent expenditures** on the other. Development or public investment expenditures are those that, like investment in general, generate a stream of income or services into the future. Government typically takes on the task of building a network of highways, and some governments, particularly in developing countries, take responsibility for providing electric power or exploitation of natural resource wealth (for example, petroleum). Education and health expenditures can also be thought of as a form of investment undertaken by government although in practice government budgets often treat them as recurrent consumption expenditures. The quality of government development investments in these areas should be judged by the same criteria that are used to judge private investments, as was discussed in Chapter 10.

Recurrent expenditures are those expenditures that a government must make year after year. They include the salaries of government employees, the purchase of office equipment, and annual payments to families living in poverty and for pensions for retirees. Most of these categories of recurrent expenditures are self-explanatory, but one category is of particular importance in developing countries largely because it is often ignored. Capital investments to build a highway are often given a high priority but the expenditures needed to maintain the highway once built are often neglected, and the highway is soon filled with potholes. This results not only from the neglect of maintenance by developing country governments but also because foreign aid agencies will frequently support a capital project but will seldom support the recurrent costs needed to keep the capital project functioning. The problem, however, is not unique to developing countries. The United States has neglected bridge and road maintenance in many parts of the country for decades and, at the time of the 2008–09 economic recession, faced the need for large maintenance and replacement expenditures, some of which were built into the stimulus program designed to get the country out of the recession.

Other common recurrent expenditures in developing (and high-income) countries are interest payments on government debt, consumer subsidies, and subsidies to loss-making state-owned enterprises. Government debt crises are the subject of Chapter 13, and here we note only that the problem with government deficits in developing countries on average is not that they are typically very large, although that is the case in some countries. The problem with chronic large deficits is that interest payments rise over time taking up an increasing share of the government recurrent cost budget either crowding out other worthwhile expenditures or leading to even larger government deficits. If the deficits are financed by borrowing abroad, foreign debt, typically in convertible currencies such as the dollar or the euro, accumulates and eats into the ability of the country to import and may eventually lead to a debt crisis. If the government borrows money domestically to cover the deficit, the interest cost in the budget will also rise. In developing countries, however, borrowing domestically often means borrowing directly from the central bank, and that is essentially the same as printing money and increasing the money supply. The reason developing countries frequently have to borrow from the central bank is that capital markets are underdeveloped and it often is not possible to sell government bonds to the general public or even to private companies. The net result is that deficits lead to money creation, and excessive money creation leads to inflation, which usually proves detrimental to the productive investment so central to economic growth.

Consumer subsidies are also not unique to developing countries. The political logic behind consumer subsidies is that certain commodities are considered essential, and government subsidizes these commodities so as to lower their price to the consumer and thus make them available to all regardless of income. In high-income countries the government typically has the ability to find out the true income of families and then target the subsidy so that it applies only to those below a predetermined poverty line—food stamps in the United States is a good example. In developing countries, however, government usually lacks the administrative capacity to discover the true income of families, although some middle-income nations are gaining this ability (see the discussion of Mexico's Oportunidades program in Chapters 6 and 8). When targeting is difficult, one option is to subsidize all sales of the commodity even though most of the subsidy will go to families that are not poor and could afford to pay the market price. General subsidies of this sort can be very expensive. When a country runs into debt and balance of payments problems and has to call for help to the International Monetary Fund (IMF), one of the first measures the IMF sets as a condition for a loan is elimination of these subsidies. Subsidies, however, are popular with the public and eliminating them typically leads to demonstrations against the government and even to major riots that threaten the existence of the government.

Even in China, where administrative capacities at the local level are quite high by developing country standards, targeting subsidies to poor families is not possible; subsidies in the 1990s and in the first decade of the twenty-first century have instead gone to designated poor counties and are available to all those in the county, including many families that are not poor. An alternative approach tried in the 1980s in Sri Lanka was to ask families to voluntarily state whether they fell below the poverty line or not. The result was that well over half the population of the country said that they fell below the poverty line even though objective data made it clear that the share below the poverty line was only a fraction of that self-reported figure. In some cases there is not even a pretense that the subsidy is designed to alleviate poverty. Countries with large oil reserves, such as Venezuela and Indonesia, have subsidized refined fuel costs to households even though the heaviest users of such fuel are the well off who can afford automobiles and motor bikes.

Subsidies to cover the losses of state owned enterprises (SOEs) grew rapidly in a great many developing countries when they first achieved independence. This was particularly so in Africa. In Tanzania alone, the number of state enterprises increased 10-fold from 1965 to 1985. By 1980, SOEs were common, and often dominant, in manufacturing, construction, banking services, natural resource industries, and agriculture. Although SOEs typically were small-scale undertakings in most developing countries before 1950, many by the beginning of the twenty-first century were among the largest firms in their countries, and some, notably in China, are among the largest enterprises in their fields anywhere in the world.

Deficits in state enterprises averaged 4 percent of the GDP across all developing countries in the mid-1970s. The problem worsened in the early 1980s, particularly in such countries as Brazil, Costa Rica, the Dominican Republic, Ecuador, Egypt, the Philippines, Turkey, and Venezuela, where SOE deficits reached between 3 and 12 percent of the GDP. In all these countries, the rest of the public sector would have generated a fiscal surplus, excluding the net transfers to the state enterprises.[1] By the late 1980s and through the first decade of the twenty-first century, the drain of SOE subsidies on government budgets has led to efforts by many developing countries to eliminate these subsidies by privatizing their SOEs. International aid agencies frequently have made SOE privatization a condition for further assistance. Privatization, however, has been a slow process, because it has been actively resisted by SOE managers and workers, not to mention politicians who use SOE employment as a patronage machine for their supporters. In countries where a large part of the private sector is controlled by minorities, as is the case with the Chinese minority in Southeast Asia or the South Asian minority in East Africa, the majority population often fears that privatization is simply a way of turning even more of modern business over to the minority.

[1] World Bank, *World Development Report 1988* (New York: Oxford University Press, 1988), p. 171.

Finally transfers from central to subnational governments conventionally are treated as recurrent expenditures even though subnational governments (provinces, departments, counties, municipalities) may use the proceeds for capital formation, such as construction of schools and hospitals. Some countries, such as Indonesia, classify some transfers as capital spending and others as consumption, so international comparisons are difficult. In a few cases, subnational governments with small transfers have access to rich sources of revenue. This is true for Bolivia, where oil-producing provinces receive large oil royalties, and for Malaysia, where the state governments of Sabah and Sarawak have earned substantial tax revenues from the export of tropical timber. In most unitary states, such as Chile, government affairs at virtually all levels are run from the capital, and subnational units of governments have few responsibilities to go with their limited sources of local revenue.

There is often a compelling argument for moving decisions about expenditures to lower levels of government. Lower levels of government are typically closer to the people being served by both investment and recurrent expenditures and thus in principle are better able to design expenditures to best meet local needs. Problems arise, however, when local governments lacking adequate tax revenues under their control finance these project and recurrent expenditures through access to bank loans. The problem can be particularly acute where the local banks are owned or controlled by local politicians. The result can be projects driven more by the political needs of local politicians than the needs of the local population and an increasing often unsustainable local government debt. In the late 1990s local Argentinian governments borrowed heavily to cover local expenditures from both domestic and international sources running up debts neither they nor ultimately the central government had the capacity to repay. Argentina defaulted on this debt in 2002 and negotiated a large-scale debt restructuring in 2005–06. Similar although less severe problems existed in both Brazil in the 1990s, but the government took steps to strictly limit the ability of local governments to invest in this way (see Box 11–1).

In many places, including many federal countries, transfer of funds from the central government to subnational units is essential because the center has monopolized the most productive sources of tax revenue. In most cases, national governments impose income taxes because subnational governments lack the resources and skill required to administer such a complex tax and could not do so effectively anyway because the income tax base easily can migrate within a country. Similarly, in the past the major source of tax revenue for some developing countries, import duties, remained a central government resource because most countries have only a few serviceable ports. Very few developing countries today, however, receive a substantial portion of tax revenue from import duties, in part because import duties have been cut sharply over the years in the various international trade negotiations that have lowered tariffs for all countries.

We have just seen that there are few easy ways to reduce government recurrent expenditure to achieve higher public savings. The scope for doing so often was

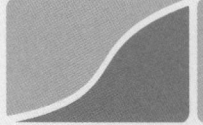

BOX 11-1 REINING IN FISCAL DECENTRALIZATION IN BRAZIL AND CHINA

BRAZIL

Brazil has a federal system of government, and the states have a substantial role in capital and recurrent expenditures. The states in the past also had banks owned by their governments, and these banks contributed in a major way to large-scale profligate state spending over many decades. There were also problems involving borrowing by the central government from the central bank. In 1996, however, the central government took steps to increase the independence of the central bank and began a program to separate the banks from control by state governments. The first phase of this effort involved an effort to privatize state-owned banks in what was called the Program to Reduce State Involvement with Banking Activities. The central government helped with the privatization process, and many of the state banks were privatized and others turned into development agencies. Then in 2000 the government passed the Law of Fiscal Responsibility that prohibited government borrowing from banks it owned or from the central bank. All new borrowing by either the central government or state governments first had to be approved by the central bank and by the senate. In 2002 governments were further prohibited from borrowing within 180 days of the end of a government's term in office. This restrained the large expenditures during the final days of an administration often designed to pay off supporters knowing that the incumbent governor or president would not have to find ways of repaying the loans involved. There were also steps taken to reduce the banks' incentive for making such loans. These efforts have played an important role both in reducing wasteful government expenditures and in reining in the chronic inflation that had plagued Brazil for decades.

CHINA

China's provincial governments are not formally independent of the central government but they have had a substantial degree of autonomy in many economic areas. Formally the largest state-owned commercial banks are national not provincial banks, but in practice local governments and the local branches of the Communist Party have had a major say in appointments to head the local branches of these national banks. The result in the 1990s was that local governments borrowed heavily from the banking system to finance local projects and to support investments of provincial- and city-owned state industrial enterprises, which led to large-scale lending partly to prop up failing state-owned enterprises that fueled bursts of inflation. Inflation was stopped but only when the central government and the central bank imposed lending quotas on state-owned banks and their branches. The government, however, did take steps to change the territory covered by the branches of the large commercial banks so that those territories did not coincide with that of the provincial and local governments, making it more difficult for local politicians to influence the selection of local bank managers.

During the large-scale investment surge that began with the 1997–98 financial crisis in Asia and elsewhere, the Chinese government began a massive state-led investment program that continued throughout the first decade of the twenty-first century, and local governments were pressured to carry out much of this investment program. Many of these investments were well thought out, but local governments lacked the tax base to pay for them and so borrowed heavily from the state-owned commercial banks and local state-owned banks. The result by 2011 was a local debt accumulation of over RMB 10 trillion, which was 25 percent of the gross domestic product (GDP). Given the weakness of the tax base of the local governments, there was a danger that the state-owned commercial banks would again be burdened by a large number of nonperforming loans requiring refinancing by the central government.[a]

[a]Anwar Shah, "Fiscal Decentralization and Macroeconomic Management," *International Tax and Public Finance* 13 (2006), 437–62.

greatest in the areas of military spending and subsidies to cover deficits of state-owned enterprises. Subsidies to state-owned enterprises, however, have been cut over the years either through privatization or by taking steps to make state enterprises competitive and profitable. Military expenditures in developing countries in the twenty-first century are still 2 percent of the GDP on average, with considerable variation across nations, which leaves some room for cutting but not a great deal. The main argument for cutting these latter expenditures is that military forces in developing countries are sometimes a greater danger to their own people than to potential enemies of the nation.

GOVERNMENT REVENUE AND TAXES

Government expenditures have to be funded or paid for. Most government expenditures are funded by revenue from taxes, including **direct taxes** (taxes on corporate or individual income and other payroll taxes such as Medicare and Social Security payments in the United States) or **indirect taxes** (sales taxes, import duties, and value-added taxes that are typically levied as a percentage of the value of a good being sold or imported), but there are other sources of funding. Mineral-rich countries often depend on royalties paid to the government by large petroleum and mineral mining companies, bonds are sometimes issued to cover the costs of a capital investment, and fees are charged for many government-provided services. Revenue can also come through aid grants from other countries or in the form of loans from international lending agencies such as the World Bank.

As incomes per capita rise, the amount of taxes collected, expressed as a share of GDP, also tends to rise, although there is considerable variation among countries as the data in Table 11-2 indicate. The taxes reported in the table do not include what are often referred to as "social contributions"—that is, taxes paid for old-age support such as the Social Security and Medicare systems in the United States. Because high-income nations have more extensive transfer programs of this kind, they also collect more in taxes to finance them. If these taxes were included in the data, the share of taxes out of GDP would rise with country income level in an even more pronounced fashion.

The relationship between the kinds of taxes collected is also associated with per capita income. For countries with low incomes and in the early stages of development, there is typically much greater reliance on international trade taxes. For the three low-income economies in Table 11-2, at least one quarter of tax revenues is obtained from taxes on international trade. As incomes rise, reliance on taxes on international trade falls off significantly. Taxes on income, personal and corporate,

TABLE 11-2 Composition of Tax Systems by Type of Tax,* 2009

| | COMPOSITION OF TAXES (PERCENT OF GDP) | | | | |
COUNTRY/ECONOMY	TOTAL TAXES	DOMESTIC INCOME TAXES	TAXES ON GOODS AND SERVICES	TAXES ON INTERNATIONAL TRADE	OTHER TAXES
Low-income economies					
Bangladesh	8.6	2.2	3.3	2.8	0.4
Cambodia	9.6	1.7	5.4	2.5	0.0
Ghana	12.5	4.2	5.4	2.9	0.0
Lower-middle-income economies					
Indonesia	11.4	5.7	4.8	0.3	0.6
El Salvador	12.5	4.7	6.8	0.9	0.0
Morocco	23.8	9.5	10.5	2.0	1.8
Upper-middle-income economies					
Colombia	11.8	4.5	5.5	0.9	0.8
Thailand	15.2	7.1	7.2	0.9	0.1
Mauritius	18.6	5.4	11.0	0.5	1.7
High-income economies					
South Korea	15.5	6.6	6.0	0.9	2.1
United Kingdom	26.0	13.3	10.1	0.0	2.5
Denmark	34.6	18.0	14.7	0.0	2.0

*Taxes refer to the central government only and are exclusive of social contributions—that is, to programs of old age support and so on.

Source: World Bank, "World Development Indicators," http://databank.worldbank.org.

BOX 11-2 TAX RATES AND SMUGGLING: COLOMBIA

In the classic case from Colombia, the import duty rate on cigarettes was over 100 percent, and it was virtually impossible to purchase duty-paid cigarettes. At such high rates, import duty collections on cigarettes were nil and the market was flooded with smuggled foreign brands. In 1969, the duty rate was reduced to 30 percent. Cigarette smuggling on the poorly policed Caribbean coast of that country continued, but duty-paid packages began to appear in the mountainous interior, and duty collections soared. Smuggling profits possible under a 30 percent duty were no longer high enough to compensate smugglers for the risks of arrest.

provide about half of the tax revenue of Denmark, Korea and the UK; far less in Bangladesh and Cambodia.

In the sections that follow, we review the different kinds of taxes and explain why some taxes are favored over others at different stages of development.

TAXES ON INTERNATIONAL TRADE

Although reliance on the taxes of foreign trade has fallen sharply in recent decades, particularly in middle-income countries, tax revenue structures in developing countries historically have depended heavily on import duties. Many low-income countries remain markedly dependent on import duties. This is particularly so for countries like the Gambia, Lesotho, Côte D'Ivoire, Togo, and Bangladesh, where as much as one quarter to one third of the total government revenue comes from taxes on imports.

For most countries, attempts to raise revenues through higher duties are unfeasible and undesirable on economic grounds. Higher import duties intensify the incentive for smuggling or evading tariffs. Various studies have shown that, for countries with already high duty rates, the incentive to smuggle increases disproportionately with further increases. Therefore, a 10 percent rise in duty rates can result in an increase in smuggling activity by more than 10 percent (Box 11–2). In mountainous countries, such as Afghanistan and Bolivia, or archipelago countries, such as Indonesia and the Philippines, borders are especially porous to smuggled imports. Singapore during the first four decades after independence did not even report its trade with Indonesia largely because it did not want Indonesia to know how much trade between the two countries went through informal (smuggling) rather than official channels.[2]

[2]Bill Guerin, "Indonesia-Singapore Gap More Than Numbers," *Asia Times,* June 27, 2003. Available online at www.atimes.com/atimes/Southeast_Asia/EF27Ae03.html, accessed February 29, 2012.

Export taxes are constitutionally prohibited in the United States and extremely rare in other industrial countries. But export taxes are not uncommon in developing countries, particularly in tropical Africa and Southeast Asia. Taxes ordinarily are imposed on exports of raw materials and have been applied on timber (Ivory Coast and Liberia), tin (Malaysia), jute (Pakistan), and diamonds (Botswana) as well as on foodstuffs, such as coffee (Colombia), peanuts (the Gambia and Senegal), cocoa (Ghana), and tea (Sri Lanka).

Over the past few decades, export taxes have declined in importance as various economic organizations, notably the World Trade Organization (WTO), have put pressure on new members and some old ones to eliminate such taxes or at least not use them to promote particular industries. Some economic groupings such as the European Union and Mercosur ban export taxes. Export taxes often are imposed in the belief that they are paid by foreign consumers. That is, the taxes themselves are thought to be exported to consumers abroad, along with the materials. But the conditions necessary for exporting taxes on exports to foreign consumers rarely are present.

Export taxes also are employed to promote nonrevenue goals, including increased processing of raw materials within natural resource–exporting developing countries. This is done by imposing high rates of export tax on unprocessed exports (cocoa beans or logs) and lower or no rates of tax on processed items fabricated from raw materials (chocolate and plywood). In principle, this use of export taxes should increase the local value added on natural resource exports and thereby generate greater employment and capital income for the local economy. Unfortunately, in many cases, the result has been that a government gives up more in export tax revenues than its country gains in additional local value added, particularly when processed raw materials are exported tax free. One study documents several instances in Southeast Asia and Africa in which the additional value added gained in heavily protected local processing of logs into plywood typically was less than half the amount of export tax revenue that would have been collected had timber been exported in the form of logs.[3]

SALES AND EXCISE TAXES

A much more promising source of government revenue is indirect taxes on domestic transactions, such as sales and excise taxes. **Sales taxes**, including **value-added taxes**, are broad-based consumption taxes imposed on all products except those specifically exempted, usually food, farm inputs, and medicine. **Excise taxes** also are taxes on consumption, but these levies are imposed only on specifically enumerated items, typically tobacco, alcoholic beverages, gambling, and motor fuel. On average, developing countries depend on domestic commodity taxes for a substantial share,

---

[3]Robert Repetto and Malcolm Gillis, eds., *Public Policies and the Misuse of Forest Resources* (New York: Cambridge University Press, 1988), chap. 10.

ranging from a bit over a quarter (the poorest countries plus the United States) to over half of total revenues (Table 11–2).

Virtually every developing country imposes some form of sales tax. In most, the tax is not applied to retail sales because of the burdensome administrative requirements of collecting taxes from thousands of small retailers. In the past, as in Chile before 1970 and in some Indian states, the tax was imposed as a gross turnover tax collected at all levels of production and distribution, with harmful implications for efficiency, income distribution, and virtually every objective of tax policy. In developing countries, administrative problems are more tractable when the sales tax is confined to the manufacturing level: A much smaller number of firms is involved, and the output of manufacturers is far more homogeneous than sales of retailers or wholesalers. For these reasons many low-income countries have used either the single-stage or the value-added form of manufacturers' tax, usually exempting very small producers. This kind of sales tax, however, involves more economic distortions than either a wholesale or a retail tax, and for that reason as well as for revenue motives, more and more middle-income countries have turned to taxes at the retail level.[4]

Increasingly, these taxes have taken the form of one or another variant of the value-added tax (VAT), widely seen as the most effective method of taxing consumption yet developed. More than 60 countries, including all members of the European Union, have adapted the VAT since it was first adopted in its comprehensive retail form in Brazil in 1967.[5] More than 40 developing countries had adopted the tax by 1994, either to replace older, outdated forms of sales taxes or to allow them to reduce reliance on harder-to-collect income and property taxes. The typical VAT tax rate varies from around 10 percent in some of the poorest countries to 15 to 20 percent in most of the others.

Excise taxes might appear to represent an ideal source of additional tax revenue. These typically are imposed on sumptuary items having relatively inelastic demand. When the price elasticity of demand for such products is very low (as for tobacco products) or relatively low (as for alcoholic beverages), an increase in excise tax rates will induce little reduction in consumption of the taxed good. If price elasticity is as low as –0.2, not uncommon for cigarettes in part because smoking tobacco has been shown to be addictive, then an additional 10 percent excise tax on this product would yield an 8 percent increase in tax revenues. Moreover, it is a hallowed theorem in optimal tax theory that taxes levied on items with inelastic demand and supply involve the smallest losses in economic efficiency, or what is the same thing, the least excess burden. **Excess burden** is defined as a loss in private welfare above

---

[4]For a full discussion of the distortions involved in different forms of sales tax, see John Due and Raymond Mikesell, *Sales Taxation: State and Local Structure and Administration* (Baltimore: Johns Hopkins Press, 1983).

[5]Carl Shoup, "Choosing among Types of VAT," in Malcolm Gillis, Carl Shoup, and Gerry Sicat, eds., *Value-Added Taxation in Developing Countries* (Washington, DC: World Bank, 1990).

the amount of government revenue collected from a tax.[6] Further, many agree, with much justification, that consumption of both tobacco and alcohol should be discouraged on health grounds.

PERSONAL AND CORPORATE INCOME TAXES

Harried ministers of finance, perceiving slack in personal and corporate income taxes, often resort to rate increases in these taxes, with no change in the tax base. The results usually are disappointing, particularly for the personal income tax. Even in middle-income countries, only a small proportion of the population is covered by the personal income tax; in contrast, the vast majority of the adult population in the United States files income tax returns each year (although just under half of all U.S. households were required to pay federal income taxes as of 2011).[7] Therefore, few developing countries can rely heavily on the personal income tax for revenues. Whereas the personal income tax accounts for over 40 percent of all federal taxation in the United States (not including Social Security and Medicare payments), rarely does the personal income tax account for close to that much of total central government revenues in developing countries. In low- and middle-income nations, when personal income taxes are applied, they are paid largely by urban elites. Not only are these groups usually the most vocal politically but they have developed such a variety of devices for tax evasion and avoidance that rate increases stand little chance of raising additional revenues. (The same is often true in high-income economies.)

Rate increases for corporate taxes are usually not productive either. In only 16 of 82 developing countries did the corporation income tax account for more than 20 percent of total taxes in the 1980s. In 2006–08, corporate taxes and personal income taxes taken together accounted for more than 30 percent of all revenue in less than half of a sample of more than 60 developing countries. And, in many of those countries, corporate tax collections often originated with foreign natural-resource firms.

NEW SOURCES OF TAX REVENUES

If higher rates on existing taxes are unlikely to raise revenues much, a second option for increasing public savings is to tap entirely new sources of tax revenues. In many developing countries, whether by accident, design, or simply inertia, many sources of tax revenue may have been overlooked entirely. Many countries have not collected taxes on motor vehicle registrations; some have not used urban property taxes as a significant source of revenue; many have not applied corporation income taxes to the income of state-owned enterprises. Kenya, for example, did not seriously tax

---

[6]For a further discussion of optimal taxation and excess burden, see Figure 11–1 and Joseph Stiglitz, *Economics of the Public Sector* (New York: Norton, 1988).

[7]Rachel Johnson, Jim Nunns, Jeff Rohaly, Eric Toder, and Roberton Williams. "Why Some Tax Units Pay No Income Tax," Tax Policy Center, Urban Institute, July 2011.

farmland, and a few countries, such as Indonesia before its 1984 tax reform, did not collect personal income taxes on the salaries of civil servants. China began to experiment with the use of urban property taxes only in the first decade of this century.

CHANGES IN TAX ADMINISTRATION

A far more significant option for increasing tax revenues is to implement changes in tax administration that permit more taxes to be collected from existing tax sources, even at unchanged tax rates. The potential for increased revenues from such action is very large and seldom realized in virtually all developing countries. Shortages of well-trained tax administrators, excessively complex tax laws, light penalties for tax evasion, corruption, and outdated techniques of tax administration combine to make tax evasion one of the most intractable problems of economic policy in developing countries.

The case studies given in Box 11–3 discuss the magnitude of the problem in India and Bolivia, which is typical of many, perhaps most, other developing countries. These examples suggest that efforts to collect a greater share of the taxes due under the current law can increase revenues substantially. But the kinds of administrative reforms required are difficult to implement and especially difficult to sustain. Even Bolivia's successful reform raised its tax ratio to only 7 percent of GDP. Korea at the beginning of its rapid development period, a country noted for its efficient and determined administration, failed in the 1960s to reach its goal of increasing collections by 40 percent through more effective enforcement, although it was able to reduce underreporting of nonagricultural personal income from 75 percent to slightly under 50 percent. Administrative reform can help and is important at any stage of development; however, better tax administration tends to improve with economic development.

FUNDAMENTAL TAX REFORM

The final policy option available for increasing tax revenues is the most difficult to implement but the most effective when it can be done. Fundamental tax reform requires junking old tax systems and replacing them with completely new tax laws and regulations. Implementing tax reform engenders enormous technical and informational, not to mention political, difficulties in all countries. In general, governments resist genuine efforts to reform the tax structure until a fiscal crisis in the form of massive budgetary deficits threatens. Even during a fiscal crisis, it is difficult to mobilize a political consensus to allow unpopular tax measures to pass. Tax policies that protect favored groups and distort the allocation of resources did not just happen; more likely, they were enacted at the behest of someone, ordinarily the privileged and the powerful.

Probably, more has been said, to less effect, about tax reform than almost any topic in economic policy. This is no less true for the United States than for the scores of developing countries where major tax reform efforts have been mounted. That the process is painful and slow is evident from the experience of several countries: In the

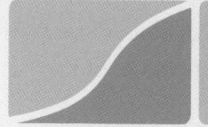

BOX 11-3 TAX ADMINISTRATION IN INDIA AND BOLIVIA IN THE 1980S

INDIA

India during the 1980s provides one of the more egregious examples of poor tax administration. During the fiscal year 1981, for example, it was found that taxes were avoided on at least 40 and possibly 60 percent of potentially taxable income. Almost 70 percent of the taxpayers covered by a survey openly admitted bribing tax officials, and three quarters of the tax auditors admitted accepting bribes to reduce tax payments. The cost of a bribe was commonly known to be about 20 percent of the taxes avoided.

BOLIVIA

In Bolivia during the same period, the tax system was chaotic. More than 400 separate taxes were levied by the national, regional, and city governments. Taxpayer records were out of date, and tax collections were recorded more than a year after they had been paid. Of 120,000 registered taxpayers, one third paid no taxes at all, while 20,000 taxpayers who did pay were not on the register. The administration had all but ceased its data processing. Administration had gotten so bad that the government was helpless to collect taxes during the hyperinflation of the mid-1980s. Tax collections fell to only 1 percent of the GDP. Faced with this chaos, the Bolivian government reformed its tax administration, simplifying it drastically. This, together with price stabilization, enabled the government to collect revenues equivalent to over 7 percent of the GDP by 1990, a low ratio by world standards but a vast improvement for Bolivia.

Sources: Omkar Goswami, Amal Sanyal, and Ira N. Gang, "Taxes, Corruption and Bribes: A Model of Indian Public Finance" (201–13), in Michael Roemer and Christine Jones, eds., *Markets in Developing Countries: Parallel, Fragmented and Black* (San Francisco: ICS Press, 1991); Carlos A. Silvani and Alberto H. J. Radano, "Tax Administration Reform in Bolivia and Uruguay" (19–59) in Richard M. Bird and Milka Casanegra de Jantscher, eds., *Improving Tax Administration in Developing Countries* (Washington, DC: International Monetary Fund, 1992).

United States, the time lag between the birth of tax innovations (tax credit for child-care expenses, inflation proofing of the tax system) and their implementation usually is at least 15 years. If anything, the lag may be slightly shorter in developing countries.

In spite of the difficulties involved, some countries were able to carry through fundamental reforms in tax structure and administration before 1980. The classic example is Japan in the 1880s, when that society began its transformation to a modern industrial power. Korea implemented a major tax reform program in the early 1960s, as did Colombia and Chile in the 1970s and Indonesia in the 1980s (see Box 11-4).

BOX 11-4 INDONESIAN TAX REFORM

In the 1970s Indonesia was a major oil exporter and received more than half of its government revenue from royalties paid by the large oil companies. The increase in petroleum prices caused by the Organization of Petroleum Exporting Countries (OPEC) in 1973 and 1979 increased these royalties to an unprecedented share of the government budget. The Indonesian minister of finance at the time, however, knew that what goes up (in this case petroleum prices) can also come down and he wanted to put Indonesia's government finances on a more stable long term basis. Non-oil sources of tax revenue, however, were based on laws that in many cases went back to the Dutch colonial period and produced limited revenue for the government and did so inefficiently.

In 1981 the ministry of finance began a major effort to completely reform and modernize the Indonesian tax system. The goal of this effort was to create a broader base for the generation of tax revenue, increase the equity of the fiscal system, and generally bring the Indonesian system in line with international best practice. The process involved the complete rewriting of the tax laws, but it also involved fundamental changes in the way taxes were administrated and enforced together with the creation of a computerized tax information system among other major changes.

A team of 25 international experts, including economists, lawyers, accountants, and data processing experts, was put together to assist 10 Indonesian government officials in this endeavor. The role of the team was to help determine what aspects of best tax practice would work best in the Indonesian context. The experts then would present their findings for a full discussion of whether the expert recommendations would in fact work in the Indonesian context in meetings attended by the minister of finance and all of the ministry officials with relevant responsibilities in this area. When this process was completed and necessary adjustments to the recommendations made, the proposal was put first to the president of Indonesia and then to parliament, which passed the legislation in late 1983. Although Indonesia had an authoritarian government at that time, powerful rent-seeking individuals both inside and outside of the government could have had a major influence on the shaping of tax reform as happens in so many countries, but in this case the recommendations that were passed largely reflected international best practice, not the special interests of rent seekers.

The key reforms were the introduction of a low-rate simplified value-added tax together with major changes in the personal and corporate income tax codes. Nonpetroleum government revenues as a result of these reforms rose from

6 percent of Indonesia's GDP just before the passage of the reforms to 10 percent of GDP by the early 1990s. This increase in revenue had much to do with the fiscal stability that Indonesia enjoyed when petroleum prices and government royalties from petroleum fell in 1986.

Source: Michael Roemer and Joseph Stern, "Indonesia: Economic Policy Reform," (63–64), in Dwight H. Perkins, Richard Pagett, Michael Roemer, Donald Snodgrass, and Joseph Stern, eds., *Assisting Development in a Changing World: The Harvard Institute for International Development, 1980–1995* (Cambridge: Distributed by Harvard University Press, 1997).

After 1980, the pace of tax reform quickened notably, in both developing and industrial countries, with many similarities in the various reform programs. Throughout much of the postwar period, tax systems commonly were fine-tuned to achieve a wide variety of nonrevenue objectives. In particular, governments in developed and developing nations alike commonly sought substantial income redistribution through the use of steeply progressive tax rates. Also, complex and largely impossible to administer systems of tax incentives were widely used in attempts to redirect resources to high-priority economic sectors and promote foreign investment, regional development, and even stock exchanges.

While fine-tuning tax systems someday may yield the desired results, it requires, at a minimum, strong machinery for tax administration and traditions of taxpayer compliance. Within developing countries, at least, there has been growing recognition that such conditions seldom prevail. Governments increasingly have turned away from reliance on steeply progressive tax rates and complicated, costly tax incentive programs.

The 1980s through the beginning of the twenty-first century saw a worldwide movement toward an entirely different type of tax system, with a shift toward vastly simplified taxes imposed at much flatter rates and with much broader bases[8] and increasingly greater reliance on consumption rather than income taxation. Tax reform programs in Bolivia, Chile, Colombia, India, Indonesia, Jamaica, and Malawi exemplify most of these trends.[9]

Two aspects of this worldwide movement in tax reform are especially salient. First, the top marginal income tax rates of 60 to 70 percent were not uncommon from 1945 to 1979. But, since 1984, country after country has slashed the top marginal rate, often substantially. Table 11–3 shows this phenomenon in a selection of developing countries. During the same period, many industrial nations, ranging from Australia and Austria through the United Kingdom and the United States also cut the top rate sharply.

---

[8]Joseph A. Pechman, ed., *World Tax Reform: A Progress Report* (Washington, DC: Brookings Institute, 1988), p. 13.

[9]A number of these cases are discussed in Malcolm Gillis, ed., *Tax Reform in Developing Countries* (Durham, NC: Duke University Press, 1989).

TABLE 11-3 Countries Reducing Highest Rates of Income Tax, 1984–2009

COUNTRY	1984–85	2009
Low-income economies		
Tanzania	75	30
Uganda	70	30
India	62	30
Ghana	65	25
Lower-middle-income economies		
Papua New Guinea	50	42
Pakistan	60	20
Philippines	60	32
Sri Lanka	55	35
Indonesia	45	35
Peru	50	30
Guatemala	42	31
Jamaica	58	25
Upper-middle-income economies		
Botswana	75	25
Brazil	60	27.5
Costa Rica	50	15
Colombia	49	33
Thailand	65	37
Argentina	45	35
Mexico	55	28
Malaysia	55	27
Chile	56	40

Sources: George J. Yost III, ed., *1994 International Tax Summaries, Coopers & Lybrand International Tax Network* (New York: Wiley, 1994); Glenn P. Jenkins, "Tax Reform: Lessons Learned," in Dwight H. Perkins and Michael Roemer, eds., *Reforming Economic Systems in Developing Countries* (Cambridge: Harvard Institute for International Development, 1991); Denise Bedell, "Personal Income Tax Rates," *Global Finance*, available at www.gfmag.com/tools/global-database/economic-data/10442-personal-income-tax-rates.html#axzz1YDeg5nMb, accessed February 2012.

In many of these cases, deep cutbacks in the highest tax rates were accompanied by reforms involving a very substantial broadening of the income tax base, through the reduction of special tax incentives, abolition of tax shelters, and the like. This pattern was especially notable in Bolivia, Colombia, Indonesia, Jamaica, and Sri Lanka, so that, even with a rate reduction, higher-income groups often ended up paying a higher proportion of total taxes than before.

Reasons for the worldwide shift toward lower tax rates on broader income tax bases are not difficult to find. First, income taxes imposed at high marginal rates have proven difficult or impossible to administrate, even in wealthy countries such as the United States. With high marginal tax rates, the incentives to evade taxes (through concealment of income) or avoid taxes (by hiring expensive legal talent to devise tax shelters) are very high. Second, the growing mobility of capital across international boundaries has meant that the risk of capital flight from a particular country increases when that country's top rates of income tax exceed those prevailing in industrial nations, where tax rates have been falling.[10] Third, the operation of the income tax systems of such developed nations as the United States and Japan has placed downward pressure on the tax rates everywhere. This is because of the *foreign income tax credit,* wherein a country like the United States allows foreign income taxes to be credited (subtracted) from U.S. taxes due on income repatriated from abroad. This credit could be used, however, up to only the amount of tax payable at U.S. rates, which was reduced from 50 to 28 percent in 1986. Finally, high marginal rates of income tax did not prove to be particularly efficacious in correcting severe inequalities in income distribution in either rich or poor countries.

The second striking feature of recent tax reforms worldwide has been the steadily growing number of countries adopting the value-added tax. Several factors account for the popularity of the VAT: The two most important are its reputation as a money machine and its administrative advantages, relative to other forms of sales taxes and income taxes.[11] The record of the VAT in generating large amounts of revenue quickly and in a comparatively painless fashion has given it a reputation as an efficient way to generate money. Although this reputation stems largely from the experience in European countries, the record in developing countries does lend some support to the alleged revenue advantages of the VAT. In Indonesia, the 4 percent share of the value-added tax in GDP in 1987 was nearly three times the share garnered in 1983 by the taxes it replaced. Notwithstanding the marked revenue success of the VAT in nations such as Brazil, Chile, and Indonesia, its reputation as a money machine for many other countries appears to have been at least slightly overstated.

In the 1980s, it was common to hear the claim that the VAT was largely self-administering. This is not so, but the tax-credit type of VAT has three principal advantages over single-stage retail and nonretail sales taxes in limiting the scope for evasion. First, the VAT is self-policing to some extent because underpayment of the tax by a seller (except, of course, a retail firm) reduces the tax credit available to the buying firm. Even so, firms that also are subject to income taxes have incentives to suppress information on purchases and sales to avoid both the value-added and income taxes. Also, this possible advantage of the VAT is diminished when evasion at the final (retail) stage of distribution is endemic. Second, cross-checking of invoices enables the tax administration to match invoices received by purchasers against those retained by sellers. The cross-check feature is a valuable aid in audit activities but no substitute for a true, systematic audit. Third, that a large share of the VAT is collected before the retail level is an advantage particularly because, in most developing countries, an abundance of small-scale retail firms do not keep adequate

---

[10]For discussion of the implications for taxation of growing international mobility of financial and physical capital, see Dwight R. Lee and Richard B. McKenzie, "The International Political Economy of Declining Tax Rates," *National Tax Journal* 42, no. 2 (March 1989), 79–87.

[11]For a full discussion of these reasons, see Alan A. Tait, *Value-Added Tax* (Washington, DC: International Monetary Fund, 1988), chap. 1.

records. In sum, the administrative advantages of the VAT are very real, if sometimes exaggerated by enthusiastic proponents.[12]

TAXES AND INCOME DISTRIBUTION

For decades, developed and developing countries alike have sought to use the fiscal system, particularly taxation, to redress income inequalities generated by the operation of the private market. Social philosophers from John Stuart Mill and eminent nineteenth-century Chilean historian Francisco Encina to twentieth-century philosophers such as John Rawls have sought to establish a philosophical basis for income redistribution, primarily through progressive taxes. No scientific basis is used to determine the optimal degree of income redistribution in any society. And across developing countries different views prevail as to the ideal distribution of income. But, in virtually all countries, the notion of **fiscal equity** permeates discussions of budgetary operations. In the overwhelming majority of countries, fiscal equity is typically defined in terms of the impact of tax and expenditure policy on the distribution of economic well-being. Progressive taxes, those that bear more heavily on better-off citizens than on poor ones, and expenditures whose benefits are concentrated on the least advantaged are viewed as more equitable than regressive taxes and expenditures.

On the tax side of the budget, the materialistic conception of equity requires that most taxes be based on the **ability to pay**. The ability to pay can be measured by income, consumption, wealth, or some combination of all three. Clearly, individuals with higher incomes over their life spans have a greater ability to pay taxes, quite apart from the moral question of whether they should do so. Indeed, the redistribution impact of taxation almost always is expressed in terms of its effects on income. However, philosophers since the time of Thomas Hobbes, a seventeenth-century English philosopher, have argued that consumption furnishes a better index of ability to pay than income; in this view, tax obligations are best geared to what people take out of society (consume) rather than what they put into society (as measured by income).

In practice, developing countries have relied heavily on these two measures of ability in fashioning tax systems. Personal and corporate income taxes employ income as the indicator; sales taxes and customs duties are indirect assessments of taxes on consumption. At a minimum, equity usually is assumed to require the avoidance of regressive taxes whenever possible. A number of tax instruments have been employed to secure greater progressivity in principle, if not in practice; all suffer from limitations to one degree or another.

---

[12]For a succinct summary of some of these issues, see John F. Due, "Some Unresolved Issues in Design and Implementation of Value-Added Taxes," *National Tax Journal* 42, no. 4 (December 1990), 383–98.

PERSONAL INCOME TAXES

The most widely used device for securing greater progressivity has been steeply progressive rates under the personal income tax. In some countries in some periods, nominal or legal marginal income tax rates have reached very high levels, even for relatively low incomes. Thus, for example, tax rates applicable to any income in excess of $1,000 in Indonesia in 1967 reached 75 percent, largely because tax rates were not indexed to rapid inflation; in Algeria in the 1960s, all income in excess of $10,000 was subject to marginal tax rates of nearly 100 percent; Tanzania imposed top marginal rates of 95 percent as late as 1981. Although, in most developing countries, marginal income tax rates are considerably lower than the preceding examples and, as is apparent from Table 11–3, have been falling, some countries still attempt to impose rates in excess of 50 percent, such as Angola, Gabon, and Cuba, but most countries with marginal rates at this level in the twenty-first century are high-income European states with large social welfare programs.

If the tax administration machinery functioned well and capital were immobile among countries, the pattern of actual tax payments of high-income taxpayers would resemble the legal, or theoretical, patterns just described. In fact, in most countries, **effective taxes** (the taxes actually collected as a percent of income) fall well short of theoretical liabilities. Faced with high income tax rates, taxpayers everywhere tend to react in three ways: (1) They evade taxes by concealing income, particularly capital income not subject to withholding arrangements; (2) they avoid taxes by altering economic behavior to reduce tax liability, whether by supplying fewer labor services, shipping capital to tax havens abroad, or hiring lawyers to find loopholes in the tax law; and (3) they bribe tax assessors to accept false returns.

For all these reasons, the achievement of substantial income redistribution through progressive income taxes has proven difficult in all countries, including the United States and the three Scandinavian nations where tax rates were long among the world's most progressive. Tax avoidance is the favored avenue for reducing tax liability in the United States, where use of the other methods can result in imprisonment. But, where tax enforcement is relatively weak, particularly where criminal penalties for evasion are absent and tax officials deeply underpaid, tax evasion and bribery are used more commonly. The scope for substantial redistribution through the income tax is, therefore, even more limited in developing countries than in the United States or Sweden.

Notwithstanding these problems, a significant share of the income of the wealthiest members of society is caught in the income tax net in many developing countries. Revenues from personal income tax collections in countries such as Colombia, South Korea, and Chile have been as high as 15 percent of total taxes and in a few others have run between 5 and 10 percent of the total. In virtually all developing countries, the entirety of such taxes is collected from the top 20 percent of the income distribution. This means, of course, that the very presence of an income tax, even one imposed at proportional rather than progressive rates, tends to reduce income inequality.

TAXES ON LUXURY CONSUMPTION

In view of the difficulties of securing a significant redistribution through income taxes, countries may employ heavy indirect taxes on luxury consumption as a means of enhancing the progressivity of the tax system. Efforts to achieve this goal usually center on internal indirect taxes, such as sales, and on customs duties on imports, but not excises on tobacco and alcohol.

Several developing countries have found that, provided tax rates are kept to enforceable levels, high rates of internal indirect taxes on luxury goods and services, coupled with lower taxes on less income-elastic items, can contribute to greater progressivity in the tax system. For revenue purposes, countries typically impose basic rates of sales taxes on nonluxuries at between 4 and 8 percent of manufacturers' values. This is equivalent to retail taxes of between 2 and 4 percent because taxes imposed at this level exclude wholesale and retail margins. Food, except that consumed in restaurants, almost always is exempted from any sales tax intended to promote redistributive goals. In developing countries, the exemption of food by itself renders most sales taxes at least faintly progressive, given the high proportion (up to 40 percent in many middle-income countries and over 50 percent in low income countries) of income of poor households spent on food. Sales taxes involving a limited number of luxury rates of between 20 and 30 percent at the manufacturers' level have been found to be workable.

The redistributive potential of sales tax rates differentiated in this way, however, is limited by the same administrative and compliance constraints standing in the way of the heavier use of income taxation in developing countries. While sales taxes are not as difficult to administer as income taxes, they do not collect themselves. A manufacturer's sales tax system employing three or even four rates may be administratively feasible in most countries, even when the highest rate approaches 40 percent. Rates much higher than that or reliance on a profusion of rates in an attempt to fine-tune the tax lead to substantial incentives and opportunities for tax evasion. Jamaica had over 15 rates before 1986, and Chile had over 20 from 1960 to 1970. In recognition of these problems, Indonesia adopted a flat-rate manufacturers' tax in 1985: The tax applied at a rate of 10 percent on *all* manufactured items and imports. The tax nevertheless was slightly progressive because it did not apply to items that did not go through a manufacturing process, including most foodstuffs consumed by low-income families.

Although the use of internal indirect taxes, such as sales taxes, can contribute to income redistribution goals without causing serious misallocation of resources, the same cannot be said for the use of customs duties. Sales taxes are imposed on all taxable goods without regard to national origin, including goods produced domestically as well as abroad. Tariffs apply only to imported goods. Virtually all countries, developed and developing, use customs duties to protect existing domestic industry. Developing countries in particular employ customs duties as the principal means of encouraging domestic industry to produce goods that formerly were imported. This strategy, called **import substitution**, is examined at length in Chapter 18.

Deliberate policies to encourage import substitution through the use of high protective tariffs, under certain conditions, might lead to results sought by policy makers. But accidental import substitution arises when tariffs are used for purposes other than protection, and this is unlikely to have positive results. Many countries, as already pointed out, use high tariffs to achieve heavier taxation of luxury consumption. Often heavy tariffs are imposed on imported luxury items for which there is no intention of encouraging domestic production. Therefore, many Latin American and some Asian countries have levied customs tariffs of 100 to 150 percent of value on such appliances as electric knives, hair dryers, sporting goods, and mechanical toys. For most countries, these items are clearly highly income elastic and apt candidates for luxury taxation.

But efforts to tax luxuries through high customs duties lead to unintended, and almost irresistible, incentives for domestic production or assembly of such products. In virtually all countries, save the very poorest, alert domestic and foreign entrepreneurs have been quick to seize on such opportunities. By the time local assembly operations are established, they usually can make a politically convincing case that the duties should be retained to enable local production to continue, even when the value added domestically is as low as 10 percent of the value of the product. Such operations, if subject to any local sales taxes, usually succeed in being taxed at the basic tax rate, usually 5 to 10 percent. By relying on tariffs for luxury taxation, the government ultimately forgoes the revenues it previously collected from duties on luxury goods, as well as severely undermining the very aims of luxury taxation.

If, instead, higher luxury rates on imports are imposed under a sales tax collected on both imports and any domestic production that may develop, unintended import substitution can be avoided. The use of import tariffs for luxury taxation—indeed, for any purpose other than providing protection to domestic industry—is one illustration of the general problem of using one economic policy instrument (tariffs) to achieve more than one purpose (protection, luxury taxation, and revenue). Reliance on import duties for revenue is subject to the same pitfalls just discussed. If it is desired to increase government revenue from imports, a 10 percent sales tax applied both to imports and any future domestic production yields at least as much revenue as a 10 percent import duty, without leading to accidental protection.

CORPORATE INCOME AND PROPERTY TAXES: THE INCIDENCE PROBLEM

Income taxes on domestic corporations and property taxes often are mentioned as possible methods for securing income redistribution through the budget. Corporate income ultimately is received, through dividends and capital gains, almost exclusively by the upper 5 to 10 percent of the income distribution. Also, ownership of wealth, which in many lower-income countries largely takes the form of land, tends to be even more concentrated than income. But, to a greater extent in developing than in developed countries, efforts to secure significant fiscal redistribution through heavier taxes on domestic corporations and property are limited both by administrative and economic realities.

Administrative problems bedevil efforts to collect income taxes from domestic firms to at least as great an extent as for income taxes on individuals. Hence, in many countries where corporate taxes on local firms have been important, as much as two thirds to three quarters of nonoil corporate taxes flow from state-owned firms, not from private firms owned by high-income individuals. Taxes on land should be subject to less severe administrative problems because it is an asset that cannot be hidden easily. However, land valuation for tax purposes has proven difficult even in Canada and the United States. It is more difficult in developing countries. Few developing countries have been able to assess property at anything approaching its true value.

Economic realities hinder efforts to achieve greater progressivity in the tax system through heavier use of corporate and land taxes because of the tendency for taxation to unintentionally burden groups other than those directly taxed. This is the **incidence problem**. The incidence of a tax is its ultimate impact, not who actually pays the tax to the government but whose income finally is affected by the tax when all economic agents have adjusted in response to the tax. The point of incidence is not always the point of initial impact. Taxes on domestic corporations may reduce the income of capitalists, who in turn might shift their investment patterns to reduce taxation. The income of the workers they employ and the prices charged to consumers may be affected as well. Ultimately, all taxes are paid by people, not by things such as corporations and property parcels.

The implications of incidence issues may be illuminated by a simple application of incidence analysis to the corporation income tax. Consider a profit-maximizing company that has no significant monopoly power in the domestic market. If taxes on the company's income are increased in a given year, then after-tax returns to its shareholders in that year are reduced by the full amount of the tax. In the short term, the incidence of the tax clearly is on shareholders. Because shareholders everywhere are concentrated in higher-income groups, the tax is progressive in the short run. If capital were immobile, unable to leave the corporate sector, the long-term incidence of the tax also would rest on shareholders and the tax would be progressive in the long run as well.

But, in the long run, capital can move out of the corporate sector. To the extent that capital is mobile domestically but not internationally, the corporate tax also is progressive in the long run. Returns on capital remaining in the corporate sector are reduced by the tax. Untaxed capital owners employed outside the corporate sector also suffer a reduction in returns, because movement of capital from the taxed corporate sector drives down the rate of return in the untaxed sector. Because the corporate tax reduces returns to capital throughout the economy, all capital owners suffer, including owners of housing assets, and in a closed economy, the long-run incidence again is progressive.

However, few if any developing economies are completely closed; indeed, capital in recent years has become much more mobile internationally. To the extent that capital can move across national borders and higher returns are available in other countries, domestic capital migrates to escape higher corporate taxes. But as capital leaves an economy, ultimately output is curtailed and the marginal productivity of workers falls. Prices of items produced with domestic capital rise. In this way, an increase in corporate taxes may be borne by domestic consumers, who pay higher prices for the reduced supply of corporate-sector goods. Domestic workers, whose income is reduced when production is curtailed, may also bear a part of the burden of the corporate tax. Hence the corporate tax may be regressive (worsen the income distribution) in the long run. Although under other plausible conditions, an increase in the corporation income tax may result in greater relative burdens on capitalists, this scenario is sufficient to illustrate that often the intentions of a redistributive tax policy may be thwarted by all the workings of the economy. Policy makers cannot be sure that all taxes imposed on wealthy capital owners ultimately are paid by them.

The foregoing discussion suggests that, whereas some tax instruments may achieve income redistribution in developing countries, the opportunities for doing so are limited in most countries, a conclusion supported by a large number of empirical studies. With few exceptions, these studies show that the failure to administer personal income taxes effectively—the failure to utilize the limited opportunities for heavier taxes on luxury consumption, overreliance on revenue-productive but regressive excise taxes, and inclusion of food in sales taxes—significantly reduces the redistribution impact of tax systems. Tax systems in developing countries tend to produce a burden roughly proportional across income groups, with some tendency for progressivity at the very top of the income scale. The very wealthy pay a somewhat greater proportion of their income in taxes than the poor, but the poor still pay substantial taxes: at least 10 percent of their income in many cases studied. Of course, in the absence of such efforts, the after-tax distribution of income may have been even more unequal. This suggests that, although difficult to implement and often disappointing in results, tax reforms intended to reduce income inequality are not futile exercises and they may prevent taxes from making the poor worse off.

The limits of tax policy suggest that, if the budget is to serve redistribution purposes, the primary emphasis must be on expenditure policy. Where redistribution through expenditures has been a high priority of governments, the results generally have been encouraging. The effects of government expenditure on income distribution are even more difficult to measure than those of taxes. But both the qualitative and the quantitative evidence available strongly indicate that, in developing countries, budget expenditures may transfer very substantial resources to lower-income households, in some cases as much as 50 percent of their income. Some of the measures using government expenditures to attack poverty were discussed in Chapter 6.

ECONOMIC EFFICIENCY AND THE BUDGET

SOURCES OF INEFFICIENCY

On the expenditure side of the budget, *social cost-benefit analysis* can be deployed to enhance efficiency (reduce waste) in government spending. On the tax side, promotion of economic efficiency is more problematic.

All taxes lead to inefficiencies to one degree or another. The objective, therefore, is to minimize tax-induced inefficiencies consistent with other goals of tax policy. In most developing societies, this objective largely reduces the necessity of identifying examples of waste engendered by taxes and purging them from the system. If a particular feature of a tax system involves large efficiency losses, called *excess burden* in public economics, and at the same time contributes little or nothing to such other policy goals as income redistribution, then that feature is an obvious candidate for abolition. A full discussion of those elements of tax systems that qualify for such treatment is properly the subject of an extended public finance monograph. We can do little more here than indicate some of the principal examples.

A major source of inefficiency in taxation is excessive costs of tax administration. In some countries and for some taxes, these costs have been so high that they call into question the desirability of using certain taxes for any purpose. This is true for certain kinds of narrow-based stamp taxes that have been used in Latin America to collect government revenue on the documentation of transfer of assets, rental agreements, checks, and ordinary business transactions. Many stamp taxes cost more to administer than they collect in revenue.

In some countries, even broad-based taxes have had inordinately high costs of collection. Sales taxes in Chile and Ecuador in the 1960s before the reform of their tax systems cost $1 in administration for every $4. Administrative costs to collect net taxes of $100 in most Organization for Economic Co-Operation and Development (OECD) countries in the early twenty-first century in contrast range from $0.42 to $2.08, with the United States at $0.47 at the low end and Japan at $1.50 at the higher end.[13] And, because taxes on capital gains are so difficult to administer everywhere, including North America, the cost of collecting this component of income taxes often exceeds the revenue in developing countries.

Many developing countries offer substantial tax incentives to encourage investment in particular activities and regions. Many of these, particularly income tax holidays for approved firms, have proven very difficult to administer and few have

---

[13]These are the average rates for 2000–02 and are taken from OECD, *Tax Administration in OECD Countries: Comparative Information Series* (Paris: Organization for Economic Cooperation and Development, 2004).

led to the desired result.[14] Given persistently pressing revenue requirements in most countries, granting liberal tax incentives may have no effect other than requiring higher rates of tax on taxpayers who do not qualify for incentives. It is a dictum of fiscal theory that economic waste (inefficiency) arising from taxation increases by the square of the tax rate employed, not proportionately. Therefore, it is not difficult to see that unsuccessful tax incentive programs involve inefficiencies for the economy as a whole that are not compensated for by any significant benefits. Largely for this reason, Indonesia abolished all forms of tax incentives in a sweeping tax reform in 1984.

Finally, some features of major tax sources involve needless waste. From the earlier discussion of the use of import duties for luxury tax purposes, it is clear that this is often a major source of inefficiency. The use of progressive tax rates in a corporation income tax is another example. Progressive rates of corporate tax, where they cannot be enforced, do little to contribute to income redistribution; and where they can be enforced, they lead to several kinds of waste. Two of the most important are fragmentation of business firms and inefficiency in business operations. The incentive for fragmentation is evident: Rather than be subject to high marginal rates of taxes, firms tend to split into smaller units and lose any cost advantages of size. Where high progressive rates are employed for company income, the tax takes a high proportion (say, 70 percent) of each additional dollar of earnings, so the incentive to control costs within the firm is reduced. For example, for a firm facing a marginal tax rate of 70 percent, an additional outlay of $1,000 for materials involves a net cost to the firm of only $300, because at the same time taxes are reduced by $700.

NEUTRALITY AND EFFICIENCY: LESSONS FROM EXPERIENCE

Experience around the world, both in developed and developing countries, seems to indicate that, in societies where efficiency in taxation matters, this objective is best pursued by reliance on taxes that are as neutral as possible. A **neutral tax** is one that does not lead to a material change in the structure of private incentives that would prevail in the absence of the tax. A neutral tax system, then, is one that relies, to the extent possible, on uniform rates: a tax on all income at a flat rate or a sales tax with the same rate applied to all goods and services. A neutral tax system cannot be an efficient tax system.

An **efficient tax system** involves a minimum amount of excess burden for raising a required amount of revenue, where the *excess burden* of a tax is the loss in total welfare, over and above the amount of tax revenues collected by the government. Figure 11–1 demonstrates how the excess burden of, say, a commodity tax is greater the more elastic the demand or the supply of the taxed item. Figure 11–1a depicts the inelastic case, good A, whereas panel b shows the elastic case, good B. Constant

---

[14]See, for example, Arnold C. Harberger, "Principles of Taxation Applied to Developing Countries: What Have We Learned?" in Michael Boskin and Charles E. McLure Jr., eds., *World Tax Reform: Case Studies of Developed and Developing Countries* (San Francisco: ICS Press, 1990).

marginal costs (MC) are assumed in both cases and at the same level for both goods to portray more starkly the contrasting results achieved in those cases. Before the tax is imposed on either good, the equilibrium price and quantity are P_a and Q_a for good A and P_b and Q_b for good B. Now, we impose a tax rate (t) on both goods. The new equilibrium (post-tax) magnitudes are P_{at} and Q_{at} for good A and P_{bt} and Q_{bt} for good B. For good A, the total amount of government revenue is the rectangle $P_aP_{at}cd$. The total loss in consumer surplus arising from the tax is the trapezoid $P_aP_{at}ce$. The excess of the loss in consumer surplus over the amount of government revenue is the conventional measure of efficiency loss from a tax, or excess burden. For good A, the excess burden is the small triangle cde. By similar reasoning, the excess burden in the case of good B is the larger triangle fgh. We see that taxes of equivalent rates involve more excess burden when imposed on goods with elastic demand.

We can see that efficient taxation requires neither uniformity nor neutrality but many different tax rates on different goods, with tax rates lower for goods with elastic demand and higher for goods with inelastic demand. This is known as the **Ramsey rule**, or the **inverse elasticity rule**. The problem is that a tax system under this rule would be decidedly regressive: The highest taxes would be required on foodstuffs, drinking water, and sumptuary items. Taxes would be lower on items such as clothing, services, and foreign travel, which tend to be both price and income elastic.

The principle of neutrality in taxation is not nearly as intellectually satisfying a guide to tax policy as efficient taxation. Nevertheless, neutral taxation is to be preferred as one of the underlying principles of taxation, along with equity, until such

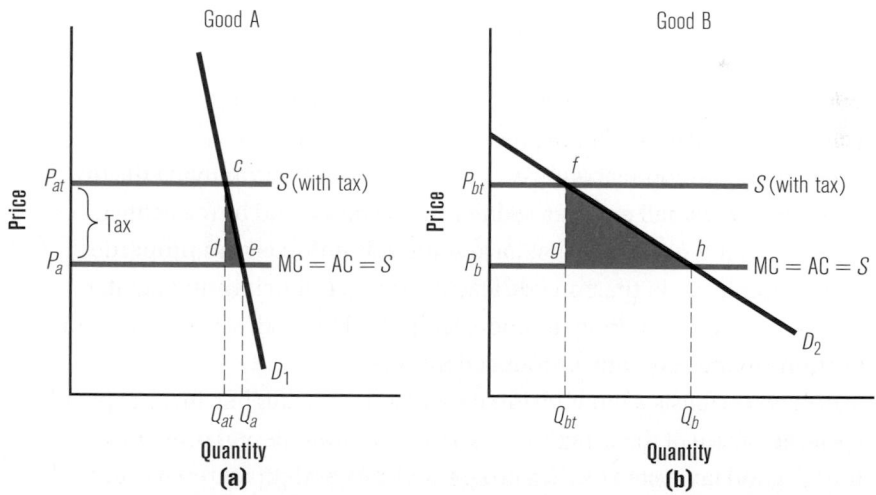

FIGURE 11-1 Taxation and Efficiency: Excess Burden of Commodity Taxes with Constant Marginal (MC) and Average Costs (AC), under Competition

(a) Case 1: Inelastic demand. (b) Case 2: Elastic demand. The shaded area in each case represents the excess burden of equal tax rates imposed on different goods. The greater the elasticity, the greater the excess burden.

time as analysts are able to identify optimal departures from neutrality—and uniformity in tax rates—in real-world settings. More intellectually satisfying tax policies must also wait until such time as administrative capacities are equal to the task of operating necessarily complicated structures of efficient or optimal taxes.

There is a paradox here. Neutral, uniform-rate taxes are less suited for efficiency goals than perfectly administered efficient taxes. Yet neutral tax systems are more likely to enhance efficiency in the economy than are efficient or optimal systems because neutral systems with uniform rates can be administered most easily and are much less vulnerable to evasion. This is not to say that neutrality has ever been or should be the overriding goal of tax policy. Governments often undertake very deliberate departures from neutral tax treatment of certain sectors or groups of society to achieve other policy goals. But, in real-world settings, these departures involve costs, not only in terms of tax administration but often in both equity and efficiency terms as well.

SUMMARY

- The expenditure side of the government budget is made up of capital or development items together with a wide variety of current use expenditures that are called *recurrent costs*. Developing country governments and donor aid programs frequently waste capital by neglecting the recurrent costs needed to maintain that capital.
- Developing countries rely mainly on indirect taxes (sales or value-added taxes and customs duties) rather than income and capital gains taxes because the latter are extremely difficult and expensive to administer in developing countries and thus produce less revenue.
- Tax reform in developing countries generally involves simplifying the tax system (one or a small number of different tax rates) and introducing taxes such as the value-added tax that have some self-enforcement properties. Greater complexity in the tax code leads to greater difficulty and greater corruption in administering the code. Simplified tax codes also reduce the distortions in the economy introduced by taxes.
- Taxation on the basis of an individual's ability to pay (higher-income people pay a larger share of their income in taxes) is a fundamental principle of equity. A good tax system is thus progressive rather than regressive, but progressive tax systems are extremely difficult to administer, particularly in developing countries, except in limited areas such as the exemption of food from sales taxes. When one looks at the actual incidence of taxes on high- and low-income earners, taxes that are designed to be progressive often turn out to be the opposite, and tax reform needs to take this into account.

12

Financial Development and Inflation

A country's **financial system** consists of a variety of interconnected financial institutions, both formal and informal. A central bank lies at the core of the organized financial system and is responsible for the control of the money supply and the general supervision of organized financial activity. Virtually everywhere, and particularly in developing countries, the commercial banking system is the most visible and vital component of the formal financial system, as acceptor of deposits and grantor of shorter-term credit. Other elements of the formal financial system include savings banks; insurance companies; and in a growing number of middle-income countries, pension funds and investment banks specializing in long-term credit as well as emerging stock exchanges. In high-income countries since the early 1990s there was the creation of a new set of institutions called *hedge funds* that played an important role in the global economic crisis of 2008–09.

Standing behind these financial institutions are a variety of government and sometimes private institutions whose role is to regulate the financial system. Typically separate agencies exist to regulate the commercial banks and the stock market, but the nature of regulation of the financial system is constantly changing. The need for regulation arises first and foremost from the fact that financial institutions exist primarily to manage the financial assets of people and companies other than the owners and managers of the financial institutions themselves. Regulation is designed to ensure that the financial assets of the public are managed responsibly without excessive risk. In the 1990s and during the first years of the twenty-first century the trend in high-income countries in North America and Europe was to reduce and even eliminate many of the regulations governing the financial system in the belief that the market would be an adequate regulator on its own. Many financial companies also developed new financial instruments that were designed to provide a service, such as insurance, that would not be subject to the standard regulations governing insurance contracts (these new instruments were called *credit default swaps*). This trend toward further liberalization of financial markets came to an abrupt end in 2009 and 2010 as the global financial crisis made it clear that markets on their own could not adequately control risky behavior of financial institutions, and a wide variety of new regulations were put in place.

The financial crisis of 2008–09 started in the United States and spread quickly to Europe, but developing countries were soon enveloped in the consequences of the global recession. The primary difference between developing and high-income countries in this context was that the developing country financial systems were simpler and made much less use of the more exotic financial instruments than did high-income countries. Commercial banks dominated the financial system in developing countries, investment banks if they existed at all were smaller and weaker, and insurance companies were in their infancy. The existence of financial systems depends on trust that they will manage a depositor's or an investor's funds well and that trust is built on a history of responsible behavior, on an effective regulatory system, and on the transparency of the operations of the financial organizations themselves. It takes decades or longer to develop trustworthy institutions and trust can be lost quickly as happened in 2008–09, but in developing countries this trust and the related effective regulation was largely confined to the commercial banks.

The limited scope of the formal financial sector in developing countries, however, left many people and small companies without ready access to credit or even to a reliable place to put their savings. In recent decades this has led to the creation of new **micro-credit institutions** designed to reach these left-out individuals, but long before formal micro-credit institutions were created, there was in virtually all developing countries an informal financial sector existing alongside the formal one. Informal financial institutions include pawnshops, local moneylenders, trade credit, and other arrangements involving the borrowing and lending of money such as intrafamily transfers and cooperative credit. In very low income countries, or even in some middle-income countries, the informal financial sector may rival the formal system in size. In almost all cases the informal sector is unregulated, although governments do interfere in its operation from time to time.

Financial policy embraces all measures intended to affect the growth, utilization, efficiency, and diversification of the financial system. In North America and western Europe, the term *financial policy* ordinarily is used as a synonym for *monetary policy*, the use of monetary instruments to reduce price instability caused by fluctuations in either internal or external markets. In the United States, these instruments include open-market operations, changes in legal reserve requirements of commercial banks, and shifts in central bank (Federal Reserve System) lending (rediscount) rates to commercial banks (these terms are explained later in this chapter). In developing countries, the term *financial policy* typically has a much broader meaning. Monetary policy is part of financial policy but so are measures intended to encourage the growth of savings in the form of financial assets, develop money and capital markets, and allocate credit among different economic sectors. Regulation to control risk, as in the 1997–98 and the 2008–09 financial crises, is also a component of financial policy.

THE FUNCTIONS OF A FINANCIAL SYSTEM

The financial system provides four basic services essential for the smooth functioning of an economy. First, it provides a medium of exchange and a store of value, called *money*, which also serves as a unit of account to measure the value of the transactions. Second, it provides channels for mobilizing savings from numerous sources and channeling them to investors, a process called *financial intermediation*. Third, it provides a means of transferring and distributing risk across the economy. Fourth, it provides a set of policy instruments for the stabilization of economic activity. When these functions are managed poorly the result on a macro level can be a financial crisis leading to a global recession, inflation, or a debt crisis. The management of inflationary pressures will be discussed in this chapter and debt crises are the subject of Chapter 13.

MONEY AND THE MONEY SUPPLY

An economy without money as a **medium of exchange** is primitive. Trade between individuals must take the form of high-cost, inefficient barter transactions. In a barter economy, goods have prices, but they are expressed in the relative prices of physical commodities: so many kilos of rice for so many liters of kerosene, so many meters of rope for so many pairs of sandals, and so on. Trading under such circumstances involves onerous information costs.

Few societies have ever relied heavily on barter because of the high costs implicit in this means of exchange. At some point, prices of goods and services begin to be expressed in terms of one or more universally accepted and durable commodities, like gold and silver or even beads and cowrie shells. The rise of commodity money diminishes the transaction and storage costs of trade but still involves problems of making exchanges across space and time. Gold and silver prices fluctuate, and the commodities, therefore, are not fully reliable as **units of account**. As specialization within an economy increases, financial instruments backed by commodities appear. In the last century, with the rise of central banking all over the world, currency evolved into *fiat* money, debt issued by central banks that is legal tender. It is backed not by commodities of equivalent value but only by the full faith and credit of the central bank.

As markets widen and specialization proceeds apace, a need arises for still another financial instrument, **transferable deposits**. In the normal course of development, *checking* or *demand deposits* (deposits that may be transferred to any economic agent at the demand of the depositor) appear first and ordinarily bear little or no interest. Rising levels of economic activity, however, create increasing needs for transaction balances; individuals will always maintain some balances in demand deposits to meet these needs but tend to economize on the levels of such deposits if no interest is paid on them. With further monetization still another financial instrument begins to grow in importance, *time deposits*, which also are legally transferable on demand but sometimes only after stated periods. Time deposits involve contractual interest payments; higher interest rates induce people to hold greater amounts of deposits in this form.

While checking (demand) and time deposits are **liabilities** (or debts) of commercial banks, they are **financial assets** for the individuals who hold them. Both demand and time deposits are known as *liquid financial assets*. Unlike *nonfinancial assets* that also can be held by households and businesses (inventories, gold, and land), demand and time deposits can be quickly and conveniently converted into their currency equivalents. *Currency*, by definition, is the most liquid of all assets. The concept of liquid financial assets is an important one in any discussion of financial policy in developing countries. For most developing countries, the movement of savers in and out of liquid financial assets may be the prime factor behind the success or failure of a financial policy. We will see that long-term shifts from tangible, or nonfinancial, physical assets to financial assets, particularly liquid assets, bodes well not only for economic growth but also for economic stability.

A country's **money supply** may be defined as the sum of all liquid assets in the financial system. While not all economists agree about what constitutes a liquid financial asset, most vastly prefer this money supply concept to those commonly employed in early postwar monetary analysis. Formerly, the money supply was conventionally defined as the sum of only two liquid financial assets: currency in circulation outside banks (C) plus demand deposits (D), which together are known as M1 (*narrow money*). However, it later became clear that, because depositors tend to view time and savings deposits (T) as almost as liquid as demand deposits, the former also should be included in any workable concept of money supply, called M2 (*broad money*). Finally, for high-income countries, specialized deposit-taking financial institutions have arisen and offer an array of options to savers other than those available in commercial and savings banks. The liabilities of these specialized institutions (O) are included in M3 (*total liquid liabilities*), the broadest measure of money. Thus

$$M1 = C + D \qquad\qquad [12\text{—}1]$$

$$M2 = M1 + T \qquad\qquad [12\text{—}2]$$

$$M3 = M2 + O \qquad\qquad [12\text{—}3]$$

For most low-income countries and many middle-income countries, liquid financial assets constitute by far the greatest share of outstanding financial assets. But, as income growth continues and the financial system matures, less-liquid financial assets assume progressively greater importance. These include primary securities such as stocks, bonds (issued both by government and firms), and other financial claims on tangible (physical) assets that are convertible into currency equivalents with only some risk of loss to the asset holder and are hence less liquid than demand or time deposits.

The evolution of financial activity follows no set pattern across countries. Differing economic conditions and policies may result in widely divergent patterns of financial growth. Nevertheless, as per capita income rises, money increases as a ratio to gross domestic product (GDP). Table 12–1 shows these patterns for broad money (M2).

TABLE 12-1   Broad Money (M2) as a Percentage of Gross Domestic Product (GDP), 1980 and 2008

COUNTRY/ECONOMY	PERCENT OF GDP	
	1980	2008
Low-income countries	19	36
Ethiopia	–	31
Tanzania	–	28
India	32	70
Bangladesh	13	55
Kenya	30	40
Nigeria	24	30
Ghana	16	24
Honduras	23	51
Lower-middle-income countries	28	54
Pakistan	39	44
Bolivia	18	55
Cameroon	21	19
Philippines	22	59
Sri Lanka	28	33
Indonesia	13	36
Peru	17	31
Egypt	52	84
Upper-middle-income countries	29	79
Colombia	24	33
Argentina	29	25
Mexico	27	26
Malaysia	71	118
Korea, Republic	29	62
High-income countries	72	113
Saudi Arabia	13	48
Japan	138	207
United States	68	83

Source: World Bank, *World Development Indicators 2011* (Washington, DC: World Bank, 2011), available at http://databank.worldbank.org/ddp/home.do.

For all income classes shown in the table, the ratio of M2 to the GDP rose substantially from 1980 through 2008. This reflects both economic growth and changing policies. Looking at country income aggregates, the ratio rises as one moves from low- to middle- to high-income economies. But the variance among countries is notable. In 2008, Kenya, a low-income economy, had a higher monetization ratio (40 percent) than either Sri Lanka (33 percent) or Mexico (26 percent) both middle-income nations. Clearly, income level is not the only determinant of financial growth.

FINANCIAL INTERMEDIATION

As financial structures become increasingly rich and diversified in terms of financial assets, institutions, and markets, the function of money as a medium of exchange, store of value, and unit of account tends to be taken for granted, except in situations of runaway inflation. As financial development proceeds, the ability of the financial system to perform its second major function, financial intermediation, grows as well. The process of financial intermediation involves gathering savings from multitudinous savers and channeling them to a much smaller but still sizable number of investors. With a few exceptions, households are the main net savers in developing countries. At early stages of economic development, a preponderant share of intermediation activities tends to be concentrated in commercial banks. As development proceeds, new forms of financial intermediaries begin to appear and gradually assume a growing share of the intermediation function. These include investment banks, insurance companies, pension funds, and securities markets.

Financial intermediation is best seen as one of several alternative technologies for mobilizing and allocating savings. The fiscal system discussed in Chapter 11 furnishes another alternative, and we see in Chapter 14 that reliance on foreign savings constitutes still another. Further, we will observe in this chapter that inflation has also been employed as a means of mobilizing resources for the public sector. Indeed, a decision to rely more heavily on financial intermediation as a means of investment finance is tantamount to a decision to rely less heavily on the government budget, foreign aid and foreign investment, and inflation to achieve the same purpose.

TRANSFORMATION AND DISTRIBUTION OF RISK

Another major service provided by a well-functioning financial system is the transformation and distribution of risk. All economic activities involve risk taking, but some undertakings involve more risk than others. Individual savers and investors tend to be risk averse; the marginal loss of a dollar appears more important to them than the marginal gain of a dollar. But the degree of risk aversion differs among individuals. When risk cannot be diversified (or pooled) across a large number of individuals, savers and investors demand greater returns (or premiums) for bearing risk and activities involving high risk tend not to be undertaken. But high-risk activities may well offer the greatest returns to the economy as a whole. A well-functioning financial system furnishes a means for diversifying, or pooling, risk among a large number of savers and investors. The system may offer assets with differing degrees of risk. Financial institutions that specialize in assessing and managing risks can assign them to individuals having different attitudes toward and perceptions of risk. The term *well-functioning financial system* needs to be emphasized here. Early in the twenty-first century, highly sophisticated financial systems in high-income countries, notably the United States, managed risk poorly and this led to the financial crisis and global recession of 2008–09.

STABILIZATION

Finally, the financial system provides instruments for the stabilization of economic activity in addition to those available under fiscal policy and direct controls. All economies experience cyclical changes in production, employment, and prices. Governments often attempt to compensate for these fluctuations through policies affecting the money supply. Because unemployment in developing countries rarely is of the type that can be cured by monetary expansion, the use of financial policy for stabilization purposes generally focuses on efforts to control inflation. As the economic crises that began in Asia in 1997 and in the United States in 2008 demonstrated, however, the financial system itself can become a major source of instability in the country. From the beginning of the twenty-first century, as a result, financial policy also has focused on more than simply whether the supply of money is growing too rapidly or too slowly. Policy makers have had to devote much attention to ensuring the integrity and stability of banks and other nonbank financial institutions to avoid a severe recession brought on by financial panic. In the discussion that follows, we focus first on the use of the financial system to control inflation and then return to the issue of how the financial system should be designed and managed to avoid panic and recession.

INFLATION

From the 1980s to the present **price inflation**, defined as a sustained increase in the overall price level, generally was regarded as a malady that in its milder forms was annoying but tolerable and in its moderate form corrosive but not fatal. Runaway inflation, also known as **hyperinflation**, however, always has been recognized as severely destructive of economic processes, with few offsetting benefits. Whereas a number of influential thinkers in the 1950s and 1960s advocated some degree of moderate inflation (for example, inflation rates between 8 and 12 percent) as a tool for promoting growth, few adherents of this view remain. Many others did not actively advocate inflation but tended to have a higher threshold of tolerance for a steadily rising general price level than now is common.

INFLATION EPISODES

Inflationary experiences vary widely among developing countries and generalizations are difficult to make. Nevertheless, postwar economic history offers some interesting national and regional contrasts in both susceptibility to and tolerance for different levels of inflation. The period before the early 1970s was one of relative price stability in developing countries. In the southern cone of Latin America, however, particularly in Argentina, Brazil, and Chile, **chronic inflation** (prices rising 20 to 50 percent per year for three years or more) was an enduring fact of economic life for much of the 1950s through the 1980s and even beyond. The experience of these countries indicates that a long period of double-digit inflation does not necessarily lead to national economic calamity in all societies. In all, about two dozen countries experienced chronic inflation from 1950 to 2008, as shown in Table 12–2, but only a few, including Tajikistan, Venezuela, and Uzbekistan, have experienced chronic inflation throughout much of the first decade of the twenty-first century.

However, a tolerable rate of inflation in one country may constitute economic trauma in another. This may be seen more readily by considering the often progressive inflationary disease, acute inflation. **Acute inflation**, defined here as inflation between 50 and 200 percent for three or more consecutive years, was experienced by 18 countries listed in Table 12–2 over the postwar period, in some cases more than once per country. For Brazil, the progression from chronic to acute inflation did not result in any noticeable slowing of that country's relatively robust economic growth, whatever it may have meant for income distribution. In Ghana, on the other hand, a decade of acute inflation coincided with a decade of decline in GDP per capita. Although it may be tempting to attribute economic retrogression in Ghana at the time to acute inflation, it is more likely that the same policies that led to sustained inflation, not the inflation itself, were responsible for declines in living standards there.[1] Since the middle of the 1990s acute inflation has been rare.

Although acute inflation has proven toxic to economic development in some settings and only bothersome in others, **runaway (hyper) inflation** almost always has had a devastating effect. Inflation rates in excess of 200 percent per year represent an inflationary process that is clearly out of control; 22 countries have undergone this traumatic experience since 1950. One major bout of runaway inflationary experience occurred in three Latin American countries: Bolivia and Argentina in 1985, Argentina again in 1988–90, and Peru in 1988–91. In Bolivia, the annual rate of inflation over

---

[1]For a diagnosis of the causes of the Ghanian economic decline after 1962, see Michael Roemer, "Ghana, 1950 to 1980: Missed Opportunities," and Yaw Ansu, "Comments" (201–30), both in Arnold C. Haberger, ed., *World Economic Growth* (San Francisco: ICS Press, 1984).

TABLE 12-2 Inflation Outliers: Episodes of Chronic, Acute, and Runaway Inflation among Developing Countries, 1948–2008 (average annual rates)

| COUNTRY | CHRONIC INFLATION (20–50 PERCENT, 3 YEARS) | | ACUTE INFLATION (50–200 PERCENT, 3 YEARS) | | RUNAWAY INFLATION (200+ PERCENT, 1 YEAR) | |
	YEAR(S)	RATE	YEAR(S)	RATE	YEAR(S)	RATE
Angola			1997–2003	143	1993–96	858
Argentina	1950–74	27	1977–82	147	1976	443
			1986–87	111	1983–85	529
					1988–91	1,400
Armenia					1990–97	700
Azerbaijan					1990–96*	590
Belarus			1997–2002	87	1990–96*	715
Bolivia	1979–81	33	1952–59	117	1983–86	1,132
Brazil	1957–78	36	1979–84	108	1985	227
					1986	145
					1987–93	831
Chile	1952–71	29			1973–76	308
	1978–80	36				
	1983–85	26				
Colombia	1979–82	26				
	1988–92	28				
Dominican Republic			1988–92	51		
Ecuador	1997–2001	49				
Georgia					1990–96*	2,279
Ghana	1986–90	32	1976–83	73		
			1995–97	75		
Indonesia					1965–68	306
Kazakhstan					1990–96*	605
Kyrgyz Republic					1990–96*	256
Latvia					1990–96*	111
Lithuania					1990–96*	179
Malawi	1998–2002	40				
Mexico			1982–88	70		
Myanmar	2001–03	29	1992	116		
Nicaragua	1979–84	33			1985–91	2,130
Paraguay			1951–53	81		
Peru	1975–77	32	1950–55	102	1988–91	1,694
			1978–87	85		
Romania			1991–93	132		
			1997–92	56		
Russia	1996–99	42			1993–95	376
Sierra Leone			1983–92	81		
South Korea			1950–55	95		
Tajikistan	2000–08	22			1990–96*	394
Turkmenistan					1990–96*	1,074
Tanzania	1980–89	27				
Turkey	1981–87	38	1978–80	69		
			1988–2002	70		

(Continued)

TABLE 12-2 *Continued*

Uganda	1990–92	37	1981–89	101		
Ukraine					1993–95	1,167
Uruguay	1948–65	26	1965–68	83		
	1981–83	34	1972–80	68		
Uzbekistan	2000-08	29	1984–92	76		
Venezuela	1987–92	40				
	1993–98	43				
	2002–08	28				
Zaire/Congo	1981–82	36	1976–80	68	1991–92	2,987
			1983–90	68	1992–95	3,206
					1996–2002	218
Zambia	1985–87	44	1988–92	113		
			1993–96	71		
Zimbabwe					2002–07	5,305[†]

[*]For a number of the former Soviet republics, the gross domestic product (GDP) price deflator data are given for the entire period 1990–96, not broken down by year.
[†]Data for Zimbabwe are not available after 2007. Some estimates place Zimbabwe's annual inflation at over 30,000 in the late 2000s.

Sources: International Monetary Fund, *International Financial Statistics Yearbook 1994* (Washington, DC: International Monetary Fund, 2004) and International Monetary Fund, *International Financial Statistics Yearbook*, 2003 (Washington, DC: International Monetary Fund, 2003); and World Bank, *World Development Indicators 2010*, at http://databank.worldbank.org/ddp/home.do accessed June 2011.

a period of several months in 1985 accelerated to a rate of nearly 4,000 percent. In Argentina, the monthly rate of price increases was 30.5 percent in June 1985 alone; on an annual basis that would have been an inflation rate of 2,340 percent. In both Bolivia and Argentina for much of 1985, workers had little choice but to spend their paychecks within days of receipt, for fear that prices would double or triple over the next week. In Peru, hyperinflation in 1989 gave birth to publications devoted only to the tracking of inflation (see Box 12–1).

In the 1990s, hyperinflation was experienced by virtually all the new republics formed after the breakup of the Soviet Union. In the first part of the 1990s, inflation reached a rate of nearly 400 percent a year in Russia over a period of several years and over 1,000 percent a year in the Republic of Georgia and Turkmenistan. In the latter two countries, civil war put heavy demands on government expenditures while reducing the ability of those governments to collect taxes, leading them to finance their activities by printing money. In Africa in the 1990s, civil war in Angola and the Congo also led to inflation rates of over 1,000 percent per year. Since the year 2000, however only the Congo (briefly) and Zimbabwe (throughout the first decade of the twenty-first century) have experienced runaway inflation. In the Congo the ongoing war in the eastern part of the country is the main cause. In Zimbabwe runaway inflation has been the result of across the board mismanagement of the economy throughout that decade.

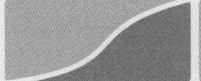

BOX 12-1 HYPERINFLATION IN PERU, 1988-90

The economic and social havoc wrought by hyperinflation is difficult to comprehend for those who have not lived through the experience. The Peruvian hyperinflation, which began in 1988 and continued until 1991, provides some rueful examples.

The inflationary process was triggered by large budgetary deficits and sustained by subsequent ongoing deficits, virtual economic collapse, and steadily rising inflationary expectations. Peru already had experienced two serious bouts with acute inflation since 1950, but the pace of inflation in 1989 was the highest in the nation's history: 28 percent per month, or about 2,000 percent per year. Moreover, inflation accelerated in the first six weeks of 1990, as prices rose by 6 percent per week, or about 1 percent per day. From January 1989 to December 1990, the value of the Peruvian currency (the inti) on the free market fell from 1,200 intis per dollar to 436,000 intis per dollar.

This hyperinflation may turn out to be one of the best documented in history: In 1988, Richard Webb, an internationally respected Peruvian economist, began to publish a magazine devoted essentially to helping producers and consumers cope with the chaos associated with runaway inflation. The magazine, called *Cuanto?* (*How Much?*) appeared monthly. It not only provided details on price developments for a large number of commodities and services but managed to extract what little humor there is in a situation in which the price of a movie ticket rises while people are waiting in line to buy it or taxi drivers must carry fare money in a burlap bag because the domestic currency collected in fares each evening is too bulky to fit in a wallet.

But precious little is funny about hyperinflation. In Peru, it was a story of government employees going without pay for weeks at a time, of indices of poverty nearly doubling from 1987 to 1989, further impoverishing the poorest 40 percent of the population. It was a story of precipitous decline in gross domestic product (GDP) and the rise of pervasive black markets in everything from dollars to gasoline to cement. It was a time when, on each payday, laborers rushed to the market to buy their weekly food supplies before they were marked up overnight. It was a tale of wide variations in price rises, in which prices for such items as pencils and chicken increased by more than 25 times from February 1989 to February 1990, but prices of light bulbs and telephone services increased "only" 10-fold.

Imagine life in Lima, the capital city, in the first few weeks of 1990, for a middle-income family trying to survive. For the first 40 days of the year, increases in the price of dying outpaced the price of living: The cost of funerals rose 79 percent, while house rent rose by 56 percent and the price of restaurant meals and haircuts increased by 44 percent. By mid-1990, the economic paralysis of Peru was virtually complete. Peru's hyperinflation ended in 1992 (although inflation remained acute at 75 percent) as government reduced its budget deficit to 1 percent of GDP.

The countries listed in Table 12–2 brought on inflation in three different ways. In one group (including Argentina, Chile, Ghana, Indonesia, Peru, Russia, and Ukraine), large budget deficits relative to GDP were financed by borrowing from the central bank. In a second group (Paraguay in the early 1950s and Brazil and Uruguay before 1974), inflation was caused by a massive expansion of credit to the private sector. And in Nicaragua, Sierra Leone, Uganda, Angola, Congo, Zimbabwe, and several of the nations created out of the former Soviet Union, political strife or civil war exacerbated the fiscal and monetary causes of inflation. Whatever the initial impetus to inflation, once it begins to accelerate, the public begins to expect inflation to continue, and this leads to even-higher, more-sustained price increases.

For developing countries as a group, Table 12–3 shows that, on average, inflation was only 13 percent a year until the oil crisis began in 1973 but jumped to 21 percent a year during the period of rising oil prices until 1981. Inflation then accelerated to more than 30 percent a year even as oil prices began falling and exceeded 50 percent a year after oil prices collapsed in 1986. In the 1990s, these high rates of inflation continued through the first half of the decade and then slowed markedly after 1995. The principal exceptions were the states of the former Soviet Union, where triple-digit inflation in many cases continued to the end of the century and in a few cases a few years more. The industrial countries, in contrast, had much lower inflation throughout and the highest price increases coincided with the rise in oil prices.

MONETARY POLICY AND PRICE STABILITY

We saw from Table 12–3 that inflation largely was conquered in Asia during the 1970s but accelerated in Latin America and Africa during and especially after the oil-price boom of the 1970s. In the 1990s, however, attempts to control inflation were more serious and widespread with the notable exception of the republics formed out of the collapse of the Soviet Union. Even in these former Soviet republics, inflation by the beginning of the twenty-first century was generally down to single digits. The only case of runaway inflation during the first decade of the twenty-first century, as already noted, was Zimbabwe, where inflation was the result of a general collapse of the economy and of a government fiscal policy in the context of a ruling elite desperately trying to hold onto power. Controlling inflation in the midst of a civil war and the collapse of government functions requires first ending the war and reestablishing a functioning government. To control inflation under more normal circumstances, monetary policy is the principal instrument used to achieve price stability.

TABLE 12-3 Inflation by Regional Groupings, 1963–2008 (percent per annum)

REGION	1963–73	1973–81	1981–92	1992–95	1995–98	1998–01	2001–08
World	26.3	13.8	17.9	19.2	6.8	4.2	4.5
Industrial countries	24.6	10.3	13.0	2.5	1.9	1.8	2.1
Developing countries	12.9	20.7	44.1	47.9	12.6	7.1	8.5
Africa	24.9	17.3	27.0	40.2	12.1	8.2	9.1
Asia	13.5	28.8	16.8	11.6	6.9	2.4	3.9
Middle East*	24.2	16.6	16.0	15.0	9.5	5.5	12.6*
Latin America and Caribbean	18.4	43.7	162.8	216.5	15.5	8.4	9.6

*The Middle East gross domestic product deflator series ends in 2007.

Sources: International Monetary Fund, *International Financial Statistics Yearbook 1994* (Washington, DC: International Monetary Fund, 1994); International Monetary Fund, *International Financial Statistics, 1998* (Washington, DC: International Monetary Fund, 1998); International Monetary Fund, *International Financial Statistics, 2003* (Washington, DC: International Monetary Fund, 2003); and International Monetary Fund, *International Financial Statistics 2010* (Washington, DC: International Monetary Fund, 2010).

MONETARY POLICY AND EXCHANGE-RATE REGIMES

Appropriate use of monetary policy in controlling inflation depends critically on the type of exchange-rate regime used by a country. Exchange-rate regimes form a continuum with fixed (pegged) exchange rates at one end and floating (flexible) exchange rates at the other. Under a **fixed-exchange-rate** system, a country attempts to maintain the value of its currency in a fixed relation to another currency, say, the U.S. dollar: The value of the local currency is **pegged** to the dollar. This is done through intervention by the country's monetary authorities in the market for foreign exchange and requires the maintenance of substantial **international reserves** (reserves of foreign currencies), usually equivalent to the value of four or more months' worth of imports.

Consider the case of Thailand, where from 1987 to early 1997 the Thai currency, the baht, was fixed at an exchange rate close to 25 baht to US$1. Because the exchange rate, if left to its own devices, would change from day to day to reflect changes in both the demand for and supply of exports and imports and capital flows, to defend the peg, the government must be prepared to use the country's international reserves to buy or sell dollars at an exchange rate of 25 to 1 to keep the exchange rate from moving. If, for example, a poor domestic rice harvest caused the nation to increase its food imports, the baht–dollar exchange rate would tend to rise (the baht would depreciate, as its dollar value falls) in the absence of any net sales of dollars from Thailand's international reserves. To sustain a fixed exchange rate, of course, the country must have sufficient foreign exchange reserves to keep on buying baht at that fixed rate. In 1997, because of large capital outflows, Thailand actually ran out of foreign exchange and had to abandon its support of the pegged rate.

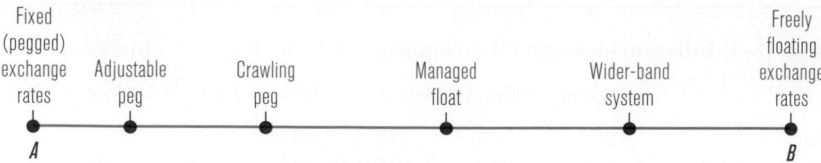

FIGURE 12-1 **Continuum of Prototypes of Exchange-Rate Regimes**

As one moves from point *A* to point *B*, both the frequency of intervention by domestic monetary authorities and the required level of international reserves tend to be lower. Under a pure fixed-exchange-rate regime (point *A*) authorities intervene so that the value of the currency vis-à-vis another, say, the U.S. dollar, is maintained at a constant rate.

Under freely **floating rates**, the authorities simply allow the value of local currency vis-à-vis foreign ones to be determined by market forces. Between the two ends of this continuum lie a number of intermediate options (Figure 12–1).[2] Closest to the floating-exchange-rate option is the *wider band* system, by which the exchange rate of a country is allowed to float or fluctuate within a predefined band of values, say, between 23 and 27 baht to US$1. But when conditions threaten to push the value of the currency beyond the band, the authorities intervene by buying or selling local currency as appropriate to stay within the band. Further along the continuum away from floating rates is the *managed float*, where the authorities are committed to defend no particular exchange rate, but they nevertheless intervene continuously at their discretion. A country with steadily shrinking international reserves, for example, might allow the value of its currency to depreciate against the value of other currencies—that is, allow the exchange rate to rise against other currencies.

Two other systems are closely related hybrids of fixed and floating rules. The *crawling peg*, used over a long period by Brazil, Colombia, and Indonesia, involves pegging the local currency against some other currency but changing this in gradual, periodic steps to adjust for any differential between the country's inflation rate and the world inflation rate. Closest to a fixed-exchange-rate system is the *adjustable peg*, involving a commitment by the monetary authorities to defend the local exchange rate at a fixed parity (peg), while reserving the right to change that rate when circumstances require.

Two very rigid forms of pegged exchange rates that a small number of countries have adopted are currency boards and dollarization. With a *currency board*, the government issues domestic currency only when it is fully backed by available foreign exchange reserves at the given exchange rate. Currency in circulation increases when additional foreign exchange becomes available (say, through increased export receipts) and decreases when foreign exchange becomes scarcer (say, through an

[2]For a full discussion of these and other types of exchange-rate regimes, see John Williamson, *The Open Economy and the World Economy* (New York: Basic Books, 1983), pp. 238–41; or Anne O. Krueger, *Exchange Rate Determination* (New York: Cambridge University Press, 1983), pp. 123–36.

increase in imports or capital outflows). This system ensures that the country will not run out of foreign exchange. However, the main instrument of adjustment becomes domestic interest rates, which increase when foreign exchange (and domestic currency) becomes scarcer, and decline when foreign exchange becomes more available. Hong Kong, Bulgaria, Argentina, Brunei, Djibouti, Estonia, and Lithuania all have or have had currency boards.

With *dollarization*, one country adopts another country's currency, as Panama did many years ago when it adopted the U.S. dollar as its currency. Most economists believe that currency boards and dollarization are appropriate in only a very limited number of developing countries that are small, very open to trade, and not vulnerable to large commodity price swings. In Hong Kong, the currency board system works reasonably well, although high interest rates and hence slower growth were required to prevent large currency outflows during and immediately after the Asian financial crisis. In Argentina at the beginning of the twenty-first century, the inability of the central government to rein in excessive local government spending caused pressures on reserves that ultimately made it impossible to maintain the peg to the dollar that was essential to the continuance of its currency board.

The currencies of all the major industrial countries have floated vis-à-vis one another since the early 1970s, with occasional intervention by national monetary authorities to prevent very sharp swings in rates. Most developing countries have adhered to either the adjustable-peg or the crawling-peg system, although an increasing number, particularly in Africa, have been adopting floating-rate systems as part of stabilization programs. Because, in practice, both pegged systems operate for particular periods like fixed-rate regimes, for our analysis, we focus most of our attention on monetary policy issues arising under fixed exchange rates in small, open economies.

SOURCES OF INFLATION

In open developing economies with fixed exchange rates, the rate of monetary expansion no longer is under the complete control of domestic monetary authorities. Rather, countries with fixed exchange rates may be viewed as sharing essentially the same money supply, because the money of each can be converted into that of the others at a fixed parity.[3] Under such circumstances, the stock of money (M), by definition, is the sum of two components: the amount of domestic credit of the banking system that is outstanding (DC) and the stock of international reserves of that country (IR), measured in terms of domestic currency. The money supply, therefore, has a domestic component and an international component, so we have

$$M = DC + IR \qquad\qquad [12-4]$$

[3]This section draws substantially on syntheses of monetary and international economics by Arnold C. Harberger. See his "A Primer on Inflation" and "The Inflation Syndrome," papers presented in the Political Economy Lecture Series, Harvard University, March 19, 1981.

Changes in the domestic money stock can occur either through expansion of domestic credit or by monetary movements that lead to changes in international reserves. That is,

$$\Delta M = \Delta DC + \Delta IR \qquad \text{[12–5]}$$

Under fixed exchange rates, a central bank of any small country can control *DC*, the domestic component, but has only very limited control over *IR*, the international component. Under such circumstances, developing countries that attempt to keep the rate of domestic inflation below the world inflation rate (through restrictive policies on domestic credit) are unable to realize this goal. If, fueled by monetary expansion abroad (growth in the world money supply), world inflation initially is running in excess of domestic inflation, the prices of internationally traded goods rise relative to those of domestic, nontraded goods.[4] Imports fall, exports rise, and the balance of payments moves toward surplus and causes a rise in international reserves. Therefore, the foreign components of the money stock rise. This is tantamount to an "importation of money" and eventually undoes the effort to prevent importation of world inflation. Again, a small country on fixed exchange rates can do little to maintain its inflation rate below that of the rest of the world. For very open countries with few restrictions on the movement of goods and capital into and out of the country, the adjustment to world inflation can be very rapid (less than a year). For less-open countries with substantial restrictions on international trade and payments, the process takes longer, but the outcome is inevitable under fixed exchange rates.

The fact that financial policy for stabilization in countries with fixed exchange rates is heavily constrained by international developments is sometimes taken to mean that changes in the domestic component of the money stock have no impact on prices in economies adhering to fixed exchange rates. On the contrary, excessive expansion in money and credit surely will result in domestically generated inflation that, depending on the rate of expansion, for a time, can be well in excess of world inflation rates. However, such a situation cannot continue for long, as excess money creation spills over into the balance of payments via increased imports and leads to a drain on international reserves and, ultimately, an inability to maintain the fixed exchange rate. As reserves dwindle, the country no longer can defend its exchange rate and devaluation becomes inevitable.[5] Inflation, therefore, can be transmitted to small, open economies through the working of the world economy or generated by domestic developments.

A growing number of developing countries have floating exchange rates (point *B* on the continuum in Figure 12–1). A floating exchange-rate regime allows countries

---

[4]This is but one of several mechanisms that led to changes in international reserves sufficient to thwart efforts by developing countries to insulate themselves from world inflation.

[5]Import controls are frequently used to stem the drain of reserves and avoid devaluation for a time. But import controls engender another set of distortions and inefficiencies, explored in Chapter 18, that eventually require more drastic measures, including devaluation.

to insulate themselves from world inflation. Under such a system, the rise in world prices attendant on world inflation would initially favor exports from the country and discourage imports. As a consequence, the current account of the country's balance of payments improves, international reserves rise, and the exchange rate soon appreciates (fewer baht are required to buy dollars, for instance). The appreciation in the country's exchange rate cancels out external price increases and prevents the importation of world inflation.

Under any exchange-rate regime, domestically generated inflation may result from excessive increases in domestic credit from the banking system to either the public or the private sector. Budget deficits of the central government, for example, must be financed by borrowing, but the embryonic nature of money and capital markets in most developing countries generally means that governments facing deficits ordinarily must resort to borrowing from the central bank. Borrowing from the central bank is equivalent to direct money creation via the printing press. The result is a direct addition to the reserve base of the monetary system, an increase in so-called high-powered money. It is important, however, to recognize that not all budgetary deficits are inflationary. We have seen that a growing economy is characterized by a growing demand for liquid assets, including money. Moderate budgetary deficits year after year, financed by the central bank, can help satisfy this requirement without leading to inflation. In general, the money stock may expand at least as fast as the growth in real income, with little or no inflationary consequences.

Earlier we saw that liquid assets normally are between 40 and 60 percent of GDP in low- and lower-middle income economies (with wide variations), equivalent to roughly three to six months of income. Therefore, the public generally is willing to hold this much in money balances. A deficit of 2 percent of GDP financed by money creation adds only marginally to the money supply and easily may be accepted by the public. But a deficit of 8 percent of GDP increases the stock of money by an amount equal to one more month of income, an amount the public may be unwilling to hold (unless nominal interest rates on deposits are greatly increased). The excess spills over into higher prices.

Use of bank credit to finance government deficits has not been the only source of inflationary monetary expansion in developing countries. Sometimes excessive growth of credit to the private sector has played a more significant role in domestically generated inflationary processes. Nevertheless, as a general rule, inflation rates that are much in excess of world inflation usually have been traceable to budgetary deficits.

For countries attempting to maintain fixed exchange rates, efforts to avoid price increases in excess of world inflation must be a matter primarily of fiscal policy, not monetary policy. If budget deficits are not held to levels consistent with world inflation, even very deft deployment of monetary policy instruments are unable to prevent rapid inflation, devaluation, or both. There still is a role for monetary policy in developing countries, but that role must be largely passive. Resourceful use of monetary policy can help by not making things worse and moderating strong inflationary pressures until the budget can be brought under control, provided the latter is done fairly quickly.

Monetary factors are causes of inflation in both fixed- and floating-exchange-rate countries. In the case of fixed exchange rates, both world monetary expansion and domestic monetary expansion generate inflation; in flexible-exchange-rate countries, inflation arises from domestic monetary sources. But, thus far, no mention has been made of so-called nonmonetary causes of inflation. It seems plausible that internal and external shocks, such as those arising from widespread crop failure in the domestic economy or a drastic increase in prices of imported energy, could have important effects on inflation in countries suffering such shocks. This is true, but the mechanism whereby nonmonetary factors may initiate or worsen inflation needs to be clearly portrayed.

Nonmonetary disturbances indeed may precipitate policy reactions that lead to domestic monetary expansion large enough to accommodate higher relative prices of food or oil and large enough to cause inflation. In the absence of accommodating monetary expansion in the face of such shocks, inflation can be contained, but at some cost. Failure to allow the money supply to expand to accommodate higher relative prices of important goods leads to increases in unemployment that most governments find unacceptable. Governments in such cases usually attempt to allow monetary expansion sufficient to avoid unwanted consequences for employment. But it is important to remember that, however advisable monetary accommodation may be on social and employment grounds, expansion in the money stock is required to fuel inflation, whatever external or internal factors may precipitate the expansion. This truth, known for centuries, is often incorrectly interpreted to mean that non-monetary factors cannot "cause" inflation. They can, but only through an expansion of the national or international stock of money or both.

CONTROLLING INFLATION THROUGH MONETARY POLICY

The array of available instruments for anti-inflationary monetary policy in developed countries include (1) open-market operations, in which the central bank can directly contract bank reserves by sales of government securities;[6] (2) increases in legal reserve requirements of banks, so that a given volume of reserves support a lower stock of money (and reduce the credit expansion multiplier as well); (3) increases in rediscount rates, so that commercial bank borrowing from the central bank becomes

---

[6]Open-market operations are used as an instrument of monetary policy in countries with well-developed financial markets. When the Federal Reserve System in the United States or a central bank in Europe wants to curtail the growth of the money supply, it sells government securities (bonds, bills) on the open market. When a buyer pays for the securities, the effect is to reduce directly the reserves of the banking system because the funds are transferred from commercial bank deposits or household cash holdings to the account of the Federal Reserve. When the Federal Reserve wants to expand the money supply, it buys securities on the open market and thus directly adds to bank reserves.

less attractive; and (4) moral suasion, by which the exhortations of monetary authorities are expected to lead to restraint in bank lending policies.

For virtually all developing countries, the first instrument (open market operations) is not available for inflation control. Securities markets typically are absent or not sufficiently well developed to allow the exercise of this powerful and flexible instrument, although some emerging market economies can now use this tool. The other three monetary policy instruments are employed, with varying degrees of success, in developing countries. In addition, developing countries often resort to two other tools employed only infrequently in developed countries: (5) credit ceilings imposed by the central bank on the banking system and (6) adjustments in allowable nominal rates of interest on deposits and loans.

RESERVE REQUIREMENTS

All central banks require commercial banks to immobilize a portion of their deposits in the form of legal reserves that may not be lent to prospective customers. For example, legal reserve requirements for Indonesian and Malaysian banks in the late 1970s were expressed as 30 percent of deposits in domestic currency in the former and 20 percent of all deposits in the latter. Banks in Malaysia were required to add 20 units of currency to reserves for every 100 units of deposits. These figures are not too far out of line with legal reserve requirements in many industrial nations, where reserve ratios of 15 percent for demand deposits and 5 percent for time deposits are common.

Increases in reserve requirements can be used to help moderate inflation. An upward adjustment in reserve requirements works in two ways: It reduces the stock of money that can be supported by a given amount of reserves, and it reduces the money multiplier. The first effect induces banks to contract credit outstanding; the second reduces the growth in the money stock possible from any future increment to reserves.[7] Changes in legal reserve requirements are usually employed only as a last-ditch measure, although China raised reserve requirements several times during the 2000–10 period, when price increases were still modest but rising. Even small changes in the required ratio of reserves to deposits can have a very disruptive impact on commercial bank operations, unless banks are given sufficient time to adjust.

CREDIT CEILINGS

In some countries, such as Indonesia from 1947 to 1983; China in 1994 to 1996 and during the first part of the twenty-first century; and at various other times in Malaysia, Sri Lanka, and Chile, credit ceilings have been used as supplementary instruments

---

[7]In its simplest form the money multiplier (m) can be expressed as
$$m = (c + 1)/(c + k)$$
where c = the ratio of currency outside banks to deposits and k = the ratio of reserves to deposits. If k is raised, then m falls.

of inflation control. The International Monetary Fund (IMF) often requires countries seeking balance-of-payments support to adopt credit ceilings as a prerequisite for assistance. General ceilings of domestic credit expansion represent a useful method of controlling growth in the domestic components of the money supply. Credit ceilings, however, do not allow full control of money-supply growth in developing countries operating under fixed-exchange-rate regimes because the monetary authorities have no control over foreign components of the money supply. Nevertheless, general credit ceilings sometimes can be usefully deployed in combating inflation in countries not experiencing major imbalances in external payments. Unfortunately, ceilings work the least well where they are needed the most because countries attempting to deal with chronic inflation are usually those experiencing the most destabilizing changes in their international reserve positions. General credit ceilings are unlikely to have much effect on inflation unless the government simultaneously takes steps to reduce the budgetary deficits that, except in major oil-exporting countries, typically are the root causes of chronic, acute, and especially runaway inflation.

Countries often supplement general credit ceilings with specific ceilings on lending to particular sectors of the economy. Indonesia attempted to fine-tune credit controls in this way from 1974 to 1983, with poor results. The system of ceilings was so detailed and cumbersome that domestic banks were unable to come close to exhausting the ceilings. Excess reserves rose. The banks had little choice but to place their excess reserves in deposits overseas, primarily in banks in Singapore. Many domestic firms in Jakarta were then forced to seek credit from Singapore banks, which held well over a billion dollars of deposits from Jakarta banks that might have been lent to domestic firms at a lower rate in the absence of credit ceilings. China, in the first part of the twenty-first century, placed ceilings on credit to real estate developers in what was believed to be an overheated real estate market but with only limited impact on investments in this area.

INTEREST-RATE REGULATION AND MORAL SUASION

In most industrial countries, the central bank can influence interest rates by varying the *rediscount rate* charged on central bank loans to commercial banks that require additional liquidity. Because the rediscount rate is central to commercial banks' operations, it is important in determining the market rate of interest on both deposits and loans. As more developing countries adopt financial reforms that free interest rates from central bank control, they are better able to use the rediscount rate as a tool for influencing market interest rates.

In developing countries that controlled rates on loans and deposits, the controlled rates have been instruments of anti-inflationary packages. The use of such interest rate adjustments have been common in Latin America, and increases in deposit rates and loan rates were major elements in the stabilization programs of South Korea and Taiwan in the mid-1960s and Indonesia in both 1968 and 1974. The objective in each case was twofold: to stimulate the demand for liquid assets and to discourage the loan demand for marginal investment projects by private-sector borrowers. The extent to which such measures can be successful depends on the interest elasticity of the demand for liquid assets and the interest elasticity of the demand for loans. In most of the cases just cited, particularly in the three Asian countries, both sets of elasticities evidently were sufficiently high because the stabilization packages succeeded to a large degree. Interest rate increases, however, were less effective in China in the 1990s and during 2000–09, largely because many firms, particularly state-owned or -controlled enterprises, are not very sensitive to the impact of higher interest costs on their investment plans.

Moral suasion by the monetary authorities, sometimes called *open-mouth operations* or *jawbone control*, is practiced no less extensively in developing than in developed countries. Warnings and exhortations to commercial banks to restrict lending or to encourage them to focus lending on particular activities have been quite common in Ghana. They also were used at various times in Malaysia, Singapore, Brazil, and elsewhere, sometimes before the imposition of credit ceilings and often to reinforce pressure on banks to adhere to ceilings. In both developed and developing countries, however, moral suasion has proven credible only when accompanied by forceful use of more tangible instruments of monetary control.

INTERNATIONAL DEBT AND COMBATING RECESSIONS

Our discussion to this point has focused on the role of monetary instruments in controlling domestic inflation because that was the dominant problem facing monetary and fiscal policy makers in developing countries since the end of World War II. In this chapter, however, we have not dealt with another major problem that has played an important role in developing countries, the role of accumulating debt obligations by many countries, particularly in Latin America and Africa. Borrowing from other countries and from international institutions such as the World Bank is also a way of financing a development program when domestic financial resources are inadequate, but it can lead to accumulating international debt to a level that the borrowing country can no longer afford. Because these international debt issues are both important and complex, we devote the next chapter to understanding the origins and solutions to developing country debt problems.

Until recently most developing countries did not have to face a problem common in high-income countries in recessions: the lack of sufficient aggregate demand to keep a country's resources of capital and labor fully employed. Developing countries frequently experienced recessions, but they were typically the result of a fall in the price of their natural resource exports or some other balance-of-payments problem. Increasing demand in these circumstances led not to the employment of unused resources but to either inflation or a worsening balance-of-payments deficit. But in 2008–09, countries that had come to rely on exports of manufactures to Europe and

North America suddenly experienced a sharp decline in the demand for their products, as a severe global recession led to a fall in incomes in high-income countries.

In the United States a standard method for getting out of a recession in previous years had been to rely on the central bank to lower interest rates, which would then lead to an increase in investment in a number of sectors, notably in housing. Even in mild recessions, however, interest rates in developing countries are seldom effective in generating increases in investment demand, largely because financial markets in these areas are undeveloped and many borrowers are not very sensitive to small changes in interest charges. In the case of the global recession of 2008–09 lowering interest rates was not very effective in either high- or middle-income countries. The only alternative for the countries affected was to turn to fiscal policy and to introduce what were called *stimulus packages,* large government expenditure programs paid for by borrowing mostly from the central bank. Among developing countries China had the largest stimulus package of well over US$500 billion if all of the components are included, and similar smaller packages were tried in Vietnam and elsewhere in Southeast Asia. These packages were made possible in part because the countries involved had built up large reserves of foreign exchange and thus did not have to fear that the increased demand would lead to large balance-of-payments deficits that could not be covered from existing foreign exchange reserves. China had enormous reserves of over $2 trillion (over $3 trillion in 2011). Many other countries in Asia, in the aftermath of the 1997–98 financial crisis that had been due in part to a lack of sufficient reserves, had built up their foreign exchange reserves as well. In the 1997–98 financial crisis, the most affected countries could not have introduced large stimulus packages to offset the impact on incomes and employment because their reserves were inadequate for even existing balance-of-payments requirements.

FINANCIAL DEVELOPMENT

Up to this point we have discussed the general role of financial systems in economic development and then turned to how financial systems can be mismanaged in a way that undermines stability in the economy and threatens growth in incomes and employment. High inflation by itself has been a major reason why the economic performance of many developing countries has suffered, and preventing inflation has often been the major focus of policy makers both within developing countries and in the international financial agencies. Controlling inflation is a major tenet of Washington Consensus–style reforms. But there is more to financial development than controlling inflation. The development of a financial system that carries out its major functions efficiently and fairly is an important and integral part of the development process.

SHALLOW FINANCE AND DEEP FINANCE

Policies for **financial deepening** seek to promote growth in the real size of the financial system, the growth of financial assets at a pace faster than income growth. In all but the highest-income developing countries, private-sector financial savings predominantly take the form of currency and deposits in commercial banks, savings and loan associations, postal savings accounts, and in some countries, mortgage banks. For most developing countries, growth in the real size of the financial system is reflected primarily in growth in the share of liquid assets in GDP. In contrast, under **shallow finance**, the ratio of liquid assets to GDP grows slowly or not at all over time and typically falls: The real size of the financial system shrinks. Countries able to mobilize large volumes of government or foreign savings can sustain high growth rates even under shallow finance policies, although even these countries may find financial deepening attractive for reasons of employment and income distribution. But, for countries where mobilization of government savings is difficult and foreign savings scarce or unwanted, deep finance may be essential for sustained income growth. This is because growth in the share of liquid assets in GDP provides an approximate indication of the banking system's ability to increase its lending for investment purposes. We will see that the hallmark of a deep financial strategy is avoidance of negative real interest rates; shallow finance, on the other hand, typically involves sharply negative real interest rates.

Growth in the real size of the financial system enhances its capacity for intermediation, gathering savings from diverse private sources and channeling these savings into productive investment. The need for financial intermediation arises because savings endowments do not necessarily correspond to investment opportunities. Individuals with the greatest capacity to save are usually not those with the entrepreneurial talents required for mounting new investment projects. Except in very simple, rudimentary economies, mechanisms are required to channel savings efficiently from savers to entrepreneurs.

If a country is restricted to self-financing by individuals or companies, many productive opportunities involving high private and social payoffs will never be seized because the resources of even the small number of very wealthy are not unlimited. Innovative, smaller-scale investors are not the only groups that fare poorly where financial intermediation is poorly developed; savers are penalized as well. Let us first examine the case in which even the most basic financial intermediaries, commercial banks, are absent. Under these circumstances, the domestic options open to savers are limited to forms of savings, such as acquisition of gold and jewelry, purchase of land and consumer durable goods, or other relatively sterile forms of investment in physical assets. Alternatively, wealthier savers may ship their savings abroad. The common feature of all such investments is that the resources devoted to them are inaccessible to domestic entrepreneurs who would adopt new technology, begin new firms, or expand production in existing enterprises.

All developing countries, therefore, have financial institutions, however embryonic, to serve as intermediaries between savers and investors, even where these intermediaries are limited to commercial banks that accept checking (demand) and time (savings) deposits from savers, to relend to prospective investors for a short term. Intermediation flourishes under deep finance, but under strategies of shallow finance intermediation is constricted and the financial system can contribute little to further the goals of economic growth. Later, we see that shallow finance may have unintended effects on employment and income distribution as well.

SHALLOW FINANCIAL STRATEGY

Shallow financial policies have a number of earmarks: high legal reserve requirements on commercial banks, pervasive nonprice rationing of credit, and most of all, sharply negative real interest rates. Countries rarely, if ever, have consciously and deliberately adopted strategies of shallow finance. Rather, the repression of the financial system flows logically from certain policies intended to encourage, not hinder, investment.

In developed and developing countries alike, policy makers often have viewed low nominal rates of interest as essential for the expansion of investment and controlled interest rate levels tightly. So long as the supply of investment funds is unlimited, low interest rates foster all types of investment activities, as even projects with low returns appear more attractive to investors. In accordance with that observation and in the belief that low interest rates are particularly essential to assist small enterprises and small farmers, governments often have placed low ceilings on nominal interest rates charged on all types of loans. These low ceilings are quite apart from special credit programs involving subsidized credit for special classes of borrowers. Because financial institutions ultimately must cover costs (or else be subsidized by governments), low legal ceilings on nominal loan rates mean low nominal interest rates on deposits as well.

As long as inflation is held in check, low ceilings on nominal loan and deposit interest rates may not retard growth, even when these ceilings are set below the opportunity cost of capital. The United States over the period 1800–1979 managed rather respectable rates of income growth, even in the presence of a set of archaic usury laws and other interest rate controls that (particularly before 1970) often involved artificially low, administered ceilings on interest rates. Even so, throughout most of the period before 1979, real interest rates in the United States remained positive; periods in which real interest rates were sharply negative were intermittent and confined to wartime (1812, 1861, 1917–18, and 1940–46).[8]

Usury laws and other forms of interest rate ceilings also have been common in developing countries. Financial officials in many developing countries, observing

---

[8]Steven C. Leuthold, "Interest Rates, Inflation and Deflation," *Financial Analysis Journal* (January–February 1981), 28–51.

gross imperfections in financial markets, have concluded that the market should not be permitted to determine interest rates. Monopoly (or oligopoly) power in financial markets, particularly in commercial banking, provides ample scope for the banks and other lenders to exercise market power in setting interest rates on loans at levels higher than the opportunity cost of capital.

There are ample observations of gross imperfections in financial systems in developing countries. Barriers to entry into banking and finance often allow a few large banks and other financial institutions to possess an inordinate degree of control over financial markets and thus exercise monopoly power in setting interest rates. Often these barriers are a direct result of government policies. Governments have prohibited new entrants into the field, adopted such stringent financial requirements for entry that only the very wealthy could amass the needed capital, or reserved permission for entry to political favorites who were attracted to banking and finance largely by the monopoly returns available when entry was restricted.

In this way, one set of government policies, entry restrictions, helps give rise to the need for extensive controls on prices charged by financial institutions. Typically, these controls take the form of interest rate ceilings imposed to limit the scope of monopoly power in the financial system. Controls by themselves do not necessarily lead to shallow finance. Rather, a combination of rigid ceilings on nominal interest rates and inflation impedes financial development and ultimately retards income growth.

Few economists believe that steeply positive real interest rates are essential for healthy growth in the real size of the financial system. The Chilean experience with very high real interest rates from 1981 to 1983 strongly suggests the opposite. There is no widely accepted answer to the question of what the required level of real interest rates is for a steady development of the financial system. The required real rate differs across countries in different circumstances. In some, financial growth may continue even at 0 or mildly negative real interest rates; for others, moderately high positive real rates of between 3 and 5 percent may be essential.

Apart from a few Latin American countries and Indonesia, most developing countries were able to keep rates of inflation at or below 5 to 6 percent before 1973. Inasmuch as nominal deposit rates typically were between 3 and 5 percent, real interest rates tended to be slightly positive or only mildly negative. When inflation accelerated in many developing countries after 1973, because few countries made more than marginal adjustments in nominal deposit rates, real interest rates turned significantly negative in a number of nations, as Table 12–4 shows for 1980. Negative interest rates endured in a few African and Latin American countries throughout the 1980s but, as the table suggests, are much less common today.

When real interest rates turn significantly negative, the maintenance of low nominal rates for promoting investment and income growth becomes counterproductive. Inflation taxes on liquid financial assets bring real growth in the financial system to a halt. Sharply negative real rates lead to shrinkage in the system, as the demand for liquid assets contracts. Contraction in the financial system results in a reduction in

TABLE 12-4 Real Lending Interest Rates, 1980s and 2008–09

COUNTRY	1980S	2008–09
Low-income countries		
Ethiopia	−18	−17
Tanzania	−18	7
India	4	4
Bangladesh	−5	8
Kenya	1	8
Nigeria	−4	19
Honduras	12	14
Lower-middle-income countries		
Bolivia	2	15
Philippines	0	6
Sri Lanka	−1	10
Indonesia	22	6
Peru	−19	18
Egypt	−4	1
Upper-middle-income countries		
Brazil	−	37
Hungary	1	6
Colombia	9	8
Malaysia	5	13
Korea	−5	2
High-income countries		
United Kingdom	−3	−1
Japan	2	3
United States	6	2

Source: World Bank, *World Development Indicators 2011* http://databank.worldbank.org/ddp/home.do, accessed June 2011.

the real supply of credit and thus constricts investment in productive assets. Under such circumstances, nonprice rationing of investible resources must occur and can take many forms. In most developing countries, only those borrowers with either the highest-quality collateral or the "soundest" social and political connections or those willing to make the largest side payments (bribes) to bank officers are successful in securing finance from the organized financial system. These criteria do not yield allocations of credit to the most productive investment opportunities.

Negative real interest rates make marginal, low-yielding, traditional types of investment appear attractive to investors. Banks and financial institutions find such projects attractive as well because they may be the safest and the simplest to finance and involve the most creditworthy borrowers. Satisfying the financial requirements of such investors constricts the pool of resources available to firms, with riskier projects offering greater possibilities for high yields. In addition, in the presence of substantial inflation, interest rate ceilings discourage risk taking by the financial institutions themselves because under such circumstances they cannot charge higher interest rates (risk premia) on promising but risky projects. Also, negative real interest rates are inimical to employment growth because they make projects with relatively high capital-output ratios appear more attractive than if real interest rates were positive. This implicit subsidy to capital-intensive methods of production reduces the jobs created for each dollar of investment, even as the ability of the financial system to finance investment is shrinking.

Negative real rates of interest tend to lower the marginal efficiency of investment in all the ways described. In terms of the Harrod-Domar model described in Chapter 4, shallow financial strategies cause higher capital-output ratios. Consequently, growth in national income and, therefore, growth in savings tend to be lower than when real rates are positive. Therefore, shallow finance retards income and employment growth even if the interest elasticity of savings is 0. And if savings decisions are responsive to real interest rates, then shallow finance has even more serious implications for income growth, as the ratio of private savings to the GDP also contracts.

DEEP FINANCIAL STRATEGY

Deep finance as a strategy has several objectives: (1) mobilizing a larger volume of savings from the domestic economy—that is, increasing the ratio of national savings to the GDP (where the interest elasticity of savings is thought to be positive and significant); (2) enhancing the accessibility of savings for all types of domestic investors; (3) securing a more efficient allocation of investment throughout the economy; and (4) permitting the financial process to mobilize and allocate savings to reduce reliance on the fiscal process, foreign aid, and inflation.

A permanent move toward policies involving positive real interest rates or, at a minimum, avoidance of sharply negative real rates is the essence of deep finance. In turn, this requires either financial liberalization that allows higher nominal rates on deposits and loans, curbing the rate of inflation, or some combination of both.

Given the difficulties involved in securing quick results in reducing inflation to levels consistent with positive real rates of interest, the first step involved in a shift from shallow to deep financial strategies ordinarily is to raise the ceilings on nominal rates for both deposits and loans. In extreme cases of acute inflation, the initial step has involved raising ceilings on nominal deposit rates to as much as 50 percent in Argentina and Uruguay in 1976 and to nearly 200 percent in Chile in 1974 (where real interest rates nevertheless remained negative until 1976). As the real rate moves toward positive levels, savers strongly tend to increase their holdings of liquid assets; this allows a real expansion in the supply of credit to investors. Available evidence suggests that countries that attempt to maintain modestly positive real interest rates over long periods tend to be among those with the highest rates of financial growth.

Where finance is deep, inflation tends to be moderate; therefore, savers are not subject to persistently high inflation taxes on liquid-asset holdings. That being the case, they are less inclined to shift their savings into much more lightly taxed domestic assets such as gold, land, or durable goods and foreign assets such as currencies or land and securities. Rather, financial resources that otherwise may have been used for these purposes flow to the financial system, where they are more accessible to prospective investors. Nonprice rationing of credit, inevitable under shallow finance, diminishes as well, and the capacity of the financial system to identify and support socially profitable investment opportunities expands. Higher-risk, higher-yielding investment projects stand a far better chance of securing finance under deep than shallow finance. Growth prospects are enhanced accordingly.

Investment finance problems, however, do not end with the provision of a growing real flow of short-term credit. As economies move to higher levels of per capita income, the pattern of investment shifts toward longer horizons. Longer-term investment requires longer-term finance. Commercial banks everywhere are ill-suited for providing substantial amounts of long-term finance, given that their deposits primarily are of a short-term nature.

Therefore, as financial and economic development proceeds, the need for institutions specializing in longer-term finance rises accordingly: insurance companies, investment banks, and ultimately equity markets (stock exchanges) become important elements in financial intermediation. The type of well-functioning commercial bank system that tends to develop under deep finance almost always is a necessary condition for the successful emergence and long-term vitality of institutions specializing in longer-term investment finance.

Earlier we observed that entry into the financial field is rarely easy, and other factors also often lead to gross imperfections in financial markets. Under such circumstances, many developing-country governments have found intervention essential to develop financial institutions specializing in longer-term finance. Intervention may take the form of establishment of government-owned development banks and other specialized institutions to act as distributors of government funds intended as a source of longer-term finance, as in Indonesia and Pakistan. In Mexico and Colombia, governments provided strong incentives for private-sector establishment of long-term financial institutions. Other governments sought to create conditions favorable for the emergence of primary securities (stocks and bonds) markets, the source par excellence for long-term finance. In cases in which these measures have been undertaken in the context of financial markets with strong commercial banking systems (Hong Kong, Singapore, Brazil, and Mexico), efforts to encourage long-term finance have met with some success. In cases in which commercial banking has been poorly developed as a consequence of shallow finance (Ghana, Uruguay before 1976) or the government has sought to "force feed" embryonic securities markets through tax incentives and other subsidies (Indonesia before 1988, Kenya, Turkey), the promotional policies have been less effective.

INFORMAL CREDIT MARKETS AND MICRO CREDIT

The discussion of financial development to this point has dealt with modern credit institutions, the formal market. But in many developing countries, as noted at the beginning of this chapter, **informal credit markets** coexist with modern financial institutions. These markets arise in many forms. In rural India, village moneylenders make loans to local farmers who have no access to commercial banks. In Ghana and other West African countries, market women give credit to farmers by paying for crops in advance of harvest, and they assist their customers by selling finished goods on credit. In South Korea, established lenders actually made loans on the street outside modern banks; this justifies their designation as the *curb* (or *kerb*) *market*. In much of rural Africa wealthy family members make loans to less fortunate kin, and all over the developing world there are cooperative arrangements to raise funds and share credit among members. Even in modern economies, pawnbrokers and others give credit outside the formal credit system.

Informal credit generally is financed by the savings of relatively wealthy individuals, such as local landowners, traders, family members who have moved into lucrative jobs or businesses, and the pooled efforts of cooperative societies. But informal lenders also may have access to the formal banking system and borrow there, to relend to customers with no access to banks. How can they do this if the banks cannot? First, because they know their borrowers so well and may have familial, social, or other ties to them, informal lenders face lower risks than distant, large banks that might loan to the same borrowers. Loan recovery rates are higher (usually much higher than found in large banks in developing countries) because those who borrow in informal markets know that the availability of loans in the future depends on repaying current loans. Second, they also face lower administrative costs in making loans. Of course, moneylenders charge very high interest rates, and this is a third reason they coexist with banks, which are often prevented by law from charging rates high enough to cover the risks and costs of loans in small amounts to very small firms and low-income borrowers.

Beginning in the 1970s, micro-credit institutions and micro-finance institutions more broadly were developed to reach populations in developing countries that had no access to credit, except in informal markets in which interest charges frequently reached annual rates of 100 percent. The best known of these new institutions was the Grameen Bank, founded in 1976 by Muhammad Yunus. Building on innovations such as Grameen, the movement to provide micro credit gained momentum and spread around the world to Africa, Latin America, and Asia where billions of people had no access to reasonable credit. The expansion in micro credit was then supplemented with programs to provide institutions designed to facilitate savings and other financial transactions by the rural poor in developing countries. **Micro finance** was the term applied to this broader set of financial transactions.

The basic idea of micro credit and micro finance was that the poor could be safe credit risks if they were organized appropriately. The Grameen Bank began by providing micro loans to poor women in the village of Jobra, Bangladesh. Today, Grameen covers virtually all of Bangladesh, with more than 2,500 branch offices and more than 20,000 employees. The Grameen Bank reports that they have over 8 million borrowers in Bangladesh; about 97 percent of whom are women, most are landless, and all are poor. Loans are made to individual women, but only through local groups that provide social pressure for repayment. Loans for micro enterprises average 28,000 taka (about US$400) and carry an annual interest rate of 20 percent. Loans are also given for other purposes, including for housing and education, at 8 and 5 percent, respectively. There is even a special program targeted at beggars, which offers very small loans at 0 interest. Today, Grameen maintains that its loans are not heavily subsidized, neither by donors nor the government of Bangladesh. The recovery rate on Grameen loans is impressive; it exceeds 97 percent and the bank reports it has earned a profit every year since it was founded. The Grameen Bank is more than a financial institution. Its loans require recipients to accept certain "social disciplines," such as cleanliness and family planning, and the bank provides such services as advice on home construction and access to education for some borrowers.[9]

A major problem with many efforts to promote micro credit, however, was that many of the institutions set up to provide such credit depended on subsidies, often quite large subsidies, either from international aid agencies or from private donations from the well to do. This was true of the Grameen Bank earlier in its history. In Indonesia in the 1980s, a government bank, the Bank Rakyat Indonesia (BRI), followed a different path. It began to provide full banking services, both loans and savings deposit facilities, to farmers, traders, and other small-scale borrowers, through their branches in over 3,000 villages. Loans are provided for either working capital or investment purposes. Today, loans range from 25,000 to 25 million rupiahs (from about $3 to $3,000), with repayment periods as short as three months and as long as two years. BRI programs—*kupedes* for the lending program and *simpedes* for the savings program—replaced a government-promoted effort that depended on heavy government subsidies and had a high rate of loan default. These new loans, in contrast, were commercially profitable without any subsidies right from the beginning.

BRI charged market rates of interest, around 30 percent a year, on its loans and paid attractive rates, about 12 percent, on deposits. These rates changed during the financial crisis of 1997–98, largely because of the high inflation in that period, but the basic rate-setting principles remained the same. In the absence of inflation, rates of 30 percent on loans may seem high, but they were considerably below the rates charged by informal money lenders. At these rates, the BRI was able to attract sufficient savings deposits to more than finance its loan program. Several million savers and borrowers mostly in rural areas gained access to the formal banking system for the first time through these BRI programs. Roughly 97 percent of the loans were repaid on time. In addition, the program became a major generator of profits for the

[9]World Bank, *World Development Report 1989*, p. 117; (New York: Oxford University Press, 1989) A. Wahid, *The Grameen Bank: Poverty Relief* (Boulder, CO: Westview Press, 1993).

BRI, something that could not be said about many of its credit programs for large-scale producers and borrowers during the 1997–98 financial crisis.[10] These loans have continued to be a major source of BRI profits in the years since the crisis.

Micro credit is sometimes promoted by its supporters as the answer to rural and urban poverty in developing countries, but as we have emphasized throughout this book, there is no single answer to how to lift the world's poor out of poverty. Micro credit and micro finance have helped poor households in Bangladesh, Indonesia, and elsewhere, but there is considerable debate over their impact on poverty (Box 12–2). While we know that some programs have done well, we do not know whether

[10]Richard H. Patten and Jay Rosengard, *Progress with Profits: The Development of Rural Banking in Indonesia* (San Francisco: ICS Press, 1991); Marguerite Robinson, "Rural Financial Intermediation: Lessons from Indonesia," Development Discussion Paper 434, Harvard Institute for International Development, October 1992.

BOX 12–2 DOES MICRO CREDIT REDUCE POVERTY?

To determine whether micro-credit loans reduce poverty, the experience of borrowers might be compared with nonborrowers. If borrowers, on average, have a lower poverty rate than do nonborrowers, we might conclude that micro credit was an effective instrument for reducing poverty, and the impact of micro credit on poverty reduction could be quantified. But this approach is problematic. We face a classic problem of *identification*. What if borrowers are systematically different from nonborrowers in some unobservable way? Maybe those who obtain micro-credit loans are more entrepreneurial or have a higher tolerance for risk. Their lower poverty rates may have more to do with these attributes than with the loans they received. Borrowers of micro credit might have sought out other types of informal credit, making it difficult to isolate the marginal impact of micro credit on poverty reduction.

Problems of identification like these can be addressed by randomized controlled trials (RCTs), which compare the impact of an intervention between an otherwise similar treatment and control group. Researchers at the Abdul Latif Jameel Poverty Action Lab (J-PAL) located at the Massachusetts Institute of Technology (MIT) conducted an RCT on micro finance in 2005 in the city of Hyderabad, India. Working with an Indian micro-finance firm, Spandana, branches were opened in half of 104 randomly selected slum neighborhoods; in the other half, branches were not opened. Spandana loans are similar to those pioneered by the Grameen Bank. They are offered to women who form groups with 6 to 10 members who are jointly responsible for the loans. Initial loans are for 10,000 rupees (about $200 at market exchange rates and $1,000 in terms of purchasing power parity [PPP]), with an annual percentage rate of 24 percent. Then 15 to 18 months after the introduction of the new branches, detailed household sur-veys were administered to almost 7,000 households living in the treatment and control neighborhoods to determine the impact of the micro-credit loans.

Because micro-finance firms other than Spandana were available throughout Hyderabad, residents of both treated and untreated neighborhoods had access to micro-credit loans. In neighborhoods where Spandana opened a new branch, 27 percent of residents took out a loan compared to 19 percent in untreated areas. This suggests that the treatment had an effect on borrowing rates. But it also indicates that between 70 and 80 percent of households did not take advantage of Spandana or any other micro-finance loans. The overwhelming majority of households either were not credit constrained or were unwilling to assume the risks associated with taking out a loan. This suggests that it may be a lack of profitable opportunities to invest borrowed funds rather than a lack of cheaper credit that constrains most poor households.

In comparing treated and untreated neighborhoods, the J-PAL study found that 7 percent of households started a new business in neighborhoods where Spandana opened a new branch compared to only 5.3 percent of households in the control areas. Access to micro credit therefore had a significant impact on the formation of new businesses. About one third of Spandana borrowers started a new business, and about one fifth spent their loans on equipment for existing businesses. The other half of borrowers used their loans for current consumption, including on food or med-icine, to buy a durable for household use (for example, a television set), or to pay down other debts. In the period covered by the survey, there was no statistically sig-nificant increase in total consumption expenditures between treatment and control areas. In other words, micro credit did not reduce poverty rates over this time period.

As the J-PAL study notes, 15 to 18 months may be too short a time to assess the long-term impact of micro credit. The new businesses started as a result of Spandana loans may need more time to earn profits and lift families above poverty. In the short term micro credit did not reduce poverty, nor was it a recipe for improving the school-ing or health of children or for empowering women. Of course, the J-PAL study is only one study, and as with all RCTs we must be careful in drawing general conclusions from any one experiment. Evidence from a variety of nonexperimental approaches finds many benefits of micro-credit loans and other micro-finance products. The authors of the Hyderabad study themselves are measured in their conclusions, noting that micro credit "may not be the 'miracle' that is sometimes claimed on its behalf, but it does allow households to borrow, invest and create and expand businesses."

Sources: Abhijit Banerjee, Esther Duflo, Rachel Glennerster, and Cynthia Kinnan, "The Miracle of Microfinance? Evidence for a Randomized Evaluation," Massachusetts Institute of Technology, June 2010; Kathleen Odell, "Measuring the Impact of Microfinance: Taking Another Look," Grameen Foun-dation Publication Series, 2010.

the hundreds and thousands of such programs around the world justify the large out-lays of outside aid that they have used. About half of the estimated $12 billion com-mitted to micro-finance organizations worldwide came as grants or concessional loans from aid agencies and donors. These resources might have been spent in other ways and had more of a poverty impact.

Micro credit often has its biggest impact when it helps individuals with limited means to start a new business and gradually expand that business. But there are many other barriers in addition to the lack of credit that can inhibit the development of new businesses and undermine the value of the credit. Many individuals borrow saying the loan is for a small business but use the money for consumption that leaves them with a debt that they may have difficulty repaying. Some borrow funds from one micro-finance organization to pay off loans they secured from another micro-finance organization. Such practices, clearly, are not sustainable for either the borrower or the lender.

Research indicates that profitable micro finance on the BRI model is not a com-plete substitute for subsidized micro finance in reaching the poorest parts of the pop-ulation. Profitable micro finance reaches large numbers of people who previously had no access to credit or appropriate vehicles for savings, but many of the programs designed to reach the poorest parts of the population in poor countries and provide other nonfinancial services along with credit also reach people that the for-profit pro-grams do not. There is clearly a role for both kinds of credit facilities.[11]

[11]For a lengthy analysis of these and many other related issues see Beatriz Armendariz and Jonathan Morduch, *The Economics of Microfinance* (Cambridge: MIT Press, 2005); Robert Cull, Asli Demirguc-Kunt, and Jonathan Morduch, "Microfinance Meets the Market," *Journal of Economic Perspectives*, 23, no. 1 (2009), 167–92. Another source that evaluates micro finance is *David Roodman's Microfinance Open Book Blog* (http://blogs.cgdev.org/open_book).

SUMMARY

- The money supply is made up of the liquid assets of an economy but the degree of liquidity of particular assets varies, leading to different, more precise definitions of the money supply.
- The rate of inflation varies greatly among developing economies. Inflation, in effect, is a tax on those who hold money balances, and a moderate rate of inflation can sometimes increase government savings and investment and not harm growth, but the higher the rate of inflation, the more people shift away from liquid assets, thus undermining the development of the financial system and harming economic growth.
- Exchange rate management is an essential component of any effort to control inflation. Exchange rate systems range from fixed exchange rates,

by which the local currency is pegged to the dollar or some other currency, to floating rates that move with market forces. In small countries with fixed-rate systems, worldwide inflation is transferred rapidly to the country with the fixed exchange rate. With floating rates, inflation arises mainly from domestic, not international, sources.

- A variety of additional mechanisms for controlling inflation are at the disposal of the central bank, all of which must, in one way or another, reduce the growth rate of the money supply. Mechanisms such as open-market operations are generally more efficient than mechanisms such as credit ceilings, but most developing countries are not in a position to conduct open-market sales and purchases of government bonds. Credit ceilings and increased bank reserve requirements are less efficient but are effective in lowering the growth of the money supply and inflation.

- Financial panics have been present throughout the last several centuries, but countries have learned how to eliminate some of the reasons for financial panic. As the experience in the late 1990s and 2007–09 of several countries around the world demonstrated, however, there are reasons why panics can still occur.

- The nominal rate of interest is the agreed-on rate between lenders and borrowers, but the real rate of interest, the nominal rate adjusted for inflation, most influences whether individuals are willing to hold liquid assets or not.

- Positive real interest rates are necessary for financial deepening, defined as the rising ratio of liquid assets to GDP. Negative real interest rates have the opposite effect. Financial deepening generally supports growth, although growth sometimes still occurs in its absence.

- As development proceeds and the economy becomes more complex and the need for long-term investment financing increases, economies require a wider variety of financial institutions. Stock markets and bond markets are one source of such long-term finance but so are insurance companies and development banks, and the latter are often supported by government for the explicit purpose of providing longer term finance.

- The formal financial system particularly in developing countries tends not to reach small businesses and individuals with limited financial resources. Informal financial markets exist to provide financing for such potential borrowers, but the interest charges on such loans tend to be very high. To counter this problem a variety of more formal efforts in the form of micro-credit institutions have arisen, providing more reasonable credit terms. The expansion of micro finance since the 1970s has been rapid, but there is still much we do not know about its overall impact on poverty.

13

Foreign Debt and Financial Crises

Beginning in 2007 (and continuing into 2011), much of the world was beset by the largest financial crisis since the Great Depression of the 1930s—a crisis originating in the United States and other advanced economies. Debt crises in several countries have played a central role. In 2010, and again in 2011, Greece, a member of the European Union was on the verge of being unable to meet its debt obligations, and there was fear the problem would spread to Portugal, Italy, and Spain. In 2010, the other members of the European Union, notably Germany, pledged up to $1 trillion to help Greece and, if necessary, the others meet their debt obligations. For the countries in crisis, devaluation of the currency, a policy often used to offset some of the negative effects of having to cut back on expenditures to repay debt, was not available because Greece, Italy, Spain, and Portugal use the common currency of the European Union, the euro. Our focus in this chapter, however, is on debt problems in developing countries, thus we will not deal further with the details of the debt problems of southern Europe and the threat these problems pose for the euro. Nonetheless, it is important to note that the global financial crisis that began in the advanced economies has had a severe impact on developing countries as both trade and financial flows have fallen rapidly in the late 2000s. The Mexican experience provides an informative case with which to begin our discussion of debt and financial crises in developing countries.

In the two decades following World War II, Mexico, like most developing countries, had few transactions with international capital markets. The country borrowed relatively little from international banks, and foreign investors only occasionally took a stake in Mexican firms. And, while it borrowed some funds from official lenders (governments and international organizations such as the World Bank), Mexico's total borrowing remained small. At the time, international capital markets were relatively undeveloped compared to today, and they were only just beginning to recover from the disruptions of the two world wars and the Great Depression. But things began to change in the late 1960s and early 1970s. Capital market instruments became more sophisticated, and the costs of international transactions fell. Bankers and other investors started to look for opportunities outside their traditional Western markets. Official lending increased as well. Mexico, along with many other countries, was eager to expand investment and accelerate growth and began to look abroad for financing. In the decades since then, Mexico's foreign borrowing has had tremendous impact, both positive and negative, on its economic growth, macroeconomic stability, job creation, and even political dynamics.

Most of Mexico's foreign financing in the early years was in the form of borrowing, especially from private creditors, as opposed to foreign direct investment. Mexico was suspicious of foreign investors and wanted to maintain ownership control of its enterprises, so borrowing was more palatable than foreign direct investment. Foreign commercial banks were more than willing to lend money to the Mexican government, state-owned companies (such as PEMEX, the state oil company), and other businesses. In 1970, Mexico's foreign borrowing from private creditors was relatively small, amounting to $350 million, or about 1 percent of the gross domestic product (GDP). But by 1980, it was borrowing nearly $15 billion a year from private creditors, about 8 percent of the GDP. More than half the debt was short term, meaning that it had to be repaid (and usually reborrowed) within one year.

At first, the borrowing seemed to help: Mexico's GDP per capita rose 4.2 percent per year between 1972 and 1981, compared with 2.6 percent during the previous seven years. But it turned out that Mexico had borrowed too much too quickly: In August 1982, it shocked the world by declaring that it could not service its debts. The country plunged into a deep economic crisis that led to a sharp reduction in investment, negative growth rates, deep strains on government finance, and considerable economic hardship for millions of Mexicans. Mexico's crisis quickly cascaded to many other developing countries that had borrowed heavily abroad, and the consequences of these crises are still playing out today in some countries. Foreign lending to Mexico plummeted after the crisis before recovering in the early 1990s, only to plunge again when Mexico faced another payments crisis in 1994 and 1995. Since the mid-1990s, Mexico's net foreign borrowing has been negative in most years, meaning that it has been repaying international lenders more than it has been borrowing.

Globally, debt flows to developing countries have followed a pattern similar to Mexico's, swinging back and forth from large inflows to large outflows and then back again. Borrowing from private commercial banks became the dominant form of international capital flows to developing countries, especially middle-income countries, in the 1970s and 1980s, surpassing official borrowing in almost every year. But debt flows fell sharply in the 1980s after the debt crises (Table 13–1). In the early

TABLE 13-1 Debt Flows to Developing Countries, 1980–2008 (billion US$)

	1980	1990	1996	2000	2008
Private debt finance	70.9	29.8	119.9	−0.4	107.9
Commercial Banks	28.7	3.2	30.7	−5.8	123.0
Bonds	1.1	1.1	49.5	17.5	10.5
Other	11.5	12.3	2.3	−4.3	−9.3
Short-term debt flows (net)	29.5	13.2	37.4	−7.9	−16.3
Official debt finance	20.5	26.4	2.8	4.9	−20.4
Bilateral	13.1	11.0	−10.4	−6.9	2.4
Multilateral	7.4	15.4	13.1	11.8	18.0
Total	91.4	56.2	122.7	4.5	128.3

Sources: World Bank, *Global Development Finance 2005* (Washington, DC: World Bank, 2005) and World Bank, *Global Development Finance 2009* (Washington, DC: World Bank, 2009); and International Monetary Fund, *International Financial Statistics*, (Washington, DC: IMF, 2009).

1990s, private debt flows grew sharply again, quadrupling in size in just six years from $30 billion in 1990 to $120 billion in 1996. But then a series of financial crises struck several emerging markets around the world, starting with Mexico in 1995; then hitting Thailand, Indonesia, Malaysia, and Korea in 1997; Russia and Brazil in 1998; and Turkey and Argentina in 2001. Debt flows collapsed, and by 2001, the $120 billion inflow of five years earlier had completely disappeared. But once the crises abated, borrowing increased again, and private debt flows rebounded to $72 billion just two years later in 2003. Official borrowing was much smaller and less volatile than private borrowing, but it fell steadily during the 1990s, and by 2003, developing countries as a whole were repaying more to official creditors than they were borrowing. For many of the poorest developing countries, grants, rather than loans, were the dominant source of foreign financing.

Even among the largest borrowers, foreign borrowing has always been small compared to domestic capital flows, in most years accounting for perhaps one fourth or less of available investable funds and only occasionally amounting to more than 3–4 percent of GDP. From the perspective of economic growth models that emphasize the role of capital formation in the growth process (such as the Harrod-Domar and Solow models), private debt flows are only modestly important. But foreign debt plays a more complex role than the basic numbers indicate. The economic impact of debt flows is magnified by their effect on macroeconomic stability, the exchange rate, interest rates, government budgets, and domestic financial institutions and their potential to trigger widespread financial crises.

This chapter explores the advantages, disadvantages, and risks associated with foreign borrowing. It describes various forms of debt, the patterns of debt flows to developing countries over the last several decades, and the basic conditions under which debt is sustainable. It examines in some detail the developing-country debt crises of the 1980s, the ongoing debt problems faced by some low-income countries, and the emerging-market financial crises of the 1990s. It then explores the main lessons that have emerged from these crises for debt management in the future. We also probe some of the tough questions that arise when countries default or no longer can pay their debt service: How much should be forgiven? How should the burden of bad loans be shared between creditors and borrowers? And what conditions, if any, should be placed on countries seeking debt forgiveness?

ADVANTAGES AND DISADVANTAGES OF FOREIGN BORROWING

Foreign debt gained a bad reputation after the crises of the 1980s, the late 1990s, and the Greek and Irish debt problems of 2010–11, in many ways deservedly so. However, prudent borrowing has been an important part of the development strategy of many countries. The United States borrowed heavily in the middle and late nineteenth century to finance its westward expansion (especially the railroads). Most countries in western Europe relied on foreign borrowing at one time or another.

From a national perspective, borrowing permits a country to invest more than it can save and import more than it can export. If the additional funds finance productive investment, they should yield sufficient returns to pay the interest and principal on the initial foreign inflows. As we saw in Chapters 3 and 4, because capital is relatively scarce in low-income countries, these countries have the *potential* to realize higher rates of return on investment and more rapid economic growth than richer countries, providing the foundation for lending from rich to low-income countries. Under these circumstances, foreign borrowing can help support growth and development at the same time as it yields attractive returns to the lender.

For countries interested in augmenting domestic saving with foreign capital, borrowing brings several advantages and disadvantages relative to foreign direct investment and other forms of capital. When a domestic firm borrows abroad, there are no controversies over foreign ownership, profit repatriation, tax holidays, and the like that arise with foreign direct investment (FDI). In addition, foreign borrowing can be undertaken much more quickly and easily than can FDI. Repayments are limited to the terms of the loan, so if an investment is highly profitable, the home country can keep the profits rather than repatriate them abroad. To simplify only slightly, as long as the rate of return on investment projects exceeds the interest rate on the debt, foreign borrowing can be a very sensible strategy to augment domestic savings, add to investment, and accelerate growth. In addition, borrowing can play a critical stabilization role for countries buffeted by balance of payments shocks. When a country's export prices suddenly collapse or its import prices rise, some temporary borrowing can help bridge the financing gap until prices rebound or the economy can adjust to the change, thus helping ease the costs of adjustment.

However, there are downsides as well. Debts must be paid, even when a project goes bad. Too much borrowing of the wrong kind or for the wrong purposes can leave developing countries vulnerable to sudden capital withdrawals and financial crises. Short-term debt, in particular, can very quickly switch from rapid inflow to rapid out-flow, which can cause sudden plunges in exchange rates and skyrocketing interest rates and wreak havoc on banks, private companies, and government budgets.

Borrowing too much to finance consumption or poorly conceived investments also can lead to trouble. Borrowing is much easier politically than raising taxes to pay for spending, especially if governments do not think they will still be in office when it is time to repay. If governments borrow to finance monuments, lavish office buildings, or fleets of expensive cars, there will be no future income stream to repay the debts. But even where governments borrow to finance investments that initially seem sound, sudden drops in export prices, rising interest rates or oil prices, or an unforeseen world recession can turn a worthwhile project into a financial loss. Governments strapped with large debt service payments sometimes face painful choices between repaying foreign lenders as promised, or maintaining spending on health, education, or other important domestic programs.

DEBT SUSTAINABILITY

How much aggregate debt can a country take on before it begins to get into trouble? There is no simple answer. A country's debts are sustainable if they can be serviced without resort to exceptional financing (for example, a special bailout by friendly donors) and without a major future adjustment in the country's income and expen-diture. But every country's situation is different. A country's ability to repay depends on a wide array of factors: the size of its debt, its trade and budget deficits, the interest rate on its debt, the mix of loans and grants it receives, its vulnerability to shocks (for example, natural disasters such as droughts or hurricanes or a fall in export prices), and the rate of growth of GDP, exports, and government tax revenues.

At a simple level, a country's debt sustainability depends on (1) how much it owes and (2) its capacity to make the required payments. But neither of these is quite as straightforward as they first seem. There are two ways to think about how much the country owes: the total stock of debt and the amount of payments due in a par-ticular year. The usual measure of the total debt stock is the sum of the face value of all debts outstanding, but this can be misleading if a significant portion of debt is subsidized. For example, the World Bank's International Development Association (IDA), the part of the World Bank that provides finance for low-income countries, provides loans with an interest rate of just 0.75 percent and 40 years to repay. Obvi-ously a $100 million loan extended on these terms creates a much smaller burden than a $100 million loan that must be repaid in 5 years with a market-determined interest rate of 7 percent. Under these circumstances it makes much more sense to calculate the net present value (NPV) of the debt. A loan extended on normal market terms would have an NPV equal to 100 percent of its face value, a grant would have NPV equal to 0, and subsidized loans would have an NPV in between, depending on the interest rate and the maturity structure (that is, the schedule to repay the loan's principal).

Debt service is the amount due for principal and interest payments in a given year. Policy makers need to know how much is due each year, but looking at just one year can be misleading because it leaves out how much is due the next year or the year after, when a big payment might be due. Thus an accurate projection of how much debt service is due when is an important component of assessing debt sustainability.

What about the second part of sustainability, a country's capacity to pay? Three measures of capacity are most common: GDP, exports, and government tax revenue. GDP is the broadest measure of the economic resources available to repay the debt. The larger a country's productive capacity and corresponding income, the greater its ability to repay debt. But if a country is repaying foreign debt, the real constraint may not be total income, but the ability to earn the dollars (or other foreign exchange) needed to repay the loans denominated in foreign currency. When Thailand, Indonesia, and Korea could not fully service their debts in late 1997, the problem was not a lack of sufficient income, but a lack of available foreign exchange. Under these circumstances, exports earned each year or the stock of foreign exchange reserves held by the central bank may be more suitable indicators of debt servicing capacity. Exports and reserves focus attention on the **external transfer problem**, the challenge of generating sufficient foreign exchange to transfer to external (foreign) creditors. But foreign exchange is not always the binding constraint either. If the government is the major debtor, an important indicator of repayment capacity is its ability to generate tax revenue that can be used to repay the debt. The importance of tax revenues points to the **internal transfer problem**, the government's challenge of raising enough revenue from households and firms to enable the government to repay the nation's debts.

DEBT INDICATORS

Analysts typically turn these broad measures into ratios, with the numerator containing either debt or debt service and the denominator showing a measure of the capacity to repay. The most common debt sustainability indicators include the following:

- *Debt/GDP*, perhaps the broadest measure of debt sustainability, compares total debt to the economy's total capacity to generate resources to repay. A closely related measure uses the net present value: *NPV debt/GDP*.

Where most debt is on market terms (for example, commercial bank loans), the difference between these two measures is small; to the extent debts are contracted on concessional (subsidized) terms, the two differ. Although each country is different, history suggests that debt distress tends to be more likely in countries where the NPV debt/GDP ratio exceeds 30 to 50 percent.[1]

- *Debt/exports* (and NPV debt/exports) compares the total debt to the capacity to generate foreign exchange. A wide range of debt/export ratios might be compatible with sustainability, reflecting the tendency for exports to vary more widely than the GDP. Analysts tend to place threshold levels for individual countries anywhere between 100 and 300 percent, most frequently around 200 percent.

- *Debt/revenue* (or NPV debt/revenue) is most relevant when the government is the largest debtor and there are concerns about its ability to generate tax revenue to repay the loans. Analysts cite ratios of anywhere between 140 and 260 percent as thresholds for individual countries.

- *Debt service/exports* has the great advantage of focusing attention on the amount owed in a single year relative to the export earnings available to make the payments, but it tells less about the overall burden of debt over time. Concern about debt distress tends to grow when this ratio exceeds 20 to 25 percent.

- *Debt service/revenue* focuses on the government's ability to generate tax revenues to make payments due in a single year. The higher this ratio, the more tax revenue that must be devoted to making debt payments and the less available for other government expenditures on health, education, infrastructure, or other purposes. History suggests that debt distress tends to appear once this ratio exceeds 10 to 15 percent.

- *Short-term foreign debt/foreign exchange reserves* focuses on the amount of debt due to be repaid within the next year compared to the available amount of foreign exchange reserves. Analysts suggest that a country is vulnerable to a rapid withdrawal of capital and a financial crisis when this ratio approaches 1:1.

These ratios reflect two broadly different ways that countries can face debt difficulties: insolvency and illiquidity. An **insolvent borrower** lacks the net worth to repay outstanding debts out of future earnings. An **illiquid borrower** lacks the ready cash to repay current debt-servicing obligations, even though it has the net worth to repay the debts in the long term. An illiquid debtor may need cash to make immediate payments, but still has the capacity to repay the debt over time, while an insolvent

---

[1]International Monetary Fund, "Debt Sustainability in Low-Income Countries: Proposal for an Operational Framework and Policy Implications," February 3, 2004. Available at www.imf.org/external/np/pdr/sustain/2004/020304.htm, accessed March 2012.

debtor does not have the income or assets to repay. The debt/GDP ratio in effect is a measure of overall solvency, indicating the value of debt relative to aggregate economic resources (in theory, ideally we would like a measure of overall wealth—the value of all assets—not just annual income, but this is extremely difficult to measure for a country). The debt service/exports, debt service/revenue, and short-term debt/reserves indicators are measures of liquidity, indicating whether a country has the capacity to make the payments due this year.

These ratios appear at first to be simplistic and mechanical, but each captures and depends on important broader features of both the debt and the economy. To see this, we examine two of the ratios in more depth: debt/exports and debt/GDP.

To explore the debt/export ratio, recall that foreign saving (F) equals the difference between imports and exports of goods and nonfactor services ($M - X$), or roughly the current account of the balance of payments. For simplicity, assume all foreign saving is in the form of borrowing. Therefore, the increase in debt in any year is

$$\Delta D = iD + M - X \qquad [13\text{-}1]$$

where ΔD represents the change in the debt stock and i is the average interest rate. For simplicity, assume that X and M grow at the same exponential rate, g_X. In that case, the stock of debt also grows exponentially at the same rate, and in the long run, the ratio of debt to exports settles at

$$D/X = a/(g_X - i) \qquad [13\text{-}2]$$

where a is the ratio of the current account deficit to exports, $(M - X)/X$, and is a constant, assuming that imports and exports grow at the same rate.[2]

Equation 13–2 tells us that the long-run ratio of debt to exports depends on the size of the current account deficit, the growth rate of exports, and the interest rate. If exports are growing faster than the average rate of interest ($g_X > i$), a country can continue to import more than it exports, meaning that a can remain positive. This should make intuitive sense: Borrowing to cover the gap between imports and exports is sustainable so long as exports are growing more than enough to cover interest payments.

Consider a numerical example. If the current account deficit as a share of exports were 8 percent ($a = 8$), the average interest rate were 5 percent, and exports were growing 9 percent a year, then the ratio of debt to exports would settle at 2 (or 200 percent). If exports grew faster than 9 percent, the debt-export ratio would fall. If, on the other hand, export growth fell to 5.5 percent, the debt/export ratio would explode

---

[2]Equation 13–1 is solved to yield equation 13–2 by letting $\Delta D = g_X D$ and substituting into equation 13–1. Then equation 13–1 becomes $g_X D = iD + M - X$, from which equation 13–2 can be readily derived (*hint:* start by dividing each side by X). The result is given by Albert Fishlow, "External Borrowing and Debt Management" (220–21) in Rudiger Dornbusch and F. Leslie C. H. Helmers, eds., *The Open Economy: Tools for Policymakers in Developing Countries* (New York: Oxford University Press, 1988).

to 1,600 percent. If it fell below the interest rate (either because export growth fell or world interest rates rose), the numerator a also would have to turn negative; that is, the current account deficit would turn to a surplus. The country could no longer run a deficit and borrow to make up the difference; instead it would have to run a surplus of exports over imports and use the balance to repay debts. This is precisely what has happened to many low-income, high-debt countries, with enormous adverse consequences in some cases.

Turning to the debt/GDP ratio, instead of examining imports and exports, a similar calculation can be made from the investment-saving perspective. Because we know from Chapter 10 that the current account balance $M - X$ is equal to the investment-saving balance $I - S_d$, equation 13-1 can be converted to the following:

$$\Delta D = iD + I - S_d = iD + vY - sY = iD + (v - s)Y \qquad [13\text{-}3]$$

In this equation, $Y = $ GDP and v and s are the investment and saving shares of GDP, respectively. As with the trade balance perspective, assume that debt and GDP grow at the same exponential rate, g_Y. Then the long-run equilibrium ratio of debt to GDP is

$$D/Y = (v - s)/(g_Y - i) \qquad [13\text{-}4]$$

In this case, if investment exceeds saving by 1 percentage point, the growth rate of GDP (expressed in current dollars) is 7 percent a year, and i averages 5 percent, the debt/GDP ratio settles at 0.5 (or 50 percent). But if GDP slips to a long-run rate of 5.5 percent, the ratio balloons to 200 percent.

Thus a country with poor overall economic performance, reflected in low export or GDP growth rates, is far more likely to get into trouble than a country with better performance. Policy makers must take these factors into account in determining how much a country can borrow and on what terms. Strong debt management, however, goes beyond these basics and includes allowing for the risk of a sudden fall in export receipts, higher interest rates, or other adverse shocks. And, as we shall see, the terms on which the debt is obtained (especially the maturity structure) can have a profound impact on vulnerability to a crisis.

FROM DISTRESS TO DEFAULT

Many developing countries have seen their debt ratios climb to uncomfortable levels at one time or another during the last two decades. Sometimes, even countries with good economic management can get into debt difficulties when they face drops in export prices or unexpected increases in import prices, say, from an increase in world oil prices. As debt-service payment burdens grow and it becomes more difficult to service the debts, countries face several important questions and trade-offs. To what extent should they continue to raise taxes and cut spending to service debts?

At what point do they try to renegotiate the terms of these loans, or in more extreme circumstances, consider outright default?

Most countries rightly see debt agreements as legal contracts in which they have an obligation to fully repay. Most want to avoid default because it can have significant negative consequences, just as filing for bankruptcy can have adverse consequences for a company. A country defaulting on its debts is likely to have much more difficulty borrowing in the future, at least for some period of time, until their prospects brighten. When creditors begin to lend again, they are likely to charge higher interest rates to compensate for the higher risks. Moreover, the process of renegotiation and restructuring can be time-consuming and costly and is something most finance officials would rather avoid. And most countries do not want the stigma and bad publicity that a default might generate.

At the same time, in extreme situations policy makers may see the costs of continuing to service their debts as outweighing the cost of default. Political leaders are willing to ask their citizens to undertake only so much austerity to repay foreign creditors. Moreover, sometimes, it might be fully appropriate for creditors to bear some of the cost of bad loans, especially if they pushed hard to provide funds for questionable projects. To the extent that creditors were partially responsible, they should absorb some of the costs through smaller repayments or even forgiveness of some of the remaining loan. Defaults are not uncommon for either private companies or public entities and certainly are not limited to developing countries (Box 13–1). Defaults occurred frequently in many Latin American and European countries during the nineteenth century and the 1930s, and Greece threatened to default in 2010 before being bailed out by the European Union, only to find itself once again facing a potential default in 2011 and 2012. Several U.S. states defaulted on their debts in the nineteenth century.

In addition, it is possible that continued repayment might undermine a country's ability to make future payment to such an extent that both the debtor *and* the creditor would be better off with some debt forgiveness. This situation is known as a **debt overhang**: The debt creates such a drag on growth that it undermines the ability of the country to make repayments.[3] Inflows of foreign financing should have a positive impact on growth, but debt service has a negative impact. As debt service grows, the negative impact becomes larger, and with debt service large enough, the overall impact on growth could be negative.

To see how this could happen, consider the following scenario. A government starts to raise taxes to repay the debt, and private companies and individuals begin to anticipate even higher taxes in the future, so they reduce investment. The growing

---

[3]Paul Krugman, "Financing versus Forgiving a Debt Overhang," *Journal of Development Economics* 29 (1988), 253–68; Jeffrey Sachs, "The Debt Overhang of Developing Countries," in R. Findlay, G. Calvo, P. Kouri, and J. Braga de Macedo, eds., *Debt, Stabilization and Development: Essays in Honor of Carlos Díaz Alejandro* (Oxford: Basil Blackwell, 1989).

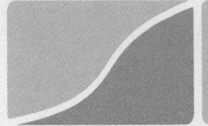

BOX 13-1 A SHORT HISTORY OF SOVEREIGN LENDING DEFAULT

In 1979, then-Citicorp chairman Walter Wriston famously pronounced that "countries don't go bankrupt." While it may technically be true that a country cannot go bankrupt, the assertion that they cannot default runs counter to the historical record. Default by governments is a practice as old as the concept of credit. Throughout history, there are many examples of countries that have refused to pay their bills or unilaterally written off debts incurred by previous governments.

The first such recorded default occurred in the fourth century B.C.E. when 10 of 13 Greek city-states with debts to the Delos temple walked away from their contractual obligations. Not long after, the island of Chios announced publicly that payments on its unsustainable debt would cease until economic conditions improved. Default in ancient times often took the form of currency depreciation, rather than a declaration of bankruptcy. For example, over the course of the three Punic Wars (241–146 B.C.E.), Rome reduced the metallic content of its monetary unit from 12 ounces to 0.5 ounce, in a series of de facto government defaults.

The practice of governmental default continued through the Middle Ages and into modern times. An eighteenth-century French minister of finance contended that "each government should default at least once every century, in order to restore equilibrium." In the nineteenth century, as the practice of lending abroad became more common, government default increased, and most European nations at least partially defaulted on their debt commitments. Some defaulted multiple times, with Spain and its seven recorded defaults leading the way. The record in developing nations was similar: Every Latin American nation without exception defaulted during the nineteenth century.

While the U.S. government avoided outright default, many individual states defaulted during this period. Some defaulted on civil war debts, while others did so on bonds issued to failed enterprises, usually railroad or bank endeavors. Arkansas and Florida each defaulted three times during the nineteenth century. And at the conclusion of the Spanish-American War in 1898, the U.S. government repudiated the debts that had been incurred by Cuba while under Spanish rule.

Germany's reparation obligations after World War I led to protracted debt difficulties that nurtured German grievances in the early 1930s. In the wave of defaults that accompanied the Great Depression of the 1930s, the international capital market collapsed, thereby leading to further widespread default. International capital flows fell sharply during the Depression and World War II, so sovereign defaults were rare in the late 1940s and the 1950s. But the international capital markets gradually revived in the 1960s and 1970s, and the debt crises of the 1980s saw a return to the sovereign defaults that had been common in the nineteenth century.

Adapted from Nancy Birdsall and John Williamson (with Brian Deese), *Delivering on Debt Relief: From IMF Gold to New Aid Architecture*, Center for Global Development and Institute for International Economics, (Washington, DC: Peterson Institute of International Economics and Center for Global Development, April 2002).

debt service burden makes lenders more reluctant to provide new finance, as they begin to fear the possibility of default. As debt burdens grow very large, the government begins to face perverse incentives against undertaking stringent adjustment measures. Economic reforms may help the country avoid default, but local citizens bear the cost of adjustment while creditors gain the benefits. Worse policies might lead to poorer economic performance but could lead to a larger debt write-off. Thus the debt burden becomes a disincentive for the very economic reforms that might be most needed. Empirical evidence on the existence of a debt overhang is mixed, but the idea has been influential in thinking about the rationale for debt restructuring and write-offs in developing countries.

Finally, while debt agreements are legal contracts, under some circumstances, governments may see the agreements as illegitimate, making default an easier option to contemplate. Debts taken on by a military dictator who took power through a coup and stole the money may not be seen as legitimate obligations by a succeeding democratically elected government. We discuss these **odious debts** later in the chapter.

THE 1980s DEBT CRISIS

The questions about default and debt restructuring are much more than hypothetical possibilities: They became very real issues for many developing countries during the last several decades. During the 1970s a large number of developing countries, especially in Latin America, borrowed extensively and accumulated large amounts of debt, so large that, by 1983, long-term debt owed by developing countries to commercial banks had grown from $19 billion to $307 billion, 16 times larger than it had been in 1970 (Table 13–2). Total debt stocks grew by a factor of 10 between 1970 and 1983, then doubled again in the 10 years that followed. But the rapid growth of debt in the 1970s and early 1980s led to trouble for some countries that had accumulated too much debt too fast. In the first half of 1982, eight countries had to reschedule their

TABLE 13-2 Long-Term Debt, All Developing Countries, 1970–2009 (billion US$)

STOCKS	1970	1983	1993	2003	2009
All sources	61	618	1,316	1,960	2,759
Official creditors	33	218	697	805	764
Private creditors	28	400	619	1,155	1,995
Of which, commercial banks	19	307	304	580	136

Sources: World Bank, *Global Development Finance 2005* (Washington, DC: World Bank, 2005); and World Bank, *Global Development Finance 2011* (Washington, DC: World Bank, 2011).

debt payments (that is, negotiate new terms to stretch out repayment). In August 1982, Mexico stunned global markets by declaring that it could not make its debt payments, signaling the beginning of a much broader series of debt crises affecting dozens of countries. From 1983 to 1987, more than $300 billion of debt repayments had to be rescheduled. Now, almost 30 years later, the effects of these crises are still reverberating in some countries, and the lessons learned are crucial for future economic management in developing countries. That much is clear from the fact that the total stock of developing country debt had grown to exceed $2.7 trillion by 2009, nearly $2 trillion of which was owed to private creditors (Table 13-2). (It is interesting to note, however, that the role of commercial banks among private creditors has declined substantially over time.)

CAUSES OF THE CRISIS

The crisis resulted from several things going wrong at once: adverse international economic shocks outside of the control of the debtor countries, poor domestic economic management, and bad lending decisions by international banks.[4]

INTERNATIONAL ECONOMIC SHOCKS In 1973, the Organization of the Petroleum Exporting Countries (OPEC) announced that it would restrict oil production, sparking a very sharp increase in world oil prices. Import values and trade deficits

[4]A huge literature examines the 1980s debt crisis. We cite some of the key works here. Jeffrey D. Sachs, ed., *Developing Country Debt and Economic Performance*, 4 vols.: Vol. 1, *The International Financial System*; Vol. 2: *Country Studies: Argentina, Bolivia, Brazil, Mexico*; Vol. 3 (with Susan Collins): *Country Studies: Indonesia, Korea, the Philippines, Turkey*; Summary vol.: *Developing Country Debt and the World Economy* (Cambridge, MA: National Bureau of Economic Research, 1989–1990). William Cline, *International Debt: Systematic Risk and Policy Response* (Washington, DC: Institute for International Economics, 1984); William Cline, *International Debt Reexamined* (Washington, DC: Institute for International Economics, 1995); Ishrat Husain and Ishac Diwan, eds., *Dealing with the Debt Crisis* (Washington, DC: World Bank, 1989); Joseph Kraft, *The Mexican Rescue* (New York: Group of Thirty, 1984).

immediately increased for oil importers around the world (including developing countries), slowed global economic growth (hampering export markets for many developing countries), and created volatility in a wide range of other commodity markets. In 1979, OPEC again cut back its production, leading to even larger increases in oil prices.

At the same time, the U.S. economy was facing a combination of slow growth and accelerating prices. With the economy under pressure, in August 1971, President Richard Nixon released the dollar from the gold standard that had determined its value since the end of World War II. This move led to a sharp deprecation of the dollar and an increase in currency volatility and uncertainty around the world. Large budget deficits emanating from spending on the Vietnam War and the sharp hike in world oil prices added to the pressure. By the end of the 1970s, U.S. inflation reached double digits, and interest rates rose very sharply, reaching 16 percent in 1981. The increase in interest rates substantially increased the interest burden for developing country debtors, whose original loans were written with variable interest rates. For a group of 15 countries in Central and South America, the rise in interest rates between 1978 and 1981 added over $13 billion to the costs of servicing their debts in 1981 alone.

DOMESTIC ECONOMIC POLICIES Even in the face of these shocks, not all debtors suffered equally. South Korea and Indonesia were among the world's largest debtors, yet sound economic policies enabled them to service their debt while continuing to grow throughout the 1980s. In particular, these countries responded by reducing their budget deficits, restraining the expansion of domestic demand, and encouraging export production. But in many other countries, reactions by policy makers exacerbated the crisis.

In the face of rising imports and trade deficits, escalating prices, and growing budget deficits, it was much easier for governments to convince themselves that the oil crisis would be short-lived rather than try to limit demand. Many believed they could borrow to cover the deficits (from either their central banks or from foreign banks) and even increase spending, rather than restrain demand and close the deficits. But this strategy, while perhaps politically expedient in the short run, could not be sustained and typically led to even higher rates of inflation and larger debts.

At the same time, some governments tried to compensate for rising import prices by maintaining an overvalued exchange rate, which restrains price increases for imports and exportable goods. This step is popular with consumers because it makes imports cheaper, but it discourages export growth and encourages capital flight. More generally, countries that had been actively promoting manufactured exports, mainly in East Asia, were in a better position to further spur exports and close their deficits than countries that followed a less open trade strategy, such as in Latin America. Ultimately, countries with overvalued exchange rates and less-active export promotion strategies faced larger current account deficits and, therefore, larger borrowing needs. Instead of improving, their debt crises just got worse.

IMPRUDENT BANK LENDING The foreign banks also bear some responsibility for making poor lending decisions. Banks were more than happy to keep lending to governments, even after the economic situation began to deteriorate and normal lending strategies suggested more prudence. Banks believed that, because the debts were **sovereign** (that is, either contracted or guaranteed by governments), they did not have to worry as much about the normal risks of default. And once the banks were heavily involved, further lending seemed a sensible way to keep debtor countries liquid enough to continue servicing earlier loans. Banks were encouraged by their own governments and the international agencies, all of which hoped that more lending would help countries grow out of the crisis, especially once the world economy recovered from its instability.

IMPACT ON THE BORROWERS

Once it became clear that many debtors would be unable to meet their obligations, the commercial banks stopped making new loans. From 1980 to 1982, private creditors provided more than $50 billion a year in new lending to developing countries; in 1987, the net resource flow was essentially zero.

The impact on the most indebted countries was severe. In effect, countries very quickly had to turn from net borrowers into net repayers of loans. We know from balance of payments accounting that net capital inflows always must equal the current account deficit, which in turn is equal to the balance of investment over domestic saving:

$$\text{Net capital inflows} = M - X = I - S_d \qquad [13\text{--}5]$$

Before the crisis, foreign borrowing (and other capital inflows) allowed the countries to finance imports in excess of exports and investment in excess of saving. But when countries began to default on the loans, banks demanded immediate repayment and reduced new lending. In the absence of other new capital inflows, countries had to reverse the signs and run a surplus of exports over imports and of saving over investment. Economic growth fell abruptly. Many governments found it difficult to raise taxes and reduce spending (to increase domestic saving), so they resorted to inflationary financing, which further destabilized the economy.

These kinds of dramatic changes were clearly evident in Mexico before and after the 1982 crisis, as shown in Table 13–3. In the five years up to and including 1981, imports exceeded exports in Mexico by the equivalent of about 2 percent of GDP and investment exceeded domestic saving by the same amount. There was strong growth in investment, GDP, and GDP per capita. But the crisis changed everything. Between

TABLE 13-3   Mexico before and after the 1982 Debt Crisis

	BEFORE THE CRISIS, 1977–81	AFTER THE CRISIS, 1982–86
Exports of goods and services (% of GDP)	9.6	16.9
Imports of goods and services (% of GDP)	11.5	10.6
Resource balance (% of GDP)	−2.0	6.3
Gross domestic investment (% of GDP)	24.7	20.4
Gross domestic savings (% of GDP)	22.7	26.7
Saving-investment gap (% of GDP)	−2.0	6.3
Gross domestic investment (real, average annual growth %)	13.0	−12.2
GDP (real, average annual growth %)	7.6	−0.6
GDP per capita (real, average annual growth %)	5.0	−2.9
Inflation, consumer prices (average annual %)	23.7	73.2

GDP, gross domestic product

Source: World Bank, *World Development Indicators*, http://databank.worldbank.org/ddp/home.do, accessed 2005.

1982 and 1986, imports fell and exports expanded sharply, providing the trade surplus necessary to pay foreign creditors. The **resource balance** (the excess of exports over imports, and the opposite of net capital inflows) shifted by a huge 8.3 percent of GDP (from −2 percent to +6.3 percent). Investment fell by over 4 percent of GDP, and domestic saving rose by a similar amount. GDP per capita fell, the budget deficit grew, and inflation skyrocketed to 73 percent per year.

These kinds of adjustments were not limited to Mexico. Between 1978 and 1981, a group of 15 heavily indebted countries imported about $9 billion more than they exported. But from 1983 to 1988, they were forced into a reverse transfer of almost $34 billion a year to service their debt. From 1970 to 1981, these countries had enjoyed per capita income growth of 2.7 percent a year, invested 25 percent of their GDP, and tolerated inflation of 39 percent a year on average. During the debt crisis, however, from 1982 to 1988, GDP growth per capita was −0.7 percent a year, investment fell to 18 percent of GDP, and annual inflation grew to 149 percent.[5]

ESCAPE FROM THE CRISIS, FOR SOME COUNTRIES

For the international commercial banks and many of the countries that had borrowed from them, especially the middle-income countries, the debt crisis of the 1980s essentially was over by the mid-1990s. For other countries (mainly low-income

---

[5]Rudiger Dornbusch, "Background Paper" (31), in Twentieth Century Fund Task Force on International Debt, ed., *The Road to Economic Recovery* (New York: Priority Publications, 1989).

countries in sub-Saharan Africa, South Asia, and Central America) that had borrowed predominantly from other governments and the international financial institutions, the debt crisis lingered unresolved into the new century.

Debt ratios improved substantially for Latin American countries from the 1980s to the 1990s and were much lower by 2005 compared to their previous high levels (Table 13-4). In most cases, improvements continued through 2009, albeit at a slower pace. Latin American debtors worked out of insolvency through debt relief agreements that involved a combination of several forms of debt restructuring and reorganization:

- *Refinancing,* involving making new loans to repay the old. In a refinancing, the amount of debt owed does not change, but the terms for repayments are eased, usually through longer repayment periods and perhaps lower interest rates.
- *Rescheduling,* closely related to refinancing, in which the original loans stay on the books, but the schedule of payments is altered to allow longer repayment periods and possibly lower interest rates.
- *Reduction,* in which the amount actually owed is reduced (that is, forgiven), either partly (a write-down) or completely (a write-off).
- *Buybacks,* whereby the debtor buys the loan from the creditor, usually for a percentage of the face value of the debt. Creditors might prefer getting an ensured payment today for part of the debt rather than taking the risk of less payment later.

TABLE 13-4 Debt Ratios, Developing Countries, 1980–2009 (percent)

	MAXIMUM OF 1980–97	2005	2009
All developing countries			
Long-term debt to GNP	43	26	22
Long-term debt to exports	203	75	75
Total debt service to exports	33	13	11
Latin American countries			
Long-term debt to GNP	60	29	24
Long-term debt to exports	343	111	111
Total debt service to exports	48	24	18
Selected countries: total debt service to exports			
Argentina	83	19	17
Bolivia	63	16	14
Brazil	82	46	23
Chile	71	15	23
Mexico	51	22	13

GNP, gross national product;.

Sources: World Bank, *Global Development Finance 2004* (Washington, DC: World Bank, 2004); and World Bank, *Global Development Finance 2011* (Washington, DC: World Bank, 2011).

- *Debt-equity swaps,* in which creditors are given equity in a company (such as a state-owned telecommunications company) in return for eliminating the debt outstanding.

Strategies to resolve the 1980s debt crisis evolved slowly in two broad stages. In 1985, nearly three years after Mexico first defaulted, U.S. Secretary of the Treasury James Baker announced what came to be known as the **Baker Plan**. This two-pronged strategy involved providing new finance to the debtor countries in return for them undertaking significant economic reforms aimed at stabilizing their economies and reducing their current account deficits. The plan did not reduce the amount of debt; it was based on the assumption that, with enough new financing and economic adjustment, the debtor countries could begin to grow and would fully repay the banks.

Financing was provided in part by the creditor banks refinancing and restructuring existing debts and partly through new funds provided by the International Monetary Fund (IMF), World Bank, and official aid agencies. The new financing provided some breathing room for the debtors because it reduced the amount of immediate adjustment necessary in the current account deficit. But adjustment was still necessary. The policy adjustment programs involved a range of steps aimed at reducing deficits in the government budget and the balance of payments, containing inflation, stimulating savings, and generating more resources for investment and debt service. These **stabilization and structural adjustment programs**, which were designed and overseen by the IMF and World Bank, typically involved devaluing the currency (or allowing it to depreciate through a float) to reduce imports and stimulate exports, cutting government expenditures, raising taxes, reducing growth in the money supply, and closing loss-making state companies.

These programs were controversial, and the austerity measures created huge burdens on the ordinary citizens of debtor countries in the form of reduced income, higher taxes and fees, reduced services from government, and other adjustments. Critics argued that, while some of these steps were necessary, the programs were not always well designed and required more austerity than was necessary while creating little burden for the creditors. Although it was hoped that this combination of new money and policy reforms eventually would allow countries to resume growth and fully repay the banks, in the end, the Baker Plan proved insufficient to resolve the debt crisis.

The key breakthrough came in 1989, when new U.S. Secretary of the Treasury Nicholas Brady unveiled a different strategy, this time incorporating the idea that the value of the debt would be written down and the commercial banks would share in some of the losses. The **Brady Plan** recognized that debtor countries needed a permanent reduction of their debt burdens to get back on sound economic footing. The strategy called for banks and debtor governments to renegotiate debts on a case-by-case basis from a menu of options, including reducing the face value of the debt, reducing the interest rate, providing new loans, and other forms of restructuring. The debtor countries issued new bonds to the banks, called **Brady bonds**, to replace the old debt. The amount of debt relief encompassed in these deals varied from country to country. Mexico's commercial bank debt was reduced by about 35 percent, whereas Costa Rica's was reduced by about 65 percent. By May 1994, Brady deals were in place covering about $190 billion in debt for 18 countries, including Poland, Ecuador, Venezuela, the Philippines, Brazil, Peru, the Ivory Coast, and other countries. Over $60 billion in debt had been forgiven. As with the Baker Plan, the new scheme included stabilization and structural adjustment programs under the auspices of the IMF and World Bank, new lending from these organizations, and bilateral debt relief.

The key to the program was the recognition by the international community and the creditor banks that by continuing to insist on full repayment, they were undermining the strength of these economies and ultimately receiving less repayment than they would under a negotiated settlement. By the early 1990s, growth had resumed and prices had stabilized. Net capital inflows, after falling to $10 billion per year between 1983 and 1989, rose to $60 billion in 1992. Debt reduction alone could not have solved the crisis, but debt reduction combined with new financing, strong adjustment efforts by the countries themselves, and especially the revival of the world economy in the early 1990s helped bring an end to the crisis, at least for some countries. A similar approach would be adopted for other heavily indebted nations almost a decade later.

THE DEBT CRISIS IN LOW-INCOME COUNTRIES

Although the debt crisis effectively ended in the early 1990s for most middle-income countries that had borrowed heavily from commercial banks, it continued for many low-income countries, especially many countries in Africa. Most of the debts of these countries are owed to either official multilateral organizations, such as the IMF and World Bank, or to donor governments, rather than to commercial banks. Thus, although the terms of the debts were more generous (and usually subsidized), the Brady Plan was not a solution for these countries because it was designed for commercial banks, ultimately providing the creditor with new bonds that it could sell on private bond markets. Different approaches were needed for these countries.

Low-income countries borrowed in the 1970s and 1980s for many of the same reasons as other developing countries. They were hit by the same set of strong international economic shocks: high oil import prices, low commodity prices, the end of the gold standard, and weak market demand in the industrialized countries. These challenges were even more difficult to meet in the poorest countries, which had a limited number of well-trained financial and economic experts, many of which had gained their independence only recently and had new and untested government institutions. The impact of these shocks was exacerbated in many countries by a prolonged period of economic mismanagement. Governments kept budget deficits high, erected significant barriers to trade, distorted market prices, and failed to provide basic infrastructure and health and education services.

Even where economic policies later improved, however, growth remained elusive, partly because many of these countries also face very difficult geographical challenges, such as being landlocked, located in the tropics (where disease is much more virulent), or located in or near the Sahara Desert. Several currently are ravaged by the HIV/AIDS pandemic, which further undermines their capacity for sustained economic growth and repayment of debt.

As with the debt crisis in Latin America, creditors sometimes added to the crisis by making loans for bad projects (many designed by the very same donors that provided the loans), although in this case the major creditors were government and multilateral agencies rather than commercial banks. In some cases industrialized country governments provided loans for poor investments and grandiose consumption projects in an attempt to win countries over to one side or the other of the cold war. Some Western loans supported corrupt governments that had little intention or capability of repaying the loans to finance presidential palaces, showcase steel mills, and other wasteful expenditures.

During the 1980s and early 1990s, the international community's strategy for the low-income countries had two components, similar to the original Baker plan: provide new finance in return for significant economic reforms in the hopes that the debtor countries could grow out of their difficulties. Beginning in 1988, the financing was augmented by partial write-downs from government creditors. Multilateral creditors, including the IMF, World Bank, and other multilateral organizations (such as the African Development Bank and Asian Development Bank) offered no write-downs until 1996.

DEBT REDUCTION IN LOW-INCOME COUNTRIES

Individual creditor governments provide debt rescheduling and debt reduction through an informal group called the **Paris Club**. The governments of the United States, the United Kingdom, Japan, Germany, France, and 14 other creditor countries coordinate to offer common terms for debt restructuring to each debtor. The first meeting was in 1956, when Argentina met with a group of its creditors in Paris. Since that time, the Paris Club has negotiated over 400 agreements with at least 80 different countries. Until 1988, all Paris Club agreements involved debt rescheduling rather than reduction. Since then, agreements typically provide debt rescheduling for middle-income countries and partial debt reduction coupled with rescheduling for low-income countries. The first debt reduction deals in 1988 provided 33 percent reduction for certain qualifying debts; by 1999, the Paris Club was providing 90 percent reduction for at least some debts owed by certain countries. Many creditor governments have gone further and provided 100 percent debt relief in some circumstances.

The arguments for providing debt relief to the poorest countries were similar but not identical to those made for the middle-income countries. The first argument was a variant of debt overhang: The debts were so large that they were impeding growth and development, partially by undermining private sector incentives but also by impeding the government's ability to make critical investments in health, education, and infrastructure.

The second argument was that the creditor governments and institutions should not have been providing so much of their financing as loans to the world's poorest countries in the first place because history suggested that accelerating growth sufficiently to repay the loans would be a major challenge. The world's poorest countries have had the most difficulty in initiating and sustaining growth, for reasons that we discussed: adverse geography, disease burdens, weak institutions, frequent climate and trade shocks, and poor policies. Providing loans to these countries rather than outright grants was based on the presumption that growth could be turned around relatively easily, providing these countries with the basis to repay their loans. But for many of the world's poorest countries, growth rates remained low, debts piled up, and many countries were able to service their loans only by receiving new loans.

The third argument is that creditors knowingly lent money to dictatorships to garner their political support, even when the dictators wasted and stole the money. Once the dictators left, the citizens of the country were left with the responsibility of repaying these debts. The Democratic Republic of the Congo, formerly Zaire, piled up large debts under the ruthless dictatorship of Mobutu Sese Seko, as Western donors happily lent him more money, even when it was obvious that most of the money was wasted or stolen. Many argue that *odious debts* (obligations accumulated by an illegitimate government in the name of a country) should be forgiven, with the costs born by the creditor (Box 13-2). The United States, which often has resisted attempts by some countries to claim odious debts, pushed hard in 2004 for other countries to forgive debts owed by Iraq. Although the United States was careful to avoid the term *odious debt* because of the legal precedent, it nonetheless argued that Iraq's debts were amassed by an illegitimate dictator and were a large impediment to future growth. In November 2004, the Paris Club agreed to cancel over $29 billion of Iraq's debts and reschedule an additional $7 billion, by far the largest debt forgiveness operation ever undertaken for a single country.

THE HEAVILY INDEBTED POOR COUNTRY INITIATIVE

By the middle of the 1990s, it was becoming increasingly clear that some of the poorest and most heavily indebted countries would not be able to repay their debts. Most of these countries almost never actually defaulted on their debt payments: Instead,

BOX 13-2 ODIOUS DEBT

Under the law in many countries, *individuals* do not have to repay if others fraudulently borrow in their name and *corporations* are not liable for contracts that their chief executive officers enter into without proper authority. The legal doctrine of odious debt makes an analogous argument that sovereign debt that is incurred without the consent of the people and that does not benefit the people should not be transferable to a successor government, especially if creditors are aware of these facts in advance. But many developing countries carry debt incurred by rulers who borrowed without the people's consent and who used the funds either to repress the people or for personal gain.

The doctrine of odious debt originated in 1898 after the Spanish American War. During peace negotiations, the United States argued that neither it nor Cuba should be responsible for debt the colonial rulers had incurred without the consent of the Cuban people and had not used for their benefit. Although Spain never accepted the validity of this argument, the United States implicitly prevailed, and Spain took responsibility for the Cuban debt under the Paris peace treaty.

Though legal scholars elaborated the details of the doctrine of odious debt, it has gained little momentum within the international legal community—still, many countries could qualify. For example, through the 1980s, South Africa's apartheid regime borrowed from private banks, devoting a large percentage of its budget to financing the military and police and repressing the black majority. The South African people now bear the debts of their repressors. Despite appeals— from the archbishop of Cape Town and South Africa's Truth and Reconciliation Commission—to have the apartheid-era debt written off, the post-apartheid government has accepted responsibility for it, perhaps out of fear that defaulting would make the country seem not to be playing by the rules of capitalism and would hurt its chances of attracting foreign investment. South Africa is not poor enough to qualify for debt relief under the HIPC Initiative.

Among other dramatic instances of odious debt, Anastasio Somoza was reported to have looted $100 to $500 million from Nicaragua by the time he was overthrown in 1979; Ferdinand Marcos amassed a personal fortune of $10 billion in the Philippines; Mobutu Sese Seko expropriated a reported $4 billion from the Democratic Republic of the Congo (then Zaire); and Jean-Claude Duvalier reportedly absconded with $900 million from Haiti. Some of the money that built these fortunes was drawn from amounts that these dictators borrowed in the name of their people. Recently, the United States successfully argued that debts accumulated by Saddam Hussein in Iraq were illegitimate and should be forgiven, although, to avoid setting a legal precedent for other countries to follow, the United States did not use the *odious debt* terminology. The international community forgave over $29 billion in Iraqi debt in 2004.

Economists Michael Kremer and Seema Jayachandran have argued for the creation of an independent institution to assess whether regimes are legitimate and declare sovereign debt incurred by illegitimate regimes odious and thus not the obligation of successor governments.

Adapted from Michael Kremer and Seema Jayachandran, "Odious Debts," *Finance and Development* 39, no. 2 (June 2002).

as the debt payments grew, the creditors lent them new money so they could repay the old, a strategy known as **defensive lending** (because the loans defend the creditor against the possibility of the debtor defaulting). But this strategy could not be sustained indefinitely, and debt levels continued to grow while growth rates remained stubbornly low.

In 1996, the international community recognized that deeper debt reduction would be necessarily. The World Bank and IMF, in conjunction with other multilateral agencies and creditor governments, launched the rather awkwardly named Heavily Indebted Poor Countries (HIPC) Initiative.[6] The HIPC include 38 countries with per capita incomes below $900 (converted using official exchange rates rather than purchasing power parity [PPP]) and with NPV debt/export ratios exceeding 150 percent.[7] Most had much higher debts. From 1982 to 1992, the NPV debt/export ratio deteriorated from an average of 266 percent to 620 percent for the HIPC. The new initiative had two key features, deeper debt relief from bilateral government creditors (initially up to 80 percent of qualifying debts, then in 1999 up to 90 percent), and for the first time ever, partial write-downs of debts owed to the multilateral agencies.

The first version of the HIPC initiative turned out to be too cumbersome and time-consuming to be effective. In the first three years, only five countries received debt relief, and the amounts involved were relatively small. In 1999 a new, enhanced HIPC Initiative was introduced to provide more relief and provide it more quickly.

To be eligible for debt reduction, a country must first establish a track record of good economic policies, as determined by the IMF and World Bank, usually

[6]For a thorough analysis of the HIPC program and related debt issues, see Nancy Birdsall and John Williamson (with Brian Deese), *Delivering on Debt Relief: From IMF Gold to New Aid Architecture* (Washington, DC: Center for Global Development and Institute for International Economics, April 2002).

[7]In certain circumstances, where countries have very open economies and the NPV/export ratio may not be appropriate (because large exports drive down the ratio), countries qualify if the NPV debt/revenue ratio is above 250 percent. For more information on HIPC, see www.worldbank.org/hipc.

including a stable macroeconomic environment, lower trade restrictions, policies to support private-sector growth, and strengthening of the financial and legal systems. Countries must develop **Poverty Reduction Strategy Papers**, detailing their plans for growth, development, and poverty reduction. Once countries establish this track record, they reach the **decision point** at which creditors provide interim relief—that is, they forgive debt payments as they fall due but do not yet forgive the stock of debt. Countries that maintain strong economic policies for an additional year or more and carry out specific reforms determined at the decision point reach the **completion point**, at which time they receive irrevocable debt reduction.

Under the program as it was conducted until 2009, countries that reach the completion point received debt reduction sufficient to reduce their NPV debt/export ratio to 150 percent, a level the IMF and World Bank deem to be the threshold for sustainable debt for low-income countries. Two features of this approach are noteworthy. First, a single threshold level is used for all countries. Basic economics would suggest that each country can sustain a different level of debt, but politically and institutionally, it was simpler for these organizations to treat all countries the same. Second, note that whereas the Paris Club forgives a percentage of debt, HIPC forgives the excess over the threshold. Thus a country with a NPV debt/export ratio of 200 percent would receive 25 percent debt forgiveness, whereas a country with a 300 percent ratio would receive a 50 percent write-off.

In 2005, the shareholders of the IMF, World Bank, and African Development Bank decided to go a step further and offer 100 percent forgiveness of all obligations owed to the three organizations for countries that reached the completion point. This step represented a major change and is the first time any of the organizations provided 100 percent forgiveness.

As of 2009, 35 HIPC had reached the post-completion point, and 12 countries were at the interim or predecision point (several mired in civil conflict were technically eligible but had made little progress). The 35 countries that reached their post-completion points had received debt relief amounting to $118 billion from the HIPC Initiative and a variety of other related bilateral and multilateral debt relief initiatives. The debt service/export ratio fell from an average of about 18 percent in 1999 to 6 percent in 2009, while debt service/revenues fell from 22 percent to 6 percent. In many countries, the benefits from the program were already evident. For example, Ghana used its savings to construct 509 new classroom blocks around the country, provide micro credit to about 43,000 farmers, and fund 560 sanitation and 141 water projects. Both Uganda (Box 13–3) and Tanzania used some of their saving to eliminate primary school fees, leading to sharp increases in school enrollment.

The HIPC Initiative demonstrates that, even after policy makers decided that some debt forgiveness is warranted, they face several key questions. These issues are more difficult in forgiving debts owed to government and multilateral institutions because market-based mechanisms are less relevant. Which countries should be eligible and which should not (that is, what are the right cutoffs for "poor" and "heavily indebted")? How much debt should be forgiven and over what time frame? Should the debtors be expected to undertake policy conditions in return for debt relief, and

BOX 13-3 DEBT RELIEF IN UGANDA

When Uganda gained its independence from Britain in 1962, there was widespread optimism that its vibrant agricultural base and diverse, talented people could provide the basis for sustained economic development. However, political instability in the late 1960s and a 1971 coup led by Idi Amin ushered in a long period of political terror and economic destruction. By the time Yoweri Museveni assumed power in 1986, Uganda was one of the poorest countries in the world. Food production had fallen by a third in 15 years; average income had declined by over 40 percent; and life expectancy was just 48 years.

The new government embarked on a broad-based economic rebuilding program that focused on rehabilitating infrastructure, restoring macroeconomic balance, lowering barriers to trade, and investing in the social sectors. In the 15 years that followed, the economy staged a remarkable recovery. Average income increased by nearly 60 percent, and the share of the population living below the poverty line fell from 56 to 44 percent. By the mid-1990s, however, Uganda had accumulated a substantial debt burden. By 1993, total external debt was more than 12 times the value of annual exports, one of the highest such ratios in the world (total debt equal to twice the value of exports is generally considered a heavy burden). Two thirds of the debt was owed to multilateral agencies, so the traditional methods for debt relief (for private sector or bilateral debt) had limited potential.

In April 1998, Uganda was the first country to become eligible for debt reduction under the Heavily Indebted Poor Countries (HIPC) Initiative. In the first formulation of the program, Uganda received about $650 million in debt relief, reducing its $3.2 billion debt stock by about 20 percent. Two years later, Uganda became the first country to qualify for the enhanced HIPC program, which offered deeper debt relief. This second phase reduced Uganda's debts by about $1.3 billion, bringing the total debt reduction to approximately $2 billion. These steps reduced Uganda's debt service payments by about $80 million per year, or about two thirds of debt service payments due. In 2005, Uganda became eligible for 100 percent forgiveness of debts owed to the International Monetary Fund (IMF), World Bank, and African Development Bank. Uganda's early success with the program was encouraging: The country sharply increased the net primary school enrollment rate from 62 to 86 percent between 1992 and 2003, raised investments in farm-to-market roads by 75 percent, and brought the share of the urban population with access to safe water from 54 percent in 2000 to 65 percent in 2003 (however, the country also increased its military spending in response to regional conflicts). Gross domestic product (GDP) per capita grew at a rate just below 3.6 percent between 1995 and 2010, increasing average income by 70 percent over that period.

This information is drawn primarily from multiple World Bank websites on the HIPC program and the country page for Uganda (look for links at www.worldbank.org).

if so, what conditions (and determined by whom)? How should the cost burden be shared? There are no obvious right or wrong answers to these questions because they involve economic, financial, political, and institutional considerations, so these issues will continue to be major challenges for policy makers in the years ahead.

EMERGING MARKET FINANCIAL CRISES

International capital flows played a central role in a series of financial crises that struck several developing countries starting in the mid to late-1990s, including Argentina, Brazil, Ecuador, Indonesia, Korea, Mexico, Russia, Thailand, Turkey, Uruguay, and Venezuela. These crises had some similarities with the 1980s and HIPC debt crises, but some critical differences as well. In most cases they struck very suddenly and ferociously, with enormous economic and financial consequences in a matter of weeks and months. Moreover, several of the worst-hit countries previously had strong economic performance and had been favorites of the international capital markets. These crises led to dramatic falls in GDP and investment, major disruptions of trade and banking relationships, widespread unemployment, and increases in poverty. They also led to widespread rethinking of both the role of foreign capital flows (especially short-term flows) and the proper timing and sequencing of financial liberalization in the development process.

At the heart of these crises were huge, sudden reversals of international private capital flows. Economies that had been receiving relatively large amounts of private capital suddenly were faced with withdrawals of lines of credit, demands to repay debts, an exodus of portfolio capital, and offshore flight by domestic investors. Table 13–5 shows both the rapid buildup in lending and the depth and speed of the subsequent reversal in capital flows for five Asian crisis economies: Indonesia, Malaysia, the Phil-

---

TABLE 13-5 Five Asian Economies:* Private External Financing before and after the Crises (billion US$)

	1994	1995	1996	1997	1998
Net private flows	40.5	77.4	103.2	−1.1	−28.3
Equity investment	12.2	15.5	19.7	3.6	8.5
Private creditors	28.2	61.8	83.5	−4.7	−36.8
Commercial banks	24.0	49.5	65.3	−25.6	−35.0
Nonbank private creditors	4.2	12.4	18.2	21.0	−1.7

*South Korea, Indonesia, Malaysia, Thailand, and the Philippines.

Source: Institute of International Finance, "Capital Flows to Emerging Market Economies," (Washington, DC: Institute for International Finance, January 1999).

ippines, South Korea, and Thailand. Net private capital flows to these five countries more than doubled *in just two years,* from $40 billion in 1994 to $103 billion in 1996. Net commercial bank lending alone nearly tripled from $24 billion to $65 billion. But, in the last six months of 1997, the private capital inflow of $103 billion suddenly turned into an outflow of $1 billion. This net reversal of capital flows of $104 billion was equivalent to about 10 percent of the combined precrisis GDPs of these five countries. Mexico suffered a similar fate during its 1994 crisis. The reversal in capital flows amounted to $40 billion over two years, equivalent to about 9 percent of GDP. Other crisis countries followed a similar pattern. With withdrawals of those magnitudes, it is little wonder these countries were plunged into crisis.

As must be the case, the reversals in capital flow immediately led to dramatic changes in trade balances, saving-investment gaps, and overall economic activity. In the five Asian crisis countries, current account balances changed from deficits averaging 5 percent of GDP in 1996 to surpluses averaging 5 percent of GDP in 1998. Economic output fell sharply in each of the crisis countries in either the year of the crisis or the year after (depending mainly on how early or late in the year the crisis struck), as shown in Table 13-6. The plunges in GDP growth in Argentina, Indonesia, and Thailand were particularly large. The poor were especially hard hit. For example, urban day laborers trying to eke out a subsistence living by loading trucks or working on construction sites suddenly were thrown out of work. Poverty rates in Indonesia doubled by official estimates from 12 percent to around 22 percent, with some unofficial estimates suggesting even higher levels.

Almost as striking as the collapse in growth was the speed of the rebound, at least in some countries. Argentina, Korea, Malaysia, Mexico, and Turkey all recorded GDP

TABLE 13-6 Gross Domestic Product (GDP) Growth before and after the Crisis

COUNTRY	YEAR OF CRISIS	REAL ANNUAL GDP GROWTH (PERCENT)			
		YEAR PRECEDING CRISIS	YEAR OF CRISIS	YEAR AFTER CRISIS	2 YEARS AFTER CRISIS
Argentina	1995	5.8	−2.8	5.5	8.1
Argentina	2001	−0.8	−4.4	−10.9	7.0
Brazil	1998	3.3	0.1	0.8	4.4
Indonesia	1997	7.6	4.7	−13.1	0.8
Korea	1997	6.8	5.0	−6.7	10.9
Malaysia	1997	10.0	7.3	−7.4	6.1
Mexico	1995	4.4	−6.2	5.2	6.8
Philippines	1997	5.8	5.2	−0.6	3.4
Thailand	1997	5.9	−1.4	−10.5	4.4
Turkey	1994	8.0	−5.5	7.2	7.0
Turkey	2001	7.4	−7.5	7.8	4.8
Venezuela	1994	0.3	−2.3	4.0	−0.2

Source: World Bank, *World Development Indicators 2004* (Washington, DC: World Bank, 2004).

growth of 5 percent or more two years after their respective crises. As we shall see, the relatively rapid recovery is at least partly a reflection of the central role played by creditor panic in many of these crises.

How did the crises happen? The affected countries had several characteristics in common. First, they tended to be middle-income and upper-middle-income countries that had been growing quickly. Second, all had received large flows of private international capital, much of it with short-term maturity structures. Third, they recently had liberalized their financial systems and had recorded a very rapid— perhaps too rapid—expansion of bank lending and other financial services. Fourth, most of the crisis countries had exchange rates heavily controlled by their central banks, often strictly fixed (or pegged) to the U.S. dollar. Fifth, some countries, but not all, had large government budget deficits financed by a combination of borrowing from local and overseas banks and bondholders. These similarities suggest that government policies contributed to the crises, especially banking, financial, and exchange rate policies. However, the quick recovery in several countries, the fact that crises struck so many countries in such a short period of time, and the consistent pattern of rapid buildup and then withdrawal of private foreign capital all suggest that flaws in the operations of international capital markets played an important role as well.

DOMESTIC ECONOMIC WEAKNESSES

Each of the crisis countries had liberalized its financial systems in the late 1980s and early 1990s and had done it in ways that inadvertently left the financial systems fragile and overextended. Entry requirements were eased for banks and other financial institutions, allowing new private banks to open. Governments removed regulations that controlled interest rates and forced banks to allocate credit to particular firms and investment projects, so banks had more flexibility in their lending and interest rate decisions. At the same time, banks were given much greater freedom to raise funds through offshore borrowing, indeed in some countries government policies actively encouraged banks to borrow from foreign banks and relend to domestic companies. In Thailand, total foreign liabilities of banks and financial institutions rose from 5 percent of GDP in 1990 to 28 percent of GDP in 1995, mostly reflecting Thai banks borrowing from foreign commercial banks. The combination of these changes led to very rapid increases in domestic lending by banks, which grew by the equivalent of more than 50 percent of GDP in just seven years in South Korea, Malaysia, and Thailand.

Of course, financial liberalization can bring about many benefits to developing countries, including the mobilization of additional resources, reduced intermediation costs, and improved allocation of credit. The problem was not financial liberalization per se but how it was done, especially how rapidly it was done. The speed and magnitude of the expansion of financial activities outstripped the government's ability to establish strong legal and supervisory institutions to safeguard the system.

Central banks did not have supervisors with the skills and authority necessary to determine which banks were vulnerable and take steps to penalize or close poorly performing institutions. Bank regulations were weak, poorly enforced, or both. In some cases, supervisors were pressured (or bribed) to overlook violations by banks with politically influential owners. As a result, some banks were undercapitalized, nonperforming loans were at high levels, and many prudential regulations were broken with no penalty. Over time, loans tended to go to weaker investment projects, and the quality of banks' loan portfolios deteriorated. This left the banks (and the financial systems more broadly) in a vulnerable situation. In Thailand, for example, extensive lending was directed at real estate, construction, and property. When property prices began to fall in late 1996, banks exposed to these markets began to weaken considerably, making these banks' foreign creditors increasingly nervous.

Exchange rate policies added to the problems. Each of the crisis countries had either fixed or heavily managed exchange rate systems; none had fully flexible currencies. Although fixed exchange rates help keep import prices stable and provide a price anchor in a highly inflationary environment, they can create three kinds of problems.

First, they tend to encourage short-term capital inflows, which are especially vulnerable to rapid withdrawals. With fixed exchange rates, investors believe there is little chance they will lose money from a rapid change in the exchange rate. A foreign investor is more likely to buy a one-month bond denominated in Mexican pesos if the investor believes there is little risk that the exchange rate will change during the month. In countries with flexible exchange rates, foreign investors must take into account the risk that a relatively small exchange rate movement quickly could wipe out any gain they realize from higher interest rates.

Second, fixed exchange rates tend to become overvalued, which makes imports cheap and undercuts the profitability of exports. Partly because of their exchange rate policies, the crisis economies generally experienced growing imports, a slowdown in export growth, and a widening of the trade deficit in the years preceding the crisis.

Third, and more subtly, once capital withdrawals begin in the early stages of a crisis, fixed exchange rates tend to help accelerate the withdrawals. Once investors recognize that withdrawals are under way, they begin to speculate against the local currency, betting that the government will have to remove the fixed exchange rate.[8] This speculation adds to the loss of reserves and the pressure on the exchange rate.

---

[8]Such speculation takes place along the lines of the following, very simplified example. A foreign investor believes that the Philippine peso will have to be devalued. The investor takes out a short-term loan of 25 million pesos from a bank in the Philippines. The investor then converts the money into dollars using the current exchange rate of 25 pesos to the dollar, yielding $1 million. If the investor is right and the exchange rate moves, fewer dollars will be required to repay the loan. For example, if the exchange rate moves to 50 pesos to the dollar, the investor need convert only $500,000 dollars to get the 25 million pesos needed to repay the loan, allowing the investor to pocket a tidy profit of the remaining $500,000. This strategy is called *shorting the peso*.

When the central bank finally runs out of reserves, it has little choice but to allow the currency to float, which usually leads to a very large depreciation. The Thai baht jumped from 25 baht to the dollar in July 1997 to 54 baht to the dollar in January 1998, and the Korean won moved from about 900 won to over 1,900 won to the dollar in just a few months before appreciating back in early 1998. It is easy to see why someone holding assets denominated in either baht or won and expecting a devaluation would have wanted to get money out of these countries as quickly as possible.

SHORT-TERM CAPITAL FLOWS

While policy weaknesses undoubtedly created vulnerabilities in these economies, to fully explain the speed and ferocity of the crises we must turn to the operations of the international capital markets and the actions of the foreign creditors.

A key reason that so much capital was able to leave these countries so quickly was that so much of it had very short-term maturity structures. A large portion of the loans to the firms, banks, and governments in the crisis countries was scheduled to be repaid in just a few months or even weeks. These **short-term loans** (with full repayment due in one year or less) were attractive to both borrowers and lenders. For the borrowers, short-term loans generally carry lower interest rates; for the lender, short-term loans carry lower risk (and require less provisioning by the supervisory authorities)[9] because the lender is not exposed over long periods of time. As long as these economies continued to grow, creditors were happy to roll over the loans when they fell due (that is, make a new loan for the same amount to repay the old loan), allowing borrowers to continue their operations. So as long as things are going well, short-term loans *appear* to pose few problems. However, as soon as there is any trouble—or more precisely, as soon as creditors think there *may* be trouble—creditors quickly withdraw their lines of credit and demand immediate repayment of loans. This is precisely what happened in East Asia: When Thailand's economy began to noticeably weaken in late 1996 and early 1997, creditors began to close off their lines of credit and demand repayment, setting off a chain of events that led to financial panic and severe economic crisis.

Economies become vulnerable to a sudden withdrawal of international capital when the short-term foreign exchange *liabilities* of the economy grow in excess of short-term foreign exchange *assets*. In that situation, economies can become *illiquid*: Roughly speaking, there may not be enough dollars (or whatever relevant foreign currency) on hand to pay all the international debts falling due. Table 13–7 shows the size of one significant type of foreign liability for the crisis countries: short-term debts

---

[9]Central banks require commercial banks to set aside (or provision) a percentage of all new loans to ensure that the bank has some capital on hand in case loans fail. The amount of provisioning varies by the perceived risk of the loan and generally is smaller for short-term loans. In part because banks do not have to provision as much for these loans, short-term loans carry lower interest rates than long-term loans.

owed to foreign commercial banks by the government, state-owned companies, commercial banks, and private corporations in each economy. The table also shows data for the main liquid foreign exchange asset of an economy: the foreign exchange reserves held by the central bank. The last column shows the key point: In each of the crisis economies, short-term foreign debts exceeded or nearly exceeded the available foreign exchange reserves. In this situation, economies are *vulnerable* to a severe crisis because if all short-term loans are called in for repayment, not enough foreign exchange is available to repay every debt.

Bear in mind that the short-term bank loans shown in Table 13–7 are just one kind of short-term foreign exchange liability. Other kinds of foreign capital also can be withdrawn quickly, including portfolio equity (that is, stock purchases), foreign-exchange bank deposits, hedging instruments, and long-term loans with clauses that

TABLE 13-7 Short-Term Foreign Debt and Reserves (million US$)

COUNTRY	PERIOD	SHORT-TERM DEBT	RESERVES	SHORT-TERM DEBT/ RESERVES
Crisis countries				
Argentina	June 1995	21,509	10,844	1.98
Argentina	June 2001	40,916	21,077	1.94
Argentina	September 2001	37,792	20,555	1.84
Argentina	December 2001	32,320	14,553	2.22
Brazil	December 1998	41,038	42,580	0.96
Indonesia	June 1997	34,661	20,336	1.70
Korea	June 1997	70,612	34,070	2.07
Malaysia	June 1997	16,268	26,588	0.61
Mexico	December 1994	33,149	6,278	5.28
Philippines	June 1997	8,293	9,781	0.85
Russia	June 1998	34,650	11,161	3.10
Thailand	June 1997	45,567	31,361	1.45
Turkey	June 1994	8,821	4,279	2.06
Turkey	June 2000	26,825	24,742	1.08
Turkey	September 2000	27,845	24,255	1.15
Turkey	December 2000	28,360	22,488	1.26
Venezuela	June 1994	4,382	5,422	0.81
Noncrisis countries				
Chile	June 1997	7,615	17,017	0.45
Colombia	June 1997	6,698	9,940	0.67
Egypt	June 1997	4,166	18,779	0.22
India	June 1997	7,745	25,702	0.30
Jordan	June 1997	582	1,624	0.36
Peru	June 1997	5,368	10,665	0.50
Sri Lanka	June 1997	414	1,770	0.23
Taiwan	June 1997	21,966	90,025	0.24

Sources: Bank for International Settlements, *The Maturity, Sectoral, and Nationality Distribution of International Bank Lending* (Basel, Switzerland: various issues); International Monetary Fund, *International Financial Statistics* (Washington, DC: various years); Joint BIS-IMF-OECD-WB Statistics on External Debt (November 30, 2004) at www.jedh.org accessed in 2005.

allow accelerated repayment, but data on these forms of capital are not available. Moreover, the withdrawals generally are not limited to foreigners: Local citizens also begin to try to convert their assets out of domestic currency and into dollars (or yen), putting further pressure on the exchange rate. Note that longer-term loans and FDI generally cannot be reversed as quickly as short-term loans and therefore are less prone to rapid withdrawals.

CREDITOR PANIC

These financial crises were at least partially the result of what are known as rational panics by the creditors. Under certain circumstances, investors may have the incentive to quickly withdraw their money from an otherwise reasonably healthy economy, if they believe that other investors are about to do the same thing. The classic example from within one economy is a bank run, in which bank depositors suddenly withdraw their funds and deplete the capital of the bank. The particular conditions under which a rational panic can occur are described in Box 13–4.

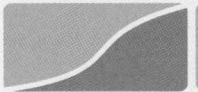

BOX 13-4 MODEL OF SELF-FULFILLING CREDITOR PANICS

Self-fulfilling creditor panics are best understood by beginning with the critical distinction between illiquidity and insolvency. An *insolvent* borrower lacks the net worth to repay outstanding debts out of future earnings. An *illiquid* borrower lacks the ready cash to repay current debt servicing obligations, even though it has the net worth to repay the debts in the long term. A *liquidity crisis* occurs if a solvent but illiquid borrower is unable to borrow fresh funds from the capital markets to remain current on debt-servicing obligations. Because the borrower is solvent, capital markets could in principle provide new loans to repay existing debts with the expectation that both the old loans and the new loans will be fully serviced. The unwillingness or inability of the capital market to provide fresh loans to the illiquid borrower is the nub of the matter.

Why might markets fail this way? The primary reason is a problem of collective action. Suppose each individual creditor is too small to provide all of the loans needed by an illiquid debtor. A liquidity crisis results when creditors as a group would be willing to make a new loan, but no individual creditor is willing to make a loan *if the other creditors do not lend as well*. One possible market equilibrium is that no individual creditor is willing to make a loan to an illiquid borrower precisely because each creditor (rationally) expects that no other creditor is ready to make such a loan.

Consider a simple illustration. Suppose that a borrower owes debt D to a large number of existing creditors. The debt requires debt service of θD in period one, and debt service of $(1 + r)(1 - \theta)D$ in period two, where r is the rate of interest charged on the unpaid balance of the loan. The debtor owns an investment project that will pay off Q_2 in the second period. (Note that for the project to be profitable, $Q_2/(1 + r)$ must be greater than the present value of total debt service payments in both periods $\theta D + [(1 + r)(1 - \theta)D]/(1 + r)$, which must be equal to D.) The debtor lacks the cash flow to repay θD because the investment project pays off only in the second period. Moreover, if the debtor defaults, the loan repayment schedule is accelerated (that is, creditors demand immediate repayment). The investment project is then scrapped, with a salvage value of $Q_1 < D$. In that case, the partial repayment of the outstanding loan from the salvage value is shared among the existing creditors on a pro rata basis.

Typically, this solvent but illiquid borrower would borrow a fresh loan, L, in the first period, use it to repay θD, and then service $(1 - \theta)D + L$ in the second period. Thus with $L = \theta D$, the total repayment due in the second period is $(1 + r)\theta D + (1 + r)(1 - \theta)D = (1 + r)D$, which by assumption is less than Q_2. In this case, then, the project remains profitable.

Suppose, however, that each individual creditor can lend at most λ, where $\lambda < D$ (that is, λ is much smaller than D). This lending limit might result from prudential standards imposed on individual bank lenders, which limit their exposure to particular debtors. If only one lender is prepared to lend in the first period, the borrower will be forced into default because it will not be able to service its debts in the first period. The new creditor lending λ in the first period would then suffer an immediate loss on its loans (indeed, it might receive nothing if repayments are prioritized such that all of the preceding creditors have priority on repayment). Obviously, a first period loan will require at least n_1 new lenders, where $n_1 = \theta D/\lambda$.

There are clearly multiple rational equilibria in this situation. In the normal case, n_1 lenders routinely step forward, the existing debts are serviced, and the future debts are also serviced. The investment project is carried to fruition. In the case of a financial crisis, each individual creditor decides not to lend on the grounds that no other creditor is making loans. The debtor is pushed into default. The debt repayments are accelerated, and the investment project is scrapped with sharp economic losses because the salvage value Q_1 is less than $Q_2/(1 + r)$. Each individual creditor, of course, feels vindicated in its decision not to lend; after all, the debtor immediately goes into default.

Source: Excerpt from "The East Asian Financial Crisis: Diagnosis, Remedies, Prospects" by Steven Radelet, et al., *Brookings Papers on Economic Activity*, No. 1, 1998. Reprinted by permission of Brookings Institution Press.

In an international context, two conditions provide the foundation for such a panic. The first is a high level of short-term foreign liabilities relative to foreign assets. In this situation, each creditor begins to recognize that, if all creditors demanded repayment, not enough foreign exchange would be available to pay everyone. The second is that some event makes creditors believe that other creditors may begin to demand repayment. The event could be a military coup, a natural disaster, a sharp fall in export prices, a fall in property prices that weakens the domestic banking system, or an event in a neighboring country that makes creditors nervous about an entire region. Once creditors believe that others might pull out, the only rational action for each creditor is to immediately demand repayment ahead of everyone else, to avoid being the last in line and left unpaid if foreign exchange reserves are depleted. This is why the very rapid withdrawals are called *rational* panics. The irony, of course, is that the simultaneous demand for repayment by all the creditors ultimately depletes reserves and brings on the very crisis that all would rather avoid. In this sense, these crises are often referred to as *self-fulfilling*: The fact that more creditors believe that a crisis is possible in itself makes a crisis more likely to actually happen.

In Asia, once Thailand's economy began to slow in late 1996 and early 1997 and banks came under increasing pressure from falling property prices, foreign creditors that had lent to Thai banks began to get nervous and withdraw their loans. Other creditors came to believe that Thailand might run out of foreign exchange reserves, devalue the baht, or both, and began to withdraw their credits. These events ultimately depleted foreign exchange reserves and forced the large depreciation of the baht that began in July 1997. The weaknesses in Thailand made creditors more nervous about its neighbors, specifically Korea, Malaysia, Indonesia, and the Philippines. A similar chain of events (with differences in the specific details and triggering events) occurred in most of the other crisis countries.

Once a panic begins, it tends to perpetuate itself for a period of time, for several reasons. First, as foreign creditors demand repayment and the exchange rate begins to depreciate, local citizens try to convert their financial assets from local to foreign currency, putting additional pressure on reserves and the exchange rate. This was a particularly large problem in Argentina, Brazil, Indonesia, and Russia. Second, the deprecations wreak havoc on the balance sheets of banks and corporations that had borrowed in foreign currency. For example, as the Indonesian rupiah jumped from about 2,500 rupiah to the dollar in mid-1997 to over 10,000 rupiah to the dollar in early 1998, Indonesian corporations with dollar debts had to come up with *four times* more rupiah to make their payments. The crippling effect of the exchange rate movement was obvious to the creditors, so the more the exchange rate fell, the faster the foreign creditors tried to withdraw any remaining loans, putting even more pressure on the exchange rate. Third, as exchange rates fall in one country, creditors begin to believe something similar will happen in neighboring countries, so they start to withdraw their funds from other emerging markets. There was no hint of trouble in

Malaysia, Indonesia, and the Philippines until the Thai baht collapsed in July 1997. Within weeks contagion had struck, and creditors were withdrawing their money from almost every country in the region.

These emerging market financial crises were not new phenomena. Similar events have been recurring in slightly different forms since the development of banks and the emergence of international capital flows several centuries ago. Economists have long recognized that financial markets (both domestic and international) tend to be prone to instability and panic. Early in the twentieth century, industrialized country governments put into place mechanisms and institutions specifically designed to reduce the frequency and severity of financial crises, including lender-of-last-resort facilities at the central bank, deposit insurance, and bankruptcy procedures, making crises much less common within these countries.

However, these key institutions generally do not exist in international financial markets, leaving these markets vulnerable to panics. When central banks face a run on their foreign exchange reserves (akin to a commercial bank facing a depositor run), no international lender of last resort stands ready to supply it with the foreign exchange it needs to remain liquid (the IMF only partially fulfills this role, as discussed later). Similarly, no international insurance mechanism akin to deposit insurance assures creditors that they will be paid if a borrower defaults. And there is no international bankruptcy court that can call for a mandatory standstill on debt service payments and oversee the distribution of assets when a country cannot meet its short-term foreign currency obligations. On each count, there is extensive debate as to whether these institutions *should* exist and, if so, how they might realistically be designed to operate effectively in an international context, where there is no single legal authority. For example, an international agency that insures creditors could lead to excessive lending to weak companies because the creditor always could rely on an insurance settlement if the company goes bankrupt. In any event, in the absence of these institutions, international financial markets continue to be prone to rapid oscillations and financial panics.

STOPPING PANICS

Once a financial panic from international capital withdrawals is under way, it is very hard to stop. There are four basic options:

1. Governments can try to convince foreign creditors and citizens to stop withdrawing funds and even supply new funding. They can reduce the demand for foreign exchange by tightening fiscal and monetary policies and, perhaps, restricting imports. They can also implement policy reforms aimed at correcting perceived weaknesses in the economy. For example, if creditors are worried about the banking sector, reforms to strengthen banks might convince creditors to begin lending again.

2. Governments can try to increase the supply of foreign exchange by borrowing from official sources (such as the IMF and World Bank), much like a commercial bank borrows from its central bank in the event of a bank run. New funds can help assure creditors that enough foreign exchange is on hand to pay everyone, if need be, and allow the economy to operate normally.

3. Governments can try to stop the creditor rush for repayment by restructuring foreign debts so they will be repaid over longer periods of time. This option may include a formal debt rescheduling, a limited standstill period during which loan repayments are postponed, or in some cases outright default.

4. The government can do nothing (intentionally or unintentionally) and let the panic run its course until all creditors have fled, foreign exchange reserves are exhausted, debts are in default, and the economy is in deep recession. At some point, even in these dire circumstances, some investors will begin to return to take advantage of low asset prices, the foreign exchange market will begin to stabilize (at a greatly depreciated exchange rate), and the economy slowly will begin to recover.

The appropriate combination of policy actions and financing depends on the root causes of the crisis and the perceptions of international creditors, but there is little doubt that both policy adjustments and financing are necessary to avoid complete collapse. The problem, of course, is that correctly diagnosing a panic and prescribing the right response is very difficult when markets are changing by the hour, little accurate information is available, and the perceptions and reactions of creditors are impossible to measure. It therefore is not surprising that both the affected countries and the international community often make mistakes when dealing with incipient crises, like the ones faced by the emerging market economies.

In most of the affected economies, once the crisis was under way, the government turned to the IMF for advice and financial assistance. The IMF was established in 1945 in the aftermath of the Great Depression and World War II to help support stability in the international monetary system, including promoting the balanced expansion of world trade, the stability of exchange rates, and orderly corrections of balance-of-payments problems.[10] It aims to prevent crises or moderate their impact by encouraging countries to adopt what it sees as sound economic and financial polices and by providing temporary financing when necessary to address balance-of-payments problems. The IMF was undoubtedly in a difficult situation in working on these crises. The policies and programs it promoted during the crises were hotly debated, with analysts divided on whether the programs initially helped ease the

---

[10]See the description of the purposes of the IMF at www.imf.org/external/pubs/ft/exrp/what.htm.

crisis or unintentionally added to the panic, at least in its early stages, by shaking the confidence of investors and further weakening the economy.[11]

The IMF's initial set of policy prescriptions, consistent with option 1, centered on tightening both fiscal and monetary policies (to reduce aggregate demand and the demand for foreign exchange) and closing weak financial institutions. Each requires a delicate balance. In countries in which the fiscal deficits were large and part of the problem (because they required significant financing) such as Argentina and Turkey, some fiscal tightening was necessary. However, in other countries, particularly those in Asia, where the fiscal balance was either a small deficit or even a surplus, tightening fiscal policy was more debatable, and some analysts believe this step may have added to the economic contraction. Tightening monetary policy and raising interest rates is even more complex. On the one hand, high interest rates might attract some foreign currency and slow capital withdrawals. On the other hand, foreign creditors might believe that high interest rates would further weaken banks and corporations, leading them to accelerate their demands for repayment. The empirical evidence on this issue is far from conclusive. Perhaps the most controversial issue was reform of financial institutions. There is no doubt that banking systems were weak and overextended and needed significant reform. However, the very abrupt closure of some of these institutions may have added to the panic in the short run, leading to an acceleration of bank runs as depositors feared their bank would be the next closed.

Actions by governments in several of the crisis economies exacerbated rather than eased the crisis. Thailand's reluctance to float its currency earlier and take steps to address the problems facing banks that were heavily exposed to property markets made the crisis more severe than it otherwise would have been. The Indonesian central bank made huge loans to try to prop up weak banks, ultimately fueling capital flight and further weakening the currency.

Turning to the second option, these programs were supported by substantial financing from the IMF and, in some cases, bilateral funding from the governments of Japan, the United States, and European countries. This financing was designed to augment the foreign exchange reserves of the crisis economies, convince creditors that sufficient funds would be available to repay everyone, and ease pressure on the exchange rate. In several cases, the amount of financing pledged by the international community was extremely large (Table 13-8). International financial commitments to Mexico, Brazil, South Korea, and Turkey all exceeded $30 billion.

---

[11]For debates on these issues, see Steven Radelet and Jeffrey D. Sachs, "The East Asian Financial Crisis: Diagnosis, Remedies, Prospects," *Brookings Papers on Economic Activity* 1 (1998), 1–90; Jason Furman and Joseph Stiglitz, "Economic Crises: Evidence and Insights from East Asia," *Brookings Papers on Economic Activity* 2 (1998), 1–136; Martin Feldstein, "Refocussing the IMF," *Foreign Affairs* 77, no. 4 (March–April 1998), 20–33; Stanley Fischer, "In Defense of the IMF," *Foreign Affairs* 77, no. 4 (July–August 1998); Timothy Lane et al., "IMF-Supported Programs in Indonesia, Korea, and Thailand: A Preliminary Assessment," IMF Occasional Paper 178 (1999); World Bank, *East Asia: The Road to Recovery* (Washington, DC: World Bank, 1998); Martin Feldstein, ed., *Economic and Financial Crises in Emerging Market Economies* (Chicago: University of Chicago Press, 2003); Nouriel Roubini and Brad Setser, *Bailouts or Bail-Ins? Responding to Financial Crises in Emerging Economies* (Washington, DC: Institute for International Economics, 2004).

TABLE 13-8 International Financing for Selected Crisis Countries

COUNTRY	IMF COMMITMENTS		BILATERAL COMMITMENTS		TOTAL COMMITMENTS		ACTUAL DISBURSEMENTS	
	BILLION DOLLARS	PERCENT GDP	BILLION DOLLARS	PERCENT GDP	BILLION DOLLARS	PERCENT GDP	BILLION DOLLARS	PERCENT GDP
Mexico (1995)	18.9	4.6	20	5.0	38.9	9.6	27.6	6.8
Thailand (1997)	4.0	2.2	10.0	5.5	14.0	7.7	11.2	6.2
Indonesia (1997)	11.3	5.0	15.0	6.6	26.3	11.6	10.8	4.7
Korea (1997)	20.9	4.0	20.0	3.8	40.0	7.7	19.4	3.7
Russia (1998)	15.1	3.5	0	0.0	15.1	3.5	5.1	1.2
Brazil (1998–99)	18.4	2.3	14.5	1.8	32.9	4.1	17.5	2.2
Turkey (1999–2002)	33.8	17.0	0	0.0	33.8	17.0	23.1	11.6
Argentina (2000–01)	22.1	7.8	1.0	0.4	23.1	8.1	13.7	4.8
Uruguay (2002)	2.7	14.5	1.5	8.0	2.7	14.5	2.2	11.8
Brazil (2001–02)	35.1	6.9	0	0.0	35.1	6.9	30.1	5.9

GDP, gross domestic product.

Source: Nouriel Roubini and Brad Setser, *Bailouts or Bail-Ins? Responding to Financial Crises in Emerging Economies* (Washington, DC: Institute for International Economics, 2004).

The amounts actually disbursed were often smaller, either because the simple announcement of the amounts available helped ease creditor concerns, the crisis began to pass before the full amounts were necessary, or sometimes because the recipient countries did not fulfill specified conditions so funds were withheld. In Mexico, South Korea, Brazil, and Turkey, the funds clearly were sufficiently large to help ease the panic; in other cases, it is less clear the amounts were sufficient. However, some analysts believe that large financing packages are harmful in the long run: Some suggest that the bailout of Mexico in 1995 made private creditors more relaxed about lending aggressively to other emerging markets and so may have contributed to the buildup in capital flows that led to other crises in 1997 and 1998. This kind of situation is known as **moral hazard**, the risk that an agreement or contract will alter the behavior of interested parties in perverse ways.[12] In this case, the agreement to bail out Mexico might have led investors to believe they could take greater risks in other emerging markets, as they would get bailed out in the event of another crisis. However, many analysts dispute whether Mexico's bail out had this effect.

Option 3 is to restructure the debts to either stretch out the maturity dates so the debts can be paid later or to write off part or all of the debt. In the most extreme cases, such as Argentina, Ecuador, and Russia, governments adopted a unilateral **standstill**—that is, they halted all debt payments—or simply defaulted. In effect, these steps effectively forced the creditors to provide financing involuntarily, what economists Nouriel Roubini and Brad Setser refer to as "bailing in" the creditors.[13] The option for default is even more complicated when the creditors are not just foreign banks but local banks or citizens who hold government bonds. When governments have borrowed from local banks, defaulting on those debts further weakens the domestic banking system and can lead to a freeze on deposits, obviously a politically unpopular step.[14]

Steps less dramatic than outright default are possible and less disruptive. Brazil and Turkey persuaded at least some of the foreign banks to roll over existing lines of credit, but these were not mandatory and many banks did not do so. More-formal restructurings are also an option. Turkey exchanged about $8 billion of short-term local currency debt, held mostly by domestic banks and residents, into longer-term dollar and lira debt. Argentina extended the maturity of about $15 billion in government debt and capitalized interest on another $15 billion in long-term debt. These deals were expensive in terms of the interest rates charged, but they provided immediate financing and avoided the disruptions of default.

Perhaps the most interesting and important debt restructuring was in South Korea. In late December 1997, under pressure from the U.S. government and the IMF,

---

[12]The classic example of moral hazard is insurance markets, where coverage against a loss might increase risk-taking behavior by the insured.

[13]Roubini and Setser, *Bailouts or Bail-Ins?*

[14]Defaulting on debts owed to foreign banks similarly can weaken those banks, but they tend to be a much smaller share of the foreign banks' balance sheets, so the impact is more limited.

the major creditors to South Korea's banks agreed to reschedule about $22 billion in debt payments that were to fall due in the first quarter of 1998. This step was taken very early in the crisis, and its preventative effect in stopping the panic was immediate: The Korean won began to appreciate, and the Korean stock market rebounded the day after the rescheduling was announced. Within weeks, the most intense part of the Korean crisis effectively was over, and the Korean economy rebounded very quickly.

Debt restructurings have several advantages. First, they at least partially share the burden of adjustment between the creditors and debtors, rather than forcing the debtor to make all the adjustments. This is not only more fair, it may have a preventative aspect: With standstills or restructuring realistic possibilities, creditors should be less likely to engage in excessive lending. Second, when debts are restructured less new finance is required from the international community (and its taxpayers). Third, because pressure to immediately repay debts is at the heart of the creditor panic, restructuring can have an immediate salutatory effect, as was the case in Korea. Debt restructurings and standstills are the centerpiece of bankruptcy proceedings in most industrialized economies, but engineering them in cross-border situations is much more difficult. Several analysts have suggested different ways to establish an international bankruptcy regime, but putting these ideas into action has proven difficult.

Panics eventually end, even when little or no action is taken to stop them, simply because foreign exchange eventually is depleted, so creditors stop demanding repayment and debt falls into default. But the resulting economic contraction can be very deep, and the financial system can be left in a shambles. In Indonesia, for example, where the financial crisis quickly cascaded into a political crisis that led to widespread rioting and destruction of property and ultimately the resignation of President Suharto in May 1998. GDP contracted by about 15 percent in 1998 before the economy finally began to stabilize in 1999, and GDP per capita did not recover to the level of 1997 until 2004.

LESSONS FROM THE CRISES

There are several things we can learn from such economic crises. First, these crises are cautionary tales about rapid financial liberalization and the difficulties involved in building strong institutions in emerging markets. The crisis economies liberalized their financial systems very quickly, without fully establishing and strengthening the institutions necessary to oversee and regulate financial transactions. Building well-functioning financial systems remains a major challenge in the development process. These crises suggest that governments should proceed carefully in liberalizing domestic financial transactions and ensuring parallel development of the requisite regulatory institutions. The financial crisis in the United States and Europe in 2008-10 further strengthened awareness of the need for caution in financial liberalization when it became apparent that even the most developed financial systems were vulnerable partly as a result of insufficient regulatory oversight of the financial system.

Second, the crises reveal the vulnerabilities of relying on a fixed exchange rate, at least for countries with large private capital inflows. The conditions under which fixed or floating exchange rates are preferable for long-run growth and development is an open question that economists have debated for two centuries, and the debate is far from resolved. Fixed rates reduce volatility in thin foreign exchange markets and can provide some certainty to skittish investors. But the crises indicate that fixed rates create vulnerability to a panic and ultimately lead to huge economic adjustments when the exchange rate no longer can be defended. Increasingly, many economists suggest that the choice for developing countries is between a very rigidly fixed rate defended with abundant foreign exchange reserves or a freely floating exchange rate. Most economists now tend to believe that the rigid fixed rate options, including a currency board or outright dollarization,[15] are appropriate in only a very limited number of developing countries and flexible exchange rates generally are the preferred choice. However, the debate on this issue is far from over and likely to continue in the years to come.[16]

Third, in terms of foreign capital inflows, there are clear differences between FDI and other long-term capital and short-term capital. Long-term capital flows are much less prone to panic and more strongly associated with long-term investment and growth. Because short-term flows create vulnerability to a panic, governments should be much more careful about, and at times possibly even discourage, short-term flows, especially while they are in the process of strengthening weak financial institutions. Some analysts support restrictions on short-term capital inflows as a temporary step to protect nascent financial systems, so long as the restrictions are limited to short-term capital (there is little support among economists for restrictions on long-term capital or outflows of any kind). Chile has been at the forefront of countries trying to encourage long-term capital flows and discourage short-term flows. During the 1990s, Chile required that foreign investors deposit a share of their investment funds in a non-interest-bearing account for one year, a step that made short-term investment much less profitable. Such restrictions reduced short-term capital flows to Chile without reducing aggregate capital flows.[17]

---

[15]Recall that, with a currency board, the government issues domestic currency only when it is fully backed by available foreign exchange reserves at the given (fixed) rate, thereby keeping the ratio of foreign currency to domestic currency constant. With dollarization, a country adopts the dollar (or another widely traded currency) as its legal currency, thereby giving up an independent monetary policy.

[16]An excellent recent survey of exchange rate policies is Michael W. Klein and Jay C. Shambaugh, *Exchange Rate Regimes in the Modern Era* (Cambridge: MIT Press, 2010).

[17]For discussions of short-term capital flows, see Richard Cooper, "Should Capital Controls Be Banished?" *Brookings Papers on Economic Activity* 1 (1999), 89–141; Jaime Cardoso and Bernard Laurens, "The Effectiveness of Capital Controls on Inflows: Lessons from the Experience of Chile," IMF Monetary and Exchange Affairs Department, 1998; Sebastian Edwards, "Capital Flows, Real Exchange Rates, and Capital Controls: Some Latin American Experiences," Department of Economics, University of California at Los Angeles, 1998; Felipe B. Larraín, ed., *Capital Flows, Capital Controls, and Currency Crises: Latin America in the 1990s* (Ann Arbor: University of Michigan Press, 2000).

Fourth, vulnerability to crises can be reduced not only by reducing short-term capital inflows but also by building up foreign exchange reserves. China and Taiwan employed just this kind of self-insurance and were able to avoid serious difficulties while crises swirled around them in 1997 and 1998, even though China, in particular, displays some of the same financial sector weaknesses evident in the crisis countries. Although China had over $30 billion in short-term foreign debt in 1997, its foreign exchange reserves were almost $150 billion. After the crises, China continued to build up its reserves, which reached an astonishing $3 trillion in 2010. Taiwan, with about $20 billion in short-term debt in 1997, had over $90 billion in reserves, so also was safe from this kind of crisis (it subsequently built its reserves to over $300 billion by 2010). Korea, whose usable reserves had dwindled to about $3 billion when its crisis erupted (compared to $70 billion in short-term debts), subsequently built up its reserves to $300 billion by 2011, effectively ensuring that it will not soon face a similar international payments crisis and have to look to the IMF for emergency financing.

Fifth, the operations of international financial markets and the immediate reactions by the official international community probably added to the severity of the crisis. As a result, there has been widespread discussion about possible reforms to the international financial architecture. These debates have proceeded on several fronts, including reforming the operations of the IMF itself, strengthening international banking standards, and establishing new international mechanisms for debt standstills and rollovers, but few fundamental changes have been made.[18] As they have been for two centuries, financial crises are likely to continue to be recurring yet difficult-to-predict phenomena affecting emerging markets around the world.

SUMMARY

- Debt flows to developing countries have oscillated widely since the 1970s. They grew rapidly until the 1980s, then fell in the aftermath of the 1980s debt crises. They accelerated again in the early 1990s, only to drop sharply after the financial crises of the late 1990s then rebound again after 2001. Middle-income countries tend to borrow from both private lenders and official creditors (such as the World Bank), whereas low-income countries borrow mainly from official sources (including IDA loans from the World Bank).

---

[18]See Roubini and Setser, *Bailouts or Bail-Ins?*; Feldstein, *Economic and Financial Crises in Emerging Market Economies;* Barry Eichengreen, *Toward a New International Financial Architecture: A Practical Post-Asia Agenda* (Washington, DC: Institute for International Economics, February 1999); Morris Goldstein, *Safeguarding Prosperity in a Global Financial System, Report of an Independent Task Force for the Council on Foreign Relations* (Washington, DC: Institute for International Economics, September 1999).

- Debt can play an important role in financing investment and stabilizing an economy buffeted by shocks, but too much borrowing, especially of the wrong kind and for the wrong purposes, can create debt problems. In particular, borrowing for consumption or weak investment projects, borrowing too much when GDP growth or export growth rates remain low, or borrowing too much on short-term debt can leave countries vulnerable to crisis.

- The debt crises of the 1980s caused major economic dislocations in many countries around the world, especially in Latin America. For countries that had borrowed heavily from private commercial banks, the debt crises by and large were resolved through Brady bonds restructurings in the late 1980s and early 1990s. However, for lower-income countries that had borrowed from official sources, debt burdens continued to grow through the 1990s. The heavily indebted poor-country initiative has begun to reduce the debt burdens for some, but not all, the countries.

- The financial crises of the late 1990s struck emerging markets that had borrowed substantial funds with short maturities and had relatively low levels of foreign exchange reserves, fixed exchange rates, and weak financial systems. The rapid withdrawal of funds caused exchange rates to plummet and interest rates to soar and caused significant damage to domestic banks, private companies, government financial accounts, and overall economic well-being.

- International capital flows are more vulnerable to these kinds of crises than domestic capital because the institutions that can help reduce risks domestically do not operate well across borders, including lender-of-last-resort facilities, deposit insurance, and bankruptcy procedures. Countries have taken steps to minimize their risks by reducing (or restricting) short-term capital flows, building up reserves, introducing more flexible exchange rates, and strengthening financial systems.

14

Foreign Aid

One of the greatest accomplishments of the past 50 years—the massive drop in the number of child deaths from 20 million children in 1960 to 8.1 million deaths last year—is an example of the tremendous progress we've made, in large part, thanks to foreign assistance. If the world comes together on a plan for financing development, the impact on health and development will be enormous. (philanthropist Bill Gates, April 2011).[1]

I have long opposed foreign aid programs that have lined the pockets of corrupt dictators, while funding the salaries of a growing, bloated bureaucracy. (U.S. Senator Jesse Helms, January 11, 2001)[2]

The two viewpoints given in the quotations opening this chapter succinctly reveal the diversity of opinions and the contours of the debates about foreign aid. Foreign aid has always been controversial. As early as 1947 Congressman (later Senator) Everett Dirksen of Illinois labeled the **Marshall Plan**, a post–World War II aid program for European reconstruction now seen as one of the most highly regarded aid programs of all time, as "Operation Rat-Hole." Prominent

[1]Bill Gates, "Staying Committed to Development," *theGatesNotes,* April 11, 2011; www.thegatesnotes .com/Topics/Development/Staying-Committed-to-Development.

[2]Jesse Helms, "Towards a Compassionate Conservative Foreign Policy." Remarks delivered at the American Enterprise Institute, January 11, 2001, available at http://aei.org/speech/foreign-and-defense-policy/ towards-a-compassionate-conservative-foreign-policy/.

economists such as Peter Bauer and Nobel laureate Milton Friedman have strongly criticized aid. Bauer believed that aid only enriches elites in recipient countries and famously quipped "aid is a process by which the poor in rich countries subsidize the rich in poor countries."[3] Friedman argued, beginning in the 1950s, that aid only strengthened and enlarged central governments, and as a result, aid did more harm than good. Critics, from both left and right, see aid as a political tool that distorts incentives, invites corruption, and entrenches corrupt dictators and elite business interests. Many believe that aid has little effect on growth and often has done more harm than good for the world's poor. They cite the widespread poverty in Africa and South Asia despite four decades of aid and point to countries that have received significant amounts of aid and have had disastrous growth records, including the Democratic Republic of the Congo (formerly Zaire), Haiti, Papua New Guinea, and Sudan. Critics call for aid programs to be dramatically reformed, substantially curtailed, or eliminated altogether.

By contrast, supporters see foreign aid as an important ingredient in fighting poverty, accelerating economic growth, and achieving other development objectives in low-income countries, especially in the very poorest countries, where people may not be able to generate the resources needed to finance investment or health and education programs. Equally prominent economists, such as Columbia University's Jeffrey Sachs and Nobel laureate Joseph Stiglitz, argue that, although aid has not always worked well, its overall record is positive, and it has been critical for poverty reduction and growth in many countries and helped prevent even worse performance in many others. Advocates argue that many of the weaknesses of aid have more to do with the donors than with the recipients, and because substantial amounts of aid are given for political purposes, it should not be surprising that it has not always been effective in fostering development. They point to a range of successful aid recipients such as Botswana, Korea, Indonesia, and Taiwan, and more recently, Ghana, Mozambique, and Uganda. They also note broader aid-financed initiatives such as the green revolution, the campaign against river blindness, and the introduction of oral rehydration therapy. They note that in the decades since aid became widespread in the 1960s, poverty indicators have fallen in many countries, and health and education indicators have risen faster than during any other 50-year period in human history.

Since its modern origins in the aftermath of World War II, foreign aid has become an important form of international capital flow from the richest to poorest countries

---

[3]Peter Bauer, *Dissent on Development* (Cambridge: Harvard University Press, 1972). For more recent critiques of aid, see William Easterly, *The Elusive Quest for Growth: Economists' Adventures and Misadventures in the Tropics* (Cambridge: MIT Press, 2001), and *The White Man's Burden: Why the West's Efforts to Aid the Rest Have Done So Much Ill and So Little Good* (New York: Penguin Press, 2006); Dambisa Moyo, *Dead Aid: Why Aid Is Not Working and How There Is a Better Way for Africa* (New York: Farrar, Straus & Giroux, 2009).

as well as a way to provide technical expertise and donate commodities such as rice, wheat, and fuel. While it plays a much less significant role in middle-income countries, it remains as much a source of debate and controversy there as in other countries. Official development assistance from Organization for Economic Co-Operation and Development (OECD) nations to low- and middle-income countries totaled close to $130 billion in 2010. Aid given to richer countries and aid provided by China, the oil-rich nations, and others add to this total. More than 40 governments around the world provide aid, and 150 countries receive at least some aid inflow. For some countries, the amounts are trivial, amounting to half of a percent of gross national income (GNI) or less. In others aid flows are substantial, totaling 20 percent, 40 percent, or even more of GNI.

This chapter explores the motivations for and impacts of foreign aid. The empirical evidence on aid effectiveness is decidedly mixed, with some research showing little or no relationship between aid and development and others showing a positive impact. On balance, the evidence suggests that on average aid has had a modest positive impact on development outcomes, but with wide variation. Aid has supported growth and development in some countries and contributed to more broad-based improvements in certain areas, such as health and agricultural technology. But, in other countries, it has had little effect and did not spur growth; in some countries, it probably held back the process of development, particularly when donors have given it to political allies with corrupt or ineffective governments that showed little or no interest in economic development.

This mixed record has led to sharp debates. Where, when, and how should aid be provided? Which countries are most likely to use aid effectively? Who should have the major responsibility for designing and implementing aid programs? What kinds of conditions should donors impose on recipients? And how can donors ensure that aid is not wasted and gets to the people who need it most and can use it most effectively?

DONORS AND RECIPIENTS

WHAT IS FOREIGN AID?

Foreign aid consists of financial flows, technical assistance, and commodities given by the residents of one country to the residents of another country for development purposes, either as grants or as subsidized loans. Aid can be given or received by governments, charities, foundations, businesses, or individuals. Not all transfers from wealthy countries to poor countries are considered to be foreign aid (or the equivalent term, **foreign assistance**). It depends on who gives it, what it is given for, and the terms on which it is provided. A commercial loan from Citibank to build an electricity generator is not aid nor is a grant from the British government to purchase military equipment. However, a grant from the British government to build an electricity generator counts as foreign aid.

An official source for definitions, data, and information on foreign aid is the Development Assistance Committee (DAC) of the OECD, an international organization with membership consisting of the governments of over 30 industrialized countries, including almost all the major donors. According to the DAC, to be counted as foreign aid the assistance must meet two criteria:

- It must be designed to promote economic development and welfare as its main objective (thus excluding aid for military or other nondevelopment purposes).
- It must be provided as either a grant or a subsidized loan.

The grants and subsidized loans that make up foreign aid are often referred to as **concessional assistance**, whereas loans that carry market or near-market terms (and therefore are not foreign aid) are categorized as **nonconcessional assistance**.[4] Distinguishing between subsidized and nonsubsidized loans requires a precise definition. According to the DAC, a loan counts as aid if it has a "grant element" of 25 percent or more, meaning that the present value of the loan (taking into account its interest rate and maturity structure) must be at least 25 percent below the present value of a comparable loan at market interest rates (usually assumed by the DAC, rather arbitrarily, to be 10 percent with no grace period). Thus the grant element is zero for a loan carrying a 10 percent interest rate, 100 percent for an outright grant, and something in-between for other loans.

Official development assistance (ODA) is the term used to describe aid provided by DAC donor governments (hence the term *official*) to low- and middle-income countries for development purposes. If a donor provides foreign aid for military purposes—as the United States does for many nations, including Egypt and Israel—this may be included in the U.S. foreign aid budget but is not included as ODA by the OECD. **Private voluntary assistance** is another and growing form of foreign assistance that also is not included in tallies of ODA because it is not official assistance. Private assistance includes grants from NGOs, religious groups, charities, foundations, and private companies. The Bill & Melinda Gates Foundation provides over $1 billion per year to support programs especially in health and education in low-income countries. World Vision, Save the Children, Care, and Oxfam International are NGOs that may be familiar to you. They collect billions of dollars each year from donations by individuals, mostly citizens of rich nations, and spend them on humanitarian and other forms of assistance in poor nations. Some estimates suggest

[4]Nonconcessional loans from donor agencies are counted as part of official development *finance* but not as official development *assistance*.

[5]Homi Kharas, "The New Reality of Aid," in L. Brainard, and D. Chollet, eds., *Global Development 2.0: Can Philanthropists, the Public, and the Poor Make Poverty History*? (Washington, DC: Brookings Institution, 2008).

that private voluntary assistance may amount to as much as one half to two thirds of ODA.[5] This is a dramatic increase from even a few decades ago.

WHO GIVES AID?

Although economic assistance from one country to another has occurred for centuries, today's foreign aid programs trace their origins to the 1940s and the establishment of the United Nations, the World Bank, the International Monetary Fund (IMF), and the Marshall Plan (Box 14–1). Historically, most aid has been given as **bilateral assistance** directly from one country to another. Some of the major bilateral aid agencies today include the U.S. Agency for International Development (USAID), the United Kingdom's Department for International Development (DFID), the Japan International Cooperation Agency (JICA), the Saudi Fund for Development, the Canadian International Development Agency (CIDA), and Swedish International Development Cooperation Agency (SIDA). Some governments have multiple bilateral aid agencies. The U.S. government has well over a dozen departments and agencies that provide bilateral aid, including USAID; the Millennium Challenge

BOX 14–1 THE MARSHALL PLAN

When World War II ended in 1945, world leaders hoped that Europe would not require much outside assistance and that the key economies (especially Britain and France) could quickly rebuild themselves. But by 1947, there had been little progress, and there was growing concern that discontent in Europe could encourage the spread of communism or fascism. U.S. Secretary of State George Marshall proposed a new approach to reconstruction at a commencement address at Harvard University on June 5, 1947, in which the United States would provide substantial amounts of funding, but only if the European nations, for the first time, could work together to draw up rational plans for reconstruction.

Despite some objections by isolationist members of the U.S. Congress, President Truman signed legislation funding the program, officially called the European Recovery Program, in April 1948. By June 1952 (when the program officially ended), the United States had provided $13.3 billion in assistance (equivalent to over $100 billion in today's dollars) to 16 countries in Europe. Almost 90 percent of the funds were provided as grants. The largest recipients in dollar terms were the United Kingdom, France, Italy, Germany, and the Netherlands. For most of the major recipients, funding exceeded 1 percent of gross domestic product (GDP). From the perspective of the United States, these were large commitments representing 1.5 percent of its GDP. The Marshall Plan was seven times larger than current U.S. official development assistance, which in 2010 was 0.21 percent of U.S. GDP.

The Marshall Plan is generally regarded as having been a huge success in helping stimulate rapid growth and recovery in Europe (although some analysts believe that recovery was already under way and would have occurred without the funding). While the Marshall Plan is often held up as a model (Marshall won the Nobel Prize for Peace, in 1953), it differed in many ways from today's aid programs. Most important, it was aimed at countries that already had relatively high incomes, highly skilled workforces, and established financial and legal institutions, characteristics absent from most low-income countries. The Marshall Plan was designed to help relatively advanced countries rebuild infrastructure and rebound to their earlier levels of productive capacity, whereas today's aid programs are aimed at the much more difficult task of initiating growth and development in countries where it (by and large) has yet to occur. Nevertheless, the Marshall Plan and its perceived success provided the foundation for today's aid programs.

Corporation; the Departments of Agriculture, Defense, Health and Human Services, State, and Treasury; and the Peace Corps.

While most bilateral aid is provided to support recipient country governments, some is disbursed to churches, research organizations, universities, private schools and clinics, and nonprofit agencies. Even private companies sometimes receive foreign assistance, such as U.S. assistance through *enterprise funds* that make investments in firms (such as in Poland in the early 1990s) or aid to micro-finance agencies, like the Grameen Bank in Bangladesh, that provide loans to small-scale entrepreneurs. Sometimes aid is provided as cash, but often it is delivered as goods (such as food aid or medicine) or services (such as technical assistance), or in the form of debt relief. An example of the latter is the nearly $5 billion in debt relief Liberia received in 2010 from the World Bank, IMF, African Development Bank, and other creditors. This was a massive sum, equivalent to almost $1,200 for every Liberian. The debt that was taken off the books had been incurred by Liberia's previous governments in the 1970s and 1980s, but 15 years of civil war had destroyed the economy, making repayment by the current government impossible.

In terms of total dollars, the United States has consistently been the world's largest donor, except for a few years in the mid-1990s, when Japan provided the largest amount of aid. In 2009, the United States provided $29 billion in ODA, with France,

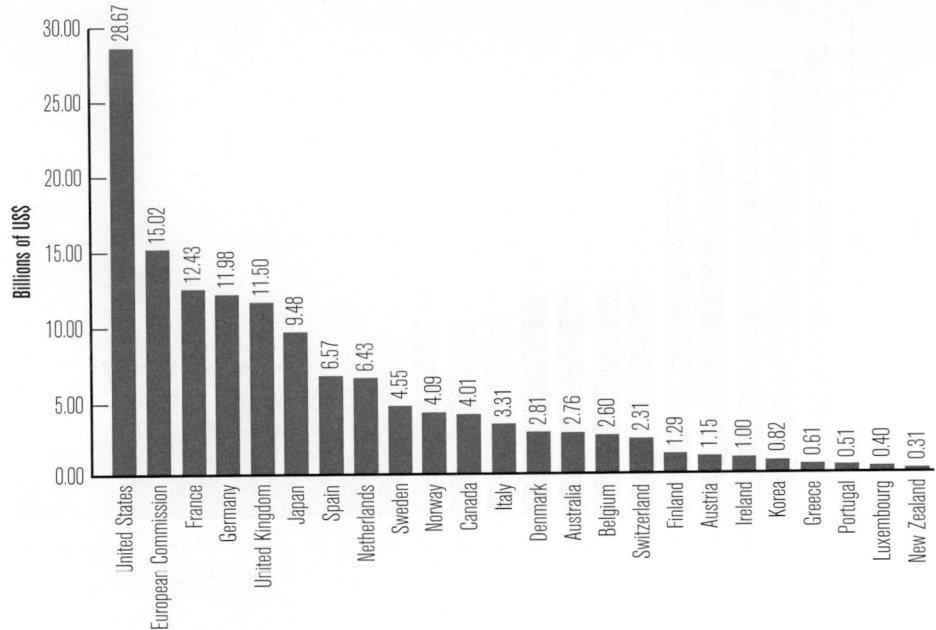

FIGURE 14-1 **Net Official Development Assistance, 2009**

Source: Organisation for Economic Co-Operation and Development Aid Statistics. Available at http://www
.oecd.org/document/49/0,3746,en_2649_34447_46582641_1_1_1_1,00.html.

Germany, and the United Kingdom the next-largest donor countries (Figure 14–1). However, when aid is measured as a share of the donor's income, a different pattern emerges (Figure 14–2). The most generous donors from this perspective are Sweden, Norway, Luxembourg, Denmark, and the Netherlands, each of which provided between 0.82 and 1.12 percent of GNI in ODA in 2009.[6] The United States is one of the smallest donors by this measure, with ODA equivalent to about 0.2 percent of U.S. income. This figure is well below its 1970 level of 0.32 percent and U.S. contributions during the 1960s, when ODA averaged 0.51 percent of U.S. income. Foreign aid makes up less than 1 percent of the U.S. federal budget. This is much smaller than the public believes: Surveys show that Americans think that the United States spends upward of 20 percent of its budget on foreign aid.[7] Although U.S. ODA levels as a

[6]Over the past decade one of the largest donors in the world measured as a share of its income was Saudi Arabia, which provided more than 1 percent of its GNI in aid. Saudi Arabia had been a much smaller donor until it increased assistance to Afghanistan and several other countries in the aftermath of the September 11 terrorist attacks on the United States. It is uncertain whether this trend will continue.

[7]Since 2001, surveys of public opinion in the U.S. consistently find that Americans overestimate the share of government spending devoted to foreign aid. In 2010, World Public Opinion.org asked a random sample of over 800 American adults, "Just based on what you know, please tell me your hunch about what percentage of the federal budget goes to foreign aid." The median response was 25 percent. A follow-up question then asks, "What do you think would be an appropriate percentage of the federal budget to go to foreign aid, if any?" The median response was 10 percent. Survey available at www.worldpublicopinion .org/pipa/pdf/nov10/ForeignAid_Nov10_quaire.pdf; accessed February 2012. Foreign aid is not alone; the public generally overestimates the relative size of most government expenditures.

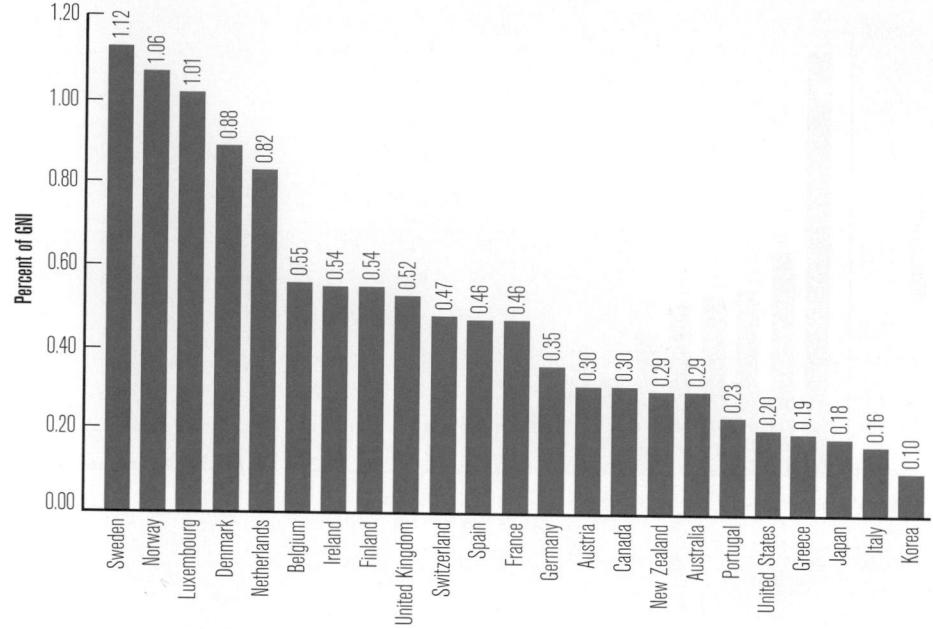

FIGURE 14-2 **Net Official Development Assistance As a Percentage of Donor GNI, 2009**

GNI, gross national income.

Source: Organisation for Economic Co-Operation and Development, Aid Statistics. Available at http://www
.oecd.org/document/49/0,3746,en_2649_34447_46582641_1_1_1_1,00.html.

share of income are small compared to other countries, the United States and other
rich countries affect poor countries in many more ways than just foreign aid: Policies on trade, technology, migration, security, and others areas are also important, as
described in Box 14-2.

In nominal terms, global ODA increased steadily from the 1960s until it reached
a peak of $60 billion in 1991, just after the end of the cold war (Figure 14-3). Aid flows
then declined for a decade before rebounding in the early 2000s. They have risen
steadily since due to an increased commitment by rich nations to assist poor ones
and to the growth in development assistance provided to Iraq and Afghanistan. In
real terms, increases in total ODA over the past decade indicate an even sharper
rate of increase from earlier trends. Measured as a share of donor income, ODA fell
throughout most of the 1980s and especially the 1990s. The 2000s reversed this trend,
with ODA as a share of GNI now on a level last achieved during the 1970s. Given the
economic problems currently facing many donor nations it is unclear if this trend
will continue. Foreign assistance may start to decline in nominal terms and as a percentage of GNI as rich nations cut back on many areas of government spending.

The values in Figures 14-1 and 14-2 include both the amounts that donors
give directly as bilateral aid and the amounts they provide indirectly as **multilateral aid**, which pools together resources from many donors. The major multilateral

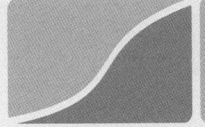

BOX 14-2 THE COMMITMENT TO
DEVELOPMENT INDEX

Rich countries affect poor countries in many ways, including through their policies on foreign aid, trade, migration, military spending, and the environment. Sometimes, these policies help poor countries; sometimes, they hurt. Open-trade policies can help provide markets for poor countries, but tariffs and quotas imposed by rich countries can keep poor countries out and slow their growth and development. To capture these broader channels beyond aid, the Center for Global Development produces an annual Commitment to Development Index that ranks 22 of the world's richest countries on the quality of their policies that affect poor countries in seven areas:

- Foreign aid, both in terms of its quantity (the amount of both government aid and private charitable contributions) and its quality, in terms of how it is given, to whom, and how much is required to be spent in the donor country.
- Trade policies, capturing tariffs, quotas, and subsidies for domestic farmers that impede trade or otherwise disadvantage poor countries trying to compete in rich-country markets.
- Foreign investment policies, including tax rates; programs that provide political risk insurance for investors against coups or other political instability; and other related policies.
- Migration, capturing the extent to which policies ease or hinder migration (particularly of unskilled rather than skilled workers) from poor to rich countries.
- Environmental policies, including greenhouse gas emissions, fishing subsidies, or other actions that lead to environmental degradation in poor countries.
- Security, including financial contributions to peacekeeping operations, naval operations that secure international shipping lanes, and penalties for certain arms exports.
- Technology, including policies that support research and development and protection of intellectual property rights, which enable creation and dissemination of innovations that help poor countries (like vaccines).

In 2010, Sweden came out on top, thanks to its large foreign aid program (relative to the size of its economy) and liberal immigration policies. Denmark ranked 2nd mostly because of its aid program. The United States ranked 11th, scoring relatively well on trade and security policies but poorly on aid programs.

South Korea, a newcomer to the Development Assistance Committee (DAC), ranked at the bottom, with weak scores on aid, environment, and migration and a strong score on technology. Japan, a more established donor, scored 2nd from the bottom with low scores in every category but technology. As with any composite ranking, the Commitment to Development Index is far from perfect, and different assumptions could change the rankings. Its intent, however, is not to be definitive in the rankings but to generate debate and discussion on the many different ways in which rich countries affect poor countries and on how the most important policies can be improved.

Source: David Roodman, a Senior Fellow at the Center for Global Development, is the architect of the index. The 2010 results are available at www.cgdev.org/section/initiatives/_active/cdi, accessed February 2012.

institutions include the World Bank; the IMF; the African, Asian, and Inter-American Development Banks; the United Nations; and the European Commission. The basic rationale for multilateral institutions is that they can provide larger amounts of aid with (presumably) lower bureaucratic costs (because donors do not have to duplicate efforts in each country) and fewer political ties (because funding decisions cannot be driven as easily by the political concerns of a single donor).

The largest multilateral agency is the **World Bank**, which began as the International Bank for Reconstruction and Development (IBRD) after its founding at a conference held in Bretton Woods, New Hampshire, in July 1944. The word *reconstruction* in the IBRD's title describes its first task, which was to help finance the reconstruction of Europe after World War II. The World Bank group today consists of five affiliated institutions operating in over 100 countries: the IBRD, the International Development Association (IDA), the International Finance Corporation (IFC), the Multilateral Investment Guarantee Agency (MIGA), and the International Centre for Settlement of Investment Disputes (ICSID). Most of the funding provided by the World Bank is *not* foreign aid. The IBRD lends to middle-income countries at market rates. It obtains its funds by borrowing on world capital markets then relends them to member countries at slightly higher rates. Because the IBRD has an excellent credit rating, it is able to borrow and relend to developing countries at cheaper rates than the recipients could obtain on their own in private markets. The IFC lends on commercial terms and takes minority equity positions in private companies. The MIGA provides guarantees to private foreign investors against loss caused by noncommercial (political) risks, and the ICSID helps settle investment disputes between foreign investors and host countries.

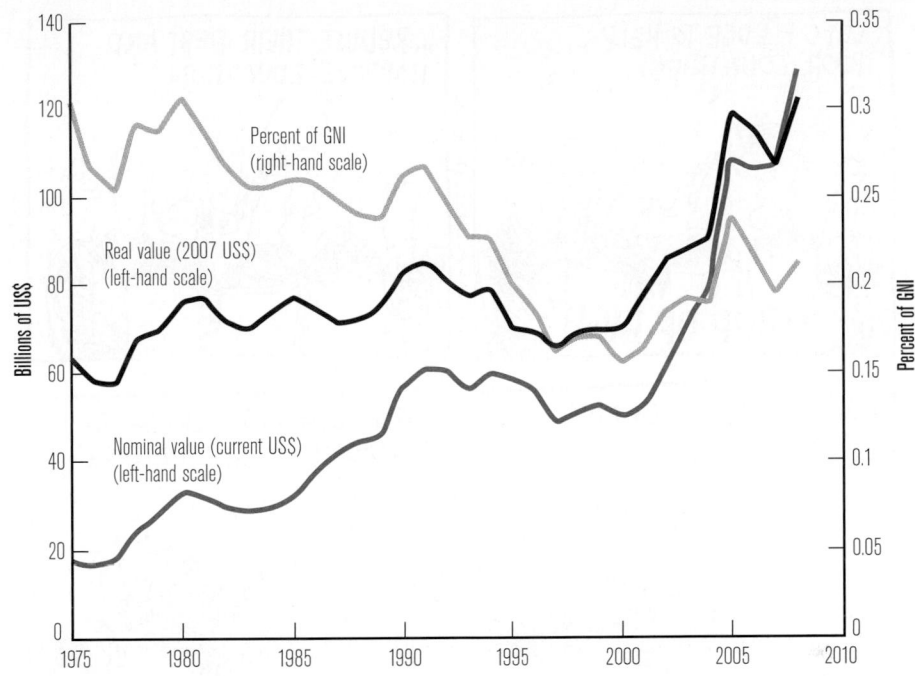

FIGURE 14-3 **Global Official Development Assistance, 1975–2008**

GNI, gross national income.

Source: World Bank, "World Development Indicators," http://databank.worldbank.org.

The only part of the World Bank that actually provides foreign aid is the IDA. Donor governments contribute funds to the IDA, which uses it to provide highly concessional loans and grants to low-income countries. Funds from the IDA are used for a wide variety of development purposes, including building roads and ports, funding agricultural research and extension, purchasing medicines and schoolbooks, and training government officials. Its standard loan terms include a "service charge" of less than 1 percent per year and a repayment period of between 20 and 40 years, including a 10-year "grace" period during which no repayment is required. To be eligible for IDA funds today, countries must have (2011) GNI per capita of less than $1,165 (although the World Bank makes a few exceptions) and not have access to borrowing on private international capital markets. About 80 countries are eligible to borrow from the IDA. Among the largest borrowers, including countries that are no longer IDA eligible but that were in the past, are India, Vietnam, Tanzania, Ethiopia, and Nigeria. The IDA has disbursed about $222 billion since 1960; annual commitments today average close to $13 billion, 20 percent of which is in the form of outright grants.

The World Bank is owned and controlled by its 187 member governments, with each member having a voting share determined by the size of its shareholding, which

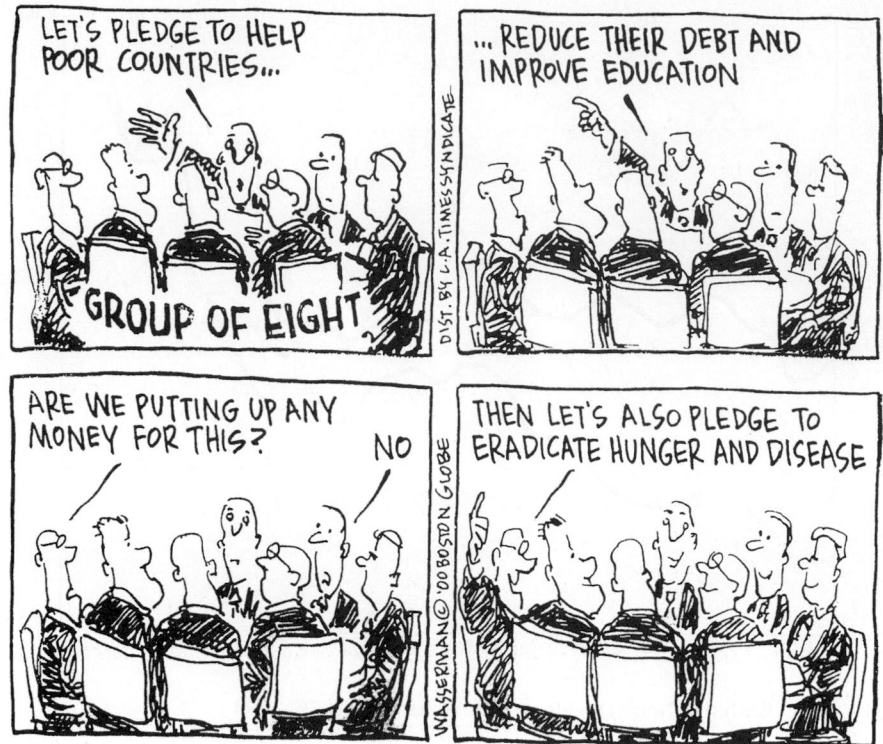

Source: "Group of Eight" cartoon by Dan Wasserman from *The Boston Globe*, January 1, 2000. Copyright © 2000 Boston Globe. All rights reserved. Used by permission and protected by the Copyright Laws of the United States. The printing, copying, redistribution, or retransmission of this Content is prohibited.

in turn is roughly commensurate with its portion of global gross domestic product. The U.S. is the largest shareholder in the IBRD (16 percent). The next-largest shareholders are Japan, Germany, the United Kingdom, and France. China and India each have about 2.7 percent of voting shares in the IBRD. There are on-going calls to reapportion voting rights away from high-income countries to low- and middle-income nations. Some progress has been made in this direction.

The **International Monetary Fund** was also founded at the 1944 Bretton Woods conference.[8] The IMF's original mission was to reestablish an international system of stable national currencies as part of an effort to rejuvenate world trade after World War II. All the IMF's early programs were in today's industrialized countries; frequent lending operations occurred with the United States, the United Kingdom, France, Germany, and other countries until the early 1970s. The IMF played a very

---

[8]The third organization that was meant to be launched at Bretton Woods was the International Trade Organization (ITO). However, the U.S. Congress failed to pass the legislation necessary to ensure U.S. participation, and the ITO never came into existence. Instead, the international community established the General Agreement on Tariffs and Trade, which was the forerunner of today's World Trade Organization (WTO).

limited role in developing countries until the late 1970s and early 1980s, when many low-income countries began to face severe balance-of-payments problems and debt crises.

Today most of the fund's operations are in low- or middle-income countries. IMF involvement in Greece and Ireland after their financial crises are important exceptions. The IMF's main purpose is to provide temporary financing to countries facing significant balance-of-payments problems stemming from a sharp fall in export prices, a rise in import prices (for example, from an increase in world oil prices), a financial crisis that leads to significant international capital flight, and other shocks. IMF funds are used to shore up the country's foreign exchange reserves and stabilize the currency, *not* to finance investment projects or consumption. The IMF is concerned primarily with helping countries achieve and maintain macroeconomic stability rather than directly supporting economic growth and development (although, of course, a stable environment is important for long-run growth). To receive IMF financing, countries must agree (sometimes controversially) to undertake policy reforms typically aimed at reducing the government budget deficit, tightening monetary policy, increasing the flexibility of the exchange rate, and quickly reducing the current account deficit to restore macroeconomic stability.

The vast majority of the IMF's financing is *not* foreign aid. For its emergency loans (called *stand-by credits*) it typically lends money for a one- to three-year period and charges market interest rates. Only about 10 percent of the IMF's outstanding loans are categorized as ODA, all of it provided to low-income countries. Although IMF programs are designed to be short term, in many instances they are renewed for many years. The IMF had continuous or nearly continuous programs beginning in the 1980s and continuing into the 2000s in Bolivia, Ghana, Malawi, the Philippines, Uganda, and several other countries.

Africa, Asia, and Latin America each have their own **regional development banks**: the African Development Bank, the Asian Development Bank, and the Inter-American Development Bank.[9] Like the World Bank, each of the major regional banks provides financing on both concessional and nonconcessional terms, depending on the income level of the borrower. Regional member countries and the major aid donors contribute to the capital of these banks, which also borrow on private capital markets to finance "hard" (nonconcessional) loans and receive contributions from aid donors for their "soft" (concessional) loan and grant operations. Other multilateral donors include the European Union (EU), the Organization of the Petroleum Exporting Countries (OPEC) Fund, and the Islamic Development Bank.

---

[9]A fourth, the European Bank for Reconstruction and Development, finances investment in eastern Europe and central Asia, but almost none of its finance is concessional.

The United Nations also has a range of foreign assistance programs that are of a considerably smaller scale than the lending programs of the World Bank or IMF. Much of this assistance comes as technical cooperation (consultants, advisers, and other expertise), primarily from the United Nations Development Programme (UNDP), the United Nations Population Fund (UNFPA), and the World Health Organization (WHO). Other United Nations agencies provide grants for development projects and humanitarian assistance, including the World Food Program (WFP), the United Nations Children's Fund (UNICEF, winner of the 1965 Nobel Prize for Peace), and the United Nations High Commissioner for Refugees (UNHCR).

WHO RECEIVES FOREIGN AID?

According to the DAC, over 150 countries and territories around the world are receiving aid. Table 14–1 shows the largest 10 recipients in 2009, each of which received more than $2 billion. Afghanistan topped the list (remember, ODA *does not* include military assistance). Total dollar amounts are important, but they do not tell the entire story. On a per capita basis, the aid flows to some of these countries are fairly small. Bangladesh received $1.2 billion in ODA, which sounds like a big number, but Bangladesh is a very populous country with over 160 million people. ODA inflows were equivalent to just a few percent of its GNI, or about $7.50 per Bangladeshi, the cost of a few kilograms of rice. But for some recipients with smaller economies, the amounts involved are quite large. Sierra Leone received $450 million in 2009 equal to 24 percent of its GNI that year. For its almost 6 million people, ODA worked out to be about $78 dollars per person, compared to a GNI per capita of $340 in the same year. For other (even smaller) countries a little bit of aid goes even farther. Tuvalu, a middle-income, island nation in the Pacific Ocean with a population of under 10,000 received $17 million in aid in 2009, which translated into 44 percent of GNI and over $1,700 per Tuvaluan. The difference in the apparent magnitudes of aid measured in nominal terms, as a share of GNI and aid per capita, reflects not only the behavior of the donors but the size of the population and income level of the recipient countries. A high aid to GNI ratio can indicate a large amount of aid, but it can also result from a low GNI or small population.

On a regional basis, sub-Saharan African countries received ODA flows averaging 4.9 percent of GNI in 2009, or $53 per person (Table 14–2). Despite the massive numbers of people living in absolute poverty in South Asia, exceeding the levels in sub-Saharan Africa, South Asia received less than 1 percent of its GNI in ODA, about $9 per person. For low-income countries around the world, donors in 2009 provided aid averaging about $47 per recipient, an increase from $14 in 2003. What happened over the those six years? Did the rich nations suddenly triple their commitment to the poorest nations? Not really. Since 2003, India graduated from low- to middle-income status, significantly raising the aid per capita amounts for low-income nations.

TABLE 14-1 Major Official Development Aid Recipients (2009)

RANK	COUNTRY	TOTAL ODA (MILLIONS OF CURRENT US$)
1	Afghanistan	6,235
2	Ethiopia	3,820
3	Vietnam	3,744
4	West Bank and Gaza	3,026
5	Tanzania	2,934
6	Iraq	2,791
7	Pakistan	2,781
8	India	2,502
9	Côte d'Ivoire	2,369
10	Congo, Dem. Rep.	2,354

RANK	COUNTRY	ODA (PERCENT OF GNI)
1	Liberia	70
2	Afghanistan	45
3	Solomon Islands	44
4	Tuvalu	43
5	Burundi	42
6	Micronesia, Fed. Sts.	41
7	Marshall Islands	32
8	Palau	28
9	Sierra Leone	24
10	Congo, Dem. Rep.	22

RANK	COUNTRY	ODA PER CAPITA (MILLIONS OF CURRENT US$)
1	Mayotte	2,751
2	Tuvalu	1,785
3	Palau	1,737
4	Marshall Islands	1,101
5	Micronesia, Fed. Sts.	1,093
6	West Bank and Gaza	748
7	Dominica	533
8	Grenada	463
9	Vanuatu	442
10	Kosovo	437

GNI, gross national income; ODA, official development assistance.

Source: World Bank, "World Development Indicators," http://databank.worldbank.org.

Generally speaking, aid is an important type of capital flow for low-income countries, but not most middle-income countries. Aid flows averaged 9.3 percent of GNI in low-income countries in 2009 but just 0.1 percent of GNI in upper-middle-income countries. As discussed in Chapter 10, in the 1990s private capital flows grew sharply in middle-income countries, more than compensating for a fall in aid. In low-income countries, private capital rose much more slowly and remained significantly smaller than aid.

TABLE 14-2 Official Development Aid Receipts by Region and Income, 2009

	MILLIONS OF US$	PERCENT OF GNI	DOLLARS PER PERSON
Sub-Saharan Africa	44,553	4.9	53
South Asia	14,607	0.9	9
East Asia and Pacific	10,276	0.2	5
Europe and central Asia	8,101	0.3	20
Middle East and North Africa	13,589	1.1	42
Latin America and Caribbean	9,104	0.2	16
Low income	36,279	9.3	47
Lower-middle income	40,482	1.1	17
Upper-middle income	13,222	0.1	5
High income	433	0.0	0.4

GNI, gross national income.

Source: World Bank, "World Development Indicators," http://databank.worldbank.org.

THE MOTIVATIONS FOR AID

What determines to whom donors provide aid and how much they give? Donors have a variety of motivations in providing aid, only some of which are directly related to economic development.

FOREIGN POLICY OBJECTIVES AND POLITICAL ALLIANCES There is little question that foreign policy and political relationships are the key determinants of aid flows. During the cold war, both the United States and the Soviet Union used aid to vie for the support of developing countries around the world. The United States provided significant amounts of aid to countries fighting communist insurgencies with little regard as to whether the aid was used for development, including Vietnam in the 1960s; Indonesia, the Philippines, and Zaire in the 1970s and 1980s; and several countries in Central America in the 1980s. The Soviet Union countered with aid to North Korea, Cuba, and countries across Eastern Europe. Both sides vied for support in newly independent countries across Africa and used aid to gain support for crucial votes in the United Nations or other world bodies. The United States and the Soviet Union are not the only countries to have used aid in this kind of competitive way: France, Germany, the United Kingdom, Taiwan, and China have used aid (among other policy tools) to try to gain support and recognition for their governments from countries around the world (Box 14–3).

Many donors provide significant aid to their former colonies as a means of retaining some political influence. Being a former colony substantially increases the probability of receiving aid flows. Between 1970 and 1994, 99.6 percent of Portugal's aid went to former colonies, whereas 78 percent of aid from the United Kingdom and

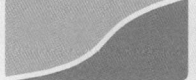

BOX 14-3 CHINA'S FOREIGN AID

China has had a small foreign aid program since the founding of the People's Republic of China in 1949. During the following three decades, China was a low-income country, with annual foreign exchange earnings of less than $10 billion a year, barely enough for China to pay for essential imports. China became a member of the World Bank in 1980 and became eligible for International Development Association (IDA) loans, with their heavily subsidized interest rates, which were available only to low-income countries. During these early decades, Chinese foreign aid involved small loans and grants mainly to friendly neighbors (North Korea for example) and to countries willing to switch formal diplomatic recognition from the Republic of China on Taiwan to the People's Republic with its capital in Beijing.

This situation began to change in the late 1980s and 1990s and changed dramatically in the first decade of the twenty-first century. China does not report the specific dollar amounts of its total aid to developing countries nor does it give a breakdown of that aid by recipient country. It is also not easy to distinguish between what is development aid in accordance with the official definition of development assistance as used by international organizations, by which the grant proportion of any assistance must be at least 25 percent of the total. Still there is no doubt that China's foreign aid had risen to billions of dollars a year by 2010. Some of this aid was in the form of outright grants, but much of it took the form of heavily subsidized loans from the Export-Import Bank of China. The official position of the Chinese government is that developing countries know best how foreign aid should be used and therefore the government never attaches conditions to its assistance, unlike the World Bank and many bilateral aid agencies that typically require the recipient country to institute particular reforms in order to receive aid.

While officially the purpose of Chinese aid is to provide unconditional funds to low-income countries to help them raise their incomes, the reality is that much of the aid is directed to countries that are important to China's own development. China's rapid industrialization over the past three decades has turned China into one of the world's largest importers of natural resource products, ranging from oil to iron and copper ore and much else. Some of the largest recipients of Chinese foreign aid have been countries in Africa that are exporters of oil or have given China the right in their country to explore for oil (Angola, Equatorial Guinea, Ethiopia, and Sudan among others). Many of these countries have repressive governments, and China often has been criticized for aiding governments that carry out repressive measures against their own people, including in the Darfur region of Sudan.

China's goal is to obtain the rights to develop and import natural resource products from whoever is willing to sell, and ownership and drilling rights are seen as a way of securing reliable sources of these products. Aid in turn helps acquire those rights. The aid finances large infrastructure construction projects, ranging from roads to government buildings and hospitals, often built by Chinese construction companies and with Chinese labor battalions. Many countries use their aid programs to support their own economic and geopolitical interests abroad so China is not unique in this respect.

Sources: State Council of China, "White Paper: China's Foreign Aid" *China Daily*, April 22, 2011; Thomas Lum, Hannah Fischer, Julissa Gomez-Granger, and Anne Leland, "China's Foreign Aid Activities Africa, Latin America, and Southeast Asia," Congressional Research Service, Washington, DC, February 25, 2009; Robert Rotberg, ed., *China into Africa: Trade, Aid and Influence* (Washington, DC: Brookings Institution Press, 2008).

between 50 and 60 percent of aid from Australia, Belgium, and France went to their former colonies.[10]

For the United States, the most important geopolitical concern outside of the cold war has been the Middle East. Since 1980, two of the largest recipients of U.S. foreign aid (which goes beyond ODA) have been Israel and Egypt because the United States provided financial support to back the Camp David peace agreement signed by those two countries in November 1979. More recently, the largest U.S. aid recipients are countries important to key national security interests, such as Afghanistan, Pakistan, and Jordan. Beginning in 2002, Iraq became the largest recipient of U.S. aid (and the largest aid recipient in the world), and its reconstruction is likely to become the largest single foreign aid program ever recorded. Aid commitments to Iraq began to decline in 2009 while increasing amounts of development assistance shifted to Afghanistan.

INCOME LEVELS AND POVERTY Income and poverty are important considerations in aid allocation, at least for some donors, although not as much as is sometimes assumed.[11] For many people in rich countries, the main rationale for aid is to help those in most need in the poorest countries. Income levels and poverty influence both the amount of aid donors provide and the extent of its concessionality. Donors generally provide their most concessional aid to the poorest countries and give fewer

[10]Alberto Alesina and David Dollar, "Who Gives Foreign Aid to Whom and Why?" *Journal of Economic Growth* (March 2000), 33–63.

[11]Alesina and Dollar, "Who Gives Foreign Aid to Whom and Why?," found that income levels were the primary motivation for aid from Denmark, Finland, Norway, and Sweden.

grants and subsidized loans for higher-income countries. Some aid programs are designed explicitly with this objective in mind. The World Bank's IDA program has an income ceiling (as do the concessional windows of the regional development banks). Once countries reach that ceiling, in most cases, they "graduate" from IDA to nonconcessional IBRD loans. Other programs have less formal graduation rules but still tend to provide less aid as incomes grow.

As incomes of the poorest countries rise, the composition of their capital inflows tends to change, with aid flows declining and private capital inflows increasing. Botswana is an example. It received aid flows equivalent to 15 percent of GNI in the early 1970s, when its income averaged less than $800 per capita, but with its average income now over $6,000, ODA amounts to only a few percent of GNI. But Botswana grew rapidly. The transition from high to low aid receipts generally takes many years because most nations do not grow as quickly as Botswana did. One study calculated that, for the most successful countries, the half-life of aid is about 12 years, meaning that aid falls to about 50 percent of its peak level after 12 years and about 25 percent of its peak after 24 years.[12] So, for many of the poorest countries, a rapid transition to private capital flows is unlikely.

COUNTRY SIZE Donors provide much more aid (either as a share of GDP or per person) to smaller countries than to large countries. If donors were concerned strictly with allocating aid to where the largest numbers of poor people live, much more aid would go to China, India, Indonesia, Bangladesh, and Pakistan. However, the very size of some of these countries sometimes daunts donors. They prefer to provide aid to smaller countries, where the difference it makes is more noticeable. Aid of $50 million would be huge in The Gambia, but would not be noticed in India. For political reasons, donors generally want to influence as many countries as possible, which tends to lead to a disproportionate amount of aid going to small countries. A vote in the UN General Assembly counts the same if it is from a small country or a large one, so donors may try to influence as many small countries as possible.

COMMERCIAL TIES Bilateral aid is often designed at least partially to help support the economic interests of certain firms or sectors in the donor country. Multilateral aid is less prone to these pressures, although by no means immune. Many analysts have concluded that commercial ties are an important determinant of Japan's aid. Food donations help support farmers that produce the crops in the United States and European Union. Many donors tie portions of their aid to purchases within the donor

---

[12]Michael Clemens and Steven Radelet, "The Millennium Challenge Account: How Much Is Too Much, How Long Is Long Enough?" Working Paper No. 23, Center for Global Development, Washington, DC, February 2003.

country. Automobiles, airline tickets, and consulting services financed by U.S. foreign aid, in most cases, must be purchased from U.S. firms. Tying aid has a long history: Much of the machinery and equipment for the Marshall Plan was purchased from U.S. companies, and all of it had to be shipped across the Atlantic on U.S. merchant vessels. Tying aid probably helps strengthen political support for aid programs within donor countries, but it adds to the costs of aid programs and makes them less effective. One study found that tying aid added 15 to 20 percent to its cost, meaning that recipients received less of a benefit from the aid notionally allocated to their country.

DEMOCRACY Historically, donors have provided foreign assistance with little regard to whether recipient country governments were authoritarian or democratic. This was particularly the case during the cold war, but since the breakup of the Soviet Union, donors have tended to increase their aid to countries that have become democracies. More aid has been aimed at strengthening fragile democracies, supporting the transition of nondemocracies to democracies, or building democratic institutions, including financing for parliaments, election monitoring systems, and groups supporting civil rights and free speech. Alberto Alesina and David Dollar, in a study covering the years 1970 through 1994, found that the typical country received a 50 percent increase in aid after switching to become a democracy.

AID, GROWTH, AND DEVELOPMENT

Many people think of foreign aid primarily as either building infrastructure (such as roads or dams) or providing emergency humanitarian relief after natural disasters, but its purposes often are more diverse. Most foreign aid is designed to meet one or more of four broad economic and development objectives:

- To stimulate economic growth through building infrastructure, supporting productive sectors such as agriculture, or bringing new ideas and technologies.
- To promote other development objectives, such as strengthening education, health, environmental, or political systems.
- To support subsistence consumption of food and other commodities, especially in emergency situations after natural disasters or humanitarian crises.
- To help stabilize an economy after economic shocks.

The extent to which aid has been successful in helping achieve these objectives is a matter of continued debate and controversy.

Despite these broader objectives for aid, economic growth has always been the main yardstick used to judge aid's effectiveness, with more aid expected to lead to

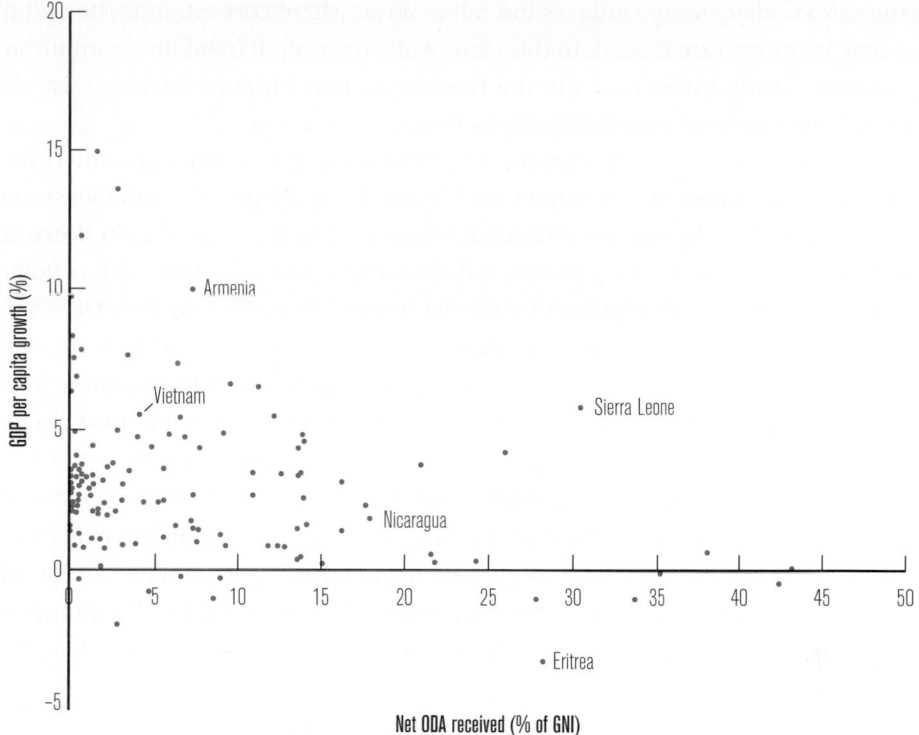

FIGURE 14-4 **Foreign Aid and Growth, 1999–2008**

GNI, gross national income; ODA, official development assistance.

Source: World Bank, "World Development Indicators," http://databank.worldbank.org.

faster growth. But, at a very broad level, there is no apparent simple relationship between aid and growth, as shown in Figure 14–4. Some countries that received large amounts of aid recorded rapid growth (Sierra Leone), whereas others recorded slow or even negative growth (Eritrea). At the same time, some countries that received very little aid did very well, whereas others did not (note the scatter of points in Figure 14–4 close to the *y*-axis.)

What does the absence of a simple relationship mean? For some analysts, it is evidence of a failure of aid to achieve its basic objectives. But for others, this simple correlation is misleading because other factors affect both aid and growth. Some countries that received large amounts of aid may face endemic disease or poor geography or may be emerging from long-standing civil conflict, in which case aid might have a positive impact on growth even if the overall growth performance remains weak. Or the causality could run in the opposite direction: Donors give more aid to countries with slow growth rates and much less to rapid growers like China. These analysts suggest that, once these other factors are taken into consideration, a positive relationship emerges. Still others conclude that aid works well under certain circumstances but fails in others. Aid might help spur growth in countries with reasonably good economic policies but fail to do so where corruption is rife and the economy is badly mismanaged. In this view, while the overall trend line is important, the variance around the trend and the reasons for that variance are also critical in understanding the true underlying relationships.

Debate on these issues has been ongoing for many years, and continues today. There is general agreement on some broad issues. Even aid pessimists (at least most of them) agree that aid has been successful in some countries (such as in Botswana or Indonesia or more recently in Mozambique and Tanzania), that aid has helped improve health by supplying essential medicines, and that aid is an important vehicle in providing emergency relief after natural disasters. Similarly, aid optimists concede that much aid has been wasted or stolen, such as by the Marcos regime in the Philippines and the Duvalier regime in Haiti, and that, even under the best circumstances, aid can have adverse incentives on economic activity. Debate continues on the overall general trends, the conditions under which aid works or does not work, and on what steps can be taken to make aid more effective. Empirical evidence is mixed, with different studies reaching different conclusions depending on the time frame, countries involved, and assumptions underlying the research. We summarize these by looking at three views on aid and growth.

VIEW 1. ALTHOUGH NOT ALWAYS SUCCESSFUL, ON AVERAGE, AID HAS A POSITIVE IMPACT ON ECONOMIC GROWTH AND DEVELOPMENT

The clearest economic rationale for aid is to promote growth by financing new investment, especially investment in public goods. Aid used to build roads, ports, electricity generators, schools, and other infrastructure augments the process of capital accumulation, which (if the investments are productive) should accelerate the rate of growth. This motivation for aid has been invoked since the Marshall Plan. Indeed, early analyses of foreign aid, such as Walt Rostow's popular 1960 book *The Stages of Economic Growth,* saw aid wholly in terms of financing investment and adding to the capital stock.[13] This idea is fully consistent with the Harrod-Domar model, which views capital formation as the main driver of growth, as well as with the Solow model, which sees capital accumulation as important for growth, albeit with diminishing returns and with a strong role for new technology. In the context of these models, aid adds to the total amount of saving, which increases investment and the capital stock, which in turn accelerates the rate of economic growth.[14]

---

[13]W. W. Rostow, *The Stages of Economic Growth: A Non-Communist Manifesto* (Cambridge: Cambridge University Press, 1960).

[14]As discussed in Chapter 4, in the Harrod-Domar model the effect is a permanent increase in the growth rate; in the Solow model it is a transitory increase in the growth rate until the economy achieves a new steady level of output.

In this view, poor countries are unable to generate sufficient amounts of saving on their own to finance the investment necessary to initiate growth, or if they do they can finance only very slow growth. As discussed in Chapter 10, saving rates tend to be low in the very poorest countries, and even where they are moderately high, the actual amount of saving is low. A country with per capita income of $200 and a saving rate of 10 percent generates saving of $20 per person per year, which cannot purchase much in terms of capital goods. In the strongest version of this view, the poorest countries may be stuck in a **poverty trap**, in which their income is too low to generate the saving necessary to initiate the process of sustained growth.[15] Total saving may be too small to compensate for depreciation, let alone add to the capital stock. In a more moderate version, the poorest countries may be able to save enough to begin to grow, but only at very slow rates. Thus aid flows provide a way to augment domestic saving and accelerate the growth process.

Aid can also support growth by building knowledge and transferring new ideas, technology, and best practices from one country to another. Some aid helps support research in low-income countries that can accelerate the pace of growth. One of the best examples is aid-funded research in the 1960s and 1970s on new varieties of seeds, fertilizers, and pesticides that helped transform agriculture in Asia through what became known as the *green revolution*. Similarly, a significant portion of aid finances advisers and technical assistance that ultimately is aimed at strengthening institutions and increasing productivity. This kind of aid, when it is effective, can be thought of as shifting the production function upward, thereby helping increase the rate of growth.[16]

The majority of studies, although far from all, find a positive relationship between aid and growth, on average, after controlling for the impact of other factors on growth.[17] In particular, beginning in the mid-1990s researchers began to investigate whether aid might spur growth, albeit with diminishing returns—that is, small amounts of aid might have a relatively large impact on growth, but each additional dollar of aid might have less effect. This may seem like an obvious point because it is the standard assumption about capital accumulation in most growth models (such as the Solow model), but it is surprising that earlier research tested only a linear relationship. Many (but not all) of the studies that allow for diminishing returns and control for other variables find a positive relationship, on average, between total aid

---

[15]See Jeffrey Sachs et al., "Ending Africa's Poverty Trap," *Brookings Papers on Economic Activity 1* (2004), 117–240.

[16]In the Solow model, the increase in the rate of growth lasts only during the transition to a new steady-state level of income.

[17]For a recent review of the research, see Michael Clemens, Steven Radelet, Rikhil Bhavnani, and Samuel Bazzi, "Counting Chickens When They Hatch: Timing and the Effects of Aid on Growth," *Economic Journal*. Published electronically December 1, 2011. http://onlinelibrary.wiley.com/doi/10.1111/j.1468-0297.2011 .02482.x/full.

and growth.[18] In terms of Figure 14–4, these studies find that other variables, such as geography, political conflict, policies, and institutions explain much of the variance in growth rates among aid recipients. They conclude that, after controlling for these variables and allowing for diminishing returns, a positive relationship between aid and growth emerges, albeit with important variance around the trend line. This view is captured by Figure 14–5a. But as we shall see, other research reached different conclusions, so the debate about the relationship between aid and growth remains open.

In addition, for defenders of View 1, aid can have a positive impact on other important development objectives that may affect growth only indirectly or affect it only after a long period of time, such as health, education, or the environment. Similarly, it can provide emergency assistance or humanitarian relief or be used to help achieve macroeconomic stability. We briefly review each of these in turn.

PROMOTING HEALTH, EDUCATION, AND THE ENVIRONMENT Nearly half of all aid flows are aimed at improving health, education, the environment, and other objectives. Aid that finances immunizations, medical supplies, medicines, bed nets (to prevent the spread of malaria), clean water, and school supplies is meant to help provide essential goods and services to people too poor to afford them. In economic terms, most of these kinds of expenditures count as additions to consumption rather than investment (although some aid for education and health, such as building schools and clinics, count as investment).

Economic growth is often a secondary, long-term objective of this kind of aid. Healthier, better-educated workers should be more productive, shifting the production function and expanding output and income. A similar argument can be made for at least some aid aimed at protecting the environment. Improving forest or fisheries management, cleaning water supplies, or reducing air pollution can improve welfare and increase productivity over time. The impact on growth, however, can take a long time to materialize. Programs to immunize children or improve the quality of primary schools do not affect labor productivity until these children join the workforce, which is many years after the aid was received.

Research on the relationship between aid and other development outcomes tends to concentrate on evaluating specific projects and interventions rather than broad cross-country trends. As with growth, in many cases, aid appears to have had

---

[18]Cross-country econometric studies that allow for diminishing returns typically do so by including both aid and aid squared as determinants of growth. This specification yields a parabola in which aid has a positive effect on growth with diminishing returns, but in theory, with enough aid, the marginal impact could be negative. However, in these studies, the data points are concentrated on the upward portion of the curve, so they do not conclude that large amounts of aid have a negative impact. See, for example, Carl-Johan Dalgaard, Henrik Hansen, and Finn Tarp, "On the Empirics of Foreign Aid and Growth," *Economic Journal* 114, no. 496 (2004), 191–216; Robert Lensink and Howard White, "Are There Negative Returns to Aid?" *Journal of Development Studies* 37, no. 6 (2001), 42–65; Henrik Hansen, and Finn Tarp, "Aid and Growth Regressions," *Journal of Development Economics* 64 (2001), 547–70.

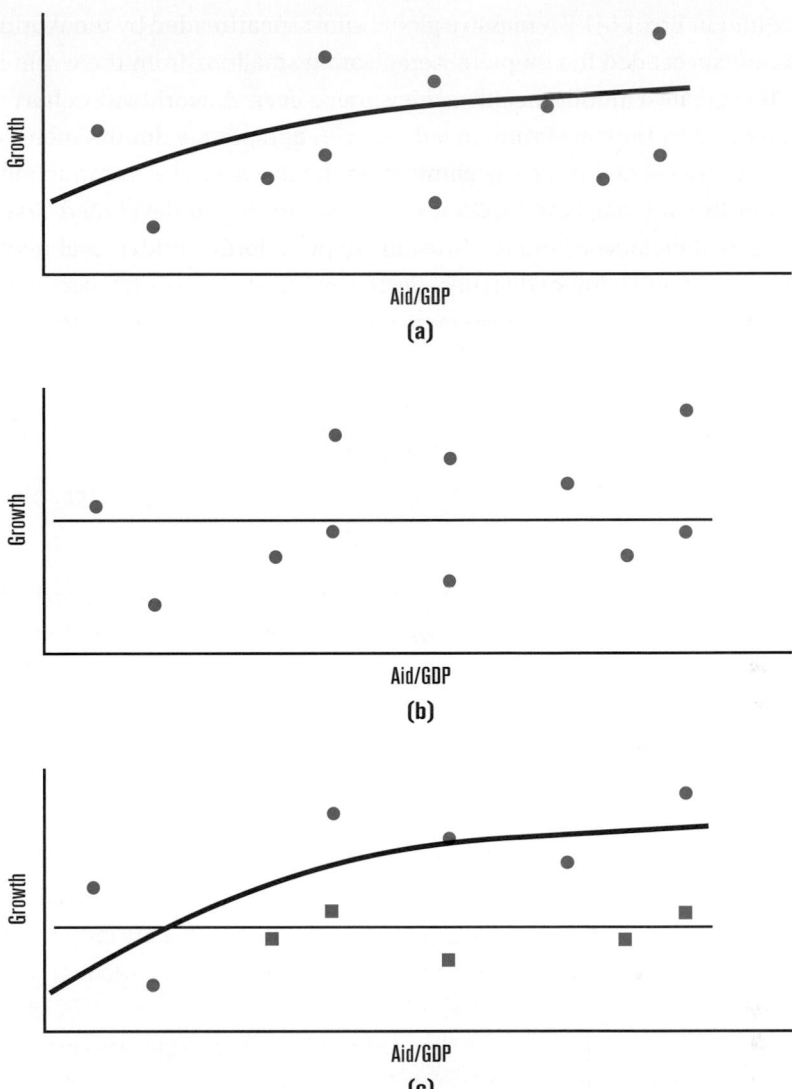

FIGURE 14-5 Three Views on Aid and Growth

(a) View 1: Aid has a positive impact on growth with diminishing returns after controlling for the impact of other variables. (b) View 2: Aid has little or no impact on growth and may have a negative impact. (c) View 3: Aid has a positive impact on growth in some circumstances (circles) but no impact in others (squares).

GDP, gross domestic product.

a strong impact on health and education, along with many interventions that failed. Perhaps the best documented are aid-financed interventions in health. A group of experts convened by the Center for Global Development documented 17 cases of large health interventions in developing countries that have been very success-ful in improving health outcomes and saving lives, several of which are discussed in

Chapter 9 and in Box 14–4.[19] A massive global effort spearheaded by the World Health Organization succeeded in completely eradicating smallpox from the world in 1977, perhaps the greatest public health achievement ever. A worldwide effort to fight polio, supported by both government aid agencies and private donors such as Rotary International, succeeded in nearly eliminating the disease. The introduction of oral rehyrdration therapy has saved millions of lives after being developed first in East Pakistan (now Bangladesh) in the 1970s. In Egypt, a donor-funded oral rehydration program helped reduce infant diarrheal deaths by an astonishing 82 percent between 1982 and 1987.

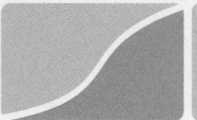

BOX 14–4 CONTROLLING RIVER BLINDNESS IN SUB-SAHARAN AFRICA

Onchocerciasis, or river blindness, is a pernicious, parasitic disease that afflicts approximately 18 million people worldwide, with well over 99 percent of its victims in sub-Saharan Africa. Spread through the bite of an infected blackfly living near fast-moving waters, river blindness causes symptoms such as disabling itching, rashes, muscle pain, skin lesions, and in its most severe cases, blindness.

In 1974, governments and donors in 11 West African countries jointly launched the Onchocerciasis Control Programme. At the time, 2.5 million of the area's 30 million inhabitants were infected with the disease, and approximately 100,000 were blind. The primary intervention was weekly aerial spraying of larvicide during rainy seasons along the region's waterways to control the disease-spreading blackflies. The aerial spraying, augmented by hand spraying of breeding grounds, persisted even through civil and regional conflicts and coups. In 1987, the program began distributing the drug ivermectin, which treats the disease's symptoms with a single annual dose.

The program was implemented through unusual cooperation between several governments and a wide range of donors. It was launched under the leadership of the World Health Organization, the World Bank, the Food and Agriculture Organization, and the United Nations Development Programme. A total of 22 donor countries contributed $560 million to support the 28-year project, with much of the financing provided through long-term commitments. The pharmaceutical company Merck & Co. donated ivermectin to the program beginning in 1987, pledging to provide it to anyone that needed it as long as they needed it, making the donation program one of the largest public—private partnerships ever

[19]Ruth Levine with Molly Kinder, *Millions Saved: Proven Success in Global Health* (Washington, DC: Center for Global Development, 2004).

created. Governments and nongovernmental organizations in the recipient countries were critical to implementing the program effectively.

The program achieved impressive success between 1974 and its conclusion in 2002: Transmission was halted completely in all 11 West African countries involved, 600,000 cases of blindness were prevented, and 18 million children born in the program area are now free from the risk of the disease. In addition to the striking health benefits, the economic impact has been impressive. An estimated 25 million hectares of arable land, enough to feed 17 million people, are now safe for resettlement. In Burkina Faso, 15 percent of the country's land that had been deserted because of onchocerciasis has been completely reclaimed, and its new residents now enjoy a thriving agricultural economy.

The program was extremely cost-effective, with a yearly cost of less than $1 per protected person. The World Bank calculated that the annual return on investment (attributable mainly to increased agricultural output) to be 20 percent, and it is estimated that $3.7 billion will be generated from improved labor and agricultural productivity.

Source: Ruth Levine with Molly Kinder, *Millions Saved: Proven Success in Global Health* (Washington, DC: Center for Global Development, 2004), chap. 6.

There have also been several successful education initiatives.[20] A girls' primary school education initiative in Balochistanm, Pakistan, led to a tripling of the number of schools, a more than doubling of girls' enrollment, and an increase in the girls' primary school completion rate from 7 to 30 percent between 1990 and 1998. In Ethiopia, a systemwide set of education reforms implemented in the 1990s with the support of USAID, the World Bank, and UNICEF led to the construction of many new schools, increasing the number of teachers and improving their training, and expanding the availability of textbooks. Between 1991 and 2001, the overall primary school enrollment ratio increased from 20 to 57 percent, and the girls' enrollment ratio jumped from 12 to 47 percent. In Indonesia, donors partially supported the construction of over 61,000 primary schools in the mid-1970s, which Massachusetts Institute of Technology (MIT) economist Esther Duflo showed led to significant increases in educational attainment and increased wages for school graduates.[21]

---

[20]For a summary of successful education interventions, see Maria Beatriz Orlando, "Success Stories in Policy Interventions towards High Quality Universal Primary Education" (Washington, DC: Center for Global Development, 2004).

[21]Esther Duflo, "Schooling and Labor Market Consequences of School Construction in Indonesia: Evidence from an Unusual Policy Experiment" *American Economic Review* 91 (September 2001).

These individual success stories only tell part of the story. There also have been many failures, where donors provided funding for health and education reforms that did not happen, for technical assistance that did not help, or for interventions that led to little change in health or education. But beyond case studies, little systematic evidence has been gathered on the circumstances under which aid-financed interventions in health and education have been successful and where they have not.

PROVIDING EMERGENCY ASSISTANCE AND HUMANITARIAN RELIEF About one tenth of all foreign aid provides emergency relief after natural disasters or humanitarian crises. Relief programs after earthquakes, floods, or other disasters typically provide food, clothing, basic medicines and drugs, and other items to help meet subsistence needs. Similarly, humanitarian aid assists people living in refugee camps and those displaced by war or other conflict. From an economic point of view, most of this aid is meant to support basic consumption rather than investment and growth, although some of it is used to rebuild ruined infrastructure and help output from collapsing further than it otherwise might following disasters.

SUPPORTING ECONOMIC AND POLITICAL STABILITY Some aid is provided to help countries facing macroeconomic instability. A fall in export prices, a rise in import prices, or an economic shock, such as a drought, flood, or earthquake, can lead to a sharp depreciation of the exchange rate, which in turn can ripple through the economy and increase the prices of traded goods and services. Aid inflows add to the supply of foreign exchange and can help moderate the pressure on the exchange rate. The IMF plays the leading role in this area, with other donors such as the World Bank providing supporting funds. Aid flows that are a response to a macroeconomic crisis or a natural disaster, as described in the previous paragraph, are inversely correlated with economic growth. Growth falls because of the crisis, and aid increases as a result. These situations account for some of the "below-the-line" cases in Figure 14–4, where aid is associated with very low or even negative GDP growth. But because aid is responding to the low growth, these cases should not be seen as examples of a failure of aid to promote growth and development.

VIEW 2. AID HAS LITTLE OR NO EFFECT ON GROWTH AND ACTUALLY MAY UNDERMINE GROWTH

How could aid have no impact or a negative impact on growth, as suggested by Figure 14–5b? One simple way is if most of it simply is wasted. If donors build large bureaucracies or spend the money on expensive technical experts from their home country that write reports no one reads, aid will not help growth. Aid that winds up in the personal off-shore bank accounts of government officials or finances a fleet of expensive cars for members of parliament creates little stimulus to growth. If aid builds a road but provides no funds for maintenance, there may be an initial burst of output, but this could be followed by a decline back to previous levels as the road deteriorates. Because donors typically like to finance capital costs of new projects but not maintenance, this is a common problem.

More insidious, if aid breeds corruption, government officials and their cronies spend their time plotting about how to siphon aid money to their own bank accounts rather than increasing output. Aid funds used to pay private contractors for construction projects or delivery of services can create opportunities for kickbacks and other illegal activities, just like any other public funds. One of the strongest critiques of aid and how it might undermine development is that it can prop up malevolent dictators and support political regimes that further impoverish rather than help the poor. U.S. aid to the Marcos regime in the Philippines during the 1970s and 1980s, for example, may have helped support an anticommunist ally but probably also lengthened the time in which his corrupt regime remained in power. The same argument can be made about aid in the 1970s and 1980s to the Central African Republic, Haiti, or Zaire.

But even if aid is not simply wasted or misused, it could have a smaller than expected impact on growth because of diminishing returns to investment as the recipient begins to reach its **absorptive capacity**. Government bureaucracies with relatively few skilled workers might have difficulty overseeing and managing larger and larger aid flows. Purchases of commodities and supplies might strain available warehouses or delivery systems. Large donations of medicines might sit unused because they cannot be delivered on time to clinics. In the long run, an increase in aid flows may help expand absorptive capacity because it can be used to train and hire more workers, expand warehouse facilities, or build infrastructure to ease bottlenecks, but in the meantime, the impact of aid may be diminished by these constraints.

Perhaps the most important way in which aid could slow growth is by undermining incentives for private sector activity. Large aid flows can spur inflation and cause a real appreciation of the exchange rate, which reduces the profitability of production of all tradable goods. Aid flows can enlarge the size of the government and related services supporting aid projects, drawing workers and investment away from other productive activities such as agro-processing, garments, or footwear exports, which have been important engines for growth in many countries. These "Dutch disease" effects are usually associated with revenues from natural resource export booms (Chapter 18), but can result from aid flows as well. Some analysts believe that large aid flows to Ghana in the late 1980s and early 1990s undermined export incentives.[22] Similarly, food aid can sometimes undermine local food production, as discussed in Box 14–5.

---

[22]See Stephen Younger, "Aid and the Dutch Disease: Macroeconomic Management When Everybody Loves You," *World Development* 20, no. 11 (November 1992), 1587–97.

BOX 14-5 FOOD AID AND FOOD PRODUCTION

For many people, it seems obvious that donating food is a good way for rich countries to help poor countries. Although sometimes that is true, under certain circumstances, donations of food can hurt local farmers by undermining the incentives
for them to produce food. If all food is produced locally (that is, there are no
imports), then an increase in food from aid donations can shift out the supply
curve for food and drive down food prices, benefiting consumers but hurting
farmers, as shown in Figure 14–6a. In an economy with no commercial imports,
food aid shifts the supply curve for food from S_1 to S_2, causing the price to fall
from P_0 to P_1. Producers react by reducing output from Q_0 to Q_1, whereas consumers increase consumption from Q_0 to Q_2, with food aid of $Q_2 - Q_1$ filling the
gap. Consumers are clearly better off (important if there is a true food shortage)
while producers are worse off.

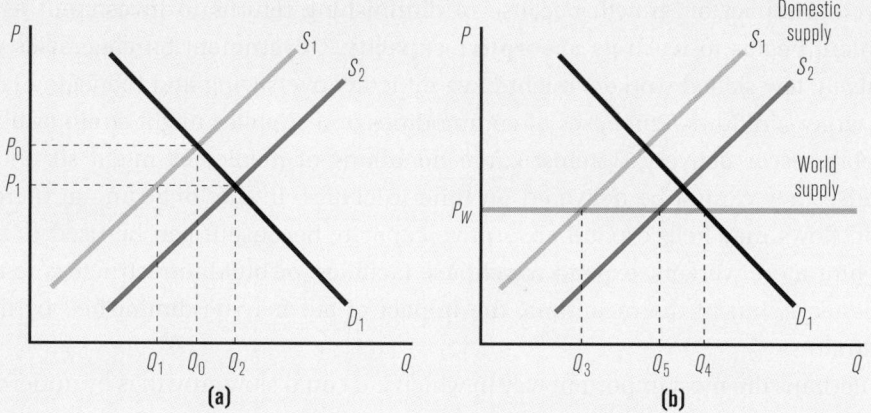

FIGURE 14-6 **Food Aid, Prices, and Production**

(a) Food aid and production in the absence of imports: Food aid lowers prices, benefiting consumers
but displacing local production. (b) Food aid and production with imports: Food aid adds to the total
supply without affecting prices or displacing production.

In an economy that produces some food but imports on the margin, the outcome is different, as shown in Figure 14-6b. With a world price of P_w, initial production takes place at Q_3 with consumption at Q_4 and imports of $Q_4 - Q_3$. In
this situation, food aid displaces imports, with imports falling to $Q_4 - Q_5$ and
food aid making up the difference $Q_5 - Q_3$. Domestic prices, food production,
and consumption do not change, with food aid, in effect, saving the economy the
cost of the displaced imported food.

AID, SAVING, AND TAX REVENUE Aid could also have a smaller-than-expected effect on growth if it has an adverse impact on saving and investment. Early analysts assumed that, because aid is a form of foreign saving, each dollar of aid would add one full dollar to investment. But this is unlikely to happen, for at least two reasons. First, as mentioned previously, not all aid is provided as investment goods or even aimed at increasing investment and growth. Second, even where aid is aimed directly at investment, the impact could be partially offset by a reduction in either private saving (through a decline in the rate of return on private investment) or government saving (through a fall in tax revenues). If a country that currently invests $100 million per year receives $10 million in new aid for investment (for example, building roads), it is highly unlikely that total investment will reach $110 million. It is far more likely that, with $10 million in new investment, some of the original $100 million will be shifted into consumption.

The impact of aid on saving is illustrated in Figure 14–7. Before the recipient country obtains aid, it can produce consumption goods and capital goods along the production possibilities frontier P. To simplify, the diagram ignores international trade and other capital inflows, so that consumption initially also must take place somewhere along the production frontier. Community tastes are defined by a set of indifference curves, of which two are shown (labeled I and II). The country's welfare is maximized if it produces and consumes at point A, where the indifference curve I is tangent to the frontier P, with consumption at C_1 and investment (and saving) at I_1.

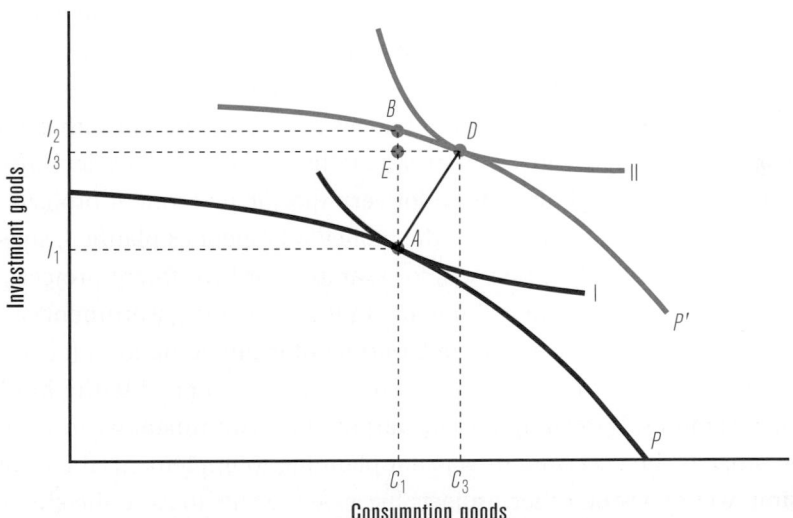

FIGURE 14-7 Impact of Aid on Investment and Consumption

Foreign aid totaling AB turns into actual new investment of only AE because the country maximizes welfare on the new frontier, P', at point D, not B. P' is not really a production frontier but a supply frontier.

Source: Adapted from Paul Mosley, "Aid, Savings and Growth Revisited," *Oxford Bulletin of Economics and Statistics* 42 (May 1980), 79–91.

Now donor countries contribute an amount AB of aid with the intention that it be used to raise investment to I_2. However, the aid moves the *consumption frontier* outward from P to P'. Now, the country maximizes its welfare at point D, the tangency between P' and indifference curve I_2, where it consumes C_3 and invests I_3. Of the aid amount AB, AE (equal to $I_3 - I_1$) is invested and "BE" (equal to $I_2 - I_3$) is consumed. Even if all the new aid money is invested as intended, some of what the country had invested before is shifted to consumption, so in effect, the aid finances an increase in both investment and consumption, with the precise impact depending on production possibilities, community tastes, and other variables left out of the figure, such as trade. Aid may finance mostly investment if $I_3 - I_1$ is a large percentage of total aid (AB), or it may mostly finance consumption if $I_3 - I_1$ is a small percentage of AB.

Why would the country react in this way and not invest all the aid it receives? Saving always requires a sacrifice of current consumption, based on the anticipation that investment will lead to increased output and greater consumption in the future. When the country receives a new inflow of aid, investment increases and the country is less willing to sacrifice that last dollar of today's consumption to finance the last dollar of investment. Thus domestic saving falls somewhat, although with the addition of foreign saving from aid total saving (and investment) rises.

When substitutions of these kinds are possible and aid effectively finances activities for which it was not originally intended, aid is said to be **fungible**. This kind of substitution could be good or bad, depending how the money is spent. If donor funds to build a school allow members of the community to save less and purchase more food, clothing, and medicine for their families, few donors would take issue. But if instead the freed-up funds are used to buy several Mercedes Benzes for the mayor and his or her staff, donors are likely to be unhappy and economic development is not served.

Aid given as a cash transfer to the budget or as program aid rather than for a specific project deliberately gives the recipient the kinds of choices demonstrated in Figure 14–7. But even if all aid is used for very specific investment projects and the donor audits projects to confirm that the money was spent as planned, substitution is possible. Project aid might be used, for example, for investment projects that the government would have made without aid. In that case, the government's resources are freed up for other purposes. If the government is intending to build an electricity generator with its own funds, then a donor decides to provide the funding, the government's money is freed up for any purpose the government wishes. Even if aid finances projects the government was not planning to implement, the government might simply cut back on other projects because it wants to raise the share of consumption for economic or political reasons.

The tendency for aid flows to "stick" as increased government expenditures, rather than result in tax relief or offsetting expenditure reductions in other areas, is sometimes called the *flypaper effect*. Several studies find that $1 in aid translates to less than $1 in government spending, typically in the range of 33 to 67 cents on the dollar. But some studies for specific countries find a strong flypaper effect, with $1 of aid translating into close to $1 of new spending. One study on Indonesia found that $1 in aid led to $1.50 in government expenditures, suggesting that aid "crowded in" government spending, perhaps by relieving constraints that were limiting government spending.[23]

Aid flows can similarly influence government revenues. A government that receives aid flows is likely to be less willing to raise marginal tax revenue from the general public, especially because taxes are not politically popular. A government without aid inflows might be willing to raise taxes to finance a new hospital, but if a donor finances the hospital, the government has much less incentive to raise the revenue. However, aid could help increase revenues if donors require governments to provide matching funds for a particular activity; if aid helped governments introduce institutional changes to strengthen the tax authority, or in the case of loans, governments knew they would need revenues in the future to repay the loans. The empirical evidence on this effect is mixed: In some countries, aid inflows corresponded with increased revenues, whereas in other cases, revenues declined.[24] Where revenues declined, the reduction may benefit ordinary citizens, who can save and consume more for their own purposes, which could help accelerate economic growth. Or it may be directed to individuals or businesses with special connections to the government.

Private saving might also be affected by aid inflows. A host of subtle influences from aid on relative prices may contribute to substitution that reduces private saving and crowds out private sector investment. Aid inflows could reduce interest rates, which in turn could reduce private saving. If investment is subject to diminishing returns, more capital in general could mean lower returns on investments and hence a greater tendency to consume rather than save in the recipient countries.

It is difficult, if not impossible, for donors to stop this substitution, although they may be able to limit it to some extent. Research suggests that aid funds are fungible, at least partially, meaning that recipients, to some extent, can substitute aid funds from their intended purpose to something else. However, the evidence suggests that aid is not perfectly fungible: Much of it goes to its intended purpose, and recipients cannot or do not transform all aid flows into other purposes.

AID DEPENDENCY Some analysts argue that aid loses some of its effectiveness when aid flows are relatively large for long periods of time, because prices, institutions, and expectations adjust to that level and, to some extent, recipients become

---

[23]See World Bank, *Assessing Aid: What Works, What Doesn't, and Why* (New York: Oxford University Press, 1998); Tarhan Feyzioglu, Vinaya Swaroop, and Min Zhu, "A Panel Data Analysis of the Fungibility of Foreign Aid," *World Bank Economic Review* 12, no. 1 (1998). For the study on Indonesia, see Howard Pack and Janet Rothenberg Pack, "Is Foreign Aid Fungible? The Case of Indonesia," *Economic Journal* 100 (March 1990).

[24]Mark McGillvary and Oliver Morrisey, "A Review of the Evidence on the Fiscal Effects of Aid," Research Paper no. 01/13 Center for Research in Economic Development and International Trade, Nottingham, UK, 2001. For a classic model on these effects, see Peter Heller, "A Model of Public Fiscal Behavior in Developing Countries: Aid, Investment, and Taxation," *American Economic Review* 65 (1975), 429–45.

dependent on aid. This situation can raise several challenges. First, the larger the amount of aid, the greater is the risk of a sudden reduction in aid. Aid flows tend to be more erratic than domestic revenues, and the degree of volatility increases with greater dependence on aid.[25] If donors suddenly reduce aid, whether because they face budget cutbacks, in response to a corruption scandal, a change in government, or for some other reason, the macroeconomic consequences can be difficult to manage. Second, large aid flows give donors substantial leverage over the recipient, so that recipients become more willing to introduce whatever conditions the donors require, good or bad, to ensure that the aid continues to be disbursed. Aid flows thus can weaken public accountability and impede the development of civil society, if the recipient government becomes more responsive to the donors than to its own citizens.

As recipients become more dependent on aid, the process of gradually reducing aid over time as development proceeds becomes more difficult. If aid finances public expenditure, a reduction of aid must be matched with either an increase in revenue or a reduction in expenditure, neither of which is particularly easy or politically popular (although raising revenue is made easier by the process of economic growth). The incentives are strong for recipients to continue to request aid for as long as possible and resist these adjustments. Egypt has been one of the world's largest aid recipients since 1980, and some observers believe that these inflows have taken the pressure off of the government to reduce wasteful expenditures and introduce other needed reforms. The downfall in 2011 of the Egyptian government of Hosni Mubarak, in part, may have been an indirect result of these consequences of aid.

Aid programs may actually weaken the institutions that society needs to enhance the process of development and reduce the need for aid. Budget institutions might be weakened by aid, especially if most aid is disbursed as projects with the money not flowing through the budget. Aid agencies need qualified accounts, economists, and financial specialists to design, monitor, and evaluate their projects. By increasing the demand for these skills, aid agencies bid up their wages, making them more expensive for everyone else, including the government (not to mention domestic firms). Aid agencies sometimes recruit the most able and promising local staff, leaving government agencies and the rest of the economy with less-qualified (and usually lower-paid) staff. In Mozambique, after the end of its civil war in the early 1990s, donors came flooding into the country and recruited many of the most-capable government workers, paying upward of five times the government salary and sometimes more than private sector salaries. But the departure of some of its most talented staff deprived the government of needed skills, and weakened government effectiveness as a result.[26]

---

[25]Aleš Bluír and Javier Hamann, "How Volatile and Unpredictable Are Aid Flows, and What Are the Policy Implications?" IMF Working Paper No. 01/167, International Monetary Fund, Washington, DC, 2001.

[26]Peter Fallon and Luiz Pereira da Silva, "Recognizing Labor Market Constraints: Government-Donor Competition for Manpower in Mozambique," in D. Lindauer and B. Nunberg, eds., *Rehabilitating Government* (Washington, DC: World Bank, 1994).

This process is not limited to the budget office: It can affect the central bank, the ministry of health (which might lose physicians or epidemiologists), the ministry of education, and other agencies. Aid agencies might be able partially to countervail these tendencies by supplying technical assistance to train government workers (although some then take other jobs) or otherwise strengthen institutional systems. Over time, there may be some benefit, as the increased wages entice more school graduates to become accountants and financial experts. In any case, aid agencies often do not take into account these possible deleterious impacts.

To some extent, the dependency can work both ways, as aid agencies become accustomed to operating large-scale programs. Donor agencies, in effect, are asked to work themselves out of their jobs by making aid less necessary and less important over time. But, like any agency, most aid agencies like to be bigger and have more aid flows to disburse. Individuals working on specific projects often like to see them continued over time; and the larger the programs, the more influence they may have over government policy choices. Promotions and other rewards often are geared to the size of the aid program they manage. Thus the incentives facing the donors sometimes encourage dependency between donor and recipient.

Proponents of View 2 point to a body of research that finds little relationship between aid and growth. Keith Griffin and John Enos were among the first to report empirical research questioning the effectiveness of aid, finding negative simple correlations between aid and growth in 27 countries. Since then, other studies concluded that there is no relationship or even a negative relationship between aid and growth,[27] in contrast to the studies cited earlier that support View 1.

VIEW 3. AID HAS A CONDITIONAL RELATIONSHIP WITH GROWTH, STIMULATING GROWTH ONLY UNDER CERTAIN CIRCUMSTANCES, SUCH AS IN COUNTRIES WITH GOOD POLICIES OR INSTITUTIONS

This perspective begins by accepting the idea that aid has had mixed results: Even where research has found a generally positive relationship, no one claims that aid has worked across all countries all the time. It recognizes that aid seems to have stimulated growth in some countries under certain circumstances but not in others and focuses on trying to decipher the key characteristics that might explain these

[27]See, for example, K. B. Griffin and J. L. Enos, "Foreign Assistance: Objectives and Consequences," *Economic Development and Cultural Change* 18, no. 2 (July 1970), 313–27; Paul Mosley, "Aid, Savings, and Growth Revisited," *Oxford Bulletin of Economics and Statistics* 42, no. 2 (1980), 79–96; Peter Boone, "The Impact of Foreign Aid on Savings and Growth," Working Paper no. 677, Centre for Economic Performance, London School of Economics, London, 1994; William Easterly, Ross Levine, and David Roodman, "New Data, New Doubts: A Comment on Burnside and Dollar's 'Aid, Politics, and Growth,'" *American Economic Review* 94, no. 3 (June 2004); David Roodman, "The Anarchy of Numbers: Aid, Development, and Cross-Country Empirics," Working Paper no. 32, Center for Global Development, Washington, DC, July 2003. For a review, see Clemens et al., "Counting Chickens When They Hatch."

differences. This view is represented by Figure 14–5c. Three "conditional" explanations have emerged, suggesting that the relationship between aid and growth might depend on the characteristics of the recipient country, the type of aid being provided, or the way in which donors provide it.

CHARACTERISTICS OF THE RECIPIENT COUNTRY The most influential of the conditional perspectives is that the impact of aid depends on the quality of institutions and policies in the recipient country. According to this view, in countries with poor macroeconomic and trade policies, high levels of corruption, and low accountability of government officials, aid is likely to have little or no impact. By contrast, in countries with reasonably good policies and institutions, aid programs can help accelerate growth. Jonathan Isham, Daniel Kaufmann, and Lant Pritchett initiated this line of research by finding that rates of return on aid-financed investments were higher in countries with strong civil liberties and other measures of governance. Craig Burnside and David Dollar took the next step by finding a significant positive relationship between aid and growth in countries with good policies and institutions and no relationship otherwise.[28] Other researchers explored the possibility that the impact of aid may differ depending on the type of government, quality of human capital, location in the tropics (presumably a proxy for health), the magnitude and frequency of export shocks, and other factors.

Although subsequent analysis cast doubt on some of these results, the idea has had an enormous influence on donor policies, probably because the conclusions of a differential effect are consistent with the experience of many development professionals. These findings have led to a shift among donors to be more "selective" in allocating foreign aid, to provide more of it to countries with relatively stronger institutions and policies, as we discuss later in the chapter.

TYPE OF AID Different kinds of aid might affect growth in different ways. One study disaggregated aid flows into those most likely and least likely to affect growth within a few years, if at all.[29] It separated aid into three categories:

- Emergency and humanitarian aid, likely to be negatively associated with growth because it increases sharply at the same time growth falls because of an economic shock.
- Aid that might affect growth only after a long period of time, if at all, and so a growth impact may be difficult to detect, such as aid for health, education, the environment, and to support democracy.

[28]Jonathan Isham, Daniel Kaufmann, and Lant Pritchett, "Governance and Returns on Investment: An Empirical Investigation," Policy Research working paper no. 1550, World Bank, 1995; Craig Burnside and David Dollar, "Aid, Policies, and Growth," *American Economic Review* 90, no. 4 (September 2000), 847–68; Paul Collier and David Dollar, "Aid Allocation and Poverty Reduction," *European Economic Review* 45, no. 1 (2002), 1–26; World Bank, *Assessing Aid: What Works, What Doesn't, and Why* (New York: Oxford University Press, 1998).

[29]Clemens et al., "Counting Chickens When They Hatch."

- Aid directly aimed at affecting growth (building roads, ports, and electricity generators, or supporting agriculture).

It found a strong relationship between the third type of aid and growth, but the relationship with the other types was less detectable. The study found some support for the proposition that the third subcategory of aid had an even stronger impact in countries with stronger institutions.

DONOR PRACTICES Many analysts argue that differences in donor practices are likely to influence aid effectiveness. Multilateral aid might be more effective in stimulating growth than bilateral aid because less of it is determined by political factors (although some argue just the opposite, that multilateral agencies tend to be too large, unfocused, and less directly accountable to taxpayers). Aid "tied" to purchases of good and services in the donor countries or used to finance conferences and international meetings might be less effective than other aid. Large aid bureaucracies add to costs and slow down disbursements, making aid less effective. Donors that coordinate with other funders and recipient governments may be more effective than those that operate completely on their own. Donors with more effective monitoring and evaluation systems might be better able to channel aid to its most productive uses, enhancing overall effectiveness. An influential view that emerged in the late 1990s is that aid might be more effective where there has been a participatory approach among government and community groups in recipient countries in setting priorities and designing aid-supported programs, a topic we return to later in the chapter. Substantial debate centers around these issues, and there is little doubt that donor practices are critical, but to date there has been very little systematic research connecting specific donor practices to aid effectiveness.

In summarizing the aid and growth research, it seems that aid has been successful in some countries but not others, with the overall trend a subject of debate. Further research is looking beneath the surface to reveal what types of aid are most effective, which are ineffective, and the precise conditions under which aid has the largest impact on growth. Just as with the evidence on the causes of economic growth more generally discussed in Chapter 3, there is still much that we do not know about the relationship between aid and growth.

DONOR RELATIONSHIPS WITH RECIPIENT COUNTRIES

The criticisms about foreign aid and the evidence that it appears to have been effective in some countries but not in others led to debates about how aid programs can be improved to more effectively support growth and development. But the challenge is not easy. Aid programs face some inherent difficulties in trying to achieve a wide range of objectives (which may differ between donor and recipient), provide financial oversight, and ensure results. In this section, we first explore some of the challenges in more depth, then turn to some specific changes that have been suggested and in some cases implemented by donors and recipients in an attempt to make aid more effective.

THE PRINCIPAL-AGENT PROBLEM

A key issue facing aid agencies is that there is only an indirect and distant relationship between the people actually providing the financing (taxpayers in donor countries) and the intended ultimate beneficiaries of aid projects (poor people living in low-income countries). Many institutions, organizations, and transactions are in between, and the decisions made along the way may not be in accord with the wishes or best interests of either the original taxpayers or the ultimate beneficiaries. All public-sector agencies and many private companies are faced with the **principal-agent problem**, but the international dimension makes it an even greater challenge for aid. Economist Bertin Martens analyzed the principal agency problem for aid agencies, and our account closely follows his.[30]

Principals in a private company (the owners), club (the members), or public administration (taxpayers) cannot make all decisions and carry out all tasks themselves, so they must delegate these responsibilities to *agents* to work on their behalf: managers, employees, elected officials, and civil servants. But agents have their own goals and motivations, which may not be the same as the principals. Agents also have more information than the principals and can use that information in ways that run counter to the principals' interests. Therefore, principals are faced with the problem of writing contracts and establishing rules that more closely align agents' interests with their own. These issues are particularly important for public-sector agencies because they tend to have multiple objectives (not just profit) and their many principals may not agree on which objective holds the higher priority. These problems make it very difficult to match incentives, such as salary, bonuses, and promotions, with performance indicators.

Most aid programs have a long, complex chain of principal-agent relationships, starting with the taxpayers who delegate authority to elected officials, who in turn become principals who delegate authority to a new set of agents, the heads of aid agencies. These relationships continue to aid agency employees, contractors, and consultants. In the recipient country, similar relationships lie between the ultimate recipients, their government, and those who actually implement programs. In most public agencies, there is considerable slippage throughout these relationships, but

---

[30]Bertin Martens, "Introduction" in Berten Martens, ed., *The Institutional Economics of Foreign Aid* (Cambridge: Cambridge University Press, 2004).

the problem is compounded in aid agencies by the physical separation of the original taxpayers and ultimate beneficiaries. In domestic public programs (such as trash collection or local schools), the taxpayers and ultimate beneficiaries are the same people, so they may have clearer information about success or failure and can reward or penalize their agents accordingly by reelecting them or voting them out of office. But this feedback loop is broken for aid agencies, as Martens points out:

> A unique and striking characteristic of foreign aid is that the people for whose benefit aid agencies work are not the same as those from whom the revenues are obtained; they actually live in different countries and different political constituencies. This [separation] blocks the normal performance feedback process: beneficiaries may be able to observe performance but cannot modulate payments (rewards to agents) as a function of performance. Although donors are typically interested in ensuring that their funds are well spent, it is extremely difficult for them to do so, since there is frequently no obvious mechanism for transmitting the beneficiaries' point of view to the sponsors.[31]

The principal-agent problem affects nearly all aspects of aid delivery, including program design, implementation, compensation, incentives, evaluation, and allocation of funding. The problem can never be fully avoided: Private companies face similar issues between owners, managers, and employees, as do private aid foundations and charities. The challenge is to design institutions and incentives to try to mitigate these problems as much as possible to clarify goals, objectives, incentives, and rewards. A key challenge for donors is how best to apply conditions to their loans to encourage recipients to act more in accord with the donors' (and possibly the ultimate beneficiaries') interests and wishes.

CONDITIONALITY

Donors often require that recipient countries adopt specific policies, or packages of policies, as prerequisites for funding; and this **conditionality** is one of the most controversial aspects of aid. Broad policy conditions are most often associated with financing from the IMF and World Bank, but all donors use them to some extent. Many bilateral donors take their lead from these two multilateral organizations and do not provide the full amount of their aid until the recipient country has met IMF and World Bank conditions. The IMF typically requires that countries adopt a more flexible exchange rate, smaller budget deficits, slower growth of the money supply, a buildup of foreign exchange reserves, privatization of certain state-owned enterprises, a reduction in import restrictions, and the implementation of broad anticorruption measures. World Bank conditions sometimes reinforce these broad policy

---

[31]Martens, "Introduction," 14.

reforms and may add some sector-specific requirements, such as liberalizing fertilizer markets before providing an agriculture loan.

In many cases, the specific policy conditions required by the IMF and World Bank are justifiable and often supported by at least some people within the recipient governments. But, other times, many people believe that IMF and World Bank conditions go too far and their conditions are harder to justify, especially when the rationale for specific reforms are less clear-cut and seen by critics as based more on ideology than hard facts and sensible economics. For example, while privatization of state-owned marketing boards, retail outlets, or trading establishments is generally not controversial, privatization of public utilities is much more open to debate. Many countries may need to impose fiscal discipline as required by the IMF, but the Fund is often accused of imposing much stricter discipline than is really necessary to achieve stability, at a cost of dampening aggregate consumption and expenditures on important social programs. Sometimes, the donors simply impose too many conditions, seemingly wanting the recipient country to fix everything at once without showing any sense of priority or feasibility. Turkey's "Letter of Intent" with the IMF in April 2003 included a table listing 131 very specific policy actions (with dozens more subcategories of actions) that the government promised to undertake as part of its program.[32] The IMF admitted that, at times, it has gone too far, as with its program in Indonesia after the financial crisis of 1997.[33]

While donors are often criticized for imposing too many conditions, they are almost as often criticized for not imposing *enough* conditions. Some advocates that criticize the IMF for imposing too much fiscal austerity also insist that it require governments to spend a minimum amount on health and education. The World Bank is often asked to add conditions to force governments to take specific actions, for example, on projects that have potential environmental consequences. This can lead to difficult dilemmas. Sometimes governments ask the World Bank to be one of many co-funders for a project, hoping that World Bank participation will provide credibility and security. In return, the World Bank typically wishes to require environmental safeguards or anticorruption measures. But because the World Bank is only one lender, its leverage may be limited. If the World Bank requires too many conditions, the government can just go ahead without them (and without the environmental safeguards), but if they ask for too few, they may find themselves funding a project with inadequate conditions.

The rationale for these conditions is straightforward: Donors believe these broad-based conditions are important for growth and development, and without them, providing aid is futile. It is easiest to see this rationale in extreme cases: If gov-

---

[32]See International Monetary Fund, "Turkey: Letter of Intent," April 5, 2003, available at www.imf.org/external/np/loi/2003/tur/01/index.htm; accessed February 2012.

[33]IMF Independent Evaluation Office, "The IMF and Recent Capital Account Crises: Indonesia, Korea, and Brazil," (Washington, DC: IMF, 2003). Available at www.imf.org/external/np/ieo/2003/cac/pdf/all.pdf.

ernment policies have led to high rates of inflation, an overvalued exchange rate, massive inefficiencies and waste of public spending, and extensive corruption, then providing aid, whatever the specific purpose, without requiring fundamental change provides no benefits and perhaps perpetuates the damage. Some even argue that the primary purpose of aid is not the money but for aid to act as a lever for the policy reforms. The conditionality debate is a microcosm of the principal-agent problem: A donor requests a recipient to take specific actions in return for receiving aid, but the recipient may have different objectives and controls sufficient information to make compliance difficult.

Cornell economist Ravi Kanbur points out two further problems with conditionality. First, it is not always clear what conditions are the most appropriate to ensure sustained growth and development. Mahbub ul Haq, an influential development adviser long associated with the UNDP, once commented that sub-Saharan Africa, "often receives more bad policy advice per capita from foreign consultants than any other continent in the world."[34] Development doctrine, as discussed in Chapter 5, has swung from a state-led approach in the 1950s and 1960s, to basic human needs in the 1970s, to a macroeconomic approach focused on open markets in the 1980s and 1990s, to a focus on institutions beginning in the mid-1990s, to a greater focus on private sector led growth in the 2000s. As a result, the list of conditions is constantly evolving.

Second, conditionality does not seem to work. Most analysts agree that governments implement reforms only when it is in their interests to do so, and donor conditions have little, if any, impact on that decision. They perhaps can spur governments to implement changes faster than they otherwise would, or provide support to reformist elements in policy debates, but cannot persuade governments to do what they really do not want to do. Many donors continue to disburse aid even when recipients fail to meet conditions, sometimes repeatedly so. Over time, recipients learn that aid flows do not necessarily depend on meeting stated conditions, a process that gradually undermines the aid institutions and the conditions they attach. Donors are faced with their own internal incentives to continue to disburse aid to support the contractors and recipients that depend on it. They also face a "Samaritan's dilemma," that withdrawing aid would create short-term pain for the very people it is aimed to help.[35]

In the end, there are no clear-cut rules for conditionality. Striking the right balance between responsible oversight and accountability, on the one hand, and ensuring against

[34]Mahbub ul Haq, "Does Africa Have a Future?" *Earth Times New Service,* January 1998.

[35]Ravi Kanbur, "The Economics of International Aid," in Serge Christophe-Kolm and Jean Mercier Ythier, eds., *Handbook of the Economics of Giving, Altruism, and Reciprocity: Applications* (Amsterdam: North Holland, 2006). Also see Jakob Svensson, "Why Conditional Aid Does Not Work and What Can Be Done About It," *Journal of Development Economics* 70, no. 2 (2003), 381–402; William Easterly, *The Elusive Quest for Growth* (Cambridge: MIT, 2002).

high bureaucratic obstacles and the imposition of unnecessary controls or unwarranted policy changes, on the other, requires flexibility, judgment, and the ability to balance multiple objectives.

IMPROVING AID EFFECTIVENESS

Since the late 1990s, as global aid flows began to rise, there has been increased discussion and debate about how aid programs could be strengthened and become more effective in supporting growth and development. These debates recognized some of the weaknesses in aid programs and resulted in some specific ideas for change. The "Paris Declaration on Aid Effectiveness and the Accra Agenda for Action" is perhaps the clearest articulation of the consensus on best practices in aid delivery.[36] In recent years, donor agencies began to put some of these ideas in practice, and some donor practices changed noticeably as a result.

COUNTRY SELECTIVITY One influential idea is that donors should be more selective about which countries they provide aid to, based on the view that aid works best in countries with good policies and institutions. In the strongest version of this view, aid should be provided *only* to countries that meet these criteria and not otherwise, with more going to countries with the highest levels of poverty. A more moderate view is that *more* aid should be allocated to countries with stronger policies and institutions but continue to provide targeted aid to some countries with relatively poor institutions, especially in postconflict situations. This proposal takes a turn on the conditionality debate: Instead of providing aid to encourage reforms, provide it to countries that already decided to implement key reforms. Economists Paul Collier and David Dollar suggested a "poverty-efficient" allocation of aid in which funding would be provided to the poorest countries with relatively stronger policies and institutions to maximize the impact of aid on global poverty reduction.[37]

Donors began to move in this direction. The World Bank uses its Country Policy and Institutional Assessment index to determine partly the allocation of its concessional IDA funds. Several European donors moved toward providing broad budget support or financing for sector-wide approaches, but only for a relatively small number of countries considered to be the most responsible. The U.S. Millennium Challenge Corporation (MCC) provides aid to only a small number of recipient countries, based largely (although not completely) on their performance on 17 indicators of policies and governance.[38] As of late 2011, the MCC had signed compacts with 23 low-income and lower-middle-income countries around the world.

[36]See the Organization for Economic Cooperation and Development (2008), "The Paris Declaration on Aid Effectiveness and the Accra Agenda for Action," available at www.oecd.org/dataoecd/11/41/34428351 .pdf; accessed February 2012.

[37]Collier and Dollar, "Aid Allocation and Poverty Reduction."

[38]Steven Radelet, *Challenging Foreign Aid: A Policymaker's Guide to the Millennium Challenge Account* (Washington, DC: Center for Global Development, 2003).

Because so much aid is allocated for political, security, and other foreign policy reasons, there are limits to how far donors are likely to go in reallocating their aid based on strict economic development criteria. This is especially true for the major bilateral donors but is true for multilateral donors as well. One frequent suggestion is for donors to more clearly separate funding primarily aimed at foreign policy goals from funding aimed at development. This would allow programs to be designed, implemented, and evaluated in different ways so donor country governments, their taxpayers, and recipients could better understand and appraise aid effectiveness.

RECIPIENT PARTICIPATION A second influential idea is that aid has been weakened by donor domination in setting priorities, designing programs and projects, choosing implementers (often consulting firms from the donor country), monitoring and evaluating results, and that aid recipients should play a much larger role in these areas. In this view, bureaucrats and activists from donor countries design too many programs, leading to a poor choice of priorities, flawed design, or weak commitment among recipients for programs they do not feel are their own. Advocates have pushed for a more participatory approach in which various groups in recipient countries (government, NGOs, charities, the private sector) play a more active role. The idea is to eliminate some of the problems in the long chain of principal-agent relationships and more tightly integrate the ultimate beneficiaries in key aspects of the aid-delivery process. This might have two benefits. First, projects might be better designed, with a more accurate view of the highest priorities and the most appropriate implementation methods to meet local needs. Second, increasing recipient participation in the design and implementation process may provide them with more ownership of the activity and a higher stake in ensuring its success. One of the first movements in this direction was the introduction of Poverty Reduction Strategy papers as the basis for World Bank and IMF debt relief and other financing. Similarly, both the Global Fund to Fight AIDS, Tuberculosis, and Malaria and the Millennium Challenge Corporation rely on a significant degree of local participation in designing and implementing the programs they finance. USAID's Feed the Future program, which aims to improve food security by supporting increased agricultural production and improved nutrition, relies on country strategies developed by local leaders and national experts.

While the participatory approach holds out promise and has been increasingly used since the early 2000s, there is no clear empirical evidence yet on the extent to which (or the circumstances under which) it improves aid effectiveness. There is a clear and inescapable tension between country ownership, on the one hand, and donor priorities and conditionality, on the other. Donors are more likely to facilitate a participatory approach in countries in which governments show a strong commitment to sound development policies and less so in countries with corrupt and dictatorial governments.

HARMONIZATION AND COORDINATION Managing aid flows from many different donors can be a constant challenge for recipient countries because different donors tend to implement their own initiatives and insist on using their own unique processes for initiating, implementing, and monitoring projects. Recipients can be overwhelmed by donor requirements to provide multiple project audits, environmental assessments, procurement reports, financial statements, and project updates. According to the World Bank, developing countries typically work with 30 or more aid agencies across a wide variety of sectors, with each sending an average of five missions a year to oversee their projects. Governments can find themselves hosting three or more aid missions a week.[39] Many recipient countries have only a limited number of skilled and highly trained technocrats; and all the donors want to meet with these top people, leaving them with much less time to deal with other pressing concerns. The government of Tanzania, which hosts several hundred aid missions each year, has introduced a "quiet time" from April to August of each year during which it asks donors to minimize meetings and missions so that the government has time to adequately prepare its annual budget.

These concerns have led to numerous suggestions and pledges for donors to more closely coordinate their activities; harmonize their accounting, monitoring, and evaluation systems; or pool their funds.[40] Some progress has been made in the form of donors providing more aid as budget support in certain countries, acting together through joint missions, and agreeing to use similar monitoring and evaluation procedures. At the same time, some newer donor initiatives appear to want to use their own new methodologies, which could compound this problem going forward.

RESULTS-BASED MANAGEMENT The emphasis on demonstrating the effectiveness of aid has led to calls for improved monitoring and evaluation and results-based management. In this view, aid programs should aim to achieve very specific quantitative targets, and decisions about renewing or reallocating aid going forward should be based on those results. There are three basic objectives. First, results-based management can help donors allocate funds toward programs that are working. Second, ongoing reviews can detect problems at an early stage and help modify and strengthen existing programs. Third, donors and recipients can better learn what approaches have worked and what have not. Stronger monitoring and evaluation helps strengthen the principal-agent relationship so that aid agencies have clearer incentives and taxpayers have better information about the impact of aid on its intended beneficiaries. USAID, for example, introduced in 2011 a new evaluation approach aimed at strengthening the impact of the agency's program on achieving specified results. There has been an explosion in empirical investigations on the impact of development interventions through randomized controlled trials, led by

---

[39]World Bank Development News Media, "Cutting the Red Tape," February 21, 2003.

[40]Ravi Kanbur and Todd Sandler, "The Future of Development Assistance: Common Pools and International Public Goods," Policy Essay No. 5, Overseas Development Council, Washington, DC, 1999.

the path-breaking work of the Jameel Poverty Action Lab at MIT. These and other similar efforts are leading to a much deeper understanding of what works and what does not work in aid-supported programs around the world.

SUMMARY

- Most aid is given by bilateral donors, but a significant portion is channeled through multilateral agencies. Global aid flows peaked in 1991, then declined in real and nominal terms until 1997, before rebounding again. Official development assistance is higher today, almost $130 billion in 2010, than ever before but not as a share of the GNI of today's developed nations. The United States currently provides the largest dollar amount of aid but is among the smallest in terms of aid as a share of its income.

- For some countries, aid flows are large and significant, while in others they are small. Sub-Saharan Africa received aid flows equivalent to about 5 percent of its income in 2009, or about $53 per person. Because of the war in Iraq, the Middle East received $42 per person in 2009, an amount much higher than the $9 per person received by South Asia, which is a much poorer region.

- For most donors, the primary motivation for providing aid is to support foreign policy objectives and political alliances. Income and poverty tend to be secondary objectives. Country size, commercial and historical ties, and the extent of democracy also play a role.

- There are three broad viewpoints on the relationship among aid, growth, and development. First, some analysts believe that aid supports growth and development by adding to investment and the capital stock, helping in the transfer of technology, supporting key health and education programs, and enhancing economic stability. Second, others believe that aid has no impact on growth and might undermine growth by distorting incentives for private production, encouraging corruption, enlarging the government, or creating aid dependency. Third, some argue that aid works under certain conditions but not others, depending on the policy and institutional environment in the recipient country, the purpose of the aid, or the donor's practices and procedures. The empirical evidence on these relationships is mixed, with different studies reaching different conclusions.

- Aid can influence both saving rates and tax revenues through a host of subtle impacts on prices, preferences, and incentives. Aid flows add to total saving and investment but less than one for one. The fungibility of aid can cause private and government saving to decline as aid increases. The impact on government revenues varies across countries, with some experiencing a decline and others an increase corresponding to higher aid flows.

- Aid agencies face a classic principal-agent problem, compounded by the fact that the original funders (taxpayers in donor countries) have only indirect and distant connections to the intended ultimate beneficiaries (poor people in low-income countries). A particular challenge for donors is how to place appropriate conditions on their aid. Donors often are criticized for putting too many, too few, or the wrong kinds of conditions on aid, and conditionality in general appears to have been largely ineffective.

- In recent years, donors began to try to make aid more effective by becoming more selective in choosing recipients, encouraging more participation by recipients in program design and implementation, coordinating more closely with each other, and managing programs based on results. It is too early to judge the effectiveness of these changes, but they are likely to affect aid programs for some time to come.

15

Managing Short-Run Crises in an Open Economy

Economic development takes place in the long term. Most of the processes discussed in the previous chapters, whether improving human welfare, increasing saving, or shifting toward manufactured exports, take years and even decades to bear significant results. If policy makers in developing countries gaze only at the far horizon, however, they are unlikely ever to reach it. Much happens in the short term, within a few months or a couple of years, to throw an economy off balance and make pursuing long-term strategies difficult and sometimes impossible. Policy makers need to emulate a ship's captain, who, always steering toward the port of destination, nevertheless must deal decisively with any storms at sea.

Among the most dangerous and likely of these storms are changes in world prices that throw the balance of payments into deficit, excessive spending that fuels inflation or unsustainable debt, and droughts or other natural disasters that disrupt production. Unless a government counteracts these economic shocks, they create greater uncertainty and higher risk for private producers and investors, who take evasive actions that reduce future investment, worsen the crisis, and cause development efforts to flounder.

During the 1970s and 1980s, the late 1990s, and in Europe in 2010–11, as pointed out in Chapters 12 and 13, many economies became unbalanced because of unstable world market conditions and their own macroeconomic mismanagement. In Chapters 5 and 11 through 13, we discussed the consequences of such **macroeconomic instability**. Countries with overvalued exchange rates and rapid inflation were unable to grow rapidly. *Stabilization programs*, many funded by the International Monetary Fund (IMF), were intended to correct these macroeconomic imbalances.

In this chapter, we develop a mechanism for analyzing the macroeconomic policies that a developing country should pursue to stabilize its economy and create a climate for faster economic growth. The model developed here incorporates the two main policy approaches for correcting macroeconomic imbalances: changing the level of domestic expenditures and adjusting relative prices. In many cases, managing economic crises specifically requires expenditure reduction (by lower government budget deficits and slower creation of money) and exchange-rate devaluation.

EQUILIBRIUM IN A SMALL, OPEN ECONOMY

Developing economies[1] have two features central to understanding how macroeconomic imbalances occur and can be corrected. First, they are **open economies**, in that trade and capital flow across their borders in sufficient quantities to influence the domestic economy, particularly prices and the money supply. Most economies are open in this sense, especially because of economic reforms in China beginning in the late 1970s and in Eastern Europe and the states of the former Soviet Union beginning in the early 1990s. Today only a few economies, such as Cuba, North Korea, and Burma, are so heavily protected and regulated (and subject to foreign embargoes) that they might not qualify as open to trade and finance.

Second, these are **small economies**, meaning that neither their supply of exports nor their demand for imports has a noticeable impact on the world prices of these commodities and services. Economists call these countries *price takers* in world markets. A number of developing countries can exert some influence over the price of one or two primary exports in world markets: Brazil in coffee, Saudi Arabia in oil, Zambia in copper, South Africa in diamonds, for example. But they almost never affect the price of goods they import, and for macroeconomic purposes, it usually is adequate to model even these countries as price takers.[2]

These two qualities, smallness and openness, are the basis for the **Australian model** of a developing economy.[3] Countries typically trade both importable and

---

[1]In developing this and the next two sections, we acknowledge an intellectual debt to Shantayanan Devarajan and Dani Rodrik, who wrote an excellent set of notes for their class on macroeconomics for developing countries at Harvard's John F. Kennedy School of Government in the late 1980s and to Richard E. Caves, Jeffrey A. Frankel, and Ronald W. Jones, who develop the open economy model in Chapter 19 of *World Trade and Payments: An Introduction* (Glenview, IL: Scott, Foresman, Little, Brown, 1990).

[2]Among developing countries, China and India are large enough that they could become exceptions to the small country rule, given continued growth in China and both greater growth and openness in India.

[3]So called because it was developed by Australian economists, including W. E. G. Salter, "Internal Balance and External Balance: The Role of Price and Expenditure Effects," *Economic Record* 35 (1959), 226–38; Trevor W. Swan, "Economic Control in a Dependent Economy," *Economic Record* 36 (March 1960), 51–66; W. Max Corden, *Inflation, Exchange Rates and the World Economy* (Chicago: University of Chicago Press, 1977). Australia also is a small, open economy.

exportable goods and services. The Australian model lumps importables and exportables together as *tradables* and distinguishes these from all other goods and services, called *nontradables*. (We use this specification again in Chapter 18's discussion of Dutch disease.)

Tradable goods and services are those whose prices within the country are determined by supply and demand on world markets. Under the small economy assumption, these world market prices cannot be influenced by anything that happens within the country and so are *exogenous* to the model (determined outside the model). The domestic (local currency) price of a tradable good is given by $P_t = eP_t^*$ where e is the nominal exchange rate in local currency per dollar (pesos per dollar for Mexico or rupees per dollar for Pakistan) and P_t^* is the world price of the tradable in dollars. Even if the supply of and demand for tradables change within an economy, the local price will not change because domestic supply and demand have a negligible influence on the world price. Yet, changes in the nominal exchange rate change the domestic price of tradables commodities. If a country **devalues** its nominal exchange rate, it increases the amount of local currency required to purchase a dollar (e increases); if a country **revalues** its nominal exchange rate it decreases the amount of local currency required to purchase a dollar (e decreases). Devaluations thus increase the local currency price of tradables (all else equal), while revaluations tend to decrease the local currency price of tradables. Because this model simplifies all tradables into one composite good, the price of tradables P_t is best thought of as an index, a weighted average of the prices of all tradables, much like a consumer price index.

Tradables include exportables, such as coffee in Kenya and Colombia, rice in Thailand, beef in Argentina, cattle in West Africa, palm oil in Malaysia and Indonesia, copper in Peru and Zambia, oil in the Middle East, and textiles and electronics in East Asia, and importables, such as rice in West Africa, oil in Brazil or Korea, and intermediate chemicals and machinery in many developing countries.

Nontradables are goods and services, such as transportation, construction, retail trade, and household services that are not easily or conventionally bought or sold outside the country, usually because the costs of transporting them from one country to another are prohibitive or local custom inhibits trade. Prices of nontradables, designated P_n, therefore, are determined by market forces within the economy; any shift in supply or demand changes the price of nontradables. Nontradable prices thus are *endogenous* to the model (determined within the model). The term P_n, like P_t, is a composite or weighted average price incorporating all prices of nontradable goods and services.

INTERNAL AND EXTERNAL BALANCE

Figure 15–1 depicts equilibrium under the Australian model. The vertical axis represents nontradables (N); the horizontal axis takes both exportables and importables and treats them together as tradables (T). The production possibility frontier shows

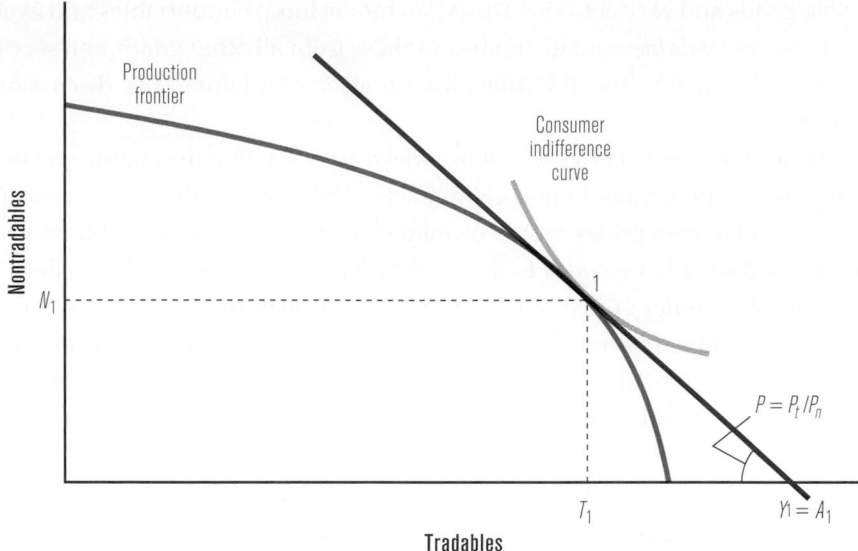

FIGURE 15-1   Equilibrium in the Australian Model

With equilibrium at point 1, the tangency of the production frontier and a community indifference curve, the country produces and consumes T_1 of tradables and N_1 of nontradables. The relative price, P, is a measure of the real exchange rate (see text).

Y_1, national income measured in tradable prices.

the menu of possible combinations of outputs of the two kinds of goods, N and T. The community indifference curves show consumer preferences between consumption of tradables and nontradables.

Equilibrium is at point 1, the tangency of a consumer indifference curve and the production possibilities frontier. At this point, the production of tradables, determined by the production frontier at point 1, is T_1, equal to the demand for tradables, determined by the indifference curve at 1, and similarly, for nontradables, supply equals demand at N_1. This is a defining characteristic of equilibrium in the Australian model: At point 1, the markets for both goods are in balance. Put another way, there is **external balance (EB)**, because the supply of tradables equals demand, and **internal balance (IB)**, because the supply of nontradables equals demand.

Point 1 simultaneously indicates the optimal (profit maximizing) combination of tradables and nontradables for producers, the optimal (utility maximizing) combination of tradable and nontradables for consumers. For both producers and consumers, this optimum occurs with respect to relative prices—in this case the relative price of tradables to nontradables. This relative price is indicated by the slope of the price line in Figure 15–1. This joint equilibrium for producers and consumers is indicated by the tangency of the indifference curve and the production possibility frontier. The tangency of the indifference curve and production frontier is jointly determined with the relative price of tradables in terms of nontradables, $P = P_t/P_n$. This relative price, P, is one way to define the **real exchange rate (RER)**, one of the important innovations of the Australian model.[4] (Box 15–1 provides a more detailed explanation of the real exchange rate.) This formulation separates out prices that are under the influence of monetary and fiscal policy and domestic market forces, P_n, from prices that can be changed only by adjustments of the nominal exchange rate, $P_t = eP_t^*$. Note that the slope of the price line that is tangent to the production possibility curve and the consumer indifference curve is the only real exchange rate consistent with equilibrium in the model.

If P rises (the price line becomes steeper in the diagram), tradables become more expensive relative to nontradables. Producers then attempt to switch along the production frontier away from N goods, toward T goods. Consumers attempt to switch in the opposite direction, up along the indifference curve to consume fewer T goods and more N goods. Therefore, a rise in P should increase the surplus of T-good production over consumption.

If the production of T goods exceeds consumption of T goods, there is an external surplus, which is identical to a surplus in the balance of trade. To see this, start with the definition of the trade balance as

$$B_t = X - M \qquad\qquad [15\text{--}1]$$

where X and M are exports and imports. Because exports are the surplus of supply over demand for exportable goods, while imports are the opposite, a surplus of demand over supply, we can write the balance of trade as

$B_t =$ value of X-goods supply $-$ value of X-goods demand $-$ (value of M-goods
        demand $-$ value of M-goods supply),
  $=$ value of X-goods supply $+$ value of M-goods supply $-$ (value of X-goods
        demand $+$ value of M-goods demand),
  $=$ value of tradables supply $-$ value of tradables demand;

or if we let the supply of tradables be S_t and demand be D_t,

$$B_t = P_t S_t - P_t D_t = P_t (S_t - D_t) \qquad\qquad [15\text{--}2]$$

In Figure 15–1, with the economy in equilibrium, consumption of tradables is equal to production, so the balance of trade is 0.

The value of income (GDP) also can be found in Figure 15–1. It is the sum of the value of output of N goods (N_1) and T goods (T_1). This value is given by Y_1, the

[4]Chapters 18 and 19 will define the real exchange rate index as RER $= R_o P_w / P_d$. The term R_o is an index of the nominal exchange rate; in this chapter we use e, the nominal exchange rate itself. The term P_w is an index of world prices, often the U.S. consumer or wholesale price index and is similar or identical to P^* as measured in practice. But P_d is a domestic consumer or wholesale price index that includes both tradable and nontradable prices, whereas P_n is an index of nontradable prices only. Thus, the Australian formulation of the real exchange rate is a more-precise definition than those given in the later chapters.

BOX 15-1 REAL VERSUS NOMINAL EXCHANGE RATES

Most anyone who has traveled outside their home country has experience with nominal exchange rates. The nominal exchange rate is simply the number of units of local currency you can buy from the country you visit with one unit of your own currency. For instance, in August 2010, you could buy just over 46 Indian rupees, or 12.6 Mexican pesos, for US$1. (Note, this implies that you could also have bought 3.65 Indian rupees with one Mexican peso.) But when you bring a dollar into India or Mexico what you really care about is not how many rupees or pesos you can buy with that dollar but rather the quantity of actual goods and services that you can buy with that dollar. This depends on the prices of goods and services in the host country in addition to the price of its currency. This distinction is the key idea underlying the concept of the real exchange rate (RER).

In the most general sense, RER is the relative price of foreign goods in terms of domestic goods. In practice, economists have developed a range of approaches to quantifying this idea. Economists working on developed economies typically measure the RER as the relative price of domestic and foreign goods. In contrast, economists working on developing countries typically measure the RER as the relative price of tradables and nontradables. Tradable commodities are goods that are *or could be* traded internationally, in contrast to nontradable goods (such as housing and many services), which are not traded internationally. A key practical distinction between these categories of goods is that there are world market prices for tradable goods, but the prices of nontradables are determined purely by local supply and demand conditions in each country.

The nominal and real exchange rates are linked together by the requirement that the relative prices of tradable and nontradable goods in the RER be expressed in the same currency units. The prices of tradables are typically expressed in U.S. dollars, whereas the prices of nontradables are expressed in units of the local currency. Thus we need to use the nominal exchange rate to convert the dollar-denominated price of tradables into units of the local currency to calculate the RER.

We can construct this RER as follows. Expressing the nominal exchange rate, e, in terms of the number of local currency units per dollar, and expressing the prices of tradables and nontradables as P_t and P_n, respectively, we can construct the RER as

$$\text{RER} = \frac{eP_t^*}{P_n} = \frac{P_t}{P_n}$$

In this equation, the asterisk on P_t in the second term indicates that the price of tradables is expressed in dollars. Multiplying this dollar-denominated price by e, the nominal exchange rate as defined above, converts the price of tradables into the same local currency units as the price of nontradables.

It is important to consider several issues related to this concept of the RER. First, note that the RER is based on price indices rather than actual nominal price levels. The RER is thus expressed relative to a base year, and changes in the relative price of tradables to nontradables, say from 1 to 1.2, would indicate percentage changes (in this case, 20 percent) relative to the base year. We refer to an increase in the RER as a *depreciation* of the local currency, and a decrease in the RER as an *appreciation* of the local currency. While this may sound counterintuitive, the rationale for these terms is that when a currency depreciates in real terms, a given quantity of foreign goods can be exchanged for a greater quantity of that country's domestic goods (and vice versa in the case of an appreciation). It is for this reason that the RER is often thought of an as an indicator of a country's international competitiveness: When a country's currency depreciates in real terms relative to its trading partners' currencies, that country's goods become less expensive to foreigners.

An important practical challenge in constructing an RER lies in the need to choose price indices for tradables and nontradables. P_t and P_n are indices of the prices of entire categories of goods. Thus constructing these price indices first requires deciding which goods (and services) belong in which category. Specific price data may also be lacking. One short cut for addressing these challenges may be to use the U.S. consumer price index in place of P_t and a similar indicator from the home country (with the same base year) in place of P_n.

Although the availability of such price indicators as the consumer price index makes them convenient, their use in constructing RERs is problematic. Theory calls for an index of nontradables prices, but the consumer price index (CPI) is typically constructed to reflect the price of a basket of consumption goods that includes both tradable and nontradable goods. The larger the share of tradable goods in that basket, the greater the divergence between what the RER tells us in theory and what we actually measure if we construct an RER using those broad price indices. In practice, aggregate price indices purely for nontradables rarely exist. Similar problems exist in choosing a price index to represent tradables prices (for use in the numerator of the RER for a given country). In this case, in which the goal is to choose a price index based to the greatest extent possible on tradables, many authors use the wholesale price index (WPI) from the United States or from a given country's trading partners. Yet this approach too is problematic because (as Lawrence Hinkle and Peter Montiel note[a]) for-

[a]Lawrence E. Hinkle and Peter Montiel, *Exchange rate misalignment: concepts and measurement for developing countries.* (Washington, DC: World Bank, 1999).

eign WPIs may not provide a very close indication of the tradables prices actually faced by consumers in the home country. There is no perfect match between the theoretical requirements and practical data availability in constructing empirical RERs. A common compromise is to use the foreign WPI to represent P_t and the domestic CPI to represent P_n.

An additional question is whether the relevant RER is purely between two specific countries (the home country and a single trading partner—that is, the bilateral RER) or between the home country and multiple trading partner countries. In general, policy makers in a given country will be more concerned with how their currency relates in real terms with all of their trading partners. In that case, it is necessary to take a (trade-weighted) average of all the bilateral RERs between the home country and its trading partners. This average is called the **real effective exchange rate (REER)**.

The central challenge for policy makers concerned with their country's international competitiveness is whether the level of the REER at any given time reflects its equilibrium value or whether it is overvalued or undervalued relative to that equilibrium. Equilibrium in this setting generally refers to the level of the REER at which a country's internal market (that is, its supply and demand for nontrable goods and labor) and its external market (that is, its supply and demand for tradable goods) are in balance.

intersection of price line P from point 1 to the T axis.[5] In national income accounting, we distinguish two concepts. Gross domestic *product*, a measure of the value of output, is given by

$$GDP = C + I + X - M \qquad [15\text{-}3]$$

where C and I are consumption and investment by both the government and the private sector. Gross domestic *expenditure*, often called **absorption**, is

$$A = C + I = GDP + M - X \qquad [15\text{-}4]$$

When, as in Figure 15-1, the economy is in equilibrium, $X = M$ and income equals absorption. Indeed, this is the other condition for equilibrium in the Australian model. From equation 15-4, we can also see that $A - GDP = M - X$, indicating

---

[5] Along the T axis, Y_1 is measured in prices of the T good, so $P_t Y_1 = P_t T_1 + P_n N_1$ or $Y_1 = T_1 + (P_n/P_t)N_1$. But $P_n/P_t = \Delta T/\Delta N$, with $\Delta N = N_1$ and $\Delta T = Y_1 - T_1$, the distance along the T axis from T_1 to Y_1. Thus the value of both goods in T prices is $T_1 + Y_1 - T_1 = Y_1$.

that any excess of expenditures over income implies a negative trade balance of equal amount. (The appendix to this chapter provides a more detailed review of balance of payments accounting.)

This exploration of the Australian model yields three results. First, macroeconomic equilibrium is defined as a balance between supply and demand in two markets: nontradable goods (internal balance) and tradable goods (external balance). Second, to achieve equilibrium in both markets, two conditions must be satisfied: Expenditure (absorption) must equal income, and the relative price of tradables (the real exchange rate) must be at a level that equates demand and supply in both markets (the slope of P in Figure 15–1). Third, this also suggests two remedies for an economy that is out of balance: A government can achieve equilibrium (stabilize the economy) by adjusting absorption, the nominal exchange rate, or both. Generally, both instruments must be used to achieve internal and external balance.

THE PHASE DIAGRAM

Using the perspective of trade theory, we tie the small, open economy model of macroeconomic management to the tools of analysis already used in this text. But the principles of stabilization can be explored from a more-useful perspective, the **phase diagram**. To develop this approach, consider the markets for tradables and nontradables from the perspective of conventional supply and demand diagrams, as in Figure 15–2.

In these diagrams, we use the real exchange rate, which is the relative price of T goods in terms of N goods (P_t/P_n), as the price in both markets. For tradable goods, that gives a conventional supply and demand diagram: As the price rises, supply increases and demand decreases. But in the nontradables market, a rise in P means a fall in the relative price of N goods, so supply decreases and demand increases. Note that, in both markets, any increase in expenditure, or absorption, A, causes an outward shift of the demand curve: At any price, consumers buy more of both goods.

To use these diagrams as a basis for macroeconomic analysis, we need to change the interpretation of the supply curve for tradables. Until now, we have assumed that all tradables are produced within the home country. But foreign investment and foreign aid can add to the supply of tradables by financing additional imports. Therefore, the supply curve should not be S_t, but $S_t + F$, where F is the inflow of long-term foreign capital in the form of aid, commercial loans, and investment.

Figure 15–2 constitutes a simple model of the small, open economy that is based on two variables: The real exchange rate, P, on the vertical axis and absorption, A, which determines the position of the demand curves. These, of course, are the conventional variables of microeconomics, price and income. But in this model, they also are the two main macroeconomic policy tools of government: The exchange rate and the level of expenditure. Because these two variables are central to macroeconomic management, it would be helpful to develop a diagram that uses them explicitly on the axes.

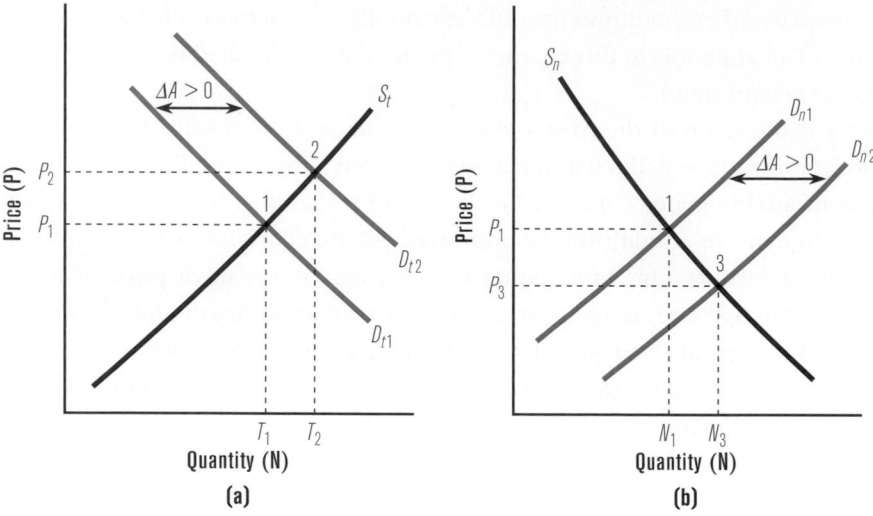

FIGURE 15-2 **Tradables and Nontradables Markets**

(a) Tradables market: The demand and supply curves for tradables S_t and D_t have the conventional slopes. (b) Nontradables market: The slopes are reversed. S_n falls as P rises (because the relative price of N is falling) and D_n rises as P rises. In both markets, demand increases when absorption (expenditure) increases, shown by and outward shift of D_t and D_n.

S, supply; D, demand; P (price) $= P_t/P_n$.

Figure 15–3 does this. It puts the real exchange rate, $P_t = eP_t^*/P_n$, on the vertical axis and real absorption, A, on the horizontal axis. The diagram also contains two curves, each representing equilibrium in one of the markets. Along the EB, or external balance, curve, the T-goods market is in balance ($S_t = D_t$). Along the IB, or internal balance, curve, the N-goods market is in balance ($S_n = D_n$).

The slopes of the two curves, EB and IB, can be derived from Figure 15–2. In the tradables market, when absorption is A_1, equilibrium is at P_1, where T_1 is produced and consumed. This equilibrium point 1 also is shown in Figure 15–3a. If absorption increases to A_2 in Figure 15–2a, the demand curve moves outward and shifts equilibrium to point 2. Note that with higher absorption, A_2, the real exchange rate, P_2, must be higher to restore equilibrium in the T-goods market. Increased absorption raises the demand for T goods. To meet this demand, it is necessary to raise output, which can be achieved only through a higher relative price of T goods, P_2. This higher price also helps regain balance by reducing the demand for T goods along the new demand curve. Point 2 is transferred to Figure 15–3a at (P_2, A_2).

In the nontradables market, when absorption is A_1, equilibrium is at P_1, where N_1 is produced and consumed. This equilibrium point 1 also is shown in Figure 15–3b. If absorption increases to A_3 in Figure 15–2b, the demand curve moves outward and shifts equilibrium to point 3. In the N-goods market, higher absorption, A_3,

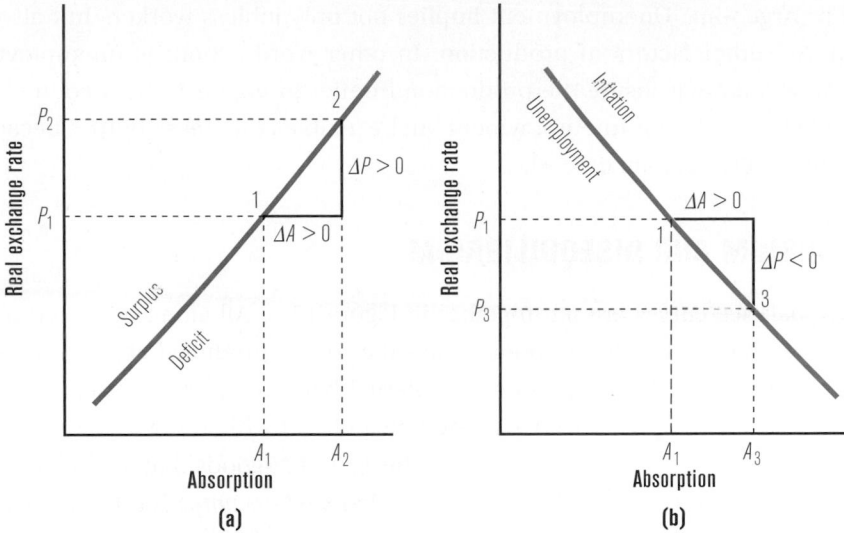

FIGURE 15-3 **The Phase Diagram**

(a) External balance (EB). (b) Internal balance (IB). The axes are the main policy variables: the real exchange rate, P, and the real absorption, A. The curves show equilibrium in the T-goods market (EB) and N-goods market (IB).

requires a lower, or appreciated, real exchange rate to restore equilibrium. Increased absorption raises demand for N goods, met by raising output, which can be achieved only through a lower relative price of T goods, P_3. This lower real exchange rate, or higher price of N goods, also helps regain balance by reducing the demand for N goods along the new demand curve. Point 3 is transferred to Figure 15–3b at (P_3, A_3).

Figure 15–3 also shows the **zones of imbalance**. In the T-goods market (panel a) for any given level of absorption, say, A_1, any real exchange rate greater than P_1 causes external surplus: The production of tradables exceeds the demand for tradables because the relative price, P, is at a more depreciated level than required for equilibrium. Any real exchange rate below (more appreciated than) P_1 causes an external deficit and the demand exceeds the supply of tradables. Therefore, the zone of surplus is northwest of EB and the zone of deficit is southeast.

In the N-goods market (Figure 15–3b), inflation is to the right of the IB curve, where the demand for N goods exceeds the supply. In that region, for any given real exchange rate, such as P_1, absorption is too high, say, A_3. To the left is the zone of unemployment, where there is an excess supply of N goods. In that region, for any given real exchange rate, say, P_3, absorption is too low, say, A_1.

The meanings of *inflation* and *unemployment* are precise in our model but not in the real world. It is best to think of inflation as being an increase in prices faster than is customary in the country in question. That rate would be quite low in Germany, Japan, or China, probably less than 5 percent a year, but quite high in

Brazil or Argentina. Unemployment implies not only jobless workers but also idle capital and other factors of production. In other words, there is unemployment when an economy is inside the production frontier in Figure 15–1. A country may have high levels of labor unemployment but be unable to increase output because it is fully utilizing its capital or land.

EQUILIBRIUM AND DISEQUILIBRIUM

The two balance curves are put together in Figure 15–4. All along the external balance curve, the demand for T goods equals the supply produced at home plus any net foreign capital inflow. All along the internal balance curve, the demand for N goods equals the supply of N goods. The only point at which there is both internal and external balance (equilibrium in both the T- and N-goods markets) is the intersection of the two curves. This is sometimes called the *bliss point*. It is the same as the tangency of the indifference curve to the production frontier in Figure 15–1 at point 1. The objective of macroeconomic policy is to adjust the exchange rate and absorption to keep an economy stable, in both external and internal balance.

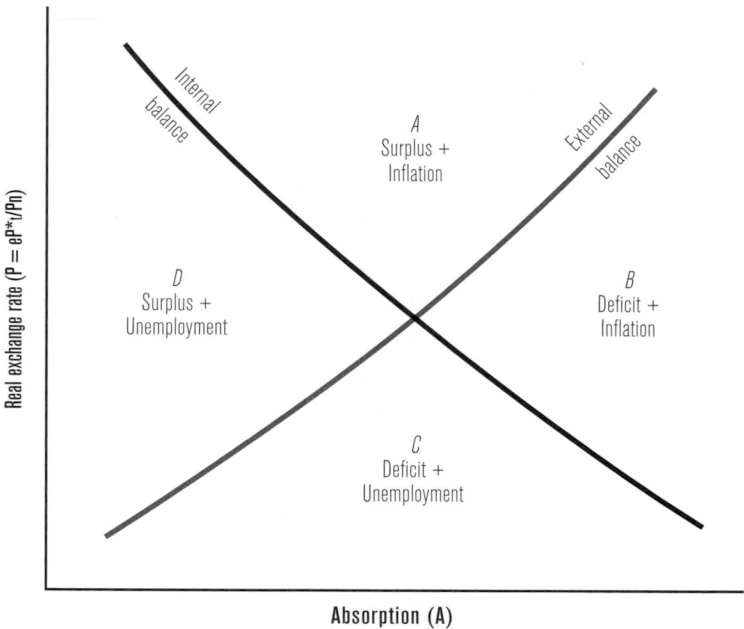

FIGURE 15-4 **Zones of Imbalance**

The economy is in equilibrium only at the intersection of the external balance (EB) and internal balance (IB) curves. Zones of imbalance are labeled. For example in zone A, the supply of T goods exceeds demand, so there is a surplus, and the demand for N goods exceeds supply, so there is inflation.

Economies spend considerable time in one of the four zones of imbalance shown in Figure 15–4. Zone *A* to the north is a region of external surplus and inflation, where the exchange rate is *undervalued*. In zone *B* to the east of equilibrium, the economy faces inflation and a foreign deficit, due principally to excessive expenditure (absorption is greater than income). To the south is zone *C*, where the exchange rate is *overvalued* (too appreciated) and there is both unemployment and an external deficit. And west of the bliss point the economy is in zone *D*, where, because of insufficient absorption, there is unemployment of all resources but a foreign surplus.

Once in disequilibrium, economies have built-in tendencies to escape back into balance. Figure 15–5 describes them separately for external balance (panel a) and internal balance (panel b). Start with an external surplus, point 1 (Figure 15–5a). The excess supply of tradables generates two self-correcting tendencies. First, the net inflow of foreign exchange adds to international reserves. If the central bank takes no countermeasures, the money supply increases and interest rates fall and induce both consumers and investors to spend more. The increase in absorption moves the economy rightward, back toward external balance. Second, the inflow of foreign exchange creates more demand for the local currency and, if the exchange rate is free to float, forces an appreciation. This is a move downward in the diagram, also toward the EB line. The net result of these two tendencies is the resultant, shown as a solid line in the diagram, heading toward external balance. If, instead, the economy starts in

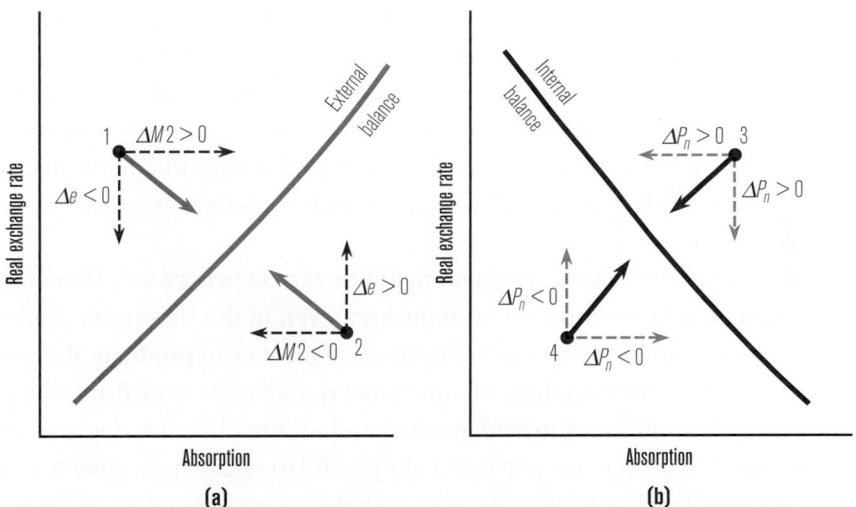

FIGURE 15–5 Tendencies toward Equilibrium

(a) External balance (EB). If the economy faces an external surplus (point 1), reserves and the money supply tend to rise while the exchange rate tends to appreciate; this drives the economy toward EB. (b) Internal balance (IB). For a deficit, if the economy faces inflation (point 3), the rise in prices leads to real appreciation of the exchange rate and a reduction in the real value of absorption; this moves conditions toward IB. Conversely for unemployment at point 4, but only if prices can fall flexibly.

external deficit at point 2, the tendencies are the opposite but the result is the same, a tendency to regain external balance.

The tendency to regain internal balance is shown in Figure 15–5b. When there is inflation (point 3), it affects both the real exchange rate and real absorption. If the nominal exchange rate remains fixed (or is not allowed to depreciate as fast as inflation), the rise in P_n causes a real appreciation. At the same time, the rise in prices can cause a fall in the real value of absorption, assuming that the central bank does not take steps to increase the money supply to compensate for inflation. Under these assumptions, the economy would move from inflation at point 3 back toward internal balance. Unemployment (point 4) would be self-correcting also if prices are able to fall as easily as they rise, but this seldom is the case.

Despite these self-correcting tendencies, in practice, they often fail to work smoothly or quickly enough because of *structural rigidities* in the economy. For instance, exchange-rate changes may take time to affect actual imports and exports, perhaps as long as two years to have a full impact. In economies like Ghana and Zambia, dominated by one or two export products such as cocoa, oil, and copper, with long gestation periods for new investment, supply elasticities for tradables may be especially low, and foreign deficits can persist for a time despite real devaluations.

Nontradables prices probably rise very quickly when demand exceeds supply, as in Figure 15–5b. But in many developing economies, inflation, once started, may resist corrective policies, and prices do not fall so easily when there is unemployment: Unions strike wage bargains that try to maintain real wages by continually raising nominal wages; banks use their market power to keep interest rates high; producers depend on imports, the prices of which are responsive only to exchange rate adjustments; and large firms with monopoly or oligopoly power keep prices up to cover costs that resist downward pressures. Such rigidities have frequently been cited to explain chronic trade deficits and inflation in Latin America, especially in Argentina and Brazil.

However, arguments about structural rigidities can be overstated. There is some flexibility in production for most export industries, even in the short term. And many producer prices are quite flexible, including those of most farm products, those in the large informal sector, and even those of some modern manufacturing firms. Nevertheless, the automatic tendencies toward external and internal balance depicted in Figure 15–5 are likely to be too slow and politically painful to satisfy most governments.

Not all the barriers to adjustment are structural. Sometimes, policies work against adjustment. When foreign reserves fall, for example, the money supply also falls automatically unless the central bank's policy is to *sterilize* these shifts by expanding domestic credit to compensate for the fall in reserves and keep the money supply from falling. Sterilization prevents the move from points 1 or 2 of Figure 15–5a toward external balance. And nominal exchange rates respond to changing market conditions only if the exchange rate is allowed to float or the government makes frequent adjustments in the nominal exchange rate to match changing economic conditions.

However, the opposite policy, a fixed nominal exchange rate, is needed if inflation in nontradables prices is to cause a real exchange-rate appreciation, as depicted at point 3 of Figure 15–5b. This fixed nominal rate is called an exchange rate *anchor* because the fixed rate alone can halt the upward drift of prices as the economy moves due south from point 3. Chile used such an anchor to slow inflation during the late 1970s (Box 15-2). If government devalues the rate to keep up with inflation,

BOX 15-2 PIONEERING STABILIZATION: CHILE, 1973-84

In the last year of the Salvadore Allende regime in Chile, when the public sector deficit soared to 30 percent of the gross domestic product (GDP) and was financed mostly by printing money, inflation exceeded 500 percent a year. In 1973, General Augusto Pinochet overthrew Allende and established an autocratic regime. An early goal of his government was to stabilize the economy. It proved to be a difficult task of many years, with important lessons for later stabilizations in Latin America.

Faced by rapid inflation and unsustainable external deficits, the government imposed a fiscal and monetary shock on the economy. The budget deficit was cut to 10.6 percent of GDP in 1974 and again to 2.7 percent in 1975. Monetary policy was tight: From the second quarter of 1975 through the middle of 1976, it has since been estimated, households and firms were willing to hold more money than was in circulation. But inflation persisted; consumer prices nearly doubled in 1977.

Despite draconian measures, prices continued to rise for two reasons. First, the peso was aggressively devalued to improve the foreign balance, the more so because of the 40 percent fall in copper prices in 1975. In 1977, the peso was worth about one-80th its 1973 value against the dollar. Second, wages in the formal sector were determined by rules that permitted adjustments based on the previous year's rate of inflation, a rule that helped perpetuate the higher rates of earlier years. It also was argued by some that the monetary policy was not stringent enough.

In 1978, the government switched gears and began using the exchange rate as its main anti-inflation weapon. At first a crawling peg was adopted with preannounced rates, the *tablita*, that did not fully adjust to domestic inflation. In 1979, the rate was fixed at 39 pesos to the dollar for three years. The appreciating real exchange rate, or *anchor*, helped control inflation, which was down to 10 percent by 1982. But it also discouraged export growth and contributed to a growing current-account deficit. At the same time, Chile liberalized its controls over foreign capital flows and attracted large inflows of loans: Net long-term capital rose from negligible amounts before 1978 to average over $2 billion a year in the following five years, equivalent to 8 percent of GDP in 1980. This inflow not only financed the growing current deficit but contributed to the real appreciation of the exchange rate.

Not until after 1984 did Chile finally achieve a semblance of both internal and external balance. It did so through a large real devaluation, approaching 50 percent, supported by tighter fiscal and monetary policies. After a decade and a half of falling income per capita, Chilean incomes grew by 5.8 percent a year from 1985 to 1991.

Source: Based on the account by Vittorio Corbo and Andrés Solimano, "Chile's Experience with Stabilization Revisited," in Michael Bruno et al., eds., *Lessons of Economic Stabilization and Its Aftermath* (Cambridge, MA: MIT Press, 1991).

Brazil's practice for many years, then real appreciation is thwarted and there is no anchor. Similarly, real absorption falls with inflation only if the government fixes its expenditure and its deficit in nominal terms and allows inflation to erode the real value of the expenditure and if the central bank restrains the money supply to grow more slowly than inflation. More typically, the fiscal authorities adjust the expenditure, while the monetary authorities adjust both the money supply and the nominal exchange rate, to fully compensate for inflation. In that case, rising prices have no impact on the real exchange rate or real absorption and an inflationary economy remains at point 3 in Figure 15–5b.

STABILIZATION POLICIES

Whether the barriers to rapid automatic adjustment are inherent in the economic structure or created by policy contradictions, in most cases, governments need to take an active role to stabilize their economies. They have three basic instruments for doing so: exchange-rate management, fiscal policy, and monetary policy.

Alternative **exchange-rate regimes** were introduced in Chapter 12. Governments can vary the exchange rate by having the central bank offer to buy and sell foreign currency at a predetermined or *fixed* official exchange rate (*e* in our nomenclature) that nevertheless can be changed from time to time or by allowing the rate to *float* in the currency market, although the central bank sometimes may intervene to influence the price. An intermediate case is the *crawling peg*, under which the central bank determines the rate but changes it frequently, as often as daily, to ensure that the official rate stays in line with domestic and world inflation; this results in a constant or slowly adjusting real exchange rate (P).

Governments have two policies that can influence the level of absorption. Fiscal policy, adjusting levels of government expenditure and taxation, directly affects the government's components of consumption and investment. It also influences private expenditure, especially consumption, which depends on *disposable income*, or income net of taxes. Monetary policy also affects private expenditure. If the central bank acts to increase the money supply, as described in Chapter 12, it increases the liquidity of households and firms, lowers interest rates, and stimulates private consumption and investment.

The power of the phase diagram is that it indicates the necessary directions for these policies, depending on the state of the economy. Figure 15–6 provides such a policy map. It shows the same external and internal balance lines as in the previous diagrams but adds a new element: four policy quadrants, I to IV, within which the policy prescription always is the same.

Take, for example, point 1, which has been placed on the external balance line but in the inflationary zone. For many years, Brazil was in this situation, with buoyant exports and balance in foreign payments but chronic inflation running from 40 to well over 100 percent a year. Because the demand for nontradables exceeds supply, we know that one necessary correction is a reduction in real absorption, monetary and fiscal *austerity*, that would reduce demand and move the economy due west from point 1. But, if that is the only policy taken, the economy would not reach internal balance until point 4, in the zone of external surplus. One imbalance is exchanged for another. To avoid generating a surplus, reduced absorption needs to be accompanied by an appreciation of the exchange rate, a move due south from point 1. The result would be a move approximately toward the equilibrium or bliss point, 0.

Note three things about this result. First, this combination of policies, austerity and appreciation, would work from any point within quadrant I to return the economy to equilibrium. That is, the same combination is needed whether the economy had inflation with a moderate external surplus or inflation with a moderate deficit, either just above or just below the EB line. If the economy starts just below external balance, with a moderate deficit, it may seem strange (*counterintuitive*) to recommend an appreciation that, on its own, would worsen the deficit. But the reduction in absorption, needed to reduce inflation, also reduces the deficit because it also lowers the demand for tradables. Indeed, it reduces the demand for tradables too much and throws the economy into surplus; this is the reason an appreciation is needed. Of course, the relative intensity of each policy is different, depending where in quadrant I the economy starts. But the basic principle holds: Anywhere in quadrant I, the right combination of policies is austerity and appreciation, the combination that moves the economy toward point 0.

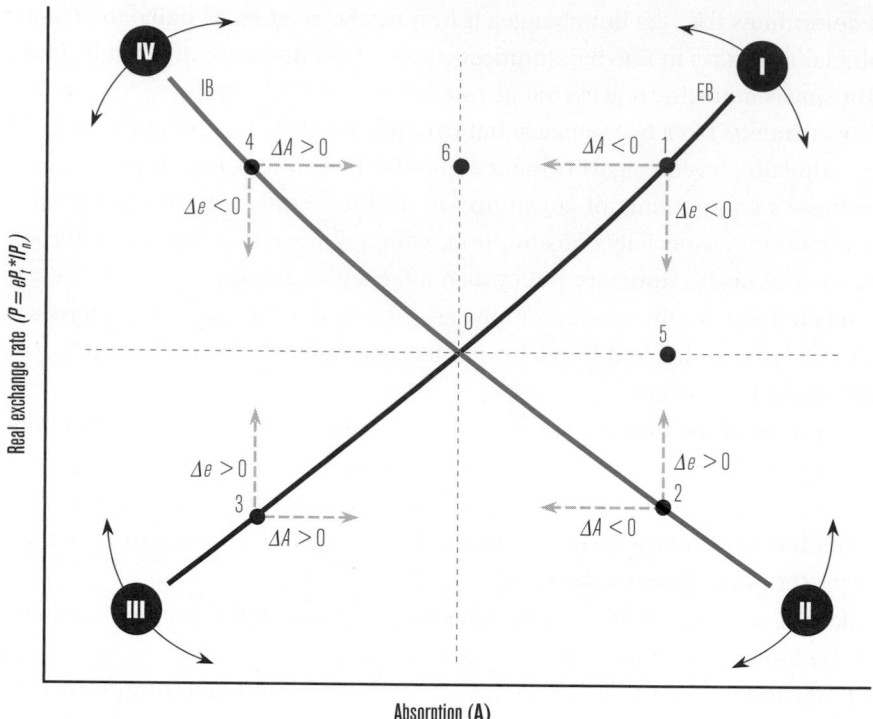

FIGURE 15-6 **Policy Zones**

From any position of disequilibrium, two policy adjustments generally are needed to restore internal and external balance. In each quadrant (I–IV) a particular combination of exchange rate and absorption policy is prescribed.

Second, in general, two policy adjustments are required to move toward equilibrium. This is a simple example of the general rule enunciated by Dutch economist Jan Tinbergen: To achieve a given number of policy goals, it generally is necessary to employ the same number of policy instruments. Here we have two goals, internal and external balance, and need adjustments in both absorption (austerity) and the real exchange rate (appreciation) to reach them both. It is not always necessary to use two goals, however. If the economy lies just to the east of equilibrium at point 5, then a reduction in absorption achieves internal and external balance simultaneously. And, if the initial situation is point 6, due north of 0, then appreciation alone does the job.

Third, we could view the policy prescription in either of two ways. Austerity is needed to reduce inflation (move west) and appreciation is used to avoid surplus (move south). Or appreciation can be targeted on internal balance (move south toward point 2) but alone would cause a deficit, so that austerity then is required to restore external balance. Therefore, no logic in macroeconomics suggests that one particular policy should be assigned to one particular goal. Economic institutions often do this anyway. In practice, the central bank might use the exchange rate to achieve external balance while the finance ministry uses the budget for internal balance. But if these two approaches are not coordinated, they may well fail to reach equilibrium.

With these principles established for quadrant I, it is fairly routine to go around the map in Figure 15–6 and see what policy responses are required:

- In quadrant II at a point like 2, with an external deficit but internal balance, exchange-rate devaluation is needed to restore foreign balance but, taken alone, would push the economy into inflation. Fiscal and monetary austerity also are needed to avoid inflation and reach equilibrium. We could reverse this assignment of policies and use austerity to achieve external balance and devaluation to stimulate the economy. Many African countries have been in this situation right up to the present, with low inflation but an insufficiency of export earnings and foreign investment to pay for the imports required for economic development.
- In quadrant III at point 3, an expansionary fiscal or monetary policy eliminates unemployment but at the cost of a foreign deficit, so devaluation is needed to reach equilibrium. Or devaluation stimulates employment and so requires expansion to eliminate the resulting surplus. This is the situation of a mature industrialized economy during a recession, with unemployed labor and capital, but it is not so common in developing countries.
- In quadrant IV at point 4, exchange-rate appreciation can eliminate the external surplus while fiscal expansion prevents unemployment. Or fiscal expansion can end the surplus while appreciation prevents a resulting inflation. A few countries in Asia, such as Taiwan and Malaysia in the 1980s, have been in this situation.

So the principles of macroeconomic stabilization are simple: If policy makers know where to place their economy on this map, they know how to move toward equilibrium. But how do policy makers know where they are? The answer lies partly in measurement, partly in art. Regularly available data on the balance of payments, changes in reserves, and inflation can help locate an economy with respect to the external and internal balance lines. Data on the nominal and real exchange rates, the budget deficit, and the money supply can indicate movements from one policy quadrant to another. Some kinds of data, such as private sector short-term borrowing abroad, however, may not be readily available to policy makers. Such was the case in Korea at the beginning of that country's financial crisis in 1997. In principle, barring such surprises as an unknown large short-term foreign debt that has to be repaid immediately, econometric models can locate the economy and indicate the policies needed to balance it. In practice, especially but not only for developing economies, such models can be too imprecise and too unstable to be wholly dependable. The art of stabilization policy comes in knowing just how hard to push on each component of policy and how long to keep pushing. In this, experience in managing a particular economy is as important a guide as the models estimated by economists.

APPLICATIONS OF THE AUSTRALIAN MODEL

Throughout this book we refer to different kinds of economic problems that are associated with developing countries, including the Dutch disease, debt crises, terms-of-trade shocks, foreign-exchange shortages, destructive inflation, and droughts or other natural catastrophes. The Australian model and its phase diagram can be used to show how these and other shocks affect macroeconomic balance and how they should be handled.

DUTCH DISEASE

In Chapter 18 we will discuss the strange phenomenon of the Dutch disease, in which a country that receives higher export prices or a larger inflow of foreign capital may end up worse off than without the windfall. The Dutch disease was first analyzed by Australian economists Max Corden and Peter Neary, using a version of the open-economy model.[6] Figure 15–7 traces the impact of a windfall gain using the phase diagram. (Box 18–1 provides an alternative exposition of Dutch disease.)

An economy in equilibrium at point 1 suddenly begins to receive higher prices for its major export or is favored by foreign aid donors or foreign investors. All the oil producers, from Saudi Arabia to Indonesia to Mexico, were in this position in the 1970s, as were coffee (and many other commodities) exporters during the boom of the mid-1970s. Egypt and Israel were rewarded with large aid programs by the United States after the Camp David accord of 1978, as was Ghana by the World Bank and others during its stabilization of the 1980s (Box 15–3). Both Chile in the late 1970s and Mexico after its stabilization in the late 1980s received large inflows of private capital, much of it a return of previous flight capital. Foreign exchange windfalls are more frequent than sometimes is supposed. In some cases, these windfalls result from new discoveries of natural resources, such as the major offshore oil reserves discovered by Ghana in 2007.

When the windfall occurs, the supply of tradable goods rises at any given price. This can be shown as a rightward shift in the supply curve in Figure 15–2a. In the phase diagram of Figure 15–7, there is a rightward shift in the EB curve. At point 1, for example, which had been in external equilibrium along EB_1, the economy now is in surplus, so the new EB curve must be to the right—for example, at EB_2. The economy cannot remain at point 1 because the inflow of reserves increases the money supply; this adds to demand and, because the windfall increases private income and government revenue, leads to greater expenditure. So absorption rises, a move

---

[6]W. Max Corden and J. Peter Neary, "Booming Sector and Deindustrialisation in a Small Open Economy," *Economic Journal* 92 (1982), 825–48.

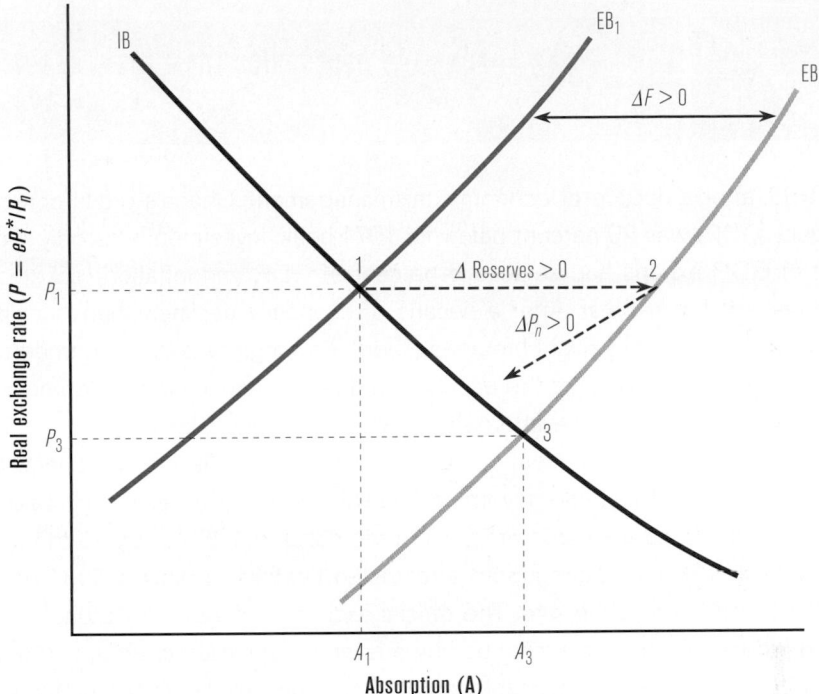

FIGURE 15-7 The Dutch Disease

An export boom or capital inflow shifts the EB curve rightward and leaves the economy at point 1 in surplus. As reserves accumulate and the money supply rises (or as the government and consumers spend the windfall), absorption rises and the economy moves eastward, into inflation. As nontradable prices rise, the real exchange appreciates. At the new equilibrium (point 3), because P is lower, the supply and demand is balanced with less production of T goods and more output of N goods than before. The loss of tradable output is what makes this a disease.

from point 1 toward point 2. This moves the economy off its internal balance, into inflation.[7]

The resulting rise in P_n has two effects: a reduction in real absorption that partially corrects the initial rise in A and, assuming the official rate is fixed, a real appreciation of the exchange rate. (The real rate also appreciates if the nominal rate is floating because the greater supply of foreign currency drives down the price of foreign currency.) Therefore, the economy first moves from point 1 toward point 2 in Figure 15-7, then begins to head in the general direction of the new equilibrium, point 3. In this case, market forces are likely to be sufficient to reach the new equilibrium, unless the

---

[7]If the windfall is an inflow of capital, this treatment is precise. In the case of a rise in export prices, however, the move from point 1 to point 2 is an approximation. Strictly speaking, a rise in export prices should raise P_t^*, a depreciation of the real exchange rate that moves the economy upward from point 1, after which the economy moves east toward EB_2.

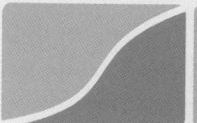

**BOX 15-3 RECOVERING FROM MISMANAGEMENT:
GHANA, 1983–91**

In 1983, after a decade of economic mismanagement, Ghana's gross domestic product (GDP) was 20 percent below its 1974 peak, investment was only 4 percent of GDP, exports had sunk to 6 percent of GDP, and inflation rocketed to 120 percent for the year. After a decade of economic decline, Ghana's military government, headed by Flight Lieutenant Jerry Rawlings, was ready to undertake drastic measures to stabilize the economy and restart economic development.

Working closely with the International Monetary Fund (IMF), Ghana focused on three deep-seated problems: exchange-rate reform, fiscal adjustment, and monetary policy. At first, the government maintained its fixed exchange rate but drastically devalued the cedi from 2.75 to the dollar in 1983 to 90 to the dollar by 1986. In 1986, Ghana adopted a restricted floating currency, using periodic auctions to determine the rate. The official exchange market was broadened in 1988, when many foreign exchange bureaus were authorized to trade currencies and virtually absorbed the parallel market in currency; by 1990, the banks were empowered to trade in an interbank currency market. This completed the move to a floating rate regime. By the end of 1992, the cedi traded at 520 per dollar.

In 1983, with fiscal revenues less than 6 percent of GDP, the urgent need was to restore revenues and control expenditures. The deficit was cut from 6.2 to 2.7 percent of GDP in the first year of austerity, and by 1985, the government had begun a major public investment program to stimulate growth. By 1988, the government had restored total expenditures to 15 percent of GDP, 20 percent of which was investment, and was running a surplus of nearly 4 percent of GDP.

Throughout the period, the money supply was constrained but inflation remained stubbornly above 20 percent a year until 1991, when it was reduced to 16 percent and real interest rates finally became positive. Because food prices play a large role in the consumer price index, investment in food production was seen as an important component of any long-run attack on inflation.

The aid donors responded handsomely to Ghana's stabilization and the accompanying economic reforms: The sum of net official transfers and net long-term capital rose from just over $100 million in 1983 to $585 million in 1991.

Stabilization helped restore economic growth. From the depression of 1983–91, GDP grew by 5.1 percent a year and investment rose to 17 percent of GDP. The improvement, although dramatic in relation to the early 1980s, still left Ghana with a lot to be done: In 1991, income per capita remained 25 percent below its 1973 level.

Source: This account is based on Ishan Kapur et al., *Ghana: Adjustment and Growth, 1983–91* (Washington, DC: International Monetary Fund, 1991).

authorities prevent appreciation and maintain real absorption and so keep the economy in an inflationary posture like point 2.

What, then, is the problem? The economy is at a new equilibrium, its terms of trade improved, its currency appreciated and so citizens have more command over foreign resources, people spending and consuming more without having to work any harder. There are two flaws in this otherwise idyllic picture. First, such windfalls generally are temporary. When export prices fall or the capital inflow dries up, the EB curve shifts back and a costly adjustment is necessary. We analyze that process in the next section.

The second problem is that, in shifting from the old to the new equilibrium, adjustments in the economy must be made. The real exchange rate P is lower, so S_t has fallen, while S_n has risen. Because the booming export sector does not retrench, nonboom tradables bear the brunt of the adjustment. Frictions in the labor market are likely to mean at least temporary unemployment as workers switch from tradable to nontradable production. If the tradable sector includes modern manufacturing, then long-term development may be set back because manufacturing is the sector likely to yield the most rapid productivity growth in the future. And if tradable industries close, it is more difficult to make the inevitable adjustment back toward point 1 when the windfall is over. This decline in nonboom-tradable production turns a foreign exchange windfall into a "disease."

What can be done to cure the disease? The government could try to move the economy back toward the old (and probably future) equilibrium at point 1. Its tools are the official exchange rate, which would have to be devalued against the tendencies of market forces, and expenditure, which would have to be reduced through restrictive fiscal and monetary policies that also reduce inflation (lower P_n or at least its growth). The resulting buildup of reserves and bank balances have to be sterilized through monetary policy so they are held as assets and not spent. It is a neat political trick to manage an austere macroeconomic policy in the face of a boom because all the popular pressures are for more spending. Not too many countries have managed it. Indonesia is among the few that have.

DEBT REPAYMENT CRISIS

When Mexico announced in 1982 that it no longer could service the debt it acquired during the oil boom of the 1970s, many other developing countries followed Mexico's lead, and the financial world entered a decade of debt crisis (Chapter 13). Most Latin American countries largely have overcome their debt problems, but many African countries continue to struggle to repay the money they borrowed, mostly from aid agencies. Although debt service insolvency encroaches gradually on an economy and can be foreseen, it often appears as a national crisis because economic management has been inept.

The formal analysis of a debt crisis is similar to that of another common phenomenon, a **decline in the terms of trade** that leads to a foreign exchange shortage, which in turn is simply the reverse of the Dutch disease. Therefore, the oil exporters, such as Indonesia, Nigeria, and Venezuela, faced a similar kind of crisis once oil prices began falling in the 1980s. We can understand the similarity between a debt crisis and a decline in the terms of trade more clearly by seeing them in their common context in the balance of payments. A decline in the terms of trade implies deterioration in the balance of trade (in which the excess of imports over exports increases). All else equal, a declining trade balance adds directly to the current account deficit. As detailed in the appendix to this chapter, one of the few ways in which countries can finance current account deficits is by borrowing abroad.[8] Indeed, many developing countries financed chronic current account deficits by borrowing abroad, in the process accumulating enormous stocks of debt (often to levels greater than their GDP). Debt crises ensue (as discussed in Chapter 13) when current account deficits become unsustainable and lenders want to be repaid.

Figure 15–8 captures this process. An economy in balance at point 1 needs to find additional resources to repay its foreign debt or needs to adjust to falling terms of trade. The supply of tradables therefore shifts to the left in Figure 15–2a; in the phase diagram, the EB curve also shifts leftward to EB_2.[9] If the crisis leads to debt relief or additional foreign aid, the curve moves less far and might settle at EB_3.

Now in foreign deficit, the economy begins losing reserves. If the government has to repay some of the debt or falling export prices cut into its revenues, the government needs to reduce its expenditures as well. Both cause a reduction in absorption. These actions move the economy toward external balance but also into unemployment. To gain the new equilibrium at point 3, it is also necessary to devalue the currency. This could be done by the central bank under a fixed rate or by the foreign exchange market under a floating rate. At the new equilibrium, the country produces more and consumes fewer tradables because P has risen. This, of course, is a loss of welfare for the populace. The surplus of S_t over D_t is used to repay the debt or simply compensates for reduced export prices.

Debt crises and the hardships they cause are not an inevitable consequence of borrowing to finance development, as was discussed in Chapter 13. If the borrowed resources are invested productively, they increase the potential output of both tradables and nontradables. Added production increases income and generates the capacity to repay the debt out of additional income, without a crisis and an austerity program. Countries such as Korea and Indonesia have been large international borrowers, but before the financial crisis of 1997–99, they escaped debt crises.

---

[8]The only other ways (beyond foreign borrowing) to finance a current account deficit are to attract foreign investment and/or to run down the central bank's stock of foreign reserves. See the appendix to this chapter for a concise summary of balance of payments accounting.

[9]Strictly speaking, we cannot analyze the fall in export prices this way, but it is a reasonable approximation for many situations. See note 7.

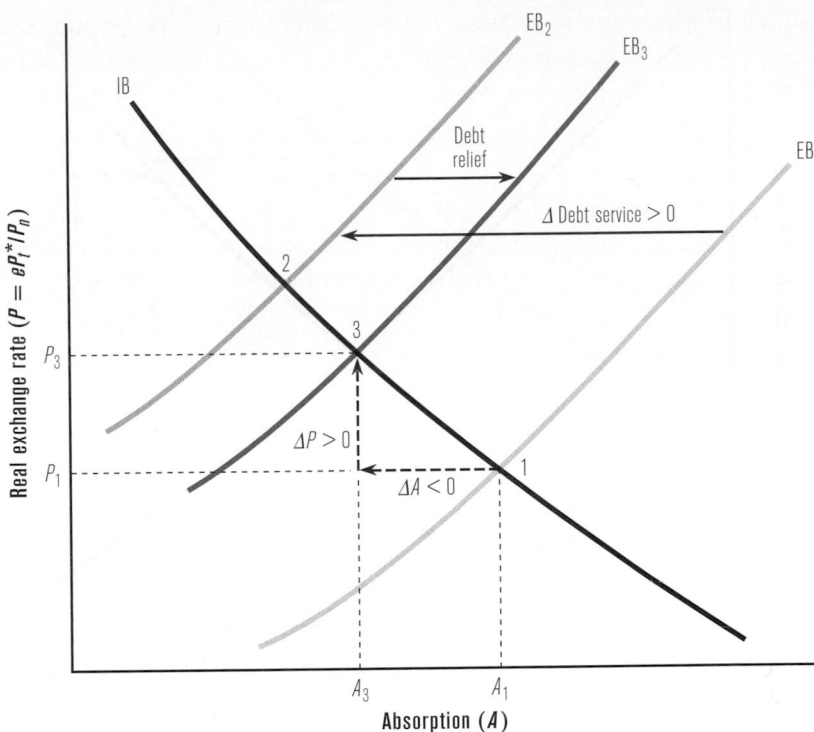

FIGURE 15-8 Debt Crisis or Declining Terms of Trade

An economy in equilibrium at point 1 suddenly needs to repay its debt (or faces falling export prices). External balance shifts from EB_1 to EB_2, although debt relief or increased foreign assistance might reshift the balance line back to EB_3. If policies accommodate the fall in reserves and income, absorption declines. A devaluing exchange rate, via central bank action or market forces, helps the economy move to its new equilibrium at point 3. With more tradables produced and less consumed, the surpluses can be used to repay the debt.

STABILIZATION PACKAGE: INFLATION AND A DEFICIT

External shock is not the only way an economy gets into trouble. Reckless or misguided government policies often are to blame. Impatient with sluggish development or intent on benefiting its constituencies, a government expands its spending and incurs a budget deficit. Unable to finance the deficit by borrowing from the public, the ministry of finance sells short-term bills to the central bank; this adds to the money supply. The economy drifts into inflation and a foreign deficit, at a point like point 1 in Figure 15-9, far from equilibrium at point 2 on the economy's original external balance curve EB_1. When economies become unstable in this way, private investors get skittish and try to invest in nonproductive assets like land or, more often, invest abroad; this deepens the external deficit. The government, recognizing the error of its ways or just hoping for some outside help to avoid painful adjustment, calls in the IMF.

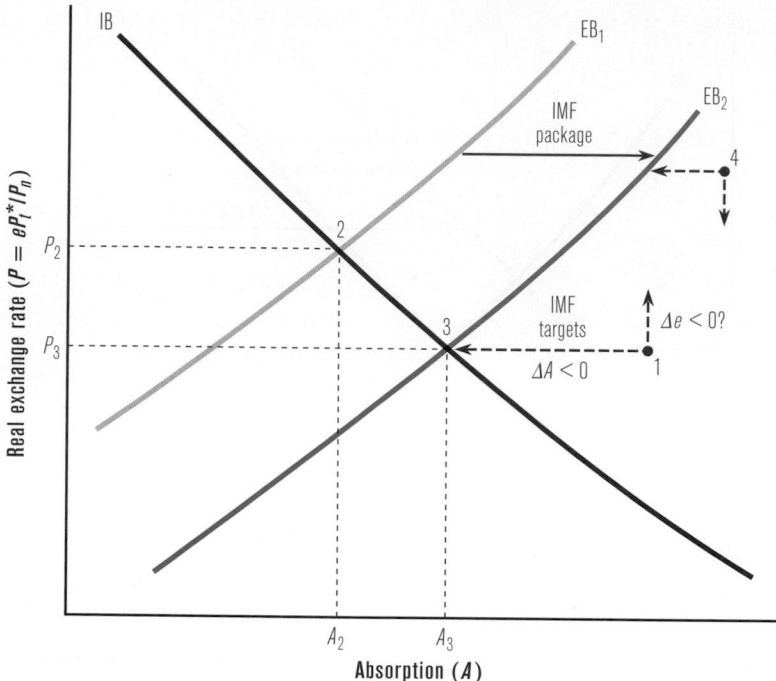

FIGURE 15-9 **Stabilization from Inflation and a Deficit**

An economy at point 1, far from equilibrium at point 2, above all needs to reduce absorption through austerity: reduced budgetary deficits and slower growth of the money supply. An International Money Fund (IMF) and donor package of aid might bring equilibrium closer by shifting the external balance to EB_2, but the aid package is conditional on the austerity program. Whether any exchange rate action is required depends on the precise initial position, point 1.

The core IMF stabilization program consists of a reduction in the government's budget deficit and programmed targets for domestic credit that, in effect, cap the growth of the money supply. Together, these measures reduce absorption in the economy and move it westward from point 1, closer to external and internal balance. IMF packages frequently include an exchange-rate devaluation as well. Whether this is needed or not depends on the precise location of the economy (point 1) relative to equilibrium (point 2). In some cases, the reduction in absorption is sufficient to reach both internal and external balance. As pictured in Figure 15–9, a small devaluation is needed to reach point 2 and avoid unemployment.

However, IMF programs usually come with substantial aid attached, not only from the fund, but from the World Bank and bilateral donors. The aid package, by adding to the economy's capacity to buy tradables, shifts the EB curve to the right, to EB_2 in the diagram, and moves equilibrium to point 3. Note two things about this aid package. First, it reduces the need for austerity to some extent, as A_3 is greater than A_2. Second, it reduces the need for devaluation of the exchange rate. Indeed, as shown, there is little or no need to devalue to move from 1 to 3. Donors and the IMF nevertheless frequently insist on devaluation. Sometimes, that may be a requirement just to reach a point like 3. In other cases, donors and the IMF may have in mind a self-sustaining stabilization that will be valid even after aid is reduced and the external balance curve moves back toward EB_1. Whatever the motive, it is important to realize that aid itself is a partial substitute for both devaluation and austerity. In essence, the aid does what higher production of tradables otherwise must do and it finances expenditures that otherwise must be cut. Ghana's experience, which fits this description, is discussed in Box 15-3. More recently, Greece has suffered a major debt crisis, the analysis of which draws on elements of both Figures 15-8 and 15-9 (Box 15-4).

BOX 15-4 THE GREEK DEBT CRISIS OF 2010-12

Problems of unsustainable debt are not limited to the poorest countries. Starting in 2010, Greece faced a debt crisis so severe as to threaten the stability of the European Union (EU). As of September 2011, it remained uncertain whether Greece would be forced to default on its foreign debts or whether other members of the EU would provide its second bailout package for Greece in two years. In May 2010, the EU and the International Monetary Fund (IMF) provided a package of loans and balance of payments support worth €750 billion (approximately $938 billion). In return, the government of Greece committed itself to an austerity program that included severe reductions in expenditures and wages, termination of tens of thousands of government jobs, and extensive tax increases. This agreement sparked widespread civil unrest in Greece, which contributed to a lack of confidence in the country's ability to implement the promised reforms and service its foreign debts.

Greece's debt problem accumulated over many years of current account deficits, the magnitude of which ballooned during the late 2000s. Greece's current account deficits as a share of GDP began mounting in the mid-1990s. Deficits on the order of 3 percent of GDP in the late 1990s more than doubled relative to GDP during 2000–05. By 2005, Greece's current account deficit was equivalent to 7.5 percent of GDP, a proportion that doubled again to nearly 15 percent by 2008. Between 2008 and 2010, Greece succeeded in reducing its current account deficit to 10.5 percent of GDP, mainly by reducing imports. Borrowing by the Greek government to finance its deficits had also grown rapidly, as the government budget deficit as a share of GDP increased from 5.7 percent in 2006 to 15.4 percent in 2009. The government's total debt shot up from €183.2 billion in 2004 (equivalent to 99 percent of GDP, or approximately $228 billion) to €330.4 billion in 2010 (equivalent to 144 percent of GDP, or approximately $438 billion). The country's general economic stagnation was further reflected in its unemployment rate, which after fluctuating around 10 percent for a decade, fell to 7.5 percent in May 2008, only to double by March 2011. Greece's GDP shrank by 6.6 percent in 2010.

By the fall of 2011, the government of Greece found itself between a rock and a hard place, as the EU debt relief package was imperiled by a threatened cutoff in response to Greece's apparent inability to meet its austerity commitments. Yet daily strikes and mounting political pressure within Greece were preventing the government (led by a socialist party, with a slim parliamentary majority) from fully implementing the promised cuts. A disorderly default was a distinct possibility, along with an exit by Greece from the euro zone.

The Australian model lends itself well to a depiction of the Greek debt crisis. The analysis shown in the figure combines elements of Figures 15–8 and 15–9. By 2005, Greece was suffering from both a balance of payments deficit and unemployment, conditions indicated by point 1. By 2010, both unemployment and the balance of payments deficit had substantially worsened, moving Greece toward point 2 (farther from both internal and external balance and far from equilibrium at point 3). It seems straightforward, based on the phase diagram, that Greece needed to reduce absorption and depreciate its real exchange rate, but there's a catch. As a member of the EU, Greece was a member of the euro zone and was thus unable to devalue its currency as a means of reducing its balance of payments deficit. The only way for Greece to induce the necessary real depreciation was to reduce P_n sufficiently. In short, austerity presented itself as virtually the only tool available to the Greek government. Pushing down wages—a central element of the Government's austerity program—would reduce P_n (because labor can be counted as a key nontradable) and help depreciate the real exchange rate. Austerity was also critical to restoring external balance because borrowing to finance the current account deficit was no longer an option for Greece.

The bailout package offered by EU member states in concert with the IMF would effectively shift the EB curve out to EB', thus reducing the amount of both real depreciation and spending cuts required to reach the new equilibrium at point 4. Herein lay the impasse encountered in the fall of 2011. Greece was widely seen as incapable of making the cuts necessary to reach equilibrium at point 3. Without the bailout package, default seemed unavoidable. Yet even the degree of austerity required to reach the postbailout equilibrium at point 4 was becoming politically impossible for the Greek government. Absent a credible commitment by the Greek government to impose the necessary spending and public employment cuts (along with substantial tax increases), the EU was unwilling to provide the bailout. The brinksmanship between Greece's govern-ment and its debtors continued into early 2012. Greece's next round of debt repayments were due in on March 20, 2012, and, absent a new bailout agree-ment, default was inevitable. In late February, just weeks before the prospective default, EU and Greek negotiators agreed on a second bailout program worth €130 billion ($169 billion) in return for renewed promises of severe austerity and greater EU influence over Greek budgets. The deal was intended to keep the Greek government solvent until 2014. Yet, Greece's continuing deep recession and political uncertainty suggested that the crisis was far from over.

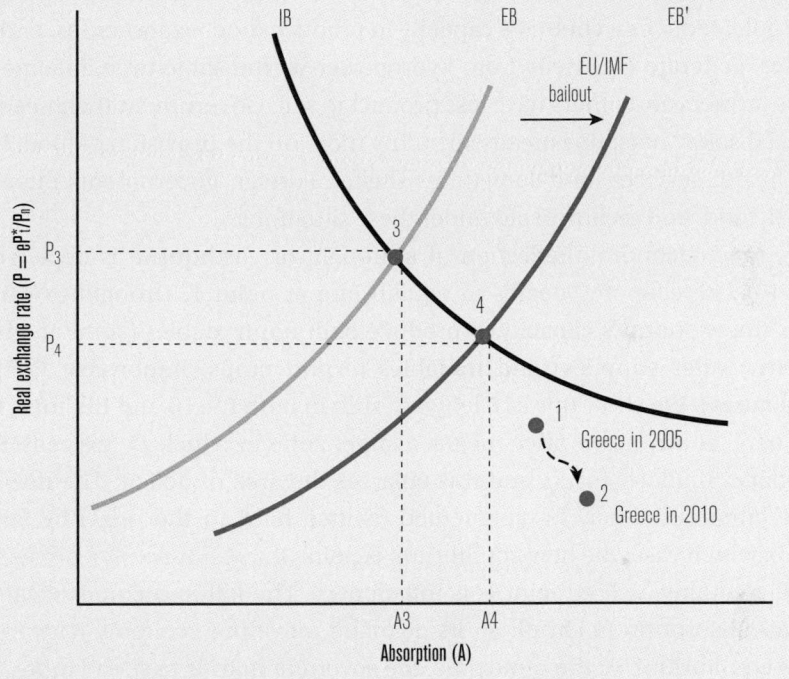

Another kind of stabilization also can be illustrated with Figure 15–9, **rapid infla-tion** (or hyperinflation). In Bolivia's hyperinflation of the mid-1980s or the chronic inflations in the past in Brazil and Argentina, external balance is a secondary con-sideration or not a major problem. Point 4 in the diagram depicts this situation. Austerity still is required to move toward equilibrium at point 2 or 3 (if there is an aid package), but devaluation only intensifies inflation. Instead, the currency must be appreciated, which also dampens inflation. One way to achieve this would be to fix the nominal rate and let the continuing (if decreasing) inflation in nontradable prices (P_n) appreciate the real rate P. This is the *exchange-rate anchor*, a device used often in Latin America, especially in Chile during the late 1970s, in Bolivia during the mid-1980s, and in Argentina during the 1990s. It has the disadvantage that a lower real rate discourages export growth. Yet investment in new exports may be part of a strategy to open the economy, diversify exports, and move the external balance curve to the right.

DROUGHT, HURRICANES, AND EARTHQUAKES

The human tragedy of drought, earthquakes, and other natural disasters in places such as Ethiopia, the West African Sahel, and Haiti in 2010 dwarfs issues of macroeconomic management. But the adept management of an economy racked by natural disaster is essential to reduce the misery of starving or displaced people. Drought, for example, reduces a country's capacity to produce food, export crops, and in some countries, generate electricity from hydropower. At the same time, income is lower because farmers and others have less product to sell. Government then needs to provide social safety nets; this means spending more on the provision of food, transportation, health services, and sometimes shelter. Foreign governments often provide financial, food, and technical aid under these situations.

The macroeconomic reflection of a drought or earthquake is depicted in Figure 15–10. The economy begins in equilibrium at point 1. Drought or earthquake reduces the economy's capacity to produce both nontradables (some foods, hydroelectricity, water supplies) and tradables (export crops, importable foods, some manufactures). We show this as a leftward shift in both the IB and EB lines: Reduced output of S_n at any given price means a larger zone in which D_n exceeds S_n; this is inflationary. Similarly for S_t, and this enlarges the area of deficit. The new external balance curve, EB_2, may be augmented (shifted back to the right) by foreign aid to EB_3, in which case, the new equilibrium is point 3.

The economy, still at point 1, is inflationary. The fall in incomes creates a tendency for absorption to shrink on its own and move the economy leftward toward the new equilibrium. At the same time, the government tries to spend more to relieve hunger, disease, and other problems. The outcome depends on the relative force of these tendencies. The impact of most natural disasters is temporary, typically lasting a year, although some African droughts have been much longer, and the Haiti earthquake of 2010 is likely to last for several years or more. It is appropriate to try to ride out such shocks with minimal adjustment, especially if foreign aid can bear much of the burden. Therefore, for example, even if an exchange-rate adjustment is called for to reach equilibrium, it is unlikely to work very well during the natural disaster and probably should be resisted. This could be said for fiscal austerity too, except that the rise in prices can deepen the suffering of those already hurt by the disaster. If the government is able to shift its expenditures so that a greater portion goes into alleviating the impact of the disaster, it may be able to relieve the worst suffering while restricting the rise of total expenditures and containing inflation.

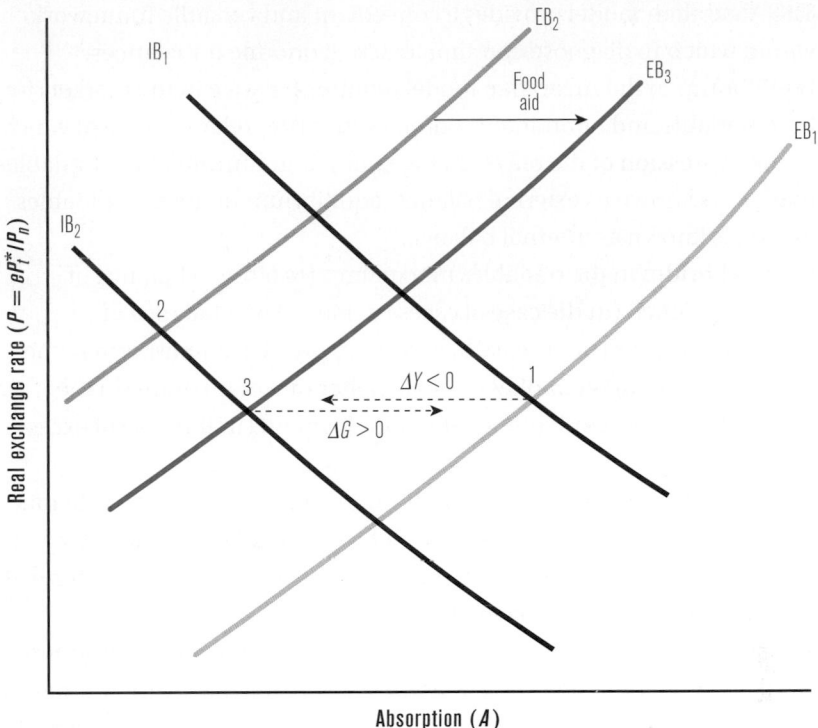

FIGURE 15-10 Drought

Drought or another natural disaster reduces the capacity to produce both nontradables and tradables, so the curves shift to the west. Disaster relief from abroad augments the external balance curve and shifts it to EB$_3$, with equilibrium at point 3. Remaining temporarily at point 1, the economy becomes inflationary. The reduction in output and therefore in income reduces absorption, but the government's need to spend more on relief tends to offset this move toward equilibrium. The outcome could be continued inflation.

SUMMARY

- Open economies may be exposed to a variety of shocks, both positive and negative, either of which may require policy responses to balance potential negative effects. In many cases, we have seen that a country's vulnerability to external shocks may be increased by its own history of poor policy choices.
- One common problem among developing countries arises from extended periods of spending more than they earn and financing the resulting current account deficits with foreign borrowing. For many developing countries, these persistent current account deficits become unsustainable, typically requiring both spending reductions and currency devaluation.

- The Australian model provides a convenient and versatile framework within which to diagnose common macroeconomic imbalances. Equilibrium in the Australian model requires balance in the markets for both tradable and nontradable commodities (the relative price of which is one expression of the real exchange rate). Equilibrium in the tradables markets is known as external balance; equilibrium in the nontradables market is known as internal balance.
- Disequilibrium in the tradables market implies either a balance of payments deficit (in the case of excess demand) or a balance of payments surplus (in the case of excess supply). Disequilibrium in the nontradables market implies either a higher rate of inflation (in the case of excess demand) or higher unemployment (in the case of excess supply).
- Considered together, these disequilibrium conditions may arise in four combinations: balance of payments deficit with inflation, balance of payments deficit with unemployment, balance of payments surplus with inflation, and balance of payments surplus with unemployment.
- The main policy tools available to regain macroeconomic equilibrium are fiscal and monetary policy interventions to change the level of domestic spending (absorption) and changes in nominal exchange rate policy aimed at altering the real exchange rate.
- Recommendations to use some combination of these policy tools to regain equilibrium must take account of the economy's natural tendencies toward equilibrium. The functionality of these natural tendencies will vary with each country's economic and policy circumstances.

APPENDIX TO CHAPTER 15: NATIONAL INCOME AND THE BALANCE OF PAYMENTS

Many macroeconomic problems and crises in developing countries have their roots in the balance of payments. Chapter 10 opens the discussion of balance of payments by describing the role of foreign savings in financing investment. Chapter 13 discusses debt crises in developing countries, and Chapter 15 provides a model for diagnosing and responding to macroeconomic crises—including debt crises. Balance of payments accounting provides a framework within which to understand many of the opportunities and risks created by opening economies to trade and financial flows.

This appendix provides a brief overview of some key aspects of balance of payments accounting.[10]

We begin by placing the balance of payments in the broader context of national income accounting. The value added from all goods and services produced domestically sums to Gross Domestic Product (GDP). In a closed economy, this exactly equals gross national expenditure, which consists of private consumption on final goods and services (C), government consumption and investment in final goods and services (G), and private investments to expand the country's capital stock (I). That is, GDP = C + I + G in a closed economy. In Chapter 15, we refer to gross national expenditure as **absorption** (A), or A = C + I + G. Adopting this notation, we can say that in a closed economy, GDP = A. In addition, in a closed economy all of gross national expenditures (or absorption) is paid to domestic entities, so GDP also equals gross national income (GNI).

When we allow for trade with other countries, it is no longer required that gross domestic product exactly equals absorption or gross national income. This is where the balance of payments comes in. Balance of payments accounting records all of the (home) country's transactions with the rest of the world, including both trade and financial flows. The main components of the balance of payments are the **current account**, the **financial account**, and the **capital account**.

We begin by incorporating the current account into national income. The current account records all foreign trade in goods (the trade balance) and services (net factor income from abroad), along with net unilateral transfers (such as foreign aid or remittances from residents working abroad). The current account also includes interest payments on foreign debts (debt service payments, but not repayment of principal on the debt). In an open economy, part of absorption may be spent on imports (M), and must be subtracted from A; conversely, some domestic production may be exported abroad (X), and the resulting payments to domestic firms are added to A. In this case, we can write the national income accounting identity as

$$GDP = C + I + G + X - M \qquad \text{[A15–1]}$$

Substituting absorption (A) in for gross national expenditure, we can re-write equation A15–1 as

$$GDP = A + X - M \qquad \text{[A15–2]}$$

---

[10]This discussion draws on Robert C. Feenstra and Alan M. Taylor, *International Macroeconomics*, 2nd edition (New York: Worth Publishers, 2012), Chapter 5 (to which the reader is referred for a more detailed treatment), as well as the IMF's *Balance of Payments and International Investment Position Manual*, 6th edition (Washington, DC: International Monetary Fund, 2011).

That is, gross domestic product equals domestic expenditure plus net exports. Rearranging the terms of equation A15-2, we can see that A − GDP = M − X. In other words, if domestic spending exceeds GDP, then our imports exceed our exports and we run a negative trade balance. The trade balance is typically the major component of the current account. As noted above, net factor income from abroad (NFIA), or income from the net export of services (e.g., wages paid to a home country resident working abroad for a foreign firm), is also part of the current account and is included in gross national income (GNI). Thus, GNI = GDP + NFIA. The difference between gross national income (GNI) and gross national disposable income (Y) is that the latter also includes the final component of the current account, net unilateral transfers (NUT). Putting these steps together, we can write

$$Y = A + (X − M) + NFIA + NUT = A + CA \qquad \text{[A15-3]}$$

where CA is the current account, which equals the sum of net exports, net factor income from abroad, and net unilateral transfers. Equation A15-3 is important. It implies that if the home country's total expenditures exceed its total receipts, the difference must be provided by running a deficit on the current account. From equation A15-3, we can see that $A − Y = −CA$. The current account balance thus serves as an indicator of whether a country's spending exceeds its income.

As discussed in Chapter 10, we can also approach the current account from the perspective of national savings. National savings is what is left over from total receipts net of private and government consumption, or $S = Y − C − G$. If we expand A in equation A15-3 to write $Y = C + I + G + CA$ and subtract $C + G$ from both sides, we arrive at the **current account identity**,

$$S = I + CA \qquad \text{[A15-4]}$$

which says that we can only save more than we invest if there is a CA surplus, and we can only invest more than we save if there is a CA deficit.

Domestic savings has two components—private savings (S_p) and government savings (S_g). Income in the private sector must be consumed, saved, or paid to the government as taxes. Thus,

$$S_p = Y − C − T \qquad \text{[A15-5]}$$

Similarly, government savings is the difference between the tax revenue collected by the government (T) and its expenditures (G), or

$$S_g = T − G \qquad \text{[A15-6]}$$

which is the government's fiscal surplus (or deficit, if $G > T$). The sum of these two equations equals our previous observation that $S = Y − C − G = S_p + S_g$, or total national savings is the sum of private savings and government savings. Substituting this idea into equation A15-4 and rearranging, we can see that

$$CA = S_p + S_g − I \qquad \text{[A15-7]}$$

Stated slightly differently, if investment is to exceed national savings, the difference must be financed from abroad, and that difference equals the current account deficit. In this sense, we can think of the current account as foreign savings. In addition, if we substitute equation A15–6 into equation A15–7, we see that

$$CA = (S_p - I) + (T - G) \qquad\qquad \text{[A15–8]}$$

which tells us that if investment exceeds private savings and/or the government runs a fiscal deficit, the current account must be in deficit by an equivalent amount.

The rest of the balance of payments story is about how the current account is financed. As noted above, in addition to the current account, the balance of payments includes the financial account (FA) and the capital account (KA). The financial account records foreign transactions involving financial assets such as stocks, bonds, and real estate ownership. The major components of the financial account (using the IMF definition) are foreign direct investment, portfolio investment, and (importantly) reserve assets (which is the stock of foreign currency—usually U.S. dollars, euros, or yen) held by the central bank. The capital account refers to the transfer of assets such as gifts to and from abroad.[11]

A fundamental principle of balance of payments accounting is that bills must be paid. This implies that the balance of payments must sum to zero, or

$$CA + FA + KA = 0 \qquad\qquad \text{[A15–9]}$$

This is the **balance of payments identity**. It implies that there are only three ways in which a country can finance a current account deficit: 1) it can borrow from abroad (from foreign governments, banks, or international lending bodies), 2) it can attract capital inflows (in the form of direct or portfolio investment), or 3) it can run down its stock of foreign reserves. If the current account is in deficit, then it must be balanced by a surplus in the financial and capital accounts (which potentially includes running down the country's stock of foreign reserves). If the balance of payments must also equal zero, what is meant when we hear about a "balance of payments deficit?" In common use, a balance of payments deficit refers to a situation in which a CA deficit is not fully balanced by a surplus in FA + KA *where FA is defined narrowly to exclude the foreign reserve assets of the central bank.* In such a case, the total balance of payments must be brought to zero by a change in foreign reserves (running them down, in this instance, to finance the remaining CA deficit).

Running a surplus in the (non-reserve) financial and capital accounts means that the home country is either borrowing from abroad or selling domestic assets to foreigners. In either case, the home country is increasing the claims by foreigners

---

[11]This narrow definition of the capital account (and broad definition of the financial account) is in accordance with the approach now taken by the IMF, along with OECD and the UN System of National Accounts. Previously, the accepted tradition was to define the capital account broadly enough to include everything that the IMF now assigns to the financial account, with the exception of the reserve assets of the central bank.

on domestic residents. Conversely, if the home country is running a current account surplus, it must also be running a deficit on the financial and capital accounts, thus increasing the claims by residents on foreigners. Since the home country's stock of net foreign assets equals the difference between claims by residents of the home country on foreigners and claims by foreigners on home country residents, the current account equals the change in net foreign assets.

PART FOUR
Agriculture, Trade, and Sustainability

16

Agriculture and Development

uring the years 2006 through 2008 the world experienced its worst food crisis since the early 1970s. Over that period, the price of corn on world markets nearly tripled, followed closely by the prices of other basic cereals. During the six months from October 2007 to April 2008 the world price of rice tripled, increasing from $335 to over $1,000 per ton. The results were immediate and sometimes violent. Food riots broke out in Bangladesh, Burkina Faso, Cameroon, Egypt, Haiti, Mozambique, and Senegal. A report from Cairo, Egypt, by Al Jazeera on March 13, 2008, recounted, "thousands of people have resorted to violence due to shortages of basic food commodities and rising food prices. At least 10 people have died . . . in riots that erupted at government subsidized bakeries." A few weeks later, on April 18, the *New York Times* reported from Port-au-Prince, Haiti, that, "Hunger bashed in the front gate of Haiti's presidential palace. Hunger poured onto the streets, burning tires and taking on soldiers and the police. Hunger sent the country's prime minister packing. Haiti's hunger, that burns in the belly that so many here feel, has become fiercer than ever in recent days as global food prices spiral out of reach, spiking as much as 45 percent since the end of 2006 and turning Haitian staples like beans, corn, and rice into closely guarded treasures." Grain prices fell in late 2008, but once again rose steeply in 2010–11.

When food prices rise dramatically, what does this imply for developing countries and the welfare of the poor? If many of the poor are farmers, do they benefit from the kinds of food price increases that have occurred in recent years? Some may benefit, if they produce and sell food in sufficient quantities; yet, most poor households are net consumers of food. Similarly, most poor countries are net importers of food. Increases in world food prices may be quite harmful. According to the Food and Agricultural Organization (FAO) of the United Nations, high food prices in 2008 pushed an additional 40 million people into hunger, raising the total to an estimated 963 million. In addition, the FAO estimates that the food import bill for developing countries increased by nearly 75 percent in 2008 as a consequence of the food price shock.[1] The implications of such events for developing countries are complex and raise central questions about the role of agriculture in both economic growth and poverty alleviation.

Agriculture has substantial implications at both the macroeconomic and micro-economic levels in most developing countries. Among countries categorized by the World Bank as low income, agriculture accounted for 25 percent of the gross domestic product (GDP) in 2008, making it the largest single sector in many countries. In addition, over 70 percent of the population of these low-income countries lived in rural areas. Even though not all rural households earn their primary income through farming, the simple observation that nearly three-quarters of the population of low-income countries was sharing one-quarter of the income suggests that poverty in the poorest countries tends to be disproportionately concentrated in rural areas. The large size of the agriculture sector, both in its share of GDP and employment, along with the likely concentration of poverty in rural areas, points to the unique opportunities that agricultural development provides. This chapter addresses the role of agriculture in economic growth and poverty alleviation; Chapter 17 looks more closely at the specific policies and institutions that governments can use to maximize those contributions.

UNIQUE CHARACTERISTICS OF THE AGRICULTURAL SECTOR

Economists Peter Timmer, Walter Falcon, and Scott Pearson identified five characteristics of the agriculture sector that distinguish it from other sectors of most developing economies: the agricultural sector's share of GDP, the agricultural sector's share of the labor force, special characteristics of the agricultural production function, that much of the agricultural sector's output is directly consumed by its producers, and agriculture's role as a resource reservoir.[2]

Agriculture is a dominant sector in many of the world's poorest countries. Table 16–1a summarizes trends in the agricultural share of GDP for major areas of

---

[1]FAO, *Crop Prospects and Food Situation*, 2008, www.fao.org/giews/, and A. Mittal, "The 2008 Food Price Crisis: Rethinking Food Security Policies," G-24 Discussion Paper No. 56, United Nations Conference on Trade and Development (UNCTAD), Geneva, June 2009.

[2]Peter Timmer, Walter Falcon, and Scott Pearson, *Food Policy Analysis* (Baltimore, MD: Johns Hopkins University Press, for the World Bank, 1983).

TABLE 16-1 The Share of Agriculture in GDP and Rural Population Share

	1965-75	1976-85	1986-95	1996-2008
(a) Share of agriculture in GDP (%)				
East Asia and Pacific	35.3	29.3	22.8	14.4
Latin America and Caribbean	13.3	10.8	8.9	6.4
South Asia	41.3	34.0	28.9	22.3
Sub-Saharan Africa	20.4	18.8	18.5	17.1
High-income countries	5.7	4.1	2.7	1.8
(b) Rural population share (%)				
East Asia and Pacific	81.1	78.0	70.8	61.2
Latin America and Caribbean	42.5	34.8	29.1	23.8
South Asia	81.1	77.8	75.0	72.2
Sub-Saharan Africa	80.4	76.1	71.6	66.4
High-income countries	33.1	29.4	26.6	23.7

GDP, gross domestic product.

Source: World Bank, "World Development Indicators," http://databank.worldbank.org.

the developing world since 1965. While it is clear that agriculture plays an important role in generating national income, it is also clear that the magnitude of that role has trended downward over time (an observation pursued in greater depth in the following section). Nonetheless, the challenge of accelerating economic growth becomes much more difficult if a large sector such as agriculture is left to lag behind the rest of the economy.

Table 16–1b demonstrates the even greater share of each region's population that lives in rural areas. Not all rural dwellers are farmers, and many farmers earn at least some of their income outside of farming. Yet, most nonfarm rural activities depend substantially on the existence of a vibrant agricultural sector. Agriculture also plays a substantial role in the consumption side of the economy. It is common among poor households in developing countries for food expenditures to make up 50 to 70 percent of total household expenditures.

The agricultural sector is also distinguished from other sectors by both the sheer number of participants and by the degree of decentralization of those participants. A farming sector may consist of hundreds of thousands, or even millions, of individual production units, all operating independently, yet all allocating resources in response to the same broad set of incentives created by government policy.

Key characteristics of the agricultural production function are also distinctive. These features include seasonality, geographic dispersion, the sources of risk, and the sources of technical change. Agricultural production is uniquely sensitive to seasonality. Most countries have distinct growing seasons, usually defined by rainfall patterns. From an economic point of view, we can think of farmers' use of seasonality as cost minimization (for example, it is much cheaper to use natural sunlight than to use electric grow lights). Yet, with the reliance on seasonality also comes strict requirements for the timing of operations. Late planting, for instance, might substantially reduce yields by failing to take advantage of the best natural growing conditions. Strict timing requirements imposed by seasonality may lead to labor shortages at critical times, such as planting and harvesting, despite widespread rural underemployment at other times of the year. If inputs such as seeds and fertilizer are not available at the right time, they may become useless. These considerations, plus the fact that agriculture is highly geographically dispersed due to its unique use of surface area as an input to production, underscore the need for efficient marketing of both inputs and outputs as a critical ingredient for agricultural development (a point discussed in more detail in Chapter 17).

Risk and uncertainty also affect production in ways that are unique to agriculture. The primary sources of risk for farmers are prices and weather. While it is true that all productive sectors must worry about the price of their output, agricultural prices tend to be particularly variable, both within and across seasons. Farmers are confronted with challenging forms of price risk, as they must commit resources (and potentially take on debt) at the time of planting despite not knowing the price they will receive for their output until months later, when they harvest their crops. This uncertainty about prices is related to weather being an additional source of risk that is unique to agriculture. Most poor farmers (especially outside of Asia) do not have access to modern irrigation systems and thus depend on rainfall. In sub-Saharan Africa only 4 percent of cropland is irrigated and in drought-prone regions, such as Africa's Sahel, weather-related risk is substantial. Too much rain can also be catastrophic, as the destruction of nearly one-fifth of Pakistan's cultivable area by the monsoon floods of 2010 demonstrated.

Productivity growth is essential for sustained agricultural development and is a critical component of overall economic development. In the long run, growth in agricultural productivity is driven by technical change. Creating and disseminating technical change in agriculture is a special challenge for policy makers. The diversity and complexity of agricultural production systems around the developing world make agricultural technologies highly context specific. A wheat variety that thrives in the Pakistani Punjab may fail miserably in Argentina. Thus substantial effort and resources are required not only to create agricultural technologies but also to adapt them to particular agroecological settings. The highly atomized and dispersed nature of agriculture in most countries then presents additional challenges for disseminating new technologies, the impact of which are nil if they are not widely adopted by farmers.

Agriculture is also unique in that producers in developing countries consume a large share of their own output. This highlights the complexity of decision making within agricultural households. Production and consumption decisions are inextricably linked. Households must consider the trade-offs inherent in allocating a mother's time to working in the field or to childcare or in deciding how much time to send children to school versus putting them to work (either on the family's own farm or as hired off-farm labor). Such decisions may have large impacts on the welfare of poor households.

Finally, agriculture differs from other sectors in having traditionally been seen largely as a reservoir of inexpensive resources (principally labor and capital) available for extraction and use in modern industry and services. In many cases, this perspective justified the neglect of agriculture by policy makers, as agriculture was perceived to be a traditional, low-productivity sector with little to contribute to industrialization. Although later approaches have challenged this view of agriculture's role in economic growth, as economies grow, agriculture tends to account for a declining share of both GDP and employment. This robust empirical regularity is part of the broader concept called **structural transformation**.

STRUCTURAL TRANSFORMATION

Structural transformation refers to the systematic changes in sector proportions as economies grow. Initially, at low levels of income, agriculture dominates both as a share of GDP and as a share of employment. As economies transition toward middle levels of income per capita, agriculture accounts for a smaller share of both GDP and employment (replaced by industry and services). This pattern is a central feature of economic development and both a cause and an effect of economic growth. In advanced economies, the farming population accounts for a negligible share of the total population. As Timmer observes, "there are more lawyers in the United States than farmers, more dry cleaning establishments than farms."[3] The relative decline of agriculture and rise of industry and services that characterize structural transformation imply an additional characteristic—namely, a substantial migration of labor from the rural to the urban economy. Finally, structural transformation is also characterized by a demographic transition (discussed in Chapter 7) in which the high birth and death rates of traditional societies are replaced by low birth and death rates (as health conditions improve with income growth).

From the perspective of the demand side of the economy, this process of structural transformation is driven by **Engel's law**, the observation by nineteenth-century statistician Ernst Engel that the proportion of income spent on food declines as income rises (that is, the income elasticity of food is positive, but less than 1). This implies that income grows faster than the demand for food, resulting in the decline of agriculture as a share of national income.

---

[3]C. Peter Timmer, "A World without Agriculture: The Structural Transformation in Historical Perspective," Wendt Lecture, American Enterprise Institute, Washington, DC, October 30, 2007, p. 5.

Structural transformation is an empirically robust phenomenon. Figure 16–1 shows the (smoothed) patterns of rural population shares and agricultural shares of GDP by region as a function of income per capita. (The same patterns are apparent in Table 16–1, which includes the average levels of these variables by decade.) It is clear from Figure 16–1 that there is a persistent, though declining, gap between the rural population share and the share of agriculture in GDP. This gap reflects the persistent, though declining, concentration of poverty in the rural economy. However, as the gap falls, labor productivity and wages across sectors tend to converge. The data in Table 16–1 show that significant gaps remain, on average, in the major regions of the developing world. Among those regions, only Latin America has approached low levels (and convergence) of rural population share and agricultural share of GDP that characterize the advanced economies. The particular path followed by any given country will vary from these norms, depending on local circumstances. Yet, the broad pattern is remarkably robust.

We can begin to consider the potential contributions of agriculture to economic growth by looking more closely at the process of structural transformation. History reflects that structural transformations broadly consist of four distinct phases.[4] The first phase begins with an increase in agricultural output per worker (average labor

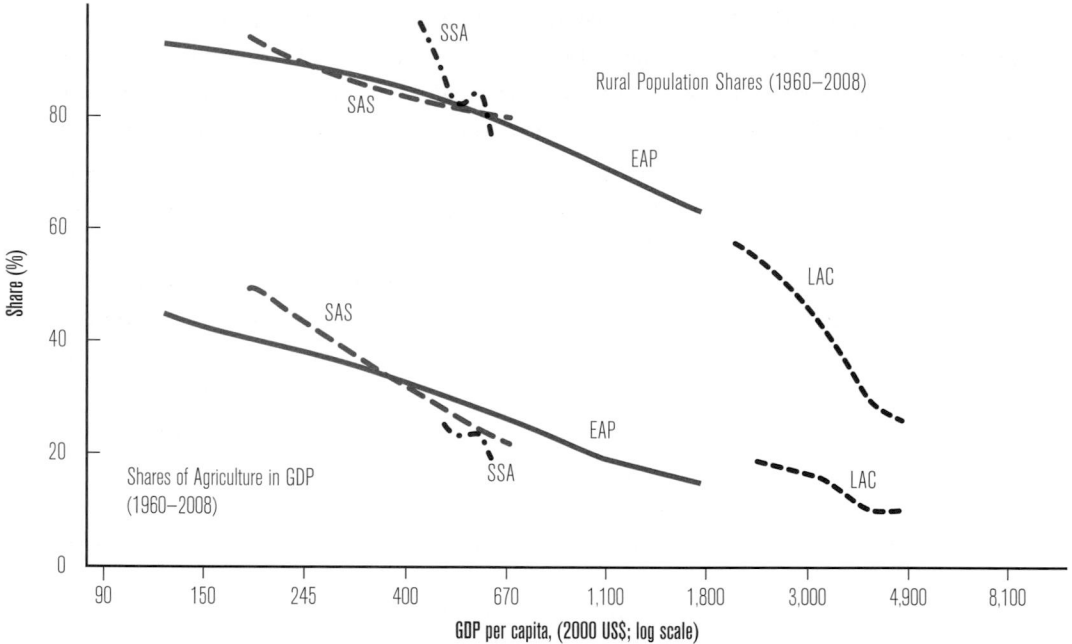

FIGURE 16-1 The Structural Transformation

EAP, East Asian and the Pacific; GDP, gross domestic product; LAC, Latin American and the Caribbean; SAS, South Asia; SSA, sub-Saharan Africa.
Source: World Bank, "World Development Indicators," http://databank.worldbank.org.

[4]C. Peter Timmer, "The Agricultural Transformation," in H. Chenery and T. N. Srinivasan, eds., *Handbook of Development Economics*, vol. 1, (Amsterdam: Elsevier Science, 1988).

productivity). This rising level of output per worker creates a surplus in the rural economy. The second phase of the structural transformation consists of the transfer of that surplus from the agricultural to the nonagricultural sector. This transfer can be implemented either directly (through taxation) or indirectly (through other forms of government intervention). This process of resource transfer is facilitated by the increasing integration of agricultural and nonagricultural factors and product market linkages, with intersectoral trade and labor migration being supported by improved infrastructure. The progressive integration of the agricultural and nonagricultural sectors is the third phase of structural transformation. Finally, the fourth phase occurs when the agricultural sector is fully integrated into the macroeconomy, at which point much of the economic distinctiveness of agriculture will have faded. This is the situation that we currently observe in the advanced economies, where agriculture and nonagriculture operate in essentially the same labor and capital markets.

The concentration of poverty in rural areas that it is implied by the gap between rural employment shares and agriculture's share in GDP also implies that average labor productivity tends to be higher in nonagricultural sectors. Indeed, it may be reasonable to believe that poverty is concentrated in rural areas *because* the level of agricultural productivity is lower than the level of productivity in nonagriculture. Williams College economist Douglas Gollin calculated the ratio of nonagricultural output per worker to agricultural output per worker in 1999–2000 for a number of countries.[5] His results are summarized in Table 16–2. Gollin's calculations confirm that average labor productivity is substantially higher in nonagricultural sectors than in agriculture. In general, the ratio of average labor productivity in nonagriculture relative to agriculture is on the order of 2.5 to 7. Countries in this range include Brazil, Côte d'Ivoire, Ghana, Indonesia, Mexico, and Pakistan. Yet, for more than a few countries, such as Burkina Faso, Burundi, China, and Thailand, this ratio is greater than 10.

If average labor productivity is often substantially higher in nonagriculture than in agriculture, then the process of structural transformation in which labor flows from agriculture to nonagriculture creates a potentially important source of economic growth. We can think of part of the benefit of structural transformation as arising from the transfer of labor from relatively low-productivity to relatively high-productivity employment. Columns 3 to 5 of Table 16–2 present Gollin's calculation of the contributions of sectoral shifts of labor to growth in total output per worker for selected countries.[6] In China, average output per worker in nonagriculture in

---

[5]Douglas Gollin, "Agricultural Productivity and Economic Growth," in Prabhu Pingali and Robert Evenson, eds., *Handbook of Agricultural Economics*, vol. 4 (Amsterdam: Elsevier, 2010).

[6]Gollin calculates the contribution of sectoral reallocation of labor to growth in aggregate output per worker as a residual. This residual is the growth in output per worker that is not explained by adding the separate contributions to growth in output per worker coming from growth in agricultural and nonagricultural output per worker. Accurate accounting for these distinct sectoral contributions requires that each sectors' contribution be weighted by the share of GDP coming from each sector. If the weighted sum is different from the actual growth in aggregate output per worker for a given country, then the difference (that is, the residual) provides an estimate of the contribution of the reallocation of labor between sectors. This type of calculation is thus quite similar in its approach to the growth accounting analysis presented in Chapter 4.

TABLE 16-2 **Ratio of Sectoral Labor Productivity, Agriculture, and Nonagriculture (1999–2000) and the Contribution of Sectoral Labor Shifts to Growth (1960–2000)**

COUNTRY	NONAGRICULTURAL OUTPUT TO AGRICULTURAL OUTPUT*	GROWTH RATE[†]	GROWTH FROM		
			AGRICULTURE	NONAGRICULTURE	SECTORAL SHIFTS
Burundi	13.91	0.005	−0.011	0	0.016
Mexico	6.28	0.01	−0.001	−0.002	0.013
Burkina Faso	29.07	0.013	0.002	0.006	0.006
Côte d'Ivoire	3.03	0.014	0.004	0	0.01
Brazil	3.37	0.017	0.002	−0.005	0.021
Ghana	2.43	0.025	0.014	0.007	0.004
Indonesia	5.07	0.028	0.001	−0.001	0.027
Pakistan	2.54	0.03	0.007	0.005	0.018
Thailand	13.07	0.043	0.004	0.007	0.032
China	11.25	0.053	0.014	−0.015	0.054

*Ratio of nonagricultural output per worker to agricultural output per worker.
[†]Output per worker

Source: Douglas Gollin, "Agricultural Productivity and Economic Growth," in Prabhu Pingali and Robert Evenson, eds., *Handbook of Agricultural Economics*, vol. 4. (Amsterdam: Elsevier, 2010), tables 4 and 5.

1999–2000 was more than 11 times greater than average output per worker in agriculture. Output per worker from 1960 to 2000 grew at 5.3 percent per year, essentially all of which was explained by shifts of workers from agricultural to nonagricultural employment. In Thailand, the labor productivity ratio was over 13. In that case, 3.2 percent of the country's 4.3 percent growth in output per worker during the four decades was explained by sectoral shifts of labor. Intersectoral labor shifts accounted for about three-quarters of the growth of output per worker in Thailand.

Our awareness of the structural transformation comes from historical observation. Yet, the notion of economies consisting of two sectors (agricultural and nonagricultural, traditional and modern, etc.) and the understanding of development as a process centered around the transfer of labor (and capital and other resources) from agriculture to nonagriculture is firmly grounded in the theoretical tradition of two-sector (or dualistic) growth models.

TWO-SECTOR MODELS OF DEVELOPMENT

Although single-sector growth models, presented in Chapter 4, have the great advantage of simplicity, they do not explore production in different sectors such as agriculture, industry, or services (such as banking or tourism); the allocation of capital, labor, and land across these different activities; or the implications for growth. Like the one-sector models, two-sector models recognize the prime importance of labor and capital in the growth process. Two-sector models can also explore differences in the levels and growth rates of productivity in different activities and the implications for relative wages (and returns on capital investment); the allocation of labor and capital across the two sectors; and the potential for migration of labor from rural (agricultural) to urban (industrial) areas. We present two-sector models here to emphasize their value for understanding the interactions between agriculture and nonagriculture during the course of development, rather than as growth models per se.

THE LABOR SURPLUS MODEL

Two-sector models have a long tradition in economic thinking. The best-known of the early models appeared in David Ricardo's *The Principles of Political Economy and Taxation*, published in 1817. In his model, Ricardo included two basic assumptions that have played an important role in two-sector models ever since.

- He assumed that agricultural production was subject to **diminishing returns** because crops require land and the supply of arable land is limited. To increase production, Ricardo felt, farmers would have to move onto poorer and poorer land, and therefore each new acre of land matched with the same amount of labor would produce less grain.
- Ricardo formulated a concept that today is called **labor surplus**. Britain in the early nineteenth century still had a large agricultural workforce, perhaps more than was necessary to produce sufficient food for all consumers. Ricardo believed that the industrial sector could draw away surplus labor from the farms without reducing total agricultural production or causing a rise in wages in either urban or rural areas.

Labor surplus, to the extent that it exists, is closely related to concepts such as rural unemployment and underemployment or disguised unemployment. Very few people in rural areas of developing countries are unemployed in the strict sense. Yet, agriculture's seasonality implies that rural employment may fluctuate from nearly full employment during planting and harvesting times to substantially lower levels of employment at other times, even though the total number of workers remains more or less constant. Economists call this **underemployment** or **disguised unemployment**.

The two-sector models we examine here focus on employment and are designed to answer several questions. How does surplus labor (or very low productivity labor) in agriculture affect industry? Can workers move to industry without causing a fall in agricultural production and thus expand total economic output? Will accelerated population growth help or make matters worse? And, what is the effect of agricultural productivity growth on intersectoral labor flows and economic growth?

The modern version of the two-sector labor-surplus model was first developed by economics Nobel laureate W. Arthur Lewis in 1954.[7] Lewis, like Ricardo before him, pays particular attention to the implications of surplus labor for income distribution and growth. Our concern here, however, is with the relationship between industry and agriculture, and for that, we use a version of Lewis's model formulated by economists John Fei and Gustav Ranis in 1964.[8]

Our starting point is the agricultural sector and the **agricultural production function**. We assume two inputs, labor and land, produce an output, such as grain. The production function in Figure 16–2 is similar to but differs slightly from the standard neoclassical production function with continuously diminishing returns to labor. Instead of showing output as a function of capital per worker, agricultural output is shown as a function of labor per unit of land. Because any increase in labor must be combined with the existing stock of land (or perhaps new land of decreasing quality), the production function exhibits diminishing returns.

The labor surplus model, however, takes diminishing returns to its extreme: It assumes that at some point, further additions of labor make zero (or even negative) contribution to output. In Figure 16–2, a rise in the labor force from *a* to *b* leads to an increase in output from *d* to *e*; an equal increase in labor from *b* to *c* leads to a smaller

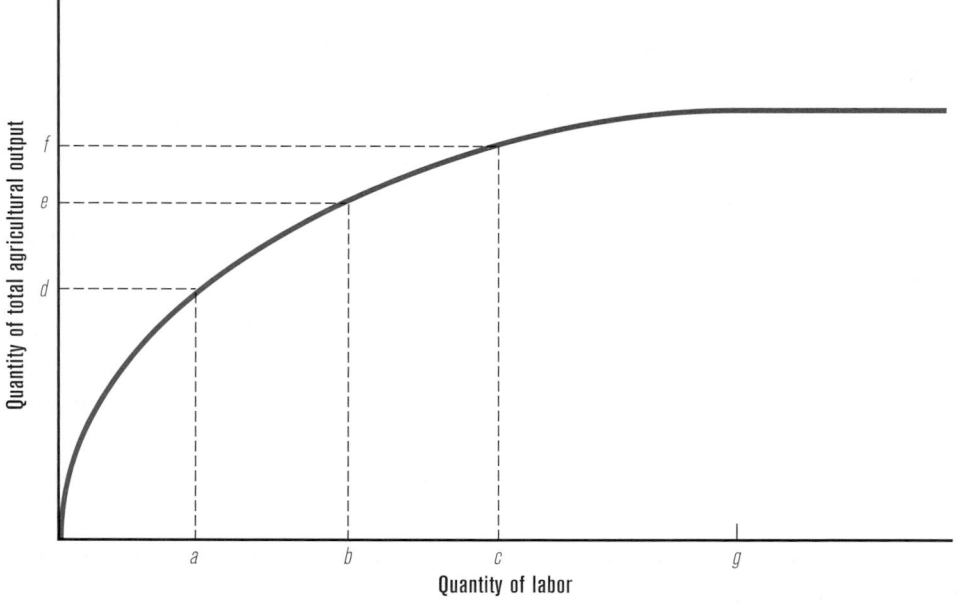

FIGURE 16-2 The Agriculture Production Function

[7]W. A. Lewis, "Economic Growth with Unlimited Supplies of Labor," *The Manchester School of Economic and Social Studies* 22 (1954), 139–91.

[8]John C. H. Fei and Gustav Ranis, *Development of the Labor surplus Economy: Theory and Policy* (Homewood, IL: Richard A. Irwin, Inc., 1964).

rise in output. At point *g*, however, further increases in the amount of labor used lead to no rise in output at all. Beyond point *g*, the **marginal product of labor (MPL)** is zero or negative, so additional labor causes no increase or reduction in output. This could happen if all arable land were fully used and so many workers were available already that adding new ones would not result in more grain being produced.

The next step is to show how rural wages are determined. The standard assumption in all labor surplus models is that rural wages do not fall below a minimum level, regardless of how many workers are available. More specifically, the usual assumption is that rural wages do not fall below the **average product** of farm labor. The logic behind this view is that a member of a farm household will not look for work outside the household unless he or she can earn at least as much as he or she would receive by staying at home. At home, total food production would be divided equally among all members of the household so each person consumes the average product of household production. A slightly different, but comparable concept is that wages are not allowed to fall below a **subsistence level**. In this view, no one would look for work off the farm for wages that were below the amount needed for a minimum level of subsistence. The minimum wage, however determined, sometimes is called an **institutionally fixed wage** to contrast it with wages determined by market forces.

If the MPL falls to zero while wages remain at some minimum level, a wedge emerges between the MPL and the wage rate. This is the key characteristic that distinguishes labor surplus models from standard neoclassical models with perfectly competitive markets (examined in the next section) in which the MPL equals the wage rate. Labor surplus models include not just the possibility that the MPL falls to zero but situations in which the MPL is above zero but less than the rural minimum wage.

These concepts are presented in Figure 16–3, which is derived directly from Figure 16–2, but with several changes. To begin with, the horizontal axis is flipped, so that moving to the right represents a decline in the number of agricultural workers. At the origin, the horizontal axis represents the point where the entire labor force works in agriculture, with no one working in industry. Next, whereas the vertical axis in Figure 16–2 represents the total agricultural product, in Figure 16–3, it is converted to represent the marginal product per unit of labor. Thus when moving to the right, as the number of agricultural workers declines, the MPL begins to increase (corresponding to Figure 16–2 in which increases in the number of workers leads to diminishing returns to labor).

The minimum or subsistence wage is represented by the dotted line *hi*. Agricultural wages remain at this level until the MPL (represented by the solid curve) rises above this minimum, which occurs at point *i*. Thereafter, agricultural wages rise, following the marginal product curve as more labor is drawn away from the sector. This curve plays a dual role: It shows both the agricultural wage and the minimum amount that industry must pay to lure workers off the farm. To hire workers away from the farm, factories have to pay at least as much as the workers are earning on the farm. Therefore, the line *hij* in Figure 16–3 can be thought of as the **supply**

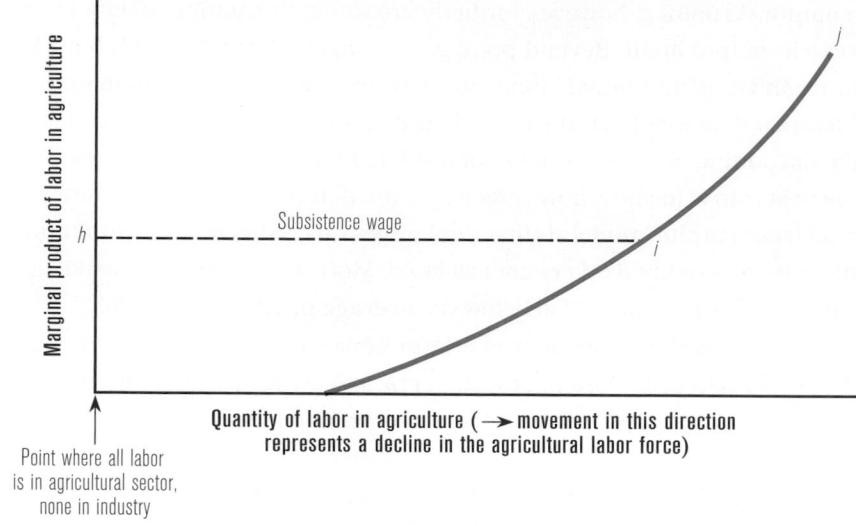

FIGURE 16-3 Modern Product of Labor in Agriculture

As the quantity of agricultural labor decreases, the marginal product increases.

curve of labor facing the industrial sector. Actually the usual assumption is that the supply curve of labor in industry is a bit above the line *hij* because factories must pay farmers a bit more than they receive in agriculture to get them to move.

The key feature of this supply curve of labor is that, unlike more common supply curves, it does not rise continuously as one moves from left to right but instead has a substantial horizontal portion. Formally, this means that the supply curve of labor up to point *i* is **perfectly elastic**. **Elasticity** is a measure of responsiveness, equal to the percentage change in one variable (in this case, the supply of labor) arising from a percentage change in another variable (in this case, wages).[9] The elasticity becomes very large when small changes in wages induce very large changes in the supply of labor. Perfect elasticity occurs when the ratio of these two percentages equals infinity. From the point of view of the industrial sector, this means that the sector can hire as many workers as it wants without having to raise wages, at least until the amount of labor is increased beyond point *i*. To the right of this point, sometimes called the *turning point*, industrial wages rise as firms draw more workers from the agricultural sector.

Figure 16-4 shows the supply and demand for labor for the industrial market. The supply curve *kk′* is taken directly from Figure 16-3 and shows the wages that industry has to pay to draw workers from agriculture. The amount 0*k* on the vertical

---

[9]More formally, this elasticity is the ratio of the percentage change in the supply of labor ($\Delta L/L$) to the percentage change in the wage rate ($\Delta W/W$): Elasticity $= (\Delta L/L)/(\Delta W/W)$. In the case of perfect elasticity, this ratio approaches infinity, which implies a flat supply curve along which employers can employ as much labor as they choose at that fixed wage.

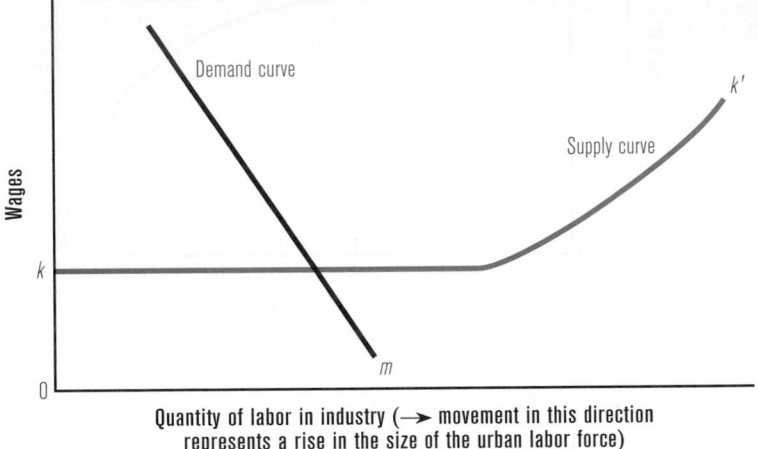

FIGURE 16-4 **The Supply and Demand for Industrial Labor**

The supply curve, *kk'*, is drawn directly from Figure 16–3. Demand, *m*, is derived from the industrial production function.

axis in Figure 16-4 is assumed to be slightly higher than the subsistence wage in Figure 16-3, as discussed previously. The supply curve turns up when the withdrawal of labor from agriculture no longer can be accomplished without a decline in the agricultural output (when the MPL rises above 0) because, at that point, the relative price of agricultural produce rises and this necessitates a commensurate rise in urban wages. In other words, because after the turning point agricultural production is falling, the price of food rises and industry must pay its workers more to compensate for the higher price of food. The demand curve for labor in industry, *m,* displays the usual downward-sloping quality and shows the wages that the industrial sector is willing to pay for different quantities of labor. This demand curve is determined by the marginal product of labor in industry and can be derived from the industrial production function. To simplify our exposition, we do not show the details of this derivation.

The final step is to combine Figures 16-2, 16-3, and 16-4 into a complete version of the model, which is shown in Figure 16-5. Figure 16-5a is the agricultural production function of Figure 16-2 with the horizontal axis flipped. An increase in the number of agricultural workers is shown as a movement from right to left from the origin (0 workers in agriculture) to point *p*, which is the initial size of the total labor force. Many versions of this model use total population rather than the labor force, and this switch has little effect if the labor force is closely correlated with total population. Figure 16-5b shows the MPL curve from Figure 16-3, and Figure 16-5c shows the supply and demand curves for labor in the industrial sector from Figure 16-4. In all three panels, a movement from left to right represents both a decline in the agricultural labor force and a rise in the industrial labor force—that is, a transfer of labor from agriculture to industry.

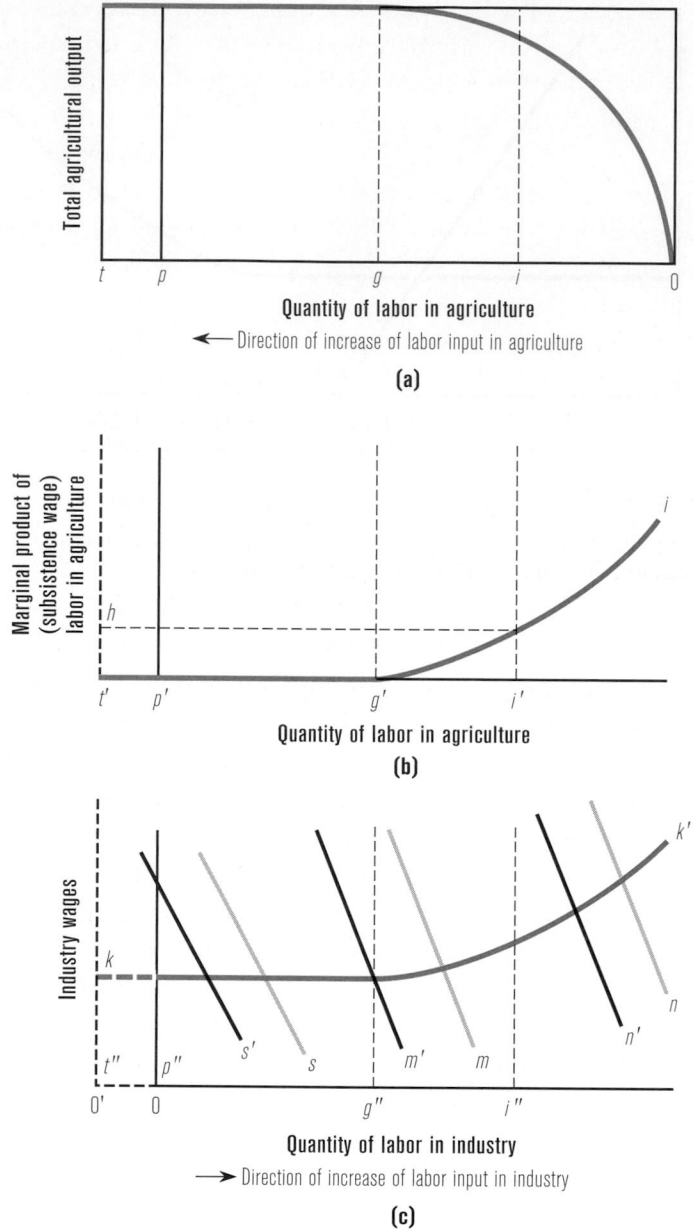

FIGURE 16-5 **The Two-Sector Labor Surplus Model**

(a) Agricultural production function. (b) Rural (agricultural) labor
market. (c) Industrial labor market. The limit imposed by the
country's population (0 to p in panel a), coupled with the agricultural
production function, allows us to analyze the effects of industry
wages on the mix between agricultural and industrial labor.

If a labor surplus economy starts with its entire population in agriculture, it can
remove a large part of that population (pg) and move it to industry or other employment with no reduction in farm output. Industry must pay those workers a wage a
bit above subsistence (the difference between the vertical distance $p''k$ in Panel c

and $p'h$ in panel b) to get the workers to move. As long as there is some way of moving the food consumed by this labor from the rural to the urban area, industrialization can proceed without reducing agricultural output, implying an increase in total GDP because the marginal product of these workers in industry is greater than zero.

As industry continues to grow, however, it eventually exhausts the supply of surplus labor. Further removal of labor from agriculture leads to a reduction in farm output. A shift in industrial labor demand to m in Figure 16–5c forces industry to pay higher wages to compensate workers for the higher price of food. The rise in the price of agricultural output relative to the price of industrial output (which has not changed) sometimes is described as the terms of trade between industry and agriculture turning against industry and in favor of agriculture. The rising price of food as workers move to industry—that is, the shift in the terms of trade against industry—accounts for the rise in the supply curve of labor between g'' and i'' in panel c.

The Fei-Ranis model can be used to explore the implications of population growth and a rise in agricultural productivity, among other things. To simplify, if one assumes a close relationship between population and the labor force, then an increase in population from p to t increases the length of the horizontal axis in all three panels. Note, however, that additional workers (or a larger population) do not increase agricultural output at all. The elastic portion of both the urban and rural labor supply curves are extended by $p't'$ and $p''t''$, respectively, thus postponing the day when industrialization causes wages to rise.[10]

Most important, if the population rises with no increase in food output, the average amount of food available per capita falls. From the standpoint of everyone but a few employers who want to keep wages low and profits high, population growth is an unqualified disaster. Wages actually may fall in the urban areas, and the welfare of the great mass of farmers certainly falls. It is a model such as this, even if only imperfectly understood, that people often have in mind when they speak of population growth in wholly negative terms.

Britain's economy displayed labor surplus characteristics during Ricardo's time. In the middle of the twentieth century China, India, Indonesia, and some countries in Africa appear to have had surplus labor, but there are few such situations today. The most recent major example of a clear application of the model is China from the 1950s through the 1970s (Box 16–1), but China's surplus labor was fully absorbed by the 1980s. More common is a situation in which a withdrawal of labor leads to a small decline in agricultural production, which brings us to the neoclassical two-sector model.

---

[10]In the industrial labor supply and demand part of Figure 16–5c, it is also necessary to move the labor demand curves to the left because the 0 point on the horizontal axis has been moved to the left. These new demand curves, s', m', and n', therefore really are the same as s, m, and n. That is, the quantity of labor demanded at any given price is the same for s' as s, and so on.

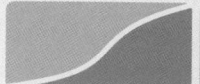

BOX 16-1 SURPLUS LABOR IN CHINA

In China, by the 1950s most arable land already was under cultivation, and further increases in population and the labor force contributed little to increases in agricultural output. Urban wages rose in the early 1950s but then leveled off and remained unchanged for 20 years, between 1957 and 1977. If allowed to do so, tens of millions of farm laborers would happily have migrated to the cities, despite urban wage stagnation. Only legal restrictions on rural–urban migration, backed by more than a little force, held this migration to levels well below what would have been required to absorb the surplus. Population growth that averaged 2 percent a year up until the mid-1970s continued to swell the ranks of those interested in leaving the countryside. In short, during this period China was a labor surplus country.

China invested in agriculture but only enough to maintain, not to raise, per capita food production. The rural–urban migration that occurred was not fast enough to eliminate the agricultural labor surplus, but it was enough to require farmers to sell more of their production to the cities. Thus the prices paid to farmers for their produce were gradually raised, while the prices paid by farmers for urban products remained constant or fell—that is, the rural–urban terms of trade shifted slowly but markedly in favor of agriculture.

To get out of this labor surplus situation, the Chinese government after 1978 had to accelerate the transfer of workers from agricultural to urban employment, take steps to keep the agricultural pool of surplus labor from constantly replenishing itself, and at the same time invest in agriculture to raise farm output. Accelerating the growth of urban employment was accomplished by encouraging production of labor-intensive consumer goods (textiles, electronics, etc.) and service industries (restaurants, taxis, etc.). To feed this increase in urban population, the government increased domestic food production by raising investment in the agricultural sector, increased food imports, and allowed a further improvement in rural–urban terms of trade that further encouraged growth in food output.

To keep the rural pool of surplus labor from replenishing itself, the Chinese government attacked the surplus at its source through a massive (and controversial) effort to bring down the birth rate. By 1980, China's population growth rate had slowed from 2 to 1.2 percent a year, and after 1997 the rate fell below 1.0 percent a year, where it has remained ever since. Rapid industrial and services growth in and around the cities and in the countryside itself has absorbed roughly 10 million new workers a year. In 1991, the workforce in agriculture reached its peak and has declined steadily since then. The agricultural labor force that accounted for 70.5 percent of total employment in 1978 reached a key milestone in 1997 when it fell to 49.9 percent, signifying that for the first time in Chinese history, less than half the people employed in the country were farmers. By 2009 the share of employment in agriculture had fallen further to under 38 percent of the total workforce, and people between the ages of 18 and 40 were mainly employed in the cities. Due to migration restrictions imposed by the government, however, their below-working-age children often remained in the rural areas with their grandparents who made up most of the over-age-40 population and most of the agricultural workforce.

THE NEOCLASSICAL TWO-SECTOR MODEL

The neoclassical model, formalized by Harvard economist Dale Jorgenson, differs from the labor surplus model in two key ways: (1) The MPL in agriculture is never zero and (2) there is no institutionally fixed minimum wage, so wages always equal the MPL.[11]

A simple neoclassical model is presented in Figure 16–6, showing the same three panels as Figure 16–5. The agricultural production function in panel a is never flat, and the marginal product of labor curve in Panel b is always rising. Correspondingly, the supply curve of labor to industry in Panel c no longer has a horizontal section. At every point, the removal of workers from agriculture reduces agricultural production and increases the MPL for those remaining in agriculture. Industry must pay an amount equal to that marginal product (plus a premium) to get workers to move. Thus, whereas in the labor surplus model industrial production can increase without reducing agricultural production (leading to an unambiguous increase in GNP), in the neoclassical model an increase in industrial production can take place only alongside a decrease in agricultural production. As labor is removed from agriculture, farm output falls, and to extract enough food from the agricultural sector to pay its workers, industry must pay higher and higher prices for good. Only if industry is in a position to import food from abroad will it be able to avoid these worsening terms of trade. If imports are not available, rising agricultural prices will lead to a higher value of output and hence higher wages for workers in agriculture. As in the labor surplus case, industry will have to pay correspondingly higher wages to attract labor. The total value of GNP rises only to the extent that industrial production rises more than agricultural output falls.

[11]Dale W. Jorgenson, "The Development of a Dual Economy," *Economic Journal* 71 (1961), 309–34.

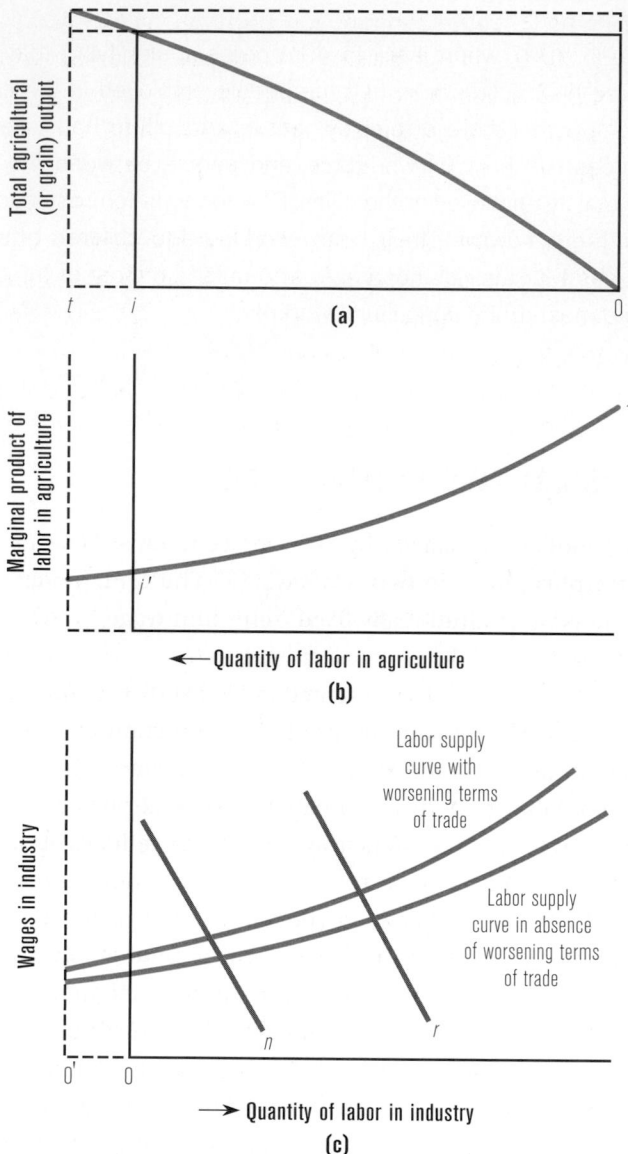

FIGURE 16-6 **Neoclassical Two-Sector Model**

(a) Agricultural production function. (b) Marginal product of labor in agriculture.
(c) Industrial labor market. The key difference between this figure and Figure 16–5 is the
agricultural production function agricultural sector, but the curve never flattens out—that is,
the marginal product of labor never falls to a minimum subsistence or institutionally fixed
wage in Figure 16–6b.

The implications of population or labor force growth in the neoclassical model
are different from what they were in the labor surplus model. An increase in population and labor in agriculture raises farm output (dashed line *t* in Figure 16–6a)

because the agricultural production function continues to rise with more labor and never flattens out. Thus, in a neoclassical model, population growth is not such a wholly negative phenomenon. The increase in labor is much less of a drain on food availability because that labor is able to produce much or all of its own requirements, and there is no surplus of labor that can be transferred without a consequent reduction in agricultural output.

If industry is to develop successfully, simultaneous efforts must be made to ensure that agriculture grows fast enough to feed workers in both the rural and urban sectors at ever-higher levels of consumption and prevent the terms of trade from turning against industry. A stagnant agricultural sector with little new investment or technological progress causes the wages of urban workers to rise rapidly and thereby cuts into profits and the funds available for industrial development. In other words, investments in improved agricultural technology or rural roads (which reduce the cost of transporting farm inputs and outputs, including food) help the industrial sector by reducing its costs. Whereas in the labor surplus model policy makers can ignore agriculture until the surplus of labor is exhausted, in the neoclassical model there must be a balance between industry and agriculture.

These dual sector models provide a clear framework in which to consider the economywide effects of productivity growth in agriculture. The best example is an extension of the two-sector model proposed by economists Mukesh Eswaran and Ashok Kotwal.[12] Eswaran and Kotwal begin by considering an economy that is closed to trade and consists of two sectors, textiles and agriculture. In this stylized economy, textiles and food are the only goods produced or consumed. Textiles are assumed to require only labor, while food production requires labor and land. Eswaran and Kotwal do not require surplus labor (and thus come closer to the neoclassical model described in Figure 16–6) but add an assumption that consumer preferences are such that people begin to consume textiles only once they are able to afford at least a subsistence level of food. It is assumed that most of the workers have not reached this subsistence level and thus will spend all incremental income on food until they reach that subsistence level of consumption. In contrast, landlords (the only other actors in this model besides workers) are richer and consume both food and textiles. The assumption that Eswaran and Kotwal share with Jorgenson, that labor markets are competitive, implies that wages are determined by the productivity of labor. Further, labor is mobile between sectors, which implies that the wage is the same in both sectors and that inducing labor to migrate from agriculture to textiles requires wages to increase. Because at an early

---

[12]M. Eswaran and A. Kotwal, "A Theory of Real Wage Growth in LDCs," *Journal of Development Economics* 42 (December 1993), 243–69, and "The Role of Service Sector in the Process of Industrialization," *Journal of Development Economics* 68 (2002), 401–20.

stage of development agricultural productivity is typically quite low, so is the wage in this economy. As wages are set in the agriculture sector, the low wage in agriculture that results from low agricultural productivity also keeps wages low (and poverty high) in the textiles sector.

Now, suppose that agricultural productivity increases. This results in both higher wages for agricultural workers and increased profits for landlords (as land also becomes more productive). This increases both the supply of and the demand for food. Landlords will also increase their demand for textiles, bidding up both textiles prices and wages. Labor will be willing and able to leave agriculture to produce those added textiles. Thus agricultural productivity growth in this simple model results in the transfer of labor from agriculture to industry while also reducing poverty (through the increased wages).

If instead the productivity increase occurs in textiles, rather than in agriculture, each industrial worker can produce more textiles. The price of textiles (in this closed economy) will fall. Yet, if most workers have yet to attain the subsistence level of food consumption (and hence consume no textiles), they receive no benefit from this change and there is no incentive for labor to migrate to industry. The wage and poverty remain unchanged, and the only beneficiaries of productivity growth in industry are the landlords, who can now consume more textiles. The implication, at least for closed economies, is that it is productivity in agriculture, not industry, that matters for poverty reduction. Whether or not surplus agricultural labor exists in any country (and therefore which version of the two-sector model is most appropriate) has long been a subject of debate (Box 16–2).

BOX 16-2 DEBATES OVER SURPLUS LABOR

The most famous debate over the existence of surplus labor was an exchange between two Nobel economics laureates, Theodore Schultz and Amartya Sen.[a] Schultz reasoned that if any country was likely to have surplus rural labor, it was India. To test whether there was surplus labor in rural India, Schultz took advantage of a sort of natural experiment—the global influenza pandemic of 1918–19 which killed approximately 50 million people, including 8.3 percent

[a]Theodore Schultz's original analysis was in his book *Transforming Traditional Agriculture* (New Haven, CT: Yale University Press, 1964). The subsequent round of exchanges between Schultz and Sen was published in *The Economic Journal* 77, no. 305 (March 1967).

of India's agricultural labor force. Schultz's test of the surplus labor hypothesis was based on the hypothesis that if there were surplus labor, the reduction in the labor force would not reduce India's agricultural output (or, by extension, the area planted). He compared the area planted just before the pandemic with the area planted just after the pandemic and found a 3.8 percent reduction in the postpandemic area planted. This reduction (which was close to Schultz's prediction of what would have happened in the absence of surplus labor) appeared to support his argument against the existence of surplus labor in agriculture.

Amartya Sen took issue with Schultz's approach. Sen made the point that surplus labor could exist within families. He gave the example of peasant families with five working members, each of whom was 20 percent idle. In that case, withdrawing one member would leave output unchanged, indicating the existence of surplus labor. But, Sen continues, if the same 20 percent reduction in labor occurred because one in five entire households disappeared while the other four remained then output would fall (at least in the short run), even if there were surplus labor within families. It is this latter scenario that Sen argues is a more apt description of the influenza pandemic. Indeed, Sen argues that the effects of the pandemic were unevenly distributed over families with a given region and between different regions in a given province, concluding that Schultz's test was inconclusive regarding the existence of surplus labor.

This debate did not end with Schultz and Sen. More recently economist Mark Rosenzweig presented rigorous microeconomic evidence of an upward-sloping supply curve for labor in developing countries (in contrast to the surplus labor model's assumption of a perfectly elastic labor supply curve, as seen in Figure 16–5, implying surplus labor).[b] Yet, economist Gustav Ranis (co-author of the Fei-Ranis model) later defended the surplus labor model. Ranis concedes that the number of contemporary developing countries with surplus labor has been declining but claims relatively recent turning points, at which certain countries ceased to have surplus labor—Taiwan in 1968, South Korea in 1973, and Thailand in 1993. Ranis contends, however, that as of 2004, China and India, as well as "other parts of South Asia, much of Central America, the Caribbean, parts of Latin America, and even some countries in sub-Saharan Africa"[c] remain in conditions that qualify as surplus labor.

[b]Mark Rosenzweig, "Labor Markets in Low-Income Countries," in H. Chenery and T. N. Srinivasan, eds., *Handbook of Development Economics*, vol. 1 (Amsterdam: Elsevier, 1988).

[c]Gustav Ranis, "Labor Surplus Economies," Center Discussion Paper No. 900, Economic Growth Center, Yale University, New Haven, CT, December 2004, p. 17.

EVOLVING PERSPECTIVES ON THE ROLE OF AGRICULTURE IN ECONOMIC GROWTH AND POVERTY ALLEVIATION

AGRICULTURE AND ECONOMIC GROWTH

If agriculture becomes a smaller share of output and employment as economies grow, how can agriculture contribute to broader economic growth? A meaningful answer to this question must delve beyond mere national income accounting relationships. In accounting terms, we can think of a country's rate of income growth as the weighted average of the growth rates of various sectors in the economy. If we adopt a dualistic perspective, in which an economy consists of agriculture and nonagriculture, the *direct* effect of growth in the agriculture sector may be large initially, but soon declines. That is, if value added in the agricultural sector is Y_A, we can write the share of agriculture in national output as $\alpha = Y_A/Y$ (where α is between 0 and 1). If the only sectors are agriculture and nonagriculture, then the share of value added from nonagriculture (Y_{NA}) in national income is $(1 - \alpha)$, and we can express the growth rate of national income as the weighted average,

$$\frac{\Delta Y}{Y} = \alpha\frac{\Delta Y_A}{Y_A} + (1 - \alpha)\frac{\Delta Y_{NA}}{Y_{NA}} \qquad [16\text{--}1]$$

where Δ indicates change. Dividing the change in the level of a variable by its level gives us its growth rate. So equation 16–1 simply states that the growth rate of national income is the weighted average of the growth rates of income in agriculture and nonagriculture, where the weights are the share of each sector's value added in national income.

We can see from this equation that the growth rate of the agricultural sector matters in a purely arithmetic accounting sense. Borrowing data for South Asia from Table 16–1, during the period 1965–75, agriculture's share of GDP (α in equation 16–1) was 41.3 percent. If governments in that region had a goal of seeing their economies grow at, say, 5 percent per year per capita, then a sector that accounted for nearly half of GDP would need to contribute. Maybe both sectors would grow at 5 percent per year per capita, in which case that would also be the weighted average growth rate. Yet, if the agriculture sector was allowed to languish because of the perception that only industrialization mattered and (taking the extreme case) thus did not grow at all (that is, if $\Delta Y_A/Y_A = 0$), then reaching a weighted average of 5 percent would require that the nonagriculture sector grow at the annual rate of 8.5 percent per year per capita, a much higher hurdle.

This simple arithmetic highlights the role of agricultural growth early in the development process when agriculture represents a large share of the economy but also suggests that agriculture's role diminishes as the sector becomes smaller over time. All we need to do is look at Table 16-1 to see that this arithmetic problem becomes less important over time. In South Asia, agriculture's share of GDP fell from 41.3 percent during 1965–75 to only 22.3 percent by the period 1996–2008. This is the structural transformation in action. The deeper questions are how does this structural transformation happen, and what is the role of agricultural growth in that process? In terms of equation 16-1, this amounts to asking whether the growth rate of nonagriculture depends to some extent on the growth rate of agriculture. Even if agriculture's direct arithmetic contribution to growth diminishes over time, agricultural growth might contribute indirectly to economic growth through its effect on growth in nonagriculture. This possibility requires us to think in greater detail about **intersectoral linkages**. Early interpretations of the dualistic development paradigm tended to ignore agriculture's potential indirect contributions to growth.

The Lewis and Fei-Ranis assumption of a very low or zero marginal product of labor in the rural economy was the dominant perspective to emerge historically from dualism. With that perspective, the post–World War II development paradigm maintained that the agricultural sector had little to contribute to the process of economic growth. This was not Lewis's own interpretation. Indeed, in introducing his model, Lewis famously wrote, "industrialization is dependent upon agricultural improvement; it is not profitable to produce a growing volume of manufactures unless agricultural production is growing simultaneously. This is also why industrial and agrarian revolutions always go together, and why economies in which agriculture is stagnant do not show industrial development."[13] It is inherent in the Lewis and Fei-Ranis models (albeit assuming closed economies) that in the absence of increasing agricultural productivity, the withdrawal of labor from agriculture eventually (in Fei-Ranis) or immediately (in the neoclassical version) results in reduced food supply, increased food prices, and thus lower real wages in industry. To continue to attract labor from agriculture under such circumstances, industrialists would have to pay continually higher nominal wages, thus undermining the incentives for continued industrial expansion. However, this was not the lesson as understood by most policy makers and early development thinkers.

The more dominant early interpretation of classical dualism was that of political economist Albert Hirschman, who wrote in 1958, "agriculture certainly stands convicted on the count of its lack of direct stimulus to setting up of new activities through linkage effects—the superiority of manufacturing in this respect is crushing."[14] This view was reinforced by the then-current assertion that primary products, such as agriculture, were doomed to suffer declining terms of trade relative to manufactured goods in international markets and thus presented few growth opportunities for poor countries. (This is the Prebisch-Singer hypothesis, discussed in more

---

[13]Lewis, "Economic Growth with Unlimited Supplies of Labor," p. 433.

[14]Albert O. Hirschman, *The Strategy of Economic Development* (New Haven, CT: Yale University Press, 1958).

detail in Chapter 18.) Widely seen, then, as a stagnant pool of underutilized labor and capital, agriculture was usually neglected in early development strategies.

The evolution of thought regarding the role of agriculture in economic growth is best understood in terms of intersectoral linkages. This perspective begins with the Lewis linkages of labor and capital flows from agriculture to nonagriculture. These are direct linkages across sectors that operate via factor markets. Ideally, labor and capital are released from agriculture as a consequence of increasing agricultural productivity. However, as discussed in Chapter 17, agricultural productivity growth is not automatic. It requires substantial investment in research and development, systems to extend new techniques to farmers, and functioning input and output markets with appropriate production incentives. In the context of early development paradigms in which agriculture was viewed as a stagnant resource reservoir, the need for such investments was not well understood. Instead, government policies often sought merely to extract labor and capital from the agricultural sector. If the development paradigm was one in which rural labor was assumed to have a zero marginal product (that is, if the production function for agricultural labor eventually became flat), labor could be withdrawn from agriculture with no reduction in output.

By the early 1960s, economists' perspectives on intersectoral linkages and agriculture's potential contributions to growth began to evolve. In a particularly influential article, agricultural economists Bruce Johnston and John Mellor listed five intersectoral linkages.[15] In contrast to the direct Lewis linkages, the Johnston-Mellor linkages were indirect. Their list of agriculture's contributions is (1) increased supplies of food for domestic consumption, (2) released labor for industry, (3) a domestic market for industrial output, (4) a supply of domestic savings, and (5) a source of foreign exchange. While the second and fourth linkages in this list built on the Lewis tradition, Johnston and Mellor set the stage for a richer understanding of agriculture's potential contributions to growth.

The first Johnston-Mellor linkage, increased food supply for domestic consumption, underscores the logic, noted earlier, that was implicit in the Lewis and Fei-Ranis approaches. A vibrant and productive agricultural sector that could both release labor and supply increasing quantities of food for domestic consumption could facilitate industrialization by helping keep food affordable for industrial workers. While affordable food is an important part of agriculture's potential contribution to poverty alleviation, it also benefits urban employers by reducing labor costs. There is a big difference, however, between government policies that keep food cheap by controlling food prices or by heavily taxing agricultural producers and government policies that keep food cheap by investing in agricultural productivity. Johnston and Mellor highlight linkages that operate not only forward, in the sense of agriculture supplying inputs and foreign exchange to nonagriculture, but also backward. The third Johnston-Mellor

---

[15] B. Johnston and J. Mellor, "The Role of Agriculture in Economic Development," *American Economic Review* 51 (1961), 566–93.

linkage, in which agriculture provides a market for domestic industrial output, can be understood as a backward linkage, one that underscores the consumption externalities that become possible when agriculture is profitable and the sector itself is growing.

Awareness of these intersectoral linkages, arising from the early contribution of Johnston and Mellor, led to numerous efforts to quantify the effects of agricultural growth on broader economic growth. These efforts generally sought to measure agriculture's contributions to growth in terms of **growth multipliers**. A growth multiplier is a number that answers the question, If a country's agricultural value added increases by $1, what is the ultimate impact on that country's aggregate GDP? If GDP is the sum of value added in agriculture and nonagriculture, then an additional $1 of agricultural output automatically adds $1 to national output. The question is to what extent intersectoral linkages operate in such a way that an additional $1 of agricultural income stimulates economic activity in nonagriculture, thus adding indirectly to national income. Growth multipliers seek to measure the sum of these direct and indirect contributions to national income.

Efforts to estimate agricultural growth multipliers based on household-level data demonstrate that it is Johnston and Mellor's backward linkage, the demand from within agriculture for domestic goods produced by the nonagriculture sector, that dominates the multiplier. The intuition is that when new resources are brought into production in the agriculture sector, farmers (and landlords) spend that incremental income. While some of those expenditures will be on additional food, some portion will also be spent on the purchase of nontradable goods produced domestically in the nonagriculture sector. The multiplier effect created by this additional rural demand will be greater under certain circumstances than under others. In particular, agriculture must make up a large share of total employment. In addition, the multiplier effect will be greater when the benefits of agricultural growth are widely shared among rural producers. This is more likely when land ownership is relatively evenly distributed. Demand-driven multiplier effects will also be larger when consumption patterns are such that large portions of the incremental demand are spent on domestically produced labor-intensive goods and services. Finally, multiplier effects will be greater when the supply of the additional goods demanded is highly elastic, which implies that the increased demand will bring forth increased supply without substantially increasing prices.[16] In practice, the origin of such income shocks, at least in Asia, was the technological improvements developed for agriculture as part of the green revolution (discussed in more detail in Chapter 17).

Efforts to quantify agricultural growth multipliers date back to the early 1980s in Asia. Economist C. Rangarajan calculated that the agricultural growth multiplier for India was 1.70, while economists Clive Bell, Peter Hazell, and Roger Slade found the

---

[16]These conditions and more technical details regarding the estimation of growth multipliers are explained in C. Delgado, J. Hopkins, and V. Kelly, "Agricultural Growth Linkages in Sub-Saharan Africa," International Food Policy Research Institute Research Report No. 107, Washington, DC, 1998.

multiplier in Malaysia to be 1.83.[17] The interpretation of these numbers is that when $1 of additional income is generated in the agricultural sector, it stimulates an additional $0.70 (or $0.83 in Malaysia) of income in nonagriculture, for a total addition of $1.70 to national income. Using similar modeling techniques, a subsequent series of studies focused on West African cases. They found agricultural growth multipliers to be even greater in Africa than in Asia, ranging from 1.96 in Niger to 2.88 in Burkina Faso, though other studies have found growth multipliers in Africa generally smaller than in Asia (more on the order of 1.30 to 1.50).[18] Applying a simpler methodology, Tufts University economist Steven Block estimated an agricultural growth multiplier for Ethiopia to be 1.54, compared to an industrial growth multiplier of 1.22 to 1.34.[19]

The Johnston-Mellor linkages also paved the way for more recent perspectives on agriculture's potential contributions to economic growth. There is strong empirical support for two additional channels through which agriculture can contribute to economic growth: a stability linkage, which connects stability in food prices with investment; and a nutritional linkage, which operates through the health of the labor force (Box 16–3).[20]

BOX 16-3 THE NUTRITION LINKAGE TO ECONOMIC GROWTH

The nutritional linkage from agriculture to economic growth is based on evidence, not from contemporary developing countries, but rather from research on eighteenth- and nineteenth-century Britain and France by Nobel Prize—winning economic historian Robert Fogel.[a] His research on the secular decline in mortality rates in western Europe combines historical detective work with nutrition, human physiology, and economic analysis. By reconstructing the distribution of

[a]Robert Fogel, "Economic Growth, Population Theory, and Physiology: The Bearing of Long-Term Processes on the Making of Economic Policy," *American Economic Review* 84, no. 3 (June 1994), 369–95.

---

[17]C. Rangarajan, "Agricultural growth and industrial performance in India," International Food Policy Research Institute, Research Report 33, Washington, DC, 1982; C. Bell, P. Hazell, and R. Slade, *Project Evaluation in Regional Perspective* (Baltimore, MD: Johns Hopkins University Press, 1982).

[18]Delgado, Hopkins, and Kelly, "Agricultural Growth Linkages in Sub-Saharan Africa," in S. Haggblade, P. Hazell, and T. Reardon, eds., *Transforming the Rural Nonfarm Economy* (Washington, DC: International Food Policy Research Institute, 2009).

[19]S. Block, "Agriculture and Economic Growth in Ethiopia: Growth Multipliers from a Four-Sector Simulation Model," *Agricultural Economics*, 20 (1999), 241–52.

[20]For a more detailed exposition of these types of linkages, see C. Peter Timmer, "Agriculture and Economic Development," in B. Gardner and G. Rausser, eds., *Handbook of Agricultural Economics*, col. 2A, (Amsterdam: Elsevier Science, 2002).

caloric intake in late-eighteenth-century Britain and France, Fogel found that the levels of caloric intake for the bottom 20 percent of the distribution were insufficient to support the physical requirements of much (if any) manual labor. In addition, he found that undernutrition of the labor force was also associated with high rates of disease and physical disability (which themselves contributed back to the problem of undernutrition). This type of chronic undernutrition also results in stunted growth (indeed, the average adult male in late-eighteenth-century Britain was about 3.5 inches shorter than in late-twentieth-century Britain). Thus chronic undernutrition in the late eighteenth century was associated, not only with increased rates of illness and disability but also with stunted growth and increased risk of death. (Because height is in part a reflection of long-term nutritional status, shorter people, on average, face a higher likelihood of premature death.)

As agricultural development in Britain and France proceeded and food supplies increased, Fogel found that nutritional status of workers also improved. The caloric intake of the bottom 20 percent of the consumption distribution increased sufficiently to permit them to work. At the same time, their improved nutritional status improved their health status, delaying illness and disability until later in life, further enhancing their ability to engage in productive labor. In short, Fogel concluded that improvements in gross nutrition account for roughly 30 percent of the growth in per capita income in Britain between 1790 and 1980. With current rates of child (under 5 years) stunting greater than 40 percent in much of sub-Saharan Africa and South Asia, this nutritional linkage may have important implications for today's developing countries. Economist Carmel Nadav provides more recent evidence, based on a sample of 97 countries, that improved nutrition contributes to economic growth.[b]

[b]C. Nadav, "Nutritional Thresholds and Growth," Department of Economics, Ben-Gurion University, Israel, 1996.

The stability linkage operates primarily at the macroeconomic level. One reason is that large fluctuations in food prices can provoke broader crises, which may undermine both political and economic stability, as the food riots of 2008 reflect. Political violence in response to rising food prices resulted in 10 deaths and nearly 500 injuries in Mozambique's capital city, Maputo, in September 2010, following a 20 percent increase in the price of bread over the course of that year. This type of instability undermines incentives for investment. (Recall from Chapter 4 the important role of investment in theories of economic growth.)

The stability of food prices may also impact national investment through another channel. In poor countries it is common for consumers to spend 50–70 percent of their income on food. In such settings, unstable food prices may directly act to destabilize savings and investment. While consumer theory might suggest that this is true for any commodity, the singularity of food in this regard derives from its large share of expenditures. Highly unstable food prices can lead farmers to save in a precautionary way to guard themselves from sudden drops in the price of their output, while consumers similarly save to guard themselves against sudden increases in food prices. This type of precautionary savings must be readily accessible (even held in cash), and those resources are thus withheld from productive investment. Food price instability can also destabilize demand for other goods and services in the economy, further undermining incentives for productive investment in the broader economy. This spillover instability arises because the demand for food is price inelastic. When food prices increase, food expenditures increase as well, reducing demand for other goods and services in the economy. The opposite occurs when food prices fall. The resulting instability in prices throughout the economy may further confuse potential investors who rely on price signals to guide their actions or lead them to allocate more investment in speculative, rather than productive, investment opportunities. As a result, the *quality* of investment may also suffer when food prices are unstable.

Empirical support for these arguments comes from several sources. Economist David Dawe presents evidence from cross-country data for the period 1970–85.[21] He finds wide fluctuations in export prices, on balance, lower investment, and slow the rate of economic growth. More specific evidence comes from Indonesia, where rice was a dominant economic sector during the 1960s and 1970s. During that time, the government of Indonesia was heavily involved in efforts to stabilize rice prices. Indonesia's rice price stabilization program during that country's first five-year plan (1969–74) generated nearly one percentage point of additional economic growth each year (or about one sixth of the country's growth over that period). As Indonesia's economy continued to grow, and its structural transformation led the rice sector to play a diminishing role, the macroeconomic benefits of rice price stabilization also diminished. Yet, the net result of these efforts over the period 1969–95 was to increase Indonesia's rate of economic growth by an average of 0.5 percentage points per year, resulting in a net increase of 11 percent greater income over that period.

AGRICULTURE AND POVERTY ALLEVIATION

Economic growth tends to reduce poverty (measured either as a head count index or a poverty gap); yet the effectiveness with which growth reduces poverty may vary from one economic setting to another. Recent research has shown that the *sectoral composition of growth* matters: On average, agricultural growth is more effective in

---

[21]D. Dawe, "A New Look at the Effects of Export Instability on Investment and Growth," *World Development* 24, no.12 (December 1996), 1905–1914.

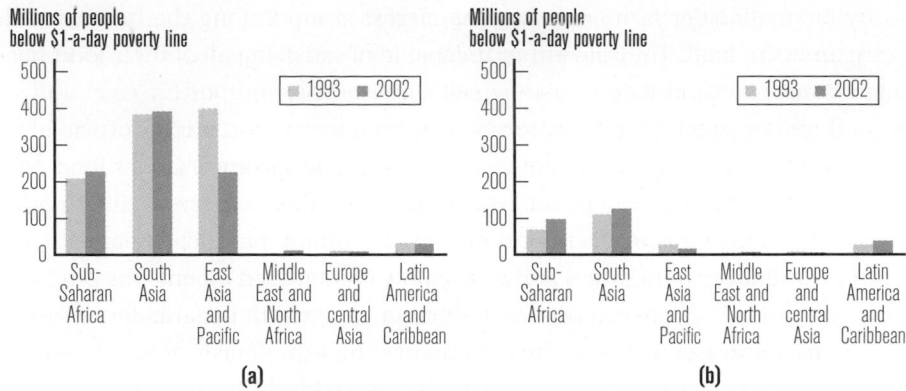

FIGURE 16–7 Number of Poor, 1993 and 2002

(a) Rural poverty. (b) Urban poverty. The number of poor rose in South Asia and sub-Saharan Africa from 1993 to 2002, measured as millions of people below the $1-a-day poverty line.

Source: Figure 1 from The International Bank for Reconstruction and Development. The World Bank: *Agriculture for Development,* 2008. Reprinted with permission.

reducing poverty than is industrial growth. This conclusion about the special potency of agricultural growth for alleviating poverty rests in part on the observation that poverty in many regions of the developing world is disproportionately concentrated in rural areas. Figure 16–7 compares the numbers of rural and urban poor in different regions for the years 1993 and 2002. For sub-Saharan Africa, South Asia, and East Asia, the numbers of rural poor vastly exceed the numbers of urban poor. Among these regions, only East Asia shows substantial reduction in the number of rural poor between 1993 and 2002; however, even in that region, the absolute number of rural poor in 2002 was about eight times greater than the number of urban poor. In countries where agriculture accounts for a large share of employment and poverty is disproportionately rural, the extent to which growth is pro-poor depends substantially on the extent to which agriculture is included in growth.

The effectiveness of the mechanisms through which agriculture helps reduce poverty also depends on the incidence of poverty among various groups in society. In reviewing recent evidence, University of California at Berkeley economists Alain de Janvry and Elisabeth Sadoulet note that for producers, the effect of agriculture in reducing poverty depends on access to assets (notably land), while for rural workers the benefits depend on their access to increased employment opportunities in agriculture and rural nonfarm activities.[22] For consumers, greater supplies of food help to reduce poverty by lowering food prices. Consumers of food might or might not also be producers. The most obvious beneficiaries of reduced food prices are pure consumers—the urban poor and rural landless. Yet, in many countries, the

---

[22]A. de Janvry and E. Sadoulet, "Agricultural Growth and Poverty Reduction: Additional Evidence," *The World Bank Research Observer* 25, no. 1 (February 2010).

majority of smallholder farmers (often the largest group among the poor) are also net consumers of food. They are either incapable of satisfying all of their food needs through their own production, or they sell some of their output for cash and buy food (and other goods). Thus, they too benefit from lower food prices (provided that the gains from reduced spending outweigh any losses to income). Lower food prices could, of course, hurt net sellers, unless productivity gains outpace declining prices. This consideration points to the importance of agricultural productivity growth, both as a driver of reduced food prices and as a source of increased income for producers. The broad association between poverty reduction and growth in agricultural productivity is reflected in Figure 16–8, which compares the experiences of South Asia and sub-Saharan Africa. In South Asia, increasing cereals yields during the 1990s accompanied decreasing incidence of poverty, while in sub-Saharan Africa relatively stagnant cereals yields accompanied a lack of progress in reducing the incidence of poverty.

While the ability of agriculture to reduce poverty is greater in settings where poverty is concentrated in rural areas, this ability also depends on certain conditions within those rural areas. The effectiveness of agriculture in reducing poverty is much stronger in settings where land ownership is more evenly distributed and where production techniques are more labor-intensive, and thus generate more employment.

How does agriculture compare with nonagriculture in its ability to reduce poverty? A number of studies have attempted to quantify the effects of growth originating in agriculture versus nonagriculture. The general consensus among these studies, based on cross-country evidence, is that growth originating in agricultural growth is on the order of three times more effective at reducing poverty than growth originating

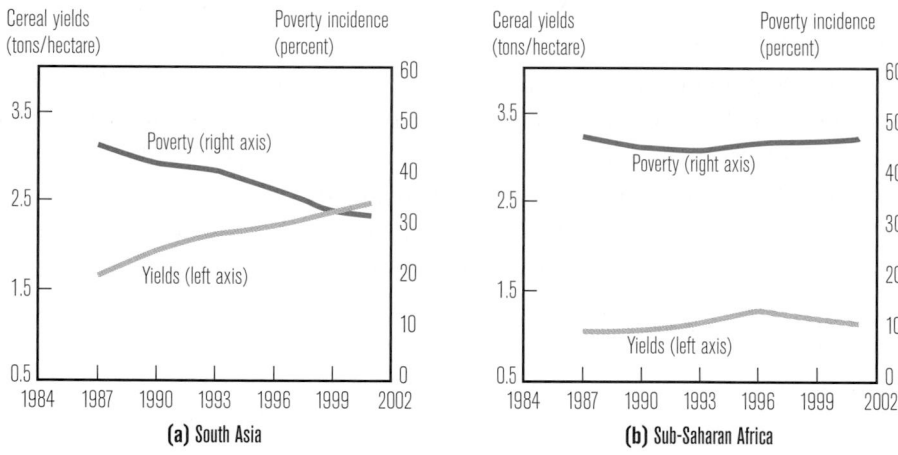

FIGURE 16-8 Cereal Yields and Poverty in South Asia and Sub-Saharan Africa, 1984–2002

Cereal yields rose and poverty dropped in South Asia but both indicators remained unchanged in sub-Saharan Africa.

Source: Figure 1.1 from The International Bank for Reconstruction and Development. The World Bank: *Agriculture for Development,* 2008. Reprinted with permission.

In nonagriculture.[23] The World Bank's *World Development Report, 2008*, which focuses on the role of agriculture in development, presents the results of a study by University of California at Berkeley economists Ethan Ligon and Elisabeth Sadoulet, who compared the effects of a 1 percent increase in GDP originating in agriculture versus nonagriculture on the expenditures of each decile of the income distribution. Based on cross-country data from 42 countries over the period 1978–2003, they estimated that growth originating in agriculture was at least three times as effective in reducing poverty as growth in nonagriculture. They also found that among the poorest people (those in the bottom decile of the income distribution), the effect of agricultural growth was approximately six times greater, whereas income growth originating in nonagriculture actually resulted in small reductions in income among the poorest households. Of course, these cross-country results do not describe the experience of any particular country, where the results will depend on a range of conditions.

AGRICULTURAL GROWTH AS A PATHWAY OUT OF POVERTY

Having established some of the theoretical connections between agricultural growth and poverty alleviation and also having considered some empirical evidence, we now turn to the question of mechanisms. For households living in poverty, what specific opportunities does agricultural growth provide for pathways out of poverty? There are three broad avenues: One possibility is for poor, subsistence-oriented farmers to increase their on-farm output for sale; a second pathway can be to engage in rural labor markets, especially for off-farm rural work; and, a third is to migrate to the urban economy. As the *World Development Report* of 2008 notes, these pathways are complementary. Nonfarm earnings can be used to invest in improved farming, and linkages within the rural economy are such that agricultural growth can both generate off-farm employment and facilitate migration. Migration, in turn, can be an important source of remittances back to rural areas that can support household consumption or investment, as has been the case in the Philippines in particular.

The 2008 *World Development Report* describes various success stories. In Tanzania the farmers that were mostly likely to exit poverty were those who diversified their production to include vegetables, fruits, and vanilla for export, in addition to traditional food crops. Similar diversification of farm output to higher-value commodities contributed to poverty reduction in Uganda and Malawi. In contrast, India and Indonesia are cited as examples in which labor markets provided an important pathway out of rural poverty for households engaged in nonfarm rural activities, such as rural services and small-scale industry. In China and Nepal, migration to cities has played a larger role. A more detailed examination of rural poverty reduction in Vietnam highlights the complementarity of these pathways out of poverty.

[23]These studies are summarized in de Janvry and Sadoulet, "Agricultural Growth and Poverty Reduction," and in *World Development Report, 2008, Agriculture for Development* (Washington, DC: World Bank, 2007).

Table 16–3 summarizes the experience between 1992–93 and 1997–98 of three categories of Vietnamese farming households who earn more than 50 percent of income from agriculture (a category that makes up 47 percent of Vietnam's rural population). This was a period in which value added in Vietnamese agriculture was growing at the rapid pace of 4.1 percent per year. The table distinguishes between subsistence-oriented farmers (6 percent of rural farming households, who sell less than 10 percent of their output), market entrant households (13 percent of farming households, who began the period as subsistence farmers but ended the period as market-oriented farmers), and market-oriented farmers (28 percent of farming households, who sell more than 25 percent of their output).

Table 16–3 shows that the market-oriented households enjoyed the greatest reduction in poverty, with rates falling from 64 percent in 1992–93 to 37 percent in 1997–98 (a reduction of 27 percentage points, or 42 percent reduction relative to the base year). This group diversified away from agriculture as a source of income, and within their agricultural earnings they also diversified away from staple crops into higher-valued crops. Market entrants tended to be poorer than the market-oriented

TABLE 16–3 **Changing Market Participation among Farming Households in Vietnam**

HOUSEHOLD CHARACTERISTICS	SUBSISTENCE ORIENTED (6%)*		MARKET ENTRANT (13%)*		MARKET ORIENTED (28%)*	
	1992–93	1997–98	1992–93	1997–98	1992–93	1997–98
Assets						
Land owned (hectares)	0.37	0.43	0.50	0.57	0.60	0.72
Education of household head (years)	4.6		6.3		6.3	
Context						
Market in community (%)	31		40		47	
Outcomes						
Real income per capita (1998 dong 1,000)	893	1,702	1,138	2,042	1,359	2,978
Share of agricultural income in total income (%)	80	62	83	66	83	73
Share of households below the poverty line (%)	86	62	73	48	64	37
Share of gross agricultural output by crop type						
Staple crops (%)	78	73	70	61	63	54
High-value crops (%)	14	13	21	31	29	39

*Number in parentheses is percent of Vietnam's rural population. These three categories of farmers collectively make up the 47 percent of the Vietnam's rural population that earns most of its income from farming.

Source: Table 3.1 from The International Bank for Reconstruction and Development. The World Bank: *Agriculture for Development*, 2008. Reprinted with permission.

households but also experienced significant reductions in their poverty rate (from 73 percent to 48 percent, a reduction of 34 percent). They too diversified away from agriculture as a source of income and away from staple crop production. Even those households that remained subsistence-oriented producers participated in agricultural growth. Yet, by comparison, the subsistence households experienced the smallest reductions in poverty rates (24 percentage points, or a 28 percent reduction) and remained heavily reliant on staple agricultural production. Agriculture thus provides a variety of pathways out of poverty. In reviewing these results, de Janvry and Sadoulet make the important point that public policies designed to reduce rural poverty (a focus of Chapter 17) must be tailored to specific types of households.[24] Market-oriented households, they note, will benefit from improved competitiveness, whereas market entrants will benefit from access to assets and markets, and subsistence-oriented farmers require improved production opportunities and access to rural labor markets. In this sample, it is clear that the beneficiaries of the greatest rate of poverty reduction among these households were the market-oriented households, whose lower initial poverty rate likely reflects greater initial access to markets. These examples from Vietnam highlight the importance of income diversification within the rural economy.

While nearly all rural households participate in agriculture, they vary widely in the shares of their income coming directly from agriculture itself. Figure 16–9 illustrates this variability across countries and regions. Nearly all rural households in Ghana, Guatemala, Vietnam, and Nepal participate in agriculture. Yet, the share of household income coming from agriculture varies widely across these illustrative countries, from a high of nearly 60 percent in Ghana, to approximately 40 percent in Vietnam. Looking within these countries, Figure 16–10 reveals fairly consistent patterns of income diversification in regard to the income distribution. In general, the poorest households are the most directly dependent on agriculture as a source of income. Agricultural wage labor also declines sharply as a share of household income as income increases, while nonagricultural income shares increase substantially. These types of income diversification may reflect strategies for coping with various risks associated with farming. It is likely that relatively wealthier households have more options for diversification than relatively poor households. Poor households, lacking land or other assets, may be forced into low-wage nonfarm employment, whereas relatively better-off rural households may have access to the capital required to take advantage of local business opportunities.

The ability of the nonfarm rural economy to provide a pathway out of poverty depends on the rate of economic growth, but also on population density.[25] India and China are examples of countries in which urban crowding, high rents, and improving infrastructure have contributed to the growth of opportunities in the nonfarm rural

---

[24]de Janvry and Sadoulet, "Agricultural Growth and Poverty Reduction."
[25]Haggblade et al., eds., *Transforming the Rural Nonfarm Economy.*

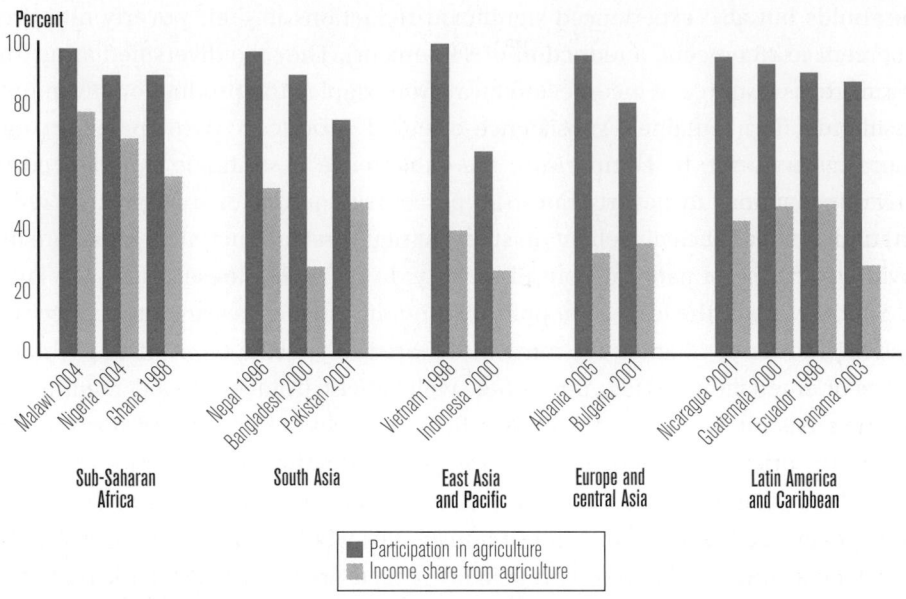

FIGURE 16-9 Percent of Households Participating in and Deriving Income from Agriculture

Source: Figure 3.2 from The International Bank for Reconstruction and Development. The World Bank: *Agriculture for Development,* 2008. Reprinted with permission.

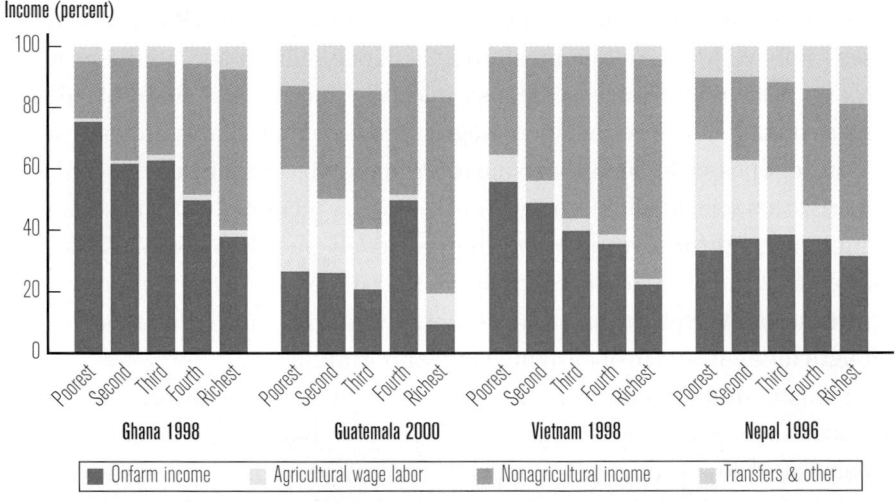

FIGURE 16-10 Sources of Income

Source: Figure 3.3 from The International Bank for Reconstruction and Development. The World Bank: *Agriculture for Development,* 2008. Reprinted with permission.

economy in a way that is much less common in sub-Saharan Africa. In most countries, the nonfarm rural economy is characterized by a high degree of heterogeneity in the scale of operations and the types of activities undertaken. Services tend to dominate manufacturing. A key point regarding the viability of nonfarm rural employment as a pathway out of poverty is that it depends on the viability of agriculture itself. Many opportunities in the nonfarm rural economy involve the processing and transportation of food, selling agricultural inputs, servicing agricultural machinery, and providing other services for which the demand arises from agriculture.

Similarly, out-migration from rural areas, although a potentially important pathway out of poverty, can reflect either a severe lack of livelihood opportunities in the rural economy or the real promise of greater welfare in urban employment. Some migration is temporary and follows agricultural seasonality, while some is permanent. From the perspective of rural development, migration can be a two-edged sword. Often, those who leave the rural economy are younger, better educated, and more skilled. Although this might reduce average labor productivity in rural areas, migrants may also be an important source of remittance income, which can contribute to improved productivity by increasing access to agricultural inputs and other productive assets.

SUMMARY

- A variety of characteristics differentiate agriculture from other sectors of the economy. These characteristics include its large share of GDP and employment, unique features of the agricultural production function, a large share of the sector's output consumed directly by its producers, and agriculture's role as a reservoir of resources.
- One of the defining characteristics of economic development is the structural transformation, during which an economy's sector proportions systematically evolve. At early stages of economic development, agriculture dominates both GDP and employment shares in the economy. Structural transformation consists of the shift of sector proportions away from agriculture toward industry and services.
- The decline in the relative size of the agricultural sector is driven, in part, by Engel's law, an implication of which is that the demand for food grows more slowly than income.
- Growth in agricultural productivity plays a critical role in facilitating the release of labor and capital from agriculture for employment in industry and services.

- Dual-sector growth models provide a stylized depiction of the interactions between the agricultural and nonagricultural sectors of the economy, specifying the conditions under which labor and capital migrate from agriculture to nonagriculture. The dominant dual-sector model, developed by Lewis and elaborated by Fei and Ranis, assumes that the defining characteristic differentiating agriculture from nonagriculture is the existence of surplus labor with low or zero marginal product.

- The Lewis and Fei-Ranis models were widely misinterpreted by policy makers in developing countries as a justification for ignoring agriculture's potential contributions to growth and concentrating investment on industrial development.

- Subsequent research demonstrated a more nuanced role for agriculture in economic growth by considering intersectoral linkages. Building on the Lewis linkages, through which agriculture supplies labor and capital to nonagriculture, Johnston and Mellor compiled a broader list of linkages, which includes agriculture's role in supplying food for nonagricultural laborers, agriculture's importance in earning the foreign exchange necessary to finance industrialization, and agriculture's role as a source of demand for the output of the nonagriculture sector.

- Intersectoral linkages also include the benefits to investment from agricultural price stabilization and agriculture's contribution to growth by supporting improved nutrition (and health) of the labor force. Agriculture provides a potent vehicle for addressing poverty, much of which is concentrated in the rural population. These contributions are direct and indirect and include both those employed in agriculture and net food consumers for whom agricultural growth reduces the price of food, often the major share of the household expenditures.

- On average, a 1 percent increase in aggregate GDP originating in agriculture has about three times the effect in reducing national poverty as a 1 percent increase in aggregate GDP originating in nonagriculture.

- Three mutually reinforcing avenues, through which agriculture can provide a pathway out of poverty, are increased on-farm output, increased engagement in rural labor markets and nonfarm rural employment, and migration to cities.

- Although many middle-income countries have grown out of their dependence on agriculture, it is clear that agriculture still has a central role to play in the development of some of today's most challenging regions, large parts of sub-Saharan Africa in particular.

17 Agricultural Development: Technology, Policies, and Institutions

The previous chapter discussed the role of agriculture in economic development, highlighting the sector's potential contributions to both economic growth and poverty alleviation. We turn now to the question of what policies and institutions are needed to maximize those contributions. Addressing that question requires a more detailed focus on the agricultural sector itself. What kinds of policies should governments adopt to promote agricultural development? Which kinds of investments are most effective? And, what kinds of institutions and rules are necessary to make the most of the policies and investments that are chosen? In short, what is required to get agriculture moving?

This chapter approaches that question by addressing the broad constraints that have limited agricultural development in general, and food production in particular, in many parts of the developing world. These constraints take many forms, and their severity varies widely across regions and countries. Some of the constraints to increasing agricultural productivity may be technological. Before the 1950s, agriculture in nearly all developing countries relied on traditional technologies and crop varieties. Traditional agriculture, while stable and well-suited to its environment, was typically characterized by low levels of productivity. Growth in agricultural output relied almost entirely on expansion of the areas under cultivation. By the 1960s, large public investments in crop science had begun to pay off in the form of seeds for improved crop varieties and packages of complementary inputs, the combination of which led to substantial increases in agricultural productivity. Yet, the benefits of this **green revolution** have been concentrated in Asia and Latin America, with comparatively little impact on agricultural development in sub-Saharan Africa.

Other constraints on agricultural development arise from unfavorable government policies (relating in particular to food prices) or from inadequate institutional support for agriculture. Both of these categories of potential constraints relate to the incentives faced by farmers. If food prices are too low, farmers may have limited incentive to expand production. In the long run, low food prices might also be a disincentive for investments in agriculture. Governments in developing countries face a fundamental dilemma in this respect: while higher food prices might provide an important incentive for farmers to increase their output, higher food prices might simultaneously increase the problems of hunger and malnutrition that are endemic in many developing countries. Farmers' incentives are also determined by institutions (that is, by the rules of the game that govern economic relations in society). Institutions governing land rights are of particular concern because farmers who own their land may have greater incentive to invest in maintaining its quality. Before exploring these issues in greater detail, we first set the scene for agriculture in developing countries by characterizing traditional agriculture and farming systems.

CHARACTERISTICS OF TRADITIONAL AGRICULTURE AND AGRICULTURAL SYSTEMS

Farms and farmers in developing countries differ widely from one another, both within and between countries. They differ in size, technology, environmental conditions, crop mix, and degree of commercialization to name but a few categories. Many farmers in poor, densely populated, countries such as Bangladesh might own no land at all and work as day laborers on other people's farms. A farmer in sub-Saharan Africa, most likely a woman, may own and cultivate several small plots totaling one to two hectares,[1] grow five or six different crops, and keep a few chickens. The current model of agricultural development in Brazil involves commercial farms of thousands of hectares, often growing soybeans for sale, coexisting with a multitude of small family farms. Given such diversity, generalizations about **traditional agriculture** are necessarily stylized. Most farms in developing countries are small-scale family farms. They consume a large portion of their own food production, though few farmers are purely subsistence farmers.[2] The livelihood, health, and productivity of farm families depend directly on the efficiency with which they allocate their scarce resources.

Traditional farms tend to be small in area, typically less than three hectares, but intensively cultivated. The demand for labor fluctuates with the agricultural seasons.

---

[1] One hectare equals 2.47 acres.

[2] This section draws on the discussion in chapters 7 and 8 in George W. Norton, Jeffrey Alwang, and William A. Masters, *Economics of Agricultural Development, World Food Systems and Resource Use*, 2nd ed. (New York: Routledge, 2010).

Labor may be in short supply during planting and harvesting time, but underemployed in other seasons. Seasonality may also bring with it wide fluctuations in food prices, as prices are at their lowest point immediately after the harvest but increase continually from that time until the next harvest. This seasonal fluctuation arises in part because traditional farms often lack adequate facilities to store their crops and must sell them shortly after harvest. The months preceding the next harvest, when prices reach their seasonal high, are often referred to as *the lean season*.

Traditional farms use traditional technologies, which typically rely on few purchased inputs (such as fertilizer, insecticides, and pesticides), grow locally indigenous crop varieties, and operate at low levels of productivity. It is widely accepted that traditional farmers allocate their resources rationally (as defined by economists) and thus do the best that they can with the few resources at their disposal. Hence the famous description by economist Theodore W. Schultz that traditional farmers are "poor but efficient."[3] Traditional farmers may also earn a significant portion of their livelihood by engaging in nonfarm rural activities, such as providing services and engaging in petty trade.

AGRICULTURAL SYSTEMS

Farming systems, characterized by technology, mix of crops and livestock, and the physical environment, vary widely across the developing world. Farming systems tend to be dominated by a small number of crops—typically a staple cereal such as rice, wheat, or corn—and many minor crops or livestock. The major types of farming systems (each of which includes a variety of subsystems) are **shifting cultivation**, **pastoral nomadism**, and **settled agriculture**. Shifting cultivation describes a system in which producers cultivate one area until its fertility is exhausted and then migrate to another plot of land. If the new areas must first be cleared of brush and the remaining brush then burned to clear the fields and increase the nutrient content of the soil, it is termed **slash and burn** agriculture. Economists George Norton, Jeffrey Alwang, and William Masters estimate that shifting cultivation is still practiced on about 15 percent of the world's cultivated area, mostly in Latin America and sub-Saharan Africa.[4] They note that shifting cultivation has been linked to soil erosion.

Pastoral nomadism, as the name implies, describes a farming system in which producers travel more or less continuously. This mobility requires that their production system be based on livestock, which the nomads shepherd across grazing areas. This system can function only in areas of low population density and is thus most frequently found in arid and semiarid agroecological zones, such as in much of the Sahel region of Africa or in the Indian state of Rajasthan. Nomadic groups typically

[3]Theodore W. Schultz, *Transforming Traditional Agriculture* (Chicago: University of Chicago Press, 1964), p. 38.

[4]Norton et al. *Economics of Agricultural Development,*" p. 150.

include five or six families traveling together with medium-size herds of livestock, perhaps 25 to 60 sheep and goats or a smaller number of camels or cattle. Increasing population densities and global climate change are particular threats to this type of farming system, which is also associated with environmental damage, resulting from overgrazing.

Settled agriculture includes a variety of systems, which as a group represent the best potential for productivity growth. Some settled agricultural systems are the following:

- *Intensive annual crops*, the most dominant system in terms of total cultivated area, typically concentrating on production of staple cereal crops (wheat, rice, and corn)
- *Mixed farming*, which builds on the interactions of crops and livestock production to manage risk and maintain soil fertility
- *Perennial crops*, generally tree crops such as bananas, coffee, cocoa, along with sugarcane, that produce for a period of years (often in combination with annual food crops)
- *Livestock systems*, producing both dairy and meat products, either through grain feeding (intensive production) or exclusively by grazing (extensive production)

Settled agriculture forms the core of efforts to modernize agriculture. The challenges are numerous, complex, and ever evolving. With cereals demand in developing countries projected to increase by nearly 50 percent between 1997 and 2020, the challenge of getting agriculture moving is urgent.[5] The starting point is a framework for diagnosing the constraints to increased productivity.

DIAGNOSING THE CONSTRAINTS TO AGRICULTURAL DEVELOPMENT

Increasing agricultural output is a high priority for most developing countries. In addition to the obvious benefit of providing greater access to food for domestic consumers, increasing agricultural output also enhances the livelihoods of those working in agriculture and related industries. In many developing countries, the agricultural

---

[5]Projections of future demand for food take into consideration not only projections of how many people will need to be fed but also projected income levels, which shape both the quantity and the type of food demanded. It is widely documented that demand for meat increases with income, and meat production implies additional demand for grain as feed. Much of this demand will be in China. Mark Rosegrant, Michael Paisner, Siet Meijer, and Julie Witcover, *Global Food Projections to 2020, Emerging Trends and Alternative Futures* (Washington, DC: International Food Policy Research Institute, 2001), p. 58.

labor force is both the largest and the poorest segment of the population. Agriculture also may involve a significant proportion of exports, as we see in such examples as cocoa exports from Ghana and coffee exports from Ethiopia. Yet, despite the substantial efforts (and ample rhetoric) that many developing countries devote to the task of increasing agricultural output, progress has often been halting and difficult. A particularly useful framework for diagnosing the constraints to increasing agricultural productivity was proposed by agricultural economist Arthur Mosher.[6]

The **Mosher framework** compares the *actual* performance of agricultural producers with their *potential* performance. Performance in this framework is represented by the output per hectare (or **yield**) of a particular commodity, often a staple cereal. Yield, even for a particular cereal, may vary widely from farm to farm in a given country. Some farmers may have better-quality land, a more conducive climate, or more regular access to water; other farmers may be closer to roads and have greater access to markets for both inputs and their output or more exposure to agricultural extension agents who teach them improved techniques. Some farmers may simply be better at farming than other farmers. The Mosher framework begins by recognizing these variations and observing the actual distribution of yields across farms, ranking them from highest to lowest. Given this distribution, the approach then addresses the question of why some yields are not higher.

What are the constraints that prevent farmers from producing more output per unit of land? The Mosher framework considers two categories of explanations: technical and economic. Figure 17–1 illustrates the sense in which we can think of technical and economic constraints as ceilings on the levels of crop yield that farmers might achieve.[7] The horizontal axis in Figure 17–1 measures the distribution of land cultivated to a particular cereal crop, and the vertical axis measures yield per hectare for that crop. Curve *a* illustrates the distribution of yields across farms, or the **achievement distribution**. These are the yields actually obtained by farmers, ordered from highest to lowest, as observed in field surveys. (This distribution would be flat if all farmers had the same yields.) Because of the differences across farms and farmers noted earlier, the achievement distribution typically slopes downward.[8]

The technical ceiling, represented by curve *t* in Figure 17–1, describes the maximum biologically possible yield given available technology. This is defined by the yield achieved by experiment stations in various regions where agricultural scientists grow the crop using the best technologies under controlled conditions.

---

[6]Arthur Mosher, *An Introduction to Agricultural Extension* (Singapore: Singapore University Press for the Agricultural Development Council, 1978).

[7]Figure 17–1 originated with Mosher, *An Introduction to Agricultural Extension*. Our discussion of this framework draws on C. Peter Timmer, Walter Falcon, and Scott Pearson, *Food Policy Analysis* (Baltimore: Johns Hopkins University Press, for the World Bank, 1983), chap. 3.

[8]Because the height of the achievement distribution measures output per hectare and the horizontal axis indicates the land area achieving each yield, the area beneath the achievement distribution measures total production.

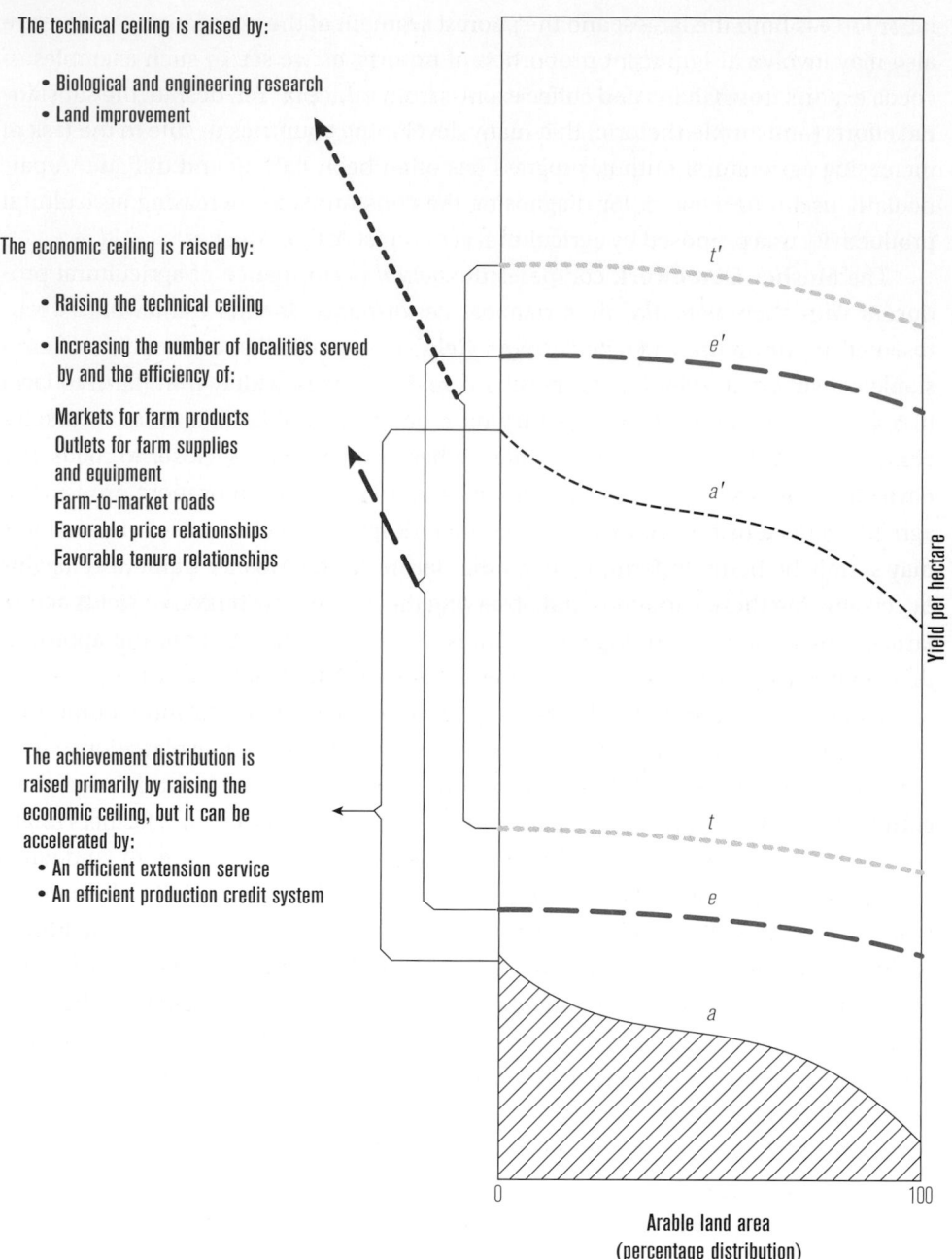

The technical ceiling is raised by:

• Biological and engineering research
• Land improvement

The economic ceiling is raised by:

• Raising the technical ceiling

• Increasing the number of localities served
 by and the efficiency of:

 Markets for farm products
 Outlets for farm supplies
 and equipment
 Farm-to-market roads
 Favorable price relationships
 Favorable tenure relationships

The achievement distribution is
raised primarily by raising the
economic ceiling, but it can be
accelerated by:
 • An efficient extension service
 • An efficient production credit system

Yield per hectare

0   100

Arable land area
(percentage distribution)

FIGURE 17-1 **The Mosher Framework**

Source: Figure 3.9 from The International Bank for Reconstruction and Development. The World Bank: *Food Policy Analysis,* 1983. The Johns Hopkins University Press for The World Bank. Reprinted with permission.

Farmers can do no better than the technical ceiling because it represents the maximum yield physically possible in a given environment. The economic ceiling, represented by curve *e*, describes the distribution of yields that are possible when all farmers maximize their profits given the opportunities available to them in a given policy environment. The economic ceiling cannot lie above what is physically possible (the technical ceiling); how far below the technical ceiling the economic ceiling lies is determined by the policy environment. Limited access to credit and the risks of uncertain weather can keep actual achievements well below the economic ceiling. As a result, the true economic ceiling (unlike the technical ceiling) cannot be observed from field data.[9] The achievement distribution, in turn, can be no higher than the economic ceiling.

Figure 17–1 also describes scenarios under which the achievement distribution and the technical and economic ceilings might be raised, thus creating space in which the achievement distribution might be raised. Improved agricultural technologies, such as improved seed varieties, can raise the technical ceiling from t to t'. This could create the possibility of raising the economic ceiling from e to e' by improving price incentives or improving the connections between farmers and markets or reforming land tenure arrangements. With the economic ceiling raised from e to e' it may then be possible to raise the achievement distribution from a to a'. Improved agricultural extension services or access to credit can contribute to raising the achievement distribution by helping farmers take maximum advantage of their technical and economic circumstances.

Figure 17–2 illustrates various relationships between the technical and economic ceilings and the achievement distribution, which may be observed in practice. *Area A* illustrates a low-productivity environment in which the achievement distribution is tightly constrained by the economic ceiling and in which the economic ceiling itself is tightly constrained by the technical ceiling. In such a setting, farmers cannot be expected to do much better, even if economic policies improve. The binding constraint in this case is the technical ceiling, which may be low owing to a lack of improved seeds. In contrast, *Area B* describes a situation in which the technical ceiling is far from binding but in which farmers are close to doing the best that they can, given what might be an unsupportive economic policy environment or poor institutions for land tenure. In *Area C*, neither the technical nor the economic ceilings are binding for most farmers, but the achievement distribution indicates that only a few farmers may be benefiting from the best available technologies. This diagnosis might point to the need for improved agricultural extension services. In *Area D*, the technical and economic ceilings are high, to the benefit of most farmers. Additional increases in yield under this scenario may require long-term investments in agricultural research to raise the technical ceiling even further.

The Mosher framework is not intended to provide a basis for detailed recommendations regarding technological development or economic policies. This framework

---

[9]Timmer et al., *Food Policy Analysis*, suggest that a general placement of the economic ceiling is possible by comparing the marginal product of fertilizer (the additional output of cereal resulting from using an additional unit of fertilizer) with the ratio of the grain price to the fertilizer price. If an additional unit of fertilizer will produce five units additional cereals output but the cost of that additional unit of fertilizer is six times the price of grain, then a rational farmer will not use additional fertilizer.

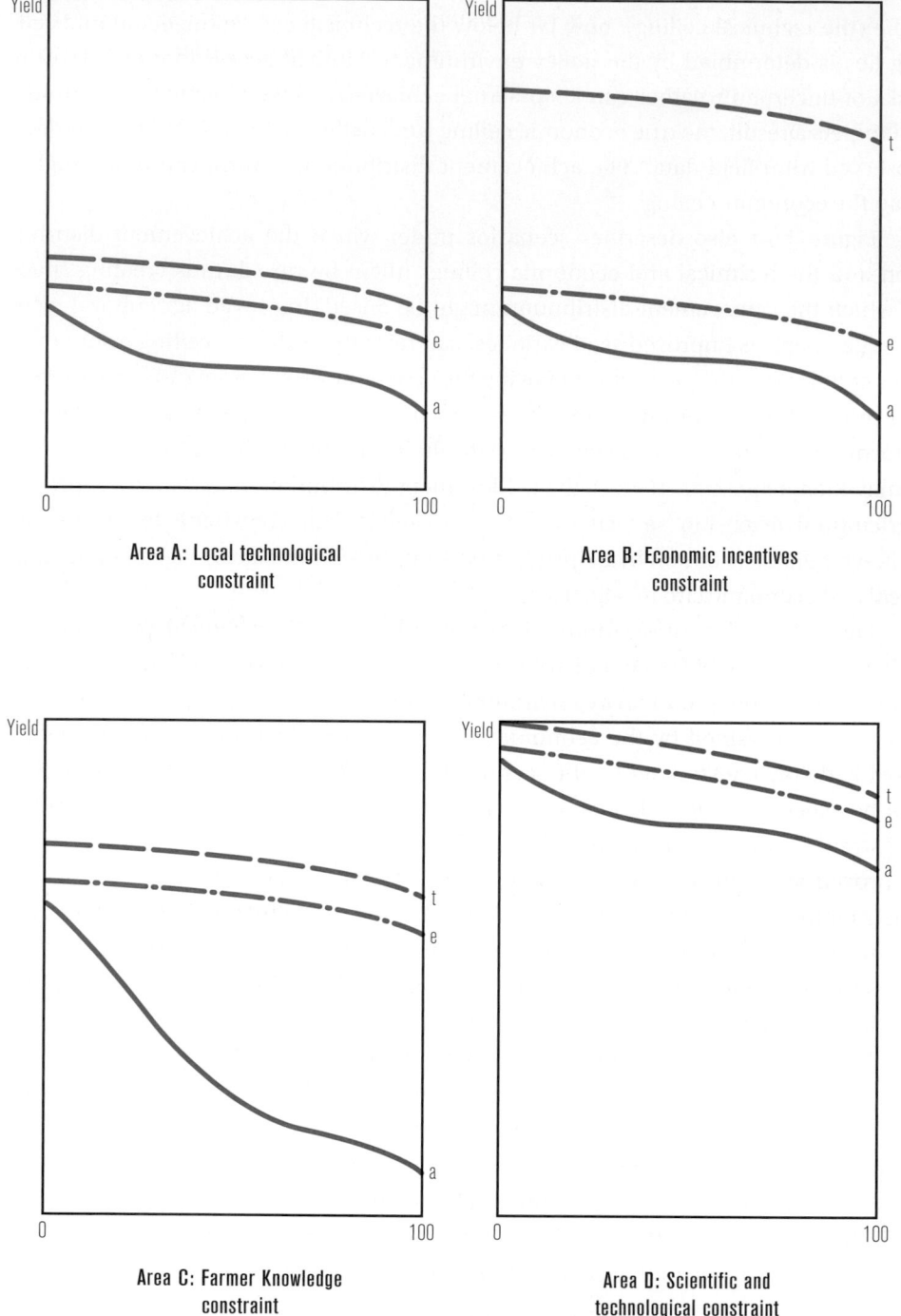

FIGURE 17-2 Possible Scenarios in the Mosher Framework

Source: Figure 3.10 from The International Bank for Reconstruction and Development. The World Bank: *Food Policy Analysis,* 1983. The Johns Hopkins University Press for The World Bank. Reprinted with permission.

provides a flexible diagnostic tool for prioritizing potential initiatives to support agricultural development and for understanding the relationships between those initiatives. The categorization of constraints as pertaining either to technology or to economic policy also provides a springboard from which to consider the challenges presented by both categories in greater detail. We begin by considering possible ways to raise the technical ceiling.

RAISING THE TECHNICAL CEILING

The height of the technical ceiling is defined in part by agroecological conditions and the agricultural potential of different areas. This is of particular concern when considering rain-fed agriculture, in which production is especially sensitive to differences in soil quality and temperature, in addition to rainfall. According to the World Bank, two-thirds of the rural population in developing countries (over 1.8 billion people) live in areas with favorable agroecological potential: about 40 percent within irrigated areas and an additional 26 percent live in areas with reliable moisture.[10] One-third of the population of the developing world (over 820 million people) live in areas with less-favorable potential, where the irrigation is scarce and rainfall is unreliable. These less-favorable areas account for 54 percent of the agricultural area but produce only 30 percent of the total value of agricultural production. Investing in irrigation is one (albeit expensive) way to raise the technical ceiling. A broader and more flexible approach to raising the technical ceiling lies in improving agricultural technology.

In the short and medium run, average technology might improve because more farms adopt improved technologies (a process known as **technology diffusion**), because the least productive farms ceased to exist, or because the best available technologies themselves improve. In the long run, however, average technology can improve only if the best technology is also improving. In this section, we consider various approaches to raising the technical ceiling on agricultural production. We examine the sources of new agricultural technologies and their impact on productivity in developing-country agriculture as well as a model of technological innovation. There has been substantial progress in developing and diffusing improved agricultural technologies, resulting in impressive gains in productivity, yet equally substantial challenges remain. Most of the gains in agricultural productivity over the past 50 years have resulted from the green revolution.

---

[10]World Bank, *World Development Report, 2008: Agriculture for Development*, (Washington, DC: World Bank, 2007), p. 54.

THE GREEN REVOLUTION[11]

The term **green revolution** refers broadly to the science-based innovations in crop breeding and farming practices, with roots dating from the 1940s, that transformed global agriculture during the second half of the last century. Agronomist Norman Borlaug is often referred to as the Father of the Green Revolution for his early scientific work in Mexico on developing **semidwarf disease resistant wheat** varieties. These new wheat varieties were an early example of **modern crop varieties (MVs)**, or **high-yielding crop varieties**, that were to become the centerpiece of the green revolution. Plants are vulnerable to a wide range of pests, diseases, and parasitic weeds that can severely reduce yields. By cross-breeding appropriate strains of wheat, Borlaug and colleagues were able to fortify the wheat then grown in Mexico against major diseases. In addition, existing wheat varieties tended to grow tall and thin as each plant competed with its neighbors for sunlight. Efforts to increase wheat yields through the application of chemical fertilizers increased the grain production of plants, but the tall thin wheat varieties tended to fall over under the added weight of grain. The creation of semidwarf wheat varieties, which had shorter and thicker stems than the traditional varieties as well as improved responsiveness to fertilizers was a solution to that problem. By the mid-1960s, similarly improved varieties of rice had also been developed and released, along with MV wheat, to farmers in Latin America and Asia.

These research programs were housed at new international agricultural research centers (IARCs). The International Maize and Wheat Improvement Center (known by its Spanish acronym, CIMMYT) was established in Mexico in 1963 (with Borlaug as its founding director), and the International Rice Research Institute (IRRI) was established in the Philippines in 1960. Both centers were supported by large grants from the Rockefeller and Ford Foundations. These were the first two centers of what is now the Consultative Group on International Agricultural Research (CGIAR), a global network of 15 research institutes. While popular accounts of the green revolution tend to focus on the early advances with MVs in the 1960s, a comprehensive review by economists Robert Evenson and Douglas Gollin suggests the green revolution remained in full swing until at least the year 2000.[12]

Part of this extended history of the green revolution is the recognition that the early successes were largely limited to wheat and rice for use in Latin America and Asia. Green revolution advances ultimately included the release of more than 8,000 MVs for 11 major crops, yet progress was uneven across both commodities and countries. Advances for certain semiarid crops, such as sorghum, millet, barley, and root crops such as cassava, did not come until the 1980s. The adoption of modern

---

[11]This section draws on R. E. Evenson and D. Gollin, "Assessing the Impact of the Green Revolution, 1960 to 2000," *Science* 300 (2003); World Bank, *World Development Report, 2008.*

[12]Evenson and Gollin, "Assessing the Impact of the Green Revolution."

Area planted with improved varieties, 2000–05, (percent of crop area).

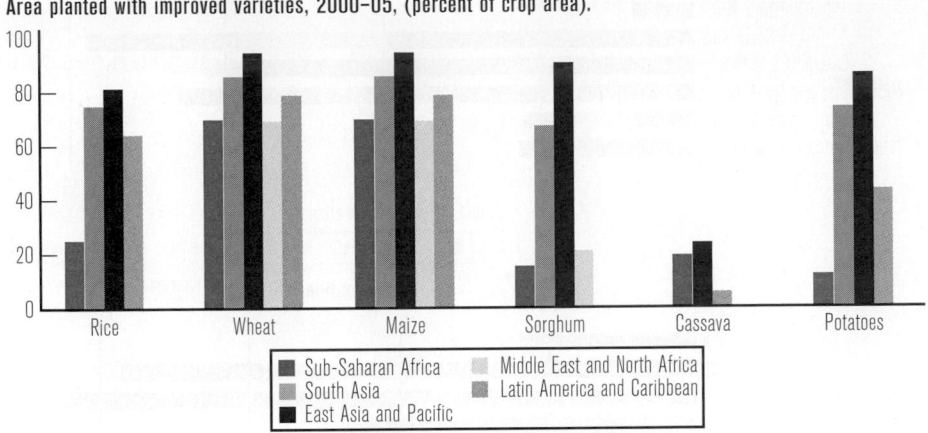

FIGURE 17-3 Modern Variety Diffusion by Crop and Region

Note: Data are provided for the period 2000–05, except for maize in some Sub-Saharan African countries where data are from 1997.
Source: Figure 7.1 from The International Bank for Reconstruction and Development. The World Bank: *Agriculture for Development,* 2008. Reprinted with permission.

varieties was widespread but unevenly distributed over time and space. Figure 17–3 illustrates the diffusion of MVs by crop and region. By the early 2000s, adoption rates across commodities in East Asia were uniformly high (exceeding 80 percent, with the exception of cassava, a root crop that plays only a small role in Asian diets). MVs for major commodities had also diffused widely through South Asia and Latin America. Yet, with the exception of wheat, adoption of MVs in sub-Saharan Africa by the early 2000s lagged far behind other developing regions. Adoption of modern varieties for rice and sorghum in sub-Saharan Africa are particularly low in comparison with other regions, even though these two crops are widely grown in the region.

Lagging adoption of MVs in sub-Saharan Africa has several explanations. One problem has been that agroecological conditions in Africa are extremely diverse—sometimes even within a single country. Another problem, particularly before the 1980s, was that the new varieties were engineered to be highly responsive to purchased inputs, such as chemical fertilizers, or (especially in the case of rice) thrived best in irrigated fields. These complementary inputs have been less common in Africa than in Asia or Latin America, limiting the ability of African farmers to benefit from green revolution innovations. Figure 17–4 demonstrates the stark disparities in input intensity across regions. By the year 2002, nearly 40 percent of cropland in South Asia was irrigated, compared to only 4 percent of the cropland in sub-Saharan Africa. Similarly, fertilizer application per hectare in sub-Saharan Africa remained but a small fraction of average fertilizer applications in other regions.

Most of the MVs were the result of genetic research performed at the international research centers. Yet the real measure of success in agricultural research is not the number of varietal releases, but their impact in farmers' fields. In the language of

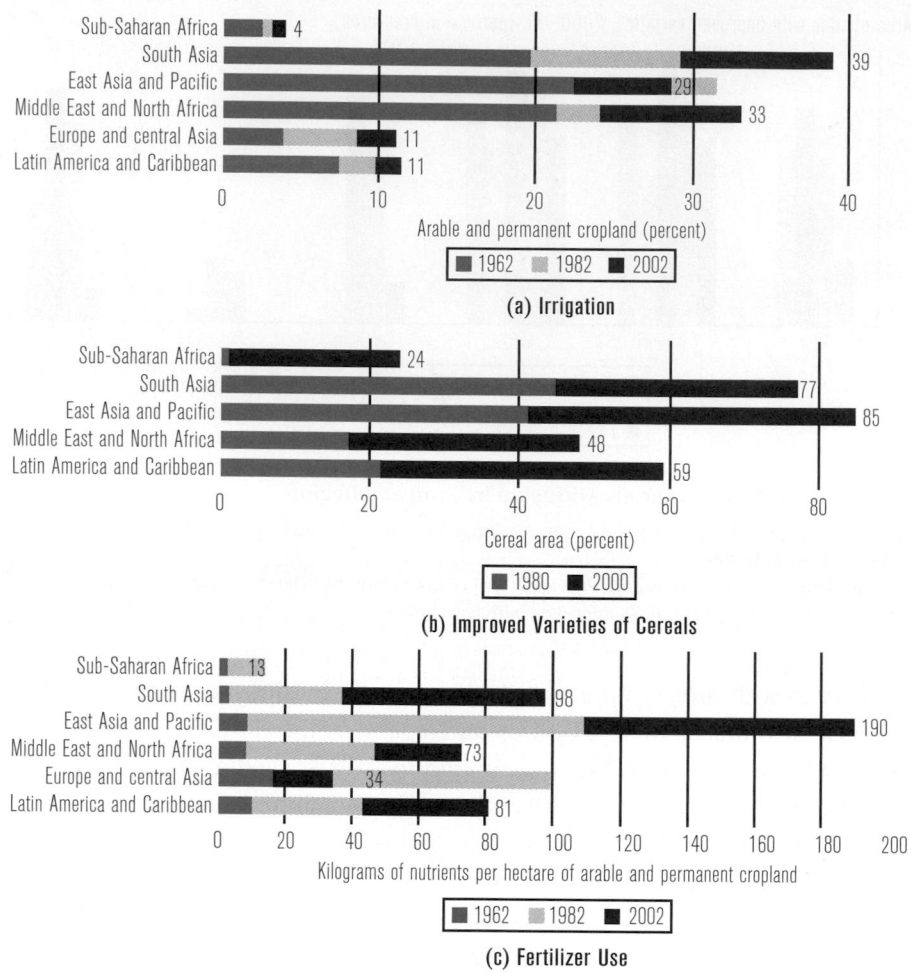

FIGURE 17-4 **Use of Agricultural Inputs by Region**

Source: Figure 2.2 from The International Bank for Reconstruction and Development. The World Bank: *Agriculture for Development,* 2008. Reprinted with permission.

the Mosher framework, new agricultural technologies may raise the technical ceiling, but it raises the achievement distribution only if those technologies are widely adopted and properly used by farmers. Table 17–1 describes growth rates by production, area, and yield for food crops by region, distinguishing between the early and late green revolution periods. The growth rate of output declined significantly from the early to the late green revolution period in every region of the developing world except for sub-Saharan Africa. These changes in the rates of output growth were driven primarily by changes in the growth rates of agricultural area, which fell in all regions except Africa.

Table 17–1 distills the growth rate of crop yield into the contributions of MVs and the contributions to yield of increases in the use of other inputs. During the

TABLE 17-1 Average Annual Growth Rates of Food Production, Area, Yield, and the Contribution of Modern Varieties

	EARLY GREEN REVOLUTION (1961–80)	LATE GREEN REVOLUTION (1981–2000)
Asia		
Production	3.65	2.11
Area	0.51	0.02
Yield	3.12	2.09
MV contributions to yield	0.68	0.97
Other input per hectare*	2.44	1.12
Latin America		
Production	3.08	1.63
Area	1.47	−0.51
Yield	1.59	2.15
MV contributions to yield	0.46	0.77
Other input per hectare*	1.12	1.38
Middle East and North Africa		
Production	2.53	2.12
Area	0.95	0.61
Yield	1.56	1.51
MV contributions to yield	0.17	0.78
Other input per hectare*	1.39	0.72
Sub-Saharan Africa		
Production	1.70	3.19
Area	0.52	2.82
Yield	1.17	0.36
MV contributions to yield	0.10	0.47
Other input per hectare*	1.07	−0.11
All developing countries		
Production	3.20	2.19
Area	0.68	0.39
Yield	2.50	1.81
MV contributions to yield	0.52	0.86
Other input per hectare*	1.98	0.95

*Refers to such factors as fertilizer and machinery. Growth rates of other inputs are taken as a residual. MV, modern crop variety.

Source: R. E. Evenson and D. Gollin, "Assessing the Impact of the Green Revolution, 1960 to 2000," *Science* 300 (2003).

early years (before 1980), as revealed by the table, MVs played a large role in driving yield growth in Latin America and Asia but made little contribution in other regions. For example, between 1961 and 1980 in Latin America, crop production grew at an annual rate of just over 3 percent, of which nearly 1.6 percent was the result of growth in yield. MVs explained over one-fourth of that 1.6 percent growth in yield. Over the same period, however, MV's accounted for only 0.097 percentage points of the

1.17 percent per year growth rate of yield in sub-Saharan Africa (thus explaining only 8 percent of the growth in Africa's crop yields).

For the developing world as a whole, crop production grew at an average rate of 3.2 percent, of which just under 0.7 percent was the result of growth in an agricultural area and 2.5 percent the results of growth in yield. The use of MVs accounted for 0.5 percentage points of the growth rate in yield, or just over one-fifth. Between 1981 and 2000, the rate of production growth for all developing countries (on average) fell to about 2.2 percent per year, whereas yield growth fell to 1.8 percent. Although yields grew more slowly after 1981, it is notable that yield growth accounted for a larger share of growth in total output post-1981, and the share of yield growth explained by MVs increased to nearly one half. Sub-Saharan Africa was the only region in which food production accelerated in the late green revolution, in part as a result of the substantially increased contribution of MVs in that period.

What would the world have been like by the year 2000 had the green revolution *not* occurred? Economists at the International Food Policy Research Institute (IFPRI; the economic policy center of the CGIAR) used a simulation model to answer this hypothetical question.[13] If no MVs had been released in developing countries, agricultural yields in developing countries would have been around 20 percent lower by the year 2000 than their actual level in that year. Cropped area in both developed and developing countries would have been 3 to 5 percent greater than their actual level, and crop prices would have been 35 to 66 percent higher. Crop production in developing countries would have been 16 to 19 percent lower than they actually were by the year 2000. The consequences of the green revolution for human welfare were enormous. The IFPRI simulation exercise indicates that had the green revolution *not* occurred, the percent of malnourished children in developing countries would have been 6 to 8 percent greater than it actually was (a difference of 32 to 42 million preschool children), and calorie consumption per capita in developing countries would have been about 14 percent lower than it actually was by the year 2000. Norman Borlaug was awarded the Nobel Peace Prize in 1970 for his pioneering contributions to the green revolution.

RECENT TRENDS IN AGRICULTURAL PRODUCTIVITY

Figure 17–5 illustrates trends in cereals yields, first comparing developed and developing countries and then distinguishing between developing regions. It is clear from Figure 17–5a that cereals yields in the developed countries are higher and have grown faster than in the developing countries. Among regions of the developing world, the differences are also striking. Although the various regions depicted in Figure 17–5b attained similar cereal yields in the early 1960s, they diverged quite dramatically

---

[13]This simulation exercise is summarized by Evenson and Gollin, "Assessing the Impact of the Green Revolution."

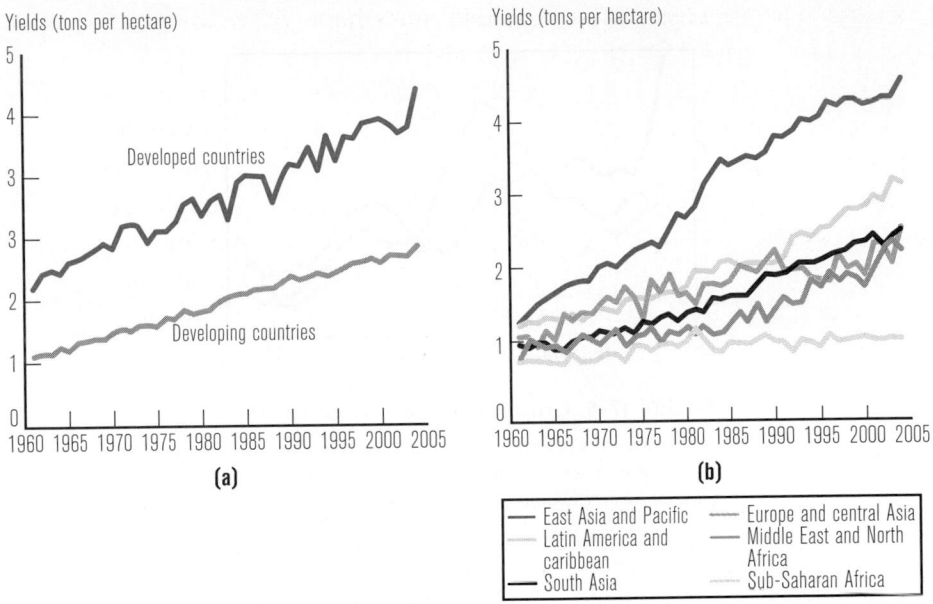

FIGURE 17-5 Cereal Yield Trends by Region

Source: Figure 2.1 from The International Bank for Reconstruction and Development. The World Bank: *Agriculture for Development,* 2008. Reprinted with permission.

by 2005. Consistent with Table 17–1, the flat trend in cereals yields for sub-Saharan Africa contrast sharply with the rapid growth experienced in East Asia, where by 2005, average yields were more than four times the level found in Africa.

While the levels of yields in cereals illustrated in Figure 17–5 increased in most regions, the *growth rates* of those increases, while remaining positive, have slowed over time. Figure 17–6 captures this disturbing global trend: The growth rate of yields in the world's major cereal crops (wheat, rice, and maize) has trended strongly downward since the 1980s. This slowdown in productivity growth may reflect that the easy gains of the green revolution's early years have been exhausted. It may also represent declining public expenditures for agricultural research and development (R&D) during the 1990s. In sub-Saharan Africa, for example, public agricultural R&D spending declined in nearly half of the 27 countries with available data, as did the R&D share of agricultural gross domestic product (GDP) for the region as a whole.[14] Yet, it is also important to recognize that agricultural innovations must be continually renewed. The stability of yield gains depends heavily on the resistance of new varieties to various pest and disease risks. As those threats evolve, agricultural technology must strive to stay one step ahead. In summarizing this problem, the World Bank's *World Development Report 2008* makes reference to the Red Queen in Lewis Carroll's *Through the Looking Glass,* who complained, "Now here, you see, it takes all the

[14]World Bank, *World Development Report, 2008.*

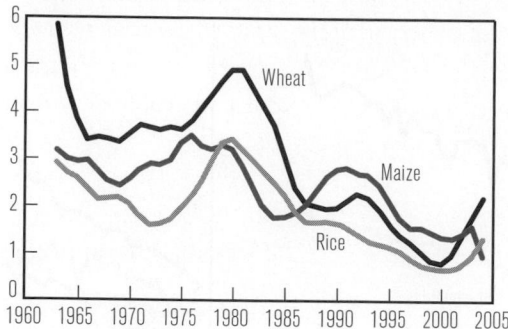

FIGURE 17-6 **Growth Rates of Cereals Yields**

Source: Figure 2.12 from The International Bank for
Reconstruction and Development. The World Bank:
Agriculture for Development, 2008. Reprinted with permission.

running you can do to keep in the same place."[15] That report then notes that one-third
to one-half of current investments and crop breeding may be aimed simply at maintaining past gains.

This discussion of agricultural productivity trends highlights the diversity of experience across the developing world, yet a consistent theme is the relative lack of progress
in sub-Saharan Africa. Figure 17–7 compares average maize yields with potential maize
yields (the so-called **yield gap**) for selected countries in sub-Saharan Africa. In each
case, average on-farm achievement falls far short of the technical ceiling implied by the
maize yields obtained on demonstration plots, reflecting the best possible conditions

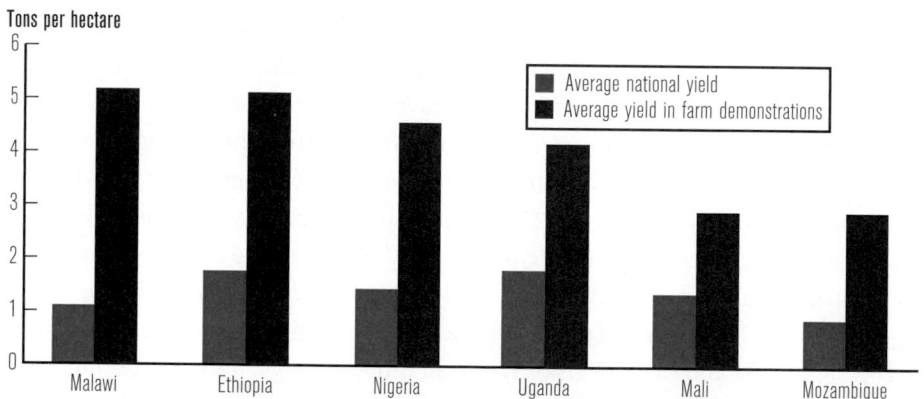

FIGURE 17-7 **The Yield Gap for Maize in Selected African Countries.**

Source: Figure 2.13 from The International Bank for Reconstruction and Development. The World Bank:
Agriculture for Development, 2008. Reprinted with permission.

[15]World Bank, *World Development Report, 2008,* p. 161.

and optimal inputs available in each country. Yield gaps in Asian agriculture tend to be much smaller, consistent with the more rapid rate of yield growth seen in Figure 17–5. The problems in sub-Saharan Africa include the greater complexity of its agricultural systems and diversity of agroclimatic conditions (both of which have increased the challenges of creating new technologies for use there), in addition to its relative lack of market infrastructure and lower levels of education. Box 17–1 introduces an important theory about how the kinds of agricultural technologies that are invented depend on economic circumstances, the theory of induced innovation.

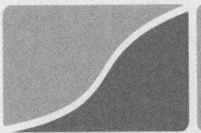

BOX 17–1 A MODEL OF INDUCED TECHNICAL CHANGE IN AGRICULTURE

The green revolution technologies that were so effective in Asia tended to emphasize biological technology. Improved seed varieties that were highly responsive to chemical fertilizers formed the core of the innovations. Biological approaches primarily work to increase output per unit of land and we can think of them as **land-saving technologies**. In contrast, mechanical innovations, such as better tractors and improved harvesting machinery, enable the cultivation of a larger area per worker. We can think of mechanical approaches as **labor-saving technologies**. Is it merely coincidence that land-saving technologies were developed for application in Asia, where labor is abundant and land relatively scarce? The broad idea that links factor endowments to the evolution of technical change is the **theory of induced innovation**.

The notion that new agricultural technologies can economize on either land or labor illustrates that multiple paths of technology development are possible. Advances in mechanical technology are motivated by the desire to reduce labor costs; advances in biological technology are motivated by the desire to increase crop output per unit of land (or animal output per unit of feed). Mechanical technology may be more appropriate in settings in which the supply of labor is constrained; biological technology might be more appropriate in settings in which the supply of land is constrained. The theory of induced innovation, popularized by economists Yujiro Hayami and Vernon Ruttan, addresses the question of which among these alternative paths of technology development is *actually* followed. Its answer is that technology evolves in response to changes in relative factor prices, economizing on the relatively scarce (and hence more costly) factors of production.[a]

[a]This theory thus portrays technical change as an endogenous process, in which realized technologies are determined by economic circumstances.

The figure below illustrates the process of induced innovation for the case of biological technology. The model builds on the concept of a **production isoquant**, which describes the various combinations of inputs (in this case, land and fertilizer) that can be combined to produce a given quantity of output.[b] The induced innovation model posits that at any given time, a large family of potential technologies could be invented. Each of these technologies can be represented by its own isoquant. We will consider the evolution of technology between two points in time (the initial point being designated "time zero," as indicated by the subscript 0, and the other point in time similarly designated as "time 1", as indicated by the subscript 1). In the figure, the isoquant i_0 might represent a particular crop variety, which could be grown in a given quantity by combining fertilizer and land in any of the combinations that lie along i_0. The more elastic (*dashed*) isoquant, i_0^*, is termed the **innovation possibility curve**.[c] In this model, the innovation possibility curve traces the envelope (or boundary) of the entire family of potential crop technologies that might be invented at that

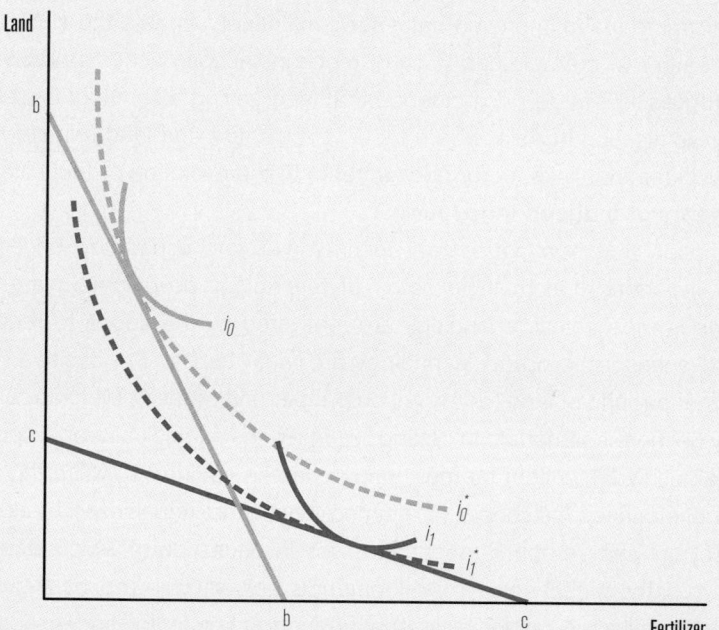

[b]We revisit this construct and provide a more detailed exposition in the discussion of producer price incentives later in this chapter.

[c]The elasticity of an isoquant refers to the ease with which producers can substitute one input for another in response to changes in relative input prices. Graphically, an inelastic isoquant will have more of an "L" shape (indicating little scope for substituting one input for another), whereas a more elastic isoquant will curve more gradually.

time zero. The line *bb* is the **isocost line**. Every point on *bb* reflects a combination of fertilizer and land use with the same total cost. Its slope reflects the relative price of fertilizer to land. The specific crop technology that gets invented in the first period (i_0) is the one that minimizes input costs with relative prices of fertilizer and land indicated by the slope of line *bb*.

Technological progress is represented by a shift over time of the innovation possibilities curve toward the origin of the graph in the figure. This reflects the idea that technological progress permits the production of a given quantity of output using a smaller quantity of inputs. Thus by time 1 in this graph, the innovation possibilities curve has shifted inward from i_0^* to i_1^*. Suppose that between time 0 and time 1 fertilizer production increases, thus reducing the relative price of fertilizer to land. This is reflected in the flatter isocost line *cc*. In response to this change in relative factor prices, the induced innovation model suggests that a new technology (depicted by isoquant i_1) is developed, a new crop variety that is more responsive to fertilizer (perhaps semidwarf wheat). This new technology will lie along the envelope of technologies that could potentially be developed at time 1, summarized by the new innovation possibilities curve, i_1^*. This particular crop variety is invented because it minimizes production costs given the new set of relative factor prices. The key intuition is that the technology *actually* invented from among potential innovations is the one that most efficiently economizes on the factor of production that has become more costly.

Source: This box draws on Yujiro Hayami and Vernon Ruttan, *Agricultural Development: An International Perspective* (Baltimore, MD: Johns Hopkins University Press, 1985).

RAISING THE ECONOMIC CEILING

The height of the economic ceiling in the Mosher framework is determined by a combination of economic incentives, farmers' access to markets, and institutions such as the rules governing land tenure. We begin by considering the impact of prices on farm-level decision making and resource allocation. The goals of agricultural development strategies may include increasing the sector's output or promoting rural welfare. In either case, a price environment that provides positive incentives to producers and makes agriculture a profitable enterprise typically calls for relatively high food prices. Such strategies are inevitably constrained by the harmful implications of high food prices for consumers, many of whom may be poor and allocate large budget shares to food, the poorest of whom may be highly vulnerable to malnutrition.

The conflicting interests of producers and consumers in regard to food prices are a central challenge for policy makers, one that is sufficiently pervasive to be termed by economists C. Peter Timmer, Walter Falcon, and Scott Pearson "the food policy dilemma."

FOOD PRODUCTION ANALYSIS[16]

Designing policies to promote agricultural development first requires an understanding of how farmers respond to price incentives. This section addresses three dimensions of decision making by farmers: what mix of crops to produce, what combination of inputs to use in production, and what quantity to produce. Poor farmers, they have to make all these decisions simultaneously. We have the luxury to examine them in turn, and then see how they combine to describe the supply curve for food. We assume in each case that farmers allocate their resources with an eye toward maximizing profits, which implies that their choices equalize marginal costs and marginal benefits.

WHAT TO PRODUCE? THE PRODUCT-PRODUCT DECISION

Farmers in developing countries rarely produce only one crop; indeed in sub-Saharan Africa it is common to see four or five different crops simultaneously planted in the same field (an approach known as **intercropping**). Whether multiple crops are grown in the same field or in different fields, farmers must decide on an optimal crop mix. Economists model this decision by considering how the opportunities made available by nature interact with market incentives. Figure 17-8 illustrates this interaction between markets and nature with a **production possibility frontier** and an **isorevenue line**. In practice farmers must determine their crop mix by choosing from among a large number of commodities. We simplify this problem by reducing it to a choice between only two commodities, for instance corn and beans. In this case, the production possibility curve, *IKLE*, describes all of the different possible combinations of corn and beans that a farmer might grow in a given field in a single season. If the farmer were to devote all of his or her resources to the production of beans alone, output would be *OE*. Similarly, if the farmer devoted all resources to the production of corn, output would be *OI*. Typically however farmers will grow some of each crop. The slope of the production possibility frontier, known as the **marginal rate of technical substitution**, thus changes at every point along the frontier. At any given point that slope equals $\Delta C / \Delta B$, where the Greek letter Δ (capital delta) indicates changes in the quantity produced of corn (*C*) and beans (*B*). The production possibilities frontier bows outward to reflect the increasing marginal cost of produc-

[16]This section draws on Timmer et al., *Food Policy Analysis*, chap. 3.

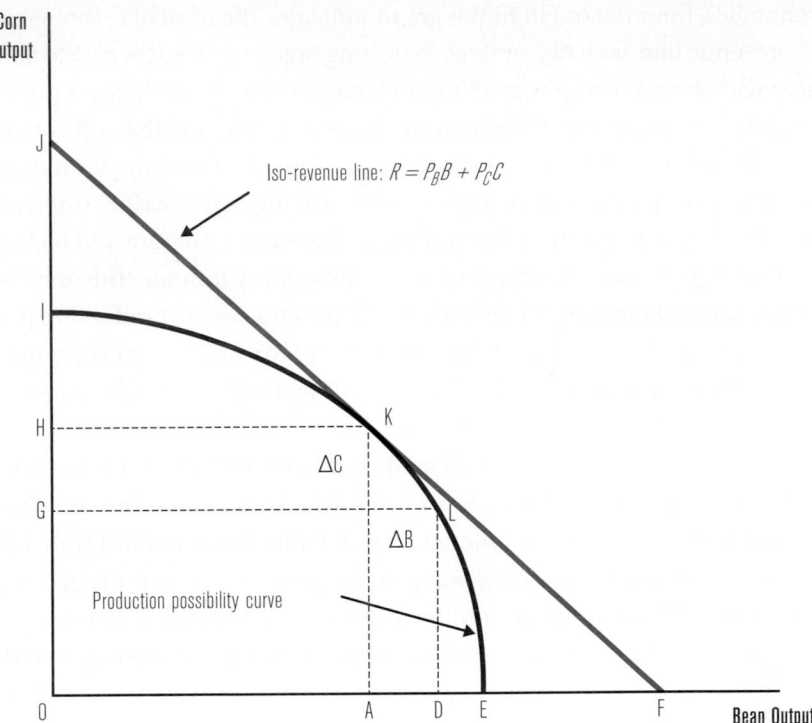

FIGURE 17-8 The Product–Product Decision

ing either commodity. This implies that a farmer who was initially growing a crop mix that included lots of beans but little corn might be able to increase corn output significantly by sacrificing a relative small quantity of bean production.

The production possibility frontier indicates all of the **technically efficient** combinations of corn and bean output. A crop mix indicated by a choice inside the production possibility frontier would be inefficient and would indicate a yield gap, as discussed earlier. A technically efficient crop mix is necessary for profit maximization (or **economic efficiency**), but it is not sufficient. The profit maximizing combination of corn and bean output can be determined only with reference to how markets value each of those crops. The total revenue generated by any particular combination of corn and bean output depends on their respective prices, P_C and P_B. The revenue generated by producing either commodity equals the price of that commodity times the quantity produced, and total revenue (R) is the sum over all of the commodities: $R = P_B B + P_C C$. For given quantities of corn and beans, this equation describes a constant level of total revenue and is known as an isorevenue line. As represented in Figure 17–8, the isorevenue line has a slope equal to $-P_B/P_C$.[17] The distance of the

---

[17]We can see that the slope of the isorevenue line is described by these relative prices by solving the revenue function for C.

isorevenue line from the origin in the graph indicates the level of revenue along any given isorevenue line, with higher lines indicating higher revenue. A profit-maximizing producer will choose a crop mix that places him or her on the highest possible isorevenue line, where *possible* is defined by the production possibility frontier. This is indicated in Figure 17–8 by the combination at point K, where the farmer produces OA quantity of beans and OH quantity of corn. The highest possible isorevenue line that the farmer can attain given the limitations imposed by nature and technology is the one that is just tangent to the production possibility frontier. This means that at point K the slope of the isorevenue line equals the slope of the production possibility frontier, that is $\Delta C/\Delta B = -P_B/P_C$. This is the only crop mix that is economically efficient among the set of technically efficient combinations defined by the production possibility frontier.[18]

We can see that the crop mix indicated by point K satisfies our requirements for profit maximization, that marginal revenue equals marginal cost by considering the implications of moving along the production possibility frontier from a point like L to K. This move would require forgoing bean production in the quantity ΔB, incurring marginal cost $\Delta B * P_B$, to produce additional corn of the amount ΔC, generating marginal revenue $\Delta C * P_C$. Setting marginal cost equal to marginal revenue would give us the expression $\Delta B * P_B = \Delta C * P_C$. Rearranging this expression, dividing both sides first by ΔB and then by P_C, gives us $\Delta C/\Delta B = -P_B/P_C$. Thus the tangency between the isorevenue line and the production possibility frontier meets our criterion for profit maximization.

Beans are an important source of protein. Suppose policy makers sought to increase the availability of protein for their population. This framework shows that they could do so by increasing the price of beans relative to the price of corn. This would increase the slope of the isorevenue line, shifting the tangency with the production possibility frontier to a point such as L, where bean output would be OD rather than OA. Similarly, many countries have recently sought to diversify their agricultural exports to include nontraditional products such as fresh vegetables. This product–product framework demonstrates that governments might promote such diversification by intervening to raise the relative prices of those nontraditional export goods. This framework should also help policy makers recognize that such a change of incentives designed to increase output of one commodity generally comes at the cost of reduced output of something else. In some cases, reducing output of something else might be the goal. Efforts to reduce poppy cultivation in Afghanistan, for instance, need to consider the relative prices local farmers face for poppy versus wheat, which is their primary alternative.

---

[18]In terms of the Mosher framework, we could think of point K as indicating a point on the achievement distribution that touches both the economic and the technical ceilings.

HOW TO PRODUCE IT? THE FACTOR–FACTOR DECISION

In addition to deciding what mix of crops to grow, farmers must also determine the least costly combination of inputs needed to produce a given quantity of output. This too is a multidimensional problem in that farmers face choices over multiple inputs, including land, labor, capital, fertilizers, water, pesticides, and insecticides. Again we simplify this problem by reducing it to two dimensions, capital and labor. Figure 17-9 illustrates farmers' factor–factor decision problem. As before, the optimal choice depends on the interaction between the constraints imposed by nature and those imposed by the market. The curve *MDEN* in Figure 17–9, known as an iso-quant, describes the different combinations of capital and labor that farmers may combine to produce a given quantity of output of a particular crop (in this illustration, 100 kilograms of rice). The slope of an isoquant changes at every point on the curve, and is given by $\Delta L/\Delta K$, where L is the quantity of labor and K is the quantity of capital employed in production. In practice, farmers may face a range of discrete choices of technique in producing that 100 kilograms of rice. Point P on the isoquant employs lots of capital and little labor and may indicate a production system built around combine harvesters or other large farm machines. In contrast, point D on the isoquant employs lots of labor and little capital and may thus rely on hand labor using small tools.

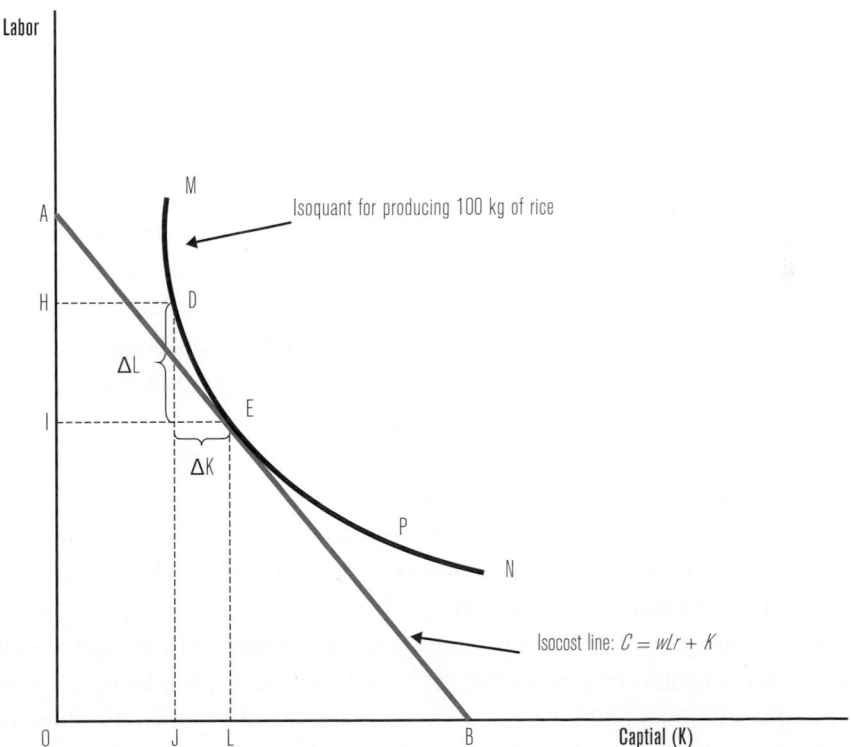

FIGURE 17-9 The Factor–Factor Decision

Every point on a given isoquant indicates a technically efficient combination of capital and labor for producing that quantity of output. Any combination of capital and labor that lies above the given isoquant would be inefficient because the same quantity of output could be produced using less of one or both inputs. Only one point among this set of technically efficient combinations of inputs is economically efficient, defined here as the minimum cost combination of inputs capable of producing a given quantity of output. Finding this optimal combination requires consideration of how the market values capital and labor. If factor markets are competitive, labor is paid a wage that reflects its marginal product. Similarly, producers must also pay for the capital (machinery) they employ. If there is a market for machinery, then the cost of renting a given machine is called the **rental rate of capital** and is analogous to the wage paid to labor. If the hourly price of labor is its wage (w) and the hourly price of capital is the rental rate paid for its use (r), then the cost of hiring a given number of workers is $w*L$ and the cost of hiring a given quantity of capital services is $r*K$, then the total cost (C) of producing 100 kilograms of rice is given by $C = wL + rK$. This cost line is called an **isocost** line because the total cost of production is the same at every point on the line. The isocost line in Figure 17–9 has a slope equal to $-r/w$, the relative factor prices.

A cost-minimizing producer will want to choose the least cost combination of capital and labor that still enables the production of a given quantity of output. In Figure 17–9, this choice corresponds to choosing the lowest isocost line that permits production of 100 kilograms of rice. This is the isocost line that is just tangent to the isoquant, point E in the graph. This unique tangency means that the slope of the isoquant is equal to the slope of the isocost line, or $\Delta L/\Delta K = -r/w$. Does this point satisfy our criterion for profit maximization that marginal cost equal marginal revenue? Imagine moving from the input mix indicated by point D to point E. Doing so would imply substituting capital in the amount ΔK for labor in the amount $-\Delta L$. The marginal cost of this substitution is $-\Delta K*r$ and the marginal benefit (savings) is $\Delta L*w$. Equating marginal cost and marginal benefit in this case implies that $-\Delta K*r = \Delta L*w$. Rearranging these terms, as above, gives us $\Delta L/\Delta K = -r/w$, indicating that the tangency of the isoquant and isocost line describes the profit-maximizing (cost-minimizing) mix of capital and labor to produce 100 kilograms of rice.

This framework also gives rise to a number of interesting policy applications. Is farm mechanization always appropriate? This framework suggests that if labor in a given country is abundant (and, by extension, inexpensive) and capital is scarce (and expensive), then a capital-intensive production technique may not be economically efficient. If policy makers want to increase rural employment, then policies such as overvalued exchange rates (that make imported capital artificially cheap) or ceilings on interest rates (potentially reducing the rental rate on capital below its equilibrium value) would be a bad idea. Such interventions would reduce the slope of the isocost line, creating an incentive for producers to shift their choice of technique in Figure 17–9 from point E toward a point like P. This would motivate an inefficient allocation of resources (adding to unemployment in this case) if these altered factor prices did not reflect society's true opportunity cost of labor and capital.

HOW MUCH TO PRODUCE? THE FACTOR–PRODUCT DECISION

Having decided what to produce and how to produce it, farmers must still decide how much to produce of any given crop. This relates directly to the decision of how much of any given input to use in production. The physical relationship that maps the quantity of inputs used to the quantity of output produced (once again, nature's constraints) is represented by the production function. In presenting the Solow growth model in Chapter 4, we introduced a production function that represented the entire economy's output. The production function in Figure 17–10 has all of the same technical characteristics as the previous ones, but now describes output for a particular crop. We can consider a two-dimensional relationship between output and a single input if we are clear that the resulting figure implicitly holds all other inputs at a constant level. A production function such as curve *EJKP* in Figure 17–10 thus maps the quantity of fertilizer used to rice yield per hectare (for given fixed quantities of all other inputs). The curve *EJKP* reflects **diminishing marginal returns** to fertilizer use. This implies that an additional unit of fertilizer applied when fertilizer use is low, such as ΔF in Figure 17–10, may bring forth a relatively large output response in rice, ΔR. Yet, the increase in rice resulting from additional units of fertilizer grows

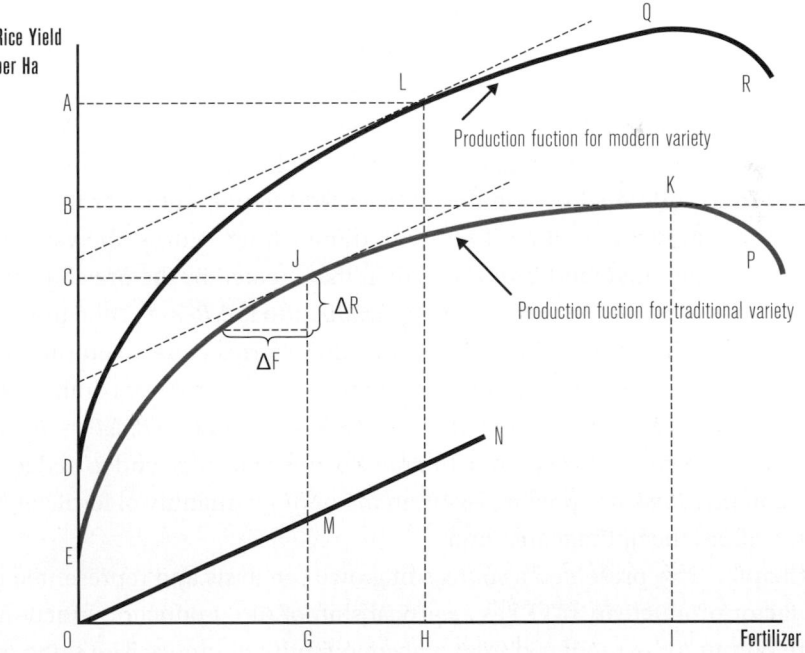

FIGURE 17-10 Agricultural Production Functions and the Factor–Product Decision

smaller with each incremental unit of fertilizer applied and ultimately may reduce rice output (as happens beyond point K in the graph) if too much fertilizer is applied. These diminishing returns to fertilizer are reflected in the decreasing slope of the production function as fertilizer use increases. The slope of the production function at any point, $\Delta R / \Delta F$, is the **marginal product** of fertilizer.

The maximum rice yield in Figure 17–10 is attained at point K, where fertilizer use is OI. Yet, the presence of diminishing returns to fertilizer makes it unlikely that OI would be the profit-maximizing quantity of fertilizer. As in the previous cases, we must consider the interaction between what nature makes possible (for a given technology) and the economic incentives signaled by the market. In this case, we must consider the market prices for rice and fertilizer. The ratio of these prices is the rate at which farmers can exchange rice for fertilizer. In Figure 17–10, the slope of line ON is given by the relative prices of fertilizer and rice, P_F / P_R (increases in the price of fertilizer make this line steeper, whereas increases in the price of rice make it flatter). How much fertilizer would a profit-maximizing farmer apply (and hence how much rice would he or she produce)? So long as the value of the additional rice produced by applying additional fertilizer is greater than the cost of that additional fertilizer, it pays to use more fertilizer.

In Figure 17–10, line ON reflects the cost of production while the production function $EJKP$ reflects revenue. Profits are maximized at the point at which the difference in height between the production function and the cost function are greatest, which we find by shifting the line ON upward (in a parallel manner) until it is just tangent to the production function (which happens at point J). A profit-maximizing farmer will thus apply quantity OG of fertilizer and produce quantity OC of rice. It is only at point J that the slope of the production function (the marginal product of fertilizer) exactly equals the relative price of fertilizer to rice, or $\Delta R / \Delta F = P_F / P_R$. Applying the criterion that marginal cost equal marginal revenue, we must compare the value of the additional rice produced by an additional unit of fertilizer with the cost of that additional unit of fertilizer. With diminishing returns, the value created by each additional unit of fertilizer is less than that created by the previous unit. The marginal revenue created by increasing rice production is $\Delta R \times P_R$, and the marginal cost of using more fertilizer is $\Delta F \times P_F$. Setting these terms equal to one another and rearranging as in the previous examples, we find that the profit-maximizing combination of fertilizer use and rice output occurs precisely where $\Delta R / \Delta F = P_F / P_R$, our expression for the tangency at point J. In practice, most farmers tend to hedge against weather and price risk by applying less than the optimal quantity of fertilizer (even if they could afford the optimal quantity).

In Chapter 3 we presented a sources of growth analysis and represented growth in total factor productivity (TFP) as a vertical shift of the production function, leading more output to be produced from a given quantity of inputs. The same concept applies to the agricultural production function depicted in Figure 17–10. TFP growth in agriculture would be reflected in a vertical shift of the production function in Figure 17–10, to curve $DLQR$. This increase in agricultural TFP reflects that a given quantity of fertilizer application results in a higher level of rice output per hectare than previously. Indeed, if rice is responsive to fertilizer, the optimal allocation of rice may increase with productivity growth, from *OG* to *OH*, even though the relative price of fertilizer to rice is unchanged.

As in the previous farm-level decision models, important policy implications arise. Governments can intervene to encourage increased food production by reducing the relative price of fertilizer to rice (or the relative price of inputs to outputs more generally). Doing so flattens the relative price line, leading to a tangency with the production function with increased fertilizer being used to produce increased rice. The choice regarding which policies to deploy is complex. Governments can lower this price ratio either by increasing the price of rice or by reducing the cost of fertilizer (or both). Either choice is likely to be both expensive and controversial. In recent years several countries have revived the strategy of subsidizing fertilizer, a previously common approach that countries were encouraged by such organizations as the World Bank to abandon as being too costly, economically inefficient, and ultimately unsustainable. (See Box 17–2 for a discussion of Malawi's renewed fertilizer subsidy scheme.) Conversely, any strategy that involves increasing food prices to incentivize farmers immediately brings us back to the food policy dilemma when we consider the impact of higher food prices on consumers, especially poor ones.

BOX 17–2 FERTILIZER SUBSIDIES IN MALAWI

"Ending Famine, Simply by Ignoring the Exports," so claimed a front page headline in the *New York Times* in describing a controversial fertilizer subsidy program in the southern African country of Malawi.[a] Malawi had long suffered from high rates of chronic hunger, and the country's average maize yields were just over one-tenth the average level in the United States. In 2007, however, Malawi attained a record-breaking maize harvest. According to the *New York Times*, "Farmers explain Malawi's extraordinary turnaround—one with broad implications for hunger-fighting methods across Africa—with one word: fertilizer." During 2004, Malawi experienced both a severe hunger crisis and a contentious presidential election in which the main parties competed in their claims about how much each would do to support farmers. A parliamentary committee recommended a nationwide program of fertilizer subsidies, which President Bingu wa Mutharika announced in June 2005.

Two initial points of contention were whether the fertilizer subsidy program would be targeted (and if so, toward which income groups) and whether it would

[a]*New York Times*, December 2, 2007.

include tobacco, one of Malawi's chief exports, along with maize, its primary consumption crop. Initially, the government decided to include only maize producers, who were unable otherwise to purchase fertilizer, so long as they were productive farmers. The program was not targeted at the smallest, least-able producers. A universal (untargeted) subsidy program was rejected by the president as being too expensive, but he later bowed to political pressure and included both maize and tobacco producers in a universal subsidy program.

The plan was to include both fertilizer and improved maize seed. In its first year, the program excluded private-sector fertilizer suppliers, but several large suppliers subsequently were included. The program was built around a voucher scheme, in which qualifying farmers would receive coupons for fertilizer, entitling them to purchase a 50-kilogram bag of fertilizer for US$6.50, or just over one-quarter of the full cost (with the government paying the remainder). During the 2005–06 growing season, the program distributed about 175,000 metric tons of fertilizer and 4,500 metric tons of improved maize seed, costing $91 million.

Malawi's record maize harvest in 2007 resulted, not only from this seed and fertilizer distribution program but also from quite favorable weather. The *New York Times* reported, "In the hamlet of Mthungu, Enelesi Chakhaza, an elderly widow whose husband died of hunger five years ago, boasted that she got two ox-cart-loads of corn this year from her small plot instead of half a cart." Malawi's maize production in 2004–05 had fallen to 1.23 million metric tons from 1.61 million the previous year. In 2005–06, the first year of the subsidy program, output increased to 2.58 million metric tons, and to 3.44 million in 2006–2007.

Adoption of the fertilizer subsidy program created a dilemma for the government of Malawi, which had counted on restoring donor confidence as the country recovered from a severe economic crisis. The donor community in general looked unfavorably on large subsidy schemes as being costly, unsustainable, and economically inefficient. The strongest donor opposition came from the International Monetary Fund (IMF) and U.S. Agency for International Development (USAID). Their concern, in addition to the economic inefficiency of subsidies, was that the scheme threatened to undermine Malawi's nascent private fertilizer marketing sector, which had emerged after the end of the government's fertilizer monopoly in the early 1990s. Other donors, such as the United Kingdom, the World Bank, and the European Union were skeptical but willing to work with the government to minimize the potential negative effects of the program. In contrast, the United Nations and many non-governmental organizations (NGOs) were openly supportive of Malawi's fertilizer subsidy program.

Precisely how much of the increased maize harvest of 2007 resulted from the fertilizer program and how much from that year's favorable rainfall remains unclear. One of the few formal attempts to estimate the subsidy's contribution to increased maize production concluded that Malawi's maize harvest was 15 to 22 percent greater as a result of the program.

Donor attitudes toward input subsidies may have softened in response to this experience. Talk now is of "smart subsidies." As economist Derek Byerlee, a co-director of the team that produced the World Bank's *World Development Report 2008: Agriculture for Development*, notes, "The World Development Report takes a pragmatic position, favoring 'smart subsidies' in select circumstances. Smart subsidies should be transparent, well targeted to the poor . . . , should help jump-start agricultural input markets and should be part of a comprehensive strategy to improve agricultural productivity." Commenting specifically on the Malawian experience, Byerlee continues, "The Bank's position is that the program should be targeted to achieve as large a set of development gains as possible. . . . Smart subsidies are important but need to be weighted against other priorities in national budgets. For example, Malawi only spends 3% of its agricultural budget on R&D—an important source of future productivity increases."[b]

[b]Interview with the World Bank Meetings Center, December 18, 2007, available at http://blogs. worldbank.org/meetings/discuss/world-development-report-2008, accessed February 2012.

Source: This box draws largely on two sources: Blessings Chinsinga, "Reclaiming Policy Space: Lesons from Malawi's 2005/2006 Fertilizer Subsidy Programme," Futures Agricultures and University of Malawi, July 2007; I. Minde, T. S. Jayne, E. Crawford, J. Ariga, and J. Govereh, "Promoting Fertilizer Use in Africa: Current Issues and Empirical Evidence from Malawi, Zambia, and Kenya," International Water Management Institute, Pretoria, South Africa and U.S. Agency for International Development, November 2008.

The expectation that higher food prices motivate increased food production ties together each of the dimensions of farm-level decision making that we have discussed. Economists summarize these multiple dimensions by considering the relationship between changes in price and changes in supply for a given crop or for agriculture in general, a relationship known as farmers' **supply response**. Figure 17–11 illustrates the theory. Figure 17–11a summarizes the relationship between input and output in terms of total revenue and total cost of production. For a given price of rice, total revenue increases by the same amount for each additional unit of output. The total revenue function ($0B$) in Panel a is thus linear with a slope equal to the unit price of rice, P_0. The total cost of producing rice also increases with the quantity produced. However the diminishing-returns characteristic of the production function implies that the total cost function ($0A$) curves upward as illustrated. Because profit is the difference between total revenue and total cost, profit is maximized in Figure 17–11a at the level of output where the vertical difference between the height of the total revenue line and the total cost curve is greatest. As in the example of the production function, we can find this point geometrically by

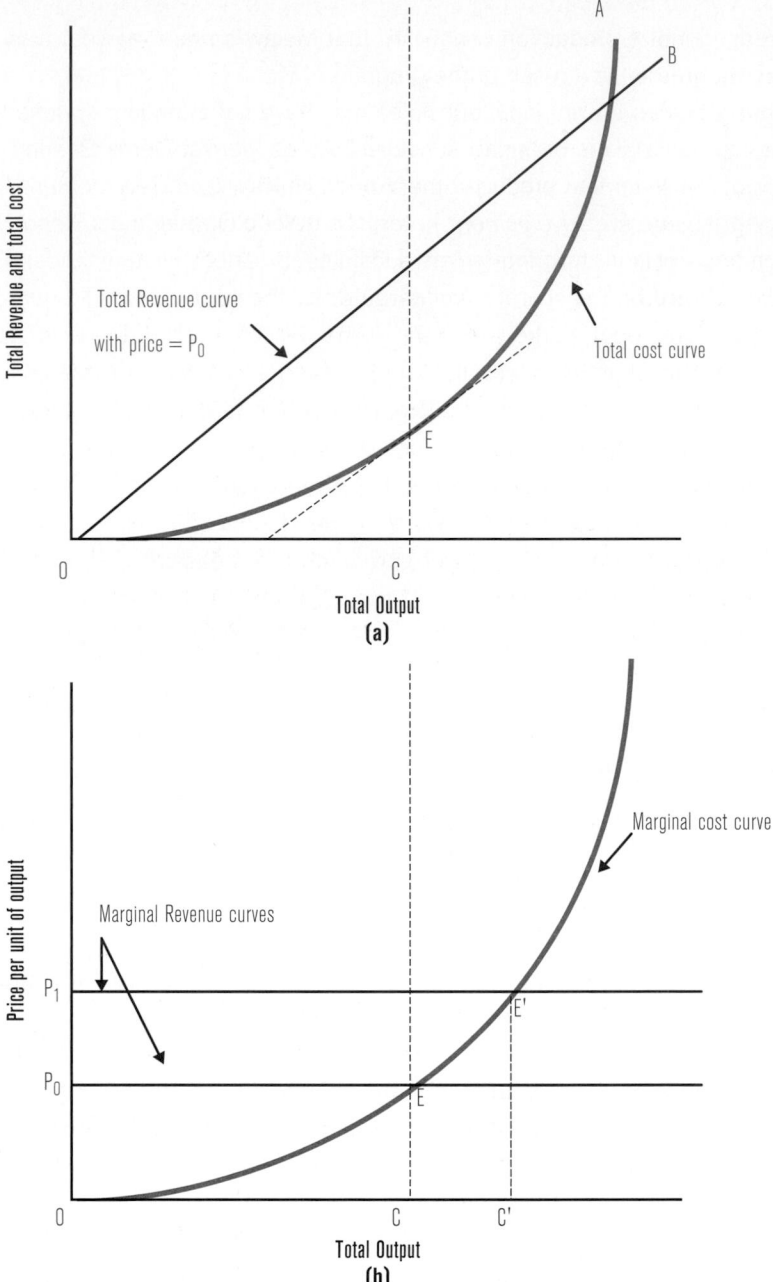

FIGURE 17-11 **The Relationship between Output and Price**

locating the tangency point between the total cost curve and a line parallel to the total revenue function. This tangency is at point E, implying that $0C$ is the profit maximizing quantity of rice.[19]

[19]We can think of a subsistence farmer tending to his or her own small plot with little more than a few hand tools as having no fixed costs, in which case the y-intercept of the total cost curve in Figure 17-11 would be zero (as drawn). A larger producer, for instance with a significant capital stock, may have fixed costs. In that case, the total cost curve would have a positive intercept, but the equilibrium condition would still be $MR = MC$.

Figure 17–11b demonstrates that rice production in the quantity $0C$ satisfies our condition for profit maximization. Panel b simply summarizes the relationships in panel a by recording the slopes of the total revenue and total cost functions at each level of output. Bear in mind that the slope at any point of a "total" function defines the analogous "marginal" function. Because the total revenue function is linear, its slope is constant so the marginal revenue function in Figure 17–11b is simply a horizontal line the height of which measures the initial price of rice, P_0. Because the total cost curve bows upward, its slope increases as a function of total output. The marginal cost curve in panel b records the slope of the total cost curve at each level output and thus also slopes upward. Figure 17–11b directly illustrates that total output equal to $0C$ is the profit-maximizing level because that is where marginal revenue equals marginal cost. If the price of rice were to increase from P_0 to P_1, the marginal revenue line would shift up as illustrated and intersect the marginal cost curve at E' instead of point E. At this higher price, the profit-maximizing quantity of output would increase to $0C'$. The marginal cost curve thus defines the supply curve.

Based on these relationships, we can summarize farmers' supply response to increased prices by the price elasticity of supply for rice:

$$\varepsilon^s = \frac{\%\Delta R}{\%\Delta P_R} \qquad [17\text{--}1]$$

where R is the quantity of rice output, and P_R is the price of rice. Estimates of the magnitude of this elasticity, calculated for agriculture more generally, vary from near zero (which would imply that producers do not increase supply in response to higher prices) to about 1.5 (which would imply that a 10 percent increase in price brings forth a 15 percent increase in supply). One reason supply elasticity might be quite low could be the existence of **nonprice constraints** to production. Farmers may lack access to the inputs necessary to increase output, either because markets are inadequate or inaccessible, input costs are too high, or credit is unavailable. Production may also be constrained by poor institutions, such as lack of secure land tenure.

One potential point of confusion in the estimation of supply elasticity lies in the question of whether this elasticity refers to a single commodity or to agriculture in general. Although the price elasticity of supply for a single commodity in a given country may be relatively high, the elasticity of supply for agriculture in general in that same country may be relatively low. Why? Recall the production possibility frontier of Figure 17–8, in which increased production of corn comes at the direct expense of reduced production of beans. Generalizing from this example, opportunities for farmers to substitute across commodities in response to changes in relative prices make such a result likely. It is also important to consider the time frame of the analysis. In the short run, many of the conditions of production are fixed; yet, in the long run conditions can change, perhaps because nonprice constraints are relaxed. As a rule of thumb, the long-run supply elasticity for given crops is approximately twice the magnitude of the short-run elasticity. From a theoretical perspective, we can think of short-run supply response as reflecting a movement along a given (static) supply curve as quantity produced responds to a change in price. Yet, it is important to note that in the long run, technical change can also contribute to farmers' supply response. In this context, we can think of technical change as reducing the marginal cost of production. This shifts the marginal cost curve downward (or, equivalently, shifts the supply curve to the right), increasing the supply of food at every price. In addition, in the long run other nonprice constraints to production response may be overcome. Improved infrastructure might provide farmers greater market access for both inputs and outputs, credit supply might increase, and farmers may learn how to improve their farming practices.

Estimates of the aggregate supply elasticity for African agriculture have tended to be low, on the order of 0.2 in the short run and 0.4 in the long run. Yet some studies of specific crops have claimed to find significantly greater elasticities. One study of Trans Nzoia, a corn-producing district in Kenya, estimated the short-run elasticity of supply of corn to be 0.53 and the long-run elasticity to be 0.76. Thus a 10 percent increase in the price of corn would result in a 5.3 percent short-run increase in corn production and a 7.6 percent increase in output in the long run.[20] Another study of food production in Tanzania found that a 10 percent increase in the price of food crops (relative to export crops) would result in a 3.9 percent short-run increase in per capita food production and a 9.2 percent long-run increase.[21]

This discussion of how agricultural producers respond to price incentives provides a foundation for understanding how policy makers might intervene to change farmers' production decisions. Whether the goal is to reduce a country's dependence on imported cereals, to increase the local supply of vegetables, to increase its supply of coffee for export, or to employ more rural labor, price policies provide a powerful, if blunt, tool for policy makers. Box 17–2 discusses fertilizer subsidies in Malawi; yet this is only one of many possible examples of how governments have tried to influence farmers' behavior. It bears repeating, however, that producer incentives are only one component of the broader realm of food policy. Food policy analysis would be relatively simple if the only goal were to increase production and maximize producers' incomes. The challenge in practice (the food policy dilemma) is how to make farming profitable while at the same time protecting poor consumers from the threat of high food prices. The prices received by farmers are lower than the prices paid by consumers. The margin between the **farm-gate price** and the **retail** price is called the **marketing margin**. This is the cost required to store, transport, and process basic farm output so that it can be purchased and used by consumers who may be far from the point of origin or who may be purchasing the food months after harvest. To the extent that these marketing margins are increased by poor infrastructure or limited access to markets, the food policy dilemma is aggravated. It is important to consider market access in conjunction with the analysis of producer incentives.

[20]Lawrence O. Moses, Kees Burger, and Arie Kuyvenhoven, "Aggregate supply Response to Price Incentives: The Case of Smallholder Maize Production in Kenya," *African Crop Science Conference Proceedings*, 8 (2007), 1271–75.

[21]Andrew McKay, Oliver Morrissey, and Charlotte Vaillant, "Aggregate Export and Food Crop Supply Response in Tanzania," DFID-TERP: CREDIT Discussion Paper 4 (No. 98/4), Center for Research in Economic Development and International Trade, University of Nottingham, Nottingham, England, 1998.

MARKET ACCESS

Poor infrastructure in much of the developing world limits farmers' access to markets and their ability both to purchase inputs and to sell the crops they produce. Farmers may see little benefit in accepting the risk of adopting modern varieties and incurring debt to buy inputs in return for the promise of increased production when markets for their produce are remote. Selling output in distant markets, particularly when transport is scarce, can be costly for farmers. Many may be limited to moving small quantities, perhaps over long distances. Production incentives are reduced when farmers face high marketing costs. The World Bank reports that 16 percent of the rural population of developing countries (about 440 million people) lives in remote areas that are at least five hours from a market town of 5,000 or more.[22] This problem varies widely across regions: in sub-Saharan Africa, the Middle East, and North Africa, nearly one-third of the population lives in these remote areas, while that is the case for 17 percent of the population of East Asia and only 5 percent of the population of South Asia. In many cases even high-potential agricultural areas lack the infrastructure necessary to connect them to markets. In Ethiopia, the World Bank reports that 68 percent of the rural population lives in areas with ample rainfall, but the average farm household lives 10 kilometers from the nearest road and 18 kilometers from the nearest public transport. These variations in quality of rural infrastructure relate to differences in both income levels and population density (as investments in public goods such as roads are more costly in low population density areas). In addition to poor infrastructure, poor institutions can also limit the agricultural supply response and more generally impede agricultural development. Box 17–3 describes the growing role of cell phones in agricultural marketing in developing countries.

BOX 17–3 CELL PHONES AND AGRICULTURAL DEVELOPMENT

Cell phones are transforming rural markets in developing countries, particularly in sub-Saharan Africa where traditional land lines were largely unknown in rural areas. By 2009, there were 10 times as many cell phones as land lines in sub-Saharan Africa, and the number continues to grow rapidly. In 1999, only 10 percent of Africans were potentially covered by mobile phone technology; yet, by 2008, this number had increased to 60 percent (though coverage remains much greater in some countries than others). This rapid growth prompted Rwandan president Paul Kagame to declare that "what was once an

---

[22]World Bank, *World Development Report, 2008*, p. 54.

object of luxury and privilege, the mobile phone, has become a basic necessity in Africa."[a] Efficient markets require easy access to information by market participants. Knowledge of market prices, wages, weather patterns, and other relevant events are critical pieces of information for farmers and traders. The rapid penetration of cell phones has greatly reduced the cost of gaining such information.

Traditionally, traders in rural African markets could learn prices in distant markets only by actually traveling to those markets. The cost and time required imposed a severe limitation on traders' knowledge of the markets in which they operated. For the traders with cell phones, information that previously required hours of travel to obtain can be learned in a short phone call or text message. Economist Jenny Aker finds that the use of cell phones by grain traders in rural Niger reduces their search costs by 50 percent.[b] She interviewed grain traders in Niger, one of whom said that with a cell phone, "in record time, I have all sorts of information from markets near and far." A second trader reported to Aker that, "[Now] I know the price for two dollars, rather than traveling [to the market], which costs $20." As a result, prices across distant markets tended to converge and consumer grain prices fell by 3.5 percent. Both traders and consumers were better off. Similarly, economist Robert Jensen finds that the availability of mobile phones in India creates substantial benefits for fish traders and consumers. There, too, prices across markets tended to converge (a sign of efficient price formation) when traders had access to mobile phones; fishermen's profits increased by 8 percent, and consumers of fish benefited from a 4 percent decline in retail prices.[c] The benefits of such rapid information sharing are particularly clear in fish markets, where the product is highly perishable. Economists Megumi Muto and Takashi Yamano note that access to mobile phones increased the likelihood that banana producers in Uganda would participate in markets by 10 percent.[d] Bananas, like fish, are highly perishable. For the marketing of such commodities, the benefits of speedy information flows are particularly clear. The *digital provide*, as Jensen called it, will surely continue its rapid expansion and transformation of rural markets around the world.

[a]Address at the Connect Africa Summit, Kigali, Rwanda, October 29, 2007.

[b]J. Aker, "Information from Markets Near and Far: Mobile Phones and Agricultural Markets in Niger," *American Economic Journal: Applied Economics* 2, no. 3 (2010), 46–59.

[c]R. Jensen, "The Digital Provide: Information (Technology), Market Performance and Welfare in the South Indian Fisheries Sector," *Quarterly Journal of Economics* 122, no. 3 (2007), 879–924.

[d]M. Muto and T. Yamano, "The Impact of Mobile Phone Coverage Expansion on Market Participation: Panel Data Evidence from Uganda," *World Development* 37, no. 12 (2009), 1887–96.

Source: This box draws on Jenny C. Aker and Isaac M. Mbiti, "Mobile Phones and Economic Development in Africa," *Journal of Economic Perspectives*, 24, no. 3 (summer 2010): 207–32.

INSTITUTIONS FOR AGRICULTURAL DEVELOPMENT

Economic historian and Nobel laureate Douglass North famously defined institutions as "the humanly devised constraints that structure human interaction. They are made up of formal constraints (rules, laws, constitutions), informal constraints (norms of behavior, conventions, and self-imposed codes of conduct), and their enforcement characteristics. Together they define the incentive structure of society and specifically economies."[23] Institutions thus define the rules of the game by which individuals in society interact with one another. In the context of agricultural development, institutions governing the ownership and transfer of land are of particular importance.

In most countries, land ownership is a key determinant of power and social status, making land allocation a highly political concern. Land (like income, wealth, and political power) is unevenly distributed. For selected countries, Table 17–2 provides data on the size of an average land holding as well as an indicator of the equity with which land is distributed within the country. The equity of land distribution is summarized in Table 17–2 by a Gini coefficient for land ownership. Recall from Chapter 6 that a Gini coefficient summarizes relative distributional equity with a number ranging between 0 and 1. The closer the Gini coefficient is to 1, the more unequal is the distribution. Several points stand out in these data. There is great variation in the size of average land holdings and the equity of land ownership across regions and countries, reflecting large differences in population density, culture, and history. Average farm sizes in Africa and Asia tend to be quite small relative to some of the larger countries in South America. In Ethiopia, the average farm size is 0.8 hectare, as compared with 469 hectares in Argentina and 740 hectares in the United States.

The Gini coefficients for land ownership in Africa tend to be on the low side, such as 0.37 in the Democratic Republic of the Congo and 0.38 in Namibia. These low Gini coefficients reflect highly equitable distributions of land ownership. Conversely, the distribution of land in South American countries is highly skewed. Gini coefficients on the order of 0.85 for Brazil and 0.93 in Paraguay indicate that a large portion of land is owned by a small number of large landowners, while the large majority of rural dwellers in those countries must divide up whatever land is left over. The highly unequal distribution of land in Latin America has such deep historical roots that special terms have evolved to describe it: **latifundia** (the term for the large estates that dominate the distribution) and **minifundia** (the small family farms on which peasant farmers struggle to feed their families).

Institutions governing land rights play a large role in shaping incentives for agricultural producers, both in terms of their level of effort and their willingness to invest in maintaining the quality of their land. Insecure land rights can undermine

[23]Douglass North, "Economic Performance through Time," in Torsten Persson, ed., *Nobel Lectures, Economics 1991–1995* (Singapore: World Scientific, 1997).

TABLE 17-2 Farm Size and Equity of Land Holdings in Selected Countries

REGION/COUNTRY	CENSUS YEAR	AVERAGE FARM SIZE (HECTARES)	GINI COEFFICIENT FOR LAND HOLDINGS
Africa			
Burkina Faso	1993	3.92	0.42
Congo	1990	0.53	0.37
Egypt	1990	0.95	0.65
Ethiopia	1989–92	0.80	0.47
Guinea	1995	2.03	0.48
Malawi	1993	0.75	0.52
Namibia	1995	2.64	0.38
Uganda	1991	4.70	0.59
North and Central America			
Bahamas	1994	11.5	0.87
Barbados	1989	190.0	0.94
Canada	1991	349.1	0.64
Honduras	1993	11.17	0.66
Panama	1990	110.0	0.87
Puerto Rico	1987	100.0	0.77
United States	1987	740.0	0.74
South America			
Argentina	1988	469.0	0.83
Brazil	1985	64.64	0.85
Colombia	1988	120.0	0.79
Paraguay	1991	77.53	0.93
Peru	1994	20.15	0.86
Asia			
India	1991	1.55	0.58
Indonesia	1993	0.87	0.46
Japan	1995	1.20	0.59
South Korea	1990	1.05	0.34
Nepal	1992	0.95	0.45
Pakistan	1990	3.78	0.57
Philippines	1991	2.16	0.55
Thailand	1993	3.36	0.47
Turkey	1991	5.76	0.61
Vietnam	1994	0.52	0.53

Source: FAO, *World Census of Agriculture* (Rome: Food and Agriculture Organization of the United Nations, 2000).

producers' incentives and limit productivity. Secure land rights can enhance agricultural productivity by creating access to credit markets through which farmers can purchase improved inputs. The rules governing land sales can influence agricultural productivity by facilitating the transfer of ownership rights to the most efficient producers.

Land rights take a variety of forms in developing countries, ranging from purely individual rights to purely collective forms of land ownership, with numerous forms in between these polar extremes. Thus at one end of the spectrum, owners have full control over who uses their land and what they produce; at the other extreme, all members of a community are entitled to use the land and benefit from the output. The most common intermediate forms of land rights are **fixed-rent tenancy** and **share cropping**. Share cropping is the dominant contractual arrangement in South Asia, while other regions of the developing world more typically rely on fixed-rent tenancy. Under tenancy, a family might rent land from a large landlord and pay a fixed cash rent. Under share cropping, the farm family rents a plot of land from the landlord, with whom the family shares a fixed portion of their output. A key difference between these systems lies in how the risks inherent in farming are divided between the landlord and the tenant. Under a fixed rent scheme, the tenant farmers bear all of the risk; their rent due on the land does not depend on the level of their output. In contrast, under share tenancy, the landlord and the tenants share the risk more evenly because the in-kind payments to the landlord depend on the tenant's level of output. Incentives for producers may also differ across types of tenancy. On large commercial farms worked by hired wage labor, owners face a complicated problem of monitoring the level of effort of their workers. In contrast, on purely communal farms, on which everyone shares the communal output, workers' incentives might be limited because an individual's rewards may not reflect that individual's efforts to maximize collective output. In terms of producer incentives, a key distinction across types of tenancy arrangements is whether the producers are **residual claimants** to the output of the farm—that is, whether their individual benefits increase with their level of effort.

Another critical distinction between different land institutions is the security and stability of producers' rights to farm particular parcels of land. A rental contract written for one or two years is certainly less secure than clear title to a given parcel. Economists Klaus Deininger and Gershon Feder summarize the costs and benefits of secure individual property rights.[24] The main benefits include (1) improved incentives to conserve and invest in the land itself; (2) the ability to transfer land ownership, possibly to those able to make the best use of the land (for instance by taking advantage of economies of scale); and (3) the ability to use land as collateral, providing farmers access to credit markets (and the potential to adopt modern varieties and inputs). The main costs are the administrative costs of actually defining land boundaries and enforcing land rights and the risk that the poorest farmers, who often depend on access to **common property resources** (such as open pastures for grazing their livestock), could be deprived of their sources of livelihood.

There is substantial evidence to support the idea that secure land rights increase both agricultural productivity and investments in land conservation (which enhance future productivity). In China, the transition from collective to private cultivation has been associated with significant increases in productivity, as individual farmers

---

[24]Klaus Deininger and Gershon Feder, "*Land institutions and land markets*," in B. L. Gardner and G. C. Rausser, eds., *Handbook of Agricultural Economics*, 1st ed. (Amsterdam: Elsevier, 2001) vol. 1, pp. 288–331.

stand to retain more of the benefits of increased effort. Longer-term investments in land conservation are also evident. In Ghana, studies have found farmers with greater tenure security are more likely to plant trees and to invest in drainage and irrigation. In Niger, farmers who owned their land applied larger quantities of manure to maintain their soil fertility than did tenant farmers. In addition, there is evidence that secure tenure rights not only induce investment in land conservation but also facilitate access to the formal credit markets necessary to finance those investments. In Thailand, land ownership titles not only increased the value of land and boosted productivity but also increased the supply of credit. Another study in Paraguay found that the benefits of land titling were roughly equivalent to 10 percent of farm income. Yet, that study also found that those benefits were strongly concentrated among the larger land owners, whereas producers with less than 20 hectares received no benefits of increased credit supply.[25]

Improving systems of **land titling** is one approach to securing tenure rights. Land titling involves providing legal documentation of land ownership. Plans to improve tenure security through titling must also consider the costs of implementation. These costs are largely administrative and include measurement and demarcation of areas, adjudication of conflicting land claims, and the cost of documentation. Land titling can also facilitate the operation of land markets, which are often underdeveloped in poor countries. Land markets, however, may not facilitate access to land by the poor if the poor lack access to credit markets. When land titling alone is insufficient to achieve social goals in regard to land rights, various forms of land reform have been attempted.

LAND REFORM

Efforts to reform land rights can take a variety of forms, including the following:

- *Reform of rent contracts* works to increase the security of tenure of the tenant farmer. Laws requiring long-term contracts that restrict the landlord's right to remove the tenant strengthen the tenant's property rights at the expense of those of the landlord without necessarily transferring income from owner to tenant.
- *Rent reduction* typically involves placing a ceiling on the percentage share of the crop that a landlord can demand as rent. If the percentage share is substantially below what prevailed in the past, the impact both on tenant welfare and the tenant family's surplus available for investment can be substantial.
- *Land to the tiller* (the former tenant) *with compensation* to landlord for loss of land is a measure that can take many different forms. Government

---

[25]These studies are summarized in Deininger and Feder, "Land Institutions and Land Markets."

might pass a law stating a ceiling on the number of acres an individual can own and so force individuals to sell all land over that limit. Or the reform law can state that only those who actually till land can own it, and all other land must be sold. A key issue in this kind of reform is whether the former landlord receives full or only partial compensation for the land that must be sold.

- *Land to the tiller without compensation* is the most radical transformation of land rights. All land not cultivated by its owner is confiscated, and the former landlord receives nothing in return. This type of reform is most commonly found in the aftermath of a major political upheaval, such as a revolution or losing a war.

The implementation of these types of land reforms becomes more complex as we move down the list, and the potential for harmful unintended consequences exists in each case. Placing ceilings on land rents is one of the least intrusive of these potential reforms. Yet rent ceilings may create incentives for landowners to evict their tenants. This was a common result in Latin America as well as in India, where similar reforms led to the loss of 30 percent of the total area operated by the poor. Conversely, Deininger and Feder report that tenancy reform in West Bengal was associated with productivity gains of 40 percent.[26] Efforts to limit the size of land holdings have generally failed. The major problem in these cases is that ceilings can be evaded, for instance, by subdividing large landholdings among family members.

Land to the tiller programs are examples of redistributive land reform. These programs involve transferring ownership of land and thus face increasing political obstacles. Experience has been mixed, with greater success under certain pre-existing circumstance. In settings in which tenants already cultivate given parcels of land that are pieces of larger landlord estates, transferring ownership of the land is administratively simple and can increase productivity by improving producers' incentives. Successful examples of this type of reform have occurred in Bolivia, Ethiopia, India, Iran, Japan, Korea, and Taiwan. Yet, experience with land reform in **hacienda** systems, by which tenants typically work most of the time on a landlord's plot of land but have their own subsistence plots, has been less positive. A common experience in Latin America when faced with the prospect of redistributive land reform was for landlords to evict their tenants or to convert them into wage laborers. In addition, land compensation schemes can be extremely costly and the task of estimating a fair compensation price for confiscated land is complicated by the poor quality of land markets in many countries. When land redistribution creates new landowners who were not previously cultivating that land, the need for complementary types of support (such as infrastructure and farmer training programs) might add substantially to the costs.[27]

---

[26]Deininger and Feder, "Land Institutions and Land Markets."
[27]Deininger and Feder, review these issues in greater detail; see "Land Institutions and Land Markets."

If land redistribution with compensation is complicated, redistribution *without* compensation is virtually impossible in the absence of a social revolution, foreign invasion, or both. The successful examples of redistributive land reform in Japan, the Republic of Korea, and Taiwan were possible only as the result of defeat in war or foreign occupation. In China and the Soviet Union, foreign invasions preceded social revolutions that destroyed the old agrarian orders and paved the way for large-scale land reform. In other cases, revolution alone created the conditions necessary for redistributive land reform. Examples include Cuba, Egypt, Ethiopia, Nicaragua, and Vietnam.

Redistributive land reform continues to be a key and controversial issue in many countries. This is particularly true in countries with highly unequal distributions of land ownership, often the result of historical legacy or ethnic discrimination. The southern African states of Zimbabwe and South Africa, for example, were settler colonies in which white minorities owned much of the prime agricultural land. Redistributive land reform has been a dominant social issue in these countries. Forced expropriation of white-owned farms in Zimbabwe began in 1999 with the support of President Robert Mugabe. Land reform in Zimbabwe has been widely criticized, not only for its violence but also because political favoritism in distributing newly seized land has contributed the failure of Zimbabwe's program to benefit most of the rural poor. In South Africa, the collapse of the Apartheid regime and the transition to democracy in 1994 brought with it high expectations among the indigenous majority for restitution in the form of land. These expectations were fueled by events in Zimbabwe. Yet, in contrast to that example, the government of South Africa has taken a more cautious approach to land reform. A desire to avoid the economic chaos that befell Zimbabwe helps explain this caution. After its election in 1994, the government of the African National Congress announced plans to redistribute 30 percent of commercial farmland to blacks by 2014; yet as of 2010, progress was limited to only 6 percent, and tensions continued to surround this issue. Redistributive land reform is also a key issue in many postconflict settings. Mozambique and Liberia, after long periods of civil war, face serious challenges of resettling large displaced populations on land since occupied by others. Land reform has also been a central issue in South America, where indigenous Indian minorities have long suffered discrimination. In Bolivia, for example, the government planned to redistribute 400,000 acres of land in 2011, a substantial increase over the 2010 level.

THE WORLD FOOD CRISIS OF 2005–08

During the years 2005–08, the world suffered its most severe food crisis since the early 1970s. The key indicator of this crisis was the rapid increase in the prices of a range of basic foods. As Figure 17–12 shows, the prices of rice, maize, and wheat increased

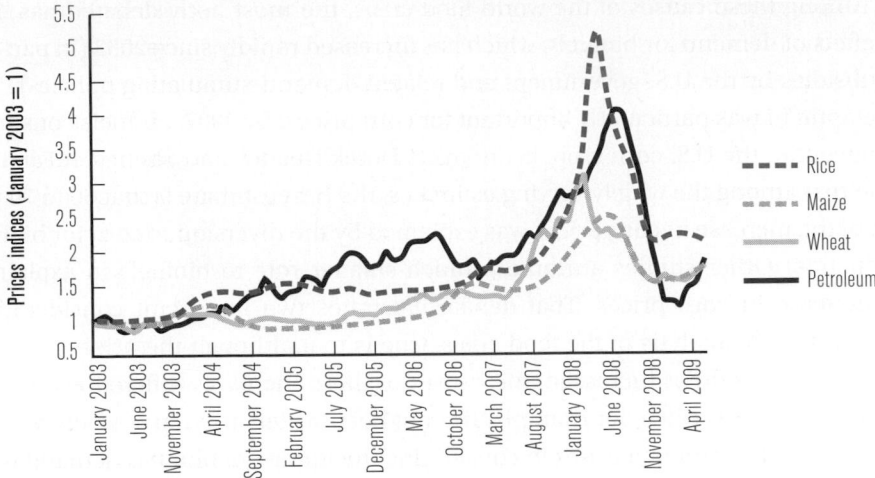

FIGURE 17-12   **Trends in the Nominal Prices of Cereals and Oil, January 2003 to May 2009**

Source: Headey, D., S. Malaiyandi, and S. Fan. 2009. "Navigating the Perfect Storm: Reflections on the Food, Energy, and Financial Crises." IFPRI Discussion Paper 00889, Figure 1. Washington, DC: International Food Policy Research Institute.

dramatically between early 2007 and mid-2008, following more gradual increases beginning in 2004. The price of maize showed the least increase, yet still reached a level by June 2008 that was two and a half times greater than it had been just two years earlier. The run up in wheat prices was even more severe, but both were outpaced by the skyrocketing price of rice during 2007–08. From October 2007 to April 2008, the world price of rice tripled (increasing from $335 to over $1,000 per ton).

CAUSES OF THE CRISIS

Explanations for the crisis include a wide range of possibilities and are the subject of continuing debate. The list of potential culprits includes both supply shocks and demand shocks: growth in demand from China and India, speculation on financial markets, hoarding and export restrictions, weather shocks, decreased productivity, low interest rates, a depreciation of the U.S. dollar, rising oil prices, declining food stockpiles, and demand for biofuels.[28] There is no definitive consensus regarding the relative contributions of these potential causes. Notably, some of these potential causes are common to all commodities (such as the effect of oil price increases and the depreciation of the U.S. dollar), whereas other causes are commodity-specific (such as supply shocks and the effect of biofuels demand).

---

[28]See D. Headey and S. Fan, "Anatomy of a Crisis: The Causes and Consequences of Surging Food Prices," *Agricultural Economics* 39 (suppl., 2008), 375–91.

Among these causes of the world food crisis, the most hotly debated has been the effect of demand for biofuels, which has increased rapidly since 2003 (in part due to subsidies by the U.S. government and related demand-stimulating policies). This development was particularly important for corn prices. By 2007, biofuels consumed 25 percent of the U.S. corn crop. Economists Derek Headey and Shenggen Fan conclude that among the widely varying estimates, the best estimate is that 60 to 70 percent of the increase in corn prices was explained by the diversion of corn for biofuels production. Other studies attribute a much smaller role to biofuels in explaining the increase in corn prices. That debate illustrates two important considerations that complicate analysis of the food crisis. One is that although the prices of a wide range of commodities increased, the causes of these increases differed across specific commodities. (Rice, for example, has not been widely used in biofuels production.) A second point that arises in considering the impact of biofuels demand is the need to consider interactions between crops. In the case of biofuels, the increased demand for corn is thought to have explained up to 40 percent of the increase in soybean prices. What's the connection? The 23 percent increase in acreage in the United States devoted to corn came at the expense of a 16 percent reduction in soybean acreage in 2007. In addition, to the extent that consumers substitute between staple gains, increased corn prices have contributed to increased demand for wheat and rice, adding to price increases for those commodities.

The explanation for the tripling of world rice prices relates more to the combustible mixture of distortionary trade interventions and panic buying. Historically, world rice markets are thin compared with those for other grains. That is, only 5 to 7 percent of global rice production is traded internationally (compared with 20 percent of wheat). This makes world rice prices relatively volatile. In addition, global rice exports are dominated by a small number of countries: Thailand, India, Vietnam, and Pakistan alone account for about 70 percent of global rice exports. So conditions in the world rice market were ripe for an implosion in November 2007, when India reacted to rising rice prices by banning exports. India's ban on rice exports set off a chain reaction in world rice markets. Importing nations, the Philippines in particular, accelerated their import orders, fearing further price increases. These orders, themselves, helped drive up prices, in response to which Vietnam, China, Cambodia, and Egypt also intervened to restrict rice exports. Figure 17–13 places these and related events on a chart of world rice prices.[29]

Commodity-specific factors also affected world wheat prices. In this case, the main culprit was a weather-induced supply shock. Australia, one of the world's leading exporters of wheat, suffered its worst drought in a thousand years in 2006, cut-

---

[29]D. Headey, S. Malaiyandi, and S. Fan, "Navigating the Perfect Storm: Reflections on the Food, Energy, and Financial Crises," Discussion Paper No. 00889, International food Policy Research Institute, Washington, DC, August 2009. For a comprehensive review of the rice crisis, see D. Dawe, ed., *The Rice Crisis: Markets, Policies and Food Security* (London: Earthscan, 2010).

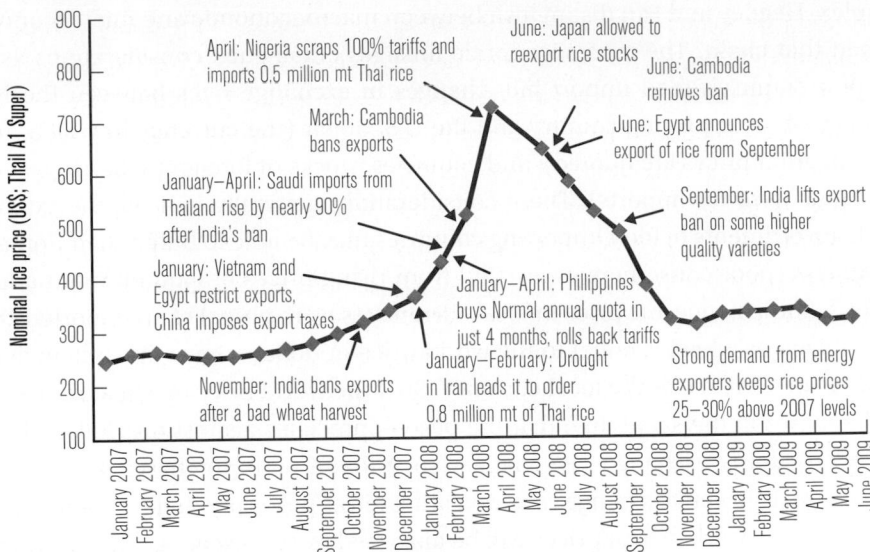

FIGURE 17-13   Events in World Rice Market

mt, metric tons.
Source: Headey, D., S. Malaiyandi, and S. Fan. 2009. "Navigating the Perfect Storm: Reflections on the Food, Energy, and Financial Crises." IFPRI Discussion Paper 00889, Figure 2. Washington, DC: International Food Policy Research Institute.

ting in half that country's wheat exports. That year's harvest in other major producing countries, including the United States, Russia, and Ukraine, were also smaller than usual.

A more general factor was the price of oil. The price of oil surged just in advance of the prices of wheat, maize, and rice. Oil prices are relevant for several reasons. For instance, chemical fertilizers are largely petroleum-based products, and most farm machinery runs on gasoline or diesel fuel. In addition, higher oil prices also increased the cost of transporting agricultural output, both within and between countries. Here too we see an interaction effect with other potential causes of the crisis: biofuels production becomes more profitable when oil prices are high. In addition, the ability of markets to respond to price increases in a range of commodities by releasing stockpiles of those grains into the market was severely constrained by the historically low levels of grain reserves at that time. Ironically, one cause of the low levels of grain reserves was the secular decline in prices before the crisis.

CONSEQUENCES OF THE CRISIS

The consequences of the world food crisis of 2005-08 are even more difficult to sort out. While our ultimate concern may be the welfare of poor households, the causal chain running from global cereals price shocks to household welfare is long and complex. Headey and Fan distinguish between macroeconomic and microeconomic links in that chain. The macroeconomic linkages entail such considerations as the size of a country's food import bill, changes in exchange rates between the local currency of an importing country and the U.S. dollar (the currency in which international grain prices are quoted), and countries' stocks of foreign exchange reserves (the funds used for imports). These considerations generally indicate the extent to which governments of food importing countries may be able to buffer their domestic consumers (poor consumers especially) from rising prices of food on international markets. For instance, the price in local currency (say, in pesos) of an imported commodity such as wheat is equal to the world price in dollars times the exchange rate (in pesos per dollar) for the local currency. So if the world price of wheat in U.S. dollars increases at the same time that the peso appreciates against the dollar (that is, if the peso–dollar exchange rate changes such that a peso purchases more dollars, resulting in a "lower" exchange rate indicating fewer pesos per dollar), then some of the increase in world wheat prices will be absorbed by this exchange rate movement and not passed along to domestic (local currency-denominated) food prices. Over the period 2003–07 countries' experiences in this regard varied widely.

Yet the welfare impacts also depend on a set of microeconomic factors that come into play once world market events have been translated into domestic food prices. At that point, changes in the relative prices of foods may motivate consumers to substitute among commodities (in favor of those that have become relatively cheaper). Opportunities for substitution away from suddenly more expensive commodities can help dampen the potential adverse effects on consumers. But these opportunities also depend on consumer preferences and the patterns of food consumption for households at different levels of income. In particular, the effect of rising food prices on household welfare depends on whether the household is a net buyer or net seller of food (as discussed earlier).

Estimates of the welfare impact of the world food crisis have also varied widely. Studies have tended to conclude that poverty (even rural poverty) tends to increase with rising food prices. This is not surprising, given that nearly all urban dwellers and a substantial proportion of rural dwellers (especially the poor) are net buyers of food (though net sellers, many of whom are still relatively poor, have benefited). While countries varied widely in the impact of the food crisis on poverty, effects also varied widely within individual countries. Economists Maros Ivanic and Will Martin concluded that on average (over the nine countries they studied) poverty rates increased by 4.5 percentage points in the short run.[30] Projecting this result to all low-income countries, they suggest that the food crisis could have increased the global poverty head count by 105 million. Their estimate is thus substantially higher than that of the Food and Agricultural Organization, which found that the food crisis increased the

---

[30]M. Ivanic and W. Martin, "Implications of Higher Global Food Prices for Poverty in Low-Income Countries," *Agricultural Economics* 39 (suppl. 2008), 405–16.

poverty head count by 40 million. These examples demonstrate both the variation in estimates of the magnitude of the impact and the broad consensus that the world food crisis hurt the poor.

SUMMARY

- A variety of characteristics distinguish agriculture from other sectors in a typical developing economy. These unique features of agriculture include its large share of GDP and employment, several technical characteristics of the agricultural production function, that much of the sector's output is directly consumed by its producers, and agriculture's role as a resource reservoir.
- Farms and farmers in developing countries differ widely from one another, both within and between countries. These differences include wide variations in farm size, technology, environmental conditions, crop mix, and degree of integration in markets. Nonetheless, it is possible to characterize traditional agriculture at a broad level of generalization as consisting of small-scale family farms producing food primarily for their own consumption, using traditional crop varieties and techniques and few purchased inputs, with low levels of productivity.
- Agricultural systems can take a variety of forms, with the major types being systems of shifting cultivation, pastoral nomadism, and settled agriculture. Most of the progress made in promoting agricultural development in recent decades has concentrated on systems of settled agriculture.
- Growth in agricultural productivity (commonly defined as the level of output per unit of land) is a central component of agricultural development. The growth rate of yields for cereal crops has been consistently high in East Asia, but quite low in sub-Saharan Africa (with the performance of other developing regions ranging between these extremes).
- Productivity growth in agriculture may be constrained by a variety of factors, including a lack of improved technology, unfavorable economic incentives, and poor-quality institutions.
- The green revolution produced new agricultural technologies and contributed significantly to agricultural productivity growth in Asia and Latin America. The benefits to farmers in sub-Saharan Africa have been more limited.
- Government policies that influence food prices play a critical role in shaping the incentives for farmers as they decide what to produce, how to produce it, and how much to produce. Meeting the goal of increasing agricultural output and productivity requires positive incentives for

farmers, typically in the form of higher food prices. Yet government efforts toward that end may be severely constrained by the negative impact of high food prices on poor consumers, many of whom may be at severe risk of undernutrition and hunger.

- Institutions governing land rights are of particular importance in shaping incentives and opportunities for farmers. Secure tenure arrangements encourage both greater levels of effort in current farm production and greater levels of investment in conserving soil resources for future production. Efforts to improve tenure security through land reform are often appealing in theory, but difficult to implement.

18

Trade and Development

n April 2009, Trinidad and Tobago hosted the fifth Summit of the Americas. The summit was viewed as a huge success, devoid of confrontation and heralded as a new beginning for relations with the region. It stood in sharp contrast to the summit held four years earlier in Mar del Plata, Argentina, when thirty-four presidents from the Western Hemisphere assembled to discuss the Free Trade Area of the Americas, an idea proposed in 1994 by Bill Clinton and supported by his successors. Mexican President Vicente Fox also backed the proposal, as did other Latin American leaders. But there were voices of dissent. Populist presidents from Argentina and Brazil had their doubts. Most critical was Hugo Chávez, the leftist leader of Venezuela, who rallied a crowd of an estimated 25,000 protesters in a stadium near the closed-door meetings proclaiming, "Each one of us brought a shovel, a gravedigger's shovel, because here in Mar del Plata is the tomb of the Free Trade Area of the Americas."

Rioting broke out after the rally, something that has happened repeatedly during official meetings about international trade. The meetings of the World Trade Organization (WTO) in Seattle in 1999 were disrupted by street protesters who felt free trade hurt workers in both developing and industrialized nations. In Cancun, Mexico, in 2003, there also were protests during the WTO meetings, both among official participants in the trade talks and by demonstrators outside. One of those demonstrators was Lee Kyang Hae, who headed South Korea's Federation of Farmers and Fishermen. Lee stabbed himself in the chest, and later died, in protest against the WTO and the more open-trade policies it advocated. Lee specifically opposed further trade liberalization of agriculture, which he believed would ruin the livelihood of many

Korean farmers. As these events demonstrate, globalization and free trade generate some of the world's most heated controversies over economic policy.

But, despite these controversies and concerns, trade among nations has been growing rapidly, and most developing countries are actively trying to expand their trade. Global trade has increased more than fivefold in the last three decades, with trade in developing countries increasing by even more. Developing nations import many more goods and services than they once did, ranging from food to pharmaceuticals to sophisticated machinery. They also export much more, not only agricultural products, oil, and other raw materials but also automobile parts, clothing, semiconductors, shoes, and toys. Revolutions in transportation (including containerized shipping), telecommunications, and production methods have facilitated this process. Supply chains have been broken up, with components made in one country and finished good assembled in another. This is true for complex products, such as automobiles, so there no longer is such a thing as "a national car." Even simple products undergo global manufacturing; a Barbie doll made in China may be assembled from plastic pellets from Taiwan, given nylon hair from Japan, and packed in a cardboard box from the United States.

Trade provides low- and middle-income nations with significant opportunities to improve welfare and accelerate growth and development. With more open trade, families and businesses have more and better choices in price, quality, and array of products than if they buy only from domestic firms. Producers have much larger markets to which they can sell. If successful, exporting firms can generate rapid job growth for large numbers of low-skilled workers, which can have a strong impact on poverty reduction. Trade also invites investment and creates the possibility for the transfer of new technologies from rich to poor countries, which can raise productivity and incomes.

But the news is not all good. Although more open trade creates many winners, it also creates losers. Firms and farmers producing at high prices for the domestic market can be forced out of business, with job losses and other disruptions. Exporters operating on world markets face the risk of rapidly falling prices or other vagaries of the world market that are out of their control. Poor weather in Nicaragua may hurt its coffee crop, sending up world prices and benefiting coffee farmers in Uganda, but a bumper crop in Vietnam can lead to a drop in prices that can leave the Ugandan farmer with much lower income. The 2008 financial crisis that precipitated a steep recession in the United States and European Union hurt exporters most everywhere in the world.

The evidence suggests that, on balance, more open trade is beneficial for developing countries and leads to more rapid growth and poverty reduction, particularly when exports are focused on labor-intensive products including agriculture and basic manufacturing. But there is plenty of controversy. Some economists argue that the contribution of trade, while positive, is smaller than many suggest and other factors are much more important in the development process. There is much debate about the key policies necessary to stimulate trade and the balance between traditional market-oriented policies and government interventions to help spur exports. Some believe that more open trade creates sweatshops and leads to a race to the bottom in wages, labor standards, and environmental outcomes. And some argue that multilateral trade negotiations are biased against poor countries, allowing rich countries to continue to protect their own agricultural and textile producers, as well as intellectual property, while forcing developing countries to open their economies.

In this chapter, we begin to examine these debates by considering recent trends and patterns in trade flows across countries. We then develop the core concept of comparative advantage and its powerful implications for international trade. Building on this essential theory, we turn to those economies whose comparative advantage lies in primary products, including food and other agricultural products; oil and natural gas; timber, minerals and other raw materials. The advantages and disadvantages of trade in such goods are then evaluated.

TRADE TRENDS AND PATTERNS

World trade has expanded dramatically over the past 50 years. Figure 18–1 shows the level of exports, expressed in current U.S. dollars, by region, from 1974 to 2007.[1] The trend in imports by region would look similar even though some nations, like the United States, import more than they export and others, like China, export more than they import. The persistence of trade deficits and surpluses do little to alter the aggregate pattern of regional trade flows.

Exports (and imports) from high-income nations continue to dominate global exchange. This may surprise you because it often seems that everything is made in China. The label, "Made in China," appears in much of our clothing, shoes, toys, and hundreds of other consumer goods. But the bulk of world trade, whether in airplanes, automobiles, computer software, machinery, pharmaceuticals, wheat, and other goods still originates and is exchanged between high-income economies. Beginning in 2009, China replaced Germany as the world's largest exporter of goods. But even as the world's largest exporting nation, China accounted for only 10 percent of world exports. Canada, not China, remains the major trading partner of the United States.

Measured at market exchange rates, the high-income economies account for almost 80 percent of world gross domestic product (GDP). Even if these nations trade a smaller percentage of their GDP than China, as many do, they still dominate world

[1]Figure 18–1 refers to merchandise exports only—that is, exports of goods, including primary products (such as agricultural goods, oil, and minerals) and manufactures, measured in current U.S. dollars unadjusted for price inflation. Trade in services, such as tourism and international transport, insurance and financial services, and call-center activities and data processing, is not included. Merchandise trade in 2007 accounted for 80 percent of total world trade.

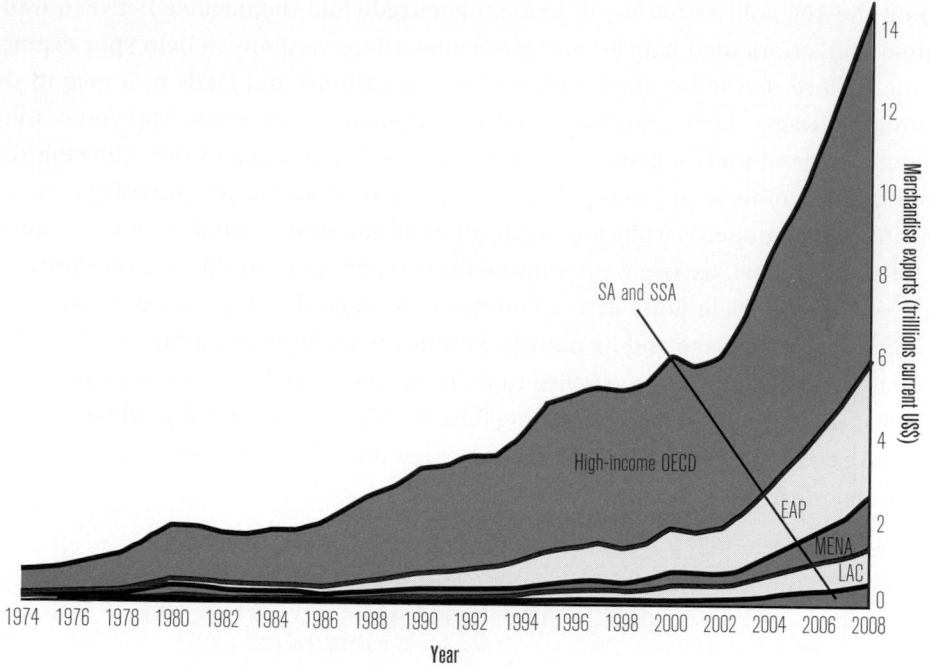

FIGURE 18-1 **Growth in World Exports by Region, 1974–2007**

EAP, East Asia and Pacific; LAC, Latin America and Caribbean; MENA, Middle East and North Africa; OECD, Organization for Economic Co-Operation and Development; SA, South Asia; SSA, sub-Saharan Africa. Exports from Europe and Central Asia are not included. Korea is included in EAP.
Source: World Bank, "World Development Indicators," http://databank.worldbank.org.

trade. Remember, GDP is the sum of all expenditures on consumption, investment, and government spending plus net exports (exports minus imports). If the high-income economies produce 80 percent of world output, it is no surprise that they also produce almost 75 percent of world exports and imports.

But there has been significant growth in exports from low- and middle-income economies. This growth can be traced back to the late 1970s, after China's reversal in policy toward a more outward-looking trade strategy. Even earlier, Hong Kong, Korea, Singapore, and Taiwan had considerable success with trade serving as an engine of economic growth. Other nations, including China, began to follow a similar model. The growth in exports from East Asia is shown in Figure 18-1 and can be seen more dramatically in Figure 18-2, which shows the share of total trade in GDP, including imports and exports of both goods and services, by region and decade. East Asia, the region with the highest rate of growth in GDP per capita over the past 30 years is also the region with the steepest increase in the ratio of trade to GDP. This ratio averaged around 20 percent in the 1970s but exceeded 75 percent in the 2000s, considerably higher than any other region. There is little doubt that trade played a central role in East Asia's achievements in both economic growth and development.

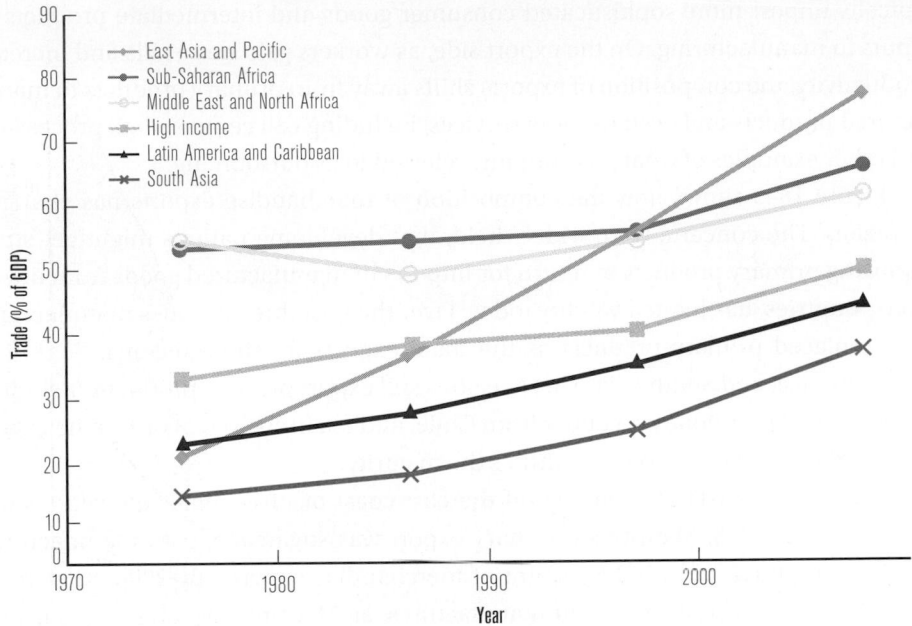

FIGURE 18-2 Importance of Trade to Economies, 1970–2007

The ratio of trade to gross domestic product (GDP) is the average value by decade by region.
Source: World Bank, "World Development Indicators," http://databank.worldbank.org.

For developing countries as a whole, imports plus exports on goods and services combined are now equivalent to over 64 percent of their total output, indicating that large portions of these economies are influenced by global markets. But there are stark regional differences in these trends, and Figure 18–2 reveals some patterns that may be less familiar. Sub-Saharan Africa is often thought to be marginalized from the global economy. This is true in terms of the region's minuscule contribution to world exports and imports. Its merchandise exports constituted 3.6 percent of the world total in 1970, falling to just 1.8 percent by 2007. But viewed from the perspective of the region, trade has always accounted for a large share of Sub-Saharan Africa's GDP. In the 1970s the trade to GDP ratio, at 53 percent, was higher than in almost any other region at that time; in the 2000s, it averaged 66 percent, second only to East Asia. The problem for the region has not been the share of trade in output but the failure of trade and GDP to grow by very much overtime. South Asia, where India's economy dominates, is the region where trade continues to play the smallest role, although that is beginning to change with a greater emphasis on both exports and imports in India and elsewhere.

As economies grow and the share of trade increases, the products imported and exported tend to change as well. On the import side, as incomes grow, countries typically import more sophisticated consumer goods and intermediate products as inputs to manufacturing. On the export side, as workers gain new skills and increase productivity, the composition of exports shifts away from primary products to manufactured products and even to some services, including call centers, data processing, and other examples of what is commonly referred to as outsourcing.

Figure 18–3 shows how the composition of merchandise exports has changed by region. The concern, once widely held, that developing nations might get stuck exporting primary products in return for imports of manufactured goods from developed countries, has limited validity today. Over the past three decades manufactures have replaced primary products as the main exports for three regions: East Asia, Latin America, and South Asia. These regions still export primary products, including natural gas from Indonesia, copper from Chile, and tea from Sri Lanka, but the export of manufactured goods now constitutes the majority.

Mauritius, an island economy off the east coast of Africa, has followed a similar pattern. In 1975, Mauritius's primary export was sugarcane, with manufactured goods accounting for only 12 percent of merchandise exports. By 2000, 81 percent of merchandise exports was from manufactures, as Mauritius became a major producer of clothing. Today, Mauritius is relying less on sugarcane and clothing and is developing exports in services, such as offshore banking, telecommunications, and

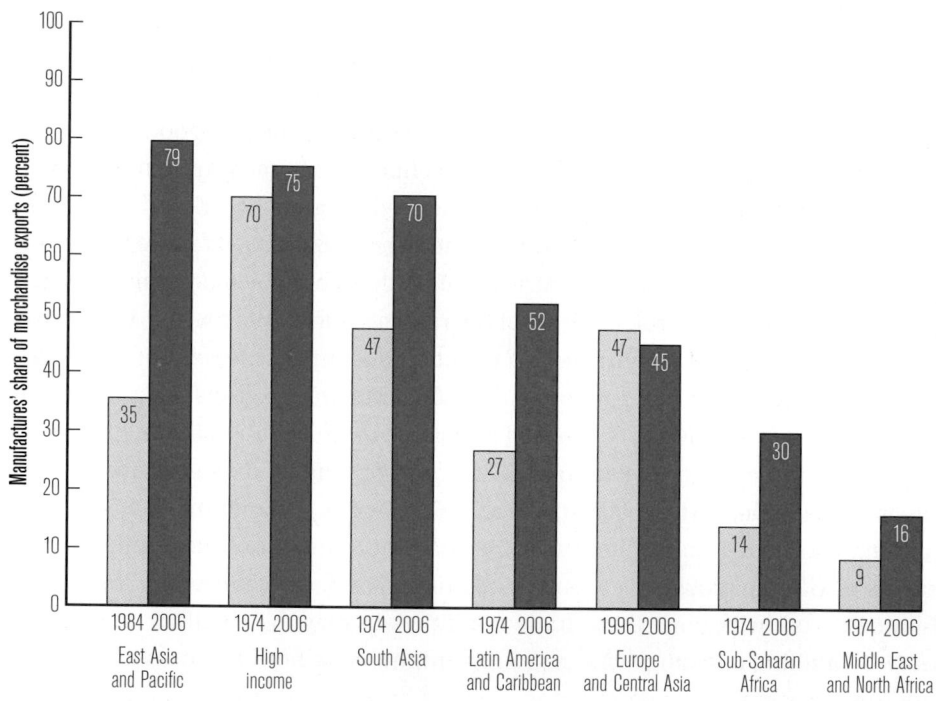

FIGURE 18-3 **Importance of Manufactured Exports by Region**

Source: World Bank, "World Development Indicators," http://databank.worldbank.org.

tourism. But on the African continent, primary products, including coffee, diamonds, groundnuts, oil, and minerals, continue to dominate merchandise trade. The impact of primary product exports on African and other economies is considered in detail later in this chapter.

For all developing regions, the majority of trade (around two thirds) continues to be with high-income economies. Since 1990, this share, not surprising, has increased significantly for the former Soviet Union and Soviet bloc. It has fallen in the Middle East as more oil exports go to other developing areas. The biggest change in Asia is that almost half of Asia's exports today are sent to other countries in Asia, including the larger high-income economies in the region (Japan, Korea, Singapore, and Taiwan). In 1980, within-Asia trade made up about one third of the region's total. Raw materials and intermediate products produced in one Asian country now are likely to be exported to a neighboring country for finishing and final export. China's dramatic rise is particularly significant. Its imports have grown almost as fast as its exports, and it is now one of the biggest markets in the world. A significant share of China's manufactured export products are assembled using components imported from other Asian economies.

WHO TRADES?

The extent to which a country trades with the rest of the world depends on many factors. Small countries, measured in this instance by population size, tend to trade more than larger ones, as they cannot efficiently produce the full range of consumer goods, intermediate products, and capital equipment demanded by consumers and businesses. Just as a small town cannot offer the same range of stores and services for shoppers as a large town, small economies cannot efficiently produce everything that households and firms would like to buy, so they tend to import more products to satisfy those demands. On the export side, as firms in small economies increase production, they are more likely to be constrained by the limited size of the market and unable to take advantage of economies of scale if they sell only locally. By exporting to global markets, they can sell larger amounts of more-specialized products. Export earnings then pay for the imports small nations demand. Producers in larger economies can sell a much larger share of their output locally without being constrained by market size. In Guyana, with a population of under 1 million, imports and exports together exceed 200 percent of GDP; in Mauritius they reach 133 percent. But in much larger Brazil and India, the ratios are 27 and 45 percent, respectively. Figure 18–4 confirms this relationship across all countries. It helps explain why sub-Saharan Africa, which has a large number of nations, half of them with populations below 10 million, has such a relatively high ratio of trade to GDP.

Trade patterns are also influenced by a country's geographical characteristics, including its access to shipping routes—especially whether it is landlocked—and its location relative to major markets. For the last several hundred years, the cheapest

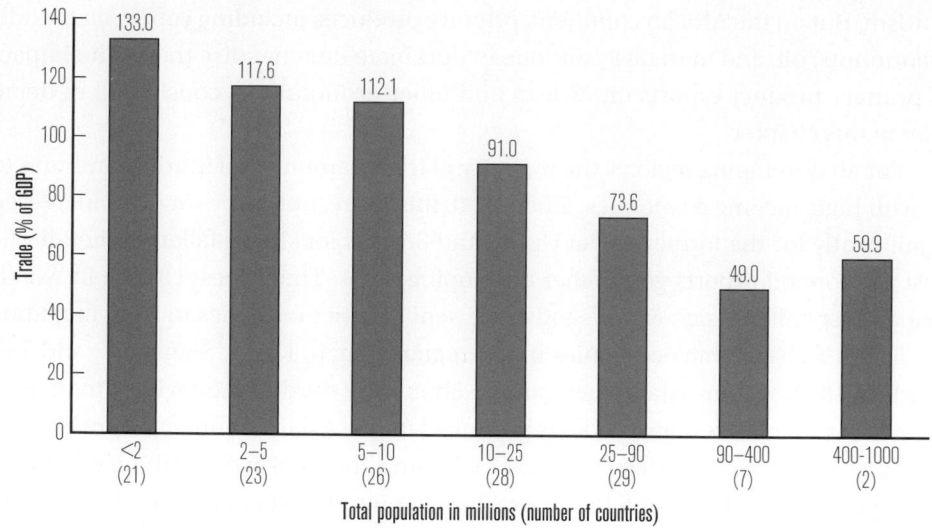

FIGURE 18-4 **Importance of Trade to Less Populous Nations**

Source: World Bank, "World Development Indicators," http://databank.worldbank.org.

and most important form of transporting goods between countries was by sea, and to this day, countries with easier access to sea-based shipping tend to have larger exports and imports than do landlocked countries. Adam Smith recognized the advantages of access to the sea for trade and commerce more than 230 years ago in *The Wealth of Nations*:

> As by means of water-carriage a more extensive market is opened to every sort of industry than what land-carriage alone can afford it, so it is upon the sea-coast, and along the banks of navigable rivers, that industry of every kind naturally begins to sub-divide and improve itself, and it is frequently not till a long time after that those improvements extend themselves to the inland part of the country.[2]

As Smith predicted, most landlocked countries trade less. Figure 18–5 identifies 44 nations that do not have a coastline. As a group, their trade to GDP ratio is 25 percent as compared to 75 percent for all other economies.[3] Less trade among the landlocked countries is a result of much higher transport costs, as they must not only pay for sea-based shipping but overland costs to and from the nearest seaport. These costs can skyrocket when relationships between neighboring countries deteriorate. Periodic conflict between Ethiopia and Eritrea has forced firms in Ethiopia to seek

---

[2]Adam Smith, *An Inquiry into the Nature and Causes of the Wealth of Nations* (New York: Modern Library, 1976), bk. 1, chap. 3, para. 3.

[3]These trade to GDP ratios are *unweighted*—for example, in the case of the landlocked nations it is the simple average of the 44 countries. When presenting most averages, by region or income group, we usually provide *weighted* averages, implicitly giving more importance to the region or group's largest economies.

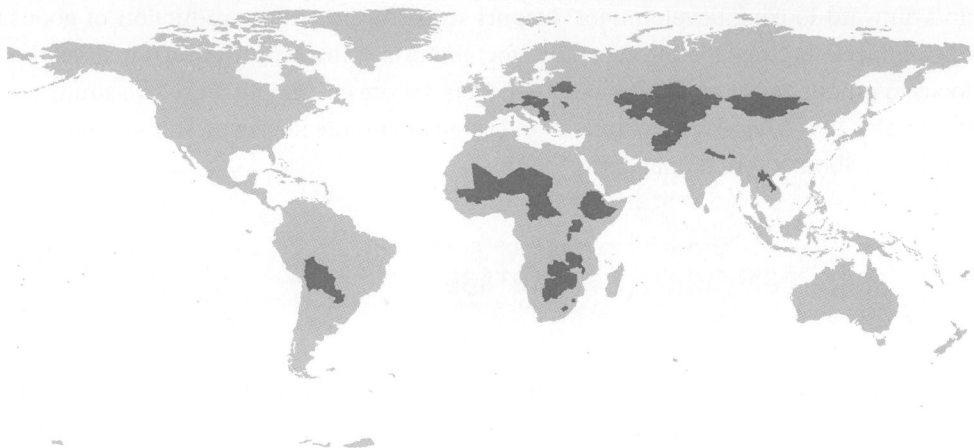

FIGURE 18-5 **Landlocked Nations of the World**

other more distant ports, for example, in Djibouti or Kenya. Landlocked Nepal almost totally depends on shipment through India. In Africa, 16 countries are landlocked, and their shipping costs have been two or three times higher than for their coastal neighbors.[4] As a result, everything that is imported is much more expensive. Similarly, exporters must pay more for shipping, raising the costs of export products and making firms less competitive on world markets.

As noted in Chapter 3, being landlocked not only reduces trade but is also associated with slower economic growth. An inability to trade more may account for this slower growth. But there are exceptions. Some landlocked high-income countries have done well, such as Austria and Switzerland, but they are located in the midst of major markets, are connected by high-quality road networks, and have had good relations with neighboring states, so shipping costs are not a major barrier. Landlocked countries that ship raw materials for which the margins between production costs and world prices are large are also in a better position to export, despite higher shipping costs. Landlocked Botswana has been very successful, as its diamonds bring in plenty of revenue to overcome higher shipping costs. Uganda's coffee, the nation's primary export, does not enjoy the same advantage. In addition to landlocked countries, countries isolated from major markets, such as Samoa and other small island countries of the Pacific Ocean, face similar issues with high shipping costs. As air shipment costs decline these disadvantages are reduced, but the vast majority of trade still takes place by sea.

In addition to size and geography, government strategies for trade and choices about trade policy determine trade outcomes. Broadly speaking, governments in developing countries have employed two different trade strategies, import substitution

---

[4]United Nations Conference on Trade and Development (UNCTAD), *Review of Maritime Transport 1995* (Geneva: United Nations Publications, 1995).

and outward-looking development. **Import substitution** is the production of goods and services that replace (or substitute for) imports. **Outward orientation** shifts the focus to producing for export for global markets. Before examining these two strategies in Chapter 19 it is necessary to understand some of the core ideas that shape economic reasoning about international trade.

COMPARATIVE ADVANTAGE

For more than 200 years, trade theorists have tried to explain why nations engage in international trade, what goods and services they trade, and how firms and consumers gain or lose. The workhorse models rely primarily on the **theory of comparative advantage**, which describes trade patterns under assumptions of *static conditions* that hold the factors of production in fixed supply and unable to cross borders. Comparative advantage has rich implications about the gains from trade. Among the most powerful results are the following:

- A country can increase its welfare by trading because the world market provides an opportunity to buy and sell goods at different prices than those that otherwise would be available to a nation that closed its economy to the rest of the world.
- The smaller the country, the greater is this potential gain from trade.
- A country often gains most by exporting commodities that it produces using its abundant factors of production most intensively, while importing goods whose production requires relatively more of scarcer factors of production.

The first implication is one of the most powerful ideas in all of economics. It is associated with the work of David Ricardo appearing in his *Principles of Political Economy and Taxation*, published in 1817. It is a testament to Ricardo's core insight that almost two centuries later comparative advantage still provides the foundation for thinking about trade between nations.

Any country can engage in and benefit from international trade, including the world's highest-cost and lowest-cost producers of any good. To see why, let us consider some examples. Mexico is the third largest trading partner of the United States. The United States is Mexico's largest trading partner. Many goods cross their borders. Among them, it is easy to understand why Mexico exports crude oil to the United States and why the United States exports aircraft to Mexico. The United States has depleted much of its oil reserves and imports oil from many countries, including Mexico. Mexico does not have an aircraft industry, nor is it likely to develop one anytime soon. That these nations would chose to trade, in essence, oil for airplanes is easy to understand. Some world trade is of this kind, by which nations trade goods that they essentially could not produce on their own. But most international trade does not have this characteristic, making the next example far more interesting.

TABLE 18-1 Production Costs and Comparative Advantage

LABOR-HOURS TO PRODUCE	MEXICO	UNITED STATES
Agricultural goods (1 ton of tomatoes)	50	40
Farm equipment (1 tractor)	300	200
Relative price (tons of tomatoes per tractor)	6	5

Mexico and the United States also trade farm equipment, say, tractors, and agricultural goods, say, tomatoes. These are goods, unlike airplanes and oil, that both nations are capable of producing. We can build a highly simplified model of trade in these goods between these two nations. The labor required to produce each product differs in the two countries, as shown in Table 18-1. By assumption, it takes fewer labor hours to produce either product in the United States. The United States is said to have an **absolute advantage** in both goods, the result, in this example, of a labor force that is more productive than Mexico's in producing both tractors and tomatoes. In our earlier case of airplanes and oil, the United States had an absolute advantage in airplanes and Mexico had one in oil. In the tractor and tomatoes example, Mexico has an **absolute disadvantage** in both goods. Yet even under the conditions described in Table 18-1, both nations are better off engaging in trade.

Without trade, Mexicans would have to produce six tons of tomatoes to buy one tractor in their home market because each tractor takes 300 labor-hours to produce compared to 50 labor-hours for one ton of tomatoes. In the United States, tractors sell for the equivalent of five tons of tomatoes because each tractor requires 200 labor-hours to produce compared to each ton of tomatoes, which requires 40 labor-hours.[5] Since each nation's **autarky prices** (domestic prices without trade) differ, there is the opportunity for mutually beneficial trade. Trade will occur when the price of tractors in terms of tomatoes lies in between the Mexican and United States autarky prices. Under free trade, the forces of supply and demand guarantee that prices will fall within this range.

Assume that both nations agree to trade one tractor for 5.5 tons of tomatoes. By selling to the United States, Mexico needs to give up only 5.5 rather than 6 tons of tomatoes to get a tractor. Thus Mexico is better off by switching its labor into producing more tomatoes and selling them to the United States. Instead of working 300 hours to produce one tractor, Mexican labor can work for 275 hours (50 hours/ton times 5.5 tons of tomatoes) and import one tractor. The 25 hours that are saved through trade can be used to produce more tomatoes and consume more of either good. The surprising result is that the United States also is better off if it buys tomatoes from

[5]This way of calculating relative prices, in Mexico tractors selling for six times the price of a ton of tomatoes and in the United States for five times, works in this oversimplified example because labor is the only input into production and production costs are the only determinant of relative prices.

Mexico and sells tractors in return, even though it can produce both tractors and tomatoes at home with fewer hours of labor. U.S. workers can spend 200 hours to produce either one tractor or 5 tons of tomatoes. If U.S. labor is shifted away from farming and into tractor production, one tractor exported to Mexico is equivalent to producing 5.5 tons of tomatoes, half a ton more than those 200 U.S. labor-hours could produce themselves. U.S. firms can produce enough tractors to satisfy domestic demand and export to Mexico, and U.S. consumers get to consume more tomatoes. Both Mexico and the United States are better off in the sense that for the same amount of effort, measured in labor-hours, they can consume more goods by engaging in trade.

Ricardo's insight was that trade would be mutually beneficial if each nation pursued the good in which it is *relatively more productive*—that is, the good in which it has a **comparative advantage**. In Mexico the opportunity cost of one tractor is six tons of tomatoes (or for one ton of tomatoes, one sixth of a tractor.) In the United States the opportunity cost of one tractor is five tons of tomatoes (or for one ton of tomatoes, one fifth of a tractor.) The United States gains by trading tractors and getting something more than five tons of tomatoes in return. Mexico gains by trading tomatoes and getting something better than one sixth of a tractor in return. The gains are the higher level of consumption trade permits. As economist Paul Krugman, who won the Nobel Prize in economics in 2008 for his pioneering work on international trade, has written, "imports, not exports are the purpose of trade. That is, what a country gains from trade is the ability to import things it wants. Exports are not an objective in and of themselves; the need to export is a burden that a country must bear because its import suppliers are crass enough to demand payment."[6]

The theory of comparative advantage may seem straightforward and intuitive, but it is often misunderstood. Whenever someone claims it is unfair for workers in high-income economies to have to compete with low-wage workers in developing nations, they are not appreciating the benefits of international trade between rich and poor nations. It is still true, as we discuss later, that trade creates winners and losers within each country; however, the theory of comparative advantage suggests that when countries trade freely, the total gains to each country outweigh the losses. Similarly, when critics refer to international trade as a competition, implying that some nations win and others lose as if trade were a zero-sum game, they are misunderstanding the mutually beneficial gains that follow from comparative advantage. And if someone says that no nation can compete with China's exports of manufactured goods they are both missing the reality of global exchange and do not understand Ricardo's basic insight.[7]

[6]Paul Krugman, "What Do Undergrads Need to Know about Trade?," *American Economic Review* 83, no. 2 (May 1993).

[7]In "Ricardo's Difficult Idea: Why Intellectuals Don't Understand Comparative Advantage," in G. Cook, ed., *The Economics and Politics of International Trade* (London: Routledge, 1998), economist Paul Krugman demonstrates how even sophisticated policy makers and commentators often miss the basic insight of comparative advantage.

THE BENEFITS OF TRADE

The core of comparative advantage is that both countries gain from trade whenever the relative prices of commodities in each country differ in the absence of trade. Once the two countries begin to trade, the relative prices of commodities begin to shift until they are the same in the two countries. This is because the model assumes no tariffs, quotas, or other barriers to free trade and it assumes that transport costs are negligible. In the example in Table 18–1, the relative price of tractors in terms of tons of tomatoes settles somewhere between five and six. The final world price that will prevail in both countries under free trade will be closer to the initial price in the market of the country whose economy is larger.

In our example, the final price in both countries would probably not settle at 5.5 tons, equidistant from the Mexican and U.S. autarky prices, but closer to 5 tons of tomatoes per tractor. This is because the U.S. economy is so much larger than that of Mexico and would exert more influence on both the supply and demand of each good. One implication is that small countries may benefit more from trade because the relative price of commodities shifts more, and therefore the gains from trade are greater. In our example, Mexico would be better off if the world price settled at 5.1 rather than 5.5 tons of tomatoes per tractor, because it would have to give up fewer tomatoes (and the labor time to produce them) for each tractor. Where world prices settle, often referred to as the **international terms of trade** (the ratio of the prices a nation receives for the goods it exports relative to the prices it receives for the goods it imports) is an important determinant of the gains from trade and is discussed in more detail later in this chapter.

The theory of comparative advantage as posed here is in the very simple form developed by Ricardo during the nineteenth century: two countries, two goods, and only one factor of production (labor).[8] Some of the complexities of the real world can be incorporated into the theory. A trading world of many countries can be handled by taking the home country, say, Kenya, and treating the rest of the world as its trading partner. Swedish economists Eli Heckscher and Bertil Ohlin expanded the theory during the first half of the twentieth century to deal with two factors of production, such as labor and capital. The Heckscher-Ohlin model leads to an extremely important result: A country tends to export products that use its abundant factors of production more intensively and imports products that require relatively more of its scarce factors.

This more general approach to comparative advantage is encapsulated in Figure 18–6. The economy of the **home country** is divided into two goods, one that will be exported (tomatoes) and one that will be imported (tractors). The country's collective utility in consuming these goods is represented by the community indifference curves.

Without trade, the home country achieves its greatest utility by producing and consuming at point *A*, the tangency of the community indifference curve IC_1 and

---

[8]Ricardo's example, fitting his era, relied on England and Portugal trading wine and cloth.

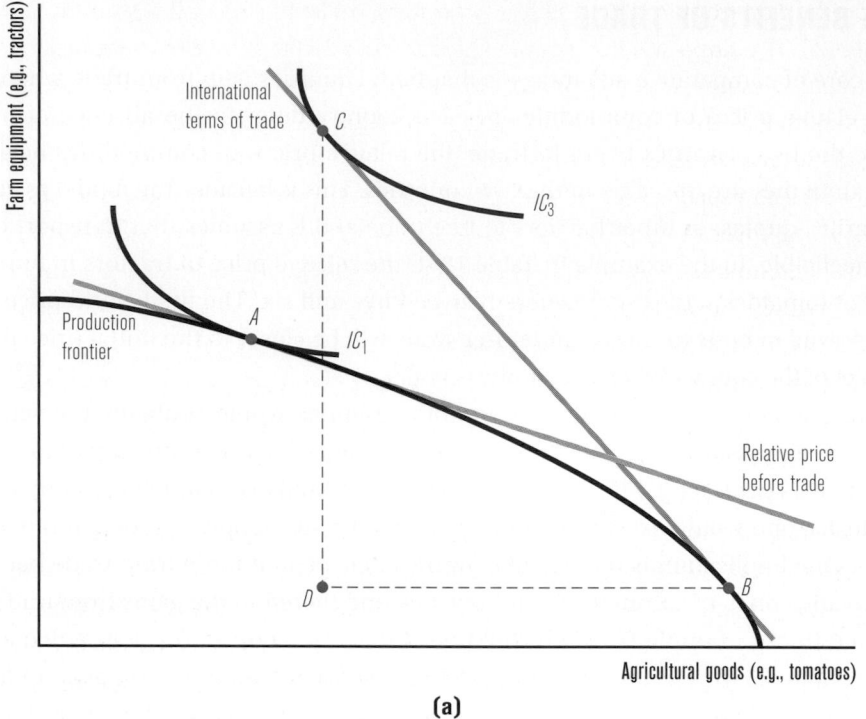

(a)

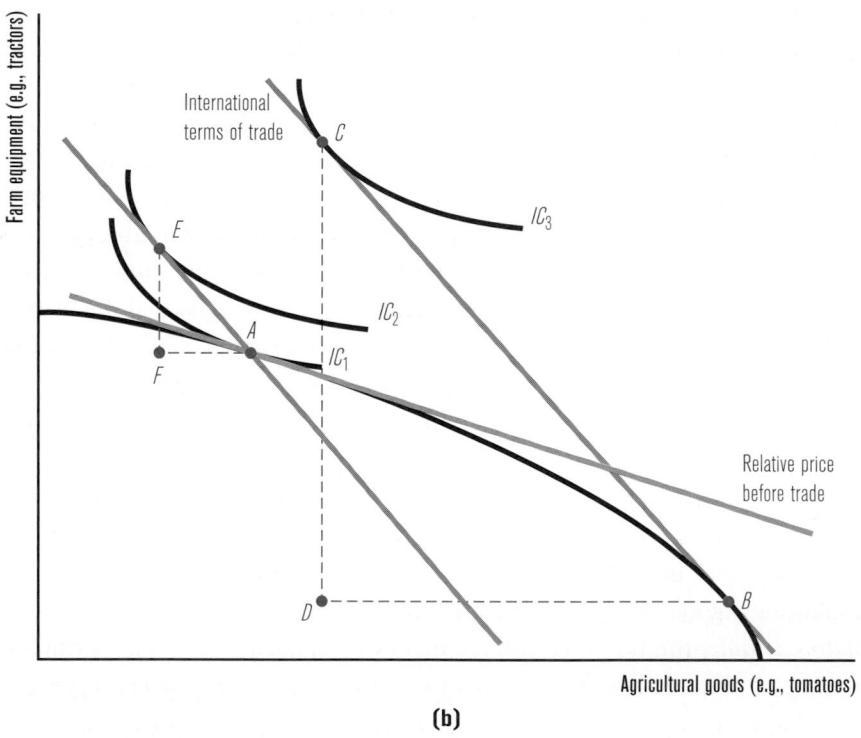

(b)

FIGURE 18-6 **Gains from Trade**

the production frontier. Because it is producing on its frontier, all resources are fully employed. The slope at *A* determines the domestic relative price of tomatoes in terms of tractors. Assume that the rest of the world is better endowed with capital than labor relative to the endowments of the home country and that world consumers have tastes broadly similar to those of the home country. Then, in world markets, the relatively higher production of tractors compared to the demand for tractors drives their prices lower than in the home country, and the relatively lower production of tomatoes compared to the demand for tomatoes drives their price higher than in the home country. Because only relative prices matter, these two statements mean the same thing: In world markets, the price of tomatoes in terms of tractors is higher than in the home country leading to the international terms of trade being steeper than the autarky price line.

This difference in relative prices between the home country and the rest of the world presents an opportunity for the home country to improve its welfare through trade. *With trade*, the country, taking advantage of its factor endowment, can produce more tomatoes and fewer tractors and can sell tomatoes on the world market at the higher relative price. By producing more tomatoes, the home country moves along its production frontier from *A* to *B*, where the international terms of trade line is tangent to the production frontier. With tomatoes to export, the country can import tractors and consume more of *both* goods and be better off. The consumption point *C* is determined by the tangency of the international terms of trade line with the community indifference curve IC_3. The country now exports *BD* tons of tomatoes and imports *CD* of tractors; the amounts for both goods equal to the difference between consumption at *C* and production at *B*. (Note that the ratio CD:BD is an exact description of the international terms of trade.) As indifference curve IC_3 is above indifference curve IC_1, the country is better off with trade than without it. Note that both with and without trade the home country produces along its production frontier and all resources are fully employed. By pursuing its comparative advantage, the home country, exerts the same level of effort because all resources are fully employed in both cases but consumes more with trade than without trade.

Figure 18–6 can be used to gain some further insight into the sources of the **gains from trade**. In Figure 18–6b, the international terms of trade line is drawn through point *A*, the equilibrium without trade. This depicts the opportunities a nation faces by trading with other nations even when it does not change production. Under such a scenario, the nation could still gain from trade benefiting from the higher prices the rest of the world is willing to pay for its export good and the lower prices the nation would pay for its imports. The country could now move from the equilibrium at point *A* to the one at point *E*, exporting *AF* tons of tomatoes in return for *EF* tractors. This exchange permits the nation to move from indifference curve IC_1 to IC_2 and be better off. (In this example, note that the ratio EF:AF = CD:BD = the international terms of trade.) The implied increase in welfare is called the **gains from exchange** because it is due only to the difference between autarky and world prices.

But facing the opportunities trade provides, a nation will also reallocate its resources as it pursues its comparative advantage. At point A producers in the home country are not maximizing profits and consumers are not maximizing utility (both of which are requirements for equilibrium in this type of general equilibrium model). It will not remain producing at point A when other nations are willing to pay more for its exports and to sell imports for less. The change in production from point A to B maximizes producers' profits and results in an additional improvement in welfare depicted in the change in consumption from point E to C, and the movement from indifference curve IC_2 to IC_3. These are the **gains from specialization**. The gains from trade are therefore made up of the gains from exchange plus the gains from specialization.

Figure 18–6 shows the gains from exchange and specialization, but trade confers many more benefits to a nation that are not illustrated by the figure. First, trade exposes domestic firms to competition. Especially in small economies, there may be a limited number of producers of particular products. This may enable them to exercise market power, supplying less and charging more for their goods. Faced with competition from imports, market power is eroded, prices fall, and consumption and welfare increases. Trade disciplines domestic firms that wield market power. Competition from foreign firms can also increase the productivity of domestic firms. Faced with competition from abroad, firms may invest less in rent seeking, gaining special favors from government to protect their market power, and more in increasing efficiency and lowering costs. In competitive markets, the most productive firms survive and in so doing improve the use of scarce resources and raise output levels.

Second, trade, especially in intermediate goods including machinery and other forms of capital, often embodies new technologies that raise productivity. In our example of trade in tomatoes and tractors, if imported tractors contain better technology (for example, higher fuel efficiency or longer-lasting tires or other parts), Mexican farmers will become more productive, producing more tomatoes per hour, because of the imported technology embodied in imports that is absent in domestic farm equipment. Referring to Figure 18–6, trade-induced productivity effects such as these would shift the home nation's production frontier outward, a graphical reflection of economic growth. These benefits are in addition to trade enabling a nation to consume beyond its production frontier.

Third, trade increases not only the amount of goods a nation can consume but also the quality and variety of goods available. Before their transition, tropical fruits, especially bananas, were viewed as an exotic luxury in countries such as East Germany and Poland. An opening to trade made such products commonplace, increasing consumer welfare. In addition to final consumption goods like bananas, trade increases the variety of other goods available, including medicines. Cellphones provide an example of the benefits trade can confer to even some of the poorest workers. Without trade, cellphones might not be available because domestic firms may not have the knowledge and technology to produce them. But because of imports, cellphones can be found in even remote areas. In India, traditional fishermen often carry cellphones with them and use them to communicate with other fishermen about where to fish and to find out about available prices for their catch at various local ports. Cellphones, a product that would have been unavailable unless imported, have eroded the market power of the fish buyers onshore and improved the livelihoods of the fishermen.

Fourth, trade also brings people into contact with one another. Whether this promotes peace, global understanding, and democracy remains an intriguing hypothesis.[9] Added to Ricardo's insight about exchange and specialization based on comparative advantage, there are many other important benefits poor nations can realize from international trade.

WINNERS AND LOSERS

Any country, whatever its size and stage of development, can benefit from trade. This is true for large countries like China and India, small countries such as Laos and Togo, high-income countries like Japan and the United States, and low-income countries such as Haiti and Mozambique. Ricardo's theory uses two goods and two nations with no restrictions on what type of nation is involved. As long as relative prices at home differ from those on world markets (or would differ in the absence of international trade), countries can increase their aggregate welfare by engaging in international trade.

Many of you may read these conclusions and remain skeptical and unconvinced. If the economic argument that trade is such a good thing is true, why is there so much opposition to globalization, the WTO, and free trade? What about sweatshops and the harsh conditions in the maquiladoras, a Spanish term used in Mexico and elsewhere that refers to factories, usually just over the border, that assemble goods for richer nations? What about the loss of jobs, factories, and a way of life throughout the old industrial belt in the European Union and United States? Trade played some role in these outcomes. Clearly the benefits of trade that stem from economic theory are missing an important part of the story.

The answer lies, in part, in the distributional consequences of trade. Comparative advantage as described by Ricardo focuses on the efficiency gains of trade, on how a given amount of resources can result in more total consumption. Although every country can gain from trade in the aggregate, *not all individuals or groups within each country necessarily gain.*

In the tomatoes for tractors example, Mexican vegetable growers gain from trade because they can sell more tomatoes at a higher price. Mexican consumers of tractors also gain, because they can now purchase imported tractors at a lower price. But, once trade begins, Mexican tractor manufacturers face competition from imports

---

[9]Douglas Irwin, *Free Trade under Fire,* 3rd ed. (Princeton: Princeton University Press, 2009), chap. 2, provides an excellent survey of the benefits of trade.

and hence sell fewer tractors at a lower price than before, whereas Mexican consumers of tomatoes must pay higher prices. (By an analogous argument, the price changes brought about by trade benefits tractor producers and tomato consumers in the United States but hurt U.S. tractor consumers and tomato growers.) If firms producing tractors (tomatoes) in Mexico (the United States) shut down in the face of imports, workers in those firms will be hurt, at least in the short run, and so may the communities in which they live. If there are such clearly defined losers from international trade, how can we be so sure that trade is a good thing?

The explanation lies in the core insight of comparative advantage. The theory tells us that the *aggregate gains* from trade outweigh the losses for the country as a whole. This is because the value of output in total rises, implying that the gains of the winners are greater than the losses of the losers. The winners gain enough to compensate the losses of the losers. But that may be cold comfort to Mexican producers of computers and consumers of tomatoes because there is no guarantee that they will be compensated for their losses. These are the distributional consequences of trade that are the seed of the political opposition to policies that promote freer trade.

The work of Heckscher and Ohlin leads to further important insights into the distributional consequences of trade.[10] If a nation's comparative advantage lies in those goods that intensively use a nation's abundant factor, than that factor gains from trade while the less abundant factor loses. If Mexico is labor abundant relative to the United States, then Mexican labor will eventually gain from trade no matter if it is employed in the production of tomatoes or tractors. This is because trade reallocates factors of production, from point A to B in Figure 18–6. Because the economy is now producing more of the labor-intensive good (tomatoes), the aggregate demand for labor rises and increases its return.[11] Of course such transitions are not seamless. Some workers, especially older ones, will find it hard to move and take on new jobs in the export sector. Trade often benefits the next generation, which is better able to take advantage of the new opportunities whether in farms now producing for export rather than subsistence, in factories making goods for overseas markets, or in call centers providing tradable services.

However suggestive the theory of comparative advantage may be for developing countries, it is only the beginning of an explanation of development through international trade. Ricardo's discussion of comparative advantage assumes *static conditions* that hold the factors of production in fixed supply and unable to cross borders. But economic growth is fundamentally a *dynamic process*. To explain growth and

---

[10]These insights are originally attributed to Wolfgang Stolper and Paul Samuelson, "Protection and Real Wages" *Review of Economic Studies* 9, no. 1 (1941).

[11]In the developed nation, which generally is capital abundant relative to its developing nation trading partner, comparative advantage lies in the capital-intensive good, and capital, not labor, is the factor that benefits from trade. This helps explain why labor in developed nations, especially less-skilled labor, and politicians who seek the vote of such groups, are often opposed to trade agreements and in favor of protecting domestic industries.

structural change we need to account for changes over time in the amount of capital, land, and labor available to producers as well as improvements in the quality or productivity of those factors. This is something comparative advantage alone cannot do. The theory of comparative advantage also does not capture the two-way relationship between trade and development. In one direction, increased trade can lead to improved welfare and higher incomes. In the other direction, advances in development go hand in hand with more highly skilled labor and higher-quality capital and machinery, opening up new opportunities for increased trade. To better understand how trade and development affect each other we need to examine some of the alternative trade strategies nations have adopted, some of which are consistent with comparative advantage and others not.

TRADING PRIMARY PRODUCTS

Most world trade involves manufactured goods. But primary products, whether agricultural raw materials, food, fuels, minerals, or ores, still represent about one third of the value of all traded goods. Figure 18–7 identifies economies that are dependent on exports of primary products, that is, where more than 75 percent of their merchandise exports is in primary products. This group includes 13 low-income, 27 middle-income, and 9 high-income economies. For most of these economies petroleum is the dominant export. But for others it might be coffee (Nicaragua), copper (Mongolia), or cotton (Burkina Faso). Given how many nations continue to depend on primary product exports, it is worth examining the role of trade in primary products on economic growth and development.

There are additional reasons for focusing on trade in primary products. First, for most developing economies, international trade often began with primary products, and subsequent thinking about the impact of trade on development has its roots in the exchange of primary products from the south for manufactured goods from the north. Second, the growth performance of resource-rich economies often has been disappointing, referred to as **the resource curse** and seemingly the opposite of the predictions of comparative advantage. The rest of this chapter considers trade in primary products as an engine of growth, its potential and its failures, as well as its broader implications for whether movements in the international terms of trade support developing economies. Trade in manufactured goods is considered in Chapter 19.

The promise of primary product exports is clear. Many low- and middle-income nations have resources that are unavailable or severely depleted in high-income economies. Tropical fruits and beverages, including bananas and coffee, cannot be grown in Europe, Japan, and North America (except in greenhouses) but are in high demand. Diamonds and oil are obvious examples of primary products in abundance in some low- and middle-income economies that face limited demand at home

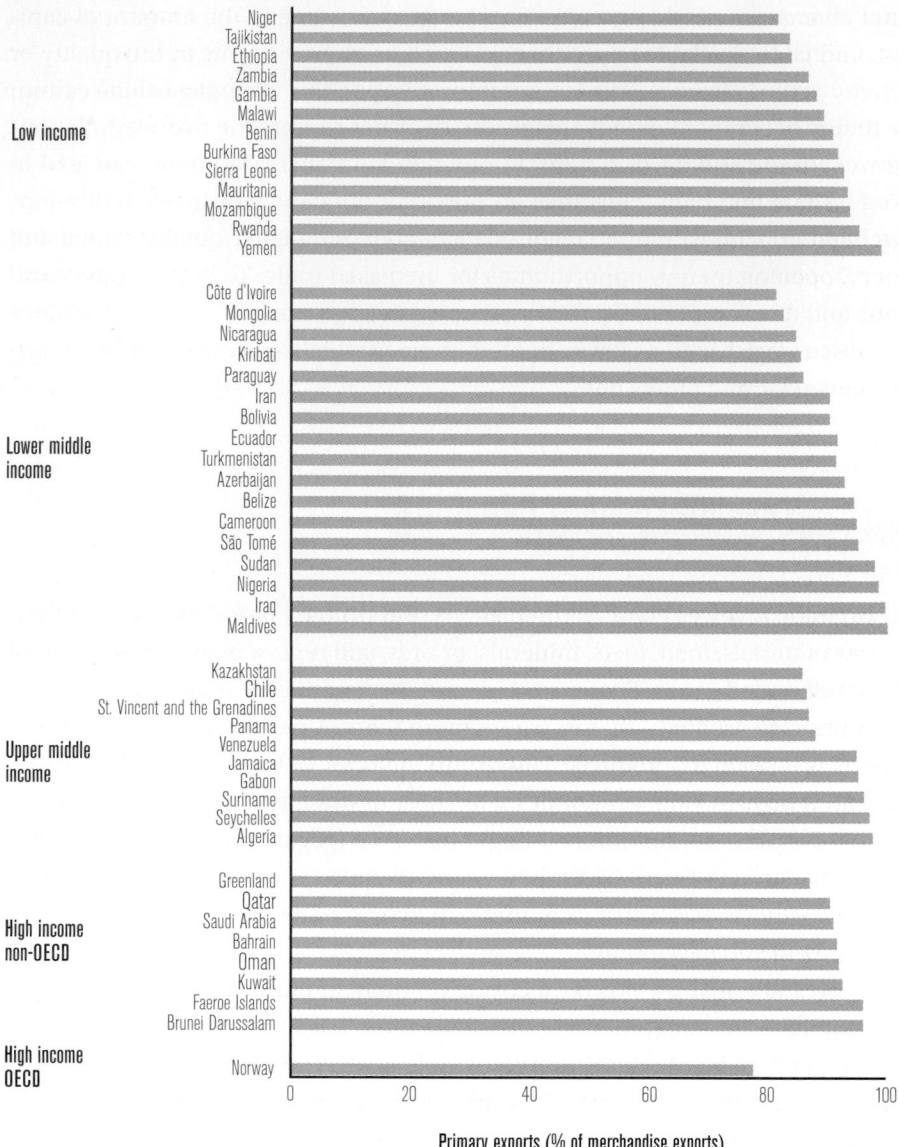

FIGURE 18-7 **The Importance of Trade in Primary Products**

OECD, Organization for Economic Co-Operation and Development. Included are countries where primary products account for 75 percent or more of all merchandise trade.
Source: World Bank, "World Development Indicators," http://databank.worldbank.org.

but significant demand abroad. Copper deposits in Chile and Zambia, coltan in the Congo (a mineral used in making the electronics for cellphones), and palm oil grown throughout Southeast Asia offer further examples.

Referring to Figure 18–6, we can substitute resource-intensive primary products on the *x*-axis and manufactures on the *y*-axis. Without trade, a nation will produce some combination of the two goods, as represented by point *A*. Once trade becomes an option, a relatively resource-rich nation will devote more of its resources to the primary goods sector, shifting capital and labor to produce more of its primary products, where it has a comparative, if not an absolute, advantage. This permits the economy to consume more, as represented by point *C*. The gains can be even greater if land or some other natural resource lies idle. If this is the case, without trade the nation might find itself in an interior point well within the production frontier. Trade creates an opportunity to take advantage of such idle resources and improve domestic consumption outcomes even more.

Burmese economist Hla Myint long ago observed that when parts of Africa and Asia came under European colonization the consequent expansion of their international trade enabled those areas to use their land or labor more intensively to produce tropical foodstuffs such as rice, cocoa, and oil palm for export. Myint applied Adam Smith's term **vent for surplus** to these cases.[12] The concept applies to a situation in which a country has the capacity to produce more than it can sell on the domestic market. Trade enables the country to employ either land or labor more fully and sell the goods produced with its "surplus" land and labor to the rest of the world. In many ways, this describes the economic development of Australia, Canada, and the United States during the nineteenth century.

In addition to helping an economy use its *current* factor endowments more intensively and more efficiently, the expansion of primary product exports can lead to the accumulation of additional factors of production, including capital and labor. Primary export–led growth can spur increases in foreign investment to complement the fixed factors of production, land, and natural resources. In the context of Figure 18–6, the country would be able to produce more because its production frontier would shift out.

Once profitable opportunities in tropical agriculture or natural resources become apparent, foreign investment is likely to be attracted to the country to exploit the country's comparative advantage. The influx of foreign investors has been a familiar story in all mineral-exporting industries and in many tropical-product industries based on plantation agriculture. Well-known historical examples include Standard Oil in Venezuela, British Petroleum in Iran, Anaconda in Chile, Alcoa in Jamaica, Firestone in West Africa, and United Fruit in Central America.[13] All these examples resulted in an increase in primary product production and exports. They also often involved political manipulation by these foreign firms in the domestic affairs of their host country, leaving a legacy that made other countries wary of foreign investment. The situation today, generally, is viewed differently, with governments able to negotiate

---

[12]Hla Myint, "The 'Classical Theory' of International Trade and the Underdeveloped Countries," *Economic Journal* 68 (1959), 317–37.

[13]Anaconda developed Chile's copper mines, Alcoa pursued Jamaica's bauxite deposits, Firestone operated rubber plantations in Liberia and elsewhere for use in tire production, and United Fruit focused on bananas throughout Central America.

better terms for the development of natural resources and the sharing of **resource rents**.[14] (Foreign direct investment was discussed in Chapter 10.)

Another potential benefit from primary product exports is the possibility of stimulating production in other, related sectors. The very notion of export-led growth implies that exports would lead to more broad-based economic growth. Several types of linkages to the rest of the economy are possible, including to upstream or downstream industries, increased production of consumer goods, enhanced infrastructure, more widely available skilled labor, and increased government revenues. Albert O. Hirschman coined the phrase **backward linkages** for the situation in which the growth of one industry (such as textiles) stimulates domestic production of an upstream input (such as cotton).[15] Expanded production of primary products also can stimulate **forward linkages** by making lower-cost primary goods available as inputs into other industries. In many developing countries, agricultural products are used as inputs to the food processing industry. Senegal and the Gambia process raw groundnuts (peanuts) into shelled nuts and cooking oil; in Indonesia, forest products are used in furniture production. Forward linkages can develop for mining and mineral products (such as, petroleum refining, plastics, or steel), but the more complex production techniques and demand for highly specialized capital and labor make it difficult for many developing countries to compete in these activities. Furthermore, developed nations often employ **tariff escalation**, imposing higher tariffs on imports of processed goods than on the raw material, making it harder for the developing nation to move up the value-added ladder.

Infrastructure linkages arise when the provision of overhead capital (roads, railroads, power, water, and telecommunications) for the export industry lowers costs and opens new production opportunities for other industries. Primary export sectors also may stimulate human capital linkages through the development of local entrepreneurs and skilled laborers. The growth of the Peruvian fishmeal industry, with its many small plants, encouraged scores of new entrepreneurs and trained many skilled workers to operate and maintain equipment. These resources then became available for subsequent development. Rubber, palm oil, and tin production for export encouraged entrepreneurs in Malaysia, and small-scale farming for export has proven an outlet for entrepreneurial talent in several African countries. But perhaps the best case for petroleum, mining, and some traditional agricultural crops is the fiscal linkage. Governments can capture large shares of the economic rents from these exports as taxes, dividends, or through leasing arrangements and use the revenue to finance development in other sectors.

---

[14]Economists use the term *rent* to refer to the excess of revenues over the costs of production plus the normal profit margin. When commodity prices rise, as in the case of petroleum exports, resource rents also tend to rise because the cost of oil drilling often does not change appreciably.

[15]Albert O. Hirschman, *The Strategy of Economic Development* (New Haven, CT: Yale University Press, 1958), chap. 6.

EMPIRICAL EVIDENCE ON PRIMARY EXPORT-LED GROWTH

Since the 1950s, some economists and the leaders of many developing countries have argued that, despite the possible benefits, primary exports cannot effectively lead the way to economic development. The most common arguments have been that the markets for primary products grow too slowly to fuel growth, the prices received for these commodities have been declining, earnings are too unstable, linkages do not work, and the fiscal windfall more often than not breeds corruption and civil strife rather than growth and development. We examine these arguments in the next section. Here, we discuss the direct empirical question, What has been the relationship between primary exports and economic growth in recent decades? A few resource-rich developing countries have performed relatively well, including Botswana, Indonesia, Malaysia, Mauritius, and some of the oil-rich states of the Persian Gulf. However, many others have grown very slowly or not at all, or have experienced increases in GDP per capita, which have been accompanied by little economic development. Such nations are Angola, Burma, Ecuador, Equatorial Guinea, Jamaica, Nigeria, and Zambia. At the same time, many of the fastest-growing Asian economies are resource poor—for example, Korea, Singapore, Taiwan, and, more recently, India and Vietnam.

Using regression analysis, economists Jeffrey Sachs and Andrew Warner examined the relationship between primary product exports and economic growth in a sample of 95 countries from around the world between 1970 and 1989.[16] They ran growth regressions that isolate the independent effects of various determinants of GDP per capita growth, including initial per capita income, openness to trade, government efficiency, investment rates, inequality, and the share of primary product exports in GDP. They found strong evidence showing that, on average and holding constant the other determinants of growth, countries with substantial primary product exports have grown much more *slowly* than resource-poor countries. They found that an increase of 10 percentage points in the ratio of primary exports to GDP was associated with a 0.7 percentage point *slower* annual rate of growth of per capita income. Figure 18–8 illustrates the basic negative relationship over a slightly longer time period (1970–96). For the 27 countries in which primary exports (in 1970) were 5 percent of GDP or less, annual per capita growth averaged 2.7 percent. By contrast, annual per capita growth averaged less than 0.5 percent in the 16 countries with primary exports equal to 20 percent or more of GDP. This

---

[16]Jeffrey Sachs and Andrew Warner, "Natural Resource Abundance and Economic Growth," NBER Working Paper No. W5398, Cambridge, MA, December 1995.

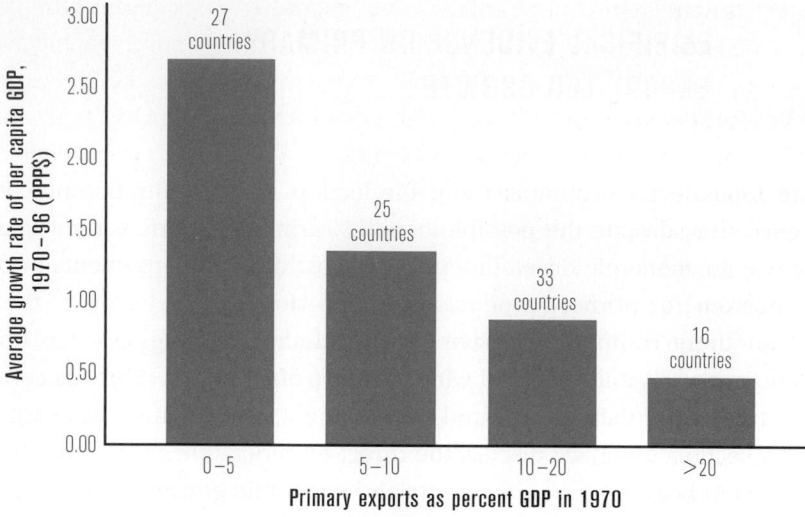

FIGURE 18-8 **Natural Resource Abundance and Economic Growth**

Countries with small amounts of primary product exports have grown more quickly than resource-abundant countries.

GDP, gross domestic product; PPP, purchasing power parity.
Source: Updated from Steven Radelet, Jeffrey Sachs, and Jong-Wha Lee, "Economic Growth in Asia," Harvard Institute for International Development, Cambridge, May 1997. Data from World Bank, *World Development Indicators* and *Penn World Tables*, mark 5.6.

represents a massive difference in the rate of economic growth and the potential for economic development.[17]

How can resource abundance be associated with slower rates of economic growth? Following the law of comparative advantage and capturing the dynamic gains from trade, primary product exports should help raise aggregate income and allow a country to increase imports and investment. There are several possible explanations for this apparent puzzle.

EXPORT PESSIMISM

Long before the growth regression results of Sachs and Warner and well before "the resource curse" became part of the vocabulary of development economics, there were reservations about primary product exports as an engine of growth for poor nations. It is worth reviewing this history because some of its themes still resonate today. What became known as **export pessimism** has its origins in work first published in the 1950s

[17]A recent study confirms these findings: "Developing countries, which in 1980 derived more than 70 percent of their export revenues from non-fuel primary commodities, increased their per capita GDP by only 0.4 percent a year between 1980 and 2006, and countries that mainly exported fuels raised their per capita GDP by 1.1 percent a year. By contrast, more-diversified exporters achieved per capita growth of 1.6 percent a year." World Bank, *Global Economic Prospects* (Washington, DC: World Bank, 2009), p. 98.

by economists Raul Prebisch, Hans Singer, and others.[18] These economists argued that, over the long run, prices for primary commodity exports on world markets tend to fall relative to prices of manufactured goods. Because at the time the Prebisch-Singer hypothesis was advanced, developing countries mostly exported primary products and imported manufactured goods, such a shift in the international terms of trade implied that, over time, developing countries would have to export more primary products to import the same amount of manufactured products. Countries relying on primary product exports, therefore, would continue to lag behind in the development process as the gains from trade would become more and more limited.

The root of the relative price movements suggested by Prebisch and Singer were traced to structural factors in the global economy. First, there is Engel's law (named after Ernest Engel, a nineteenth-century German statistician who first proposed the idea) that the demand for staple foods grows more slowly than income. For high-income countries, the income elasticity of demand for food is below one half, implying that the demand for food (including food imported from developing countries) tends to lag far behind income growth. At the same time, the demand for manufactured goods is income elastic, causing demand and hence prices to grow relatively more rapidly for such goods. The implication is that developing nations would wind up earning relatively less for their exports and paying relatively more for their imports.

Second, technological change in manufacturing also works against the demand for raw materials and the nations that produce them. New technologies and improved machinery help firms reduce wastage so that less raw material is needed in the production process. Modern looms waste less cotton yarn, new mining techniques are more efficient, and so forth. Perhaps even more significant, new technologies allow for the substitution of synthetics for raw materials. Synthetic rubber long ago replaced natural rubber in automobile tires and other applications; fiber optics has substantially reduced the use of copper in wire; and automobiles use fiberglass instead of steel, decreasing the demand for iron ore. There is widespread evidence that industrial production has grown more rapidly than the consumption of raw materials.

Third, Prebisch argued that manufacturing firms in developed countries tended to have market power, whereas primary producers in developing countries faced much greater competition. As a result, prices for manufactures were less flexible than those for primary goods. With productivity growth, primary producers would face lower prices due to competition from other producers, but this would not happen to the same degree with manufactured goods. In manufactures, productivity growth might raise profits rather than lower prices. This reasoning provided one more reason why poor nations might expect declining terms of trade and export pessimism.

---

[18]United Nations (Raul Prebisch), *The Economic Development of Latin America and Its Principal Problems* (Lake Success, NY: United Nations, 1950); Hans W. Singer, "The Distribution of Trade between Investing and Borrowing Countries," *American Economic Review* 40 (May 1950), 473–85. See also the later reflections of these two economists in G. Meier and D. Seers, eds., *Pioneers in Development* (Washington, DC: World Bank, 1985).

Prebisch, Singer, and the others concerned about trade and development based some of their findings on characteristics of the global economy that existed in the first half of the twentieth century and no longer hold. They also did not focus on such commodities as diamonds, natural gas, oil, tropical woods, and other primary products that face either relatively income elastic demand, shrinking supply, or few synthetic substitutes. They did not expect primary producers to be able to transition to manufactured goods as have many low- and middle-income economies. Nor did they envision the fierce global competition in manufactured goods that exists today or the cartels that influence the prices of some primary product markets. The export pessimism they expressed half a century ago, which went on to influence the trade strategies of many nations, is mostly rejected today. Too many low- and middle-income nations have benefited from exports as an engine of growth. But Prebisch and Singer's attention to the terms of trade and its implications for developing nations remains an important issue, one worthy of further examination.

DECLINING TERMS OF TRADE?

Concern over the direction of the terms of trade is easy to understand within the context of the theory of comparative advantage; but it is *not* a critique of that theory. Figure 18–9 reproduces Figure 18–6a and adds a decline in the terms of trade. The

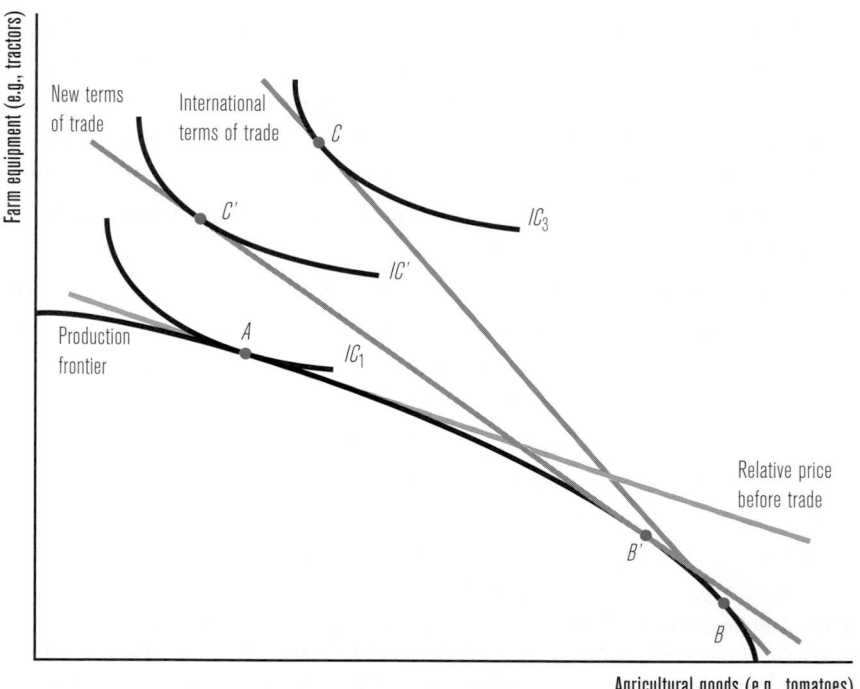

FIGURE 18-9 **Declining Terms of Trade**

counterclockwise rotation in the world price line indicates that the relative price of the exported good (tomatoes) has fallen relative to the price of the imported good (tractors). With these price changes, the nation exporting agricultural goods is worse off than before. It captures fewer gains from specialization, now producing at *B'* rather than at *B*, and lower gains from exchange and finds itself on a lower community indifference curve, *IC'*.

According to Figure 18–9, any country experiencing a decline in its terms of trade still realizes gains from trade. The nation is better than if it returned to autarky at point *A* and did not engage in any trade. But it would obviously prefer the initial terms of trade that permitted consumption at point *C* rather than at point *C'*. While the shift in the terms of trade in the figure diminishes the gains from trade for the nation exporting agricultural goods, the opposite would be true for the nation importing tomatoes and exporting tractors. For this nation, which in the Prebisch-Singer view would be a developed economy, the gains from trade would increase. No wonder some export pessimists called for a new international economic order, which would improve the benefits the developing nations received from global trade. Such concerns continue to be expressed by those both attending and protesting at meetings of the WTO.

In the simple two-good, two-country model the impact of the terms of trade on the gains from trade is straightforward. The empirical record, in a world of multiple products and nations, is somewhat less so. We begin by looking at trends in commodity prices. Figure 18–10 presents the trend from 1960 to 2009, in an index of commodity prices compiled by the United Nations Conference on Trade and Development (UNCTAD). The index refers to a broad range of commodities, excluding oil but including everything from coffee, cotton, timber, and tobacco to nickel and zinc. Food products account for about two thirds of the value of the index. Two trends are apparent. There has been a general secular decline in the price of non-fuel commodities over the past 50 years. The fluctuation in commodity prices is an even more pronounced trend.[19]

To capture movement in the terms of trade for primary product exporters, we need to know more than the trend in commodity prices. What about the price of imports? The terms of trade for these nations can be constructed by dividing a commodity price index, capturing the price of exports, by an index for the unit value of manufactures meant to reflect the price of imports. Trends in such a terms of trade index look similar to those depicted in Figure 18–10. Relative to manufactures, non-fuel

---

[19]These trends are reinforced if one looks at even longer time periods. Paul Cashin and C. John McDermont analyzed the behavior of commodity prices from 1862 to 1999, using a data set on industrial commodity prices compiled by *The Economist*. They found a downward trend in real commodity prices of 1 percent per year over the 140-year period. What was more pronounced was the degree of price volatility that increased over time. They concluded that the downward trend in commodity prices was "of little practical policy relevance." It was the variability in prices that had profound consequences for achieving macroeconomic stability. Paul Cashin and C. John McDermont, "The Long Run Behavior of Commodity Prices: Small Trends and Big Variability," IMF Staff Working Papers 49, no. 2 (2002).

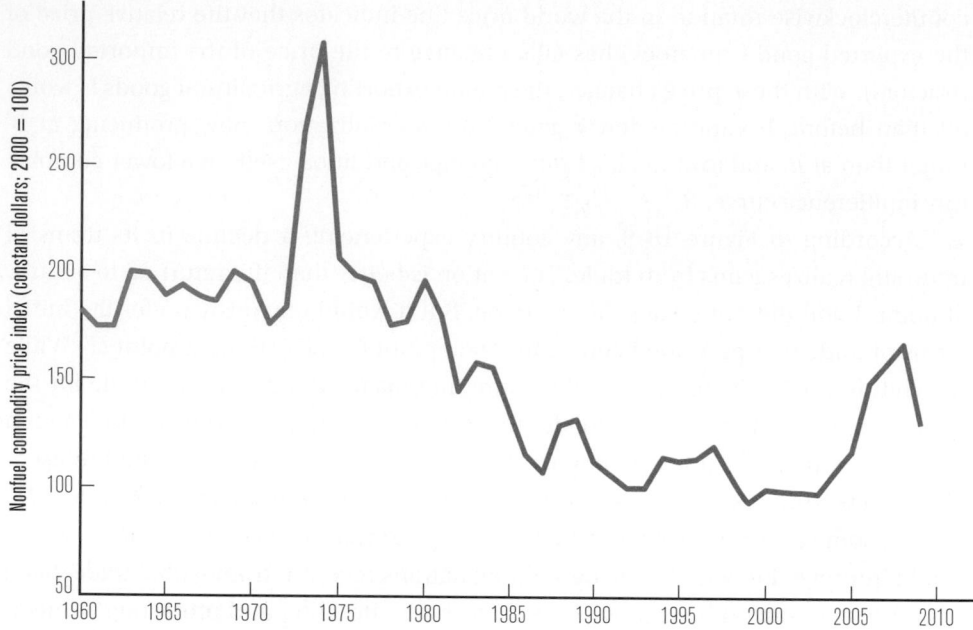

FIGURE 18-10 Nonfuel Commodity Price Trends, 1960–2009

Sources: United Nations Conference on Trade and Development, UnctadStat http://unctadstat.unctad.org/ReportFolders/reportFolders.aspx; International Monetary Fund, Primary Commodity Prices, *Index of Non-Fuel Primary Commodities,* available at www.imf.org/external/np/res/commod/index.aspx.

commodity prices have declined since the 1960s. Even more pronounced is the pattern of relative commodity booms and busts. In the 1970s there was a brief but sharp upturn in commodity prices; another commodity price boom began after 2003 but ended, at least temporarily, with the global recession in 2008.

Although the Prebisch-Singer hypothesis is properly addressed by looking at commodity data, the overall terms of trade for a country (including all products) is what really matters for its development. A commonly used measure of relative prices of traded goods is the **net barter terms of trade**, T_n. The term T_n is the ratio of two indexes: the average price of a country's exports (P_e), whether they are primary products or manufactures, and the average price of its imports (P_m). Figure 18–11 shows two different series of the net barter terms of trade since 1960. When oil exporters are included, the terms of trade of all developing countries rise dramatically after 1972 and remain high, despite the fall of oil prices during the 1980s and early 1990s. But the terms of trade for non-oil-exporting developing countries decline over the period by almost 30 percent. Over these decades, there is support for the Prebisch-Singer hypothesis about declining terms of trade facing non-oil exporting developing nations, though the experience of individual countries varies around this average trend.

More important, evidence on the poor long-run growth and development performance of most primary product exporters involves factors other than

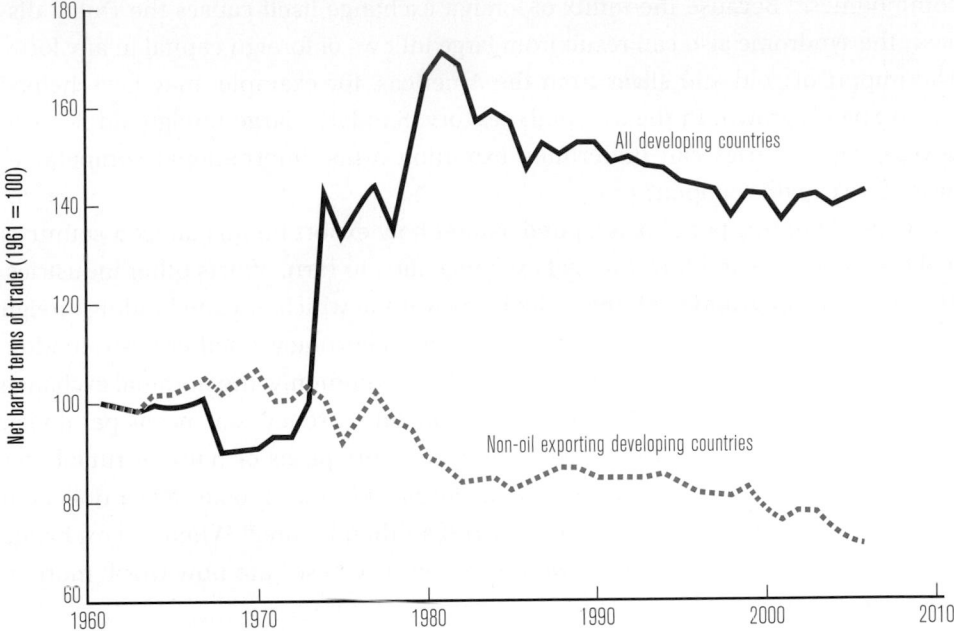

FIGURE 18-11 **Net Barter Terms of Trade, 1961–2006**

Source: IMF, *International Financial Statistics Yearbook 1987* (Washington, DC: IMF, 1987); IMF, *International Financial Statistics Yearbook 1996* (Washington, DC: IMF, 1996); and IMF, *International Financial Statistics Yearbook 2007* (Washington, DC: IMF, 2007).

movements in the terms of trade. For oil exporters and non-oil exporters alike, commodity price trends alone do not account for the resource curse. Other explanations are needed.

DUTCH DISEASE

Prebisch and Singer worried about declining terms of trade. But *improvements* in a nation's terms of trade brought on by booming primary export prices may be even more perilous for an emerging economy. The problem has been labeled **Dutch disease**, named after the experience of the Netherlands after 1960, when major reserves of natural gas were discovered. The ensuing export boom and the balance-of-payments surplus promised new prosperity. Instead, during the 1970s, the Dutch economy suffered from rising inflation, declining export of manufactures, lower rates of income growth, and rising unemployment. The oil boom of the 1970s and early 1980s produced similar paradoxes in a number of countries, including Mexico, Nigeria, and Saudi Arabia. Coffee booms in some African economies have followed a similar path. It is too early to tell if the commodity boom of the 2000s will leave a similar legacy, although there are indications that some of the mistakes of the past are not being repeated.

Economists began to realize that Dutch disease might be a very general phenomenon, applicable to all countries that enjoy export booms of primary commodities.[20] Because the influx of foreign exchange itself causes the Dutch disease, the syndrome also can result from large inflows of foreign capital in any form. The import of gold and silver from the Americas, for example, may have helped retard Spain's growth in the sixteenth century. Similarly, large foreign aid flows to developing countries can undermine exporting firms' international competitiveness. How can this happen?

One key to this paradox is to understand how export booms affect a country's real exchange rate and how the real exchange rate, in turn, affects other industries. The official or **nominal exchange rate** is the price at which anyone holding foreign exchange, such as dollars, can convert it into local currency whether pesos in Mexico, naira in Nigeria, or rupiah in Indonesia. Most commonly, the nominal exchange rate is quoted in local currency per unit of foreign currency, say, pesos per dollar. When the exchange rate rises (that is, there are more pesos or naira or rupiah per dollar), the domestic currency is said to *depreciate* because it takes fewer dollars to buy the same amount of pesos, naira, or rupiah than before.[21] When the exchange rate falls, the domestic currency *appreciates* because pesos are now worth more in dollars than before.

The real exchange rate starts with the nominal exchange rate then incorporates the prices of tradable goods and **nontradable goods** to analyze how changing prices and exchange rates affect the incentives for production and consumption. Economists call any good that is or could be imported or exported a tradable, whether apparel or automobiles, oil or soybeans. Prices for tradable goods generally are determined on world markets and, in most cases, are not affected by domestic conditions in developing countries, each of which tends to be small relative to the size of the global market. Nontradables are goods produced domestically and not imported or exported. Prices for nontradables are determined by supply and demand conditions in the domestic market. Examples include construction, electricity, local transportation and personal services, the prices of which depend almost entirely on local conditions as these goods and services are not traded across borders. Even some manufactured goods or farm products, which are heavily protected and not subject to competition from imports, can be considered nontradables.

---

[20]Early theoretical work on the Dutch disease appears in W. Max Corden and S. Peter Neary, "Booming Sector and Deindustrialization in a Small Open Economy," *Economic Journal* 92 (December 1982), 825–48. Our late co-author, Michael Roemer, applied this theory to developing countries in "Dutch Disease in Developing Countries: Swallowing Bitter Medicine" (234–52), in Matts Lundahl, ed., *The Primary Sector in Economic Development* (London: Croom-Helms, 1985). A recent survey of the literature on Dutch disease and, more generally, the resource curse, is Frederick van der Ploeg, "Natural Resources: Curse or Blessing?" *Journal of Economic Literature* 49 (June 2011).

[21]The language on exchange rate changes sometimes is confusing. When the nominal exchange rate rises, it takes more domestic currency (naira) to buy foreign currency (dollars). Equivalently, this means that it takes fewer dollars to buy naira. In this latter sense, the naira is said to depreciate, or lose value, when the exchange rate rises.

The real exchange rate most commonly is defined as,

$$\text{RER} = (E_o \times P_T)/P_N \qquad\qquad [18\text{-}1]$$

where RER is an index of the real exchange rate, E_o is an index of the official (nominal) exchange rate, P_T is an index of the prices of tradable goods expressed in foreign currency (such as, U.S. dollars), and P_N is an index of the domestic price of nontradables expressed in local currency (such as, pesos.) Note that the RER is an index of prices, like the terms of trade, not a price itself. Also note that, because P_T is expressed in foreign currency, by multiplying by E_o, the numerator $(E_o \times P_T)$ becomes a domestic currency index of tradable's prices. Therefore, the RER can be thought of as the ratio of the price of tradable goods to the price of nontradable goods, all expressed in domestic currency. An increase in the RER—because of either an increase in the nominal exchange rate (more pesos per dollar), a rise in the dollar prices of tradable goods on world markets (more dollars per barrel of oil), or a fall in nontradables prices (fewer pesos for water, a haircut or school fees)—suggests that the relative price of tradables in domestic markets has risen. Such a shift should encourage firms to produce more tradable goods and discourage the consumption of tradable goods. Following the language of nominal exchange rates, a rise in the RER is referred to as a *real depreciation* of the peso, naira, or rupiah, and a decline in the RER is called a *real appreciation*. Official devaluations, which raise the peso price of dollars (E_o), cause the real rate to depreciate, at least initially. The same is true for an increase in world tradable prices. An increase in nontradables prices has the opposite effect, causing the RER to appreciate.[22] Thus while the nominal exchange rate tells you how many pesos you can buy with a dollar, the real exchange rate is an index describing the quantity of actual goods and services you can buy with a dollar when you trade with Mexico. When a country's RER appreciates (depreciates) that country becomes less (more) competitive in international export markets.

The Dutch disease is a wolf in sheep's clothing because it typically starts with what looks like a good thing: A boom in a country's raw material exports. But the boom in exports can cause a sharp appreciation of the RER, in two ways. First, the influx of foreign exchange from higher export earnings creates a surplus of foreign currency. Unless the central bank tries to maintain the official exchange rate at its former level, this increase in the supply of foreign exchange causes the market exchange rate to fall and the currency to appreciate in value. This is because the export windfall of dollars entering the country must typically be converted into local currency, and this increase in the demand for pesos bids up the dollar price of pesos, lowering the nominal exchange (E_o), causing a real appreciation of the peso relative to the dollar. Second, higher income from booming primary exports also spurs faster domestic price inflation. It does this because the additional income creates greater demand

---

[22]For a comprehensive discussion of the real exchange rate, see Sebastian Edwards, *Real Exchange Rates, Devaluation and Adjustment: Exchange Rate Policy in Developing Countries* (Cambridge: MIT Press, 1991).

for all goods and services in the economy. To the extent that this demand spills over into more imports, there is an outflow of foreign exchange but no inflation, because the price of imports is not much affected by demand in a single country. But prices for nontradable goods and services are likely to increase. Due to a limited supply of nontradables, especially in the first months or years of the boom, the greater demand results in higher prices for nontradables. (By way of an example, think of how a commodity boom could lead to rising domestic land and real estate prices.) From equation 18–1 we know that both the appreciation of the domestic currency and the rise in nontradable prices cause the RER to appreciate.

To understand how the real exchange rate becomes the key to the Dutch disease paradox, consider the impact of the real exchange rate on export industries *other than the booming primary export sector.* Booming commodity prices, stimulate more rapid domestic inflation and cause the RER to appreciate, rendering *other* exports less competitive and hence less profitable. Therefore, the disease is the deleterious effect of a commodity boom on other export sectors. Producers of tradables, both nonprimary product exporters and import competitors, face rising costs in their purchases of nontradable goods and services, including the wages of their workers. But they cannot charge higher prices because they compete with foreign producers, either as exporters or as import competitors. These farmers and manufacturers face a profit squeeze that causes some of them to reduce production and employment. The boom in primary exports and nontradables is partly offset by a contraction in other tradable industries. If the contracting industries have more long-run potential for productivity growth, the short-run benefits of the commodity price boom will have negative long-term growth consequences.

If it is relatively easy to move capital and labor between the booming commodity sector and other activities, and the booming sector can employ all the factors of production released from other, now less-profitable activities, then the commodity boom poses no major problem. As prices for the primary export product rise, labor and capital can move into the booming sector, and the economy is better off as a result. If the boom ends, the factors of production can move back to their previous activity. But this usually is not the case. If the booming sector is highly capital intensive (such as petroleum), few new jobs are created, so unemployment may go up (although the indirect employment effects of the boom in construction and other activities can mitigate this effect). More insidiously, when the boom ends (and booms always end), it is likely to be very difficult to move the factors of production back to their previous employment. Manufacturing activities cannot just restart overnight or, in many cases, can farming. In addition, the boom can lead to social or migratory shifts that are hard to unwind. Nigeria's oil boom in the 1970s encouraged rural workers to migrate to urban areas to look for new, high-paying construction and civil service jobs. When the oil boom ended, few urban workers wanted to return to rural areas. Many other oil exporters suffered similar fates when petroleum prices fell. (Box 18–1 illustrates the sectoral shifts common to Dutch disease.)

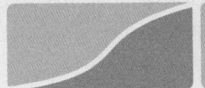

BOX 18-1 DUTCH DISEASE: A GEOMETRIC PRESENTATION

Dutch disease is best illustrated in an economy consisting of three sectors. Two of these sectors are tradables, the booming sector (B) and the lagging sector (L); the third sector is nontradables (N). Output in each sector is produced using a factor of production specific to that sector (for instance land in agriculture) and labor. Workers are assumed to move freely between sectors, implying that the equilibrium wage rate is the same in all three.

Suppose that the country experiences a positive trade shock, for example the discovery of large reserves of offshore oil as occurred in Ghana in 2007. We can understand the potential consequences of this shock by considering its effects on supply and demand in each of the economy's three sectors. The figure "Booming Tradables" illustrates the initial shock as a rightward shift in the supply curve in the booming tradables sector, from S_B to S'_B. This results in an increase in the quantity exported at the world price P_B by ΔX_B. (The positive trade shock could also occur due to a sudden increase in the world price of the booming sector export good, P_B, which would similarly increase the quantity of exports.) The country enjoys a windfall of new income.

Most likely, some of this windfall will be spent on nontradables. This spending effect is illustrated by the rightward shift in the demand curve for nontradables, from D_N to D'_N, in the figure "Nontadables." (Remember, although this small country takes the prices of tradable goods as given by world markets, the price of its nontradable goods is determined exclusively by supply and demand within the country.) This spending effect increases the price of nontradable goods from P_N^0 to P_N^1, shifting the equilibrium from point a to b. The spending effect generates inflation, and by increasing the price of nontradables relative to the price of tradables also causes the real exchange rate to appreciate. Inflation and real appreciation are the initial symptoms of Dutch disease.

Meeting the additional demand for nontradables requires that workers migrate from the lagging tradables sector into nontradables. Additional workers also migrate from the lagging tradables sector into the booming tradables sector. This outflow of workers from the lagging sector is shown in "Lagging Tradables" as a leftward shift in the supply curve from S_L to S'_L, increasing the quantity imported at the world price P_L by ΔM_L. Similarly, there may be a net outflow of workers from the nontradables sector into the booming sector, resulting in a leftward shift in the supply curve for nontradables, illustrated in "Nontradables" as a shift from S_N to S'_N. These shifts are called the "resource movement effect." This creates an excess demand for nontradables at equilibrium point b, causing still more domestic price inflation and more appreciation of the real

Booming Tradables

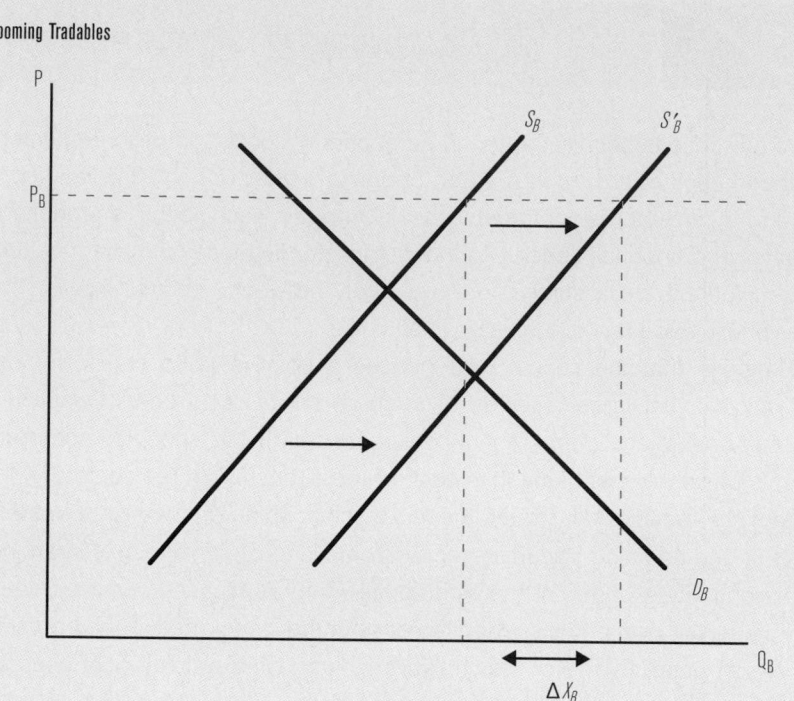

Nontradables

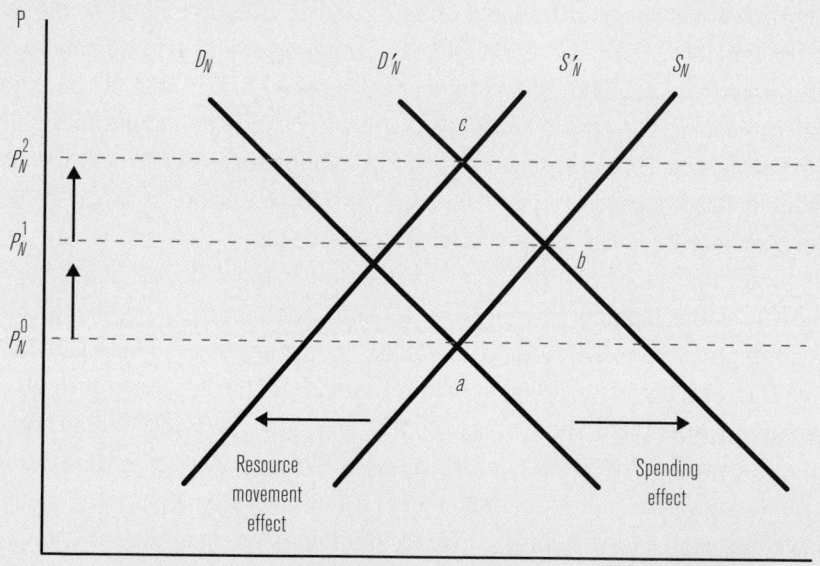

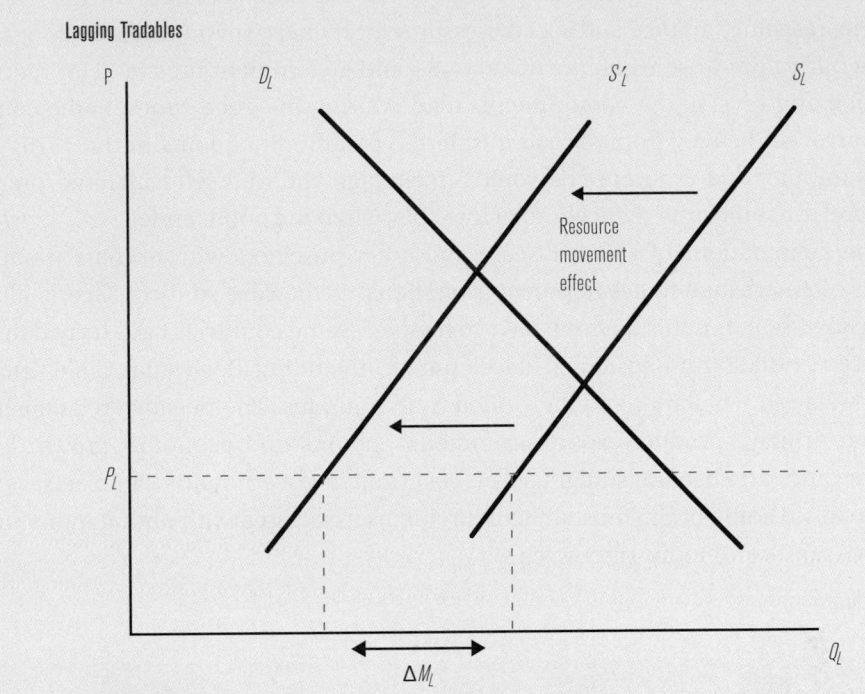

exchange rate as the nontradables market reaches a new equilibrium at point c, with the price of nontradables now increasing to P_N^2.

While the net impact of these effects on the quantity of nontradables is ambiguous, the quantity produced in the lagging sector falls. This is an important part of why the Dutch disease is considered an illness. Once workers leave that sector, they may never return, even after the boom ends. In practice, the lagging sector in many episodes of Dutch disease in developing countries is agriculture.

Source: Based on W. M. Corden, "Booming Sector and Dutch Disease Economics: Survey and Consolidation," *Oxford Economic Papers* 36, no. 3 (November 1984).

Because mineral and other primary sectors typically pay high taxes, commodity booms can lead to a swelling of government revenue. This *fiscal linkage* can be used to stimulate development, especially if the additional revenue is invested in public services, such as infrastructure, education, and health, or to promote efficient investment in tradable sectors, notably agriculture and manufacturing, that have been rendered less competitive by the primary export boom. Although some governments use their fiscal resources effectively during commodity booms, the record has often been dismal, with significant resources wasted on frivolous projects. Precisely when fiscal resources are generously available, finance ministers have the most difficult time resisting political and social pressures for higher expenditures. Once again, the big difficulties arise when the boom ends, and government must quickly reduce spending and reverse the commitments made during the good times. Some countries borrowed heavily from abroad during the commodity booms of the 1970s on the assumption that export prices would remain high and were left with large foreign debts and a significantly reduced capacity to pay when the boom ended.

The depredations of Dutch disease and other problems with primary product exports often are fatal to development aspirations, as the case study of Nigeria illustrates (Box 18-2). But this does not have to happen. Some countries have turned their resource windfalls into sustained development, including Botswana, Chile, Indonesia, Malaysia, Thailand, and the United Arab Emirates. The negative relationship between primary product exports, commodity booms and economic growth is a tendency, not an absolute straightjacket. Determined governments can take several steps to avoid some of the most difficult problems associated with abundant natural resources and commodity price cycles.

BOX 18-2 NIGERIA: A BAD CASE OF DUTCH DISEASE

In 1973–74, the oil embargo imposed by Arab countries, followed by the activation of the Organization of the Petroleum Exporting Countries (OPEC) as an effective cartel, quadrupled the price of petroleum on world markets. In 1979–80, the price doubled again, so that by the end of 1980 the terms of trade for oil exports, relative to the price of imports, was nearly seven times the level in 1972. In Nigeria, higher export prices generated an oil windfall, which added 23 percent to nonmining gross domestic product (GDP) in the middle 1970s and again in the early 1980s. Looking back, Nigeria's oil revenues did little to promote economic development.

Nigeria's political history has been marked by intense competition among ethnic groups, including the Biafran war of the late 1960s. One of the major battlegrounds of this strife, which continues today, has been the incidence of taxation and government expenditure. Under this kind of pressure, the Nigerian government spent its oil windfall. Public investment rose from 4 to 30 percent of nonmining GDP, and the average pay for civil servants was doubled in 1975. Much of the newfound revenue was squandered on wasteful projects; some disappeared into the offshore bank accounts of powerful members of the government and military. The second oil windfall only whetted fiscal appetites even more: From 1981 to 1984, the budget deficit averaged 12 percent of nonmining GDP.

Fiscal excesses exacerbated the tendency of export windfalls to create inflation. Prices rose while the central bank kept the nominal exchange rate fixed, so that, by 1984, the real exchange rate had appreciated to nearly three times its level in 1970–72. Over the decade ending in 1984, Nigeria's non-oil exports fell almost 90 percent in nominal terms, a classic if extreme symptom of Dutch disease. Agriculture suffered worst. Because rural constituencies were politically weak, little of the oil windfall was invested in agriculture, while vast amounts were spent, and wasted, on infrastructure and industry. From 1973 to 1984, the quantity of agricultural exports fell by more than two thirds, while agriculture output per capita and total caloric consumption per capita both declined. From 1972 to 1981, growth in nonmining GDP was a respectable 5.3 percent, but this was only 60 percent of the growth rate during the five years before the oil price boom.

Oil prices declined during the 1980s and did not rise significantly again until the 2000s. Throughout this period, Nigeria oil revenues per capita kept growing even as Nigeria's population increased from almost 50 to 125 million people. But despite rising oil revenues, Nigeria experienced little economic growth and saw its poverty rate more than double and inequality soar. All these difficulties cannot be explained by Dutch disease alone, although during some time periods an appreciating real exchange rate contributed to the nation's woes. It can be argued that Nigeria might have been better off without oil.

Source: Henry Bienen, "Nigeria: From Windfall Gains to Welfare Losses?" (227–60), in Alan Gelb, ed., *Oil Windfalls: Blessing or Curse?* (New York: Oxford University Press for the World Bank, 1988); Frederick van der Ploeg, "Natural Resources: Curse or Blessing?" *Journal of Economic Literature* 49, no. 2 (June 2011).

The best prevention for Dutch disease effects is to avoid or reverse the initial real appreciation of the currency. In most cases, this requires a devaluation of the currency, accompanied by strong restraints on government spending and money creation by the central bank, both aimed at curbing inflation. The government needs to resist demands for expansion and save its newfound revenues until there is time to plan sensible, well-targeted projects with high returns. More-successful governments channel new investments into health, education, and infrastructure development that improve overall well-being, enhance productivity, and open up economic opportunities outside the primary goods sector. Such an investment policy accomplishes two things. First, it harnesses export windfalls to finance sound, long-term development. Second, by delaying the new expenditures, the government acts *countercyclically* and so helps stabilize the economy by spending less during the most inflationary period of the export boom and more after the boom has faded. Indonesia pursued some of these strategies in the 1970s and 1980s and, facing the same increase in prices for oil exports as did Nigeria, had far better growth and development outcomes (Box 18-3). Early evidence on the commodity boom of the 2000s suggests that better macroeconomic management has been pursued by many primary product exporters as they attempt to minimize Dutch disease. On average, fiscal spending by resource dependent economies has been

BOX 18-3 INDONESIA: FINDING A CURE

At first, the oil boom affected Indonesia much as it did Nigeria. The 1973–74 boom added 16 percent to nonmining gross domestic product (GDP) and the 1979–80 price surge raised the windfall to 23 percent. From the first windfall, the government spent more than 60 percent. From 1974 to 1978, the real exchange rate appreciated an average 33 percent over its preboom level, a bit more than in Nigeria at that time. Yet the outcome was very different in Indonesia. Throughout the boom period, the government was required to balance its budget each year, and because all controls had been removed from foreign exchange transfers, stringent management of the money supply was necessary to protect foreign exchange reserves. These self-imposed restraints limited the impact of the windfalls on inflation.

The Indonesian government adopted two policies that took advantage of oil windfalls for national development goals. First, investment in agriculture had a high priority, especially the goal of achieving self-sufficiency in rice production. The government financed irrigation systems, encouraged the adoption of new rice varieties, subsidized fertilizer and pesticide sales, provided credit to farmers, invested in rural health and education facilities, and built roads and other infrastructure in rural areas. By 1982–83, Indonesia's total food output per capita was a third above its 1970 level—a performance far above average for all developing and industrial countries over the period. The second policy was to devalue the exchange rate enough to avoid real appreciation. Major devaluations were imposed in 1978, 1983, and 1986, after which the rate was managed flexibly to maintain its real value. At the end of the oil boom period in 1984, the Indonesian real exchange rate had *de*preciated 8 percent from its 1970–72 average. Consequently, over the period from 1971 to 1984, the quantity of non-oil exports grew by over 7 percent a year, and from 1972 to 1981, nonmining GDP expanded by over 8 percent a year.

Shrewd policy played a major role in effecting an early cure for incipient Dutch disease. The government also placed great stress on integrating the multitude of ethnic groups of this diverse country and avoided the conflicts over fiscal resources that paralyzed Nigeria. It undertook a series of reforms that laid the basis for rapid growth. Import tariffs were substantially reduced, the banking sector was opened to foreign competition, and new regulations were set up to create an active stock market. These reform measures served to align Indonesia more closely to the global economy. The result was a period of rapid growth. Between 1988 and 1996 GDP, measured at constant U.S. dollars, grew at an annual rate of 6.8 percent, reducing poverty levels from the 1976 level of 54 million to 22.5 million by 1996. Indonesia, which at one time had been considered a laggard among the East Asian economies, was now considered a development miracle. Part of its success was due to policies that avoided succumbing to Dutch disease.

Source: Bruce Glassburner, "Indonesia: Windfalls in a Poor Rural Economy," in Alan Gelb, ed., *Oil Windfalls: Blessing or Curse?* (New York: Oxford University Press for the World Bank, 1988).

more prudent and the RERs of these countries have appreciated less than in past commodity booms.[23]

Still, primary commodity exporters tend to grow more slowly than more diversified economies. Policies of restraint, essential to stabilization, are seldom popular and often vigorously opposed by political pressure groups. Although the judicious use of commodity revenues is easy to prescribe and essential for an economy's health, the advice often is not taken in sufficient doses to affect a cure. The relationship between primary commodities and governance is considered next.

THE RESOURCE TRAP

Indonesia and Nigeria are both populous countries that export oil. Oil represents both an opportunity and a challenge to these economies. As described in Boxes 18–2 and 18–3, Indonesia managed earlier resource booms well and prospered; Nigeria did not. The same can be observed when comparing Botswana and Sierra Leone, two countries that export diamonds or Chile and Zambia, two copper exporters. The populations of Botswana, Chile, and Indonesia have experienced economic development; those of Nigeria, Sierra Leone and Zambia have not. Clearly, governance and politics played a large role in these different outcomes. Managing Dutch disease and making productive use of export revenues was not simply a technical matter but one of political will and effective governance.

[23]World Bank, "Dealing with Changing Commodity Prices," in World Bank, *Global Economic Prospects* (Washington, DC: World Bank, 2009), discusses recent trends. It notes that countries experiencing a commodity boom for the first time, often because of newly discovered resources (Chad, Equatorial Guinea, Sudan, Yemen) or recent statehood (Azerbaijan and Kazakhstan), are showing the same kind of macroeconomic volatility that characterized more established producers during earlier booms. Those developing economies with prior experience with commodity price cycles appear to be better managing the macroeconomic consequences of the current boom.

To understand the relationship between primary product exports and governance, it is useful to turn to the work of British economist Paul Collier, who has written extensively on commodity exports and economic development. Some of his early work was on the consequences of the coffee price boom of the late 1970s on Kenya's economic development. In 2007, Collier published *The Bottom Billion*, the title of which refers to the populations of 58 countries, mostly in Africa, whose people are "living and dying in fourteenth century conditions." What distinguishes these economies from other developing nations is their failure to grow over the past three to four decades. Some have experienced long-term economic stagnation; others have seen per capita incomes decline. Collier argues that these economies have fallen into one of several **traps** that have prevented them from growing. Dependence on natural resource exports is directly implicated in his analysis.

Collier specifically identifies a natural resource trap, which incorporates problems we already have discussed. Dutch disease and the appreciation of the RER can crowd out nonprimary product exports with more long-term growth potential. Price volatility during the boom often leads to public expenditures wasted on white elephant projects, expansions in civil service employment motivated more by political patronage than service delivery, or outright theft by corrupt officials. Commodity booms often are also associated with increased foreign borrowing and the accumulation of debt. If borrowed funds are spent wisely, this is a good strategy. If the borrowed funds are misspent, then during the inevitable and subsequent bust in commodity prices and government revenues, the economy faces a debt burden and must service its debt often by cutting essential development expenditures. Underlying these problems of commodity price cycles and macroeconomic mismanagement is poor governance, which according to Collier and others, is tied to the resource revenues themselves.

Simply stated, resource revenues worsen governance. Evidence for this is provided by the World Bank, which has developed indexes of corruption. Oil and mineral exporters, on average, have more corruption than agricultural exporters, who in turn are more corrupt than diversified exporters (the latter include economies that export a range of fuel, non-fuel primary commodities and manufactures).[24] Corruption then acts as a tax, often a large one, on economic activity. It encourages rent-seeking behavior rather than productive investment and growth suffers accordingly. Collier closes the circle among dependence on resource revenues, widespread corruption and poor governance, and a lack of economic growth by explaining why resource revenues breed corruption. Revenue from oil, diamonds, minerals, and certain other commodities reduce the need to tax citizens.[25] The government secures revenues by nationalizing the resource industry or by making leasing arrangements

---

[24]World Bank, "Dealing with Changing Commodity Prices," p. 109.

[25]Not all primary commodities are equally vulnerable to these problems. The more concentrated production and revenues, the easier it is for the state to appropriate resource revenues. This is what makes oil, diamonds, gold, silver, uranium and other minerals, and some plantation crops different from cotton, rice, fish, and livestock exports.

with multinational extractors. Either way, the revenues bypass the population in a way that ordinary tax collection does not. If citizens are not directly taxed they may be less likely to hold public officials accountable.

When resource rents are available, political patronage often becomes the means of political competition, far more effective in garnering votes or remaining in power than by improving the provision of public services or fostering national development. Collier argues that resource revenues can pollute governance in autocratic regimes and democracies alike, and can be inimical to development in both low-income countries (Congo, Sierra Leone) and middle-income nations (Russia, Venezuela.) He worries that when resource revenues worsen governance, the trap is hard to break free from.

In addition, Collier describes a **conflict trap** that ensnares the bottom billion. Civil wars have been endemic, particularly in sub-Saharan Africa. Collier argues that the existence of mineral wealth significantly increases the likelihood of civil war, as greed motivates many rebel groups and mineral wealth itself helps finance conflict. Competition over the control of valuable natural resources for export certainly played (and in some instances continues to play) a role in the civil wars in Angola, Congo, Sierra Leone, and Sudan. The expression *blood diamonds*, stems from some of these conflicts. In Fiji, Collier argues, control over the valuable mahogany and other tropical wood concessions, was central to the armed insurgency that took place in 2000 and temporarily overthrew the elected government. According to Collier, low income, slow growth, and dependence on primary commodity exports significantly increase the probability that a nation will experience a civil war.

BREAKING THE RESOURCE CURSE

Collier paints a bleak picture, far bleaker even than that of Prebisch and Singer, of the prospects for the resource-rich nations among the bottom billion. His critics agree that correlations between resource abundance and poor development outcomes are relatively robust, but find far less statistical support for the causal channels Collier identifies.[26] And even if a resource trap exists, there are examples of nations that have escaped. If Botswana leveraged diamond revenues into rapid growth, so can Angola. If Indonesia, despite its own pervasive corruption, managed its oil revenues well, then so can Nigeria. The resource curse, if one exists, can be overcome. Some recent approaches include the use of sovereign wealth funds and wider adoption of the Extractive Industries Transparency Initiative (EITI) and similar international charters.

Sovereign wealth funds refer to the accumulation of foreign assets, usually financed by primary product export earnings. These funds are distinct from the foreign reserve holdings of central banks that are intended to help with short-term macroeconomic stabilization. By keeping resource earnings in assets denominated in foreign currencies, RER

---

[26]See William Easterly's review of *The Bottom Billion*, "An Ivory Tower Analysis of Real World Poverty," *The Lancet* 307 (October 27, 2007) 1475–76.

appreciation and Dutch disease can be reduced. The funds also can be used countercyclically and smooth the expenditure flows that follow from commodity price cycles and can provide a national nest egg for when non-renewable commodities are depleted. But they are not a substitute for good governance. Sovereign wealth funds can be mismanaged or abused just like any other source of government revenue. Venezuela, for example, has borrowed heavily against its sovereign wealth fund minimizing its potential benefits.

EITI, launched in 2002 by the British government, is an attempt to impose some accountability on both international companies engaged in oil and mining and on governments who receive payments for these natural resources. Without an international charter like EITI, negotiations for drilling or mining rights are often held behind closed doors and beyond public scrutiny. As Collier puts it, such deals often are good for the companies and for the minister doing the negotiations but not for the country.[27] EITI is an international coalition of governments, companies, multilateral organizations, and civil society that creates a global standard for the verification and publication of both company payments and government revenues obtained from oil, gas, and mining. It requires firms in extractive industries to disclose payments for oil and mineral rights, governments to disclose receipt of payments, and independent international audits of these transfers. The hope is that greater transparency will reduce corruption and make governments more accountable in their use of resource revenues. In 2009, oil-rich Azerbaijan became the first country validated as compliant with all EITI requirements. More than two dozen other low- and middle-income nations are following Azerbaijan's lead and 40 of the world's largest oil, gas and mining companies are participating in the EITI process.

EITI is one example of an international charter Collier recommends as a means of improving accountability and governance among the bottom billion. He also recommends the use of verifiable international auctions for granting mineral rights. This would complement EITI and further reduce the back-room deals that govern the award of many such contracts. On the expenditure side, there also needs to be transparency in how government revenues are spent. In Uganda, the ministry of finance reported how much money was released to a given locality. Local media outlets were informed and individual schools were sent a poster informing them of what they should expect to receive. One study found that these steps increased the flow of resources to their intended recipients from only 20 to 80 percent of the initial allocation.[28] Collier believes that a package of international standards and charters can

[27]From, "Paul Collier on *The Bottom Billion*," TED, May 2008, available at www.ted.com/talks/paul_collier_shares_4_ways_to_help_the_bottom_billion.html.

[28]Ritva Reinikka and Jakob Svensson, "The Power of Information: Evidence from a Newspaper Campaign to Reduce Capture," World Bank Policy Research Working Paper No. 3239, Washington, DC, March 2004. See also Paul Hubbard, "Putting the Power of Transparency in Context: Information's Role in Reducing Corruption in Uganda's Education Sector," Working Paper Number 136, Center for Global Development, Washington, DC, December 2007, which argues that the improved flow of resources to intended beneficiaries was the product of many reforms in government practice, including but not solely the result of, more transparent information.

impose some checks and balances on bad governance and help transform natural resource exports from a curse to a means for promoting economic development.

David Ricardo would probably recognize some contemporary debates about trade between nations. He would still argue on behalf of the potential benefits of trade for improving aggregate output and welfare. The gains from trade are as real today as they were in the early nineteenth century. But trade is not a panacea. As the discussion of primary product exports demonstrates, economic growth and development entails far more than just the pursuit of comparative advantage.

SUMMARY

- World trade has grown rapidly in recent decades. Trade between high-income economies still dominates world commerce, with developing nations (including China) accounting for about one quarter of the total. With imports and exports from low- and middle-income economies growing more quickly than their GDPs, trade has contributed to a rise in globalization and to the importance of trade for most nations.

- The share of trade in GDP tends to be higher the smaller the economy and the better its access to seaports and major world markets. Landlocked nations, of which there are 44, tend to trade less and grow more slowly than nations with coastlines. As economies grow, the composition of trade tends to change, with exports shifting from primary products toward manufactured goods.

- Comparative advantage, an idea developed by David Ricardo, allows two countries to gain from trade with each other, even when factor inputs are more productive for all products in one country than the other. By pursuing comparative advantage, countries experience gains from exchange and gains from specialization, and are able to raise national income.

- Beyond these gains, trade encourages competition and reduces the market power of domestic firms, facilitates the adoption of new technologies, can spur investment, and increases the quality and variety of goods available. But trade is not without costs; there are both winners and losers. In the short run, firms and their workers in the export sector see their business expand and in the import-competing sector contract. Trade tends to benefit a nation's abundant factors of production with the gains of the winners surpassing the losses of the losers.

- Most world trade involves manufactured goods, but primary products continue to dominate the exports of many low- and middle-income economies. Unfortunately, many of these economies have suffered from a resource curse, by which a dependence on oil and other primary good exports often has been associated with economic stagnation and even decline.

- Pessimism about primary product exports and development has a long history. In the 1950s, economists such as Prebisch and Singer argued that the terms of trade steadily and systematically would turn against primary products. This, they argued, was because of structural features in the global economy, including that demand for these exports typically grow more slowly than for manufactures.

- Today, the arguments of Prebisch and Singer no longer are seen as explaining the resource curse. More often, the problem is not steadily declining terms of trade but the cycles of price booms and busts in some commodities. This can lead to the phenomenon known as Dutch disease, by which a country rich in natural resources suffers slower growth. Dutch disease most often is associated with an appreciation of a nation's real exchange rate, which harms growth in other sectors, especially in nonprimary good exports.

- Beyond Dutch disease, lies an even more troubling explanation for the resource curse. Resource revenues tend to worsen governance in a way that export earnings from manufactured goods do not. In weak states lacking good institutions, resource rents can perpetuate civil wars, fuel endemic corruption, and undermine the necessary checks and balances required for good governance.

- Nations can and have overcome the resource curse by pursuing prudent macroeconomic policies and by taking the necessary steps to prevent waste and corruption in the use of primary export revenues. International charters like the EITI are a mechanism for supporting the improved governance of oil and other resource exporters.

19

Trade Policy

I n 2009, the Pew Research Center, conducted a survey of global attitudes. It sampled populations in 55 countries. One question asked, "What do you think about the growing trade and business ties between your country and other countries—do you think it is a very good thing, somewhat good, somewhat bad or a very bad thing for our country?" Over 2,000 people were surveyed in India and 96 percent replied that trade was "very good" or "somewhat good." In China and South Korea, 93 and 92 percent, respectively, felt the same way. The percentages in Nigeria and Brazil were 90 and 87. Somewhat lower approval ratings of international trade were voiced in France (83 percent), Russia (80 percent), Japan (73 percent), and the United States (65 percent). In every country surveyed, a majority of respondents thought trade was "very" or "somewhat good."

Given the benefits of international trade discussed in the previous chapter, it is not surprising that trade is positively viewed by the general population. It can raise national income, result in lower prices for many goods, and increase product quality and variety. In some nations, exports are perceived of as the engine of economic growth. But a favorable view toward trade is not the same as support for free trade. Trade may be viewed favorably at the same time that workers and firms call for protection from imports. Politicians in rich and poor countries often find it in their interest to support trade protection. In many nations, policies that favor exports over imports are pursued, a strategy reminiscent of the mercantilism that Adam Smith and David Ricardo argued against hundreds of years ago.

World trade may today be more open than at any time in the past 50 or even 100 years, but the trade strategies that nations adopt continue to mix openness with elements of protection or other forms of support for individual firms and sectors. The ideal trade strategy to promote economic growth and development remains a subject of continued debate, influenced by both economic theory and real world experience.

There exists a continuum of trade strategies a nation might pursue. At one end is economic isolationism, sometimes referred to as autarky, by which a nation elects to be self-sufficient. Japan pursued something close to this strategy before its opening to the West in the 1850s after the arrival of Commodore Matthew Perry and the black ships of the U.S. Navy. More recent examples include Albania (1976–91) after the principles set forth by Communist leader Enver Hoxha, and Burma (1962–88) under the ideology of military ruler Ne Win. Today, North Korea comes closest to pursuing a strategy of autarky. Its official state ideology, *juche*, includes economic self-sufficiency as a key element. But even North Korea engages in some limited international trade, exporting minerals, animal products and, allegedly, illicit goods such as missiles, narcotics and counterfeit cigarettes to secure critical imports of fuel and food, as well as luxuries for the nation's elite.

At the other end of the continuum from autarky is free trade. Free trade refers to the unfettered movement of goods and services across national borders. It implies that goods move as freely between nations as they do within nations. Once again, there are few examples. Hong Kong, especially before its return to Chinese sovereignty in 1997, is cited as having been one of the world's most open economies with few barriers to trade or support of one industry over another. Today, free trade characterizes the internal trade among members of the European Union (EU). But trade between EU members and the rest of the world is subject to numerous barriers, including tariffs, quantitative restrictions, and subsidies. Free trade agreements, such as the North American Free Trade Agreement (NAFTA) between Canada, Mexico, and the United States, often include restrictions on the exchange of some goods between member nations. It took 15 years for NAFTA to eliminate restrictions on trade in corn, sugar, and other commodities. U.S. anti-dumping duties have been applied to cement from Mexico and softwood lumber from Canada, whereas Mexico has imposed similar duties on high fructose corn syrup from the United States. Trade between NAFTA members in these and other commodities has been less free than internal trade within each nation's borders.

If autarky and free trade are rare and at opposite ends of the continuum of trade strategies, then most nations must adopt trade strategies that fall somewhere in between. The policy debate centers on how inward looking or how outward oriented an economy should be. The pendulum of which approach to follow has swung back and forth. The historical development of all advanced economies, whether Britain, Japan, or the United States, included periods of trade protection followed by a more open approach. A relaxation of restraints on trade characterized the early twentieth century only to be reversed after World War I and the Great Depression. The infamous Smoot-Hawley tariffs, passed into law in 1930 by the U.S. Congress, set off a round of retaliatory tariffs in other countries that contributed to a dramatic reduction in global commerce and a prolonged decline in world output. After World War II, many nations signed the 1947 Global Agreement on Tariffs and Trade (GATT), resulting in a reduction in tariffs and other trade barriers and an expansion in international trade.

In the developing world, Latin America's primary export markets were severely disrupted by the Great Depression and by the scarcity of commercial shipping during World War II. Having built up domestic manufacturing capacity during this period, Argentina, Brazil, Colombia, Mexico, and other countries systematically erected barriers to keep out competing imports after the war. In Asia and Africa, most countries adopted inward-looking strategies in the 1950s and 1960s, as newly independent states wanted to develop their own industrial capacity and distance themselves from their former colonial rulers. By the 1960s, import substitution was the dominant strategy of economic development.[1] But this strategy did not live up to its promise and by the 1980s had generally been abandoned in favor of more outward-looking approaches. The early export-oriented emerging economies of East Asia (Hong Kong, Korea, Singapore, and Taiwan) had demonstrated the advantages of an export orientation.

Broadly speaking, governments in developing countries have employed two different trade strategies, import substitution and export orientation. Import substitution (IS) is the production of goods and services that replace (or substitute for) imports. Because new firms in developing countries often are unable, at least initially, to compete on world markets, import substitution protects domestic firms from international competition by erecting trade barriers that make imported products more expensive or more difficult to purchase, with the aim that over time firms will become more efficient and competitive. **Export orientation** shifts the focus to producing for global markets. This strategy is designed to make producers internationally competitive by relying on market forces; strengthening key institutions; and, in some cases, using subsidies, managed exchange rates, and other policy instruments. The core idea behind import substitution is that newly developing industries cannot survive at first without some protection from imports, giving them the chance to learn and grow. In contrast, the core idea behind an outward-looking trade strategy is for firms to compete internationally to gain access to new technologies, increase efficiency, and enlarge the scope of their potential market. We consider each strategy in turn.

IMPORT SUBSTITUTION

The basic idea of IS is straightforward. For sustained economic development, countries need to shift from primary production to manufacturers to prevent prolonged specialization in low-productivity activities. Some early proponents saw IS as both

[1]Recall the arguments of Raul Prebisch and Hans Singer discussed in the previous chapter. Their concerns and explanations for declining terms of trade facing developing nations provided some of the intellectual support for the import substitution trade strategies that many governments pursued.

a trade strategy and as a way to structurally transform an economy and referred to it as import substitution industrialization (ISI). Proponents of IS argue that firms are unlikely to be able to compete in manufactures immediately and require government assistance to get started. Ideally, the first step is to identify products with large domestic markets, as indicated by substantial imports, and relatively simple production technologies that can be mastered quickly, rather than products requiring advanced machinery and highly skilled labor. Governments then introduce either tariffs or quotas to increase the price of competing imports. **Tariffs** are taxes imposed on imports at the border; **quotas** are quantitative limits on specified categories of imports. These protective barriers by raising the price of imports, reduce the quantity of imports in the domestic market, and allow domestic manufacturers to charge higher prices, compensating them for higher production costs and making their operations profitable. The strategy comes at a cost to consumers and other firms, who must pay the higher prices with commensurate welfare and profit losses as a result.

This stylized approach (focus on relatively simple products with large domestic markets) implies that consumer goods, such as processed foods, beverages, textiles, clothing, and footwear, should be the first targets. By contrast, capital goods should not be heavily protected because they require more sophisticated skills and raising their costs hurts all downstream industries and investors that buy capital goods. Nevertheless, many developing countries have used IS to protect steel, machinery, and other capital goods, usually with little success.

Today, most economists are critical of the IS strategy, but there are valid arguments in favor of this approach, the most compelling of which is the concept of an **infant industry**. Entrepreneurs opening new production facilities in a developing country must compete against firms from industrialized countries that have long experience and have mastered both production technologies and marketing. The managers and workers of the new, or infant, industry must learn to use these technologies efficiently to compete. This process of learning by doing can take several years. Advocates of IS argue that without some form of assistance these investments are unlikely to take place and developing countries will be unable to learn the skills needed eventually to compete with imports on equal footing. For this strategy to work, an infant industry must "grow up" to be capable of eventually competing without protection against imports. This suggests that tariffs should be *temporary* and decline toward zero over time, as productivity increases and production costs fall. For this strategy to be economically worthwhile, the eventual (and discounted) benefits to society of establishing the new industry should exceed the current costs to the economy of protection.

To more fully understand IS and trade strategies in general, we first explore the impact of tariffs, quotas, and subsidies on imports, production, and consumption. We then examine the relationship between exchange rate policy and trade, before returning to an overall evaluation of IS.

PROTECTIVE TARIFFS

The most direct effect of a protective tariff, whether it is imposed by a developing or a developed economy, is to raise the domestic price of the good above the world price. For the importing country, the world price is the cost at the port of entry, usually called the *c.i.f. price* (including cost, insurance, and freight) or *border price*. If we assume the country is small relative to the world market and that the imported good is a perfect substitute for the good produced domestically, then the country faces a world supply curve that is perfectly elastic at the world price. We also assume that the domestic market is competitive, permitting us to represent the domestic market using standard supply and demand curves. In Figure 19–1, at the world or border price, P_w, consumers demand Q_1 and local producers produce Q_2; the balance, $M_1 = Q_1 - Q_2$, is imported. If an **ad valorem** (that is, percentage) tariff, t_0, is placed on the good, the percentage increase in the domestic price, $t_0 = (P_d - P_w)/P_w$, is referred to as the **nominal rate of protection**.[2] The tariff reduces quantity demanded to Q_3 and increases domestic production to Q_4, the latter being the goal of import protection. Imports are reduced to $M_2 = Q_3 - Q_4$.

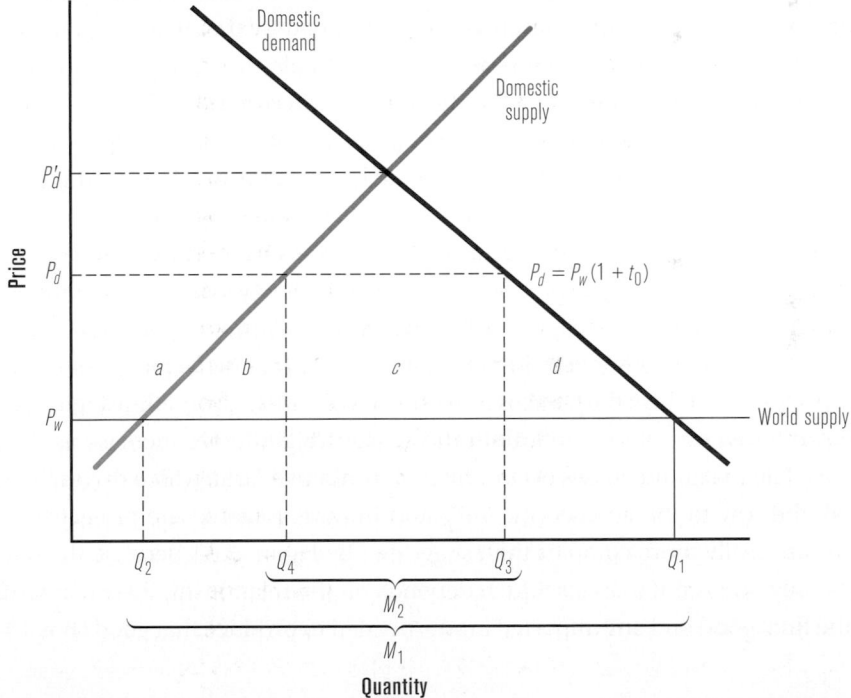

FIGURE 19-1 Nominal Tariff Protection

[2]Tariffs sometimes are applied not in percentage terms but as specific duties—for example, instead of, say, 25 percent of the c.i.f. price, 15 pesos or 75 rupees are added to the c.i.f. price. When a specific duty, t_d, is applied, the nominal rate of protection is t_d/P_w.

The increase in domestic output from Q_2 to Q_4 has two effects. First, it increases the *producers' surplus* by an amount given by trapezoid a, which captures the extent to which producers receive a price, P_d, that exceeds their marginal cost of production, represented by the domestic supply curve. Second, the increase in production entails a *resource cost*, given by triangle b, because it uses labor, machinery, and raw materials that could be used more efficiently to produce something else. The resource cost can best be understood by thinking about the opportunity cost of increased domestic production. Without the tariff, the nation can import an amount equal to Q_2 to Q_4 by paying the world price and costing, $P_w(Q_4 - Q_2)$. To produce this added amount at home costs more. The cost equals the additional cost of all these units, which is the area under the supply curve from Q_2 to Q_4; an amount equal to: $P_w(Q_4 - Q_2) + b$. Because it costs more to produce at home than to import, the society is using its resources inefficiently. Society could have used its resources to import the same quantity of the good, Q_2 to Q_4, and applied the extra resources represented by triangle b, to produce and consume something else.

Consumers pay for protection both by the higher price, P_d, they pay on all purchases and by reducing consumption from Q_1 to Q_3. Part of what they pay is transferred to the government as tariff revenue that can be used by society for other purposes. This amount is a transfer within society rather than a loss. Tariff revenue is equal to the new quantity of imports, M_2, multiplied by the increase in the import price resulting from the tariff, represented by rectangle $c = (t_0 P_w) \times M_2$. The total cost to consumers is represented by the loss of *consumer surplus*, the difference between consumer demand and the market price, equal to area $a + b + c + d$. The loss to consumers is only partially compensated by the gains to either producers (trapezoid a) or the general public (through the tariff revenues represented by rectangle c). Area $b + d$, two triangles representing welfare losses not compensated by gains to anyone, called the *deadweight loss*, represents the efficiency loss to the economy.

We already identified area b as a loss resulting from the inefficiency of producing the good at home rather than importing it; area d is the inefficiency resulting from higher prices that reduce the choices available to consumers, sometimes referred to as the *consumption cost* of the tariff. Both these deadweight losses increase as the tariff rate rises. The maximum losses occur under a prohibitive tariff, which drives the world price all the way to the autarky price, P'_d, and imports to zero. The protective effects of tariffs are really more complex than suggested by Figure 19–1 because the diagram focuses only on output markets. Much depends on the relationship between tariffs on both the final good and any imported inputs needed to produce that good (Box 19–1).

IMPORT QUOTAS

Industries also can be protected through **quantitative restrictions** on imports, usually in the form of quotas. With quotas, the government determines in advance the quantity of imports it wants to allow, whereas with tariffs, the quantity of imports depends

BOX 19-1 EFFECTIVE RATES OF PROTECTION

How much do tariffs affect producer's incentives to shift production? The tariff rate on competing imports gives us a clue but does not tell the whole story. The tariff rate determines the nominal rate of protection, which focuses on the effect of tariffs on *output* prices. But producers also care about the effect of tariffs on *input* prices and, ultimately, on the margin between revenues and input costs. Whereas a tariff on competing imports helps raise profits, tariffs on intermediate goods reduces them.

The **effective rate of protection (ERP)** measures the protection afforded by the entire structure of tariffs on inputs and outputs.[a] It focuses attention on the impact of trade policies on *value added*, the difference between the selling price of the good and the unit cost of intermediate goods.[b] Value added can be measured in domestic prices as the difference between the domestic price of the product (P_d) and the domestic cost of material inputs per unit of output (C_d), while the value added at world prices is the difference between the world price of the product (P_w) and the costs of inputs valued at world prices (C_w). The ERP is the ratio between the two:

$$ERP = \frac{\text{Value added (domestic prices)}}{\text{Value added (world prices)}} - 1 = \frac{P_d - C_d}{P_w - C_w} - 1$$

The key difference between domestic prices and world prices is tariffs (and other trade barriers such as quotas that can have similar effects on prices). The tariff on competing imports (t_0) raises the domestic price of the product above the world price, $P_d = P_w(1 + t_0)$, while the average tariff on inputs (t_i) raises the costs of producing it, $C_d = C_w(1 + t_i)$. Thus domestic prices and costs can be expressed in terms of world prices and tariffs:

$$ERP = \frac{P_w(1 + t_0) - C_w(1 + t_i)}{P_w - C_w} - 1 \text{ or } ERP = \frac{P_w t_0 - C_w t_i}{P_w - C_w}$$

[a]The concept of the effective rate of protection is due to Max Corden, "The Structure of a Tariff System and the Effective Protection Rate," *Journal of Political Economy* 74 (June 1966), 221–37.

[b]Within this margin, the manufacturer must pay all the factors of production: wages, rents, interest on borrowed capital, and profit. Together these payments are equal to the value added.

Because the denominator is the value added calculated at world prices, the ERP measures the impact of all tariffs on the value added, rather than on prices. The measurement of ERP easily can be extended to include quotas, subsides, or other policies that influence output and input prices and thus the value added. To see the powerful insights from the ERP concept, suppose a producer manufactures a product that sells for $100 and costs $60 to produce on world markets, so that value added is $40. Consider the impact on value added of three stylistic cases of tariff policy:

- *The tariff on output is exactly the same as the tariff on inputs.* Say both t_0 and t_i equal 10 percent. You might think there would be no impact, but there is one. The sales price rises to $110 and domestic costs increase to $66, so value added increases by 10 percent to $44. A uniform tariff, 10 percent in this case, provides effective protection on value added of 10 percent, exactly equal to the nominal rate of protection.
- *The tariff on output is higher than the tariff on inputs.* If $t_0 = 10$ percent but $t_i = 0$, the domestic price rises to $110 and the valued added rises from $40 to $50. Thus the ERP $= 25$ percent, much higher than the nominal rate of protection of 10 percent. More generally, if t_0 is greater than t_i, the ERP exceeds the nominal rate of protection. Note the key point here: What seems like a small tariff can have a huge impact on the margin between costs and prices and thus a big impact on producers' incentives to reallocate resources away from sectors with no protection to those with protection. Tariff structures in many countries tend to follow this pattern, escalating from relatively low rates on inputs to higher rates on finished products. Under these circumstances, ERPs of 100 percent are not uncommon.
- *The tariff on output is lower than the tariff on inputs.* If there is no tariff on competing imports but a 10 percent tariff on inputs ($t_i = 10$ percent), domestic costs rise to $66 but output prices remain at $100. Thus value added falls to $34 and the ERP is a *negative* 15 percent. Although a tariff structure that undermines investment incentives seems unlikely, it is actually fairly common, particularly for agriculture and export products. Governments like to keep food prices low to keep urban consumers happy and so are reluctant to impose duties on food imports. Therefore, protective tariffs on fertilizer, seeds, or irrigation equipment undermine the profitability of agriculture and switch investment out of agriculture. As for exports, governments cannot use tariffs to raise output prices because exporters sell on world markets. A tariff on inputs raises exporters' costs and reduces incentives to invest in export industries. This pattern of protection is a critical problem undermining the international competitiveness of exporting firms in many developing countries.

on the reactions of producers and consumers to higher prices, as captured by the elasticities of supply and demand. A quota that limits imports to the same quantity as a tariff has many of the same effects. In Figure 19–1, a quota limiting imports to M_2 forces the domestic price up to P_d, increases domestic production to Q_4, and decreases consumption to Q_3, just as with the tariff. The quota permits M_2 units of imports at every possible price, in essence, shifting the domestic supply to the right by an amount, M_2. Equilibrium in the market occurs at the intersection of domestic demand and domestic supply augmented by the quota. In Figure 19–1 this occurs at price P_d and quantity Q_3, identical to the effects of the tariff t_0. The loss in consumer surplus, the deadweight losses, and the gain in producer surplus are also the same for quota, M_2, as for ad valorem tariff, t_0.

But in two critical respects import quotas have different effects from tariffs. First, the government does not necessarily collect revenue equal to area c. To enforce the quota it must issue licenses to a limited number of importers, giving them the right to purchase up to M_2 of imports. If the government simply gives away the licenses with no fee (which many governments do, using the licenses as patronage for politically well-connected importers), license holders earn a windfall profit equal to the area of rectangle c. This is because the importer can purchase the goods at price P_w on the world market and sell them at P_d domestically. This windfall, often called a **quota rent**, can be substantial, so importers expend a great deal of effort to obtain them, including possibly offering large bribes, in effect sharing the quota rent with the right government official. (Under a tariff, importers can also bribe customs officials to avoid collection of all of the required tariffs.) Alternatively, and preferably, the government could sell the import licenses at auction. Assume the government decides to auction 1,000 import licenses, each license entitling the holder to import $M_2/1{,}000$ units of the good. Potential importers would be willing to pay up to an amount $c/1{,}000$ for each of these licenses because that is the amount of the potential revenue windfall they could earn. A well-functioning auction could yield the government the same revenues as a tariff, although the distribution of quotas often is seen as more costly to administer than tariffs.[3]

Second, market dynamics that shift the domestic supply and demand curves or the world price have very different impacts with tariffs and quotas. Consider a fall in the world price P_w. With a tariff, both P_w and P_d fall, giving consumers the benefit of the lower price. Consumption increases, domestic production declines, and imports rise to fill the gap. Under a quota, however, imports cannot rise unless the quota is increased. Domestic production and consumption remain unchanged, and the domestic price remains at P_d. The lower world price simply increases the quota rent, with the benefit going directly to import license holders. Put more generally, under

---

[3] Distributing quota rents can be complex. The U.S. government uses quotas as both an instrument of protection for the U.S. sugar industry and as a tool of foreign policy. The United States has protected its domestic sugar industry since the 1930s, resulting most years in much higher prices for sugar in the domestic market than in the world market. U.S. quotas are allocated to sugar-exporting nations, with Brazil, Dominican Republic, and Philippines receiving the largest amounts. The governments of these nations then decide how to allocate the valuable quota rents. In essence, the U.S. government, through its use of quotas, takes some of the money U.S. consumers pay for higher-priced sugar and gives that money to other nations.

most (but not all) circumstances because tariffs allow changes in imports on the margin, domestic producers and consumers react on the margin to market changes as they would in an open economy; with quotas, they react on the margin as they would in a closed economy. Because of these consequences of quotas, economists prefer tariffs, and trade reforms and international trade agreements often start with the elimination of quotas or at least conversion to their equivalent tariffs.

TRADE PROTECTION AND POLITICS

From the partial equilibrium model of a tariff (or quota) developed in Figure 19–1, it seems almost illogical for trade protection ever to be used. Consumers lose consumer surplus equal to $a + b + c + d$ because of the tariff but producers and government gain only $a + c$. A general equilibrium approach reaches similar conclusions. (Box 19–2). If the costs of protection outweigh the benefits, why would a government employ such measures?

The infant industry argument acknowledges that domestic costs of production, captured by the domestic supply curve, are higher than production costs elsewhere. That is precisely why trade protection is needed. It enables the new industry to gain experience, bringing costs down, causing the domestic supply curve to fall, and eventually making the domestic industry competitive. Short-run costs, according to this line of reasoning, are worth paying for expected productivity growth and any positive spillover effects once the infant industry matures.

Another and in some ways better explanation for the widespread use and persistence of trade protection involves its distributional consequences and the incentives such protection creates. Consider Thailand's 60 percent tariff on imported beer. With the tariff, domestic producers can sell more beer and can sell it at a higher price. The tariff keeps lower-priced beer from Laos and Vietnam out of Thailand. Domestic breweries earn more revenue and greater producer surplus. They employ more workers because the tariff expands production beyond the level comparative advantage warrants. But consumers lose. They face fewer alternatives and pay a higher price for beer. In the aggregate, according to our models, consumers lose more than producers gain. To explain the persistence of the tariff, what may really matter is the extent of *individual* gains and losses.

With the tariff, individual consumers have to pay a few more baht (the Thai currency) for a bottle of beer. They would prefer to pay less, but the amounts involved for consumers are small relative to their total expenditures. It is hard to imagine mobilizing the public to protest over the beer tariff. For Thai beer producers the incentives are different. They are relatively few in number and the potential gains from a tariff are large. Millions of Thai beer drinkers each pay a bit more for beer, but these losses when aggregated become the gains shared by only a few firms. It is easy to imagine these firms mobilizing to seek political support or the favor of influential government

BOX 19-2 THE TWO-COUNTRY MODEL WITH A TARIFF

We can also examine the impact of a tariff using the two-country, two-good, two-factor model developed in Chapter 18. Mexico is again trading tomatoes and tractors with the United States (or with the rest of the world.) Mexico has comparative advantage in tomatoes and imports tractors. If Mexico engages in no trade, it consumes and produces at A; with free trade it produces at B and consumes at C. Trade increases utility from the level at IC_1 to that at IC_3.

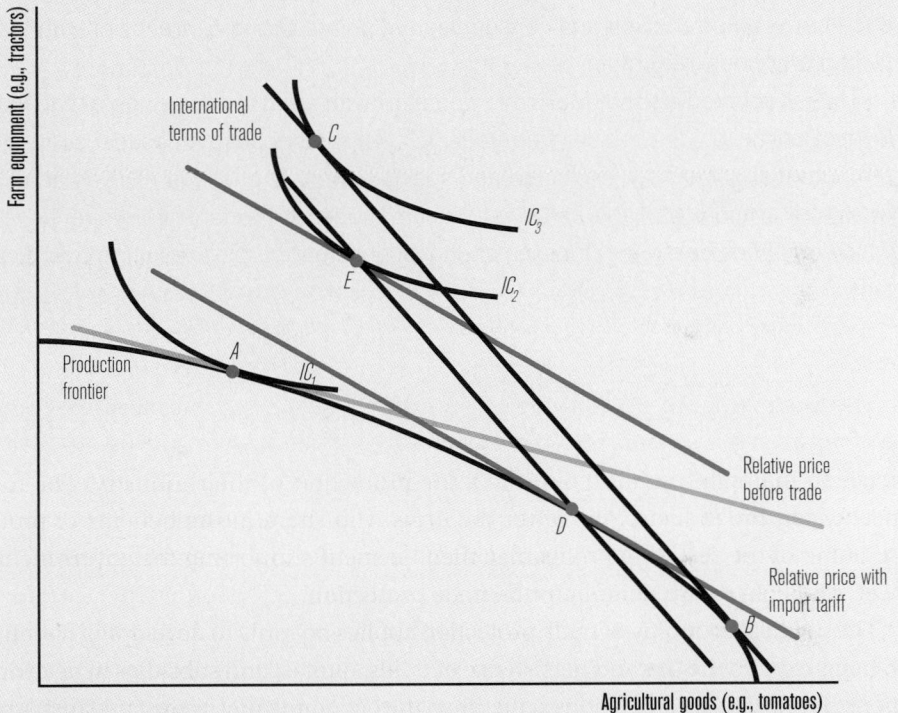

Assume Mexico embarks on an import substitution strategy and decides to protect its tractor industry with a tariff, t_0. The tariff changes the slope of the price line facing domestic producers. Before the tariff, the slope is, Px/Py; after the tariff it is, $Px/[Py(1 + t_0)]$. This causes the price line to rotate and become flatter. Because of the tariff, it becomes more profitable to produce tractors in Mexico and resources move out of tomatoes. Production moves from B to D. If the tariff is high enough, a so-called prohibitive tariff, the price line will rotate by even more and relative prices will be the same as under autarky. The economy will neither import nor export and will produce and consume at A with a corresponding loss in utility.

Assuming the tariff is not prohibitive and Mexico's trading partner does not retaliate with a tariff on tomato imports, how much will Mexico import and export, and where will it consume? Assuming Mexico is a small economy and a price taker on world markets, then the international terms of trade remain unchanged and are now drawn through point D. To find consumption, recognize that Mexican consumers, like Mexico's producers, no longer face international prices; they now face relative prices, which include the tariff the government placed on tractors. The economy consumes at E, a point on the international terms of trade line that is also at the tangency between the price line including the tariff and IC_2. In the figure, both imports and exports, identified by the difference between production and consumption at points D and E, are lower with the tariff than under free trade.

The model predicts that Mexico is worse off with a tariff, consuming at a lower level of utility, IC_2, than under free trade, IC_3. This is because it has lost some of the potential gains from exchange and specialization. The loss in utility is analogous to the findings of the partial equilibrium model of the tariff in Figure 19–1, which identifies deadweight losses and lost consumer surplus resulting from the tariff.

officials to maintain the tariff and the trade protection of their industry. The more concentrated the industry, the fewer the firms who share in the benefits of protection. Some of the resulting profits may then be spent supporting the government in power, which, in return, maintains the trade protection.

The political economy of trade protection applies not only to developing nations. It also helps explain the use and persistence of tariffs, quotas, and subsidies in developed nations. The political calculations rather than the economic merits explain Japan's protection of its rice farmers and the European Union's protection of its dairy industry. Politics in the United States explains trade protection for everything from steel to sugar. Because of domestic political interests, it often is difficult to remove trade protections once they are introduced. One solution is to include tariff reductions as part of multilateral treaties. In the case of the Thai beer tariff, it expired in 2010 as part of the ASEAN Free Trade Area, a regional trade treaty among nations in Southeast Asia.

PRODUCTION SUBSIDIES

Direct subsidies are an alternative to tariffs or quotas as a means of protecting domestic manufacturers. Many high-income economies use large subsidies to support agricultural production and protect it from global competitors, often at the expense of potential competitors from developing countries. Emerging economies use subsidies as well, often to shelter more capital-intensive manufacturing from import competition. The impact of subsidies is similar to tariffs in some ways: A 20 percent protective tariff on imports and a 20 percent subsidy on output have identical effects on producer surplus. But the effects on consumers and the government budget can be quite different.

A subsidy of s_0 percent, equal to the earlier tariff of t_0, effectively moves the supply curve from S to S', as shown in Figure 19–2. Production shifts out from Q_2 to Q_4, but prices do not change, so consumers still purchase Q_1 at the original price P_w. Thus a big advantage of using subsidies is that there is no loss of consumer surplus. The total cost of the subsidy is $a + b$, but in this case, the funds come from the government budget rather than being imposed only on consumers of the particular good. Producers are equally happy with a subsidy or an equivalent tariff. As with the tariff, they gain producer surplus a, with a resource loss of b. Thus the deadweight loss is only triangle b, which is smaller than the amount $b + d$ with a tariff or quota.

If protection is to be employed, economists generally prefer subsidies over tariffs (and tariffs over quotas) because consumers are able to purchase more of the good while society pays no more for production than under an equivalent tariff. The cost is borne by taxpayers as a whole, not just the consumers of the product. Subsidies usually appear as an expenditure item in the government's budget, so there is an annual accounting for the costs of protection. Unfortunately, government officials tend to prefer quotas or tariffs over subsidies, precisely because the costs do not appear on

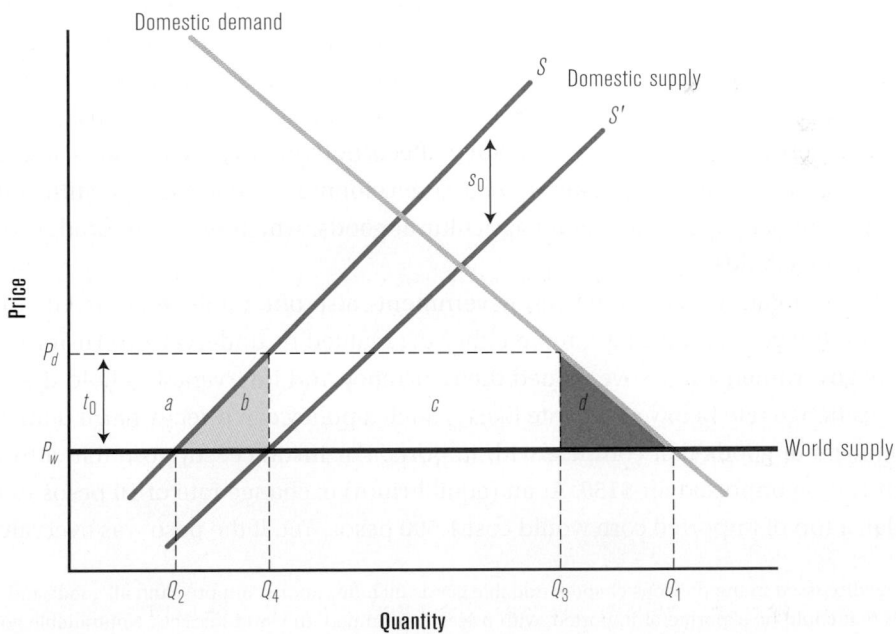

FIGURE 19–2 **The Impact of Subsidies on Firms Competing with Imports**

the budget and are less obvious to society as a whole. Subsidies also suffer from the same problem facing tariffs and quotas. What sectors warrant protection, whatever the form? How does a government decide which industry to support? How long must the subsidy last? While there are examples of governments identifying and supporting industries that went on to be successful, there are even more examples of when this approach failed. "Picking winners" is never easy.

EXCHANGE-RATE MANAGEMENT

Tariffs, quotas, and subsidies are only some of the tools policy makers can use to influence trade. One of the most powerful instruments they can employ is the exchange rate, which often affects more transactions than any other single price in an economy and directly affects the domestic prices of everything traded. Tariffs, quotas, and subsidies are used to support very specific products and sectors by changing the relative price between those products and all other products. The exchange rate, by contrast, has a uniform effect on the prices of all tradable goods but alters the price between tradables and nontradables.[4]

Figure 19–3 illustrates the market for foreign exchange, in which exporters supply and importers demand foreign currencies. The vertical axis is the exchange rate measured in local currency; for example, pesos per dollar. With a floating exchange rate system, a rate of e_e is an equilibrium rate that clears the market. IS strategies have a tendency to cause the domestic currency to appreciate. Tariffs and quotas on imports reduce the demand for foreign exchange at every possible exchange rate. In Figure 19–3, this leads to a shift in the demand curve and to a new equilibrium exchange rate, e_e'. The new exchange rate acts like a tax on exports because it now costs more foreign exchange to buy a unit of domestic currency or, equivalently, a dollar's worth of exports now returns fewer pesos. This is an important insight. Anytime a government uses trade protection it affects both imports *and* exports. Many IS strategies were designed to foster industrial development but at the same time often hurt traditional exports, including agricultural goods, which often are produced by poorer households.

In formulating trade strategies, governments also often intervene directly to fix their exchange rate, causing it to be either overvalued or undervalued. Historically, many governments have overvalued their currency and intervened to hold the official exchange rate below e_e at a rate like e_0. Such a policy can directly harm domestic producers of goods that compete with imports. For instance, suppose that a ton of corn can be imported for $150. At an (equilibrium) exchange rate of 10 pesos to the dollar, a ton of imported corn would cost 1,500 pesos. Yet, if the peso was overvalued

---

[4]As discussed in the previous chapter, tradable goods include exports, imports, and all goods and services that could be exported or imported, with prices determined on world markets. Nontradable goods are produced locally and not subject to competing imports, with prices determined by local supply and demand conditions.

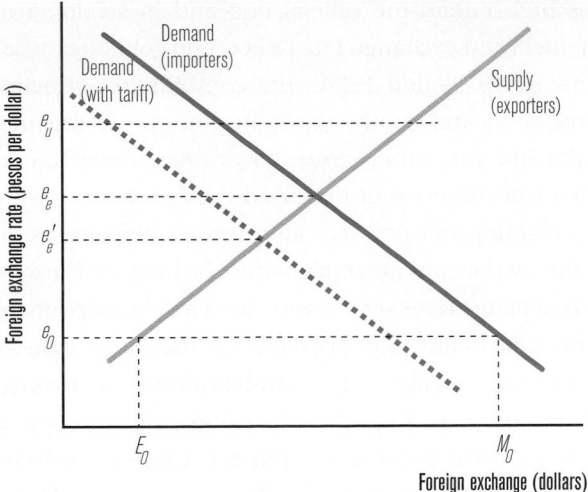

FIGURE 19-3 Overvalued and Undervalued
Exchange Rates

relative to its equilibrium, say at the rate of 8 peso per dollar, that same ton of imported corn would cost only 1,200 pesos. This might make consumers happy, but local corn farmers would have to compete against artificially cheap imports, resulting in a 20 percent decrease in their earnings. At the same time, anything exported and sold in dollars earns fewer pesos. The result is an increase in import demand and a fall in exports. As contradictory as it might at first seem, IS strategies often employed overvalued exchange rates as a policy instrument. The goal was not to make *all* imports cheaper because the intent of IS is to protect domestic industries. Overvalued exchange rates were used to make capital goods and other critical imports, such as food or fuel, cheaper in terms of domestic currency. Nonessential imports are kept out of the domestic market via high tariffs and quantitative barriers. Ironically, there can even be a vicious circle in which tariffs lead to overvalued exchange rates, which reduce the cost of imports and thus create a need for even higher tariff rates to compensate.

A quick look at Figure 19-3 identifies some of the problems associated with employing overvalued exchange rates. Like any price ceiling, it creates excess demand. At e_0 the excess demand for foreign exchange equals, $M_0 - E_0$. Because the foreign exchange market now fails to clear, it becomes necessary to ration foreign exchange, requiring licenses and the administrative controls to oversee them. Such licenses easily become a source of rent seeking and corruption. Overvalued exchange rates also give rise to black markets for foreign exchange.[5] This is because overvaluation creates chronic excess demand for foreign currencies. Incentives are created to deal foreign

[5]In the 1970s and 1980s, travelers to many developing nations, including the authors of this text, invariably were asked by taxi drivers from the airport if they wanted to exchange money, a sure sign of an overvalued exchange rate and the black markets they encouraged.

exchange at rates higher than the official one and in so doing may frustrate the intended goals of the IS and exchange rate policy, and generate more rent seeking.

As recently as the 1970s and 1980s, the combination of overvalued exchange rates and pervasive tariffs and quotas was quite common. Some of this was because of IS strategies. But in many other cases, governments overvalued their exchange rates primarily to lower the price of imported goods for those who were politically well connected, including the political elite, urban consumers, and the military. Today, following one of the core precepts of the Washington Consensus discussed in Chapter 5, official exchange rates set at overvalued levels are relatively uncommon.

Some governments follow the opposite strategy and intervene to hold the exchange rate above e_e at a rate like e_u. They **undervalue their currency**. This approach makes all imports more expensive and, at the same time, makes exports more profitable by increasing their price in domestic currency. Undervalued exchange rates help stimulate exports and provide protection to firms competing with imports by raising the price of competitive products. They have been used in some East Asia economies, most notably China, as part of more outward-looking strategies. We evaluate their use later in the chapter.

OUTCOMES OF IMPORT SUBSTITUTION

Import substitution has the potential to be an effective strategy for certain sectors over a limited period of time. Almost all countries have tried it at one stage or another, and many have achieved some success. Even Latin America, which is often cited for the failures of IS, had more rapid growth in the 1960s and 1970s under IS regimes than it did for the next 20 years as it moved in the direction of more liberal trade. But in Latin America and elsewhere, all too often, the basic conditions for prolonged success are not met. In many countries, IS protected too many activities and remained in place for too long. Developing countries are littered with infants that never grew up and were never able to compete internationally, such as the petrochemical industry of Colombia, the automobile industry of Malaysia, and the textile industry of Kenya. Firms in these industries have tended to require protection indefinitely, at continuous cost to the rest of society. Sometimes IS fails because of an initially poor choice to protect the wrong kinds of activities (the microcomputer industry in Brazil); often it stems from the reluctance of governments to remove the protection given to politically well-connected industrialists.

Most developing countries have relatively small internal markets, either because per capita incomes are low or populations are relatively small. This makes them poor candidates for IS because the domestic market quickly becomes saturated. The next step, expansion to export markets, may never happen because of low productivity growth which may itself be the result of the trade protection intended to help the industry. Facing a small domestic market there may be little domestic competition and few incentives to innovate. A limited market means that firms cannot take advantage of economies of scale and may produce at less than their minimum efficient size. And by reducing their commercial links with the rest of the world, import-substituting countries limit their exposure to new technology and ideas.

IS has had some limited success in bigger economies with large internal markets, at least for a short period of time. But even the very large economies of China and India had more success when they stopped looking only inward—for the Chinese economy after the reforms that began in 1978 and for India after 1991. Of course, these reforms entailed more than a change in trade strategies, and it is difficult to pinpoint the specific contribution of the change in trade policy.

Ironically, many countries that try IS run into balance-of-payments problems from growing trade deficits. Even though the strategy is designed to replace imports with domestic production, not all imports can be replaced (especially capital goods). Because the strategy effectively discourages exports, foreign exchange earnings lag, especially because IS often is accompanied by an overvalued exchange rate. Therefore, many countries following this strategy have had to borrow heavily and found it difficult to meet their debt service requirements. Better macroeconomic management could have avoided these problems, but the instruments of IS did not help.

Underlying the protective regime also is a set of incentives that reward political lobbying, corruption, and bribery more than economic efficiency and competitiveness. When higher domestic costs, reduced import prices, or better-quality foreign goods erode the competitive position of domestic firms, a natural reaction is for these firms to turn to the government for enhanced protection. This option blunts the competitive instincts of entrepreneurs, who normally would have to cut costs, improve quality, and thus raise productivity. In this environment, the most successful managers are those who have the political skills or connections with which to bargain effectively, or simply bribe, officials who determine tariff rates, administer import quotas or distribute foreign exchange. The pursuit of such unearned benefits is known as *rent-seeking behavior*. Rent seeking also hurts economies by diverting real resources from productive uses.

EXPORT ORIENTATION

Since the late 1980s, many countries have shifted the balance of their trade policies away from IS toward more export-oriented trade policies, in which firms compete on global markets. This strategy has many names, including *outward orientation, openness, export promotion,* and *export orientation.*[6] The idea is to introduce policies that

---

[6]Joining a free trade area, as Mexico did with Canada and the United States under the North America Free Trade Agreement (NAFTA) can also be seen as a move toward greater outward orientation. However, some free-trade areas or other types of economic integration can be more like import substitution if the combined economies are small and members build tariff walls around themselves, reducing trade with nonmembers.

encourage firms to produce products that are competitive on world markets, especially labor-intensive manufactured exports and agricultural products but also competitive substitutes for imports. The key difference with IS is that this strategy uses global competition to encourage investment, productivity gains, learning, and new technology to support growth.[7]

In the typical pattern, in the early stages, firms manufacture and export relatively simple labor-intensive products, such as textiles, clothing, shoes, toys, electronic equipment, and furniture. Some countries also export agricultural products and labor-intensive agroprocessing goods, such as fresh vegetables, fruit juices, or cut flowers, and increasingly certain services including data entry, basic accounting, and call centers. Then, over time, as workers learn new skills and gain access to improved technology, firms begin to shift to more-sophisticated products (which pay higher wages to match greater productivity and skills). As the country's comparative advantage gradually shifts, the mix of exports changes as well to include more-advanced electronic devices, automobile parts, higher-end clothing, steel, and many other consumer and capital goods.

The shift toward more outward-oriented policies among developing countries began in the 1960s with the Four East Asian Tigers: Hong Kong, Korea, Singapore, and Taiwan. They demonstrated that developing countries could compete on world markets by carving out niche markets in producing labor-intensive manufactured products. Their rapid growth in trade was accompanied by accelerating economic growth, reductions in poverty, and other advancements. Following their example, most of the very rapidly growing developing countries in recent decades have introduced some form of this strategy, including Chile, China, Indonesia, Malaysia, Mauritius, Poland, Thailand, Tunisia, and Vietnam. India's growth rate also accelerated in the 1990s as it shifted to a more outward-oriented strategy.

But not all countries that have shifted to policies that are more outward oriented achieved the success they had hoped for. Bolivia introduced many steps to open its economy, and while growth has recovered from the negative rates that prevailed in the early 1980s, it has averaged only about 1.5 percent since the late 1980s. Many of the countries formed by the breakup of the Soviet Union pursued more open trade strategies but realized little growth in either trade or output, especially during the 1990s. Without the other elements that encourage investment and entrepreneurship, including institutions that protect property rights and enforce the rule of law, trade reforms alone had minimal impact. In the 1990s, Zambia implemented reforms that resulted in one of the most liberal trade regimes in all of Africa. But the hoped for growth in exports did not follow. Part of the problem was macroeconomic instability, including high inflation and a volatile real exchange rate. Under

---

[7]For an overview of the shift in thinking about trade policy and development between the 1960s and 1990s, see Anne O. Krueger's presidential address to the American Economic Association: "Trade Policy and Economic Development: How We Learn," *American Economic Review* 1, no. 87 (March 1997).

such conditions, firms were reluctant to invest in new ventures whether in exports or import-competing sectors.[8]

REMOVING THE BIAS AGAINST EXPORTS

Policies that favor imports, including tariffs and overvalued exchange rates, implicitly are biased against exports. Recent decades have seen a retreat from such policies. As shown in Figure 19-4, there has been a clear global trend to reduce average tariffs. In South Asia, average tariffs fell from over 50 percent in 1987 to under 15 percent by 2007. Tariffs in all regions fell. Some changes in individual countries have been dramatic. In Costa Rica, the average statutory tariff was 55 percent in 1980 and only 6.2 percent in 2007; in Turkey it fell from 44 to 1.9 percent over the same time period. Currencies officially set at overvalued rates once common are also now rare.

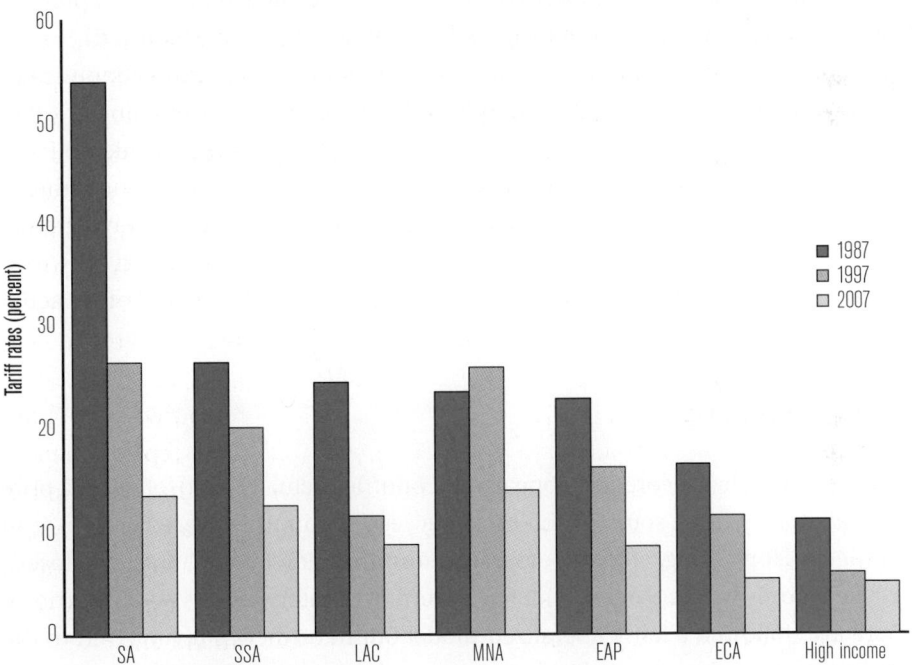

FIGURE 19-4 Average Unweighted Tariff Rates by Region

EAP, East Asia and the Pacific; ECA, Europe and central Asia; LAC, Latin America and the Caribbean; MNA, Mideast and North Africa; SA, South Asia; SSA, sub-Saharan Africa.
Source: World Bank, "Trends in Average Applied Tariff Rates in Developing and Industrial Countries, 1981–2007," available at http://econ.worldbank.org/WBSITE/EXTERNAL/EXTDEC/EXTRESEARCH/0,,contentMDK:21051044~pagePK:64214825~piPK:64214943~theSitePK:469382,00.html.

[8]World Bank, "Trade Liberalization: Why So Much Controversy?" in *Economic Growth in the 1990s: Learning from a Decade of Reform* (Washington, DC: World Bank, 2005).

The basic steps toward full-fledged liberalization aimed at removing the bias against exports will sound familiar:

- Remove quotas and tariffs and other forms of protection, especially on capital and intermediate goods.
- Allow the currency to float with a market-determined exchange rate, and ensure macroeconomic stability through prudent monetary and fiscal policies.
- Reduce unnecessary regulatory burdens, bureaucratic costs, and red tape that add to business costs.
- Keep factor markets flexible, especially for labor and credit, with market determined wages and interest rates.

In a full liberalization strategy, these steps are augmented with general approaches to strengthen infrastructure (especially roads, ports, electricity supplies, and telecommunications to connect firms with the rest of the world and reduce production costs), invest in education and public health (to ensure a well-educated, healthy, and productive workforce), and improve governance (so that property rights are respected).

These basic policies will not surprise any student of neoclassical economics or simply someone who has been reading this textbook. Outward orientation is often seen as synonymous with broader market-based and liberalized economic policies. The neoclassical approach does not prescribe a bias toward exports but rather a regime that is neutral in its treatment of exports, import substitutes, and nontraded goods. In this view, the strategy is not aimed at exports per se, but export growth is likely to follow because the distortions that inhibited exports and favored other activities are removed.

FAVORING EXPORTS

While liberalization has theoretical appeal, few countries actually have followed a pure neoclassical strategy, and some of the most successful countries were far from it in some respects. Hong Kong, at least before its return to China in 1997, was the closest, where the economy was very open, with few government interventions and distortions. Singapore also followed a fairly liberalized model but nevertheless diverged from the neoclassical norm in that many of its largest export industries are government-owned service firms in telecommunications, port services (including one of the world's best-run airports), and air transport (the world-renowned Singapore Airlines).[9] Korea was much more interventionist. It erected stiff protective barriers against many imports,

---

[9]Hong Kong and Singapore often are compared. They are both city-state, island economies that have transitioned to high-income status and relied heavily on trade to do so. Hong Kong, however, has come considerably closer to free trade than more interventionist Singapore. See Lawrence Krause, "Hong Kong and Singapore: Twins or Kissing Cousins?" *Economic Development and Cultural Change* 36, no. 3 (April 1988).

especially consumer goods. A visitor could literally see the effect. In the 1980s one could stand for hours at one of the busiest street corners in Seoul, where many lanes of traffic intersect, and not see a single imported car. The streets were choked with automobiles, but only those produced by Daewoo, Hyundai and a few other large Korean conglomerates. Tariff and other barriers kept Fords, Toyotas, VWs and every other international brand out of the domestic market.

Korea's government also controlled interest rates at below-market levels, directing cheap credit to favored industries and firms, including exporters. What made the approach outward-looking is that interventions were used to induce, and sometimes force, firms to meet ambitious export targets. Success or failure was dictated to a large degree by the ability to compete on world markets, rather than domestically.[10] Korea went beyond simple outward orientation and neutrality and introduced a bias toward exports. In contrast to an inward-looking regime, a Korean firm could not take advantage of protection or other preferential treatment unless it met stringent export targets. Korean car manufacturers, for example, became competitive on global markets and began to export while selling to a protected local market. Some of the tools of protection were used to help fledgling exporters who were learning by doing: adopting new technologies, learning how to master them, reducing costs of production, finding and entering markets overseas, and eventually competing on equal terms with foreign firms.[11] But not all firms succeeded. Korea's drive to expand its heavy and chemical industries in the 1980s met with more limited success.

The strong bias and intervention to support exporters followed in Korea was not the rule for all the Asian exporters. Indonesia, Malaysia, Taiwan, and Thailand used a more mixed approach.[12] Heavily protectionist and interventionist in certain areas, some of the industries explicitly supported never became internationally competitive, such as Malaysia's Proton automobiles and Indonesia's IPTN aircraft. What was more successful were the policies that insulated export industries from the distortions of the home market and permitted firms to buy inputs and sell output at close to world market prices, as the neoclassical strategy dictates, permitting a wide range of exporting firms to become competitive in international markets.

China has been more interventionist and pursued outward-oriented policies far from free trade and the full-fledged liberalization described earlier. As economist Dani

---

[10]See Marcus Noland and Howard Pack, *Industrial Policy in an Era of Globalization: Lessons From Asia* (Washington, DC: Institute for International Economics, March 2003).

[11]For a wonderful description of how Korean firms implemented "learning by doing" read Ira Magaziner and Mark Patinkin, "Fast Heat: How Korea Won the Microwave War," *Harvard Business Review* 67 (January–February 1989).

[12]The revisionist school on Korea, questioning the neoclassical approach, was led by Alice Amsden, *Asia's New Giant: South Korea and Late Industrialization* (New York: Oxford University Press, 1989). Taiwan's interventionist strategy is documented by Robert Wade, *Governing the Market: Economic Theory and the Role of Government in East Asian Industrialization* (Princeton, NJ: Princeton University Press, 1990). The World Bank attempted to reconcile neoclassical and revisionist thinking in its much-discussed book, *The East Asian Miracle: Economic Growth and Public Policy* (Washington, DC: World Bank, 1993).

Rodrik has put it, "China's policies resemble more those of a country that messed up big time than those of a country that became a formidable competitive threat in world markets to rich and poor countries alike."[13] In 1993 after a decade and a half of rapid export and economic growth, average tariffs still remained at 40 percent, the sixth highest level in the world at that time. (By 2007, six years after joining the World Trade Organization [WTO], Chinese tariffs had fallen below 10 percent.) But even more than its prior tariff regime, China, along with Korea and Taiwan in earlier years, used and still uses exchange rate policy to favor exporters by undervaluing its currency.

By pegging the exchange rate above the market-clearing rate, imports become more expensive and exports more profitable. This policy contributed to China's rapid export growth, its large trade surplus, and the resulting accumulation of foreign exchange reserves. An undervalued currency acts as an indirect subsidy for Chinese exporters. Like all subsidies, it comes at a cost, making imports more expensive and thus reducing consumption and consumer welfare for the average Chinese. Reserve accumulation can be helpful to a point, but reserves, by definition, are resources that a society puts aside and does not use for current consumption or investment. They are subject to exchange rate and other risks and may lose their value, as demonstrated during the financial crisis of 2008.

The costs of China's exchange rate policy also have external ramifications. China frequently is cited as engaging in unfair trade practices because of the way it manages its exchange rate. Legislation has been proposed in the U.S. Senate to impose tariffs on Chinese goods equal to the extent of undervaluation of its currency, a quantity that is subject to some debate. Some, including Ben Bernanke, chairman of the U.S. Federal Reserve Bank, have a different concern. They argue that China's huge foreign reserves, a consequence of its exchange rate policy, were part of the underlying causes of the 2008 global financial crisis. These reserves, Bernanke suggests, contributed to the global economic imbalances that drove interest rates down and created the conditions that encouraged the huge risk taking and subsequent collapse of financial institutions in search of higher returns. Continuation of such policies also is seen as an impediment to restoring the global imbalances that remain today and that may limit global economic recovery (Box 19-3).

BUILDING EXPORT PLATFORMS

Another approach taken in almost all of the countries that have achieved rapid export growth was to establish specialized export platform institutions that enabled exporters to import and sell at close to world market prices, even in the presence of more widespread distortions. The platforms took a variety of forms, including export processing zones (EPZs), bonded warehouses, duty exemption programs, and science and

[13]Dani Rodrik, "What's So Special About China's Exports?" *China in the World Economy* 14, no. 5 (September–October 2006).

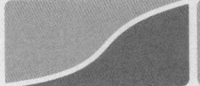

BOX 19-3 IS CHINA'S EXCHANGE-RATE POLICY UNFAIR?

China has been criticized by some for maintaining an undervalued exchange rate that makes its exports more profitable; others argue that the currency is not seriously misaligned. China for a decade kept its currency, the renminbi (RMB), fixed against the U.S. dollar at a rate of 8.28 yuan to $1. Then in 2005 China introduced a managed float. and the yuan rose in value to 6.83 to $1. As the world moved into recession in 2007 and 2008, China again fixed its exchange rate ending further revaluation. Despite fixing the exchange rate, however, Chinese exports fell sharply in 2009 due to declining world demand for Chinese manufactures. With the beginning of recovery from the world recession in 2010, China's exports recovered rapidly and it announced in June of that year that it would allow its currency to float; it was expected that the Chinese currency would appreciate in value.

Several pieces of evidence suggest that the RMB was still undervalued in mid-2010—that is, kept at above the market clearing rate, as with exchange rate, e_u, in Figure 19–3. China's current account surplus (exports minus imports of both goods and services) had grown to 8 percent of gross domestic product (GDP) in 2008 and remained at a very high level of 4 percent in 2009, as predicted by Figure 19–3. Normally, a current account surplus is matched by an outflow of foreign capital, as countries invest the proceeds abroad. But China attracted net capital *inflows* of an additional 1.7 percent of GDP in 2009. Because this current account surplus has existed for many years (since 1994) China accumulated very large foreign exchange reserves of US$2.45 trillion as of the end of the second quarter of 2010, equivalent to roughly two years of imports.

China's exchange rate is not the only policy that affects these balances. The government maintains an array of restrictions on capital flows, which tend to discourage outflows of capital. In the absence of these controls, the surpluses would not be so large. Even taking these arguments into account, many economists still conclude that the RMB is undervalued, perhaps by 15 to 25 percent.[a]

An undervalued RMB makes Chinese exports more profitable, and indeed exports rose fourfold between 2000 and 2009, much of it through importing components from other countries in the region and assembling finished products for export. This export growth is a key reason for China's overall economic growth and its impressive reduction in poverty, as many unskilled workers have found jobs in the special economic zones (SEZs; much like export processing

[a]Morris Goldstein and Nicholas Lardy, *The Future of China's Exchange Rate Policy: Policy Analyses in International Economics 87* (Washington, DC: Institute for International Economics, 2009).

zones, discussed later in this chapter). Moreover, the buildup in reserves also allows China to maintain macroeconomic stability, as it is unlikely to face the kind of capital account crisis many of its neighbors faced in the late 1990s, as described in Chapters 12 and 13. China's buildup in reserves is partly a defensive move in response to these crises.

But the policy of maintaining an undervalued exchange rate has its costs, especially the longer it is in place. Restraining consumption reduces the welfare of ordinary Chinese by making imports of consumer goods more expensive. Foreign exchange reserves equivalent to two years of imports are also far greater than China requires to defend against a future run on its currency as happened elsewhere in Asia in 1997 and 1998. These large reserves are also mainly invested in government bonds (one third of China's reserves are invested in U.S. Treasury bonds), which in recent years have paid a low rate of interest.

But perhaps most important the undervalued exchange rate brings threats of protectionism from trading partners: Individual U.S. senators have proposed putting a high tariff on all Chinese imports unless China revalues the RMB substantially. China's exchange rate policy has become a convenient scapegoat for the U.S. trade deficit, even though China's exchange rate contributes relatively little to the U.S. deficit compared to other factors more in the control of the United States, particularly its budget deficit and low personal saving rate. Undervalued exchange rates and a rapid growth of exports do not usually lead to threats of retaliation when a country's total foreign trade is small as was the case in China in the 1970s when its total exports were under US$10 billion a year. In those years, threats of protection were made against the much larger exports of Japan, which was also believed to have an undervalued currency. But in 2009 China passed Germany to become the largest exporting country in the world and hence the focus of all those concerned about the impact of rising imports on their domestic industries.

China's exchange rate policy has contributed to its rapid economic growth and poverty reduction in recent years, and its large reserve holdings help stabilize the economy and reduce the chances of a major capital account crisis. An undervalued exchange rate also helped China postpone the date when exporters of products depending on cheap labor, because of rising Chinese wages, would have to give way to exporters in other countries where wages are lower. But, over the longer run, there will be little extra benefit for China to continue to accumulate reserves at the expense of consumption and possible protectionist retaliation. China, like Japan and the other East Asian exporters of manufactures who depended for a time on undervalued exchange rates, is likely to let its exchange rate rise to a point at which the renminbi no longer is undervalued.

technology parks. These institutions are designed to create an enclave for fledgling export industries, where they can be insulated from the controls and price distortions of the protected domestic market and be better able to compete on world markets.[14]

EPZs are located physically or administratively outside a country's customs' barrier, typically as fenced-in areas near a port, that provide exporters access to duty-free imports, reduced business regulations, expedited customs clearance, and reasonable infrastructure. Bonded warehouses essentially are single-factory EPZs that can be located anywhere, yet still have many of the other advantages of EPZs. These factories are called *bonded warehouses* because firms usually post a bond as a guarantee against any duties that might be applicable to imports diverted to the domestic market, and if they sell output locally instead of export it, they are liable to pay the import duties. Duty exemption systems allow qualifying firms to import their inputs duty free. Science and technology parks are like EPZs, but with infrastructure specially suited for electronics, pharmaceuticals, biomedical products, or other products related to science and technology.

The basic idea is straightforward. Potential exporters face a variety of challenges, including high tariffs or quotas on their inputs, poor infrastructure, and red tape. The neoclassical solution is to remove all import tariffs and quotas, improve infrastructure, and reduce red tape. The problem is that, for a variety of institutional and political reasons, no country realistically can implement all these steps quickly. Most governments lack the large number of trained personnel to take on so many issues at once, and political forces are likely to fight certain steps, like reducing tariffs. It can take many years for a country to build the infrastructure and introduce all the policy changes needed for firms throughout the economy to become competitive. The export platform approach is to allow one part of the economy to be competitive, while steps are taken over time to introduce economywide changes. Providing an enclave allows some firms, mainly producing labor-intensive manufacturers, to become competitive on world markets before all the required steps are in place for the economy as a whole.

Most of the successful exporting countries established at least one, and in most cases more than one, of these programs. Malaysia relied mainly on EPZs that provided reliable infrastructure and allowed exporters (mainly in electronics) to import and export without being taxed; the government also established bonded warehouses and a duty exemption system for other exporters. Indonesia established an agency in the Ministry of Finance that granted exemptions from import licensing restrictions and drawbacks (rebates) for duties paid on imported inputs. The vast majority of Tunisia's manufactured exporters operate as bonded warehouses, whereas Mauritian exporters are located mainly in export processing zones. China's special enterprise

---

[14]See David L. Lindauer and Michael Roemer, eds., *Asia and Africa: Legacies and Opportunities in Development* (San Francisco: ICS Press, 1994), esp. chaps. 1 and 11. Also see Steven Radelet, "Manufactured Exports, Export Platforms and Economic Growth," CAER Discussion Paper No. 42, Harvard Institute for International Development, Cambridge, MA, September 1999.

zones, located up and down the coast, have been the source of most of its manufactured exports. In the Dominican Republic, exports from EPZs increased by a factor of five during the 1990s, and by the end of the decade accounted for over 80 percent of all exports. EPZ employment reached nearly 200,000 people by the end of the 1990s, about 17 percent of the Dominican workforce. About 60 percent of employees are women, a pattern that is typical of many EPZs.[15]

Export platforms have not always been successful. When they are located far from ports in an attempt to spur development in isolated areas, production costs usually are too high for firms to compete. If firms in export platforms still face high regulatory costs or must wait long periods of time for goods to clear customs, they will not be successful on global markets. And export platforms cannot overcome poor macroeconomic management that leads to high inflation, overvalued or volatile exchange rates. Egypt's EPZs have not spurred faster export growth because they still face high production costs. Kenya's bonded warehouses began to expand in the 1980s, but when macroeconomic policies deteriorated and the currency became overvalued in the 1990s, 60 of 70 bonded warehouses closed. Export platforms, whatever their forms, are no silver bullet, but they provide examples of how innovative institutions shaped to a country's specific needs can help support market-based growth.

TRADE STRATEGY AND INDUSTRIAL POLICY

Almost all nations recognize the importance of increased integration into the global economy and the need to look outward. But an outward orientation is not the same as free trade or laissez-faire. Policy neutrality regarding production for exports versus the domestic market has been the exception rather than the rule. The debate revolves less around inward versus outward orientation and more around the use of **industrial policy**, a broad set of interventions including, but not limited to, undervalued exchange rates and EPZs, which governments may use to favor one set of economic activities over another.

Most economists remain wary of industrial policies. They recognize the various and pervasive market failures that constrain the growth of new firms and activities, from credit markets unwilling to finance new products to the lack of complementary inputs to service export initiatives, but are unsure governments are up to the challenge of improving the situation. Governments tend not to have the knowledge and information to figure out what firms really need, and more often than not industrial policies breed corruption or promote inefficiency. Such economists recognize that there are examples of success with industrial policy. POSCO, a Korean steel producer, was formerly a state-owned enterprise that grew behind high trade barriers into one

---

[15]Staci Warden, "A Profile of Free Trade Zones in the Dominican Republic," Harvard Institute for International Development, Cambridge, MA, 1999.

of the world's largest and most efficient private steel corporations. Farmed salmon in Chile, today a highly successful industry, was initiated and fostered by a quasi-public agency. But for each of these positive examples, there are many more where industrial policy has failed from airplanes in Indonesia to tanneries in Ethiopia.

Harvard University economist Rodrik, takes the opposite view. He acknowledges the failures of past strategies. Import substitution, planning, and state ownership of enterprises were tried and, in some cases, succeeded for a while but in the end failed to generate sustained economic growth and development. But liberalization and full reliance on market forces *also* delivered less than what was hoped for, especially in Latin America and sub-Saharan Africa. Even where there has been success, cursory examination of the economic miracles of past decades reveals how far they were from the neoclassical ideal and how central a role government played in favoring exports, specific sectors, and even specific industries and firms. In East Asia and Latin America it was the combination of private initiative and public interventions to support exports that characterized most cases of successful trade and development strategies.

Rodrik and others see the role of government as extending beyond the traditional areas of ensuring macro stability, providing public goods, and resolving externalities (such as pollution). Government also has a coordinating role to play in facilitating the structural change inherent in the development process. Economies need to move away from traditional products and to diversify their economies, but this is not easy to do. As Rodrik puts it, the problem is one of "self-discovery." Comparative advantage and factor endowment theory offer important insights into the benefits and direction of trade, but they alone are insufficient to explain the specific goods different nations export. Labor abundant economies may all export labor-intensive goods, but why did entrepreneurs in Bangladesh specialize in T-shirts and in Pakistan in soccer balls? Why is Korea the dominant exporter of microwaves while Taiwan, an economy with similar factor endowments, exports none but dominates in bicycles? In each of these examples individual entrepreneurs figured out that they could succeed in a particular product. Their success was then imitated by others and the industry expanded.

Rodrik argues that in most developing countries, governments need to do something to encourage this process of self-discovery.[16] Entrepreneurs need to determine which existing goods and technologies from abroad can be adapted to local conditions and successfully exported in global markets. But they may be reluctant to do so for many reasons. For one, the gains of their individual efforts may be undercut by the inevitable imitation that will follow their success. In this instance, self-discovery presents a classic public good problem: Information on what products a firm might successfully export is both nonexcludable and nonrival; therefore, not enough of this information will be forthcoming. Government intervention can help. Some form of protection or subsidy must accrue to the initial investor, and not the copycats, to

---

[16]Dani Rodrik, *One Economics, Many Recipes: Globalization, Institutions, and Economic Growth* (Princeton, NJ: Princeton, 2007), 4.

encourage the self-discovery that may be absent on its own. Other coordination problems may be resolved by government action, for example, in the setting of product standards for exports or relieving infrastructure constraints.

Rodrik is not alone in his support of industrial policy as part of a developing nation's trade policy. In their exhaustive review of the literature on trade and industrial policy for a recent volume of the *Handbook of Development Economics*, economists Ann Harrison and Andrés Rodríguez-Clare do not go as far as Rodrik does in supporting hard industrial policies, including trade protection in the form of tariffs, quotas, and subsidies. But they do see a need for soft industrial policies aimed at resolving the coordination problems that nations face trying to break into established export markets. They argue for partnerships between the public and the private sectors in identifying and resolving the binding constraints facing entry into in new markets.[17]

TRADE, GROWTH, AND POVERTY ALLEVIATION

The promotion of exports and the use of industrial policy is not the only area where there is disagreement among development economists over trade policy. A lively debate remains over the centrality of trade in generating economic growth and of the consequences of increased trade for alleviating poverty. This may seem surprising given the many theoretical reasons discussed in the previous chapter for how trade can improve factor productivity and encourage economic growth and for why trade favors a nation's abundant factor and, in the case of poor labor abundant economies, is expected to reduce poverty. The empirical evidence, however, is less straightforward. We begin by discussing the empirical evidence on trade and growth; in the next section, we turn to the evidence on trade and poverty alleviation.

Hundreds of academic papers have been written examining the relationship between trade and growth. It is important to understand why it is so difficult to establish an empirical pattern linking trade, trade policy, and economic growth. Problems of reverse causality, omitted variable bias and the measurement of trade policy confront the economist trying to sort out the underlying relationship. (If you have taken a course in econometrics some of these common problems may be familiar to you.)

Economists Jeffrey Frankel and David Romer tackle the difficult issues of the direction of causality and omitted variable bias in a paper aptly titled, "Does Trade Cause Growth?"[18] A strong positive relationship between trade and per capita income does not prove that the former is the *cause* of the latter. It is entirely plausible

---

[17]Ann Harrison and Andrés Rodríguez-Clare, "Trade, Foreign Investment, and Industrial Policy for Developing Countries," in Dani Rodrik and M. R. Rosenzweig, eds., *Handbook of Development Economics*, vol. 5 (Amsterdam: North Holland, 2009).

[18]Jeffrey Frankel and David Romer, "Does Trade Cause Growth?" *American Economic Review* 89, no. 3 (June 1999).

that the causation runs the other way: Income and productivity growth, by increasing productive capacity and reducing costs, can make a country more competitive in world markets and lead to faster growth of manufactured exports. Also possible is that both export growth and economic growth are simultaneously caused by something else, such as improved macroeconomic policies, more stable political systems, reduced corruption, or increased savings. If one does not fully account for these factors (the omitted variables) it is possible that trade statistically is picking up their influence even if it is not the causal determinant of higher income levels.

Frankel and Romer address these issues by tracing the portion of trade due to geographical characteristics (such as a country's size, its location relative to its trading partners, and whether it is landlocked), which tend to be weakly correlated or uncorrelated with other possible determinants of growth. They show that this geographical component of trade has a large and positive effect on income. The study supports the direction of causality running from trade to growth but acknowledges the result is not highly significant; a finding echoed in subsequent studies. Causality is hard to untangle because, to a large extent, export growth and economic growth probably support each other in a virtuous circle: Exporting countries have greater access to new machinery and technology that support growth, while faster economic growth provides the means to finance investments in the new machinery, technology, and infrastructure that support exports.

The study by Frankel and Romer uses the ratio of exports plus imports to gross domestic product (GDP) as their measure of trade. This is a common way of measuring *trade volumes*. In the survey article by Harrison and Rodríguez-Clare cited earlier, the authors reviewed hundreds of articles, many that relate trade volumes to either income levels or growth rates while adjusting for other possible determinants of growth and employing a wide range of econometric specifications. They conclude that there is a strong correlation between increasing trade shares and country performance, ceteris paribus. This is not a surprising finding. Although trade may not be a panacea, one would be hard pressed to think of any successful low- or middle-income nation where trade has not become a large part of its economy.

Trade *volumes*, however, are not the same as trade *policies*. Trade policies, whether reducing tariffs, managing the exchange rate, or creating EPZs, are the instruments governments have at their disposal. Trade volumes are a consequence of these and other policies. For the policy maker, understanding the impact of alternative trade policies on growth would be of great value. But this is not easy to determine. Harrison and Rodríguez-Clare's exhaustive survey finds no significant correlation between lower tariff levels on final goods and country performance. Does this suggest that trade liberalization is a bad idea? Certainly not.

The problem is what alternative measures of trade policy can tell us. Measuring the links between specific trade policies and growth is complex because a range of policies affect trade and countries often employ instruments of import protection combined with policies for export promotion. Looking at any one policy in isolation from others can provide ambiguous results, as no single policy can fully reflect a country's range of trade policies. Consider import tariffs: China, Korea, Malaysia, and other countries kept tariffs high on many products, while some other countries that reduced average tariff rates were not rewarded with rapid export growth. But the most successful countries did more than just lower average tariffs. The exact policy combination differed, although they all had the common element of zero tariffs on imported inputs and capital goods for exporters, and they took other steps to reduce costs for exporters and to integrate firms with the global economy. Because the policy mix differed, it is that much harder to measure for research purposes and to prescribe the precise steps that other countries might want to take.[19]

An alternative approach is to examine combinations of trade policies. An often cited example is a study by Jeffrey Sachs and Andrew Warner.[20] They consider the economic growth performance of 79 countries around the world during the period 1970–89 and find that countries with more open policies and less-biased exchange rates grew about 2 percentage points faster than did closed economies. As we have highlighted throughout the text, 2 percentage points added to the growth rate is a huge amount with the potential to rapidly alleviate poverty and transform a society. Can greater openness to trade deliver this much? The Sachs-Warner measure of trade policy considered a country to be "open" if it passed five criteria: (1) its average tariff rate was less than 40 percent, (2) its nontariff barriers (such as, quotas) covered less than 40 percent of imports, (3) the premium on the unofficial parallel market exchange rate did not exceed 20 percent, (4) there were no state monopolies on major exports, and (5) it was not a socialist economy. This is a broad interpretation of what openness entails and goes well beyond trade policy.

It is not surprising that the Sachs and Warner study has been subjected to a lot of scrutiny and debate. One of the key criticisms concerns their index of openness and their conclusions about trade policy. Poor management of the exchange rate (item 3) is more likely a call to improve macroeconomic policy than to liberalize trade. Similarly, reliance on state monopolies (item 4) and the socialist economy criteria (item 5) may have more to do with governance than with trade per se. Several researchers have found that it is precisely these items (items 3, 4, and 5) in the Sachs-Warner openness index that explain most of the difference in growth performance during the 1970s and 1980s. Reducing trade barriers (items 1 and 2) had little independent explanatory power.[21] Today, socialism, state monopolies over exports, and gross

[19]Lant Pritchett, "Measuring Outward Orientation in LDCs: Can It Be Done?" *Journal of Development Economics* 49, no. 2 (1996), 307–35.

[20]Jeffrey Sachs and Andrew Warner, "Economic Reform and the Process of Global Integration," *Brookings Papers on Economic Activity* 1 (1995), 1–118.

[21]The seminal articles in this debate are Ann Harrison and Gordon Hanson, "Who Gains from Trade Reform? Some Remaining Puzzles," *Journal of Development Economics* 59, (1999), 125–54; Francisco Rodríguez and Dani Rodrik, "Trade Policy and Economic Growth: A Skeptic's Guide to the Cross-National Evidence," in Ben S. Bernanke and Kenneth Rogoff, eds., *NBER Macroeconomics Annual 2000* (Cambridge: NBER, 2001). An updated version of the Sachs and Warner approach covering a much longer time period, 1950–98, finds results confirming the original study. See Romain Wacziarg and Karen Welch, "Trade Liberalization and Growth: New Evidence," *World Bank Economic Review* 22 (2008), 187–231.

overvaluation of exchange rates have generally disappeared. The Sachs and Warner findings appear to offer little guidance on how to conduct trade policy.

A skeptical reader might conclude that economists know little about the impact of trade and trade policy on economic growth and that it does not matter what strategy a nation pursues. This is the wrong conclusion to draw. Economists believe that increased trade confers benefits but that the steps necessary to stimulate economic growth and increased trade go beyond simply reducing tariffs and quotas and include strong macroeconomic management (such as a sensible exchange rate policy), steps to strengthen key economic and governance institutions, and policies that more broadly improve the environment for investment and productivity growth. The institutional innovations needed to spark both trade and growth may be different from those prescribed by a pure neoclassical model, and innovations that work in one country may not be easily replicable in others. Different paths to trade reform have been successful in different settings. One approach is not suited to all nations. But even those who are most skeptical about the relationship between trade and growth do not suggest that openness to trade is an ill-advised strategy or that broad trade barriers are conducive to long-run growth.

TRADE REFORMS AND POVERTY ALLEVIATION

Once again it will be useful to distinguish between trade volumes and trade policies and their respective impacts on the poor. We know from the previous section that increases in the share of exports (or of exports plus imports) out of GDP are well correlated with economic growth. In Chapter 6 we presented evidence that growth generally is good for the poor. If average incomes rise, as long as income inequality does not increase by too much, the incomes of the poor will also rise, lifting many above the poverty line. Taken together, this suggests that increasing trade is associated with poverty alleviation. The expansion of exports and increased foreign direct investment has brought a decline in poverty in many countries across all continents. This is most apparent in Asia's success stories of development. Over the past two decades, China, India, Indonesia, and Thailand have experienced rapid growth in exports and a decline in poverty. Simulations conducted in the early 2000s concluded that a global move toward freer trade could lift more than 300 million people out of poverty within 10–20 years through trade's impact on income growth.[22]

The mechanisms by which increased trade can reduce poverty are relatively straightforward. A more outward orientation reduces poverty by increasing the demand for labor. Trade in unskilled labor-intensive products, whether in agriculture or manufacturing, has the potential to create substantial employment opportunities for members of households living below or near the poverty line. Many of

---

[22]William Cline, *Trade Policy and Global Poverty* (Washington, DC: Center for Global Development, 2004); World Bank, "Market Access and the World's Poor," in *Global Economic Prospects and the Developing Countries 2002: Making Trade Work for the World's Poor* (Washington, DC: World Bank, 2002).

these workers tend to be young women in their late teens and 20s. This is what happened in many of the more outward-oriented economies in East Asia and elsewhere. New job opportunities increased the wage income of poor households and reduced the number of individuals living in poverty. Many of the poor also benefited as consumers. Trade reduces the price of imports, including that of necessities, and can increase the real incomes of poor households. Trade can also raise government revenues and improve social spending directed at the poor.

But trade has other impacts as well. In Chapter 18 we discussed how trade produces both winners and losers. Trade creates new employment opportunities in the expanding export sector but also eliminates jobs as some domestic firms find themselves unable to compete with cheaper imports. Trade can lower the prices of goods; this is beneficial to the consumer of the good but can harm the producer. After the NAFTA agreement between Canada, Mexico, and the United States, corn exports from the United States to Mexico increased, helping poor, often urban households who now faced lower food prices but hurting some small-scale Mexican corn producers who now received lower prices for their crops. Because of these varied effects, the impact of trade, especially of trade reforms, on the poor is varied and complex.

Recent case studies on a number of countries help identify the ways in which trade policy impacts poverty.[23] After Colombia joined the WTO in 1981, the nation's policy makers drastically lowered tariff and nontariff barriers in manufacturing. In 1984, the average tariff on Colombian manufactured good was 50 percent; by 1998 it had fallen to 13 percent. Workers in import-competing sectors, where tariffs tended to be the highest, suddenly faced significant price competition. These workers started to experience rising levels of unemployment and/or of informal employment, falling incomes and increasing poverty. But other Colombians had the opposite experience. Those working in the expanding export sector gained more formal sector jobs, increased incomes, and lowered rates of poverty. Something similar happened in India. After the trade reforms of the early 1990s, the rural poor gained less than the urban poor, and the more dependent a rural district was on trade the smaller the decline in poverty. What the results from Colombia and India demonstrate is that not all poor people are the same and that one set of policies may affect different groups of poor households differently, even within the same country.

The results also seem to contradict the basic theoretical arguments for why trade should help the poor in developing nations. Theories that identify factor endowments as the basis of comparative advantage, discussed in Chapter 18, predict that opening to trade favors a nation's abundant factor. If poor nations are abundant in unskilled labor, poor households should gain from trade as the economy moves to export more labor-intensive goods. This has happened throughout much of East

[23]Ann Harrison, ed., *Globalization and Poverty* (Cambridge: NBER, 2007). See in particular the chapters on Colombia by Pinelopi Goldberg and Nina Pavcnik, on India by Petia Topalova, and on Mexico by Gordon Hanson.

Asia. Why are the findings different in Colombia and India? One reason is that factor endowment models assume that labor is mobile between sectors. If workers can easily move out of the contracting import-competing sector and into the expanding export sector, they should experience the gains from trade. What the studies on Colombia and India reveal is that if workers cannot easily relocate, often because of labor regulations that constrain the expansion of new jobs, then the gains from trade may not be transmitted in the ways the factor endowment model predicts.[24] Whether this is a short-run outcome or a long-run one is something not yet understood. Parents may be unable to take advantage of new opportunities, but maybe when their children grow up they will be better able to respond to the new opportunities trade provides.

The studies on Colombia and India do not suggest that trade reform in these economies was a bad idea. What they do suggest is that trade reforms *alone* often cannot be relied on to reduce poverty. Complementary policies have to be pursued. In Colombia and India, policy reforms were needed to improve worker mobility across sectors and regions. In Zambia, trade reforms were not enough to help farmers exploit new export opportunities. They also needed help accessing credit and obtaining extension services to aid them in growing nontraditional crops. Also needed are social safety nets to catch those who are hurt by trade reforms because they are unable to adjust to new market opportunities. In rich and poor settings alike, increased integration with the global economy produces winners and losers. Most economists argue that the gains of globalization far outweigh the losses, but that does not mean everyone gains. Some will be worse off, sometimes requiring safety nets to help them as their nation transitions to a more integrated global economy.

KEY ISSUES ON THE GLOBAL TRADE AGENDA

INCREASED GLOBAL COMPETITION AND THE RISE OF CHINA (AND INDIA)

The benefits for an individual developing country from greater outward orientation may be smaller in the future than those achieved by the original Four East Asian Tigers. When Hong Kong, Korea, Singapore, and Taiwan began to compete on global markets, there was little competition from other developing countries, so their firms were able to expand and multiply quickly. Today, many more developing countries have adopted this strategy, including the population giants China and India, generating concerns

---

[24]Trade models that assume that factors are not perfectly mobile between sectors are referred to as *specific-factor models* and are an alternative to the Heckscher-Ohlin model discussed in the previous chapter.

about tougher competition and falling prices for export products. As new highly efficient producers enter a market, prices often fall in the short run, as new entrants create
overcapacity and drive out higher cost producers. Examples include semiconductors
when prices fell in the mid-1990s as world productive capacity grew rapidly and coffee
when prices dropped after Vietnam started producing, hurting some traditional coffee
exporters such as Ethiopia and Honduras. After the expiration of global agreements to
manage world trade in clothing, China's expansion into garment exports put pressure
on firms as far away as tiny Lesotho in southern Africa. There is no question that some
firms and some nations lose while others gain in a world of globalized trade.

The long-term evidence, however, suggests that world trade can expand very
quickly and accommodate many new firms. Since 1950, world exports grew much
more quickly than world output, and exports of manufactured products grew most
quickly of all. The United States was a huge force in world markets, accounting for
25 percent of world output after World War II, much larger than China today, and
there was concern that U.S. firms would dominate all trade. But while the reduction
of trade barriers by the United States and its European allies put pressure on some
firms as world prices dropped, the changes created many new opportunities for other
firms. Similarly, in today's world, as more countries trade and transport and telecommunication costs continue to drop, the opportunity for firms to specialize increases.
Global production networks allow firms from many different countries to contribute
to the production of one finished good, with each firm specializing in a particular
phase of the production process. Many exports from China are assembled and finished products built with components imported from other countries. A computer
from China might include a screen made in Malaysia, a circuit board from Singapore,
and a keyboard made in the Philippines.

As developing countries open to world markets, they also become consumers
for other country's exports, not just competitors. Trade is a two-way process. China
and India are rapidly increasing their imports as well as their exports and are becoming two of the largest markets in the world for other countries. China is now one of
Indonesia's top five export markets importing oil and gas, timber, fish, and even some
electronics products. China recently edged out the United States as Brazil's major
trading partner. China is also aggressively establishing trade with nations throughout
sub-Saharan Africa and today runs an overall trade deficit (imports exceed exports)
with the region.

Still many nations worry that with the expansion of China's trade, and to a lesser
extent India's, that there is little room for their exports of labor-intensive goods in the
global economy. Low-income economies believe they cannot match the combination of low wages and high productivity in China's factories. There is more than a little truth to such fears. The explosion of Chinese garment exports has driven firms in
many nations, previously operating behind the protection afforded by the 1995 global
Agreement on Textiles and Clothing, out of business. But this is also a static view of
trading opportunities. Wages in China are increasing as the average productivity of

Chinese workers rises. News stories increasingly report labor shortages, rising wages, and growing numbers of strikes by Chinese workers. These are all signs of a growing scarcity of labor, a result fully expected and hoped for as China develops. This also means that China's comparative advantage is changing, creating new opportunities for lower wage economies. Reebok, New Balance, and other manufacturers of running shoes, for example, are expanding in Indonesia in response to rising wages in China.

Some middle-income nations, like Mexico, face similar problems that may be more challenging. Relative to the United States, Mexico's factory endowment is unskilled labor. But Mexican wages are too high relative to those of China, and its relative productivity level not high enough, to compete with China in many goods destined for the U.S. market. Its comparative advantage, in part, lies with its locational advantage. Proximity to U.S. markets means goods from Mexico can get to the United States in a fraction of the three weeks typically needed to ship goods across the Pacific. This especially favors heavier products such as auto parts for which shipping costs are higher. Mexico's gains from trade certainly are limited by China's export drive but comparative advantage still works and the basic rationale for an outward-oriented strategy remains.

DOES OUTWARD ORIENTATION CREATE SWEATSHOPS?

Some critics argue that outward orientation leads to a global sweatshop economy, in which corporations pit workers around the world against each other in a race to the bottom to see who will accept the lowest wages, benefits, and environmental standards. It is understandable how someone looking at the factories that produce shoes and textiles in low-income countries could reach this conclusion. By rich world standards, the wages are very low, often only a few dollars a day or less. Workers labor for long hours in repetitive tasks, often with only limited breaks. In many cases, the conditions are deplorable. This is also true for firms producing for local markets, for agricultural workers, and others.

Low wages are a reflection of the extent of poverty in low-income countries. Wages are set not by what firms pay in other countries but by the productivity of local workers (which establishes the demand for labor) and the wages paid to workers' next-best opportunity (which determines the supply of labor). As we have seen, billions of the world's population live on less than $2 a day. Many toil in backbreaking work in agriculture to try to feed their families, and others work in market stalls, as servants, dock laborers, or in other difficult positions. Many have no job and little or no income at all. A 25-year-old woman machine operator in a textile firm in Nairobi earns about one 13th of what her counterpart earns in Amsterdam or Taipei.[25] This huge gap in pay is not because the Kenyan worker is exploited by her employer or because the Dutch or Taiwanese workers are 13 times more skilled. It is because pay differences across countries reflect differences in the average level of *economywide*

---

[25]Union Bank of Switzerland, *Prices and Earnings* (Zurich: UBS AG, 2009).

productivity. Workers in Kenya have less physical and human capital to work with and, on average, output per worker is low. Therefore, the market-determined wage is going to be substantially lower than in high-productivity Taiwan or the Netherlands.

For many people, the opportunity to work in a steady factory job for a few dollars a day is a big improvement over other options and can represent an important first step in rising above subsistence living and out of poverty. Without such options, poverty could be worse, rather than better. Efforts to substantially and immediately raise wages to industrialized-country standards could backfire. Firms forced to pay well above the marginal product of labor hire fewer workers, substitute machines for workers, or simply decide to relocate their operations, making workers even worse off. No one advocates that factory jobs with relatively low wages (by global standards) should be seen as the end goal. Rather, it should be seen as the first step on what ideally will be a dynamic path on which job skills, wages, and standards of living can grow steadily over time. The United States, Japan, and the nations in the European Union all went through a phase of very low wages and difficult working conditions during their transition from agrarian economies to industrialized nations. This is not meant to glorify this phase. It suggests only that there are no shortcuts to achieve economic development. Wages rise as the average productivity of the economy rises, the result of productive investments in both capital and people. Success stories in recent years are those nations that grew rapidly and were able to get through the very low wage and difficult working conditions phase quickly.

The image of a race to the bottom suggests that wages steadily *fall* in countries that compete to attract foreign firms that export to world markets. Sometimes wages fall at first for some workers, as uncompetitive protected firms close down and where wages effectively were subsidized by consumers who paid a higher price for protected products. But the typical pattern in countries that shift to outward orientation is not a steady fall in wages; instead, wages rise over time as workers gain new skills and factories become more productive. Evidence suggests that, in countries that attract foreign direct investment, multinational corporations tend to pay higher average wages and have better average working conditions than do domestic firms engaged in the same activities. Nike subcontractors in Indonesia paid nearly three times the average annual minimum wage, and workers in foreign-owned apparel and footwear factories in Vietnam rank in the top 20 percent of the population by household expenditure. In Mexico, export-oriented firms pay upward of 50 percent higher wages than similar nonexporting firms. Pay for workers in EPZs generally is higher than for similar activities outside of zones.[26]

The concern about the race to the bottom goes beyond wages and includes working conditions and labor standards. Advocates of stronger labor standards argue

[26]Drusilla Brown, Alan Deardorff, and Robert Stern, "The Effects of Multinational Production on Wages and Working Conditions in Developing Countries," Working Paper No. 9669, National Bureau of Economic Research, Cambridge, MA, April 2003; Theodore H. Moran, *Beyond Sweatshops: Foreign Direct Investment and Globalization in Developing Countries* (Washington, DC: Brookings Institution Press, 2002), p. 7; Edward Graham, *Fighting the Wrong Enemy: Antiglobal Activists and Multinational Enterprises* (Washington, DC: Institute for International Economics, 2000), chap. 4.

that they are necessary to guard against corporations imposing poor working conditions, such as excessively long hours, short breaks, gender discrimination, and poor ventilation and other health and safety hazards. Opponents argue that the imposition of stricter standards raises producer costs and discourages investment, thereby hurting workers by costing them their jobs. Despite the sometimes polemic debate, there is ample middle ground. Some standards are widely shared. The International Labour Organization (ILO) refers to these as **core standards**: abolishing forced labor; ending discrimination based on gender, race, ethnicity, and religion; eliminating child labor where it is harmful to the child; and permitting freedom of association of workers and the right to collective bargaining. For other improvements in conditions, which often are referred to as **cash standards**, the costs to producers are often small, including providing reasonable work breaks and improving safety conditions (such as unlocking doors, supplying fire extinguishers, and improving ventilation). In other words, some working conditions can be improved without adding significantly to costs and discouraging investment.

There is no question that working conditions are worse in low-income countries than in richer countries, and this is the case not just for firms engaged in trade but for those selling in protected domestic markets and for agriculture. The goal is to improve those conditions over time. Does outward orientation and greater trade make these conditions worse or better? The evidence is not complete, but overall it suggests that working conditions generally improve as economic growth proceeds in outward-oriented countries.[27] This outcome is not always the case. There are situations in which investors threaten to go elsewhere if workers are allowed to unionize or individual workers advocating for better conditions lose their jobs, as is the case with nonexporting firms. But in countries that expanded trade over a sustained period of time, such as Korea, Indonesia, Malaysia, and Mauritius, working conditions improved and are much better than they were in the late 1980s and early 1990s.[28] There is evidence that working conditions are improving across China as factories increasingly compete for workers.

In countries where there is little investment and growth, worker conditions tend to stagnate. Export-oriented firms tend to include a large share of foreign investors, and most studies show that worker conditions tend to be better in foreign-owned factories compared to similar domestically owned factories. This hardly suggests that advocacy efforts are misplaced. Better conditions in foreign-owned firms are partly in response to advocacy: Multinational firms respond to adverse publicity about poor worker conditions and attempt to bring about improvements (Box 19–4). But it is hard to find systematic evidence of a decline in worker standards and a race to the bottom as countries become more open and expand trade.

---

[27]Kimberley Ann Elliot and Richard B. Freeman, *Can Labor Standards Improve under Globalization?* (Washington, DC: Institute for International Economics, 2003); Brown et al., "The Effects of Multinational Production."

[28]The evolution of wages and working conditions in Korea is discussed in David L. Lindauer et al., *The Strains of Economic Growth: Labor Unrest and Social Dissatisfaction in Korea* (Cambridge, MA: Harvard Institute of International Development, 1997).

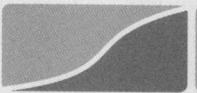

BOX 19-4 LABOR ACTIVISTS AND LABOR OUTCOMES IN INDONESIA

Anti-sweatshop campaigns and other forms of labor activism pressure firms in developing nations to improve working conditions, especially firms producing brand name goods for export. No company wants their subcontractors exposed as operating sweatshops because consumers in advanced economies may respond to such negative publicity by buying fewer products. Public relations campaigns targeting Nike, the Gap, and others have been effective in getting these corporations to impose codes of conduct on the factories that produce their footwear and apparel. But are the workers in these factories always helped by such actions? By raising labor costs are jobs lost? How often do firms close down in the face of labor activism? Are such firms foot-loose and able to relocate to countries where there is less activism and attention to labor standards?

Whether labor activists wind up helping or hurting the workers they intend to aid is an empirical question. Ann Harrison and Jason Scorse investigated this question using econometrics for Indonesia during the 1990s. They employ a "difference in difference" approach, which permits the researcher to separate out underlying trends from the behavior of a treatment versus a control group. Harrison and Scorse were interested in how wages and employment changed over time in districts where there was a concentration of firms exporting textiles, footwear, and apparel (TFA). They compare these changes with districts in which there was a concentration of firms producing for the domestic market or engaged in products other than TFA.

Indonesia provided an excellent opportunity to study the impact of labor activists because of Jeff Ballinger, a U.S. labor activist, who in the 1990s exposed the harsh working conditions and poor pay of workers in Indonesia's footwear industry. Ballinger targeted plants that produced running shoes for Nike, reasoning that by drawing attention to Nike, pressure could be brought to bear on other footwear and clothing producers. In a 1992 article in *Harper's* magazine, Ballinger published the pay stub of Sadisah, an Indonesian worker in a Nike subcontractor. In one week she worked 63 hours and earned 76,120 ruppiah ($37.46 at the market exchange rate.) Ballinger noted that it would take Sadisah 44,492 years to earn the $20 million Michael Jordan earned for his endorsement of Nike products. Ballinger's story and subsequent exposés were reported by many U.S. newspapers, magazines, and television networks.

Harrison and Scorse concluded that Ballinger's efforts were successful: "wages increased systematically more for exporting and foreign TFA plants in districts where activists concentrated their efforts." Equally important, they found no adverse total employment effects—that is, employment growth in targeted

TFA districts was not hurt relative to employment growth in non-TFA districts. This somewhat counterintuitive finding is explained, in part, by the very low share of Indonesian labor costs, around 5 percent, of the final retail sales price of a Nike shoe. It is also explained by the very low wages that TFA workers received at the start of the period. Mostly young women worked in these factories, and they received wages well below those of other manufacturing workers, making it easier for Nike and its contractors to absorb the increases in their pay. The evidence on labor activism in Indonesia appears to be win–win: Low-paid workers received higher wages and did not suffer any job loss. But the authors of the study are quick to point out that these results may be temporary, not permanent, because Nike shifted some of its outsourcing to other low-cost producers, including Cambodia and Vietnam. High-end running shoes are also a somewhat unique product and labor activism on goods with less brand name identity and smaller profit margins may not have the same effects.

Sources: Ann Harrison and Jason Scorse, "Improving the Conditions of Workers?: Minimum Wage Legislation and Anti-Sweatshop Activism," *California Management Review* 48, no. 2 (2006); Ann Harrison and Jason Scorse, "Multinationals and Anti-Sweatshop Activism," *American Economic Review* 100, no. 1 (March 2010); Kimberly Ann Elliott and Richard B. Freeman, "White Hats or Don Quixotes?: Human Rights Vigilantes in the Global Economy," in Richard Freeman, Joni Hersch and Lawrence Mishel, eds., *Emerging Labor Market Institutions for the Twenty-First Century* (Chicago: University of Chicago Press, 2004).

EXPANDING MARKET ACCESS

Implementing a more-open trade strategy is successful only if there are markets in which developing country exporters can sell their products, and the most important markets remain those in the European Union, Japan, and the United States. Generally speaking, these countries have low trade barriers, with relatively low average tariffs and quotas by world standards. But their largest trade barriers and greatest protection are precisely on the products in which low-income countries have a comparative advantage: textiles, apparel, and agriculture. Although the world's richest countries advocate for free markets and recommend that poor countries shift toward greater outward orientation, they also maintain trade barriers that impede that process. A key question is whether industrialized countries will react to their own macroeconomic problems and to the greater competition on world markets from China, India, and many other developing countries by maintaining protectionist measures or by imposing new ones. Or will the advanced economies allow even greater market access to goods produced in developing countries.

Limits on market access are reflected in tariff revenues. In most years, the United States collects more tariff revenue on exports from poor countries than rich countries. Consider U.S. imports from Bangladesh and France. In 2009, Bangladesh paid $563 million in tariffs to the United States, whereas France paid half as much, $285 million. This alone is regressive, with the poorer nation paying more than the richer one. But the implicit tax rate of these tariffs is even more striking. Bangladesh exported only $3.7 billion worth of goods to the United States, including underwear and towels; France exported nearly *10 times* as much, $34 billion, including wine and airplanes. The implied average tariff on French products is under 1 percent; on Bangladesh over 15 percent.[29]

Tariff peaks refer to relatively high tariffs amid generally low tariff levels. For industrialized countries, tariffs of 15 percent and above are generally recognized as tariff peaks and often are applied to imports from developing nations. The United States charges a 32 percent tariff on acrylic sweaters, a Bangladeshi export, but no tariff on artwork imported from France. **Tariff escalation** refers to having no or low import duties on raw materials and higher duties on the finished goods that use these raw materials. For example, the United States does not charge a tariff on cocoa beans, but charges more than 25 cents a pound on imports of certain kinds of chocolate. Tariff escalation makes it harder for firms in developing countries to compete in the markets for some finished goods. Such mercantilist practices were denounced by Adam Smith over 200 years ago but remain features of developed nation trade policies.

High-income nations have worked to reduce protection on most manufactured goods, including imports of textiles and apparel. For decades, textile and clothing imports were restricted via a complex system of quotas and tariffs under an agreement imposed by the industrialized countries called the Multi-Fiber Agreement (MFA), later amended as the Agreement on Textiles and Clothing (ATC). Under these arrangements, each industrialized country allowed only a certain amount of imports of textiles and clothing from each developing country. Some exporters, like China, Indonesia, and Thailand, easily filled their quota and were not allowed to export more. This helped other developing countries, as investors began to look at countries like Bangladesh, Lesotho, Mauritius, and Sri Lanka to locate production facilities and export to the industrialized countries.[30] But, because of the quotas, the rich countries imported far less overall than they would have with open markets, which drove up domestic prices, hurting domestic consumers while protecting domestic textile and apparel makers (and their workers) at the expense of firms and workers in developing countries. Most of these multilateral arrangements expired during the

---

[29]Edward Gresser, "U.S. Trade Preference Programs: Options for Reform," Senate Committee on Finance, March 9, 2010.

[30]Cambodia is another country that benefited from the quota system. But it adopted a unique position, in part, because of pressure from the U.S. government. Cambodian garment exporters agreed to follow strict guidelines on worker rights, hoping that the United States and other developed nation consumers would be willing to pay more for garments certified to have been produced in factories complying with a number of nonwage labor standards. With the end of the system of managed trade in garments, it remains uncertain whether consumers in industrialized countries will pay more for Cambodian products or simply shop for the lowest-priced goods available.

past decade but national tariff and nontariff barriers on textiles and apparel imports remain, leaving firms in developing countries at a significant disadvantage.

Agriculture is another heavily protected sector, in rich and poor nations alike, and one that probably raises more controversy than any other economic sector. Canada, the EU, Japan and the United States provide substantial protection to their agricultural producers through both tariff and nontariff barriers and direct subsidies to producers. As shown in Table 19–1, the estimated magnitude of protection is quite large, ranging from a tariff equivalent of about 20 percent in the United States to over 80 percent in Japan. According to this analysis, in Canada, the EU, and Japan high trade barriers on agriculture are much more significant than production subsidies; the opposite holds in the United States.

A wide range of products is protected, including cotton, dairy products, maize, peanuts, rice, soybeans, sugar, and wheat. Sugar is among the most distorted markets in the world, with the industrialized countries subsidizing domestic producers and imposing strict quotas to limit imports. In recent years, U.S. consumers have paid as much as three times the world price of sugar because of U.S. sugar quotas, subsequently affecting the price of everything from candy to processed foods to soft drinks produced in the United States. But it is not only U.S. consumers who are supporting domestic sugar producers, growers of sugar cane in the Caribbean, Central America, and elsewhere are deprived from earning more by the limits placed on exports to the United States and other developed nation markets.

Trade protection provides farmers in industrialized countries with a significant advantage over potential competitors, and weakens the incentives for increased production in developing countries. Production and export subsidies also encourage *increased production* in the industrialized countries, which adds to world supply putting downward pressure on world prices. One World Bank estimate suggests that the protection by the developed economies depresses world rice prices by 33 to 50 percent, and for sugar and dairy products, by 20 to 40 percent.[31] When farmers in developing countries receive lower prices, they produce less and earn less for the amount they produce, reducing their total income.

TABLE 19–1 **Overall Protection in Agriculture (percent tariff equivalent)**

TYPE OF PROTECTION	UNITED STATES	CANADA	EUROPEAN UNION	JAPAN
Tariffs	8.8	30.4	32.6	76.4
Subsidies	10.2	16.8	10.4	3.2
Total	19.9	52.3	46.4	82.1

Source: William Cline, *Trade Policy and Global Poverty* (Washington, DC: Center for Global Development, 2004).

[31]World Bank, *Global Economic Prospects and the Developing Countries 2002.*

Large agricultural interests in the industrialized countries lobby hard to maintain their protection. Rural states and provinces often have considerable political power, far greater than their share of total population might warrant. The outcome is continued protection of agriculture even though trade barriers and production subsidies are costly to consumers and taxpayers. In 2006, according to a study by the Organization for Economic Co-Operation and Development (OECD), government policies in rich countries that supported agriculture transferred close to $300 billion worth of income to farmers, amounting to almost one third of all farm earnings. In one often-cited calculation, the average Japanese cow gets $7.50 a day from various government subsidies and other forms of protection, whereas a cow in Europe receives $2.50 a day.[32] This is at a time when over 1 billion people in the developing world live on less than $1 a day.

The combined impact of industrial country tariffs, quotas, and subsidies is significant. The elimination of industrialized country barriers would likely add more to the GDP of poor countries than they receive in foreign aid. Two studies find that the elimination of these barriers would lift an additional 300 million or more people out of poverty.[33] It is unlikely that the industrialized countries will reduce these barriers on their own. The hope has long been that they would do so in the context of multilateral trade negotiations.

MULTILATERAL TRADE NEGOTIATIONS AND THE WTO

With the outbreak of World War I, a long epoch of globalization came to an end as the industrialized countries began to erect high trade barriers, a trend reinforced by the onset of the Great Depression. With the end of World War II, this pattern began to change. Industrialized country leaders began to reduce tariffs, and they looked for ways to accelerate and consolidate the process. The result was a shift toward **multilateral trade negotiations**, involving many nations simultaneously negotiating reductions in tariffs. The idea was that, with a large international effort in which participants would pledge to reduce their tariffs if other countries did the same, each individual country would be better able to overcome narrow interest groups at home that opposed trade liberalization. These discussions led to a proposal in 1948 to establish the International Trade Organization (ITO) as a sister organization to the International Monetary Fund (IMF) and World Bank. Although the ITO was never established, in large part because of the opposition of the U.S. Congress, multilateral trade negotiations expanded and flourished in the ensuing decades through a less-formal institution known as the **General Agreement on Tariffs and Trade (GATT)**. Between 1947 and 1994, eight rounds of multilateral trade negotiations took place

---

[32]Nicholas Stern, "Dynamic Development: Innovation and Inclusion," Munich Lectures in Economics, Center for Economic Studies, Ludwig Maximilian University, November 19, 2002.

[33]World Bank, *Global Economic Prospects and the Developing Countries 2002*; Cline, *Trade Policy and Global Poverty*.

through the GATT, covering mostly tariffs but later including nontariff barriers and other trade related issues.

The Uruguay Round of trade negotiations (so named because its initial meeting took place in Punta del Este, Uruguay, in September 1986) was completed in 1994. It was by far the largest trade negotiation ever held, with 123 countries taking part. Developing countries had high hopes at the outset of the Uruguay Round because it was the first in which a large number of them were allowed to participate and it was the first in which industrialized countries, with great reluctance, agreed to include agricultural subsides. Discussions led to what later was called the *grand bargain* between rich countries and low- and middle-income ones. This approach represented a significant shift from the traditional GATT approach on reciprocity. Instead of each country agreeing to open its markets on certain goods if the others did the same, the Uruguay Round featured an implicit deal in which the richer countries agreed to certain steps in some areas in return for the developing countries agreeing to steps in other areas, many of which went way beyond traditional border barriers.

The industrialized countries promised (1) significant reduction in tariffs on manufactured goods, (2) the end of the Multi-Fiber Agreement that had restricted trade in textiles and garments, and (3) reductions in agricultural protection with a commitment to even larger reductions in the next round. For their part, developing countries promised (1) reductions in their own tariffs; (2) agreement on new rules on investment, trade in services, and trade-related intellectual property rights (TRIPs; intended to prevent the use of patented material and the production of generic copy-cat products without permission); and (3) support of a new organization, the **World Trade Organization (WTO)**, to replace the GATT. The WTO, established on January 1, 1995, would serve as a central institution for global trade negotiations aimed at establishing a system of rules for fair, open, and undistorted competition and as a forum for settling disputes among members.

Despite increased access in some industrialized country markets, many developing countries eventually were deeply disappointed in the Uruguay Round. There were three broad concerns. First, the industrialized countries' pledge to reduce subsidies for agriculture generally did not materialize. Second, the new agreements on investment, services, and TRIPs were much more complicated than simply reducing tariffs or quotas, and as a result, the developing countries had to build domestic institutional and legal expertise, which required significant time and money. These changes were a large burden on many low-income countries that had a scarcity of highly skilled legal and administrative expertise. The industrialized countries promised to provide technical assistance to help with the transition but often did not fully follow through. Third, the TRIPs agreement resulted in developing countries paying higher prices for medicines and pharmaceutical products covered by patents. For many goods and services, protecting property rights and rewarding those that invest in research and development makes sense, but paying high market prices and preventing the sale of cheaper generic brands became a particularly contentious issue around medicines, particularly those used for treating HIV/AIDS. Only 10 years later was there the beginnings of serious discussion about how to make these drugs more affordable for low-income countries, as discussed in Chapter 9.

For many, the Uruguay Round came to be considered a bum deal rather than a grand bargain,[34] and the unhappiness contributed to the raucous demonstrations against the WTO in Seattle in 1999 and at other subsequent WTO meetings. A new round of trade negotiations under the WTO began in 2001. Called the Doha Round because the first meetings were held in Doha, Qatar, they also were referred to as "the development round" intended to serve the needs of the developing nations. Negotiations were difficult from the start and collapsed in 2008, although attempts to restart the talks continue.

The Doha Round began with an ambitious agenda, not uncommon in any round of trade negotiations. Agricultural trade protection and subsidies once again were on the table and remained one of the major reasons for the failure to reach an agreement. Under discussion was an opening up of international trade in services, everything from accounting to banking to shipping—activities that often are highly regulated and closed to foreign firms. Developed nations are particularly interested in liberalizing trade in these sectors where they often have comparative advantage. Nonagricultural market access (NAMA), covering manufactures and some primary goods, was intended to deal with problems of tariff peaks and escalation. Rich nations also wanted more discussion of trade facilitation, in essence, improved customs practices, which are an ongoing source of corruption and delay in many developing nations. More transparency in government procurement and new rules on competition policy, a form of global antitrust policy, were also part of the list of items to be discussed.

Many high-level meetings were held not only in Doha but in Cancun, Hong Kong, and often in Geneva, home to the WTO. The agenda progressively narrowed, and while progress was made, including on licenses for cheaper generic drugs, most meetings ended badly without agreement on major issues. The collapse in 2008 had much to do with where the trade round started: agricultural protection. There were divisions among the developing nations. Big agricultural exporters like Brazil had different interests than India, with its large and still relatively protected rural sector. But the real divide remained between rich nations and poor ones. The final straw was a dispute among the United States, China, and India. Developing nations rightly complain about the production and export subsidies farmers in rich nations receive, but developing nations, including China and India, also protect their farmers, relying mostly on trade barriers. WTO rules permit developing nations to impose tariffs, in this case on agricultural goods to protect their farmers, in the event of an import surge or sharp fall in crop prices. Disagreement over the use of this **special safeguard mechanism** could not be resolved. The United States wanted the trigger for when the

---

[34]Sylvia Ostry, "Why Has Globalization Become a Bad Word?," the Alcoa-Intalco Works Distinguished Lecture, Western Washington University, October 25, 2001.

safeguard kicked in to be set high; China and India wanted it to be set low. More fundamental, the Doha Round collapsed because many of the developing nations felt it was time for the rich nations to make large concessions, especially in agriculture, and for the poor nations to give little in return. To many economists this was a disappointing outcome because developing nations stood to gain a lot from dismantling their own trade barriers.

Earlier trade rounds collapsed only to start up again. This may happen with the Doha Round too. In the meantime, trade negotiations have not stood still. Nations have turned away from multilateral talks and entered into bilateral and regional agreements. In 2001, there were only 49 such agreements in place; by 2009 there were 167. The disadvantage of such agreements is that they do not permit the forces of *global* comparative advantage to work and can promote inefficient firms protected by a bilateral or regional agreement. Such agreements also create a confusing mix of rules and administrative requirements firms must comply with because nations sign different agreements with different trading partners. This diverts the attention of scarce managerial capacity and can impede productive investment. Bilateral and regional deals also take the pressure off of governments to compromise on multilateral agreements, like the Doha Round. To their credit, however, regional trade pacts may be better than no trade pact at all. Despite the failures to date in concluding the Doha Round, the world appears to be moving in the direction of greater market access and expanded trade, but there is no guarantee that this trend will continue.

TEMPORARY MIGRATION: ANOTHER DIMENSION OF INTERNATIONAL TRADE

The General Agreement on Trade in Services (GATS) establishes rules for WTO member nations on trade involving services such as banking, telecommunications, and tourism. Mode IV of the GATS refers to the temporary movement of people from one country to another to perform a service, which in principle could involve an actor, accountant, construction worker, or many others. The abiding principle is nondiscrimination: WTO member nations do not restrict trade, in this case of a service, based on country of origin. What is unique about Mode IV is that it involves not the movement of goods but of people, and controlling immigration is probably where nations are most protectionist. The freer movement of people across national borders is not on the agenda of most nations, especially the developed ones.

Agreements on Mode IV are highly limited but raise a critical issue: What role should increased immigration between rich and poor nations play in promoting economic development? The argument is a compelling one. There is no easier way of improving the lives of poor people than to permit them to migrate to a developed nation where wages are higher and employment opportunities better. It is far easier for a poor person to migrate to a rich nation than it is to bring economic development to where the poor person lives.

Harvard economist Lant Pritchett argues that there is no tool in the arsenal of economic development that has more potential to alleviate poverty than a significant increase in the amount of migration between developing and developed nations. The gains from further trade liberalization, or from increases in foreign aid, pale in comparison to those of even modest increases in the flow of labor between nations. One set of estimates suggests that complete trade liberalization would increase developing nation GDP by around $100 billion annually; an increase in temporary migration equal to 3 percent of the labor force of the OECD nations (about 18 million people) would raise the welfare of those moving by much more: $170 billion per year. Pritchett offers another compelling calculation, comparing the benefits of microfinance to temporary migration. The average annual microloan in Bangladesh is about $360 and the average lender receives his or her first loan at age 23. If one further assumes a generous 18 percent return to such loans, a lifetime of such borrowing yields about $700 in net present value.[35] If a low-skilled Bangladeshi man were permitted to work in the United States, he would earn this amount in only *four weeks*! Imagine the benefits if he were able to work one or more years. Think of the remittances thousands of such workers would send back home.

The benefits of migration should be obvious. The wage gap between workers in rich and poor nations is enormous. Pritchett provides a conservative estimate: Low-skilled workers across 42 low- and middle-income nations working in the United States would, on average, increase their annual earnings by $13,000 (purchasing power parity; PPP). They would be employed in activities in which many immigrants, both legal and illegal, already are employed, as laborers in construction and on farms, kitchen workers in restaurants, gardeners, providers of daycare or care for the elderly, and in other jobs that many natives often find too "dirty, dangerous, or difficult." A focus on increased global labor mobility among relatively unskilled workers also deflects concerns about brain drain and its potential impact on the migrant's country of origin.[36]

The benefits of permitting more temporary migration are clear but so is the opposition. Some of this opposition can be muted by calling for an increase in *temporary* not permanent migration. Temporary migrants would not be on a path to citizenship with all the implications that entails. They would be limited mostly to economic opportunities. Citizens of rich nations still worry that immigrants will lower native wages and take away native jobs; engage in criminal activity; and be a

---

[35]The calculation is from Lant Pritchett, "The Cliff at the Border," in R. Kanbur and M. Spence, eds., *Equity and Growth in a Globalizing World* (Washington, DC: World Bank, 2010). Pritchett fully develops the economic and moral argument for greater global labor mobility in *Let Their People Come: Breaking the Deadlock in International Labor Mobility* (Washington, DC: Center for Global Development, 2006). Estimates of the potential benefits of temporary migration are presented in World Bank, "Labor Mobility and the WTO: Liberalizing Temporary Movement," in *Global Economic Prospects 2004: Realizing the Development Promise of the Doha Agenda* (Washington, DC: World Bank, 2004).

[36]Brain drain itself is a controversial idea. The problem of brain drain is disputed in a case study of health workers from West Africa in Michael Clemens, "Do Visas Kill?: Health Effects of African Health Professional Emigration," Center for Global Development Working Paper 114, Washington, DC, 2007.

burden to taxpayers, contributing little in taxes while using public services such as schools, hospital emergency rooms, and state-provided welfare payments. There is an element of truth in each of these concerns but careful analysis tends to show that these costs, if they exist at all, tend to be small, especially relative to the huge gain in the well-being of the immigrant himself or herself. Unskilled immigrants tend to depress the wages of unskilled natives by only a few percentage points and do not increase the unemployment of natives with similar skills. Immigrants are less likely to commit crimes because the costs are greater; they face not only jail sentences but also deportation. Immigrants pay taxes and tend not to be a net fiscal drain in aggregate terms although they can be on local communities. Much of the opposition to increased immigration is based on misperceptions of its costs to natives and on matters of culture. Throughout the world, in rich and poor nations alike, people often have a visceral and negative response to those who are foreign. Overcoming this response, even in the name of reducing global poverty, is a formidable challenge.

SUMMARY

- There exists a continuum of approaches toward international trade that nations can adopt. At one end is autarky or economic isolation; at the other is free trade. In practice, most nations fall somewhere along this continuum, exercising some degree of inward-looking versus outward-oriented policies.
- Almost all countries have used import substitution at various times. Implementing this approach often meant using trade barriers, including tariffs and quotas, and overvalued currencies. Such interventions can prove costly to an economy. In theory, IS can allow domestic firms to learn production techniques, improve efficiency, and eventually compete on world markets. However, despite some exceptions, this strategy often leads to weak technology, low efficiency, and slower growth.
- Many developing countries began to shift to more outward-oriented trade strategies in the 1980s. Outward orientation allows firms to become more specialized, sell to larger global markets, and import leading technologies. Most countries that follow this strategy begin with labor-intensive manufacturing and agriculture, with the goal of moving to more-sophisticated products over time. Concerns that this strategy leads to a race to the bottom in wages and labor standards are generally not supported by the evidence.
- Outward orientation often is associated with policies that favor exports. This might include production subsidies such as access to cheap credit for exporters, undervalued exchange rates, or EPZs. Nations like China and Korea

that have pursued outward-looking strategies have also protected domestic firms from import competition, often conditional on export success.

- A lively debate remains over the use of both trade and industrial policy to foster rapid economic growth. Full liberalization of markets does not characterize the experience of some of the world's most successful economies, whereas many attempts at trade liberalization have delivered less than expected. At the same time, it is easy to point to both successes and failures when governments intervene to pick firms or sectors to support. Some partnership between the public and private sector is probably needed to alleviate the binding constraints on economic growth.

- Evidence suggests a strong positive relationship between trade and growth. Countries with larger amounts of trade tend to record faster growth. But the direction of causality is not certain. The evidence is even less clear relating trade policies and growth. This, in part, is due to difficulty in measuring trade policy. Some critics suggest that trade may be less important than other factors, such as strong institutions and an overall climate that supports investments, in explaining rapid growth. But few suggest that a lack of openness is conducive to growth.

- Economies that have experienced rapid growth in exports, especially of labor-intensive products, have witnessed decreases in poverty. But trade liberalization alone may have a differential impact on the poor. As import prices fall and export prices rise, some of the poor may be hurt by a more open economy, often because their mobility from contracting to expanding sectors of the economy is impeded.

- Many issues remain on the global trade agenda. Some worry about the impact of China and India, the two most populous nations in the world, on the opportunities for other economies. Most evidence suggests that there is room in the global economy for all nations.

- Protectionist policies in the industrialized countries continue to impede exports from developing countries, especially in textiles, apparel, and agriculture. It remains to be seen whether the industrialized countries will maintain these barriers or even erect new ones as competition from developing countries increases or whether multilateral negotiations will lead to reductions in these barriers and increased opportunities for developing countries.

- While multilateral negotiations surrounding trade issues continue, including the ill-fated Doha Round, nations are seeking bilateral and regional agreements to increase their access to markets. One dimension of trade negotiations that has received relatively little attention is to increase the movement of people across borders. Some economists believe that an increase in temporary migration between rich and poor nations could be one of the most effective instruments available for addressing global poverty.

20

Sustainable Development

The path to development followed by today's advanced economies was fueled by technologies intensive in their use of energy and natural resources and prodigious in their production of environmental pollutants. Is this the same path today's poor countries must follow? What are the potential conflicts between development and the environment? According to scientist Jared Diamond, the potential consequences of such a conflict include nothing short of societal collapse.[1] Citing both ancient and recent examples, Diamond argues that unintended ecological suicide ("*ecocide*") was a primary cause of the demise of major civilizations throughout history, ranging from the Maya to the Vikings to modern-day states like Somalia and Rwanda. Diamond elaborates,

> The processes through which past societies have undermined themselves by damaging their environments fall into eight categories, whose relative importance differs from case to case: deforestation and habitat destruction, soil problems (erosion, salinization, and soil fertility losses), water management problems, overhunting, overfishing, effects of introduced species on native species, human population growth, and increased per capita impact of people. . . . The environmental problems facing us today include the same eight that undermined past societies, plus four new ones: human-caused climate change, build up of

---

[1] Jared Diamond, *Collapse: How Societies Choose to Fail or Survive* (London: Penguin Books, 2005). Diamond defines *collapse* as "a drastic decrease in human population size and/or political/economic/social complexity, over a considerable area, for an extended time" (p. 3).

toxic chemicals in the environment, energy shortages, and full human utilization of the Earth's photosynthetic capacity.[2]

Concerns about the Earth's ability to support continued human development date back at least to the eighteenth century. In 1798, British economist and demographer Thomas Malthus, in his famous *Essay on the Principle of Population*, predicted that continued population growth would bring the world to disaster. Malthus based his analysis on two premises: "That food is necessary to the existence of man," to which Malthus applied the assumption that the production of food would grow arithmetically, and "That the passion between the sexes is necessary and will likely remain nearly in its present state," from which Malthus extrapolated that population would grow geometrically.[3] He concluded "The power of population is so superior to the power of the Earth to produce subsistence for man, that premature death must in some shape or other visit the human race."

Some recent thinking has echoed Malthus. In 1972, the Club of Rome published *The Limits to Growth*, a report by a team of analysts based at the Massachusetts Institute of Technology. This study predicts that "If the present growth trends in world population, industrialization, pollution, food production, and resource depletion continue unchanged, the limits to growth on this planet will be reached sometime within the next 100 years." Among other projections, the report suggests that, based on then-current reserves, the world would exhaust its supply of oil by 1992.

While these and other dire predictions have so far proved false, the question of whether today's developing countries can (or should) follow a historical development path similar to that followed by today's advanced countries, with potentially serious environmental impacts, remains valid. The depletion of both renewable and nonrenewable resources, especially fossil fuels, and the threat of environmental damage pose challenges on a scale unimaginable in the time of Malthus. Concern over the sustainability of economic development and growth has expanded to emphasize global climate change. Scientists point to increasing atmospheric concentrations of **greenhouse gases** such as carbon dioxide (CO_2), which may dangerously raise global surface temperatures by trapping solar radiation in the earth's atmosphere. As we discuss in the final section of this chapter, the potential negative consequences of global warming for development are immense. Various forecasts indicate potential reductions of grain yields of up to 50 percent in Africa, extinction of valuable plant and animal species, increased disease and water stress, and the displacement of millions of poor residents of low-lying coastal zones as the melting polar ice caps cause sea levels to rise. There are even widely expressed fears that the entire nation of the Maldives, a

---

[2]Diamond, *Collapse: How Societies Choose to Fail or Survive*, pp. 6–7. By "photosynthetic capacity," Diamond is referring to the limited capacity of Earth to support crop growth. He cites calculations that by the late 1980s, humankind had either used, wasted, or diverted about half of the Earth's capacity to produce crops.

[3]An arithmetic progression is 1, 2, 3, 4, 5, 6; a geometric progression is 1, 2, 4, 8, 16, 32.

collection of 1,200 coral islands in the Indian Ocean, 80 percent of which rise no more than one meter above sea level, could simply disappear by the year 2100.

WILL ECONOMIC GROWTH SAVE OR DESTROY THE ENVIRONMENT?

The relationship between economic growth and the environment is complex and dynamic. One important mediating variable is technology. When Malthus foretold of "premature death" for the human race, he excluded the possibility that technical change in agriculture would boost productivity, permitting food supplies to outpace population growth.[4] Technical change also affects the efficiency with which we use renewable and nonrenewable resources as well as the level of environmental damage caused. Increased automobile fuel efficiency and the more recent development of electric cars are only two among many examples of how technical change can help reduce environmental impacts. Our assumptions about the role and pace of technical change are critical in shaping our conclusions about whether economic growth is good or bad for the environment.

The relationship between levels of pollution and levels of income is generally thought to follow an inverted-U shape, with pollution rising as income increases from low levels but falling once income passes some intermediate level. Because this inverted-U pattern is similar to the relationship between inequality and national income famously posited by economist Simon Kuznets (introduced in Chapter 6), this empirical relationship between pollution and national income is called the **environmental Kuznets curve**. This relationship is depicted in Figure 20–1 as the "conventional EKC." Economist Susmita Dasgupta and colleagues describe the basic intuition underlying this relationship,

> In the first stage of industrialization, pollution in the . . . world grows rapidly because people are more interested in jobs and income than clean air and water, communities are too poor to pay for abatement, and environmental regulation is correspondingly weak. The balance shifts as income rises. Leading industrial sectors become cleaner, people value the environment more highly, and regulatory institutions become more effective.[5]

Statistical estimations of this relationship have suggested that pollution peaks at levels of income per capita between $5,000 and $8,000, and declines as income grows above that range.

[4]The Club of Rome's *Limits to Growth* (New York: Universe Books, 1972) study recognized the potential impact of technical change but assumed that its pace would be insufficient to overcome ensuing environmental constraints.

[5]Susmita Dasgupta, Benoit Laplante, Hua Wang, and David Wheeler, "Confronting the Environmental Kuznets Curve," *Journal of Economic Perspectives* 16, no. 1 (winter 2002), 147.

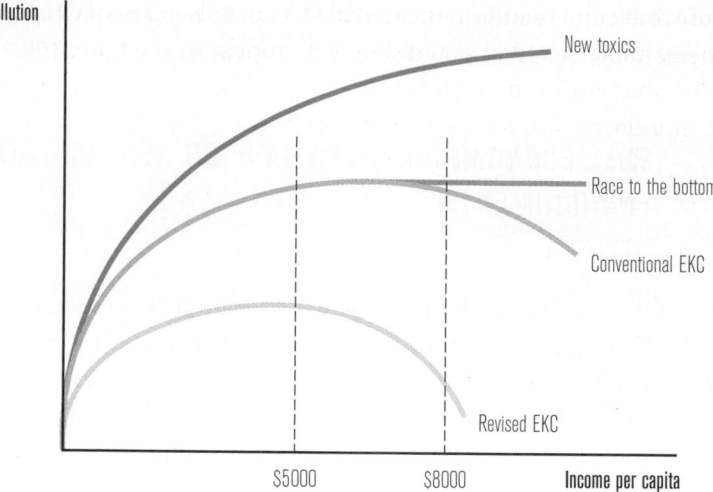

FIGURE 20-1 **Potential Paths for the Environmental Kuznets Curve (EKC)**

Source: "Confronting the Environmental Kuznets Curve," by Smita Dasgupta, Benoit Laplante, Hua Wang, and David Wheeler. *Journal of Economic Perspectives*, Vol. 16, No. 1, Winter 2002: 147–168, p. 148. Reprinted by permission of the American Economic Association.

Dasgupta notes, however, that estimates of the conventional environmental Kuznets curve have been criticized as misleading snapshots of a dynamic process. If, for example, free trade and globalization create a "race to the bottom", as countries compete by lowering their environmental standards, then the curve may simply flatten out (as depicted in Figure 20–1). Or if income growth and industrialization merely create new environmental hazards, it's possible that the environmental Kuznets curve could rise over time (the "new toxics" path). Conversely, Dasgupta and colleagues cite recent and more optimistic evidence that the environmental Kuznets curve has been shifting downward as growth becomes less polluting and the turning point occurs at increasingly lower levels of income (the "revised EKC"). Thus the relationship between pollution and economic growth remains a subject of debate, one with high stakes, given that current income levels in most of the developing world remain far below the turning point of even the "revised" EKC.

Moreover, we cannot simply infer that increasing levels of income *cause* pollution to first rise and then fall. Alternative explanations for the inverted-U pattern include the natural progression from clean agrarian to polluting industrial to clean service sector domination of the economy, the beneficial effects of greater institutional development and better public policies in advanced economies, and advances due to technical change. It has also been suggested that wealthier countries have reduced their pollution levels by exporting their pollution-intensive production activities to developing countries. If true, this would call into question the ability of today's poor countries to follow the inverted-U pattern, suggesting a path similar to the "race to the bottom" or even the "new toxics." If it were simply the case that economic growth automatically reduced pollution, we would have little else to worry about in the long run, and policy makers could focus exclusively on promoting growth. This is not the case. The fact that earlier predictions of environmental catastrophe proved overly dire is no guarantee against future environmental catastrophes.

Diamond (along with many economists), skeptical about the environmental Kuznets curve, poses this choice more starkly, asserting,

> because we are rapidly advancing along this non-sustainable course, the world's environmental problems *will* get resolved, in one way or another, within the lifetimes of the children and young adults alive today. The only question is whether they will become resolved in pleasant ways of our own choice, or in unpleasant ways not of our choice, such as warfare, genocide, starvation, disease epidemics, and collapse of societies.[6]

The first step in assessing the sustainability of development lies in defining what we mean by *sustainability* and thinking about how to measure it. How will we recognize sustainable development when we see it? What is it in particular that is to be sustained?

CONCEPT AND MEASUREMENT OF SUSTAINABLE DEVELOPMENT

Among the myriad academic and popular definitions of sustainable development, the most widely cited is that of the World Commission on Environment and Development (commonly known as the Brundtland Commission, 1987), which defined it as "development that meets the needs of the present without compromising the ability of future generations to meet their own needs."[7] While highlighting the notion of intergenerational equity, the Brundtland Commission's concept of sustainable development remains vague, and in particular fails to define "needs." For instance, "needs" might be interpreted to require the maintenance of only a bare minimum standard of living, though most of us might hope for more than such a low standard for our children. The Brundtland Commission's definition is also vague with respect to the question of what it means for future generations to meet their needs. This concept could imply that the well-being of future generations remains above some (undefined) minimum standard, that future well-being be equal to present well-being, or that each generation's well-being be equal to or greater than the well-being of the previous generation. Recent discussions of sustainable development by economists

---

[6]Diamond, *Collapse: How Societies Choose to Fail or Survive,* 498.

[7]World Commission on Environment and Development. *Our Common Future* (Oxford: Oxford University Press, 1987), p. 43 (also known as the Brundtland report).

have tended to define a sustainable path as one along which intergenerational well-being does not decline.

Operationalizing the standard that the well-being of future generations not decline requires a clear definition of well-being and some means of measuring it. For instance, in Chapter 2 we addressed the question of happiness as a measure of well-being, with the paradoxical finding that happiness is not monotonically tied to income. In practice, economists often use income as a proxy for the level of development. For the purpose of measuring the potential well-being of future generations, however, we need to expand that concept to equate well-being with the economy's **wealth**. Economists have shown that the only way for intergenerational well-being not to decline is for per capita wealth not to decline. Non-declining wealth *per capita* requires that the growth rate of wealth be greater than or equal to the growth rate of population.[8] But what do we mean by *wealth*?

This concept of sustainable development requires a broad concept of wealth. Economics Nobel Laureate Kenneth Arrow and colleagues define wealth as "the social worth of an economy's entire productive base. Because the productive base consists of the entire range of factors that determine intergenerational well-being, we . . . refer to wealth as *comprehensive wealth*."[9] **Comprehensive wealth** (also referred to as **total wealth**) is made up of **produced capital** (buildings, roads, machinery and equipment), **natural capital** (minerals and fossil fuels, forests, agricultural land, and protected areas), and **intangible capital** (a broad category that includes human, social, and institutional capital).[10] Comprehensive wealth differs from the more familiar concept of gross domestic product (GDP) in a critical way that highlights the concept of sustainability: GDP includes, besides the production of goods and services, the value of asset liquidation as part of national output. When Chile or Zambia mine and export copper, the depletion of this natural resource counts toward each nation's GDP, but growth based on the depletion of natural resources may not be sustainable. This type of resource use diminishes comprehensive wealth.

Measuring the different categories of capital is a challenge. The value of each type of capital is a function of its price, yet we observe prices only for goods and services that are traded in markets. This is a special problem in the case of natural capital for which markets are often missing. Water is an example of a vital and limited natural resource, the majority of which is used as an input for agriculture. Often there

---

[8]The growth rate of any ratio is the growth rate of the numerator minus the growth rate of the denominator. Wealth per capita is the ratio (wealth to population). Thus the growth rate of wealth per capita is the growth rate of wealth minus the growth rate of population. If the population growth rate exceeds the growth rate of wealth, then wealth per capita declines.

[9]Kenneth J. Arrow, Partha Dasgupta, Lawrence H. Goulder, Kevin J. Mumford, and Kirsten Oleson, "Sustainability and the Measurement of Wealth," National Bureau of Economic Research Working Paper 16599, Cambridge, MA: NBER, December 2010, p. 2.

[10]This discussion draws on World Bank, *The Changing Wealth of Nations, Measuring Sustainable Development in the New Millennium* (Washington, DC: World Bank, 2011).

is no well-defined market for water use. Yet, depletion of water resources is a major concern, and the failure to price water to reflect its opportunity cost may exacerbate this depletion. The damage caused by air and water pollution, including the damage to human health, is also difficult to value precisely. Various ecosystem services (such as the supply of wild foods, cultural and recreational uses, and the aesthetic value of natural landscapes) also often lack market prices and are difficult to incorporate explicitly in wealth accounting. The same is true for such public goods as biodiversity and carbon storage. In part because of even more severe challenges to measurement, intangible capital is typically measured as a residual, the difference between total wealth and the sum of produced and natural capital. Total wealth is calculated as the present value of future consumption that is sustainable. In making these estimates, the World Bank applies a discount rate of 1.5 percent over a period of 25 years. This calculation of total wealth is thus independent of the value of the three forms of capital, allowing intangible capital to be calculated as the residual.

Table 20–1 provides wealth and per capita wealth data for different country groups in 1995 and 2005. Global wealth between these years increased by 34 percent. Over that same period, global population increased by 17 percent, resulting in a 17 percent increase in global wealth per capita. The largest absolute increases in per capita wealth were in the high-income nations, but every income group experienced gains. Table 20–1 also provides insights into both the composition of total wealth and changes in that composition as a function of income level. Intangible capital makes up the largest category of wealth at all levels of income and in both years. Yet there is a clear pattern of change in the composition of total wealth: low-income countries rely substantially on natural capital compared with high-income countries, with most of the difference lying in the relative proportions of intangible capital. This cross-sectional pattern is also apparent over time, as increased wealth in the low-income countries is associated with a shift in the composition of total wealth from natural capital to intangible capital. This decreasing reliance on natural capital as a component of total wealth is consistent with the structural transformation introduced in Chapter 16. Thus, notes a World Bank study, "For countries dependent on nonrenewable natural capital, transforming natural capital to other forms of wealth is the path to sustainable development."[11]

For many developing countries fortunate enough to have large endowments of natural resources, it is precisely the failure to make this transformation that threatens the sustainability of their development paths. Nigeria provides a prime example of this problem. Oil has dominated Nigeria's economy since the discovery in the late 1950s of the country's enormous reserves, accounting for nearly all of its export revenue and over one third of GDP. The government of Nigeria has financed much of its operations with oil revenue, continually drawing down this nonrenewable resource. Yet, Nigeria remains poor and underdeveloped relative to its potential because it has

---

[11]The World Bank, *The Changing Wealth of Nations,* p. 6.

TABLE 20-1 Wealth and Per Capita Wealth by Type of Capital and Income Group, 1995 and 2005 (constant 2005 US$)

INCOME GROUP	1995						2005					
	TOTAL WEALTH (US$ BILLIONS)	PER CAPITA WEALTH (US$)	INTANGIBLE CAPITAL (%)	PRODUCED CAPITAL (%)	NATURAL CAPITAL (%)	TOTAL WEALTH (US$ BILLIONS)	PER CAPITA WEALTH (US$)	INTANGIBLE CAPITAL (%)	PRODUCED CAPITAL (%)	NATURAL CAPITAL (%)
Low income	2,447	5,290	48	12	41	3,597	6,138	57	13	30
Lower middle income	33,950	11,330	45	21	34	58,023	16,903	51	24	25
Upper middle income	36,794	73,540	68	17	15	47,183	81,354	69	16	15
High income OECD	421,641	478,445	80	18	2	551,964	588,315	81	17	2
World	504,548	103,311	76	18	6	673,593	120,475	77	18	5

OECD, Organization for Economic Co-Operation and Development.

Source: Table 1.1 from The International Bank for Reconstruction and Development. The World Bank: *The Changing Wealth of Nations: Measuring Sustainable Development in the New Millennium*, 2011. Reprinted with permission.

failed to transform Its natural capital into either manufactured or intangible capital (such as a more highly educated labor force). Indeed, there is a simple rule of thumb (known as the **Hartwick rule**) that suggests that a sustainable development path for countries that depend on nonrenewable resources requires the rents from those resources to be continually invested rather than consumed.[12] Nigeria is hardly alone among developing countries in having depleted its endowment of natural resource abundance while failing to develop accordingly. In addition to other oil exporters, such countries as the Democratic Republic of the Congo, Zambia, and Zimbabwe have all failed to develop to the potential available through their natural resource endowments.[13] In contrast, diamond-rich Botswana has been among the world's fastest-growing economies. Mexico and Peru have also succeeded in transforming natural capital into manufactured capital.

The tradeoffs are somewhat more complicated for countries in which the natural capital endowment is based on renewable resources, such as forest land. In these cases, property rights and other supporting institutions can play important roles in limiting harvests to sustainable levels. Deforestation in the Amazon exemplifies the overexploitation of a renewable natural resource. In this, and many other cases, the overutilization of renewable resources happens because the lack of market prices for such resources often leads them to be undervalued and threatened. The reliance of low-income countries on natural capital comes with the risk that the depletion of natural capital may cause permanent losses of biodiversity and other ecosystem services.

SAVING FOR A SUSTAINABLE FUTURE

Comprehensive wealth defines the current generation's well-being and constrains the well-being of future generations. A sustainable path of development (a path along which the well-being of each generation is at least equal to that of the previous generation) requires the creation of wealth at a rate at least equal to the rate of population growth. Wealth creation results from savings and investment over time. From one period to the next, the increase in comprehensive wealth equals **adjusted net saving (ANS)**, sometimes called **genuine saving**, defined as "gross national savings adjusted for the annual changes in the volume of all forms of capital."[14] We can measure countries' ANS by starting with the familiar concept of gross saving (S), which is simply total income minus total consumption. Maintaining wealth requires saving

---

[12]Specifically, the portion of the rents that should be invested under the Hartwick rule is equivalent to the depreciation of the capital stock, a proportion that approaches the full rent as the resource becomes progressively depleted.

[13]Chapter 18 discusses the pitfalls associated with countries' reliance on natural resource exports for their trade strategy.

[14]The World Bank, *The Changing Wealth of Nations*, p. 37. The only theoretical difference between the increase in comprehensive wealth and adjusted net savings is that the former includes capital gains (which arise from changes in the real price of assets).

sufficiently to offset depreciation of existing assets. In standard national accounting, this idea is captured by measuring **net saving (NS)**, defined as gross saving minus the depreciation of made capital (D_m):

$$NS = S - D_m \qquad\qquad [20-1]$$

But focusing on depreciation of only made capital is too limited, and in principle the concept should be expanded to include depreciation of natural capital (D_n), including the depletion of energy stocks, dwindling mineral assets, and damage from air pollution. This gives rise to the measurement of ANS:

$$ANS = S - D_m - D_n \qquad\qquad [20-2]$$

This corrected definition of net saving suggests that, if enough is saved each year to cover the depreciation of both made and natural capital, the economy can sustain its wealth and its level of consumption. In principle, this idea could be extended to include other assets as well, including human capital, knowledge, and social assets. However, measurement difficulties and lack of data make this extension difficult in practice, so we restrict our discussion here to made and natural capital. We can interpret ANS as an indicator of sustainability of an economy's development path. If ANS is declining (particularly if it is declining over consecutive years), this indicates that the economy's path is unsustainable, that it's depleting the productive base on which the welfare of future generations depends. Because some forms of capital are inevitably excluded from the calculation of ANS, its interpretation in practice requires caution and judgment. Research by economists Susana Ferreira, Kirk Hamilton, and Jeffrey Vincent has shown that ANS does predict future economic performance in a cross section of countries, but only if ANS is adjusted to account for the depletion of natural resources.[15]

Figure 20–2 illustrates ANS trends by developing region since 1970. While the data indicate substantial variability, several broad observations stand out. Both East Asia and South Asia have high and increasing rates of ANS compared with Latin America (for which the rate of ANS has been relatively low but positive over time) and sub-Saharan Africa (for which the rate of ANS has been low, trending downward, and negative after 2005). The unsustainable path reflected for sub-Saharan Africa is dominated by large oil-exporting countries, such as Nigeria, which (as noted above) fuels its economy through the gradual depletion of its oil reserves without converting that natural capital into other forms of capital. The positive trends in East and South Asia are dominated by the large and rapidly growing economies of China and India, which by comparison have relied less on the depletion of natural resources and more on the expansion of their stocks of physical and human capital. Box 20–1 extends the

---

[15]Susana Ferreira, Kirk Hamilton, and Jeffrey Vincent, "Comprehensive Wealth and Future Consumption: Accounting for Population Growth," *World Bank Economic Review* 22, no. 2 (2008), 233–48.

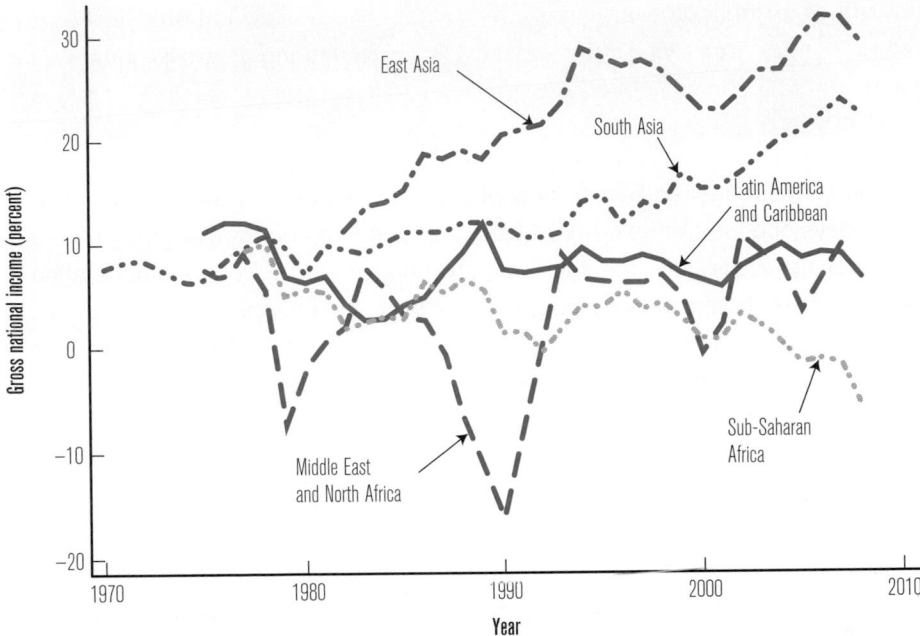

FIGURE 20-2 **Adjusted Net Saving for Developing Regions, 1970–2008**

Data exclude particulate emission damage.

Source: World Bank, "World Development Indicators," http://databank.worldbank.org.

analysis of ANS as an indicator of sustainability to incorporate the effects of population growth, illustrating these concepts with the case of Ghana, where ANS was positive while ANS per capita was negative.

To summarize, the concept of sustainable development has been defined in numerous ways; yet the most popular definition, that of the Brundtland Commission, highlights the requirement that consumption by today's generation must be accompanied by sufficient conservation of resources so as not to reduce the consumption potential of future generations. Knowing whether we are meeting this standard requires clear definitions and specific metrics. Economists' efforts to measure the sustainability of development have focused on net saving as an indicator of whether resource use by the current generation is expanding or contracting the potential creation of wealth by future generations. Experience to date is mixed. While some countries and regions have succeeded in rapidly expanding the potential wealth of future generations, others have been consuming rather than investing their resource base. These latter regions thus appear to be following unsustainable development trajectories. In many cases, the unsustainable depletion of natural resources and environmental damage through pollution are a result of market failure. The following section defines and illustrates this concept.

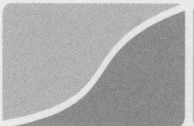

BOX 20-1 THE MALTHUSIAN EFFECT OF POPULATION GROWTH ON ADJUSTED NET SAVINGS IN GHANA

Adjusted net savings (ANS) is a concept that we can use to measure sustainability. As developed in the text, ANS tracks changes in a country's comprehensive wealth. Sustainability requires that wealth be nondecreasing from one generation to the next; yet from a welfare perspective, wealth must be measured per capita. If the population is growing, then maintaining per capita wealth at a constant level requires that comprehensive wealth grows at the same rate as population. From this perspective, it is entirely possible that development would not be sustainable in the per capita sense, even if comprehensive wealth is increasing. In other words, a negative rate of ANS reduces both total and per capita wealth; yet the converse is not necessarily true—a positive rate of ANS need not imply increases in wealth per capita. Some countries may add to their total wealth but not enough to compensate for population growth. To determine whether the rate of ANS is sufficient to increase wealth per capita, we must adjust that rate to take account of population growth. This requires subtracting from ANS the amount by which ANS must increase each year simply to keep up with population growth—the so-called **Malthusian term**. If the remaining difference is positive, then wealth per capita increases. If the remaining difference between actual ANS and the amount of ANS needed to maintain per capita wealth is negative, then wealth per capita decreases. This difference is the **adjusted net saving gap**. As a percent of gross national income, this saving gap tells us how much the rate of ANS would need to increase to keep wealth per capita constant over time.

Ghana provides an example of a country in which comprehensive wealth grew absolutely but fell per capita. Measuring saving and wealth in per capita terms requires a small modification to the accounting framework developed in the chapter. Because most of what we termed intangible capital consists of human capital (and is thus reflected in the population itself), we must exclude intangible capital from our calculation of comprehensive wealth per capita to avoid double counting (now that population enters the formula directly). For lack of data, we also exclude the value of carbon emissions per capita from our calculation of ΔANS.

The table on the following page details the calculation of changes in wealth per capita in Ghana for the year 2000, when Ghana's population grew by 1.7 percent. The left-hand column of the table decomposes tangible wealth per capita into its subcategories. The right-hand column shows the composition of adjusted net savings, subtracting the consumption of fixed capital and resource depletion from the sum of gross national saving and educational expenditures. Ghana's ANS per capita was $16. The Malthusian term equals the population growth rate times comprehensive wealth per capita, or $0.017 \times \$2022 \approx \$34$. Even though Ghana's ANS per capita was positive, the country's per capita wealth fell by $16 − $34 = −$18. Stated differently, the growth rate of Ghana's total wealth was $16/$2022 = 0.8 percent which was less than the 1.7 percent rate of population growth. This suggests an unsustainable long-run trajectory for Ghana.

Tangible wealth ($ per capita)		Adjusted net saving	
Subsoil assets	65	Gross national saving	40
Timber resources	290	Education expenditure	7
Non-timber forest resources	76	Consumption of fixed capital	19
Protected areas	7	Energy depletion	0
Cropland	855	Mineral depletion	4
Pastureland	43	Net forest depletion	8
Produced capital	686		
Total tangible wealth	2,022	Adjusted net saving	16
Population growth	1.7%	Δ Wealth per capita	−18

Source: Table 5.1 from The International Bank for Reconstruction and Development. The World Bank: *Where is the Wealth of Nations? Measuring Capital for the 21st Century*, 2006. Reprinted with permission.

MARKET FAILURES

The term *market failure* describes situations in which market prices deviate from scarcity values and individuals and companies make decisions that maximize their own profits but cause losses for others and society as a whole. A central theme of this chapter is that, within a single country, correcting those market failures and establishing properly working, efficient markets can be among the most powerful and effective mechanisms to promote efficient resource use, reduce environmental degradation, and generate sustainable development. At first blush, that proposition may seem counterintuitive. The point, however, is that environmental degradation often occurs because market participants do not take into account the full costs of their actions on the environment. For example, prices of goods produced in a factory may not include the costs to society of the air pollution generated by that factory. Government policies and interventions aimed at incorporating these costs into market decisions help improve environmental outcomes, make markets work better, and bring broader benefits to society.

Prominent among the market failures affecting resources are externalities—*costs* borne by the population at large but not by individual producers and *benefits* that accrue to society but cannot be captured by producers (see also Box 5–1). The most important externalities are those caused by the depletion or degradation of natural resources, including the environment. If resources are depleted at rates faster than they can be replenished or substituted by human-made capital, development will be unsustainable, either nationally or globally. If markets fail in this fundamental way, how can they promote sustainable development? To resolve this apparent conflict, we first need to analyze in greater depth the reason that markets fail to allocate natural resources efficiently.

EXTERNALITIES AND THE COMMONS

During the eighteenth century, as the Industrial Revolution began in England, cows still grazed on the commons of many villages in England and its American colonies. The essence of a village commons was **open access**, free of charge, to any member of the village. The first villagers to take advantage of open access had ample grazing for their livestock; their only cost was the time it would take to herd their animals to the commons, allow them to graze, and herd them home. But the amount of land was fixed and soil fertility and climate limited the quantity of grass. As more villagers used the commons, the grass became sparse, so the animals took longer to feed or, in the case of open rangeland, herders were forced to travel farther to find forage, so that everyone's costs rose. The rising average cost to each herder eventually discouraged grazing on the commons. But the new entrants did not have to pay compensation for the rising costs imposed on each of the previous entrants and more grazing took place than was in the interests of the village as a whole. Eventually, because no one incorporated the full cost of their grazing into their decisions, overgrazing destroyed the commons as a useful source of feed for everyone.

The dilemma of the commons is a widespread phenomenon, applicable to any limited resource to which access is unlimited. Grazing on open range, whether in the U.S. West or the African savanna, has the same outcome. Open access to timberlands or access at fees well below the social cost results in overlogging and the destruction of native forests in Brazil, Ghana, Indonesia, and many other tropical countries. Open access to fishing grounds in the North Atlantic, in Peru's Pacific waters, and in some inland lakes in Africa has already depleted fish stocks beyond their ability to regenerate. Free use of water from a stream benefits upland farmers, who have first access to the water, at the expense of downstream farmers, who get less water. Even traffic congestion in cities like Bangkok, Mexico City, and New York fits the description of a common property: City streets, to which access is free, are the common resource; each new vehicle causes worse traffic jams, forcing all previous entrants into longer, more costly commutes.

The earth's environment is composed of several common resources: air and the atmosphere, fresh water and the oceans, the earth's soils, and the diverse plant and animal species that live in this biosphere. Access to the environment typically is free. When manufacturers and farmers vent their waste into the air or water or create toxic dumps in the ground, they create health problems for the affected population, reduce the value of land in the affected area, destroy recreational potential, and generally reduce the welfare of people who value a clean environment. When lumber companies cut down a rain forest, they destroy the habitat of plant and animal species that are of value to others, including local populations that may harvest them or citizens or tourists who simply like to see them. Deforestation in the tropics significantly reduces biodiversity, perhaps eliminating potential new sources of pharmaceuticals or industrial products as well. They also may alter local climates, change patterns of water availability to surrounding farmers, and cause soil erosion. When we include the environment as a common resource, then much private activity generates external costs and market failure becomes a very general phenomenon. On a grand scale, we might think of the earth's entire atmosphere as a commons beset by the negative externality of greenhouse gas emissions, resulting in global climate change.

External costs and benefits are at the core of the common resource problem. A new producer creates higher costs for all previous entrants or all producers impose external costs on the general population. In either case, in the absence of regulation, taxes, or property rights for environmental quality, external costs are not borne by the producers who cause them and the prices of their products do not reflect the social costs of production. Thus more of these resource-depleting or -polluting goods and services are produced and consumed than would be the case if prices reflected external costs. Hence societies pollute more than their people would choose if markets reflected all social costs.

Figure 20–3 shows this process. In a market with competitive producers, the supply curve S represents private marginal costs, PMC. Market equilibrium occurs at price P_1 with output Q_1. But, if this is a polluting industry, the external costs make the social marginal cost, SMC, higher. If these costs were reflected in the market, the price would jump to P_2 and demand, and therefore output, would be reduced to Q_2. As less of the offending product is grown or manufactured, there would be less environmental degradation.

Designing responses to problems of the commons requires a closer look at what we mean by *the commons*, more formally referred to as **common-pool resources (CPRs)**. CPRs have two characteristics: It is difficult to exclude anyone from using them, and use by one person reduces the availability of that resource for use by others. Potential solutions to the types of problems noted earlier depend more specifically on the nature of property rights governing the CPR. Most of the problems of CPRs arise when property rights are defined as open access regimes, where there

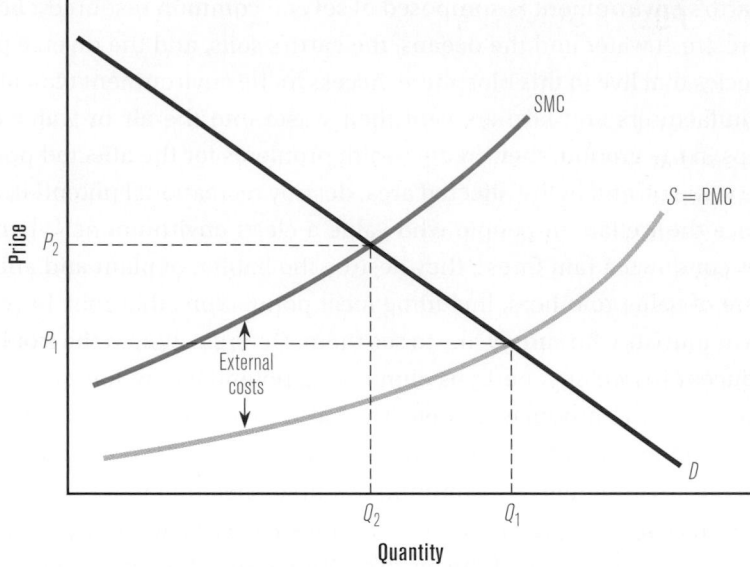

FIGURE 20-3 **External Diseconomies**

Polluters impose costs on others. If these external costs were reflected in the firms' costs, the social marginal cost curve (SMC) would prevail, the market price would be P_2, and output would be Q_2. But because the firms do not bear these costs, their private marginal cost curve (PMC) is lower, so more of the polluting product (Q_1) is produced and consumed.

are no property rights at all. Yet, other CPRs may be characterized by the existence of group property rights, individual (or firm) property rights, or government property rights. In such settings, tragedies of the commons are not inevitable. Economics Nobel Prize winner Elinor Ostrom shows that a wide range of institutions for governing and managing CPRs can, and have, evolved for CPRs that are not simply open access resources. Farmer-managed irrigation systems in Nepal are one among many examples of locally determined rules for conserving natural resources. Ostrom and colleagues find that particular settings are most conducive to the evolution of successful informal rules for managing CPRs. These settings are environments where the resource degradation is not yet too severe and where users have good information about conditions, situations in which users depend on the resource as a main source of their livelihoods and are interested in sustainability of the resource, and settings in which national governments facilitate local organization (rather than attempt to impose rules from outside the community).[16]

[16]Elinor Ostrom, *Governing the Commons: The Evolution of Institutions for Collective Action* (New York: Cambridge University Press, 1990). See also Joanna Burger, Christopher B. Field, Richard B. Norgaard, Elinor Ostrom, and David Policansky, "Revisiting the Commons: Local Lessons, Global Challenges," *Science* 284, no. 5412 (April 1999), 278.

POLICY SOLUTIONS

The market failures that lead to overexploitation of natural resources stem from external costs that are not borne by producers. Even in a well-functioning market economy, externalities require government intervention to make markets work better and to reach efficient market outcomes. Governments can bestow property rights on private users, regulate access to common resources, impose taxes (or pay subsidies) that reflect external costs (or benefits), and issue tradable access rights. There is also recent experience with informal regulation by local communities in the absence of formal government regulation. We discuss each of these options in turn.

PROPERTY RIGHTS

Common properties generate external costs because no one owns or controls the right to exploit them. For some resources, a simple solution would be to confer ownership, which economists call **property rights**, on a single individual or company. As long as the owner is a profit-maximizer and sells output in a competitive market, the socially optimal outcome is achieved without further government intervention. Property rights, to be effective, must be exclusive and well defined, leaving no doubt to the owners and possible competing claimants about what has been conferred and to whom. Rights need to be secure, so that the risk of loss through legal challenge or expropriation is reduced and enforceable through the judicial system. Ownership must be valid over a long-enough horizon that the owners have a stake in the long-term, sustainable exploitation of the resource. Longevity converts the resource into an asset for the producer, who can reap the benefits from investments in improving and sustaining its productivity. And the rights must be transferable, so the owner can realize the benefits of the resource asset by selling the property at any time.

The implications of clearly assigned property rights for market-based pollution abatement were formalized in 1960 by Nobel economist Ronald Coase. The **Coase theorem** posits that under certain circumstances (in particular, zero transaction costs), clear assignment of property rights leads bargaining in free markets to attain optimal levels of externalities. It is important that the Coase theorem also suggests that this result is independent of the specific allocation of those property rights.[17] A stylized example of the Coase theorem could be a situation in which an upstream factory dumps effluent waste into a river, which then flows downstream and destroys a fishery. When the river itself belongs to neither the factory nor the fisherman, this negative externality persists. The Coase theorem suggests that if either the factory or the fisherman is assigned property rights to the river, free bargaining between the two parties will result in the optimal level of pollution.

---

[17]R. H. Coase, "The Problem of Social Cost," *Journal of Law and Economics* 3 (1960), 1–44.

GOVERNMENT REGULATION

As an alternative to conveying private property rights, governments themselves can act as the owners of common resources and directly regulate their use. Governments can limit the quantity of a hunter's kill, a fisher's catch, a logger's haul, a rancher's herd, or a polluter's emissions. And they can regulate the kinds of equipment that can or must be used: Some kinds of fishing nets, boats, or navigation equipment have been banned; hunters may be restricted in their choice of weapons; polluters are required to install equipment that scrubs gas emissions and treats wastewater.

Quantity regulations raise two issues. First, how do the regulators know the optimal levels of access and output? If property rights can be conveyed, efficient outcomes are approached through market forces and no government judgments are needed. But if regulation replaces the market, regulators need to estimate the characteristics of both producers' costs and users' demand for the products of a common resource. To get a sense of these information requirements, consider the regulation of air pollution. The external costs of pollution are manifest in the reduced welfare of others: poor health, unsightly environment, lower property values, fewer and more expensive recreational possibilities, and possibly reduced productivity and income. If these costs could be measured, they would be depicted by a curve such as marginal external cost (MEC) in Figure 20–4, which shows the marginal external cost of pollution (measured along the horizontal axis). Those who believe that the costs of pollution are higher than normally recognized or who put a high premium on reducing pollution argue,

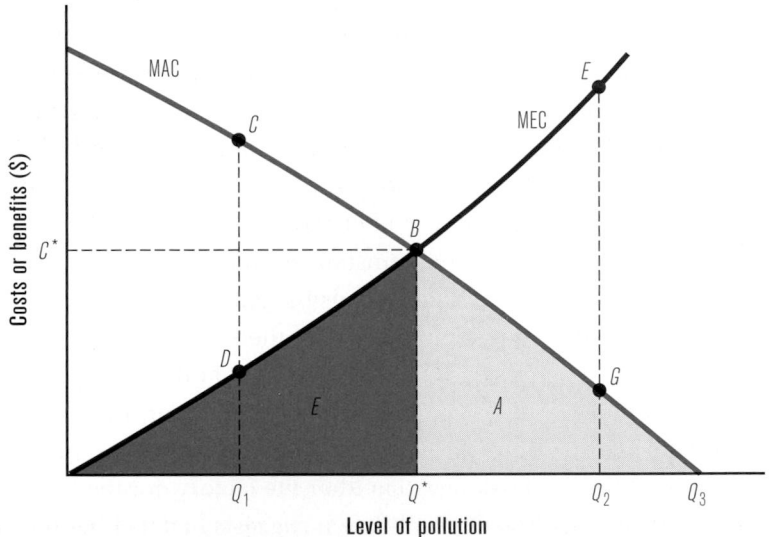

FIGURE 20-4 Optimal Level of Pollution

The marginal external cost of pollutants, borne by the population, is given by MEC; the marginal cost of abatement, borne by the firm, is MAC. The total cost to society (area $E + A$) is minimized and pollution is optimal at Q^*, where MEC = MAC.

in effect, that the MEC curve should be shifted up. Wherever it is located, any reduction in pollution (a movement to the left on the horizontal axis) means a reduction in the cost to society from pollution or, equivalently, an increase in the marginal external benefit of abatement.

However, there is a cost to abating pollution. The polluting firm, say, a petrochemical plant, can reduce its effluents either by changing its production process, installing abatement equipment such as gas scrubbers and water treatment plants, or reducing output. The marginal cost of abatement (MAC) function traces these marginal abatement costs. At any point along MAC, the cost shown is that of the lowest-cost method of abatement. Moving from right (high pollution) to left (lower pollution), MAC rises because it becomes increasingly costly to clean up air or water the stricter are the standards or the lower the level of contamination. It is important to recognize that these costs of abatement, although borne by the petrochemical firm, also are costs to society because they involve either less consumption of petrochemicals or savings spent on abatement that otherwise might have been spent on investment in other goods or services people want. These abatement costs thus have equal weight to the benefits gained by reducing pollution.

Society's (and government's) aim should be to minimize the combined costs of pollution and its abatement. This is achieved at Q^* in Figure 20–4, where MEC = MAC. At this point $Q_3 - Q^*$ of pollution has been abated (assuming for convenience that Q_3 is the maximum amount of pollution), and Q^* of pollution remains. Because these are marginal cost curves, the total external cost of pollution is the area E under MEC from 0 to Q^*. And the total cost of abatement is given by the shaded area A under the MAC curve between Q^* and Q_3. With less pollution, such as Q_1, the marginal abatement cost exceeds the marginal external cost of pollution and the total cost of additional abatement, the area of the trapezoid Q_1Q^*BC, exceeds the net gain from reduced pollution, Q_1Q^*BD. If more pollution is permitted, such as Q_2, the additional external cost, Q^*Q_2EB, exceeds the reduced cost of abatement, Q^*Q_2GB.

Therefore, society is better off with some pollution than with none, because abating the last unit of pollution is expensive relative to its benefits. Similarly, society gains from some exploitation of natural resources, even nonrenewable ones. But how do the regulators, who wish to achieve this optimal level of pollution, know what it is? To find Q^*, they have to know all the external costs of pollution, as a function of the levels of contaminants in the air, water, and soil. In addition to these estimates of direct economic costs, finding Q^* requires having a method for estimating the values people place on environmental amenities such as clean air, water, and soil. The costs in some cases are substantial. A recent collection of studies from the World Bank estimate the costs of environmental degradation in the Middle East and North Africa.[18] As summarized by country and by resource category in Table 20–2, these costs are

---

[18]Leila Croitoru and Maria Sarraf, eds., *The Cost of Environmental Degradation: Case Studies from the Middle East and North Africa* (Washington, DC: World Bank, 2010).

TABLE 20-2 **Cost of Environmental Degradation in the Middle East and North Africa (percent GDP)**

	ALGERIA	EGYPT	LEBANON	MOROCCO	SYRIA	TUNISIA
Air pollution	1.0	2.1	1.0	1.0	1.3	0.6
Lack of access to water supply and sanitation	0.8	1.0	1.1	1.2	0.9	0.6
Land degradation	1.2	1.2	0.6	0.4	1.0	0.5
Coastal zone degradation	0.6	0.3	0.7	0.5	0.1	0.3
Waste management	0.1	0.2	0.1	0.5	0.1	0.1
Subtotal	3.6	4.8	3.4	3.7	3.3	2.1
Global environment (CO_2 emissions)	1.2	0.6	0.5	0.9	1.3	0.6
Total	4.8	5.4	3.9	4.6	4.6	2.7

GPD, gross domestic product.

Source: Leila Croitoru and Maria Sarraf, eds., *The Cost of Environmental Degradation: Case Studies from the Middle East and North Africa* (Washington, DC: World Bank, 2010).

estimated to range from approximately 3 percent to 5 percent of GDP. Various studies of the cost of environmental degradation in China suggest a figure up to 13 percent of GDP. Such studies, however, confront a range of limitations (data in particular), and their results are generally not directly comparable (due to the use of differing methodologies). Their results are best interpreted as providing orders of magnitude.

In the absence of precise cost estimates, regulators must set somewhat arbitrary standards based on studies estimating the impact of pollutants on human health, animal survival, forest die back (from acid rain) and regeneration, and presumed climate changes.

TAXES, SUBSIDIES, AND PAYMENTS FOR ENVIRONMENTAL SERVICES

A third option is that, in principle, the government also could achieve optimal rates of resource use by imposing taxes that reduce the incentive for producers to use common properties or manufacture polluting products. A tax might be imposed on output that represents the external costs of production, so that the private marginal cost schedule shifts up to equal the social marginal cost schedule.[19] This might take the

---

[19]In Figure 20–3, the tax would shift the PMC schedule up to coincide with the SMC schedule.

form of a tax on each ton of steel or petrochemicals at a rate representing the external cost of pollution or a tax on gasoline to cover the costs of both pollution and traffic congestion. If the tax is on output or level of effort, the incentive is to reduce production of the good with external costs. If the tax can be levied on the externality itself, there is an additional incentive to invest in reducing external costs. For example, a tax on the quantity of pollutants would give petrochemical plants an incentive to abate pollution, because the tax then is reduced. In general, attempts to tax pollutants have had limited success (and even less success in high-income countries than in developing and transitional economies). Monitoring is difficult (and expensive), charge rates generally are set too low, and tax avoidance can be relatively easy. Malaysia began to implement pollution taxes in the 1970s, and China now operates the world's largest pollution tax system, though its effectiveness is disputed.[20] Box 20–2 describes efforts to tax water pollution in Colombia.

BOX 20-2 TAXING WATER POLLUTION IN COLOMBIA

Until the mid-1990s, Colombia's efforts to curb water pollution had relied exclusively on a traditional command-and-control approach in which regional environmental regulatory authorities were responsible for issuing permits for the discharge of wastewater. These permits were intended to limit the quantity of discharges and to require that they meet specific effluent standards. These regional regulatory authorities, known as CARs (which stands for *Corporaciónes Autónomas Regionales*), had issued permits to less than one third of all discharges by 2002 and were lax in their monitoring and enforcement of discharge standards.

Beginning in 1997, Colombia tried a new approach to reducing water pollution based on economic incentives, a per unit tax of pollution emitted. The implementation of this tax was specified in Decree 901, which directed that CARs first produce inventories of all facilities discharging wastewater and then set five-year pollution reduction goals for each water basin in their jurisdiction. The CARs would then set tax rates per unit of effluent based on a minimum fee determined by the Ministry of Environment, and then monitor the facilities' discharges on a regular basis.

Implementation of this water pollution tax encountered several barriers. Implementation was uneven across CARs, with only nine of Colombia's 33 CARs

[20]Jeffrey R. Vincent and Rozali Mohamed Ali, *Managing Natural Wealth: Environment and Development in Malaysia* (Washington, DC: Resources for the Future, 2005).

fulfilling all of the program requirements by 2003. In addition, less than half the polluting facilities were actually charged the tax, and collection rates from those facilities averaged only 27 percent between 1997 and 2002. Municipal sewage authorities were particularly reluctant to pay their taxes, sparking complaints of unfairness by private firms. Implementation of the pollution tax was also hindered by confusion surrounding the continued existence of the previous command-and-control system of permits.

Despite these impediments, a number of Colombia's water basins achieved significant reductions in wastewater discharges. The extent to which this achievement can be attributed to the discharge fee program is difficult to assess. The confusion lies in the fact that before 1997, nearly all of the CARs lacked the regulatory and enforcement capacity necessary to effectively implement *any* pollution reduction program. Once charged with the added responsibilities of creating inventories of polluting facilities and developing monitoring systems (with substantial technical support from the Ministry of Environment), the CARs' ability to enforce the old emissions standards was also enhanced. The discharge fee system was more transparent than the previous approach, requiring regular reporting by the CARs. In addition, the new fee system created economic incentives for better performance by the CARs themselves, which were allowed to keep fee revenues.

Source: Allen Blackman, "Incentives to Control Water Pollution in Developing Countries, How Well Has Colombia's Wastewater Discharge Fee Program Worked and Why?," *Resources* (Spring 2006) [Resources for the Future, Washington, DC].

Taxes that internalize external costs have two important advantages over regulation. First, they allow the producer to choose the method of reducing access to a common resource so that rents are not dissipated in wasteful expenditures forced by regulators. The cost savings with this flexibility can be substantial. Second, taxes can generate substantial revenues for the government. These kinds of revenues can be used to fund environmental programs or in other ways to compensate citizens for the harm caused by pollution and other environmental degradation.

The inverse of this discussion is also true. Some externalities are positive. Positive externalities exist when an activity creates social benefits that are external to the firm. Examples might include the invention of new technologies that spill over into other firms or sectors, or the provision of improved health or training for workers, or the pollination of neighboring orchards by bees from an apiary. Because these benefits are external to the firm, marginal social benefits exceed marginal private benefits, and markets undersupply them. In such cases, subsidies (which are simply negative taxes) may be justified to encourage optimal production of positive externalities. Such programs, however, run the risk of subsidizing activities that might have happened even in the absence of the subsidy.

Payments for environmental services (PES) are an extension of the idea of subsidizing the production of positive externalities. Economist Sven Wunder has defined PES as a voluntary transaction by which a well-defined environmental service is purchased by a buyer of that service from a provider conditional on the provision of the service.[21] Such arrangements effectively create markets that had been missing for external environmental benefits. For instance, forest conservation may provide little direct benefit to farmers, whose private costs and benefits might then favor cutting down forests to expand their fields. Yet, downstream populations must then forego the benefits created by forests, such as biodiversity and carbon storage. PES systems create markets through which potential beneficiaries of environmental services pay potential providers of those services. In this example, PES could be made to farmers to induce them not to destroy forest land for agricultural expansion. The buyers of environmental services might be the actual users of the services (for instance, a producer of hydroelectric power might pay upstream land users to conserve water). In other instances, governments (or even international financial institutions such as the World Bank) might pay providers for environmental services on behalf of users of those services.[22] Examples of user-financed PES programs are payments for watershed services in Pimampiro, Ecuador; payments for biodiversity and watershed services in Los Negros, Bolivia; and payments for carbon sequestration in Ecuador. Examples of government-financed PES programs are China's Sloping Land Conservation Program, Mexico's Payments for Hydrological Environmental Services program, and South Africa's Working for Water program.[23] PES programs exemplify practical efforts to implement the Coase theorem, as do the idea of marketable permits to pollute.

MARKETABLE PERMITS

A fourth intervention is to create a property right where none exists by issuing **marketable permits**, granting the holders the right to harvest a common resource up to a given limit or giving producers a license to pollute the environment up to specified amounts. Although environmentalists sometimes scoff at the notion of a *right* to pollute or exploit resources, this idea recognizes that zero pollution is usually not optimal because of the costs involved in achieving that goal. These permits may be

[21]Cited in Stefanie Engel, Stefano Pagiola, and Sven Wunder, "Designing Payments for Environmental Services in Theory and Practice: An Overview of the Issues," *Ecological Economics* 65 (2008), 663–74.

[22]Engel et al., Designing Payments for Environmental Services in Theory and Practice," p. 666.

[23]These programs are reviewed in Sven Wunder, Stefanie Engel, and Stefano Pagiola, "Payments for Environmental Services in Developing and Developed Countries," *Ecological Economics* [Special ed.] 65, no. 4 (May 2008), 663–852.

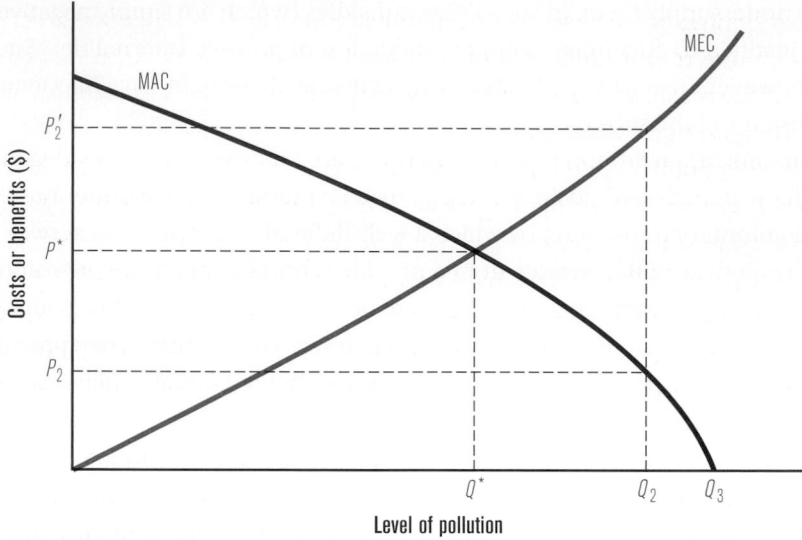

FIGURE 20-5 Marketable Permits to Pollute

The marginal cost of abatement (MAC) schedule shows the demand for pollution rights. If rights are issued to pollute up to Q_2, these are worth P_2 to polluters, but the public places a value of P_2' on reducing pollution. This could be the basis for a bargain to reduce pollution to the optimal level, Q^*.

MEC, marginal external cost.

the most efficient way to reduce pollution and resource overuse, and this approach has been a major innovation of the past decade. The U.S. sulfur dioxide reduction scheme relies on tradable rights, and both Iceland and New Zealand revived fishing stocks by assigning fishing rights at a sustainable level and allowing fishers to trade their quotas freely.

Figure 20–5 shows how a pollution permit works.[24] The MAC and MEC curves are copied from Figure 20–4. Say that the government knows the optimal level of pollution and auctions off emissions permits totaling Q^*. Any firm polluting without a permit, if detected, would be fined or shut down. (Thus permits have the same enforcement requirements as regulations or taxes.) If MAC represents the cost of pollution abatement for all firms in the market, they would bid up the price of permits to P^*. The MAC schedule (moving from right to left) shows that firms can reduce pollution from Q_3 to Q^* at costs less than P^*. Additional reductions in pollution would cost more than P^*. Therefore, the MAC schedule is the demand curve for permits. Either the government can issue a given number and observe the auction price paid for them or it can set a price and issue whatever number of permits is demanded by polluters.

[24]This figure is adapted from David W. Pearce and R. Kerry Turner, *Economics of Natural Resources and the Environment* (Baltimore: Johns Hopkins Press, 1990), 319–20.

In developing and transitional economies, where policy dependence on market forces is a more recent phenomenon, marketable permits have been less common, though are increasing in frequency. Examples are transferable quotas for fisheries in Chile (beginning in 1991) and South Africa (beginning in 1997). Chile also implemented an auctioning system for bus permits in its capital city, Santiago, starting in 1991, and a system of tradable quotas for the emission of total suspended particulates (TSP) from stationary sources in Santiago the following year. A review of Chile's TSP trading program found it to have had limited success due to several problems with its implementation.[25] One problem was that the enabling law itself was vague in regard to the way that permits would be allocated across firms. The program also initially overestimated the emissions target, which was subsequently reduced. By issuing permits totaling too high a level of emissions, effectiveness was limited. Effectiveness was further limited by the long period of time acquired for approval by the government for the sale of pollution permits between firms. These technical and institutional impediments to implementing Chile's marketable permit program indicate the challenges facing countries that choose this approach.

INFORMAL REGULATION

Informal regulation of pollution does not rely on traditional government-generated regulation. In place of formal regulation, such programs often rely on the public disclosure of information about firms' and factories' environmental performance to local stake holders (for instance people living near a factory or a firm's customers). Potential benefits of informal regulation are its low cost and its lack of reliance on formal regulatory institutions. These characteristics make informal regulation of pollution especially attractive in developing countries, which are typically short of both funds and highly evolved regulatory institutions. Public disclosure potentially empowers communities to pressure polluters to improve their environmental performance. The effects of such pressure might operate directly on the firm or indirectly if increased community awareness of the problem and its source leads to greater demand for formal intervention. In some circumstances, public disclosure can even bring pressure from capital markets for firms to alter their behavior. Public disclosure programs take one of two forms: registries of plants' emissions (without rating environmental performance), and programs that use plants' emissions data to rate environmental performance.[26] Chile and Mexico are among at least 20 countries with pollution registries, and performance ratings programs exist in China, Ghana, India, and several other developing countries.

---

[25]Jessica Coria and Thomas Sterner, "Tradable Permits in Developing Countries: Evidence from Air Pollution in Chile," *Journal of Environment & Development* 19, no. 2 (2010), 145–70.

[26]For an excellent survey, see Allen Blackman, "Alternative Pollution Control Policies in Developing Countries," *Review of Environmental Economics and Policy* 4, no. 2, (Summer 2010), 234–53.

The effectiveness of public disclosure types of informal environmental regulation, in practice, may depend on characteristics that may or may not be present in developing countries. For instance, in the absence of a credible threat of more stringent formal regulation, informal regulation may have less traction. In addition, capital markets may have little leverage in settings dominated by small firms with little reliance on outside investors. Further, information does not always flow freely in every country. Despite these contingencies, reviews of the effectiveness of public disclosure programs have found them to be effective in reducing pollution. These effects tend to be greater in cases in which the initial violations were the most flagrant. Yet, to date, rigorous evidence of successful ratings programs comes only from Indonesia, the Philippines, Vietnam, and China.[27]

POLICY FAILURES

Although some government intervention is necessary to correct for the market failures associated with natural resources, it is equally true that, all over the world, government policies frequently contribute to wasteful use of resources and the degradation of the environment. Too much intervention or intervention of the wrong kind can be just as costly as too little intervention. We have seen that, when production has external costs, one approach is to internalize those costs by raising production costs through taxing output or granting marketable property rights. But, instead, governments commonly subsidize or otherwise reduce the costs the production of commodities that degrade natural resources and often compromise property rights in ways that encourage rapacious exploitation. Examples are not hard to find.

Forestry policy has been especially destructive in many tropical countries. For many years Brazil subsidized ranching and other activities that encroached on the Amazon rain forest. Through at least the first five years of the twenty-first century, the area deforested each year in the Brazilian Amazon was equivalent in size to the state of New Jersey. Approximately two thirds of the deforested land in Brazil in recent decades has been used for cattle ranches, and most of the remaining third has been cleared for subsistence farming. More recently, commercial agriculture has also been an important source of deforestation in Brazil. Tax policies favorable to pasture land encouraged deforestation. Brazil has reformed some of these environmentally harmful tax incentives and stepped up efforts to regulate deforestation. At the end of 2010, the government of Brazil announced that the rate of deforestation in the Amazon for the previous year was 67 percent lower than the average rate of deforestation for the period 1996–2005. Time will tell if this improved trend proves durable. Box 20–3 describes the policy failures underlying the rapid rate of deforestation in Indonesia.

---

[27]Blackman, "Alternative Pollution Control Policies in Developing Countries," pp. 241–42.

BOX 20-3 POLICY FAILURES AND DEFORESTATION IN INDONESIA

Over the course of the twentieth century, Indonesia's forested area was cut by nearly 50 percent, mostly the result of commercial logging. In May 2010, the government of Indonesia introduced a moratorium on new logging contracts. Yet, for decades before 2010, Indonesia's rapid rate of deforestation was in some measure the result of government policy, more specifically, the failure of government policy. Four main categories of policy failure are to blame: policies supporting the buildup of excess capacity in the wood processing industry, conversion of forested areas into agricultural land, inefficient collection and use of rents collected from the forestry sector, and the absence of effective property rights in many forested areas.

Beginning in the 1970s, government policy in Indonesia supported the expansion of the timber processing industry by restricting the export of raw timber. This depressed domestic timber prices, thus subsidizing timber processors. The resulting overcapacity stimulated the demand for raw timber, much of it logged illegally. Government-subsidized loans to the timber processing industry heightened these incentives.

Substantial tracts of forest were also clearcut to create space for large oil palm plantations. This process accelerated during the 1990s and is cited as having contributed to the massive forest fires of 1997–98. In addition, the government was promoting migration from densely populated Java to the outer islands and cleared additional forest land to accommodate the migrants' farming activities.

The government was also inefficient in its collection of rents from the forestry sector. By law, the government was supposed to levy fees based on both forest area harvested and the number of units harvested. These fees were to be used for replanting the harvested areas. In practice, rent collection was limited, estimated to be between 24 and 36 percent of total economic rents in 1997–98, resulting in substantial windfall profits for the logging industry.

All of these problems have been made worse by the absence of secure property rights. By law, the state controls all forest areas. This means that the actual users of those lands have minimal incentive to invest in the long-term maintenance of that resource. Accelerated deforestation is one symptom of this problem.

Source: Raymond Atje and Kurnya Roesad, "Who Should Own Indonesia's Forests? Exploring the Links between Economic Incentives, Property Rights and Sustainable Forest Management," Economics Working Paper Series 76, Center for Strategic and International Studies, Jakarta, 2004.

Trade policy has been equally destructive. Ghana, Indonesia, and Malaysia, for example, placed bans on log exports as a means of promoting wood-processing industries. Export bans drive down the domestic price of tropical hardwood and so make it very profitable for sawmills and plywood mills to purchase logs and export semifinished products. But these industries are usually inefficient and consume resource rents through higher production costs. Because timber companies cannot export tropical hardwoods, such as ebony and mahogany, as logs, these valuable species are used along with low-value timber to make inexpensive products, such as plywood sent to Japan to make forms for pouring cement. The role of self-imposed log export bans in destroying rain forests should be a warning to northern countries that want to preserve tropical forests by imposing their own import bans on these logs.[28]

Energy pricing is another common policy failure. In oil-rich countries like Nigeria and Venezuela, energy has been kept cheap in an attempt to stimulate industrialization and diversification, and Indonesia subsidized kerosene ostensibly to help the rural poor. This policy has multiple adverse effects. It encourages wasteful domestic consumption and reduces the country's petroleum and gas reserves and its export-earning potential. It encourages the use of cars and minibuses and so adds to congestion. Cheap energy promotes industry ill-suited to the country's endowments. Firms and consumers have little incentive to adopt energy-saving technology. Because burning oil is an important source of air pollution, all these overuses contribute to environmental degradation. Similarly, some oil importers, such as Argentina, China, Egypt, and India, have subsidized petroleum products by as much as 50 percent of the world price and so encouraged imports they cannot afford, industries that cannot compete in world markets, and environmental degradation that market pricing would have discouraged.[29]

Infrastructure investment is a third area of widespread policy failure. In forestry and energy pricing, governments typically underprice the resource and fail to force private operators to account for external costs. In infrastructure investment, governments often create new external costs and fail to account for them in project planning. Environmental groups have focused much of their ire on investments in power dams, irrigation and flood control systems, roads, and power plants that damage their environments. Dams that flood their upstream areas displace local populations, who sometimes do not fare as well in new locations, and destroy natural habitat. Egypt's huge Aswan Dam controls the floodwaters of the Nile. But before the dam, those floodwaters had beneficial effects, replenishing soil and leaching out unwanted salts, so the dam may have reduced agricultural productivity over the long run. This

---

[28]On forest policies, see Robert Repetto and Malcolm Gillis, eds., *Public Policies and the Misuse of Forest Resources* (Cambridge: Cambridge University Press, 1988); Jeffrey Vincent, "The Tropical Timber Trade and Sustainable Development," *Science* 256 (1992), 1651–55.

[29]Bjorn Larsen and Anwar Shah, "World Fossil Fuel Subsidies in Global Carbon Emissions," Working Paper WPS 1002, World Bank, Washington, DC, October 1992, esp. chart 1.

does not mean that dams are necessarily bad ideas but rather the full costs are not always recognized up front and incorporated into prices.

The problem of common pool resources, policy responses to externalities, and policy failures are particularly important for the poor. The world's poor are disproportionately concentrated in fragile environments, and their livelihoods depend disproportionately on natural resources (especially open access and other forms of common property resources). The interactions between poverty and the environment are complex, yet they are central to an understanding of sustainable development.

POVERTY-ENVIRONMENT LINKAGES

Economic growth, poverty alleviation, and environmental sustainability are three primary goals for development. As Figure 20-6 suggests, these goals are intrinsically linked to one another through a complex set of interactions. In characterizing this

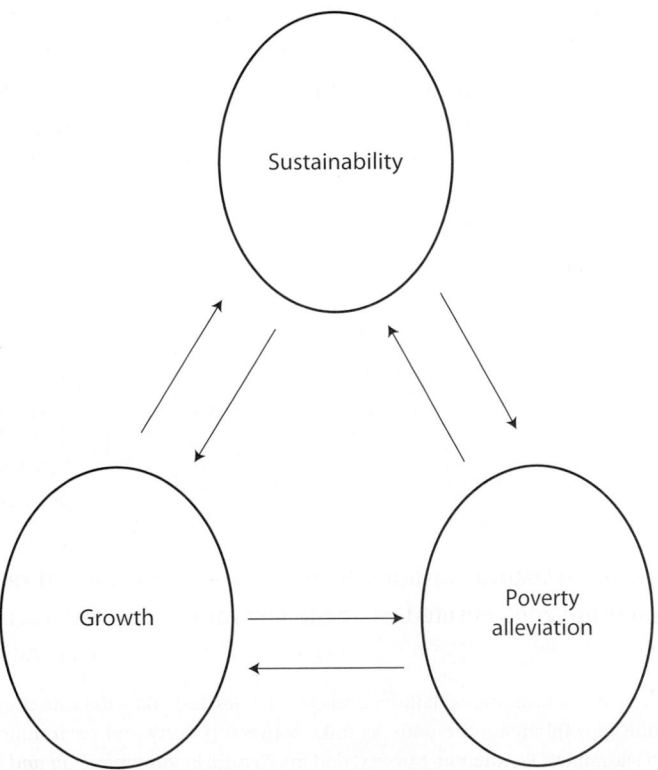

FIGURE 20-6 The Critical Triangle of Development Goals

Source: Vosti, S. A. and T. Reardon. 1997. *Sustainability, Growth, and Poverty Alleviation: A Policy And Agroecological Perspective*, Figure 1.1. Washington, DC: International Food Policy Research Institute.

"critical triangle of development goals," economists Stephen Vosti and Thomas Reardon note that these goals are highly compatible with one another *in the long run*. It is easy to see that a robust and healthy natural resource base will better support growth in agricultural productivity, which in turn can play a critical role in poverty alleviation and economic growth. However, in the short run countries may confront difficult tradeoffs among these goals. If activities of the poor contribute to the degradation of the commons, efforts to preserve the environment by limiting access to the commons might aggravate poverty. The nature and severity of these tradeoffs may vary widely across different combinations of circumstances, though institutional failures and resulting externalities of the types discussed earlier provide a unifying theme.[30] This section focuses on the bidirectional linkages between poverty alleviation and environmental sustainability.

The complex relationship between poverty and environmental degradation arises because severe poverty in the world is disproportionately rural, and rural livelihoods depend heavily on natural resources, especially land and water. The reliance of the poor on natural resources centers on agriculture but also includes livestock, fisheries, and forest resources. Degradation of these resources directly threatens livelihood strategies of many of the world's poor. The Millennium Ecosystem Assessment Board, in its 2005 report *Ecosystems and Human Well-Being*, notes that "Over the past 50 years, humans have changed ecosystems more rapidly and more extensively than in any comparable period of time in human history, largely to meet rapidly growing demands for food, fresh water, timber, fiber, and fuel. This has resulted in a substantial and largely irreversible loss of the diversity of life on earth." The report further suggests that

> The changes that have been made to ecosystems have contributed to substantial net gains in human well-being and economic development, but these gains have been achieved at growing costs in the form of the degradation of many ecosystem services . . . and the exacerbation of poverty for some groups of people. These problems, unless addressed, will substantially diminish the benefits that future generations obtain from ecosystems. The degradation of ecosystem services could grow significantly worse during the first half of this century and is a barrier to achieving the Millennium Development Goals.[31]

The problems of natural resource degradation particularly threaten the poor because the poor are concentrated in fragile environments, which are more vulner-

---

[30]A deeper discussion of institutional failures and externalities, including the causes and consequences of rapid population growth among the poor, as links between poverty and environmental degradation appears in Partha Dasgupta, "Population, Poverty, and the Natural Environment," in Karl-Goran Mäler and Jeffrey Vincent, eds., *Handbook of Environmental Economics*, vol. 1 (Amsterdam: North Holland, 2003), chap. 5.

[31]Millennium Ecosystem Assessment, *Ecosystems and Human Well-Being: Synthesis.* (Washington, DC: Island Press, 2005), p. 1.

able to degradation. Examples of fragile environments are areas with thin soil cover that are vulnerable to erosion, tropical forests, and coastal estuaries. About one quarter of the world's population lives on fragile land, yet the distribution of this population varies widely by region. While only 11 percent of the population of wealthy countries (Organization for Economic Co-Operation and Development; OECD) live on fragile lands, this proportion increases to about 25 percent in South and East Asia, and jumps to nearly 40 percent in sub-Saharan Africa and the Middle East. These percentages increase substantially when we consider the rural poor in particular. About 66 percent of the world's rural poor live on fragile lands, with the proportion rising to approximately 75 percent of the rural poor in sub-Saharan Africa, West Asia and North Africa.[32]

There are numerous examples of the value of environmental services in the livelihood strategies of the poor. Environmental services include such diverse functions as the supply of water and food, carbon sequestration, crop pollination, and recreation. Mangroves, coral reefs, forests and forested watersheds, and flood plains are among the key environmental features that figure prominently in the livelihood strategies of poor people around the world. Coastal mangroves, for instance, can be a valuable source of forest and fishery products. Economists Saudamini Das and Jeffrey Vincent have shown that mangroves buffered coastal villages in Orissa, India, from a super cyclone in 1999. The storm surge from that cyclone killed 10,000 people, but deaths were significantly reduced in villages protected by mangrove forests.[33]

Tropical rain forests are a prominent example of a diminishing natural resource of substantial economic value. Rain forests provide benefits that are both local and global in scope. The global environmental benefits of tropical rain forests include carbon sequestration (discussed later in the chapter), rainfall recycling, and flood control. Conversely, the loss of rain forests can impose important negative externalities, including increased buildup of carbon dioxide, increased smoke, and reduced rainfall, a particular concern in the Amazon. While these effects are quite broad, even global, the effect of tropical rain forests on the poor depend more on rain forests' local impact.

Direct harvesting of timber products is the most obvious local service and also the most problematic. The challenge with timber is to limit harvesting to sustainable yields. Overharvesting of timber resources, both legal and illegal, contributes significantly to deforestation, though deforestation for agricultural expansion may be even greater (whether by large commercial farms in Brazil and Indonesia or by small-

[32]Edward Barbier, "Poverty, Development, Environment," *Environment and Development Economics* 15 (2010), 635–60, tab. 1(b).

[33]Saudamini Das and Jeffrey Vincent, "Mangroves Protected Villages and Reduced Death Toll during Indian Super Cyclone," *Proceedings of the National Academy of Science* 106 no. 18 (2009), 7357–60.

holder farmers in Africa and mainland Southeast Asia).[34] In doing so, it also reduces the value of other local rain forest services. The World Bank estimates that nontimber forest products directly support the livelihoods of approximately 400 million people and indirectly support the livelihoods of approximately 1 billion people.[35] Nontimber forest products include food, fibers, dyes, minerals, and latex and have a total value in international trade of at least $9 billion per year (excluding medicinal products, which are valued at greater than 10 times that figure). Fuel wood is also a critical forest service, particularly for the poor; although it provides less than 7 percent of world energy use, fuel wood accounts for 40 percent of energy use in sub-Saharan Africa (and 90 percent of the use of wood in Africa).[36] Tropical forests are also critical to managing watersheds, helping regulate water flows, cleaning and filtering the water, and preventing the deterioration of soil quality. Tropical rain forests have also been an important component of tourism (ecotourism in developing countries is growing rapidly), are a vital source of biodiversity, and are thought to contain more than half of the land-based species on the planet.

The value of such services is particularly important to the world's poor. Economists have identified three different functions of forest income in rural livelihoods: (1) safety nets because forest products might help to compensate for other production shortfalls, (2) support for current consumption such as food and fuels as noted earlier, and (3) a source of income growth and potential pathway out of poverty. In a review of 51 case studies from 17 developing countries, economist Paul Vedeld and colleagues found that forest environmental income made up an average of 22 percent of total income, with an average absolute value of $678 per household. The proportion of forest income in total income was greatest among the poor, with fuel woods and wild foods together accounting for 70 percent of total forest income.[37] Yet, the ability to derive livelihoods from natural resources also depends on the quality of those resources themselves. Barbier cites evidence from India that poor households in villages near high-quality forests derived up to 40 percent of their income from forest resources, whereas similar households in villages near poor-quality forests derived closer to 10 percent of their income from forest products.[38]

While these data and examples demonstrate the broad association between poverty and the quality of environmental resources, the challenge lies in understanding the mechanisms through which poverty and the environment interact. Early studies, such as the Brundtland Commission, depicted a simple vicious circle in which "poor

---

[34]Kenneth M. Chomitz et. al., *At Loggerheads? Agricultural Expansion, Poverty Reduction, and Environment in the Tropical Forests* (Washington, DC: World Bank, 2007).

[35]World Bank. *Sustaining Forests: A Development Strategy* (Washington, DC: World Bank, 2004).

[36]Mandar Trevedi, Stavros Papageorgiou, and Dominic Moran, *What Are Rainforests Worth?* Forest Foresight Report Number 4, Global Canopy Program, Oxford, UK, 2008.

[37]Paul Vedeld et al., "Forest Environmental Incomes and the Rural Poor," *Forest Policy and Economics* 9 (2007), 869–79.

[38]Barbier, "Poverty, Development, Environment," p. 645.

people are forced to overuse environmental resources to survive from day to day, and their impoverishment of their environment further impoverishes them, making their survival ever more uncertain and difficult."[39] Subsequent studies suggest a more nuanced view.

Reardon and Vosti provide a useful framework for understanding poverty-environment links in rural areas.[40] Reardon and Vosti summarize their conceptual framework with the flowchart presented in Figure 20–7. Their approach relates four blocks of variables: asset categories of the rural poor, income-generating activities and land use at the household and village levels, categories of natural resources (including soil and water), and conditioning factors such as markets, prices, and infrastructure (or more broadly, institutions) that mediate interactions between the first three blocks of variables.

In this framework, each category of assets represents a potential form of poverty. Asset categories include natural resources that are both privately and commonly held (soil, water, biodiversity), human resources (health, education, labor), on-farm resources (physical and financial), off-farm resources (physical and financial), and community-owned resources (roads, common pasture lands) as well as social and political capital (political power). Households can be poor in any of these categories. Reardon and Vosti emphasize that asset-specific poverty can spill over in various ways to result in environmental degradation. If, for example, land ownership is required to obtain credit, then a household that is poor in land may be precluded from making investments to improve their farm and nonfarm capital (including soil protection). As a consequence, such households may be unable to intensify their farming activities or work away from the farm, perhaps forcing them to rely on expanding their farming activities into fragile lands. Even though a given household may not be poor in the conventional welfare sense, it may still lack sufficient resources to invest in improving the resource base.

The Reardon-Vosti conceptual framework also distinguishes between categories of environmental resources. Soil, water, biodiversity, and air may be either helped or harmed by household activities, depending in part on the value of those resources to rural households. Yet, a potential problem arises when the value of such resources to society at large differs from their value to poor rural households. Reardon and Vosti illustrate this point with the example of a large tree that society may value as a carbon sink but which a poor rural household may see as either timber for sale or a source of ash to enhance soils. As in many such cases of negative environmental externalities,

---

[39]World Commission on Environment and Development, *Our Common Future* (New York: Oxford University Press, 1987), p. 27 as cited by Barbier, "Poverty, Development, Environment."

[40]Thomas Reardon and Stephen A. Vosti, "Poverty-Environment Links in Rural Areas of Developing Countries," in T. Reardon and S A. Vosti, eds., *Sustainability, Growth, and Poverty Alleviation, A Policy Perspective* (Baltimore: Johns Hopkins University Press, for the International Food Policy Research Institute, 1997).

the issue is one of missing markets. In this case there may be no market for the service of the tree as a carbon sink.

Figure 20–7 illustrates how these four blocks of variables interact with one another. Households pursue their food security and livelihood goals based initially

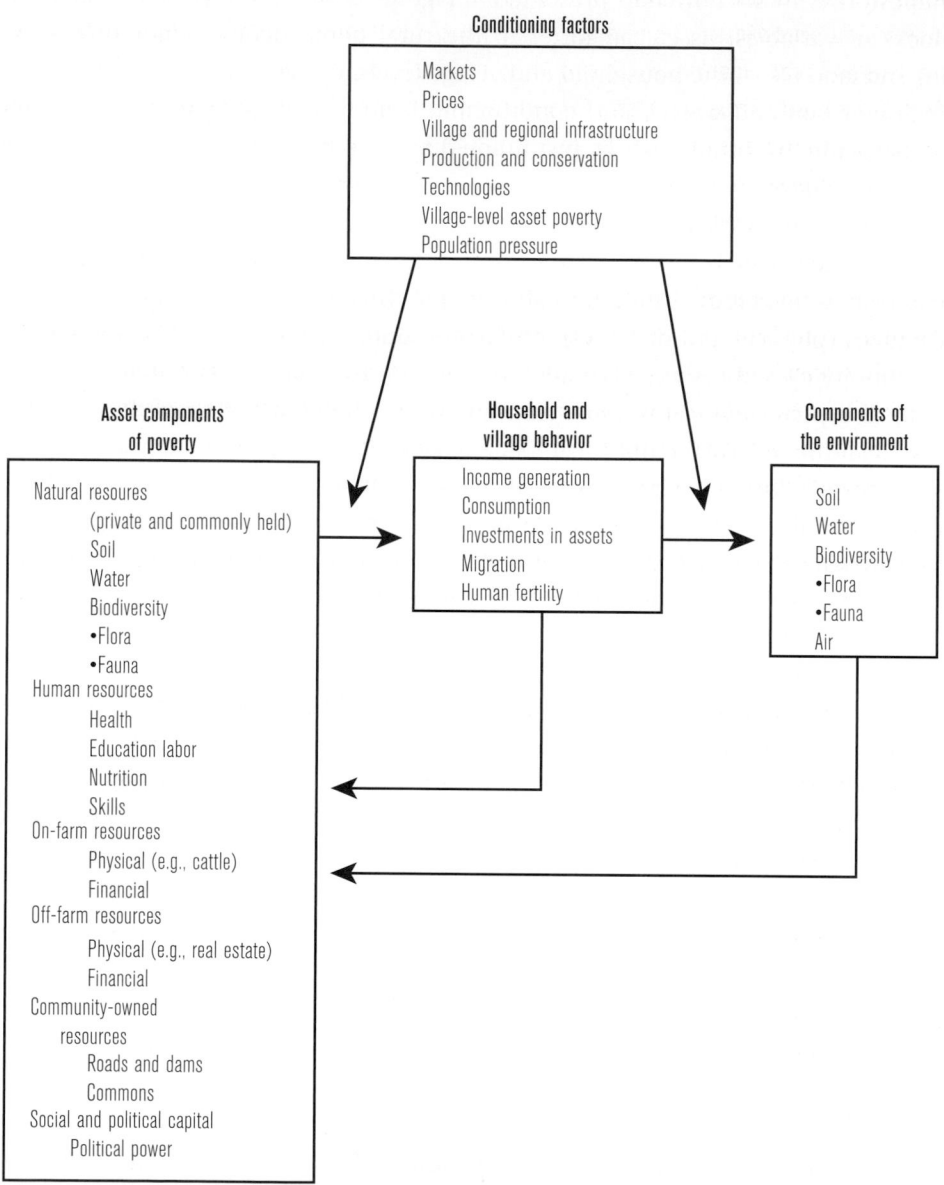

FIGURE 20-7 Conceptual Framework for Poverty–Environment Links

Source: Vosti, S. A. and T. Reardon. 1997. *Sustainability, Growth, and Poverty Alleviation: A Policy And Agroecological Perspective*, Figure 4.1. Washington, DC: International Food Policy Research Institute.

on their stock of assets. Their ability to use these assets in pursuing their objectives depends on a variety of conditioning factors, including accessibility of markets, prices, infrastructure, available technologies, and population pressure. For the poor, community assets and the availability of common pool resources may also play a large role. These factors shape household decisions regarding how to allocate their assets in pursuing their livelihood objectives. For example, the incentives for households to allocate their labor between agricultural and nonagricultural activities (such as working on others' farms) may depend on the relative prices of agricultural output versus local wage rates. Technological choices available to the rural poor may also be limited. Thus subsistence-oriented farmers may be unable to adopt modern inputs to increase yields, forcing them to expand the area cultivated onto fragile lands to increase their agricultural output. Each of these choices has environmental implications. Area expansion might require cutting trees. Working in off-farm activities might reduce pressure on the land, yet might also create incentives to reallocate investment funds away from on-farm land conservation. Diversification of farming activities to include livestock husbandry also has environmental implications, particularly because grazing is often done on public land, where overgrazing is common and can lead to soil erosion and degradation. It does not necessarily follow, however, that it is the poor who contribute the most to this type of environmental degradation. Reardon and Vosti note that it is typically wealthier households that own larger herds and potentially cause greater harm to the environment. The sum total of these environmental effects of household income-earning and investment activities, both positive and negative effects, in turn define the natural resource and asset base available to households in the future.

Reardon and Vosti provide several examples of the complex interactions between poverty and the environment, stressing in particular the dependence of these interactions on the specific type of asset poverty and the specific environmental context. Rwanda is one of the most densely populated countries in Africa. Most of the poor are farmers with little land and few animals. Their primary asset is their own labor. Lacking capital and credit, they are often prevented from investing in soil conservation and unable to intensify their farming practices by purchasing chemical fertilizers and other modern inputs. In such circumstances farmers' main strategy for increasing agricultural output may be simply to increase their own labor input. Yet, in the absence of complementary inputs, potential yield increases are limited, with the likely consequence that the limited land resources of poor farmers in Rwanda quickly become depleted. The result may be a vicious circle in which resource-constrained farmers have little choice but to exhaust their own land, thus increasing their own poverty.

Reardon and Vosti provide a quite different example from the Brazilian rain forest, where the poor may be rich in biodiversity but poor in terms of soil quality and access to capital and labor. Once again, the problem is one of missing markets, in this case a market for biodiversity. The broad range of asset poverty confronting poor farmers in the Brazilian rain forest may constrain them to cut down trees to expand their farmland and to burn those trees to generate nutrients for the poor-quality soil. Farmers thus substitute biophysical processes for markets to meet their needs. Breaking this cycle may require new agricultural technologies to increase the productivity of existing farmland, improved off-farm opportunities, and the creation of markets for forest cover and biodiversity. Reardon and Vosti note that much of the alarming deforestation of the Brazilian Amazon has been not the result of poverty but rather the response by large landowners to fiscal and other incentives.

The links between poverty and the environment are thus strongly conditional on given circumstances, in particular the specific nature of poverty; the range of available environmental resources; and the institutional, technological, and market conditions governing the choices and activities of households, both poor and rich. Reducing poverty may protect the environment when poverty is driving unsustainable mining of resources. Yet poverty alleviation might contribute to other sources of environmental degradation, such as overuse of agricultural chemicals. At the same time, environmental improvements might reduce poverty that results from the dependence of poor farmers on a depleted resource base. Yet environmental improvement achieved by barring the poor from common pool resources could increase poverty. The conceptual framework presented in this section suggests that a nuanced understanding of the categories of asset poverty and local conditioning variables is necessary to simultaneously reduce poverty and protect the environment. These challenges are writ large in the case of global climate change.

GLOBAL CLIMATE CHANGE

Global climate change may represent the greatest single challenge to sustainable development. While its causes are a subject of debate and predictions of its consequences are uncertain, there is broad scientific consensus regarding the existence of global climate change. As summarized by the Intergovernmental Panel on Climate Change (IPCC) in its fourth assessment report, "Warming of the climate system is unequivocal, as is now evident from observations of increases in global average air and ocean temperatures, widespread melting of snow and ice and rising global average sea level."[41] The IPCC report notes that the last years of the twentieth century and the first years of the twenty-first century include 11 of the 12 warmest years since 1850 (when systematic recording of global surface temperatures began). Changes in sea level and snow cover are consistent with the evidence of increasing global surface temperatures. Figure 20–8 illustrates long-term changes in global mean surface air temperatures, underscoring the rapid temperature increases since the mid-1970s.

[41]IPCC, 2007: Climate Change 2007: Synthesis Report. Contribution of Working Groups I, II and III to the Fourth Assessment Report of the Intergovernmental Panel on Climate Change [Core Writing Team, Pachauri, R.K and Reisinger, A. (eds.)]. IPCC, Geneva, Switzerland, p. 104.

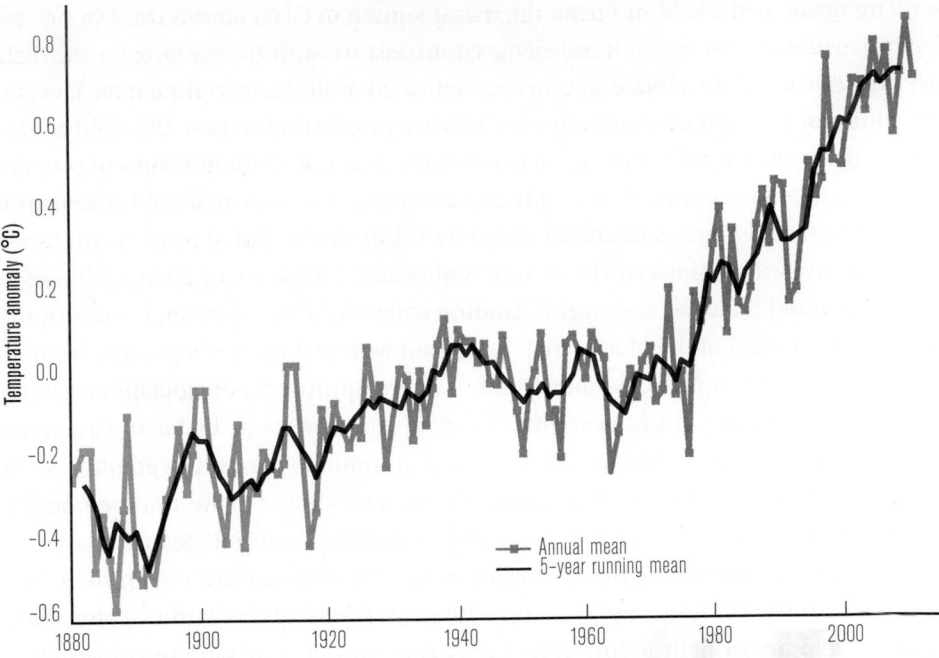

FIGURE 20-8 **Changes in Global Annual Mean Surface Air Temperature**

Source: National Aeronautics and Space Administration, Goddard Institute for Space Studies, available at http://data.giss.nasa.gov/gistemp/graphs_v3/Fig.A.gif.

The current effects of climate change are apparent from observations of a broad range of natural systems. The IPCC reports major impacts on hydrological systems, such as increased runoff from glacier- and snow-fed rivers and warming of lakes and rivers. They also cite the impact of climate change on biological systems—for example, earlier timing of spring events such as bird migration and reproduction and geographic (poleward) shifts in the ranges of plants and animals in addition to the effects changing aquatic biological systems have on fish migrations and changes in algal, plankton, and fish abundance as well as the health of coral reefs.

Global climate change is driven primarily by the accumulation of greenhouse gases (GHGs) in the earth's atmosphere, where they trap heat. The main GHGs are carbon dioxide (CO_2), methane (CH_4), nitrous oxide (N_2O), and halocarbons. Global concentrations of GHGs have increased substantially since 1750, a result of human activities, according to the IPCC. Agriculture and fossil fuels use have been the leading contributors.[42] Climate change is a central concern for sustainable development owing to the role of human economic activity in the emission of GHGs and the ensuing physical and economic implications of potential changes in the earth's natural resource base.

[42]Intergovernmental Panel on Climate Change, *Climate Change 2007*, p. 37.

The developed world has been the major source of GHG emissions. Average per capita carbon emissions in developing countries are approximately one third the level produced by developed countries. Figure 20-9 illustrates per capita levels of CO_2 emissions as a function of countries' relative population sizes. The height of each bar in Figure 20-9 indicates per capita emissions, and the width indicates population (so the area of each country's bar indicates total emissions). The top 10 countries in terms of CO_2 emissions account for over two thirds of the global total. It is interesting to compare emissions in the United States and China. As of 2006, China overtook the United States as the world's leading source of CO_2 emissions, contributing just over 22 percent of the global total compared with just under 20 percent from the United States. Per capita emissions in the U.S. are approximately four times greater than those in China, yet China compensates for this difference by having a population just over four times greater. International arguments about how to address the problem often start with this observation. There is no simple answer to the question of how efforts to limit climate change should be divided between lifestyle changes in the heavily carbon-emitting rich countries versus creating and paying for the means for poor countries to grow and develop without replicating the carbon dependence of the development path followed by the rich countries. Carbon emissions clearly

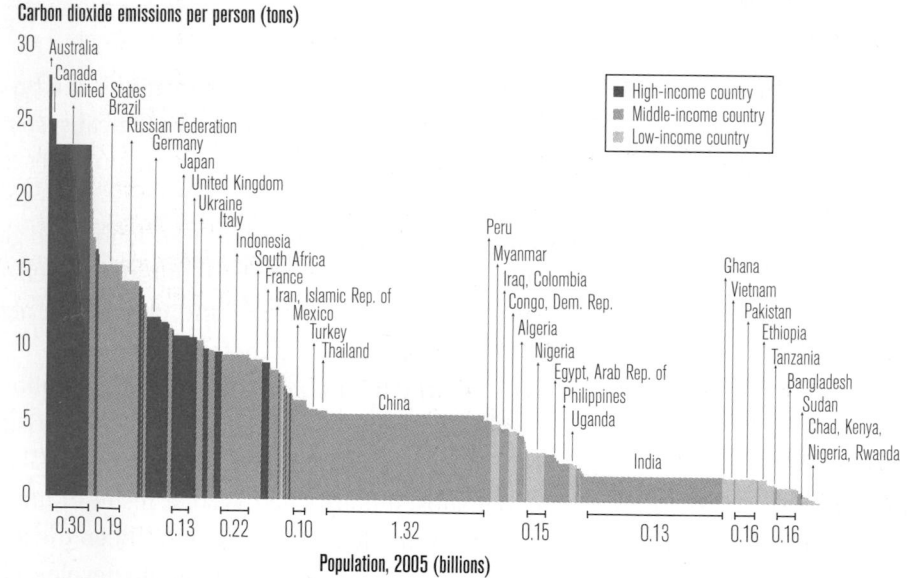

FIGURE 20-9 **Per Capita Carbon Dioxide Emissions As a Function of Population Size**

The width of each column depicts population and the height depicts per capita emissions, so the area represents total emissions. Per capita emissions of Qatar (55.5 tons of carbon dioxide equivalent per capita), UAW (38.8), and Bahrain (25.4)—greater than the heights of the y-axis—are not shown. Among the larger countries, Brazil, Indonesia, the Democratic Republic of Congo, and Nigeria have low energy-related emissions.
Source: World Bank, *World Development Report 2010: Development and Climate Change.* (Washington, DC: World Bank, 2009), fig. 1.1.

increase with national income. While technological change has the potential to reduce this association, continued income growth around the world seems likely to result in substantial momentum in global emission trends.

While there is growing evidence that some negative impacts of climate change have already occurred, much of the concern about global climate change and its threats to development and human welfare lies in the possible future effects of climate change.[43] Unfortunately, as noted by sportsman Yogi Berra, "It's tough to make predictions, especially about the future." Predictions regarding the future course of global climate change and its effects on human activity are highly uncertain, and scenarios vary widely. The IPCC itself presents six alternative scenarios for temperature change (in °C at 2090–99 relative to 1980–99) ranging from 1.8 to 4.0.

The severity of these impacts varies widely by region as well as within regions. As a general matter, the poor are the most vulnerable; their lives are more exposed to nature and their livelihoods more dependent on it. Africa is particularly at risk. According to the IPCC, global warming of only 1.5°C could increase the number of Africans exposed to water stress by 75 to 250 million; a 2.5°C increase could add 350 to 600 million Africans exposed to water stress and reduce yields from rain-fed agriculture by up to 50 percent. Effects within Africa will vary. For instance, the IPCC predicts that by 2080, arid and semiarid land in Africa will increase between 5 and 8 percent. In Asia, the IPCC projects decreased availability of fresh water in central, south, east, and southeast regions. A 1.5°C increase in average temperatures could decrease wheat and maize production in India by 2 to 5 percent, while an increase of 3°C could decrease China's rice production by 5 to 12 percent. The densely populated river delta regions of South, East, and Southeast Asia are predicted to suffer increased flooding, which will then increase morbidity and mortality from waterborne diseases. In Latin America, global warming greater than about 2.5°C could increase the number of people suffering water stress by 80 to 180 million. Tropical areas of Latin America face the loss of significant biodiversity; indeed, the IPCC suggests that global warming on the order of 4°C could lead to the extinction of up to 45 percent of Amazonian tree species. Increases in temperature and decreases in soil water are projected to transform tropical forest areas in eastern Amazonia into savannas. While soybean yields in the temperate zones of Latin America may increase with global warming, the IPCC predicts increased food insecurity and decreased water availability throughout the region.[44] Global climate change thus poses a direct and fundamental challenge to development. This challenge is complicated by the overarching need

---

[43]For instance, evidence that climate change resulting from greenhouse gases and other forms of air pollution have significantly reduced the growth rates of rice harvests in India since the mid-1980s is presented in Maximilian Auffhammer, V. Ramanathan, and Jeffrey Vincent, "From the Cover: Integrated Model Shows That Atmospheric Brown Clouds and Greenhouse Gases Have Reduced Rice Harvests in India," *Proceedings of the National Academy of Sciences* 103 (2006), 19668–72.

[44]Auffhammer et al., "From the Cover," p. 50.

to reduce poverty and hunger while avoiding doing so at the expense of continued environmental degradation that might ultimately undermine development itself.

There is great momentum in climate change. The current stocks of GHG emissions in the atmosphere are sufficient to drive continued climate change for decades, even if all future emissions were to cease immediately. According to the World Bank,

> Immediate action is needed to keep warming as close as possible to 2°C. That amount of warming is not desirable, but it is likely to be the best we can do. . . . From the perspective of development, warming much above 2°C is simply unacceptable. But stabilizing at 2°C will require major shifts in lifestyle, a veritable energy revolution, and a transformation in how we manage land and forests.[45]

While estimates vary in their magnitude, there is no doubt that substantial reductions in global carbon emissions relative to the steep trajectory based on business as usual will be required to limit global warming to 2°C.

From an economic perspective, the emission of GHGs into the atmosphere is an example of a negative externality, "the biggest market failure the world has seen," in the words of economist Nicholas Stern.[46] The key distinctions, in Stern's view, between more common externalities and GHG emissions are that GHG emissions are global in both impact and origin, some of the effects may be quite long term, the scientific understanding of the process of global warming and its long-term future impacts is uncertain, and the impacts are potentially immense and irreversible.

Even without agreeing on the details, most analysts agree that responding to the potential threats from global climate change requires simultaneous action on two fronts: **mitigation** and **adaptation**. Mitigation refers to the actions taken to reduce the extent of future climate change, and adaptation refers to the actions required to adjust human activities to the environmental changes that occur. Greater expenditures on mitigation tend to be associated with lower expenditures required for adaptation, and vice versa. Evaluating the tradeoffs between economic growth and environmental protection is a complex and highly controversial exercise. Issues to be resolved with respect to mitigation include choice of a stabilization target for surface temperature increases, when to begin changing behaviors and economic activities to attain that target, whose behaviors and activities to change, the cost of mitigation, and critically, who pays those costs.

Estimates by economists that weigh the costs against the benefits of mitigating climate change vary substantially and have a big impact on conclusions regarding the optimal timing and degree of mitigation. Such calculations are sensitive to a

---

[45]World Bank, *World Development Report 2010: Development and Climate Change* (Washington, DC: World Bank, 2009),p. 3.

[46]Nicholas Stern, "The Economics of Climate Change [Richard T. Ely Lecture]," *American Economic Review: Papers and Proceedings* 98, no. 2 (2008), p. 1. Stern is also the lead author of a major international study of the economics of climate change, *The Economics of Climate Change: The Stern Review* (Cambridge: Cambridge University Press, 2007).

variety of necessary assumptions and choices by analysts. Key parameters are the time horizon covered by the analysis, the sensitivity of global climate increases to given changes in CO_2 concentration, the costs of mitigation, likely damages from climate change, and the choice of the discount rate (important for comparing present versus future costs or benefits). Strong assumptions are required for all of these parameters in order to calculate the **optimal target** for CO_2 concentrations. *Optimal* in this context refers to the concentration level that would result in the least reduction in the present value of global consumption.

Cost–benefit analysis is an essential tool in efforts to design policy responses to global climate change, yet cost–benefit analysis alone cannot resolve the debate. Even if all scientists agreed on the sensitivity of global climate increases to given changes in CO_2 and all economists agreed on the costs of mitigating the associated damages, cost–benefit analysis would still be limited by its inability to assign values to nonmarket environmental goods and services. In addition, choosing the appropriate discount rate to apply to future costs and benefits is a particularly critical component of cost–benefit analysis. Policy prescriptions arising from cost–benefit analyses are highly sensitive to the choice of discount rate, yet there has been little agreement about what rate to apply or even how to choose one. The higher the discount rate, the lower the weight given to the future in comparison with the present. The sensitivity of cost–benefit analysis of climate change mitigation to the choice of discount rate arises because the costs of mitigation occur in the short run while the benefits occur primarily in the long run. One complicating factor is that if incomes grow over time, then future generations would be better able to pay the costs of climate damage, potentially justifying the choice of a lower discount rate today. Ethical concerns are even more complicated, as the discussion is essentially about tradeoffs between the welfare of present and future generations. Is it right to place less importance on the welfare of future generations (as discounting implies)? Conversely, what level of mitigation cost is ethically assigned to the current generation when the benefits are both uncertain and in the distant future?

Two prominent economic studies of climate change have reached quite different conclusions in regard to the optimal timing and extent of mitigation actions, largely owing to their divergent choices of discount rates. The *Stern Review*, which assumes a low discount rate (along with a high sensitivity of climate change to CO_2 emissions and low mitigation costs), concludes that large-scale and immediate interventions to mitigate climate change are essential.[47] In contrast, a study by economist William Nordhaus, which assumes a higher discount rate (along with a lower sensitivity of climate change to CO_2 emissions and higher mitigation costs), argues for more limited and more gradual efforts to mitigate climate change.[48] We can interpret these differing

---

[47] *The Stern Review.*

[48] William Nordhaus, *A Question of Balance: Waiting the Options on Global Warming Policies.* (New Haven, CT: Yale University Press, 2008).

approaches in terms of their targets for future global climate change. While the more aggressive efforts at mitigation tend to target a 2°C increase in average global temperature, the more gradual approach implies a target closer to 3°C increase. The incremental cost of achieving the lower target (a form of **climate insurance**) is estimated to be only about 0.5 percent of global GDP.[49] Part of the reason the incremental cost of achieving the lower target is not greater is that the lower mitigation cost associated with the higher limit on climate change is partially offset by the greater future costs of adaptation required to address the greater future damage resulting from increased temperatures.

Much of this debate over the urgency and appropriate extent of mitigation hinges on the analysts' choice of discount rates. Critics have assailed the *Stern Review* as having stacked the deck in favor of urgent and substantial mitigation by its choice of a low discount rate. In reviewing this debate, economist Martin Weitzman suggests that the *Stern Review* might be "right for the wrong reasons." For Weitzman, the primary argument in favor of more aggressive mitigation of climate change is not about consumption smoothing and discount rates. He argues that our fundamental uncertainty regarding future impacts of climate change is paramount and that even if utter catastrophe is a low-probability event, mitigation provides an important form of insurance.[50]

Adaptation to climate change refers to deliberate actions taken to reduce the impacts of climate change. In its fourth assessment report, the IPCC summarizes planned adaptation measures by sector. In response to expected water shortages resulting from climate change, potential adaptation measures include expanded rainwater harvesting, improved water storage and conservation techniques, and desalination. The primary constraint to these types of adaptations is financial. Agricultural systems might adapt to climate change by adjusting planting dates, altering crop varieties and the mix of crops produced, and by improving the control of soil erosion by planting more trees. These changes will require both training and technological support for farmers. As discussed in Chapter 17, institutional support for farmers in the form of improved land tenure arrangements may also be necessary to create incentives for improved soil management. Protecting coastal zones from the effects of rising sea levels is another important dimension of adaptation to climate change. The construction of seawalls and storm surge barriers, and the creation of marshlands and wetlands as coastal buffer zones may be critical to protect vulnerable populations in low-lying coastal areas. In this case, land availability and financing may be the primary constraints. Additional measures, such as improved energy

---

[49]This difference, as summarized in World Bank, *World Development Report 2010*, p. 8, is calculated as the difference between each model's predicted net present value of global GDP versus the net present value of global GDP, assuming no climate change.

[50]Martin Weitzman, "The Stern Review of the Economics of Climate Change [Review]," *Journal of Economic Literature* 45, no. 3 (2007), 703–24.

efficiency and increased use of renewable energy resources are also important planned forms of adaptation to climate change.

The costs and benefits of adaptation at the global level are difficult to estimate precisely, in part owing to the uncertainties noted in this chapter. Two dimensions of the cost are clear. The capacity for adaptation depends significantly on a country's level of development. Adaptive capacity is thus highly unequally distributed around the world. It is also clear that lesser efforts at mitigation in the short run will result in higher costs of adaptation in the long run.

The wide-ranging assumptions (especially regarding the ceiling for global temperature increase) required to estimate the cost of either mitigation or adaptation produce widely ranging results. The estimates for annual mitigation costs in the year 2030 range from \$139 to \$175 billion (in 2005 US\$).[51] The financing requirements can be substantially greater because of the high up-front capital costs of mitigation projects, a potential barrier to participation by developing countries. The range estimated for annual adaptation costs is wider. Estimates for the short term (2010–15) range from \$4 billion to greater than \$100 billion, and estimates for the medium term (2030) range from \$15 billion to \$100 billion. At the high end, this funding requirement is less than 0.2 percent of the world's GDP. As of 2010, donor funding commitments for adaptation and mitigation totaled only \$9 billion, far short of the estimated requirements.

Global progress in efforts to mitigate and adapt to climate change requires international cooperation. Fears of reduced rates of economic growth and questions of fairness between countries and of how to share the substantial costs have impeded international cooperation to date. Since 1992, international climate negotiations have taken place within the United Nations Framework Convention on Climate Change (UNFCCC), which sets targets for stabilizing atmospheric concentrations of GHGs. The Kyoto Protocol, adopted in 1997 and implemented in 2005, supplemented the original convention. Difficult negotiations failed to secure U.S. participation. Subsequent efforts, such as the Bali Action Plan, adopted in 2007 through the UNFCCC, the 2009 United Nations Climate Change Conference held in Copenhagen (the 15th conference of parties to the Kyoto Protocol), the 2010 United Nations Climate Change Conference held in Cancun, Mexico (the 16th conference of parties to the Kyoto Protocol), and the 2011 United Nations Climate Change Conference held in Bonn, Germany, reflect the continuing difficulties associated with organizing international cooperation in this vital area.

The issues at stake in international climate negotiations are central to the topic of sustainable development. This chapter began by raising the question of whether today's developing countries have the option of following the same energy- and resource-intensive development path previously established by today's wealthy

---

[51]These estimates are drawn from World Bank, *World Development Report 2010*, table 6.2.

economies. The argument that this path is not sustainable is manifest largely in its implications for the continued atmospheric accumulation of GHGs and climate change. In the context of global climate negotiations, the specific questions revolve around who should pay to fix this problem. Specifically, the Kyoto Protocol set targets for reducing global GHG emissions. These targets are binding only on the relatively wealthy countries (the so-called Annex I countries under the UNFCCC). Unfortunately, 13 years after adoption of the Kyoto Protocol (and 5 years after it came into force), official pledges of emissions reductions offered at Cancun amounted to only 60 percent of the reductions required to limit the rise in global temperature to 2°C.

The position taken by developing countries (ironically led by China, the world's leading emitter of CO_2) is that they should continue to be exempt from commitments to reduce emissions. For the developing countries it is a matter of fairness. After all, they argue, it was the developed countries that largely created the problem over a period of many decades, while the developing countries are both most at risk and least capable of bearing the costs of mitigation and adaptation. On their side, developed countries (the United States in particular) continued to push back, contending that developing countries too should be bound by emissions reduction targets. Despite its signature by President Clinton, the U.S. Senate never ratified the Kyoto Protocol (a legal requirement for U.S. accession to the treaty). This refusal to ratify was based on "the disparity of treatment between the Annex I Parties and Developing Countries," and the fear that a legally binding commitment to reduce GHG emissions would undermine the U.S. economy's international competitiveness. China in particular, with its large trade surplus with the United States, became a focus of U.S. dissatisfaction with the Kyoto Protocol. In essence, the U.S. position rests on the lack of requirement for China to reduce its total emissions, despite the much greater level of per capita emissions in the United States. Ultimately, these issues are highly politicized within both the developed and developing countries, and therein lies a central and continuing impediment to international negotiations on climate change.

SUMMARY

- Natural resource constraints and the cumulative effect of negative environmental externalities raise the possibility that the energy- and resource-intensive path toward development followed by today's advanced economies may no longer be available for today's developing countries. Long-term development must be environmentally sustainable.
- There is a general consensus, based on historical data, that economic growth from a low starting point is associated with increasing levels of pollution; yet beyond some intermediate level of income, economic growth is associated with decreasing levels of pollution. This inverted-U pattern is

known as the environmental Kuznets curve. (The association may not be causal.)

- Sustainable development has been defined as "development that meets the needs of the present without compromising the ability of future generations to meet their own needs."
- Comprehensive wealth (as distinct from GDP) is an accounting approach that incorporates the use of both natural resources and human capital. Changes over time in comprehensive wealth are measured by adjusted net saving. One economic indicator of sustainability is that comprehensive wealth not decline from one generation to the next. This requires that adjusted net saving grows more rapidly than population.
- Much of the negative environmental effect of economic activity results from externalities, social costs not included in private firms' profit-maximizing decisions. Such externalities are particularly prevalent in settings with common property resources.
- Categories of policy solutions to the problem of negative externalities include the creation of property rights where none previously existed, government regulation, taxation of the polluting activity, the creation of marketable permits to pollute, and informal regulation.
- The relationship between poverty and environmental degradation is complex. Most people living in fragile environments are poor, and poor people more frequently rely on the environment for their livelihood. A nuanced understanding of the categories of asset poverty and local conditioning variables is necessary to simultaneously reduce poverty and protect the environment.
- Global climate change may represent the greatest single challenge to sustainable development. We can think of the accumulation of greenhouse gases as a negative externality, and the earth's atmosphere as a global commons.
- Though details of the potential consequences of global climate change are shrouded in uncertainty, it seems clear that concerted international efforts to mitigate climate change are urgent if future economic development is to be sustainable.

Index

Note: Figures are noted with *f*; tables are noted with *t*; boxed topics are noted with *b*.

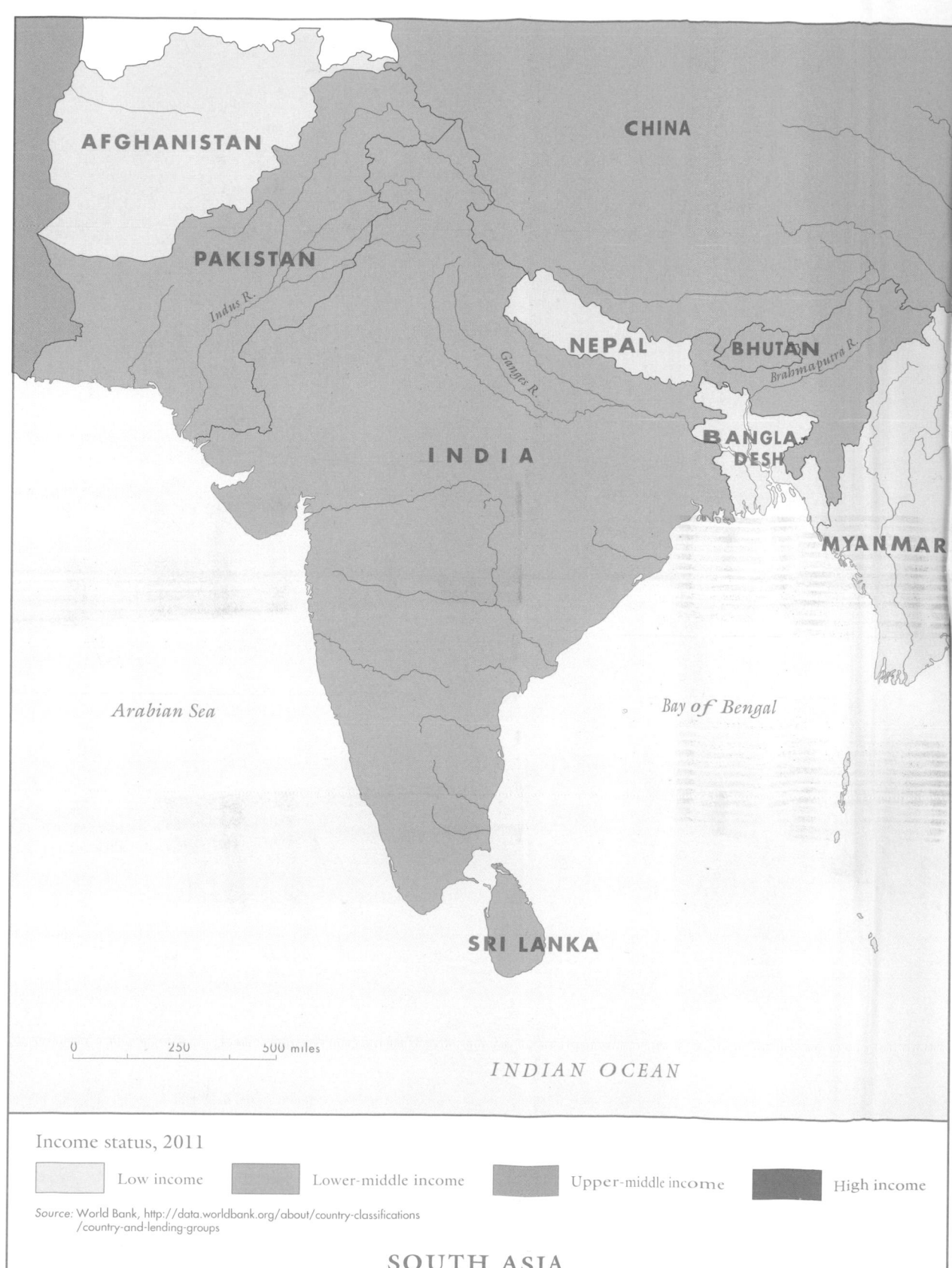

AFGHANISTAN

CHINA

PAKISTAN

Indus R.

NEPAL

BHUTAN

Brahmaputra R.

Ganges R.

INDIA

BANGLA-
DESH

MYANMAR

Arabian Sea

Bay of Bengal

SRI LANKA

0   250   500 miles

INDIAN OCEAN

Income status, 2011

Low income   Lower-middle income   Upper-middle income   High income

Source: World Bank, http://data.worldbank.org/about/country-classifications
/country-and-lending-groups

SOUTH ASIA